APPLIED THERAPEUTICS FOR CLINICAL PHARMACISTS

APPLIED THERAPEUTICS FOR CLINICAL PHARMACISTS

Second edition

edited by:

Mary Anne Koda-Kimble, Pharm.D.
Associate Clinical Professor of Pharmacy
Vice-Chairwoman, Division of Clinical Pharmacy
School of Pharmacy
University of California
San Francisco

Brian S. Katcher, Pharm.D.
Lecturer in Pharmacy
School of Pharmacy
University of California
San Francisco

Lloyd Y. Young, Pharm.D.
Assistant Professor of Clinical Pharmacy
College of Pharmacy
Washington State University
Pullman

APPLIED THERAPEUTICS, Inc.
San Francisco

Applied Therapeutics for Clinical Pharmacists

Copyright © 1978 by Applied Therapeutics, Inc.

Applied Therapeutics, Inc.
P.O. Box 31-747
San Francisco, California 94131

Earlier edition copyright © 1975 by Applied Therapeutics, Inc.

Printed in the United States of America

Library of Congress Catalog Card Number: 78-72533

ISBN 0-915486-02-4

Fourth printing, September 1980

Typesetting by Pacific Typography, Emeryville, California
Artwork primarily by Denis Ko Production Art, San Francisco, California
Printing by the Haddon Craftsmen, Scranton, Pennsylvania

Published by:
Applied Therapeutics, Inc.
P.O. Box 31-747
San Francisco, California 94131

TO OUR STUDENTS
WHO NEVER LET US FORGET
THERE IS MORE TO LEARN

PREFACE TO THE SECOND EDITION

The first edition of this text evolved from our early clinical pharmacy teaching programs at the University of California and Washington State University. These programs and others throughout North America have since grown and matured considerably; this is reflected in the second edition in the expanded list of contributors and chapter titles. Furthermore, all of the retained chapters have been thoroughly revised and updated.

The objectives of this text are stated in the preface from the first edition and they remain the same. This book is designed to illustrate the appropriate clinical application of pharmacology and pharmacokinetics to specific patient problems. We still feel that this is best accomplished through the use of case history presentations, pertinent questions and well-referenced responses, since this approach brings into focus the nature of the decision making process. Although this textbook is primarily aimed at educating pharmacists for their new, more active roles in health care, it should be of value to medical students, physicians, and nurse practitioners as well.

Mary Anne Koda-Kimble
Brian S. Katcher
Lloyd Y. Young

PREFACE TO THE FIRST EDITION

In the past decade, new roles for the pharmacist have emerged. More and more frequently the pharmacist is placed in increasingly responsible positions within the health care delivery system. In this capacity (s)he is able to have a significant influence on the quality of health care delivered to the patient. M. Silverman and P. Lee have skillfully assessed the current and future role of the pharmacist in *Pills, Profits and Politics.*[1]

" . . . It is the pharmacist who can play a vital role in assisting physicians to prescribe rationally, who can help see to it that the right drug is ordered for the right patient at the right time, in the right amounts and with due consideration of costs and that the patient knows how, when and why to use both prescription and non-prescription products.

"It is the pharmacist who has been most highly trained as an expert on drug products, who has the best opportunity to keep up-to-date on developments in this field and who can serve both physician and patient as a knowledgeable adviser. It is the pharmacist who can take a key part in preventing drug misuse, drug abuse and irrational prescribing."

Many schools of pharmacy have made substantial curriculum changes to prepare their graduates for these responsibilities. Although traditional pharmacy courses have imparted factual information about drugs, they have not enabled the student to apply these facts to the drug therapy of patients. Similarly, traditional pharmacology and medical textbooks do not provide the professional with sufficient information to make a judgment regarding the selection and dosing of a particular product for a specific patient. To arrive at this decision, the clinician must consider a number of patient factors including age, renal and hepatic function, concurrent disease states and medications and allergies. (S)he must also consider drug product factors including bioavailabilty, pharmacokinetics, efficacy, toxicity, risk to benefit ratio, and cost.

We have found that students have most difficulty in **integrating** and **applying** the multiple components of their education to formulate the safest, most rational drug regimen for a given patient. We have also observed that although the student is able to enumerate the adverse effects of a drug, (s)he is unable to **recognize** or monitor for these effects should they occur in his/her patient.

This text is an outgrowth of the clinical pharmacy courses taught at the University of California and at Washington State University. The major objective of these courses is to enable the student to practice effectively in the clinical setting. Lectures on the pathophysiology and medical management of disease states are supplemented with conferences where students are challenged with drug therapy questions frequently asked by physicians and by case histories which require drug therapy assessment and the selection of appropriate alternatives. The objective of these conferences and this text is to enable the student to identify relevant factors in drug treatment such as the probability of whether or not a specific drug is responsible for a patient's symptoms; the clinical significance of a drug interaction; why a specific drug is not achieving therapeutic blood levels; the dose for a patient with multiple disease states.

The success of the conference portion of our courses was a major determinant of the format used for this text: case histories which simulate the actual practice situation and frequently asked therapeutic questions are followed by well-referenced responses.

The authors have drawn much information from their own clinical experiences. *It remains the responsibility of every practitioner to evaluate the appropriateness of a particular opinion in the context of the actual clinical situation and with due consideration of any new developments in the field.* Although the authors have been careful to recommend dosages that are in agreement with current standards and responsible literature, we suggest the student consult several appropriate information sources when dealing with new and unfamiliar drugs.

Mary Anne Koda-Kimble
Lloyd Y. Young
Brian S. Katcher

[1]Silverman, M. and Lee, P.R.: *Pills, Profits and Politics*, University of California Press, Berkeley, 1974, p. 192.

CONTRIBUTORS

R. Jon Auricchio, Pharm.D.
Assistant Professor of Clinical Pharmacy, College of Pharmacy, Washington State University, Pullman.

Steven L. Barriere, Pharm.D.
Assistant Clinical Professor of Pharmacy, School of Pharmacy; Clinical Pharmacist, Infectious Disease Service, University of California, San Francisco.

C. A. Bond, Pharm.D.
Assistant Clinical Professor of Pharmacy, School of Pharmacy, University of Wisconsin, Madison.

Thomas J. Cali, Pharm.D.
Assistant Professor of Clinical Pharmacy, Philadelphia College of Pharmacy and Science, Philadelphia.

Moses S. Chow, Pharm.D.
Assistant Clinical Professor, School of Pharmacy, University of Connecticut, Storrs; Director, Drug Information Service, Hartford Hospital, Hartford, Connecticut.

Unamarie Clibon, Pharm.D.
Assistant Professor of Pharmacy, College of Pharmacy, University of Texas, San Antonio; Clinical Teaching Coordinator, Audie-Murphy Veterans Administration Hospital, San Antonio, Texas.

Richard Grant Closson, Pharm.D.
Assistant Clinical Professor of Pharmacy, School of Pharmacy; Clinical Pharmacist, Ambulatory Care Clinic, University of California, San Francisco.

James H. Coleman, Pharm.D.
Assistant Professor of Clinical Pharmacy in Psychiatry, College of Medicine, University of Tennessee, Memphis; Clinical Pharmacist — Specialist in Psychiatry, Veterans Administration Medical Center, Memphis, Tennessee.

Joel O. Covinsky, Pharm. D.
Associate Professor of Clinical Pharmacy, Schools of Pharmacy and Medicine, University of Missouri, Kansas City; Docent Clinical Pharmacist, Truman Medical Center Hospital, Kansas City, Missouri.

Gary C. Cupit, Pharm.D.
Assistant Clinical Professor of Pharmacy and Pediatrics; Director, Drug Information Analysis Service, School of Pharmacy; Clinical Pharmacist, Pediatric Service, University of California, San Francisco.

Richard F. deLeon, Pharm.D.
Associate Clinical Professor of Pharmacy; Associate Director of Pharmaceutical Services; Assistant Dean for Pharmaceutical Services; Director of Central Services, University of California, San Francisco.

Betty J. Dong, Pharm.D.
Assistant Clinical Professor of Pharmacy, School of Pharmacy, University of California, San Francisco; Clinical Pharmacist, Division of Family Practice, San Francisco General Hospital, San Francisco.

Julia K. Elenbaas, Pharm.D.
Assistant Professor of Clinical Pharmacy, School of Pharmacy, University of Missouri, Kansas City; Assistant Coordinator, Western Missouri Area Health Education Center Drug Information Service, Kansas City, Missouri.

Robert M. Elenbaas, Pharm.D.
Assistant Professor of Clinical Pharmacy, Schools of Pharmacy and Medicine, University of Missouri, Kansas City; Clinical Pharmacist, Department of Emergency Health Services, Kansas City General Hospital, Kansas City.

James C. Eoff, III, Pharm.D.
Associate Professor and Vice-Chairman, Department of Pharmacy Practice, College of Pharmacy, University of Tennessee Center for the Health Sciences, Memphis.

William E. Evans, Pharm.D.
Director, Clinical Division of Pharmacy, St. Jude Children's Research Hospital, Memphis, Tennessee.

Ronald P. Evens, Pharm.D.
Assistant Professor of Clinical Pharmacy, School of Pharmacy, University of Texas, Austin; Director of Drug Information Services, University of Texas Health Science Center at San Antonio.

John T. Frank, Pharm.D.
Assistant Clinical Professor of Pharmacy, School of Pharmacy, University of Southern California, Los Angeles; Assistant Director of Pharmacy, Cedars-Sinai Medical Center, Los Angeles, California.

John G. Gambertoglio, Pharm.D.
Assistant Clinical Professor of Pharmacy, School of Pharmacy; Clinical Pharmacist, Kidney Transplant Unit, University of California, San Francisco.

Mark A. Gill, Pharm.D.
Assistant Clinical Professor of Pharmacy, School of Pharmacy, University of Southern California, Los Angeles.

Patrick D. Ginn, Pharm.D.
Clinical Instructor of Pharmacy, School of Pharmacy, University of California, San Francisco; Director, Drug Information Analysis Center, Valley Medical Center, Fresno, California.

Lawrence J. Hak, Pharm.D.
Assistant Professor of Clinical Pharmacy, School of Pharmacy, University of North Carolina, Chapel Hill; Clinical Pharmacist, North Carolina Memorial Hospital, Chapel Hill.

Philip D. Hansten, Pharm.D.
Associate Professor of Clinical Pharmacy, College of Pharmacy, Washington State University, Pullman.

Linda L. Hart, Pharm.D.
Assistant Professor of Clinical Pharmacy, College of Pharmacy, University of Utah, Salt Lake City.

Robert J. Ignoffo, Pharm.D.
Assistant Clinical Professor of Pharmacy, School of Pharmacy; Oncology Clinical Pharmacist, Clinical Pharmacy and Cancer Research Institute, University of California, San Francisco.

Darryl S. Inaba, Pharm.D.
Assistant Clinical Professor of Pharmacy, School of Pharmacy, University of California, San Francisco; Director of Operations — Drug Detoxification, Rehabilitation and After-Care Project, Haight-Ashbury Free Medical Clinic, San Francisco.

Brian S. Katcher, Pharm.D.
Lecturer in Pharmacy, School of Pharmacy, University of California, San Francisco.

Steven R. Kayser, Pharm.D.
Associate Clinical Professor of Pharmacy; Supervisor, Inpatient Clinical Pharmacy Services; Clinical Pharmacist, Anticoagulation Clinic, University of California, San Francisco.

Mary Anne Koda-Kimble, Pharm.D.
Associate Clinical Professor of Pharmacy; Vice Chairwoman, Division of Clinical Pharmacy, School of Pharmacy; Clinical Pharmacist, Diabetic Clinic, University of California, San Francisco.

Nancy E. Korman, Pharm.D.
Assistant Clinical Professor of Pharmacy, School of Pharmacy, University of California, San Francisco; Clinical Pharmacist, Veterans Administration Hospital, San Francisco, California.

Donald T. Kishi, Pharm.D.
Associate Clinical Professor of Pharmacy; Vice Chairman, Division of Clinical Pharmacy, School of Pharmacy; Clinical Pharmacist, Neurology Service, University of California, San Francisco.

Louis C. Littlefield, Pharm.D.
Assistant Professor of Pharmacy, College of Pharmacy, University of Texas at Austin/University of Texas Health Science Center at San Antonio.

Richard J. Mangini, Pharm.D.
Research Pharmacist for the Mediphor Drug Interaction Project and Minerva Project, Division of Clinical Pharmacology, Department of Medicine, Stanford University Hospital, Palo Alto, California.

Anthony S. Manoguerra, Pharm.D.
Assistant Clinical Professor of Pharmacy, School of Pharmacy, University of California, San Francisco; Director of Professional Services, San Diego Poison Information Center at the University of California Medical Center, San Diego.

Scott D. Matthiessen, Pharm.D.
Staff Pharmacist, Inpatient Pharmacy, University of California, Hospital and Clinics, Los Angeles.

Robert K. Maudlin, Pharm.D.
Assistant Professor of Clinical Pharmacy, College of Pharmacy, Washington State University, Pullman; Assistant Clinical Professor of Family Medicine, University of Washington School of Medicine; Education Director, Family Medicine, Spokane.

Gail W. McSweeney, Pharm.D.
Assistant Clinical Professor of Pharmacy, School of Pharmacy; Clinical Pharmacist, Surgery Service, University of California, San Francisco.

Gary M. Oderda, Pharm.D.
Associate Professor of Clinical Pharmacy, School of Pharmacy, University of Maryland, Baltimore; Director, Maryland Poison Information Center, Baltimore.

J. Robert Powell, Pharm.D.
Assistant Professor of Pharmaceutical Sciences, College of Pharmacy, University of Arizona, Tucson.

Michael A. Riddiough, Pharm.D.,M.P.H.
Congressional Fellow, Health Program, Office of Technology Assessment, United States Congress, Washington, D.C.

Sam K. Shimomura, Pharm.D.
Associate Clinical Professor of Pharmacy; Drug Information Specialist, School of Pharmacy; Clinical Pharmacist, Medicine Service, University of California, San Francisco.

John K. Siepler, Pharm.D.
Assistant Professor of Pharmacy Practice, College of Pharmacy, University of Illinois, Chicago.

Glen L. Stimmel, Pharm.D.
Assistant Clinical Professor of Pharmacy and Psychiatry, Schools of Pharmacy and Medicine, University of Southern California, Los Angeles.

Michael E. Winter, Pharm.D.
Associate Clinical Professor of Pharmacy; Co-Director of Clinical Pharmacokinetics Laboratory, School of Pharmacy, University of California, San Francisco.

Lloyd Y. Young, Pharm.D.
Assistant Professor of Clinical Pharmacy, Washington State University, Pullman.

Table of Contents

Chapter 1

Interpretation of Clinical Laboratory Tests

John T. Frank
Philip D. Hansten
Mary Anne Koda-Kimble

The ability to interpret and apply clinical laboratory data to drug therapy has become a day to day function of the hospital pharmacist. Laboratory results are monitored by pharmacists to assess the therapeutic and adverse effects of drugs; to determine the proper dose of drugs; to assess the need for additional or alternate drug therapy; and to prevent misinterpretation of these tests because of drug interference. In some medical centers with advanced pharmacy programs, pharmacists are ordering laboratory tests and using the results to alter the drug therapy of anticoagulants, antibiotics, theophylline preparations, and antiarrhythmics.

While the analyses of serum, urine, and other fluids are routinely used to manage hospitalized patients, the cost of obtaining this data has increased the overall cost of health care enormously. The pharmacist must recognize this fact and request only those tests which in his/her opinion will substantially benefit the patient. There is little justification to frequently order multi-organ baseline studies in the absence of any suspected problem.

The results of clinical laboratory tests falling within a predetermined range of values are termed "normal" and those outside this range are called "abnormal." However, other factors must be taken into consideration. Sometimes age, sex, time since last meal, drugs, or other factors affect the range of normal values for a given test. It is important to note that the normal limits are somewhat arbitrary, and abnormal laboratory values are not necessarily of diagnostic significance. Similarly, a normal value can actually be "abnormal" depending upon the disease state and conditions in the body. For example, serum calcium is partially bound to plasma proteins, and its level is dependent upon the level of these plasma proteins. If plasma proteins are low, serum calcium will generally be below the lower limit of normal. Thus, a finding of a normal calcium in a patient with very low plasma proteins is essentially an "abnormal" result, even though the value falls within the predetermined normal range. Another important consideration with respect to normal values is that different clinical laboratories may use different methods for performing various tests. When different methods are used, the ranges of normal values may be different. Also, a given laboratory may change their methods or equipment resulting in possible changes in normal values. Therefore, one should use the normal value tables published by the laboratory when interpreting these tests, not those published in reference texts.

There are several common sources of laboratory error:

a. *Spoiled specimen* — improper handling, improper preservation, or undue delay in performing the test may invalidate the results obtained. For example,

if a blood sample is allowed to hemolyze, a spurious hyperkalemia may result because erythrocytes are rich in potassium as compared to plasma (11,18).

b. *Specimen taken at wrong time* — the levels of many substances in biological fluids can fluctuate depending upon the time of day, relation to meals, and other factors. Thus, specimens obtained at improper times can yield misleading tests results.

c. *Incomplete specimen* — this is most likely to occur in studies requiring 24-hour urine collections due to the difficulty in remembering to save each voiding.

d. *Faulty reagents* — reagents improperly prepared or deteriorated (more likely with infrequently done tests) may produce erroneous results.

e. *Technical errors* — the technologist may make an error in reading an instrument or making a calculation. Patient names and samples may get mixed up, or results may be transcribed incorrectly.

f. *Diet* — certain foods contain substances which can appear in biological fluids and interfere with various laboratory tests.

g. *Procedures* — some of the procedures performed can alter laboratory test results. For example, digital examination of the prostate can elevate serum acid phosphatase and electroconversion can cause elevations in serum creatine phosphokinase (CPK).

h. *Medication* — drugs may alter the results obtained in laboratory tests by the following mechanisms:

1) Drugs may interfere with the testing procedure. An example of this would be ascorbic acid-induced false negative results for urine glucose (glucose oxidase methods).

2) Drugs may actually alter laboratory values by virtue of their pharmacologic and toxic properties. An example of this would be the elevation of serum uric acid caused by thiazide diuretics.

Several sources are available which include information concerning the effects of drugs on results of clinical laboratory tests (6,16,20).

Laboratory error must always be considered when the result does not correlate with that which would be predicted for any given patient.

There are between 400 and 500 different laboratory tests which may be performed. A discussion of all of these is clearly beyond the scope of this chapter, and only routine or frequently ordered laboratory tests will be covered here. Tests used to diagnose special diseases will be discussed in greater depth in corresponding chapters.

Finally, a word of caution. Therapists should not become so engrossed in the patient's "numbers" that the patient himself is overlooked. Always remember to *treat* the patient and *observe* laboratory tests; do not treat laboratory values.

CASE HISTORY – HEMORRHAGE: A 19-year-old male was admitted to a surgical floor following blunt trauma to the abdomen sustained in an automobile accident. The surgeon started an IV and ordered serial hematocrits. At the same time blood samples were drawn and sent to the laboratory for typing and cross matching, a complete blood count (CBC), and other tests.

1. Why was the hematocrit ordered rather than the hemoglobin or red blood cell count?

The hematocrit (normal: 45%) and hemoglobin (15 gm/dL) are indirect measurements of the red blood cell (RBC) count and are decreased in cases of hemorrhage and anemia. The hematocrit or packed cell volume (PCV) is the percentage of whole blood volume occupied by the RBCs. It is the preferred test in this patient, because it can be rapidly performed at the bedside. The RBC count and hemoglobin determinations must be performed in the laboratory which incurs some delay in obtaining the results. Also, the RBC count is the least accurate of the three tests because dilution and sampling are required to obtain the results.

Trauma patients frequently suffer from internal hemorrhage which can be detected by a drop in the serum hematocrit before other symptoms of internal bleeding become apparent, such as a fall in blood pressure or auscultation of fluid in the gut.

2. In the above case, serial hematocrits were performed every 15 minutes and lower values were reported each time. The last determination revealed a hematocrit value of 21% (normal 40-50%) and the patient was taken to surgery for an emergency laparotomy. He received 16 units of whole blood during surgery. Post-operatively, the patient was oozing blood from his incision sites. What is the probable cause of bleeding?

Stored banked blood rapidly loses the activity of its clotting factors and platelets. Blood filters are used to filter out platelet clumps while the blood is being infused. The result is an iatrogenic thrombocytopenia (low platelets) with prolonged bleeding times.

Other common causes of thrombocytopenia include: bone-marrow suppressant drugs (most often antineoplastic agents), acute allergic reactions, massive exchange transfusions, and folate and B-12 deficiencies.

3. A 27-year-old Caucasian male was started on chloramphenicol 1 gm IV q 8 h by IV piggyback. The patient's physician ordered a daily reticulocyte count. What is the reason for monitoring the reticulocyte count? How can a reticulocytosis be interpreted?

Reticulocytes are immature red blood cells which normally account for only 0.1 to 1.0% of the total number of RBCs. Changes in bone marrow function (accelerated or reduced cell production) will be reflected in the reticulocyte count before any change is seen in the RBC count. Reticulocytes have a short life span (a few days), whereas mature RBCs survive approximately four months.

The RBC count (hematocrit, hemoglobin) must be considered when interpreting the reticulocyte count since it is the absolute count rather than the percent of RBCs which more accurately reflects bone marrow function. A corrected value may be obtained using the following formula:

$$\text{Corrected Reticulocyte Count} = \text{Observed Value} \times \frac{\text{Patient's Hct, RBC count, or Hgb}}{\text{Normal Value of Lab Test Used}}$$

Since chloramphenicol is a known bone marrow suppressive agent, a decreased "retic" count will serve as an early warning parameter for the toxic effects of chloramphenicol. Likewise, other drugs which suppress the bone marrow can be monitored in this manner. Also see chapter on *Anemias.*

An elevated reticulocyte count will be observed when RBC production is increased. Reticulocytosis commonly occurs in response to acute blood loss, hemolysis, and corrective drug therapy. Therefore, response to replacement therapy in the case of folic acid, B-12, and iron deficiency anemias can be monitored with the reticulocyte count (13a).

4. A 58-year-old chronic alcoholic was admitted to the medical ward for observation following a brawl. As part of the standard work-up, red blood cell indices were performed with the following results:

Mean Corpuscular Volume (MCV):
108 cubic microns (80-95)
Mean Corpuscular Hemoglobin (MCH):
38 micrograms (27-31)
Mean Corpuscular Hemoglobin Concentration (MCHC):
34 gm% (32-36)

What is the value of the RBC indices? How should they be interpreted in this patient?

The RBC indices characterize the size and color of the *average* red blood cell and are derived from the patient's hemoglobin, hematocrit and RBC count. Basically, the MCV and MCH are calculated by dividing the hematocrit and hemoglobin respectively by the RBC count. The MCHC is calculated by dividing the hemoglobin by the hematocrit. All of these values are multiplied by a factor of 10 to obtain the correct units. The MCHC is the most accurate index, because the RBC is not included in its calculation. A small RBC or a cell with a low MCV is described as *microcytic.* A large RBC or a cell with a high MCV is described as *macrocytic.* Cells which have small amounts or concentrations of hemoglobin are pale and are described as *hypochromic.* Anemias of various etiologies have cells with characteristic appearances, and it is for this reason that the indices are frequently useful in helping to establish the diagnosis and treatment of anemias. It is important to re-emphasize that the indices describe the *average* cell and cannot take the place of direct observation of a blood smear. For example, the MCV may be normal in a patient with a "mixed" (i.e. microcytic and macrocytic) anemia.

The MCH and MCV are both increased and the MCHC is normal in macrocytic anemias associated with B-12 or folic acid deficiency. This characteristic picture is illustrated in the alcoholic patient described who is likely to have a dietary folic acid deficiency. Iron deficiency produces a microcytic, hypochromic anemia in which all three indices are decreased. Finally, anemias characterized by normal indices (*normochromic, normocytic*) generally occur in association with acute blood loss, hemolysis, bone marrow failure, and chronic disease. Refer to the chapter on *Anemias* for a more in-depth discussion of these anemias (13a,14,19).

5. A 23-year-old patient on the gynecology service developed a low blood pressure and a temperature of 39.4°C (103°F) on the seventh day after a cesarean section. The results of the WBC count and differential were reported from the laboratory as follows:

WBC	33,000	(Normal 5-10,000/mm³)
Neutrophils ("segs", "polys")	76%	(Normal 55-69%)
Bands ("stabs")	13%	(Normal 0-3%)
Lymphocytes	10%	(Normal 20-40%)
Monocytes	0	(Normal 0-9%)
Eosinophils	1%	(Normal 1-3%)
Basophils	0	(Normal 0-1%)

On the basis of these tests and other findings, the physician diagnosed pelvic inflammatory disease. Are these results consistent with a bacterial infection?

Yes, white blood cells are the host's chief defense system, and the neutrophil is the main component of that system. Typically, in bacterial infections, there is an increased WBC count, an increase in the proportion of neutrophils and a "shift to the left." The latter term indicates a greater proportion of bands (neutrophil precursors) or less mature WBC forms. Because the number of neutrophils is increased, the percentage of other types of white cells are proportionately decreased.

As the infection progresses, the percentage of band cells will decrease, because there is also an increase in the number of neutrophils which have a longer half-life. This decrease in bands does not necessarily indicate improvement. A decrease in the percentage of neutrophils with a drop in the total WBC count is characteristic of effective antibiotic therapy. Significant drops in the WBC count may be observed within the first 24 hours after starting antibiotics.

6. What are the major causes of eosinophilia?

Eosinophils are usually increased by allergic reactions. The pharmacist should become suspicious of an allergic drug reaction whenever the absolute eosinophil count exceeds 300 cells (3% of 10,000 WBC's). Eosinophils may increase before, after, or concurrent with other evidence of allergy such as a rash. An elevated count without other evidence of allergy is not generally considered sufficient cause to discontinue a suspected medication.

Dermatologic conditions (e.g. pemphigus), parasitic infections, Loeffler's syndrome, certain infections like scarlet fever, and diseases of the hemopoietic system like Hodgkin's disease are associated with increased eosinophil counts.

CASE HISTORY – CHF, HYPONATREMIA, AND EDEMA: A 73-year-old female was admitted to the CCU of the medical center. She had been treated at the hospital several months earlier for congestive heart failure (CHF). An admitting serum electrolyte screen revealed a serum sodium value of 123 mEq/L. The patient had evidence of pulmonary edema and severe (4+) pedal edema.

7. Should this patient be given sodium chloride to return her serum sodium value to normal?

No, one of the most common forms of hyponatremia is that occurring with edema. The concentration of sodium per liter of serum is low, but this occurs because the volume of serum is increased relative to increases of sodium. The usual treatment for this type of hyponatremia is salt and water restriction plus diuretics. Also see chapter on *Congestive Heart Failure.*

8. What other types of hyponatremia are there?

Generally speaking, hyponatremia can be either dilutional (as in the case presented) or depletional. *Dilutional hyponatremia* occurs whenever the extracellular fluid compartment expands without an equivalent increase in sodium. This type is associated with cirrhosis, congestive heart failure, nephrosis, or the administration of osmotically active solutes such as salt poor albumin or mannitol.

Depletional hyponatremia occurs when the serum sodium is low in the absence of edema. Causative factors include mineralocorticoid deficiencies, salt losing renal disease, and replacement of sodium containing fluid losses with non-saline solutions. Also see chapter on *Fluid and Electrolyte Disorders.*

9. How significant is an increase in serum sodium (hypernatremia) and what are some of the causes?

Sodium is the major extracellular cation of the body and has a major role in maintaining serum osmolarity. Changes in sodium concentration at either extreme can represent life threatening emergencies. Sodium concentrations of 170 mEq/L or more are considered life threatening.

One of the most common causes of hypernatremia encountered today is dehydration. It most often occurs in the very young and the very old (the "nursing home prune syndrome") as a result of hypotonic fluid loss. The diagnosis is generally made on the basis of physical findings. The increase of serum sodium above normal can be used to estimate the volume requirement of water to rehydrate the patient.

CASE HISTORY – DIABETIC WITH KETOACIDOSIS AND POTASSIUM IMBALANCE: A 27-year-old juvenile-onset diabetic was admitted to the hospital in diabetic coma with a blood sugar of 380 gm/dL (normal 100 gm/dL). Urine output was 135 ml/hr (normal 50 ml/hr), and the urine was 4+ positive for sugar and acetone. Stat emergency chemistry results showed a blood pH of 7.31 and a serum potassium level of 4.1 mEq/L (normal 3.8-5.2 mEq/L).

10. Should the pharmacist monitoring this patient be concerned about the "normal" potassium level?

Yes. Treatment of the patient's diabetic coma without supplemental potassium could result in a life threatening hypokalemia with resulting cardiac arrest.

Potassium is the body's chief intracellular cation (intracellular concentrations of potassium approximate 150 mEq/L), and because of the body's energy systems, only a fraction of the intracellular stores are present in the serum. When the pH of the blood is acidic, potassium shifts out of the cell due to the presence of increased intracellular hydrogen ion. Because the patient is acidotic, a higher than normal serum potassium level would be expected. However, because there has been a significant loss of total body potassium, the serum level appears normal. If the patient's acidosis and hyperglycemia are corrected without replacing potassium (both effects cause a shift of K+ into cells), severe hypokalemia may occur (2). Also see the chapters on *Fluid and Electrolyte Disorders* and *Acid-Base Disorders.*

11. If the complications of hypokalemia are primarily related to the heart, what are the complications of hyperkalemia, and what is considered to be a high potassium level?

The main complication of hyperkalemia is also related to the heart. Potassium levels of 6.5 mEq/L or more should be considered cause for immediate treatment. Above 6.5 mEq/L, cardiac findings may progress rapidly to complete heart block and cardiac arrest. Short term improvement in hyperkalemia can be achieved by administering glucose and insulin or administering bicarbonate. The eventual approach to therapy is to eliminate excess potassium, not just shift it into cells. Therefore the administration of a potassium exchange resin or dialysis is considered standard treatment. Also see chapter on *Fluid and Electrolyte Disorders.*

12. What are some common causes of hyperkalemia and hypokalemia?

As presented in the case, hyperkalemia can occur due to an increase in hydrogen ions. The other most common cause of hyperkalemia in hospitalized patients is renal failure. Hidden sources of exogenous potassium should not be administered to these patients; for example, a 20 million unit dose of potassium penicillin G contains 34 mEq of potassium, an amount sufficient to raise the potassium level of a renal failure patient.

High potassium results are sometimes spurious. If a blood sample has hemolyzed in the test tube, the intracellular potassium will leak out of the RBCs and a falsely high serum potassium level will be reported. A frequent cause of hypokalemia is failure of patients to take supplemental potassium while on potassium wasting diuretics. Hypokalemia is also seen in patients with hypochloremic conditions. Also see chapter on *Fluid and Electrolyte Disorders.*

13. How does a low chloride affect the potassium level?

Sodium is passively absorbed with chloride in the proximal tubule of the kidney. In the presence of hypochloremia (normal 98-108 mEq/L) greater than normal amounts of sodium reach the distal tubule where the kidney's mechanism for conserving sodium is to exchange it for hydrogen (with a resulting increase in generated bicarbonate) and potassium. A hypochloremia can therefore lead to a hypokalemic metabolic alkalosis. The treatment of this condition is the replacement of potassium with potassium chloride.

14. What are the usual causes of hypochloremia and hyperchloremia?

Hyperchloremia can occur as a result of some types of renal disease. It also occurs in dehydration and as result of excessive saline administration. Hypochloremia often occurs as a result of excessive gastric suctioning, vomiting, and the over-use of diuretics.

CASE HISTORY – PANCREATITIS: A 38-year-old male Caucasian was admitted to the surgical ward with a chief complaint of acute abdominal pain. The patient has a long history of gall bladder disease. Physical examination revealed a very distressed, anxious patient. The patient was hypotensive, his deep tendon reflexes were hyperactive, and his urine output was diminished.

Emergency laboratory tests revealed the following abnormal results:

Serum amylase	680 Somogyi units/100 ml (Normal 60 - 180)
Serum calcium	7 mg% (Normal 9 - 11 mg%)
Hematocrit	60%

The resident surgeon made the diagnosis of acute pancreatitis.

15. Why would pancreatitis cause a high hematocrit?

A number of diseases, including pancreatitis, produce a loss of extracellular fluid. In the case of pancreatitis, fluid is sequestered in the gut and, as a result, intravascular volume is reduced and RBCs are concentrated. Whenever fluid is sequestered in other than the intracellular and extracellular compartments, the area of fluid accumulation is referred to as a "third space." In the above case, fluid was **third spaced** in the gut with resulting intravascular hemoconcentration.

16. Why is this patient's serum calcium low?

In acute pancreatitis, lipases act on body fats to produce a physiologic soap. The addition of calcium to an emulsified fat produces an insoluble (hard) soap. The hypocalcemia that occurs in acute pancreatitis can be life threatening. Constant infusions of calcium are sometimes employed in therapy.

17. What factors regulate the body's calcium?

In the normal adult there are 1-2 Kg of calcium of which 98% is in the skeleton. The calcium found in the serum is approximately 50% bound to serum protein. The unbound calcium is the form that plays a critical role in regulating neuromuscular function. Because of the relationship between serum proteins and calcium, patients with hypoproteinemias may have a lower than normal serum value but still have a normal circulating unbound calcium fraction. Endrocrine, renal, gastrointestinal, and nutritional factors regulate the body's calcium stores. Also see the chapter on **Fluid and Electrolyte Disorders.**

18. What was the significance of the amylase determination in this case? What drugs can elevate the serum amylase?

Amylase is an enzyme found in the pancreas and parotid glands and is elevated when either of these tissues is inflamed, injured, or destroyed. In this case, the high amylase is due to a pancreatitis. It should be pointed out that there is no absolute correlation between the severity of disease and the measured serum level of an enzyme, since enzymes are also released from living tissue. Also, in patients with advanced disease, there may be insufficient viable tissue to produce high enzyme levels despite widespread involvement of the organ.

Drugs which constrict the sphincter of Oddi, such as the narcotics may increase the intrapancreatic ductal pressure and increase the serum amylase. See the chapter on **General Care: Pain.** Also, drugs which produce a pancreatitis (e.g. diuretics, alcohol, corticosteroids) or parotitis (e.g. iodides) may increase the serum amylase (6).

CASE HISTORY – SEPSIS AND ELEVATED BUN: A 66-year-old male patient was admitted to the hospital in a coma. An initial diagnosis of septic shock was made. On the second hospital day a blood urea nitrogen (BUN) level of 46 mg% was reported by the laboratory, (normal 7 - 18 mg%). The patient's drug therapy included gentamicin and methicillin.

19. What is the significance of an elevated BUN?

Urea is the end product of protein metabolism. The concentration of urea nitrogen in the blood is dependent on several factors, including renal function. Because BUN levels vary inversely with renal function, the BUN is often used as a screening test to determine renal function.

20. Is BUN an accurate indicator of renal function? What factors alter the BUN?

Blood urea nitrogen is an insensitive test of renal function because it is affected by so many other factors:

a. *Renal Function:* Urea is filtered by the glomerulus and variably reabsorbed by the tubules. Therefore, alterations in either of these functions will influence the blood level.

b. *Catabolism:* Protein breakdown which occurs in catabolic states may increase the BUN. Drugs such as tetracycline and corticosteroids have catabolic effects.

c. *Gastrointestinal Bleeding:* A common cause of high BUN levels is GI hemorrhage. The blood in the gut is a rich source of protein, and its breakdown results in high BUN levels.

d. *Nutrition:* Diets very high or very low in protein can increase or decrease BUN levels.

e. *Hydrational Status:* In the presence of dehydration, greater than normal amounts of BUN are reabsorbed from the kidney tubule, producing higher than normal blood levels. These elevated levels are also caused by a hemoconcentration effect (10).

21. Can it be determined whether or not an elevated BUN is caused by an intra-renal defect or one of the other factors listed above?

The normal ratio of BUN: Creatinine is approximately 10:1. In renal failure, both values should increase proportionately so that the ratio remains the same. If factors other than renal failure are contributing to an elevated BUN, this normal ratio will be exceeded. Of course, the patient's history and physical signs and symptoms are also used to determine whether or not any of the other factors are causing the elevation (10).

22. An 83-year-old woman is admitted to the hospital following a stroke. On the eighth hospital day she develops evidence of pneumonia and is started on gentamicin 80 mg q 8 h and penicillin. Her serum creatinine has been reported as 1.2 mg% on each of the last three laboratory tests (normal 0.7 mg% - 1.3 mg%). What is the significance of a serum creatinine level? Can the glomerular filtration rate (GFR) be estimated from a serum creatinine value?

Creatinine is an end product of muscle metabolism and has a relatively constant rate of formation which is dependent on the muscle mass of each individual. It is primarily eliminated by glomerular filtration and is therefore a relatively sensitive indicator of renal function. Each time the serum creatinine doubles, the GFR decreases by one-half. This general rule of thumb only holds for steady state creatinine levels.

The serum creatinine of 1.2 mg% reported for this patient does not necessarily indicate that she has normal renal function. Elderly individuals frequently have less muscle mass and lower baseline serum creatinine levels. Thus, a serum creatinine of 1.2 mg% in an 83-year-old individual probably represents significant renal impairment. An additional consideration is that the dose of gentamicin may require some adjustment in this patient (10).

23. A 21-year-old motorcycle enthusiast was hospitalized following a traffic accident. An initial serum creatinine, drawn on admission, was 0.9 mg%, and a second level, drawn four hours later, was 1.3 mg%. The surgeon wished to start the patient on tobramycin and nafcillin. The pharmacist was asked to help determine the dose of tobramycin. The pharmacist noted that the creatinine results were within the normal limits (WNL) and that the patient was young and athletic. He therefore recommended a normal loading and maintenance dose of tobramycin. Was the pharmacist's conclusion about this patient's renal function accurate? How should he have assessed renal function?

Creatinine serum levels, like drug serum levels, rise or fall to a new "steady state" level when elimination is altered. Therefore, a rise from 0.9 mg% to 1.3 mg% in only four hours may indicate severe renal impairment.

It is important to re-emphasize the importance of treating the patient, not the laboratory values. A decreased urine output or grossly bloody urine are examples of signs of inadequate renal function.

As an alternative, the pharmacist could recommend the usual loading dose and request a twelve-hour creatinine clearance measurement to determine future maintenance doses of tobramycin. If the hospital has the resources to measure drug serum levels, the dose could also be individualized using this data.

CASE HISTORY – HEMOLYSIS: A 42-year-old male with a two year history of hypertension controlled with methyldopa was admitted to the hospital following an episode of orthostatic hypotension. Admitting laboratory results showed a hematocrit of 27%. Because the patient had a long history of alcoholism, liver function tests were performed. The following laboratory results were obtained:

Bilirubin (Total/Direct) 3.5/0.6 mg% (Normal 1.2/0.4)
Alkaline Phosphatase 4 Bodansky Units (Normal 2 - 5)
SGOT 42 Units (Normal 5 - 40)
SGPT 38 Units (Normal 5 - 35)

24. Describe the formation, transport, metabolism, and excretion of bilirubin. See Figure 1.

Bilirubin is primarily a breakdown product of hemoglobin and is formed in the reticuloendothelial system (Step 1). It is then transferred into the blood (Step 2) where it is almost completely bound to serum albumin. (Step 3). When the bilirubin arrives at the sinusoidal surface of the liver cells, the free fraction is rapidly taken up into the cell (Step 4) and converted primarily to bilirubin diglucuronide (Step 5). This conjugated form is then excreted in the bile (Step 6) and appears in the intestine where bacteria convert the majority of it to urobilinogen (Step 7), with a very small amount of the bilirubin being reabsorbed. Most of the urobilinogen is destroyed or excreted in the feces (Step 13), but some is reabsorbed into the blood (Step 8). A portion of this small amount of urobilinogen in the blood is then reabsorbed into the liver (Step 9) and subsequently excreted in the bile (Step 12); the other portion is excreted into the urine (Step 10). The mechanism by which conjugated bilirubin in the liver cell is transferred to the blood (Step 14) is not well understood. However, with many types of liver disease this conjugated form of bilirubin (direct acting) is present in increased concentrations in the blood. When this concentration exceeds 0.2 to 0.4 mg%, bilirubin will begin to appear in the urine (Step 11). Unconjugated bilirubin (indirect acting) is not water soluble and is highly bound to serum albumin. Both of these factors account for its lack of excretion into the urine (15).

25. The physician made a diagnosis of hemolytic anemia, possibly secondary to methyldopa. What are the causes of an elevated bilirubin, and how do the reported liver function tests help support the diagnosis of hemolysis?

There are three major causes of increased bilirubin levels in adults:

a. *Hemolysis:* When RBCs are broken down at a fas-

ter than normal rate, there is an increased formation of indirect bilirbubin. If the liver is conjugating and eliminating bilirubin normally, the total bilirubin will increase out of proportion to the direct bilirubin. This was evident in the case presented.

b. *Hepatocellular damage:* In conditions where the liver itself is unable to conjugate bilirubin, the total bilirubin will again rise out of proportion to the direct. Therefore, in the case presented, the diagnosis cannot be confirmed by the bilirubin levels alone.

c. *Cholestasis:* When an obstruction to bile flow occurs in the absence of severe liver impairment, the

Fig. 1: Bilirubin Metabolism

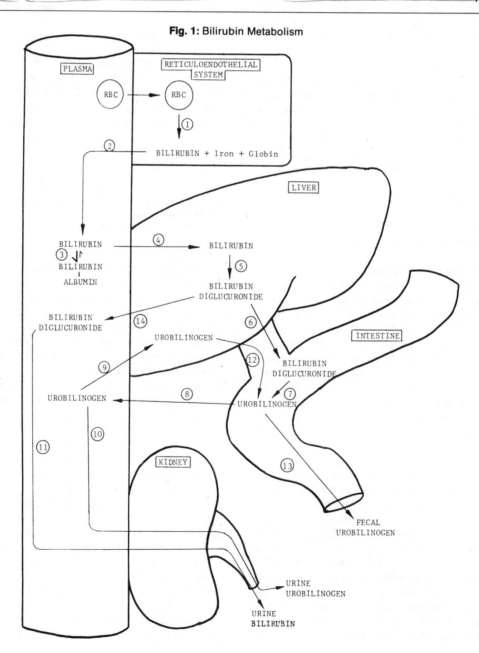

total bilirubin will increase with a far greater proportion of direct bilirubin being present. The remaining liver function tests reported were measurements of enzyme levels which are influenced by hepatic disease. Alkaline phosphatase is an enzyme found in high concentration in the bone, liver, and placenta. Because this enzyme is excreted by the liver into the bile, it is useful in differentiating cholestasis from other forms of jaundice. High alkaline phosphatase levels occur in conditions where there is an obstruction to bile flow. Diseases of tissues where alkaline phosphatase is found in high concentrations will also give rise to high serum levels.

In the case reported, the absence of either a high alkaline phosphatase or direct bilirubin would indicate that there is not cholestatic component to the patient's disease.

26. What is the importance of the serum alkaline phosphatase, SGOT, and SGPT in the assessment of liver function? Where are these enzymes found?

Alkaline phosphatase is found primarily in liver and bone, with the intestine and kidney also contributing to serum levels of the enzyme. Serum levels are elevated consistently in obstructive hepatic disease and are accompanied by elevations in serum bilirubin. Metastatic bone disease, rapid bone growth, and osteomalacia (e.g. that induced by phenytoin) are other common causes of an elevated alkaline phosphatase level. The normal level in this patient is evidence for the absence of obstructive liver disease.

Serum glutamic oxaloacetic transaminase (SGOT) and serum glutamic pyruvic transaminase (SGPT) are enzymes found in the liver as well as in muscle, brain, and other tissues and are important in amino acid and carbohydrate metabolism. As discussed earlier, enzyme levels increase in the serum when the tissues containing these enzymes are injured. For example, when there is severe hepatocellular destruction, as may occur in hepatitis, the SGOT and SGPT levels are elevated to between 500 and 3000 international units. In cholestatic jaundice (obstructive liver disease) the elevations are generally much lower (between 100 and 400 units).

In the case presented, the absence of markedly elevated levels, along with an increased indirect bilirubin level suggests the possibility of hemolysis as a probable diagnosis. Additional tests, not routinely performed, will confirm the diagnosis suggested by the routine liver function tests.

CASE HISTORY– PROSTATIC CARCINOMA: A 60-year-old man with carcinoma of the prostate was admitted to the hospital for a hypophysectomy. An adrenalectomy had already been performed, and he was receiving diethylstilbesterol and corticosteroids.

Lab Results:

Acid Phosphatase (Prostatic)	*0.26 U/100 ml*	*(Normal 0-0.7/100 ml)*
Acid Phosphatase (total)	*1.28 U*	*(Normal 0.1-0.73)*
Total Bilirubin	*0.8 mg%*	*(Normal 0.2-1.0)*
Alkaline Phosphatase	*20 U/ml*	*(Normal 2-5)*
Lactic Dehydrogenase (LDH)	*330 U/ml*	*(Normal 100-225)*

27. Why was an acid phosphatase determination done on this patient?

Prostatic tissue contains high concentrations of acid phosphatase, and patients with carcinoma of the prostate that has extended beyond the capsule usually have elevated serum levels of this enzyme. In this patient it was already known that the carcinoma was metastatic, and the acid phosphatase level was performed as an aid in determining *extent* of disease rather than the *nature* of the disease.

Both "prostatic" and "total" acid phosphatase were determined, because acid phosphatase is found in platelets and erythrocytes as well as the prostate. Thus the enzyme of prostatic origin is more specific for prostatic disease (4).

28. What is the most likely cause of the elevated alkaline phosphatase in this patient? Why can we rule out obstructive hepatic disease as a primary cause?

Since this patient has a normal total serum bilirubin, significant hepatic obstruction is not likely. The most likely cause of the elevated serum alkaline phosphatase in a patient of this type is carcinoma metastatic to bone.

29. How can a serum leucine aminopeptidase (LAP) determination distinguish between bone and hepatobiliary disease as a cause of an elevated serum alkaline phosphatase?

Serum LAP levels generally parallel those of serum alkaline phosphatase in hepatobiliary disease, while LAP is usually normal in bone diseases; thus, in this patient we might expect a normal serum LAP (4).

30. Why is the serum lactic deydrogenase (LDH) elevated in this patient? In what other types of conditions is the LDH elevated? How can the diagnostic specificity of the serum LDH be increased?

Patients with metastatic carcinoma tend to have elevated serum LDH values, and in carcinoma of the prostate, the levels of this enzyme have been used as a guide to chemotherapy. LDH is found in a wide variety of tissues; thus, elevations of serum levels can occur following disease in many different organs and tissues. This fact has limited the diagnostic usefulness of serum LDH determinations.

Serum LDH can be divided electrophoretically into five different isoenzymes. Since different tissues contain different proportions of these enzymes, isoenzyme separation can increase the usefulness of serum LDH in the diagnosis of some disorders. For example, the myocardium, erythrocytes and kidney contain primarily isoenzymes one and two while the liver and skeletal muscle are high in isoenzyme five (4,8).

31. What would you expect the serum aldolase level to be in this patient?

The serum aldolase resembles the LDH in being a rather ubiquitous enzyme in human tissues and is elevated in many of the same disorders. In carcinomas, one would expect similar elevations in both serum LDH and serum aldolase (4).

32. What are the major causes of creatine phosphokinase (CPK) elevations?

Creatine phosphokinase is an enzyme which is found primarily in muscle tissue. It is the first enzyme to rise following an acute myocardial infarction and can be elevated following strenuous exercise or muscle injury. Intramuscular injections of irritating drugs (i.e. digoxin, diazepam, chlorpromazine, phenytoin, and several antibiotics) can elevate this enzyme and confuse diagnosis. Other drugs, such as amphotericin B and clofibrate can cause direct muscle damage and elevate CPK levels (6).

REFERENCES

1. Collins RD: *Illustrated Manual of Laboratory Diagnosis, Indications and Interpretations.* Lippincott, Philadelphia, 1968.
2. Costrini, NV and Thomson, WM (eds): *Manual of Medical Therapeutics,* Ed. 22. Little Brown and Co., Boston, 1977.
3. Damm C: *Handbook of Clinical Laboratory Data.* The Chemical Rubber Company, Cleveland, Ohio, 1965.
4. Davidsohn I et al: *Todd-Sanford Clinical Diagnosis by Laboratory Methods,* Ed 15, WB Saunders, Philadelphia, 1974.
5. Dyke SC: *Recent Advances in Clinical Pathology.* Little Brown and Co. Boston, 1968.
6. Hansten PD: *Drug Interactions,* Ed 3. Lea & Febiger, Philadelphia, 1975.
7. Harper HA et al: *Review of Physiological Chemistry,* Ed 16. Lange Medical Publications, Los Altos, CA, 1977.
8. Henry RJ and Professional Staff of Bioscience Laboratories: *Specialized Diagnostic Laboratory Tests,* Ed 9, Bio-Science Laboratories, Van Nuys, Ca 1972.
9. Hoffman WS: *The Biochemistry of Clinical Medicine,* Ed 3. Year Book Medical Publishers, Chicago, 1964.
10. Kassirer J: Clinical evaluation of kidney function-glomerular function. NEJM 285:385, 1971.
11. Krupp MA et al: *Physician's Handbook,* Ed 18. Lange Medical Publications, Los Altos, Ca., 1976.
12. Levinson SA and MacFate RP: *Clinical Laboratory Diagnosis,* Ed 7. Lea & Febiger, Philadelphia, 1969.
13. Martin HF: *Normal Values in Clinical Chemistry.* Marcel Dekker Inc., New York, 1975.
13a. Rapaport SI: *Introduction to Hematology,* Harper & Row, New York, 1971.
14. Ravel R: *Clinical Laboratory Medicine,* Ed 2. Yearbook Medical Publisher Inc., Chicago, 1973.
15. Schmid R: Bilirubin metabolism in man. NEJM 287:703, 1972.
16. Sunderman FW: Drug interference in clinical biochemistry. Critical Review of Clinical Laboratory Science 1:427, 1970.
17. Thorn GW et al (eds): *Harrison's Principles of Internal Medicine,* Ed 8. McGraw Hill, NY, 1977.
18. Wallach J: *Interpretation of Diagnostic Tests,* Ed 2. Little, Brown and Co., Boston, 1974.
19. Widmann FK: *Goodale's Clinical Interpretation of Laboratory Tests,* Ed 7. FA Davis Co., Philadelphia, 1973.
20. Young DS et al: Effects of drugs on clinical laboratory tests. Clin Chem 18:1041, 1972.

Chapter 2

Clinical Pharmacokinetics

Michael E. Winter

In recent years, drug concentrations in biologic fluids have gained increased acceptance as a guide for drug therapy. Pharmacokinetics and biopharmaceutics are useful in predicting plasma levels as well as the changes in plasma levels which occur over time.

This chapter is a review of the basic principles of pharmacokinetics and assumes that the reader has had some formal education in this area. It should be emphasized, however, that although plasma levels are useful in the evaluation of therapy, they constitute only one parameter, and should not be used as the sole criterion for treatment.

Pharmacokinetic calculations should be considered only as a guide to the determination of dosage regimens. For example, if a calculated regimen appears unreasonable, a re-evaluation would be necessary. There is always the possibility that there has been a mathematical error or that the pharmacokinetic parameters utilized in the calculations are incorrect for the patient in question. In the latter instance, even the most elegant calculation is invalid.

This last point is an important one. Because many of the pharmacokinetic parameters available in the literature are based on a relatively small number of patients or normal volunteers (43,47,67), values obtained from the experimental data are, at best, estimates for those which might be expected in any given patient. This problem, as well as the variations which exist between subjects, emphasizes the need to obtain accurate plasma-level measurements and to re-evaluate pharmacokinetic parameters for each patient.

This chapter will describe the basic pharmacokinetic parameters first, then explain how these parameters may be used in the clinical setting. A more indepth discussion of these principles may be found in other references (51,63).

The case examples here focus on only a few of the drugs for which pharmacokinetic data are available. Although specific drugs are used in each case, it is important for the reader to recognize that the fundamental principles illustrated may be applied to many other drugs. Review articles which list pharmacokinetic parameters for a number of drugs (8,47) are useful; however, the reader is encouraged to seek out the original literature to determine the degree of intersubject variability and to evaluate the methodology and data from which such review material was obtained.

The first part of this chapter reviews the following pharmacokinetic parameters, the factors affecting them, and their use:

   a. Bioavailability (F) — extent of absorption
   b. Desired plasma concentration (Cp)
   c. Volume of Distribution (Vd) — major determinant of loading dose
   d. Clearance (Cl) — major determinant of maintenance dosing
   e. Elimination rate constant (Kd)—major determinant of time to reach steady state or for drug elimination, or for dosing interval

The second portion of the chapter will apply and interpret pharmacokinetic data in specific clinical situations.

BIOAVAILABILITY (F)

The rate of drug administration can be expressed by the following equation:

F x dose/τ = Rate in (R$_i$)   **(Eq. 1)**

where F is the bioavailability or fraction of the dose which is absorbed and tau (τ) is the dosing interval or time over which the dose is given.

When the salt of a drug is administered, F represents the bioavailability of the salt because the dose is usually expressed as the amount of salt which is administered. To determine F for the parent compound it is necessary to multiply this figure by the fraction of the total molecular weight which the active drug represents.

The *first-pass effect* may also affect bioavailability. That is, even though a drug is absorbed, it may be metabolized before it ever reaches the systemic circulation. Lidocaine is an example of a drug with a first-pass effect that is so great that oral administration is not practical (6). In the case of propranolol, a significant amount of drug is metabolized so that a much larger oral dose is required to achieve the same pharmacologic response as that obtained from an intravenous dose. The propranolol issue is further complicated by the presence of an active metabolite, 4-hydroxypropranolol (44).

The *dosage form* and *route of administration* may be important factors in determining the bioavailability of a drug. For example, the fraction of orally administered digoxin that is absorbed can depend not only on the source or manufacturer, but also on the dosage form. The average F for tablets is 0.62 while it is 0.77 for elixirs (18). Intravenous digoxin has an F of 1.0 since all of the dose reaches the systemic circulation.

Although the rate of absorption can be important when a rapid onset of drug action is required, it generally is not of concern when a drug is administered chronically. Rate becomes important only if it is so slow that it limits the absolute bioavailability of the drug.

1. What is the administration rate for digoxin 0.25 mg (250 mcg) given once daily as tablets? As the elixir?

As tablets:
  F x dose/τ = 0.62 x 250 mcg/day = 155 mcg/day

As elixir:
  = 0.77 x 250 mcg/day = 192 mcg/day

2. If a patient taking 0.25 mg digoxin daily as the tablet requires intravenous administration of the drug, what would an equivalent dose be?

Assuming F is 0.62 for oral tablets and 1.0 for an IV solution, the equivalent dose would be equal 155 mcg/day. Since the value of F is only an estimate, a reasonable dose would be approximately 150 mcg/day IV.

3. What is the equivalent dosage of oral theophylline for a patient receiving IV aminophylline at a rate of 80 mg/hr?

Although all of the drug that is administered intravenously reaches the systemic circulation, only 80% of aminophylline is the active compound theophylline; the remaining fraction is the ethylenediamine salt. Therefore, the bioavailability of theophylline from aminophylline would be 0.8. If it is assumed that oral theophylline is totally available, the equivalent oral dose would be:

  F x dose/τ = 0.8 x 80 mg/hr = 64 mg/hr

If oral aminophylline were to be given, the equivalent dose would be 80 mg since the ethylenediamine salt would be present in both the IV and oral dosage forms.

DESIRED PLASMA CONCENTRATION (Cp)

In the clinical setting, the drug concentration in plasma (Cp), which is used as a guide for therapy, represents drug that is bound to plasma protein plus drug that is unbound or free. It is the free or unbound form of the drug that is in equilibrium with the receptor site and is the pharmacologically active moiety. Decreased plasma protein binding can present a problem if the usual ratio of free (active) drug to total drug concentration in the plasma is increased. In such cases a greater pharmacologic effect can be expected for any given Cp (25).

The fraction of drug that is free is usually expressed as **alpha (α):**

(Eq. 2)

$$\alpha = \frac{\text{Free drug concentration}}{\text{Total drug concentration}} = \frac{\text{Cp free}}{\text{Cp bound + Cp free}}$$

There are two factors which control alpha. One is the binding affinity of the drug for the plasma protein (frequently albumin), and the second is the amount of plasma protein available for binding (25). In most cases alpha is independent of the drug concentration as long as saturation of the binding sites is not approached. Changes in the concentration of binding protein, however, will affect the bound concentration, but generally, not the free concentration, resulting in an altered alpha or fraction of the total drug concentration which is free.

If the albumin concentration is decreased, that drug which is released will not remain in the plasma exclusively, but will equilibrate with the tissue compartment resulting in a very minor increase in Cp free as long as Vd is relatively large (see Fig. 1).

The smaller alpha is, the greater will be the significance of altered plasma protein binding. In general, if alpha is normally less than or equal to 0.1 (i.e., 10% or less free), there is a good possibility that protein binding changes will be clinically significant; if alpha is greater than or equal to 0.5 (50% or more free), it is unlikely that plasma protein binding changes will be of any consequence.

As a general rule, if alpha increases in any given situation, the clinician should reduce the desired Cp by the same proportion (25).

4. What should the therapeutic plasma level for phenytoin be in a uremic patient? How is this value derived?

A number of studies have documented the fact that the protein binding of phenytoin is altered in the uremic patient. The alpha for phenytoin in uremics has been estimated to be in the range of 0.2 to 0.3; the alpha for patients with normal renal function is approximately 0.1 (1,45). Therefore, therapeutic phenytoin levels of 10 to 20 mcg/ml represent free drug concentrations of 1 to 2 mcg/ml in the non-uremic patient. If the fraction free is increased for any given plasma level by a factor of 2.5 ($\alpha = 0.25$), plasma levels (total drug) in the range of 4 to 8 mcg/ml should result in free phenytoin levels of 1 to 2 mcg/ml in uremic patients.

Unfortunately, it is not known how rapidly this change in protein binding occurs, and it may, in part, be due to the reduced serum albumin concentrations which are frequently observed in uremic patients.

The relationship between the plasma concentration of a drug and the plasma protein concentration may be expressed by the following equation:

$$\frac{Cp'}{Cp_{adjusted}} = (1-\alpha) \times \frac{P'}{P} + \alpha \qquad \textbf{(Eq.3)}$$

This equation can be used to estimate how significantly, altered plasma albumin levels will affect the desired therapeutic drug concentration. Cp' and P' represent the patient's observed drug plasma level and albumin concentration respectively; α and P represent the average, "normal" values for alpha and albumin concentration (usually 4 gm/100 ml); and $Cp_{adjusted}$ is the plasma concentration of drug that would have been observed if albumin had been normal. (Also see Question 58).

5. What would the adjusted phenytoin concentration be for a patient with normal renal function who has an observed plasma level of 5.5 mcg/ml and an albumin concentration of 2.0 gm/100 ml?

Using the normal alpha of 0.1 for phenytoin, and an albumin concentration of 4 gm/100 ml, the adjusted phenytoin concentration would be approximately:

$$Cp_{adj} = \frac{Cp'}{(1-\alpha) \times \dfrac{P'}{P} + \alpha} = \frac{5.5\ \text{mcg/ml}}{(1-0.1)\dfrac{2\text{gm/100ml}}{4\text{gm/100ml}} + 0.1}$$

$$Cp_{adj} = \frac{5.5\ \text{mcg/ml}}{0.9 \times 0.5 + 0.1} = \frac{5.5}{0.55} = 10\ \text{mcg/ml}$$

That is, the Cp that would have been observed if the albumin were "normal" would be approximately 10 mcg/ml, and the pharmacologic effect that one would expect from the observed 5.5 mcg/ml would be equal to the adjusted level of 10 mcg/ml. The free level in both instances would be 1.0 mcg/ml. In general, adjustments are not necessary for increased or moderate reductions in albumin levels, and using albumin concentration in Eq. 3 is appropriate only when the drug in question is bound primarily to albumin. Many of the basic drugs, e.g., quinidine and lidocaine, are bound

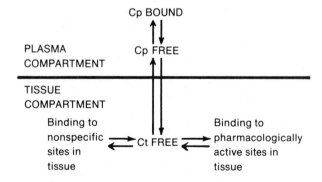

Fig. 1: *Equilibrium between free and bound drug concentrations.* It is assumed that only Cp FREE can cross into the tissue compartment or site of pharmacologic activity.

primarily to globulin proteins, making adjustments for albumin concentration inappropriate. Adjustment for changes in globulin binding is difficult, because the basic drugs are usually bound to a specific globulin which is only a small part of the total globulin concentration.

VOLUME OF DISTRIBUTION (Vd)

The *volume of distribution* for a drug or the "apparent volume of distribution", does not necessarily refer to any real volume (51) and is simply the size of the compartment necessary to account for all the drug in the body if it were present at the same concentration everywhere as in the sample measured. The equation for the volume of distribution is expressed as follows:

$$Vd = \frac{Ab}{Cp} \quad \text{or} \quad Cp = \frac{Ab}{Vd} \qquad \textbf{(Eq. 4)}$$

where Vd is the apparent volume of distribution, Ab is the amount of drug in the body, and Cp is the plasma concentration of drug. Since the volume of distribution is the factor which accounts for all of the drug in the body, it can be used to estimate the *loading dose* necessary to rapidly achieve some desired plasma concentration:

$$\textbf{Loading dose} = \frac{Vd \times Cp}{F} \qquad \textbf{(Eq. 5)}$$

where Cp is the desired plasma level and F represents the fraction of the dose administered that will reach the systemic circulation.

Apparent volume of distributions which are larger than the plasma compartment (>3L) only indicate that the drug is also present in tissues or fluids outside that compartment. The actual sites of distribution cannot be determined from this value.

The apparent volume of distribution is a function of the lipid versus water solubilities and of the plasma and tissue protein binding properties of the drug. Factors which tend to keep the drug in the plasma (increase Cp), such as low lipid solubility, binding to plasma protein, or decreased tissue binding, reduce the apparent volume of distribution. It follows then that factors which decrease Cp, such as decreased plasma protein binding, increased tissue binding, and increased lipid solubility, increase the apparent volume of distribution.

It is important to remember, however, that plasma levels (Cp) represent both the free or pharmacologically active and inactive or bound drug. Therefore, plasma protein binding changes which alter the apparent volume of distribution will also alter the desired plasma concentration in the opposite direction so that the loading dose is generally not changed. (See Eq. 5) (25). This assumes that the major portion of the drug is actually outside the plasma compartment and the amount of drug bound to plasma protein is a small percentage of the total.

6. Estimate the loading dose of digoxin for a 70 kg man which would be necessary to attain a plasma level of 1.5 ng/ml (mcg/L).

If one assumes that the apparent volume of distribution is approximately 7.3 L/kg (49) and the bioavailability of the tablets is 0.62, the calculated loading dose would be:

$$\frac{7.3 \text{ L/kg} \times 70 \text{ kg} \times 1.5 \text{ mcg/L}}{0.62} = 1236 \text{ mcg or } 1.236 \text{ mg}$$

A reasonable approximation would be 1.25 mg given orally as tablets. The usual clinical approach would be to give the loading dose in divided doses (0.25-0.5 mg per dose) every six hours and observe the patient before each successive dose is administered. In addition, clinicians frequently use a bioavailability factor greater than 0.62 (e.g. 0.7 or 0.75) to guard against overshooting the desired level.

7. What would an appropriate intravenous loading dose of phenytoin be for a 70 kg uremic patient who has a normal plasma albumin concentration?

Odar-Cedarlof (45) indicated that although plasma phenytoin levels following a single intravenous dose in uremic patients were one-half of those observed in normal patients, the fraction free (alpha) increased from 0.12 to 0.25. Therefore, the lower plasma levels which were one-half of normal produced the same free or pharmacologically active concentration. Also, the volume of distribution increased by approximately two-fold (0.65 L/kg to 1.44 L/kg). This information indicated that the phenytoin loading dose would be the same for uremic and non-uremic patients, assuming no change in bioavailability. (see Eq. 5).

Loading dose = $(2 \times Vd) (\frac{1}{2}Cp_{desired})$ = no change in LD

8. How will decreased tissue binding affect the apparent volume of distribution of a drug?

Decreased tissue binding will increase the Cp by allowing more of the drug to remain in the plasma. It will also decrease the apparent volume of distribution (13). If the desired plasma level remains unchanged, a smaller loading dose will be required. (See Fig. 1, Question 18, and Eq. 5.)

$$\frac{Vd \cdot Cp}{F} = \text{loading dose}$$

9. What is a two compartment model?

If one thinks of the body as a single compartment, pharmacokinetic calculations are relatively simple. However, there are some situations when it is more appropriate to consider the body as two, and occasionally more than two compartments. The first compartment can be thought of as a rapidly equilibrating

volume, usually made up of blood and those organs or tissues which have high blood-flow. This first compartment has a volume referred to as Vp or $V_{initial}$. The second compartment requires a somewhat longer time period to equilibrate with the drug. Its volume is referred to as Vt or tissue volume (51). The half time of the distribution phase is referred to as the **alpha (α) half-life,** and the half time of drug elimination from the body is referred to as **beta (β) half-life.** The sum of Vp and Vt is the **apparent volume of distribution (Vd).** See Fig. 2. Drug is assumed to enter and be eliminated from Vd in Vp.

10. What is the significance of a two compartment model in the calculation of a loading dose?

Because some time is required for drug to distribute into Vt, a rapidly administered dose calculated from Vd (Vp + Vt) would result in an initial Cp larger than predicted because of the smaller initial volume of distribution (Vp). This has significance in two cases. The first is when a target organ in which the drug may have a toxic or therapeutic effect appears as though it were located in Vp, e.g., lidocaine. In this instance the concentration of drug in the target organ could be much higher than expected and produce toxicity. This problem can be circumvented by calculating the total loading dose based on Vd; then, either administering the

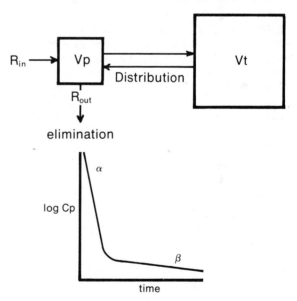

Fig. 2: *Volumes of distribution for a two-compartment model. Vp is the initial volume of distribution. Vt represents the tissue volume of distribution. Note that drug elimination (R_{out}) is assumed to occur in Vp. The lower graph shows how a drug administered into Vp follows a biphasic decay pattern. The initial decay half-life (α t½) is usually due to drug being distributed into Vt. The second decay half-life (β t½) is usually due to drug being eliminated from the body.*

loading dose at a rate slow enough to allow for distribution into Vt, or giving sufficiently small increments of the total loading dose so that the Cp in Vp does not exceed some presumed critical concentration (4,42).

The second situation occurs when the target organ is in the second compartment, Vt (e.g. digoxin). In this case, Cp can be rather high initially, as long as the distributed or equilibrated drug concentration is within therapeutic concentrations. If plasma samples for these drugs are obtained before distribution is complete, the reported level will not reflect the tissue concentration at equilibrium. In general, these samples cannot be used to predict therapeutic or toxic effects of the drug (66).

The problem of distribution is most significant when the drug is given by the intravenous route. It is not a problem when a drug is given orally, because the rate of absorption is usually slower than the rate of distribution from Vp into Vt; an exception to this rule is digoxin.

CLEARANCE (Cl)

How one achieves a desired plasma concentration by giving a loading dose has already been discussed. To maintain that concentration, the drug must be replaced at a rate equal to its loss. The pharmacokinetic parameter which accounts for drug loss from the body is clearance. *Clearance* can best be thought of as the intrinsic ability of the body or its organs of elimination (usually kidneys and liver) to remove drug from the blood or plasma. Clearance is expressed as a volume per unit of time. It is important to recognize that clearance by itself does not indicate how much drug is being removed, it only represents the volume of blood or plasma which would be completely cleared of drug if it were present. The amount of drug removed depends on the concentration of drug as well as the clearance.

$$R_o = Cl \times Cp \qquad \text{(Eq. 6)}$$

where R_o is rate of drug removal and Cl is clearance. At steady state (ss) the rate of drug removal (R_{out} must equal the rate of drug administration (R_{in}):

$$R_{in} = R_{out}$$

If we substitute $Cl \times \overline{Cpss}$ for R_{out} where $\overline{Cpss}$ is equal to the average Cp at steady state:

$$R_{in} = Cl \times \overline{Cpss} \qquad \text{(Eq. 7)}$$

The clearance can then be calculated from a known rate of drug administration and a steady state plasma level.

$$\frac{R_{in}}{Cpss} = Cl \qquad \text{or} \qquad \frac{R_{in}}{Cl} = \overline{Cpss} \qquad \text{(Eq. 8)}$$

11. What is the apparent clearance of lidocaine in a patient who is receiving an intravenous infusion of 2 mg/min and has a steady state plasma level of 3 mg/L?

Since the plasma level represents steady state, and at steady state R_{in} is equal to R_{out}, Eq. 8 can be used to calculate the lidocaine clearance in this patient:

$$\frac{2 \text{ mg/min}}{3 \text{ mg/L}} = Cl = 0.667 \text{ L/min}$$

The lidocaine clearance is therefore 0.667 L/min (667 ml/min), if one assumes that the bioavailability of lidocaine is 1.0 (100%) when it is administered intravenously.

12. What pharmacokinetic parameters are used to estimate the maintenance dose of a drug?

If Eq. 1 is combined with Eq. 6, the following equation can be derived:

$$F \times dose/\tau = Cl \times \overline{Cpss} \qquad \text{(Eq. 9)}$$

$\overline{Cpss}$ represents the average steady-state concentration which is desired. Therefore, the maintenance dose can be estimated if the clearance, $\overline{Cpss}$, dosing interval, and the fraction absorbed are known.

$$\text{Maintenance Dose} = \frac{Cl \times \overline{Cpss} \times \tau}{F} \qquad \text{(Eq. 10)}$$

13. How should clearance be adjusted when the patient's weight is not the average 70 kg usually reported in the literature?

In general, clearance is best adjusted on the basis of body surface area rather than body weight (64). This concept is also used to correct creatinine clearance to a normalized body surface area of 1.73 m². Body surface area can be calculated from Eq. 21, or, it can be obtained from various charts and nomograms (52,56). If body weight is reasonably close to the average 70 kg (1.73 m²), an adjustment based on weight will not incur any great error.

14. Can clearance be affected by changes in plasma protein binding?

Like the volume of distribution, the value assigned to clearance does not necessarily represent any real volume per unit time. This can be seen if clearance (see Eq. 8) is expressed as:

$$Cl = \frac{rate_{in}}{Cpss}$$

As previously discussed, Cp represents both free and bound drug. Because only the unbound drug can be metabolized or eliminated, the clearance calculated in patients with decreased plasma protein binding may be increased, but the *amount* of drug cleared per unit time remains the same (see Eq. 8 and Eq. 6):

$$\frac{\text{Rate}_{in}}{\text{Cpss}} = \text{Cl}$$

$$\text{Cl} \times \overline{\text{Cpss}} = \text{Rate}_{out} \text{ (no change)}$$

This relationship will remain true as long as the amount of drug cleared does not exceed that which is unbound as the blood or plasma passes through the eliminating organ. Some drugs, however, are metabolized or excreted so efficiently that some (perhaps all) of the drug bound to plasma protein re-equilibrates with plasma after the initial free drug is removed and is then metabolized or excreted (70). In this situation the plasma protein is acting as a "transport system" for the drug, carrying it to the eliminating organs. In such cases, the plasma level will increase until the amount of drug presented to the eliminating organ, then cleared, is equal to the rate of drug administration.

The *extraction ratio* for a drug will indicate whether the plasma proteins are acting as a transport system for metabolism, or as "innocent by-standers". The extraction ratio can be thought of as the fraction of the drug presented to the eliminating organ which is cleared after a single pass through that organ. One way to get a rough estimate of the extraction ratio is to divide the blood or plasma clearance of a drug by the blood or plasma flow to the eliminating organ. If the extraction ratio exceeds alpha, or binding constant, then the plasma proteins are acting as a transport system, and clearance will not increase proportionately to a change in alpha. If, however, the extraction ratio is less than alpha, it is probable that clearance will appear to increase by the same proportion that alpha changes. This approach does not take into account other factors such as the binding and elimination from red blood cells, or changes in metabolic function, but it may serve as a useful guide.

15. Can cardiac output affect drug clearance?

Decreased cardiac output affects the ability of the liver to remove drugs by decreasing hepatic blood flow. This becomes significant for drugs with high extraction ratios (60). Congestive heart failure can also produce passive liver congestion thereby decreasing its metabolic ability. This would affect those drugs with low extraction ratios whose clearances are not flow-limited (54).

16. What are the major organs of drug elimination and metabolism, and how can clearance be adjusted for changes in their function?

Generally, drug elimination occurs through two routes: as unchanged drug through the kidney (renal clearance) and by metabolism in the liver (metabolic clearance). These two routes of clearance are as-sumed to be independent of one another and additive (51).

$$\text{Cl}_{total} = \text{Cl}_{metabolism} + \text{Cl}_{renal} \qquad \textbf{(Eq. 11)}$$

where Cl_{total} is total clearance, $\text{Cl}_{metabolism}$ is clearance by metabolism, and Cl_{renal} is clearance by the renal route. Since the kidneys and liver function independently, it is assumed that a change in one does not affect the other. This enables one to estimate Cl_{total} in the presence of renal or hepatic failure of both. If one knows the fraction of Cl_t which is comprised of the metabolic (Cl_m) and renal (Cl_r) routes respectively, the clearance for the affected route can be reduced proportionately before the Cl_t is calculated. Since metabolic function is difficult to quantitate, this approach is most often used when there is decreased renal function:

$$\text{Cl}_{adjusted} = \text{Cl}_m + (\text{Cl}_r \times \text{fraction of normal renal function re-maining}) \qquad \textbf{(Eq. 12)}$$

Equation 12 can be used to estimate the maintenance dose in renal failure by substituting the adjusted Cl_t into Eq. 10. This assumes, of course, that the metabolites are not active and Cl_m is not affected by renal failure.

A change in the ability of an eliminating organ to function is most significant when it constitutes the major route of drug elimination. However, as the major elimination pathway becomes further and further compromised, the "minor" pathway becomes a more significant proportion of the total clearance. For example, a drug which is usually 67% eliminated by the renal route and 33% by the metabolic route will be 100% metabolized in the event of complete renal failure; the total clearance, however, will only be one-third of the normal value.

ELIMINATION RATE CONSTANT (Kd)

The two situations thus far discussed include the estimation of a loading dose determined by the apparent volume of distribution and the maintenance dose determined by the apparent clearance. When a loading dose is not given or a maintenance dose is given on an intermittent basis, it may be desirable to predict how the plasma level will change with time. The change will be a function of the clearance and the volume of distribution and is frequently expressed as the elimination rate constant, Kd.

$$\text{Kd} = \frac{\text{Cl}}{\text{Vd}} \qquad \textbf{(Eq. 13)}$$

The *elimination rate constant* is expressed as a fraction per unit of time and represents the fraction of the volume of distribution which will be cleared per unit of time. For example, a drug with a clearance of l0 L/day and a Vd of 100 L would have an elimination rate constant of 0.1 days^{-1}, i.e.,

$$\frac{10\ L/d}{100\ L} = 0.1\ day^{-1}$$

The elimination rate constant (Kd) is the rate of elimination at an instant in time, and if the plasma level is decaying, the *amount* of drug removed per day will become less and less, although the *fraction* of the total amount of drug remaining in the body which is removed will remain constant. This essentially defines **first-order elimination kinetics** where the fraction eliminated remains unchanged, or clearance and Vd are constant. The amount eliminated per unit time can be viewed as $Cl \times Cp = R_{out}$ where Cl is constant and Cp is continuing to decrease. Because the rate of decline is a first-order process, it can be made linear by plotting the logarithm of the plasma level versus time (see Fig. 3). The plasma level decay can be described by the following equation:

$$Cp = Cp° \times e^{-kdt} \qquad \text{(Eq. 14)}$$

where Cp° and Cp are the plasma concentrations at the beginning and end of the time interval t, and e^{-kdt} is the fraction of Cp° remaining at time t. If Cp is equal to ½Cp° then by definition t is equal to **t½ (half-life).** The relationship between k_d and t½ can be derived from Eq. 14:

$$Cp = Cp° \times e^{-kdt}\ or,$$

$$\ln \frac{Cp}{(Cp°)} = -Kdt$$

if Cp = ½Cp°, then

$$\ln(½) = -Kd\ t\ (or\ t½\ since\ Cp = ½Cp°)\ or,$$

$$-.693 = -Kdt½\ or,$$

$$Kd = \frac{.693}{t½} \qquad \text{(Eq. 15)}$$

Also, if $\frac{Cl}{Vd}$ is substituted for Kd (Eq. 13) in Eq. 15, the following equation for t½ can be derived:

$$t½ = \frac{.693\ Vd}{Cl} \qquad \text{(Eq. 16)}$$

Half-life is therefore, dependent upon and determined by the pharmacokinetic variables, Cl and Vd, not vice versa. It is frequently assumed that because Eq. 13 can be rearranged to

$$Cl = Kd\ Vd \qquad \text{(Eq. 17)}$$

that clearance is determined by Kd (or half-life) and Vd; however, this is conceptually incorrect. In other words, one cannot make any assumptions about the Vd or clearance of a drug based upon knowledge of the half-life alone. If the half-life of a drug is prolonged, for example, the clearance may be increased, decreased or the same depending upon the Vd.

Loading doses can be calculated from Vd alone, and maintenance doses can be calculated from clearance. However, the half-life, without one of the other two parameters, does not enable one to estimate either the loading or maintenance dose.

17. When is the half-life an important pharmacokinetic parameter?

Half-life is an important variable to consider when one needs to answer questions with regard to time such as: *"How long will it take to reach steady-state on a constant dosing regimen?" "How long will it take for all of the drug to be removed from the body?"* These questions can be answered if it is realized that one half-life is required to reach 50%, two half-lives to reach 75%, three half-lives to reach 87.5%, and four half-lives to reach 93.75% of the new steady state. In most clinical situations, it is sufficient to wait three to four half-lives before it is assumed that a new steady state has been reached or that most of the drug has been eliminated from the body. This concept does not take into consideration the absolute magnitude of change or the plasma levels which are observed at the beginning and end of this time period. Therefore, to accept approximately 90% of a new steady state level as satisfactory is an arbitrary decision which may, on occasion, have to be altered.

The half-life may also be used to *estimate the appropriate dosing interval* (τ) during maintenance therapy. If no more than a 50% change in plasma level between doses is desired, the dosing interval (τ) should be made less than or equal to the half-life. The maintenance dose can then be calculated from Eq. 10. The plasma levels will be above the average steady-state plasma level for approximately the first half of the dosing interval and below the average steady-state plasma level during the second half of the dosing interval.

A more exact estimate of the peak or **maximum plasma level at steady state (Cpss max)** can be ob-

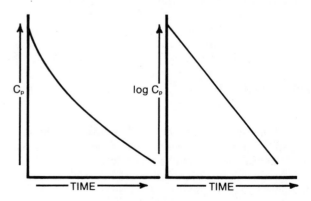

Fig. 3: *First order elimination when Cp or log Cp is plotted vs. time.*

tained from the formula:

$$Cpss_{max} = \frac{\frac{F \times dose}{Vd}}{(1-e^{-kd\tau})}$$ (Eq. 18)

where F × dose/Vd is the maximal change in plasma concentration (Δ Cp) and $(1-e^{-kd\tau})$ is the fraction lost during the dosing interval τ. The **minimum or trough plasma level at steady state ($Cpss_{min}$)** could then be estimated by the following equations which are derived from Eq. 14 and a definition of $Cpss_{min}$.

$$Cpss_{min} = Cpss_{max} \times e^{-kd\tau}$$
or
$$Cpss_{min} = Cpss_{max} - \frac{F \times dose}{Vd}$$ (Eq. 19)

In certain situations, the dosing interval is much longer than the half-life and, for all practical purposes, all of the drug is eliminated during a dosing interval. Therefore, each new dose is essentially a new loading dose. Antibiotics are commonly dosed in this manner because the therapeutic index is usually so large that wide fluctuations in plasma levels are acceptable and the therapeutic effect requires that the plasma level be above some minimal concentration for only a brief period of time relative to the entire dosing interval.

Some authors have suggested that the elimination rate constant (Kd) be adjusted in a manner similar to clearance (see Eq. 11) to determine doses for patients in renal failure (10,67). They make the assumption that clearance is proportionate to Kd if the Vd remains constant. Because clearances by various routes are additive (see Eq. 10), so are the elimination rate constants (see Eq. 13):

$Kd_{adjusted} = K_{metabolic} + (K_{renal} \times$ fraction of normal renal function remaining) (Eq. 20)

The adjusted Kd is then multiplied by the normal volume of distribution to estimate the adjusted clearance:

$Cl_{adjusted} = Kd_{adjusted} \times Vd_{normal}$ (Eq. 21)

$Cl_{adjusted}$ is used to estimate the maintenance dose in renal failure (see Eq. 10):

$$\text{Maintenance dose} = \frac{Cl_{adjusted} \times Cpss \times \tau}{F}$$

This approach satisfactorily estimates the adjusted clearance, but it may be a poor estimate of half-life if Vd is altered in renal failure (67). If Vd is altered in renal failure, one must still use the normal value for Vd in Eq. 21 since Kd was adjusted with the assumption that Vd was unchanged. The most direct method of calculating an adjusted clearance is to use the clearance values initially as described in Eq. 12.

CLINICAL APPLICATION OF PHARMACOKINETIC PRINCIPLES

The basic pharmacokinetic parameters: clearance, volume of distribution, and elimination-rate constant or half-life, will now be applied to specific clinical situations. Although the following situations are based on drugs which are actually used in the clinical setting, the reader should place major emphasis on the pharmacokinetic concepts, rather than the characteristics of the specific drug used in the example.

When confronted with a pharmacokinetic problem, it is important to first assess when the last dose of the drug was given and how long the patient has been taking the drug. If steady state exists, clearance is the primary pharmacokinetic parameter one should consider. If a change in plasma level has resulted from the administration of a single dose, the volume of distribution should be considered. And, if one must predict the change in plasma level which will occur with time, both clearance and volume of distribution (i.e. Kd or t½) will be needed to solve the problem. Data should not be fitted into a formula without first determining whether the formula is appropriate to solve the problem.

18. J.P. is a 68-yr-old 70 kg woman with congestive heart failure (CHF) and chronic renal failure (C_{cr} 25 ml/min). It is decided that a loading dose of digoxin is to be administered. What must you consider in calculating the estimated loading dose?

If it is assumed that the desired steady state plasma level is 1.5 mcg/L (ng/ml), the loading dose can be calculated using Eq. 5:

$$L.D. = \frac{Vd \times Cp}{F}$$

Several studies (28,55) have documented that the apparent volume of distribution of digoxin is smaller (4.7 L/kg) for patients with renal failure, especially those patients with creatinine clearances below 30 ml/min (22). However, although some patients have a volume of distribution which is one-half of normal, others show no change at all. A reasonable approach might be to use the average value for patients in renal failure of approximately 330 L (4.7 L/kg) (49). If the dose is to be given orally as tablets, bioavailability must also be considered.

$$L.D. = \frac{330 L \times 1.5 mcg/L}{0.62} = 798 \text{ mcg or approx. } 0.75 \text{ mg.}$$

This approach assumes that a plasma level of 1.5 mcg/L is an appropriate pharmacokinetic endpoint. One author believes that since there is decreased tissue binding of digoxin in patients with renal failure, the desired plasma level should be increased to insure therapeutic tissue levels (65). This theory implies that the total amount of drug in the body (Ab), not Cp, would be a more appropriate pharmacokinetic end-point. Since there are no studies which correlate the total amount of drug in the body with toxicity, and since there is no indication that renal failure patients can "tolerate" higher than average plasma digoxin levels, it is this author's opinion that "normal" therapeutic digoxin plasma levels should be used as the pharmacokinetic endpoint.

19. What would be an appropriate maintenance dose of digoxin for J.P.? How long would it take to reach steady state?

Maintenance doses are designed to replace the amount of drug lost during the dosing interval, and can be determined using Eq. 10:

$$M.D. = \frac{Cl \times \overline{Cpss} \times \tau}{F}$$

Digoxin clearance can be estimated using a variation of Eq. 12 (28,55):

$$Cl_t = Cl_r + Cl_m$$

$$\text{Digoxin } Cl_t = 1.0 \times C_{Cr} + 40 \text{ ml/min}$$

If the metabolic clearance of digoxin is reduced by one-half in CHF (28,55), clearance for this patient may be estimated as follows:

$$\text{Digoxin } Cl_t = 1.0 \times 25 \text{ ml/min} + 20 \text{ ml/min} = 45 \text{ ml/min}$$

If the units are changed from ml/min to L/day, the clearance equals:

$$\frac{52 \text{ ml/min} \times 1440 \text{ min/day}}{1000 \text{ ml/L}} = 64.8 \text{ L/day}$$

and the daily maintenance dose can be estimated as follows:

$$M.D./day = \frac{64.8 \text{ L/day} \times 1.5 \text{ mcg/L} \times 1 \text{ day}}{0.62}$$

$$M.D. = 156.8 \text{ mcg/day}$$

Thus, 1¼ tablets of 0.125 mg digoxin should be administered daily. Many clinicians would prefer to give only 0.125 mg daily to insure that the clearance has not been overestimated, and then adjust the dose upward if necessary.

To insure that steady state has been reached, the patient must receive a constant dose for three to four half-lives. The half-life can be estimated by using Eq. 13:

$$\frac{Cl}{Vd} = Kd = \frac{0.693}{t\frac{1}{2}}$$

or by Eq. 16:

$$t\frac{1}{2} = \frac{Vd \times 0.693}{Cl}$$

As can be seen, the t½ will be a function of both the clearance and volume of distribution.

If the average Vd is 7.3 L/kg, then an estimated t½ is:

$$t\frac{1}{2} = \frac{511 \text{ L} \times 0.693}{75.6 \text{ L/day}} = 4.68 \text{ days}$$

It will therefore take 4 × 4.7 days or 18.8 days to reach steady state. If, however, the VD is only 330 L as estimated in Question 9, the half-life will only be:

$$t\frac{1}{2} = \frac{330 \text{ L} \times 0.693}{75.6 \text{ L/day}} = 3.03 \text{ days}$$

and it will only take 4 × 3.0 days or 12 days to reach steady state. Therefore, it will take 12 to 18 days to reach steady state. However, since all of the calculations were based on average literature values, this is only an estimate.

20. A patient who has been on the same dose of digoxin for 15 days comes to the clinics for follow-up and is found to be doing well. A digoxin plasma level drawn on the morning of her visit is reported as 2.4 ng/ml. If the upper limit for the therapeutic level is 2.0 ng/ml, how can you account for the level being in the toxic range?

Since this level supposedly represents $\overline{Cpss}$, one must evaluate each of the factors which may alter steady state (Eq. 9):

$$F \times dose/\tau = Cl \times \overline{Cpss}$$

or

$$\overline{Cpss} = \frac{F \times dose}{Cl \times \tau}$$

a) F: the patient may be absorbing more than the average of 62%.

b) Dose: the patient may be taking more than the prescribed dose, although taking less than the prescribed dose occurs more commonly (54).

c) τ: the patient may be taking the proper dose more often than prescribed.

d) Cl: the patient's clearance or ability to eliminate the drug may be less than it was estimated to be. If this were the case, this may not be a steady state level, as the half-life would be longer (see Eq. 16).

e) $\overline{Cpss}$: the assay could be in error, interfering substances may be present, or the plasma level may have been drawn during the distribution phase of the drug.

Plasma levels obtained during the distribution phase of digoxin are higher than anticipated because the drug is absorbed from the gastrointestinal tract faster than it is distributed into the tissues. Since the myocardium responds to digoxin as though it were in the tissue compartment (V_t), plasma levels obtained before distribution is complete do not correlate with pharmacologic effects of the drug (53,66). Most authors recommend that digoxin plasma levels be obtained just before the next dose is given, or that a minimum of six hours be allowed to elapse after taking a dose before the sample is obtained (66). Since the alpha or distribution t½ is approximately 35 minutes (30), only two hours are required to see maximum response following intravenous administration of digoxin. However, Shapiro found that distribution occurred at about four hours following an intravenous dose of the drug (53).

21. Outline a reasonable plan to determine the cause of a higher than predicted digoxin level?
a) Ask the patient whether the daily digoxin dose was taken before or after the blood sample was obtained.
b) Determine the patient's compliance. This is difficult but must be attempted.
c) Determine if any drugs interfered with the digoxin assay. Literature reports of interference by drugs having a steriod nucleus similar to that of digoxin are applicable only to the specific antibody and radioimmunoassay used in the particular report, and may not apply to the specific assay used to determine the patient's digoxin plasma level. Therefore, the laboratory measuring the serum level would have to be contacted about the possibility of assay interference (32,58).
d) Reschedule a second digoxin plasma level, but be certain that it is drawn a minimum of six hours after a dose. Preferably, obtain the sample in the morning before the daily dose is taken.
e) Evaluating the patient's Cl and F is difficult and costly because such evaluation would require hospitalization of the patient. It would only result in the obvious conclusion of reducing the dose if it was decided that, in fact, the level was too high. This approach would only be used under the most unusual of circumstances.

22. In 1966, Doherty and Perkins (11) evaluated the kinetics of digoxin in hyperthyroid, hypothyroid and euthyroid patients. Fig. 4 is a representation of one of the graphs from this study. Using the graph, discuss the implications of thyroid disease on loading dose, maintenance dose, and the time required to reach steady state, relative to the euthyroid state. Assume that the same C̄pss is desired in all patients.
Loading dose: Since hypothyroid patients have higher plasma levels, they must have a decreased apparent volume of distribution. Therefore, a decrease in the loading doses would be appropriate. Hyperthyroid patients have lower plasma levels and would require larger loading doses for the same reasons.
Time to reach steady state: The slope of all the decay curves are the same. Therefore, the half-lives and elimination-rate constants are equal, and the time required to reach steady state will be the same for hyperthyroid, hypothyroid and euthyroid patients re-

ceiving digoxin.
Maintenance dose: Since Kd is the same in all patients, the clearance and volume of distribution must both change by the same proportion and in the same direction (see Eq. 13):

$$\frac{Cl}{Vd_{(variable)}} = Kd_{(same\ in\ all\ patients\ studied)}$$

Therefore, hypothyroid patients must have a decreased clearance as the volume of distribution is decreased. The reduction in clearance would necessitate a reduction in maintenance doses. Hyperthyroid patients must have an increased clearance as the Vd is increased; therefore, an increase in maintenance dose would be indicated if C̄pss is to remain the same as for euthyroid patients.

It is important to re-emphasize, however, that although Kd and Vd were used to estimate clearance, the latter is an independent variable which like Cl, is affected by thyroid disease. However, since both clearance and Vd were affected in the same direction, and to the same degree, the half-life (Kd) did not change.

23. J.R., a 10 kg child, is admitted to the hospital for an acute attack of asthma. His theophylline level obtained on admission was reported to be 5 mcg/ml. What dose of aminophylline is needed to rapidly increase the plasma level to 15 mcg/ml (mg/L)? (Also see chapter on *Asthma*)
Since the patient has a plasma concentration of 5 mg/L and the desired level is 15 mg/L, an increase of 10 mg/L is necessary. The apparent volume of distribution is approximately the same for children as for

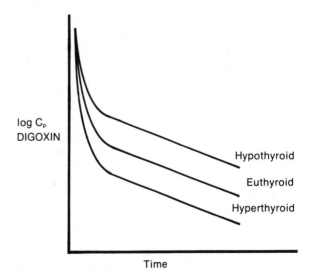

Fig. 4: *Distribution and elimination of digoxin when administered by the intravenous route to hypothyroid, hyperthyroid, and euthyroid patients. (Ref. 11)*

adults, or about 0.4 to 0.5 L/kg (36). Therefore, J.R.'s Vd can be estimated to be:

$$Vd = 10 \text{ kg} \times 0.45 \text{ L/kg} = 4.5 \text{ L}$$

If the desired Cp is 10 mg/L and 80% of aminophylline contains the active ingredient, theophylline (i.e., F = 0.8), the loading dose can be estimated using Eq. 5:

$$L.D. = \frac{4.5 \text{ L} \times 10 \text{ mg/L}}{0.8} = 56.25 \text{ mg}$$

24. What would be an appropriate maintenance infusion to keep the plasma level at 15 mg/L?

Because the patient is a child and weighs considerably less than the average 70 kg adult, an estimate of the clearance may be most accurate if it is done on the basis of body surface area.

The surface area can be estimated in the following way (63):

Body Surface Area (BSA) = 0.088 × (weight in kg)$^{0.728}$

(Eq. 22)

$$BSA = 0.088 \times 10 \text{ kg}^{0.728} = 0.47 \text{ m}^2$$

This is approximately 27% of the average BSA for a 70 kg adult (1.73 m²). Since theophylline clearance for a 70 kg adult asthmatic is 4.73 L/hr (41), J.R.'s clearance is approximately 1.28 L/hr. This is about twice the clearance one would have estimated based on weight (14%). Using this clearance, the maintenance dose of aminophylline can be calculated using Eq. 10:

$$M.D. = \frac{1.28 \text{ L/hr} \times 15 \text{ mg/L} \times 1 \text{ hr}}{0.8} = 24 \text{ mg/hr aminophylline}$$

or

19.2 mg/hr theophylline

The above dose is somewhat above the usually suggested aminophylline dose of 5 to 10 mg/kg/6 hr (16). Therefore, it may be desirable to initiate a lower maintenance dose and increase it as necessary. (Recent unpublished data indicate a better clearance estimate would be 2.8 L/hr/70 kg, resulting in a dosage estimate within the suggested range.)

25. Why is it necessary to compare the estimated pediatric dose, which is based on extrapolated pharmacokinetic data, with literature values?

The assumption used in the above calculations is that the pediatric patient is as fully developed metabolically as an adult, and the capabilities of his clearing organs are proportional to his body surface area. If, however, the child's liver or kidneys are not fully developed, the assumption that a child is essentially a small adult is invalid. This situation occurs when theophylline is administered to premature infants. In these subjects, a prolonged half-life of approximately 30 ± 6.5 hrs, is associated with a very low blood clearance of 17.58 ± 2.34 ml/kg/hr (2). Note that this is a blood clearance; a plasma clearance would be even lower (an average adult plasma clearance is 63 ml/kg/hr) (41). Therefore, in comparing the calculated results with those actually observed in patients, it can be determined whether or not the assumptions made were valid.

26. Once the infusion rate, as calculated in Question 24, is begun, how long would it take to reach steady state?

Since this calculation involves a time factor, or asks the question "how long?", the pharmacokinetic parameters of clearance and volume of distribution must be used to determine the half-life (see Eq. 16):

$$t\frac{1}{2} = \frac{0.693 \times 4.5 \text{L}}{1.28 \text{ L/hr}} = 2.44 \text{ hr}$$

Once the half-life has been determined, it can be multiplied by four to determine how long it will take to reach steady state:

4 × 2.5 hr = 10 hr to reach steady state

Although the predicted half-life is much shorter than the average adult value of 5 to 6 hours (41), it is compatible with the average theophylline half-life for children of 3.0 hours (39).

27. Since the calculated half-life is shorter than usual, what must be considered when the child is changed to oral medication?

Since the half-life is relatively short, one must either be satisfied with wide swings in the plasma levels during the usual six-hour dosing interval or shorten the dosing interval. The Cpss$_{max}$ can be estimated using Eq. 18, if one assumes that the bioavailability of theophylline is 100%:

$$\text{Theophylline Cpss}_{max} = \frac{\dfrac{19.2 \text{ mg/hr} \times 6 \text{ hr}}{4.5 \text{ L}}}{(1 - e^{-0.693/2.5 \text{ hr} \times 6 \text{ hr}})}$$

$$= \frac{25.6 \text{ mg/L}}{0.81} = 31.59 \text{ mg/L}$$

The trough level can be estimated using Eq. 19:

Theophylline Cpss$_{min}$ = 31.59 mg/L − 26 mg/L = 6 mg/L

In this case not only is there a wide swing in the plasma level, but the peak levels are well above 20 mg/L which is usually accepted as the upper limit of the therapeutic range.

28. Calculate an appropriate dose and dosing interval which will keep the theophylline plasma level for J.R. between 5 mg/L and 20 mg/L.

Although elaborate calculatons could be made, an easy way to estimate the interval is to determine how many half-lives it takes for the plasma level to drop from 20 mg/L to 5 mg/L. In this case, it will take exactly two half-lives: one to go from 20 mg/L to 10 mg/L, and a second to go from 10 mg/L to 5 mg/L. Therefore, the dosing interval should be two half-lives or five hours.

To increase the plasma concentration from 5 mg/L to a level of 20 mg/L, one must essentially give a small loading dose every five hours (see Eq. 5):

$$\text{Dose/5 hr} = \frac{V_d \times \Delta C_p}{F}$$

$$\text{Dose/5 hr} = \frac{4.5 \text{ L} \times 15 \text{ mg/L}}{0.8} = 84.5 \text{ mg/5 hr}$$

29. E.B., a 62-year-old 75 kg man, was admitted to the hospital during an acute asthmatic attack. He had been receiving 200 mg of aminophylline po every six hours as an outpatient. In the hospital he is started on 1 mg/kg/hr aminophylline IV. Theophylline levels were obtained on admission and 15 hours later. They were reported as 15 mg/L and 25 mg/L (mcg/ml) respectively. Does the theophylline value of 25 mg/L represent a steady state level?

To determine if this is a steady state level, one must estimate the half-life or elimination rate constant. To calculate Kd, the clearance and volume of distribution must be evaluated.

First, assume 25 mg/L does represent $\overline{C}_{pss}$ and calculate the apparent clearance using Eq. 8:

$$Cl = \frac{\text{Rate}_{in}}{\overline{C}_{pss}}$$

$$Cl = \frac{0.8 \times 75 \text{ mg aminophylline/hr}}{25 \text{ mg/L theophylline}} = 2.4 \text{ L/hr}$$

Next, assume that the patient's Vd is approximately equal to that reported in the literature (0.45 L/kg) and estimate Kd or t½ using Eq. 16:

$$t\frac{1}{2} = \frac{0.693 \ V_d}{Cl}$$

$$t\frac{1}{2} = \frac{0.693 \times 75 \text{ kg } 0.45 \text{ L/kg}}{2.4 \text{ L/hr}} = 9.75 \text{ hours}$$

Since less than two half-lives have elapsed since the infusion was started, and a significant increase in plasma level was observed (10 mg/L), the assumption that steady state had been reached was incorrect. Also, it is evident that the steady state level which will be achieved on the 1 mg/kg infusion will be higher than the observed 25 mg/L and that the true half-life is longer than 9.75 hours. The eventual $\overline{C}_{pss}$ could be estimated; however, calculations based on an increase in plasma levels during an infusion are difficult because they depend on an accurate plasma level measurement and a constant infusion rate, two conditions which are difficult to meet in the clinical setting.

30. Determine the aminophylline dose which will be required to achieve a plasma theophylline level of 15 mg/L.

Clearly, in this patient an infusion rate of 75 mg/hr is too large; however, since we cannot ascertain the true $\overline{C}_{pss}$, it is difficult to make an accurate estimate of the dose until additional pharmacokinetic data are gathered.

One approach would be to obtain a theophylline plasma level then stop the infusion for approximately one half-life (in this case about 10 hours), and obtain a second theophylline plasma level. This would more accurately estimate this patient's half-life (Kd). Then using the literature value for Vd, a clearance can be calculated using Eq. 17 (Cl = KdVd). Once the clearance has been determined, the dose can be estimated using Eq. 8.

It is important to emphasize that if the second plasma level obtained is greater than 50% of the initial plasma level (i.e. the time interval is less than one half-life) then there is more likely to be a large error in interpretation. If this is the case, this method should not be used as the sole criterion for an estimation of half-life.

31. Assume the plasma level had increased to 32 mg/L before the infusion was discontinued and 12 hours later the observed plasma level was 16 mcg/ml. Estimate the infusion rate needed to maintain a $\overline{C}_{pss}$ of 15 mg/L?

If the estimated Cp of 32 mg/L was a steady state level, we could calculate a clearance and then determine the maintenance dose which would result in a $\overline{C}_{pss}$ of 15 mg/L using Eq. 10. A second approach would be to estimate the elimination rate constant or half-life using Eq. 14.

In this case, the t½ is 12 hours, since the observed plasma level at that time was exactly one-half of that observed just before the infusion was discontinued. Once Kd has been determined the clearance can be estimated using the literature values for Vd (see Eq. 17):

$$Cl = Kd \times Vd$$

$$Cl = \frac{0.693 \times 0.45 \text{ L/kg} \times 75 \text{ kg}}{12 \text{ hrs}} = 1.96 \text{ L/hr.}$$

The infusion rate of aminophylline required to maintain a level of 15 mcg/ml can be estimated using Eq. 10:

$$\text{M.D.} = \frac{Cl \times \overline{C}_{pss} \times \tau}{F}$$

$$\text{M.D.} = \frac{1.96 \text{ L/hr} \times 15 \text{ mg/L} \times 1 \text{ hr}}{0.8} = 36.75 \text{ mg/hr}$$

32. Design an oral dosage regimen that would keep the plasma level within the desired range of 10 mg/L to 20 mg/L.

Since the half-life is 12 hours, any dosing interval of less than 12 hours should result in peak levels that are less than twice the trough levels. For example, by using the hourly rate of administration calculated in Question 31 of 36.75 mg/hr, and a dosing interval of 6 hours, $Cpss_{max}$ can be calculated (see Eq. 18):

$$Cpss_{max} = \frac{\dfrac{F \times dose}{Vd}}{1 - e^{-Kd_\tau}}$$

$$Cpss_{max} = \frac{\dfrac{0.8 \times 36.75 \ mg/hr \times 6 \ hr}{0.45 \ L/kg \times 75 \ kg}}{1 - e^{-0.693/12 \ hrs \times 6 \ hrs}} = \frac{5.23}{1 - 0.7} = 18.9 \ mg/L$$

If a calculator or graph paper are not available to determine the value of $(1 - e^{-0.693/12 \ hr \times 6 \ hr})$, a first estimate of e^{-Kdt}, or the fraction remaining at time t can be made by assuming that the elimination rate is relatively constant over the first half-life. The rate of plasma level decline will then be directly proportional to the fraction of the half-life. In this case, one-half of one half-life or half of 0.5 will equal 0.25; in other words, 25% is lost in one-half of a half-life. Thus, plasma levels will fall 25% during the six hours after each peak. This estimate is close to the actual decline of 29%. As long as only an estimate is needed, and the time interval is less than a half-life, this approach is probably satisfactory in most clinical situations.

33. P.O., a 52-year-old male, is seen in the clinic for congestive heart failure, mild renal failure, and a history of atrial fibrillation. He is presently receiving quinidine sulfate 300 mg every six hours and digoxin 0.25 mg alternating with 0.125 mg daily. A quinidine plasma level is ordered to be drawn one hour after his next dose. Is this the optimal time for the plasma level to be drawn?

In general, peak plasma levels are difficult to interpret, as they are subject to error if the actual peak occurs later than anticipated. Trough levels, on the other hand, will also be affected by absorption rate, but to a much lesser degree (see Fig. 5). Trough levels obtained just before the next dose are, therefore, more useful as a routine monitoring parameter in plasma level evaluation. Levels drawn at other times should be avoided unless there is a specific reason to do so, (e.g. in the case of an acute toxicity).

34. If the trough levels were obtained on your suggestion and the reported quinidine level was 2.5 mg/L (mcg/ml), how would the type of assay affect your pharmacokinetic calculations?

The type of assay used is important because some are less specific than others and measure a larger proportion of the supposedly inactive metabolites (9). The plasma levels reported using the non-specific assay are higher than those reported by the method measuring only active drug. This is especially important in renal failure since the concentration of metabolites is increased (24). Results from a less specific assay would be expected to result in a decrease in the calculated volume of distribution (see Eq. 4):

$$Vd = \frac{Ab}{Cp}$$

and decrease in the calculated clearance (see Eq. 8):

$$Cl = \frac{R_{in}}{Cpss}$$

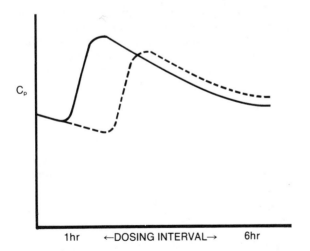

Fig. 5: *Schematic representation of the effect of delayed absorption (---) on plasma level measurements.* Note the magnitude of the error at one hour compared to six hours.

Fig. 6: *Plasma level time curve for intravenous bolus (–) and oral (. . . . .) administration, when $\tau = t\frac{1}{2}$.* Note the dampening effect of oral dosing on $Cpss_{max}$ and $Cpss_{min}$.

The half-life would be affected by the assay performed if the ratio of quinidine metabolites to active drug changes significantly with the disease state. Although similar half-lives are observed in patients with normal renal function by both methods (7.2 vs. 7.0 hours), the observed quinidine half-lives in renal failure are 6.6 hours and 11.7 hours for the specific and non-specific assay respectively. The prolonged half-life calculated using the results of the non-specific assay can be explained by the fact that quinidine metabolites accumulate to a greater extent in renal failure than does the parent compound. The essentially unaltered half-life for the parent compound is compatible with the fact that only a small fraction of drug is cleared by the renal route (20%) (62).

35. Assuming the assay used was relatively specific and the metabolites are pharmacologically inactive, estimate this patient's quinidine clearance and half-life.

First, assume the $Cp_{trough} = \overline{Cp}ss$. This approach is usually satisfactory as long as the dosing interval is less than or equal to the half-life since it incurs a maximum 30% error. With oral dosing and delayed absorption, the error will be even less. See Fig. 6.

If one assumes that the absolute bioavailability of the quinidine base is 72% (61) and remembers that 82% of quinidine sulfate is the base, then the patient's estimated clearance based on Eq. 8 is:

$$Cl = \frac{R_{in}}{\overline{Cp}ss}$$

$$= \frac{F \times dose/\tau}{\overline{Cp}ss}$$

$$= \frac{(0.82 \times 0.72) \times 300 \text{ mg/6 hr}}{2.5 \text{ mg/L}} = 11.8 \text{ L/hr}$$

If a literature value of 3 L/kg is used for the volume of distribution (62), the apparent half-life using Eq. 16 would be:

$$t\frac{1}{2} = \frac{0.693 \text{ Vd}}{Cl} = \frac{0.693 \times 3 \text{ L/kg} \times 70 \text{ kg}}{11.8 \text{ L/hr}} = 12.33 \text{ hr}$$

The apparently long half-life indicates that $\tau < t\frac{1}{2}$ and our original assumption that $Cpss_{min}$ is reasonably close to $\overline{Cp}ss$ appears to be correct.

36. What would be your approximation of $Cpss_{max}$?

The $Cpss_{max}$ could be estimated by adding $Cpss_{min}$ to the change in plasma level which would occur following administration of 300 mg quinidine sulfate (see Eq. 19):

$$Cpss_{max} = Cpss_{min \text{ (observed)}} + \frac{F \times dose}{Vd}$$

$$Cpss_{max} = 2.6 \text{ mg/L} + \frac{0.82 \times 0.72 \times 300 \text{ mg}}{3 \text{ L/kg} \times 70 \text{ kg}} = 3.5 \text{ mg/L}$$

This approach assumes that absorption is immediate and that little or no elimination occurs during the absorptive phase. Oral dosing slows absorption and dampens the curve making the peak somewhat lower than predicted. See Fig. 6.

37. Many literature sources cite a "therapeutic" range of 4–8 mg/L for quinidine. Since this patient's level is 2.5 mg/L, should his dose be increased?

Since the plasma level was measured by a more specific assay, lower "therapeutic" levels should be expected. The usual therapeutic range for quinidine by the double extraction method (Cramer and Isaksson) is 2 to 5 mg/L (24). The clinical condition of the patient should also be considered.

38. B.E., a 63-year-old 70 kg woman, was admitted to the coronary care unit with a diagnosis of acute myocardial infarction. Her previous history indicates that she is a long-standing diabetic with moderate renal failure (C_{Cr} = 30 ml/min). On the second hospital day frequent premature ventricular contractions are noted, and 375 mg of procainamide po every six hours is started.

Pharmacokinetic data reported for procainamide in the literature are as follows (27): Cl = 540 ml/min; t½ = 3.0 hrs; Vd = 2 L/kg; F = 0.75 to 0.95; and fraction cleared unchanged = 50%. Will 375 mg po every six hours achieve adequate procainamide levels in this patient with renal failure?

The clearance in this patient can be estimated using Eq. 12:

$$Cl_t = Cl_m + (Cl \times \text{fraction of renal function remaining})$$

Since the fraction of the drug that is cleared unchanged is normally 50% and the patient has approximately 30% of her renal function, the total clearance would be:

$$Cl_t = 270 \text{ ml/min} + (270 \times 0.3) = 351 \text{ ml/min}$$

$$Cl_t = 350 \text{ ml/min or } \frac{350 \text{ ml/min} \times 60 \text{ min/hr}}{1000 \text{ ml/L}} = 21 \text{ L/hr}$$

$\overline{Cp}ss$ may be estimated using Eq. 9:

$$\overline{Cp}ss = \frac{F \times dose/\tau}{Cl}$$

$$\overline{Cp}ss = \frac{0.8 \times 375 \text{ mg/6 hr}}{21 \text{ L/hr}} = 2.53 \text{ mg/L}$$

Since the therapeutic levels for procainamide are 4–8 mg/L, it appears as though the levels which will be achieved with this dose are inadequate.

39. How long will it take to reach steady state procainamide levels?

First estimate the half-life using Eq. 16:

$$t\frac{1}{2} = \frac{0.693 \times 2 \text{ L/kg} \times 70 \text{ kg}}{21 \text{ L/hr}} = 4.62 \text{ hours}$$

Since steady state is approached in 3 to 4 half-lives, it will take 18.5 hours to reach steady state.

40. Why is the metabolism of procainamide important in this patient?

Usually drug metabolites are pharmacologically inactive; however, N-acetyl-procainamide (NAPA), a metabolite of procainamide, is pharmacologically active (12,13) and has been estimated to be as potent as procainamide on a milligram for milligram basis. It is approximately two-thirds active when plasma concentrations are compared (12).

Patients have been identified with NAPA plasma levels that are five to six times the procainamide levels (12). A number of factors appear to contribute to increased NAPA concentrations including renal failure and acetylation phenotype. Patients who are phenotypically rapid acetylators, and who have good renal function, appear to convert 28% of the administered procainamide to NAPA, while slow acetylators convert an average of 15% to NAPA (14).

41. What effect will B.E.'s renal failure have on the disposition and $\overline{C}pss$ of the active metabolite, NAPA? The pharmacokinetic parameters for NAPA are as follows (59): Cl = 11.4 L/hr or 190 ml/min; Vd = 1.4 L/kg; t½ = 6.0 hours; fraction eliminated unchanged (renal) = 0.8; and fraction metabolized = 0.2.

Since 80% of NAPA is cleared unchanged, the effect of renal failure on the clearance is significant. The clearance for NAPA can be calculated using Eq. 13:

$$NAPA\ Cl_t = Cl_m + Cl_r\ (\text{fraction of renal function remaining})$$
$$NAPA\ Cl_t = 38\ ml/min + (152\ ml/min \times 0.3) = 83.6\ ml/min$$

The clearance is therefore reduced to 44% of normal:

$$\frac{83.6\ ml/min}{190\ ml/min} \times 100\%$$

If the R_i (i.e. metabolic conversion from procainamide to NAPA) is constant, the steady state concentration of NAPA will increase by a factor which is the inverse of the clearance change, since the product of Cl and $\overline{C}pss$ must equal the rate in at steady state (see Eq. 7):

$$R_i = 0.44\ Cl \times 1/0.44\ \overline{C}pss$$

In summary, the $\overline{C}pss$ for NAPA would increase by a factor of $\frac{1}{0.44}$ or 2.27.

42. What fraction of procainamide (PA) is converted to NAPA in this patient? Assume he is a fast acetylator.

A fast acetylator with normal renal function converts

28% of procainamide to NAPA. Thus, the clearance for PA in such a patient can be respresented by an expansion of Eq. 12 which accounts for the multiple metabolic pathways for PA:

$$PA\ Cl_t = PA\ Cl_{m(other)} + PA\ Cl_{m(NAPA)} + Cl_r \times \text{fraction renal function remaining}$$
$$= 0.22 + 0.28 + 0.50 = 1.0$$

This patient has a Cl_{cr} of 30 ml/min. Therefore, his clearance for procainamide is represented as follows:

$$PA\ Cl_t = 0.22 + 0.28 + (0.5 \times 0.3)$$
$$= 0.65$$

Since the fraction of PA cleared by the kidneys is decreased in this patient, the fraction cleared by metabolism to NAPA is increased from 0.23 to 0.43 ($\frac{0.28}{0.65}$) of the total clearance.

43. Estimate the $\overline{C}pss$ for NAPA in this patient.

First, estimate the rate in for NAPA, i.e. the rate of metabolic conversion from PA to NAPA. Since the fraction of PA which is cleared as NAPA is 0.43 (see Question 42), the rate in for NAPA can be estimated using Eq. 7 and Eq. 9:

$$Rate_{in(NAPA)} = 0.43 \times (F \times \frac{dose\ PA}{\tau})$$
$$= 0.43 \times (0.85 \times \frac{375\ mg}{6\ hour})$$
$$= 22.9\ mg/hour$$

Using Eq. 8 and the NAPA Cl_t calculated in Question 41, the $\overline{C}pss$ for NAPA can be determined:

$$\overline{C}pss(NAPA) = \frac{R_i(NAPA)}{Cl_t(NAPA)}$$
$$= \frac{22.9\ mg/hr}{\dfrac{83\ ml/min \times 60\ min/hr}{1000\ ml/L}}$$
$$= \frac{22.9\ mg/hr}{4.95\ L/hr}$$
$$= 4.6\ mg/L$$

44. What is your revised estimate of the time required to reach steady state for the antiarrhythmic activity of procainamide and NAPA?

Since NAPA has the longest half-life, its elimination rate will be the major determinant of the time required to reach steady state. NAPA's half-life can be estimated using Eq. 16:

$$t½ = \frac{0.693\ Vd}{Cl}$$
$$= \frac{0.693 \times 1.44\ L/kg \times 70\ kg}{4.95\ L/hr} = 13.72\ hrs$$

If four half-lives are required to reach steady state, it will take 55 hours to achieve steady state levels. To be more exact, it will take 55 hours to reach steady state after procainamide levels have reached a plateau, because the rule of three to four half-lives to steady state only applies to situations where the rate-in is constant, and the rate-in of NAPA would continue to increase until the procainamide levels have reached steady state. However, because NAPA would start to form following the first procainamide dose, there probably would not be a great error in using 55 hours.

45. Does the now recognized presence of NAPA make procainamide levels useless?

No, not completely, but it does point out the need for an assay that will measure both compounds. The original guidelines of 4 to 8 mg/L (27) for procainamide levels are probably adequate if the patient has good renal function because NAPA was probably present when the therapeutic levels were established. The presence of the active metabolite NAPA may, however, explain why therapeutic effects have been observed in the presence of low procainamide levels. NAPA's long half-life may also account for the successful use of PA in dosing intervals which are longer than the half-life of procainamide. There are as yet no studies in humans documenting NAPA's toxicity, although one study in animals did suggest that NAPA was less toxic than procainamide (12). In one study where NAPA was administered to human subjects, levels as high as 17.2 mg/L were not associated with any apparent toxicities (39). Because the number of patients was limited and only a single dose was given, it is probably not yet valid to assume that NAPA is less toxic than procainamide.

46. A 65-year-old 60 kg white male was admitted to the coronary care unit with diagnosis of myocardial infarction, heart failure, and premature ventricular contraction (PVCs). He has prior history of alcoholism and cirrhosis. A 50 mg bolus of lidocaine was given and a lidocaine infusion was started at a rate of 2 mg/min. The patient was controlled initially, but fifteen minutes after the bolus was given, the ventricular contractions were observed again, and a second bolus of 25 mg was given and the infusion rate increased to 3 mg/min. The patient's response was good, but he complained of feeling dizzy about eight hours after the infusion had been started. The following day, approximately 25 hours after the infusion was begun, the patient had a grand mal seizure, and the lidocaine was discontinued. Using the data below as a guide, evaluate the peak plasma level achieved after the first 50 mg bolus of lidocaine.

Lidocaine pharmacokinetic parameters in various diseases (60):

	$\alpha t\frac{1}{2}$ (min)	$\beta t\frac{1}{2}$ (hr)	Vp (L/kg)	Vd (L/kg)	Cl (ml/min)
Normal	8.3	1.8	0.53	1.32	10
Heart failure	7.3	2.0	0.30	0.88	6.3
Liver disease	8.8	5.0	0.61	2.31	6.0

Lidocaine is a drug that exhibits two-compartment kinetics with the therapeutic or target tissue (myocardium) appearing as though it were located in the initial compartment (Vp). Therefore, when a bolus dose is given, calculations of plasma levels should be based on Vp, not on Vd. Therefore Eq. 5 may be rearranged to:

$$Cp = \frac{F \times loading\ dose}{Vp}$$

Since the Vp appears to increase in liver disease and decrease in congestive heart failure, two estimates of Cp should be made because it is uncertain which effect predominates:

$$Cp = \frac{50\ mg}{0.61\ L/kg \times 60\ kg} = 1.37\ mg/L\ in\ liver\ disease$$

$$Cp = \frac{50\ mg}{0.3\ L/kg \times 60\ kg} = 2.78\ mg/L\ in\ heart\ failure$$

The anticipated range for the peak plasma concentration of lidocaine is therefore between 1.4 and 2.8 mg/L.

47. For this patient, was increasing the infusion rate appropriate when the second lidocaine bolus was given?

No. PVCs recurred 15 minutes after the initiation of therapy but 3 to 4 elimination half-lives (β) are required to evaluate the efficacy of the infusion. The reappearance of the PVCs within 3 to 4 distribution half-lives (α) indicates that the initial bolus was inadequate after it had distributed. Increasing the infusion rate would have been appropriate only if the arrhythmia had recurred after distribution was complete.

48. Since the half-life of lidocaine is essentially unchanged in congestive heart failure, is it true that the infusion rate need be adjusted in this patient on the basis of his liver disease alone?

No. The half-life is useful only to determine when something will happen. In this case steady-state plasma levels should be reached in approximately six to eight hours for both normal and congestive heart failure patients, while 15 to 20 hours would be required for patients with liver disease.

Because $t\frac{1}{2}$ is a function of Vd as well as clearance, it can only be used to determine the maintenance dose when the volume of distribution is constant.

Lidocaine is a good example of a drug for which Vd is not constant, resulting in half-lives which do not directly reflect the change in clearance. Therefore one cannot estimate maintenance doses from half-life data alone.

49. What would be the anticipated steady-state lidocaine level at the time the patient had the seizure?

If we assume only a 40% reduction in clearance due to either congestive heart failure or the liver disease, the elimination clearance would be:

6 ml/min/kg × 60 kg = 360 ml/min = 0.36 L/min.

Rearranging Eq. 9 so that steady state lidocaine levels can be calculated:

$$\overline{Cpss} = \frac{F \times dose/\tau}{Cl}$$

$$\overline{Cpss} = \frac{1.0 \times 3 \text{ mg/min}}{0.36 \text{ L/min}} = 8.33 \text{ mg/L}$$

The estimated $\overline{Cpss}$ of 8.3 mg/L is probably conservative because it is reasonable to assume that a patient with both liver disease and heart failure will have a smaller clearance than would a patient with only one of these problems. If both diseases reduced the clearance by 40%, the patient would have a total lidocaine clearance of 0.216 L/min and the steady-state plasma levels would be approximately:

$$\overline{Cpss} = \frac{3 \text{ mg/min}}{0.36 \times 0.6 \text{ L/min}} = 13.9 \text{ mg/L}$$

As levels above 9 mg/L are associated with seizures (4,60), the plasma levels estimated and the observed clinical response would appear to be consistent with each other.

50. Given that the patient has disease states which tend to both decrease (congestive heart failure) and increase (liver disease) the volume of distribution for lidocaine, would you estimate the Vd to be larger or smaller than normal?

One cannot say for certain. However, because this patient's seizure occurred approximately 25 hours after the infusion was started, it would appear that the half-life was longer than average, corresponding to a Vd which was larger than average (see Eq. 16).

51. R.M., a 32-year-old 80 kg male, was admitted to the hospital with apparent phenytoin toxicity. Prior to admission he had been followed in the neurology clinic, and because of poor seizure control, his phenytoin was increased from 300 mg daily to 500 mg daily. Phenytoin plasma levels resulting from the 300 mg daily dose were 9 mg/L. On admission, the plasma phenytoin level was reported as 37.5 mg/L. Renal and hepatic function appeared normal. Assume these are steady-state levels and that the pa-

tient has complied with therapy. Does the four-fold increase in plasma level seem reasonable for a less than two-fold increase in daily dose?

Although most drugs appear to be eliminated by a first-order process (clearance is constant), phenytoin exhibits capacity-limited kinetics (5,38,40), which means that for a given increase in daily dose of phenytoin, the plasma level will show a greater than proportional rise at steady-state. Phenytoin is primarily metabolized to p-hydroxy-phenyl-phenylhydantoin (HPPH) by an enzyme system which appears to follow Michaelis-Menten kinetics (5,31,38).

The relationship between rate-in (daily dose) and the steady-state plasma level ($\overline{Cpss}$) is expressed in Eq. 9:

$$F \times dose/\tau = Cl \times \overline{Cpss}$$

With phenytoin it appears that clearance can be expressed as:

$$Cl = \frac{V_{max}}{Km + Cpss} \qquad \text{(Eq. 23)}$$

where V_{max} is the maximum rate of HPPH production and Km (Michaelis-Menten constant) is the phenytoin concentration which will one-half saturate the metabolic enzyme system. If equations 9 and 23 are combined, the following is derived (38,40):

$$F \times dose/\tau = \frac{Vm}{Km + Cpss} \times \overline{Cpss} \qquad \text{(Eq. 24)}$$

The significance of this equation is that if Cpss is small compared to Km, the clearance approaches Vm/Km and appears to be constant or first-order. However, as $\overline{Cpss}$ approaches or exceeds Km, the clearance decreases, resulting in a disproportionate rise in $\overline{Cpss}$. The value of Km reported in the literature ranges from 2.2 mg/L (33) to 11.5 mg/L (38). Since the values of Km are very near or below the usually accepted therapeutic range of 10 to 20 mg/L, one should expect to see large increases in plasma level resulting from moderate or small increases in daily dose as the therapeutic range is approached.

At least two authors suggest that nomograms are useful in estimating appropriate dose adjustments (38,50); however, others feel that the variability of V_{max} and Km is so great that each individual patient should be evaluated separately (33,37), recognizing the potentially sensitive relationship between the daily dose and steady-state plasma levels. Aspirin (salicylic acid) is another drug which exhibits capacity-limited kinetics; however, it is much more difficult to deal with kinetically as it has five major pathways of elimination, some of which are first-order and others which are capacity-limited (35).

52. How could one estimate the Vm and Km values

for phenytoin in an individual patient?

The relationship between daily dose and $\overline{C}pss$ can be made linear by plotting daily dose (rate-in) versus daily dose divided by $\overline{C}pss$ (clearance) for at least two steady-state plasma levels. The graph for R.M. is plotted in Fig. 7, where the rate-in intercept is V_{max} and the slope of the line formed by plotting R_{in} versus clearance is the negative value of Km or 633.3 mg/day and −10 mg/L respectively.

53. Using the data from Fig. 7, calculate the daily phenytoin dose necessary to achieve a steady-state plasma level of 15 mg/L.

Using the V_{max} of 633 mg/day, and 10 mg/L as the Km, the daily phenytoin dose could be estimated using Eq. 24:

$$F \times dose/\tau = \frac{Vm \times \overline{C}pss}{Km + \overline{C}pss}$$

If one assumes F = 1.0 and τ = 1 day, the daily dose can be calculated as follows:

$$\text{Daily dose} = \frac{633 \text{ mg/day} \times 15 \text{ mg/L}}{10 \text{ mg/L} + 15 \text{ mg/L}} = 379.8 \text{ mg/day}$$

54. Since 379.8 mg is an impractical dose of phenytoin, what would the $\overline{C}pss$ be if 350 mg or 400 mg/day were selected as the daily dose?

Rearrange Eq. 24 to express $\overline{C}pss$ as:

$$\overline{C}pss = \frac{Km \times daily\ dose}{Vm - daily\ dose} \qquad \text{(Eq. 25)}$$

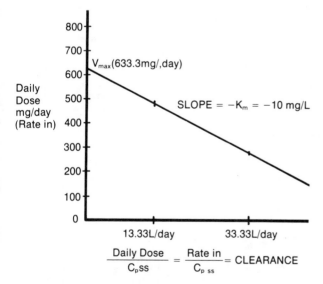

$$\frac{\text{Daily Dose}}{C_p ss} = \frac{\text{Rate in}}{C_{p\ ss}} = \text{CLEARANCE}$$

Fig. 7: *Relationship between daily dose of phenytoin and* $\overline{C}pss$. *The slope of the line is the negative value of Km, and the point of intersection with the daily dose plot is the* V_{max}.

For a daily dose of 350 mg, the $\overline{C}pss$ would be:

$$\overline{C}pss = \frac{10 \text{ mg/L} \times 350 \text{ mg/day}}{633 \text{ mg/day} - 350 \text{ mg/day}} = 12.4 \text{ mg/L}$$

And, for a daily dose of 400 mg, the $\overline{C}pss$ would be:

$$\overline{C}pss = \frac{10 \text{ mg/L} \times 400 \text{ mg/day}}{633 \text{ mg/day} - 400 \text{ mg/day}} = 17.17 \text{ mg/L}$$

55. Estimate the clearance at steady state if the daily dose of phenytoin is equal to V_{max}.

According to Fig. 7, the clearance would be zero. This in turn would indicate that $\overline{C}pss$ approaches infinity as one daily dose approaches V_{max} (see Eq. 25). In reality, the patient would stop taking the phenytoin when the levels were high enough to produce significant toxicity and steady state would not be achieved. In addition, 1-5% of phenytoin is eliminated renally by a first-order process (31). This becomes more significant as Cp increases and clearance by the metabolic route decreases.

56. What would the phenytoin half-life be for R.M. on admission?

Although the usual reported half-life of phenytoin is approximately 22 hours (3), one would not expect the half-life to be constant, as clearance changes with the plasma concentration of phenytoin. If (Vm/Km + $\overline{C}pss$) is substituted for Cl in Eq. 16, a formula for phenytoin half-life is derived:

$$t\frac{1}{2} = \frac{0.693\ Vd}{V_{max}} (Km + \overline{C}pss) \qquad \text{(Eq. 26)}$$

On the basis of Eq. 26 it can be predicted that the half-life will be longer as phenytoin concentrations increase, an observation that has been previously confirmed (17). In this patient, using a Vd = 0.65 L/kg (45) and the calculated estimate of Vm and Km, the half-life can be estimated as follows:

$$t\frac{1}{2} = \frac{0.693 \times (0.65 \text{ L/kg} \times 80 \text{ kg})}{633 \text{ mg/day}} (10 \text{ mg/L} + 37 \text{ mg/L})$$

$$= 2.68 \text{ days (64 hours)}$$

57. Will the plasma level be one-half of 37 mg/L after 64 hours if no further doses are given?

No. As the plasma level decreases, the half-life becomes shorter, so that the plasma level will be even less than 18.5 mg/L 64 hours after the last dose has been withheld. The assumption in this estimation is that there is no further absorption from previously administered phenytoin.

58. Would renal failure alter the daily dose of phenytoin necessary to achieve a therapeutic effect?

Assuming the liver function does not change, one

would not anticipate the necessity of dose adjustment with changing renal function because the renal route is not a significant pathway of phenytoin elimination (1,31). However, Km is a plasma concentration (mg/L) measured as total drug (bound and free), indicating that the change in protein binding affinity which occurs in renal failure (1,45) should result in a lower Km value. In renal failure, the change in desired "therapeutic" plasma level will be proportional to the Km change, assuming there is no accumulation in renal failure of a competitive inhibitor for phenytoin metabolism.

59. Why does changing from oral to intramuscular phenytoin result in a sudden and dramatic decrease in phenytoin levels?

Phenytoin is a relatively insoluble compound which crystallizes within the muscle following intramuscular administration (69). It appears that the phenytoin crystals are slowly absorbed, resulting in an initial reduction in the phenytoin dosage (absorption) rate. In addition, because of the capacity-limited phenytoin metabolism, the drop in plasma level will be more than proportional to the reduction in absorption from the intramuscular injection. This was well demonstrated by Wilder (68) when a change from oral to intramuscular administration resulted in an initial decrease in the phenytoin plasma level of 40 to 60%, while the HPPH elimination, which should be proportional to the amount of drug absorbed, decreased by only 16%.

60. The estimation of a patient's renal function is often an integral step in the application of pharmacokinetics to drug therapy. How can creatinine clearance be estimated from serum creatinine?

If the daily production of creatinine, creatinine clearance, and serum creatinine is analogous to the relationships between rate of drug administration, drug clearance, and drug plasma level, creatinine clearance can be evaluated in a manner similar to drug clearance (see Eq. 8).

$$R_{in} = Cl \times \overline{Cpss}$$

where Cl is creatinine clearance (C_{Cr}) and $\overline{Cpss}$ is the steady state serum creatinine concentration ($SrCr_{ss}$).

Usually the R_{in} or daily creatinine production is assumed to be approximately 20 mg/kg/day for males between the ages of 30 and 50 and decreases with age. The R_{in} appears to be somewhat less for females and also decreases with age (19,57). A serum creatinine of 1 mg/100 ml appears to correspond to a creatinine clearance of approximately 100 mg/min (57). If the R_{in} is held constant, the fraction of normal creatinine clearance would be the inverse of serum creatinine.

$$\frac{1}{Sr\ Cr_{ss}} = \text{fraction of normal renal function}$$

Therefore C_{Cr} may be estimated according to the following formula:

$$C_{Cr} = 100\ ml/min \times 1/SrCr_{ss}\ (ml/min) \qquad \text{(Eq. 28)}$$

61. Estimate the creatinine clearance for a 38-year-old male with a serum creatinine of 3 mg/100 ml.

Using Eq. 28, the C_{Cr} may be estimated to be:

$$C_{Cr} = 100\ ml/min \times \tfrac{1}{3} = 33\ ml/min$$

62. Is the creatinine clearance affected by the size of the patient?

Although it does not appear in Eq. 28, the normal creatinine clearance (100 ml/min) is based on a patient with the body surface area of 1.73 m² (70 kg). Even though the daily production of creatinine would be expected to increase with body size, so would creatinine clearance (kidney size). Therefore, a serum creatinine of 1.0 mg/100 ml for a patient larger or smaller than 1.73 m² should represent a creatinine clearance greater or less than 100 ml/min. Body surface area (BSA) could be compensated for by modifying eq. 28 in the following way:

$$C_{Cr} = (100\ ml/min \times 1/Sr\ Cr_{ss})\ (Patient's\ BSA/1.73\ m^2)$$

$$\text{(Eq. 29)}$$

The patient's BSA can be obtained from a graph (52,56) or estimated from Eq. 22.

63. What is the creatinine clearance for an 85-year-old 70 kg man with a serum creatinine of 1.0 mg/100 ml?

Usually, as patients age, their muscle mass represents a smaller proportion of their total weight. Therefore the R_{in} for creatinine is decreased on a mg/kg basis.

The following equation attempts to compensate for the decreased muscle mass in elderly patients (19).

$$\textbf{Men:}\ \frac{98 - 0.8\ (age - 20)}{Sr\ Cr} = C_{Cr}\ (ml/min)$$

$$\text{(Eq. 30)}$$

$$\textbf{Women:}\ 0.9\ \frac{98 - 0.8\ (age - 20)}{Sr\ Cr} = C_{Cr}\ (ml/min)$$

The creatinine clearance for this patient is :

$$\frac{98 - 0.8(85 - 20)}{1.0\ mg/100\ ml} = 46\ ml/min$$

Note that Eq. 30, like Eq. 28, should be adjusted if the patient has a BSA considerably different from 1.73 m², and that any patient with a muscle mass significantly different from the average population should not be evaluated by this technique.

64. If a patient suddenly loses some portion of renal function, what period of time would be required to achieve a new steady-state serum creatinine so that renal function can be estimated?

Since this is a problem concerning "how long?", both creatinine clearance and the volume of distribution (50 L) will determine the time required to achieve steady state (15). If Vd is assumed to be constant, the time for 95% of steady state to be achieved in patients with 50, 25, and 10% of normal renal function has been estimated to be 1.07, 2.5, and 6.7 days respectively (7). Even though an estimate of creatinine clearance cannot be made for a non-steady-state serum creatinine, it should be recognized that a rapidly increasing serum creatinine does indicate very poor renal function.

65. Since serum creatinine can be influenced by both the rate of creatinine production and creatinine clearance, why not always get a direct creatinine clearance measurement?

Although a measurement of creatinine clearance is generally regarded as the best way to evaluate renal function, it does have limitations. The cost of doing a creatinine clearance is considerably greater than a serum creatinine, and a minimum of 12 hours, preferably 24 hours, is required for the urine collection. Frequently the urine collection is inaccurate because some has been accidentally discarded, or the time of collection is shorter or longer than requested (23).

The adequacy of the urine collection should always be checked by comparing the expected creatinine production with the amount actually collected. If the amount collected differs significantly from the predicted production, it is likely that the reported creatinine clearance is inaccurate.

REFERENCES

1. Adler DS et al: Hemodialysis of phenytoin-quantitation in a uremic patient. Clin Pharmacol Ther 18:65, 1975.
2. Aranda JV et al: Pharmacokinetic aspects of theophylline in premature newborns. NEJM 295:413, 1976.
3. Arnold K et al: The rate of decline of diphenylhydantoin in human plasma. Clin Pharmacol Ther. 11:121, 1969.
4. Benowitz N: Clinical application of the pharmacokinetics of lidocaine. In Cardiovascular Drug Therapy, ed by K. Melmon, FM Davis, Philadelphia, pp 77-101.
5. Bochner F et al: Effects of dosage increments on blood phenytoin concentrations. J Neurol Neurosurg Psych 35:873, 1972.
6. Boyer RW et al: Pharmacokinetics of lidocaine in man. Clin Pharmacol Ther 12:105, 1971.
7. Chiou WL et al: Pharmacokinetics of creatinine in man and its implications in the monitoring of renal function and in dosage regimen modifications in patients with renal insufficiency. J Clin Pharmacol 15:427, 1975.
8. Chow MS et al: Pharmacokinetic data and drug monitoring: 1. Antibiotics and antiarrhythmics. J Clin Pharmacol 15:405, 1975.
9. Cramer G et al: Quantitative determination of quinidine in plasma. Scand J Clin Invest. 15:553, 1963.
10. Dettli L: Individualization of drug dosage in patients with renal disease. Med Clin North Am 58:977, 1974.
11. Doherty et al: Digoxin metabolism in hypo and hyperthyroidism. Ann Intern Med 64:489,507, 1966.
12. Elson J et al: Antiarrhythmic potency of N-acetyl-procainamide. Clin Pharmacol Ther 17:134, 1975.
13. Gibaldi M et al: Drug distribution and renal failure. J Clin Pharmacol 12:201-204, 1972.
14. Gibson FP: Acetylation of procainamide in man and its relationship to isonicotinic acid-hydrazide acetylation phenotype. Clin Pharmacol Ther 17:395, 1975.
15. Goldman R: Creatinine excretion in renal failure. Proc Soc Exp Biol Med 85:446, 1954.
16. Headings DL: The Harriet Lane Handbook 7th ed. Yearbook Med Pub Inc. Chicago, 1975, p. 178.
17. Houghton et al: Rate of elimination of tracer doses of phenytoin at different steady state serum phenytoin concentrations in epileptic patients. Br J Clin Pharmacol 1:155, 1974.
18. Huffman DH et al: Absorption of digoxin from different oral preparations in normal subjects during steady state. Clin Pharmacol Ther 16:310, 1974.
19. Jellife RW: Creatinine clearance: Bedside estimate. Ann Intern Med 70:604, 1973.
20. Jenne W et al: Effect of congestive heart failure on the elimination of aminophylline (abstr.) J Allergy Clin. Immunol 53:80, 1974.
21. Jusko WJ et al: Myocardial distribution of digoxin and renal function. Clin Pharmacol Ther 16:449, 1974.
22. Jusko WJ et al: Pharmacokinetic design of digoxin dosage regimens in relation to renal failure. J Clin Pharmacol 14:525, 1974.
23. Kassirer JP: Clinical evaluation of kidney function-glomerular function. NEJM 285:385, 1971.
24. Kessler KM et al: Quinidine elimination in patients with congestive heart failure or poor renal function. NEJM 290:706, 1974.
25. Koch-Weser J et al: Binding of drugs to serum albumin. NEJM 294:311, 1976.
26. Koch-Weser J: Pharmacokinetics of procainamide in man. Ann NY Acad Sci 169:370, 1971.
27. Koch-Weser J et al: Procainamide dosage schedules, plasma concentrations, and clinical effects. JAMA 215:1454, 1971.
28. Koup JR et al: Digoxin pharmacokinetics: role of renal failure in dosage regimen design. Clin Pharmacol Ther 18:9, 1975.
29. Koysouko R et al: Relationship between theophylline concentrations in plasma and saliva of man. Clin Pharmacol Ther 15:454, 1974.
30. Kramer WG et al: Pharmacokinetics of digoxin: comparison of a two and a three compartment in man. J Pharmacokinet Biopharm. 2:299, 1974.
31. Kutt H et al: Diphenylhydantoin, metabolism, blood levels, and toxicity. Arch Neurol 11:642, 1964.
32. Lader S et al: The measurement of plasma digoxin concentration: a comparison of two methods. Eur J Clin Pharmacol 5:22, 1972.
33. Lambie DG et al: Therapeutic and pharmacokinetic effects of increasing phenytoin in chronic epileptics on multiple drug therapy. Lancet 2:386, 1976.
34. Lee WK et al: Antiarrhythmic efficacy of N-acetyl-procainamide in patients with premature ventricular contractions. Clin Pharmacol Ther 19:508, 1976.
35. Levy G et al: Limited capacity of salicyl phenolic glucuronide formation and its effect on the kinetics of salicylate elimination in man. Clin Pharmacol Ther 13:258, 1972.
36. Levy G et al: Pharmacokinetic analysis of the effect of theophylline on pulmonary function in asthmatic children. Ped Pharmacol Ther 86:789, 1975.
37. Lund L et al: Phenytoin dosage nomograms (letter). Lancet 2:1305, 1975.
38. Martin E et al: The clinical pharmacokinetics of phenytoin in man. To be published.
39. Maselli GL et al: Pharmacologic effect of intravenously administered aminophylline in asthmatic children. J Pediatr 76:777, 1970.
40. Mawer GE et al: Phenytoin dose adjustments in epileptic patients. Br J Clin Pharmacol 1:163, 1974.
41. Mitenko PA et al: Pharmacokinetics of intravenous theophylline.

Clin Pharmacol Ther 14:509, 1972.

42. Mitenko PA et al: Rapidly achieved plasma concentration plateaus with observation on theophylline. Clin Pharmacol Ther 13:329-335, 1972.

43. Mitenko PA et al: Rational intravenous doses of theophylline. NEJM 289:600, 1973.

44. Niles AS et al: Clinical pharmacology of propranolol. Circ 52:6, 1975.

45. Odar-Cedarlof I et al: Kinetics of diphenylhydantoin in uremic patients: Consequence of decreased protein binding. Eur J Clin Pharmacol 7:31, 1974.

46. Ohnhaus EE et al: Protein binding of digoxin in human serum. Eur J Clin Pharmacol 5:34, 1972.

47. Pagliaro LA et al: Critical compilation of terminal half-lives, percent excreted unchanged, and changes of half-life in renal and hepatic dysfunction for studies in humans with references. J Pharmacokinet Biopharm 3:333, 1975.

48. Piafsky KM et al: Disposition of theophylline in acute pulmonary edema (abstr). Clin Res 22:726A, 1974.

49. Reuning RH et al: Role of pharmacokinetics in drug dosage adjustment: 1. Pharmacologic effect kinetics and apparent volume of distribution of digoxin. J Clin Pharmacol 13:127, 1973.

50. Richens A et al: Serum phenytoin levels in management of epilepsy. Lancet 2:247, 1975. (Error corrected in Lancet 2:1305, 1975.)

51. Rowland M: Drug administration and regimens. In *Clinical Pharmacology and Basic Principles of Therapeutics,* ed by K Melmon and H Morelli, Macmillan New York, 1972, pp 21-60.

52. *Scientific Tables, Documentia Geigy,* 7th ed, by Diem K and Lentner C Ciba-Geigy, Ltd., Switzerland, 1972.

53. Shapiro W et al: Relationship of plasma digitoxin and digoxin to cardiac response following intravenous digitalization in man. Circ 42:1065, 1970.

54. Sheiner LB et al: Instructional goals for physicians in the use of blood level data and the contribution of computers. Clin Pharmacol Ther 16:260, 1974.

55. Sheiner LB et al: Modeling of individual pharmacolinetics for computer-aided drug dosage. Comput Biomed Res 5:441, 1972.

56. Shirkey HC: Posology, In *Pediatric Therapy,* 5th ed, ed by Shirkey HC, Mosby, St. Louis, 1972, p. 32.

57. Siersback-Nielson K et al: Rapid evaluation of creatinine clearance (letter) Lancet 1:1133, 1971.

58. Smith TW et al: Clinical value of the radioimmunoassay of the digitalis glycosides. Pharmacol Rev 25:219, 1973.

59. Strong JM et al: Pharmacokinets in man of the N-acetylated metabolite of procainamide. J Pharmacokinet Biopharm 3:223, 1975.

60. Thompson PD: Lidocaine pharmacokinetics in advanced heart failure, liver disease, and renal failure in humans. Ann Intern Med 78:499, 1973.

61. Ueda CT et al: Absolute quinidine bioavailability. Clin Pharmacol Ther 20:260, 1976.

62. Ueda CT et al: Disposition kinetics of quinidine. Clin Pharmacol Ther 19:30, 1976.

63. Wagner JG: *Biopharmaceutics and Relevant Pharmacokinetics.* Drug Intelligence Publications, Illinois, 1971.

64. Ibid. pp 18-25.

65. Wagner JG: Loading and maintenance doses of digoxin in patients with normal renal function and those with severely impaired renal function. J Clin Pharmacol 14:329, 1974.

66. Walsh FM et al: Significance of non-steady state serum digoxin concentrations. Am J Clin Pathol. 63:446, 1975.

67. Welling PG et al: Prediction of drug dosage in patients with renal failure using data derived from normal subjects. Clin Pharmacol Ther 18:45, 1975.

68. Wilder BJ et al: A method for shifting from oral to intramuscular diphenylhydantoin administration. Clin Pharmacol Ther 16:507, 1974.

69. Wilensky AJ et al: Inadequate serum levels after intramuscular administration of diphenylhydantoin. Neurology 23:318, 1973.

70. Wilkinson GR: A physiological approach to hepatic drug clearance. Clin Pharmacol Ther 18:377, 1975.

71. Willich CW et al: Therophylline-induced seizures in adults. Ann Intern Med 82:784, 1975.

Chapter 3

Fluid and Electrolyte Disorders

Lawrence J. Hak

Table of Abbreviations

ADH	antidiuretic Hormone
BUN	Blood urea nitrogen
D5W	5% Dextrose in Water
ECF	Extracellular Fluid
E_{osm}	Effective Osmolality
FBS	Fasting blood sugar
GI	Gastrointestinal
ICF	Intracellular fluid
mg%	milligrams per 100 ml
mOsm	milliosmols
NS	normal saline
OAS	Osmotically active substance
P_{osm}	Plasma osmolality
TBW	total body water

1. J.B. is a 26-year-old 75 kg male who on a routine physical exam had a laboratory report as follows: Na 142, K 4.0, Cl 101, CO₂ 24, Ca 10 mg%, BUN 26 mg%, Cr 0.9 mg%, glucose 85 mg% and a serum osmolality of 285 mOsm. These lab values are all within normal limits and vary little from day to day. What are the physiologic mechanisms which function to maintain body fluids and electrolytes within these narrow constraints?

The internal environment of the body is maintained mainly by renal mechanisms which regulate fluid and electrolyte balance and by cell membranes which maintain the intracellular electrolyte composition.

The electrolyte composition of intracellular fluid (ICF) and extracellular fluid (ECF) is quite different as shown in the table below:

	ECF	ICF
Na	142 mEq/L	10 mEq/L
K	4 "	140 "
Cl	103 "	2 "
HCO₃	25 "	8 "
Mg	3 "	35 "
Ca	5 "	3 "
P (HPO₄)	2 "	95 "

Cell membranes are normally impermeable to anions and either actively retain or extrude cations (70). Most cell membranes are permeable to both Na and K which diffuse passively following concentration gradients. Therefore, in order to maintain an ICF Na concentration of 10 mEq/L with an ECF concentration of 140 mEq/L, Na must be actively extruded from the ICF (60); the reverse is true for K. This process is accomplished through the Na-K-ATPase system located on the cell membrane (49,103,123).

2. What determines the solute concentration of various body compartments?

The solute concentration of body fluids varies in the usual range of 280 to 300 mOsm/kg water (70). By os-

motic processes water moves across a semipermeable membrane from an area of lower concentration of particles to an area of higher concentration until the concentration on on each side of the membrane is equal, at which time water movement will cease (43). Since all cell membranes are freely permeable to water (23), addition of solute to one compartment will cause the movement of water between compartments to eliminate osmotic gradients (57).

Thus, the osmolality of the ICF will always be equal to the osmolality of the ECF even though the solute composition of each compartment is significantly different (70).

3. How might one estimate the osmolality of intravenous solutions and body fluids?

The osmolality of any solution may be calculated using the following formula:

$$mOsm/L = \frac{mg/L}{M.W.} \times \text{number of particles}$$

Example: normal saline (0.9% NaCl)

$$mOsm/L = \frac{9000}{58.5} \times 2 = 308 \text{ mOsm/L}$$

Example: 5% dextrose

$$mOsm/L = \frac{50,000}{180} \times 1 = 278 \text{ mOsm/L}$$

For univalent ions a mEq = mOsm. Since over 90% of the ECF cations are sodium (81), and each cation is accompanied by an anion, plasma osmolality (Posm) may be estimated using the following equation.:

$$Posm = 2\,(PNa) + \frac{BUN\ (mg\%)}{2.8} + \frac{FBS\ (mg\%)}{18}$$

Thus, in a patient with a serum Na of 142, BUN of 26, and glucose of 85, an estimation of plasma osmolality would be:

$$Posm = 2\,(142) + \frac{26}{2.8} + \frac{85}{18}$$

$$= 298 \text{ mOsm/L}$$

Since urea, like water, is freely permeable to most cell membranes it will not affect fluid shifts between compartments and therefore is not considered in calculating effective osmolality (Eosm), thus:

$$Eosm = 2\,(PNa) + \frac{FBS}{18}$$

From the above equation, it can be seen that glucose and urea contribute very little to plasma osmolality. Therefore, with the exception of patients with hyperglycemia, the effective osmolality of body fluids can be estimated simply by multiplying the serum sodium by two.

4. What is meant by electrochemical equivalents and what is a milliequivalent?

Electrolytes in solution combine according to their electrical charge (ionic valence) rather than according to their molecular or atomic weights. The standard of reference for electrical equivalence is one atomic weight of hydrogen; thus, an equivalent of any ion is that amount which will replace or combine with one atomic weight or one gram of hydrogen. The equivalent weight of any substance may be calculated by dividing the gram molecular weight by the valence. A milliequivalent weight then is equal to the equivalent weight divided by 1000.

The principles of equivalence can best be illustrated by the following examples which were adapted from Schroeder (97).

Formulas:

$$\text{Eq Wt} = \frac{\text{Molecular Weight (gm)}}{\text{valence}}$$

$$\text{mEq Wt} = \frac{\text{Eq Wt (gm)}}{1000}$$

$$\text{mEq/L} = \frac{\text{mg/100 ml} \times 10 \times \text{valence}}{\text{Molecular Weight}}$$

mEq Wt of various substances:

Na = .023	HCO₃ = .061
K = .039	NaCl = .0585
Ca = .020	KCl = .0746
Mg = .012	NaHCO₃ = .084
Cl = .0355	

Problems:

a. A diet containing 100 mEq of Na would contain (X) gm of Na and (Y) gm NaCl.

$$\text{mEq} = \frac{\text{Wt (gm)}}{\text{mEq Wt}}$$

$$100 \text{ mEq} = \frac{X \text{ gm}}{.023}$$

$$X = 2.3 \text{ gm Na} = 100 \text{ mEq Na}$$

$$100 \text{ mEq} = \frac{Y \text{ gm}}{.0585}$$

$$Y = 5.85 \text{ gm NaCl} = 100 \text{ mEq Na}$$

b. How many mEq of Calcium are in 5 gm of anhydrous CaCl₂

$$X \text{ mEq} = \frac{5 \text{ gms}}{.0555}$$

$$X = 90 \text{ mEq Ca in 5 gm calcium chloride}$$

c. How many mEq/L are contained in normal saline?

$$\text{mEq/L} = \frac{\text{mg/100 ml} \times 10 \times \text{valence}}{\text{molecular weight}}$$

$$\text{mEq/L} = \frac{900 \times 10 \times 1}{58.5}$$

$$= 154 \text{ mEq/L of Na}$$

$$= 154 \text{ mEq/L of Cl}$$

d. How many mEq/L of Ca are in a liter of solution which contains 10 mg/100 ml CaCl₂ · 2H₂O?

$$\text{mEq/L} = \frac{\text{mg/100 ml} \times 10 \times \text{valence}}{\text{molecular weight}}$$

$$= \frac{10 \times 10 \times 2}{147}$$

$$= 1.36$$

In referring to normal plasma electrolyte concentration, milliequivalents are generally used for substances which are highly ionized in plasma, for example, sodium, potassium, chloride, and bicarbonate. Calcium and phosphorus are usually reported as milligrams per cent rather than milliequivalents per liter, because calcium is approximately 40% bound to plasma proteins and other nonionizable substances. Since bound calcium is not ionized, it is not electrochemically equivalent.

Plasma assay procedures for calcium do not differentiate between bound and ionized forms; therefore, the laboratory reports calcium as milligrams per 100 ml. Similarly, phosphorus is found in serum in multiple forms, such as H_2PO_4, HPO_4, PO_4. Because it is not possible to provide a valence for the phosphorus, the total phosphorus is measured and reported as milligrams per cent rather than as milliequivalents.

5. How is body water distributed in a 75 kg male?

Normally total body water **(TBW)** in males represents approximately 60% of body weight (22). This percentage varies according to the relative amount of fat present, since fat cells contain negligible amounts of water. In females TBW approximates 50% of body weight (22). Thus, in a 75 kg male TBW equals 45 liters. This fluid is distributed into two compartments. Two-thirds (30 liters) is intracellular fluid **(ICF)**. The **ECF** is further subdivided with approximately 75% (11.25L) in the interstitial space and 25% (3.75L) in the intravascular space (70). It therefore follows that two-thirds of the body's osmotically active substances **(OAS)** are found in the ICF with the remaining one-third in the ECF.

Since the quantity of OAS in the ICF is relatively fixed, the ICF volume is determined by water balance. Salts of Na comprise greater than 90% of the OAS of the ECF fluid; therefore, ECF volume is controlled by Na balance (70).

6. How much water is required daily for a 70 kg male to maintain normal body functions? What conditions require additional fluid replacement?

The minimum daily water requirement is approximately 1300 ml, while approximately 2300 ml are needed for maximal body function. These water requirements may be broken down as follows:

	Minimal	Maximal
Insensible Loss:		
Respiration	500 ml	500 ml
Sweat	500 ml	500 ml
Urine	500 ml	1500 ml
	1500 ml	2500 ml
Water production from catabolism	−200 ml	−200 ml
	1300 ml	2300 ml

To maintain renal function, a minimum urine production of 20 ml/hr is required. Maximal renal efficiency occurs with a urine output of about 1500 ml per 24 hours.

An increase in insensible water loss occurs when there is an elevation of body or environmental temperature. About 500 ml are needed for each 5° rise in environmental temperature above 85°F and an additional 500 ml is required for a body temperature of 103°F. There is a 10% increase in fluid requirement for each °C rise in body temperature.

Supplemental fluids will also be required when there are excess gastrointestinal (GI) losses or when there is "third spacing" of body fluids. Patients with colostomies, enterocutaneous fistulas, diarrhea or vomiting and those on nasogastric suction will require both fluid and electrolyte replacement. "Third spacing" represents the abnormal sequestration of body fluids in a space which generally does not contain substantial volumes of fluid. Conditions associated with third space loss include peritonitis, burns, intestinal obstruction and ascites.

7. What volume changes would occur in body fluid compartments if you were to administer the following solutions to a 75 kg male: 2 liters of NS; 3 liters of D5W?

Because Na and Cl ions are confined to the ECF compartment and saline is isosmotic with normal body fluids, the entire two liters of solution will remain in the ECF and total body osmolality will not change.

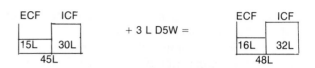

As glucose solutions are administered, endogenous insulin secretion will cause the glucose to enter the ICF where it will either be metabolized or stored as glycogen. In either case, the ICF concentration of OAS will not significantly change and the net effect on body fluids of giving D5W will be the same as if sterile water was administered. Thus, since two-thirds of the body's OAS are in the ICF and one-third in the ECF, two liters of water will enter the ICF, one liter will remain in the ECF and total body osmolality will decrease.

8. J.B. is a 26-year-old 75 kg male diabetic with the following laboratory values: Na 142, K 4.0, Cl 101, CO_2 24, BUN 26 mg%, Cr 0.9 mg% and glucose 85. If J.B. neglected to take his insulin, what fluid shifts would occur if his serum glucose acutely rose to 500 mg%? What would happen to his serum sodium?

Initially, a serum Na of 142 mEq/L would provide an estimated plasma osmolality of 284 mOsm/L and a total body osmotically active solute of 12,780 mOsm (45L × 284 mOsm/L). If his serum glucose acutely rose to 500 mg%, his ECF osmolality would increase by 27.7 mOsm/L (500/18 mg%) to 312 mOsm/L and his total body solute would increase, by 416 mOsm (27.7 mOsm/L × 15L ECF) to 13,196 mOsm. If his total body water did not change, osmotic forces would move water from the ICF to the ECF until a new equilibrium was attained. Total body osmolality will increase to:

$$\frac{13,196 \text{ mOsm}}{45 \text{ L}} = 293 \text{ mOsm/L},$$

and the new ICF would be:

$$30 \text{ L} \times \frac{284 \text{ mOsm/L}}{293 \text{ mOsm/L}} = 29 \text{ L}.$$

His new ECF volume would be:

$$\frac{(15 \text{ L} \times 284 \text{ mOsm/L}) + (27.7 \text{ mOsm/L} \times 15 \text{ L})}{293 \text{ mOsm/L}} = 16 \text{ L}.$$

In addition, his serum Na would decrease to 133 mEq/L:

$$142 \text{ mEq/L} \times \frac{15 \text{ L}}{16 \text{ L}} = 133 \text{ mEq/L}.$$

9. What additional homeostatic mechanisms would occur as J.B.'s body fluid osmolality began to increase?

(a) The osmoreceptors in the thirst center, sensing an increase in body fluid osmolality, stimulate thirst and cause an increased oral intake of fluid (130).

(b) The osmoreceptors in the supraoptic nuclei of the hypothalamus send stimuli to the posterior pituitary causing the release of antidiuretic hormone (ADH) which promotes water reabsorption in the distal tubule and collecting duct of the nephron (44,59,115). However, as the serum glucose rises above the renal threshold for glucose reabsorption (180 mg%), an osmotic diuresis occurs preventing maximal ADH-stimulated water reabsorption. In addition, as the osmotic diuresis increases tubular fluid volume, the tubular fluid concentration of Na will be less than that of the tubular epithelial cells and peritubular spaces so that sodium will passively diffuse back into the tubular fluid causing a natriuresis. Ultimately, deficits of both total body Na and water will occur.

10. How should J.B.'s fluid and electrolyte imbalances be corrected?

Insulin should be administered to enhance the uptake and utilization of glucose by cells and to alleviate hyperosmolality. Intravenous normal saline or 1/2 NS is required initially to replace ECF volume lost through osmotic diuresis. This is particularly important if the patient is exhibiting signs and symptoms consistent with dehydration (poor skin turgor, increased pulse rate, and postural hypotension). Eventually, ½ NS or D5½NS will be required to completely restore normal fluid balance.

11. B.A. is a 55-year-old 85 kg male who on routine physical examination was found to have the following lab values: Na 130, K 4.0, Cl 96, CO₂ 20. What conclusions can one draw from this patient's serum Na. What factors may cause a false hyponatremia?

The serum Na concentration says nothing about total body sodium content, nor sodium balance, although it may provide an estimate of body osmolality (81). Situations where the reported value for serum Na may not reflect the true value include:

(a) *Hyperglycemia* — Glucose, an OAS in the ECF will draw fluid into the ECF space resulting in a dilutional hyponatremia. A general rule to follow is that for each 100 mg per 100 ml increment from normal serum glucose, serum Na will decrease by 1.6 mEq/L (16,48,50).

(b) *Hyperlipemia* — In this situation the Na concentration of plasma water may be normal but the lipids reduce the quantity of water per unit volume of plasma, resulting in a pseudohyponatremia (31).

12. What are the common mechanisms by which true hyponatremia occurs?

Hyponatremia may result from a total body deficit of Na or an excess of total body water (31,110). In the latter case, total body Na may be normal or even increased; however, excess TBW produces a dilutional hyponatremia.

Na Deficit: True Na depletion hyponatremia results when losses of Na exceed losses of water. Clinically, this occurs when there is an excessive loss of GI fluids (vomiting, diarrhea), adrenal insufficiency, salt wasting nephritis, or an excessive use of diuretics (31,81). Initially, the loss of Na causes a decrease in ECF volume. Homeostatic mechanisms result in thirst (130), increased proximal tubule reabsorption of Na and water, and secretion of aldosterone and ADH.

In response to the thirst stimulus, fluids (usually low in Na content) are ingested. Approximately 2/3 of this electrolyte free water passes osmotically into the ICF. The portion remaining in the ECF worsens the hyponatremia without sufficiently restoring volume while the ADH prevents the kidney from producing dilute urine in spite of the hyponatremia. The patient presents clinically with hypotension, azotemia, oliguria and an absence of edema.

Excess of Total Body Water: The most common cause of hyponatremia is an altered renal excretion of water (81) combined with excessive water intake. Under normal conditions when a quantity of water exceeds body requirements the kidney excretes electrolyte-free water (52). Generation of free water is accomplished by reabsorption of solute (NaCl) in the distal portion of the ascending loop of Henle—a portion of the collecting duct which is impermeable to water (55) and in the collecting duct where water permeability is determined by the relative presence or absence of ADH (52). In the absence of ADH, the ascending limb, distal tubule and collecting duct are impermeable to water while reabsorption of NaCl continues. The electrolyte free water remaining in the tubule and collecting duct is excreted in the urine, and, free water is cleared. In the presence of ADH, the ascending limb remains water tight but the distal tubule and collecting duct become permeable to water and reabsorption occurs. It follows, then, that in order for the kidney to excrete free water, three factors must be operable: (a) sufficient NaCl must be delivered to the ascending limb and distal tubule in order to generate free water, (b) mechanisms necessary to decrease ADH secretion must be intact, and (c) there must be sufficient functioning renal mass for appropriate quantities of water to be excreted. If any one or combination of any of the above conditions are absent (e.g. inappropriate secretion of ADH, congestive heart failure, liver failure) excess accumulation of body water and, thus, dilutional hyponatremia will result.

13. How can one differentiate between hyponatremia resulting from true sodium depletion and that resulting from the accumulation of excess water with or without sodium?

Although the symptoms are similar for both dilutional and salt depletion hyponatremia, it is important to determine the etiology since the treatment of these disorders differs considerably. A patient with true sodium depletion hyponatremia will usually present with prerenal azotemia, an elevated hematocrit, hypotension, a rapid, thready pulse, and cool, clammy skin as a result of vasoconstriction. All of the mentioned signs and symptoms are related to depletion of vascular volume. Mucous membranes will usually be dry, and tissue turgor will be decreased (31). In the patient with dilutional hyponatremia, these indices will usually be normal.

Therapy of the patient with true salt depletion hyponatremia is accomplished by replacement of sodium either orally or intravenously as isotonic saline. In severe cases, intravenous administration of hypertonic saline may be necessary (31,132). The sodium deficit should be calculated on the basis of total body water. The therapy of patients with dilutional hyponatremia will differ depending upon the underlying pathophysiologic mechanism of the disease process and the clinical presentation. Although therapy must be individualized for each patient, sodium and/or water restriction is generally instituted.

14. What are the signs and symptoms of hyponatremia?

Whether the hyponatremia is the result of salt depletion or is dilutional, the net effect is a decrease in effective extracellular OAS and a relative overhydration of the intracellular space. This produces symptoms of weakness, nausea, difficulty in concentration, headache and somnolence. In severe cases, seizures may occur (31).

15. A 40-year-old female with long standing pyelonephritis and hypertension was brought to the emergency room just after having a grand mal seizure. She was unresponsive on arrival. For the past 3 days prior to admission (PTA) she had experienced nausea, vomiting, diarrhea and fever and had been drinking large amounts of fluids and cola although she ate little food. Her admission laboratory values were Na 110, Cl 86, CO_2 18, BUN 97, Cr 7.1. Her weight was 60 kg which was not different from her normal weight. What is the most likely explanation for her serum Na? How should it be treated?

As a result of vomiting, diarrhea, and chronic pyelonephritis this patient lost considerable quantities of ECF. As she replaced her volume loss with electrolyte free water, there was a decrease in ECF osmolality and water moved into the intracellular space until osmotic equilibrium occurred. Thus, calculations of salt replacement must take into account the movement of total body water. If one assumes that her TBW is 30L (50% of body weight in females) and that her normal serum Na is 140 mEq/L, the sodium deficit may be calculated.

Na Deficit (mEq) = (normal serum Na − actual serum Na) × TBW

Na Deficit (mEq) = (140-110) × 30

Na Deficit = 900 mEq

Because of the acuteness of this situation, half of her Na deficit (450 mEq) should be replaced with hypertonic saline (3%) over eight hours, i.e.,

$$\frac{450 \text{ mEq}}{512 \text{ mEq/1000 ml}} = 880 \text{ ml of 3% saline}$$

Replacement of 450 mEq of Na should raise her ECF Na concentration enough to relieve the symptoms of hyponatremia. The remainder of her deficit may be replaced slowly over several days. Sufficient fluid and Na to replace insensible water loss and urine output should also be provided.

16. S.T. is a 62-year-old male with a long standing history of atherosclerotic cardiovascular disease (ASCVD) and two previous myocardial infarctions (MI's). He presents to the hospital with 4+ pitting edema in the pretibial and sacral areas, severe shortness of breath and two pillow orthopnea. His blood pressure was 130/95; his pulse was 92 and his respiratory rate was 24. Initial lab values were as follows: Na 133, K 3.3, Cl 95, CO_2 32, BUN 44, Cr 1.3, serum glucose 95. What are the pathophysiologic mechanisms of this patient's hyponatremia and what would be an appropriate therapeutic regimen for him?

This patient is a classic presentation of hyponatremia resulting from congestive heart failure (124). The pathophysiologic mechanisms are as follows. In congestive heart failure, cardiac output is decreased, resulting in decreased perfusion of the kidneys. This apparent decrease in intravascular volume sets off several homeostatic mechanisms within the kidney.

a. There is an increased proximal tubular reabsorption of sodium and water which results in a decreased delivery of sodium to the diluting segments of the nephron and impairs the kidney's ability to generate and excrete free water.

b. The decrease in volume sensed by the juxtaglomerular cells causes a release of renin and ultimately an increased secretion of aldosterone. This results in an increased reabsorption of sodium and water in the distal tubules.

c. As a result of a decrease in cardiac output, cardiac return is diminished. The volume receptors in the left atrium (42, 44), sensing a decrease, set off a stimulus for the secretion of anti-diuretic hormone (41, 58, 103). The net effect of the renal response to decreased cardiac output is an increased reabsorption of both sodium and water. The excess secretion of ADH results in a dilutional hyponatremia even in the presence of excess total body sodium. Therapy for this patient includes: salt and water restriction, digitalis, and diuretics. (See *Congestive Heart Failure* chapter.)

17. Discuss the distribution and elimination of potassium.

A normal 70 kg male has a total body potassium of approximately 3500 mEq (82, 123), most of which is located intracellularly (98). Only about 50 mEq of potassium is in the ECF under normal conditions and the average concentration is 4 mEq/L. The average total body ICF concentration of K is 143 mEq per liter of cell water with almost 90% being found in muscle cells (128).

For adults, the usual daily dietary intake of potassium equals output and ranges from 50-150 mEq. Normally, more than 90% of the potassium which is ingested is excreted in the urine; only small amounts are found in the sweat and feces (79, 98, 122). The kidneys will increase potassium excretion in response to augmented intake. However, renal conservation of potassium is not as efficient as that for sodium, and even in the presence of a total body deficit there is an obligatory loss of 10 mEq or more per day.

18. Relate the major body functions of potassium with the symptomatology observed in hyper- and hypokalemia.

One of the major functions of potassium is to maintain the excitability of neuromuscular tissue (123). The resting membrane potential is a function of and varies directly with the ratio of intracellular to extracellular potassium (21, 127). Since the normal intracellular potassium concentration is approximately 140 mEq/L, and the extracellular concentration is 3.5 mEq/L, it is evident that small alterations in intracellular potassium concentration do not significantly affect the ratio and therefore, the resting membrane potential. However, small alterations of even one milliequivalent per liter of extracellular potassium significantly affect the ratio and therefore, the resting membrane potential. Acute changes in extracellular K would have the following consequences (39, 40, 127): Acute hypokalemia would be associated with an increased resting membrane potential, thus requiring a greater than normal stimulus to obtain an action potential. Clinically, one would observe weakness and paralysis. Hyperkalemia, on the other hand, would result in a decreased resting membrane potential and an enhanced state of excitability; cardiac arrhythmias are a common consequence of this disorder. If the alteration in extracellular potassium occurs slowly so that equilibration between intracellular and extracellular K can occur, the ratio will not change and excitability disturbances will not be observed (79).

Potassium also plays an important role in carbohydrate and protein metabolism and enzymatic reactions (122). Physiologic concentrations of intracellular potassium are required for glycogen synthesis in the liver as well as skeletal muscle. Insulin secretion is blunted in hypokalemic patients (11, 38), and the thiazide-induced hyperglycemia seen in latent diabetes may be ameliorated by potassium repletion (11, 90, 121, 131). Small reductions in intracellular potassium concentration result in significant reductions of protein synthesis. Several enzyme systems (77, 84, 114, 123, 125) require potassium, including adenosinetriphosphatase, which hydrolyzes adenosene triphosphate (ATP). This process releases energy for numerous metabolic processes (4, 26, 54).

19. What factors may falsely elevate a patient's serum potassium?

The normal range for serum potassium is generally considered to be 3.5 to 5 mEq/L (131), although a range of 3.8 to 4.5 mEq/L may be more appropriate (112). Artifactual elevations of serum potassium may result from hemolysis within the collection tube or leakage of potassium from cells when samples are not promptly separated (134). Prior exercise or trauma to tissue in the area where the blood sample is obtained will also falsely elevate potassium levels. In addition, diseases associated with thrombocytosis may falsely elevate potassium levels as platelets release potassium within the collection tube (79). A general rule to follow is that errors in blood sample collection and analysis result in elevated K levels, while low levels are usually correct.

20. Does the serum potassium always reflect a patient's total body potassium status?

Apparent excesses or deficits in serum K may occur even though total body K is normal because under certain circumstances there can be shifts of K between the intracellular and extracellular compartments.

Acute alterations in acid-base balance will alter serum levels of K without necessarily changing total body stores (99). For each decrease in the plasma pH of 0.1 unit there is an increase in the serum potassium of 0.63 mEq/L (122, 123). The administration of glucose and insulin will shift serum potassium intracellularly.

Scribner and Burnell (100) estimate that when sudden shifts of K between compartments do not occur, a loss of 100 to 200 mEq of total body K is required to reduce the serum K by 1 mEq/L if the initial serum K was above 3 mEq/L. When the initial serum K is below 3 mEq/L a total body K deficit of 200 to 400 mEq will be necessary to lower serum K by 1 mEq per liter.

21. An 18-year-old female came to the emergency room with a four day history of anorexia, nausea, and

vomiting which she attributed to the "stomach flu." Physical examination revealed poor skin turgor and dry mucous membranes. Laboratory values at that time included the following: Na 134, K 3.0, Cl 90, HCO₃ 32. Discuss all the possible etiologies of this patient's hypokalemia.

Potassium depletion occurs in situations where potassium losses are in excess of intake. This occurs most commonly when there are excessive gastro-intestinal losses (vomiting, diarrhea, NG aspiration) (122), because the gastric and intestinal secretions contain potassium concentrations of 5 to 20 mEq/L.

Metabolic alkalosis resulting from the loss of acid gastric fluid will cause renal wasting of potassium. Although the mechanism for this is unclear, several possibilities exist. First, as a result of the metabolic alkalosis, less H will be available at distal tubular exchange sites and one might presume that potassium might preferentially occupy the transport site; however, there is no evidence to demonstrate competition between H and K ions for secretory sites (98). Another possibility is that alterations in acid-base balance modify the active transport of potassium intracellularly in the distal tubular cells, thus altering the size of the intracellular potassium pool. Potassium secretion is thought to vary directly with the size of the intracellular pool (65). Lastly, as extracellular volume is lost via the GI tract, homeostatic mechanisms which conserve volume will come into play. An increased secretion of aldosterone will increase renal K loss. Ultimately renal losses of K in this situation will considerably exceed that lost in the GI fluids.

The metabolic alkalosis observed in this patient will also cause serum potassium to shift intracellularly. (Also see the chapter on *Edema*.)

An obvious cause of hypokalemia which is often overlooked occurs in patients who take nothing by mouth. This also occurs in hospitalized patients if sufficient K is not included in intravenous fluids to replace urinary losses. Also, if such patients receive sufficient quantities of glucose and/or amino acids to increase the intracellular potassium capacity but only receive enough K to replace urinary losses, total body K deficits and hypokalemia will ensue.

22. What are some other causes of hypokalemia? (Also see *Congestive Heart Failure* chapter.)

Certain renal diseases, especially those associated with tubular defects, result in potassium deficits and hypokalemia (7, 64, 74). The inability to secrete H into the urine appears to be the basic defect resulting in increased K secretion at the sodium exchange sites. Patients usually present with systemic acidosis, potassium deficits and hypokalemia. An example of such a case is renal tubular acidosis. (See *Diseases of the Kidney*.)

Primary hyperaldosteronism (3) also results in potassium deficits. These patients differ from those with tubular defects in that they usually present with metabolic alkalosis, rather than acidosis. They usually have hypertension and have normal renal function in spite of excess urinary losses of potassium (14, 91).

Secondary hyperaldosteronism is caused by a decrease in extracellular volume (dehydration, diuretics) or a decrease in effective extracellular volume (cirrhosis with ascites, nephrotic syndrome, congestive heart failure, etc.) and results in a depletion of total body potassium.

Case A: A 15-year-old boy sustained a crush injury when a tractor he was driving overturned and pinned him for a period of four hours. He was referred to University Hospital for treatment of his acute renal failure secondary to the crush injury. Nasogastric suction was started and was productive of coffee ground material. The abdomen has remained flat and tense with questionable bowel sounds. An EKG revealed tall, peaked T waves. His vital signs were within normal limits with the exception of a temperature of 38.5.

Pertinent laboratory values on admission were as follows: K 6.8 mEq/L, HCO₃ 13 mEq/L, Creatinine 9.6 mg%, BUN 128 mg%, Hct 28%, WBC 18,000 with 85% Polys, Total protein 5.4, Albumin 2.3 gm%, and Calcium 8.2 mg%.

His current medication include: Pen G 10 MU IV qd, Amphogel per ng 30 cc prn, Sodium Bicarbonate 50 mEq IV x 1, D 20 W, Kanamycin 500 mg IM bid and blood transfusions as needed.

23. Discuss the EKG changes which may be caused by changes in serum potassium.

Electrocardiogram findings are often valuable in assessing serum potassium levels (71, 111). As the serum K exceeds 5.5 mEq/L, peaking of T waves is the first EKG change seen. Depressed ST segments follow with increasing K concentrations. As the K concentration exceeds 6.5 mEq/L, widening of the QRS complex is usually present. When the K concentration exceeds 7 mEq/L the P wave amplitude usually decreases and the P-R interval is usually prolonged. With hypokalemia, the EKG shows flattening or inversion of the T waves and depression of the ST segment with low voltage. A baseline EKG prior to alterations in serum K is of great value in interpreting EKG changes. For example, cardiac ischemia or a myocardial infarction may cause flattening or inversion of T waves in the presence of normal serum K. Likewise, hyperkalemia may return inverted T waves to normal in spite of cardiac ischemia.

24. In the above patient, what are the possible etiologies of hyperkalemia?

There are several factors contributing to this patient's high serum potassium.

Since a majority of the total body potassium is located intracellularly, a high serum potassium may result from any situation where there is substantial tissue or cellular damage or from a severe catabolic state. The crush injury in this patient contributes substantially to the hyperkalemia.

The metabolic acidosis will cause a shift of intracellular potassium to extracellular spaces.

Severe renal failure is a major cause of this patient's hyperkalemia (108) because the kidney is the primary route of potassium elimination.

The patient is receiving a large load of exogenous potassium in the presence of compromised renal function. The sources include the potassium in the penicillin G, blood transfusions, and that absorbed from gastrointestinal blood losses (coffee ground material).

25. What modes of therapy are available for the emergency treatment of this patient's hyperkalemia?

Calcium should be administered initially to reverse the EKG changes. Calcium salts antagonize the cardiac toxicity of potassium. The IV infusion of one gram of calcium gluconate over 5 to 10 minutes may provide improvement in EKG abnormalities caused by hyperkalemia (94). However, this therapy probably should not be used in digitalized patients as calcium potentiates the effect of cardiac glycosides and toxicity may ensue.

The intravenous administration of sodium bicarbonate has been shown to be of value in rapidly lowering serum K levels especially in patients who are acidotic (99). The usual dose is 50 mEq IV over several minutes with repeated doses administered every 15 to 20 minutes as needed (94). Alternatively, a 5% solution of sodium bicarbonate may be administered by constant IV infusion (99).

The intravenous administration of glucose and insulin may be the most effective mode of emergency treatment for hyperkalemia (71). The infusion of 60 to 100 grams of glucose together with 20 to 25 units of regular insulin (94) rapidly lowers serum K as K moves intracellularly with glucose and is stored with glycogen (71). This therapy will lower serum K for up to 12 hours (94).

(Also see the chapter on *Diseases of the Kidney*.)

26. What factors function to maintain calcium balance?

The quantity of total body calcium varies according to skeleton size and bone density with greater than 99% of body calcium being found in the skeleton (62). The remaining calcium is distributed both intracellularly and extracellularly, and the concentration in these compartments is similar (27).

The normal serum concentration of calcium is maintained within the narrow range of 9 to 11 mg/100 ml. This concentration reflects a dynamic equilibrium between calcium intake, turnover, and excretion from the body (67, 75, 88). Under normal conditions about 40% of serum calcium is bound to serum protein, 50% is ionized, and about 10% is ultrafiltrable but unionized, i.e., as phosphate, bicarbonate, and citrate complexes (27, 75, 88, 117). The physiologically active ionized fraction is in equilibrium with the unionized and bound fractions, and the constancy of serum levels results from a sensitive regulatory mechanism involving parathyroid hormone (PTH) and calcitonin (1). The gastrointestinal absorption of calcium is mainly regulated by vitamin D (18).

Since a large proportion of serum calcium exists in the bound form, changes in serum albumin may affect serum calcium levels even though the concentration of the physiologically active ionized form may be within normal limits. For every 1 gm% decrease in serum albumin, the serum calcium decreases by 0.8 mg%.

The amount of calcium absorbed into the body is dependent on dietary intake and the efficiency of intestinal absorption. Although intestinal absorption of calcium can occur by passive diffusion, quantities greater than 2 gm of elemental calcium per day are required (12, 72). At the usual dietary intake of approximately 400 mg to 800 mg per day, passive absorption of calcium is negligible, and vitamin D stimulated intestinal active transport of calcium is required to maintain calcium balance (6, 17, 80, 103). (See section on chronic renal failure for a more detailed discussion of the metabolism of vitamin D.)

27. What role does calcium play in normal body functions?

The role of calcium in normal body functions has been reviewed by Maggia and Hunemaun (75). These include the maintenance of cellular membrane excitability, nerve tissue excitability, and contractility of skeletal, smooth, and cardiac muscle. Calcium also functions as a co-factor in the activation of various enzyme systems including those of the pancreas and coagulation system. Calcium ion concentration also affects the secretory activity of endocrine and exocrine glands. Hypercalcemia stimulates gastric secretion which may explain the increased incidence of peptic ulcer disease in conditions associated with hypercalcemia. In addition, hypercalcemia exerts multiple effects on renal function, including a reduction in glomerular filtration rate and defective conservation of water by either interfering with ADH or decreasing the activity of the counter-current multiplier system. Hypercalcemia also interferes with tubular function resulting in decreased ammonia production and acid excretion, and increased excretion of sodium, potassium, glucose, phosphate, and amino acids (23, 75).

Calcium has also been demonstrated to play a role in the contraction of vascular smooth muscle (47). Whether this direct effect results in hypertension seen with hypercalcemia or whether the hypercalcemic effects on renal function result in hypertension is unknown at this time (20, 120).

28. A 65-year-old man was admitted to the hospital in a coma. He had been in his usual state of good health until approximately two months prior to admission when he began to experience generalized fatigue and epigastric pain which was not relieved with antacids. His symptoms continued until the day of admission when he became confused and rapidly went into coma. On admission his blood pressure was 165/95, pulse 82, and respirations 21. His physical exam was within normal limits with the exception of a palpable liver 3 cm below the right costal margin; he was responsive only to deep pain. Initial laboratory data included Na 144, K 3.5, Cl 100, CO_2 21, BUN 40, Calcium 16 mg/100 ml, P 1.9 mg/100 ml. Over the next ten days the patient was treated with saline and furosemide, which resulted in lowering his serum calcium to 8.1 mg/100 ml. On the eleventh hospital day the patient developed GI bleeding and died. Autopsy revealed carcinoma of the esophagus with metastases to the liver, local lymph nodes, and bone. The parathyroid glands were normal. What is the most likely etiology of hypercalcemia in this patient? What are some other causes of hypercalcemia?

Hypercalcemia frequently occurs in patients with a variety of neoplasms (76, 86). Although the exact mechanism by which hypercalcemia occurs is not known, humoral substances which stimulate osteoclastic bone resorption appear to play a major role. Examples of these substances are polypeptides with parathyroid hormone-like activity (93, 104), vitamin D-like sterols (37), prostaglandins (53, 113) and osteoclast-activating factors (OAF) (76).

In addition to neoplastic disease, hypercalcemia is also associated with sarcoidosis, Paget's Disease, milk alkali syndrome, vitamin D intoxication and hyperthyroidism. Under normal physiologic conditions the plasma concentration of calcium is a major factor in the regulation of parathyroid hormone (PTH) release, and there is an inverse linear relationship between plasma calcium levels and circulating levels of PTH. Thus, serum calcium levels function as a homeostatic feedback control in PTH secretion. Conversely, in patients with parathyroid adenomas or parathyroid hyperplasia, the normal negative feedback control is lost and increased secretion of PTH continues in spite of elevated serum calcium levels.

29. What are the signs and symptoms of hypercalcemia?

Essentially, every organ system is affected by increased circulating levels of calcium. Multiple psychiatric disturbances may occur with the symptoms often being proportional to the degree of hypercalcemia, although this is not always the case. Tiredness, lethargy, apathy, and depression or agitation, nervousness, and insomnia may occur. Neurotic behavior, psychomotor retardation, agitated depression and paranoia have all been reported to occur with hypercalcemia and are reversible as the elevated levels of calcium are returned to normal. Headaches and generalized muscle weakness are common. Gastrointestinal manifestations include anorexia, nausea, and vomiting (121). Increased acid and pepsin secretion occur, and there is an increased incidence of ulcers in patients with hyperparathyroidism (126).

Acute hypercalcemia may result in hypertension which reverses as the serum calcium levels return to normal. Chronic hypercalcemia is often accompanied by hypertension. However, in this situation the elevated pressure is the result of hypercalcemia-induced renal failure and does not return to normal when serum calcium levels are decreased. Electrocardiographic changes which may occur with hypercalcemia include a decreased QT interval and shortened or absent S-T segment (111). A variety of cardiac arrythmias may occur during hypercalcemia (116). The inotropic effect of digitalis glycosides is enhanced by calcium and digitalis toxicity may be aggravated by hypercalcemia. Precipitation of calcium in the cornea and conjunctiva often occurs in patients with chronic hypercalcemia.

30. What drugs are used to treat hypercalcemia? What are their mechanisms of action?

a. *Saline and Furosemide*: (See chapter on *Edema*.)

b. *Glucocorticoids* are widely used in the initial therapy of hypercalcemia although the exact mechanism by which they lower serum calcium remains unknown. Most patients with myeloma, lymphoma, or leukemia will respond to prednisone 40 to 60 mg daily (56) — possibly due to the antitumor effect of the steroids (10). These agents also exert an anti-vitamin D effect which may decrease both bone resorption and gastrointestinal absorption of calcium (10). Ultimately, the tumor must be controlled to produce a permanent reduction in the serum calcium.

c. *Mithramycin*, an antibiotic that has antitumor activity especially in the treatment of embryonal cell carcinoma of the testis (51), has recently become a mainstay in the therapy of malignant hypercalcemia. Although the exact mechanism of action of mithramycin is unknown, it has been proposed that it acts through inhibition of RNA synthesis (51). PTH directly stimulates bone resorption possibly by initiating the development of osteoclast differentiation (96). A process which is related to an increased synthesis of RNA within the osteoclast (51). Thus, it is likely that mithramycin exerts its activity by inhibition of the effect of PTH on the osteoclast. Also, small doses of mithramycin have been shown to block the hypercalcemic action of pharmacologic doses of vitamin D (83).

Cumulative doses of mithramycin, like those used in tumor therapy, are quite toxic and may cause fever, nausea, vomiting, and dermatitis (51). Hemorrhage resulting from vascular damage, thrombocytopenia and altered platelet function, and depression of factors II, V, VII, and X (73) may occur in over 50% of the patients (51). Hepatic dysfunction occurs regularly and is associated with elevated levels of SGOT, SGPT, and LDH; the morphologic finding is usually central lobular necrosis (51).

Severe renal damage, although less frequent, does occur with cumulative doses; mild renal damage with proteinuria is common (51). Although serious toxicity limits the use of mithramycin as a tumor agent, the doses used to treat hypercalcemia (25 to 150 mcg/kg/week) are well tolerated (25, 106). The drug may be administered by IV bolus or by IV infusion over 24 hours. Gradual decreases in serum calcium levels occur usually within 48 hours after administration of mithramycin. The duration of the effect is variable and repeated doses may be required every 3 to 7 days.

(d) *Phosphates*: (See below).

31. E.M. is a 50-year-old female with the diagnosis of primary hyperparathyroidism who at this time refuses surgery. Although she has been relatively asymptomatic, she consistently has serum calcium levels ranging between 11.5 to 12.5 mg/100 ml. What measures should be used to control this patient's hypercalcemia?

When surgery is not feasible, adequate salt and water intake must be assured to prevent dehydration, which will decrease the renal excretion of calcium and accentuate the hypercalcemia by decreasing the extracellular volume. Agents which may cause hypercalcemia (vitamin D, thiazides, antacids, etc.) should be avoided. Also, careful use of digitalis glycosides is necessary to prevent calcium potentiated digitalis toxicity. Immobilization of the patient should be minimized as this accelerates bone resorption. Restriction of calcium in the diet is usually of no benefit as most of the calcium is coming from the bones; however, milk products which contain vitamin D should not be taken (10). If these measures are unsuccessful, oral phosphates should be added to the regimen in a dosage of 1 to 3 grams of elemental phosphorus per 24 hours (46). Antacid preparations should not be taken concomitantly as these agents bind phosphate in the gut.

32. What is the mechanism by which phosphate salts lower serum calcium?

Although inorganic phosphates lower serum calcium when administered orally or by IV infusion, the mechanism(s) by which they do so is unclear since the renal excretion of calcium actually decreases during therapy (36, 45). Several investigators (36, 45, 69) propose precipitation of $CaHPO_4$ as the mechanism, while others (9) believe phosphate administration promotes bone formation. The available evidence supports the theory that calcium is removed from the blood and deposited as a phosphate precipitate in soft tissue and bone. Although clinical complications generally do not occur, hypotension and actue renal failure have been associated with the rapid administration of intravenous phosphate solution (102).

33. When it is observed, what are the signs and symptoms of hypocalcemia?

The major manifestation of hypocalcemia is tetany. Earliest symptoms are numbness of the fingers and tingling or burning in the extremities. As hypocalcemia progresses, muscle cramps may occur, followed by visible muscle spasms of the extremities. In severe cases generalized convulsions are observed (121).

A widened S-T segment is seen on EKG, and impaired cardiac contractility leading to cardiac enlargement and heart failure is seen with hypocalcemia (111, 121). Thinning and loss of body hair usually occurs with chronic hypocalcemia. In addition the skin becomes dry and keratotic, resembling eczema.

Hypocalcemia occurs in malabsorptive states and in primary and secondary hypoparathyroid states. Also see chapter on *Diseases of the Kidney* for a discussion of the treatment of hypocalcemia associated with chronic renal failure. Acute shifts of unionized calcium onto protein which may follow rapid correction of acidosis may also be associated with the symptomatology described above.

34. F.C. is a 36-year-old black male with end stage renal failure (CCr 4 ml/min) who is currently being managed by diet and drug therapy while awaiting admission into a chronic hemodialysis program. His regimen includes a 20 gm protein Giovanetti diet, Titralac 10 ml tid ac, Basaljel Extra Strength 10 ml po tid pc, Lasix 120 mg po q am and multivitamins once daily. He was brought to the emergency room where he appeared to be uremic, with drowsiness and a clouded sensorium. Initial laboratory values were Na 139, K 4.2, Cl 102, CO₂ 18, BUN 74, Cr 12.5, and glucose 89. EKG revealed a prolonged P-R interval and a broadening QRS complex. On questioning the patient and his family it was concluded that adherence to both diet and prescribed drug regimens was excellent; however, the patient had been constipated for the past two weeks and had been taking milk of mag-

nesia several times a day for the past week. A stat serum magnesium level was drawn and found to be 7.2 mEq per liter. How does the kidney handle magnesium normally and in renal failure?

Normally, circulating levels of ionized magnesium are available for glomerular filtration and are probably reabsorbed in the early portion of the distal tubule by an active process (2). Tubular secretion has not been documented (78). Under conditions of magnesium deprivation, the normal kidney will conserve magnesium and the daily excretion may be as low as 1 mEq (19, 30). Hypomagnesemia may be seen in patients with pyelonephritis, nephrosclerosis and renal tubular acidosis (107, 118) probably because of a defective tubular reabsorption. Patients with azotemia often have elevated levels of magnesium due to decreased renal elimination of the ion (89). The degree of hypermagnesemia generally correlates with the magnitude of azotemia (119). Thus, the administration of magnesium containing compounds such as antacids or laxatives to uremic patients is likely to produce hypermagnesemia. This patient's clouded sensorium and EKG findings are consistent with hypermagnesemia (118).

35. A 35-year-old male was admitted to the hospital after a generalized convulsion. He has had regional enteritis for the past 10 years requiring surgery on two occasions for removal of diseased bowel. The most recent surgery was four weeks prior to his seizure. Since that surgery he has had continual diarrhea and food intake has been poor. On admission he was confused and had multiple focal seizures. His serum calcium was 7.6 mg/100 ml. Intravenous administration of calcium returned his serum calcium level to normal; however, his state of consciousness did not improve and he experienced another seizure. At this time his serum magnesium level was 0.9 mEq/L and intravenous administration of magnesium was be-

gun. On the next day, his CNS symptoms had cleared, his neuromuscular irritability had disappeared and his appetite was improved. Discuss the usual causes, clinical manifestations and treatment of hypomagnesemia.

Symptomatic magnesium deficiency is uncommon, and when it does occur it is usually seen in conditions where decreased intake or absorption of magnesium is present in conjunction with increased losses (121). Malabsorption syndrome, Kwashiorkor and protein calorie malnutrition, and alcoholism are conditions associated with decreased intake or absorption. Conditions associated with impaired conservation of magnesium include hypercalcemia, hyperaldosteronism, diabetic acidosis, hyperthyroidism, diuretic therapy, and inappropriate secretion of antidiuretic hormone (34).

The clinical manifestations of magnesium depletion include tremors, seizures which are usually generalized but sometimes focal, confusion, tetany which does not respond to calcium infusions, and bizarre involuntary movements of the extremities with facial twitching. Cardiovascular signs include tachycardia, flattening or inversion of T waves and premature atrial or ventricular beats (121).

Guidelines for the treatment of magnesium deficiency have been suggested by Fink (29). When azotemia is not present, an initial loading dose of 49 mEq of magnesium may be administered IV over three hours followed by an additional 49 mEq IV every 12 hours until the deficiency is corrected. If the intramuscular route is preferred, as much as 98 mEq per 24 hours may be administered in divided doses every 2 to 4 hours for the first day, followed by 33 to 49 mEq per day in divided doses until the deficiency is corrected. When azotemia is present, reduced dosage may be required and serial magnesium determinations must be monitored closely.

REFERENCES

1. Aurbach JD et al: Polypeptide hormones and calcium metabolism. Ann Intern Med. 70:1243, 1969.
2. Barker ES et al: Studies on renal excretion of magnesium in man. J Clin Invest 38:1733, 1959.
3. Barrett PKM et al: Conn's syndrome. Proc Roy Soc Med 51:720, 1958.
4. Bernstein J et al: Role of the sodium pump in the regulation of liver metabolism in experimental alcoholism. Ann NY Acad Sci 242:560, 1974.
5. Black DAK: Potassium Metabolism in *Clinical Disorders of Fluid and Electrolyte Metabolism,* Ed by Maxwell MH and Kleeman, CR, McGraw-Hill, New York, 1972, p. 121.
6. Brickman AS et al: 1,25 dihydroxy-vitamin D-3 in normal man and patients with renal failure. Ann Intern Med 80:161, 1974.
7. Burnett CH et al: An analysis of some features of renal tubular dysfunction. Arch Intern Med 102:881, 1958.
8. Butler AM et al: Parenteral fluid therapy I. estimation and provi-

sion of daily maintenance requirements. NEJM 231:585, 1944.
9. Carrol E. et al: Stimulation of bone formation by inorganic phosphate and inhibition of bone resorption by thyrocalcitonin. J Clin Invest 46:1043, 1967.
10. Chopra D et al: Hypercalcemia and malignant disease. Med Clin N Amer 59:441, 1975.
11. Chowdhury FR et al: Chlorthalidone-induced hypokalemia and abnormal carbohydrate metabolism. Horm Metab Res 2:13, 1970.
12. Clarkson EM et al: The effect of a high intake of calcium carbonate in normal subjects and patients with chronic renal failure. Clin Sci 30:415-1966.
13. Clementsen HJ: Potassium therapy. A break in tradition. Lancet 2:175, 1962.
14. Conn JW: Primary aldosteronism, a new clinical syndrome. J Lab Clin Med 45:3, 1955.
15. Corsa L et al: The measurement of exchangeable potassium in man by isotope dilution. J Clin Invest 29:1280, 1950.
16. Crandall ED: Serum sodium response to hyperglycemia. NEJM 290:465, 1974.
17. DeLuca HF: Vitamin D endocrinology. Ann Intern Med 85:367, 1976.

18. DeLuca HF: The kidney as an endocrine organ for the production of 1,25-dihydroxyvitamin D, a calcium-mobilizing hormone. NEJM 289:359, 1973.
19. Dunn MJ et al: Magnesium depletion in normal man. Metabolism 15:884, 1966.
20. Earll JM et al: Hypercalcemia and hypertension. Ann Intern Med 64:378, 1966.
21. Eckel RE et al: Membrane potentials in K-deficient muscle. Am J Physiol 205:307, 1963.
22. Edelman IS et al: Anatomy of body water and electrolytes. Amer J Med 27:256, 1959.
23. Edelman IS: Exchange of water between blood and tissues, characteristics of deuterium oxide equilibration in body water. Am J Physiol 171:279, 1952.
24. Edelman IS et al: Body composition: Studies in the human being by the dilution principle. Science 115:447, 1952.
25. Edwards CRW: Mithramycin treatment of malignant hypercalcemia. Brit Med J 3:167, 1968.
26. Epstein FH et al.: Role of sodium, potassium-ATPase in renal function. Ann NY Acad Sci 242:519, 1974.
27. Epstein FH: Calcium and the kidney. Am J Med 45:700, 1968.
28. Felig P: Diabetic ketoacidosis. NEJM 290:1360, 1974.
29. Fink EB: Therapy of magnesium deficiency. Ann NY Acad Sci 162:901, 1969.
30. Fitzgerald MG: Experimental study of magnesium deficiency in man. Clin Sci 15:635, 1956.
30b. Fletcher RF et al: A case of magnesium deficiency following massive intestinal resection. Lancet 1:522, 1960.
31. Fuisz RE: Hyponatremia. Medicine 42:149, 1963.
32. Gennari FJ et al: Osmotic diuresis. NEJM 291:714, 1974.
33. Gill JR: Edema. Ann Rev Med 21:269, 1970.
34. Gitelman HJ et al: Magnesium deficiency. Ann Rev Med 20:233, 1969.
35. Glabman S et al: Micropuncture study of the effect of acute reduction in glomerular filtration rate on sodium and water reabsorption by the proximal tubules of the rat. J Clin Invest 44:1410, 1965.
36. Goldsmith RS et al: Inorganic phosphate treatment of hypercalcemia of diverse etiologies. NEJM 274:1, 1966.
37. Gordon GS et al: Osteolytic sterol in human breast cancer. Science 151:1226, 1966.
38. Gorden P: Glucose intolerance with hypokalemia failure of short-term potassium depletion in normal subjects to reproduce the glucose and insulin abnormalities of clinical hypokalemia. Diabetes 22:544, 1973.
39. Grob D et al: Potassium movement in patients with familial periodic paralysis. Relationship to the defect in muscle function. Amer J Med 23:356, 1957.
40. Grob D et al: Potassium movement in normal subjects, effects on muscle function. Amer J Med 23:340, 1957.
41. Gupta PP et al: Role of atrial afferents in the tachycardia and increased antidiuretic hormone levels of moderate hemorrhage. Federation Proc 25:571, 1966.
42. Gupta PD et al: Responses of atrial and aortic baroreceptors to non-hypotensive hemorrhage and to transfusion. Am J Physiol 211:1429, 1966.
43. Hays RM: Dynamics of body water and electrolytes, Maxwell and Kleeman (eds.), Clinical Disorders of Fluid and Electrolyte Metabolism, McGraw-Hill, 1972.
44. Hays RM: Antidiuretic hormone. NEJM 295:659, 1972.
45. Hebert LA et al: Studies of the mechanism by which phosphate infusion lowers serum calcium concentration. J Clin Invest 45:1886, 1966.
46. Hill CS et al: Drug therapy of hypercalcemia in cancer patients. Drug Therapy 3:19, 1973.
47. Hiroaka M et al: Role of calcium ions in the contraction of vascular smooth muscle. Amer J Physiol 214:1084, 1968.
48. Jenkins PG et al: Hyperglycemia-induced hyponatremia. NEJM 290:573, 1974.
49. Katz AI et al: Physiologic role of sodium-potassium-activated adenosene triphosphatase in the transport of cations across biologic membranes. NEJM 278:253, 1968.
50. Katz MA: Hyperglycemia-induced hyponatremia — Calculation of expected serum sodium depression. NEJM 289:843, 1973.
51. Kennedy BJ: Metabolic and toxic effects of mithramycin during tumor therapy. Amer J Med 49:494, 1970.
52. Klahr S et al: Renal regulation of sodium excretion. Arch Intern Med 131:780, 1973.
53. Klein DC et al: Prostaglandins: Stimulation of bone resorption in tissue culture. Endocrinology 86:1436, 1970.
54. Knox WH et al: Mechanism of action of aldosterone with particular reference to (Na K)-ATPase. Ann NY Acad Sci 242:471, 1974.
55. Kokko JP: Membrane characteristics governing salt and water transport in the loop of Henle. Federation Proc 33:25, 1974.
56. Lazor MZ et al: Mechanism of adrenalsteroid reversal of hypercalcemia in multiple mycloma. NEJM 270:749, 1964.
57. Leaf A et al: The mechanism of the osmotic adjustment of body cells as determined in vivo by the volume of distribution of a large water load. J Clin Invest 33:1261, 1954.
58. Leaf A et al: An antidiuretic mechanism not regulated by extracellular fluid toxicity. J Clin Invest 31:60, 1952.
59. Leaf A et al: The normal antidiuretic mechanism in man and dog: Its regulation by extracellular fluid toxicity. J Clin Invest 31:54, 1952.
60. Leaf A: Cell swelling. A factor in ischemic tissue injury. Circulation 48:455, 1973.
61. Leyssac PP: The in vivo effect of angiotension and noradrenalin on the proximal tubular reabsorption of salt in mammalian kidneys. Acta Physiol Scand 64:167, 1965.
62. Lutwak L et al: Current concepts of bone metabolism. Ann Intern Med 80:630, 1974.
63. MacLeod SM: The rational use of potassium supplements. Postgrad Med 57:123, 1975.
64. Makler RF et al: Potassium — losing renal disease. Quart J Med 25:21, 1956.
65. Malnic G et al: Potassium transport across renal distal tubules during acid base disturbances. Am J Physiol 221:1192, 1971.
66. Martinez-Malonado M et al: Diuretics in nonedematous states. Physiological basis for the clinical use. Arch Intern Med 131:797, 1973.
67. Massry SG et al: Excretion of phosphate on calcium. Arch Intern Med 131:828, 1973.
68. Massry SG et al: Effect of NaCl infusion on urinary Ca and Mg during reduction in their filtered loads. Am J Physiol 213:1218, 1967.
69. Massry SG et al: Inorganic phosphate treatment of hypercalcemia. Arch Intern Med 121:307, 1968.
70. McCurdy DK: Hyperosmolar hyperglycemic nonketotic diabetic coma. Med Clin N Amer. 54:683, 1970.
71. Merrill JP et al: Clinical recognition and therapy of acute potassium intoxication. Ann Int Med 33:797, 1950.
72. Meyrier A et al: The influence of high calcium carbonate intake on bone disease in patients undergoing hemodialysis. Kidney Internat 4:146, 1973.
73. Monto RW et al: Observations on the mechanism of hemorrhagic toxicity in mithramycin (NSC-24559) therapy. Cancer Res 29:697, 1969.
74. Mudge GH: Clinical patterns of tubular dysfunction. Am J Med 24:785, 1958.
75. Muggia FM et al: Hypercalcemia associated with neoplastic disease. Ann Intern Med 73:281, 1970.
76. Mundy GR et al: Bone-resorbing activity in supernatants from lymhoid cell lines. NEJM 290:867, 1974.
77. Muntwyler E et al: Muscle electrolyte composition and balances of nitrogen and potassium in potassium-deficient rats. Am J Physiol 174:283, 1953.
78. Murdaugh HV Jr et al: Magnesium excretion in dog studied by stop-flow analysis. Am J Physiol 198:571, 1960.
79. Newmark SR et al: Hyperkalemia and hypokalemia. JAMA 231:631, 1975.
80. Norman AW: 1, 25- Dehydroxy-vitamin D-3: A kidney-produced steroid hormone essential to calcium homeostasis. Amer J Med 57:21, 1974.
81. Orloff J et al: Hyponatremia. Circulation 19:284, 1959.
82. Potassium formulations and therapy. The Medical Letter on Drugs and Therapeutics 11:77, 1969.
83. Parsons V et al: Effect of mithramycin on calcium and hydroxyproline metabolism in patients with malignant disease. Brit Med J 1:474, 1969.
84. Pitts BJR: The relationship of the K-activated phosphatase to the Na, K-ATPase. Ann NY Acad Sci 242:293, 1974.
85. Porter RS: Serum potassium concentration. Hosp Pharmacy 11:151, 1976.
86. Powell D et al: Nonparathyroid humoral hypercalcemia in patients with neoplastic diseases. NEJM 289:176, 1973.

87. Pullen H et al: Intensive intravenous potassium replacement therapy. Lancet 2:809, 1967.

88. Raisz LG: Calcium, phosphate, magnesium and trace elements in *Clinical Disorders of Fluid and Electrolyte Metabolism,* Maxwell and Kleeman eds McGraw-Hill Book Company, NY, p. 347, 1972.

89. Randall RE et al: Hypermagnesemia in renal failure: Etiology and toxic manifestations. Ann Intern Med 61:73, 1964.

90. Rapoport MI et al: Thiazide-induced glucose intolerance treated with potassium. Arch Intern Med 113:405, 1964.

91. Relman AS et al: Electrolyte balance and acid-base metabolism in primary aldosteronism. J Clin Invest 36:923, 1957.

92. Relman AS et al: The kidney in potassium depletion. Am J Med 24:764, 1958.

93. Riggs BL et al: Immunologic differentiation of primary hyperparathyroidism from hyperparathyroidism due to nonparathyroid cancer. J Clin Invest 50:2079, 1971.

94. Rovner DR: Use of pharmacologic agents in the treatment of hypokalemia and hyperkalemia. Ration Drug Ther 6:1, 1972.

95. Rundo J et al: Total and "exchangeable" potassium in humans. Nature 175:774, 1955.

96. Ryan WG et al: Effects of mithramycin on Paget's disease of bone. Ann Intern Med 70:549, 1969.

97. Schroeder R: The meaning of milliequivalents. Minnesota Pharmacist 10:10, 1969.

98. Schultze RG: Recent advances in the physiology and pathophysiology of potassium excretion. Arch Intern Med 131:885, 1973.

99. Schwartz KC et al: Severe acidosis and hyperpotassemia treated with sodium bicarbonate infusion. Circulation 19:215, 1959.

100. Scribner BH et al: Symposium: water and electrolytes interpretation of the serum potassium concentration. Metabolism 5:468, 1956.

101. Seftel HC et al: Early and extensive potassium replacement in diabetic acidosis. Diabetes 15:694, 1966.

102. Shackney S et al: Precipitous fall in serum calcium, hypotension, and acute renal failure after intravenous phosphate therapy for hypercalcemia. Report of two cases. Ann Intern Med 66:906, 1967.

103. Share L et al: Cardiovascular receptors and blood liter of antidiuretic hormone. Am J Physiol 203:425, 1962.

104. Sherwood LM et al: Production of parathyroid hormone by nonparathyroid tumors. J Clin Endocrinol Metab 27:140, 1967.

105. Skou JC: Enzymatic basis of active transport of Na and K across cell membrane. Physiol Rev 45:596, 1965.

106. Slayton RE et al: New approach to the treatment of hypercalcemia — the effect of short-term treatment with mithramycin. Clin Pharmacol Ther 12:833, 1971.

107. Smith WO et al: Serum magnesium in renal diseases. Arch Intern Med 102:5, 1958.

108. Steinmetz PR et al: Hyperkalemia in renal failure. JAMA 175:689, 1961.

109. Stephens FI: Paralysis due to reduced serum potassium concentration during treatment of diabetic acidosis: Report of case treated with 33 grams of potassium chloride intraveneously. Ann Intern Med 30:1272, 1949.

110. Strauss MB et al: Surfeit and deficit of sodium: A kinetic concept of sodium excretion. Arch Intern Med 102:527, 1958.

111. Surawicz B: Relationship between the ECG and electrolytes. Am Heart J 73:814, 1967.

112. Tarail R et al: The ultrafilterability of potassium and sodium in human serum. J Clin Invest 31:23, 1952.

113. Tashjian AH Jr et al: Prostaglandins, calcium, metabolism and cancer. Fed Proc 33:81, 1974.

114. Tobin T et al: Studies on the two phosphoenzyme conformations of NaK-ATPase. Ann NY Acad Sci, 242:120, 1974.

115. Verney EB: Croonian lecture: The anti-diuretic hormone and the factors which determine its release. Proc R Soc Lond 135:25, 1947.

116. Voss DM et al: Cardiac manifestations of hyperparathyroidism with presentation of a previously unreported arrhythmia. Amer Heart J 73:235, 1967.

117. Walser M: Ion association VI. Interactions between calcium, magnesium, inorganic phosphate, citrate, and protein in normal human plasma. J Clin Invest 40:723, 1961.

118. Wacker WEC et al: Magnesium, in *Mineral Metabolism: An advanced treatise: Vol. 2. The elements, Parts A-B.* Part A edited by CL Comar and F Bronner, Academic Press, New York, p. 483, 1964.

119. Wacker WEC et al: Magnesium metabolism. NEJM 278:772, 1968.

120. Weidmann P et al: Blood pressure effects of acute hypercalcemia. Ann Intern Med 76:741, 1972.

121. Weiner M et al: Signs and symptoms of electrolyte disorders. Yale J Biol Med 43:76, 1970.

122. Welt LG et al: The consequences of potassium depletion. J Chron Dis 11:213, 1960.

123. Welt LG et al: A primer on potassium metabolism in *Clinician: Potassium in Clinical Medicine,* MEDCOM, Inc., New York, p. 13, 1973.

124. Weston RE et al: The pathogenesis and treatment of hyponatremia in congestive heart failure. Am J Med 29:558, 1958.

125. Wilde WS: Potassium. In *Mineral Metabolism,* Vol. II, Comor and Bronner, eds. Academic Press, New York 1962, p. 73.

126. Wilder WT et al: Peptic ulcer in primary hyperparathyroidism. Ann Intern Med 105:536, 1960.

127. Williams JA et al: Effects of nephrectomy and KCl on transmembrane potentials, intracellular electrolytes, and cell pH of rat muscle and liver in vivo. J Physiol 212:117, 1971.

128. Woodbury DM: Physiology of body fluids, in *Physiology and Biophysics,* Richard Patton, Eds, 20th ed., Saunders, Philadelphia, 1973.

129. Woodbury DM et al: Effects of aldosterone and desoxycorticosterone on tissue electrolytes. Proc Soc Exp Biol 94:720, 1957.

130. Wolf AV: Aometric analysis of thirst in man and dog. Am J Physiol 161:75, 1950.

131. Wolf, FW et al: Further observations concerning the hyperglycemic activity of benzothiadiazines. Diabetes 13:115, 1964.

132. Wynn V: The osmotic behavior of the body cells in man. Lancet 2:1212, 1957.

133. Yendt, ER: Disorders of calcium, phosphorus, and magnesium metabolism in *Clinical Disorders of Fluid and Electrolyte Metabolism,* Maxwell and Kleeman, Eds, McGraw-Hill, New York 1972, p. 401.

134. Zervas M et al: Normal laboratory values. NEJM 290:39, 1974.

Chapter 4

Acid-Base Disorders

Thomas J. Cali
Mary Anne Koda-Kimble

In man, extracellular fluid concentration of hydrogen ion is maintained at an almost constant level. Arterial blood pH varies from 7.38 to 7.42 in a healthy person; venous blood and interstitial fluid pH vary between 7.33 and 7.37, (32) and intracellular pH is generally believed to vary from 4.5 to 7.4 depending upon the rate of metabolism, and local tissue blood flow (11).

Acidosis causes central nervous system (CNS) depression, which may lead to coma or death (53), while alkalosis causes CNS excitation and is likely to result in a convulsive disorder or tetany. Arterial pH can vary from 6.8 to 7.7 and still be compatible with life.

The pH can be calculated from the following equation:

$$ \text{Eq. 1} $$
$$ pH = pK + \log \frac{HCO_3^-}{H_2CO_3} = 6.1 + \log \frac{HCO_3^-}{(.03)(PCO_2)} $$

An important concept illustrated by this equation is that it is the *ratio* of HCO_3^- to H_2CO_3, not their absolute concentrations, that determines the pH. It therefore follows that if both the HCO_3 and PCO_2 are increased or decreased proportionately, the *ratio* remains fixed and the pH is *not* affected.

The serum bicarbonate is primarily regulated by the kidneys, while the PCO_2 is under pulmonary control. The body compensates to preserve the ratio of HCO_3 to PCO_2. Changes in the ratio resulting from increased or decreased HCO_3 are *metabolic* disturbances, while changes in the ratio caused by increased or decreased PCO_2 are *respiratory* disturbances.

Acid-base disturbances cannot be assessed on the basis of a serum bicarbonate or respiratory rate alone. To illustrate, an elevated serum bicarbonate is consistent with both metabolic alkalosis and chronic respiratory acidosis; similarly, hyperventilation is consistent with both respiratory alkalosis and metabolic acidosis. Therefore, the patient's laboratory studies, signs and symptoms cannot be assessed without taking the patient's medical history into account.

1. List and discuss the significance of the major laboratory tests used to assess acid-base balance.

CO₂ Content; CO₂ Combining Power; Serum bicarbonate (Normal 23-28): Ninety-five percent of the value obtained as *CO_2 content* is HCO_3. If a CO_2 content is 20 mM/L, the corresponding HCO_3 level is 19 mEq/L in venous blood. The *CO_2 combining power* is a measure of HCO_3 in the plasma after equilbration of plasma with a PCO_2 of 40 mmHg. *Bicarbonate* reported with blood gases represents the actual HCO_3 concentration in arterial blood as calculated from the Henderson-Hasselbach equation. Bicarbonate ion changes in the same direction as CO_2 content in acid-base disorders. The CO_2 content is the most commonly used test (23).

Arterial pH (Normal 7.38-7.42): Arterial blood must be collected in a glass, heparinized syringe and the pH must be determined immediately. Arterial pH is essential in determining the severity of the disorder and in monitoring the therapy of mixed disorders (23).

Arterial PCO₂ (Normal 35-45 mmHg): The PCO_2 measures the partial pressure of carbon dioxide in arterial blood. It indicates the level of respiratory acid and its contribution to total hydrogen ion activity. An increase in PCO_2 is consistent with respiratory acidosis, while a decrease in PCO_2 is consistent with respiratory alkalosis (23).

Serum Chloride (Normal 96-106 mEq/L): The serum chloride level may indicate acid retention or base excretion by the kidney. Hypochloremia may increase proximal tubular reabsorption of bicarbonate, leading to metabolic alkalosis. Hyperchloremia may reflect the addition of hydrogen ion with chloride ion in the ECF

and is consistent with metabolic acidosis (23).

Urinary pH: People with an average dietary intake excrete urine that is acidic. In acid-base disorders, the urinary pH usually changes with renal compensation. In metabolic acidosis, renal excretion of acid increases, lowering urine pH. In acute metabolic alkalosis, the renal transport maximum (Tm) for bicarbonate is exceeded and urine becomes alkaline. If metabolic alkalosis is chronic, urinary pH may be normal. Patients with acute metabolic alkalosis and hypokalemia reabsorb bicarbonate ion in the distal and proximal tubule, perpetuating the alkalosis and producing paradoxical aciduria (23).

Arterial PO₂ (normal 80-90 mmHg): Acidosis shifts the oxygen-hemoglobin dissociation curve downward and to the right, decreasing oxygen-hemoglobin binding and increasing tissue delivery of oxygen (16). Alkalosis has the opposite effect. An alkalotic patient with a PO_2 of 70 mmHg could be oxygenating tissues appropriately.

2. Summarize the effects of the four primary acid-base disorders on pH, hydrogen ion concentrations, PCO₂, and HCO₃.

	pH	(H⁺)	PCO₂	HCO⁻₃
Metabolic acidosis	↓	↑	↓	↓
Metabolic alkalosis	↑	↓	↑	↑
Respiratory acidosis	↓	↑	↑	↓
Respiratory alkalosis	↑	↓	↓	↑

Note: Dotted arrows indicate compensatory changes.

CASE HISTORY – HYPERCHLOREMIC METABOLIC ACIDOSIS: R.G., a 54-year-old male is being seen in the ophthalmology clinic. Three days prior to this visit, therapy was begun with acetazolamide sustained release capsules for chronic open angle glaucoma. The patient has returned to clinic complaining of shortness of breath, polyuria and polydipsia. Laboratory studies reveal:

Na⁺	136 mEq/L	PO₂	96 mmHg
K⁺	6.1 mEq/L	PCO₂	36 mmHg
Cl⁻	108 mEq/L	pH	7.22
CO₂	15 mM/L		

3. Assess this patient's acid-base disorder.

The low CO_2 content and pH are both consistent with metabolic acidosis and the low PCO_2 (increased respiratory rate) is consistent with respiratory alkalosis or compensated metabolic acidosis. The normal unmeasured anion concentration and high serum chloride level, together with the history and evidence above, indicate that the patient has metabolic acidosis with respiratory compensation secondary to acetazolamide therapy.

4. How does acetazolamide induce metabolic acidosis?

The formation of carbonic acid from carbon dioxide and water is catalyzed by carbonic anhydrase (CA) in the cells of the proximal tubules. Following the dissociation of carbonic acid to hydrogen ion and bicarbonate, the hydrogen ion is secreted (in exchange for sodium) into the tubule, and the bicarbonate is reabsorbed (with sodium) into the blood stream. Acetazolamide inhibits CA, thereby decreasing the generation, and ultimately the secretion, of acid and the reabsorption of sodium. A mild metabolic acidosis results.

5. What treatment is indicated for this patient? Would sodium bicarbonate be indicated on an acute basis?

Acetazolamide produces a naturesis and diuresis by decreasing the intracellular generation of hydrogen ion which is normally exchanged for tubular sodium. This effect will diminish in 7 to 10 days as CA activity increases; therefore, the patient should be instructed to continue therapy and maintain adequate hydration.

Sodium bicarbonate would not be indicated, nor would it be effective in an acute situation. Normally, filtered bicarbonate is buffered and completely resorbed in the proximal tubule. However, since acetazolamide decreases proximal tubular hydrogen ion availability, any additional bicarbonate filtered by the glomerulus would be excreted in the urine and would have no permanent systemic effect.

6. The patient was placed on sodium bicarbonate, 650 mg four times daily and was given a three month's supply. Is the patient at risk of developing metabolic alkalosis from chronic ingestion of oral sodium bicarbonate. How is bicarbonate normally handled by the body?

Normally, the maximum tubular reabsorption (T_m) for bicarbonate is 25 mEq/L, and any excess bicarbonate is eliminated in the urine. Therefore, alkalosis rarely occurs secondary to exogenous bicarbonate ingestion unless the T_m for this anion is increased.

Examples of factors which increase the T_m include chloride or potassium depletion and situations which increase sodium reabsorption. In the latter instance, sodium is exchanged for hydrogen ion, thereby generating excess bicarbonate which must be reabsorbed. Volume contraction and the administration of glucocorticoids are other examples of factors which increase sodium and, indirectly, bicarbonate reabsorption (49,50,52).

7. Why is R.G.'s serum potassium elevated?

Up to 50% of the hydrogen ion is buffered by intracellular organic anions and protein. In acidosis, excess hydrogen ion moves intracellularly; to maintain electroneutrality, sodium and potassium are displaced into the extracellular fluid compartment. Therefore, hyperkalemia is commonly observed in acidotic individuals. Clinicians use a general rule of thumb that for every 0.1 unit pH change from the normal value of 7.4, one can expect a reciprocal change in the serum potassium value of 0.6 mEq/L (14a,44).

8. R.G. has a hyperchloremic metabolic acidosis with a normal anion gap. What disorders or drugs are associated with this imbalance?

Metabolic acidosis characterized by an increased chloride level and a normal anion gap is commonly referred to as *hyperchloremic metabolic acidosis*. There are three major causes: an excessive acid load, large losses of alkaline body fluids, and diminished acid excretion by the kidneys. See Table 1. Rapid volume expansion with intravenous fluids can also cause a mild metabolic acidosis through dilution of plasma bicarbonate (3,19a).

Table 1
COMMON CAUSES OF HYPERCHLOREMIC METABOLIC ACIDOSIS

I. **Excess Acid Load**
   A. Hyperalimentation (see chapter on *Hyperalimentation*)
   B. Acidifying Agents
      1. Ammonium chloride
      2. Arginine HCl
      3. Lysine HCl

II. **Large Losses of Alkaline Body Fluids**
   A. Diarrhea, ileostomy, colostomy
   B. Excessive cathartic use
   C. Pancreatic fistula

III. **Decreased Renal Excretion of Acid**
   A. Renal Tubular acidosis (see chapter on *Diseases of the Kidney*)
   B. Carbonic anhydrase inhibitors
      1. Acetazolamide
      2. Sulfamylon
   C. Uremia (occasionally)

9. J.G., a 35-year-old male with known chronic glomerulonephritis, is admitted to the hospital complaining of dyspnea. Initial laboratory data reveals:

Na^+	138 mEq/L	PO_2	88 mmHg
K^+	5.4 mEq/L	PCO_2	34 mmHg
Cl	96 mEq/L	pH	7.27
CO_2	17 mM/L	Glucose	110 mg/dl
		BUN	148 mg/dl

Assess the patient's acid-base status.

The patient has impaired renal function which causes retention of titratable acid. The serum CO_2 content is low, and is consistent with metabolic acidosis. The low PCO_2 is consistent with respiratory alkalosis and/or respiratory compensation for metabolic acidosis; the low pH is also consistent with metabolic acidosis.

10. What is the anion gap or unmeasured anions? Calculate from the previous question, the anion gap for J.G.

The principle of electroneutrality dictates that the sum of all positive charges in the extracellular fluid (ECF) be exactly neutralized by an equal number of negative charges. The serum sodium and potassium account for 95% of all cations present in the ECF. Chloride and bicarbonate represent the anionic components but account for only 85% of ECF anions. Therefore, the sum of the measured anions does not fully equal the sum of the measured cations. This difference, measured in mEq/L is termed the anion gap.

Anion Gap =   Eq. 2
(Serum Na^- + Serum K^+) − (Serum Cl^- + Serum HCO_3^-)

Since the serum concentration of potassium is relatively low, the above formula can be shortened:

Anion Gap = (Serum Na^+)− (Serum Cl^- + Serum HCO_3^-)
          = 12−14 mEq/L   Eq. 3

Under normal conditions the unmeasured anions representing anionic protein, sulfates, phosphates, and anionic groups of organic ions, total approximately 12−14 mEq/L (19a,44). An elevated anion gap gives the clinician a clue to the etiology of a metabolic acidosis. For example, it can be consistent with lactic acidosis, salicylate intoxication, diabetic ketoacidosis, and methanol intoxication. For J.G. the anion gap is equal to:

138 − (96 + 16) = 26 mEq/L

This is consistent with the chronic metabolic acidosis which occurs in patients with renal failure since the elimination of organic acids is decreased.

CASE HISTORY – LACTIC ACIDOSIS: A 56-year-old, 65 Kg male with diabetes mellitus has been taking phenformin HCl 50 mg twice daily for two years. On the morning of admission, he vomited and complained of back pain. In the emergency room, he was alert with a supine blood pressure of 130/85, a pulse of 80/min and a respiratory rate (RR) of 32/min. He became progressively less responsive. Laboratory studies revealed:

Na-139 mEq/L	*CO_2 content-3 mM/L*	*pH-7.0*
K-5.1 mEq/L	*BUN-72 mg/dl*	*PCO_2-14 mmHg*
Cl-106 mEq/L	*Glucose-86 mg/dl*	*HCO_3-4 mEq/L*

A urinalysis revealed a pH of 5.0 and trace ketones. There were no salicylates or crystals.

11. Assess this patient's acid-base status.

This patient has a severe metabolic acidosis (pH 7.0; HCO_3 4 mEq/L; CO_2 content 3 mM/L; urine pH 5.0) with a large anion gap (139 − (106 + 2) = 31 mEq/L) and respiratory compensation (RR 32/min; PCO_2 11 mmHg). These findings could be consistent with diabetic ketoacidosis, but this is unlikely in view of the normal glucose level and the small amounts of ketones in the urine (21). The latter could be indicative of mild starvation ketosis. If one considers the fact that this patient has some degree of renal impairment and is ingesting phenformin, the history and laboratory values are more consistent with lactic acidosis (14,46). See Question 12.

12. Review the association of phenformin HCl with lactic acidosis. What are some other causes of lactic acidosis?

Phenformin HCl therapy is associated with an increase in basal lactate levels (46,67), and with inhibition of renal excretion of up to 50% of an acid load (56).

In a retrospective evaluation of lactic acidosis by Conlay (14) 5 of 6 cases were associated with phenformin. Brach and associates (7) reported a series of 10 fatalities from lactic acidosis, 8 of these 10 were associated with phenformin. Since 1959, approximately 240 cases of phenformin induced lactic acidosis with a fatality rate of approximately 50% were reported to the FDA (2a). Estimates of deaths from lactic acidosis associated with phenformin range from several dozen to more than a thousand annually. Alcohol intake, renal disease and any condition which can predispose to hypoxic situations (e.g. shock) may potentiate phenformin lactic acidosis. However, lactic acidosis has occurred in some phenformin-treated patients even in the absence of risk conditions and even at relatively low doses. The following drugs and conditions have been associated with lactic acidosis (10):

a. Shock — all types (47,34,41)
b. Diabetes Mellitus (15)
c. Phenformin (45,61,68,14,46)
d. Leukemia (22)
e. Glycogen storage disease (35)
f. Ethanol (59,63)
g. Exercise (9,66)
h. Epinephrine (31)
i. Severe anemia (60)

13. Should this patient's acidosis be treated? What are the goals of therapy and what are the dangers of correcting the acidosis too rapidly?

This patient's acidosis is severe (pH< 7.1) and deserves immediate therapy. When the serum bicarbonate falls to 5 mEq/L or less, the situation is very serious, since at this level, maximum respiratory compensation ($PCO_2 \approx 15$ mmHg) has occurred, and small changes in the bicarbonate will result in large changes in the pH. The goal of therapy is to increase the pH to greater than 7.2 or to increase the bicarbonate by 4–6 mEq/L over 6–12 hours. The bicarbonate may then be increased to a level of approximately 15 mEq/L over the next 24 hours. Blood gases should be monitored every 2-3 hours to assess the patient's response to therapy (38).

Rapid and full correction of the acidosis is unnecessary and may be dangerous for the following reasons. Compensatory hyperventilation may persist 36-48 hours after acidosis has been corrected placing the patient in jeopardy of a respiratory alkalosis. Second, the methods for determining the doses of the alkalinizing agents are, at best, estimates and these agents may in themselves produce a metabolic alkalosis. Rapid correction has also been said to aggravate cerebrospinal fluid acidosis resulting in deterioration in the condition of such patients (51). Severe hypokalemia can occur, because potassium is redistributed from extracellular to the intracellular spaces. Finally, tetany resulting from rapid shifts of free, ionized calcium onto serum protein can occur when there is an acute increase in pH (38). It should also be kept in mind that since many of the agents used to treat metabolic acidosis are sodium salts, volume overload and pulmonary edema are potential complications of therapy.

14. What agents and methods are available for the treatment of metabolic acidosis? What are their advantages and disadvantages?

First, every effort should be made to identify and correct the underlying etiology of the metabolic acidosis (e.g. shock, diabetic ketoacidosis, diarrhea). If metabolic acidosis is severe or if it persists, consideration should be given to the use of alkalinizing agents. Sodium bicarbonate, sodium lactate, sodium acetate, THAM, and hemodialysis have all been used successfully in the treatment of metabolic acidosis.

Sodium bicarbonate provides the bicarbonate ion directly and is generally the agent of choice except in patients who are extremely susceptible to volume overload.

Sodium lactate and *sodium acetete* are used to treat metabolic acidosis because they are metabolized to bicarbonate; however, since their effectiveness depends on their conversion to bicarbonate, $NaHCO_3$ remains the agent of choice. Sodium lactate should not be used to treat lactic acidosis, because lactate metabolism is impaired in these individuals and bicarbonate is not likely to be generated (54).

THAM (Tris-hydroxymethyl-amino methane), or tromethamine, buffers hydrogen ion and generates bicarbonate in the following manner (42):

$$\text{THAM}$$
$$H_2O + CO_2 \rightleftharpoons H_2CO_3 \rightleftharpoons \text{THAM } H^+ + HCO_3^- \qquad \text{Eq. 4}$$

Although THAM lowers PCO_2, it depresses ventilation and can aggravate hypoxia in patients with chronic obstructive pulmonary disease (42). THAM is highly alkaline, and administration may result in local vascular spasm, pain, phlebitis or thrombosis (6). There are two theoretical advantages of THAM over bicarbonate. First, in a patient who will not tolerate a sodium load, THAM may expand ECF volume less than sodium bicarbonate (6). Secondly, THAM may penetrate cells more rapidly than sodium bicarbonate (55). This latter effect is probably unnecessary, actually may be detrimental (1), and is unproven. Since THAM has no proven advantage over bicarbonate and has additional side effects, sodium bicarbonate is still preferred.

Although *dialysis* has been used in the management of metabolic acidosis, peritoneal dialysis is considerably less effective in removing lactate than hemodialysis, because peritoneal dialysates contain lactate (69,20). Dialysis is of particular value if the metabolic acidosis is caused by a dialysable substance. Additionally, dialysis may be useful to maintain the desired fluid balance in a patient who is unable to accommodate the sodium load which accompanies sodium bicarbonate administration.

15. Discuss the use of methylene blue in the treatment of lactic acidosis.

Lactic acid is an end product of anaerobic glucose metabolism and is formed by the reduction of pyruvic acid:

$$\text{Pyruvic acid} + NADH_2 \rightleftharpoons \text{lactic acid} + NAD \qquad \text{Eq.5}$$

$$\text{Lactic acid} = \text{Pyruvic acid} \times \frac{K[NADH_2]}{[NAD]} \qquad \text{Eq. 6}$$

Therefore, lactate production is dependent upon both the concentration of pyruvate and on the ratio of $NADH_2$ to NAD (reduced nicotinamide adenine dinucleotide to nicotinamide adenine dinucleotide). Hypoxia increases the relative amounts of $NADH_2$ and lactate accumulates because it cannot be oxidized.

Methylene blue (tetramethylthionine chloride) can function as a hydrogen ion donor:acceptor (46). Since lactic acidosis is often associated with an increased ratio of $NADH_2$ to NAD, methylene blue would theoretically be of benefit because it can generate NAD.

$$\text{Methylene blue} + NADH_2 \longrightarrow \text{Methylene blue H} + NAD$$
$$\text{Eq. 7}$$

The newly generated NAD could then combine with lactic acid and shift Eq. 5 to the left (65). However, the clinical use of methylene blue has been limited, and results have not been dramatic.

16. What is the role of sodium nitroprusside in the treatment of idiopathic lactic acidosis?

Inadequate perfusion to an area results in local hypoxia and a switch to anaerobic glycosis with subsequent lactic acidemia (37). Sodium nitroprusside increases venous capacitance and decreases arteriolar resistance. Theoretically, these effects should increase perfusion to hypoxic tissue or increase lactate metabolism by increasing hepatic perfusion. However, the literature describes only one case in which idiopathic lactic acidosis was successfully reversed by sodium nitroprusside (64).

17. How can the dose of sodium bicarbonate be estimated? Determine an initial dose of bicarbonate for this patient.

Clinicians have used the following formula to estimate the initial doses of sodium bicarbonate. It is based upon the premise that the volume of distribution (Vd) for bicarbonate is approximately 50% of body weight.

Eq. 8

$$\frac{\text{Bicarbonate}}{\text{Dose (mEq)}} = 0.5 \times \text{Body Weight (Kg)} \times \frac{\text{Desired Increase in}}{\text{Serum } HCO_3 \text{ (mEq/L}}$$

If the initial goal of therapy is to increase the serum bicarbonate by 6 mEq/L, the dose for this patient can be calculated as follows:

$$\frac{\text{Bicarbonate}}{\text{Dose (mEq)}} = 0.5 \times 65 \times 6 \text{ mEq/L} = 195 \text{ mEq}$$

18. Four hours after the sodium bicarbonate was administered, repeat arterial blood gases revealed that the patient had not responded as predicted (HCO_3 7 mEq/L). The patient was judged to be "alkali resistant." What are some causes of bicarbonate resistance?

Patients may require higher than predicted doses of bicarbonate when there is a high rate of production of endogenous acid (e.g. lactic acidosis or ketoacidosis) and when there are large, continuous losses of bicarbonate (e.g. severe diarrhea).

In some patients, large amounts of hydrogen ion are sequestered intracellularly. In these individuals, large amounts of bicarbonate move into the cells and the volume of distribution is increased. This Vd apparently diminishes as the acidosis is corrected (54).

Although clinically untested, Garella (24) recommends that an initial dose of bicarbonate be based upon a Vd equal to 100% of body weight if the HCO_3 is less than 5 mEq/L. This method should be used very cautiously if the acidosis is produced by an anion which can eventually be metabolized to bicarbonate (e.g. lactate).

CASE HISTORY – METABOLIC ALKALOSIS: M.S. is a

63-year-old, 104 lb female with a long history of hypertension and congestive heart failure. For the past six months, she has been bothered by dependent edema despite intermittent therapy with digoxin and hydrochlorothiazide 50 mg every other day. On admission, supine BP was 160/80 mmHg, pulse was 88/min and regular, respiratory rate was 28/min and temperature was normal. Physical examination revealed neck vein distension at 45°, cardiomegaly, and an S_3 gallop. A liver edge was palpated 3 cm below the left costal margin and she had bilateral thigh and ankle edema.

She was treated with bedrest, salt restriction, digoxin 0.25 mg daily and furosemide 80 mg twice daily. By the next morning she had lost six pounds and her supine blood pressure was 105/60 mmHg. Her laboratory values were as follows:

	On Admission		Hospital Day 2	
Na	137	mEq/L	135	mEq/L
K	3.6	mEq/L	2.9	mEq/L
Cl	98	mEq/L	90	mEq/L
CO₂	28	mM/L	33	mM/L
BUN	31	mg/dl	48	mg/dl
Creatinine	1.0	mg/dl	1.1	mg/dl
pH	–	–	7.5	
PCO₂	–	–	42	mmHg

19. Assess the patient's acid-base status on hospital day two. What is the etiology of this patient's acid-base imbalance?

The elevated CO_2 content, low serum chloride and increased pH are all consistent with a metabolic alkalosis. The normal PCO_2 is further indication that the alkalosis is of metabolic, not respiratory origin.

The alkalosis in this patient is almost certainly an effect of over-diuresis as indicated by the weight loss, decreased blood pressure, elevated BUN, decreased chloride, and decreased potassium.

Diuretics may produce alkalosis by several mechanisms. First, diuretic-induced hypochloremia causes a greater proportion of sodium to be reabsorbed in exchange for hydrogen ion; thus, the proximal tubular reabsorption of bicarbonate is increased. Secondly, if a patient is made hypokalemic by diuretics, a greater portion of sodium will be reabsorbed in exchange for hydrogen ion (rather than K) in the distal segment of the tubule. Finally, extracellular fluid contraction in itself can produce metabolic alkalosis. Also see Question 8 and chapter on Edema.

Although metabolic alkalosis is usually associated with both chloride and potassium deficits, chloride depletion is the critical factor in most cases of metabolic alkalosis. In the presence of metabolic alkalosis and profound hypochloremia, reabsorption of filtered chloride is almost complete, and a urinary chloride determination will demonstrate virtually no chloride in the urine (i.e. less than approximately 10 mEq/L). If more than 10 mEq/L of chloride is found in the urine in the absence of diuretics, it is likely that the potassium deficiency is contributing to the alkalosis (25).

20. What are the major causes of metabolic alkalosis?

Loss of acid from the body is by far the most common cause of metabolic alkalosis. This occurs when there are excessive losses of upper gastrointestinal fluid (e.g. vomiting and naso-gastric suction) and when hydrogen ion excretion (or bicarbonate reabsorption) by the kidneys is increased. This may occur as a result of corticosteroid or diuretic therapy and in patients with hyperaldosteronism or Cushing's disease. Rarely, alkali therapy will cause a metabolic alkalosis (42,44).

21. Besides discontinuing or adjusting the diuretic therapy, how should this patient be managed? How should correction of the acid-base imbalance be monitored?

In general, metabolic alkalosis should be managed by correcting the underlying cause. Any fluid deficits (19) and ion disturbances which are present should also be corrected.

Hypochloremia must be corrected, since a significant portion of sodium which is filtered by the kidney will be reabsorbed through cation (K+ and H+) exchange as long as there is a chloride deficit. This can be accomplished by replacing fluid losses with sodium chloride, and to some extent by correcting the potassium deficit with potassium chloride. As chloride is replaced, the patient will undergo a bicarbonate diuresis and the alkalosis will be corrected (12,13). Also see chapter on *Edema*. Fluids should be replaced gingerly in this patient in view of the fact that she was admitted in congestive heart failure and has a history of hypertension (38).

If therapy is appropriate, serial laboratory values should reflect an increasing serum potassium as well as an increasing serum chloride. The CO_2 content should be decreasing at this time. The urine chloride should be monitored to determine adequacy of chloride replacement (44), urine chloride concentrations of 60−100 mEq/L are indicative of ECF chloride repletion. Serial blood gases should be monitored if necessary. Other important parameters to monitor in this patient include her weight, blood pressure and signs and symptoms of congestive heart failure.

22. What are the roles of hydrochloric acid and arginine HCl in the management of metabolic alkalosis?

When the alkalosis is severe (i.e. that characterized by tetany associated with convulsions or severe respiratory depression), an acid such as arginine monohydrochloride, ammonium chloride, and dilute (0.1N − 0.2N) hydrochloric acid may need to be administered (32a,70). However, ammonium chloride is limited by its CNS toxicity, and dilute hydrochloric acid must generally be administered through a central vein.

Since bicarbonate has an apparent volume of distribution approximately equal to 50% of total body weight (3), the dose of acid required can be approximated according to the following formula:

Eq. 9

$$\text{Dose (in mEq)} = 0.5 \times (\text{Weight in Kg}) \times \binom{\text{Bicarbonate Decrement}}{\text{Desired}}$$

For example, if the serum bicarbonate level in a 70 Kg patient is 39 mEq/L and one wishes to decrease this to 29 mEq/L, the calculation is:

Acid required = (.5) (70) (10) = 350 mEq

If this amount of acid (arginine monohydrochloride) is administered in addition to fluid volume, sodium chloride, and potassium chloride, the serum bicarbonate should decrease to 29 mEq/L in approximately 12-24 hours.

23. An elderly male is admitted to a hospital with chronic obstructive pulmonary disease (COPD) and increasing pulmonary failure. Laboratory data on admission include:

	Venous		Arterial
Na	138 mEq/L	pH	7.33
K	5.0 mEq/L	PCO_2	68 mmHg
Cl	98 mEq/L	PO_2	60 mmHg
HCO_3	40 mEq/L		

Assess this patient's acid-base disorder. What are some common causes of this disorder, and what are the body's normal compensatory mechanisms?

The patient's history and blood gases (acidic pH, hypoxia, and hypercapnia) are consistent with chronic respiratory acidosis. The markedly elevated serum bicarbonate level could be consistent with a primary metabolic alkalosis but most likely represents the presence of compensatory metabolic alkalosis in this patient. Since it takes several days for maximal renal compensation to occur in response to hypercapnia, *acute* respiratory acidosis is accompanied by a rather small elevation in serum bicarbonate. If serum bicarbonate levels are greater than 30 mEq/L in this situation, a superimposed metabolic alkalosis should be suspected (8,42). Acutely, hemoglobin and tissue buffers are responsible for defending the body against excessive hydrogen ion concentrations.

Any drug or condition which produces hypoventilation can cause respiratory acidosis. Examples of these include central nervous system depressant drugs, generalized pulmonary diseases, disorders affecting the respiratory muscles, diseases of the central nervous system, and extreme obesity (8,42,44).

24. After treatment with mechanical ventilation, the following studies were obtained:

	Venous		Arterial
Na	138 mEq/L	pH	7.50
K	4.8 mEq/L	PCO$_2$	45 mmHg
Cl	95 mEq/L	PO$_2$	95 mmHg
HCO$_3$	42 mEq/L		

Assess the patient's current acid-base abnormality. What are the goals of therapy when treating respiratory acidosis?

The mechanical respirator has corrected the respiratory acidosis as evidenced by the normal PO$_2$ and PCO$_2$. However, since it takes several days for renal compensatory mechanisms to return to normal, this therapy has placed the patient in uncompensated metabolic alkalosis. Although the patient is unable to correct this metabolic imbalance by hypoventilation because he is on a respirator, bicarbonate diuresis will eventually occur.

The patient's respirator should be adjusted to a slower rate to maintain the PCO$_2$ greater than 45 mmHg, while at the same time avoiding a hypoxic level that would compromise respiratory function. The CO$_2$ content should be monitored and as a bicarbonate diuresis begins, the patient's ventilation can be increased in keeping with the objectives of his pulmonary disease therapy.

Generally, the goal of therapy is to correct the underlying disorder and improve ventilation; immediate restoration of a normal pH is unnecessary and may result in complications as illustrated in the above case. It should also be emphasized that the production of alkalosis is particularly undesirable in patients with chronic pulmonary disease because it depresses respiratory drive (8,42).

CASE HISTORY – RESPIRATORY ALKALOSIS: A 28-year-old female was admitted to the labor room of University Hospital. Physical examination revealed a pregnant woman who was having 60 second contractions every three to four minutes. Her cervix was dilated to 7 cm and the head of the fetus was engaged. She was under full control using the La Maze breathing technique. Several hours later her contractions became much stronger and recurred every 30-60 seconds. She complained of numbness and tingling around her lips, lightheadedness, and cramping in her calves. She was panting and blowing to control her labor pains and to keep herself from "bearing down."

25. Assess this patient's acid-base status. What other conditions are associated with this particular acid base imbalance? Which laboratory values would be consistent with your prediction? How should it be treated?

This patient has all the signs and symptoms (perioral paresthesia, lightheadedness, muscle cramps) of acute respiratory alkalosis which was caused by voluntary hyperventilation. The pathogenesis of these symptoms is unclear but is probably related to changes in cerebral circulation and ionic calcium levels which occur in alkalosis. Generally, any condition that stimulates respiration increases the elimination of carbon dioxide and can potentially produce respiratory alkalosis (3,42,44). These include mechanically assisted ventilation, central nervous system disease involving the medullary respiratory center, any hypoxic condition (e.g. anemia, residence in high altitudes, pulmonary embolism), cirrhosis, hypermetabolic conditions (e.g. hyperthyroidism, fever, gram-negative sepsis), salicylate intoxication, and psychogenic hyperventilation.

When there is an acute drop in the PCO$_2$, bicarbonate is consumed to make carbonic acid which is converted to CO$_2$ and expired. The low PCO$_2$ value increases the HCO$_3$:PCO$_2$ ratio (see Eq. 1) resulting in a respiratory alkalosis. Thus, acute respiratory alkalosis is characterized by an elevated pH, a decreased PCO$_2$, and a modest decrease in the serum bicarbonate. Even when the PCO$_2$ decreases acutely from 40 mmHg to 15 mmHg, the accompanying drop in serum bicarbonate only amounts to 7–8 mEq/L. A serum bicarbonate which is less than 15 mEq/L suggests the presence of a concurrent metabolic acidosis (8).

The treatment of respiratory alkalosis is directed at correction of the underlying problem. In this case, for example, the patient should simply be instructed to take some deep breaths and to breathe a bit more slowly. Psychogenic hyperventilators can be instructed to place a bag over their nose and mouth and rebreathe the carbon dioxide. It is rarely necessary to administer respiratory suppressants or 5% carbon dioxide (8,42). The morbidity and mortality associated with respiratory alkalosis has been correlated with PCO$_2$ values as illustrated by the summary results of a retrospective study of 114 patients with respiratory alkalosis (43). Shock and sepsis occurred more frequently in Group 1 patients.

	PCO$_2$	Mortality
Group 1	15 mmHg	88%
Group 2	20–25 mmHg	77%
Group 3	25–30 mmHg	73%
Group 4	35–45 mmHg	29% (p < .001)

26. What are two common errors in the laboratory evaluation of acid-base disturbances?

When evaluating laboratory data, clinicians must remember that they are treating a *patient* and not abnormal laboratory values. Patients must always be evaluated clinically, and if laboratory data are inconsistent with the overall clinical picture, other confirmatory tests should be performed. Laboratory data concerning acid-base balance can be especially misleading in patients with two ongoing primary disturbances. A highly abnormal CO_2 (greater than 40 mM/L), with a relatively normal pH, may be manifested in the presence of concurrent metabolic alkalosis and respiratory acidosis, and does not reflect a medical emergency. These two disorders tend to move CO_2 in the same direction, but pH in opposite directions as follows:

metabolic alkalosis = ↑ CO_2 content ↑pH

respiratory acidosis = ↑ CO_2 content ↓pH

Likewise, concurrent metabolic acidosis and respiratory acidosis could result in an extremely low pH (less than 7.0) and a relatively normal CO_2 content due to off-setting effects:

metabolic acidosis = ↓CO_2 content ↓pH

respiratory acidosis = ↑CO_2 content ↓pH

The relatively normal CO_2 content in this situation is grossly misleading, as the pH may be so depressed as to be considered a medical emergency. Since CO_2 content is usually among the first laboratory data received, the above distinction is essential.

27. In general, how does the therapy of mixed disorders differ from that of primary disorders? Name some clinical situations where mixed acid-base disorders occur frequently.

Generally, the same principles used to treat primary disorders may also be applied to the therapy of mixed acid-base disorders. However, if mixed disorders exert the same effect on pH, a medical emergency generally exists, and therapy must be vigorous. On the other hand, if the mixed disorders exert opposite effects on pH, overzealous therapy may produce an uncompensated disorder and thereby create a medical emergency.

Concurrent metabolic and respiratory acidosis occurs following a cardiac arrest (4) and must be treated vigorously with sodium bicarbonate. Respiratory acidosis and metabolic alkalosis occur in patients with chronic obstructive pulmonary disease, and concurrent metabolic acidosis and respiratory alkalosis occur in patients who are intoxicated with salicylates (33) or those with the hepatorenal syndrome or septic shock.

28. A one and one-half-year-old child is admitted to the emergency room with a history of salicylate ingestion. The following laboratory studies were obtained and a diagnosis of metabolic acidosis and respiratory alkalosis was made.

Na	140 mEq/L	pH	7.30
K	5.0 mEq/L	PCO_2	20 mmHg
Cl	95 mEq/L	HCO_3	9.5 mEq/L
CO_2	10 mM/L		

The patient was placed on a mechanical respirator. Several hours later the PCO_2 was 45 mmHg and the pH was 6.95. Assess the patient's acid-base disorder at this time.

Initially the patient had metabolic acidosis and respiratory alkalosis with a relatively normal pH. Improved ventilation removed the respiratory alkalosis leaving pure uncompensated metabolic acidosis with a pH of 6.95 and placed the patient in grave danger. See chapter of *Poisonings* for further information on the treatment of salicylate intoxication.

29. How can the PCO_2 be used to determine whether a patient with metabolic acidosis also has a primary respiratory acid-base disorder?

The degree of respiratory compensation (PCO_2) for any given degree of metabolic acidosis can be predicted according to the following formula (2):

$$PCO_2 = 1.54 \times HCO_3 + 8.36 \pm 1.1 \qquad \text{Eq. 10}$$

For example, the PCO_2 for an acidotic patient with a HCO_3 of 12.5 mEq/L should be approximately 28 mmHg ± 1.1. If the measured PCO_2 is significantly higher than this calculated PCO_2, the patient has a complicating primary respiratory acidosis. If the measured level is significantly lower than the calculated value, a complicating primary respiratory alkalosis is present.

REFERENCES

1. Adler S et al: Intracellular acid-base regulation. II, The response of muscle cells to changes in CO_2 tension of extracellular bicarbonate concentration. J Clin Invest 44:8, 1965.
2. Albert MS: 'Quantitative displacement of acid-base equilibrium in metabolic acidosis. Ann Int Med 66:312, 1967.
2a. Anon: Phenformin: New labeling and possible removal from market. FDA Drug Bull 7:6, 1977.
3. Beeson PB et al: *Textbook of Medicine,* 14th edition, Philadelphia, WB Saunders Company, 1975.
4. Bishop RL et al: Sodium bicarbonate administration during cardiac arrest. JAMA 235:506, 1976.
5. Bleich HL: Computer evaluation of acid-base disorders. J Clin Invest 48:1689, 1969.
6. Bleich HL et al: Tris buffer (THAM) an appraisal of its physiologic effects and clinical usefulness. NEJM 274:782, 1966.
7. Brach BB et al: A review of deaths due to suspected lactic acidosis at a large metropolitan hospital. South Med J 68:202, 1975.

8. Brackett NC Jr et al: Acid-base response to chronic hypercapnia in man. NEJM 280:124, 1969.

9. Bruce RA et al: Anaerobic metabolic response to acute maximal exercise in male athletes. Amer Heart J 67:643, 1964.

10. Cady LD Jr et al: Quantitation of severity of critical illness with special reference to blood lactate. Crit Care Med 1:75, 1973.

11. Carter NW: Intracellular pH. Kidney Internat 1:341, 1972.

12. Cohen JJ: Correction of metabolic alkalosis by the kidney after isometric expansion of extracellular fluid. J Clin Invest 47:1181, 1968.

13. Cohen JJ: Selective chloride retention in repair of metabolic alkalosis without increasing filtered load. Amer J Physiol 218:165, 1970.

14. Conlay LA: Phenformin and lactic acidosis. JAMA 235:1575, 1976.

14a. Costrini NV and Thomson WM (eds): Manual of Medical Therapeutics, Ed 22. Little Brown and Co., Boston 1977.

15. Daughaday WH et al: Lactic acidosis as a cause of non ketotic acidosis in diabetic patients. NEJM 267:1010, 1967.

16. Davenport HW: The ABC of Acid-Base Chemistry, Sixth Edition. The University of Chicago Press, 1974.

17. Davidson MB et al: Phenformin, hypoglycemia, and lactic acidosis: Report of attempted suicide. NEJM 275:886, 1966.

18. De Strihou CVY et al: The "carbon dioxide response curve" for chronic hypercapnia in man. NEJM 275:117, 1966.

19. Earley LE et al: Sodium metabolism. NEJM 281:72, 1969.

19a. Emmett ME et al: Clinical use of the anion gap. Medicine 56:38, 1977.

20. Ewy GA et al: Lactic acidosis associated with phenoformin therapy and localized tissue hypoxia. Ann Intern Med 59:878, 1963.

21. Felig P: Diabetic ketoacidosis. NEJM 290:1360, 1974.

22. Field M et al: Lactic acidosis in acute leukemia. Clin Res 11:193, 1963.

23. Fleischer WR: Laboratory assessment of acid-base imbalance. Geriatrics P. 96, 1974.

24. Frick PG et al: The treatment of severe metabolic alkalosis with intravenous N/10 or N/5 hydrochloric acid. Ger Med Mon 9:242, 1964.

25. Garella S et al: Saline-resistant metabolic alkalosis or "chloride-wasting nephropathy." Ann Int Med 73:31, 1970.

26. Garella S et al: Severity of metabolic acidosis as a determinant of bicarbonate requirements. NEJM 289:121, 1973.

27. Giebisch G et al: The extrarenal response to acute acid base disturbances of respiratory origin. J Clin Invest 34:231, 1955.

28. Goldberg M et al: Computer-based instruction and diagnosis of acid-base disorders. A systematic approach. JAMA 223:269, 1973.

29. Goldring RM et al: Respiratory adjustment of chronic metabolic alkalosis in man. J Clin Invest 47:118, 1968.

30. Goldstein MD et al: Influence of graded degree of chronic hypercapnia on the acute carbon dioxide titration curve. J Clin Invest 50:208, 1971.

31. Greene NM: Effect of epinephrine on lactate, pyruvate and excess lactate production in normal human subjects, J Clin Lab Med 58:682, 1961.

32. Guyton AC: Textbook of Medical Physiology, 5th edition, Philadelphia, WB Saunders Company, 1976.

32a. Harken, AH et al: Hydrochloric acid in the correction of metabolic alkalosis. Arch Surg, 110:819, 1975.

33. Hill JB: Salicylate intoxication, NEJM 288:1110, 1973.

34. Hopkins RW et al: Hemodynamic aspects of hemorrhagic and septic shock. JAMA 191:731, 1965.

35. Howell RR et al: Glucose-6-phosphatase deficiency glycogen storage disease. Pediat 29:553, 1962.

36. Huckabee WE: Abnormal resting blood lactate II: Lactic acidosis. Amer J Med 30:840, 1961.

37. Huckabee WE: Lactic acidosis. Am J Cardiol 12:663, 1963.

38. Kassirer JP: Serious acid-base disorders. NEJM 291:773, 1974.

39. Klahr S et al: Acid-base disorders in health and disease. JAMA 222:566, 1972.

40. Knatterud GL et al: A study of the effects of hypoglycemic agents on vascular complications in patients with adult onset diabetes: V evaluation of phenformin therapy. Diabetes 24 (Suppl 1): 65, 1975.

41. Maclean LD et al: Patterns of septic shock in man — A detailed study of 56 patients. Ann Surg 166:543, 1967.

42. Makoff DL: Acid-base metabolism in Clinical Disorders of Fluid and Electrolyte Metabolism, 2nd ed., edited by Maxwell MH., Kleeman CR., New York, McGraw-Hill Book Co., 1972, pp. 297.

43. Mazzara JT et al: Extreme hypocapnia in the critically ill patient. Am J Med 56:450, 1974.

44. McCurdy DM: Mixed metabolic and respiratory acid-base disturbances: Diagnosis and treatment. Chest, 62 (suppl):35S, 1972. (suppl):35S, 1972.

45. Milisci RE et al: Phenformin-induced lactic acidosis. Am J Med Sci 265:447, 1973.

46. Olivia PB: Lactic acidosis. Am J Med 48:209, 1970.

47. Peretz DI et al: Lactic acidosis: a clinically significant aspect of shock. Can Med Ass. J 90:673, 1964.

48. Pierce NF: The ventilatory response to acute base deficit in humans. Ann Int Med 72:633, 1970.

49. Pitts RF: Control of renal production of ammonia. Kidney Internat 1:297, 1972.

50. Pitts RF: Physiology of the Kidney and Body Fluids, 3rd edition, Chicago Yearbook Medical Publishers, Inc. 1974.

51. Plum F et al: Acid-base balance of cisternal and lumbar cerebrospinal fluid in hospital patients. NEJM 289:1346, 1973.

52. Rastegar A et al: Physiologic consequences and bodily adaptations to hypercapnia and hypopcapania. Chest 62 (suppl): 28S, 1972.

53. Relman AS: Metabolic consequences of acid-base disorders. Kidney Internat 1:347, 1972.

54. Relman AS et al: Profound acidosis resulting from excessive ammonium chloride in previously healthy subjects: a study of two cases. NEJM 265:848, 1961.

55. Robin ED et al: Intracellular acid-base relations and intracellular buffers. Ann NY Acad Sci 92:539, 1961.

56. Rooth G et al: Renal response to acid load after phenformin. Br Med J 4:256, 1973.

56a. Rosenfeld.

57. Schwartz WB: Lactate versus bicarbonate, a reconsideration of the therapy of metabolic acidosis, Am J Med 32:831, 1962.

58. Schwartz WB: Medicine and the computer. NEJM 283:1257, 1971.

59. Seligson D et al: Some metabolic effects of ethanol in humans. Clin Res Proc 1:86, 1953.

60. Siebert DJ et al: Assessment of tissue anoxemia in chronic anemia by the arterial lactate pyruvate ratio and excess lactate formation. J Lab Clin Med 69:177, 1967.

61. Steiner DF et al: Respiratory inhibition and hypoglycemia by biguanides and decamethylenediguanide. Biochem et Biophys Acta 30:329, 1958.

62. Strauss FG et al: Phenformin intoxication resulting in lactic acidosis. Johns Hopkins Med J 128:278, 1971.

63. Sullivan JF et al: Renal excretion of lactate and magnesium in alcoholism. Am J Clin Nutr 18:231, 1966.

64. Taradash MR et al: Vasodilator therapy of idiopathic lactic acidosis. NEJM 293:468, 1975.

65. Tranquada RE et al: Methylene blue in the treatment of lactic acidosis. Clin Res 11:230, 1963.

66. Turrell ES et al: The acid-base equilibrium of the blood in exercise. Am J Physiol 137:742, 1942.

67. Varma SK et al: Hyperlactataemia in phenformin-treated diabetes. Br Med J 1:205, 1972.

68. Walker RS et al: Mode of action and side effects of phenformin hydrochloride. Brit Med J 2:1567, 1960.

69. Waters WC III et al: Spontaneous lactic acidosis. Am J Med 35:781, 1963.

70. Williams SE: Hydrogen ion infusion for treating severe metabolic alkalosis. Brit Med J 2:1189, May 15, 1976.

Chapter 5

Hyperalimentation

Gail W. McSweeney
Gary C. Cupit

Hyperalimentation (HA), or total parenteral nutrition (TPN), is a method of providing complete nutritional support by the intravenous route. Attempts to accomplish this were made as early as 1930 but they were largely unsuccessful because of the instability of the solutions available and the inability of scientists to overcome the technical problems. However, in 1966, Stanley Dudrick and his co-workers at the University of Pennsylvania developed a method for inserting and maintaining a catheter in the superior vena cava that could be used for the delivery of large quantities of a hypertonic protein-dextrose solution. Two years later, the first reports of successful parenteral therapy appeared in the literature, first with Beagle dogs and then with infants and adults (20,21,81); hyperalimentation had become feasible. This therapy is primarily used to restore or maintain adequate nutritional status for two reasons: ① to allow the patient to survive a long, devastating illness, and ② to enable the patient to heal more rapidly and efficiently. Hyperalimentation is an extremely complex procedure and should not be attempted unless other alternatives have been determined to be unsatisfactory; it can result in life-threatening complications.

1. What are the indications for hyperalimentation (HA) therapy? Characterize the patient who is a candidate for hyperalimentation therapy.

The indications for HA fall into several broad categories (see Table 1), but it should be reserved for those patients who cannot meet their nutritional needs adequately by the oral route and who will not be expected to resume oral alimentation within a very few days. In a general sense, the type of patient who is a realistic candidate for HA is one who has lost 10% of body weight due to injury or illness, is in negative nitrogen balance (converting body protein to glucose for metabolism), and who is not expected to eat or take tube feedings soon. A patient will not begin to reverse these factors for 5 to 7 days after the institution of therapy. Therefore, it should not be considered unless it is anticipated that HA will be continued for at least 7 to 10 days. HA therapy may continue for months or years.

Table 1
Indications for Hyperalimentation Therapy

A. Disruption of gastrointestinal
function or continuity
  1. Congenital anomalies of the newborn
  2. Fistulas
  3. Malabsorption
  4. Complete obstruction
  5. Ulcerative or granulomatous colitis
  6. Pancreatitis
B. Hypermetabolic states
  1. Severe burns
  2. Major or multiple trauma
  3. Neoplastic disease
  4. Peritonitis
C. Acute renal failure
D. Anorexia nervosa

2. Describe the procedure which must be followed to insert a subclavian catheter for administration of a HA solution.

Because the solutions are hypertonic, they must be administered into a large vein. This is generally accomplished by insertion of a catheter into the subclavian vein with the tip of the catheter lying near the right atrium. This technique allows immediate dilution of the nutrient solution by an enormous quantity of blood as soon as it enters the body and decreases or prevents irritation of the vein itself. The catheter must be inserted using strict aseptic technique. The operator wears a cap, mask, gloves and gown and, after putting the patient in Trendelenberg position, prepares a sterile field around the area of insertion. The skin is scrubbed vigorously in a circular, outward motion with Betadine solution, defatted with acetone and then scrubbed with Betadine again. With the patient's head turned to the opposite side, the skin is infiltrated with a local anesthetic at the inferior margin of the midclavicle and through the subcutaneous tissue along the anticipated course of the venipuncture needle. A 14 gauge, 5 cm long needle is attached to a 5 cc syringe after removing the plastic catheter. The needle is advanced, bevel side down, from the skin passing under the clavicle and aiming its tip at the anterior margin of the trachea in the suprasternal notch. Continuous negative pressure is exerted on the syringe so that when the tip enters the subclavian vein there will be prompt filling with blood. The patient is then asked to perform a Valsalva maneuver while the syringe is removed and replaced with the plastic catheter. This catheter is then threaded down the vein until its tip lies just above the right atrium. An X-ray to ensure proper placement of the catheter is obtained before HA therapy is begun to rule out pneumothorax, arterial puncture, air embolism or cardiac tamponade. A solution of 5 or 10% dextrose in water can be used to keep the line open in the interim (49).

3. What are the components of a hyperalimentation solution? Are there any advantages of one protein source over another?

The solutions used for parenteral nutrition are designed to approximate the normal diet and are composed of all the required nutritional components currently known and available for use. The primary ingredients are protein and dextrose (glucose). Originally, the protein source was a breakdown product of beef, a hydrolysate, but the incidence of allergic reactions was significant and amino acid availability was difficult to assess. For these reasons, the solutions currently used are casein (milk) hydrolysates and free amino acid combinations (see Table 2). In patients with a normal ability to assimilate protein, i.e., those without significant hepatic or renal impairment, the hydrolysates and the amino acid solutions produce equivalent positive nitrogen balance (78). The major calorie source in HA solutions is glucose which, in addition to providing 4 calories per gram (anhydrous), is necessary for its protein sparing effect and for its stimulation of insulin. Insulin, while producing its effects on carbohydrate metabolism, has direct positive influence on amino acid transport, protein anabolism, and growth hormone activity (57,69). The other components, vitamins, minerals, and electrolytes will be discussed later.

4. Why do the solutions have such a high dextrose concentration relative to the protein?

In order to incorporate amino acids into protein and achieve anabolism, large quantities of calories are needed. Glucose spares amino acids and stimulates the release of insulin which promotes the incorporation of amino acids into protein. The commercially available HA solutions have calorie to nitrogen ratios that range from 150 to 200 calories of glucose per gram of nitrogen. Since protein is 16% nitrogen by weight, one gram of nitrogen is equivalent to 6.25 grams of protein. These figures were based upon analyses of an oral diet which varies according to the availability of foods, taste and custom. The ratio selected, therefore, is not necessarily an optimal combination for the complete utilization of nitrogen for anabolism.

Chen (14) demonstrated that until a level of 450 calories of glucose per gram of nitrogen was reached, nitrogen losses did not decrease below the obligatory level found in urine and feces. This study implies that this level is optimal because none of the infused protein is eliminated. Although this figure is attractive, the work was done in children with gastrointestinal anomalies and does not evaluate the protein needs in the septic, debilitated or catabolic adult, nor does it address the specific needs for anabolism. The most convenient way to evaluate nitrogen utilization in the patient on HA is to follow the urine urea nitrogen; if the amount of amino acid infused is in excess of that needed by the body for other uses or per unit glucose,

Table 2
Amino Acid and Electrolyte Content of Commercially Available Protein Solutions for Hyperalimentation

	TRAVAMIN or AMIGEN 10% (500 ml)	TRAVASOL 8.5% (500 ml)	FRE AMINE II 8.5% (500 ml)	AMINOSYN 3.5% (680 ml)	NEPHRAMINE 5.1% (250 ml)
PROTEIN SOURCE	Casein	Soybean	Soybean	Soybean	Soybean
Peptides	Yes	No	No	No	No
Grams	50 gm	42.5 gm	39 gm	33.3 gm	12.7 gm
Utilizable	85% (42.5 gm)	100% (42.5 gm)	100%	100%	100%
AMINO ACIDS	mg/100 ml	mg/100 ml	mg/100 ml	mg/100 ml	mg/100 ml
Leucine	820	526	770	313	880
Phenylalanine	400	526	480	147	880
Methionine	260	492	450	133	880
Lysine	520	492	620	240	640
Isoleucine	520	406	590	240	560
Valine	620	390	560	267	650
Threonine	380	356	340	173	400
Tryptophan	70	152	130	53	200
Histidine	260	372	240	100	—
Arginine	320	880	310	327	—
Non-essential amino acids	Yes	Yes	Yes	Yes	No
NITROGEN					
Grams	6.5	7.15	6.25	5.34	1.46
Utilizable	5.4	100%	100%	100%	100%
ELECTROLYTES	mEq/L	mEq/L	mEq/L	mEq/L	mEq/L
Na	60	—	10	—	6
K	31	—	—	3.6	—
Ca	10	—	—	—	—
Mg	4	—	—	—	—
Cl	44	17	—	—	—
MPO$_4$	60	—	20	—	—
Acetate		2.6	—	20	—
MIXING					
Kit	No	No	Yes	No	No
Individual	Yes	Yes	Yes (special)	Yes	Yes

then the amino acids will be transaminated or broken down for gluconeogenesis. If this occurs, the unneeded nitrogen will become evident in an elevation of this laboratory value and therapy should be adjusted by either increasing the glucose or decreasing the protein.

5. What is the maximum number of calories that can be given to a patient on hyperalimentation? What factors alter glucose utilization?

The rate of glucose metabolism is greatest in the infant, adolescent and young adult, often approaching 1.2 gm/kg/hr, but in the average, non-diabetic adult, the figure is closer to 0.5 gm/kg/hr. Significantly altered utilization occurs in diabetics and patients with shock, sepsis, severe stress, or pancreatic disease. Glucose tolerance can also be altered by increased sympathetic tone caused by elevated levels of circulating catecholamines. This condition occurs in stressed patients (e.g. trauma or surgical). In situations such as these, the administration of exogenous insulin may improve the patient's glucose utilization, but it is important to be aware that this addition will not suppress endogenous production. Because the usual negative feedback mechanisms seen with hormonal control do not function in this situation, hypoglycemia may occur if the clinical picture changes and the patient's relative insulin resistance decreases. Continuous re-evaluation must be made of glucose utilization (41,77).

6. How should a patient on hyperalimentation be monitored? How can nitrogen balance be monitored in patients with hepatic and/or renal failure?

All initial laboratory and clinical data should be obtained as recommended in Table 3. After this, the frequency for review of a specific parameter depends on the patient, but there are some guidelines. Electrolytes can change very rapidly and should be monitored daily until the patient is stabilized; thereafter follow-up values should be obtained two to three times weekly depending on the confidence in continued stability (i.e., no acute changes in renal, fluid or acid-base status). After stabilization, a hematology panel, liver and renal function tests and other parameters which change more slowly should be obtained weekly. Initially, while the glucose load is changing, the blood sugar should be monitored daily and the urine sugars should be evaluated four times a day to avoid hyper- or hypoglycemia. Thereafter, if urine sugars can be depended upon to accurately reflect the patient's status, they should continue to be checked at least twice daily to detect any changes in glucose tolerance. This change could be the first sign of another complication, such as sepsis. A pump should be used to regulate the infusion rate so that if glucose tolerance changes in a previously well controlled patient, it will

Table 3
Monitoring Protocol for
Total Parenteral Nutrition

(1) Baseline Studies:
Hemoglobin
Hematocrit
RBC indices
Platelet count
Sodium
Potassium
Chloride
Bicarbonate
Calcium
Phosphate
Magnesium
Fe and Fe binding capacity
Fasting blood sugar
BUN
Creatinine
Uric acid
Total protein
Albumin
Prothrombin time
Bilirubin
SGOT
Alkaline phosphatase
Urinalysis
Chest X-ray
EKG

(2) Daily Studies During Stabilization (5-7 days):
Urine glucose every six hours
　　　(with simultaneous blood sugars for the
　　　　　first 24-48 hours to establish
　　　　the renal threshold for glucose).
Blood glucose
Serum electrolytes
Accurate records of fluid intake and output
Body weight

(3) Routine Studies Following Stabilization:
Daily:
　　Fluid intake and output
　　Body weight
　　Urine glucose
Three times weekly:
　　Sodium
　　Potassium
　　Chloride
　　Bicarbonate
Once weekly:
　　CBC
　　Platelet count
　　Prothrombin time
　　BUN
　　Creatinine
　　Calcium
　　Phosphate
　　Magnesium
　　RBC indices
Once monthly:
　　Repeat baseline studies

not be dismissed as a simple change in the flow rate. Weight must be followed to assess the anabolic effects of HA. However, the weight will not reflect new muscle mass for about five days because the initial increases will reflect a slightly positive fluid balance. The BUN is a good indicator of nitrogen utilization and is much easier to obtain than elaborate nitrogen balance studies which probably do not provide more clinically useful information. A rising BUN in a patient with stable renal function that exceeds a BUN:Creatinine ratio of 10:1 indicates a pre-renal azotemia which means that too much protein per unit of glucose is being infused.

7. Describe the composition of the initial solution. How should it be administered?

Therapy must be initiated slowly with regard to the glucose load because the pancreas needs time to equilibrate to this new demand for insulin. Ordinarily, patients can be started on 1000 cc/day of a 25% dextrose-protein solution. The rate is gradually increased over several days as glucose tolerance permits (68). The amount of protein given per liter should be the final concentration planned for the patient (e.g. FreAmine II 4.25%, Travamine 5%), since there is no equilibration period needed for the protein load. The initial protein solution should be reduced in patients with hepatic or renal impairment, and the BUN should be followed closely to assess the patient's level of function in assimilating and/or excreting nitrogen.

The initial electrolytes to be added must be calculated by adding or subtracting any amounts necessitated by contributing abnormalities in the patient or the special electrolyte requirements of hyperalimentation to normal replacement values. Ions involved in glucose utilization and intracellular electrolytes will be needed in quantities out of proportion to normal replacement values. Potassium is needed to transport glucose across cell membranes, and is also a major intracellular cation. Consequently, in the manufacture of new muscle mass, quantities needed by the patient may be three to four times the usual replacement value; magnesium and phosphate needs will also rise for the same reason. However, the requirements for sodium and calcium which are largely extracellular cations, will remain close to replacement values because the vascular volume is not significantly altered by hyperalimentation or anabolism (9,17,18,71,82) See Table 4 and Question 8.

8. Discuss the electrolyte complications and requirements observed in patients on hyperalimentation therapy.

The electrolytes which are of greatest concern in patients on hyperalimentation are primarily the intracellular ions. It is these cations and anions which are needed in large quantities due to the dextrose load and the expansion of the intracellular space resulting from anabolism.

Low levels of **phosphate** have been clearly as-

Table 4
General Guidelines for Protein, Glucose, Fluid and Electrolyte Requirements

Basic requirements per 24 hours (divided among 3 liters):

Water	2,500-3,500 ml
Calories	2,500-3,500
Protein	100-150 gms
Nitrogen	16-25 gms
Carbohydrate	525-750 gms
Sodium	100-200 mEq
Potassium	50-200 (varies greatly)
Magnesium	10-30 mEq
Phosphate	20-25 mEq/1000kcal
Calcium	5-25 mEq
MVI	1 vial in 1 liter/day

Variable Requirements:

*Folate 1 mg/day	Do not order in the same bottle with MVI because of incompatability.
*Vitamin K	Add once a week or prn as dictated by laboratory data.
*Vitamin B_{12}	Give prior to the initiation of hyperalimentation therapy.
Insulin	May be added to the bag or given subcutaneously on a sliding scale. If 3+ to 4+ glycosuria persists, consider reduction in hyperalimentation solution rate.

*NOTE: For more reliable results, these drugs should not be added to the hyperalimentation fluid.

sociated with symptoms of confusion, neuromuscular irritability, hemolytic anemia, and impaired leucocyte function. At levels below 1 mg%, impairment of erythrocyte structure and function occur. In red blood cells, ATP and 2,3-diphosphoglycerate (DPG) are generated by anaerobic metabolism of glucose and are dependent on the availability of PO_4 from the extracellular fluid. Low levels of ATP and 2,3-DPG increase the affinity of oxygen for hemoglobin and can produce tissue hypoxia. ATP is also necessary for maintenance of the erythrocyte membrane and very low levels can shorten the red blood cell life span. The requirement for phosphate appears to be a function of the glucose calories infused. It is recommended that 20 to 25 milliequivalents of phosphate per 1000 calories be administered (46,70).

Requirements for **calcium** increase only slightly during hyperalimentation, but it must be monitored carefully because of its relationship to phosphate levels. If the serum level is normal, the daily calcium requirement is 10 to 25 milliequivalents. Calcium and phosphate form an insoluble complex when mixed and the lower the concentrations of glucose and protein, the more readily it will precipitate. In an HA solution of 25% dextrose and 4 to 5% protein, 15 mEq of calcium and 45 mEq of phosphate can usually be mixed without complexation. However, it is simpler to put the ions in alternate bottles at slightly higher concentrations.

Because **potassium** is an intracellular ion, 20 to 40 mEq per 1000 calories may be required in addition to the usual replacement amounts in patients on HA. Serum levels of this cation can change rapidly, especially in the presence of fistulae, diarrhea, and acid-base imbalances. Therefore, daily levels should be obtained until the patient is stable and daily requirements can be accurately and confidently determined (9,17,18).

Magnesium requirements may reach 10 to 20 mEq per day but the serum level should be followed closely, especially in elderly patients or those with impaired renal function as it can accumulate and lead to muscle flaccidity and apnea.

9. What special considerations must be taken when hyperalimentation is prescribed for a patient in renal or hepatic failure?

The excess endogenous nitrogen pool in patients with renal failure can be used to manufacture non-essential amino acids for anabolic purposes if sufficient non-protein calories and essential amino acids are given. For such patients the glucose concentration in the TPN solution can be increased and the amino acid concentration can be reduced or changed to one containing only essential amino acids, such as Nephramine which contains 1.7% protein and 46.7% dextrose. Laboratory parameters must be followed closely to arrive at the best solution.

In those with severe hepatic decompensation, the protein load must be greatly reduced, as the patient can no longer efficiently break down peptides or transaminate amino acids to provide the specific ones needed for anabolism. Furthermore, excess exogenous nitrogen can precipitate coma in such individuals. A reduced concentration of the free essential and nonessential amino acid solutions containing relatively larger amounts of branched chain amino acids will probably promote anabolism and cause less azotemia and encephalopathy. Solutions for use in impaired hepatic function are now under investigation (1, 2, 7, 8, 19, 33, 45, 66).

10. What are the complications of hyperalimentation therapy? How are they manifested and how may they be corrected?

The complications of HA can be considered in several broad categories: disorders of glucose and amino acid metabolism, electrolyte abnormalities (see Question 8), sepsis, and several other more specific problems such as elevation in liver enzymes, prolongation of the prothrombin time and anemia.

Hyperglycemia occurs most frequently when the initial infusion rate is too rapid and the patient has not had sufficient time to produce an adequate amount of endogenous insulin. Less frequently, there has been a change in the glucose tolerance of a previously controlled patient. The consequences include dehydration secondary to osmotic diuresis and hyperosmolar, nonketotic, hyperglycemic coma in non-diabetics. The latter condition has a mortality rate of 50% and is preventable if the patient is monitored carefully. In diabetics, the sequence of events is the same with the addition of ketoacidosis. Treatment includes fluids to correct the dehydration, correction of electrolyte abnormalities and the possible addition of potassium and insulin to lower the blood sugar (17). Also see Question 7.

If the hypertonic infusion is discontinued abruptly, there is some danger of a **rebound hypoglycemia** secondary to the persistence of endogenous insulin from prolonged stimulation of the islet cells, but this rarely occurs. The body can equilibrate in about 60 minutes and return to baseline hormone levels, but this process may take longer in the debilitated, stressed patient who is most commonly the candidate for hyperalimentation. For this reason, it is recommended that the infusion be discontinued slowly over 24 to 36 hours, or as glucose tolerance permits (68).

The disorders of amino acid metabolism are not as predictable, preventable, or manageable as are those of glucose. **Hyperchloremic metabolic acidosis** can be caused by the generation of HCl from metabolism of arginine and lysine, or from the addition of chloride with added electrolytes in an amount which is excess of the amount of sodium added to the TPN solution. The latter problem is observed when, for example, large amounts of potassium as well as sodium chloride are given to patients who are in renal failure, dehydrated, or to those who are severely debilitated. The problem can be prevented or corrected by substituting some or all of the chloride with phosphate or acetate which is metabolized to bicarbonate. Bicarbonate should not be added to hyperalimentation solutions because it produces pH, compatibility, and carbon dioxide production problems. Acetate corrects acidosis without causing the aforementioned problems and is completely converted to bicarbonate in vivo. Lactate salts are commercially available but are not recommended because only 50% of the salt is metabolized to bicarbonate and they may even cause lactic acidosis in patients with hepatic failure who are unable to metabolize lactate (18,49).

Hyperammonemia is a problem that is most often seen in the neonate but it does occur in adults with hepatic failure. It occurs most frequently following the administration of the hydrolysates which contain 20 to 40 mMoles of free ammonia or ammonium ion per 100 cc; the crystalline amino acid solutions contain only minute amounts. The inability to handle ammonia seems to be related to the ammonia-urea cycle (Fig. 1). In the presence of a relative deficiency of arginine, and probably ornithine and aspartic acid, the liver cannot convert ammonia to the excretable urea. If arginine is added to the HA solution the hyperammonemia will be corrected. Since arginine is an acid producing substance, signs and symptoms of acidosis must be carefully monitored and corrected if present.

The amino acid profiles of the commercially available protein solutions reflect the composition of naturally occurring proteins such as milk and egg albumin. While these solutions work well in patients with a normal ability to transaminate amino acids, they can create **plasma amino acid imbalances** in patients who have difficulty handling some of these substances. Specifically, patients with advanced liver disease have difficulty utilizing phenylalanine, methionine, and tryptophan, and levels of leucine, isoleucine, and valine are depressed (all of these are essential amino acids). While much research remains to be done, it is becoming apparent that elevated levels of some amino acids may be toxic and may interfere with the metabolism of others. For example, an excess of phenylalanine may inhibit the transfer of tyrosine across the blood-brain barrier. This is an important phenomenon as tyrosine is necessary for the synthesis of normal brain catecholamines (23,53).

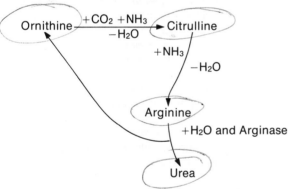

Fig. 1. Urea Formation from Ammonia.

Sepsis is a complication which may be minimized by scrupulously adhering to aseptic technique in the insertion and care of subclavian catheters and in the manufacture and administration of solutions. Also, the subclavian catheter should be used exclusively for the administration of the hyperalimentation solution (81). Even a small deviation from accepted procedure can introduce contaminating organisms into an environment where they can multiply rapidly. Exposure to exogenous organisms is, however, not the only hazard. Patients on nutritional therapy are frequently on broad-spectrum antibiotics and steroids as well. These drugs can impair host defense mechanisms and disrupt normal flora to the extent that organisms nor-

mally present can proliferate and become infectious. The tip of the intravenous catheter lying in the vena cava, constantly bathed in a hyperosmolar solution also provides a nidus for bacterial or fungal growth.

The manifestations of sepsis due to TPN can include chills, fever, and leucocytosis, but this condition may manifest itself merely as a change in glucose tolerance in a previously stabilized patient. When these changes occur, the patient should be evaluated for any other sites of infection before the HA solution is discontinued and the catheter removed. Re-insertion of the intravenous line itself is hazardous and should not be done more often than necessary. Only when other sites of infection have been eliminated should the line be removed and the catheter tip cultured to identify any organism that may be present. The sepsis will usually resolve without the use of antibiotics once the nidus for growth has been removed (17,18,41).

Elevations in liver enzymes are discussed in Question 11. Any change or increase in bilirubin may represent a manifestation of the underlying, or a new disease state and should be evaluated for this possibility.

Since there is no vitamin K present in the HA solutions or the commercially available multiple vitamin preparations for parenteral use, a **prolongation of the prothrombin time** may develop in a few days. Patients should be checked weekly, or more often if necessary. A supplement of Vitamin K_3 10 mg intramuscularly will usually correct any abnormality which is observed (32).

Anemia is seen commonly in patients who are ill enough to require parenteral nutrition, but it should be evaluated for specific etiology and corrected, if possible. Folic acid, cyanocobalamin (B_{12}), and, occasionally, iron will have to be given during therapy as the base solutions and vitamin additives do not contain them.

11. A patient on hyperalimentation for several weeks developed minor elevations in liver enzymes. What is a possible etiology of this observed abnormality?

When hydrolysates were used exclusively as the protein source, it was postulated that these abnormalities were due to unutilizable peptide fragments; however, the introduction of free amino acid solutions did not alter this pattern. When liver biopsies showed fatty infiltration of the hepatocytes, another postulate was that the large quantities of glucose being administered were being made into fat rather than being completely incorporated into new muscle mass. More recent work by Richardson and Sgoutas (62) indicates that this condition is due to an essential fatty acid deficiency in patients maintained on fat-free solutions for long periods of time; they have demonstrated reversal of the infiltration and enzyme elevation with administration of linoleic acid, the essential fatty acid.

Fatty liver is also seen in protein depleted patients who cannot manufacture the lipoprotein necessary to transport fat out of the liver. It is important to note that these elevated enzymes are not accompanied by an elevated bilirubin.

CASE A; FATTY ACID DEFICIENCY:

S.K. is a 44-year-old man who was admitted to the hospital two months ago with a history of intermittent abdominal pain which was occasionally associated with bloody emesis. A diagnosis of peptic ulcer was made and surgery was performed to correct the condition (Bilroth II). The postoperative course was complicated by a paralytic ileus, failure of the abdominal wound to heal and several enterocutaneous fistulas. The patient was started on total parenteral nutrition (TPN) consisting of dextrose 25%, synthetic amino acids 3%, electrolytes, and vitamins. After one week of therapy, the fistulas were improved; however, after five weeks of therapy, the patient's skin became dry and scaly. At first, this condition was confined to body folds, but it became more generalized over the next few days. At this point, linoleic acid comprising 4% of the patient's total caloric intake was added in the form of Intralipid 10%. After approximately 14 days, the scaling disappeared.

12. What is essential fatty acid (EFA) deficiency?

Essential fatty acid deficiency may be defined in both clinical and chemical terms. Clinically, it is manifested by scaly skin lesions, sparse hair growth, thrombocytopenia and poor wound healing (60,79). Chemically, linoleic (tetraene) acids with 2, 3 and 4 double bonds at the specific positions of the carbon chain are polyunsaturated essential fatty acids (59). In the absence of EFA's, there will be a decrease in dienes and tetraenes and an increase in monoenes (oleic acid). These would lead to failure of the formation of arachidonic (tetraene) and other polyunsaturated fatty acids that are necessary for the normal structure and function of cell membranes. These alterations in specific types of EFA's may be monitored by following the ratio of triene to tetraene fatty acids present in the plasma. According to Holman (42,43) the ratio of triene:tetraene rises above 0.4 in essential fatty acid deficiency.

13. How long does it take for a person to develop the symptoms of EFA deficiency?

In both children and adults, it appears that the triene:tetraene ratio becomes elevated above 0.4 within one to two weeks of initiating fat-free total parenteral nutrition (59,63,64). However, even in the face of these chemical changes, clinical symptoms may not be manifested for three weeks to six months after the institution of fat-free therapy.

14. How may these changes be prevented or reversed?

Requirements for the content of EFA in a nutritional program for infants and adults have not been agreed upon at this time. It is generally recommended for infants that the minimum and optimum intake of linoleic acid be 1% and 4% of the total calories, respectively (44,76). In addition, it has been shown that when linoleic acid approached 4 to 5% of total caloric intake, the efficiency of caloric utilization increased (76). Adults also appear to require an intake of linoleic acid equal to approximately 4% of their total caloric intake (63).

Administration of linoleic acid to patients on fat-free nutritional programs may be accomplished by several methods. The most direct method would be to administer the fats intravenously with a preparation such as soybean oil emulsion (Intralipid 10%). This preparation is approximately 50% linoleic acid. Therefore, if an adult patient were receiving 3,000 calories daily from a total parenteral nutrition program, only 4% of these calories, or 120 calories, need be supplied as linoleic acid daily. This would correspond to approximately 220 ml of Intralipid daily, since it is only 50% linoleic acid.

Another method is available for those patients who can tolerate a limited oral intake. This consists of the oral administration of safflower oil to supply needed linoleic acid (63). Safflower oil contains 70% linoleic acid (74). Only 20 ml of 100% safflower oil daily will supply the necessary EFA's. This assumes that 100% absorption occurs. Patients with gastrointestinal disease may require larger amounts.

The most novel approach to the correction of EFA deficiency comes from the work of Press, Hartop and Profley (61). They showed that cutaneous application of sunflower seed oil to one forearm resulted in sufficient absorption to correct EFA deficiency and could serve as an alternative method of preventing it. The usefulness of this approach has not been finally determined but it may have some merit as a means of preventing or mitigating the onset of EFA deficiency. It is much less expensive and more readily available than the parenteral soybean emulsion.

CASE B; FAT EMULSION THERAPY:

J.G. is a 47-year-old, 60 kg black female admitted for treatment of second and third degree burns over 50% of her body surface area. Her past medical history indicates that she has had a myocardial infarction resulting in mild congestive heart failure for the last seven years. This has been adequately controlled with furosemide, 80 mg, twice daily. All other medical and surgical history was negative.

Fluid and electrolyte treatment was begun immediately and continued for the first week of hospitalization. Complications of her management included:

a. Congestive heart failure requiring digitalization.
b. Massive fluid losses.
c. Hypoproteinemia (albumin less than 2.5 gm%).
d. Gastrointestinal bleeding secondary to stress ulcer.

On her seventh day of hospitalization, TPN therapy in conjunction with soy bean oil emulsion (Intralipid) was considered.

15. What are the indications for Intralipid therapy?

Parenteral fat emulsions are used as a source of essential fatty acids for depleted patients (see Questions 10, 11 and 12) and as a concentrated source of calories for patients who cannot tolerate dextrose concentrations greater than 25% or whose fluid intakes must be restricted. Examples include patients with ascites, renal failure, or congestive heart failure.

16. How is Intralipid metabolized when it is given by the intravenous route? Should heparin be added to the solution?

Studies in dogs and humans (36) have shown that the fat particles, one micron in size, are cleared rapidly from the bloodstream by a mechanism similar to the clearance of chylomicrons. The rate of clearance of free fatty acids from the serum is directly related to the dose of carbohydrates administered concomitantly. Interestingly, the triglyceride clearance remains constant, regardless of the quantity of infused carbohydrate (58).

The reticuloendothelial system (RES) also plays a role in the metabolism of fat emulsions (55). After the RES phagocytizes the fat emulsions, intracellular lipoprotein lipase hydrolyzes triglycerides to free fatty acids and glycerol. One investigator (16) recommends the addition of small amounts of heparin to stimulate lipoprotein lipase and aid in the clearance of fat. However, many other studies have shown this to be unnecessary (73,80,82).

17. When is the use of Intralipid contraindicated? Under what circumstances should it be used with caution?

Intralipid should not be used in patients with pathologic hyperlipidemia, lipoid nephrosis, or acute pancreatitis accompanied by hyperlipidemia. It must be given cautiously to patients with severe liver damage, pulmonary disease, or blood coagulation disorders (51). Care must also be taken when the danger of fat embolism exists and in infants with hyperbilirubinemia (38).

18. What baseline studies are needed, and how frequently should they be monitored?

In addition to the normal baseline tests for TPN discussed in Question 6, patients on fat emulsions should be monitored in the following manner. Serum triglyceride and cholesterol levels should be drawn before therapy is initiated and at weekly intervals thereafter. Lipemia must clear after daily infusions. Baseline liver function tests should be obtained and repeated at weekly intervals. Finally, platelet counts should be drawn twice weekly in adults. In newborns they should be obtained daily for the first week of therapy, every other day for the second week and then three times weekly thereafter.

19. Describe the proper administration of fat emulsion.

Before Intralipid therapy is initiated, a comprehensive nutritional program that includes carbohydrates and protein must be established. When instituted, the Intralipid emulsion must be piggybacked into either the central venous line or the peripheral administration line. It must not be mixed with electrolyte or other nutrient solutions, and no additives of any nature (e.g. drugs or vitamins) should be added to the fat emulsion. The emulsion can be infused with amino acid-carbohydrate mixtures by means of a Y-connector located near the infusion site. Filters must not be used with the fat emulsion since the particle size is larger than the filter pores.

In adults, the fat emulsion infusion is begun initially at one milliliter per minute for the first 30 minutes. Then, if no adverse reactions occur, the infusion rate may be increased so that the infusion is completed in not less than four hours. On the first day of therapy, patients should receive no more than 500 ml of 10% fat emulsion. Doses after the first day may be increased to a maximum of 2.5 gm/kg of 10% fat emulsion.

In children, the initial rate of fat emulsion should be 0.1 ml per minute for 15 to 30 minutes. If no reactions occur, the rate may be increased to 1 gm/kg in no less than four hours. The daily dose may then be incrementally increased to a maximum of 4 gm/kg (16).

Under no circumstances should the calorie contribution of fat exceed 60% of the patient's total daily caloric intake. The remaining 40% or more should consist of carbohydrate and amino acids to promote efficient anabolism.

Recently, the relationship between the non-protein caloric sources and the utilization of protein has been studied (28,31,48) to determine whether fat or carbohydrate promoted the more efficient utilization of nitrogen. One group (48) preferred the use of fat emulsions alone with amino acids on the theory that if serum glucose and insulin levels were decreased, more fat would be utilized and lean body mass would be spared. This has not been substantiated by a large clinical trial.

20. What acute reactions and side effects are noted in patients on fat emulsion infusions? Are there any long-term effects of fat emulsion therapy?

The most frequent acute response is the *febrile response*. This occurred in almost 3% of patients in one series (37), and in 28% of another (25). Other secondary reactions are chills, shivering, vomiting, and pain in the chest and back. Thrombophlebitis occurs rarely when fat emulsion is administered by the peripheral route and is estimated to occur in 1% of patients.

Long-term or delayed reactions that occur in patients receiving fat emulsion infusions include enlarged liver and spleen, thrombocytopenia, and transient elevation in liver function tests. When fat comprises a larger than recommended percentage of the infused calories, a syndrome of overloading may develop. This is manifested by focal seizures, fever, leucocytosis, and shock.

Another long-term toxicity that is receiving increasing attention is the deposition of fat pigment in the liver in patients maintained on long-term therapy. This deposition has been documented in both animal (52) and human (53) studies. However, the appearance of this pigment in hepatic cells is not directly associated with measurable changes in hepatic function, nor is there evidence of permanent structural damage. No correlation was found in one of these studies (53) with either age, clinical diagnosis, rate, or total dose of fat emulsion. The effect of fat emulsions on hepatic function remains difficult to assess in the clinical situation because infusions of protein, carbohydrate or both will also induce structural changes in the liver over long periods of time. Hepatic function should be monitored once or twice weekly while patients are receiving fat emulsions.

CASE C; PEDIATRIC TOTAL PARENTERAL NUTRITION:

M.W. is a three-week-old, 42 kg infant who was born with congenital omphalocoele with evisceration of the stomach, approximately one-third of the liver and portions of the intestine. On the day of delivery, the infant was taken to surgery where closure of the omphalocoele was performed with placement of a Dacron graft over the abdominal cavity. After surgery the patient was fed by a nasogastric tube. Feedings were interrupted after approximately ten days when signs of necrotizing enterocolitis developed. Nutrition during the next ten days was accomplished by peripheral administration of dextrose 10% in water. On day 21 you are consulted about the appropriate use of hyperalimentation in this patient.

21. How does total parenteral nutrition in the pediatric patient differ from that in the adult?

The pediatric nutritional requirements are summarized in Table 5. Guidelines for the management of children on TPN solutions are similar to adult recommendations.

One way in which the nutrition of infants can be managed effectively is by the **peripheral route** (24). By this method, it is possible to infuse solutions with lower osmolalities than those administered by the central route. When the osmolality is decreased, it is necessary to infuse greater quantities of solution to maintain an adequate caloric intake. For example, solutions given to newborns are generally 2 to 4% amino acids and 20 to 25% glucose when given by the central route. These are generally infused at a daily volume of 100 ml/kg. By the peripheral route, solutions are usually 1 to 2% amino acids and 10 to 12% glucose. However, daily infusion volumes are often 150 to 250 ml/kg. The recent addition of fat emulsions to the parenteral nutrition solutions makes the peripheral route more attractive. This method is relatively safe if the peripheral lines are rotated frequently, and complications associated with the central venous route are avoided. In the past, the caloric content of peripheral nutrition solutions were increased by the addition of ethyl alcohol which has a caloric value of 7 cal/gm (6). However, the unpredictable blood alcohol levels (61) and hepatotoxicity (68) were major drawbacks to the use of this substance.

The metabolic complications of parenteral nutrition in infants are similar to those observed in adults. However, two areas differ: hyperammonemia and metabolic acidosis.

Hyperammonemia in the pediatric patient is confined to the newborn age group. Etiologies for this abnormality include: (a) high free ammonia levels of hydrolysates; (b) an amino acid imbalance produced by nitrogen sources; (c) subclinical liver diseases; (d) an arginine deficiency; (e) hepatic immaturity; and (f) hepatic dysfunction due to nutritional depletion (40,49). The hydrolysates contain 20 to 40 mM/100ml of free ammonia (29) while the free amino acid solutions contain 0.1 to 1 mM/100 ml (49).

When hyperammonemia is asymptomatic it is best managed by decreasing the amount of nitrogen being infused. The amounts can then be gradually increased by titrating the infused protein against serum ammonia levels.

Symptomatic hyperammonemia, as evidenced by lethargy, decreased responsiveness, twitching movements of the extremities, and even grand mal seizures, is best treated by discontinuing the protein infusions. Acute treatment includes the institution of dextrose solutions with electrolytes. Arginine may be cautiously administered in a dose of 2 to 3 mM/kg (40). When ammonia levels have been reduced and when clinical symptoms have dissipated, the nitrogen source may be restarted. Again, the serum ammonia levels are monitored to arrive at the correct dose of nitrogen. If it is evident that the amount of infused protein is insufficient for growth, arginine supplementation may be necessary. Generally, 1 mM/kg/day is used to maintain adequate nitrogen intake without increasing serum ammonia levels (40). If the amount of arginine HCl necessary to maintain normal ammonia levels produces acidosis, then NaHCO₃ may be added or the arginine can be administered as the glutamate salt.

The problem of **metabolic acidosis** in infants on amino acid solutions is one that has generated considerable confusion as to etiology. Infants receiving a fibrin hydrolysate (39) showed no significant deviation of acid-base status, while those receiving synthetic amino acid mixtures developed mild hyperchloremic metabolic acidosis.

A variety of explanations have been proposed for the development of this acidosis (41). Some have implicated the titratable acidity of the parenteral nutrition solutions (13); however, the titratable acidity of a solution does not indicate how it will be handled *in vivo*. In fact, it has been shown (39) that protein hydrolysates, which do not cause acidosis, have three to four times the acidity of the synthetic amino acid solutions which do cause acidosis. This can be explained by considering the fate of two acidic solutions (41). For example, if one measures the pH and titratable acidity of 0.1 M lactic acid and 0.1 M hydrochloric acid, these solutions have identical titratable acidities. However, the infusion of lactic acid into a normal individual will not produce a metabolic acidosis because it is metabolized to carbon dioxide and water. Infusion of an equal amount of hydrochloric acid, on the other hand, would result in an acidosis since it is not metabolized and is excreted slowly by the kidney.

Chan (12) proposed that there is an excessive endogenous production of organic and sulfuric acids. However, this study has been criticized because the assay used for sulfur excretion was poor and because the acid intake in the infusate was not considered (41).

Most likely, the synthetic amino acids contain a potential acid load which is not present in the hydrolysates (41). In the fibrin and casein hydrolysates, inorganic cations exceed inorganic anions. This anion gap is balanced by glutamate, aspartate and negatively charged peptides, which are metabolized to bicarbonate. However, the crystalline amino acids have cation gaps which are equivalent to their content of arginine HCl and lysine HCl. These substances generate hydrochloric acid on metabolism.

The acidosis that is observed with these preparations is not a serious problem. Its management or prevention consists of the health professional being aware of the salts of the various electrolytes that are added to the parenteral solution. If chloride salts are substituted with the lactates, acetates, phosphates, or gluconates, this problem can be controlled. Maintaining a Na to Cl ratio of 1 to 1 and using other salts will alleviate the acidosis.

The future use of TPN in pediatric patients centers around the provision of better amino acid mixtures for children. Infants should receive greater amounts of amino acids that are essential for them including histidine, cystine and probably tyrosine (41,75). Additionally, an essential to nonessential amino acid ratio of 1 to 1 is necessary since it has been shown that tissue proteins have this ratio (3).

Table 5
Pediatric Nutritional Requirements

Ingredient*	Amount Required
Protein	2.0 — 2.5 gm/kg/day
Glucose	25 — 30 gm/kg/day
Sodium	3 — 5 mEq/kg/day
Potassium	2 — 3 mEq/kg/day
Phosphate	0.25 — 0.5 mEq/kg/day
Magnesium sulfate	0.25 mEq/kg/day
Calcium gluconate	0.25 — 0.5 mEq/kg/day
Multiple vitamins (MVI)	0.25 — 0.5 ml/kg/day

*The requirements of the individual ingredients may vary depending on the patient's serum values obtained prior to the initiation of therapy. Adjustment should be made based on frequent determinations of the patient's electrolyte status.

22. How can a program of TPN be utilized in the infant with poor renal function? Are there specific solutions available for the management of patients on dialysis or restricted protein intakes?

Intravenous nutrition with amino acids in the traumatized patient has been proven to be of value in reducing the net protein catabolism. However, the solutions of synthetic amino acids, protein hydrolysates, or casein hydrolysates all contain considerable amounts of nonessential amino acids. These solutions are unsuitable for uremic patients because they can produce an excess of urea and prevent the utilization of the urea pool for protein synthesis (7).

Rose and Dekker demonstrated that protein-depleted rats can utilize urea as a source of nonessential nitrogen in protein synthesis (67). Giordano proved that uremic patients can achieve the same utilization of urea when they are orally fed a diet consisting of synthetic essential amino acids (33). The value of this regimen has been shown to be effective in humans when they receive parenteral infusions (1,4,8,56). The amino acid content of these essential amino acid solutions is listed in Table 6.

The major difference between the two solutions is the addition of histidine and arginine to the Abbott renal formula. Recent studies have shown that the addition of arginine and histidine is necessary for improved nitrogen balance in uremic patients (7,54), and it also has been shown that optimal utilization of nitrogen is obtained when the ratio of nonprotein calories to grams of nitrogen is at least 425:1 (14).

This level of caloric intake usually corresponds to a solution composed of glucose 47% and essential amino acids 1.5%. Hopefully, this mixture will allow optimal utilization of exogenous nitrogen and re-utilization of endogenous urea. An infusion providing the patient with a total caloric intake of 60 to 80 Cal/ kg/day is attempted. Problems of hyperglycemia are managed by the use of crystalline insulin or by de-creasing the glucose concentration of the infusates. Rises in BUN are corrected by decreasing the concen-tration of infused protein or by increasing nonprotein calories, or both.

Table 6
Amino Acid Content of Essential
Amino Acid Formulas

Amino Acid (gm/100 ml)	Nephramine(a)	Abbott Renal Formula(b)
L-Isoleucine	0.56	0.47
L-Leucine	0.88	0.73
L-Lysine	0.80	0.54
DL-Methionine	0.88	0.73(c)
L-Phenylalanine	0.88	0.73
L-Threonine	0.40	0.33
L-Tryptophan	0.20	0.17
L-Valine	0.65	0.53
L-Histidine	0.0	0.43
L-Arginine	0.0	0.60
TOTAL	5.25	5.27

(a) McGaw Labs, Glendale, CA 91201
(b) Abbott Labs, North Chicago, Illinois 60064
(c) Abbott Renal Formula contains only L-Methionine

23. How is the patient who is receiving TPN best returned to oral feeding?

Long-term insult and disuse of the gastrointestinal tract will result in a degree of atony and may also alter normal secretory functions. Therefore the return to oral feeding must be gradual, beginning with easily digested products.

The low-residue, chemically defined diets (for example, Vivonex and Precision LR) are good to begin with because they are absorbed passively, do not re-quire mechanical and biochemical alteration, and do not generate a large amount of feces. Small quantities, adjusted to the isotonicity of the extracellular fluid, are given. The strength and amounts are gradually in-creased as the patient is able to tolerate oral feedings. Diarrhea may result if the patient is advanced too rapidly. Once the patient is able to tolerate the full strength hypertonic (600 mOsm) solution, the diet may be advanced slowly until the patient's previous dietary regimen has been reinstituted.

The intravenous solution may be continued, in re-duced amounts, during the initial stages of oral feed-ing to maintain good nutritional status. Since the hypertonic glucose solutions can suppress the appe-tite, it may be necessary to reduce the amount given at the outset of oral feeding to encourage the patient to eat and increase his oral intake to adequate levels (11,64,65).

24. What are some other uses for amino acid solu-tions besides hyperalimentation?

Amino acid solutions have been used as protein sparing therapy in previously well-nourished post-operative patients who are suddenly without nutri-tional support. While the exact mechanism has yet to be determined, it appears that the administration of protein alone, without glucose or fat, will reduce the degree of negative nitrogen balance that is seen in this situation and will cause the patient to switch more quickly from protein breakdown to fat breakdown for the generation of calories. Although this does not pre-vent catabolism, the goal of therapy is to minimize the breakdown of lean muscle and to help the stressed patient heal rapidly and efficiently. The research in-formation available in the literature does show small reductions in muscle wasting, but does not specific-ally address the issue of clinical differences in patient well-being or survival (10,26,31,45).

REFERENCES

1. Abel RM et al: Essential L-amino acids for hyperalimentation in patients with disordered nitrogen metabolism. Am J Surg 128:317, 1974.
2. Abel RM et al: Intravenous essential amino acids and hypertonic dextrose in patients with acute renal failure. Am J Surg 123:631, 1972.
3. Abitbol CL et al: Plasma amino acid patterns during supplemen-tal intravenous nutrition of low-birth-weight infants. J Ped 86:766, 1975.
4. Abitbol CL et al: Total parenteral nutrition in anuric children. Clin Nephrol 5:153, 1976.
5. Aguirre A et al: The role of surgery and hyperalimentation in the therapy of gastrointestinal-cutaneous fistulae. Ann Surg 180:393, 1974.
6. Benda GI et al: Peripheral intravenous alimentation of the small premature infant. J Ped 81:145, 1972.
7. Bergstrom J et al: Intravenous nutrition with amino acid solu-tions in patients with chronic uremia. Acta Med Scand 191:359, 1972.
8. Bergstrom J et al: Parenteral nutrition in uremia. Acta Anaes-thesiol Scand (Suppl) 55:147, 1974.
9. Bernard RW et al: Total body potassium measurements as a guide to intravenous alimentation. Ann Surg 178:559, 1973.
10. Blackburn GL et al: Peripheral intravenous feeding with isotonic amino acid solutions. Am J Surg 125:447, 1973.
11. Bury KD et al: Use of a chemically defined liquid elemental diet for the nutritional management of fistulas of the alimentary tract. Am J Surg 121:174, 1971.
12. Chan JC et al: Hyperalimentation with amino acid and casein hydrolysate solutions: mechanism of acidosis. JAMA 220:1700, 1972.

13. Chan JC et al: pH and titratable acidity of amino acid mixtures used in hyperalimentation. JAMA 220:1119, 1972.

14. Chen WJ et al: Amino acid metabolism in parenteral nutrition with special reference to the calorie: nitrogen ratio and the blood urea nitrogen level. Metabolism 23:1117, 1974.

15. Copeland EM et al: Intravenous hyperalimentation as an adjunct to cancer chemotherapy. Am J Surg 129:167, 1975.

16. Coran AG et al: Total intravenous feeding of infants and children without the use of a central venous catheter. Ann Surg 179:445, 1974.

17. Dudrick SJ et al: Parenteral hyperalimentation: metabolic problems and solutions. Ann Surg 176:259, 1972.

18. Dudrick SJ et al: Principles and practice of parenteral nutrition. Gastroent 61:901, 1971.

19. Dudrick SJ et al: Renal failure in surgical patients. Treatment with intravenous essential amino acids and hypertonic dextrose. Surgery 68:180, 1970.

20. Dudrick SJ et al: Long-term parenteral nutrition with growth, development and positive nitrogen balance. Surgery 64:134, 1968.

21. Dudrick SJ et al: Can intravenous feeding as the sole means of nutrition support growth in the child and restore weight loss in the adult? Ann Surg 169:974, 1969.

22. Fischer JE et al: Hyperalimentation as primary therapy for inflammatory bowel disease. Am J Surg 125:165, 1973.

23. Fischer JE et al: Plasma amino acids in patients with hepatic encephalopathy. Am J Surg 127:40, 1974.

24. Fox HA et al: Total intravenous nutrition by peripheral vein in neonatal surgical patients. Pediatrics 52:14, 1973.

25. Freuchen I et al: Parenteral nutrition in surgical patients. Acta Chir Scand (Suppl) 325:55, 1964.

26. Freeman JB et al: Evaluation of amino acid infusions as protein sparing agents in normal adult subjects. Am J Clin Nutr 28:477, 1975.

27. Freeman JB et al: Metabolic effects of amino acids vs dextrose infusion in surgical patients. Arch Surg 110:916, 1975.

28. Gassaniga AB et al: Nitrogen balance in patients receiving either fat or carbohydrate for total intravenous nutrition. Ann Surg 182:163, 1975.

29. Ghadimi H et al: Biochemical aspects of intravenous alimentation. Pediatrics 48:955, 1971.

30. Greenberg GR et al: Protein sparing therapy in postoperative effects of added hypocaloric glucose or lipid. NEJM 294:1411, 1976.

32. Greene HL et al: Vitamins in total parenteral nutrition. Drug Intell Clin Pharm 6:355, 1972.

33. Giordano C: Use of exogenous and endogenous urea for protein synthesis in normal and uremic subjects. J Lab Clin Med 62:321, 1963.

34. Hallberg D: Therapy with fat emulsions. Acta Anaesthiol Scand 55:131, 1974.

35. Hallberg D:Elimination of exogenous lipids from the blood stream. An experimental methodological and clinical study in dog and man. Acta Physiol Scand (Suppl) 65, 254:1, 1965.

36. Hallberg D et al: Fat emulsions for complete intravenous nutrition. Postgrad Med J 43:307, 1967.

37. Hargreaves T: Effect of fatty acids on bilirubin conjugation. Arch Dis Child 48:446, 1973.

38. Heird WC et al: Metabolic acidosis resulting from intravenous alimentation mixtures containing synthetic amino acids. NEJM 287:943, 1972.

39. Heird WC et al: Hyperammonemia resulting from intravenous alimentation using a mixture of synthetic L-amino acids: A preliminary report. J Ped 81:162,1972.

40. Heird WC et al: Total parenteral nutrition; the state of the art. J Ped 86:2, 1975.

41. Holman RT: The ration of trienois-tetraenois acids in tissue lipids as a measure of essential fatty acid requirement. J Nutr 70:405, 1960.

42. Holman RT: Essential fatty acid deficiency, Progress in the Chemistry of Fats and Other Lipids. Vol. 9, Oxford, Pergamon, 1971, p. 275.

43. Holman RT et al: The essential fatty acid requirement of infants and the assessment of their dietary intake of linoleate by serum acid analysis. Am J Clin Nutr 14:70, 1964.

44. Host WR et al: Hyperalimentation in cirrhotic patients, Am J Surg 123:57, 1972.

45. Hoover HC et al: Nitrogen sparing intravenous fluids in postoperative patients. NEJM 293:172, 1975.

46. Hypophosphatemia-Medical Staff Conference, University of California, San Francisco, West J Med 122:482, 1975.

47. Jeejeeboy KN et al: Metabolic studies in total parenteral nutrition with lipid in man: comparison with glucose. J Clin Invest 57:125, 1976.

48. Johnson JD et al: Hyperammonemia accompanying parenteral nutrition in newborn infants. J Ped 81:154, 1972.

49. Johnson C et al: Parenteral hyperalimentation. Drug Intell Clin Pharm 9:493, 1975.

50. Kapp JP et al: Platelet adhesiveness and serum lipids during and after Intralipid infusions. Nutr Metab. 13:92, 1971.

51. Koga Y et al: Effect of complete parenteral nutrition using fat emulsion on liver. Ann Surg 181:186, 1975.

52. Koga Y et al: Hepatic intravenous fat pigment in infants and children receiving lipid emulsion. J Ped Surg 10:641, 1975.

53. Kopple JD et al: Nitrogen balance and plasma amino acid levels in uremis patients fed an essential amino acid diet. Am J Clin Nutr 27:806, 1974.

54. Lemperle G: Depression and stimulation of host defense mechanisms after severe burns. Plast Reconstr Surg 45:435, 1970.

55. Leonard CD et al: Parenteral essential amino acids in acute renal failure. Urology 6:154, 1975.

56. Long CL et al: Comparison of fibrin hydrolysates and crystalline amino acid solutions in parenteral nutrition. Am J Clin Nutr 27:163, 1974.

57. Mac Fadyen BV et al: Triglyceride and free fatty acid clearances in patients receiving complete parenteral nutrition using a ten percent soybean oil emulsion. Surg Gynecol Obstet 137:813, 1973.

58. Meng HC: Fats. Symposium on Total Parenteral Nutrition, Jan. 17-19, 1972. American Medical Association, Chicago 1972.

59. Paulsrud JR et al: Essential fatty acid deficiency in infants induced by fat-free intravenous feeding. Am J Clin Nutr 25:897, 1972.

60. Peden VH et al: Intravenously induced infantile intoxication with ethanol. J Ped 83:490, 1973.

61. Press, M et al: Correction of essential fatty acid deficiency in man by the cutaneous application of sunflower seed oil. Lancet 1:597, 1974.

62. Richardson TJ et al: Essential fatty acid deficiency in four adult patients during total parenteral nutrition. Am J Clin Nutr 28:258, 1975.

63. Riella MC et al: Essential fatty acid deficiency in human adults during total parenteral nutrition. Ann Int Med 83:786, 1975.

64. Rocchio MA et al: Use of chemically defined diets in the management of patients with high output gastrointestinal cutaneous fistulas. Am J Surg 127:148, 1974.

65. Rocchio MA et al: Use of chemically defined diets in the management of patients with acute inflammatory bowel disease. Am J Surg 127:470, 1974.

66. Rose WC et al: Urea as a source of nitrogen for the biosynthesis of amino acids. J Biol Chem 223:107, 1956.

67. Rubin E et al: Fatty liver, alcoholic cirrhosis produced by alcohol in primates. NEJM 290:128, 1974.

68. Sanderson I et al: Insulin response in patients receiving concentrated infusions of glucose and casein hydrolysate for complete parenteral nutrition. Ann Surg 179:387, 1974.

69. Sgoutas DS et al: The effect of intravenous hyperalimentation on erythrocyte lipids. Proc Soc Exper Biol Med 1974.

70. Sheldon G et al: Phosphate depletion and repletion. Ann Surg 182:683, 1975.

71. Shils ME: Minerals in total parenteral nutrition. Drug Intell Clin Pharm 6:385, 1972.

72. Solassol CL et al: New techniques for long term intravenous feeding: an artificial gut in 75 patients. Ann Surg 179:519, 1974.

73. Sonderjelm L et al: Progress in the Chemistry of Fats and Other Lipids 9 (Part 4) 1970, p. 555.

74. Sturman JA et al: Absence of cystathionase in human fetal liver: is cystine essential? Science 169:74, 1970.

75. Tahiro T et al: The effect of fatty acid deficiency during intravenous hyperalimentation in pediatric patients. J Pediatr Surg 10:203, 1975.

76. VanWay CW et al: An assessment of the role of parenteral alimentation in the management of surgical patients. Ann Surg 177:104, 1973.

77. Vinnars E et al: Comparative nitrogen balance studies with an amino acid solution based on nutritional studies against protein based solutions. Acta Anaesthiol Scand (Suppl) 53:76, 1973.

78. White HB et al: Blood lipid alterations in infants receiving intravenous fat-free alimentation. J Pediatr 83:305, 1973.

79. Wilmore DD et al: Clinical evaluation of a 10% intravenous fat emulsion for parenteral nutrition in thermally injured patients. Ann Surg 178:503, 1973.

80. Wilmore, DD et al: Safe long term venous catheterization. Arch Surg 98:256, 1969.

81. Yeo MT et al: Total intravenous nutrition. Arch Surg 106:792, 1973.

Chapter 6

General Care: Anxiety and Insomnia

Brian S. Katcher

A discussion of sedatives and hypnotics is appropriate to the topic of General Care, since 85% of the prescriptions for these drugs are written by non-psychiatrists (139); insomnia is the second most common indication for drug therapy in hospitalized patients (127); anti-anxiety drugs account for about half of the prescriptions filled in retail pharmacies (11); and 15% of the U. S. population was treated with minor tranquilizers during the past year (139). Diazepam (Valium) is the most widely used drug in medical practice, and its popularity accounts for the dramatic increase in psychoactive drug prescriptions over the past decade (16,17).

The widespread use of prescription sedatives, alcohol, or marijuana to alleviate boredom, loneliness, frustration, and stress constitutes a major health problem (27,133). A thorough analysis of this problem is beyond the scope of this chapter which will focus on the appropriate clinical use of sedatives. However, the significant social costs of widespread psychoactive drug use must be borne in mind whenever these drugs are given to patients.

A great variety of drugs have been used for daytime sedation and sleep, but in nearly every case the benzodiazepines are the drugs of choice. The benzodiazepines (Table 1) are more consistently effective, less likely to interact with other drugs, less likely to cause adverse respiratory or hemodynamic effects, safer in overdose, and have less abuse potential than barbiturates and most other sedatives. Although barbiturates were the most commonly used sedatives ten years ago, they have recently been described as obsolete (8) and archaic (101). It has been suggested that barbiturate use be limited to induction of anesthesia and a few conditions such as epilepsy or hyper-

bilirubinemia where phenobarbital is particularly effective (5,6). This attitude is unduly restrictive, but these drugs deserve to be used less. Meprobamate (Miltown, Equanil), glutethimide (Doriden), methaqualone (Quaalude), and methyprylon (Noludar) share most of the disadvantages of the barbiturates.

1. A.M. is a 35-year-old 50 kg woman who complains of recent onset of neck and shoulder pain, nervousness, occasional insomnia, and general feelings of lack of well-being. A thorough physical examination reveals no objective signs of disease. She admits that stresses from her job may be playing a causative role in her symptoms. What is the role of psychoactive drug treatment in this patient?

This patient has many signs and symptoms which are consistent with ***anxiety.*** Anxiety, often manifested as insomnia, is among the most prevalent symptoms seen in medical practice. A precise definition is impossible, but some experience of anxiety is familiar to everyone, and in most circumstances it need not be considered as particularly pathological. Its manifestations include a diverse range of unpleasant mental and physical states. A few examples are:

Psychic: apprehension, irritability, nervousness, mild depression, inadequacy, indecision, and worry.

Somatic: tremor, insomnia, restlessness, headache, constipation, diarrhea, nausea, muscle tension, and palpitations.

A rational approach to therapy begins with the realization that the causes of anxiety are psychological. Therefore, psychological approaches should be the mainstay of therapy. Simply talking with the patient or suggesting other non-drug methods of alleviating her insomnia may help. Minor tranquilizers will provide only symptomatic relief. There is some controversy as to when minor tranquilizers should be used and what factors account for their well documented widespread use. Some of the arguments opposing and supporting the liberal use of minor tranquilizers follow.

Excessive Use: Prescribing drugs for minor emotional upset reinforces the notion of "illness" and fosters dependency. The drug industry has promoted psychoactive drugs in such a manner as to define more and more facets of human behavior as medical problems requiring drug treatment (114,131). If usage continues to increase at the present rate, everyone will be taking minor tranquilizers by the year 2000 (17). When people use drugs to cope, they decrease their development of non-drug coping strategies. The more people use drugs, the less they will be able to manage without them (27).

Appropriate Use: Alleviation of suffering by the direct treatment of symptoms is traditional medical practice. Since minor emotional disturbance is common, the wide use of these drugs is not inappropriate (42). Furthermore, in spite of the wide use of minor tranquilizers, epidemiologic evidence indicates that patients have extremely conservative attitudes toward these drugs and rarely use them every day (118).

If a minor tranquilizer is prescribed for this patient, it should not be the primary means of treatment, and supply should be limited.

2. A decision is made to give the above patient fifty doses of a minor tranquilizer to be taken as needed while she works out her problems. Which anxiolytic drug is the best choice?

The benzodiazepines are the drugs of choice for anxiety. Because of the subjective nature of anxiety, assessments of clinical response vary from study to study. However, comprehensive reviews of hundreds of double-blinded controlled studies demonstrate that diazepam (Valium), chlordiazepoxide (Librium), oxazepam (Serax), and other benzodiazepines are clearly more effective than barbiturates, meprobamate, or hydroxyzine (52,96).

Phenothiazines and tricyclic antidepressants have been promoted for use in anxiety. They are effective, but significant side effects and severe toxicity in suicide attempts make them poor choices. The more sedating tricyclic antidepressants are promoted for their combined antianxiety and antidepressant effects. However, most clinically encountered depression is a symptom of anxiety and is classified as "secondary or reactive depression" (see chapter on Affective Disorders). These mild depressive symptoms respond equally well to either tricyclic antidepressants or benzodiazepines, but a purely psychological approach should be tried first. Propranolol (Inderal) and other beta-adrenergic blocking agents have been tried experimentally as antianxiety agents. Results have been favorable, particularly in mediating the somatic effects of anxiety (166,169). However, the side effects of beta blockade will limit general application in anxiety states.

Any of the benzodiazepines would be appropriate for this patient. Diazepam is most popular probably because its lipophilic structure favors rapid passage into the central nervous system (see Question 10). This rapid action also makes it a good hypnotic, and its long half-life after redistribution provides residual anxiolytic effects the following day. Oxazepam has a short half-life and is easier to titrate in debilitated and older patients. The benzodiazepines are compared in Table 1. They are all equally effective.

TABLE 1
COMPARISON OF BENZODIAZEPINES

Generic Name	Trade Name	Usual Daily Dose	T½ (β)	Metabolites	Plasma Protein Binding (91,98,161,164)	Lipophilic Nature by n-Heptane/Water Partition Coefficient at pH 7.4 (172)
diazepam	Valium	6 to 40 mg	20-80 hrs	active	98%	150
desmethyldiazepam	see Fig. 1		50-100 hrs	active	97%	6
chlorazepate	Tranxene	15 to 60 mg	see desmethyl-diazepam	active		
chlordiazepoxide	Librium	15 to 100 mg	6-30 hrs	active	96%	0.2
oxazepam	Serax	30 to 120 mg	5-10 hrs	inactive	87%	0.01
lorazepam	Ativan	2 to 6 mg	12 hrs	inactive		
flurazepam	Dalmane	hypnotic only 15 or 30 mg	extremely short but active metabolite 50-100 hrs	active		

See also Fig. 1 for metabolic relationships.

3. A.M., who was described above, is given a prescription for "Diazepam (Valium) 10 mg, 50 tabs, Sig: ½ to 1 tablet as needed." How will the pharmacokinetic properties of this drug affect its dosing?

Diazepam is rapidly absorbed after oral administration (93), and blood levels can be correlated with clinical effects (36,71,91). Its half-life is age-dependent and is about 20 hrs in a 20-year-old and increases in a linear fashion to 90 hrs at age 80. This increase in half-life is due to an age-related increase in the volume of distribution (98). Steady state levels for any given dosage schedule will be the same regardless of age, but older subjects will take longer to reach steady state, and the peaks and troughs of their blood level curves will be less extreme than those of younger subjects. This 35-year-old woman will have a diazepam half-life of nearly 40 hrs. The effects of the first doses will wane in a few hours due to extensive tissue distribution, so frequent dosing may be required in the beginning. She should take only half-tablet doses at first, because subjects unfamiliar with the drug are more likely to experience motor and cognitive impairment during the distributional phase (64,71). Larger doses at night will help her sleep and contribute to the cumulative effect.

In evaluating the effect of any given total daily dose, it must be remembered that each dose will have a cumulative effect until steady state (four half-lives) is reached. In this case it will take more than a week to reach plateau drug levels. (Also see Question 24). Thus, a dosing pattern that is successful at the end of three days may cause excessive sedation if continued for a total of eight days. It is also important to consider that the metabolites of diazepam (Fig. 1) are active, and desmethyldiazepam also has a long half-life.

In many cases patients will take only an occasional dose or regular doses for two or three days. Such sporadic dosing is entirely correct, since symptomatic effect is being titrated against clinical need.

4. What other factors might affect this patient's response to diazepam?

Sedation from diazepam and chlordiazepoxide occurs significantly more frequently in non-smokers than in smokers and is correlated with the number of **cigarettes** smoked. Although induction of benzodiazepine metabolism was suggested (21,104), pharmacokinetic studies demonstrate that the disposition of diazepam is not affected by smoking (98). Therefore, the interaction between nicotine and benzodiazepines must occur within the central nervous system. Excessive coffee **(caffeine)** consumption has been suggested as a frequent cause of anxiety (44) and may antagonize the benzodiazepines in a similar manner. Regular users of **ethanol** are less sensitive to the effects of all sedatives, but ethanol will obviously have an additive sedative effect. Furthermore, ethanol enhances the absorption of diazepam (68a).

5. A clinician states that he always has excellent results when he prescribes phenobarbital (PB) or meprobamate for anxiety. He feels diazepam (Valium) is too expensive, and he has not had good results with it. Comment.

A recent double-blinded multicenter comparison of phenobarbital (134 mg daily mean), diazepam (20 mg

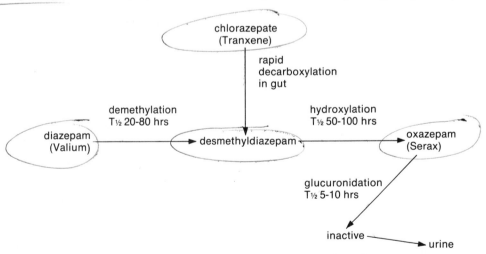

Fig. 1. Active Metabolites of Several Benzodiazepines. Desmethyldiazepam is an important pharmacologically active metabolite. Although the principal metabolites of chlordiazepoxide are desmethylchlordiazepoxide and demoxam, desmethyldiazepam was recently found to also be a major metabolite (37). Note that oxazepam has a short half-life without active metabolites; its chloro-analogue is lorazepam.

daily mean), and placebo in 241 ambulatory patients indicates that diazepam is superior to PB and that phenobarbital is only slightly more effective than placebo (30). Similar results have been observed elsewhere (52,96). An analysis of 26 controlled double-blind trials comparing meprobamate with placebo raised significant doubts as to its efficacy (45).

The explanation for this physician's clinical experience can be found in his attitudes toward these drugs. Placebo gives about a 50% successful response, compared with 70% for an effective drug when both are given with a neutral attitude. Since the placebo works as often as it fails, favorable attitudes toward ineffective or slightly effective drugs are reinforced. A positive attitude will then increase the response to these agents. Similarly, this physician's poor experience with diazepam can also be attributed to his attitude. In a study attempting to compare two antianxiety drugs with placebo in patients undergoing psychotherapy, 82% of the patients chose not to complete the study because the therapists discouraged the use of drugs. Consequently, the drug aspect of the study had to be discontinued even though 87% of the patients ultimately improved (165). Thus, attitude is an important determinant of minor tranquilizer response.

Meprobamate can cause serious physiological dependence after doses of 3.2 to 6.4 gm per day for 40 or more days (22,62). Both phenobarbital and meprobamate are more hazardous in suicide attempts than the benzodiazepines. Therefore, the benzodiazepines are the drugs of choice for anxiety. Cost is no longer an issue, since in many cases generic chlordiazepoxide can be used.

6. A 54-year-old well compensated cirrhotic male is nervous and restless. His laboratory data include: total bilirubin 2.8 mg%, alkaline phosphatase 120 IU/ml, SGOT 64 kU/ml, and plasma albumin 3.1 gm/100 ml. Can he be given diazepam (Valium)?

The half-life of diazepam in twenty-one patients with acute viral hepatitis, cirrhosis, or chronic active hepatitis was twice as long as age matched controls. This increase in half-life is due to a substantial decrease in hepatic extraction and occurs in spite of the increase in free drug available for metabolism due to lowered serum albumin (98). Therefore, with repeated doses diazepam will accumulate to abnormally high levels. Furthermore, the clearance of desmethyldiazepam is also decreased in liver disease (97a). Sedatives, particularly chlordiazepoxide, are frequent precipitating factors in hepatic coma (40). Chlordiazepoxide (60) and diazepam (93,162) share similar metabolic pathways, and both accumulate more than normally in liver disease. Flurazepam has not been studied well enough to allow comment. The hepatic

metabolism of other sedatives is discussed in the chapter on Diseases of the Liver.

Quantitative recommendations for dose reduction of diazepam are difficult, because the degree of impaired plasma clearance of diazepam cannot be correlated to any of the standard liver function tests (98,156). Another benzodiazepine, oxazepam (Serax), was eliminated normally in eleven patients with cirrhosis or acute viral hepatitis compared with age matched control subjects (161). Oxazepam is conjugated to a glucuronide metabolite that is pharmacologically inactive and is excreted by the kidney. Apparently, glucuronidation is less impaired in hepatocellular disease than are metabolic processes catalyzed by other enzymes. Interestingly, two of the cirrhotic patients in this study demonstrating normal disposition of oxazepam also participated in the earlier study on diazepam cited above (98).

Thus, oxazepam is an excellent choice for this patient. A dose of 15 mg every four hours as needed would be a reasonable start, although dosage must be individualized. It should be noted that cirrhotics can be exquisitely sensitive to sedatives. Nervousness due to impending hepatic coma or the early stages of alcohol withdrawal were ruled out in this patient, but these considerations should be applied to similar situations.

7. While the order for oxazepam (Serax) is being written for the above patient, it is decided that he requires the more immediate effects of a parenteral dose. Since oxazepam is only available in an oral dosage form, the intern plans on giving an intravenous dose of diazepam (Valium). He points out that accumulation is not a consideration for the first dose of drug. Are there any other considerations for this patient?

His albumin is low, and hypoalbuminemia can alter drug response. Diazepam is about 98% bound to plasma protein (91,98), and albumin is quantitatively the most important source of plasma binding for drugs (102). Small decreases in the plasma protein binding of highly bound benzodiazepines can result in large increases in the concentration of free drug. The amount of drug that gets into the central nervous system (CNS) is dependent upon the unbound or free portion in the plasma (91,164). Thus, subjects with low albumin have been found to have higher cerebrospinal fluid concentrations of chlordiazepoxide than normal subjects given the same dose (164).

The clinical significance of this phenomenon is supported by epidemiologic evidence from the Boston Collaborative Drug Surveillance Program. Unwanted CNS depression attributed to diazepam was significantly more frequent in patients with low serum albumin, and the incidence of this excess sedation was inversely proportional to albumin concentration, irrespective of the cause of hypoalbuminemia. The incidence of unwanted sedation from diazepam in the 1202 patients studied ranged from 2.9% in patients with serum albumin concentrations of 4.0 gm/100 ml or greater to 9.3% in patients having serum albumin levels less than 3.0 gm/100 ml. A similar trend was noted with chlordiazepoxide but did not reach statistical significance (48).

The protein binding of various benzodiazepines is compared in Table 1. Oxazepam is only 87% protein bound, and therefore it is little affected by changes in serum albumin. This topic is discussed further in the chapter on Clinical Pharmacokinetics where phenytoin is used as an example. In this case, it should be noted that the above epidemiologic evidence is based primarily on oral dosing, and the magnitude of free serum drug peaks should be even greater with intravenous administration.

This patient can be given intravenous diazepam even though he will be more sensitive than a healthier subject. Intravenous diazepam, 5 mg over 5 min, in 23 patients with relatively well compensated liver disease, produced electroencephalographic and clinical changes comparable to those seen in normal subjects; serum albumins were not reported (132). Diazepam is often used in high doses for cirrhotics undergoing alcohol withdrawal, and it is generally well tolerated. Limiting the dose to 2-5 mg and carefully observing clinical response should prevent any problems in this situation.

8. A student observes that diazepam (Valium) is frequently given intravenously (IV) to patients in the hospital. What precautions should be observed, and how safe is this route of administration?

Injectable diazepam is formulated with 40% propylene glycol and 10% ethyl alcohol because of its poor solubility in water. Addition of 10 mg (2 ml) of this formulation to 100 ml of 5% dextrose in water (D5W) produces *precipitation.* Visible precipitation is noted when this formulation is injected at a rate of 5 mg/min into an IV line of D5W running at 20 ml/min or normal saline running at 15 ml/min (105). Therefore, it should not be mixed with IV fluids or other drugs and must be injected directly into the vein. The rate of administration should be not greater than 5 mg (1 ml) per minute. Faster administration increases the risk of propylene glycol induced hypotension and arrhythmias (160). Small veins, such as the dorsum of the hand or wrist, should be avoided because of the greater risk of thrombophlebitis (110).

Of 173 hospitalized patients receiving IV diazepam, adverse reactions occurred in 6 patients. Three of these were *life threatening reactions* and included respiratory depression, hypotension, or coma. All oc-

curred in severely debilitated patients, some of whom were already experiencing CNS depression from other drugs. As a whole, the population studied was far from healthy; nearly 25% died while in the hospital. Twenty percent of the patients in this study were in their eighth decade or older. Therefore, it may be concluded that adverse reactions to IV diazepam are relatively infrequent even in the seriously ill. Hepatic decompensation, advanced cardiac or pulmonary disease, or concurrent administration of other CNS depressant drugs warrants special caution. (47)

A series of 1500 administrations of IV diazepam in a healthier population receiving the drug prior to gastrointestinal endoscopy resulted in thrombophlebitis as the only reported adverse reaction. *Thrombophlebitis* was associated with the use of small veins, and the overall incidence was 3.5 per cent (110). No IV injection is completely without hazard, but IV diazepam is relatively safe.

9. A patient recovering from abdominal surgery has an acute anxiety reaction while his incision is being examined. How effective would an intramuscular injection of diazepam be in this situation?

Because its poor water solubility requires special formulation for a parenteral dosage form, precipitation of diazepam may occur at the site of injection and cause slow or incomplete absorption (57). Many studies (10,41,71,90,121,162) have shown that oral administration results in faster and higher blood levels, with associated quicker and greater clinical effects, than the same dose given intramuscularly (IM). Therefore, an oral dose would be a better choice for this situation. If more immediate results are required, the IV route should be used.

10. Describe the parenteral dosage form of chlordiazepoxide (Librium). Does it offer any advantages over parenteral diazepam (Valium)?

Parenteral chlordiazepoxide is packaged as a powder that must be dissolved immediately prior to administration. Isomerization to a less active compound occurs in solution and in the presence of light. Therefore, any excess solution must be discarded. The 2 ml intramuscular diluent packaged with each ampule of chlordiazepoxide powder contains 20% propylene glycol, 4% polysorbate 80, 1.5% benzyl alcohol, 1.6% maleic acid and sodium hydroxide to adjust the pH to approximately 3. Like diazepam, absorption after IM injection is slower and less complete than after the same dose given orally (49). Also, IM injections are painful and increase serum creatine phosphokinase (58).

Chlordiazepoxide can be given intravenously by dissolving the powder with 5 ml sterile water for injection or normal saline and administering the solution over one minute. The manufacturer claims that a solution prepared with the IM diluent has been safely given intravenously, but it is not recommended because of air bubbles which form when this diluent is mixed with the powder. The intravenous solution cannot be given IM, because it is extremely painful.

Chlordiazepoxide is less lipid soluble than diazepam (Table 1). Therefore, it would be expected to enter the central nervous system (CNS) at a slower rate. A study comparing plasma and cerebrospinal fluid (CSF) concentrations of chlordiazepoxide after a 100 mg oral dose noted that plasma (free) and CSF levels equilibrated gradually over a two hour period (164). A somewhat analogous study with diazepam demonstrated complete equilibrium between free drug in plasma and drug in CSF within less than an hour after a 10 mg IM dose (91). Obviously, there were some differences between these two studies, but the evidence is adequate to conclude that chlordiazepoxide enters the CNS at a slower rate than diazepam. The marked preference that former heroin addicts express for oral diazepam over equipotent doses of chlordiazepoxide is, perhaps, further evidence of the more rapid passage of diazepam into the CNS (73). Thus, an intravenous dose of diazepam would be expected to have more immediate effect than an intravenous dose of chlordiazepoxide.

Therefore, parenteral chlordiazepoxide offers no advantage over diazepam. It is less rapidly acting, and preparation of the parenteral solution is inconvenient.

11. J.W. is a 76-year-old woman who has been hospitalized with a broken hip. She is alert and well oriented, but she is anxious. How should she be sedated?

Older subjects have greater inherent CNS sensitivity to sedatives. Other factors which may *increase* their response include decreased albumin, hepatic metabolism, renal function, and body weight. In contrast, an increased apparent volume of distribution will delay and prolong response (31). Chronological age is not a consistently reliable indicator of sensitivity to sedatives. Therefore, the degree of dosage reduction must be determined empirically (157).

Although diazepam is effective in geriatric patients (33), a significant increase in fatigue and decrease in memory have been observed in individuals taking 12 mg daily for two weeks (152). Muscle weakness and hypotension have also been observed (157). Still, the benzodiazepines are a better choice than the barbiturates, which frequently cause confusion and paradoxical excitement, or the phenothiazines, which are more effective in controlling symptoms of senility but have greater cardiovascular effects.

The incidence of excess sedation from diazepam or chlordiazepoxide increases significantly with age (21). Diazepam metabolism is little affected by age, but the apparent volume of distribution is progressively increased with age. The half-life increases in a linear fashion by approximately one hour for every year of age after the second decade (98). Thus, dosage is particularly hard to titrate in older individuals. Oxazepam is the best choice for geriatrics (125a), because its half-life is inherently short (Table 1) and is not affected by age (161).

Chloral hydrate is sometimes used as a hypnotic in the elderly because of its low potency. Fifteen milligrams of flurazepam (Dalmane) is widely used as hypnotic for elderly patients; however, larger doses should be used with caution, because patients over 70 years of age are at great risk of experiencing adverse reactions from 30 mg per day or more (60a). Oxazepam can be used as a hypnotic by giving two or three times the dose that is effective for daytime sedation.

12. Mrs. Jones is having a prescription for diazepam (Valium) filled at the community pharmacy. When told to be careful while driving, she becomes alarmed. She replies that she is dependent upon the use of her automobile. What basis is there for the pharmacist's warning?

Although the benzodiazepines have more specific antianxiety activity than barbiturates, meprobamate, or antihistamine sedatives, and thus cause less sedation, all of these drugs cause some general central nervous system depression. An extensive review of the effects of diazepam on psychomotor and cognitive functions (97) demonstrated measurable effects on a variety of laboratory parameters, but, as with other reviews of the effects of minor tranquilizers on performance (14,123), results were inconclusive and difficult to extrapolate to clinical situations. It has been suggested that neurotics may actually become better drivers while being treated with minor tranquilizers (14,72,117), but most laboratory studies use healthy volunteers as subjects. Also, most studies are short term and subjects are given a single dose or only a few doses.

A recent double-blind study using neurotic outpatients as subjects demonstrated that psychomotor performance was impaired by diazepam, 5 to 10 mg three times a day for two weeks as compared with placebo. Both drug and placebo groups improved with time, and differences between the diazepam and placebo groups tended to decrease over the two-week period even though drug blood levels were continually rising (146). Apparently, familiarity with the test and the drug effect improved performance. Thus, an activity as familiar as driving may be little affected by diazepam in subjects who are familiar with its effects.

However, the knowledge that alcohol consumption is associated with at least 50% of highway fatalities in the U. S. dictates some caution with all psychoactive drugs (72). At present there is no epidemiologic evidence correlating traffic accidents with minor tranquilizer use.

In spite of the limited useful information available, it can be concluded that diazepam does impair psychomotor performance to some degree, and this impairment is most significant in subjects unfamiliar with the drug. Mrs. Jones can drive her car, but she should be particularly cautious at first. She should not drive after consuming alcoholic beverages, because alcohol significantly increases psychomotor impairment caused by diazepam (97,116).

13. A 26-year-old woman in her eighth week of pregnancy has just read a magazine report identifying diazepam (Valium) as a cause of cleft lip and cleft palate. Because she has used the drug several times a week for the past six months, she is now seeking abortion counseling. How should she be advised? Are any of the other minor tranquilizers teratogenic?

Several retrospective studies have shown an association between oral clefts and maternal exposure to diazepam during the first trimester of pregnancy. When birth records from the Finnish Register of Congenital Malformation were analyzed, 27 of 599 mothers of children with oral clefts had taken benzodiazepines during the first trimester, as opposed to 13 of 590 matched control mothers of normal children (154,155). First trimester maternal exposure to diazepam was found in 6.1% (6 of 99 cases) of oral clefts in a Norwegian hospital, as compared with a 1.1% first trimester exposure rate among normal births reported by the Medical Birth Registry of Norway (1). Two hundred and seventy-eight mothers of infants with birth defects were interviewed in Atlanta. Exposure to diazepam during the first trimester was four times more frequent among mothers of children with cleft lip with or without cleft palate than among women who gave birth to infants with other defects (147). The associations noted in these studies could have been due to chance, but it is interesting that similar associations were noted by three separate groups of investigators. However, in a retrospective study in Hungary of 1377 birth defects, there was no difference in the frequency of diazepam exposure among mothers who delivered babies with oral clefts and those who delivered babies with other birth defects (35).

In a prospective study involving 19,044 live births there was a higher rate of birth anomalies for mothers exposed to meprobamate or chlordiazepoxide during the first 42 days of pregnancy. The rate of anomalies after exposure to meprobamate or chlordiazepoxide

was 12.1 per 100 and 11.4 per 100 respectively, whereas the rate of anomalies in children born of mothers taking no drug was 2.6 per 100. These data suggest that meprobamate and chlordiazepoxide may be teratogenic when taken during the first six weeks of pregnancy. Most of the birth defects involved the cardiovascular system; there were no cleft lips or palates (126). On the other hand, in a follow-up study of more than 50,000 pregnancies and their outcomes in twelve university hospitals from 1958 to 1966, there was no correlation between maternal use of meprobamate or chlordiazepoxide during any month of pregnancy and birth defects (68).

Although these studies are not conclusive, several of them suggest an association between in utero exposure to minor tranquilizers and fetal abnormalities. Therefore, the FDA has warned:

Since the use of these drugs during the first trimester of pregnancy is rarely a matter of urgency, benefit-risk considerations are such that their use during this period should almost always be avoided (7).

It should be noted that each of the studies cited above involved relatively small numbers of patients exposed to the drug, and other factors may have been responsible for the birth defects. This woman who is seeking abortion counseling should be told that casual relationships have yet to be established. Even if a four-fold increase in risk for cleft lip, with or without cleft palate, does exist, the absolute increased risk (from 0.1% to 0.4%) is very low. To place this risk in perspective, the overall risk of major anomalies at birth is 2% (148).

Since analogies to thalidomide will no doubt be made, it should be noted that the likelihood of birth defects from thalidomide taken between 35 and 50 days after menstruation is close to one hundred per cent (115). This woman's child is not at great risk. Even if the increased risk is real, it is so low that the effects of a two-fold increase in diazepam consumption by women in their first trimester of pregnancy would escape detection by the largest national defect monitoring program (148). Nevertheless, minor tranquilizers may be low level teratogens and should be avoided early in pregnancy.

14. N.L. has been taking chlordiazepoxide (Librium), 10 mg three times a day for the past two weeks. He has become increasingly argumentative with his wife, and at work he insulted his employer of ten years with unprecedented hostility. Could this be a drug effect?

The drug should be discontinued. Isolated cases of hostility induced by chlordiazepoxide and diazepam have been reported, but the occurrence of this side effect is infrequent (52). Oxazepam appears to be free of this side effect (151). This hostility reaction is different from the behavioral disinhibition that may be caused by any sedating drug.

In animals this effect occurs with chlordiazepoxide and diazepam but not with pentobarbital (112). Laboratory studies of college students have demonstrated that chlordiazepoxide, but not oxazepam, increases hostility as an inner affective state (43,103,149,150). These increases in hostility require sensitive psychological tests to be detected, but they are real and reproducible. Overt hostility is noted only in response to a frustrating stimulus (150).

Clinical reports of benzodiazepine-induced hostility are limited. It has been suggested that the psychopharmacological effects observed in college students in a laboratory setting cannot be extrapolated to anxious patients. When chlordiazepoxide was compared with placebo in 225 anxious neurotic outpatients, chlordiazepoxide was significantly more effective in reducing hostile, irritable, and anxious symptomatology. None of the drug treated patients experienced increased hostility (144).

This behavioral side effect is rare, although subclinical tendencies may exist. The precise incidence is unknown.

15. L.H. is a 55-year-old man who has just been admitted to the Coronary Care Unit with a myocardial infarction. His pain is being treated with intravenous morphine. Should he receive a sedative as well?

This is a clear indication for sedation. Complete rest is of great importance, and anxiety is a frequent occurrence (25). Morphine should be used only for pain and not for sedation because of possible adverse hemodynamic effects. The benzodiazepines may reduce the need for narcotics in these patients (61), and they are more effective and cause less cardiovascular effects than other sedatives (51,52).

If a decision is made to use oral anticoagulants, dosing will not be altered by prior or concomitant administration of benzodiazepines. This is not true for most other sedatives. For example, phenobarbital can induce the enzymes that metabolize oral anticoagulants to such a degree that the dosage requirement of oral anticoagulant may be doubled. If oral anticoagulant dosage is established while the patient is taking phenobarbital, prothrombin times will be markedly increased when the phenobarbital is stopped, and hemorrhage may occur (100). Antihistamines are the only other group of sedatives that can be safely used with oral anticoagulants, but they are considerably less effective than the benzodiazepines.

16. Phenobarbital 30 mg prn is ordered for a patient who is being stabilized on warfarin (Coumadin). How many doses will be required before metabolism is induced? Can a few doses per day be taken safely?

Two days of phenobarbital 210 mg per day significantly decreased the half-life of warfarin in 13 of 21 subjects (32). Induction may occur with only a few doses. Administration of phenobarbital for a week or more will stimulate microsomal enzymes in almost all subjects, but the degree of effect will vary from subject to subject; recovery time also varies, but two to three weeks is sufficient for most patients (100). A safe minimum dose cannot be recommended. Three weeks of treatment with only 60 mg per day has been demonstrated to have substantial effect (34). There is also some evidence that barbiturates may decrease the absorption of oral anticoagulants (2). Phenobarbital should be avoided in patients receiving oral anticoagulants.

17. N.W. is a 65-year-old 70 kg male with chronic obstructive pulmonary disease (COPD) recovering from a severe upper respiratory infection. On the day before his planned discharge from the hospital he observes the first parts of a successful but traumatic treatment of a cardiac arrest in his roommate. N.W. is now very anxious. His pH is 7.4, and his arterial blood gases are PO_2 65 mm Hg (normal 95-100) and PCO_2 50 mm Hg (normal 40). How hazardous are sedatives in this situation?

Although the benzodiazepines cause less respiratory depression than other sedatives, their use in patients with respiratory disease must be approached with considerable caution, since they can precipitate respiratory failure.

In a study of six patients with COPD with mean P_aO_2 of 60 mm Hg and a P_aCO_2 of 49 mm Hg there was no change in arterial blood gases or pulmonary function after five days of oral diazepam, 10 mg qid (106). Ten patients with COPD given diazepam in doses of 0.11 mg/kg IV, showed slight respiratory depression: mean P_aO_2 fell from 67 to 65.6 mm Hg and P_aCO_2 rose from 38 to 41.4 mm Hg (26). Large doses of diazepam, 0.5 mg/kg, in eighteen patients with COPD also produced slight respiratory depression: mean P_aO_2 fell from 70 to 65 mm Hg and P_aCO_2 rose from 43 to 49 mm Hg; these changes are comparable to those seen during sleep in this patient population (141). Although there was considerable variation in response among patients, these data suggest that a few oral doses of a benzodiazepine will be safe in this patient if he is carefully observed. Diazepam should be used for the initial dose because of its rapid onset. Oxazepam would be a good choice for subsequent doses, because its short-half life will allow effects to dissipate rapidly when it is stopped.

The hazard of respiratory depression from sedatives, including benzodiazepines, should not be dismissed. Diazepam decreases the ventilatory response to hypoxia even in healthy subjects (109). Chlordiazepoxide 10 mg tid po for three days can cause significant deterioration in patients already in respiratory failure (128). Furthermore, hypoxia is a frequent cause of anxiety in obstructive pulmonary disease; in such cases, the use of sedatives is both inappropriate and dangerous.

18. What is insomnia, and when should it be treated with hypnotic drugs?

Individuals vary widely in their sleep requirements. Most adults average about seven and a half hours sleep per night, but some healthy subjects require less than three hours, while others require more than nine. Sleep tends to become more fragmented with age (75,77).

Insomnia is therefore subjective; it is the individual experience of inadequate sleep. It is experienced as difficulty in falling asleep, difficulty in staying asleep, or premature awakening. These problems may occur separately or in concert. (83)

There are many causes of insomnia; hypnotic drugs alleviate the symptoms but do not correct the underlying defect (46). Medical causes of insomnia, such as pain, nocturia, hypoxia, or pulmonary congestion, should receive more specific treatment. Severe psychiatric illnesses, such as schizophrenia or primary (endogenous) depression, often manifest with symptoms of insomnia. In these cases, specific treatment with phenothiazines or tricyclic antidepressants is more rational than hypnotics which may cause further deterioration. Drug-induced insomnia, such as that caused by caffeine, or the early morning effects of a previous evening's excess with alcoholic beverages, or an evening dose of diuretic, is easily remedied without hypnotics.

The physical and emotional discomfort experienced in hospitalization is a common cause of insomnia and constitutes a valid indication for hypnotic drug therapy. Insomnia is the second most common indication for drug therapy in hospitalized patients (127). Temporary insomnia caused by stressful life events is normal (130); a few doses of hypnotic are often considered rational and safe (50,129). Chronic insomnia is generally the result of an underlying emotional disturbance, and psychiatric evaluation is preferable to hypnotic drug treatment (77,83).

19. B.W. is a 53-year-old 75 kg male who is entering the hospital for repair of an inguinal hernia. Which hypnotic should he receive if he is unable to sleep during his hospital stay?

In this case there is little basis for selection of any particular hypnotic. When given in equipotent doses for a few nights all nonproprietary hypnotics are equally effective in promoting and maintaining sleep, and all have similar potential for hangover (46,50, 111,174). However, in most circumstances, as illustrated in the questions below, flurazepam (Dalmane) is the hypnotic of choice (55).

20. L.M. is a 58-year-old 68 kg man who is entering the hospital for a total hip replacement. Which hypnotic should he receive during his hospital stay?

Since he will be in the hospital longer than a few nights, he should receive a hypnotic that remains effective with continued use. Sleep laboratory studies have demonstrated that chloral hydrate 1 gm and glutethimide (Doriden) 500 mg begin to lose their effectiveness after a few nights and are ineffective after 10 nights (81). Similar studies have demonstrated that pentobarbital (Nembutal) 100 gm and secobarbital (Seconal) 100 mg are ineffective after two weeks of continued use (84,87). Flurazepam (Dalmane) 30 mg, on the other hand, is effective when given nightly for as long as four weeks (84). Other hypnotics have not yet been evaluated for long term effectiveness.

Therefore, flurazepam (Dalmane) is the drug of choice for this patient; a 30 mg dose is consistently effective (53,55).

21. A 66-year-old woman is being stabilized on warfarin (Coumadin). It is noted that she received a 100 mg dose of secobarbital last night. Will her prothrombin time be affected?

It is unlikely that this single dose will have any effect. One or two doses of barbiturate hypnotic produced no alteration in the prothrombin times of 27 patients taking oral anticoagulants (153). Animal studies indicate that secobarbital and pentobarbital are less potent stimulators of microsomal enzymes than phenobarbital (170). However, repeated doses of secobarbital significantly increase the rate of warfarin metabolism (145). Therefore, the drug should be discontinued. Glutethimide (Doriden) is a potent inducer of microsomal enzymes. The effect of chloral hydrate on oral anticoagulant dosing is discussed in the chapter on Thrombosis.

If this patient requires a hypnotic, she should be given a benzodiazepine or an antihistamine sedative. Diphenhydramine (Benadryl) 50 mg is sometimes used in this situation. Fifty mg is an effective dose (74,159) and doubling this does not improve the hypnotic efficacy of this agent (168). There is a similar lack of dose-response with hydroxyzine (Vistaril, Atarax) (24). Fifty mg of either of these antihistamines are approximately equal to 60 mg of pentobarbital (24,168), an appropriate dose for this 66-year-old woman. If she requires greater hypnotic effect, flurazepam (Dalmane) 30 mg should be given.

22. What are the sleep stages and REM, and what is their significance in the clinical use of hypnotics?

When the normal sleep of a young adult is studied under laboratory conditions with an electroencephalogram (EEG), the following patterns are noted. When the subject falls asleep, the EEG tracings are of low amplitude and high frequency. As sleep progresses, the amplitude increases and the frequency decreases. This process is described in terms of stages, beginning with stage 1 and progressing to stage 4, the deepest stage, which is characterized by high amplitude low frequency waves. Once stage 4 is reached, the pattern reverses, and stages 3, 2, and 1 are seen. Return to stage 1 is usually followed by a period of *rapid eye movements (REM)*. REM sleep is associated with dreaming and is sometimes referred to as D sleep. This entire cycle occurs over an interval of about ninety minutes and is repeated four or five times during a single night's sleep. Stage 4 is often absent in subsequent cycles. Stage 4 sleep also decreases with age. About 25% of normal sleep is spent in REM sleep (83).

Most hypnotics decrease REM sleep. On subsequent nights with repeated administration, this suppression is attenuated but remains below the baseline level. When the hypnotic is stopped, there is a marked increase in REM sleep well above normal baseline levels. This **REM rebound** has been associated with increased dreaming, nightmares, and frequent wakening (65,77,82,83,137). Patients experiencing these symptoms may continue to take hypnotics in an attempt to prevent insomnia and disturbed sleep caused by hypnotic withdrawal; thus, a "sleeping pill" habit is created.

REM rebound has been demonstrated after three nights of treatment with pentobarbital (Nembutal), glutethimide (Doriden), methyprylon (Noludar), and methaqualone (Quaalude, Sopor) 300 mg but not 150 mg (79,80). Flurazepam (Dalmane) 15 and 30 mg and chloral hydrate 500 and 1000 mg cause small amounts of REM suppression, but significant REM rebound has not been demonstrated with these drugs (67,77,80,86). Flurazepam 60 mg causes significant REM suppression, but REM rebound does not occur (80), probably because of the half-life of its active metabolite is long. One study demonstrated significant REM suppression with 800 mg chloral hydrate, but significant rebound was not noted (38). Ethyl alcohol depresses REM, and rebound may occur during the later part of the night (99).

This information is based on sleep laboratory studies on a relatively small number of subjects, most of whom were young healthy males. The nature of sleep laboratory studies is such that patient samples must be small. Huge amounts of polygraph data are produced by a single subject in a single night, and the entire readout must be scored manually by a technician. Although there are clinical reports to substantiate this phenomenon (77,82,137) and reviews on drug dependency give credence to it (78,95,138), some authorities (111,129) suggest that withdrawal insomnia is not a frequent complication in the clinical use of barbiturate and other REM suppressant hypnotics. However, it is a good argument against their use. Therefore, flurazepam and chloral hydrate have an advantage over other hypnotics.

It has been suggested that some medical conditions, such as coronary artery disease and duodenal ulcer, may benefit from the effects of REM suppressant hypnotics, but findings are inconsistent. Furthermore, REM suppression abates with continued use, and the effects of REM rebound when hypnotics are discontinued have not been evaluated. Also, the clinical importance of any particular stage of sleep has not yet been determined. However, REM rebound is of concern because it may be a factor in inducing dependence on barbiturates and other REM suppressant hypnotics (83).

23. E.W. is a 54-year-old woman who brings the following prescription to her community pharmacist: Nembutal 100 mg, #60, Sig: i hs for sleep. On consulting her medication profile it appears that she has been taking secobarbital, pentobarbital, or glutethimide at an average rate of two doses per night for the last three months since the profile was begun. When asked about this, she explains that she is unable to sleep without medications. Her sleeping problem began nearly two years ago when she was hospitalized for a cholecystectomy. She continued to take the sleeping pills that were given to her on discharge from the hospital, because they had helped her, and she felt they would insure the rest needed for a good recovery. She has stopped taking them on several occasions, but each time she has been plagued by difficulty in falling asleep and frequent wakenings. She has maintained a supply from several physicians at her insistence that normal sleep is impossible without them. She attributes the problem to a unique hormonal imbalance not fully appreciated by any physician she has seen. Comment.

Sleeping pill withdrawal insomnia is well documented (77,82,137), but the incidence is unknown. The mechanism of induction of this dependence is outlined in the previous question. Symptoms similar to those experienced by this patient have been produced experimentally in healthy subjects (77).

At this point hypnotics are merely preventing withdrawal symptoms. In a sleep laboratory study which compared ten patients who had consumed hypnotics regularly over periods ranging from months to years with ten insomniac controls, the group taking drugs had equal or greater difficulty in falling and staying asleep than the insomniac controls (82).

E.W. should not be withdrawn abruptly because of the unpleasant effects that would occur. One therapeutic dose should be withdrawn every five or six nights, and she should be informed that increased dreaming, vivid dreams, and possibly nightmares may occur, but this effect is transient. If complete withdrawal is difficult, flurazepam may be substituted (82).

This case illustrates the importance of monitoring and limiting the duration of hypnotic use. Patients who are encouraged to limit their hypnotic use are significantly more likely to do so than those who are given no instructions (29). REM suppressant hypnotics should be avoided in outpatients. Flurazepam is the hypnotic of choice.

24. H.H. is a 40-year-old 60 kg woman who has been experiencing insomnia since last week when her husband was diagnosed with leukemia. A friend gave her a secobarbital (Seconal) 100 mg capsule, and although it gave her a good night's sleep, it left her dizzy the following day. Would chloral hydrate be a good choice for this patient? How does hypnotic dosage affect response?

Chloral hydrate's reputation as a short-acting drug is based on the relatively low potency of the 0.5 to 1 gm doses that are generally used; these doses will induce sleep but will not reliably maintain it. Larger doses may cause gastrointestinal upset. Although sleep laboratory studies have shown chloral hydrate 500 mg to be both effective (67) and ineffective (80) in normal subjects, controlled (74) and epidemiologic (159) studies in hospitalized patients indicate that 0.5 gm is an effective dose. However, chloral hydrate 1 gm is less effective than secobarbital 100 mg (142). Therefore, chloral hydrate in doses of 0.5 to 1 gm is a mild hypnotic that is effective early in the night but exerts little effect later in the night; it rapidly becomes ineffective with continued use (79,81). Thus, it offers no advantage over a small dose of flurazepam; furthermore, the latter drug is effective with prolonged use and has a larger therapeutic index.

H.H.'s experience with secobarbital illustrates the importance of dosage. Dose may be as important in determining the duration of action of a hypnotic as the choice of drug. On this basis, it has been suggested that the classification of hypnotics as short, intermediate, or long acting may be misleading (120,174). Most hypnotics are metabolized relatively slowly, and redistribution contributes to termination of their effect. For example, secobarbital is a short to intermediate acting barbiturate, but its half-life is 29 hours (28). A 50 mg dose may have been satisfactory for this patient, but rapid loss of effectiveness (Question 20), risk of habituation due to REM suppression and rebound

(Questions 22 and 23), and high suicide potential make barbiturates poor choices for outpatients.

Diazepam has a long half-life and active metabolites, but because it is rapidly redistributed from the CNS to other tissues, it is a short-acting drug. Therefore, 10 mg will induce sleep but will not cause a hangover. Larger doses will have a greater effect later in the night and will help maintain sleep. The hypnotic efficacy of diazepam and flurazepam have not been directly compared, but 10 mg of diazepam is probably about equal to 15 mg of flurazepam. These doses of flurazepam are about half as expensive.

Although flurazepam produces residual effects with the same frequency as equipotent doses of barbiturate and other hypnotics, the subjective quality of the hangover is considerably less unpleasant (20,63). Continued effectiveness with repeated use, ability to produce a good approximation of normal sleep, low suicide potential, and residual antianxiety effect are additional factors supporting the use of flurazepam. She should be given 15 mg capsules with instructions to take one and repeat in an hour if needed. She should be cautioned that food will delay absorption and thereby decrease early night effectiveness and increase the likelihood of hangover (76). Alcohol will increase the residual effects of flurazepam (125), and, of course, no sedative should be taken in conjunction with large amounts of ethanol. Flurazepam has a very short half-life, but its principal metabolite is active and has a half-life of 50 to 100 hours (53). Therefore, previous use will affect response. Flurazepam 30 mg is more effective on the second night than on the first night of administration, and when it is stopped after repeated use, it is still effective on the first withdrawal night (86).

25. A middle-aged man asks the community pharmacist to recommend a mild sedative. He was laid off his job last month, and ever since then, he has been having difficulty sleeping and is sometimes anxious during the day. What recommendations can be made?

Non-prescription sedatives, usually containing methapyrilene and scopolamine are widely used, but their effectiveness is questionable. In a double-blind trial in anxious outpatients seen in general medical practice Compoz was significantly less effective than low doses of chlordiazepoxide and no different from placebo (143). Sominex, which is methapyrilene 25 mg and scopolamine 0.25 mg, contains more drug per tablet than most non-prescription sedatives, but two tablets were no different from placebo in sleep laboratory studies of subjects with chronic insomnia (88). Methapyrilene 50 mg has been shown less effective than diphenhydramine 50 mg and no different from placebo as a hypnotic in hospitalized patients (168).

Products containing a combination of antihistamine and analgesic have been shown more effective than placebo in subjects with pain and insomnia (163,167), and one study found such a combination effective as a hypnotic in subjects without pain (177). These products are at best only marginally effective. Most health professionals think of bromides only in their historical context, but they are still available in proprietary remedies, and reports of bromide intoxication continue to appear in the literature (122).

There is little basis for recommending non-prescription sedatives. The effects of exercise or a hot bath or shower are more beneficial. An interesting sleep laboratory study (23) demonstrated a hot milk beverage to be significantly more effective than a lactose capsule identified as a folk remedy in subjects 42 to 66 years of age. The warm beverage was less effective in younger subjects.

REFERENCES

1. Aarskog D: Association between maternal intake of diazepam and oral clefts. Lancet 2:921, 1975.
2. Aggeler PM: Effect of heptabarbital on the response to bishydroxycoumarin in man. J Lab Clin Med 74:229, 1969.
3. Anon: Antianxiety drugs in organic and functional syndromes. Medical Letter 14:93, 1972.
4. Anon: Diazepam (Valium) in hypertension. Medical Letter 16:96, 1974.
5. Anon: Are our barbiturates really necessary? Brit Med J 3:285, 1975.
6. Anon: Barbiturates on the way out. Brit Med J 3:725, 1975.
7. Anon: Teratogenicity of minor tranquilizers. FDA Drug Bulletin 5:14, 1975.
8. Anon: Are barbiturates obsolete as hypnotics and sedatives? Drug Ther Bull 14:7, 1976.
9. Ayd FJ: Oxazepam: an overview. Dis Nerv Syst 36 (sect 2):14, 1975.
10. Baird ES et al: Delayed recovery from a sedative: correlation of the plasma levels of diazepam with clinical effects after oral and intravenous administration. Brit J Anaesth 44:803, 1972.
11. Balter MB et al: Cross-national study of the extent of antianxiety/sedative drug use. NEJM 290:769, 1974.
12. Barraclough BM: Barbiturate prescribing: psychiatrists' views. Brit Med J 2:927, 1976.
13. Benson WH: Comparative evaluation of diazepam (Valium) and phenobarbital. J M A Georgia 60:276, 1971.
14. Berger FM et al: The effect of antianxiety tranquilizers on the behavior of normal persons, in *Psychopharmacology of the Normal Human* (Evans and Kline, ets). Chas C Thomas, Springfield, Ill 1969.
15. Bielman P et al: Flurazepam: study of its hypnotic properties in normal subjects. Int J Clin Pharmacol 6:13, 1972.
16. Blackwell B: Psychotropic drugs in use today. The role of diazepam in medical practice. JAMA 225:1637, 1973.
17. Blackwell B: Minor tranquilizers: use, misuse or overuse? Psychosomatics 16:28, 1975.
18. Blackwell B: Rational drug use in the management of anxiety. Rational Drug Ther 9:1, June 1975.
19. Blackwell B: A critical review of oxazepam: efficacy and specificity. Dis Nerv Syst 36(sect 2):17, 1975.
20. Bond JA et al: The residual effects of flurazepam. Psychopharmacol 32:223, 1973.
21. Boston Collaborative Drug Surveillance Program: Clinical depression of the central nervous system due to chlordiazepoxide in relation to cigarette smoking and age. NEJM 288:277, 1973.
22. Braun J et al: Anxiety, neurosis, depressive disorder and meprobamate addiction. West J Med 123:115, 1975.
23. Brezinova V et al: Sleep after a bedtime beverage. Brit Med J 2:431, 1972.
24. Brown CR et al: The oral hypnotic bioassay of hydroxyzine and pentobarbital for nighttime sedation. J Clin Pharmacol 14:210, 1974.
25. Cassem NH et al: Psychiatric consultation in a coronary care unit. Ann Int Med 75:9, 1971.
26. Catchlove RFH et al: The effects of diazepam on respiration in patients with obstructive pulmonary disease. Anesthesiol 34:14, 1971.
27. Chambers CD et al: *Chemical Coping.* Spectrum Publications, New York 1975.
28. Clifford JM et al: Absorption and clearance of secobarbital, heptabarbital, methaqualone, and ethinamate. Clin Pharm Ther 16:376, 1974.
29. Clift AD: Factors leading to dependence on hypnotic drugs. Brit Med J 3:614, 1972.
30. Cohen J et al: Diazepam and phenobarbital in the treatment of anxiety: a controlled multicenter study using physician and patient rating scales. Curr Ther Res 20:184, 1976.
31. Cooks J et al: Pharmacokinetics in the elderly. Clin Pharmacokinetics 1:280, 1976.
32. Corn M: Effect of phenobarbital and glutethimide on biological half-life of warfarin. Thromb Diath Haem 16:605, 1966.
33. Covinton JS: Alleviating agitation, apprehension, and related symptoms in geriatric patients. Southern Med J 68:719, 1975.
34. Cucinell SA et al: Lowering effect of phenobarbital on plasma levels of bishydroxycoumarin and diphenylhydantoin. Clin Pharm Ther 6:420, 1965.
35. Czeizel A: Diazepam, phenytoin, and aetiology of cleft lip and/or cleft palate. Lancet 1:810, 1976.
36. Dasberg HH et al: Plasma concentrations of diazepam and its metabolite N-desmethyldiazepam in relation to anxiolytic effect. Clin Pharm Ther 15:473, 1974.
37. Dixon R et al: N-desmethyldiazepam: a new metabolite of chlordiazepoxide in man. Clin Pharm Ther 20:450, 1976.
38. Evans JI et al: Sleep and hypnotics: further experiments. Brit Med J 3:310-313, 1974.
39. Faraj BA: Hypertyraminemia in cirrhotic patients. NEJM 294:1360, 1976.
40. Fessel JM: An analysis of the causes and prevention of hepatic coma. Gastroent 62:191, 1972.
41. Gamble JAS et al: Plasma diazepam levels after single dose oral and intramuscular administration. Anaesthesia 30:164, 1975.
42. Gardner EA: Implications of psychoactive drug therapy. NEJM 290:800, 1974.
43. Gardos G et al: Differential actions of chlordiazepoxide and oxazepam on hostility. Arch Gen Psych 18:757, 1968.
44. Greden JF: Anxiety or caffeinism: a diagnostic dilemma. Am J Psychiat 131:1089, 1974.
45. Greenblatt DJ et al: Meprobamate: a study of irrational drug use. Am J Psychiat 127:1297, 1971.
46. Greenblatt DJ et al: The clinical choice of sedative-hypnotics. Ann Int Med 77:91, 1972.
47. Greenblatt DJ et al: Adverse reactions to intravenous diazepam: a report from the Boston Drug Surveillance Program. Amer J Med Sci 266:261, 1973.
48. Greenblatt DJ et al: Clinical toxicity of chlordiazepoxide and diazepam in relation to serum albumin concentration: a report from the Boston Collaborative Drug Surveillance Program. Europ J Clin Pharmacol 7:259, 1974.
49. Greenblatt DJ et al: Slow absorption of intramuscular chlordiazepoxide. NEJM 291:1116, 1974.
50. Greenblatt DJ et al: Rational use of psychotropic drugs: hypnotics. Amer J Hosp Pharm 31:990, 1974.
51. Greenblatt DJ et al: Benzodiazepines. NEJM 291:1011 and 1239, 1974.
52. Greenblatt DJ et al: *Benzodiazepines in Clinical Practice.* Raven Press, New York 1974.
53. Greenblatt DJ et al: Flurazepam hydrochloride. Clin Pharm Ther 17:1, 1975.
54. Greenblatt DJ et al: Pharmacokinetics in clinical medicine: oxazepam versus other benzodiazepines. Dis Nerv Syst 36(sect 2): 6, 1975.

55. Greenblatt DJ et al: Flurazepam hydrochloride, a benzodiazepine hypnotic. Ann Int Med 83:237, 1975.

56. Greenblatt DJ et al: Influence of magnesium and aluminum hydroxide mixture on chlordiazepoxide absorption. Clin Pharm Ther 19:234, 1976.

57. Greenblatt DJ et al: Intramuscular injection of drugs. NEJM 295:542, 1976.

58. Greenblatt DJ et al: Serum creatine phosphokinase concentrations after intramuscular chlordiazepoxide and its solvent. J Clin Pharmacol 16:118, 1976.

59. Greenblatt DJ et al: Clinical pharmacokinetics of lorazepam. Clin Pharm Ther 20:329, 1976.

60. Greenblatt DJ et al: Clinical pharmacokinetics of chlordiazepoxide, in Pharmacokinetics of Psychoactive Drugs (Gottschalk and Merlis, eds). Spectrum Publications, New York 1976.

60a. Greenblatt DJ et al: Toxicity of high-dose flurazepam in the elderly. Clin Pharmacol Ther 21:355, 1977.

61. Hackett TP et al: Reduction of anxiety in the coronary-care unit: a controlled double-blind comparison of chlordiazepoxide and amobarbital. Curr Ther Res 14:649, 1972.

62. Haizlip TM et al: Meprobamate habituation. NEJM 258:1181, 1958.

63. Harper CR et al: Aviator performance and the use of hypnotic drugs. Aerospace Med 43:197, 1972.

64. Hart J et al: The effects of low doses of amylobarbitone sodium and diazepam on human performance. Brit J Clin Pharmacol 3:289, 1976.

65. Hartmann E: Pharmacological studies of sleep and dreaming: chemical and clinical relationships. Biol Psychiat 1:243, 1969.

66. Hartmann E et al: The effects of long term administration of psychotropic drugs on human sleep: the effects of chlordiazepoxide. Psychopharmacolog 33:233, 1973.

67. Hartmann E et al: The effects of long term administration of psychotropic drugs on human sleep: the effects of chloral hydrate. Psychopharmacolog 33:219, 1973.

68. Hartz SC et al: Antenatal exposure to meprobamate and chlordiazepoxide in relation to malformations, mental development, and childhood mortality. NEJM 292:726, 1975.

68a. Hayes SL et al: Ethanol and oral diazepam absorption. NEJM 296:186, 1977.

69. Heinonen J et al: The effect of diazepam on airway resistance in asthmatics. Anaesthes 27:37, 1972.

70. Hemminki E: Diseases leading to psychotropic drug therapy. Scand J Soc Med 2:129, 1974.

71. Hillestad L et al: Diazepam metabolism in normal man. Clin Pharm Ther 16:479 and 485, 1974.

72. Hollister LE: Psychotherapeutic drugs and driving. Ann Int Med 80:413, 1974.

73. Inaba DS: Personal communication, Haight Ashbury Free Medical Clinic, San Francisco.

74. Jick H et al: Clinical effects of hypnotics; a controlled trial. JAMA 209:2013, 1969.

75. Johns MW: Sleep and hypnotic drugs. Drugs 9:448, 1975.

76. Johnson PC et al: Nonfasting state and the absorption of a hypnotic. Arch Int Med 131:199, 1973.

77. Kagan F et al: Brook Lodge Conference on Hypnotics. Spectrum Publications, New York 1975.

78. Kales A et al: Drug dependency; investigations of stimulants and depressants. Ann Int Med 70:591, 1969.

79. Kales A et al: Hypnotics and altered sleep-dream patterns; all night EEG studies of glutethimide, methyprylon, and pentobarbital. Arch Gen Psychiat 23:211, 1970.

80. Kales A et al: All-night EEG studies of chloral hydrate, flurazepam, and methaqualone. Arch Gen Psychiat 23:219, 1970.

81. Kales A et al: Hypnotic drugs and their effectiveness; all-night EEG studies of insomniac subjects. Arch Gen Psychiat 23:226, 1970.

82. Kales A et al: Chronic hypnotic-drug use; ineffectiveness, drug-withdrawal insomnia, and dependence. JAMA 227:513, 1974.

83. Kales A et al: Sleep disorders. NEJM 290:487, 1974.

84. Kales A et al: Effectiveness of drugs with prolonged use: flurazepam and pentobarbital. Clin Pharm Ther 18:356, 1975.

85. Kales A et al: Shortcomings in the evaluation and promotion of hypnotic drugs. NEJM 293:826, 1975.

86. Kales A et al: Sleep laboratory studies of flurazepam: a model for evaluating hypnotic drugs. Clin Pharm Ther 19:576, 1976.

87. Kales A et al: Effectiveness of intermediate-term use of secobarbital. Clin Pharm Ther 20:541, 1976.

88. Kales J et al: Are over-the-counter sleep medications effective? All-night EEG studies. Curr Ther Res 13:143, 1971.

89. Kane FJ: Current use of hypnotic drugs — is it rational? Southern Med J 63:376, 1970.

90. Kanto J: Plasma concentrations of diazepam and its metabolites after peroral, intramuscular, and rectal administration. Int J Clin Pharmacol 12:427, 1976.

91. Kanto J et al: Cerebrospinal-fluid concentrations of diazepam and its metabolites in man. Acta Pharmacol Toxicol 36:328, 1975.

92. Kaplan SA et al: Blood level profile in man following chronic oral administration of flurazepam hydrochloride. J Pharm Sci 62:1932, 1973.

93. Kaplan SA et al: Pharmacokinetic profile of diazepam in man following single intravenous and oral and chronic oral administrations. J Pharm Sci 62:1789, 1973.

94. Katz RL: Sedatives and tranquilizers. NEJM 286:757, 1972.

95. Kay DC: Sleep and some psychoactive drugs. Psychosomatics 14:108, 1973.

96. Klein DF et al: Review of minor tranquilizer literature, in Diagnosis and Drug Treatment of Psychiatric Disorders. Williams & Wilkins, Baltimore 1969.

97. Kleinknecht RA et al: A review of the effects of diazepam on cognitive and psychomotor performance. J Nerv Ment Dis 161:399, 1975.

97a. Klotz U et al: Disposition of diazepam and its major metabolite desmethyldiazepam in patients with liver disease. Clin Pharmacol Ther 21:430, 1977.

98. Klotz U et al: The effects of age and liver disease on the disposition and elimination of diazepam in adult man. J Clin Invest 55:347, 1975.

99. Knowles JB et al: Effects of alcohol on REM sleep. Q J Stud Alcohol 29:342, 1968.

100. Koch-Weser J et al: Drug interactions with coumarin anticoagulants. NEJM 285:487 and 547, 1971.

101. Koch-Weser J et al: The archaic barbiturate hypnotics. NEJM 291:790, 1974.

102. Koch-Weser J et al: Binding of drugs to serum albumin. NEJM 294:311 and 526, 1976.

103. Kochanski GE et al: The differential effects of chlordiazepoxide and oxazepam on hostility in a small group setting. Am J Psychiat 132:861, 1975.

104. Koppelman MS: Metabolism of benzodiazepines. NEJM 288:917, 1973.

105. Korttila K et al: Polyethylene glycol as a solvent for diazepam: bioavailability and clinical effects after intramuscular administration, comparison of oral, intramuscular and rectal administration, and precipitation from intravenous solutions. Acta Pharmacol Toxicol 39:104, 1976.

106. Kronenberg RS et al: The use of oral diazepam in patients with obstructive lung disease and hypercapnia. Ann Int Med 83:83, 1975.

107. Lader M: The nature of anxiety. Brit J Psychiat 121:481, 1972.

108. Lader MH et al: Residual effects of hypnotics. Psychopharmacolog 25:117, 1972.

109. Lakshminarayan S et al: Effect of diazepam on ventilatory responses. Clin Pharmacol Ther 20:178, 1976.

110. Langdon DE et al: Thrombophlebitis with diazepam used intravenously. JAMA 223:184, 1973.

111. Lasagna L: Hypnotic drugs. NEJM 287:1182, 1972.

112. Leaf RC et al: Chlordiazepoxide and diazepam induced mouse killing by rats. Psychopharmacolog 44:23, 1975.

113. Lehmann HE et al: Pharmacotherapy of Tension and Anxiety. Chas C Thomas, Springfield Ill 1970.

114. Lennard HL et al: Hazards implicit in prescribing psychoactive drugs. Science 169:438, 1970.

115. Lenz W: Malformations caused by drugs in pregnancy. Amer J Dis Child 112:99, 1966.

116. Linnoila M et al: Drug interaction on psychomotor skills related to driving: diazepam and alcohol. Europ J Clin Pharmacol 5:186, 1973.

117. Linnoila M: Effect of drugs and alcohol on psychomotor skills related to driving. Ann Clin Res 6:7, 1974.

118. Manheimer DI et al: Popular attitudes and beliefs about tran-

quilizers. Am J Psychiat 130:1246, 1973.

119. Marjerrison G et al: Comparitive psychophysiological and mood effects of diazepam and dipotassium chlorazepate. Biol Psychiat 7:31, 1973.

120. Mark LC: Archaic classification of barbiturates. Clin Pharm Ther 10:287, 1969.

121. McCaughey W et al: Comparison of the sedative effects of diazepam given by the oral and intramuscular routes. Brit J Anaesth 44:901, 1972.

122. McDanal CE et al: Bromide abuse: a continuing problem. Am J Psychiat 131:913, 1974.

123. McNair DM: Antianxiety drugs and human performance. Arch Gen Psychiat 29:611, 1973.

124. Mellinger GD et al: Patterns of psychotherapeutic drug use among adults in San Francisco. Arch Gen Psychiat 25:385, 1971.

125. Mendelson WB et al: The morning after: residual EEG effects of triazolam and flurazepam, alone and in combination with alcohol. Curr Ther Res 19:155, 1976.

125a. Merlis S et al: The use of oxazepam in elderly patients. Dis Nerv Syst 36(sect 2):27, 1975.

126. Milkovich L et al: Effects of prenatal meprobamate and chlordiazepoxide hydrochloride on human embryonic and fetal development. NEJM 291:1268, 1974.

127. Miller RR: Drug surveillance utilizing epidemiologic methods; a report from the Boston Collaborative Drug Surveillance Program. Amer J Hosp Pharm 30:584, 1973.

128. Model DG: Effects of chlordiazepoxide in respiratory failure due to chronic bronchitis. Lancet 2:869, 1974.

129. Modell W: Updating the sleeping pill. Geriatrics 29:126, 1974.

130. Moriarty JD: Insomnia: often a therapeutic challenge. Dis Nerv Syst 36:279, 1975.

131. Muller C: The overmedicated society: forces in the marketplace for medical care. Science 176:488, 1972.

132. Murray-Lyon LM et al: Clinical and electroencephalographic assessment of diazepam in liver disease. Brit Med J 4:265, 1971.

133. National Commission on Marijuana and Drug Abuse: *Drug Use in America: Problem in Perspective,* final report, US Government Printing Office 1973.

134. Nelson, MM et al: Associations between drugs administered during pregnancy and congenital abnormalities of the fetus. Brit Med J 1:523, 1971.

135. Nicholson AN et al: Effect of N-desmethyldiazepam (nordiazepam) and a precursor, potassium chlorazepate, on sleep in man. Brit J Clin Pharmacol 3:429, 1976.

136. O'Reilly RA et al: Determinants of the response to oral anticoagulant drugs in man. Pharmacol Rev 22:35, 1970.

137. Oswald I et al: Five weeks to escape the sleeping-pill habit. Brit Med J 2:1093, 1965.

138. Oswald I: Dependence upon hypnotic and sedative drugs. Brit J Psychiat (spec pub 9): 272, 1975.

139. Parry HJ et al: National patterns of psychotherapeutic drug use. Arch Gen Psychiat 28:769, 1973.

140. Peck AW et al: Residual effects of hypnotic drugs: evidence for individual differences on vigilance. Psychopharmacol 47:213, 1976.

141. Rao S et al: Cardiopulmonary effects of diazepam. Clin Pharm Ther 14:182, 1973.

142. Rickels K et al: A comparative controlled clinical trial of seven hypnotic agents in medical and psychiatric inpatients. Am J Med Sci 245:142, 1963.

143. Rickels K: Over-the-counter daytime sedatives; a controlled study. JAMA 223:29, 1973.

144. Rickels K et al: Chlordiazepoxide and hostility in anxious outpatients. Am J Psychiat 131:442, 1974.

145. Robinson DS et al: Interaction of commonly prescribed drugs and warfarin. Ann Intern Med 72:853, 1970.

146. Saario I et al: Modification by diazepam or thioridazine of the psychomotor skills related to driving: a subacute trial in neurotic outpatients. Brit J Clin Pharmacol 3:843, 1976.

147. Safra MJ et al: Association between cleft lip with or without cleft palate and prenatal exposure to diazepam. Lancet 2:478, 1975.

148. Safra MJ et al: Valium: an oral cleft teratogen? Cleft Palate J 13:198, 1976.

149. Salzman C et al: Chlordiazepoxide, expectation and hostility. Psychopharmacolog 14:38, 1969.

150. Salzman C et al: Chlordiazepoxide-induced hostility in a small group setting. Arch Gen Psychiat 31:401, 1974.

151. Salzman C et al: Is oxazepam associated with hostility? Dis Nerv Syst 36(sect 2):30, 1975.

152. Salzman C et al: Psychopharmacologic investigations in elderly volunteers: effect of diazepam in males. J Amer Geriat Soc 23:451, 1975.

153. Samuelsson SM et al: Do barbiturates influence the prothrombin-proconvertin level during anticoagulant therapy? Scand J Clin Lab Invest 17:73, 1965.

154. Saxen I: Associations between oral clefts and drugs taken during pregnancy. Int J Epidemiol 4:37, 1975.

155. Saxen I et al: Association between maternal intake of diazepam and oral clefts. Lancet 2:493, 1975.

156. Schenker S et al: The effect of parenchymal liver disease on the disposition of sedatives and analgesics. Med Clin N Amer 59:887, 1975.

157. Shader RI et al: *Psychotropic Drug Side Effects.* Williams & Wilkins, Baltimore 1970.

158. Shader RI et al: Benzodiazepines: safety and toxicity. Dis Nerv Syst 36(sect 2):23, 1975.

159. Shapiro S et al: Clinical effects of hypnotics; an epidemiologic study. JAMA 209:2016, 1969.

160. Sharer L et al: Intravenous administration of diazepam: effects on penicillin-induced focal seizures in the cat. Arch Neurol 24:169, 1971.

161. Shull HJ et al: Normal disposition of oxazepam in acute viral hepatitis and cirrhosis. Ann Int Med 84:420, 1976.

162. de Silva JAF et al: Blood level distribution patterns of diazepam and its major metabolites in man. J Pharm Sci 55:692, 1966.

163. Smith GM et al: Use of subjective responses to evaluate efficacy of mild analgesic-sedative combinations. Clin Pharm Ther 15:118, 1974.

164. Stanski DR et al: Plasma and cerebrospinal fluid concentrations of chlordiazepoxide and its metabolites in surgical patients. Clin Pharm Ther 20:571, 1976.

165. Stone WN et al: Impact of psychosocial factors on the conduct of combined drug and psychotherapy research. Brit J Psychiat 127:432, 1975.

166. Stone WN et al: Anxiety and β-adrenergic blockade. Arch Gen Psychiat 29:620, 1973.

167. Sunshine A: A comparative study of Excedrin PM and placebo. J Clin Pharmacol 14:166, 1974.

168. Teutsch G et al: Hypnotic efficacy of diphenhydramine, methapyrilene, and pentobarbital. Clin Pharm Ther 17:195, 1975.

169. Turner P: Beta-adrenoceptor blockade in hyperthyroidism and anxiety. Proc Roy Soc Med 69:375, 1976.

170. Valerino DM et al: Effects of various barbiturates on hepatic microsomal enzymes. Drug Metab Disp 2:448, 1974.

171. Valzelli L: *Psychopharmacology.* John Wiley & Sons, New York 1973.

172. Van der Kleijn E: Protein binding and lipophilic nature of ataractics of the meprobamate- and diazepam-group. Arch Internat Pharmacodyn 179:225, 1969.

173. Wang RIH et al: Hypnotic efficacy of lorazepam and flurazepam. Clin Pharm Ther 19:1976.

174. Way WL et al: Sedative-hypnotics. Anesthesiol 23:170, 1971.

175. Wheatley D et al: Psychiatric aspects of hypertension. Brit J Psychiat 127:327, 1975.

176. Winstead MK et al: Diazepam use in military sick call. Military Med 141:180, 1976.

177. Wolff BB: Evaluation of hypnotics in outpatients with insomnia using a questionnaire and a self-rating technique. Clin Pharm Ther 15:130, 1974.

178. Woodward JA et al: Patterns of symptom change in anxious depressed outpatients treated with different drugs. Dis Nerv Syst 36 (sect 2):125, 1975.

179. Yamamoto J et al: The treatment of severe anxiety in outpatients: a controlled study comparing chlordiazepoxide and chlorpromazine. Psychosomatics 14:46, 1973.

Chapter 7

General Care: Pain

Ronald P. Evens
Mary Anne Koda-Kimble

Pain is an unpleasant sensation disturbing a patient's comfort, thought, sleep, or normal daily activity and is only *symptomatic* of an underlying disease process. When obtaining a patient's subjective description of pain, clinicians commonly organize their questions into a *PQRST* mnemonic. The letter P represents *palliative* or *precipitating* factors (e.g. exertion, diet, emotions, stress, infection, antacids, and posture). The letter Q represents the *quality* of pain (e.g. sharpness, dullness, knife-like, crushing, waxing, waning or pulsating). The letter R represents region or *radiation* of pain (e.g. substernal region radiating to the left arm). Many conditions may produce pain in the same regional area, e.g. substernal pain may be secondary to angina pectoris, myocardial infarct, pleuritis, esophagitis, cholecystitis, bone fracture, or muscle strain. The letter S deals with the patient's subjective descriptions of the *severity* of the pain (e.g. awakened at night by the pain, or takes the patient's breath away). The letter T concerns the *temporal* nature of the pain (e.g. day or night, relationship to meals or activities, acute or chronic).

This chapter will emphasize the clinical use of potent analgesics. The relative efficacy of the mild analgesics will also be discussed; however, the major side effects of these agents are considered in depth elsewhere in this text.

POTENT ANALGESICS:

1. What are the characteristics of an ideal analgesic study? Why are analgesics so difficult to evaluate?

Since the sensation, transmission, perception, and reaction to pain are highly variable, the measurement of pain is necessarily subjective and this creates difficulties in evaluating analgesic efficacy. To exemplify this point, Beecher (12) reviewed 15 double-blind clinical trials and found that placebos produced satisfactory pain relief in 35% ± 2% of 1082 patients suffering from a variety of painful states. Furthermore, in one study, 52% of 199 patients with headaches were effectively treated with a placebo. Lasagna (51) has reviewed the pitfalls of analgesic studies extensively. The following are major points to consider in reviewing any analgesic study (54,56,74):

a. A new analgesic should be compared to both a placebo and a drug standard (e.g. morphine sulfate 10 mg/70 kg or acetylsalicylic acid 600 mg) to validate its efficacy.

b. Once analgesic efficacy has been established, equianalgesic doses must be employed before conclusions can be reached with regard to the comparative side effects of any two agents.

c. Trial designs should incorporate double blinding, randomization and cross-over techniques to minimize bias.

d. A large, homogeneous population suffering from a similar type and degree of pain should be studied (e.g. post-operative, post-partum, cancer, or headache pain).

e. Factors which alter pain perception and its relief should be minimized (e.g. co-administration of CNS depressants, prior administration of other analgesics, sociological population differences).

2. What general pharmacotherapeutic principles should be considered in the treatment of pain?

a. If possible, treat the etiology of the pain and remove or minimize exacerbating factors.

b. Do not mask the presence of progression of the underlying pathologic process by altering the neurologic examination of obliterating the character of the pain which is essential in establishing a diagnosis.

c. Give sufficient doses of an analgesic as frequently as needed to alleviate the pain. See Question 7.

d. Individualize the dose and route of administration by taking into consideration the patient's weight, severity of pain, presence of concomitant conditions which may predispose the patient to the adverse effects of these agents, organ function, and patient convenience.

e. Make every attempt to avoid the co-administration

of drugs which will potentiate the CNS depressant and cardiovascular effects of the potent narcotic agents.

f. Provide positive empathetic and psychological support (6,12,27,41,54,84).

3. What is the optimal analgesic dose of morphine?

An intramuscular dose of 10 mg/70 kg of morphine sulfate can provide significant analgesia in two-thirds of patients with severe pain. A larger dose, 15 mg/70 kg, may provide relief for 75% of patients but will be accompanied by an increased incidence of side effects.

Ten milligrams of morphine is the standard of reference used in evaluating the efficacy of other potent analgesics. When any comparison is made between potent analgesics with regard to incidence or degree of side effects, it is imperative that these be made with equianalgesic doses. Although 10 mg/70 kg is considered to be the standard dose, it is important to recall that individual dose requirements vary according to the severity of pain, response to pain, weight, and the presence of concomitant disease states. Thus, usual analgesic doses range from 8 mg or less to 15 mg (49,51,84).

4. What parenteral doses of the major narcotic analgesics will produce the same level of analgesia as 10 mg/70 kg of morphine administered subcutaneously? What is the duration of analgesic action of these agents?

See Table 1.

5. In general, none of the narcotic analgesics are as effective orally as they are parenterally. Compare the parenteral to oral ratios of the more commonly used narcotics. What considerations must be taken into account when evaluating the relative potencies of the two routes of administration?

Oral administration generally produces a slower onset of activity, a lesser degree of pain relief, and a longer duration of action. Therefore, oral agents are not particularly useful for rapid alleviation of acute, severe pain. Oral and parenteral routes may be compared in terms of peak analgesic effect or total analgesic effect (areas under the time-action curves). The potent analgesics with reasonable oral activity are listed in Table 2. The oral potency of other analgesics have not been studied or are considered to have minimal efficacy by this route (8,9,37,38,51,85).

CASE A (Questions 6-10): A 30-year-old male was admitted to the surgery ward with a chief complaint of severe periumbilical pain which was followed by nausea and vomiting. A diagnosis of acute appendicitis was made and the patient was scheduled for an emergency appendectomy.

Table 1
COMPARATIVE DOSES AND DURATIONS OF ACTION OF COMMON POTENT ANALGESICS

Drug	Trade Name	SC or IM Dose Equivalent to 10 mg/70 kg Morphine Sulfate (in milligrams)	Duration Of Action (in hours)
Alphaprodine	Nisentil	40-60	½-2
Anileridine	Leritine	25-40	2-6
Codeine*	—	120	3-6
Fentanyl	Sublimaze	0.2	1½
Hydromorphone	Dilaudid	1.5	4-5
Levorphanol	Levo-Dromoran	2-3	4-8
Meperidine	Demerol	75-100	2-4
Methadone	Dolophine	7.5-10	3-8
Methotrimeprazine**	Levoprome	15-20	
Morphine	—	10	3-7
Oxycodone***	Percodan, Percocet	10-15	3-6
Oxymorphone	Numorphan	1-1.5	4-6
Pentazocine	Talwin	45-60	2-3

*Doses this high are rarely given parenterally. Even this dose has a lower analgesic ceiling than MS. Doses of 60 mg are given parenterally for mild to moderate pain.

**A phenothiazine.

***Commercially available in combination with other ingredients.

References: 10,11,18,26,27,38,51,54,60,84

Table 2
ORAL ANALGESIC POTENCY OF
MAJOR NARCOTIC ANALGESICS

Drug	Parenteral: Oral Dose Ratio In Terms of Total Relief	Parenteral: Oral Dose Ratio In Terms of Peak Analgesic Effect
Morphine	1:6	1:12
Codeine	1:2	1:3
Oxycodone	1:2	—
Methadone	1:2	—
Meperidine	1:3	1:4
Pentazocine	1:3	1:4

The patient's past medical history was significant in that five years prior to admission (PTA) he had a goiter removed; he is currently treated with 0.2 mg thyroxine daily. He also had an acute psychotic episode eight years PTA following the ingestion of sweets laced with LSD at a New Year's party. He currently takes no drugs of abuse.

Following surgery, he was given 2 mg of morphine sulfate intravenously. Since he complained of itching along the arm, codeine 60 mg IM q4h was ordered once he returned to the ward. This produced an itchy wheal at the site of injection and a generalized pruritis, and he was switched to meperidine 50 mg plus promethazine 50 mg every four to six hours prn pain. The next morning the medical student responsible for the case noted the history of drug abuse, discontinued the meperidine and promethazine and ordered pentazocine 60 mg IM every six hours prn pain. That evening the patient had to be restrained because he was found choking the patient who shared his room because he thought the man had turned into a gorilla.

6. Was this patient allergic to morphine and codeine? What drugs can be given to a patient who is allergic to morphine?

Narcotic agents can release histamine. This pharmacologic effect manifests itself clinically as a local itchy wheal at the site of injection, itching along the vein when the narcotics are administered intravenously (46), and a transient, generalized pruritis which is not accompanied by a rash. These phenomena are not always reproducible and are not considered to be true drug allergies. However, if a patient is truly allergic to morphine (e.g. rash, difficulty breathing), codeine should not be administered since it has a similar chemical structure and it is estimated that 10% is demethylated to morphine. Methadone, pentazocine, and meperidine are examples of potent analgesics which have chemical structures which are substantially different from that of morphine (38,40).

These should be tried since there will be less likelihood of cross-sensitivity.

7. Assess the meperidine order for this patient.

The dose of meperidine is very likely to be inadequate for this patient since a dose of 75-100 mg is equianalgesic with 10 mg of morphine. Furthermore, the specified dosing interval is more consistent with the duration of action of morphine than for meperidine. Frequently, clinicians prefer meperidine because it is their understanding that it is not as addicting as the other narcotics. Unfortunately, there is no basis for this reasoning (11,51,84) and this, together with a lack of knowledge of the effective dose range and duration of action of this agent, frequently results in inadequate analgesic coverage.

Clinicians should not exercise undue caution in prescribing narcotic analgesics for fear of "addicting" patients. In a survey by Marks and associates (57), a majority of physicians underestimated the effective dosage range, overestimated the duration of action, and exaggerated the dangers of addiction for medical inpatients receiving meperidine. Patients should not suffer pain needlessly as hospital-induced narcotic addiction is a rare problem. The Illinois State Drug Abuse Center showed in 1971 that only three of 1900 cases of addiction were possible complications of previous medical treatment (57). This does not mean to imply, however, that physical dependence does not occur (see *Drug Abuse* chapter for definitions of physical dependence and addiction). Approximately 50% of patients who have received therapeutic doses of narcotic analgesics several times daily for one to two weeks will experience some mild degree of sleep disturbance and rhinorrhea after abrupt withdrawal; however, these symptoms are not usually recognized as being a consequence of narcotic administration. In the hospital, the drug is administered in a defined context and the patient does not have the same stimuli for addiction as in the nonmedical social setting where contact with friends, sights, and sounds associated with drug taking powerfully reinforce the rituals leading to abuse.

The patient's thyroid function should also be considered since hypothyroid individuals are said to be more sensitive and hyperthyroid individuals less sensitive to the analgesic and toxic effects of narcotics (16,38). It is very likely that this patient is clinically euthyroid and the dose will not need to be adjusted.

8. What is the rationale for the co-administration of promethazine with meperidine? What particular precautions must be taken when these drugs are administered together?

Phenothiazines are often given in conjunction with narcotics to "enhance" the analgesic effect of these drugs. However, all phenothiazines have an antanalgesic effect initially which may be followed by varying degrees of antanalgesia or analgesia depending on the drugs used. Promethazine (Phenergan), in particular, has a significant antanalgesic effect after one hour, and one study showed that it had no potentiating effects on the analgesia produced by meperidine.

Dundee (21) divided the phenothiazines into three groups. Those with slight analgesic activity after one hour were, in general, those with a dimethylaminopropyl side chain. These include promazine (Sparine), triflupromazine (Vesprin), propiomazine (Largon), trimeprazine (Temaril), and methotrimeprazine (Levoprome). Promethazine (Phenergan) is an important exception. Those with a slight antanalgesic effect after one hour were those with a piperazine side chain. These include perphenazine (Trilafon), prochlorperazine (Compazine), trifluperazine (Stelazine), thiethylperazine (Torecan). Those with significant antanalgesia after one hour included thioridazine (Mellaril) and promethazine (Phenergan).

In addition, one must also consider the fact that phenothiazines may enhance the hypotensive, sedative, and respiratory depressant effects of the narcotic agents. One study performed in normal subjects demonstrated that although 25 mg of chlorpromazine alone had variable effects on respiration, the addition of the same dose to 100 mg of meperidine resulted in a greater degree and duration of respiratory depression than meperidine alone. Maximum respiratory depression occurred one hour after meperidine alone was administered and one-half of the effect disappeared three hours later. However, when meperidine was given in conjunction with 25 mg of chlorpromazine, maximum respiratory depression occurred 1.5 hours following administration and remained maximally depressed three hours later. One patient, although normal, exhibited extreme sensitivity to these effects (respiratory rate of 1-2/minute) which lasted two hours (49). Such combinations should be used with extreme caution in patients whose respiratory capacity is already compromised. Since respiratory depression may be prolonged, phenothiazines should be administered only with every other dose of the narcotic (21,35,46,49).

9. Could pentazocine have caused this patient's unusual behavior? What is the incidence of dysphoria secondary to pentazocine compared to that associated with morphine?

Numerous case reports of visual and auditory hallucinations and other psychic reactions have been attributed to pentazocine following both parenteral and oral doses (3,13,28,29,42). For example, four patients exhibited dysphoric hallucinations which were manifested as multicolored flashing of patterns or animals,

with or without concomitant auditory changes (28). Their onset followed only one or two doses of 30 mg IM or 50 mg PO. In a comparative evaluation of morphine 10 mg IM vs. pentazocine 40-50 mg IM, hallucinations occurred in 7 of 49, and 24 of 65 patients respectively (3). In another study, psychic changes occurred following 13 of 114 doses of pentazocine (40 mg) as opposed to only 2 of 116 doses of morphine (10 mg) (13). These studies indicate that there is a much higher incidence of dysphoria associated with the use of pentazocine than with morphine. Therefore, pentazocine should be avoided in patients predisposed to psychological disturbances.

10. Which side effects of narcotics are of particular importance in a post-operative patient? How can these effects be monitored?

Post-operative patients are often subjected to other CNS depressants which can potentiate the respiratory depressant effects of narcotics. Furthermore, respiratory depression and inhibition of the involuntary cough reflex predisposes the patient to atelectasis post-operatively. However, failure to cough and breathe properly are most often due to the pain associated with recent surgery. Therefore, it is best to administer the analgesic and to make certain that the patient is prompted to cough and breathe deeply several times during the day since voluntary coughing and breathing reflexes are not depressed by the narcotics.

Narcotics may also contribute to post-operative urinary retention and paralytic ileus by increasing smooth muscle tone and by decreasing the propulsive movements of the gastrointestinal tract. There is little or no evidence to indicate that equianalgesic doses of narcotics differ with respect to their effects on the gastrointestinal tract.

Finally, hypotension which may be caused by excessive fluid or blood loss during and after the surgical procedure may be exacerbated by the peripheral dilatory effects of the narcotic agents. Therefore the respiratory rate, blood pressure, urinary output, and bowel sounds must be monitored closely in post-operative patients receiving narcotics.

11. What are the primary factors which must be considered in the selection of a potent analgesic for use in labor? Which potent analgesics are most frequently used and why?

The ideal analgesic for a woman in labor should: (a) provide adequate pain relief; (b) have no effect on the course or duration of labor, and (c) affect fetal vital signs minimally during labor and at birth (38, 70a, 70b, 78). If possible, all CNS depressants should be avoided during labor to avoid any compromise in fetal vital functions. However, if the contractions are very hard, erratic, and prolonged early in the course of labor (i.e. minimal cervical dilation), a short-acting analgesic may be useful to blunt the labor pain and to sedate the mother so that she may regain control over her contractions (if she is using the Lamaze or similar technique) and to conserve her energy for the actual delivery.

Meperidine and its congener, alphaprodine, are frequently used in obstetrics because they are short-acting, appear to affect the course of labor minimally and because in equianalgesic doses they depress fetal respiration to a lesser extent than morphine or methadone (20,38,71,76). The lack of effect on fetal respiration may well be related to the short duration of action, since it is less likely that the fetus will be delivered during the period of maximal respiratory depression if these drugs are administered well before delivery.

Pentazocine also appears to have minimal effects on the fetus and labor, but it is not superior to meperidine (53,65).

12. A 65-year-old man with a 10-year history of angina pectoris has an acute myocardial infarction. Pentazocine 45 mg IV is prescribed. Are there any contraindications to the use of this agent in this situation? Which potent analgesic should be used?

This dose of pentazocine is an effective analgesic in this situation (25); however, pentazocine has several hemodynamic effects which increase the work load on the myocardium and increase myocardial oxygen consumption. Intravenous doses of 30 and 60 mg increase the mean aterial pressure, heart rate, pulmonary artery pressure and left ventricular end diastolic pressure (39,40,63,72). Furthermore, pentazocine can produce idiosyncratic hypotensive episodes (6/149 doses in one trial) which could be disastrous in such a patient (25).

Morphine, on the other hand, produces no change or a decrease in the same parameters (2,52,73) so that myocardial wall tension and oxygen consumption may ultimately be decreased. Other properties in its favor are that it has a longer duration of action when given intravenously than does pentazocine (73) and it produces minimal heart rate and orthostatic blood pressure changes (24,89). The sedative and emetic effects of the two agents are comparable (2,25,73).

In summary, although both agents are effective analgesics, pentazocine has greater cardiovascular toxicity and could actually exacerbate an acute myocardial infarction (1,47,81). Methadone (73) and meperidine (52,73) affect the cardiovascular system in a manner similar to morphine.

13. The pharmacy has received an order for morphine sulfate, 500 mg in 500 cc D-5-1/4NS for the operating room. How and why are such large quantities of morphine used. What are the major complications associated with the use of these doses of morphine?

Intravenous solutions of morphine sulfate in total doses of 0.5-8.0 mg/kg have been used alone, or together with nitrous oxide, for anesthesia in patients undergoing open heart surgery such as that for aortocoronary bypass (5,67,77). Arens et al (5) have given total doses as high as 900 mg (average 240-420 mg) in conjunction with nitrous oxide. The usual initial dose ranged from 1.5 to 3.0 mg/kg IV and was administered over a 10 to 15 minute period. Patient response was assessed by observing pupillary changes, level of consciousness, respiratory rate, and a variety of cardiovascular parameters.

The primary problems associated with the use of large parenteral doses of morphine are related to its effects on the cardiovascular, respiratory, and central nervous systems. The observed effects on the cardiovascular system have been variable. A decrease and an increase in the blood pressure (5,55,67,77), an increase in cardiac output (5,55), an increase in the pulmonary artery pressure, and an increase in central venous pressure (55) have been observed. Respiratory depression was profound and necessitated ventilatory assistance for up to 8-12 hours post-operatively in some cases (15). Post-operative central nervous system irritability, manifested by jerky movements precipitated by external stimuli, and episodes of psychosis and disorientation were observed in 21% of the patients in one study (5).

CASE B (Questions 14-17): A 24-year-old hemophiliac male is admitted to the emergency room with several minor lacerations, a possible concussion, shock secondary to internal bleeding, and painful hemarthrosis secondary to a motorcycle accident. Morphine sulfate 10 mg SC was ordered and he was transferred to the medical ward for further evaluation. There, the patient was given several units of blood and antihemophilic factor. He was also given 50-100 mg of meperidine intramuscularly every four hours as needed for pain. On the 25th hospital day, it was noted that the patient continues to use four to six doses of meperidine per day. A decision is made to switch him to 60 mg of parenteral pentazocine for fear of addiction.

14. Is there any particular danger in administering morphine to this patient?

Narcotic analgesics are generally avoided in patients with head injury for the following reasons:

a. The pupillary changes, nausea, and general central nervous system clouding may mask or confuse the diagnosis.

b. Head injury potentiates the respiratory depressant effects of narcotics.

c. Narcotics induce carbon dioxide retention which in turn causes vasodilation of the cerebral arteries and an increase in the intracranial pressure. This may be disastrous in a situation where cerebral spinal fluid pressure is already elevated (11,38,43).

15. If a narcotic is to be administered, what is one route of choice for this patient?

Subcutaneous and intramuscular morphine are poorly and unpredictably absorbed in patients with hypovolemic shock because the peripheral circulation in these individuals is poor. Furthermore, repeated doses of drug given by these routes may accumulate, only to be released once the circulation is restored. Therefore, intravenous administration is the route of choice. It is also important to recall that patients with reduced blood volume secondary to hemorrhage, dehydration and other causes are particularly susceptible to the hypotensive effects of narcotics (11,38,66).

16. Was the physician's fear of meperidine addiction legitimate in this patient?

Drug addiction, or compulsive drug use, and physical dependence may occur independent of one another (see chapter on *Drug Abuse*). Although there is evidence that very few drug abusers were addicted as a result of legitimate medical treatment with narcotics (57), there is no question that meperidine has addiction liability (4,31,32,88). There is insufficient information provided in this case to determine whether or not this individual has a propensity for drug addiction. However, there is little question that he may have developed some degree of physical dependence which may produce signs and symptoms of withdrawal if meperidine is discontinued. As little as two to three weeks of continuous daily drug administration produces physical dependence and a withdrawal syndrome (31,69) within hours of discontinuation. Symptoms consisting of lacrimation, rhinorrhea, perspiration, tremors, gooseflesh, anorexia, and mydriasis occur and last for about two days (31).

17. What are the dangers of administering pentazocine to this patient at this point?

Although pentazocine is a mild narcotic antagonist (1/50 nalorphine), 80 mg has been known to precipitate abstinence in morphine-dependent addicts. The drug can also induce mild abstinence in patients who have been given narcotics for chronic pain. If pentazocine is instituted, the dose should be increased gradually and the patient should be observed closely for symptoms of abstinence (8,58). If possible, the meperidine should be withdrawn gradually; a drug-free period of two days prior to the institution of pen-

tazocine has also been suggested (38).

18. Although B.A. is suffering from severe pain secondary to the melanoma on her leg, she often refuses her morphine because it makes her extremely nauseous and occasionally causes her to vomit. Can this side effect of morphine be avoided?

Morphine and its derivatives induce nausea and vomiting by stimulating the chemoreceptor trigger zone (CTZ). Although the CTZ is stimulated initially, subsequent doses of morphine generally suppress the vomiting center. Because the incidence of nausea (40%) and vomiting (15%) increases in ambulatory patients, it is generally agreed that a vestibular component is also involved (90).

If the patient is receiving analgesics on a regular basis, it is doubtful that she will have difficulties with subsequent doses. However, if nausea persists, phenothiazines, which suppress the CTZ, are recommended. Antihistamines are generally ineffective in the treatment of narcotic induced nausea and vomiting. Although promethazine's antiemetic properties are primarily accredited to its antihistaminic effects, it seems quite conceivable that promethazine would suppress emesis at both the vestibular apparatus and the CTZ. It may, therefore, be worthwhile to try this drug in the ambulatory patient. One must remember that the phenothiazines in conjunction with narcotics may potentiate the sedative, respiratory depressant, and orthostatic hypotensive effects of these drugs. The antiemetic effects of promethazine are long-acting (24-30 hours) and once daily administration would be adequate (11,38,86). (Also see Question 8 in the chapter *General Care: Nausea & Vomiting*.)

19. A patient is admitted for severe, intermittent right upper quadrant pain accompanied by nausea, vomiting, and clay colored stools. The differential diagnosis is biliary colic versus acute pancreatitis. An order is written for morphine sulfate 10 mg IM every 3 to 4 hours if needed for pain. Are any of the other potent analgesics preferred in this situation?

Morphine can produce spasm of smooth muscle, including the sphincter of Oddi, and this may increase intrabiliary pressures sufficiently to induce biliary colic. Also, the resulting back pressure may increase the serum amylase 5-10 times the control value which could confuse the diagnosis. This effect may last for 24 hours (51,68).

Meperidine was initially introduced as an anticholinergic before it was found to have potent analgesic properties. It has been said, therefore, that the drug does not share morphine's spasmogenic effects on the biliary tract. Opinions are conflicting, but studies directly measuring intrabiliary pressures indicate that meperidine definitely does have a spasmogenic effect on the sphincter of Oddi and can increase biliary pressure. This effect may not be as great or prolonged as that produced by morphine (5 to 10 cm vs ≥ 10 cm), however, and some say it is not as predictable (34,51).

The effects of pentazocine on the gastrointestinal tract are variable, but a few small studies indicate that in equianalgesic doses, pentazocine has the same propensity to induce smooth muscle spasm as do the narcotics. In one study, 40 mg of pentazocine given intramuscularly induced spasm of the sphincter of Oddi and an elevation of the serum amylase in two out of five subjects. In three patients with T-tubes placed in the common bile duct, 30 mg of pentazocine given intramuscularly produced spasm of the sphincter of Oddi forty minutes after administration which lasted two to three hours. There was no elevation of serum amylase in these patients (19,33).

In summary, meperidine and pentazocine increase biliary pressure, but not as predictably or to the same degree as morphine. In this situation they are the preferred drugs and should be administered after serum amylase levels are drawn.

20. B.A. is a 54-year-old white male with cirrhosis of the liver, severe ascites, and mild jaundice. His stools are generally benzidine positive and he occasionally has bright red blood per rectum secondary to hemorrhoids. He had been placed on oral neomycin intermittently for a flapping tremor and a decreased sensorium which developed when the protein content of his diet was increased. He is currently alert and receiving only a stool softener, spironolactone 50 mg each day, and neomycin. He develops severe right upper quadrant pain for which morphine sulfate is ordered. What must be considered when administering narcotics to this type of patient?

Morphine is metabolized in the liver and could theoretically accumulate in patients with decreased liver function. One study shows that in patients with liver disease, 8 mg of morphine sulfate can induce EEG changes similar to those which occur with impending hepatic encephalopathy. These changes were not induced in normal subjects and were particularly noticeable in patients who had a history of (a) hepatic encephalopathy, (b) jaundice and ascites, or (c) gastrointestinal bleeding complicating their liver disease. These changes could not be correlated with alkalosis, hypokalemia or increased blood ammonia levels. The mechanism by which morphine induces these changes is unknown. Because morphine and other narcotic analgesics can induce hepatic coma, they are contraindicated in patients with signs of impending coma (36).

Meperidine is 95% metabolized primarily through demethylation and de-esterification in the liver at a rate of 10-22% per hour (17). In subjects without hepatic disease, the half-life is biphasic with a rapid alpha phase of 3.3-7.1 minutes and a slow beta phase of 3.1-3.7 hours following an IV dose (59). Its plasma clearance is about 0.84 liters/minute and its average steady state volume of distribution is 196 liters.

In hepatic insufficiency, meperidine elimination is slowed considerably. Following a 0.8 mg/kg single IV dose of meperidine the beta half-life in eight normal subjects vs 10 cirrhotic patients was 3.2 ± 0.8 hours vs 7± 1 hours, respectively (48). The plasma clearance was reduced from 1.3 liters/minute to 0.66 liters/minute. Liver function tests did not correlate with plasma clearance. Similar depressed drug elimination was evident in two matched groups of 15 normal subjects and 14 acute viral hepatitis patients after a 0.8 mg/kg IV dose. In this study the beta half-life was 3.4 ± 0.8 hours in the control group and 7 ± 2.7 hours (4.4−14.3 hours) in the patients with hepatitis. The plasma clearance in the two groups was 1.3 ± 0.5 liters/minute and 0.65 ± 0.2 liters/minute respectively (61). As the hepatitis resolved, drug elimination returned to normal. Therefore, prolonged drug activity may be expected in this cirrhotic patient and the dosing interval as well as the dose may require adjustment.

21. A 65-year-old male is admitted to the hospital with a broken hip. He has a history of asthma and chronic obstructive pulmonary disease secondary to heavy smoking. Morphine 10 mg IM is ordered to alleviate his hip pain. Why should morphine be used with caution in this patient? Are there any other potent analgesics which could be used in this situation?

Morphine and other narcotic agents depress respiration in therapeutic doses and should be used cautiously in patients with compromised respiratory function for the following reasons (11,38,87a):

a. Narcotics decrease the rate of respiration, the tidal volume and minute volume (38,90). Additionally, they decrease the respiratory response to an increased pCO_2 and hypoxia (99), both of which may be the primary drives for ventilation in the severely decompensated patient. They can also produce irregular and periodic breathing patterns (90).

b. Narcotics depress the involuntary cough reflex and cough is an important factor in the elimination of bronchial plugs which may predispose these patients to infections.

c. Theoretically, narcotics could precipitate bronchial constriction through the release of histamine.

In equipotent doses, other narcotics produce the same degree of respiratory depression as does morphine (22,28,73,79).

In equianalgesic doses pentazocine produces respiratory depression equal to or greater than that produced by morphine. Furthermore, because pentazocine is a weak narcotic antagonist, respiratory depression is not antagonized by levallorphan or nalorphine (45,46,58). Naloxone, a pure narcotic antagonist which is void of any agonistic activity, will antagonize the respiratory depressant effects of pentazocine. Doses of 16 mcg/kg or less reduce the respiratory depression by 60%. Mechanical respirators may also be used until the effect of the drug has waned (41a, 80).

There are very few alternative analgesics for such a patient. If pain is extremely severe, one may choose to use a low dose of narcotic to make the pain more tolerable while closely monitoring respiratory function. Alternatively, one might consider methotrimeprazine, a phenothiazine derivative, which produces less respiratory depression than equianalgesic doses of morphine. See Question 24.

22. M.S. is a 47-year-old woman with metastatic breast cancer involving multiple osseous sites that produce excruciating persistent pain, intensified by ambulation. At doses of 600-1200 mg, aspirin and acetaminophen provide minimal relief. The resident is planning to use narcotic analgesics and asks what is the oral drug of choice.

In terminal cancer, pain is a chronic problem throughout the limited life expectancy of the patient. The chronicity of the pain and the related fear of dependence should not preclude the regular prescription of narcotic agents; this patient's daily activity is severely compromised by the pain, and the relatively poor prognosis alters the usual concern about the consequences of addiction. Also, the associated factors of anxiety and insomnia can exaggerate the patient's pain level. Therefore, anxiolytic agents and bedtime sedatives are useful adjuncts to analgesia (16a,18,84a).

The guidelines in selecting an analgesic agent for terminal cancer pain include disease and drug factors: (a) stage of neoplastic progression — e.g. second or third stage in this patient with disseminated cancer; (b) pain severity — e.g. continual nature in this patient; (c) cause of pain — e.g. osseous tissue destruction and possibly nerve compression; (d) occupational life expectancy — e.g. ambulation of 4-6 hours/day; (e) prior therapy — e.g. inadequate non-narcotic analgesia with tolerance to their initial benefit at maximal doses; (f) adjunctive therapy to minimize the complicating problems that increase pain awareness; (g) proposed new drug activity — relief potential, duration of effect, oral bioavailability, and side effects (84a).

Following the use of non-narcotic agents and adjunctive therapy, the agents most frequently recommended include methadone 10-20 mg, pentazocine 50-100 mg, levorphanol 2-4 mg, and oxycodone 10-20 mg with aspirin (Percodan). The analgesic activity at equipotent doses of these four agents is comparable (54). Methadone and levorphanol have the longest duration of activity (3-8 hours), followed by oxycodone (3-6 hours) and pentazocine (2-3 hours); thus, less frequent drug administration is possible with the former agents. Oral bioavailability favors methadone, levorphanol and oxycodone (about 50%) over pentazocine (about 35%). The most significant side effects following such chronic daily consumption are sedation, constipation, and respiratory depression, which are comparable with these agents but may require dosage reduction to the most balanced situation between analgesia and adverse effects. Dependence liability is present with each agent (least with pentazocine) but does not present a practical problem in this terminal cancer case with severe pain (18,54). Therefore, methadone, levorphanol or oxycodone should be initiated in the doses recommended above with adjustments over days to weeks to individualize therapy. Tachyphylaxis may occur, requiring subsequent increase in dosage. Brompton's mixture, a combination of narcotic and stimulant in a hydroalcoholic vehicle, is becoming widely used in the control of chronic cancer pain; it is discussed in Question 23.

23. A 55-year-old male with terminal, metastatic throat cancer has been taking 20-30 Percodan tablets daily for control of his cancer pain. Because he has developed symptoms of salicylate toxicity the following solution is ordered:
Methadone . . . 10 mg/5 cc
Cocaine . . . 10 mg/5cc
Ethanol . . . 5%
Honey to taste
Sig: Rinse and swallow 5 cc prn pain. What is the rationale of the foregoing combination of ingredients? What evidence exists for its efficacy? How stable is this mixture?

The above represents one physician's version of Brompton's Mixture, also known as Brompton's Cocktail and Val Stick Solution. The basic formula most frequently includes a narcotic such as heroin, morphine or methadone; a central nervous system stimulant such as cocaine or dextroamphetamine; alcohol, in concentrations ranging from 0-40%; and a flavored vehicle such as syrup or chloroform water. The precise formulation varies from institution to institution.

Although heroin and morphine have been used frequently, the University of Rochester uses methadone instead because of its greater by the oral route activity (87). Way and Adler (85a) describe oral morphine's absorption as erratic and poor. A 10 mg oral morphine dose was indistinguishable from a placebo, and doses from 20 to 120 mg possessed only minimal activity.

The CNS stimulant was originally added to counteract the sedative effects of the narcotic and to potentiate the analgesic activity of the narcotic (87). Apparently, many cancer victims requiring large doses of narcotic do not wish to be totally sedated for the remainder of their lives. It may also counteract narcotic-induced respiratory depression. *Cocaine* is degraded in the gastrointestinal tract and is, therefore, poorly absorbed. Therefore, swishing the solution in the mouth may increase absorption through the oral mucosa. The local anesthetic properties of the drug may also alleviate pain associated with oral or throat cancer; the liquid is also easier to swallow than a solid dosage form. Because cocaine is poorly absorbed, others have replaced this ingredient with *dextroamphetamine*. There is also some evidence that a combination of dextroamphetamine and morphine has greater analgesic activity than morphine alone (22a).

If taken in sufficient quantities, *alcohol* can alter the mood, add to the sedative qualities of the narcotic and improve the palatability of the mixture. The sedative effects may be desirable when the CNS stimulant properties of the mixture predominate.

Phenothiazines sometimes are added to Brompton's mixture or are given separately to alleviate the nausea associated with the use of this mixture, to tranquilize the patient, and to potentiate the analgesic effects. When phenothiazines and narcotics are administered concomitantly, one must also consider the potentiation of other narcotic side effects as discussed in Question 8.

The *stability* of the "standard" solution as described in Martindale's Pharmacopoiea (15) (morphine HCl 15 mg; cocaine HCl 10 mg, alcohol 1.8 ml, syrup 3.5 ml, and chloroform water qs 10 ml) has been studied. At 22° C, 10% degrades over eight weeks. Elevated temperatures reduce the stability as 10% degrades over 4 weeks at a temperature of 30° C and over 2 weeks at a temperature of 37° C. If chlorpromazine or prochlorperazine is added, the shelf life is decreased by two weeks (83).

Brompton's mixture has primarily been used in cancer patients. Uncontrolled studies and the experience of clinicians seem to indicate that it is efficacious in alleviating pain (62,64,82,83) and that very little tolerance to the analgesic effect occurs. That is, the average single dose every four hours was relatively low once the initial pain was relieved. In one study (82) each dose was less than or equal to 10 mg of morphine for 60% of the patients; in another (62), the average dose of morphine was less than 20 mg for 78% of the patients. In all studies phenothiazines and other CNS depressants were given concomitantly to achieve optimal pain relief.

Side effects associated with the use of this mixture include nausea, vomiting, insomnia, agitation, sedation and constipation. All of these may be minimized by the judicious addition of phenothiazines, sedatives, and stool softeners to the supportive therapy. If tolerance to the analgesic effect occurs, the concentration of narcotic in the preparation should be increased and the quantity of stimulant per dose should remain the same. Also, when long acting narcotics are used, one must keep in mind that tolerance to the respiratory depressant effects may not parallel development of tolerance to the analgesic effects. Therefore, the patient's respiratory function must be followed closely.

24. Compare methotrimeprazine with morphine in terms of analgesic potency and side effects.

Methotrimeprazine, a congener of chlorpromazine, has potent analgesic properties. A dose of 15 mg IM is equianalgesic with 8 mg of morphine when used in the treatment of cancer pain, and the drugs are comparable with respect to both total and peak analgesic effects. Methotrimeprazine (MTZ) is not addicting and produces less respiratory depression than equianalgesic doses of morphine. The greater incidence of side effects occurring with MTZ is primarily due to its sedative effects. Sedation occurred in 39% of those patients receiving MTZ as opposed to 12% of those receiving equianalgesic doses of morphine. Pain at the injection site occurred with 13% of doses given. Dry mouth with nasal stuffiness or dryness occurred with 5% of doses. Nausea and vomiting occurred in 29% of those patients receiving morphine sulfate and in only 5% of those receiving MTZ. Methotrimeprazine produces a greater incidence of orthostatic hypotension than does morphine: when 10-15 mg of MTZ was given to healthy males, 70% experienced syncope when rapidly tilted into an upright position. It should therefore be used with extreme caution in ambulating patients (7,30,70).

25. J.S. is a 75-year-old man with extreme pain due to severe disabling osteoarthritis and vertebral disc degeneration. During an episode of exacerbation of the back pain, a dose of 8 mg of morphine produced complete relief to the surprise of the clinician. Characterize the response of older subjects to pain and to analgesics.

Aged patients experience greater relief of pain with narcotic analgesics. In a study of 712 patients receiving 10 mg of morphine or 20 mg of pentazocine, analgesia in patients over 50 years of age was superior to that experienced by younger subjects. Pain intensity was reduced, and relief was augmented in these older patients (14). In contrasting 200 young subjects (20-30 years old) and aged patients (54-97 years old), artificial pain from a light dolorimeter resulted in significantly lower pain perception and higher reaction thresholds in the older patient sample (75). Furthermore, it has been demonstrated that older subjects obtain higher plasma levels of meperidine after an IM injection than do younger subjects; decreased tissue binding seems to account for these higher plasma levels (18b).

MILD ANALGESICS:

26. What is the optimal analgesic dose of aspirin? Does the degree of analgesia correlate with salicylate blood levels?

It is commonly assumed that a 650 mg dose of aspirin produces maximum analgesic activity; however, there are studies which show an extension of the dose-response curve. In one study, increments of dose from 25 mg to 1800 mg increased the pain relief provided by aspirin for postpartum pain. Whether or not a significant increase in the incidence of side effects accompanied these high doses was not studied (128).

The level of analgesia correlates poorly with blood salicylate levels; therefore, studies which claim superiority of one product over another using these values should be interpreted cautiously. Acetylsalicylic acid levels correlate best with analgesic activity (93).

27. Aspirin is accepted as the standard of comparison for mild analgesics. How does the analgesic effect of 650 mg of aspirin compare with codeine, codeine/aspirin combination, dextropropoxyphene, acetaminophen, and placebo?

The following summarizes the conclusions of several reviews and clinical studies which compare the efficacy of the mild analgesics (92, 93, 107, 112, 120, 121, 124, 125, 129, 151):

Codeine 32 mg & ASA 650 mg>
Codeine 60 mg (orally) ≥
ASA 650 mg = Acetaminophen 650 mg ≥
Dextropropoxyphene 65 mg >
Dextropropoxyphene 32 mg = Placebo

The relative efficacy of propoxyphene has been extremely controversial and is the subject of many studies. Two literature reviews of 25 double-blind propoxyphene studies concluded that 65 mg of propoxyphene was equivalent or inferior to acetaminophen 650 mg, aspirin 650 mg, and codeine 65 mg in the relief of cancer, portpartum, postoperative and mixed painful situations (120,121). Moertel and associates treated 57 ambulatory patients with mild to moderate cancer pain in a cross-over comparison and determined that pain relief was achieved in 62% of patients receiving ASA 650 mg, 50% of patients receiving acetaminophen 650 mg, 60% of patients receiving codeine 60 mg, 43% of patients receiving propoxyphene 65 mg, and 32% of patients receiving a placebo; propoxyphene and placebo were statistically

inferior to ASA (124). Acetaminophen 650 mg was superior to propoxyphene with regard to pain intensity score, relief-from-pain score, and global evaluation when used in the treatment of 100 women with episiotomy pain; acetaminophen was effective in 62% of the patients whereas propoxypene was effective in 34% (107).

28. A 43-year-old man with a history of peptic ulcer disease enters the emergency room with a chief complaint of severe upper abdominal distress and black stools. He describes a recent increase in aspirin intake of 16 tablets daily to control his severe headaches. Characterize aspirin-induced gastrointestinal (GI) side effects.

Aspirin has three major gastrointestinal effects which may or may not be related to one another: dyspepsia, occult blood loss, and acute gastrointestinal hemorrhage.

Dyspepsia, which does not necessarily correlate with blood loss, occurs in one out of 15 patients taking aspirin, but only one out of 20 experience this effect consistently (92). Ten to twenty percent of patients taking anti-inflammatory doses of aspirin experience dyspepsia (93). Since this effect is very likely due to local irritation from particulate ASA, ingestion with large quantities of warm water or antacids may alleviate this symptom in some patients. Both maneuvers increase the dissolution rate of the aspirin tablets.

Aspirin ingestion is associated with a 6 to 11 fold increase in daily *GI blood loss* in normal subjects (94,113,114,115). When 600 mg of ASA was given to normal subjects four times daily, 73% lost 5 cc of blood from the gastrointestinal tract each day. The daily GI blood loss from a control group was 0.5cc. Although there was little variation in the daily blood loss caused by a given dose of aspirin in any given individual, the variation between individuals was great; some individuals lost as much as 115 cc of blood after ingesting a similar dose of aspirin (130,145).

The amount of blood which is lost may be dose-related. In one study, 300 mg qid produced an average daily blood loss of 4.6 cc; 600 mg qid produced a loss of 8 cc; and 900 qid produced a loss of 11.2 cc (130). Also, the same dose administered twice as frequently can increase the blood loss. ASA 600 mg qid caused a 4.3 cc blood loss as compared to a 10.3 cc blood loss caused by ASA 300 mg administered 8 times daily (130). The concomitant ingestion of alcohol may also increase the blood loss from aspirin (101).

The amount of blood loss is apparently unrelated to the presence or absence of dyspepsia (142), a previous history of peptic ulcer disease or GI hemorrhage (102), salicylate levels (106,130), or achlorhydria (97). However, in patients who are already bleeding (as opposed to those with a past history of GI hemorrhage), both aspirin and sodium salicylate can increase the amount of blood loss 4 to 10 fold (102). Interestingly, the ingestion of aspirin with food or milk (142) or the co-administration of corticosteroids does not alter the incidence or degree of occult blood loss.

The bleeding is primarily due to a local erosive effect of aspirin. Gastroscopic studies show local changes ranging from slight hyperemia to intense congestion with local hemorrhage in as many as 80% of patients ingesting aspirin (103,145). Apparently, saturated solutions which form around particles of ASA entrapped in the mucosal folds promote cellular damage, mucosal erosion, and hemorrhage. Disruption of mucosal permeability has also been demonstrated following the gastric instillation of aspirin solutions (144).

Occult blood loss can be minimized by administering enteric coated (145) or buffered aspirin (113) or by the concurrent administration of antacids (145). However, it should be recalled that the absorption of enteric coated tablets may be erratic or delayed (92,145), an undesirable feature for individuals seeking rapid relief of pain.

Finally, *acute gastrointestinal hemorrhage* precipitated by aspirin appears to be a phenomenon which is separate from its ability to cause dyspepsia or occult blood loss. This is exemplified by a case report of a 67-year-old man who presented with tarry stools and hematemesis following the ingestion of 650 mg of aspirin three to four times daily for a fever. Gastroscopy revealed multiple hemorrhagic sites in the gastric mucosa, and therapy with ice water lavage and whole blood replacement brought the acute episode under control within four days (143). Even though patients with a history of peptic ulcer disease do not necessarily exhibit occult blood losses greater than the normal population, their susceptibility to massive hemorrhage precipitated by aspirin must always be considered (97,149).

29. A 35-year-old woman with hemophilia (factor VIII level of <1%) developed severe headaches and treated herself with three Stanback prn. Soon thereafter she noticed an increased frequency and severity of bruising following minor trauma. What is the content of this product? Could it have caused the bruising in this patient? What could you recommend for her headache?

Stanback contains 324 mg of aspirin, 16 mg of caffeine and 97 mg of salicylamide per tablet. The aspirin in this product inhibits platelet aggregation and depresses platelet adhesiveness; this effect prolongs the bleeding time and may contribute to the easy bruisability observed by this patient.

Aspirin apparently alters platelet function through irreversible acetylation of platelet membranes (148). This abolishes or causes a severe delay in the second wave of aggregation stimulated by both epinephrine and collagen; the first wave is unaltered (119). As little as 150 mg effectively acetylates all circulating platelets (127), and in one study a daily dose of 300 mg produced the same degree of altered platelet aggregation as did 3600 mg (147). The effect of a single dose is detectable for 7 days which is the time required for a turnover in the platelet population. Platelet adhesiveness is also affected by drugs other than aspirin (e.g. dipyridamole, Anturane).

Aspirin's effect on platelet function is reflected in a prolongation of the bleeding time. A 5-10 fold increase has been observed following daily doses of 325-2925 mg of aspirin, and this alteration may take 4-10 days to return to normal. Single doses of 1000 mg have also been observed to increase the bleeding time (105,109).

Individuals with bleeding disorders, such as this patient with a factor VIII deficiency, experience a 2-4 fold elevation in the bleeding time approximately two hours after aspirin administration (109,132). Severe hemophiliac patients may exhibit an eight fold prolongation in the bleeding time following a single dose of 1000 mg of aspirin (109,139,140).

Sodium salicylate (139,140), acetaminophen (110,118), propoxyphene (95,110), pentazocine (95), and codeine (95) do not alter platelet function or bleeding times in hemophiliac subjects and can be considered for use in this patient.

30. A 25-year-old man ingested 60 acetaminophen (Tylenol) 325 mg tablets approximately 5 hours prior to admission. Describe acetaminophen-induced hepatotoxicity. What is the treatment of choice?

Following an acute intoxication, acetaminophen produces dose-dependent hepatic damage (96). Biochemical evidence of liver cell destruction peaks in two to three days as evidenced by an elevation in the SGOT (over 1250 IU), serum bilirubin, and prothrombin time. Jaundice and a palpable liver appear by the third to fourth day, and without therapeutic intervention, hepatotoxicity progresses to fulminant hepatic failure by the third to fifth day. Further patient deterioration to coma and death may ensue within 4-18 days. Liver biopsy specimens reveal a centrilobular, diffuse necrosis of the hepatocytes with a variable inflammatory reaction. Apparently the half-life of acetaminophen is prolonged to approximately 7 hours (normal: 2-3 hours) in patients with liver damage, and this produces acetaminophen levels which are 5-10 times higher than would be expected 12 hours following the ingestion (133,134).

Animal studies indicate that an active intermediate metabolite of acetaminophen is the hepatotoxic entity, since metabolic enzyme induction potentiates the toxicity and enzyme inhibition prevents hepatic damage. This potentially toxic intermediate metabolite is normally conjugated by glutathione. In acetaminophen overdose, glutathione stores are insufficient, and the intermediate metabolite accumulates to toxic levels. Depletion of glutathione stores prior to the administration of acetaminophen results in more severe hepatic necrosis, while pre-administration of glutathione precursors such as cysteine reduces acetaminophen-induced hepatic damage (122,135).

Because they possess a sulfhydryl (−SH) group similar to that of glutathione, cysteamine (CA), cysteine, penicillamine, and dimercaprol were studied in animals to ascertain whether or not they would protect against acetaminophen hepatotoxicity (146). If a sufficient dose was administered, CA, cysteine, and glutathione reduced mortality and prevented hepatic enzyme elevations when given within one hour of the overdose. Only cysteine was effective at two and four hour intervals between the time of overdose and treatment. When CA and cysteine were administered 61% and 80% of glutathione hepatic levels were maintained respectively, while a 95% depletion of glutathione was observed in untreated animals following the administration of acetaminophen.

Prescott et al (135) successfully prevented or reduced the severity of hepatotoxicity in humans by infusing 2 gm of cysteamine initially followed by 1.2 gm over 20 hours to five patients who had ingested between 8 and 50 gm of acetaminophen. When cysteamine was not used, 100% of patients with acetaminophen levels greater than 300 mcg/ml, 70% of patients with levels between 250-300 mcg/ml, 56% of patients with levels between 150-250 mcg/,ml, and 20% of patients with levels of less than 150 mcg/ml developed hepatotoxicity. In seven other clinical trials involving 102 patients, cysteamine substantially reduced the liver damage in most cases (100, 104, 108, 136, 137, 138, 141). Complete protection occurred only if CA was administered within 10 hours of the overdose. Although one study concluded that CA was not efficacious when compared to supportive care alone, the data indicate that there was a significant reduction in serum transaminases and bilirubin levels following CA treatment. Furthermore, their publication failed to describe their CA protocol, making evaluation of the study difficult (98).

The primary limitation to cysteamine administration is severe, persistent nausea, vomiting and sedation which may last for up to 24 hours following treatment (98,100,104,135,136,138,141). Therefore, other compounds with sulfhydryl groups or glutathione precursors have been tried to avoid this debilitating reaction. Dimercaprol (42 mg/kg over 48 hours) when administered within 12 hours of ingestion protected the liver in 6 of 10 patients as compared to 8 of 10 patients who received cysteamine (100). Methionine, a precursor of glutathione, moderately reduced liver damage in 5 patients (138). Penicillamine also produced a lesser protective effect than cysteamine.

Since cysteine has been effective in maintaining hepatic glutathione levels and reducing hepatotoxicity. N-acetylcysteine (NAC,Mucomyst), a commercially available product, has been used to treat acetaminophen overdoses. Increases in SGPT were prevented in mice following an acetaminophen dose of 1200 mg/kg. Animal survival following NAC therapy was dose related: single doses of 600-1000 mg/kg were effective in 93-100% and 300 mg/kg were effective in 60% (131).

There are two case reports of acetaminophen toxicity treated with oral NAC (117,129a). There was a substantial delay before therapy was initiated in both instances, and both patients developed hepatotoxicity. However, both individuals survived, and this was attributed to the NAC therapy. In one instance NAC was diluted in a cola soft drink and 140 mg/kg was given initially followed by 70 mg/kg every 8 hours for three days. No toxicity was noted (129a).

Cysteamine remains the therapy with the greatest proven success in acetaminophen intoxications, although its toxicities, lack of availability in this country, and parenteral route of administration are disadvantages in comparison with N-acetylcysteine. If cysteamine is not available, NAC should be tried, although further clinical trials are required to substantiate the limited experience with this agent. (Also see the chapter on *Poisonings*.)

31. A 28-year-old woman is brought into the emergency room by her husband with symptoms of lethargy following a suicide attempt with propoxyphene. On physical examination, she presents with miosis, tachycardia (105 beats/minute), and a respiratory rate of 11/minute. What are the symptoms of propoxyphene intoxication? What is the treatment of choice?

Propoxyphene is a structural analog of methadone, and central nervous system depression is the predominant effect following the acute ingestion of large doses. One report described 10 patients who had ingested between 700 and 2000 mg of propoxyphene. The predominant manifestation of intoxication was respiratory depression, followed by coma, convulsions and death (153). Other case reports describe similar symptoms: lethargy, respiratory depression, miosis, tachycardia, coma, hypotension and convulsions (111,116,150,152,153).

Naloxone, a narcotic antagonist, is effective in reversing the symptomatology of propoxyphene intoxication and does not produce any adverse effects (111,116,150,152). The recommended dose of naloxone for all narcotic overdose situations is 0.005 mg/kg IV (99). A dose of 0.8 mg IV has induced pupillary dilatation, an increase in the respiratory rate from 2 to 20/minute, and consciousness within one minute (150). Single doses of 0.2 to 0.8 mg have similarly reversed the depression (116,150), but multiple doses are usually required to maintain the response (111,116,150). If a single 0.4 mg does does not produce a rapid response, this should be repeated within minutes until reversal occurs (111,152). Up to 2.4 mg IV has been required to achieve a respiratory response; even then, subsequent doses were required within three hours to maintain consciousness (152).

REFERENCES

Potent Analgesics:

1. Alderman EL: Analgesics in the acute phase of myocardial infarction. JAMA 229:1646, 1974.
2. Alderman EL et al: Hemodynamic effects of morphine and pentazocine differ in cardiac patients. NEJM 287:623, 1972.
3. Alexander JI et al: Central nervous system effects of pentazocine. Br Med J 2:224, 1974.
4. Anslinger HJ: Demerol. JAMA 132:43, 1946.
5. Arens JF et al: Morphine anesthesia for aortocoronary bypass: Procedures Anesth Analg 51:901, 1972.
6. Batterman RC: Pain relief with analgesic agents. Dis Mon 1, 1968 (Aug).
7. Beaver WT et al: A comparison of the analgesic effects of methotrimeprazine and morphine in patients with cancer. Clin Pharmacol Ther 7:436. 1966a.
8. Beaver WT et al: A comparison of the analgesic effects of pentazocine and morphine in patients with cancer. Clin Pharmacol Ther 7:740, 1966b.
9. Beaver WT et al: A clinical comparison of the analgesic effects of methadone and morphine administered intramuscularly and of orally and parenterally administered methadone. Clin Pharmacol Ther 8:415, 1967.
10. Beaver WT et al: A clinical comparison of oral and intramuscular administration of analgesics: pentazocine and phenazocine. Clin Pharmacol Ther 9:582, 1968.
11. Beaver WT: The pharmacologic basis for the choice of an analgesic. I. Potent Analgesics. Pharmacol Phy 4:1, 1970.
21. Beecher HK: The powerful placebo. JAMA 159:1602, 1955.
13. Bellville JW et al: Evaluating side effects of analgesics in a cooperative clinical study. Clin Pharmacol Ther 9:303, 1968.
14. Belleville JW et al: Influence of age on pain relief from analgesics. JAMA 217:1835, 1971.
15. Blacow NW (ed): *Martindale – The Extra Pharmacopoeia*, 26th Ed, 1972. London Pharmaceutical Press, pg 1105.
16. Benedict EB: Morphine in myxedema. JAMA 94:1916, 1930.
16a. Brule G: Clinical use of narcotic analgesics in terminal cancer. Int J Clin Pharmacol 9:180, 1974.
17. Burns JJ et al: The physiological disposition and fate of meperidine in man and a method for its estimation in plasma. J Pharmacol Exp Ther 114:289, 1955.
18. Catalano RB: The medical approach to management of pain caused by cancer. Sem Oncol 2:379, 1975.
18a. Chan K et al: The effect of ageing on plasma pethidine concentration. Brit J Clin Pharmacol 2:297, 1975.
19. Danhof IE: Pentazocine effect on gastrointestinal motor function in man. Am J Gastroent 48:295, 1967.
20. DeVoe SJ et al: Effects of meperidine on uterine contractility. Am J Ob Gyn 105:1004, 1969.
21. Dundee JW et al: Alterations in response to somatic pain associated with anaesthesia. XV. Further studies with phenothiazine derivatives and similar drugs. Br J Anaesth 35:597, 1963.
22. Forrest WH et al: Respiratory effects of alphaprodine in man. Ob Gyn 31:61, 1968.
22a. Forrest WH et al: Dextroamphetamine with morphine for the treatment of postoperative pain. NEJM 296:712, 1977.
23. Gould WM: Central nervous disturbance with pentazocine. Br Med J 1:313, 1972.
24. Grendahl H et al: The effect of morphine on blood pressure and cardiac output in patients with acute myocardial infarction. Acta Med Scand 186:515, 1969.

25. Grossman JA et al: A clinical trial of pentazocine analgesia in acute myocardial infarction and acute coronary insufficiency. Curr Ther Res 13:505, 1971.
26. Halpern LM: Treating pain with drugs. Minn Med 57:176, 1974.
27. Halpern LM et al: 'Analgesics' in *Drugs of Choice 1976-1977*, 1976, (Modell W editor), CV Mosby Co, St. Louis, p. 195.
28. Hansbrough ET: Hallucinations following pentazocine. Missouri Med 67:602, 1970.
29. Hemphill RE: Hallucinations from pentazocine. S Afr Med J 47:1984, 1973.
30. Helrich M et al: Circulatory response to tilting following methotrimeprazine and morphine in man. Anesth 25:662, 1964.
31. Himmelsbach CK: Studies of the addiction liability of Demerol. J Pharmacol Exp Ther 75:64, 1942.
32. Himmelsbach DK: Further studies of the addiction liability of Demerol. J Pharmacol Exp Ther 79:5, 1943.
33. Hinshaw J et al: Pentazocine a potent non-addicting analgesic. Am J Med Sci 251:57, 1966.
34. Hopton DS et al: Action of various new analgesic drugs on the human common bile duct. Gut 8:296, 1967.
35. Houde RW et al: Analgetic power of chlorpromazine alone and in combination with morphine. Fed Proc 14:353, 1955.
35a. Huskisson EC: Measurement of pain. Lancet 2:1127, 1974.
36. Jackson GL et al: Analgesic properties of mixtures of chlorpromazine with morphine and meperidine. Ann Intern Med 45:640, 1956.
37. Jaffe JH: Opiate dependence and the use of narcotics for the relief of pain. Mod Treat 5:1121, 1968.
38. Jaffe HJ et al: Narcotic analgesics and antagonists, in the pharmacologic basis of therapeutics, 5th ed. (Goodman LS and Gilman A, Eds.), MacMillan, New York, 1975, p 245.
39. Jewitt DE et al: Increased pulmonary arterial pressures after pentazocine in myocardial infarction. Br Med J 1:795, 1970.
40. Jewitt DE et al: Cardiovascular effects of pentazocine in patients with acute myocardial infarction. Br Heart J 33:145, 1971.
41. Jick H et al: A new method for assessing the clinical effects of oral analgesic drugs. Clin Pharmacol Ther 12:456, 1971.
41a. Kallos T et al: Naloxone reversal of pentazocine-induced respiratory depression (letter). JAMA 204:932, 1968.
42. Kane FR et al: Mental and emotional disturbance with pentazocine use. S Med J 68:808, 1975.
43. Keats AS: Effect of nalorphine and morphine on the cerebral spinal fluid pressure in man (Abstract 1228). Fed Proc 13:374, 1954.
44. Keats AS et al: Potentiation of meperidine by promethazine. Anesth 22:34, 1961.
45. Keats AS et al: Studies of analgesic drugs. VIII. A narcotic antagonist analgesic without psychotomimetic effects. J Pharmacol Exp Ther 143:157, 1964.
46. Keats AS et al: Respiratory effects of narcotic antagonists. J Pharmacol Exp Ther 151:126, 1966.
47. Kerr F et al: Analgesia in myocardial infarction. Br Heart J 36:117, 1974.
48. Klotz U et al: The effect of cirrhosis on the disposition and elimination of meperidine in man. Clin Pharm Ther 16:667, 1974.
49. Lambersten CJ et al: The separate and combined respiratory effects of chlorpromazine and meperidine in normal men controlled at 46 mm Hg alveolar pCO_2. J Pharm Exp Ther 131:381, 1961.
50. Lasagna L et al: The optimal dose of morphine. JAMA 156:230, 1954.
51. Lasagna L: The clinical evaluation of morphine and its substitutes as analgesics. Pharmacol Rev 16:47, 1964.

52. Lee G et al: Comparative effects of morphine, meperidine and pentazocine on circulatory dynamics in patients with acute myocardial infarction. Am J Med 60:949, 1976.

53. Levy DL: Obstetric analgesia. Pentazocine and meperidine in normal primiparous labor. Ob Gyn 38:907, 1971.

54. Loan WB et al: Strong analgesics: Pharmacological and therapeutic aspects. Drugs 5:108, 1973.

55. Lowenstein E et al: Cardiovascular response to large doses of IV morphine in man. NEJM 281:1389, 1969.

56. Lutterbeck PM et al: Measurement of analgesic activity in man. Int J Clin Pharmacol 6:315, 1972.

57. Marks RM et al: Undertreatment of medical inpatients with narcotic analgesics. Ann Intern Med 78:173, 1973.

58. Martin WR: Opioid antagonists. Pharmacol Rev 19:463, 1967.

59. Mather LE: Meperidine kinetics in man. Intravenous injection in surgical patients and volunteers. Clin Pharmacol Ther 17:21, 1975.

60. Matts SGF: Analgesics. Br J Clin Pract 27:359, 1973.

61. McHorse TS et al: Effect of acute viral hepatitis in man on the disposition and elimination of meperidine. Gastroent 68:775, 1975.

62. Melzack R et al: The Brompton mixture: Effects on pain in cancer patients. Can Med Assoc J 155:125, 1976.

63. Miller HC et al: Effect of pentazocine on pulmonary circulation. Lancet 2:1167, 1972.

64. Mount BM et al: Use of the Brompton mixture in treating the chronic pain of malignant disease. Can Med Assoc J 115:122, 1976.

65. Mowat J et al: Comparison of pentazocine and pethidine in labour. Br Med J 2:757, 1970.

66. Murphee HB: Clinical pharmacology of potent analgesics. Clin Pharmacol Ther 3:473, 1962.

67. Nagashima H et al: Neuroleptanesthesia with morphine for aortocornary bypass surgery. Anaesthetist 23:313, 1974.

68. Nossell HL: The effect of morphine on the serum and urine amylase and the sphincter of Oddi. Gastroent 29:409, 1955.

69. Noth PH et al: Demerol: A new synthetic analgetic spasmolytic and sedative agent I. Clinical observations. Ann Intern Med 21:17, 1944.

70. Pearson JW et al: Effect of methotrimeprazine in respiration. Anesthes 24:38, 1963.

70a. Pearson JW: Analgesia for obstetric and gynecologic patients. Mod Treat 5:1164, 1968.

70b. Ricciarelli EAM et al: Opioids and obstetrics. Clin Ob Gyn 17:259, 1974.

71. Riffel HD et al: Effects of meperidine and promethazine during labor. Ob Gyn 42:738, 1973.

72. Scott ME et al: Circulatory effects of IV pentazocine in patients with acute myocardial infarction. Curr Ther Res 13:81, 1971.

73. Scott ME et al: Effects of diamorphine, methadone, morphine and pentazocine in patients with suspected acute myocardial infarction. Lancet 1:1065, 1969.

74. Sechzer PH: Demand method evaluation of analgesics. Curr Ther Res 19:343, 1976.

75. Sherman ED et al: Sensitivity to pain in the aged. Can Med Assoc J 83:944, 1960.

76. Sliom CM: Analgesia during labor: A comparison between dihydrocodeine and pethidine. S Afr Med J 44:317, 1970.

77. Stanley TH et al: Comparison of blood requirements during morphine and halothane anesthesia for open-heart surgery. Anesthes 41:34, 1974.

78. Steel GC: Obstetric analgesia. Int Anesth Clin 11:75, 1973.

79. Takki S et al: A comparison of pethidine, piritramide and oxycodone in patients with pain following cholecystectomy. Anaesth 22:162, 1973.

80. Telford J et al: Narcotic and narcotic antagonist mixtures (review). Anesthes 22:465, 1961.

81. Todres D: The role of morphine in acute myocardial infarction. Am Heart J 81:566, 1971.

82. Twycross RG: Clinical experience with diamorphine in advanced malignant disease. Int J Clin Pharmacol 9:184, 1974.

83. Twycross RG et al: Euphoriant mixtures. Br Med J 4:552, 1973.

84. Vandam LD: Analgetic drugs — The potent analgetics. NEJM 286:249, 1972.

84a. Ventafridda V et al: Considerations in the use of analgesic drugs in different states of neoplastic disease. Int J Clin Pharmacol 9:174, 1974.

85. Wang RIH: Pain and principles for its relief. Mod Treat 5:1083, 1968.

85a. Way EL et al: The biological disposition of morphine and its surrogates — 1. Bull WHO 25:227, 1961.

86. Watt R et al: Prophylaxis and treatment of nausea and vomiting. Pharmacol Physicians 2:12, 1968.

87. Weintraub M: Potentiation of narcotic analgesics with central stimulant; The use of modified Brompton's mixture. Clinical Pharmacology Reports, 5:9, 1976. A publication of the Univ. of Rochester, Dept. of Pharmacology and Toxicology.

87a. Weil JV et al: Diminished ventilatory response to hypoxia and hypercapnia after morphine in normal man. NEJM 292:1103, 1975.

88. Wiedner H: Addiction to merperidine hydrochloride. JAMA 132:1066, 1946.

89. Zelis R et al: Morphine: effects and determinants of myocardial oxygen consumption in man. Clin Rev 17:121, 1971 (Abst.).

90. _____: Narcotic analgesics-II. Adverse effects. Br Med J 2:587, 1970.

Mild Analgesics:

92. Beaver WT: Mild analgesics: A review of their clinical pharmacology, Part I. Am J Med Sci 250:577, 1965.

93. Beaver WT: Mild analgesics: A review of their clinical pharmacology, Part II. Am J Med Sci 251:576, 1966.

94. Beirne JA et al: Gastrointestinal blood loss caused by tolmetin, aspirin, and indomethacin. Clin Pharmacol Ther 16:821, 1974.

95. Binder RA et al: Treatment of pain in hemophilia. Am J Dis Child 127:371, 1974.

96. Clark R et al: Hepatic damage and death from overdose of paracetamol. Lancet 1:66, 1973.

97. Dixon AJ (ed), Salicylates, An International Symposium. J and A Churchill, Ltd. London, 1963.

98. Douglas AP et al: Controlled trial of cysteamine in treatment of acute paracetamol (Acetaminophen) poisoning. Lancet 1:111, 1976.

99. Driesbach RH: Handbook Of Poisoning, 8th Ed, Lange Medical Publications, Los Altos, Ca, 1974, p 285.

100. Gazzard BG et al: Controlled trial of cysteamine and dimercaprol in the prevention of liver damage after paracetamol overdose. Gut 16:839, 1975.

101. Goulston K et al: Alcohol, aspirin and GI bleeding. Br Med J 4:664, Dec. 14, 1968.

102. Grossman MI et al: Fecal blood loss produced by oral and IV administration of various salicylates. Gastroent 40:383, 1961.

103. Hahn KJ et al: Morphology of gastrointestinal effects of aspirin. Clin Pharmacol Ther 17:330, 1975.

104. Harvey F et al: Action of cysteamine in paracetamol poisoning Lancet 2:1082, 1974.

105. Hirsh J et al: Relation between bleeding time and platelet connective tissue reaction after aspirin. Blood 41:369, 1973.

106. Holt PR: Measurement of GI blood loss in subjects taking aspirin. J Lab Clin Med 56:717, 1960.

107. Hopkinson III JA et al: Acetaminophen versus propoxyphene hydrochloride for relief of pain in episiotomy patients. J Clin Pharmacol 13:251, 1973.

108. Hughes RD et al: Cysteamine for paracetamol poisoning. Lancet 1:536, 1976.

109. Kaneshiro MM et al: Bleeding time after aspirin in disorders of intrinsic clotting. NEJM 281:1039, 1969.

110. Kasper CK et al: Bleeding times and platelet aggregation after analgesics in hemophilia. Ann Int Med 77:189, 1972.

111. Kersh ES: Treatment of propoxyphene overdosage with naloxone. Chest 63:112, 1973.

112. Koch-Weser J: Acetaminophen. NEJM 295:1297, 1976.

113. Leonards JR et al: Effect of pharmaceutical formulation on gastrointestinal bleeding from aspirin tablets. Arch Int Med 129:457, 1972.

114. Leonards JR et al: Gastrointestinal blood loss from aspirin and sodium salicylate tablets in man. Clin Pharmacol Ther 14:62, 1973.

115. Leonards JR et al: Gastrointestinal blood loss during prolonged aspirin administration. NEJM 289:1020, 1973.

116. Lovejoy FH et al: The management of propoxyphene poisoning. J Ped 1:98, 1974.

117. Lyons L et al: Treatment of acetaminophen overdosage with

N-acetyl-cysteine. NEJM 296:174, 1977.

118. Mielke Jr CH et al: Use of aspirin or acetaminophen in haemophilia. NEJM 282:1270, 1970.

119. Mielke Jr CH et al: Aspirin as an antiplatelet agent: Template bleeding time as a monitor of therapy. Am J Clin Path 59:236, 1973.

120. Miller RR et al: Propoxyphene hydrochloride: A critical review. JAMA 213:996, 1970.

121. Miller RR: Propoxyphene: A review. Am J Hosp Pharm 34:413, 1977.

122. Mitchell JR et al: Acetaminophen-induced hepatic necrosis: I— Role of drug metabolism. J Pharmacol Exp Ther 187:185, 1973.

123. Mitchell JR et al: Acetaminophen-induced hepatic necrosis: IV — Protective role of glutathione. J Pharmacol Exp Ther 187:211, 1973.

124. Moertel CG, et al: A comparative evaluation of marketed analgesic drugs. NEJM 286:813, 1972.

125. Moertal CG et al: Relief of pain by oral medications. JAMA 229:55, 1974.

126. O'Brien JR: Effect of anti-inflammatory agent on platelets. Lancet 1:894, 1968.

127. O'Brien JR: Effects of salicylates on human platelets. Lancet 1:779, 1968.

128. Parkhouse J et al: The clinical dose response to aspirin. Br J Anaesth 40:433, 1968.

129. Parkhouse J: Simple analgesics. Drugs 10:336, 1975.

129a. Peterson, RG et al: Treating acute acetaminophen poisoning with acetylcysteine. JAMA 237:2406, 1977.

130. Pierson RN et al: Aspirin and GI bleeding, chromate blood loss studies. Am J Med 31:259, 1961.

131. Piperno E et al: Reversal of experimental paracetamol toxicosis with N-acetylcysteine. Lancet 2:738, 1976.

132. Praga C et al: Effect of aspirin on platelet aggregation and bleeding time in haemophilia and Von Willibrand's disease. Acta Med Scand (Suppl.) 525:219, 1971.

133. Prescott LF et al: Plasma-paracetamol halflife and hepatic necrosis in patients with paracetamol overdosage. Lancet 1:519, 1971.

134. Prescott LF et al: The effects of hepatic and renal damage on paracetamol metabolism and excretion following overdosage: A pharmacokinetic study. Br J Pharmacol 49:602, 1973.

135. Prescott LF et al: Successful treatment of severe paracetamol overdosage with cysteamine. Lancet 1:588, 1974.

136. Prescott LF et al: Cysteamine for paracetamol overdosage. Lancet 1:988, 1974.

137. Prescott LF et al: Cysteamine for paracetamol poisoning. Lancet 1:357, 1976.

138. Prescott LF et al: Cysteamine, methionine, and penicillamine in the treatment of paracetamol poisoning. Lancet 2:109, 1976.

139. Quick AJ: Salicylates and bleeding: The aspirin tolerance test. Am J Med Sci 252:265, 1966.

140. Quick AJ: Acetylsalicylic acid as a diagnostic aid in hemostasis. Am J Med Sci 254:392, 1967.

141. Scott CR et al: Cysteamine treatment in paracetamol overdose. Lancet 1:452, 1975.

142. Scott JT et al: Studies of GI bleeding caused by corticosteroids, salicylates, and other analgesics. Q J Med 30:167, 1961.

143. Shambaugh Jr GE: Gastric bleeding and aspirin. JAMA 218:1573, 1971.

144. Smith BM et al: Permeability of the human gastric mucosa. Alteration by acetylsalicylic acid and ethanol. NEJM 285:716, 1971.

145. Smith MJH and Smith PK: The Salicylates, a Critical Bibliographic Review. Interscience Publication, NY 1966.

146. Strubelt O et al: The curative effects of cysteamine, cysteine, and dithiocarb in experimental paracetamol poisoning. Arch Tox 33:55, 1974.

147. Stuart RK: Platelet function studies in human being receiving 300 mg of aspirin per day. J Lab Clin Med 75:463, 1970.

148. Sutor AH et al: Effect of aspirin, sodium salicylate and acetaminophen on bleeding. Mayo Clin Proc 46:178, 1971.

149. Tainter ML and Ferris AJ: Aspirin in Modern Therapy. Bayer Co. Division of Sterling Drug Inc, NY, 1969.

150. Tarala, R et al: Treatment of dextropropoxyphene poisoning. Br Med J 2:550, 1973.

151. Vandam LD: Analgesic drugs — The mild analgesics. NEJM 286:20, 1972.

152. Vlasses, PH et al: Naloxone for propoxyphene overdosage. JAMA 229:1167, 1974.

153. Young, DJ: Propoxyphene suicides. Report of nine cases. Arch Int Med 129:62, 1972.

Chapter 8

General Care: Fever

Louis C. Littlefield

1. How is body temperature regulated and what physiologic alterations during infectious processes produce fever?

Under normal conditions, body temperature is controlled about a specific "set-point" temperature by a neuronal regulatory mechanism within the hypothalamus and is the summation of heat production and heat dissipation. The preoptic area of the hypothalamus and adjacent regions of the anterior hypothalamus contain receptors which are heat sensitive and neurons which are capable of altering physiologic processes to increase heat loss and decrease heat production during hyperthermic states. In contrast, when cold receptors in the posterior hypothalamus are stimulated, signals are transmitted to the hypothalamic temperature control center to alter physiologic functions to increase heat production and decrease heat dissipation (21).

In the majority of hyperthermic states, fever is believed to result from a pyrogen-mediated elevation in the set-point temperature (62). While exogenous pyro-gens, such as a gram negative endotoxin or an antigen-antibody complex, may act directly to produce an elevation of body temperature, most experimental evidence supports the concept that an endogenous pyrogen acts upon the hypothalamus to elevate the body's set-point temperature (1). Endogenous pyrogen has been shown to exist in a precursor form in neutrophils, polymorphonuclear leukocytes, and bone marrow-derived phagocytic cells (monocytes, histiocytes and Kupffer cells) and is released during phagocytic processes. The primary means of heat conservation is cutaneous vasoconstriction which prevents the conduction of body heat from internal body compartments to the skin. Another method of conserving heat is decreased sweating, a phenomenon which generally accompanies hyperthermic states. One of several methods may be used by the body to increase heat production. First, a primary motor center for shivering is located in the posterior hypothalamus and, in response to an elevated set-point temperature, can produce an increased skeletal muscle tone throughout the body. Although significant increases in body temperature may be achieved without actual shivering, once muscle tone exceeds a critical level, clinically detectable shivering ensues, increasing heat production. A second method of increasing heat production which may be of particular importance to the newborn infant, is augmented cellular metabolism in mitochrondrially-rich brown fat stores induced by sympathetic stimulation.

2. What is the clinical definition of fever and what methods for measuring temperature are available?

In all normal persons there exists a diurnal temperature variation, the peak occurring in the late afternoon or early evening, the nadir in the early morning between three and five o'clock. This two to three degree variation in body temperature appears to be independent of sleep habits and eating and working patterns, although exercise and emotional stress have been shown to produce significant temperature elevations. The average oral temperature recording is considered to be 98.6° F (37° C), although the normal range may vary anywhere from 97.7 to 99.5° F in older children and adults and may be even higher in infants (24). Therefore, the clinical definition of fever is generally accepted to be an oral temperature above the range of 99.5 to 100.5° F (8). If rectal temperatures are properly recorded, the readings are generally 0.5 to 1° F higher than oral temperatures, whereas axillary temperatures are generally 1° F lower than oral readings (55).

The most accurate determination of body temperature is generally obtained by measuring rectal temperature. Although safer and easier to measure, axillary temperatures may be less accurate. For the patient who is fully cooperative and does not have an acute respiratory illness, oral temperature recordings may be the most convenient. Accurate and consistent body temperature measurements can be obtained by following some simple guidelines. First, due to the variability in accuracy between thermometers of different manufacturers, it is suggested that, whenever feasible, the same thermometer be used throughout a patient's illness. Rectal temperatures should be obtained by inserting a security bulb thermometer 5 cm (2 inches) into the patient's rectum for a period of three minutes. Accurate oral temperature recordings generally require five to ten minutes, during which time the patient should not breathe through the mouth in order to avoid spuriously low values. Also, it is important to remind patients not to take an oral temperature just after the mouth has been artificially heated or cooled. Axillary temperatures should be recorded after the thermometer has been in place for three to five minutes.

3. When should fever be treated?

Although the role of fever during infectious pro-

cesses has been studied throughout the time spanned by modern medicine, it is not well established whether fever is an essential host defense mechanism or a normal, yet questionably significant, biological response to infection (27). The possible beneficial role of fever in host responses has been reviewed and, in general, there is no solid evidence to support the concept that fever enhances specific mechanisms of resistance (4).

The child with fever deserves special attention due to numerous factors affecting diagnostic and therapeutic decisions. As a general rule, the younger the child, the more subtle are the clinical manifestations of life threatening infections (36, 41). Therefore, the newborn infant (birth to two months of age) with fever deserves aggressive diagnostic evaluation and therapeutic monitoring. In contrast, the child older than one year of age with the same fever and negative clinical findings can usually be followed on an outpatient basis, offering the parents reassurance of the probably benign course of the illness (55).

Fever-triggered seizures (also see chapter on **Epilepsy**) remain a concern of the pediatrician, although the risk of developing seizures, in an otherwise normal patient, is extremely low until the body temperature exceeds 104 - 106° F (40). In one recent review of high fevers seen in a private pediatric practice, among 101 patients without a prior history of seizures, convulsions occurred in only 12 out of 108 episodes of fever greater than 104° F (60). In addition, the majority of febrile seizures in nonepileptic patients occur before antipyretic therapy is begun; therefore, only a relatively small percentage of patients at risk for febrile seizures may benefit from aggressive antipyretic therapy (40).

Another factor affecting decision-making processes is whether or not the febrile course should be preserved for diagnostic and follow-up purposes. Since there does not appear to be a relationship between elevation of body temperature and personal discomfort (13), low grade fevers (less than 102° F) may be best managed without therapeutic intervention.

4. What would be the most effective means of reducing body temperature in a patient with a fever of 105° F?

The overall effectiveness of existing treatment modalities can be determined by examining controlled studies designed to identify the onset, potency, and duration of antipyretic action for each modality. The work of Steele and associates (56) demonstrated the superiority of acetaminophen in combination with ice water sponging or sponging with hydroalcoholic solutions in rapidly achieving a reduction of body temperature. These authors also point out that the two groups of patients so treated appeared to experience the greatest amount of personal discomfort. In addition, the toxic potential (e.g. coma) of topically applied alcohol solutions mitigates against its use in febrile patients (17, 38, 54). Hunter was unable to confirm the antipyretic effectiveness of acetaminophen and tepid water sponging used in combination (23). Since the greatest rate of temperature reduction in Steele's study occurred between 40° C (104° F) and 38.9° C (102° F), Hunter's grouping together of all patients with temperatures exceeding 39° C (102° F) does not allow one to evaluate the antipyretic effectiveness of each treatment modality at higher body temperatures.

Several well controlled studies have compared the antipyretic effectiveness of aspirin and acetaminophen (6, 14, 57, 59). In general, these studies have shown that (a) these two agents are comparable with respect to onset, peak and duration of antipyretic action when administered in equal doses, and (b) the two drugs are comparable to tepid water sponging with respect to duration of action although sponging may act more rapidly to reduce elevated body temperature.

In summary, the most effective means of lowering body temperature is not necessarily the most comfortable or safest. In addition to liberal fluid intake, which is required to replace increased fluid losses accompanying febrile episodes, the combined use of tepid water sponging and an oral antipyretic appears to be an effective and acceptable means of reducing body temperature.

5. During pediatric work rounds in the neonatal ICU, the intern asks you for a specific therapeutic recommendation for a 3-day-old infant with a temperature of 102.8° F. What recommendation would you make and on what basis?

From the previous comments, it is apparent that this child deserves a septic workup if poor feeding, irritability, jaundice, apnea, or respiratory distress is also present (41). Simple measures, such as removing the child's blankets and heavy clothing, maintaining a normal room temperature and/or increasing air circulation within the room may be sufficient to allow for body temperature reduction.

If the above measures are not effective, then tepid water sponging would be preferred over aspirin or acetaminophen. The primary reasons in support of this statement are the relative efficacy of tepid water sponging in reducing fever and the decreased ability of the newborn to eliminate either of the above drugs. Information obtained from newborn infants whose mothers had received aspirin just prior to delivery indicates that the neonate has a decreased salicylate elimination potential due to decreased biotransformation processes and renal excretion (32). The newborn infant has a longer half-life of the terminal, near-exponential phase of salicylate elimination relative to adults, indicating a lower V_{max}/K_m ratio of saturable metabolic processes.

Similarly, a study of 12 healthy full-term infants, two to three days of age, has shown a decrease in the elimination rate constant for acetaminophen (mean = 0.208 hr^{-1}) (33) as compared to that reported for adults (mean = 0.315 to 0.368 hr^{-1}) (10, 43, 48) accompanied by an increase in biological half-life to 3.5 ± 0.85 hours (average ± SD). A second study including three full-term infants, one to two days of age, did not find a significant increase in biological half-life (39) although it did confirm decreased acetaminophen glucuronide formation and increased acetaminophen sulfate formation as reported by Levy and associates (33).

From the above data, it may be concluded that a single dose of acetaminophen or aspirin may be given, but repeated doses would be difficult to schedule without knowing precise elimination rate characteristics. (Question 10 gives additional information which should be considered before recommending aspirin for a newborn infant.)

6. The mother of a three-year-old 14.6 kg male child calls a pharmacy for advice regarding the treatment of her son's fever of 103.6° F. She states that she has acetaminophen (Tylenol) drops in the house which she purchased for her 13-month-old daughter and also has adult strength aspirin. In addition to previously discussed cooling measures, what specific drug and dosage recommendation would you make?

There are several methods which could be used to calculate an appropriate antipyretic dose of aspirin or acetaminophen for this patient. One method that is frequently quoted is one grain of aspirin per year of age repeated every four to six hours. However, a three-year-old child within two standard deviations of an average body weight for age may weigh anywhere from 11.9 to 17.3 kg (11). This rather large range of probable body weight supports the generalization that pediatric doses are more appropriately determined according to the patient's body weight rather than age. Shirkey recommends an antipyretic dose of 65 mg/kg/day for aspirin (28) which is within the range of 10-20 mg/kg/dose recommended by Done (13). Since previously cited studies have documented equivalent antipyretic activity of aspirin and acetaminophen, an appropriate dose of either agent for this patient would be approximately 150 mg every four to six hours as needed.

A comparison of the adverse and toxic effects of the two agents reveals that therapeutic doses of acetaminophen, in contrast to aspirin, are remarkably free from adverse effects. Even following mild accidental or therapeutic overdoses with acetaminophen, there are virtually no clinical manifestations present. In contrast, the early signs and symptoms of salicylism (nausea, vomiting, irritability, hyperpnea and hyperthermia) may closely resemble the clinical manifestations of the disease for which the drug is being used. Therefore a reasonable tendency on the part of parents may be to continue aspirin administration rather than to discontinue it. Following larger accidental or therapeutic overdoses (greater than 200 mg per kg body weight), acetaminophen's propensity to produce hepatocellular destruction may actually make it a more toxic substance than salicylates when compared on a mg per mg basis. Therefore, although acetaminophen may possess fewer side effects than aspirin at therapeutic doses, it appears to possess a greater toxic potential following ingestion of large single doses (19, 20, 50, 52).

Although acetaminophen may be more expensive than aspirin, it seems that its characteristics of equivalent antipyretic effectiveness and reduced toxic potential at doses within the therapeutic range make it more desirable for use in this patient. An exception to this recommendation would exist if the patient would benefit from the more potent anti-inflammatory activity of aspirin.

A final word of caution must be offered with respect to the numerous liquid dosage forms of acetaminophen which are currently marketed. Commonly available concentrations include 60 mg/0.6 ml, 120 mg/2.5 ml and 120 mg/5 ml (25); therefore, the pharmacist must exercise caution in recommending an appropriate acetaminophen dose in terms of milligrams and milliliters to be administered.

7. Is there any evidence supporting the concomitant administration of aspirin and acetaminophen?

A study reported by Steele and associates has demonstrated that the concurrent administration of acetaminophen and aspirin produces a more sustained antipyresis than that which can be attained with either agent alone (57). On the basis of this study of 120 pediatric patients, there were no apparent differences between aspirin alone, acetaminophen alone, or combined therapy within the first two hours of observation. However, after four to six hours, those receiving both drugs had sustained temperature suppression, while those receiving a single antipyretic were noted to have gradual increases in their body temperatures. Although the authors suggested that the concurrent administration of acetaminophen and aspirin may reduce the toxic potential of aspirin since the dose could be repeated every six hours or more rather than every four hours, a more simplistic approach would be an elimination of aspirin altogether. The authors also suggested that since aspirin and acetaminophen are detoxified by similar metabolic processes, it is possible that the additive antipyretic effects may reflect accumulation of one of the drugs. Although Levy and Yamada (30) have demonstrated a competitive inhibition between acetaminophen and salicylamide biotransformation, orally administered sodium salicylate did not result in a competitive inhibition between acetaminophen and

salicylate biotransformation (31). Since all cited studies were designed as single dose experiments, other explanations must be sought to explain the additive antipyretic effects of the two agents.

8. A 23-year-old male with allergic rhinitis and bronchial asthma asks whether he should take aspirin or acetaminophen for a fever secondary to a cellulitis. Questioning of the patient reveals no history of acute allergic symptoms following previous aspirin administration.

A number of allergic reactions to aspirin have been described in the literature including asthma, urticaria, angioedema, rhinitis and even anaphylaxis (42, 49). Asthmatic episodes may occur within minutes after ingestion of aspirin-containing products and may range in severity from mild, brief exacerbations to severe protracted attacks accompanied by cyanosis, coma, and rarely, death (12, 15, 29). Recent literature evaluating the incidence of aspirin intolerance estimates that as many as 28% of children and 16% of adults with bronchial asthma may show a significant deterioration of pulmonary function testing following aspirin ingestion (37, 51). Since antibodies to aspirin have not been found in the serum of aspirin-sensitive subjects (53) and since many of the substances which can also produce exacerbations of asthmatic symptoms are prostaglandin synthetase inhibitors, there is continued interest and research in progress to associate a selective prostaglandin synthetase inhibition with aspirin's ability to cause increased lower airway obstruction (61).

Although the patient did not give a positive history of an acute allergic reaction following aspirin ingestion, he is at a relatively high risk that some detectable decrease in airway patency may occur; therefore, he should be advised to avoid aspirin-containing products.

9. Can aspirin or acetaminophen be used as an antipyretic/analgesic agent in a patient with a glucose-6-phosphate dehydrogenase (G-6-PD) deficiency?

Until recently aspirin has been reported to be a hemolytic agent in patients with erythrocyte glucose-6-phosphate dehydrogenase deficiency (22, 26, 58). Criticism of previously reported cases of aspirin-induced RBC hemolysis has been raised by Glader (18) who points out that infections and other clinical conditions, known to produce RBC hemolysis, are often present in those patients receiving salicylates. In vitro and in vivo studies with aspirin and its oxidant metabolite, gentisic acid, confirm that gentisic acid possesses oxidant activity, but only at concentrations which would be produced with blood salicylate levels of 500-3500 mg/dl. Therefore, salicylate concentrations up to

350 mg/dl have no apparent effect on G-6-PD deficient cells. In support of his *in vitro* data, Glader challenged 22 patients with G-6-PD deficiency with a four day course of aspirin at doses of 50 mg/kg/day and found no evidence of increased hemolysis (18).

Acetaminophen's effects on G-6-PD deficient RBC's have also been studied and the general conclusion is that it does not increase the rate of RBC hemolysis (16).

10. What is the relative effectiveness of aspirin or acetaminophen when administered as a rectal suppository?

In spite of the paucity of information regarding adequate bioavailability and clinical response, aspirin and acetaminophen suppositories are frequently used for patients who cannot tolerate oral medications. A study by Nowak and associates reported that both the rate and total amount of aspirin absorbed from a suppository dosage form is less than that which is reported for oral dosage forms (44). A general trend noted in this study was that a rectal retention time of five hours or less resulted in a total urinary salicylate recovery of 54-64% while a retention time greater than ten hours resulted in a total urinary salicylate recovery of 82-98%.

Variations in the amount of acetaminophen absorbed from commercially available suppository vehicles have also been reported (47). At equivalent mg/kg doses, the oral dosage formulations produce higher serum levels and result in a greater total amount absorbed than is reported for rectal suppositories.

Although some antipyretic/analgesic effects could be derived from the administration of aspirin or acetaminophen suppositories, the decreased rate of absorption and total amount absorbed may result in unpredictable therapeutic outcomes.

11. A 6-year-old child with a 24 hour history of severe vomiting and diarrhea is brought to the emergency room for evaluation. Physical examination reveals a temperature of 104° F, a respiratory rate of 25/min and a blood pressure of 90/60. Her mucous membranes are dry and her skin is cool to the touch. What are the risks of administering aspirin to a patient with fever and dehydration? Can tepid water sponging be used safely in this patient?

In addition to aspirin's ability to inhibit the action of endogenous pyrogen on hypothalamic thermoregulatory centers, it acts on vascular smooth muscle to produce peripheral vasodilation, thereby increasing heat dissipation (19). This peripheral site of action may be undesirable in a patient with moderate to severe dehydration accompanied by intravascular volume depletion. Since dehydration by itself may produce an elevation of body temperature (55), restoration of intravascular volume with liberal fluid intake (2000-3000 ml/m²/day) may be sufficient. However, if fever remains after these measures have been implemented, oral antipyretic therapy could be instituted.

Similarly, warnings against the routine use of tepid water sponging in dehydrated patients have been issued (2). In such patients who are already peripherally vasoconstricted due to intravascular volume contraction, tepid water sponging may actually increase the degree of vasoconstriction and thereby increase heat retention. The clinical clue used to identify these patients is a temperature gradient between central and peripheral compartments as manifested by a febrile patient who is cool to the touch.

12. A 26-year-old pregnant woman who is within a few days of expected time of delivery calls a pharmacy late one evening to verify whether or not it is acceptable for her to take aspirin for fever and a "head cold." What is your response?

To answer this question, one must consider the effects of aspirin upon the mother and fetus. In a retrospective study of 103 patients who took daily salicylate doses in excess of 3,250 mg for at least the last six months of gestation (34), revealed that those who took aspirin had an average gestational period which was seven to ten days longer than the control groups; labor time was approximately five hours longer than the control groups; and greater estimated blood loss at the time of delivery. Similar effects of salicylates on prolongation of gestation and labor were also reported by Collins and Turner(7).

At least two separate studies have reported suppression of collagen-induced platelet aggregation in 80% (9) to 100% (5) of newborn infants whose mothers ingested aspirin within seven days of time of delivery. This platelet effect coupled with aspirin's ability to interfere with prothrombin synthesis adds a risk factor to both mother and fetus. Another factor to consider is the ability of the salicylates to displace bilirubin from albumin binding sites, resulting in increased concentrations of free bilirubin in the serum (35, 45, 46).

Therefore, since acetaminophen has not been associated with any of the previously described unwanted effects on the mother or fetus, it would serve as an acceptable alternative for the symptomatic treatment of this patient.

REFERENCES

1. Atkins E: Pathogenesis of fever. Physiol Rev 40:580, 1960.
2. Aynsley-Green A et al: Tepid sponging in pyrexia. Brit Med J 2:393, 1975.
3. Aynsley-Green A et al: Use of central and peripheral temperature measurements in care of the critically ill child. Arch Dis Child 49:477, 1974.
4. Bennett IL et al: Fever as a mechanism of resistance. Bact Rev 24:16, 1960.
5. Bleyer WA et al: Studies on the detection of adverse drug reactions in the newborn: II. The effects of prenatal aspirin on newborn hemostasis. JAMA 213:2049, 1970.
6. Colgan MT et al: The comparative antipyretic effect of N-acetyl-P-aminophenol and acetylsalicylic acid J Pediat 50:552, 1957.
7. Collins E et al: Salicylates and pregnancy. Lancet 2:1494, 1973.
8. Cone TA: Diagnosis and treatment: Children with fevers. Pediatrics 43:290, 1969.
9. Corby DG: The effects of antenatal drug administration on aggregation of platelets of newborn infants. J Pediat 79:307, 1971.
10. Cummings et al: A kinetic study of drug elimination: The excretion of paracetamol and its metabolites in man. Br J Pharmacol 29:150, 1976.
11. Diem K and Lentner C (eds): Scientific Tables, 7th edition, Geigy Pharm., 1974, p. 695.
12. Dysart BR: Death following ingestion of five grains of acetylsalicylic acid. JAMA 101:446, 1933.
13. Done AK: Antipyretics. Pediat Clin N Amer 19:167, 1972.
14. Eden AN et al: Clinical comparison of three antipyretic agents. Amer J Dis Child 114:284, 1967.
15. Francis N et al: Death from ten grains of aspirin. J Allergy 6:504, 1935.
16. Fraser IM et al: Effects of drugs and drug metabolites on erythrocytes from normal and glucose-6-phosphate dehydrogenase-deficient individuals. Ann NY Acad Sci 151:777, 1968.
17. Garrison RF: Acute poisoning from use of isopropyl alcohol in tepid sponging. JAMA 152:317, 1958.
18. Glader BE: Evaluation of the hemolytic role of aspirin in glucose-6-phosphate dehydrogenase deficiency. J Pediat 89:1027, 1976.
19. Goodman LS and Gilman A (Eds): The Pharmacological Basis of Therapeutics, 5th edition, Macmillan Publ. Co., 1975, pp. 325-347.
20. Goulding R: Acetaminophen poisoning. Pediatrics 52:883, 1973.
21. Guyton AC: Textbook of Medical Physiology, 5th edition, W.B. Saunders Co., 1976, pp 961-969.
22. Hochstein P: Glucose-6-phosphate dehydrogenase deficiency: Mechanisms of drug-induced hemolysis. Exp Eye Res 11:389, 1971.
23. Hunter J: Study of Antipyretic therapy in current use. Arch Dis Child 48:313, 1973.
24. Iliff A et al: Pulse rate, respiratory rate and body temperature of children between two months and 18 years of age. Child Develop 23:238, 1952.
25. Kastrup, E.K. (Ed.): Facts and Comparisons, Facts and Comparisons, Inc., St. Louis, Mo., p. 248b-249b.
26. Kellermeyer RW et al: Hemolytic effect of therapeutic drugs: Clinical considerations of the primaquine-type hemolysis. JAMA 180:128, 1962.
27. Klastersky J et al: Is suppression of fever or hypothermia useful in experimental and clinical infectious diseases? J. Infect Dis 121:81, 1970.
28. Koch-Weser J: Acetaminophen. NEJM 295:1297, 1976.
29. Lamson RW et al: Some untoward effects of acetylsalicylic acid. JAMA 99:107, 1932.
30. Levy G et al: Drug biotransformation interactions in man III: acetaminophen and salicylamide. J Pharm Sci 60:215, 1971.
31. Levy G et al: Drug biotransformation interactions in Man V: acetaminophen and salicylic acid. J Pharm Sci 60:608, 1971.
32. Levy G et al: Kinetics of salicylate elimination by newborn infants of mothers who ingested aspirin before delivery. Pediatrics 53:201, 1974.
33. Levy G et al: Pharmacokinetics of acetaminophen in the human neonate: Formation of acetaminophen glucuronide and sulfate in relation to plasma bilirubin concentration and d-glucaric acid excretion. Pediatrics 55:818, 1975.
34. Lewis RB et al: Influence of acetylsalicylic acid, an inhibitor of prostaglandin synthesis, on the duration of human gestation and labor. Lancet 2:1159, 1973.
35. Maisels MJ: Bilirubin: On understanding and influencing its metabolism in the newborn infant. Pediat Clin N Amer 19:447, 1972.
36. McCarthy PL et al: The serious implications of high fever in infants during their first three months. Clin Pediat 15:794, 1976.
37. McDonald JR et al: Aspirin intolerance in asthma. J Aller Clin Immunol 50:198, 1972.
38. McFadden SW et al: Coma produced by topical application of isopropanol. Pediatrics 43:622, 1969.
39. Miller RP et al: Acetaminophen elimination kinetics in neonates, children, and adults. Clin Pharmacol Ther 19:284, 1976.
40. Millichap JG: A critical evaluation of febrile seizures. J Pediat 56:364, 1960.
41. Moffett HL: Pediatric Infectious Diseases: A Problem-Oriented Approach, J.B. Lippincott Co., 1975, p. 338.
42. Moore-Robinson et al: Effect of salicylates in urticaria. Br Med J 4:262, 1967.
43. Nelson E et al: Kinetics of the metabolism of acetaminophen by humans. J Pharm Sci 52:864, 1963.
44. Nowak MM et al: Rectal absorption from aspirin suppositories in children and adults. Pediatrics 54:23, 1974.
45. Odell GB: Studies in kernicterus: I. The protein binding of bilirubin. J Clin Invest 38:823, 1959.
46. Palmisano PA et al: Salicylate exposure in the perinate. JAMA 209:556, 1969.
47. Pagay SN et al: Effect of vehicle dielectric properties on rectal absorption of acetaminophen. J Pharm Sci 60:600, 1971.
48. Prescott LF et al: The comparative metabolism of phenacetin and N-acetyl-P-aminophenol in man, with particular reference to effects on the kidney. Clin Pharmacol Ther 9:605, 1968.
49. Prickman LE et al: Hypersensitivity to acetylsalicylic acid (aspirin). JAMA 108:445, 1937.
50. Proudfoot AT et al: Acute paracetamol poisoning. Brit Med J 4:557, 1970.
51. Rachelefsky GS et al: Aspirin intolerance in chronic childhood asthma: detected by oral challenge. Pediatrics 56:443, 1975.
52. Rumack BH et al: Acetaminophen poisoning and toxicity. Pediatrics 55:871, 1975.
53. Samter M et al: Intolerance to aspirin (Clinical studies and consideration of its pathogenesis). Ann Int Med 68:975, 1968.
54. Senz EH et al: Coma in a child following use of isopropyl alcohol in sponging. J Pediat 53:323, 1958.
55. Shirkey HC (Ed.): Pediatric Therapy, 5th ed., C.V. Mosby Co., 1975, pp 331-335.
56. Steele RW et al: Evaluation of sponging and of oral antipyretic therapy to reduce fever. J Pediat 77:824, 1970.
57. Steele RW et al: Oral antipyretic therapy: Evaluation of aspirin-acetaminophen combination. Amer J Dis Child 123:204, 1972.
58. Swanson M: Drugs, chemicals and hemolysis. Drug Intel Clin Pharm 7:6, 1973.
59. Tarlin L et al: A comparison of the antipyretic effectiveness of acetaminophen and aspirin. Amer J Dis Child 124:880, 1972.
60. Tomlinson WA: High fever: Experience in private practice. Amer J Dis Child 129:693, 1975.
61. Vane JR: The mode of action of aspirin and similar compounds. J Aller Clin Immunol 58:691, 1976.
62. Youmans GP et al: The Biologic and Clinical Basis of Infectious Diseases, W.B. Saunders Co., 1975, pp. 99-104.

Chapter 9

General Care: Nausea and Vomiting
Scott D. Matthiesen

There is perhaps no more frequent sign or symptom of illness than nausea and vomiting. Although nausea is a very subjective feeling and thus difficult to evaluate and treat, the presence of vomiting strongly suggests an active organic disease and spurs the physician on to rapid diagnosis and treatment.

Vomiting can be due to a wide range of etiologies including infection, neoplasm, radiation, uremia, pregnancy, anesthesia, severe pain, and very commonly, an adverse reaction to drug therapy. Certainly, ideal control of vomiting is treatment of the underlying cause; however, since this is not always immediately possible, palliative treatment with anti-emetic drugs is often indicated.

The benefits gained from preventing emesis are a reduction in the risks of aspiration and electrolyte abnormalities, as well as alleviation of the obvious distress that accompanies vomiting. Unfortunately, the anti-emetic agents available today are less than ideal drugs for the control of vomiting, both in effectiveness and in absence of toxicity. As a result, the risks versus benefits of anti-emetic therapy must be weighed carefully and the choice of anti-emetic made on sound pharmacologic as well as clinical grounds.

1. Discuss the physiology of the vomiting reflex.

The initiation of vomiting ultimately requires involvement of a nucleus of cells located in the reticular formation of the medulla, below the floor of the fourth ventricle. In close proximity to this vomiting center, resting on the floor of the fourth ventricle is another nucleus of cells called the chemo-trigger zone (CTZ). The CTZ receives input from the cerebral cortex, hypothalamus, vestibular center, and, in addition, is capable of reacting to non-neural, blood-born stimuli such as bacterial toxins and drugs. The vomiting center has inputs from the CTZ and afferent fibers coming from the gastrointestinal tract via the vagus. Thus, the act of vomiting can be initiated in either of two ways. First, the CTZ, receiving cortical, vestibular, hypothalamic, or chemical stimuli, is depolarized thus activating the vomiting center which sends impulses down the vagal efferents to the GI tract. Secondly, the vomiting center can be activated without CTZ mediation, by vagal stimulation through irritation of so-called mucosal receptors in the gastrointestinal (GI) tract; these afferent impulses initiate emesis by a reflex arc mechanism.

Propagation of emesis involves an enormously complex coordination of skeletal and smooth muscle. Not by coincidence then, the vomiting center is surrounded by the centers for inspiratory and spastic respiration, the vasomotor center, the vestibular, and the salivary centers. Apparently, this intimate association allows perfect coordination to occur. It may also explain why vomiting is an all or none response which

cannot be aborted by the most drastic physiologic pharmacologic manipulations. Consequently, termination of vomiting depends solely on the removal or interruption of stimuli reaching the CTZ or vomiting center.

Although this model (6) is over twenty years old, surprisingly little new information has been uncovered since. If these mechanisms are accepted, then pharmacologic agents capable of a) depressing sensitivity of the CTZ and/or vomiting center to chemical or neural stimuli, or b) blocking afferent impulses through selective anticholinergic action, will in theory be therapeutically effective anti-emetics.

2. By what mechanisms do phenothiazines inhibit the vomiting reflex?

In routine pharmacologic screening of chlorpromazine, the phenothiazine prototype, a number of investigators described its unique ability to inhibit apomorphine induced emesis in dogs (10,19). Later studies clarified the mechanism of this anti-emetic action by administering chlorpromazine together with a variety of agents whose site of emetic action was known at the time. They demonstrated that chlorpromazine prevented emesis normally induced by apomorphine and other drugs acting on the CTZ, but not that induced by oral copper sulfate and agents whose emetic action is on the vomiting center (11). Accordingly, these investigators concluded that the protective action of chlorpromazine was due to a direct action solely on the CTZ. A later study also provided evidence that in small doses, chlorpromazine's anti-emetic effect was primarily due to its action on the CTZ; however, it was also shown that much higher doses afforded significant protection from oral copper sulfate induced vomiting as well (25). Therefore, the anti-emetic action of chlorpromazine may be dose related, with low doses selectively depressing the CTZ and higher doses also depressing the vomiting center; however, it must be emphasized that all these studies were performed in animals.

3. Does the mechanism of action or anti-emetic potency differ among the various phenothiazines?

A number of studies have shown that most phenothiazines block apomorphine induced emesis (12,38,48) and, although some studies claim increased ability to depress the vomiting center with some agents (12), these phenothiazines should be considered to have the same mechanism of action.

The potency of these agents differ widely. The order of increasing anti-emetic potency for the phenothiazines (based on apomorphine inhibition tests) is chlorpromazine (Thorazine), triflupromazine (Vesprin), prochlorperazine (Compazine) and thiethylperazine (Torecan), perphenazine (Trilafon), and fluphenazine (Prolixin). Whether this variation in activity is due to an increasing affinity for an emetic receptor on the CTZ, or an increasing ability to depress the vomiting center as well as the CTZ, remains to be clarified (32,44).

Promethazine (Phenergan) has no action against apomorphine induced emesis and thus is not thought to have any action on the CTZ. Promethazine probably owes its anti-emetic action to its anticholinergic properties (25).

4. Which phenothiazine is most appropriate for initial empirical anti-emetic therapy? What are the most common side effects encountered when phenothiazines are used as anti-emetics?

Obviously, this is an inappropriate question considering the vast range of clinical settings in which an anti-emetic would be indicated. On the other hand, it is probably the question most frequently asked a pharmacist in regard to anti-emetics.

This type of question is best answered by considering the risks versus benefits of therapy. Clinically, the anti-emetic activity of all the phenothiazines is equal in the treatment of nausea and vomiting due to infection, uremia, cancer, radiation, anesthesia, or drug toxicity (12,31,32,38,56,59,64). Therefore, the choice of phenothiazine for initial anti-emetic therapy must be made on the basis of their relative potentials for side effects at equipotent doses.

The structure-activity relationships of the phenothiazines has been extensively reviewed (36). Although the list of side effects is long, an examination of the clinical studies using these drugs as anti-emetics reveals that only sedation, hypotension, and extrapyramidal effects are of significant consequence.

Sedation is reported in 50-80% of the patients receiving aliphatic phenothiazines as anti-emetics, with chlorpromazine having the highest incidence (32,44,58). Hypotension occurs with the next greatest frequency, again with chlorpromazine being the greatest offender (44,58). Although this side effect is rare with the piperazine analogs (prochlorperazine and thiethylperazine), the concomitant use of a narcotic increases the incidence to that of chlorpromazine. Although relatively rare at anti-emetic doses, extrapyramidal effects occur more frequently with the more potent piperazine phenothiazines perphenazine and fluphenazine (31,64), and the risk of this effect eliminates these agents for first-line, empirical anti-emetic therapy.

On the basis of these observations, the recommended phenothiazines for initial anti-emetic therapy in situations where the duration of therapy is expected to be short, are prochlorperazine and thiethylperazine. If chronic therapy is planned, chlorpromazine may be considered as well, because

tolerance appears to develop to the sedative and hypotensive effects of this agent (44).

5. A patient returns to the surgical ward after a thyroidectomy. In addition to his thyroid problem, the patient has a history of grand mal seizures. He has been maintained on phenytoin (Dilantin) 300 mg daily for 5 years, but due to surgery all medications have been stopped for 24 hours. Soon after the operation he experiences one episode of vomiting and still complains of nausea. Standing chart orders read "Compazine 10 mg IM q 4 hrs prn nausea." What should be considered?

There are two considerations in this patient. The first is the use of phenothiazines in a patient with a seizure disorder. Although animal and retrospective human studies have shown that high doses of phenothiazines, such as those used to treat schizophrenia, can decrease the electroconvulsive threshold and cause seizures in patients with convulsive disorders (7,41,60), the risk of using phenothiazines in anti-emetic doses in such patients should be considered low. In this patient, however, as serum phenytoin levels decrease due to his npo status, the risk of precipitating a seizure with phenothiazines increases.

Secondly, it must be realized that one or two episodes of vomiting frequently occur in patients as they recover from anesthesia. The mechanical action of vomiting poses a small risk in a patient recovering from a thyroidectomy, as opposed to one recovering from a gastrectomy, and the use of anti-emetics should be viewed in this light. In this patient parenteral phenytoin and a non-phenothiazine anti-emetic, such as benzquinamide (Emete-con), should be given.

6. An 8-year-old child awakes nauseated following a tonsilectomy. After checking the chart, a nurse administers 10 mg Compazine intramuscularly. Fifteen minutes later the child is found in an extremely rigid position with his head deviated far to the left and eyes rotated upward. He is apparently unresponsive to verbal or physical stimuli. What action should be taken?

This child is suffering from one of the bizarre adverse reactions typically associated with phenothiazine administration, namely an acute dystonic reaction of oculogyric crisis (4,26). Although reports of this reaction are most common following the administration of anti-psychotic doses of phenothiazines, it may rarely occur in patients given anti-emetic doses. Patients should be observed frequently following the administration of the first dose. This reaction is more likely to occur in the very young and older age groups.

Fortunately, rapid and effective treatments are available. Diazepam (Valium) 10 mg IV or diphenhydramine (Benadryl) 50 mg IV may be given to reverse this side effect (30,51).

7. A 44-year-old male is admitted to initiate levodopa therapy for Parkinsonism. He is begun on 1 gm bid. Shortly thereafter he complains of nausea and vomits twice. The physician orders Compazine 10 mg IM q 4 hrs prn nausea. What should be considered?

This situation illustrates the inappropriate and perhaps harmful use of phenothiazines as anti-emetics. It is likely that the patient's nausea is due to the rapid initiation of levodopa therapy in high doses. As pointed out in the chapter on Parkinsonism, nausea is a frequent side effect of levodopa and is often controlled by initiating therapy with small doses which are more frequently spaced or possibly given with meals.

In addition, the administration of a phenothiazine can exacerbate this patient's Parkinsonism and may actually block the beneficial effects of levodopa by blocking dopaminergic receptors in the extrapyramidal system (17,67). Although any phenothiazine capable of producing extrapyramidal side effects should be avoided in patients with Parkinsonism, it is difficult to make their use in anti-emetic doses a strict contraindication.

Recently, benzquinamide (Emete-con) has been reported to produce extrapyramidal side effects (27). Acute dystonic reactions have been reported when this agent was used in normal anti-emetic doses, therefore it too should be avoided in patients with Parkinsonism.

8. How can the nausea and vomiting secondary to narcotics be treated?

Morphine and its analogs have a profound and complicated effect on the CTZ and vomiting center in man. The nausea and vomiting produced by these drugs is most often related to CTZ stimulation and can effectively be blocked by narcotic antagonists, phenothiazines with CTZ depressant activity, and benzquinamide (33,39). The emetic action of all narcotics appears to be dose-related as nausea and vomiting occur with all when compared at equianalgesic doses (39).

In addition to CTZ stimulation, narcotic analgesics affect the neural pathways between the vomiting center and the vestibular nucleus, increasing the sensitivity of the vomiting center to vestibular stimulation (28). Indeed, nausea and vomiting from opiates are relatively uncommon in recumbent patients as opposed to those who are ambulatory. This suggests then that agents useful in motion sickness (see Question 11) may be useful in reducing narcotic induced nausea, especially in ambulatory patients.

In contrast to stimulation of the CTZ, narcotic analgesics depress the vomiting center once therapeutic drug levels are obtained, thus making it unlikely that further doses spaced 4-6 hours apart will elicit continuous vomiting episodes. On the other hand, patients using opiates on a prn basis may experience nausea after each dose.

The anti-emetic of choice for narcotic induced vomiting would be benzquinamide (Emete-con) since, unlike phenothiazines, it does not potentiate narcotic induced hypotension or respiratory depression (13,45,52,57). The drawback to using this drug is it is only available in a parenteral dosage form. When an oral or rectal dosage form is more desirable, prochlorperazine (Compazine) or thiethylperazine (Torecan) would be the drugs of choice.

In patients who experience nausea and vomiting from narcotics only when ambulatory, promethazine (Phenergan), cyclizine (Marezine), or meclizine (Antivert) should be of value by decreasing the vestibular stimulation reaching the vomiting center. The differences between these drugs are minimal, although meclizine has a significantly longer duration of action, making it more suitable for prophylactic use.

9. Is prochlorperazine or benzquinamide the more efficacious anti-emetic in post-operative patients?

Benzquinamide (Emete-con), is a non-phenothiazine anti-emetic which was developed to challenge the role of the phenothiazines in the control of post-operative vomiting. When comparing such a drug with phenothiazines one must consider its efficacy and safety. It must have an equal or greater ability to prevent emesis and, more importantly, should not lower the blood pressure, prolong sleeping time, or depress respiration to the same extent as the phenothiazines.

Since benzquinamide has been shown to block apomorphine induced emesis as well as prochlorperazine, it can be assumed that it has the same mechanism of action (37). This is borne out by clinical studies that have shown benzquinamide to be at least equal to prochloperazine in reducing the incidence of post-operative vomiting (23,42,46).

Investigations into the cardiovascular actions of benzquinamide have shown that the drug consistently *raises* mean arterial pressure an average of 10 mm Hg; heart rates were inconsistently affected, but a tendency toward increase was seen. Both alpha and beta blocking agents inhibited these effects, as did pretreatment with reserpine (13,52).

Two studies compared the effects of benzquinamide and prochlorperazine, with and without meperidine, on respiratory depression by examining their effect on the CO_2 stimulation test (45,57). The well known respiratory depressant action of meperidine was demonstrated as was the superadditive effect of prochlorperazine combined with meperidine. No respiratory depression was caused by benzquinamide and that observed following the administration of benzquinamide and meperidine was less than that seen with meperidine alone.

It must be concluded from this information that benzquinamide is as effective and possesses fewer adverse effects than prochlorperazine in the postoperative setting.

10. What is the place of trimethobenzamide (Tigan) in anti-emetic therapy?

The use of trimethobenzamide, introduced over fifteen years ago, is still controversial. Initial use of trimethobenzamide was based on the fact that it is structurally related to the antihistamines which possess anti-emetic activity (8). Pharmacologic studies have shown this agent is capable of inhibiting apomorphine-induced emesis in dogs and does not have significant tranquilizing, cardiovascular, or respiratory actions at anti-emetic doses (37). Initially, investigators (1) concluded that trimethobenzamide, in contrast to placebo, reduced the "average severity" of vomiting significantly in patients with cancer and uremia. A close examination of the results in patients receiving both trimethobenzamide and placebo (cross-over) shows that the placebo gave complete relief in 30% of the patients and trimethobenzamide was effective in 60%. Although this is a two-fold increase in effectiveness, it should also be noted in actuality only 30% of the patients were relieved of their vomiting by trimethobenzamide, while studies with phenothiazines (32,56) show efficacy in approximately 80% of patients not benefiting from placebos.

A study of 2,000 post-operative patients (18), found trimethobenzamide 50% more effective than placebo in reducing the incidence of nausea and vomiting and concluded it to be a good choice as a post-operative anti-emetic. However, the term anti-emetic implies prevention of vomiting and nowhere in this study was there discussion of a reduction in the number of vomiting episodes. Basing the efficacy of an anti-emetic on the patient's subjective evaluation of "nausea" is invalid.

In another study (47), trimethobenzamide was less effective than placebo in reducing the incidence of vomiting in the post-operative period, and data collected over a 24 hour period suggested that use of trimethobenzamide is followed by a rebound *increase* in emesis.

Other studies have also failed to supply sufficient evidence for efficacy although the incidence of side effects is low (2,3,5,65). Therefore, trimethobenzamide cannot be recommended as an effective anti-emetic.

11. Describe the pathophysiology of motion sickness, and explain why antihistamines and sympathomimetics are the drugs of choice in its treatment.

Of the many possible mechanisms involved in the poorly understood syndrome of motion sickness, that put forth by Wood and Graybiel (66) appears to be the most plausible. As a result of stimulation of the labyrinth system, impulses are carried via a balanced network of cholinergic and adrenergic fibers to the vestibular network located near the vomiting center. When there is strong stimulation, the vestibular nucleus is bombarded with an abnormal number of impulses which could radiate through the adjacent cholinergic-mediated reticular system to the vomiting center. The evidence supporting this mechanism is largely based on the pharmacology of those drugs which are effective in preventing motion sickness: the antihistamines and amphetamines.

Although antihistamines block apomorphine induced emesis (9) in extremely high doses, their beneficial action in motion sickness is apparently mediated through a different mechanism since the more potent apomorphine blocking agents, the phenothiazines are ineffective (16,29). It is more likely that these drugs inhibit the cholinergic-mediated spread of impulses from the vestibular nucleus to the vomiting center (34,35). That the effect is not related to the antihistaminic properties is supported by the fact that agents with greater ability to block histamine then diphenhydramine were shown to afford no protection against motion sickness (16). Indeed, all of the drugs effective in the treatment of motion sickness possess significant anticholinergic properties as evidenced by their common side effects of dry mouth, cycloplegia, tachycardia, constipation, and sedation.

The efficacy of the amphetamines can be explained by the theoretical balance between sympathetic and parasympathetic fibers terminating on the vestibular nucleus. Presumably, prevention of motion sickness can be accomplished if the norepinephrine-mediated system is favored since it appears to shunt vestibular impulses *away* from the vomiting center. This phenomenon may be due to the fact that anatomical, sympathetic fibers from the vestibular nucleus pass by the vomiting center at a distance greater than do the cholinergic fibers. In any case, a supra-additive effect is achieved when an anticholinergic is given together with an amphetamine (66).

12. The mother of a 12-year-old child who consistently becomes "car sick" asks for your recommendation for treatment. How should a patient be initiated on medication for the control of motion sickness?

Because response is unpredictable, treatment should be initiated with a drug and dose that produces minimal side effects. Promethazine (Phenergan), diphenhydramine (Benadryl), dimenhydrinate (Dramamine), cyclizine (Marezine), and meclizine (Antivert) are equal in efficacy, but diphenhydramine may cause excessive sedation. Another factor to be taken into consideration is cost. An example of this is Dramamine whose only active component is diphenhydramine (Benadryl) (15,50), yet a 50 mg tablet containing 25 mg diphenhydramine is twice as expensive as 25 mg Benadryl.

If the initial drug is ineffective or the side effects are bothersome, switching to another agent or adjusting the dose may be effective. Some patients will not be controlled by any of these drugs. In these instances atropine, scopolamine, or a combination of a mild anticholinergic and small doses of dextroamphetamine may be tried (66). If the latter is used, an increased risk of cardiovascular side effects must be anticipated. Because they are less effective after motion sickness has developed, these drugs must be administered 30-60 minutes before vestibular stimulation is anticipated; all except for meclizine must be given at 4-6 hour intervals to maintain effect. Meclizine is often effective when given only once or twice daily.

13. A 24-year-old woman who has missed two menstrual periods complains of severe nausea which occurs in the morning and evening. She thinks she is pregnant and needs something for her morning sickness. What is the etiology of morning sickness, and what treatments best control this syndrome? Have any of these agents been found to be teratogenic?

Morning sickness refers to the nausea and vomiting which occurs in the first months or pregnancy. Approximately 50% of the pregnant population will experience these symptoms which may actually occur at any time of day. The cause is unknown, but neurological, endocrine, metabolic, and psychological factors have all been proposed (22). Hyperemesis gravidarum is an extension of simple morning sickness in which vomiting results in metabolic disturbances and even death. The treatment of hyperemesis gravidarum is quite different from that of morning sickness and will not be discussed.

Drugs were commonly used to treat morning sickness until 1961 when thalidomide was found to be teratogenic. Understandably, the use of drugs in pregnancy, especially for mild nausea and vomiting, has fallen off sharply in recent years. Presently, the agents used to treat morning sickness include pyridoxine (vitamin B_6), antihistamines, phenothiazines, sedatives, and combinations of these drugs. Which, if any, of these agents are both effective and

safe is difficult to determine due to the limited number of controlled clinical studies and the high percentage of placebo response obtained.

Lask (40), found that promethazine relieved morning sickness in 47 of 60 patients and six more obtained partial relief. In his control group of ten women with morning sickness, however, symptoms disappeared in three and diminished in four. Meclizine was found to be more effective than placebo in one study (20), and similar results have been obtained with diphenhydramine (40), dimenhydrinate (14), and hydroxyzine (62); however, in all studies the placebo response was about 50%. One of the more frequently prescribed combination products containing dicyclomine, doxylamine, and pyridoxine (Bendectin) was compared with placebo in 110 women (24); 94% taking the combination had some relief of their symptoms, but 65% receiving placebo also responded. Lastly, a phosphorated carbohydrate mixture (Emetrol) of levulose and dextrose with phosphoric acid added to adjust the pH has been stated to be ''probably more effective than a placebo'' (43); however, studies evaluating its effectiveness have been criticized for poor design (53). The mechanism of action of this product is purported to be a delaying in gastric emptying time as a result of the high osmotic pressure of the solution.

Review articles (18,63,68) have not uncovered statistically significant evidence of potential for teratogenicity with the use of promethazine, dicyclomine, doxylamine, cyclizine, or meclizine. Meclizine has been implicated in the past (63), but subsequent studies have not produced further evidence against it. Indeed, in 1966 the FDA had required that meclizine and cyclizine carry labels warning against their use in pregnant women based on teratogenicity studies in animals. However, subsequent epidemiologic studies have shown no increase in embryo deaths or malformed children born to women using these drugs during pregnancy and consequently the FDA warning has since been removed (61).

In conclusion, promethazine and the more common antihistamines have shown equal effectiveness and risk, and the choice of agent should depend on cost. Pyridoxine is probably no better than placebo; however, if used as such, a 50% response can be expected. The benefits of the combination products are slight and hardly worth the astronomical cost. These agents are usually administered twice a day in the morning and at bedtime. The nightime dose is designed to protect against symptoms which occur the next morning. For this purpose meclizine may be best suited due to its longer duration of action.

Finally, it must be emphasized that drug therapy for morning sickness should never be considered first line therapy. Psychological reassurance and dietary advice are often quite effective. Most women do best with frequent small carbohydrate meals and plenty of fluids.

REFERENCES

1. Abrams WB et al: Clinical evaluation of Tigan. NY State J Med 59:4217, 1959.
2. Bardfeld PA: A controlled double-blind study of trimethoben-zamide, prochlorperazine, and placebo. JAMA 196:796, 1966.
3. Bellville JW et al: Postoperative nausea and vomiting: Antiemetic efficacy of trimethobenzamide and perphenazine. Clin Pharmacol Ther 1:590, 1960.
4. Berk BZ: Reaction to prochlorperazine? Lancet 1:776, 1969.
5. Blatchford E: Comparison of antiemetic effects of cyclizine, trimethobenzamide, and atropine. Canad Anesth Soc J 8:159, 1961.
6. Borrison HL et al: Physiology and pharmacology of vomiting. Pharmacol Rev 5:193, 1953.
7. Boston Collaborative Drug Surveillance Program: Drug induced seizures. Lancet 2:627, 1972.
8. Boyd EM et al: Agents affecting apomorphine induced vomiting. J Pharmacol Exp Ther 119:390, 1957.
9. Boyd EM et al: Antihistamines and apomorphine induced emesis. Canad J Med 31:320, 1953.
10. Boyd EM et al: Prevention of apomorphine induced vomiting by chlorpromazine. Fed Proc 12:303, 1953.
11. Brand TD et al: Aniemetic activity of chlorpromazine in the dog and cat. J Pharmacol Exp Ther 110:86, 1954.
12. Browne E et al: Vomiting mechanisms: trial of a new antiemetic — thiethylperazine. So Med J 54:953, 1961.
13. Burstein CL: Benzquinamide: a cardiovascular stimulant useful during general anesthesia. Anesth Analg 42:429, 1963.
14. Carlinger PE: Treatment of nausea and vomiting of pregnancy with Dramamine. Science 110:215, 1949.
15. Chen S et al: Influence of diphenhydramine on apomorphine induced emesis. J Pharmacol Exp Ther 98:245, 1950.
16. Chin HI et al: Motion Sickness. Pharmacol Rev 7:33, 1955.
17. Colzias GC: L-DOPA in parkinsonism. NEJM 281:272, 1969.
18. Coppolino CA et al: Tigan as an antiemetic in the immediate post-operative period. JAMA 180:326, 1962.
19. Courvossier S et al: Pharmacodynamic properties of chlor-promazine. Arch Internat de Pharmacodyn et de Therap 92:305, 1953.
20. Diggory PLC et al: Use of meclizine for relief of nausea and vomiting of pregnancy. Lancet 2:370, 1962.
21. Ekslain EF: Prochlorperazine as a pre and post anesthetic adjunct: pilot study. Wisconsin Med J 58:357, 1959.
22. Fairwheather DVI: Nausea and vomiting in pregnancy. Amer J Obstet Gyn 102:135, 1968.
23. Finn H: Antiemetic efficacy of benzquinamide. NY State Med J 71:651, 1971.
24. Geiger CJ: Bendectine in the treatment of nausea and vomiting in pregnancy. Obstet Gyn 14:688, 1959.
25. Glaviano VV et al: Dual mechanism of antiemetic action of chlorpromazine in dogs. J Pharmacol Exp Ther 114:358, 1955.
26. Gott PH: Drug reaction simulating tetanus. NEJM 224:167, 1966.
27. Grove WR et al: A benzquinamide induced extrapyramidal reaction. Drug Intell Clin Pharm 10:638, 1976.
28. Gutner LB et al: The effects of potent analgesics upon vestibular function. J Clin Invest 31:259, 1952.
29. Hanford B: Drugs preventing motion sickness at sea. J Pharmacol Exp Ther 111:447, 1954.
30. Hilson D et al: Diphenhydramine in the treatment of oculogyric crisis. Brit Med J 1:381, 1968.
31. Homburger F: Perphenazine as an antiemetic in cancer and other diseases. JAMA 167:1240, 1958.
32. Homburger F et al: Chlorpromazine in nausea and vomiting due to cancer. NEJM 251:820, 1954.
33. Jaffe JH et al: Narcotic analgesics and antagonists. In The Pharmacologic Basis of Therapeutics, Goodman and Gilman eds, 5th ed, Macmillan, New York 1975, p. 252.
34. Jaju BP et al: Effects of belladonna alkaloids on the vestibular system. Amer J Physiol 21:1248, 1970.
36. Jarvick ME: Drugs used in the treatment of psychiatric disorders. In The Pharmacological Basis of Therapeutics, Goodman and Gilman eds, 4th ed, Macmillan, New York 1970, p. 155.
37. Klein RL et al: Inhibition of apomorphine induced vomiting by benzquinamide. Clin Pharmacol Ther 11:530, 1970.
38. Laffen RJ: Comparison of fluphenazine with other phenothiazines in inhibiting apomorphine induced vomiting. J Pharmacol Exp Ther 131:130, 1961.
39. Lasagna L: The clinical evaluation of morphine and its substitutes as analgesics. Pharmacol Rev 16:47, 1964.
40. Lask S: Treatment of nausea and vomiting in pregnancy with antihistamines. Brit Med J 1:652, 1953.
41. Logothetis J: Spontaneous epileptic seizures and EEG changes in phenothiazine therapy. Neurology 17:869, 1967.
42. Lutz H et al: Antiemetic effects of benzquinamide in postoperative vomiting. Curr Ther Res 14:178, 1972.
43. Medical Letter on Drugs and Therapeutics 16:45, 1974.
44. Moyer JH: Chlorpromazine as a therapeutic agent. Arch Int Med 95:202, 1955.
45. Mull TD et al: A comparison of the ventilatory effects of two antiemetics: benzquinamide and prochlorperazine. Anesthesiol 40:581, 1974.
46. Pitts NE: A clinical pharmacological evaluation of benzquinamide: a new antiemetic agent. Curr Ther Res 11:325, 1969.
47. Purkis IE: The action of thiethylperazine, a new antiemetic, compared with perphenazine, trimethobenzamide, and a placebo in suppression of postoperative nausea and vomiting. Canad Anesth Soc J 12:595, 1965.
48. Rosenkilde H et al: A comparison of some phenothiazine derivatives in inhibiting apomorphine induced vomiting. J Pharmacol Exp Ther 120:375, 1957.
49. Schalleck W et al: Antiemetic activity of trimethobenzamide. J Pharmacol Exp Ther 126:270, 1959.
50. Schmidt J et al: Dimenhydrinate and diphenhydramine and apomorphine induced emesis. J Pharmacol Exp Ther 106:412, 1952.
51. Schnell RG: Drug induced dyskinesia treated with intravenous diazepam. J Florida Med Assoc 59:22, 1972.
52. Scriabine A et al: Some cardiovascular actions of benzquinamide. J Pharmacol Exp Ther 144:131, 1964.
53. Shapiro S: Unpublished data from the Boston Collaborative Drug Surveillance Program (testimony before OTC Panel) 1974.
54. Smith PK: Treatment of airsickness with drugs. Amer J Med 4:649, 1948.
55. Smithells RS: Meclizine and fetal abnormalities: a prospective study. Brit Med J 1:217, 1964.
56. Smithy G et al: Prochlorperazine for the treatment of nausea and vomiting in patients with cancer and other diseases. NEJM 256:27, 1957.
57. Steen SN et al: The effects of benzquinamide and prochlorperazine separately and combined on the human respiratory system. Anesthesiol 36:519, 1972.
58. Stephens CR et al: Control of nausea and vomiting with chlorpromazine: incidence of side effects. Arch Int Med 96:794, 1955.
59. Taylor C et al: Thiethylperazine: a clinical investigation of a new antiemetic drug. Canad Anesth Soc J 10:51, 1963.
60. Tedeschi D et al: Effects of various phenothiazines on minimal electroshock seizure threshold and spontaneous motor activity of mice. J Pharmacol Exp Ther 123:35, 1958.
61. The Federal Register 40:12935, March 21, 1975.
62. Turner HJ: Double-blind evaluation of hydroxyzine as an antiemetic in pregnancy. J Reprod Med 7:36, 1971.
63. Watson CI: Evidence of teratogenicity with meclizine. Brit Med J 2:1446, 1962.
64. Weiss S et al: Symptomatic relief of nausea and vomiting with perphenazine; a preliminary report. Amer J Gastroent 29:173, 1958.
65. Wolfson B et al: Investigation of Tigan in preventing postoperative nausea and vomiting. Anesth Analg 41:172, 1962.
66. Wood CD et al: Theory of motion sickness based on pharmacologic reactions. Clin Pharmacol Ther 11:621, 1970.
67. Yahr MD et al: Drug therapy of parkinsonism. NEJM 287:20, 1972.
68. Yerushalmy G et al: Evaluation of the teratogenic effect of meclizine in man. Amer J Obstet Gyn 93:553, 1965.

Chapter 10

General Care: Constipation & Diarrhea

Linda L. Hart

Changes in bowel habits are common medical complaints. During 1974, $223,520,000 was spent in the U.S. on laxatives and other elimination aids due to a preoccupation with the size, frequency, and consistency of stools (8).

One individual's diarrhea can be another's constipation, since no exact definitions exist for these terms. Constipation is defined as infrequent or difficult evacuation of feces (1). Diarrhea is defined as increased frequency and/or fluid content of bowel movements (91). Questions must be asked of the patient to determine the extent of the variation from normal habits. In one study, 99.3% of healthy adults and 98.25% of patients had a defecatory pattern which was between the limits of three stools per day and three stools per week (28).

Laxatives have no role in the management of constipation due to intestinal pathology. All laxatives are contraindicated in patients with cramps, colic, nausea, vomiting, and other symptoms of appendicitis or any undiagnosed abdominal pain (40). Bulk laxatives have an established role in the treatment of diverticular disease (86) and the irritable colon syndrome (65). Laxatives are also indicated in the treatment of certain poisonings and in the preparation of patients for radiologic or endoscopic examinations. Previously, laxatives were used in conjunction with some anthelminthic drugs. Laxatives are of only secondary importance in the management of functional constipation. In functional constipation it is important that the cause be recognized and corrected. Traditionally, laxatives have been recommended as a part of the therapeutic regimen for patients with a variety of medical disorders that are accompanied by constipation or that might be aggravated by the patient straining or passing hard feces (40). (See Questions 6, 7, 8, 10, 11, 12, 13 for recommendations concerning the uses of laxatives.)

Classically, laxatives have been categorized as stool softeners or emollients, bulk-forming, saline, and stimulant or irritant. The use of a stool softener or bulk-forming laxative will result in the elimination of a soft formed stool. The full effect is not achieved for about 3 days. Stimulant or saline laxatives result in a more fluid evacuation usually within a few hours (40).

All *stimulant laxatives* can cause griping, intestinal cramps, increased mucous secretion, and excess fluid and electrolyte loss. Therefore, they should only be used occasionally (2). Stimulant laxatives recognized as safe and effective by the FDA Panel on Laxatives (2) include castor oil, bisacodyl, aloe, cascara sagrada, danthron, senna preparations, phenolphthalein, and dehydrocholic acid. Individual effective doses of a stimulant laxative may vary from 4 to 8 fold. The action may be seen within 3 hours, within 6 hours, or after 24 hours (40).

All *saline laxatives* may cause serious electrolyte disturbances and water loss. Thus, they should be used only occasionally. Safe and effective saline laxatives include magnesium citrate, magnesium hydroxide, magnesium sulfate, disodium phosphate, monosodium phosphate, sodium biphosphate, and sodium phosphate (2). Reliable clinical comparison of the saline laxatives is lacking, and estimates of relative efficacy may be wrong by a factor of 2 or more (40). Systemic absorption of the saline laxatives does occur (see Questions 10, 11).

Bulk-forming laxatives are not absorbed from the gastrointestinal tract and increase the frequency of bowel movements and soften stools by holding water in the fecal mass. The FDA Panel on Laxatives (2) classified the following bulk-forming laxatives as safe and effective: psyllium preparations, dietary bran, karaya gum, polycarbophil, semisynthetic cellulose derivatives, and malt soup extract. Bulk-forming laxatives are indicated in the management of irritable bowel syndrome (see Question 6), diverticulosis (see Question 7), and in the presence of anorectal disease (see Question 13). The distinctive features of the individual bulk-forming laxatives are of limited practical significance. Choices are frequently dictated by other ingredients in the product.

The *emollient laxative* mineral oil, although classified as safe and effective by the FDA Panel on Laxatives (2), is considered obsolete by many authorities (15). Other stool softeners or emollients that were classified as safe and effective by the FDA Panel on Laxatives (2) include dioctyl sulfosuccinate (see Question 9), and glycerin and sorbitol. Glycerin, when adminis-

tered as a suppository, is effective in producing a bowel movement usually within 30 minutes with minimal side effects such as rectal discomfort, rectal burning or griping, and cramping pain. Sorbitol is safe and effective for short term use in the dose of 120 ml administered rectally. Despite the FDA classification, clinicians still view sorbitol as an osmotic diarrhetic rather than an emollient or stool softener.

1. A previously healthy elderly patient complaining of acute constipation of 10 days duration needs a laxative. What could be causing this patient's constipation? What should be ruled out before a recommendation is made?

Normal defecation requires a complex interaction of nervous reflexes, smooth and skeletal muscle contractions, and voluntary initiation. The sudden occurrence of constipation in a normal individual may indicate the development of an abnormality in the innervation or musculature of the intestine or of associated reflexes and accessory muscles (73). Such abnormalities may be caused by severe infections, particularly of the central nervous system, acute mesenteric circulatory catastrophe, renal colic, cerebral vascular accidents, painful anal lesions, ingestion of certain drugs, cancer of the colon, diverticular disease, or fecal impaction. Digital examination of the rectum or proctocoscopy may be necessary for proper diagnosis. A low pressure barium enema is indicated if the cause of the constipation has not been found (9, 74).

Constipation may be associated with a host of medical disorders including hypothyroidism, hyperparathyroidism and other hypercalcemic states, tuberculosis, urinary tract disease, lead poisoning, congestive heart failure, a major psychosis, a profound depression, parkinsonism, and diabetes (9). Because constipation is associated with so many medical diseases, it is rarely used as a diagnostic criterion.

Constipation may also result from the ingestion of drugs such as narcotic analgesics, anticholinergics, diuretics, and various inorganic ions such as iron, aluminum, and calcium (9). A careful drug history should be obtained from this patient to exclude any drug related causes for his acute constipation. For the treatment of drug induced constipation see Questions 11, 14, 15. Various laxatives would be contraindicated in patients with certain medical problems. Therefore, it is important to know the medical history of this patient before recommending a laxative. (See Questions 10, 11, 12, 13.)

2. A patient who is otherwise healthy and taking no medication complains of chronic constipation, malaise, and bloating. This patient is purchasing a laxative. Can these symptoms be caused by his constipation?

Contrary to the many advertisements for laxative products, no known ill effects occur if the bowel is not evacuated daily. Indigestion, bloating, anorexia, the passage of flatus, lower abdominal discomfort, malaise, headache, and other symptoms which are attributed to constipation by the lay public are not caused by constipation. Nor is there any evidence to support the claim that regularity promotes health as the advertisements would have us believe. Defecation does not rid the body of toxic products which, if allowed to accumulate, will result in poisoning of the individual (9). A nineteen year old male who had no bowel movements for four month intervals without symptoms has recently been reported (89).

3. A patient has been taking Ex-Lax (97.2 mg yellow phenolphthalein) daily for the past two years. What are the general effects of chronic laxative ingestion and the specific adverse reactions due to laxatives?

A condition known as "cathartic colon" has been demonstrated in patients who have taken laxatives chronically. The findings on barium enema are predominately right sided and consist of a dilated terminal ileum, contracted cecum, loss of haustration in the ascending colon, and regions of apparent stricture formation. Ulceration is usually not a predominant feature. Pathologically, there is loss of intrinsic innervation, atrophy of smooth muscle coats, excess adipose tissue in the submucosal layer, and thickening of the muscularis mucosae. The anthraquinone containing laxatives have been shown to cause melanosis coli which is pigmentation of the bowel wall with degeneration of the mesenteric plexus. The stimulant laxatives, but not bulk and emollient laxatives, have been implicated as a cause of cathartic colon (25). The length of time necessary for the development of this condition appears to be quite long. Case reports of cathartic colon describe patients who have ingested laxatives for fifteen to forty years and at greatly increased dosages (25, 115).

Since this patient is ingesting a phenolphthalein containing product, the many adverse effects of phenolphthalein should be discussed. Fixed-drug eruptions, Stevens-Johnson syndrome, and lupus erythematous have been reported due to phenolphthalein. The skin lesions may persist and/or leave residual pigmentation (68, 104). Phenolphthalein containing laxatives change the color of alkaline urine to pink.

Patients who ingest laxatives chronically may show electrolyte disturbances. Hypernatremia (41), hypokalemia (45), and hypocalcemia (44, 72) have resulted from laxative use. Laxatives may cause malabsorption and steatorrhea (109). Factitious diarrhea due to laxative ingestion is not uncommon (29). Various other adverse reactions to specific agents used as laxatives have been reported. Mineral oil may cause lipid

pneumonitis if aspirated (103). Calomel has led to mercury intoxication (31). Podophyllin is said to be teratogenic (23, 62). Oxyphenisatin was removed from the market because of hepatotoxicity (36, 73, 97). The anthraquinones are excreted into the milk of lactating women but in insufficient quantities to cause laxation in the infant (48).

4. A 70 year old man complains of chronic constipation. His wife died about one year ago and the man is living alone. He states that he dislikes cooking and frequently his meals consist of soup and tea. The pharmacist recommends Metamucil, one tablespoonful twice a day, and increased fluid intake. Is the recommendation appropriate? What alternative laxatives may be chosen?

Inadequate dietary intake has been cited as a cause of constipation. A diet high in undigestable fiber, including such foods as fruits (prunes, figs), fresh vegetables (salads), and coarse grains (rolled oats, whole wheat, and bran), should be prescribed for the man and appropriate referral to a social agency should be made to insure compliance. A bulk-forming laxative may be used temporarily to relieve his anxiety about his constipation or may be used chronically if his diet cannot be modified. The clinician should instruct the patient to ingest a glassful of liquid with each dose of bulk-forming laxative to minimize the risk of obstruction of the gastrointestinal tract which on rare occasions has resulted from these agents (108). The patient should be told that the laxative effect of the bulk-forming agents may appear in 12 to 24 hours but that the full effect may not be seen until the second or third day of therapy (40). He should also be told that flatulence may occur, and increasing his fluid intake may relieve this complaint (40).

Although the pharmacist recommended Metamucil, available evidence does not justify the choice of one bulk-forming laxative over any other product of the same class. The most important factors to consider in choosing a preparation would be palatability, cost, and convenience. Products which contain more than 15 mEq (345 mg) of sodium in the maximum daily dose such as Metamucil Effervescent should not be used by a patient whose ingestion of sodium is severely restricted because of congestive heart failure, hypertension, or renal failure. Some bulk-forming laxatives such as L.A. Formula contain 50% glucose which may be clinically significant in a diabetic patient.

5. The elderly gentleman's daughter states that she has recently read an article discussing the amount of fiber that should be included in the diet and that by eating fiber many diseases will be prevented or cured. She asks your opinion concerning this matter.

Recent epidemiologic studies indicate that the low

fiber content in the refined foods consumed in highly civilized countries may contribute to the high prevalence of constipation (21), diverticular disease (86), the irritable bowel syndrome, appendicitis (19), and colonic cancer (20, 56) in these countries. Attebury and associates (10) reported a laxation rate of once every five to seven days in subjects maintained on a chemically defined minimum residue diet. Painter (87) reported that dietary fiber in the form of a high residue diet given for four years to seventy patients with diverticular disease was 85% effective in relieving or abolishing symptoms. The evidence for the association between the consumption of a diet low in fiber content and the occurrence of appendicitis and colonic cancer is not convincing at this time (76). The average American diet contains approximately 4 grams of fiber. It is recommended that 6 to 16 grams of fiber be included in the diet each day. Bran has been suggested as a source of dietary fiber (2). One half cup of 100% bran flakes contains 2 grams of fiber. One slice of whole wheat bread contains approximately 1.2 grams of fiber.

6. A 33 year old female advertising executive complains of chronic constipation and abdominal distress which is relieved by defecation. The stools are hard and frequently contain mucous. What is the diagnosis of this patient and how should she be treated?

This is a typical case of the spastic colon presentation of irritable bowel syndrome which is a common functional disorder associated with anxiety. The other presentation of this syndrome is known as nervous diarrhea. A patient may have either of the manifestations of the irritable bowel syndrome or the symptoms may alternate. The irritable colon syndrome may account for as many as 70% of the patients referred to gastroenterologists (57). The changes in bowel habits may be precipitated by or related to emotional stress. Many patients with irritable bowel syndrome are "bowel conscious" and may abuse laxatives. This aggravates their clinical condition and distorts the medical history. The disturbed motor function of the intestine in these individuals correlates well with emotional upsets. Otherwise, the physical examination of these individuals is within normal limits (74).

The treatment of irritable bowel syndrome now includes the recommendation of a high residue diet and the administration of bulk-forming laxatives as was suggested for the patient in Question 4. Katz (65) reported that 73-82% of patients suffering from various disorders, including irritable colon syndrome, achieved improvement in laxation when treated with a bulk-forming laxative.

Anticholinergic drugs are frequently prescribed for the symptoms of the irritable bowel syndrome. A recent review of 400 papers on eighteen of the most commonly prescribed anticholinergic agents failed to reveal any well-controlled studies showing that these drugs are effective for irritable bowel syndrome when given orally (57). It was shown in a double-blind trial that the symptoms of irritable bowel syndrome respond to placebo; six percent of the patients preferred placebo, and 47% of the patients had no preference between placebo and a belladonna-phenobarbital drug (98).

7. What are diverticulosis and diverticulitis? What are the causes and symptoms? How should diverticular disease be treated?

In Western countries diverticula can be found in 20% of all people over 50 years of age (74). Diverticulosis describes a condition where the colonic mucosa herniates through the circular muscle layer of the colon at the site of the penetrating arterial branches. Diverticulitis is the presence of inflamed diverticula. Diverticula develop because of defects in the circular muscle layer because of weakness and/or increased intraluminal pressure. The most prominent finding in diverticular disease is thickening of the longitudinal and circular muscle layers. The reason for the muscle thickening may be increased intracolonic pressure which has been related to the low amount of fiber in Western diets (see Question 5) (75, 100). Most patients with diverticula are asymptomatic. Symptoms and complications of diverticular disease are more common in elderly patients. Symptoms in diverticulosis include abdominal pain, flatulence, constipation or diarrhea, and blood in the stool. Symptoms in diverticulitis include lower abdominal pain, signs of peritoneal irritation, fever, constipation, malaise, and rectal bleeding. There is no evidence that the treatment of diverticulosis reduces the incidence of complications or alters the clinical course, although symptoms may be controlled (100). A high fiber diet is recommended for the treatment of diverticular disease (see Question 4). Low residue diets and medications such as morphine which increase intracolonic pressure should be avoided (see Question 14). In acute diverticulitis the patient should be hospitalized, given nothing by mouth, and intravenous fluids and electrolytes should be administered. Antibiotic therapy should be based on appropriate cultures. Analgesics may be required. Surgery is indicated for repeated bouts of acute diverticulitis, bowel obstruction, the development of fistulas, and hemorrhage (75, 100).

8. A patient without any concomitant diseases is scheduled for a barium enema tomorrow. What agents may be used to prepare the colon for this examination? Does any laxative regimen offer an advantage over any other laxative regimen?

Before a barium enema is performed, it is necessary that the colon be cleared of fecal contents. Therefore, a preparation that will accomplish this objective with the least discomfort to the patient should be recommended. The use of many of the regimens to prepare the colon for either endoscopic or radiologic examination seems to be based on tradition rather than scientific evidence.

Margulis conducted a survey and found that castor oil was the most commonly used laxative for this indication. The dose of castor oil varied from 30 ml to 90 ml, although 60 ml as a single oral dose was preferred in adults (71). Pancreatic lipase hydrolyzes castor oil to ricinoleic acid which stimulates the excretion of water and electrolytes into the bowel (24). Because of its action on the small intestine, castor oil results in a complete evacuation of the bowel within two hours. Since the onset of action of castor oil is so short, it should not be given at bedtime (40). Many patients complain about the taste of castor oil so an emulsion of castor oil is offered as a more palatable alternative. However, in this survey 120 ml of castor oil emulsion (Neoloid) was not thought to be as effective as 60 ml of plain castor oil (71).

Patients given castor oil in preparation for a barium enema also are given "enemas until clear" just prior to the examination. In a study of 102 patients given enemas, 40% were unable to retain any enema solution, 60% required three or more enemas, and only one-fourth of the study films were considered excellent (85). The enema itself causes hyperemic changes in the mucosa and increased mucous secretion. Therefore, it is recommended that the examination not be performed until at least 30 minutes after the last enema (71). There are reports of rectal irritation that lasted as long as 3 weeks after soap enemas as well as reports of anaphylaxis, rectal gangrene, and serious fluid loss secondary to acute colitis after soap enemas (92). It is recommended that soap enemas not be used.

Another regimen used to prepare patients for barium enema examination is known as the hydration technique (11). On the day before the examination the patient is given a low residue diet for lunch, a clear liquid dinner, and frequent glasses of water. After dinner the patient is given 11 ounces of magnesium citrate solution and at bedtime 15-20 mg of bisacodyl orally. On the morning of the examination the patient eats no breakfast and a bisacodyl suppository is inserted one hour prior to the examination. In one study (11), radiologic examinations were rated as good for 84.5% of the patients prepared with this regimen, and for 61.8% of patients prepared with castor oil and cleansing enemas. All patients treated with castor oil complained of cramps and expressed a dislike of the enemas. With the hydration technique, 1.5% of patients experienced adverse effects.

Full doses of saline laxatives lead to a semifluid or watery bowel evacuation in three hours or less. The saline laxatives have long been assumed to act by the attraction of water into the intestine by the hyperosmolar concentration of poorly absorbed ions. However, recent evidence suggests that the mechanism of action may involve the release of the hormone cholecystokinin-pancreozymin (CCK-PZ) which stimulates the motor and secretory activity of the GI tract (50). A saline laxative may cause serious electrolyte disturbances and water loss and it is recommended that saline laxatives be administered with enough water to prevent any net loss of fluids. For these reasons, this regimen has the patient ingest a glassful of water every 1-2 hours on the day prior to the examination. Magnesium citrate is used in this regimen to grossly clear the colon and facilitate the action of bisacodyl.

Bisacodyl is a stimulant laxative which in contact with colonic mucosa promotes evacuation by inducing mass movements in the colon through its action on the mucosa or submucosal plexi of the large intestine. The drug is considered to be a contact laxative, because application of topical anesthetics to the mucosa blocks its action. In animal studies bisacodyl inhibits sodium-potassium ATP-ase thereby limiting sodium and water reabsorption in the small intestine. Bisacodyl may also inhibit the reabsorption of tyrosine and glucose, causing water to be retained by the hyperosmolar colonic contents (38). The enteric coated tablets should not be chewed and should not be taken within one hour of antacids or milk. The effect of bisacodyl when given orally is seen in 6 to 12 hours; when administered rectally, the effect occurs within 15 to 60 minutes (40).

9. Dioctyl sodium sulfosuccinate is a frequently prescribed laxative. Is this agent safe and effective? When is it indicated? What is the effective dose?

The FDA Panel on Laxatives (2) classified dioctyl sodium sulfoxuccinate (DSS) as safe and effective. DSS does produce softening of the stool (55, 90) and *in vitro* studies attribute the mechanism of action of DSS to its detergent properties which reduce the surface tension and allow water and fats to penetrate the fecal mass. More recent evidence shows that DSS causes an increase in cyclic adenosine monophosphate (cyclic AMP) in the mucosal cells of the colon which stimulates the excretion of water and electrolytes into the colon (35). The maximal effect of DSS may not be achieved for 24 to 48 hours (40). DSS does not cause significant toxicity (2); however, because of the possibility of DSS increasing the gastrointestinal or hepatic cell absorption of other drugs, the FDA Panel on Laxatives (2) recommended that it be used only occasionally and no longer than daily for one week. This warning was prompted by the association of DSS with the hepatotoxicity of oxyphenisatin and dantrol (36, 73, 97, 110, 114). Although this association has not been proven, the Panel wanted to focus on the possibility of a cause and effect relationship. It is recommended that DSS be used as a single ingredient laxative and that patients chronically ingesting DSS be monitored for hepatotoxicity.

DSS is indicated in constipation due to hard stools and in conditions where painful or difficult defecation should be avoided (see Questions 10, 11, 12, 13). DSS may be used in conditions where stimulant laxatives are contraindicated. According to Palmer (88), it is senseless to prescribe stool softeners in elderly patients with hypotonic constipation which is characterized by the late arrival of feces at every point along the colon and a decrease in water absorption. In these patients, the colon is partially full from one end to the other with a soft putty like stool. The toneless abdominal wall cannot expulse the feces.

There is controversy over the effectiveness of DSS in preventing constipation. Goodman and associates (46) reported that 200 mg DSS qd was not effective in altering the incidence of constipation in a group of elderly hospitalized patients. Whether a larger dose is more effective remains to be determined. However, it appears that the recommended dose is too low to achieve therapeutic results. It is suggested that therapy be instituted at 200 mg/day and dose adjustments be made at 2 day intervals until the therapeutic endpoint is reached. Larger doses may be necessary at the beginning of therapy. The usual dosage range is from 200 to 600 mg (40) although doses of 1500 mg have been prescribed. No comparative clinical studies exist for the various dioctyl sulfosuccinate salts on the market.

10. A patient with a long history of congestive heart failure due to hypertension recently suffered a myocardial infarction. Now the patient complains of constipation. How should this patient be treated?

Because defecation has been demonstrated to change hemodynamics, straining at stool may be dangerous if a thrombus is present in a heart chamber, in the veins of the legs, or in the pelvic area. Death from emboli, ventricular rupture, and cardiogenic shock have been attributed to straining in patients who have suffered a myocardial infarction (33). For these reasons, it is recommended that these patients be placed on a laxative regimen. Bowel movements do not usually occur and are not encouraged in the first three days after the infarction.

In this situation, the sodium content of various laxatives would prevent their use. Metamucil Effervescent could not be used because it contains 250 mg (11 mEq) sodium per dose. The amount of sodium contained in recommended doses of phosphate salts ranges from 88 to 176 mEq. The amount of sodium absorbed from the phosphate enema varies from 1.6 to 31 mEq (118). There is risk of serum sodium elevation by either route of administration with these laxatives. The preference of the potassium or calcium salt of dioctyl sulfosucci-

nate does not appear to be based on sound judgment. The amount of sodium (approximately 5 mg) in 100 mg of DSS is of doubtful clinical significance in a patient on the usual sodium restricted diet.

This patient could be treated with 240 mg DSS daily; Dennison (33) subjectively evaluated the results of 103 patients so treated as excellent. Others recommend for myocardial infarction patients milk of magnesia 30 ml at bedtime, bisacodyl, or glycerin suppositories. No well-controlled trials support the recommendation of one laxative regimen over any other in this situation.

11. Mr. B.B. is a 56-year-old patient with chronic renal failure. Medications which Mr. B.B. is taking include clonidine 0.3 mg bid, aluminum hydroxide gel 30 ml qid, calcium carbonate 600 mg qid, ferrous sulfate 300 mg tid, multivitamin one qd, and folic acid 1 mg qd. What laxative might you recommend for his constipation? Are any of the drugs that he is taking contributing to his constipation?

This patient should be treated with either a bulk-forming laxative or dioctyl sulfosuccinate which will increase the water content of the fecal material. If the patient is not severely fluid restricted, liberalization of his fluid intake may help to alleviate his constipation. If the diet can be modified to increase fiber content, this may also help. The sodium content of the laxatives should be kept to a minimum as in patients with congestive heart failure or hypertension. Since approximately 15 to 30% of ingested magnesium is absorbed, which may result in toxicity in the presence of renal insufficiency, magnesium containing laxatives should be avoided. Elevated serum phosphate levels and decreased serum calcium have been reported with the prolonged use of phosphate containing laxatives or enemas in patients with renal failure, so these laxatives should not be used (71).

Many renal patients require drugs which contain inorganic ions such as aluminum hydroxide, calcium carbonate, and ferrous salts. All of these preparations are constipating, the mechanism of which is attributed to the astringent properties of the ions. A 49 year old female undergoing hemodialysis for chronic renal failure developed perforation of the colon and died of septicemia and peritonitis. The perforation probably resulted from chronic constipation which was aggravated by aluminum hydroxide that was used to lower hyperphosphatemia (44). Five cases of intestinal obstruction due to antacid gels were reported by Brettschneider (17). Another case of intestinal obstruction due to impacted aluminum hydroxide tablets which were not chewed was reported by Potyk (93). Constipation is seen occasionally during clonidine therapy. One case report of ileus attributed to clonidine therapy recently appeared (13). The mechanism of this adverse effect is currently unknown. Polystyrene resin

(Kayexalate) which is used to reduce hyperkalemia in renal patients is associated with a high incidence of constipation.

12. A lady who is 8 months pregnant asks a pharmacist to recommend a laxative.

Constipation is a common complaint in pregnancy. During the last trimester, the large uterus may inhibit the expulsive forces of the abdominal and diaphragmatic muscles. Hemorrhoids and painful anal lesions may result in a voluntary suppression of the defecatory reflex. Iron therapy may contribute to the development of hard stools. Stool softeners or bulk-forming laxatives are preferred in the treatment of the constipation of pregnancy. Irritant laxatives should be avoided.

These laxatives may be continued into the postpartum period where constipation is due to ileus secondary to bowel dilation in a decompressed abdomen, perineal pain, and laxness of the anal sphincter and abdominal muscles (80).

13. A patient who suffers from hemorrhoids needs a laxative. What laxatives should be recommended?

Patients with anorectal disease including hemorrhoids, fissures, and fistulas should use either a softener or a bulk-forming agent if a laxative is indicated. Dioctyl sulfosuccinate, a psyllium preparation, or one of the cellulose containing products should be recommended. This patient should avoid mineral oil, because the bacteria laden oily film that coats the rectum has been associated with infections and delayed healing of the rectal wounds (15).

14. Mrs. C.R. is suffering from metastatic breast carcinoma. To relieve her severe pain she is receiving injections of morphine sulfate 10 mg every 4 hours. What is your recommendation for the treatment of her constipation?

One half of the constipating effects of the narcotic analgesics are said to be due to the delay of gastric emptying for as much as 12 hours. One fourth of the constipating effects are due to a decrease in propulsive peristalic waves in the colon which move the feces over short distances, an increase in the tone of colon, and an increase in non-propulsive contractions of the colon which results in increased resistance to the forward movement of material in the colon. As the movement of stool is retarded, the contact time for reabsorption of water from the fecal mass is increased, and the feces become desiccated. The remainder of the constipating effects are due to increased tone in the anal sphincter and decreased sensitivity to the defecation reflex because of central nervous system depression (58).

The treatment of the constipation should be aimed at decreasing the pressure within the colon which is retarding the movement of fecal material and at preventing the reabsorption of water from the feces. A bulk-forming laxative will accomplish both of these objectives. The pressure in the colon is proportional to the tension in the muscle walls and is inversely proportional to the radius of the bowel lumen. This relationship is known as the Law of LaPlace and is shown by the following formula: $P = t/r$. Bulk-forming laxatives, by increasing the radius of the bowel lumen, will decrease the pressure. Also, bulk forming laxatives hold water in the stool. This patient should be started on the usual dose of one of the bulk-forming laxatives such as 15 ml psyllium twice a day, and an evaluation of the response should be made in two to three days for dosage adjustment.

This patient must be carefully monitored for the development of an impaction which results from excessive dehydration of feces due to prolonged retention in the rectum or rarely, the sigmoid colon. The symptoms of impaction include cramping, lower abdominal pain, and paradoxical diarrhea as watery stools are passed around the hardened mass. The recommended treatment of fecal impaction includes softening with an oil-retention enema or an enema of 5 ml of 1% dioctyl sodium sulfosuccinate diluted to 100 ml with water. Alternatively, the mass may be broken manually and then evacuated with an enema of water or saline (117).

15. Mr. R.A. is a patient with a history of chronic depression for which he is receiving amitriptyline 300 mg per day. What is your recommendation for the treatment of this patient's constipation? How frequently is constipation caused by tricyclic antidepressants?

Again, as in all other cases of constipation, modifications of diet are indicated to increase fiber content, and fluid intake. Also, a change in daily life style such as increased exercise and an uninterrupted bowel routine are recommended. If these measures do not achieve the desired results, then a bulk-forming laxative or dioctyl sulfosuccinate in sufficient dose (200 to 500 mg) is recommended.

A 54 year old woman treated with 25 mg amitriptyline three times a day for 4 weeks developed paralytic ileus (43). Diamond (34) reported a 4% incidence of constipation in his patients with gastrointestinal complaints treated with 10 to 25 mg imipramine four times a day. He noticed that patients who had constipation as a complaint prior to therapy had more complaints of constipation during therapy. The severity of the constipation is unquestionably related to the age of the patient and the dosage, so elderly patients and patients receiving higher doses should be monitored more closely (6).

The tricyclic antidepressants as well as the phenothiazines, antihistamines, and anticholinergics are constipating because of their anticholinergic action. Anticholinergics retard the massive contractions which propulse the bolus of feces over long distances or move a large volume of material. These massive contractions are associated with eating or gastric emptying and are the reason that many people move their bowels following a meal (57).

16. What drug interactions have been attributed to laxatives?

Cellulose derivatives are said to bind digitalis, nitrofurantoin, and salicylate, although the clinical significance of this interaction has not been elucidated (2). Mineral oil may decrease the absorption of fat soluble vitamins. Steigmann and co-workers (110) found that a dose of mineral oil greater than 2.5 ml when given with meals significantly decreased the plasma level of vitamin A. However, 30 ml when given at bedtime did not affect the plasma vitamin A level. Javert and Macri (59) found that the effects of mineral oil ingestion on prothrombin levels varied with individual patients as well as the frequency of dosing. On intermittent dosage, 33% of the patients developed decreased prothrombin levels, and 70% of the patients developed decreased prothrombin levels while ingesting mineral oil daily for one to two weeks. The timing of the dose, 15 to 30 ml, in relation to meals was not stated in this study. It is recommended that patients taking oral anticoagulants avoid mineral oil (84). DSS enhances the absorption of mineral oil which has been associated with granuloma formation in lymph nodes, the liver, and intestinal mucosa (15). The concomitant ingestion of these two agents is not recommended. Prescot reported that sorbitol accelerates the absorption of acetaminophen and phenacetin, although no specific data regarding his interaction were given (94).

17. What laxative products are unsafe and/or ineffective?

The FDA Panel on Laxatives (2) found calomel, degraded carrageeman (Irish Moss), podophylum resin, and other resins such as colocynth, elaterin, gamboge, ipomea, and jalap to be unsafe an/or ineffective as laxatives. Combination products which contain nonlaxative ingredients that do not contribute to laxation and which greatly increase the risk of side effects (belladonna alkaloids) or for which there is no medical or scientific rationale (bismuth subnitrate, capsicum, ginger, ipecac powder, multivitamins, minerals, and caroid-papain) were recommended for removal from the market unless or until further study supports their use. The Panel was unable to classify products containing agar, bran tablets, native carrageeman, guar gum, aloin, bile salts, ox bile, d-calcium pantothenate, frangula, prune concentrate, prune powder, chinese rhubarb, sodium oleate, tartaric acid, and poloxalkol due to lack of pertinent data.

18. A 19-year-old college student asks the pharmacist to recommend a product for the treatment of his diarrhea. What could be causing the diarrhea? What questions should the pharmacist ask before making a recommendation?

The causes of diarrhea are multiple. Viruses, bacteria, such as enteropathogenic *Escherichia coli, Shigella* and *Salmonella,* and parasites, such as *Endamoeba histolytica* account for the majority of acute infectious diarrhea in the United States today. The ingestion of toxins as in food poisonings or the ingestion of chemicals or drugs may also cause acute diarrhea. Acute diarrhea may be the presenting symptom in any systemic infection, a variety of gastrointestinal diseases including regional enteritis, ulcerative colitis, and disturbances of gastrointestinal secretion and motility, in numerous endocrine abnormalities, and in lymphosarcoma. At times history, physical examination, gross and microscopic examination of the stool, bacteriologic studies, radiologic examination, and proctoscopy are necessary for the accurate diagnosis of diarrhea (74).

The pharmacist should obtain a detailed history regarding the diarrheal episode, including the onset, duration, characteristics of the stool such as the presence of blood, pus, and mucous, associated symptoms, previous travels, ingestion of possibly contaminated foods, ingestion of drugs, and knowledge of other people with similar symptoms.

19. The college student then states that the diarrhea developed suddenly and the stools are watery but do not contain blood. The student states that he does not have a fever, but he is suffering from loss of appetite, abdominal cramps, and nausea and vomiting. Many of the people living in the same dormitory have had similar symptoms which have lasted approximately 48 hours. What antidiarrheal agent can the pharmacist recommend?

This is the classical picture of acute self-limiting diarrhea which is probably due to viral enteritis. Opiates are safe and effective as antidiarrheal agents in acute self-limiting diarrhea which does not exceed 2 days duration. The dose of opium taken one to four times a day is 15 to 20 mg for adults, and 5 to 10 mg for children 6 to 12 years old. The recommended dose of paregoric is 4 ml, and 1 to 2.5 ml up to four times a day, for adults and children respectively (2). Such agents are available in all but 13 states without a prescription. Other narcotics such as codeine in a dose of 15 to 30 mg every 6 hours or diphenoxylate 2.5 to 5 mg four times a day could be used in adults in place of opium, but these require a prescription in all states.

If this patient is in a state where products containing opium are not available over-the-counter (OTC), there is no OTC antidiarrheal agent that can be rationally recommended. The FDA Panel on OTC Antidiarrheal Agents (2) concluded that adequate and reliable scientific evidence is not available at this time to permit final classification of the active ingredients listed:

Adsorbents	activated attapulgite, activated charcoal, kaolin, pectin
Anticholinergics	atropine sulfate, homatropine methylbromide, hyoscyamine sulfate
Astringents	hydrated alumina powder, bismuth salts, calcium hydroxide, phenyl salicylate, zinc phenosulfonate
Other active ingredients	calcium carbonate, lactobacilli acidophilus, lactobacilli bulgaricus, sodium carboxymethylcellulose, and bismuth subsalicylate

The Panel also recommended that products containing rhubarb fluid extract, aminoacetic acid (glycine), potassium carbonate and scopolamine hydrochloride (hyoscine hydrochloride) be removed from the market because of lack of "scientific or even sound theoretical basis for the claimed efficacy." (2)

20. A patient has heard that various antidiarrheal agents may be removed from the market and questions the reasons for this since these products have always proven to be effective for him. What is your response to this patient?

These agents have been used in acute self-limiting diarrhea which would have resolved in 2 to 3 days whether the condition was treated or not. There is some controversy as to whether the treatment of acute infectious diarrhea with antidiarrheal agents actually results in a prolongation of the symptoms. Since it is believed that diarrhea is a defense mechanism to rid the body of the infecting agent, some authorities are questioning the treatment of acute infectious diarrhea with opioids or diphenoxylate (37).

21. A patient with peptic ulcer disease is being treated with 10 ml Mylanta II one and three hours after meals. The patient has developed incapacitating diarrhea. What should be done for this patient?

This is an example of drug-induced diarrhea. The magnesium in the antacid is acting as a laxative. Although this product, like many antacids, is a combination of magnesium and aluminum which have opposite effects on the bowel, many patients experience diarrhea or constipation on antacid therapy. It is suggested that an equally effective dose (80 mEq available neutralizing capacity) of a more constipating antacid such as aluminum hydroxide be substituted for one or more doses of Mylanta II. It is often necessary for the patient to experiment with dosage substitution until bowel habits are normalized. (see also chapter on *Peptic Ulcer Disease)*

22. A 65 year old woman with metastatic bronchogenic carcinoma has been treated with oral clindamycin for 6 days. The patient now has profuse nonbloody diarrhea (greater than 5 stools per day). On examination the stool is found to contain many polymorphonuclear leukocytes and is guaiac positive. Drug-induced colitis is suspected. Is this patient's history consistent with the diagnosis of clindamycin colitis? What other drugs have been implicated as causing colitis? What is your recommendation concerning the therapy of this patient?

Prior to 1970 the most commonly incriminated antibiotic as a cause of colitis and diarrhea was tetracycline. Between 1960 and 1974, 32 cases of colitis associated with lincomycin were reported (54). The incidence of diarrhea is estimated to be up to 50% in patients receiving lincomycin (64, 95). The Upjohn Company estimates the incidence of serious clindamycin-associated colitis to be between 1 in 50,000 to 1 in 100,000 (65). However, Tedesco (111) reported a 21% incidence of diarrhea in patients receiving clindamycin. Approximately one half of these patients in this study had pseudomembranous colitis, although none were seriously ill and all recovered. Kabins and Spira (63) reported a 17% incidence of colitis in patients treated with clindamycin in September and October of 1974 and a 44% mortality rate.

Previously, this adverse reaction was thought to occur more frequently in older female patients with serious underlying disease. However, two recent reviews (54, 113) report age ranges of 25-81 years and 15-87 years respectively, and 87% and 72% respectively of the patients were without serious underlying diseases. These reviews also reported a higher incidence of colitis in female patients. Neither review found any correlation between the total oral dose or duration of therapy with the onset, severity, or duration of the diarrhea. Hoberman (54) reported a time interval between the initiation of clindamycin and the onset of diarrhea from 3 days after beginning therapy to 7 days after discontinuing the drug. In both reviews the majority (16/16 and 46/47) of patients presented with diarrhea but not grossly bloody stools. Abdominal cramping, fever, leukocytosis, and nausea and vomiting accompanied the diarrhea. Examination of the bowel showed pseudomembranous colitis in 9 of 16 patients in Hoberman's review (54) and 36 of 47 patients in the review by Tedesco (113). The remainder of the patients were diagnosed as having nonspecific colitis. If the antibiotic was discontinued, the fever and cramping usually resolved in 48-72 hours and the diarrhea subsided in 4 to 14 days (113). Both reviews emphasize the necessity of promptly discontinuing the antibiotic if diarrhea occurs.

The etiology of antibiotic associated colitis is unknown. Current theories of pathogenesis include alterations in gut flora, with a decrease in anerobic organisms, direct toxicity to the colonic mucosa by the antibiotic or a toxic metabolite, and a familial predisposition (49).

Clindamycin should be immediately discontinued. There is a graver prognosis if the drug is continued after the onset of the diarrhea or if diarrhea occurs after the drug has been discontinued (26). Intravenous fluids with electrolytes should be instituted to maintain hydration and electrolyte balance. It is recommended that diphenoxylate and opiates be avoided (82), although one review of clindamycin-associated colitis did not find the administration of diphenoxylate/atropine deleterious (113). Ramirez-Ronda (96) states that the most severe complications occurred when clindamycin was continued after onset of diarrhea and when opiates or Lomotil (diphenoxylate plus atropine) was prescribed as symptomatic therapy. Since the precipitation of toxic megacolon by the administration of opiates or anticholinergic agents in cases of ulcerative colitis has been reported, such a hazard may also exist in pseudomembranous colitis (81). The use of steroids in this disorder remains controversial. One recent article reports that the administration of cholestryamine stopped the diarrhea in two patients with clindamycin-associated colitis (18).

23. A 23 year old American Black man complains to you of bloating, cramping abdominal pain, flatulence, and diarrhea which he associates with the ingestion of certain foods, particularly milk. He asks for a recommendation for treatment. What questions would you ask? What is the most likely cause of his symptoms? What is your recommendation for treatment?

The same type of history would have to be obtained in this situation as was obtained in Question 18. However, since the patient attributes his symptoms to the ingestion of certain foods, a more complete dietary history is necessary. It appears that this patient is suffering from lactase deficiency. This patient is in a high risk group for lactase deficiency, as it is present in 60-90% of American Negros, Africans, and Asians. A high incidence (60-67%) is also reported in Jews and American Indians. The incidence of lactase deficiency in Caucasians in the United States is 10 to 20% (14). Adults with lactase deficiency were able to drink milk as infants. The onset of their symptoms usually occurs in adolescence or early adult life as in this patient. Lactase deficiency is not an allergic or hypersensitivity reaction to milk proteins. The absorption of dietary carbohydrate depends on the presence of disac-

charidases in the intestinal brush border. When these enzymes are absent, the carbohydrate cannot be absorbed. Osmotic diarrhea is caused by an accumulation of non-absorbable solutes in the gut lumen which inhibits the absorption of water and electrolytes. Also, there is movement of water from the plasma into the gut lumen because of the net osmotic effect (42). This results in the symptoms described by this patient. Lactase deficiency is also seen in nontropical and tropical sprue, regional enteritis, cystic fibrosis, and ulcerative colitis and is commonly temporarily seen after a bout of acute infectious diarrhea (47). The treatment of diarrhea due to lactase deficiency is avoidance of milk. The patient should be instructed to avoid milk until the symptoms subside. Then he might reintroduce milk in his diet in small quantities, the amount of milk necessary to produce symptoms may vary from one to four glasses. Medications should not be recommended (69).

24. A 52 year old male patient who recently underwent a partial gastrectomy, pyloroplasty, and vagotomy as treatment for his 20 year history of peptic ulcer disease asks your advice concerning the treatment of his diarrhea. About 15 minutes after a meal, this patient complains of dizziness, palpitations, sweating, weakness, and diarrhea. What is the most probable cause of this patient's symptoms? What is your recommendation for treatment?

This patient probably has the post-gastrectomy dumping syndrome which is characterized by a feeling of fullness or distress in the epigastrum, a general sensation of warmth, sweating, tachycardia, weakness, lightheadedness and syncope. The symptoms usually occur 5 to 30 minutes after a meal (32, 53). The syndrome occurs because the reservoir function of the stomach is compromised and the hyperosmolar contents are propelled too rapidly into the small intestine (42). The initial vasomotor symptoms (dizziness, lightheadedness, tachycardia, flushing, sweating, and a reduction in systolic blood pressure) occur within 5 to 10 minutes postprandially and last from 20 minutes to one hour. These symptoms are associated with elevated serum levels of bradykinin (30, 70). The second set of symptoms (borborygmi, nausea, vomiting, diarrhea, weakness, and abdominal distress) occur within 15 to 20 minutes after the meal and last from 20 to 50 minutes. These symptoms are well correlated with an increase in serotonin in the plasma (70).

Between 20 and 40 per cent of patients who have had surgery for peptic ulcer disease suffer from the dumping syndrome immediately after the operation. The symptoms decrease in severity until only 5 to 10% suffer persistent disability (107). Medical management is usually effective in controlling the symptoms. The patient should be placed on an "anti-dumping diet" which is high in protein and low in carbohydrate. The diet should be consumed as at least 6 small feedings per day. All concentrated forms of carbohydrates, such as desserts, sugar, and jellies, should be avoided. Fluids should be restricted at mealtimes. Some patients improve symptomatically when given anticholinergic agents. The patient should be instructed to lie flat after meals until the symptoms are controlled (107). Cyproheptadine has been reported to have antibradykinin, antihistamine, and antiserotonin activity. This drug has been used in dumping syndrome patients in doses of 4 to 8 mg before meals with varying success in relieving the symptoms (60, 61). However, only case reports or studies of a small number of patients have been reported; no well-controlled trials have been reported to date in the literature. If medical management is ineffective in controlling the symptoms, surgery should considered.

25. Mrs. J. B. and her family are going to Mexico City for the holidays. She wants to take something to prevent the trip from being ruined by "turista." The travel book suggests EnteroVioform. Mrs. J.B. asks you to sell her this medication. What is "turista"? How can it be avoided and treated?

EnteroVioform is the trade name for iodochlorhydroxyquin, one of the family of halogenated hydroxyquinolines. In the United States this drug is available only by prescription, but many of the antidiarrheal agents that can be purchased without a prescription in other countries contain one of the halogenated hydroxyquinolines. Except for one poorly designed study with iodochlorhydroxyquin, there is no evidence that this drug has any prophylactic or therapeutic value in traveler's diarrhea. Well designed studies have shown it to be ineffective (77). The use of iodochlorhydroxyquin has been associated with the development of peripheral neuropathy and myelopathy. Symptoms include minimal dysesthesia and visual disturbances. The development of toxicity has been dose related with 1% of patients developing toxicity after ingesting 750-1500 mg of iodochlorhydroxyquin for less than two weeks, while toxicity occurred in 35% of those ingesting this dose for greater than two weeks. If the dose was increased to 1500-2250 mg for one to three weeks, 44% of the patients developed toxicity (83). Because of the lack of evidence of efficacy and its possible toxicity, it is recommended that this drug not be used (5).

Turista is a common name for traveler's diarrhea which is characterized by an acute onset of 10 to 20 episodes watery diarrhea per day. It is frequently accompanied by abdominal cramps, nausea, vomiting, anorexia, malaise, chills, or fever. The disease usually occurs within 7-10 days of arrival and 40-50% of Americans visiting Mexico City can expect to contract the problem. The diarrhea usually will last from 1-5 days, or in more severe cases, one week (77). It is now estimated that from 1/2 to 3/4 of the cases of traveler's diarrhea are caused by enteropathogenic *E. coli* (5, 78). The enterotoxin produced by this organism produces a secretory diarrhea. The small intestine actively secretes ions from the base of the villi. The intestinal secretion results from stimulation of adenyl cyclase which leads to a high intracellular concentration of cyclic AMP. Solutes, especially bicarbonate and chloride, which are followed by water are secreted into the gut lumen from the blood. Secretory diarrhea is also caused by this mechanism with cholera, *Clostridium welchii* toxin, theophylline, prostaglandins, and bile salts (42).

Mrs. J. B. and her family should be advised to avoid tap water, iced beverages, and uncooked foods. All water should be purified by boiling or with 2-4 drops of 4-6% chlorine bleach, 5-10 drops of 2% tincture of iodine or the use of Halazone tablets according to directions. Bottled carbonated beverages and beer are considered safe, but all bottled water is not sterile. If one personally peels fruit, it is safe. The entire family should avoid swimming in water that might be contaminated with sewage (77).

If one of the family develops diarrhea, fluid and electrolyte replacement is the most important therapeutic modality. A solution which contains 3.5 gm NaCl, 2.5 gm NaHCO3, 1.5 gm KCl, and 20 gm glucose per liter is recommended. This solution is available commercially abroad as Choloral or Vitor SA. Fruit juices, cola, ginger ale, and carbonated beverages with added salt may be used if an electrolyte solution is unavailable (77). Antibiotics should only be prescribed when there is evidence of systemic spread or in confirmed cases of infection with *Salmonella typhi, Shigella shigae* or *Shigella flexnerri* (116). Evidence suggests that retarding gut motility may predispose the patient to bacteremia in Salmonella infections, or may delay the clearance of the infecting organism from the body as in Shigellosis (37). (see also Question 20). There is no evidence that antimotility medications favorably alter the clinical course of acute intestinal infections. Therefore, Mrs. J. B. should be told not to use Lomotil, Paregoric, or any of the other available antimotility agents (77). If the patient has blood or mucous in the stool or tenesmus, the infecting agent may be an invasive organism, and a stool culture should be obtained (77).

26. A mother of an 18 month old infant requests a medication for the treatment of her child's diarrhea. What questions should be asked of the mother, and what is your recommendation for treatment?

As in all cases of diarrhea a detailed history of the diarrhea including onset, duration, and characteristics of the stool should be obtained. Inquiries concerning associated symptoms such as fever, vomiting, the recent administration of any drugs, an estimation of weight loss, and any recent changes in diet are essential.

If the diarrhea has been present for less than 2 days, there is no blood, pus or mucous in the stools, there are no serious associated symptoms, and the child does not show evidence of moderate or severe dehydration, the child probably has mild self-limiting diarrhea. Moffet (79) found the causative organisms to be viruses in 23% of cases of infantile diarrhea. Ryder and co-workers (102) cultured enteropathogenic E. coli from the stools of 72% of symptomatic infants and from 25% of asymptomatic infants.

Maintaining hydration and electrolyte balance is the most important goal of therapy. All solid fluids and milk should be withheld. Clear fluids may be given for 24 hours (52). An electrolyte solution such as Pedilyte is preferred to the usual home remedies such as jello water, cola, and ginger ale in order to avoid diluting the infant's electrolytes. The mother should be discouraged from preparing an electrolyte solution at home (16). Kaolin has no appreciable effect on fluid and electrolyte loss, though the stools appear firmer (52). The administration of antibiotics does not alter the clinical course of the diarrhea even if the stool culture is positive (52). The administration of Lomotil is dangerous and is contraindicated (101). This drug may decrease the frequency of bowel movements without decreasing the fluid and electrolyte loss into the bowel. Thus, the depletion of extracellular fluid and electrolytes may be masked (3). In children the atropine effects of urinary retention, dry mucous membranes, thirst, and flushing can occur even at the doses contained in Lomotil (0.025 mg/tablet) (4). The ingestion of as few as 6 Lomotil tablets has led to the death of one 2 year old child (99). Ileus occurred in a 2 1/2 year old child treated with Lomotil, although the dose and duration of therapy was not stated (22). If the child does not respond to the withholding of the regular diet and the administration of electrolyte solution, he should be referred to a physician.

At times infantile diarrhea is protracted because of the loss of the brush border from the intestinal villi resulting in a loss of the enzymes which split disaccharides such as lactose. In this situation the child has loose frothy stools when milk is reintroduced into the diet. A non-lactose containing formula should be substituted for three weeks (52).

27. A diabetic patient complains about having nocturnal diarrhea. He has juvenile onset diabetes of 22 years duration which has resulted in retinopathy, nephropathy, and peripheral neuropathy. What should be recommended for the treatment of this patient's diarrhea?

Profuse watery bowel movements which are some-times urgent, often preceded by abdominal cramping, and occurring most frequently at night are associated with diabetes. Usually the patients are male and peripheral neuropathy is most consistently associated with the complaint of diarrhea. On questioning, the patient may also complain of orthostatic hypotension, steatorrhea, and impotence. The pathogenesis of the diarrhea may involve autonomic neuropathy, an intestinal overgrowth of bacteria, pancreatic exocrine deficiency, and/or absorptive defects. Diarrhea may occur unnoticed during sleep, and daytime incontinence is also common. There are unexplained and unexpected remissions and exacerbations of diabetic diarrhea (106).

Unfortunately, the treatment of diabetic diarrhea is usually unsuccessful. Bulk-forming laxatives and anti-motility agents are worth a trial. Sometimes the diarrhea responds to the administration of antibiotics such as ampicillin or tetracycline. If steatorrhea is present, it usually does not respond to pancreatic enzyme replacement (106). Condon reported 4 patients with intractable diarrhea due to vagotomy or diabetes who responded to the administration of 4 gm of cholestyramine three times a day (27).

28. What drugs have been reported to cause clinically significant diarrhea without causing colitis?

Diarrhea is listed as an adverse reaction to many drugs. If the antibiotics that cause colitis, the antimetabolites, and the antacids are excluded, it appears that there are few drugs which cause clinically significant diarrhea. For the change in bowel function to be defined as clinically significant, there must be greater than five diarrheal episodes per day. The administration of ampicillin results in mild to severe diarrhea. In a study of 400 children who were given ampicillin orally, severe diarrhea occurred in 3 and mild to moderate diarrhea occurred in 119 (12). Tedesco (112), in a prospective study of 200 adult patients, found that bowel habits changed in 16%, but diarrhea occurred in only 4.5%. Neither study (12, 112) found the diarrhea to be related to dose or route of administration.

Diarrhea is a common adverse effect of propranolol. Five of 28 patients developed diarrhea while taking 40 to 160 mg propranolol daily (51). Diarrhea is said to be the most common gastrointestinal side effect seen with guanethidine therapy. The diarrhea is said to be explosive and unpredictable (7). One patient of 64 developed diarrhea while on guanethidine therapy 12.5 mg to 60 mg daily (105). Eleven of 49 patients treated for mild to moderate hypertension with guanethidine 5 to 60 mg per day complained of diarrhea (39). Diarrhea is said to be common with methyldopa therapy and may be accompanied by abdominal cramps (7).

Perhaps the problem of drug-induced diarrhea may be placed in perspective by observing the incidence of diarrhea in a healthy population; Kulkarni et al (67) in a prospective study found that one of 25 healthy persons complained of diarrhea.

1. Anon: Dorland's Illustrated Medical Dictionary, 24th ed, WB Saunders Co, Philadelphia, 1965, p. 338.
2. Anon: Proposal to establish monographs for OTC laxative, antidiarrheal, emetic and antiemetic products. Federal Register 40: 12902-12934, March 21, 1975.
3. Anon: Lomotil. Med Let 11:46, 1969.
4. Anon: Lomotil for diarrhea in children. Med Let 17:104, 1975.
5. Anon: Traveler's diarrhea: new developments. Med Let 18:86, 1976.
6. Anon: CNS stimulant and antidepressant drugs. In Side Effects of Drugs Vol VI, edited by L. Meyler and A. Herxheimer. Williams and Wilkins Co, Baltimore and Excerpta Medica Foundation, Amsterdam, 1968, p. 10.
7. Anon: Hypotensive drugs. In Side Effects of Drugs Vol VI, edited by L Meyler and A Herxhemier. Williams and Wilkins Co, Baltimore and Excerpta Medica Foundation, Amsterdam, 1968, p. 207.
8. Anon: Special report, what the public spent for drugs, cosmetics, tolletries in 1974, Product Management, p. 37, Aug 1975.
9. Almay T: Constipation. In Gastrointestinal Diseases, edited by MH Sleisenger and JS Fordtran. WB Saunders Co, Philadelphia, 1973, pp 320-325.
10. Atterbury HR et al: Effect of a partially chemically defined diet on normal human fecal flora. Am J Clin Nutr 25:1391, 1972.
11. Barnes MR: How to get a clean colon with less effort. Radiol 91:948, 1968.
12. Bass JW et al: Adverse effects of orally administered ampicillin. J Pediatr 83:106, 1973.
13. Bauer GE et al: Pseudo-obstruction due to clonidine. Br J Med 1:169, 1976.
14. Bayless TM et al: Lactose intolerance and milk drinking habits. Gastroent 60:605, 1971.
15. Becker GL: The case against mineral oil. Am J Dig Dis 19:344, 1952.
16. Bosso JA: Topics in pediatric clinical pharmacy. Utah Pharm Dig 84:3, 1975.
17. Brettschneider L et al: Intestinal obstruction due to antacid gels. Gastroent 49:291, 1965.
18. Burbige EJ et al: Pseudomembranous colitis, associated with antibiotics and therapy with cholestryramine. JAMA 231:1157, 1975.
19. Burkitt DP: The aetiology of appendicitis. Br J Surg 58:695, 1971.
20. Burkitt DP: Possible relationships between bowel cancer and dietary habits. Proc Roy Soc Med 64:964, 1971.
21. Burkitt DP et al: Dietary fiber and disease. JAMA 299:1068, 1974.
22. Caplan LH et al: Antidiarrheal drug effect simulating intestinal obstruction. Am J Gastroent 42:540, 1964.
23. Chamberland MJ et al: Toxic effect of podophyllin application in pregnancy. Br Med J 3:391, 1972.
24. Chingell C: The effects of phenolphthalein and other purgatives on rat intestinal Na/K adenosine triphosphatase. Biochem Pharmacol 17:1207, 1968.
25. Clain J et al: Cathartic colon with unusual histological features. S Afr Med J 48:216, 1974.
26. Cohen LE et al: Clindamycin-associated colitis, JAMA 223:1379, 1973.
27. Condon JR: Cholestyramine and diabetic and post-vagotomy diarrhea. Br J Med 4:423, 1973.
28. Connell AM et al: Variations in bowel habits in two population samples. Br Med J 2:1095, 1965.
29. Cummings JH et al: Laxative-induced diarrhea, a continuing clinical problem. Br Med J 1:537, 1974.
30. Cuschieri A et al: Kinin release after gastric surgery. Br Med J 3:565, 1971.
31. Davis LE et al: Central nervous system intoxication from mercurous chloride laxatives. Arch Neurol 30:428, 1974.
32. Davis RL et al: Hormonal basis for the dumping syndrome. Rocky Mount Med J 71:94, 1974.
33. Dennison AD: Use of dioctyl sodium sulfosuccinate in cardiovascular disease correction of bowel function. Am J Cardiol 1:400, 1968.
34. Diamond S: Amitriptyline in the treatment of gastrointestinal disorders. Psychosomat 5:221, 1964.
35. Donowitz M: Effect of dioctyl sodium sulfosuccinate on colonic fluid and electrolyte movement. Gastroent 69:941, 1975.
36. Dujoune CA et al: Toxicity of a hepatotoxic laxative preparation in tissue culture and excretion in bile in man. Clin Pharmacol Therap 13:602, 1972.
37. Dupont HL et al: Lomotil therapy of induced shigellosis. Clin Res 21:598, 1973.
38. Ewe K: Effect of laxatives on intestinal water and electrolyte transport. Eur J Clin Invest 2:283, 1972.
39. Ferguson RK et al: Patient acceptance of guanethidine as therapy for mild to moderate hypertension. Circul 54:32, 1976.
40. Fingl E: Laxatives and cathartics. In The Pharmacologic Basis of Therapeutics, 5th ed, edited by Goodman LS and Gilman A. Macmillan Co. New York, 1975, pp 977-985.
41. Fonkalsurd E et al: Hypernatremic dehydration from hypertonic enemas in congenital megacolon, JAMA 199:584, 1969.
42. Fordtran JS: Diarrhea. In Gastrointestinal Disease, edited by MH Sleisenger and JS Fordtran. WB Saunders Co, Philadelphia, 1973, pp 304-308.
43. Gardner DR et al: Ileus after amitriptyline. Br Med J 1:1160, 1963.
44. Ghose MK et al: Spontaneous Colonic Perforation: A complication in a hemodialysis patient. JAMA 214:145, 1970.
45. Goldfinger P: Hypokalemia, metabolic acidosis and hypocalcemic tetany in a patient taking laxatives. J Mt Siani Hosp 36:113, 1969.
46. Goodman J et al: Dioctyl sodium sulfosuccinate — an ineffective prophylactic laxative. J Chron Dis 29:59, 1976.
47. Greenberger NJ et al: Disorders of absorption. In Harrison's Principles of Internal Medicine. 7th ed McGraw Hill, San Francisco, 1974, p. 1471.
48. Greenhalf JO et al: Laxatives in the treatment of constipation of pregnant and breast feeding mothers. Practitioner 210:259, 1973.
49. Harrod MJ et al: Familial pseudomembranous colitis and its relation to lincomycin therapy. Am J Dig Dis 20:808, 1975.
50. Harvey RJ et al: Saline purgatives act by releasing cholecystokinin. Lancet 2:185, 1973.
51. Hebb AR et al: A new beta-blocking agent, propranolol, in the treatment of angina pectoris. Canad Med Assoc J 98:246, 1968.
52. Hatcher G: Diarrhea. Br Med J 1:571, 1976.
53. Hinshaw DB et al: Preoperative and postoperative "dumping" studies in patients with peptic ulcer. Am J Surg 122:269, 1971.
54. Hoberman LJ et al: Colitis associated with oral clindamycin therapy, a clinical study of 16 patients. Am J Dig Dis 21:1, 1976.
55. Hyland CM et al: DSS as a laxative in the elderly. Practitioner 200:698, 1968.
56. Irving D et al: Fibre and cancer of the colon. Br J Cancer 28:462, 1973.
57. Ivey KJ: Are anticholinergics of use in irritable colon syndrome. Gastroent 68:1300, 1975.
58. Jaffe JH and Martin WB: Narcotic analgesics and antagonists. In The Pharmacologic Basis of Therapeutics, 5th ed, edited by LS Goodman and A Gilman. Macmillan Co, New York, 1975, p 253.
59. Javert ET et al: Prothrombin concentration and mineral oil. Am J Obstet and Gyn 42:409, 1941.
60. Johnson LP et al: Serotonin antagonist in experimental and clinical "dumping". Ann Surg 156:537, 1962.
61. Johnson LP et al: Treatment of dumping with serotonin antagonists. JAMA 180:493, 1962.
62. Joneja MG et al: Effects of vinblastine and podophyllin on DBA mouse fetuses. Toxicol and Appl Pharmacol 27:408, 1974.
63. Kabins SA et al: Outbreak of clindamycin — associated colitis (letter). Ann Inter Med 83:830, 1975.
64. Kaplan K et al: Lincomycin. Pediatr Clin North Am 15:313, 1958.
65. Katz LJ et al: A clinical evaluation of certain bulk and irritant laxatives. Gastroent 20:149, 1952.
66. Kratochuil C: Letter to physicians, The UpJohn Company. Kalamazoo, Michigan, Aug 16, 1974.
67. Kulkarni RD et al: Baseline (spontaneous) symptoms in healthy persons, a prospective study. J Clin Pharmacol 15:442, 1975.

68. Lewin KJB: Phenolphthalein reactions simulating disseminated (systemic) lupus erythematosus. Lancet 2:461, 1962.
69. Low-Beer TS et al: Diarrhea, mechanism and treatment. Gut 12:1021, 1971.
70. MacDonald JM et al: Serotonin and bradykinin in the dumping syndrome. Am J Surg 117:204, 1969.
71. Margulis AR: Examination of the Colon, In *Alimentary Tract Roentgenology,* 2nd ed. Vol 2, edited by AR Margulis and HJ Burhenne, CV Mosby Co, St Louis, 1973, p 932.
72. McConnell TH: Fatal hypocalcemia from phosphate absorption from laxative preparation. JAMA 216:147, 1971.
73. McHardy G et al: Jaundice and oxyphenisatin. JAMA 211:83, 1970.
74. Mendeloff A: Constipation, diarrhea, and disturbances in anorectal function. In *Harrison's Principles of Internal Medicine,* 7th ed, McGraw Hill, San Francisco, 1974, pp 215-218.
75. Mendeloff A et al: Diseases of the colon and rectum. In *Harrison's Principles of Internal Medicine,* 7th ed, McGraw Hill, San Francisco, 1974, pp 1490-1491.
76. Mendeloff AI: A critique of fiber deficiency. Am J Dig Dis 21:109, 25:762, 1976.
77. Merson MH et al: Traveler's diarrhea. JAMA 234:201, 1975
78. Merson MH et al: Traveler's diarrhea in Mexico. NEJM 294:1299, 1976
79. Moffet HL et al: Epidemiology and etiology of severe infantile diarrhea. J Pediat 72:1, 1968.
80. Mundow L: Dantron/poloxalkol and placebo in puerpural constipation. Brit J Clin Pract 29:95, 1975
81. Norland CC et al: Toxic dilation of colon. Med 48:229, 1969.
82. Novak E et al: Unfavorable effect of atropine-diphenoxylate (Lomotil) therapy in lincomycin caused diarrhea. JAMA 235:1451, 1976
83. Oakley GP: The neurotoxicity of halogenated hydroxyquinolines. JAMA 225:395, 1973.
84. O'Reilly RA et al: Oral anticoagulant drugs in man. Pharmacol Rev 22:35, 1970.
85. Padilla G et al: Variables affecting the preparation of the bowel for radiologic examination. Nurs Rev 21:305, 1972.
86. Painter NS et al: Diverticular disease of the colon, a deficiency disease of western civilization. Br Med J 2:450, 1971.
87. Painter NS et al: Unprocessed bran in treatment of diverticular disease of the colon. Br Med J 2:137, 1972.
88. Palmer ED: Presbycolon problems in nursing homes. JAMA 235:1150, 1976.
89. Pelot D et al: Constipation of prolonged duration. Am J Gastroent 63: 252, 1975.
90. Phelps DK: Effect of DSS on bowel function in mental patients. J Indiana State Med Assoc 51:646, 1958.
91. Phillips SF: Diarrhea, a current view of the pathophysiology. Gastroent 63:495, 1972.
92. Pike BF et al: Soap colitis. NEJM 285:217, 1971.
93. Potyk D: Intestinal obstruction from impacted antacid tablets. NEJM 283:134, 1970.

94. Prescott LF: Pharmacokinetic drug interaction. Lancet 2:1239, 1969.
95. Price DJ et al: Trial of phenoxymethylpenicillin, phemethicillin, and lincomycin in treatment of staphylococcal sepsis in a casualty department. Br Med J 3:407, 1968.
96. Ramirez-Ronda CH: Incidence of clindamycin-associated colitis (letter). Ann Intern Med 81:860, 1974.
97. Reynolds TB et al: Puzzling jaundice, probable relationship to laxative ingestion. JAMA 211:86, 1970.
98. Rhodes JB et al: Clinical assessment, double blind drug trials and computer analysis of patients with moderately severe irritable colon syndrome. Gastroent 64:829, 1973.
99. Riely ID: Lomotil poisoning. Lancet 1:373, 1969.
100. Rogers, AI: Colonic diverticular disease. Hoechst Roussel Pharmaceuticals Inc. Sommerville NJ, 1975.
101. Rosenstein G et al: Warning, the use of Lomotil in children. Peds 51:132-134, 1973.
102. Ryder RW et al: Infantile diarrhea produced by heat-stable enterogenic Escherichia coli. NEJM 295:849, 1976.
103. Salm R et al: A case of chronic paraffin pneumonitis. Thorax 25:762, 1970.
104. Savin JA: Current causes of fixed drug eruptions. Br J Dermatol 83:546, 1970.
105. Seedat YK et al: Further Experiences with guanethidine, a clinical assessment of 103 patients. S Afr J Med 40:140, 1966.
106. Sleisenger MH Roseman DM: Systemic diseases and the gut. In *Gastrointestinal Diseases,* edited by MH Sleisenger and JS Fordtran. WB Saunders Co, Philadelphia, 1973, p 385.
107. Smith FW Jeffries GH: Late and Persistent post gastrectory problems. In *Gastrointestinal Diseases,* edited by MH Sleisenger and JS Fordtran, WB Saunders Co, Philadelphia, 1973, pp 822-825.
108. Souter WA: Bolus obstruction of gut after use of hydrophilic colloid laxatives. Br Med J 1:166, 1965.
109. Stanley MD et al: Comparative effects of cholestyramine, Metamucil and cellulose on bile salt excretion in man. Gastroent 62:816, 1972.
110. Steigman FH et al: Critical levels of mineral oil affecting the absorption of vitamin A. Gastroent 20:587, 1952.
111. Tedesco FJ et al: Clindamycin-associated colitis, a prospective study. Ann Intern Med 8:429, 1974.
112. Tedesco FJ: Ampicillin associated diarrhea, a prospective study. Am J Dig Dis 20:295, 1975.
113. Tedesco FJ: Clindamycin-associated colitis, a review of the clinical spectrum of 47 cases. Am J Dig Dis 21:26, 1976.
114. Tolman KG et al: Possible hepatotoxicity of doxidan. Ann Intern Med 84:290, 1976.
115. Urso FP et al: The cathartic colon. Radiol 116:557, 1975.
116. Viranuvetti V: Management of traveler's diarrhea. Drugs 6:406, 1973.
117. Wightman KJR et al: Assessment of symptoms in *Gastroenterology,* edited by A Bogoch, McGraw Hill, San Francisco, 1973, p 32.
118. Zumoff B et al: Rectal absorption of sodium from hypertonic sodium phosphate solutions, Sloan Kettering Institute for Cancer Research, New York, NY.

Chapter 11

Essential Hypertension

Lloyd Y. Young
Michael A. Riddiough

with Hypertensive Emergency Section by
R. Jon Auricchio

CASE A: F.W., a 39-year-old black man, first became aware of his hypertension about 8 to 9 years ago following a routine blood pressure examination during a community flu immunization program. He was referred to a physician at that time, and a complete hypertensive workup was initiated. A diagnosis of essential hypertension was considered to be the most likely and medications were prescribed. The medications made him lethargic and he discontinued therapy on his own. He failed to return to his physician until approximately three years prior to this admission when he noted some diffuse chest pains, dizziness, and visual symptoms. Once again antihypertensive medications were prescribed and the symptoms abated even though the medications were taken only sporadically. Approximately one year later, this gentleman was seen in a university medical clinic with a blood pressure of 210/130 mm Hg and was hospitalized.

Physical examination at that time, demonstrated an alert, obese, young man in no severe acute distress. The supine and sitting blood pressure was 210/130, with a pulse of 100, and a respiratory rate of 16. Fundoscopic examination revealed the disc to be flat. A-V nicking was present with mild venous engorgement as was moderate venous tortuosity and marked arteriolar narrowing. No exudates or hemorrhages were seen on examination.

The serum creatinine was 2.0 mg/100 ml with an endogenous creatinine clearance of 41 ml/minute. Other laboratory evaluations were non-remarkable, although the electrocardiogram revealed left ventricular hypertrophy. His blood pressure was stabilized and discharge medications from that hospitalization included hydrochlorothiazide 50 mg daily, KCl 10% solution 15 ml daily, hydralazine 100 mg four times daily, methyldopa 250 mg four times daily, and guanethidine 10 mg three times daily.

He took these medications regularly and his blood pressure averaged about 130/95 mm Hg at the time of his first clinic visit approximately one month after his hospitalization. However, on this regimen weakness, marked lethargy, inability to concentrate, postural hypotension and impotence developed. As a result he again took his medications sporadically with the exception of one tablet of hydrochlorothiazide daily. His hypertension was uncontrolled for about two years until this admission.

Yesterday he was home sitting in a chair when he noticed a numbness beginning in his hand, radiating up his arm, down his left side, and involving his left facial area. On physical examination, the blood pressure was 195/115 supine and 198/110 standing; the pulse was irregular, with frequent premature beats, and a rate of about 90; respirations were normal; and the weight was 200 pounds.

Fundoscopic examination demonstrates papilledema and exudates bilaterally with blurred disc margins. Arteriolar spasm is moderately severe and significant AV nicking with tortuous arterioles are present. Examination of the heart indicates an irregular rhythm with premature contractions occurring as often as every third to fourth beat. There is a suggestion of left ventricular heave. He does have documented left ventricular hypertrophy on ECG with a strain pattern and left axis deviation. Laboratory data include a hematocrit of 35%, 4+ proteinuria with several red and white blood cells in the urine sediment, BUN 35 mg/100 ml, serum creatinine 3.8 mg/100 ml, uric acid 10.1 mg/100 ml, fasting blood sugar 145 mg/100 ml, and cholesterol 275 mg/100 ml.

He states that he has occasionally been dizzy and has had sexual difficulties in "getting it on" while taking his medications as directed, therefore he has only been taking his hydralazine a couple times each day in a sporadic manner. He also describes 3 or 4 episodes of precordial chest pains in both the right and left side which does not radiate to his arms or his neck. The chest pain is sometimes associated with exertion. He claims in addition to suffer from a chronic mild cough especially in the mornings; there is no hemoptysis.

Social history indicates that he has smoked 1.5 packs of cigarettes per day for the last 19 years. Previous attempts to decrease or quit smoking have caused nervousness. He is a social drinker and has a cocktail nightcap each night. He sleeps poorly at night and drinks 6 to 8 cups of coffee daily in order to "keep going."

His mother is 59 years of age and also suffers from hypertension. A maternal uncle, five maternal aunts, and his maternal grandmother were known to be hypertensive. Two paternal uncles were also hypertensive.

1. This 39-year-old black man first became aware of his hypertension about eight to nine years ago during a community flu immunization program. How prevalent is hypertension?

Hypertension is the most common cardiovascular abnormality encountered in medicine. It affects an estimated 23 million Americans or about 10 to 15% of the adult population in the United States. A random sample of adults 18 to 79 years of age conducted by the U.S. Department of Health, Education, and Welfare in the early 1960's indicated that 15% of whites and 27% of blacks have hypertension as defined by World Health Organization criteria (63,199). Subsequent epidemiological surveys have confirmed these prevalence figures. If borderline hypertensives (systolic pressures 140 to 160 mm Hg, and diastolic pressures of 90 to 95 mm Hg) are included, as in the Framingham, Massachusetts survey of a predominantly white, middle class community, then 41% of men and 48% of women could be classified as hypertensives (133).

Although the statistics concerning the prevalence of hypertension are alarming, the majority of Americans with elevated blood pressures, remain either undetected, untreated, or inadequately treated (230). Other surveys indicate that about one-half, or approximately 12 million hypertensives in the United States are unaware that they have hypertension, and of those who are aware, fewer than half are receiving treatment for their hypertension. The really dismal statistic however, is that only one-half of those being treated are being adequately treated (186,204). Thus, ½ of ½ of ½ means that only one-eighth of the 23 million hypertensives, or only about 3 million hypertensives are being adequately treated in the United States. There still does not appear to be improvement in these statistics despite the national concern for this disease.

In reviewing these statistics it becomes abundantly clear that hypertension is highly prevalent, and the discovery of this disease during a routine examination is not at all unusual. The fact that this patient's high blood pressure has remained uncontrolled for most of the 8 to 9 years is also not totally surprising, although it is inexcusable.

2. F.W. is diagnosed as having essential hypertension. What is essential hypertension?

The term essential hypertension, formerly termed benign essential hypertension, refers to all cases of hypertension for which no cause can be found. It is certainly not benign nor is it essential. It is however, the major category of hypertension because approximately 90% of patients with persistent elevations of blood pressure are considered to have essential hypertension.

Essential hypertension itself is affected by many etiological factors primarily because of the complex interplay of various physiological variables. Chemical mediators such as renin, neural mediators such as baroreceptors, volume factors, tissue perfusion, vessel elasticity, blood viscosity, cardiac output, and vascular caliber all interact in response to hemodynamic and physiological demands. Each of these etiological factors provides varying degrees of blood pressure elevations at various times. Nevertheless, whatever the cause, a sustained elevation of blood pressure is associated with increased morbidity and mortality.

3. What is the nature of the morbidity and mortality associated with essential hypertension? What did this patient experience?

Although the vast majority of hypertensives are asymptomatic (226), they are nevertheless subject to greatly increased risks of strokes, heart attacks, kidney failure, and heart failure.

Effects on the Brain: Hypertension, unequivocally more than any other factor, predisposes individuals to the development of atherothrombotic brain infarcts which are the most common variety of stroke (102). With long-standing hypertension, multiple large infarcts or hemorrhages can cause brain tissue destruction. With accelerated hypertension, encephalopathy, cerebral edema, infarcts, and hemorrhages appear rapidly. It is estimated that the risk of stroke is five times higher in hypertensives as compared to normotensives (102); and the mortality rate from stroke is four to five times higher in blacks than in whites (199). Cerebrovascular accidents are probably responsible for up to 10 to 15% of deaths attributed to hypertension.

Effects on the Heart: A number of long-term studies have confirmed the relationship of hypertension to accelerated atherosclerosis and coronary artery disease. Left ventricular hypertrophy occurs as a result of cardiac compensation for the excessive workload on the left ventricle which must pump the usual amount of blood against an increased peripheral resistance. This increased heart size and subsequent increased myocardial oxygen requirement may exceed the capacity of the coronary circulation and result in angina pectoris. Myocardial infarction and congestive heart failure account for the majority of deaths secondary to hypertension (54). Furthermore, the mortality rate from hypertensive heart disease is substantially higher in blacks than in whites.

Effects on the Kidney: Abnormalities in renal function usually do not occur until late in the course of essential hypertension. Nevertheless, approximately 10% of the deaths secondary to hypertension result from renal failure.

Effects on the Eye: Disturbances in vision can be due to cerebral lesions but are usually due to hemorrhage into the retina or vitreous. Retinal lesions can produce scotomata and blurred vision. Even blindness may occur in the presence of papilledema (54,72,166).

The *Keith-Wagener* classification of hypertensive retinopathy commonly is used to provide a simple method for serial evaluation of the hypertensive patient. Repeated eye examinations can be used to observe the progression of hypertensive vascular effects, because the retina is the only tissue in which the arteries and the arterioles can be examined directly.

KW I —   Minimal arteriolar narrowing.

KW II —   AV nicking and above: Generally indicates chronic hypertension of 10 years duration or more.

KW III — Hemorrhages, exudates and above: Generally indicates accelerated phase of hypertension.

KW IV —   Papilledema and above: Generally indicates malignant hypertension. Therapy is urgent. The term "malignant" is used because mortality is 100% within two years if the patient is not treated (54).

It cannot be determined if F.W. did in fact suffer a cerebrovascular accident based upon the data which were provided in the case, although the numbness which radiated up his arm involving his left side and left facial area raises the index of suspicion. End organ heart damage may be reflected by the irregular rhythm with frequent premature contractions, the left ventricular hypertrophy, and the questionable chest pains. The effects of hypertension on the kidney may be evidenced by the incremental increases of serum creatinine as well as by the 4+ proteinuria, and the increased BUN. The end organ effects on the vasculature are perhaps mirrored by the papilledema and exudates seen on fundoscopic examination which were not present on earlier evaluations.

4. What symptoms of hypertension are manifested by this patient?

Hypertension is usually not associated with any symptoms which alert individuals to its presence. It can only be detected by the direct measurement of blood pressure. Although headaches and nose bleeds are occasionally cited as symptoms of high blood pressure, the United States Health Examination Survey of 6672 subjects indicated that the occurrence of headaches, epistaxis, and tinnitus could not be statistically related to systolic or diastolic blood pressures (225).

Symptoms do not commonly accompany hypertension, and as a result, patients frequently neglect to follow antihypertensive medication regimens. If patients fail to adhere to therapeutic plans, they usually feel better because they no longer need to tolerate uncomfortable medication side effects. Furthermore, patients who already have adapted to a higher level of blood pressure oftentimes are lethargic (like F.W.) when blood pressure is lowered. Therefore, it is not surprising that a substantial number of hypertensives fail to comply to therapy.

5. F.W. has consistently failed to take his antihypertensive medications for the past 8 to 9 years. How can patient compliance to therapy be improved?

The subject of compliance, or more appropriately noncompliance, is a popular topic of discussion and concern. Previously, clinicians generally assumed that once a patient's disease state had been documented and a therapeutic plan initiated, that the patient would adhere to it. It was a false assumption. Over 50 studies demonstrate that the single greatest contributing fac-

tor to therapeutic failures is the inability of patients to follow a directed course of therapy. Not only have these studies shown that 25 to 59% of patients fail to take medications as directed, but also that 4 to 35% of these patients were using their medications in a manner which posed serious threats to their health (202). As a result, many clinicians began patient education programs for their hypertensive patients. The basic assumption underlying the value of patient education was that an informed and well-guided patient should be able to make a valuable contribution to the success of his/her own treatment. However, in contrast to expectations, recent studies demonstrate that general information about hypertension, by itself, has almost no effect on patient compliance to medication nor on long-term blood pressure control (139,183).

Half of the 230 hypertensive Canadian steel workers in Sackett's study (183), were randomly assigned to receive an educational program designed to teach facts about hypertension; end-organ damage; the benefits of therapy; the need for compliance; and simple general suggestions for pill-taking. This program was highly effective in teaching these men about hypertension and its management, as evidenced by the fact that 85% of the men in the test group mastered the health information, in contrast to 18% in the control group (183). Unfortunately, statistical analyses failed to reveal any association between compliance and knowledge. The conclusion of this study is not that all health education is meaningless, but rather that patient education by itself, without behavior modification messages, is inadequate. Such a finding is really not surprising when one considers the numbers of cigarette smokers who already are aware of the dangers associated with smoking.

McKenney, a pharmacist, went beyond merely providing patients with information about hypertension and the need for compliance. With each individual patient, he discussed specific details of the medication program, clarified directions, sought out complications, assessed patient responses to therapy, and recommended changes to the physician when indicated. Compliance increased from 25 to 79%, and the number of patients achieving normotension increased from 20 to 79% (139). However, six months after the discontinuation of this program, patient compliance decreased to 42%. Two points can be concluded from this study. The first is that efforts to improve compliance must be continuous when managing life-long diseases. The second point is that methods aimed at improvement of compliance must focus on the patient as an individual. McKenney was successful only if he spent time with each individual patient to make sure that the patient was receiving the optimum in drug therapy. Whenever therapy is prescribed without due consideration for the individual characteristics of each and every patient, therapeutic results always will be inadequate.

Other effective strategies in improving compliance to antihypertensive medications include home monitoring of blood pressure (181); provision of all diagnostic and therapeutic services at the work site (4), although augmented convenience has not been uniformly effective (183); use of a specially trained nurse (62), pharmacist (38), or paramedical personnel (181); and a number of behaviorally oriented procedures such as reinforcing high compliance by rewarding it (182). Whatever strategy is chosen is unimportant. What is important is that utilization of a specific individually-directed compliance strategy generally increases patient compliance (169), and such strategies must be employed because hypertensives do not take their medications.

It is also of interest that F.W. was evaluated and treated unsuccessfully at a university medical clinic. His experience at that clinic was probably not much different than the findings of Alderman and Ochs (5) that the present-day general medical clinic cannot satisfy the needs of most hypertensive patients. Half of all clinic patients were lost to follow-up within the first year, and adequate decreases in blood pressure control were achieved by less than 25% of the patients. Furthermore, this study found no clinic changes with regard to work-up, chart procedure, or effective treatment resulting from the classic Veterans Administration studies (216,218) which clearly documented the value of antihypertensive therapy.

New methods of health care delivery to the hypertensive population must be explored. Since hospital clinics provide almost 20% of all ambulatory care (5), the first step in improving hypertensive care is to recognize that the traditional clinic is inadequate to provide effective long-term treatment (59).

6. What variables predispose this patient to hypertension, and what variables are predictive for a more severe prognosis?

This patient's *family history* is highly suggestive of familial hypertension. The concept of genetic influences on blood pressure regulation is well established in the literature (168,189) and clinicians recognize that hypertension and its complications commonly occur in families. Although familial aggregation of blood pressure is well documented in children of natural families (238), such a correlation is not as strong in adopted children (199). Nevertheless, it is estimated that a child with two hypertensive parents has a 60% chance of becoming hypertensive during a lifetime (187). Thus, hypertension clearly has a familial tendency. However, it should be noted that families share not only common genes, but also a common environ-

ment which cannot be ignored. It is reasonable therefore, to conclude that hypertension is determined by genetic factors which in turn are modified by various environmental factors such as the level of socioeconomic class (157) and high salt intake (108,195).

Race is also a significant index of risk in hypertension. Vital statistics indicate that hypertension is not only more prevalent in blacks, but also that the mortality risk in black patients with hypertension is almost double that of white patients (63). Furthermore, if hypertension is evident in blacks at an early age, the mortality rates are even more dramatically increased. Reportedly, blacks under the age of fifty with hypertension have six to seven times higher rates of mortality than whites of comparable age (63).

The younger the *age* of the patient at the onset of hypertension, regardless of race, the greater is the reduction in life expectancy. According to life insurance data, men with blood pressures of 150/100 mm Hg and who are 50 to 59 years of age have twice the death rate over the next 20 years as do comparable normotensives; but at ages 30 to 39, the 20 year mortality increases to five times that of normal. Therefore, when hypertension occurs at an early age, even modest elevations of blood pressure are associated with greatly increased risks.

Sex is also an important prognosticator of hypertensive disease as men suffer more severe consequences of hypertension than women. The mortality data are approximately twice as high in men as in women.

Obesity is associated with both increased prevalence and incidence of hypertension and changes in weight are associated with changes in blood pressure (199). Overweight men, who lose 15% of their body weight, are able to decrease their systolic pressures by 10%; however, if men gain 15% of their weight, systolic pressures will be increased by an average of 18% (210). Apparently, increases in body weight result in higher blood pressures and more hypertensive cardiovascular disease (105). Since obese individuals with normal blood pressures do not suffer substantially increased risks of cardiovascular disease (105), it perhaps can be concluded that obesity leads to hypertension which then elicits excessive vascular complications (112).

Although control of obesity in white Americans could potentially decrease the prevalence of hypertension, clinicians have been minimizing the value of weight loss in the treatment of high blood pressure. The general lack of long-term success in the treatment of obesity, coupled with the conviction that reductions in blood pressure with weight loss are probably due entirely to a concomitant reduction in salt intake (42), probably account for the apathy concerning weight reduction as an adjunctive modality for the therapy of hypertension. However, renewed interest in weight reduction for obese hypertensives has been generated by a controlled study which demonstrated an average decrease of 26 mm Hg systolic and 20 mm Hg diastolic in a group of obese hypertensives. These patients lost about 9.5 kg of body weight over a period of two months, were not taking any antihypertensive medications, and were not salt restricted. The results were even more dramatic in another group of obese hypertensives who also lost weight and who were previously uncontrolled in spite of antihypertensive medications. No significant changes in blood pressure or weight occurred in this study's control group (176).

F.W. has a strong *family history* of hypertension and is a *young obese black man* who was first informed of his hypertension when he was about 30 years of age. He also drinks about 6 to 8 cups of **coffee** daily. In a double-blind, randomized, cross-over study of the effects of a single dose of caffeine in nine young healthy non-coffee drinkers, the mean blood pressure rose 14/10 mm Hg one hour after ingestion. The amount of caffeine administered (250 mg) was comparable to the amount in two to three cupfuls of coffee. The caffeine increased not only the blood pressure by approximately 14% but also increased plasma renin activity by 57%, plasma norepinephrine by 75%, and plasma epinephrine by 207%. These effects lasted throughout the four hours of this study (179). Considering the fact that the thiazide diuretics probably decrease diastolic pressures by about 10 mm Hg maximally, it would seem that caffeine should be considered as an important etiologic variable in the development of hypertension.

To be concerned only with this patient's hypertension without regard to the effects of his excessive cigarette **smoking** seems somewhat cavalier, because both hypertension and cigarette smoking have the potential for end-organ damage. The mortality rates from coronary disease among men age 45 to 54, who smoke more than 20 cigarettes a day, are three times higher than similar aged nonsmokers (123). The Center for Disease Control estimates that 25% of approximately 648,540 heart disease deaths in the United States each year are the result of cigarette smoking (33). Furthermore, retrospective and prospective studies demonstrate that cigarette smoking is responsible for approximately 70% of chronic bronchitis and emphysema cases. Likewise, the statistics for lung cancer and other carcinomas are equally impressive.

✳Cigarette smoking also increases epinephrine and norepinephrine release, as well as systolic and diastolic blood pressures. In one study, the mean systolic pressures increased from 108 mm Hg to a maximum of 120 mm Hg and the mean diastolic pressures increased from 67 mm Hg to a maximum of 70 mm Hg during smoking. Control groups were not similarly affected (40).

This patient is apparently knowledgeable concerning the undesirable effects of cigarette smoking because of his previous attempts to discontinue his 1.5 pack/day habit. He was unsuccessful in his attempts because of nervousness, but smokers are not more calm than non-smokers; Schachter (184) speculates that perhaps smoking is not so much anxiety-reducing, as not smoking (or insufficient nicotine) is anxiety-increasing. It would be beneficial if this patient could be taught to self-initiate relaxation responses (17).

This patient's prognosis is not good because significant end-organ damage has already developed. Even with minimal damage to the eyes, heart, or kidneys, mortality increases. In the classic Veterans Administration study, the incidence of major complications over a time span of approximately three years, was 2.5 fold higher in patients with end-organ damage than in patients not exhibiting such problems (219). F.W. already exhibits significant target organ deterioration as evidenced by physical examination of his heart, eyes, and kidneys.

7. What are the effects of treatment on the morbidity and mortality of hypertensive patients?

Reduction of elevated blood pressure, whatever, the cause, unequivocably lowers morbidity and mortality. The Veterans Administration's classic study of 143 men with initial diastolic pressures averaging 115 through 129 mm Hg had to be terminated because of the high incidence of morbidity in the untreated hypertensive group. Of the 70 untreated patients, 38% developed a complication in less than 16 months as compared to only 3% of the treated hypertensives (218). Four deaths out of 70 patients (5.7%) and severe complications such as myocardial infarction, cerebral thrombosis, congestive heart failure, transient ischemic attacks, cerebral hemorrhage, increasing azotemia, and grade IV retinopathy occurred in the placebo treated group. Only two serious complications occurred in all of the 73 treated patients.

Phase II of the Veterans Administration Study Group followed 380 male hypertensives with diastolic blood pressures averaging 90-114 mm Hg. Treatment in this study decreased the risk of developing morbidity over a five year period from 55% to 18% (216). The majority of patients who benefited from treatment either had systolic pressures above 164 mm Hg or diastolic pressures above 104 mm Hg. Hypertensives with diastolics ranging from 90 to 104 mm Hg did not benefit as dramatically perhaps due to the fact that end-organ complications appear considerably more slowly, and longer term follow-up would be necessary to uncover such sequelae. In general, the higher the pre-treatment blood pressure, the greater the benefit of treatment. Therapy effectively allays the development of congestive heart failure, stroke, and other hypertensive complications, but is relatively ineffective in preventing the atherosclerotic complications of coronary heart disease (216,218).

8. The Veterans Administration studies (216,218) concerning the effect of treatment on morbidity and mortality were based upon arbitrarily defined ranges of diastolic blood pressures. Likewise, the report of the Joint National Committee on Detection, Evaluation, and Treatment of High Blood Pressure based their recommendations and findings on diastolic pressures. Are systolic pressures of significance?

Although elevated systolic blood pressures occur in elderly patients and in individuals with high output states such as anemia and thyrotoxicosis, they are generally dismissed and regarded as innocuous. Clinicians maintain that diastolic pressures are more diagnostic because they better reflect mean blood pressures and are more closely correlated with the increased peripheral resistance component of hypertension. Such concepts are now being reconsidered in light of epidemiological studies (103,173) which document a stronger association of coronary heart disease with systolic than with diastolic blood pressures in some groups of patients. Systolic pressures serve as well, or better than, diastolic pressures in predicting the probability of thrombotic strokes, coronary heart disease, left ventricular hypertrophy, and congestive heart failure (117).

There is simply no evidence to confirm the misconception that elevations of systolic blood pressures in the aged, or any other population are innocuous. Some investigations even speculate that systolic pressure elevations may actually increase atherogenesis rather than merely reflect atherosclerotic changes in arteries. Although more studies are needed, it is evident that elevated systolic pressures should not be totally ignored.

9. What should be the goal of antihypertensive therapy for patients like F.W.?

The ultimate goal of antihypertensive therapy is to prevent morbidity and deaths due to hypertensive disease. This goal is achievable if elevated blood pressures are lowered and maintained at acceptable levels. However, the need to attain normotension must be balanced against potential drug toxicities and unnecessary or intolerable drug side effects. It is counterproductive to expect patients to tolerate incapacitating or extremely discomforting drug side effects simply to treat what patients usually perceive as an asymptomatic disease.

According to the Joint Commission (48), "the first goal of antihypertensive therapy is to achieve and maintain diastolic pressure levels at less than 90 mm

Hg with minimal adverse effects." This certainly appears to be a desirable goal. Insurance records show that even minimal or borderline hypertension is associated with a shortened life expectancy. An untreated blood pressure of 140/95 mm Hg decreases life expectancy by nine years, and a blood pressure of 150/100 mm Hg cuts 16.5 years off the normal life expectancy (91,204). Furthermore, the VA study (217) of hypertensives with diastolic blood pressures averaging 90 to 114 mm Hg demonstrated that treatment clearly decreased morbidity and mortality.

While a diastolic blood pressure of less than 90 mm Hg may be optimal for longevity, there is no evidence to suggest that the benefits versus risk ratio justifies the aggressive pursuit of this goal. The majority of VA patients who did benefit from therapy had diastolic pressures greater than 104 mm Hg (217). Furthermore, the prevention of hypertensive morbidity may not depend upon a complete normalization of blood pressure.

In one study (48), renal, cardiac, and fundoscopic changes as well as mortality were not significantly different between patients whose blood pressures were normalized as compared to those whose blood pressures were lowered to 20 and 33% of normal (65). Apparently, considerable therapeutic benefits result whenever the blood pressure can be lowered, even if the pressure is not lowered to normal. Additionally, upon closer scrutiny of the data from the VA study (204), about one-third of the treated patients whose pre-treatment diastolic pressures were greater than 105 mm Hg continued to have elevated blood pressures (mean of 98 mm Hg) but experienced considerably less morbidity.

Of the poorly-controlled treated patients with mean blood pressures of 98 mm Hg, 14.9% later developed myocardial infarctions, strokes, or cardiovascular deaths as compared to 9.7% of the well-controlled treated patients with mean blood pressures of 76 mm Hg. However, the difference between these two groups was not statistically significant. In the untreated control group, 28.9% experienced statistically significant increases in cardiovascular complications. Therefore, it is not necessary to demand a blood pressure lowering to normal levels. This conclusion does not mean that such a goal should not be attempted. However, whenever the goal of a normal blood pressure cannot be achieved without disturbing side effects, clinicians can accept the compromise that even partial reduction of blood pressure significantly modifies the risks of hypertensive end-organ damage.

Perhaps this latter philosophy could have been of help to F.W. At one time, his blood pressure was lowered to 130/95 mm Hg; however, he also developed weakness, marked lethargy, inability to concentrate, postural hypotension, and impotence. Thus, it is not surprising that he voluntarily refused to comply to his medication regimen.

10. At what level of blood pressure and with what medications should therapy be initiated?

Virtually all patients with repeatedly confirmed diastolic blood pressures of greater than 105 mm Hg or higher should definitely be treated. This recommendation by the Joint Commission (148) is based upon data from the Veterans Administration Study Group (217, 218) of compliant, male, veterans 30 to 73 years of age. Not all hypertensives are compliant, nor are all hypertensives male veterans. However, it is reasonable to extrapolate this data to all hypertensives until other contradictory data become available.

"Treatment of patients with diastolic pressures from 90 to 104 mm Hg should be individualized" (148). Elevated systolic blood pressure, presence of target organ damage, family history of hypertensive complications, smoking, male gender, elevated blood cholesterol level, and diabetes are other risk factors which the Joint Commission (148) suggests should influence the decision to initiate therapy. These factors are known to be risk factors for atherosclerotic complications. Therefore, it seems prudent to consider these factors, although their relationship to the benefits of antihypertensive therapy has not been reported (99).

In view of insurance actuarial data and the Veterans Administration studies, it seems reasonable to initiate therapy in all patients with diastolic pressures greater than 90 mm Hg. Any elevation in blood pressure is undesirable. Although the evidence regarding treatment of patients with diastolics of 90 to 104 mm Hg is not at all impressive, and is not in many instances statistically significant, one should heed the adage of where there is smoke, one must suspect a fire. Perspectives, however, must be maintained. It is not reasonable to aggressively extinguish a suspected fire only to discover that extensive water damage has destroyed the very possessions which were to be protected. In other words, the cure should not be worse than the disease.

Either the thiazide diuretics and/or non-pharmacological interventions should be initiated in almost all patients with diastolic pressures of 90 to 100 mm Hg after baseline laboratory data are collected. The thiazides are effective antihypertensives, and side effects are minimal in most instances. They achieve a smooth control of the blood pressure without significant cerebral or postural effects, and they also potentiate other antihypertensive drugs. Thus, it seems reasonable to initiate therapy with hydrochlorothiazide 50 mg daily and to increase this regimen to twice daily if needed. Any other thiazide or thiazide-like diuretic in comparable doses would also be useful. If patients continue to be asymptomatic and without evidence of eye ground or other end-organ changes, additional drug therapy would be overly aggressive in most patients based upon currently available evidence.

Non-pharmacological interventions should also be initiated for patients as an adjunct to, or in lieu of, the thiazide diuretics for asymptomatic patients with diastolic pressures in the range of 90 to 100 mm Hg. Dietary salt limitations and weight reduction for obese patients should be considered (see Question 6). If the physician or other primary care practitioner has experience with an effective meditation or other relaxation technique, and if such experiences are compatible with the patient's lifestyle and beliefs, application should be attempted. Several investigators (1,217,203) have concluded that regular practice of rest and relaxation techniques does lower arterial pressure, especially in the early stages of hypertensive disease. However, it would seem that relaxation techniques would be applicable only to a very small select population. It is difficult enough to get patients to comply to taking medications twice a day, much less expect them to meditate for 20 minutes twice daily. Nevertheless, if such practices are embraced by patients, encouragement would be appropriate (170).

11. How can different drug combinations be selected rationally?

The effective management of hypertension often requires the concurrent administration of two or more drugs. Because medications have different mechanisms of actions, antihypertensive drug therapy should be formulated with the aim of affecting different blood pressure regulatory mechanisms. For example, it is not rational to choose two sympathoplegic agents without having first considered the combination of a diuretic or a vasodilator in combination with a single sympathoplegic agent.

Rational therapeutics would suggest a stepped-care approach to treatment. Such an approach (e.g. Table 1) begins therapy with a small dose of an antihypertensive drug that is gradually increased until the maximal antihypertensive effect which can be expected is exerted, or until side effects appear. Then other drugs are added, as needed, one after the other until a predetermined therapeutic goal is attained. In this manner, the best, and least toxic drugs are utilized to the fullest extent before the other less satisfactory agents are added. Use of fixed dosage antihypertensive combination products is not recommended because such usage does not permit individualized titration of single drugs.

Although the flow chart of antihypertensive drug therapy in Table 1 offers several choices in each category, the following choices are advocated for reasons to be apparent in later sections of this chapter:

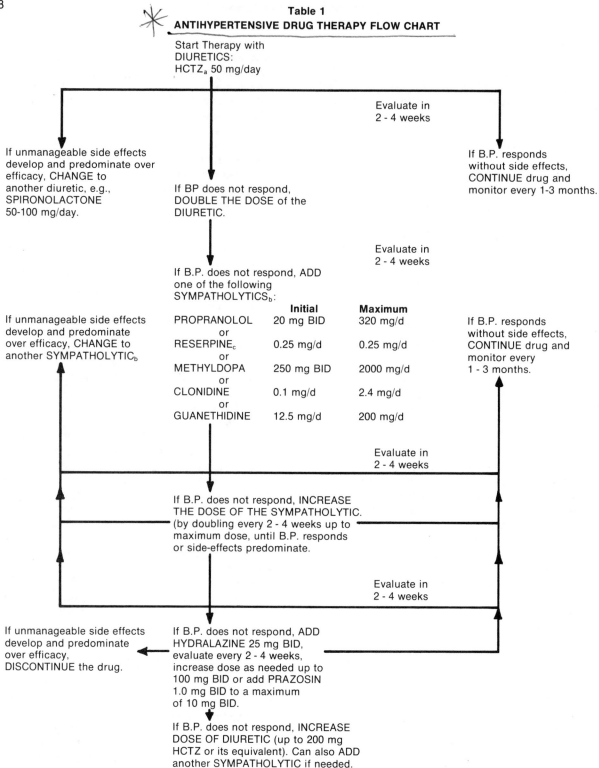

138

Table 1
ANTIHYPERTENSIVE DRUG THERAPY FLOW CHART

Start Therapy with DIURETICS: $HCTZ_a$ 50 mg/day

Evaluate in 2 - 4 weeks

If unmanageable side effects develop and predominate over efficacy, CHANGE to another diuretic, e.g., SPIRONOLACTONE 50-100 mg/day.

If BP does not respond, DOUBLE THE DOSE of the DIURETIC.

If B.P. responds without side effects, CONTINUE drug and monitor every 1-3 months.

Evaluate in 2 - 4 weeks

If B.P. does not respond, ADD one of the following $SYMPATHOLYTICS_b$:

	Initial	Maximum
PROPRANOLOL	20 mg BID	320 mg/d
or		
$RESERPINE_c$	0.25 mg/d	0.25 mg/d
or		
METHYLDOPA	250 mg BID	2000 mg/d
or		
CLONIDINE	0.1 mg/d	2.4 mg/d
or		
GUANETHIDINE	12.5 mg/d	200 mg/d

If unmanageable side effects develop and predominate over efficacy, CHANGE to another $SYMPATHOLYTIC_b$

If B.P. responds without side effects, CONTINUE drug and monitor every 1 - 3 months.

Evaluate in 2 - 4 weeks

If B.P. does not respond, INCREASE THE DOSE OF THE SYMPATHOLYTIC. (by doubling every 2 - 4 weeks up to maximum dose, until B.P. responds or side-effects predominate.

Evaluate in 2 - 4 weeks

If unmanageable side effects develop and predominate over efficacy, DISCONTINUE the drug.

If B.P. does not respond, ADD HYDRALAZINE 25 mg BID, evaluate every 2 - 4 weeks, increase dose as needed up to 100 mg BID or add PRAZOSIN 1.0 mg BID to a maximum of 10 mg BID.

If B.P. does not respond, INCREASE DOSE OF DIURETIC (up to 200 mg HCTZ or its equivalent). Can also ADD another SYMPATHOLYTIC if needed.

a. Can use any thiazide in dose equivalent to hydrochlorothiazide (HCTZ) 50 mg.

b. The choice of sympatholytic is usually based upon minimizing side effects in the individual patient.

c. Do not increase reserpine dosage above 0.25 mg/day. Change to another sympatholytic.

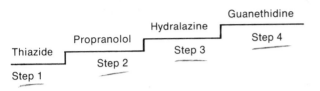

Step 1: Thiazide
Step 2: Propranolol
Step 3: Hydralazine
Step 4: Guanethidine

12. After F.W.'s first hospitalization one of his discharge medications was hydrochlorothiazide 50 mg daily. Is this an adequate antihypertensive dose for F.W.?

A close association exists between the blood pressure lowering effects and the diuretic effects of thiazides. Thus, thiazides and thiazide-like drugs exert their antihypertensive effects at doses which enhance sodium excretion (22).

As effective diuretics, thiazides may induce the excretion of approximately 5% of the total sodium load which has been glomerularly filtered (52). If less sodium is filtered, less sodium will be presented to the distal tubules where thiazide diuretics are effective. Therefore, the thiazides are ineffective diuretics in patients with creatinine clearances less than 30 ml/min (9). F.W.'s creatinine clearance at this time was 41 ml/minute. Although hydrochlorothiazide will still be effective, it will be less so than if his creatinine clearance was normal. Additionally, large doses of sympatholytics or vasodilators can produce substantial sodium and fluid retention. Since he was receiving 400 mg of hydralazine, 1000 mg of methyldopa, and 30 mg of guanethidine daily, it would have been reasonable to increase his hydrochlorothiazide dosage to a maximum.

The maximum effective antihypertensive dose of hydrochlorothiazide usually approximates its maximum effective diuretic dose, and is generally about 150 to 200 mg/day. Further increases in dose do not provide greater hypotensive activity. Although the serum concentration was doubled in a study of 19 patients who received 450 mg/day of hydrochlorothiazide, the blood pressure reduction was not greater than in those receiving only 150 mg/day (140).

In another study of 37 patients with hypertension, chlorthalidone, a thiazide-like diuretic, produced similar hypotensive effects with four different doses. The reduction in blood pressure was maximal in 25 of the patients on a dose of 25 or 50 mg of chlorthalidone, but maximal blood pressure reduction was only observed in the remaining 12 patients when 100 to 200 mg doses were given. The likelihood of response of these individuals to a given chlorthalidone dose could not be predicted and was not affected by the severity of hypertension. When 50 mg/day or less of chlorthalidone was used, two-thirds of the hypertensive pa-

tients responded maximally with only minor concomitant changes in serum potassium, chloride, and uric acid. The patients who required higher doses experienced more frequent biochemical disturbances (211). Likewise, a reduction in dosage from 50 mg daily of chlorthalidone to 50 mg three times a week produced no significant changes in diastolic pressures, although hyperuricemia and hypokalemia were more significant with the higher dosage regimen (15). The results from these studies seem to suggest that diuretic antihypertensive activity is less dose dependent than the effect on serum potassium and serum uric acid.

13. Laboratory data obtained during this hospitalization indicate that end-organ hypertensive disease has progressed. F.W.'s serum creatinine has increased from 2.0 mg/100 ml, which was noted during his first hospitalization, to 3.8 mg/100 ml. Furosemide is added to the hypertensive regimen. The hydrochlorothiazide is not discontinued with the thought being that the thiazides have antihypertensive effects independent of their diuretic actions. How do the thiazides lower blood pressure, and should hydrochlorothiazide be continued in this patient with significant renal impairment?

The exact mechanism of antihypertensive action of the thiazide diuretics is unknown despite extensive use in the treatment of hypertension. Initially, thiazides reduce circulating blood volume and cardiac output. However, after two weeks of continuous therapy, the thiazide diuretic phase gradually diminishes and the blood volume and cardiac output almost return to normal. Therefore, the long-term antihypertensive effects of diuretics may be independent of prolonged volume depletion.

Postulated theories concerning thiazide actions abound in the literature. Some claim impaired vascular responsiveness to endogenous catecholamines (66); others claim an altered sodium content of arterial walls; or even altered sodium metabolism. Irrespective of the ultimate mechanism, the thiazides relax peripheral vascular smooth muscle and reduce elevated blood pressures (44).

This patient's serum creatinine of 3.8 mg/100 ml can be estimated (129) to correspond to a creatinine clearance of approximately 22 ml/min. It is unlikely that the thiazides will be effective diuretics in patients with this degree of renal dysfunction, and the addition of furosemide is appropriate for this patient. The hydrochlorothiazide should be discontinued, because a functioning kidney with the ability to respond with a natriuresis is necessary for the antihypertensive action of thiazides. To evaluate this very aspect, twelve stable renal failure patients on maintenance hemodialysis were studied after being treated with hydrochlorothiazide, metolazone, and placebo in four-week treatment cross-over periods. Therapy did not induce a diuresis in these patients with non-functioning kidneys, and the blood pressure was not lowered (16).

14. Are thiazide diuretics and furosemide (Lasix) equally effective in reducing blood pressures in non-edematous hypertensives with normal renal function?

The fact that furosemide is a very useful and potent diuretic does not necessarily mean that it modifies arteriolar tone to the same extent as the thiazide diuretics. The superiority of furosemide as an antihypertensive agent in patients with normal renal function remains controversial.

In a double-blind controlled study involving 20 hypertensive ambulatory patients, hydrochlorothiazide 50 mg twice daily was twice as effective as 40 mg of furosemide twice daily in lowering blood pressure (8). In another study, Healy and associates (88) reported that furosemide 40 mg twice daily did not reduce blood pressure at all in nine subjects on long-term therapy; whereas 100 mg daily of chlorthalidone (Hygroton) was an effective antihypertensive. Nevertheless, clinical experience does indicate that furosemide is an effective antihypertensive medication, and studies can be found to document its effectiveness.

The effectiveness of the thiazides as antihypertensives is well established and not at all controversial in patients with normal renal function. Since the thiazides are less expensive and less toxic than furosemide, they are to be considered the antihypertensive diuretics of choice for patients without renal impairment. The vast majority of patients requiring diuretics can be well managed with the thiazides and have little to gain from the availability of new and more powerful agents.

Thus, the choice of hydrochlorothiazide for F.W. when his kidneys were functioning adequately was appropriate, as was the choice of furosemide when his kidney function deteriorated.

15. Does this patient's laboratory data implicate any diuretic-induced side effects?

A high serum **uric acid,** like F.W.'s 10.1 mg/100 ml, is not uncommon during either thiazide or furosemide therapy; approximately 40 to 50% of such treated patients will develop serum uric acid levels above 7.0 mg/100 ml. This asymptomatic hyperuricemia can occur within a few days of therapy, but the serum uric acid generally returns to normal levels when the diuretics are discontinued. An increased prevalence of hyperuricemia has also been associated with hypertension independent of medication intake (47,115).

Probenecid can be used to lower serum uric acid

levels and is not known to significantly affect blood levels of antihypertensive medications. Likewise, allopurinol 300 mg/day can prevent the hyperuricemia induced by diuretics and can maintain serum uric acid below pre-diuretic levels (154). These hypouricemic agents should not be administered on a prophylactic basis. Only some patients will develop hyperuricemia, and asymptomatic hyperuricemia is generally not treated (126). Also see the *Gout and Hyperuricemia* chapter.

Prolonged thiazide, chlorthalidone, quinethazone, furosemide, and ethacrynic acid therapy may produce a mild **hyperglycemia,** particularly in patients with latent diabetes (124,153). The glucose intolerance is usually mild and generally subsides after therapy. There is some evidence that potassium supplementation may correct the abnormal glucose tolerance caused by thiazide diuretics (175).

The mechanism of diuretic-induced hyperglycemia is unknown, but theories include a direct effect on tissue glucose metabolism; reduction of islet cell secretion of insulin; and finally, the production of acute pancreatitis (also see *Diabetes* chapter). Thus, F.W.'s fasting blood sugar may well reflect a diuretic-induced hyperglycemia.

The thiazide diuretics (6), chlorthalidone (7), and theoretically furosemide are associated with increases in serum **cholesterol** and **triglycerides.** In one study, the mean increase in serum cholesterol of 11 mg/100 ml in a group of 39 diuretic-treated patients on a special diet was not large, but the increase appears more dramatic when it is compared to the control group data from 35 patients who decreased their serum cholesterol by about 11 mg/100 ml. The diuretic-treated group also demonstrated a 34 mg/100 ml increase in serum triglyceride concentration. These changes could not be explained by hemoconcentration, and the mechanism of elevated serum lipids induced by these diuretics remains a mystery. Regardless of the mechanism, elevated serum lipids are associated epidemiologically with coronary heart disease. As a result, the increased probability of developing coronary atherosclerosis resulting from these mean serum lipid increases could possibly offset the benefit gained from lowering blood pressure in an otherwise healthy 35-year-old man (6). Considering the controversy concerning therapy of hyperlipidemia and its influence on morbidity and mortality, this patient should not be treated with lipid lowering agents. He definitely should continue the diuretic component of his antihypertensive regimen.

16. Upon discharge from his first hospitalization, F.W. received a prescription for KCl 10% with directions to take 20 mEq/daily in addition to his other antihypertensive medications. Should potassium

supplements be routinely prescribed for all hypertensives who are treated with thiazides or furosemide?

The reported incidence of hypokalemia in ambulatory patients receiving thiazides for hypertension ranges from 10 to 40% (106,136,180). The variability in these estimates is due to differences in diagnostic criteria, methodology, and duration of study. Some authors measure total body potassium concentrations while others measure serum potassium concentrations; however, the correlations between these two measurements are often poor (180). The serum potassium concentration is not a good measure of total body potassium, because it is affected by other parameters such as total body weight, pH of the serum, and state of hydration. On the other hand, the clinical manifestations of potassium deficiency (fatigue, drowsiness, dizziness, confusion, EKG changes, muscle weakness and pain) correlate better with serum concentrations than with the total amount in the body. Losses of body potassium that are not reflected in decreases of the serum potassium are generally not of clinical significance. Therefore, it is primarily the fall in extracellular potassium concentration that creates clinical problems, despite the fact that 98% of total body potassium is intracellular (118,180).

Although the estimates concerning long-term thiazide induced hypokalemia range from 10 to 40%, most clinicians feel that the 10% figure is probably more reflective of their experiences. Thus, it seems rather aggressive to prescribe prophylactic potassium chloride supplements to all hypertensives receiving thiazides if approximately 90% of these patients will not need such supplementation. All of the potassium chloride preparations taste bad, cause some degree of gastrointestinal distress, and create problems with patient compliance which often carries over to other antihypertensive medications as well. Furthermore, potassium supplementation has been associated with hyperkalemia and other adverse reactions in 5.8% of patients receiving supplementation (232). Since it is relatively rare for low doses of thiazides to cause clinically significant hypokalemia in patients who are receiving it for long term antihypertensive therapy (118), potassium supplementation is not advocated for all thiazide-treated patients. Exceptions include those on digitalis or those who have pre-existing medical problems that may require supplementation, such as congestive heart failure, cirrhosis with ascites, and nephrosis.

17. If potassium supplementation is deemed necessary, what therapeutic interventions can be employed in the ambulatory setting?

Hypokalemia can be corrected with oral potassium chloride in liquid preparations, as slow release potassium chloride tablets, as well as with the potassium sparing diuretics, spironolactone or triamterene. If spironolactone is chosen, 50 to 100 mg daily is usually adequate for most mild cases of potassium insufficiency resulting from 100 mg/day doses of hydrochlorothiazide or its equivalent. Triamterene daily doses should be 100 to 200 mg. Although triamterene is usually less expensive than spironolactone, unlike spironolactone, it is without significant antihypertensive properties. Both spironolactone and triamterene should be used with extreme caution in patients receiving concomitant potassium supplements and in patients with renal dysfunction, because hyperkalemia can occur. Furthermore, individual patient responses to the potassium conserving actions of these two agents are not always predictable, and moderately severe hypokalemia would best be corrected with potassium chloride.

Potassium rich foods such as dried fruits, fresh bananas, and orange juice are expensive, high in calories, high in sugar content, and usually inadequate for all but the very mildest cases of hypokalemia. Diabetics, obese hypertensives, and other overweight patients should not be encouraged to utilize these foodstuffs as potassium supplements without due consideration for the above factors.

Reports of hyperkalemia resulting from abuse of salt substitutes (81) has led to speculation concerning the use of such substitutes as viable therapeutic agents. One teaspoonful of Morton's LITE-SALT contains about 37 mEq of potassium and 3.0 grams of sodium chloride (41). When used in conjunction with other true salt substitutes like Neocurtasal or Adolph's Salt Substitute, this form of potassium supplementation is not only palatable but inexpensive. The LITE-SALT can be used at the dining table, and the salt substitutes can be used in cooking and also can be sprinkled over a dinner salad as well. Patients with renal impairment, cardiac failure, or patients receiving spironolactone and triamterene must be cautioned concerning the use of salt substitutes (178).

18. Discuss the hormonally related side effects of spironolactone. How does the clinician assess the role of this drug as the etiological factor?

Spironolactone may induce gynecomastia. This condition is characterized by the excessive development of male mammary glands and is occasionally associated with lactation. Although more common bilaterally, unilateral gynecomastia can also develop. The series of patients reported with this condition is too small to provide a proper estimate of an overall incidence, but gynecomastia is not an uncommon complaint. At least 24 cases of spironolactone-induced gynecomastia have been described in the literature (78).

Four of seven men (56%) in one trial developed gynecomastia while receiving 50 to 150 mg of daily spironolactone. In these cases, the breasts were enlarged and invariably accompanied by bilateral pain, tenderness, and lumpiness. The breast itself was not necessarily pendulous, but tender masses approximately 2 to 4 cm in diameter and 1 to 2 cm in depth could be palpated. Unfortunately, 3 of these 4 men were also receiving digitalis preparations, which are also associated with gynecomastia. However, the gynecomastia in these men abated within 1 to 14 months after cessation of spironolactone despite continuation of the digitalis products (37).

Thirty percent (eight out of twenty-eight) of Sherlock's (196) male patients who were being treated with chlorothiazide and spironolactone for fluid retention and hepatic cirrhosis developed gynecomastia. However, cirrhosis of the liver itself may cause hyperestrinism and may result in gynecomastia because the liver is responsible for the metabolism of estrogen.

The mechanisms by which drugs in general, and spironolactone in particular, cause gynecomastia are unknown. Studies imply that spironolactone affects testosterone biosynthesis in man, but the resultant circulating testosterone and estradiol levels do not adequately explain the estrogen-like side effects. Spironolactone also is known to act as an antiandrogen by inhibiting androgen binding to receptor sites (128). Others (23) speculate that spironolactone suppresses gonadotropin release. Furthermore, it should be noted that spironolactone and the digitalis glycosides are both structurally similar to steroid hormones.

Spironolactone is also associated with other endocrine abnormalities. Not only did Spark and Melby (200) note that virtually all men receiving spironolactone in daily doses of 400 mg for 3 to 5 weeks developed gynecomastia, but that others claimed decreased libido and 30% became impotent. All of the women in this study experienced menstrual irregularities, and some also developed breast engorgement. These adverse effects all disappeared upon cessation of spironolactone therapy. Amenorrhea is also known to occur with standard doses of spironolactone (122).

In assessing the role of spironolactone in the development of these problems, clinicians must evaluate two basic parameters. First, a temporal relationship must be established between the onset of symptoms and the initiation of drug use. However, the onset of symptomatology sometimes may be quite delayed. Secondly, other possible causes must be ruled out because gynecomastia, impotence, decreased libido, and amenorrhea have other possible etiologies. For example, digitalis, methyldopa, and twenty-two other drugs and hormones have been associated with development of gynecomastia, as have a host of other clinical conditions (78) including liver disease. Impotence has been related to several drugs (see Question 40), and amenorrhea also has multiple possible etiologies.

19. Is spironolactone preferred over the thiazide diuretics in patients with low renin essential hypertension?

Suppressed plasma renin activity (PRA) is observed in about 25% of patients with essential hypertension (34,79,201). Primary aldosteronism is also associated with low plasma renin activity and with hypertension as well. These two factors have led to speculations as to whether low renin hypertension is caused by excess mineralocorticoid activity. Since spironolactone (Aldactone) antagonizes the pharmacological actions of aldosterone as well as other mineralocorticoids (127), it has been used to test this hypothesis.

In these studies, hypertensives with low plasma renin activity and normal aldosterone production responded well to spironolactone (2,31,79,201). Since these early initial reports, a number of other studies have produced conflicting results (21,25,60). It now appears that low renin essential hypertensives also respond well to thiazide and other diuretics. These results suggest that volume may be the critical factor rather than mineralocorticoid excess. Still other studies note that hypertensive patients respond to diuretics independently of their renin status.

The entire concept of modifying therapy based upon renin studies leaves much to be desired. Until renin studies are refined and until there is a general consensus based upon reproducible studies, traditional antihypertensive therapy should be followed. At this point in time, spironolactone offers no major advantage over other diuretics in the management of essential hypertension.

20. How do antihypertensive medications affect plasma renin activity (PRA)?

All antihypertensive medications can affect PRA determinations and can do so through various mechanisms. Thiazides (20,206), chlorthalidone (51), spironolactone (131), and loop diuretics all increase PRA by either altering sodium content in the macula densa cells and/or by reducing plasma volume. Hydralazine (212), diazoxide (49), and all other vasodilating antihypertensive medications elevate PRA perhaps by altering renal perfusion pressure, resulting in renin production because of reflex sympathetic discharge. Clonidine (11) probably lowers PRA through its central sympathetic inhibitory action. Guanethidine elevates PRA in sodium depleted patients, but lowers PRA in patients in normal sodium balance (80,119). Methyldopa (191) most likely depresses PRA through a central action. Propranolol (27) very effectively inhibits PRA through its ability to block beta receptors. Potassium administration also tends to reduce PRA. In each instance, the antihypertensive activity of these medications is probably totally independent of their effects on PRA.

Clinicians must be aware of these effects of antihypertensive medications on PRA in order to correctly interpret PRA determinations.

21. Can plasma renin activity (PRA) predict the pathogenesis of essential hypertension?

In 1972, John Laragh and associates (119) grouped essential hypertensive patients into different categories based upon renin and aldosterone determinations. Of 219 essential hypertensives, 27% had subnormal plasma renins, 57% had normal renin activity, and 16% had abnormally high renins. Since hypertensives could be grouped into three different biochemical categories, essential hypertension clearly is not a homogeneous disease.

When these three categories of hypertensives were each inspected as a group, some surprising facts were discovered. For example, Brunner and Laragh (26) noted that strokes and myocardial infarctions did not occur in patients with low renin hypertension. In contrast, patients with high or normal renin had an 11% frequency of heart attacks and a 14% frequency of strokes over a nine year period. Furthermore, the high renin group of essential hypertensives exhibited more azotemia, proteinuria, hypokalemia, optic fundi deterioration, and higher mean diastolic pressures. These investigators attributed this high incidence of cardiovascular complications in patients with essential hypertension and normal or high renin activity to a vasculotoxic effect of renin (119).

Other investigators have also grouped essential hypertensives into three categories consisting of low, normal, and high renin activity, and noted that the percentages of patients in each group were similar to Laragh's groupings. However, with one exception (36), others have not been able to verify the prognostic implications of Laragh's PRA determinations. As a result, Laragh's multitude of publications have been carefully re-evaluated and constructively criticized (107). Nevertheless, his work is impressive. Thus, despite much intensive research and debate, the precise relationship between renin levels, hypertension, and pathogenesis is still uncertain. At present, one can only safely conclude that all hypertensives should be treated regardless of their renin status.

If the presently unfulfilled promise of renin profiling eventually bears fruit, therapy can be more rationally chosen based upon the ability of antihypertensive medications to affect the renin levels as discussed in Question 20.

22. Currently, the use of reserpine is often debated with convincing arguments favoring both its virtues and its liabilities. What are its documented liabilities and how can they be assessed?

The most clinically significant reserpine-induced problem is *mental depression* which may be severe enough to require hospitalization or even terminate in suicide. In a review of 16 studies involving 724 reserpine-treated patients, an overall 20% incidence of depression was noted when this medication was used in daily doses of 0.25 mg to 10.0 mg (74). The exact incidence of depression associated with the use of small antihypertensive doses, such as 0.25 to 0.5 mg daily is not reported, but it is known to occur commonly. However, the severity of depression is generally related to dosage and duration of therapy.

Supposedly, the people most vulnerable to reserpine-induced depression are the so-called "sedentary intellectuals" or people who perform daily tasks requiring sophisticated thought integration. These people usually present with subtle symptomatology such as mildly impaired thought processes, early morning awakening, alterations in diet or weight, and a flat affect; however, more severe symptoms such as suicidal tendencies may also become apparent. The precise mechanism whereby reserpine induces these changes is not known, but most likely it involves depletion of central amines like 5-hydroxytryptamine, dopamine, and norepinephrine. Depletion of brain amines occurs very slowly when reserpine is used in the small doses commonly prescribed. Thus, the onset of psychic changes is insidious, and it is often extremely difficult to relate behavioral changes to the medication. Patients with suspected or known depressive tendencies should not receive this drug. Reserpine must be discontinued and should never be reinstituted in patients who develop reserpine-associated depression.

Other central nervous system side effects which commonly occur include bizarre dreams, somnolence, insomnia, and hallucinations (197). Barbiturates, but not benzodiazepines, may increase the incidence of these reserpine-induced side effects (165).

Nasal congestion commonly accompanies reserpine administration due to depletion of vasoconstricting amines in the nasal vasculature. If treatment is necessary, small infrequent doses of oral decongestants such as pseudoephedrine may be used, although chronic use is to be avoided. If the nasal congestion is bothersome, alternate antihypertensive therapy should replace the reserpine.

Peptic ulceration and *carcinogenicity* are discussed in subsequent questions.

23. A 50-year-old mildly hypertensive male is hospitalized with a two week history of abdominal pains

which are relieved by foods and antacids and a chief complaint of black tarry stools and hematemesis. The patient has been on reserpine 0.25 mg/day for ten years. Can this low dose of reserpine cause a peptic ulcer?

Reserpine primarily produces gastrointestinal ulcerations by stimulating the secretion of excessive hydrochloric acid. This parasympathetic mediated secretory response to reserpine is dose-related and usually occurs only when reserpine is given parenterally or in very large oral doses (116,177). In standard doses, oral reserpine, usually does not stimulate gastric secretion significantly; however, intravenous doses greater than 1.0 mg markedly stimulate gastric secretory activity. Even though gastric secretion may be increased with large doses, the incidence of ulceration and gastrointestinal bleeding secondary to reserpine is very low. Moser (149) claims that ulceration is almost non-existent with the small doses commonly used in the treatment of mild hypertension. Hollister (94) noted only three cases of ulcers among six hundred patients receiving large doses of rauwolfia preparations. Nevertheless, some patients may be unusually sensitive to rauwolfia compounds, because perforation and hemorrhage have occurred with reserpine doses of less than 1.0 mg per day (228). Thus, it is best to avoid reserpine in patients with gastrointestinal problems.

24. A 53-year-old female patient has been taking reserpine 0.25 mg daily for the past 20 years. She has been reading a popular magazine concerning reserpine usage and the development of breast cancer. She truculently asks "would you continue taking this drug if you were me?" What is an appropriate response?

In 1974 reports from the Boston Collaborative Drug Surveillance Program (BCDSP), Oxford University, and the University of Helsinki suggested that the statistical risk of breast cancer was three times greater in reserpine-treated women over 50 years of age who received this drug for more than one year than in women not taking reserpine (10,19,90). Unfortunately, all three studies were performed by restrospective chart reviews, thereby minimizing the value of case controls. Also, these three studies can be criticized because of inborn patient selection biases. Patients with breast cancer may simply have had better accessibility to health care facilities, because patients in higher socioeconomic classes are known to have higher incidences of breast cancer. Other epidemiological risk factors were also not considered. Although three independent studies seem to represent confirmatory findings, closer consideration uncovers a strong possibility of investigator bias, because the BCDSP requested close colleagues from Oxford and

Helsinki to confirm their findings. These studies have not been confirmed, and actually have been refuted (133).

Nevertheless, popular lay magazines have dramatized reserpine's supposed association with breast cancer because of the popularity of this subject matter. As a result, clinicians will be queried concerning the continued use of reserpine by women excessively fearful of developing cancer.

Until more data become available, the following is our approach to dealing with reserpine-treated women. The choice of continuing therapy is left to the patient after she is adequately informed of the available data. If asked to decide for patients, we conservatively recommend discontinuance of therapy. Furthermore, reserpine is not initiated in women patients, and all women desiring to continue reserpine treatment are taught breast self-examination for cancer.

Although the three studies initiated by the BCDSP are only preliminary and have been refuted, it seems prudent to discontinue the use of reserpine. Since reserpine is a mild antihypertensive with multiple side effects, and since other agents are available, it is difficult to justify the use of reserpine in women in light of its possible carcinogenicity.

25. A 45-year-old hypertensive black male taking methyldopa presents with a chief complaint of fever of unknown origin of five weeks duration characterized by recurring chills, nausea, vomiting and diarrhea. Three weeks prior to admission he was hospitalized with a temperature of 105° F, but workup then was unremarkable. He became afebrile on the eighth hospital day and was discharged. However, three days later the same symptoms recurred. Has methyldopa been implicated in drug-induced fevers?

One of the major adverse reactions to methyldopa is a drug-induced fever that may occur in 1 to 3% of patients. It is usually associated with myalgia, malaise, nausea, vomiting, or diarrhea (149,158). Less commonly, it may also be associated with other allergic manifestations such as skin rash, eosinophilia, or hepatic symptoms. The onset of fever generally occurs between the ninth to the nineteenth day. However, after a challenge dose, the fever occurs within six to twelve hours (73). Frequently, patients are hospitalized and the fever seems to abate when treated with penicillin. This phenomenon is explainable because outpatient medications are often discontinued when patients are hospitalized.

26. A 55-year-old hypertensive presents in her physician's office with fever, chills, malaise, nausea, slight scleral icterus, and a mildly pruritic rash. The diagnosis is that of influenza. Routine laboratory

evaluations show that all findings are within normal limits except for an SGOT value of 800 units. She was told to return home and rest, but to revisit her physician if her symptoms did not subside. She was also instructed to continue with her antihypertensive medications consisting of hydrochlorothiazide 50 mg twice daily and methyldopa 500 mg twice daily. Is it possible that she suffers from drug-induced disease?

Methyldopa administration has been associated with numerous cases of hepatic injury, and over 100 cases have been reported since 1960. The majority of these cases involve a slight hepatitis with only transient abnormalities in liver function tests. These cases are commonly without clinical symptoms, but at least seven cases of fatal hepatic necrosis (29,134,207), one case of granulomatous hepatitis (147) and several cases of chronic active hepatitis (188,207) have been reported. A review of over 2000 patients reported an overall incidence of methyldopa-induced hepatic dysfunction of approximately 2.8% (96). Surprisingly, 75% of serious methyldopa hepatic reactions occurred in women, but more women may take methyldopa than men.

Methyldopa-induced hepatic injury may occur from two days (147) to as long as 26 months after treatment is initiated, but most cases occur within 4 to 16 weeks after initiation of therapy. The hepatitis is considered to be an allergic type reaction as it is not dose-related. Some patients have developed this toxicity while receiving very small doses (e.g. 250 mg/day), while others may take more than three grams daily for years and never experience this adverse reaction. Histological examination of liver tissue generally reveals varying degrees of non-specific damage, although fat droplets and eosinophils may be seen.

Clinically, methyldopa hepatotoxicity is indistinguishable from viral hepatitis. This patient presented with the typical signs and symptoms of chills, fever, fatigue, malaise, nausea, and a pruritic rash. Other signs and symptoms include vomiting, diarrhea, right upper quadrant pain, jaundice, and hepatosplenomegaly. Positive ANA, direct Coombs', and LE preparations sometimes can be demonstrated. Virtually all patients survive this reaction if they are not rechallenged, and if they are reasonably healthy. Recovery is usually complete 2 to 8 weeks after discontinuation of the medication.

Baseline transaminases should be obtained prior to initiation of methyldopa therapy and again at 4 to 8 weeks so that this reaction can be recognized early. Also it should be noted that the Babson method of SGOT determinations can be falsely elevated by methyldopa interference with the test (164).

27. What is the significance of a Coombs' test, and what is its relationship to methyldopa?

A positive direct Coombs' test indicates the presence of an antibody attached to a red cell membrane and is a characteristic feature of autoimmune hemolytic anemia. It does not indicate the kind or the source of the antibody, and hemolysis may or may not be present. Various drugs such as penicillin, quinine, or quinidine, and diseases such as rheumatoid arthritis, leukemia, or ulcerative colitis occasionally result in a non-specific positive direct Coomb's test (222).

Three different mechanisms of immunohemolytic anemia secondary to drug administration have been found. Penicillin in the range of 20 million units per day can produce the haptene type of hemolytic anemia with a positive direct Coombs' reaction. The penicillin becomes firmly bound to the red corpuscle and acts as a haptene to stimulate antibody formation. The antibody then reacts only with the penicillin-coated red corpuscles resulting in a positive direct Coombs' with hemolytic anemia. Quinidine and quinine can produce the "innocent bystander type" of drug-induced hemolytic anemia without at first attaching to the red cell membrane surface. These drugs can stimulate antibody formulation and the drug-antibody complex then attaches to the red cells and damages them. A third mechanism for the development of a positive Coombs' test is the methyldopa type of immunohemolytic anemia. In this type of reaction, the antibodies do not react with the drug itself or the drug-coated corpuscles but rather with antigens of the patient's own red cells. A possible hypothesis for this mechanism is that the drug or one of its metabolites becomes incorporated into the red corpuscles, perhaps at the formative normoblast or reticulocyte stage, thereby causing a subtle alteration of the red cell antigens (32,222). Approximately 20% of patients who take methyldopa may develop a positive reaction to the direct Coombs' test. Carstairs reports that of 65 patients taking 1 gram or less per day of methyldopa, 11% had a positive test; of 86 patients taking 1-2 grams per day, 19% had a positive test; and of 51 patients taking more than 2 grams per day, 36% had a positive test. This dose-related incidence of a positive Coombs' test secondary to methyldopa is further substantiated by Louis and associates' (130) study of 110 patients. The majority of these patients developed the positive Coombs' test between the sixth and twelfth month of methyldopa therapy; only rarely were there exceptions to this time span.

Although the incidence of a positive Coombs' may be high with methyldopa therapy, the actual incidence of hemolytic anemia is really very low. None of Carstairs' 202 patients exhibited overt hemolytic anemia despite a 20% incidence of a direct positive Coombs'. Moreover, Louis' review of 110 patients also showed no evidence of hemolytic anemia although

15% presented with a positive direct Coombs' test. It is estimated that of those patients who do have a positive Coombs' test secondary to methyldopa, only 0.1-0.2% of these patients will develop an autoimmune hemolytic anemia (45,235).

Two preliminary observations by Chen and Ooi (35) and Burn-Cox (28) indicate that Chinese may be exempt from the positive Coombs' test caused by methyldopa.

28. How do the biopharmaceutic and pharmacokinetic characteristics of propranolol affect the dosing of this drug in hypertension?

Individuals require different doses of propranolol to achieve optimal antihypertensive effects. While these differences in doses between individuals are due in part to the nature of hypertension, biopharmaceutic and pharmacokinetic factors are also partially responsible.

Propranolol is well absorbed orally; however, up to 20-fold differences in plasma concentrations may result when a standardized single oral dose is given to different subjects (56,192). This variation is primarily due to individual differences in hepatic extraction of the drug. Also, "first pass" elimination can remove as much as 50 to 70% of an oral dose (57). Additionally, a two-fold difference in the plasma protein binding of propranolol further contributes to inter-individual dosage variations.

Serum levels of 50 to 100 ng/ml of freely available propranolol are probably required to effectively block beta receptors. Such levels usually can be achieved with oral doses ranging from 80 to 320 mg daily (194), although some hypertensives may require higher levels and larger doses (57). Serum propranolol levels, however, fluctuate widely not only between different individuals, but intra-individually as well (215).

The plasma half-life of propranolol varies between 3.5 to 6.0 hours; however, chronic oral administration increases the serum half-life because of saturation of hepatic sites and clearance mechanisms. The duration of antihypertensive action of propranolol may exceed the plasma half-life, because effective blood pressure control can be achieved with twice daily dosing (76,172).

Due to these significant pharmacokinetic differences, clinicians must titrate propranolol therapy to each individual's needs. Doses as small as 40 mg/day may prove toxic (172), while doses as high as 2000 mg have been needed to produce an antihypertensive effect.

29. How effective is propranolol in hypertension, and how does it lower blood pressure?

Numerous studies indicate that propranolol has a definite place in the treatment of hypertension when used alone or in combination with other antihypertensives (220). When administered to essential hypertensives, it produces a substantial fall in blood pressure in about 30 to 90% of patients (171,221,237). Factors which enhance its effectiveness include proper patient selection, use of adequate doses, concomitant use of diuretics, addition of vasodilators if needed, and moderate dietary sodium restrictions. Propranolol is well accepted in the treatment of labile hypertension, systolic hypertension associated with hyperkinetic circulatory states, high renin hypertension, hypertension with sympathetic excesses, renovascular hypertension, and essential hypertension of varying degrees of severity.

Although propranolol is known to be effective, the mechanisms underlying its antihypertensive activity are not at all established. Most speculations on its mechanism of antihypertensive action revolve around the effects of beta-blockade on the four primary physiological determinants of blood pressure (i.e. the central nervous sytem, kidney, heart, and peripheral vasculature). Propranolol probably lowers blood pressure by affecting all of these anatomical structures, albeit to different degrees in different patients due to differences in the underlying pathology of each structure.

Some postulate that the blood pressure lowering effect of propranolol is due to a reduction in cardiac output which parallels the observed decreases in heart rate (68,120,132). Other postulate that propranolol's antihypertensive effect is at least partially due to interference with the central nervous system (56,92,98,145). Still others, notably John Laragh's group at Columbia-Presbyterian, fervently claim that it lowers blood pressure by decreasing plasma renin activity (27,93,119).

Whatever the ultimate mechanism, propranolol produces good control of blood pressures. Generally, it does not produce postural or exercise hypotension; does not predictably interfere with sexual function; does not sedate; does not cause gastrointestinal distress; does not affect mental acuity; does not cause nasal stuffiness; and is much more acceptable from a patient's point of view than more conventional therapy.

30. A 49-year-old hypertensive, insulin-dependent diabetic is being treated by a neurologist for severe migraine headaches. His hypertension is being treated with hydrochlorothiazide 100 mg daily and with methyldopa 1500 mg daily. These medications maintain his blood pressure in the range of 140-150/90-95 mm Hg and have not permitted further cardiac deterioration beyond left ventricular hypertrophy. His past medical history includes chronic obstructive pulmonary disease and a prior history of childhood asthma. Up to five Cafergot sublingual tablets per

attack have not controlled his migraine headaches, and propranolol 20 mg bid is added. It is hoped that the propranolol will not only alleviate the headaches, but will also permit reduction or discontinuation of the methyldopa. What special problems will propranolol present to this patient?

Propranolol must be used with caution in this patient, as potential side effects may be particuarly devastating in this setting. First of all, this medication can mask the warning symptoms of hypoglycemia. Although most reports involve insulin-dependent diabetics, like this patient, those diabetics treated by oral diabetic medications and dietary restrictions may also be vulnerable. Propranolol also has a direct dual effect on blood sugar. It may cause hyperosmolar nonketotic diabetic coma, or it may cause severe hypoglycemia. Therefore, propranolol is not recommended for use in diabetic patients unless unique indications exist and close patient monitoring is possible. Also see Diabetes chapter.

Secondly, propranolol should be used with caution in patients with asthma or chronic obstructive pulmonary disease. This medication can cause spasms in the pulmonary tree and a bronchoconstriction which may be more resistant to treatment because of prolonged beta-2 receptor blockade.

Propranolol also can aggravate or precipitate congestive heart failure. Although patients with preexisting cardiac decompensation may be especially prone to this reaction, restoration of cardiac function with digitalis and diuretics may permit the use of propranolol. This patient exhibits left ventricular hypertrophy, but is not in failure. Therefore, his risk of developing this adverse reaction is not unduly increased. Initial doses, however, should be small (e.g. 10 mg tid) and increased slowly (e.g. 10 to 20 mg/daily at one to two week intervals).

Although other sympatholytic antihypertensive agents may also depress myocardial contractility, their liabilities are substantially less than that of propranolol. In this patient the combination of propranolol and methyldopa could be a problem. Therefore, he should be taught to record his own radial pulse and report reductions into the 40 to 50 beats-per-minute range.

Another problem which may arise in this particular patient is the development of peripheral vasoconstriction not unlike that of Raynaud's phenomenon (137). Based upon currently available data, it is not clear whether the combination of ergotamine (in Cafergot) and propranolol would synergistically produce this problem (13,46).

Due to these potential problems, the use of propranolol in this patient would probably be unwise. While data are limited, clonidine has been used to treat migraine headaches (156,190,231). Although clonidine may be a reasonable alternative, it can also potentiate insulin-induced hypoglycemia in man (90), and might cause vasoconstriction as well (234).

31. What is the rationale for using propranolol and hydralazine in combination for the treatment of essential hypertension?

Since the vast majority of hypertensive patients manifest an abnormal elevation of systemic vascular resistance, a logical approach to antihypertensive therapy would be to use drugs which lower blood pressure by direct dilation of the arterial bed. Vasodilator drugs such as hydralazine (Apresoline), and minoxidil (an investigational agent) directly relax arteriolar smooth muscle and have far greater effects on resistance than capacitance vessels. These agents not only reduce the increased peripheral vascular resistance characteristics of hypertension, but do so without producing side effects of postural hypotension, weakness, lethargy, and sexual dysfunction, which are so commonly observed with sympatholytic agents. The antihypertensive effect achieved by these agents, however, is limited by reflex increases in sympathetic discharge that increase heart rate and cardiac output inappropriately. Thus, hydralazine is said to be contraindicated in patients with a myocardial infarction or angina pectoris. In order to offset the cardiac stimulating properties of hydralazine, reserpine or guanethidine are oftentimes administered concomitantly, because in high doses, these agents cause a bradycardia and a decrease in cardiac output. However, the sympatholytic agents cause a generalized sympathoplegia that interferes with reflex mechanisms necessary to maintain blood pressure during postural changes and exercise (236).

Since the beta-adrenergic blocker, propranolol, inhibits cardiac adrenergic stimulation, decreases cardiac output, and is an effective antihypertensive agent, it would seem logical to combine beta blockade with a vasodilating drug. In a study of 23 patients on a stabilized diuretic regimen with moderate to severe, difficult to control, essential hypertension, the combination of propranolol and hydralazine was evaluated. Propranolol was initiated first in doses of 20 mg every six hours and this dose was increased to 40 mg every six hours after two days in most patients. Beta-blockade was confirmed by an isoproterenol infusion test and then hydralazine was added to therapy in an initial dose of 25 mg every six hours which was increased to a maximum of 400 mg per day. Propranolol lowered the mean supine blood pressure from 188/118 to 162/102 mm of Hg and lowered the heart rate from 94 to 72 beats per minute. Addition of hydralazine further reduced the mean supine blood pressure to 134/88 mm Hg. Only two patients failed to achieve diastolic pressures lower than 100 mm Hg on this combination therapy, yet the diastolic pressures were lowered in them by 31 and 41 mm Hg. The effective antihypertensive action was not associated with postural hypotension, tachycardia, other hemodynamic disturbances, impairment of renal function or adverse symptoms in any patient (236).

Similar dramatic responses in blood pressures were obtained when propranolol was used in combination with the new piperidino-pyrimidine vasodilator, minoxidil (71). Moreover, a comparative study of minoxidil and hydralazine in combination with beta-blockers and diuretics demonstrated greater therapeutic efficacy with minoxidil (75).

32. Many drugs have been reported to induce a syndrome resembling systemic lupus erythematosus (e.g. procainamide, isoniazid, phenytoin), but hydralazine appears to be associated with a high incidence of this syndrome. What is the incidence of hydralazine-induced lupus? Describe this syndrome.

Hydralazine (Apresoline) was first noted in 1953 to induce a syndrome clinically and serologically similar to systemic lupus erythematosus (SLE). Since then, more than 200 cases have been reported. Hydralazine-induced lupus develops in 8 to 13% of patients receiving relatively large doses. This observation led to the initial recommendation that hydralazine dosages be maintained below 400 mg/day to minimize this toxicity. However, Alarcon-Segovia and associates (3) reported nineteen patients who developed lupus even though their doses were less than 200 mg per day. SLE has occurred following dosages as small as 75 mg daily for less than one month. Nevertheless, the consensus remains that the likelihood of developing lupus, as a result of hydralazine, increases with large doses and with long duration of therapy. A possible contributing factor to hydralazine-induced lupus is the rate at which the drug is metabolized. Hahn and co-workers (83) report that the patients in their series who developed hydralazine lupus were slow acetylators of the drug.

The clinical manifestations of hydralazine-induced lupus resemble those of SLE and include polyarthritis, fever, dermatitis, lymphadenopathy, hepatosplenomegaly, serosites, antinuclear antibodies, leukopenia, and LE cells (83). However, unlike spontaneously occurring SLE, nephritis, central nervous system involvement, and cardiac manifestations are uncommon in this syndrome induced by hydralazine (30).

Circulating antibodies to hydralazine have been reported, suggesting that hydralazine-induced lupus is, in part, a hypersensitivity response (83). As with all drug-induced cases of lupus, clinical manifestations are generally reversible upon cessation of hydralazine therapy. However, clinical manifestations may continue for 7 to 8 years after drug administration is stopped.

33. F.W.'s episodes of chest pain which were possibly related to exertion (see Case A) are thought to be due to hydralazine. Although reflex tachycardia secondary to hydralazine would have been averted if F.W. complied to his therapeutic regimen, it has been decided to replace hydralazine with the new vasodilator, prazosin. Since prazosin is a vasodilator, what is the basis for advertisements claiming lack of reflex tachycardia?

Prazosin is a quinazoline derivative that supposedly produces direct arteriolar vasodilation in addition to exerting sympatholytic activity. This latter action may be due to some type of alpha-adrenergic blockage unlike that of other alpha blockers (38). The drug reduces total peripheral resistance, increases cardiac index, produces mild to moderate increases in heart rate, does not reduce glomerular filteration rate nor renal plasma flow, and reportedly lowers plasma renin activity (87).

Although prazosin has both vasodilating and sympatholytic actions, most (97,113) recommend that it primarily be considered as a vasodilator. Its place in therapy, therefore, will be in those situations where hydralazine is now currently used. It is estimated that 1 mg of prazosin is equipotent to about 20 mg of hydralazine, although prazosin may be effective in patients refractory to hydralazine.

Since prazosin is both a vasodilator and a sympatholytic, it shares the liabilities of both. Pitts (167) reports weight gain and a 4% incidence of edema in a study of 924 patients; both phenomena are most likely due to sodium and fluid retention. Dizziness following exertion or upon standing most commonly occurs after the first dose or following a large increase in dose and probably is due to alpha-adrenergic blockade. This "first dose" effect can be alleviated by commencing with a lower dose and by giving the first dose prior to retiring in the evening. While postural hypotension is common with some hypotensive drugs, loss of consciousness is not (87). As many as 16% of patients may experience dizziness and faintness after the first dose of this drug. Sudden collapse with loss of consciousness occurs within 30 to 90 minutes of the initial dose in about 1% of patients (70). Reflex tachycardia reportedly is not as common or severe as that caused by hydralazine, although cardiac palpitations have been noted in several studies. A few cases of anginal attacks have been associated with the use of prazosin (109).

34. Based upon its mechanism of action, as well as its biopharmaceutic and pharmacokinetic prop-

erties, how should guanethidine be dosed in ambulant patients?

Guanethidine concentrates in the neurosecretory granules in post-ganglionic sympathetic nerve endings. At this site, it depletes norepinephrine from storage granules, as well as blocks norepinephrine release upon physiologic nerve stimulation (143). The net result of these actions is inhibition of sympathetic reflexes, with a resultant decrease in blood pressure due primarily to venous pooling.

Oral absorption of guanethidine ranges from 3 to 60% (142,174). Approximately 30% of the absorbed drug is excreted unchanged renally, and 60% appears in the urine as inactive metabolites. While individual responses vary greatly, serum plasma levels of 8 ng/ml usually correlate well with effective antihypertensive responses. Individual differences may be due to expanded plasma volumes or individual patient variations in absorption, metabolism, distribution, or excretion patterns (223). The estimated elimination half-life is 5 hours (193), while its effective duration of action is at least 24 hours. The drug remains in the body for several days. Guanethidine has a long onset of action; minimal effects may be seen within three days while maximal effects may take 3 to 6 weeks.

Shand (193) and McAllister (138) report a method of rapidly initiating guanethidine therapy by administering large divided doses (50 to 100 mg, up to tid) for 1 to 3 days, followed by daily maintenance doses of $^1/_5$ to $^1/_7$ of the total loading dose. While these investigators report effective antihypertensive responses in 14 hospitalized patients with minimal side effects, the value and safety of such administration techniques must be questioned in the treatment of ambulant patients. The more conservative use of 10 to 12.5 mg initial doses, adjusted to the patient's response in 10 to 12.5 mg increments every 1 to 2 weeks is more rational. When combined with effective diuretic therapy, 25 to 50 mg daily is the usual therapeutic dose, although up to 150 mg may be needed.

35. Mr. Smith is a hypertensive patient who consistently refills his prescriptions for hydrochlorothiazide (Hydrodiuril) and guanethidine (Ismelin). Today he presents with a prescription for amitriptyline (Elavil) 25 mg tid to treat his depression caused by an impending dissolution of marriage. Discuss this situation.

Norepinephrine is synthesized from tyrosine and is stored in intra-axonal granules which protect it from inactivation by monoamine oxidase (MAO). Following a stimulus, norepinephrine is released from nerve terminals into the synaptic cleft where it can then initiate a synaptic transmission. After release, norepinephrine is either inactivated by circulating catechol-o-methyl transferase (COMT), or is recaptured and transported back into the storage granules by an amine concentrating pump mechanism located in the neuronal membrane. This specialized re-uptake mechanism is not entirely specific, and the storage granules will accept other amines if they have a betahydroxyl or a dihydroxybenzene group (155). Thus, other amines such as tyramine, amphetamine, ephedrine, and guanethidine share this re-uptake pump.

Drugs like guanethidine block adrenergic neurons because they are concentrated within them by this membrane transport system. The necessity of this transport system for guanethidine's antihypertensive activity is demonstrated by the loss of guanethidine's effectiveness when its uptake is inhibited. This is the basis of the significant drug-drug interaction with Elavil, because tricyclic antidepressants block this amine uptake and thereby antagonize the antihypertensive effect of guanethidine (144).

Furthermore, the cause of Mr. Smith's depression may be drug-induced in that guanethidine can interfere with sexual performance in a large percentage of patients by causing impotence or failure of ejaculation. It has been claimed that 63% of men studied had this side effect (14). Vejlsgaard (214) reports this side effect in twelve out of forty patients (34%); Oates and associates (159) noted it in two out of five (40%) patients.

36. A concerned pharmacist calls Mr. Smith's physician to discuss the tricyclic antidepressant's interference with guanethidine's antihypertensive action. The physician wishes to know the clinical significance of this drug interaction.

Reports indicate that desipramine (Pertofrane) and protriptyline (Vivactil) can antagonize the antihypertensive effects of guanethidine within two days. This effect persists for four to five days after discontinuing these antidepressants. Meyer and associates (144) report a case involving a forty-seven year old male who was adequately treated with guanethidine 75 mg/day. Subsequent to the initiation of amitriptyline 25 mg three times daily, the guanethidine dose was progressively increased until 300 mg/day was needed to maintain adequate blood pressure control. Eventually, the amitriptyline was discontinued and the guanethidine dose was gradually decreased until the patient could be maintained on 87.5 mg/day. To further investigate the drug interaction, this same patient was given a five day course of amitriptyline 50 mg three times daily; again the effects of guanethidine did not return until eighteen days after the discontinuation of amitriptyline. A period of six months was required before the antagonism was completely overcome.

Therefore, this interaction is indeed clinically significant. Because this depression is apparently reactive in nature, it can be treated with benzodiazepines and/or with psychotherapy (see chapters on *General Care: Anxiety and Insomnia* and *Depression*).

37. A 65-year-old hypertensive diabetic has been effectively treated with hydrochlorothiazide (HCTZ) 50 mg bid and guanethidine 25 mg daily for 15 years. Due to an unexplained recent loss of diabetic control, the HCTZ was discontinued. Two weeks later, his blood pressure rose to 170/110 mm Hg and a twelve pound weight gain was noted. HCTZ therapy was reinstituted and the guanethidine dose was increased to 75 mg/daily. Within one week, his blood pressure dropped to 140/76 mm Hg. He experienced fainting spells upon arising too quickly and developed explosive diarrhea as well. How could these symptoms be alleviated?

Like all non-diuretic antihypertensive agents, guanethidine produces sodium and fluid retention which results in some loss of antihypertensive activity (198). Therefore, guanethidine should always be administered concurrently with a diuretic.

Due to its peripheral venous pooling action, guanethidine commonly produces orthostatic hypotension characterized by dizziness, lightheadedness, weakness and, occasionally, fainting. In order to minimize this problem, doses should be slowly titrated to the patient's level of tolerance. Individuals who are physically active, elderly, or who have autonomic insufficiency (e.g. some diabetics) are particularly vulnerable. Techniques for minimizing this problem include arising slowly from sitting or prone positions and flexing one's arms and legs prior to standing. Potentiating factors include ingestion of vasodilating chemicals such as alcohol, entering a warm room, vigorous exercise, prolonged standing, and taking hot showers. Patients should be cautioned about these factors when guanethidine therapy is initiated and when doses are increased.

The sympatholytic action of guanethidine often results in a relative excess in parasympathetic innervation of the gastrointestinal (GI) tract. As a result of this imbalance, GI motility is increased and loose stools or explosive diarrhea may occur. Possible methods of correction include dividing a single daily dose into two doses, or adding small doses of an anticholinergic agent.

In this case, the dose of guanethidine should not have been increased prior to assessing the effect of the reinstituted HCTZ. Vigorous lowering of blood pressure, especially in the elderly, may precipitate strokes or myocardial infarctions.

38. Describe the antihypertensive action of clonidine (Catapres). How does its efficacy compare with other sympatholytics? Does it possess unique properties?

Clonidine has been marketed in the United States for only a few years, but has been extensively used in Europe, the United Kingdom, and Australia. It has an imidazoline structure and is chemically related to the alpha adrenergic blockers, tolazoline and phentolamine. Its mechanism of action, however, differs from all other antihypertensive agents. It activates post-synaptic alpha-adrenergic receptors in the cardiovascular control center located in the medulla oblongata (162). Clonidine also suppresses renin release (82). Other possible central mechanisms are being researched (213). The net effect of clonidine is a reduced outflow of sympathetic activity from the central nervous system, resulting in diminished sympathetic stimulation of the heart, kidney, and peripheral vasculature. Consequently, this drug decreases both cardiac output and peripheral vascular resistance (114).

Clonidine is well absorbed orally. Its onset of action is 30 to 60 minutes, and peak serum levels (usually correlated with maximum effectiveness) occur within 2 to 4 hours. Clonidine does not significantly alter renal hemodynamics (161), and the drug can be used safely in patients with impaired renal function.

Clonidine is most effective when combined with a diuretic, since it produces sodium and fluid retention. Due to its unique mechanism of action, clonidine may prove to be valuable when other sympatholytic agents are ineffective or produce unacceptable side effects. Initial dosing should start at 0.1 mg bid and be increased at weekly intervals by 0.1 to 0.2 mg daily. Although the manufacturer's recommended maximum daily dose is 2.4 mg, doses of 0.4 to 0.6 mg per day usually suffice.

39. A 38-year-old school teacher has been taking clonidine 0.2 mg twice daily for two weeks, along with HCTZ 100 mg daily. Her severely elevated blood pressures (180/120 mm Hg) have returned to normal (140/90 mm Hg); however, she has been somnolent at work and continually has a dry mouth with accompanying parotid gland pain. She related her discomfort to her medications and discontinued them. Twenty-four hours later, she became restless, agitated, developed headaches, insomnia, and began sweating. Upon visiting the local emergency room, she was again hypertensive (170/115). Can you explain her symptoms? How should her problems be treated in the emergency room?

Most of the side effects of clonidine (sedation, dry mouth, sodium and fluid retention, orthostasis, and sexual difficulties) resemble those of methyldopa. Of these, sedation, dry mouth, and fluid retention are quite common. Additionally, a 10% incidence of parotid gland pain has been cited (82).

The most serious problem associated with clonidine use is an adrenergic syndrome that can result from abrupt clonidine withdrawal. Produced by excessive catecholamine release, this syndrome is characterized by agitation, headache, abdominal pain, insomnia, sweating and sometimes nausea and vomiting. Rapid blood pressure elevations may accompany these symptoms, and hypertensive crises have been reported (213). The incidence of this reaction is not known, and its severity may be reduced if the patient continues to take other antihypertensive drugs. It has occurred upon cessation of doses of 0.2 mg daily (114). Slow withdrawal of clonidine therapy over 3 to 7 days, usually circumvents this problem. Symptoms and moderate blood pressure elevations usually subside upon reinstating clonidine therapy. Crisis situations require vigorous treatment with potent antihypertensives. Phentolamine, with the possible addition of propranolol is advocated (114), although nitroprusside has also been used effectively (213). Sole use of propranolol is not recommended, as it only corrects the symptoms and may in fact potentiate the vasoconstrictive action of circulating catecholamines (161).

40. A 38-year-old accountant has recently experienced dissolution of his marriage, moved to a new town, and started a new job. His blood pressure repeatedly has been in the 150-160/100-110 mm Hg range and has not responded to hydrochlorothiazide 100 mg daily. Additional sympatholytic therapy is being considered. Considering the nature of his work and his social situation, which side effects of the sympatholytics should be avoided? Which agent(s) should be recommended?

Three major types of side effects should be particularly avoided in this case. These are mental depression, other disturbing central nervous system effects, and sexual difficulties. While often overlooked as serious problems, these side effects commonly occur with some of the sympatholytic agents and can interfere with one's sense of well being. **Mental depression:** Because the use of reserpine is commonly associated with depression, it should be avoided in this patient (see Question 22). Other sympatholytics also are associated with depression. Depression occurs in about 4 to 13% of patients treated with methyldopa, in up to 10% of those treated with clonidine, up to 21% of those taking guanethidine, and rarely with propranolol (197). Although these percentages are based upon inconsistent diagnostic criteria, depression should be considered a potential hazard of any sympatholytic antihypertensive.

Disturbing CNS Effects: Reserpine, methyldopa, and clonidine commonly produce somnolence. Reported incidence rates for the latter two drugs range from 40 to 80%. This effect often subsides within a few weeks, although it may be prolonged for months. It can reappear when doses are increased, or when therapy is reinstated. Repeated observations of this effect in a given patient may reflect medication noncompliance and reinstitution of therapy a few days prior to the clinic visit. Tiredness, nightmares, insomnia and visual hallucinations are rarely reported with the use of methyldopa, clonidine, and propranolol (197). Forgetfullness has been reported in 9 patients taking methyldopa (61). Since these side effects can impair a person's ability to normally perform daily activities, they should be assessed by close objective clinician observation.

Sexual Dysfunction: An inability to achieve or maintain an erection is commonly associated with methyldopa treatment; reported estimates range from 2-33% (100,152). Guanethidine can prevent ejaculation or cause retrograde ejaculation; one investigator estimates a 60% incidence rate (121). Clonidine reportedly produces fewer sexual problems than either methyldopa or guanethidine, although this may merely reflect less intense clinician observation. Reserpine rarely produces sexual difficulties, and propranolol is thought to be relatively free of such effects.

Detection and management of drug-induced sexual disorders is difficult due to client and clinician discomfort in discussing this subject and the multifaceted determinants of sexual functioning. At least 90% of perceived sexual dysfunctions in men are psychologically based. For this reason alone, it may be important to accurately assess the etiological role of a drug when sexual problems occur. Temporal relationships between the initiation of a drug's usage and the onset of the perceived problem should be evaluated. If a drug-compliant patient awakes with an erection, the drug is usually not the causative factor. Other causes of sexual dysfunctions should be assessed, e.g. alcohol intoxication, depression, diabetes or misconceptions about sexual performances. Practically speaking, however, once a male patient associates his self-perceived sexual inability with the use of a drug, the clinician has only one course of action — to provide positive psychological support, which may include instruction in human sexuality, and to change to another drug, preferably propranolol and possibly clonidine.

Considering Mr. N's situation and our desire to avoid inducing any of the problems cited above, propranolol appears to be the drug of choice, barring any contraindications to its use.

Hypertensive Emergency

R. Jon Auricchio

CASE B: A.L. is a 46-year-old white male who presents to the emergency room in acute respiratory distress. Two days prior to admission (PTA), he developed shortness of breath which worsened on exertion. Over the two day period, he also developed a severe headache unrelieved by aspirin; substernal chest pain; anorexia; and nausea.

Past medical history includes a five year history of angina which two months PTA resulted in hospitalization for an acute inferior myocardial infarction. He denies any history of diabetes, hypertension or renal disease.

Physical examination reveals a well-nourished, slightly obese (80 kg) male in acute respiratory distress who looks older than his stated age. HEENT is within normal limits. The patient is oriented X 3. Neck examination reveals normal appearing carotids without venous distention. There are decreased breath sounds bilaterally with rales present at both bases. The abdomen is soft and non-tender without hepatosplenomegaly. Cardiac examination reveals an S_3 gallop without murmurs and the PMI is normal. There are no heaves or thrills. Vital signs: Pulse 100/min, Respiratory rate 34/min, BP 190/135 mm Hg.

Laboratory values include the following: Na 141 mEq/L; K 5.2 mEq/L; Cl 98 mEq/L; BUN 75 mg%; Cr 5 mg%; WBC 11 × 10^3 with a normal differential; RBC and RBC indices are within normal limits.

Urinalysis: hematuria, RBC casts, 3+ protein, specific gravity 1.021.

Chest X-ray reveals cardiomegaly and a "ground glass" appearance consistent with pulmonary edema.

Impression: Pulmonary edema secondary to acute left ventricular failure, R/O MI, hypertensive emergency, and acute glomerulonephritis.

41. What do the terms hypertensive crisis or hypertensive emergency refer to and in what clinical situations is it encountered?

The terms hypertensive crisis (emergency) refer to clinical situations in which a marked elevation of arterial pressure, if not treated promptly, carries a high rate of morbidity and mortality. These episodes are usually characterized by an acute and marked elevation of arterial pressure, arteriolar spasm, necrotizing arteriolitis, and secondary organ damage (249,262). Hypertensive emergencies generally occur in patients

with pheochromocytoma, renal vascular disease, or accelerated essential hypertension (262). Acute life-threatening elevations of blood pressure can also occur in previously normotensive individuals during the course of acute glomerulonephritis, head injury, severe burns, eclampsia, or in patients receiving monoamine oxidase inhibitors who ingest foods rich in tyramine.

Rapid, severe blood pressure elevation is not always the hallmark of a hypertensive emergency. Indeed, even moderate elevations of arterial pressure in the context of a variety of disease states demand prompt treatment. Specific examples include acute left ventricular failure, intracranial hemorrhage, dissecting aortic aneurysm, and post-operative bleeding at suture sites.

42. How frequently are hypertensive emergencies encountered?

Hypertensive crisis is most commonly encountered as a complication during the accelerated phase of inadequately controlled essential hypertension (1). Although the incidence of hypertensive crisis is unknown, it has been estimated that of the population of patients with essential hypertension, approximately 1 to 7% will develop hypertensive crisis (277, 188). Several authors have noted a greater frequency in the 40- to 60-year age range and a slight predominance of males over females (256,261,278,282).

43. What symptoms does this patient display which are consistent with hypertensive crisis?

Symptoms associated with hypertensive crisis are highly variable and result from damage to specific organ systems. The primary sites of damage are the central nervous system, heart, kidneys, and eyes. Therefore, symptoms of hypertensive crisis merely reflect the degree of injury of these organ systems.

Central nervous system (CNS) damage may present solely as a severe headache or can be accompanied by dizziness, nausea, vomiting, and anorexia. Mental confusion with apprehension is indicative of more severe disease, as is nystagmus, localized weakness, or a positive Babinski sign. CNS damage may be rapidly progressive and result in coma or death. If a cerebrovascular accident has occurred, slurred speech or motor paralysis may be present.

Cardiac complications of hypertensive crisis may be manifested by congestive heart failure or angina pectoris. The reader is referred to those chapters for descriptions of the common signs and symptoms associated with both diseases. Myocardial infarctions may also be precipitated and most frequently manifest themselves with symptoms of shortness of breath, diaphoresis, loss of consciousness, and a severe crushing substernal chest pain that often radiates to the axillary region.

Ocular symptomatology of hypertensive crisis is usually related to changes in visual acuity. Complaints of blurring of vision or loss of eyesight are frequently associated with the fundoscopic findings of hemorrhages, exudates, and sometimes papilledema.

Renal complications are generally noted by laboratory examination and may include findings such as hematuria, proteinuria, pyelonephritis, as well as an elevated serum BUN and creatinine.

This patient's symptoms are consistent with damage to the CNS, heart, and kidneys. The occipital headaches, accompanied by nausea and anorexia, suggest a mild degree of CNS involvement. Cardiovascular damage perhaps can be implied by the increased frequency of anginal episodes and the sudden onset of shortness of breath and dyspnea on exertion. These symptoms may well represent acute left ventricular failure. Chest X-ray evidence of pulmonary edema in conjunction with the bibasilar rales also are consistent with a failing heart. The elevated serum creatinine and BUN and the grossly abnormal urinalysis are suggestive of renal damage. All these signs and symptoms are compatible with an acute elevation of arterial pressure.

44. What are the goals of treatment of this disease?

Hypertensive emergencies require immediate hospitalization and administration of medications to reduce arterial pressure. Effective therapy greatly improves the prognosis, reverses symptoms, and arrests the progression of end-organ damage (254,269,298). Treatment reverses the vascular changes in the eyes and slows or arrests the progressive deterioration in renal function (266). The damaged vessels begin to heal and mortality decreases (254,269,279,298). Whether treatment can completely reverse end-organ damage is related to two factors, how soon treatment is begun and the extent of the damage at the initiation of therapy (266,280,296). Without treatment, the two year mortality approaches 90% (259,260,261,282).

The drug of choice for hypertensive emergencies depends upon the clinical situation. If encephalopathy, acute left ventricular failure, dissecting aortic aneurysm, or other serious conditions are present, the blood pressure should be promptly lowered with parenteral antihypertensive medications such as nitroprusside, trimethaphan, or diazoxide. If a slower blood pressure reduction over several hours or days is acceptable, parenteral reserpine, hydralazine, or methyldopa may be used.

The rate of blood pressure lowering must be individualized. Too rapid a decrease can reduce blood flow to the brain and kidneys and could precipitate a stroke. This is especially true in the elderly and those suffering from cardiovascular disease. In addition, patients who have chronically elevated blood pressures are less likely to tolerate abrupt reductions in their blood pressures, and the amount of reduction appropriate for these patients is somewhat less. Thus, absolute guidelines cannot be stated. However, for most patients a reduction of 5 to 10 mm Hg every 5 to 10 minutes is appropriate, and a diastolic pressure of 100 mm Hg is often an appropriate therapeutic endpoint.

45. What antihypertensive medication would be the most appropriate for the patient described in Case B and why?

The acute elevation of blood pressure in conjunction with the left ventricular failure and the pulmonary edema in this patient represent a hypertensive emergency. The arterial pressure should be promptly lowered with parenteral medications which have an onset of action within minutes of starting treatment. Antihypertensive medications which cause cardiostimulation should be avoided, because this patient has severe coronary disease, and has recently suffered an acute myocardial infarction.

Although nitroprusside (Nipride), trimethaphan (Arfonad), and diazoxide (Hyperstat) all decrease total peripheral resistance, diazoxide produces the greatest degree of cardiostimulation. Diazoxide has marked positive inotropic and chronotropic myocardial effects, may increase the heart rate by 30%, and significantly increases cardiac output. Nitroprusside and trimethaphan decrease cardiac output, stroke volume, left-end diastolic pressure, venous return, and only slightly increase the heart rate (240). Since diazoxide markedly increases cardiac output and heart rate (286), it has the potential to increase myocardial oxygen demand and precipitate an ischemic attack. In a study of 14 hypertensive patients who received diazoxide and who had no prior history of angina or myocardial infarction, 50% developed ST-T wave changes on EKG; 43% developed substernal discomfort with pain or tightness; 35% developed substernal discomfort with ST-T wave changes; and one patient experienced a myocardial infarction (265). Other investigators have also reported an association of myocardial infarctions with diazoxide (257,265).

In light of the strong possibility that diazoxide may precipitate an anginal or ischemic attack in this patient, either trimethaphan or nitroprusside would be an appropriate choice. Of these two agents, nitroprusside is usually preferred because trimethaphan can cause constipation, paralytic ileus, and urinary retention (250,276,298).

46. How should nitroprusside be administered, and what dosage should be used to initiate treatment for this patient?

Nitroprusside is a rapidly-acting, potent antihypertensive agent effective within seconds after intravenous administration (281). Upon discontinuation of nitroprusside therapy, all antihypertensive activity abruptly ceases, and the drug is cleared from the body within the ensuing two minutes. As a result, nitroprusside must be administered by constant intravenous infusion and should be used with a constant rate infusion pump.

Since nitroprusside dosage varies with patients and clinical situations, the dosage must be titrated to the desired decrease in blood pressure. Initial infusion rates of 0.5 mcg/kg/min of nitroprusside are commonly used; the rate of infusion is then adjusted to produce the desired hypotensive effects. Rates of 0.3 to 8.0 mcg/kg/min usually will be effective (275), but higher dosages are occasionally needed, and as much as 800 mcg/kg/min has been safely used (258).

The filling of coronary vessels is dependent upon both systolic and diastolic pressures. Thus, excessive lowering of arterial pressure in patients with compromised coronary circulations may exacerbate myocardial ischemia. Since this patient already has a history of impaired coronary circulation, it would be prudent to initiate nitroprusside therapy with a low dose such as 0.5 mcg/kg/min. The rate can be increased by 0.5 mcg/kg/min increments if necessary, and the patient should be monitored for signs and symptoms of chest pain.

47. How should nitroprusside be prepared?

Nitroprusside is available in amber vials containing 50 mg of sodium nitroprusside dihydrate. The contents of the vial should be mixed with 2 to 3 ml of 5% dextrose in water (D5W) and then diluted in 500 ml of sterile D5W to produce a final concentration of 100 mcg/ml.

Light inactivates nitroprusside and produces a color change from red to blue. Since degradation of nitroprusside by light is a major problem, a fresh solution should be prepared every four hours, and an opaque material such as tin foil should be wrapped around the infusion bottle.

48. An infusion of nitroprusside was started for this patient at an initial rate of 0.5 mcg/kg/min and was increased to 2 mcg/kg/min over 10 minutes. At this latter dose, the blood pressure decreased to 130/100 mm Hg. The patient's respiratory rate is decreasing, and his shortness of breath seems to be lessening; however, the patient is diaphoretic and his facial muscles are twitching. Are these side effects of nitroprusside, and is it essential to discontinue therapy? What are the major side effects of nitroprusside?

Nitroprusside is a remarkably safe drug when used

properly. The incidence of toxic reactions to this drug is quite low, and side effects generally are acute in onset and result from too rapid intravenous administration (242,251,281,292). Some acute problems with nitroprusside include nausea, vomiting, diaphoresis, nasal stuffiness, muscular twitching, dizziness, weakness, and severe hypotensive overshoot. Fortunately, all of these symptoms can be quickly reversed by decreasing the rate of nitroprusside infusion. It is certainly conceivable that the symptoms being experienced by this patient are caused by the nitroprusside, especially in light of the rapid four-fold increase in his nitroprusside infusion rate over a ten minute span. Thus, this patient's nitroprusside intravenous rate should be decreased temporarily. Therapy need not be discontinued.

With chronic or prolonged nitroprusside administration, other problems may be encountered and are presumably due to a build up of thiocyanate ion, a major metabolite. Symptoms of thiocyanate toxicity vary but usually consist of fatigue, weakness, tinnitus, psychosis, and rarely hypothyroidism. Almost exclusively, chronic toxicities have occurred in patients with severely impaired renal function, and caution is advised when used in this setting.

Routine monitoring of serum thiocyanate levels should be considered when the drug is used for more than 2 to 3 days or when it is used in patients with renal failure or hypothyroidism. The serum level at which toxicity occurs is not well defined. Some claim that toxicity occurs when thiocyanate levels are between 3 to 15 mg% (242); others recommend discontinuing the nitroprusside if thiocyanate levels reach 10 mg% (251). The manufacturer states that nitroprusside administration may be continued for prolonged periods as long as thiocyanate levels are kept below 10 mg% (272).

Practically, routine monitoring of serum thiocyanate levels is probably unnecessary except when the drug is to be used for prolonged periods (more than 2 to 3 days) in patients with severe renal failure. Several authors have reported no toxicity or buildup of thiocyanate ion in patients with normal renal function receiving the drug for up to 32 days (251,258,274).

CASE C: M.G. is a 59-year-old white female who is hospitalized for a complete medical work-up. Her chief complaint is a one week history of lethargy accompanied by four episodes of nausea and vomiting followed by the acute onset of low back and abdominal pain. Her past medical history includes adult onset diabetes mellitus (AODM) of 10 years duration, a 5 year history of essential hypertension, and an aorto-femoral bypass graft 3 years ago. Significant findings on physical examination include a pulse of 95 beats/minute; a blood pressure of 210/140 mm Hg;

hemmorrhages and papilledema; and 2+ pulses in the inguinal region with a bruit on the left. The SMA-12 panel was non-remarkable except for a plasma glucose of 170 mg%. It has been concluded that immediate lowering of her blood pressure with diazoxide would be appropriate.

49. Would the use of diazoxide create any special risks which must be monitored in this patient?

Diazoxide predictably induces hyperglycemia by several postulated mechanisms (252,283). Decreased peripheral glucose utilization, direct stimulation of catecholamine release, and inhibition of insulin release (287), have all been proposed to explain the hyperglycemia.

Although hyperglycemia is a frequent side effect, it is usually transient and consists only of mild elevations in serum glucose. In one study of 700 patients treated with diazoxide, a mild transitory elevation of serum glucose occurred in 40% of non-diabetics and in 75% of diabetic subjects 1 to 4 hours after treatment was initiated. In the diabetic group, glucose elevation was more prolonged and lasted from 24 to 48 hours (246). In another study of 41 patients who received diazoxide, the mean glucose values increased only about 6 mg% during the first 48 hours. Occasionally, however, serious hyperglycemic hyperosmolar coma with serum glucose levels as high as 942 mg% has been reported (243,255,285,293). Most of the severe hyperglycemic cases occurred in patients with renal impairment, adult-onset diabetes, liver disease, and in patients recovering from general anesthesia.

Patients at special risks for diazoxide-induced hyperglycemia should be monitored by serum glucose measurements. If substantial hyperglycemia develops, insulin or perhaps oral hypoglycemic agents may be appropriate. Also see the *Diabetes* chapter.

50. Show should diazoxide be administered and how should it be dosed?

Diazoxide must be administered by rapid intravenous injection as both the intensity and duration of the antihypertensive activity increases with the rate of the injection (283). In fact, slow intravenous injection may not result in an appreciable change in arterial pressure (270), because most of the drug would be heavily bound to protein sites and hence, be unable to reach receptor sites on arteriolar smooth muscle. At 37°C and normal albumin concentrations, 91% of diazoxide is bound in human plasma (284).

Different rates of administration have been advocated, but in general the intravenous injection should take no longer than ten seconds. The drug should be given undiluted via a peripheral vein using extreme caution to avoid extravasation because the high alkalinity (pH 11.6) of the solution is very irritating to tissues.

Currently, the recommended diazoxide dosage needed to achieve adequate lowering of elevated blood pressure is 5 mg/kg or 300 mg with a repeat dose in 30 minutes if the patient has failed to respond (245,263,289). Although this 300 mg traditional dose of diazoxide is well accepted, investigators now seem to be experimenting with alternate dosing schemes. In one study (268), diazoxide doses of 150 mg were equally effective as the traditional larger dose; and in another report (241), doses of 3 mg/kg effectively reduced blood pressure by 30 mm Hg in children. Both of these studies suggest that smaller standard doses may be equally effective and may mitigate the risk of hypotensive overshoot.

Other recent studies suggest that blood pressure lowering can be individualized and titrated by repeated small injections of the drug. Velasco gave initial doses of 25 to 50 mg and subsequent doses of 25 mg every ten minutes for up to eight doses. Effective control was achieved and excessive hypotension was not experienced (295). In accord with this concept, data indicate a linear relationship between blood pressure lowering and the log dose administered (241, 295). Thus, it may be possible to relate the required dosage to the pre-treatment blood pressures. Such newer concepts may well alter the way in which diazoxide is used in the future.

51. M.G. is given 300 mg of diazoxide over 10 seconds intravenously. When should peak effects occur and how often should the blood pressure be monitored?

The hypotensive effects of diazoxide usually begin within 1 to 5 minutes and peak effects usually occur within 3 to 5 minutes (253,264,281). However, the duration of hypotensive action is unpredictable. As a general rule, clinicians can expect diazoxide to be effective for 3 to 12 hours although its effects be as brief as two hours or as long as 72 hours (247,281,291).

The patient's blood pressure should be monitored every five minutes for the first 15 to 30 minutes. After this time, the arterial pressure gradually returns to normal (262,264).

52. Thirty minutes after the first dose of diazoxide, an appreciable decrease in blood pressure was not detectable. A second dose of 150 mg was administered over 10 seconds to M.G., and again she did not respond. How often is diazoxide ineffective in the treatment of hypertensive emergencies?

McDonald (267) administered 91 doses of diazoxide to 41 patients and observed that it was effective in 55%, transiently effective in 10%, and ineffective in 35%. In another study (268) of 101 severe hypertensives, 78.5% of initial diazoxide doses were effective in decreasing diastolic blood pressures to less than 100 mm Hg or in decreasing the diastolic pressure by 30 mm Hg for more than one hour in duration. These initial doses were transiently effective (i.e. decreasing diastolic pressures according to the above criteria for less than one hour) in 7.7% of the cases, and ineffective in 13.8%. A significant percentage of patients (17.8%) were refractory to diazoxide and needed to be treated with another agent despite proper diazoxide administration techniques.

Diazoxide is an effective drug in most types of hypertensive emergencies, but it may not always produce the desired response in a significant number of instances. Additionally it has a variable duration of action and doses are difficult to titrate to the desired hypotensive effect. As a result, nitroprusside is more often considered to be the drug of choice for hypertensive emergencies.

53. Should diuretics be administered concomitantly with diazoxide?

Although diazoxide is a congener of the thiazide diuretics, it possesses neither chloruretic or natriuretic properties. Indeed, marked sodium and water retention are the rule and lead not only to edema formation, but also to a neutralizing of its hypotensive action (239,247,248). The exact mechanism for this effect is unproven, but may be due to an activation of the renin system or to a direct anti-natriuretic effect on renal tubules (239).

To overcome these sodium retaining properties, diuretics should be administered concomitantly. The more potent loop diuretics are the preferred agents and doses of 100 to 200 mg/day of furosemide are common (262). Diuretic therapy should be instituted prior to initiation of diazoxide.

REFERENCES

1. Abboud FM: Relaxation, autonomic control and hypertension. NEJM 294:107, 1976.
2. Adlin EV et al: Spironolactone and hydrochlorothiazide in essential hypertension; blood pressure response and plasma renin activity. Arch Intern Med 130:855, 1972.
3. Alarcon-Sergovia D et al: Clinical and experimental studies on the hydralazine syndrome and its relationship to systemic lupus erythematosus. Med 46:1, 1967.
4. Alderman MH et al: Detection and treatment of hypertension at the work site. NEJM 293:65, 1975.
5. Alderman MH et al: Treatment of hypertension at the university medical clinic. Arch Intern Med 137:1707, 1977.
6. Ames RP et al: Elevation of serum lipids during diuretic therapy of hypertension. Am J Med 61:748, 1976.
7. Ames RP et al: Increase in serum lipids during treatment of hypertension with chlorthalidone. Lancet 1:721, 1976.
8. Anderson J et al: A comparison of the effects of hydrochlorothiazide and of furosemide in the treatment of hypertensive patients. Quart J Med 40:541, 1971.
9. Anderson RS et al: Diuretics. In *Clinical Use of Drugs in Renal Failure*, CC Thomas, Springfield, Ill., 1976, p 145-158.
10. Armstrong B et al: Retrospective study of the association between use of rauwolfia derivatives and breast cancer in English women. Lancet 2:672, 1974.
11. Baer L et al: Suppression of renin and aldosterone by clonidine. Ann Intern Med 74:830, 1971.
12. Ball P et al: Effects of prazosin in patients with hypertension. Clin Pharmacol Ther 20:138, 1976.
13. Baumrucker JF: Drug interaction: propranolol and Cafergot. NEJM 288:916, 1973.
14. Beckman H: *Dilemmas in Drug Therapy*, W. B. Saunders Co., Philadelphia, PA, 1967, p 176.
15. Bengtsson C et al: Effect of different doses of chlorthalidone on blood pressure, serum potassium, and serum urate. Brit Med J 1:197, 1975.
16. Bennett WM et al: Do diuretics have antihypertensive properties independent of natriuresis? Clin Pharmacol Ther 22:499, 1977.
17. Benson H: Systemic hypertension and the relaxation response. NEJM 296:1152, 1977.
18. Berglund G et al: Propranolol given twice daily in hypertension. Acta-Med Scand 194:513, 1973.
19. Boston Collaborative Drug Surveillance Program: Reserpine and breast cancer. Lancet 2:669, 1974.
20. Bourgoigne JJ et al: Renin-angiotensin-aldosterone system during chronic thiazide therapy of benign hypertension. Circ 37:27, 1968.
21. Bravo EL et al: Spironolactone as a non-specific treatment for primary aldosterone. Circ 48:491, 1973.
22. Brest AN et al: Mechanisms of antihypertension drug therapy. JAMA 211:480, 1970.
23. Bridgman JF et al: Drug induced gynecomastia. Brit Med J 2:520, 1974.
24. Brodsky JB et al: Acute postoperative clonidine withdrawal syndrome. Anesthesiol 44:519, 1976.
25. Brooks CS et al: Diuretic therapies in low renin and normal renin essential hypertension. Clin Pharmacol Ther 22:14, 1977.
26. Brunner HR et al: Essential hypertension: renin and aldosterone, heart attack, and stroke. NEJM 286:441, 1972.
27. Buhler FR: Propranolol inhibition of renin secretion. NEJM 287:1209, 1972.
28. Burns-Cox CJ: Negative Coombs'. Lancet 2:673, 1970.
29. Cacace LG et al: Alpha-methyldopa hepatitis. Drug Intel Clin Pharm 10:144, 1976.
30. Carey RM et al: Pericardial tamponade: A major manifestation of hydralazine-induced lupus syndrome. Am J Med 54:84, 1973.
31. Carey RM et al: The syndrome of essential hypertension and suppressed plasma renin activity: normalization of blood pressure with spironolactone. Arch Intern Med 130:849, 1972.
32. Carstairs KC et al: Incidence of a positive direct Coombs' test in patients on alphamethyldopa. Lancet 2:133, 1966.
33. Center for Disease Control: The effects of smoking on health, Morbid Mortal Weekly Report 26:145, 1977.
34. Channick BJ et al: Suppressed plasma renin activity in hypertension. Arch Intern Med 123:131, 1969.
35. Chen BT et al: Negative Coombs' in Chinese. Lancet 1:87, 1971.
36. Christlieb AR et al: Renin: a risk factor for cardiovascular disease? Ann Intern Med 81:7, 1974.
37. Clark E: Spironolactone therapy and gynecomastia. JAMA 193:163, 1965.
38. Constantine JW et al: Analysis of the hypotensive action of prazosin. *Hypertension: Mechanisms and Management*. Onesti, Kim, Moyer (eds). Grune and Stratton, New York, 1973 p 429-444.
39. Cranston EL et al: Effect of triamterene on elevated arterial pressure. Am Heart J 70:455, 1965.
40. Cryer PE et al: Norepinephrine and epinephrine release and adrenergic mediation of smoking-associated hemodynamic and metabolic effects. NEJM 295:573, 1976.
41. Cummins RO et al: Potassium in salt substitutes. NEJM 292:1082, 1975.
42. Dahl LK: Salt and hypertension. Am J Clin Nutr 25:231, 1972.
43. Davidov M et al: Antihypertensive properties of furosemide. Circ 36:125, 1967.
44. deCarvalho JGR et al: Hemodynamic correlates of prolonged thiazide therapy: comparison of responders and nonresponders. Clin Pharmacol Ther 22:875, 1977.
45. deTorregrosa MV et al: Coombs' positive drug-induced hemoly-

tic anemia. Am J Clin Path 53:490, 1970.

46. Diamond S: Propranolol and ergotamine tartrate. NEJM 289:159, 1973.

47. Dollery CT et al: Hyperuricaemia related to treatment of hypertension. Brit Med J 2:832, 1960.

48. Dorph S et al: The visceral changes in hypertension and their response to drug treatment. Acta Med Scand 187:411, 1971.

49. Doyle AE et al: Plasma renin levels and vascular complications in hypertension. Brit Med J 2:206, 1973.

50. Doyle AE: Use of beta-adrenergic blocking drugs in hypertension. Drugs 8:422, 1974.

51. Drayer JLM et al: Intrapatient comparison of treatment with chlorthalidone, spironolactone, and propranolol in normorennemic essential hypertension. Am J Cardiol 36:716, 1975.

52. Earley LE et al: Thiazide diuretics. Ann Rev Med 15:149, 1964.

53. Elkington SG et al: Hepatic injury caused by L-alpha-methyldopa. Circ 40:589, 1969.

54. Engelman K et al: Elevation of arterial pressure. In Harrison's *Principles of Internal Medicine,* Chapter 35, 8th ed. McGraw-Hill, New York, 1977, p 188-192.

55. Ibid.

56. Esler M et al: Pathophysiologic and pharmacokinetic determinants of the antihypertensive response to propranolol. Clin Pharmacol Ther 22:299, 1977.

57. Evans GH et al: Disposition of propranolol: drug accumulation and steady-state concentrations during chronic oral administration in man. Clin Pharmacol Ther 14:487, 1973.

58. Feisal KA et al: Effect of chlorothiazide on forearm vascular responses to norepinephrine. J Appl Physiol 16:549, 1961.

59. Freis ED: The mismanagement of hypertension. Arch Intern Med 137:1669, 1977.

60. Ferguson RK et al: Spironolactone and hydrochlorothiazide in normal renin and low-renin essential hypertension. Clin Pharmacol Ther 21:62, 1977.

61. Fernandez PG: Alpha methldopa and forgetfulness (Letter). Ann Intern Med 85:128, 1976.

62. Finnerty FA: The nurse's role in treating hypertension. NEJM 293:93, 1975.

63. Freis ED: Age, race, sex, and other indices of risk in hypertension. Am J Med 55:275, 1973.

64. Freis ED: How far should blood pressure be lowered in treating hypertension? JAMA 232:1017, 1975.

65. Freis ED: The treatment of hypertension and why, when, and how. Am J Med 52:664, 1972.

66. Frohlich ED et al: Altered vascular responsiveness: initial hypotensive mechanism of thiazide diuretics. Proc Soc Exp Biol Med 140:1190, 1972.

67. Frohlich ED: Mechanism of beta blockade hypotension, NEJM 287:1247, 1972.

68. Frohlich ED et al: The paradox of beta-adrenergic blockade in hypertension. Circ 37:417, 1968.

69. Frohlich ED: Use and abuse of diuretics. Am Heart J 89:1, 1975.

70. Gifford RW: Clinical application of new antihypertensive drugs. Clev Clin Q 42:255, 1975.

71. Gilmore E et al: Treatment of essential hypertension with a new vasodilator in combination with beta-adrenergic blockade. NEJM 282:521, 170.

72. Gilmore HR: The treatment of chronic hypertension. Med Clin N Amer 55:317, 1971.

73. Glontz GE et al: Methyldopa fever. Arch Intern Med 122:445, 1968.

74. Goodwin FK et al: Depressions following reserpine: A re-evaluation. Semin Psychiat 3:435, 1971.

75. Gottlieb TB et al: Combined therapy with vasodilator drugs and beta-adrenergic blockade in hypertension. Circ 45:571, 1972.

76. Greenblatt DJ et al: Adverse reactions to propranolol in hospitalized medical patients. Am Heart J 86:478, 1973.

77. Greenblatt DJ and Shader RI: On the psychopharmacology of beta adrenergic blockade. Current Ther Res 14:615, 1972.

78. Greenlaw C: Spironolactone induced gynecomastia. Drug Intell Clin Pharm 11:70, 1977.

79. Gunnels JC et al: Hypertension, adrenal abnormalities, and alterations in plasma renin activity. Ann Intern Med 73:901, 1970.

80. Guthrie GP et al: Renin and the therapy of hypertension. Sahmbhi.

81. Haddad A et al: Potassium in salt substitutes. NEJM 292:1082, 1975.

82. Haeusler G: Clonidine-induced inhibition of sympathetic nerve activity: no indication for a central presynaptic or an indirect sympathomimetic mode of action. Arch Pharmacol 286:97, 1974.

83. Hahn BH et al: Immune responses to hydralazine and nuclear antigens in hydralazine-induced lupus erythematosus. Ann Intern Med 76:365, 1972.

84. Hansson L et al: Blood pressure crisis following withdrawal of clonidine, with special reference to arterial and urinary catcholamine levels and suggestions for acute management. Am Heart J 85:605, 1973.

85. Hansson L et al: Propranolol therapy in essential hypertension: observations on predictability of therapeutic response. Int J Clin Pharmacol 10:79, 1974.

86. Harris AL: Clonidine withdrawal and blockade (Letter). Lancet 1:596, 1976.

87. Hayes JM et al: Experience with prazosin in the treatment of patients with severe hypertension. Med J Aust 1:562, 1976.

88. Healy JJ et al: Body composition changes in hypertensive subjects on long term oral diuretic therapy. Brit Med J 1:716, 1970.

89. Hedeland H et al: The effect of insulin induced hypoglycemia on plasma renin activity and urinary catecholamines before and following clonidine in man. Acta Endocrinol 71:321, 1972.

90. Heinonen OP et al: Reserpine use in relation to breast cancer. Lancet 2:675, 1974.

91. Herting RL et al: The physiologic and pharmacologic basis for the clinical treatment of hypertension. Med Clin N Amer 51:25, 1967.

92. Holland BO et al: Propranolol in the treatment of hypertension. NEJM 294:930, 1976.

93. Hollifield JW et al: Proposed mechanisms of propranolol's antihypertensive effect in essential hypertension. NEJM 295:68, 1976.

94. Hollister LE: Hematamesis and melena complicating treatment with rauwolfia alkaloids. Arch Intern Med 99:218, 1957.

95. Hoobler SW et al: Clonidine hydrochloride in the treatment of hypertension. Am J Cardiol 28:67, 1971.

96. Hoyumpa AM Jr et al: Methyldopa hepatitis, Am J Dig Dis 18:213, 1973.

97. Hua ASP et al: Studies with prazosin: A new effective hypotensive agent. Med J Aust 1:559, 1976.

98. Ibrahim MM et al: Hyperkinetic heart in severe hypertension. A separate clinical hemodynamic entity. Am J Cardiol 35:667, 1975.

99. Ingelfinger JA et al: Therapy for hypertension. How much of what drug for whom? JAMA 238:1369, 1977.

100. Johnston P et al: Treatment of hypertension with methyldopa. Br Med J 1:133, 1966.

101. Jose A et al: Suppressed plasma renin activity in essential hypertension: roles of plasma volume, blood pressure, and sympathetic nervous system. Ann Intern Med 72:9, 1970.

102. Kannel WB et al: Epidemiologic assessment of the role of blood pressure in stroke, the Framingham study. JAMA 214: 301, 1970.

103. Kannel WB et al: Systolic versus diastolic blood pressure and risk of coronary heart disease: The Framingham study. Am J Cardiol 27:335, 1971.

104. Ibid.

105. Kannel WB et al: The relation of adiposity to blood pressure and development of hypertension: the Framingham study. Ann Intern Med 67:48, 1967.

106. Kaplan NM: *Clinical Hypertension.* Medcom Press, New York, 1973.

107. Kaplan NM: The prognostic implications of plasma renin in essential hypertension. JAMA 231:167, 1975.

108. Kawasaki T et al: The effect of high-sodium and low-sodium intake on blood pressure and other related variables in human subjects with idiopathic hypertension. Am J Med 64:193, 1978.

109. Kellaway GSM: Adverse drug reactions during treatment of hypertension. Drugs 2 (Suppl):91, 1976.

110. Kellett RE et al: The treatment of moderate hypertension with catapress. *Catapress in Hypertension.* Conolly (ed), Butterworth. London, 1970.

111. Kelly KL: Beta-blockers in hypertension: a review. Am J Hosp Pharm 33:1284, 1976.

112. Keys A et al: Coronary heart disease: overweight and obesity as risk factors. Ann Intern Med 77:15, 1972.

113. Kincaid-Smith P: Vasodilator's in the treatment of hypertension. Med J Aust(Suppl) 1:7, 1975.

114. Kobinger W: Pharmacologic basis of the cardiovascular actions of clonidine. *Hypertension: Mechanisms and Management.* Onesti, Kim and Moyer(eds), Grune and Stratton, New York, 1973, pg 369-380.

115. Kinsey D et al: Incidence of hyperuricemia in 400 hypertensive patients. Circ 24:972, 1961.

116. Kirsner JB et al: The effect of reserpine upon basal gastric secretion in man. Arch Intern Med 99:390, 1957.

117. Koch-Weser J et al: The therapeutic challenge of systolic hypertension. NEJM 289:483, 1973.

118. Kosman ME: Management of potassium problem during long-term diuretic therapy. JAMA, 230:743, 1974.

119. Laragh JH et al: Renin, angiotensin and aldosterone system in pathogenesis and management of hypertensive vascular disease. Am J Med 52:633, 1972.

120. Lawrence T et al: Beta-adrenergic receptor blocking drugs. Med Clin N Amer 57:944, 1973.

121. Leishman AW et al: Hypertension and guanethidine after five years. Angiology 18:705, 1967.

122. Levitt JI: Spironolactone therapy and amenorrhea. JAMA 211:2014, 1970.

123. Lew EA: High blood pressure, other risk factors and longevity: the insurance viewpoint. Am J Med 55:281, 1973.

124. Lewis PJ et al: Deterioration of glucose tolerance in hypertensive patients on prolonged diuretic therapy. Lancet 1:564, 1976.

125. Lewis PJ et al: Mechanism of beta-blockade hypotension. NEJM 288:689, 1973.

126. Liang MH et al: Asymptomatic hyperuricemia: the case for conservative management. Ann Intern Med 88:666, 1978.

127. Liddle GW: Aldosterone antagonists. Arch Intern Med 102:998, 1958.

128. Loriaux DL et al: Spironolactone and endocrine dysfunction. Ann Intern Med 85:630, 1976.

129. Lott RS et al: Estimation of creatinine clearance. Drug Intell Clin Pharm 12:140, 1978.

130. Louis WJ: Methyldopa and haemolytic anaemia. Med J Aust 2:104, 1967.

131. Lowder SG et al: Prolonged alteration of renin responsiveness after spironolactone therapy. NEJM 291:1243, 1974.

132. Lydtin H: Propranolol therapy in essential hypertension. Am Heart J 83:589, 1972.

133. Mack TM et al: Reserpine and breast cancer in a retirement community. NEJM 292:1366, 1975.

134. Maddrey WC et al: Severe hepatitis from methyldopa. Gastroenterol 68:351, 1975.

135. Mann NM: Gynecomastia during therapy with spironolactone. JAMA 184:778, 1963.

136. Manner RJ et al: Prevalence of hypokalemia in diuretic therapy. Clin Med 79:15, 1972.

137. Marsden CW et al: Raynaud's phenomenon as a side effect of beta-blockers. Br Med J 2:176, 1976.

138. McAllister RG: Guanethidine in antihypertensive therapy: experience with an oral loading regimen. J Clin Pharmacol 15:771, 1975.

139. McKenney JM et al: The effect of clinical pharmacy services on patients in essential hypertension. Circ 48:1104, 1973.

140. McLeod PJ: Effects of large and small doses of hydrochlorothiazide in hypertensive patients. Clin Pharmacol Ther 11:733, 1970.

141. McMartin C et al: The absorption and metabolism of guanethidine in hypertensive patients requiring different doses of the drug. Clin Pharmacol Ther 12:73, 1971.

142. Ibid.

143. Melmon KL: The clinical pharmacology of commonly used antihypertensive drugs. *Cardiovascular Drug Therapy,* Melmon K(ed). FA Davis, Co, Phila, 1974, pp 175-197.

144. Meyer JF et al: Insidious and prolonged antagonism of guanethidine by amitryptyline. JAMA 213:1487, 1970.

145. Meyers MG et al: Brain concentration of propranolol in relation to hypotensive effect in the rabbit with observations on brain propranolol in man. J Pharmacol Exp Ther 192:327, 1975.

146. Michelakis AM et al: The effect of chronic adrenergic receptor blockade on plasma renin activity in man. J Clin Endocrinol Metab 34:386, 1972.

147. Miller AC et al: Methyldopa-induced granulomatous hepatitis. JAMA 235:2001, 1976.

tion and treatment of high blood pressure. JAMA 237:255, 1977.

149. Moser M: Use and abuse of antihypertensive drugs. Gen Pract 35:87, 1967.

150. Mroczek WL et al: Lack of association between plasma renin and history of heart attack or stroke in patients with essential hypertension. Lancet 2:464, 1973.

151. Mroczek WJ et al: Prolonged treatment with clonidine: comparative antihypertensive effects alone and with a diuretic agent. Amer J Cardiol 30:536, 1972.

152. Newman RJ: Sexual dysfunction due to methyldopa. Br Med J 4:106, 1974.

153. Nickerson M: Ch 33: Antihypertension. In *The Pharmacological Basis of Therapeutics* 4th ed. Goodman L and Gilman A (eds). The Macmillan Co., New York, 1970, p 728-744.

154. Nicotero JA et al: Prevention of hyperuricemia by allopurinol in hypertensive patients treated with chlorothiazide. NEJM 282:133, 1970.

155. Nies AS et al: Recent concepts in the clinical pharmacology of antihypertensive agents. Calif Med 106:388, 1967.

156. Nurick S: Clonidine in migraine. Lancet 1:901, 1972.

157. Oakes TW et al: Social factors in newly discovered elevated blood pressure. J Health Soc Behav 14:198, 1973.

158. Oates JA: Antihypertensive drugs that impair adrenergic neuron function. Pharmacol for Physicians 1:1, 1967.

159. Oates JA et al: The relative efficacy of guanethidine, methyldopa and pargyline as antihypertensive agents. NEJM 273:729, 1965.

160. Onesti G et al: Clonidine: a new antihypertensive agent. Am J Cardiol 28:74, 1971.

161. Onesti G et al: Antihypertensive effect of clonidine. Circ Res (Suppl II) 18-19:53, 1971.

162. Page LB et al: Drugs in the management of hypertension. Amer Heart J 91:810, 92:114, 92:252, 1976.

163. Page LB et al: Medical management of primary hypertension (a three-part series). NEJM 287:960, 1972, 287:1018, 1972, 287:1074, 1972.

164. Pearson M et al: Aldomet interference with the Babson method of SGOT analysis. Med J Aust 2:84, 1972.

165. Pfeiffer HJ et al: Clinical toxicity of reserpine in hospitalized patients. Am J Med Sci 271:269, 1976.

166. Pickering G: Ch 8, 15, 17, 20, in *High Blood Pressure* 2nd ed. J & A Churchill Ltd. 1968.

167. Pitts NE: The clinical evaluation of prazosin, a new antihypertensive agent. *Prazosin-Evaluation of a New Antihypertensive Agent.* Cotton(ed). Excerpta Medica, Amsterdam, 1974, pp 149-163.

168. Platt R: Heredity in hypertension. Lancet 1:889, 1963.

169. Podell RN et al: Hypertension and compliance: implications for the primary physician. NEJM 294:1120, 1976.

170. Pollack AA et al: Limitations of transcendental meditation in the treatment of essential hypertension. Lancet 1:71, 1977.

171. Prichard BN et al: Treatment of hypertension with propranolol. Brit Med J 1:7, 1969.

172. Ibid.

173. Rabkin SW et al: Predicting risk of ischemic heart disease and cerebrovascular disease from systolic and diastolic blood pressures. Ann Intern Med 88:342, 1978.

174. Rahn KH et al: Comparison of antihypertensive efficacy, intestinal absorption, and excretion of guanethidine in hypertensive patients. Clin Pharmacol Ther 10:858, 1969.

175. Rapaport MI et al: Thiazide-induced glucose intolerance treated with potassium. Arch Intern Med 113:405, 1964.

176. Reisin E et al: Effect of weight loss without salt restriction on the reduction of blood pressure in overweight hypertensive patients. NEJM 298:1, 1978.

177. Roth JL: Role of drugs in the production of gastroduodenal ulcer. JAMA 187:418, 1964.

178. Riddiough MA: Preventing, detecting, and managing adverse reactions of antihypertensive agents in the ambulant patient with essential hypertension. Am J Hosp. Pharm 34:465, 1977.

179. Robertson D et al: Effects of caffeine on plasma renin activity, catecholamines and blood pressure. NEJM 298:181, 1978.

180. Rovner DR: Use of pharmacologic agents in the treatment of hypokalemia and hyperkalemia. Ration Drug Ther 6:1, 1972.

181. Sackett DL et al: Hypertension control, compliance and science. Am Heart J 94:666, 1977.

182. Sackett DL: Patient and therapies: getting the two together. NEJM 298:178, 1978.

183. Sackett DL et al: Randomised clinical trial of strategies for im-

proving medication compliance in primary hypertension. Lancet 1:1205, 1975.

184. Schachter S: Pharmacological and psychological determinants of smoking. Ann Intern Med 88:104, 1978.

185. Schneider EM et al: Gastric secretion as influenced by rauwolfia alkaloids, Ann Intern Med 47:640, 1957.

186. Schoenberger JA et al: Current status of hypertension control in an industrial population. JAMA 222:559, 1972.

187. Schoenberger JA: Management of essential hypertension. Med Clin N Amer 55:11, 1971.

188. Schweitzer IL et al: Acute submassive hepatic necrosis due to methyldopa. Gastroenterol 66:1203, 1974.

189. Schweitzer MD et al: Genetic factors in primary hypertension and coronary disease. J Chron Dis 45:1093, 1962.

190. Shafar J et al: Evaluation of clonidine in prophylaxis of migraine (double-blind trial and follow-up). Lancet 1:403, 1972.

191. Shakil M et al: Effect of methyldopa on plasma renin activity in man. Circ Res 25:543, 1969.

192. Shand DG: Individualization of propranolol therapy. Med Clin N Amer 58:1063, 1974.

193. Shand DG: A loading-maintenance regimen for more rapid initiation of the effect of guanethidine. Clin Pharmacol Ther 18:139, 1975.

194. Shand DG: Propranolol. NEJM 293:380, 1975.

195. Shaper AG: Cardiovascular disease in the tropics III, blood pressure and hypertension. Brit Med J 3:805, 1972.

196. Sherlock S et al: Complicatons of diuretic therapy in hepatic cirrhosis. Lancet 1:1049, 1966.

197. Simpson FO: Hypertension and depression and their treatment. Aust NZ J Psychiat 7:133, 1973.

198. Smith AJ: Clinical features of fluid retention complicating treatment with guanethidine. Circ 31:485, 1965.

199. Smith WM: Epidemiology of hypertension. Med Clin N Amer 61:467, 1977.

200. Spark RF et al: Aldosteronism in hypertension the spironolactone response test. Ann Intern Med 69:685, 1968.

201. Spark RF et al: Hypertension and low plasma renin activity: Presumptive evidence for mineralocorticoid excess. Ann Intern Med 75:831, 1971.

202. Stewart RB et al: A review of medication errors and compliance in ambulant patients. Clin Pharmacol Therap 13:463, 1972.

203. Stone RA et al: Psychotherapeutic control of hypertension. NEJM 294:80, 1976.

204. Taguchi J et al: Partial reduction of blood pressure and prevention of complications in hypertension. NEJM 291:329, 1974.

205. Tarazi RC et al: Beta-adrenergic blockade in hypertension. Practical and theoretical implications of long term hemodynamic variations. Am J Cardiol 29:633, 1972.

206. Tarazi RC et al: Long term thiazide therapy in essential hypertension: evidence for persistent alteration in plasma volume and renin activity. Circ 41:709, 1970.

207. Thomas E et al: Spectrum of methyldopa liver injury. Am J Gastroent 68:125, 1977.

208. Thompson FD et al: Beta-blockade in the presence of renal disease and hypertension. Brit Med J 2:555, 1974.

209. Tobian L: How to treat benign essential hypertension. Gen Pract 37:125, 1968.

210. Tobian L: Hypertension and obesity. NEJM 298:46, 1978.

211. Tweeddale MG et al: Antihypertensive and biochemical effects of chlorthalidone. Clin Pharmacol Ther 22:519, 1977.

212. Ueda H et al: Observations on the mechanism of renin release by hydralazine in hypertensive patients. Circ Res 26:(& 27 Suppl.2)201, 1970.

213. VanZwieten PA: The central action of antihypertensive drugs, mediated via central alpha-receptors. J Pharm Pharmacol 25:89, 1973.

214. Vejlsgaard V et al: Double blind trial of four hypotensive drugs. Brit Med J 2:598, 1967.

215. Vervloet E et al: Propranolol serum levels during 24 hours. Clin Pharmacol Ther 22:853, 1977.

216. Veterans Administration Cooperative Study Group on Antihypertensive Agents: Effects of treatment on morbidity in hypertension II: results in patients with diastolic blood pressure averaging 90 through 114 mm Hg. JAMA 213:1143, 1970.

217. Ibid.

218. Veterans Administration Cooperative Study Group on Antihypertensive Agents: Effects of treatment on morbidity in hypertension: results in patients with diastolic pressures averaging 115 through 129 mm Hg. JAMA 202:1028, 1967.

219. Veterans Administration Cooperative Study Group on Antihypertensive Agents: Effects of treatment on morbidity III: Influence of age, diastolic blood pressure, prior cardiovascular disease. Further analysis of side effects. Circ 45:991, 1972.

220. Veterans Administration Cooperative Study Group on Antihypertensive Agents: Propranolol in the treatment of essential hypertension. JAMA 237:2303, 1977.

221. Waal HJ: Hypotensive action of propranolol. Clin Pharmacol Ther 7:588, 1968.

222. Wallerstein RO: Ch 9: Blood, in Current Diagnosis and Treatment, Krupp MA and Chafton MJ eds. Lange Medical Publication, Los Altos, CA, 12th ed. 1973, p 262-64.

223. Walter IE et al: The relationship of plasma guanethidine levels to adrenergic blockade Clin Pharmacol Ther 18:571, 1975.

224. Weber MA et al: Treatment of hypertension with an antihypertensive agent possessing vasodilator activity. Med J Aust (Suppl) 1:9, 1975.

225. Weiss NS: Relation of high blood pressure to headache epistaxis, and selected other symptoms. NEJM 287:631, 1972.

226. Ibid.

227. Wertheimer L et al: Furosemide in essential hypertension: a statistical analysis of three double blind studies. Arch Intern Med 127:934, 1971.

228. West WO: Perforation and hemorrhage from duodenal ulcer during the administration of rauwolfia serpentina: report of five cases. Ann Intern Med 48:1033, 1958.

229. Wilber JA et al: Hypertension — A community problem. Am J Med 52:653, 1972.

230. Ibid.

231. Wilkenson M: Drugs for the treatment of migraine. Pharmaceut J 210:276, 1973.

232. Wilkinson PR et al: Total body and serum potassium during prolonged thiazide therapy for essential hypertension. Lancet 1:759, 1975.

233. Wilkinson PR et al: Twice-daily propranolol treatment for hypertension. J Intern Med Res 2:220, 1974.

234. Winchester JF et al: Iatrogenic Raynaud's phenomenon. Brit Med J 3:113, 1971.

235. Worlledge SM et al: Autoimmune hemolytic anemia associated with alphamethyldopa. Lancet 2:135, 1966.

236. Zacest R et al: Treatment of essential hypertension with combined vasodilation and beta-adrenergic blockade. NEJM 286-617, 1972.

237. Zacharias FJ et al: Propranolol in hypertension. Am Heart J 83:755, 1972.

238. Zinner SH et al: Familial aggregation of blood pressure in children. NEJM 284:401, 1971.

HYPERTENSIVE EMERGENCIES:

239. Bartorelli C et al: Hypotensive and renal effects of diazoxide — a sodium-retaining benzothiadiazine compound. Circ 27:895, 1963.

240. Bhatia SK et al: Hemodynamic comparison of agents useful in hypertensive emergencies. Am Heart J 85:367, 1973.

241. Boerth RC et al: Dose response relation of diazoxide in children with hypertension. Circ 56:1062, 1977.

242. Cacace L et al: Treatment of hypertensive emergencies with sodium nitroprusside. Drug Intell Clin Pharm 4:187, 1970.

243. Charles S et al: Nonketoacidotic hyperglycemia and coma during intravenous diazoxide therapy in uremia. Diabetes 20:501, 1971.

244. Donferth E: Hyperglycemia after diazoxide administration (letter). NEJM 285:1487, 1971.

245. Drug Commentary. Dept. of Drugs. Evaluation of diazoxide. JAMA 224:1422, 1973.

246. Finnerty F Jr.: Hyperglycemia after diazoxide administration (Reply). NEJM 285:1487, 1971.

247. Finnerty FA et al: Clinical evaluation of diazoxide: A new treatment for acute hypertension. Circ 28:203, 1963.

248. Finnerty FA: Relationship of extracellular fluid volume to the development of drug resistence in the hypertensive patient. Am Heart J 81:563, 1971.

249. Freis ED: Hypertensive crisis. JAMA 208:338, 1969.
250. Frohlich ED: Inhibitor of adrenergic function in the treatment of hypertension. Arch Int Med 133:1033, 1974.
251. Gifford RW: Hypertensive emergencies and their treatment. Med Clin N Am 45:441, 1961.
252. Gifford RW: Treatment of hypertensive emergencies in *Hypertension: Mechanisms Management. The XXVI Hahnemann Symposium* edited by G Orestic K Kim and J Moyer, New York, Grune & Stratton, 1973, pp 809-817.
253. Hamby WM et al: Intravenous use of diazoxide in the treatment of severe hypertension. Circ 37:169, 1968.
254. Harrington M: Results of treatment in malignant hypertension: A seven year experience in 94 cases. Brit Med J 2:969, 1959.
255. Harrison B et al: Severe nonketotic hyperglycemia precoma in a hypertensive patient receiving diazoxide. Lancet 2:599, 1972.
256. Heptinstall RH: Malignant hypertension: A study of 51 cases. J Path 65:423, 1953.
257. Kanada S et al: Angina-like syndrome with diazoxide therapy for hypertensive crisis. Ann Int Med 84:696, 1976.
258. Katz RL: Sodium nitroprusside for controlled hypotension and hypertensive emergencies edited by LC Mork and SH Ngai, *Highlights of Clinical Anesthesiology,* Harper and Row, New York, New York, 1971, pp 48-54.
259. Keith NM et al: Some different types of essential hypertension: Their course and progress. Am J Med Sci 197:332, 1939.
260. Keith NM et al: The syndrome of malignant hypertension. Arch Int Med 41:141, 1928.
261. Kincaid-Smith P et al: The clinical course and pathology of hypertension with papilledema. Q J Med 27:117, 1958.
262. Koch-Weser J: Hypertensive emergencies. NEJM 290:211, 1974.
263. Koch-Weser J: Diazoxide. NEJM 294:1271, 1976.
264. Koch-Weser J: Vasodilator drugs in the treatment of hypertension. Arch Int Med 133:1017, 1974.
265. Kumar GK et al: Side effects of diazoxide. JAMA 235:275, 1976.
266. McCormack LJ et al: Effects of antihypertensive treatment in the evolution of renal lesions in malignant nephrosclerosis. Am J Pathol 34:1011, 1958.
267. McDonald WJ et al: Intravenous diazoxide therapy in hypertensive crisis. Am J Cardiol 40:409, 1977.
268. Miller WE et al: Management of severe hypertension with intravenous injections of diazoxide. Am J Cardiol 24:870, 1969.
269. Mroczek W et al: The value of aggressive therapy in hypertensive patients with azotemia. Circ 40:893, 1969.
270. Mroczek WJ et al: The importance of the rapid administration of diazoxide in accelerated hypertension. NEJM 285:603, 1971.
271. Nickerson M et al: Antihypertensive agents and the drug therapy of hypertension. In *The Pharmacological Basis of Therapeutics,* L Goodman and A Gilman, 5th ed, edited by. MacMillan Publishing Co., New York, 1975, pp 713-715.
272. Nipride package insert, Roche Laboratories, 1974.
273. Nourok DS et al: Hypothyroidism following prolonged sodium nitroprusside therapy. Am J Med Sci 248:129, 1964.
274. Page IH et al: Cardiovascular actions of sodium nitroprusside in animals and hypertensive patients. Circ 11:188, 1955.
275. Palmer RF et al: Sodium nitroprusside, NEJM 292, 1975.
276. Patton W et al: The methonium compounds. Pharmacol Rev 4:219, 1952.
277. Perera GA: Hypertensive vascular disease: Description and natural history. J Chron Dis 1:33, 1955.
278. Perera GA: The accelerated form of hypertension: A unique entity? Trans Assoc Am Phy 71:62, 1958.
279. Perry HM et al: Studies on the control of hypertension VIII. Mortality, morbidity and remissions during 12 years of intensive therapy. Circ 33:958, 1966.
280. Pickering G: Reversibility of malignant hypertension. Lancet 1:413, 1971.
281. Romankiewicz J: Pharmacology and clinical use of drugs in hypertensive emergencies. Am J Hosp Pharm 34:185, 1977.
282. Schottstaedt WF et al: The natural history and cause of malignant hypertension with papilledema. Am Heart J 45:331, 1953.
283. Sellers EM et al: Influence of intravenous injection rate in protein binding and vascular activity of diazoxide. Ann NY Acad Sci 226:319, 1973.
284. Sellers EM et al: Protein binding and vascular activity of diazoxide. NEJM 281:1141, 1969.
285. Shin B et al: Hyperglycemic hyperosmolar nonketotic coma following diazoxide, anesthesia and operation. Anesth Analg 56(4):506, 1977.
286. Sonnenblick EH et al: Oxygen consumption of the heart. Newer concepts of its multifactorial determination. Am J Cardiol 22:328, 1968.
287. Speight TM et al: Diazoxide: A review of its pharmacological properties and therapeutic use in hypertensive crisis. Drugs 2:78, 1971.
288. Spivak JL et al: Hypertensive crisis. In *Manual of Clinical Problems in Internal Medicine,* 1st ed, edited by JL Spivak and HV Barnes, Brown and Co, Boston, Mass 1974. pp 10-12.
289. The Medical Letter on Drugs and Therapeutics. Diazoxide. Med Lett 15:53, 1973.
290. Thirlwell MP et al: The effect of diazoxide on the veins. Am Heart J 83:512, 1972.
291. Thompson AE et al: Clinical observations on an antihypertensive chlorothiazide analogue devoid of diuretic activity. Can Med Assoc J 87:1306, 1962.
292. Tuzel I: Sodium Nitroprusside: A review of its clinical effectiveness as a hypotensive agent. J Clin Pharmacol 14:494, 1974.
293. Updike SJ et al: Acute diabetic ketoacidosis? A complication of intravenous diazoxide administration for refractory hypertension. NEJM 280:768, 1969.
294. Vaamonde CA et al: Hypertensive emergencies. Med Clin N Am 55:325, 1971.
295. Velasco M et al: A new technique for safe and effective control of hypertension with intravenous diazoxide. Curr Ther Res 19:185, 1976.
296. Veterans Administration cooperative study group on antihypertensive agents: II. Results in patients with diastolic blood pressures averaging 90 through 114 mm Hg. JAMA 213:1143, 1970.
297. Vidt D: Management of hypertensive emergencies. Clin Med 82:35, 1975.
298. Woods J et al: Management of malignant hypertension complicated by renal insufficiency. NEJM 277:57, 1967.
299. Zitowitz L et al: Some acute cardiovascular actions of diazoxide a non-diuretic antihypertensive benzothiodizine. Fed Proc 21:114, 1962.

Chapter 12

Congestive Heart Failure

Mary Anne Koda-Kimble

Congestive heart failure (CHF) is a syndrome (that is, a group of symptoms) which results when the right, left or both ventricles fail to pump sufficient blood to meet the body's needs. An estimated two million people in the United States currently have CHF and 2-5 cases per 1000 persons are diagnosed yearly. The Framingham Heart Disease Epidemiology Study (65) reported that over a 16 year period 3.5% of women in the population studied developed congestive heart failure. This corresponded to an annual rate of 2.3 and 1.4 cases per 1000 males and females respectively. There was a clear correlation between the incidence of CHF with both sex and age. Males were clearly predisposed to CHF; by the sixth decade, the incidence among men was five times that of the fourth decade. It is apparent that as the size of our geriatric population increases, CHF will become a more frequently encountered clinical entity. Despite early diagnosis and optimal medical management by today's standards, the prognosis of these patients is not much better than it is for those with cancer. In the Framingham study 60% of men and 40% of women died within 5 years of the diagnosis of CHF.

The increasing prevalence of this disease in our society taken together with the facts that digitalis is one of the most commonly prescribed drugs and that the incidence of digitalis toxicity has increased 2.5-14 times over 30 years makes this topic extremely pertinent to us today (5,51,71).

The two major classes of drugs used in the treatment of CHF are digitalis glycosides and diuretics. This chapter will emphasize the proper use of digitalis glycosides — more specifically, digoxin. The reader is referred to the chapter on *Edema* for a thorough discussion of the diuretics.

The following case history is typical for a congestive heart failure patient and will serve as a basis for the questions which follow.

CASE HISTORY: A.J. is a 58-year-old black male who is admitted with a chief complaint of increasing shortness of breath and weight gain. Approximately two years prior to admission the patient noted the onset of DOE after one flight of stairs, orthopnea, and ankle edema. Since that time the patient's symptoms have progressed in spite of intermittent hydrochlorothiazide therapy. Approximately three weeks prior to admission the patient noted the onset of episodic bouts of PND. Since then he has been able to sleep only in a sitting position. In the past three weeks the patient has noted a productive cough, nocturia (2-3 times/night) and a mild, dependent edema.

The patient's other medical problems include a four year history of peptic ulcer disease; a two year history of rheumatoid arthritis which has been managed well with phenylbutazone; chronic headaches; and hypertension which has been poorly controlled with guanethidine and propranolol. There is also a strong family history for diabetes mellitus.

Physical examination revealed a dyspneic, cyanotic, tachycardic male with a blood pressure of 160/100 mm Hg, pulse of 100/min, and a respiratory rate of 28/min. He was 5'11" and 80 kg. His cervical veins were distended. On cardiac exam an S_3 gallop was heard; his PMI was at the sixth ICS 12 cm from the MSL. His liver was enlarged and tender to palpation and a positive HJR was observed. He was noted to have 3+ pitting edema of the extremities and sacral edema. Chest examination revealed inspiratory rales and rhonchi bilaterally.

The pharmacist's medication history revealed the following:

Present medications: Hydrochlorothiazide, 50 mg qod; Propranolol, 80 mg tid; Guanethidine, 50 mg daily; Phenylbutazone, 100 mg qid; Maalox, 30 cc alternating with Amphogel, 30 cc q 2 hr while awake. Allergies: Oral penicillin resulted in a total body rash in 1960. He has had no penicillin since. Adverse reactions: ASA causes nausea and burning of his stomach. He claims no dietary restrictions.

Admitting laboratory values included the following (normal values for the University of California are in *parentheses):*

Hematocrit, 39.4% (45); White Blood Count, 3500/mm³ (5-10,000); Sodium, 132 mEq/L (136-144); Potassium, 3.2 mEq/L (3.5-5.3); Chloride, 90 mEq/L (96-106); Bicarbonate, 30 mEq/L (23-28); Magnesium, 1.2 mEq/L (1.7-2.7); Fasting Blood Sugar (FBS), 120 mg/100 ml (65-110); Uric Acid, 8.0 mg/,100 ml (3.5-7.0); Blood Urea Nitrogen (BUN), 40 mg/100 ml (10-20); Creatinine, 2.0 mg/100 ml (0.5-1.2); Alk Phos 120 U (40-80); SGOT 100 U (40). Chest x-ray revealed bilateral pleural effusions and cardiomegaly.

1. Discuss the etiology of CHF.

There are two major types of heart failure. **High output failure** results when the heart fails to pump enough blood to meet the metabolic demands of the tissues. This may occur in a hyperthyroid patient whose metabolic demands are greater or in a severely anemic patient whose tissues require a greater volume of blood to supply normal metabolic needs. **Low output (congestive) failure** is the more common of the two and will be the major emphasis of discussion. This form occurs when the heart is unable to pump all the blood with which it is presented. Many factors may contribute to the development of CHF. These include those which (a) increase cardiac workload, (b) impair myocardial contractility, and (c) impair the filling of the right ventricle.

Cardiac workload is increased if the blood volume which the heart must pump *(preload)* is increased. This can occur following the too rapid administration of blood plasma expanders and osmotic diuretics or by the administration of large amounts of sodium or sodium retaining agents. A malfunctioning aortic valve which results in regurgitation of blood into the left ventricle can also increase the volume of blood which must be pumped. Hypertension or atherosclerotic disease increases arterial impedence *(afterload),* thereby increasing the workload on the heart. Hypertension is a major etiologic factor in the development of CHF. The Framingham group (65) found that 75% of the patients who developed congestive heart failure had prior histories of hypertension. In another study the risk of developing CHF was six times greater for hypertensive than for normotensive patients (41). Cardiac anomalies, as for example narrowing of the aortic valve, and severe lung disease are also sources of increased resistance.

Myocardial contractility is decreased when there are fewer or poorly functioning myocardial fibers. This usually results from primary cardiac disease of which rheumatic heart disease, coronary artery disease, myocardial infarction, cardiomyopathies and persistent arrhythmias are examples. Occasionally, drugs such as propranolol or daunomycin induce CHF by decreasing myocardial contractility (see Question 3).

2. Identify those factors which specifically contribute to the etiology of this patient's heart failure.

a. Hypertension (see Question 1).
b. Age (see Introduction).
c. Drugs (see Questions 1 and 3): Propranolol — decreases myocardial contractility; see *Angina* chapter. Guanethidine — mild sodium retention; blocks cardiac dependent sympathetic tone. Antacids — large sodium load. Clinicians should be aware that many pharmaceutical manufacturers have changed their antacid formulations to minimize the sodium content (e.g. Maalox) so that this is becoming much less of a concern for CHF patients. See *Peptic Ulcer Disease* chapter. Phenylbutazone — sodium retention with increased plasma volume; see *Rheumatoid Arthritis* chapter.

3. By what mechanisms do drugs contribute to the exacerbation or induction of congestive heart failure? Discuss the clinical significance of drug-induced congestive failure.

Drugs which produce expansion of the intravascular volume or decrease cardiac contractility should be avoided or used with caution in patients with congestive heart failure.

Drugs may produce volume expansion by several mechanisms. They may (a) increase retention of sodium and water by the kidney, (b) increase the intravascular osmotic pressure causing a redistribution of interstitial and intracellular water into intravascular space and (c) increase total body sodium and water by their high sodium content. Only rarely have these drug effects been quantitated. In many cases one can only rely on what he knows about the pharmacology of the drug and on scattered case reports. A listing of these drugs together with a comment on the clinical significance of their effects in patients with congestive heart failure follows.

Amphetamines — Smith et al (78a) report a case of amphetamine-induced cardiomyopathy manifested as severe CHF in a 45-year-old female. The patient had a history of depression, narcolepsy and cataplexy for which she was treated with high dose dextroamphetamine (100 mg/day; 2 mg/kg) intermittently for five years and continuously for 7 years. An attempt to withdraw the amphetamine resulted in deterioration of her cardiac status. The authors point to the similarity between this case and the myocarditis associated with pheochromocytoma and refer to ischemia and myocardial hypertrophy induced by sympathomimetic amines in animals.

Androgens — Sodium retention and edema may result from the chronic administration of these substances.

Glucocorticoids — Those with significant mineralocorticoid effects cause sodium retention through stimulation of sodium reabsorption in exchange for potassium in the distal convoluted tubule of the kidney (see *Glucocorticoid* chapter). Those with minimal mineralocorticoid effects (e.g. prednisone in low to moderate doses or dexamethasone) should be used in preference to hydrocortisone in CHF patients.

Daunomycin — This cancer chemotherapeutic agent, which has been used in the treatment of acute myelocytic leukemia, has a direct dose-related cardiotoxic effect that may occur several months after therapy has been terminated (average 80 days) (92a). This commonly presents as myocardial infarction (29), arrhythmia and other ECG changes (92a), and congestive heart failure (92a). ECG changes may occur early in therapy and are not predictive of the highly fatal (79% mortality), therapy-resistant congestive heart failure (92a). Initially, when high doses were used (greater than 35 mg/kg or 950 mg/m²), the incidence of cardiotoxicity was estimated to be 10%. When daunomycin doses were confined to less than 600 mg/m², the incidence dropped to less than 3% in a group of 2000 patients (6). A recent analysis of 5,613 patients receiving daunomycin revealed that the incidence of cardiomyopathy was 1.5% at a total dose of 600 mg/m² and 12% at a dose of 1000 mg/m². Children appear to be more susceptible to the congestive heart failure: the overall incidence was 1.6% for children and 0.6% for adults (92a).

Diazoxide — The mechanism by which this drug induces sodium and water retention has not been clarified. It may increase the proximal tubular reabsorption of sodium (2,91). Sodium retention caused by this agent is significant and predictable. Potent, loop diuretics are frequently used in conjunction with this agent to prevent volume expansion, edema, weight gain, CHF and resistance to its hypotensive effects (46).

Estrogens — These agents frequently produce sodium retention, edema and weight gain (see *Oral Contraceptive* chapter).

Guanethidine — Sympatholytic agents decrease cardiac output thereby diminishing GFR and increasing sodium retention (78,97). Guanethidine has anther theoretical disadvantage for CHF patients in that it deprives the failing heart of the sympathetic drive it requires to maintain cardiac output. Clinically, exacerbation of CHF does not appear to be a problem with this agent (16).

Licorice — Contains glycerrhyzic acid which has a structure closely resembling the mineralocorticoids. Glycerrhyzic acid which has been used experimentally in the treatment of peptic ulcer disease induces cardiac asthma or edema in up to 20% of the patients in whom it is used (13). Symptomatic CHF was produced following the ingestion of 700 gm of licorice over a period of one week (13).

Table 1
**SODIUM CONTENT OF MEDICINALS —
SELECTED ADULT MEDICATIONS WITH AN
EXTRAORDINARILY HIGH SODIUM CONTENT
(50 mg/DOSE)**

Drug	Unit	mg Na/ unit
I. Parenteral Products		
Amcillin S	1 g/inj	62
Dynapen	63 mg/5 ml	67
Geopen	5 g	680
Keflin	1 g vial	62
Methicillin	1 g vial	55
Omnipen N	2 g vial	124
Penbritin-S	1 g vial	66
PenG Na (Squibb)	5 mu/vial	233
Polycillin	1 g vial	68
Principen N	1 g/inj	70
Prostaphlin	4 g vial	144
Staphcillin Buff	1 g vial	61
Unipen Inj.	1 g vial	73
II. Oral Liquids		
Dristan Cough Formula	5 ml	59
Phenergan Expectorant (plain or VC)	5 ml	51
Phospho-Soda	5 ml	554
Vicks Cough Syrup	5 ml	54
Vicks Formula 44 Syrup	5 ml	68
III. Oral Solid Dosage Forms		
Alka-Seltzer	tab	521
Bisodol Powder	10 g	1540
Bromo Seltzer	80 g/capful	717
Erythrocin Filmtab	250 mg	70
Fizrin	pkt	673
Kayexelate Powder	15 g	550
Nervine Effervescent	tab	544
Panteric Granules	teaspoonful	161
Pasna Pak Granules	6 g pkt	600
Pasna Tri-Park Granules	5.5 g pkt	490
Rolaids	tab	53
Sal Hepatica	rounded tsp	1000
Sodium Salicylate	10 gr tab	97
IV. Food Supplements		
Carnation Slender	10 oz can	440
Lytren	1 oz	189
Meritene Powder	1 oz	113
Vivonex-100	6 doses	2385
V. Miscellaneous		
Fleets Enema	4.5 oz	5000*

* Average absorption = 275-400 mg/enema. (25e,65c,101)

Lithium carbonate — Although the diuretic effect of this agent is well known, it is *occasionally* associated with sodium retention, edema, and rarely, CHF (17,88). It is important to note that a low sodium diet may result in retention of lithium (67).

Methyldopa — See guanethidine.

Osmotic agents — The rapid intravenous administration of slowly diffusable substances capable of exerting osmotic activity may result in acute volume overload and the exacerbation of congestive heart disease. Such agents include mannitol, albumin, urea, hypertonic glucose and/or saline.

Phenylbutazone — This drug may increase the blood volume by up to 50%. Several cases of CHF which have been exacerbated by this drug exist in the literature. (See *Rheumatoid Arthritis* chapter.)

Propranolol — See *Angina* chapter.

Salicylates — Large, anti-inflammatory doses of aspirin can cause vasodilation and dilution of blood with tissue fluids resulting in a decreased hematocrit and increased blood volume. These doses also cause sodium retention by a mechanism yet to be elucidated. This may become clinically significant in arthritics taking large, chronic doses of aspirin who also have underlying carditis (90). In a series of 50 arthritic patients, 9 (18%) developed symptoms of congestive heart failure after 3-8 days of therapy. Six of these cases were mild and of short duration (3). Salicylates containing large amounts of sodium should also be avoided in these patients.

Sodium Containing Drugs — See Table 1 (18). For antacids see *Peptic Ulcer Disease* chapter.

4. Discuss the pathogenesis of CHF. What are the compensatory mechanisms which develop in response to a failing myocardium?

When the heart begins to fail, the body puts into play several complex compensatory mechanisms in an attempt to maintain cardiac output and oxygenation of vital organs (10,16). These include cardiac dilatation, cardiac hypertrophy, an increased sympathetic tone, and sodium and water retention. An understanding of these compensatory mechanisms is essential to the understanding of the signs and symptoms of congestive heart failure. Most patients do not present in overt congestive failure but in some degree of compensated failure. Many of their symptoms, therefore, reflect the presence of these compensatory mechanisms.

Cardiac dilation results when the ventricles fail to pump the entire volume of blood with which they are presented. If the rate at which blood is delivered remains the same but the rate at which it is pumped to other tissues diminishes, it is apparent that a residual amount of blood will begin to accumulate in the ventricles. Thus, end diastolic volume increases, myocardial fibers are stretched, and the ventricle(s) become dilated. Within certain limits, the amount of pressure which can be exerted by a muscle fiber for a given degree of contraction increases as its length increases (Starling's Law). Therefore, even if the degree of fiber shortening remains unchanged, the volume of blood ejected with each contraction (cardiac output) increases in an enlarged ventricle. Theoretically, as cardiac dilatation progresses, cardiac output could decrease (descending limb of the Starling Curve), but this is rarely observed clinically.

Cardiac hypertrophy is a long-term adaptation to an increased diastolic volume and represents an absolute increase in muscle mass.

A diminished cardiac output (CO) results in decreased tissue perfusion. In an attempt to increase CO, there is a reflex **activation of sympathetic (SANS) tone.** Cardiac output increases as a result of the inotropic and chronotropic effects of the catecholamines. Also, there is vasoconstriction in the skin, gastrointestinal and renal circulation so that perfusion to vital organs (CNS and myocardium) is maintained. Both the decreased cardiac output of CHF and vasoconstriction secondary to sympathetic tone decrease renal blood flow. This in turn sets off a complex chain of events leading to **sodium and water retention** and eventually increased blood volume. Increased SANS tone increases renal vascular resistance and decreases glomerular filtration rate (GFR). As GFR decreases more sodium is reabsorbed in the proximal tubule. Additionally, glomerular filtrate may be preferentially shunted to nephrons with long loops on Henle thereby increasing the surface area for sodium reabsorption (10). Renin is released in response to decreased renal perfusion leading to a corresponding increase in angiotensin formation. Angiotensin has two effects favoring sodium and water retention: its vasoconstricting effects may further decrease GFR and it stimulates the secretion of aldosterone, a hormone which increases sodium reabsorption at the distal tubule. A diminished effective circulating plasma volume also stimulates the release of antidiuretic hormone (ADH) resulting in the subsequent retention of free water.

5. List the signs, symptoms, and laboratory abnormalities of congestive heart failure exhibited by this patient. Relate them to the pathogenesis of the disease and to right or left heart failure if possible.

The signs and symptoms of CHF are conveniently divided into those which are attributable to left ventricular failure and right ventricular failure. These are more easily understood if the student clearly understands the flow of blood through the heart and systemic circulation since congestion of blood occurs behind the failing ventricle. Symptoms of **left** heart failure then, can be attributed to the following.

(a) **Decreased tissue perfusion** results in weakness, fatigue, and cyanosis.

(b) There are symptoms related to the **presence of compensatory mechanisms.** An increased end diastolic volume produces **left ventricular hypertrophy** (LVH) and an S3 gallop. This may be observed on chest x-ray or diagnosed on the ECG. The point of maximal impulse (PMI) corresponding to the apex of the left ventricle is displaced laterally or downward. Its normal location is at the 5th intercostal space (ICS) less than 10 cm from the midsternal line (MSL). The increased sympathetic (SANS) tone is responsible for the **tachycardia,** sweating, pallor and cyanosis. In the recumbent position, SANS tone is diminished, renal perfusion is increased and edema fluid is mobilized, resulting in **nocturia.** Sodium and water retention cause **weight gain** and **edema.**

(c) **Shortness of breath (SOB), dyspnea on exertion (DOE),** a productive cough, rales, pleural effusions on x-ray and cyanosis are all due to **pulmonary congestion. Paroxysmal nocturnal dyspnea (PND)** or cardiac asthma is characterized by severe shortness of breath which awakens the patient from sleep. It is alleviated by an upright position. It results from pulmonary vascular congestion which is allowed to advance to pulmonary edema and bronchospasm. Pulmonary rales, pleural effusions and chest x-ray findings indicative of vascular congestion in the upper lung fields are also typical of left ventricular failure.

As left heart failure progresses, pulmonary venous pressure increases until the right ventricle is unable to empty completely. Pure right heart failure (RHF) or cor pulmonale may also occur following a pulmonary embolism or secondary to severe pulmonary disease. Symptoms of **right** heart failure can be related to systemic venous hypertension and hypervolemia. These include the following.

(a) **Dependent pitting edema** results from increased venous and capillary hydrostatic pressure which causes a redistribution of fluid from the intravascular to interstitial spaces. Ankle and pretibial edema are common findings in ambulatory patients because fluid tends to localize in the dependent portions of the body secondary to gravitational forces. **Sacral edema** may be present in patients at bed rest.

(b) **Hepatomegaly,** hepatic tenderness, and ascites result from hepatic congestion and increased portal pressure.

(c) Congestion of the gastrointestinal tract makes the patient **anorexic.**

(d) Increased jugular venous pressure (JVP) results in **jugular venous distention** (JVD). Normally there is no JVD when the patient is sitting at a 30 degree angle. The presence of **hepatojugular reflux** (HJR) is also indicative of an increased JVP. The HJR is positive if there is JVD when pressure is applied over the liver for 1 minute.

6. What therapeutic maneuvers and drugs are used in the management of congestive heart failure? What is the rationale for their use? What is the goal of therapy?

The medical management of congestive heart failure includes correction of underlying disease states (e.g. hypertension), bed rest, a sodium restricted diet, digitalis glycosides and diuretics (16). More recently, vasodilators have been used to manage CHF unresponsive to traditional therapy. See Question 28. The ultimate goal of therapy is to abolish disabling symptoms and improve the quality of the patient's life. None of the aforementioned measures are curative and it has been dishearteningly demonstrated that despite treatment, the five year survival of these patients is not prolonged (41).

Bedrest or restriction of physical activity decreases the metabolic demands of the failing heart and minimizes gravitational forces contributing to the formation of edema. Renal perfusion is also increased in the prone position resulting in diuresis and eventual mobilization of edema fluid.

A **sodium restricted diet** may be instituted to decrease blood volume and to offset the abnormal renal retention of sodium observed in congestive heart failure. If the ability of the kidney to excrete sodium is not severely compromised, it is possible to approach normal balance by restricting the intake of sodium to match excretion. Even though less than one gram is required to meet physiologic needs, the normal American diet contains 10 grams of sodium chloride. A severely salt restricted diet (less than 500 mg Na or 1.3 gm NaCl is unpalatable and poorly adhered to. Dietary sodium can be cut to 2-4 gm of NaCl by eliminating cooking salt. This diet is much more reasonable from the patient's point of view in that it is much more palatable and therefore more easily adhered to. It is convenient to remember that 1 gram of sodium is equivalent to 2.5 grams of salt (NaCl) and that one level teaspoonful of salt weighs approximately 6 grams.

As mentioned previously, the two major drug classes used in the management of CHF are digitalis glycosides and diuretics. Correction of the underlying defect is the most rational approach to the treatment of any disease. Therefore, digitalis which improves cardiac contractility, cardiac output, and renal perfusion represents a rational choice in the pharmacologic management of congestive heart failure. Not infrequently, the edema of moderate to severe cases of CHF may be unresponsive to therapeutic doses of digitalis and sodium restriction. To the extent that excessive volume may be increasing the workload of a compromised heart, diuretics may be useful. Additionally, if volume overload is symptomatic (e.g. pulmonary congestion, venous stasis and thrombosis of the extremities), diuretics should be initiated. It is important to emphasize that vigorous diuretic therapy carries the risk of volume depletion and diminished cardiac output.

7. What are the goals of diuretic therapy in a congestive heart failure patient?

Initially, the goal of diuretic therapy is to remove the

edema without causing intravascular depletion. The rate at which edema can be removed is limited by its rate of mobilization from the interstitial to the intravascular fluid compartment. Therefore, if diuresis is too vigorous intravascular volume depletion may result (24). Various authors have proposed that diuretics be administered on an intermittent basis so that periods of diuresis are followed by rest periods during which diuretic-induced volume and electrolyte changes are given an opportunity to recover. Intermittent dosing may take the form of every other day therapy, single daily dose therapy, or several consecutive days of therapy followed by short rest periods (26,45,73). Such regimens, of course, must be individualized to the patient's response which is measured by monitoring the improvement of signs and symptoms, weight changes, as well as fluid intake and output. Once edema is removed, therapy is aimed at maintaining sodium balance in such a way that reaccumulation does not occur. A program of moderate sodium restriction coupled with diuretic and digitalis therapy generally results.

8. Which diuretics are used for the treatment of CHF? What factors must be considered in the selection and use of diuretic agents in the CHF patient?

Thiazide diuretics are the most commonly employed diuretic agents in the management of congestive heart failure. Aside from differences in duration of action, at maximum therapeutic doses there is essentially no difference in potency or toxicity among these compounds (23). The choice of agent within this class, therefore, is governed primarily by cost and bioavailability. Hydrochlorothiazide, for example, is much better absorbed than is chlorothiazide (see Edema chapter).

The effectiveness of diuretics is dependent upon the amount of sodium delivered to their site of action. Proximal tubular reabsorption of sodium is increased in patients with congestive heart failure, and in some instances the avidity for sodium at this site may render thiazide diuretics minimally effective. In these cases the use of furosemide or ethacrynic acid, which work more proximally than the thiazides should be considered (24). Used alone, spironolactone and triamterene are weak diuretics and are minimally effective in the treatment of symtomatic edema (9). However, their effects are additive with the thiazides and they are sometimes used in lieu of potassium supplementation.

Loop diuretics (ethacrynic acid and furosemide) are the only agents which may be effective in the presence of any significant degree of renal failure (serum creatinine 3-8 mg percent) (26). This may be due to their ability to decrease renal vascular resistance and redistribute renal blood flow. It should be pointed out, however, that in the long run these agents are also

capable of inducing azotemia secondary to contraction of the vascular volume and decreased glomerular filtration rate.

Spironolactone and triamterene should be avoided in patients with renal failure (BUN 40 mg percent) since hyperkalemia may develop from their use (26).

Diuretic therapy is considered in great detail in the Edema chapter.

9. Examine the laboratory values in Case History A. Which of the abnormal values listed may be attributed to hydrochlorothiazide? Are any of these significant in a patient taking digitalis?

The mild hypochloremic alkalosis and hypokalemia observed in this patient are quite likely a result of thiazide therapy which has not been supplemented with potassium chloride (24). Hypokalemia predisposes to digitalis toxicity and is of particular concern in a patient who is to be given a loading dose of digitalis. Vigorous diuresis may also produce absolute hyponatremia; however, in this patient dilutional hyponatremia secondary to abnormal sodium and water retention is a more likely explanation (note presence of edema). Magnesium depletion also predisposes to digitalis toxicity and can be a complication of long term diuretic therapy (4,74,85). Also see Question 25.

Mild hyperglycemia and asymptomatic hyperuricemia are most likely related to thiazides (24) (see chapters on Edema; Diabetes).

10. The patient is to be given a digitalis preparation. What effects does digitalis have on the heart? How does it improve a patient with congestive heart failure?

Digitalis has two major pharmacologic actions on the heart. The first is that of increasing the force of contraction of both the normal and abnormal heart (inotropic effect). Although the mechanism of this effect has not been clarified, it is currently thought that digitalis enhances excitation contraction coupling by releasing free calcium ions within the cardiac cell. Free intracellular calcium potentiates the interaction of actin and myosin, the major contractile proteins of muscle tissue (47,50,82). Digitalis also has electrophysiologic effects on the heart which appear to be distinctly separate from and independent of its positive inotropic effects (50a,62,99). The mechanism of these effects is also unclear but is thought to be due to an inhibition of the sodium pump which maintains intracellular electronegativity by actively transporting sodium out of the cell (47,48,82). The electrophysiologic effects of digitalis vary in different areas of the heart and are also modified by the vagotonic actions of the drug. These effects account for the therapeutic effectiveness of digitalis in the treatment of rapid atrial rhythms associated with rapid ventricular response (80). (See *Cardiac Arrhythmias* chapter). Additionally, disturbances in conduction and rhythm observed with toxic doses are mediated through alteration of the myocardium's electrical function.

Although the final experimental evidence is lacking, it appears that these two effects of digitalis are independent of each other and this fact has several important clinical implications: (a) the practice of dosing a patient to toxicity to achieve the therapeutic benefits of inotropism is invalid since enhanced contractility may be observed before toxicity is reached (44,99); (b) suppression of digitalis induced arrhythmias does not simultaneously obliterate the inotropic effect of the drug; and (c) because inotropic effects are observed at low doses of digitalis, patients who are sensitive to the toxic effect of the drug may still benefit from doses which were previously considered subtherapeutic (62).

Digitalis increases the force of contraction of the failing heart. As a result, cardiac output is increased and the compensatory mechanisms previously outlined are no longer required. End diastolic volume is decreased and heart size is reduced. Elevated venous pressure and pulmonary congestion are also eventually alleviated. As tissue perfusion improves, sympathetic tone is lowered to normal levels. Subsequently, diuresis and a drop in heart rate are observed. Because it improves the primary defect which led to the development of the syndrome, digitalis represents a rational choice in the pharmacologic management of congestive heart failure (16,80).

Both the vagal and direct effects of digoxin account for its suppression of conduction in the AV node. The decreased conduction velocity and prolonged refractory periods in this area of the heart are the basis for the prolonged PR interval which may be observed following digitalis therapy. Conduction in the ventricles is enhanced giving rise to a shortened QT interval. Refractory periods are also decreased so that the tissue is more vulnerable to ectopic beats. At the same time digitalis suppresses the automaticity of normal pacemakers, it increases the automaticity within the atria and ventricles giving rise to ectopic pacemakers. (15,33,82).

11. What are the therapeutic endpoints of digitalis therapy? How is a patient on digitalis monitored?

As noted previously (Question 10), the practice of dosing a patient to toxicity and then "backing off" is both dangerous and irrational.

For years, clinicians have been plagued by the fact that no sharp therapeutic endpoint exists for digitalis therapy. Nonspecific ECG changes (ST depression and T wave abnormalities and shortening of the QT interval) do not correlate with toxic or therapeutic effects of the drug (15,80). In general, the clinician must look for improvement of signs and symptoms. The patient begins to subjectively and objectively improve; he is less dyspneic and complains of less orthopnea; venous distension and signs of pulmonary congestion diminish or disappear; diuresis (monitored through urinary output; weight loss) and diminished heart rate may be observed, although the response of heart rate to digitalis may be variable depending upon the patient's underlying disease. Ankle edema does not mobilize immediately and is a poor therapeutic endpoint to use (15,64).

Although digoxin and digitoxin levels are currently available a "therapeutic level" has not been clearly defined. It has been observed that most patients who are taking digitalis and are not digitalis toxic have serum levels in the range of 0.5-2.0 ng/ml (12,81,94). However, it is important to remember that inotropic effects occur with very small doses so that clinical evaluation ultimately remains the best therapeutic guide.

12. What baseline information should be obtained prior to the administration of digitalis?

Before a patient is given a loading dose of digitalis, it is essential to ascertain whether or not the patient has taken any form of digitalis within the past two to three weeks. Dissipation of digitalis activity may require days to weeks depending upon the half-life of the particular digitalis preparation ingested. It is apparent that the loading dose will have to be decreased if the patient already has some digitalis remaining in his body (see Question 23 for sample calculations).

Cardiac arrhythmias may be the only sign of digitalis toxicity. Therefore, a baseline electrocardiogram is essential if the clinician is to distinguish between a cardiac arrhythmia arising from digitalis toxicity and that resulting from underlying heart disease.

Finally, the clinician should be cognizant of the presence of any disease states, drugs, or physiologic disturbances which could increase the patient's susceptibility to digitalis intoxication (see Question 25). It is worthwhile to determine serum potassium levels and to correct deficiencies prior to therapy. Renal function should also be evaluated if the digitalis preparation to be administered is dependent upon the kidney for its elimination (15).

13. A 58-year-old male is admitted for elective cholecystectomy. He also has a three year history of CHF which has been well controlled with digoxin 0.25 mg daily. After surgery, the patient is placed on an NPO regimen and is given digoxin by the intramuscular (IM) route. On hospital day 3 the patient

experiences **severe pressing chest pain which radiates to his left arm. An ECG is done and serial serum enzymes are ordered to rule out MI. Comment.**

Patients who are hospitalized and placed on a nothing by mouth (NPO) regimen are frequently given medications by the parenteral route. There is some evidence for the delayed or incomplete absorption of intramuscular digoxin; its availability appears intermediate between that of IV and PO digoxin (11,28). Doses should be adjusted downward by 20% if the patient is to receive the drug by this route for more than one or two doses.

There are few indications for the use of IM digoxin. Absorption from the injection site is poor, and when equivalent doses are administered, the urinary recovery of digoxin is 17% higher from intravenous injections when compared to the intramuscular route.

Additionally, peak serum levels following IM injection are actually lower and occur later than comparable oral doses (22); serum-tissue equilibration requires 10-12 hours as opposed to the 6 hours required for the oral route. Greenblatt (27) noted that IM injection of undiluted digoxin was consistently followed by intense muscular pain and fasciculations. Pain was disabling for two hours and subsided over the next several hours; however local tenderness and pain on motion persisted for two days. Digoxin-induced creatine phosphokinase (CPK) elevations are of great importance in this patient. Although any IM injection can cause mild elevations of serum CPK (2-6X), digoxin can increase control levels by 15-17 times 8 hours after its injection (27).

The intravenous route is the preferred parenteral method of administration. However caution is warranted when digoxin is given intravenously. Too rapid administration may result in acute myocardial toxicity caused by a direct effect of the drug. Additionally, the commercially available preparaton contains 40% propylene glycol; rapid administration of this cardiotoxic compound may also result in acute myocardial depression. It is therefore recommended that the commercial preparation be given at a maximum rate of 1cc per minute, or preferably that it be diluted with 10cc of normal saline for injection and then administered as a slow infusion (27).

14. A 62-year-old male with a one year history of congestive heart failure is examined in the clinic. Although previously well controlled on a sodium restricted diet and digoxin 0.25 mg, he has become progressively dyspneic and edematous over the past month. A repeat digoxin level is reportedly 0.3 ng/ml. A digoxin level taken previously was 0.7 ng/ml. What are some explanations for these events?

Patient compliance must definitely be taken into consideration. Weintraub et al (96) determined that the mean serum digoxin concentration for noncompliant patients was 0.7 ng/ml while that for compliant patients was 1.2 ng/ml. Scheiner et al (77) found that serum digoxin levels were lower in out-patients than in in-patients. They postulate that this difference may be attributable to poor compliance. Thirty-four percent of the patients in the first study cited were noncompliant, but this was felt to be a conservative figure since the patient's word was taken as fact. Those patients taking two or more drugs were less likely to comply.

Digoxin bioavailability should also be considered. Since the prescription is written generically, it is quite possible that the patient received a less bioavailable brand the last time he filled his prescription. Variability in the bioavailability of digoxin preparations has been the subject of several reports (28,34,56,87,94,95). Wagner points out the difficulties in comparing the results of these studies. Among these are the differences in methods, sampling times, and standards for comparison. Several articles (72,87,94) discuss the major pitfalls in designing bioavailability studies. It is not surprising therefore, that there are conflicting reports of digoxin bioavailability in the literature. Nevertheless, it is possible to make some generalizations. The availability by the intravenous route is greater than or equal to that of the intramuscular route (28); oral administration of the solution produces higher serum levels than does administration of the tablets. The fraction of drug available (F) from the intramuscular injection varies from 0.7-1.0 (22,28); that of the solution varies from 0.65-0.9 (20,22,37); and that of the tablet varies from 0.5-0.8 (22,34). The average F for the tablets is 0.62 and it is 0.77 for the elixir (34a). Additionally, it has been demonstrated that the availability of oral tablets varies from manufacturer to manufacturer (56) and in some instances from lot to lot. It should be pointed out that although this study is highly suggestive of inter-manufacturer variability, that it unequivocally demonstrates only differences in *rate,* not *extent* of absorption. The studies of Greenblatt et al (28) show a high correlation between the area under the serum concentration vs eight hour time curve and the more valid urinary excretion methods. Variations in manufacturing techniques can alter the dissolution rates and bioavailability of these products (76,89,94). Until FDA specifications are clearly defined, it is suggested that the clinician use the Lanoxin brand of digoxin.

Other patient factors (diseases and drugs) may diminish the bioavailability of digoxin and should also be considered (see Question 15).

Altered digoxin metabolism is rare but should be considered. Luchi et al (59) report a patient who required 1.0-2.0 mg digoxin daily to control atrial fibrillation. Although her half-life for digoxin was the same as the controls, she metabolized a greater percent of digoxin to cardioinactive products.

Concurrent metabolic abnormalities may decrease the responsiveness to digoxin. **Hypocalcemia** has been reported as a cause of digitalis resistance (15b) as has **hyperthyroidism** (see chapter on *Diseases of the Thyroid*).

15. What factors alter the availability of digoxin?

Administration of digoxin with **meals** affects the rate but not the extent of absorption (72,98). That is, the peak concentrations are lower and delayed but the steady state serum concentrations are equivalent.

Alteration of the absorption of digoxin following oral administration in patients with **malabsorption** syndromes has also been studied (31). It was found that poor and erratic absorption occurred in patients with malabsorption states such as sprue, short-bowel syndrome and rapid intestinal transit. Mean steady state serum levels for 0.25 mg digoxin daily were significantly less than those of controls (0.4 vs 1.2 ng/ml). This difference was even more significant in view of the fact that the malabsorbers had a much lower mean body weight (31). Hall et al (30) also studied digoxin bioavailability in malabsorptive states but were unable to demonstrate large differences in serum digoxin concentrations. Their patients were administered a more soluble form of digoxin and their malabsorbers had poorer renal function than did the controls.

Antacids and **kaolin-pectin** decreased the bioavailability of a single dose of digoxin (0.75 mg) in normal subjects (10a). Sixty ml doses of aluminum hydroxide, magnesium hydroxide, magnesium trisilicate, and kaolin-pectin taken concurrently with tablets of digoxin (Lanoxin) decreased the six-day total urinary excretion. The percents of total dose recovered were as follows: control-40%; aluminum hydroxide-30.7%; magnesium hydroxide-27%; magnesium trisilicate-29%; and kaolin-pectin-23%.

Bowel hypermotility secondary to **laxatives** may result in low steady state digoxin levels. A single case is reported in the studies of Heizer et al (31). The effect of **neomycin** on digoxin absorption was studied by Lindenbaum et al (55). They found that single doses of neomycin (0.1-3 gms) administered in conjunction with digoxin depressed and delayed peak serum concentrations. Steady state serum concentrations of digoxin when administered daily with 2 gms neomycin for 8 days were significantly lower than those achieved when digoxin was given alone (e.g. 0.82 ng/cc vs 0.58 ng/cc). Nonabsorbable bile acid binding resins (Cholestyramine; Cuemid; Questran and a polymer of tetraethylene pontamine, Colestipol) bind both digoxin and digitoxin. Digoxin does not bind as extensively as does digitoxin. *In vitro* studies in the pres-

ence of duodenal juice show that 1 mg of cholestyramine binds 2.8 ± 0.42 ng. Once absorbed, digoxin probably does not undergo sufficient enterohepatic circulation for cholestyramine to alter steady state serum levels (1b). This has been confirmed by the *in vivo* studies of Hall et al (30a) which indicate that chronic cholestyramine therapy produces only a small increase in the stool output of digoxin. However, Bigger and Strauss (7) logically recommend that administration of digoxin precede that of the resin by 1½ hours.

Sulfasalazine (39d) and **phenytoin** (49a) have also been reported to decrease the bioavailability of digoxin.

16. Discuss the clinical significance and basis for the interaction of digitoxin with other drugs.

Digitoxin differs from digoxin in several respects (see Question 18). These differences become important when considering drug interactions with digitalis preparations. Unlike digoxin, a significant fraction of digitoxin is metabolized to more polar compounds which are readily excreted into urine and bile. Thus, drugs which induce hepatic enzymes (e.g. phenylbutazone [PBZ], phenytoin [DPH], and phenobarbital [PB]) can theoretically increase the metabolic degradation rate of digitoxin. Solomon et al (86) noted that steady state serum levels of digitoxin were lower in two patients. One was ingesting PBZ, the other DPH along with the digitoxin. The ingestion of PB (60 mg tid x 12 weeks) lowered serum digitoxin levels by 50%. Doses of 60 mg qid for 8 weeks decreased the plasma half life by 25%. Patients taking any of these drugs in combination with digitoxin may require higher doses of the latter. Conversely, if these drugs are discontinued, the patient should be monitored for emerging digitalis toxicity.

Digitoxin is protein bound to a greater degree than digoxin (97% vs. 23%) (83). *In vitro* experiments have demonstrated that high concentrations of drugs which also have a high affinity for albumin (PBZ, clofibrate, warfarin, tolbutamide, sulfadimethoxine) are capable of displacing digitoxin from proteins. Therapeutic doses of these drugs do not produce levels which displace digitoxin to a significant extent (7).

Twenty-five percent of a given dose of digitoxin enters the enterohepatic circulation (20). Thus drugs which interrupt enterohepatic recycling by binding digitoxin in the GI tract and preventing its reabsorption may shorten its half life and lower steady state serum concentrations of the drug. On this basis anion exchange resins (Colestipol and Cholestyramine) have been administered to patients who have taken overdoses of digitoxin (1b). These investigators found that the administration of Colestipol (10 gm initially followed by 5 gm every 6 hours) shortened the plasma half life of digitoxin from 9.3 days to an average of 2.75 days. Additionally, clinical signs of toxicity disappeared in 24-30 hours in treated patients whereas symptoms of toxicity persisted for 3 days in the untreated controls. Cholestyramine would be expected to have effects similar to that of Colestipol but to a lesser degree. *In vitro* studies indicate that duodenal juice decreased the binding capacity of cholestyramine for digitoxin.

17. Both the liver and the gastrointestinal tract are congested in patients with heart failure. Does the patient with CHF absorb or metabolize drugs any differently than do normal subjects?

There are very few studies which directly address this question. Some drugs which have been studied include digitoxin, lidocaine and quinidine.

There may be only a slight delay in the absorption or no difference in the absorption of *digitalis* in a patient with CHF when compared to that of a normal subject (64).

The half-life of *lidocaine* is prolonged in patients with CHF. Both the volume of distribution and plasma clearance of the drug may be decreased in these patients so that the loading and maintenance doses will have to be adjusted (92) (also see chapter on *Cardiac Arrhythmias*).

The volume of distribution and clearance of *quinidine* appear to be decreased by 30-40% in patients with CHF (16a), although the half-life is generally unchanged (16a, 42). For this reason, both the loading and maintenance doses of quinidine should be empirically decreased in patients with CHF. Since the data are incomplete, subsequent dose adjustments should be made on the basis of clinical evaluation of the patient, ECG's and serum levels.

The half life and clearance of *theophylline* appear to be decreased in patients with CHF (31a,39c) in that usual doses produce unexpectedly high serum levels and symptoms of toxicity in this group of patients. (Also see chapter on *Asthma*).

18. What are the major pharmacokinetic differences between the most commonly used digitalis preparations: digoxin, digitoxin, digitalis leaf, deslanoside, and ouabain? (17,79)

Digoxin is a polar glycoside which is adequately but incompletely absorbed. The absorption of liquid preparations is virtually complete (80-90%) whereas that of oral tablets varies from 50%-85% (see Question 14). The rapid onset of action (30-60 minutes) of digoxin corresponds with peak plasma levels. Maximum effects from a single dose are observed 5-6 hours after administration, a time when distribution is virtually complete. Digoxin has a volume of distribution of 290

L/m² or approximately 7.3 L/kg lean body weight (69). Only 23% is protein bound (83). Digoxin has an intermediate half life between ouabain and digitoxin of 1.8 days and elimination is by first order kinetics (48b,82). Thirty-five percent of the total amount of drug in the body will be eliminated in a 24 hour period. Glomerular filtration of unchanged drug is the primary route of elimination (20% daily). Non-renal mechanisms, primarily hepatic metabolism, are responsible for the daily elimination of 14% (37). Very little digoxin (6.8%) enters the enterohepatic circulation (20).

Digitoxin—is the least polar and most lipid soluble of the glycosides discussed. It has the slowest onset of action (1-2 hours) and peak effect (4-12 hours) and the longest half life (5-7 days) of all the digitalis glycosides (20,73,89). Only 11.4% of the total body stores are eliminated daily (39). It is more completely absorbed (100%) than is digoxin and undergoes enterohepatic circulation to a greater degree (26%). Digitoxin is 90-95% protein bound (83). Its elimination occurs primarily via hepatic metabolism and renal excretion of metabolic by-products, 92% of which are inactive and 8% of which are active. Digoxin is the major active metabolite.

Digitalis leaf—USP digitalis leaf is composed primarily of three glycosides: digitoxin, gitoxin, and gitalin. Digitoxin is the most important of these compounds and is responsible for the majority of the pharmacologic activity of the mixture. The onset and duration of action of digitalis leaf are therefore identical to that of digitoxin. The use of powdered digitalis leaf has been largely replaced by the purified crystalline preparations (digoxin; digitoxin). More accurate standardization of active drug content and an insignificant difference in cost have made these latter preparations the agents of choice.

Ouabain—Ouabain has the most rapid onset (5-10 minutes) and shortest half life (21 hours) of the digitalis glycosides. Its peak effects occur in 30-120 minutes.

Ouabain is absorbed very poorly from the gastrointestinal tract and is therefore only available for intravenous use. Like all the digitalis glycosides, its elimination from the body follows first-order kinetics. Because the kidneys comprise the primary route of excretion for ouabain, a decrease in renal function will result in a decrease in its rate of elimination and a prolonged half life (73,79). The kinetics of ouabain in patients with varying degrees of renal dysfunction have not been extensively studied and definitive data are not available. It might be best, therefore, to avoid its use in such patients.

The clinical situations in which ouabain would be the glycoside of choice are rather limited. The time to onset of action and peak effect following an intravenous dose of ouabain is not a great deal shorter than is that for digoxin. In most circumstances where prompt action is required, digoxin will suffice. Ouabain is the agent of choice in the relatively rare case where a few minute's delay in increasing cardiac output would be life threatening.

Deslanoside—Deslanoside is almost identical to digoxin in chemical structure. Unlike digoxin, however, it is very poorly absorbed from the gastrointestinal tract and is therefore recommended only for parenteral use. The elimination half life (33 hours), time to onset of action (10-30 minutes) and peak effect (1-2 hours) of deslanoside are not significantly different from those of digoxin. Deslanoside offers no real advantages over digoxin (79).

NOTE: The pharmacokinetic parameters for digoxin and formulas useful for individualized dosing regimens are summarized in Table 2. These will be referred to in Questions 19-23.

Table 2: Summary of Pharmacokinetic Parameters for Digoxin

Half-life	1.5-2 days (closer to 2 days)
Bioavailability(F)	
Tablets	0.62 (0.5-0.85)
Elixir	0.77
Volume of Distribution(Vd)	290 L/m² or 7.3 L/kg
Usual safe digitalizing dose (adults)	0.01-0.02 mg/kg
Therapeutic levels	0.5-2.0 ng/ml (varies from lab to lab)

19. A 50-year-old, 70 kg male is found to have mild congestive heart failure on a routine medical check up. Electrolytes and renal function are within normal limits and a baseline ECG is obtained. The patient is to be treated with digoxin. Compute the patient's digitalizing and maintenance dose.

Normally, a loading (digitalizing) dose is administered when a patient is initiated on digitalis preparations. This corresponds to the total amount of drug which has accumulated in the body at steady state (Ab). Determination of the loading dose is highly empirical and frequently depends upon the clinical experience of the clinician. However several methods may be used to determine the digitalizing dose. In all cases, an assessment of the patient is essential.

Method I. The digitalizing or loading dose (LD) may be estimated using the patient's weight. Jelliffe (38) notes that an oral digitalizing dose ranging from 0.01-0.02 mg/kg produces therapeutic levels and carries a minimal risk for toxicity. The incidence of arrhythmias rose to 30-40% when total body glycoside stores were greater than 0.03 mg/kg. Since the patient has mild CHF it is reasonable to start with a low dose.

$$\text{Digitalizing Dose} = 0.01 \text{ mg/kg} \times 70 \text{ kg} = 0.7 \text{ mg}$$

The maintenance dose (MD) simply replaces that amount of drug which is lost in one dosing interval (τ) which is one day in the case of digoxin. Using a formula derived by Jeliffe (36), it is possible to estimate the percent of the loading dose which is lost per day:

$$\text{\% eliminated daily} = 14 + \frac{\text{Ccr}}{5}$$

where 14 represents the fraction of digoxin eliminated by the metabolic route and Ccr/5 or creatinine clearance/5 represents the fraction eliminated by the kidneys. Since this patient's renal function is normal, we can assume his Ccr is 100 ml/min. The fraction of the loading dose which is lost daily would therefore be approximately 35% and the maintenance dose (MD) would be 0.25 mg daily:

$$
\begin{aligned}
\text{MD} &= \text{LD} \times \text{fraction lost daily} \\
&= 0.7 \text{ mg} \times 0.35 \\
&= 0.25 \text{ mg daily}
\end{aligned}
$$

Method II. Based on his or her clinical experience, the clinician may arbitrarily decide that a maintenance dose of **x** mg would resolve the patient's symptoms. Let us assume that the therapeutic maintenance dose for this patient is felt to be 0.125 mg daily. Then 0.125 mg represents 35% of the digitalizing dose:

$$
\begin{aligned}
\text{Digitalizing Dose} &= \frac{\text{Maintenance Dose}}{\text{Fraction eliminated daily}} \\
&= \frac{0.125 \text{ mg}}{0.35} \\
&= 0.35 \text{ mg}
\end{aligned}
$$

Method III. Finally, the digitalizing dose may be based upon the serum level one wishes to achieve. For example, let us assume that the clinician wishes to achieve a steady state plasma digoxin concentration of 1.0 mcg/L. Then, using Eq. 5 in the *Clinical Pharmacokinetics* chapter, it is possible to estimate the loading dose required to attain this level:

$$\text{Loading Dose (LD;Ab)} = \frac{Vd \times Cp}{F}$$

If digoxin is to be administered orally, the loading dose for this patient would be:

$$
\begin{aligned}
\text{LD} &= \frac{7.3 \text{ L/kg} \times 70 \text{ kg} \times 1.0 \text{ mcg/L}}{0.62} \\
&= 824 \text{ mcg or } 0.82 \text{ mg}
\end{aligned}
$$

Again, if one assumes that the patient eliminates 35% of the total amount of digoxin in his body each day (see Method I), the maintenance dose would be:

$$
\begin{aligned}
\text{MD} &= 0.82 \text{ mg} \times 0.35 \\
&= 0.287 \text{ mg daily}
\end{aligned}
$$

Since all of the pharmacokinetic parameters used above are based upon average literature values, an approximation of this maintenance dose can be given by alternating a dose of 0.25 mg with 0.375 mg (average 0.312 mg daily).

Alternatively, one can calculate the MD based upon an estimate of **digoxin clearance.** This can be computed in two ways. By rearranging Eq. 13 in the *Clinical Pharmacokinetics* chapter, one can see that clearance (Cl) is equal to the product of the elimination rate constant (Kd) and the volume of distribution (Vd):

$$Cl = KdVd$$

Kd is equal to 0.693/t½ (see Eq. 15 in *Clinical Pharmacokinetics* chapter). If it is assumed that this patient has a normal t½ (1.8 days) and an average Vd, his clearance would be:

$$Cl = \frac{0.693}{1.8 \text{ days}} \times 7.3 \text{ L/kg} \times 70 \text{ kg}$$
$$= 196.7 \text{ L/day}$$

Another method of estimating digoxin clearance is to use an equation derived by Koup et al (48a):

$$Cl_{digoxin} = 1.3 \times Ccr + 40 \text{ ml/min}$$

where (1.3 × Ccr) represents the renal clearance of digoxin and 40 ml/min represents the metabolic clearance of digoxin for a *70 kg man*. The value for the metabolic clearance may have to be decreased to 20 ml/min in patients with severe congestive heart failure. Also see Eq. 12 in *Clinical Pharmacokinetics* chapter. For this patient:

$$Cl_{digoxin} = 1.3 \times 100 \text{ ml/min} + 40 \text{ ml/min}$$
$$= 170 \text{ ml/min or } 244.8 \text{ L/day}$$

The units of L/day were obtained by multiplying 170 ml/min by 1440 min/day and dividing by 1000 ml/L.

To calculate the maintenance dose based upon the clearance for digoxin, use Eq. 10 in the *Clinical Pharmacokinetics* chapter:

$$MD = \frac{Cl \times Cpss \times \tau}{F}$$

Using the clearance value obtained by the first method (Eq. 15):

$$MD = \frac{197 \text{ L/day} \times 1.0 \text{ mcg/L} \times 1 \text{ day}}{0.62}$$
$$= 0.316 \text{ mg/day}$$

Using the clearance value obtained using koup et al's equation (Eq. 12):

$$MD = \frac{245 \text{ L/day} \times 1.0 \text{ mcg/L} \times 1 \text{ day}}{0.62}$$
$$= 0.395 \text{ mg/day}$$

It is apparent that there is some discrepancy in the various methods used to calculate the maintenance dose (0.287 mg *vs* 0.395 mg *vs* 0.316 mg). In the experience of clinicians practicing in the pharmacokinetics laboratory at the University of California, the equation derived by Koup et al tends to overestimate digoxin clearance. Since there is some evidence to suggest that the renal clearance of digoxin may vary between 0.4-1.8 times the creatinine clearance (29a), our consultants use a factor of 1.0 rather than 1.3 to predict a renal digoxin clearance. The principle used by Koup et al to calculate clearance appears to be the most valid since it obviates the need to estimate the volume of distribution which can vary widely among patients (40,48a,70). Jeliffe's approach is fallacious in that it inherently assumes that the Vd for all subjects is constant and it is now recognized that Vd's vary, especially in patients with renal failure. However, in general, his formula gives a reasonable first estimate in the actual clinical setting, and this may be related to the fact that his methods are derived from data garnered from congestive heart failure patients with and without renal failure rather than healthy subjects.

20. Assume that the above patient is to be given a digitalizing dose of 0.015 mg/kg. How rapidly should the dose be administered?

The speed with which a loading dose of digitalis is administered depends primarily on the clinical situation. Slow initiation of digitalis therapy with maintenance doses of digoxin (60) in lieu of a loading dose is considered the method of choice for ambulatory, non-acute patients with no renal dysfunction. Its main advantage over rapid digitalization is that it does not require continuous monitoring of the patient and is thus very suitable to the ambulatory care setting. The main disadvantage, however, is that a considerable length of time is required to accumulate maximum body glycoside stores and achieve therapeutic effects. Also, should the patient develop digitalis toxicity it would be more difficult to determine the exact amount of drug he has in his body. Additionally, changes in renal function will affect the time required to reach plateau.

The length of time required to achieve plateau concentrations of a drug administered on a routine basis at maintenance doses is dependent on the elimination half-life of that drug. It will take four half-lives to reach 93% of plateau levels. Thus, a patient with normal renal function placed on a daily dose of 0.25 mg of digoxin will require about 7.0 days to reach maximum glycoside concentrations (4 × 1.8 days = 7.2 days). However, if the same patient were anephric (t½ = 4.4 days) it would take 17 days to reach plateau and the maximum concentration would be approximately 2½ times that of a normal patient receiving the same dose.

If digitoxin were administered in such a manner it would require approximately 25 days to reach steady state in patients with normal kidney function and up to 45 days for patients with renal insufficiency. It is therefore impractical to digitalize patients with digitoxin in this manner.

When using the slow method of digitalization the clinician should remember to avoid increasing doses before maximum effects are observed. It would be fallacious to increase a patient's maintenance dose after three days, for example, if no clinical improvement were observed.

In this patient the daily maintenance dose which will be required to achieve a steady state glycoside store of 1.0 mg (0.015 mg/kg × 70 kg) is 0.35 mg (1.0 mg × 35% eliminated/day).

The patient should be very near steady state when he returns to the clinic in one week. These doses were not adjusted for oral availability, because the loading dose recommended by Jelliffe (10-20 mcg/kg) was based upon the *oral* dose ingested by patients to achieve therapeutic levels (39a).

21. A patient with moderate to severe CHF is admitted to the hospital for treatment. He is to be digitalized with 1.0 mg digoxin. How rapidly should he be digitalized? (Assume renal function is normal.)

Administration of the total loading dose of digitalis within a 24-hour period is probably the method of choice for hospitalized patients. This method has several advantages: the patient is very quickly brought to maximum therapeutic effect; symptoms of toxicity are less likely to be delayed, more likely to be observed and more easily correlated to drug concentrations within the body; and diminished renal function does not affect the time required to reach maximum drug level and therapeutic effect.

An initial dose of 0.5 mg should be given. Six to eight hours later the patient should be evaluated for clinical improvement and signs of digitalis toxicity. If none exist he should be given a dose of 0.25 mg. In another six hours he should again be evaluated for signs of toxicity and if there are no contraindications a final dose of 0.25 mg should be administered. Thus, within a 12-hour period the patient has been digitalized to a level of one mg. Each fraction of the digitalizing dose is separated by a six hour period so that tissue distribution can occur. Additionally, one should be able to observe the full clinical effects of the preceding dose if this dosing interval is used (70,95a).

Daily losses should be replaced by administration of a daily maintenance dose in order to sustain this level of digitalization (one mg). Since 35% of digoxin is eliminated each day in patients with normal renal function, the daily maintenance dose for this patient would be 0.35 mg. The above regimen could be administered either parenterally or orally. If the digitalizing dose is administered intravenously then one would have to increase the *oral* maintenance dose to account for its poor availability (e.g. oral M.D = 0.35 mg/62% absorbed).

If the patient presented here had developed signs and symptoms of digitalis toxicity after receiving a total dose of only 0.75 mg, further digoxin administration would have been discontinued. Assuming that the drug had been administered properly, we would now know that this patient becomes digitalis toxic when the total amount in his body is 0.75 mg. In the future, it would be possible to avoid any therapeutic regimen which resulted in body glycoside stores of 0.75 mg or more.

22. A 50-year-old female with normal renal function is given 0.125 mg digoxin × 7 days. On a return clinic visit it is felt that she continues to have debilitating symptoms of CHF. Estimate her serum digoxin concentration (weight = 50 kg). If we wish to increase her serum concentration to 1.4 ng/ml, what will her new maintenance dose be?

Since this patient has been taking the same dose of digoxin for 7 days and since her renal function is normal, her digoxin level should be at steady state. Using Eq. 9 in the *Clinical Pharmacokinetics* chapter, one can estimate the average steady state serum concentration of a drug if the clearance and fraction absorbed are known:

$$\overline{C}pss = \frac{F \times Dose}{\tau \times Cl}$$

For this patient, the clearance for digoxin can be estimated to be (see Question 19):

$$Cl_{digoxin} = (1.0 \times 100 \text{ ml/min} + 20 \text{ ml/min}) \frac{50 \text{ kg}}{70 \text{ kg}}$$

$$= 85.7 \text{ ml/min or } 123 \text{ L/day}$$

Note that the metabolic clearance was adjusted for CHF and that the total clearance was adjusted for the weight of the patient. If a value of 0.7 is used for F, the $\overline{C}pss$ could then be estimated to be:

$$\overline{C}pss = \frac{0.7 \times 125 \text{ mcg}}{1 \text{ day} \times 123 \text{ L/day}}$$

$$= 0.71 \text{ mcg/L or ng/ml}$$

To increase her serum concentration to 1.4 ng/ml, one would simply double her maintenance dose. This is determined by setting up a proportionality equation:

$$\frac{Current \text{ MD}}{Current \text{ } \overline{C}pss} = \frac{New \text{ MD}}{Desired \text{ } \overline{C}pss}$$

If the clinician wishes to achieve a more rapid response, the patient could be given a loading dose to attain the higher serum concentration. Assuming the patient's current digoxin level is 0.7 mcg/L and the desired level is 1.4 mcg/L, a net increase of 0.7 mcg/L must be achieved. The Vd for this patient must be estimated before the oral loading dose which will be required to produce this increment can be estimated (see Question 10-Method III):

$$Vd = 7.3 \text{ L/kg} \times 50 \text{ kg} \times 365 \text{ L}$$

$$LD = \frac{0.7 \text{ mcg/L} \times 365 \text{ L}}{0.7}$$

$$= 365 \text{ mcg}$$

23. A 70 kg male whose CHF has been well controlled on digoxin 0.5 mg daily x 2 years is admitted with a 3 day history of intestinal flu. The patient is treated with fluid and electrolyte replacement. On the morning of hospital day 2 it is decided to digitalize the patient to his former level. The patient has not taken digoxin for 4 days. Calculate his current body stores of digoxin (Ab). What would the loading dose for this patient be? His creatinine clearance is 100 ml/min. Assume F (oral availability) = 0.7.

It is possible to calculate the maximum amount of digoxin stored in the body at steady state (i.e. just after he has taken a daily dose) using a modification of Eq. 9 in the *Clinical Pharmacokinetics* chapter (see Question 19-Method I):

$$Ab \text{ max} = \frac{(F)(Dose)}{\text{fraction eliminated daily}}$$

$$= \frac{0.7 \times 0.5 \text{ mg}}{0.35} = 1.00 \text{ mg}$$

The formula which describes the exponential elimination of digoxin is:

$$Ab = Ab \text{ max } e^{-kdt}$$

where (e^{-kdt}) represents the fraction remaining after time (t). Therefore the amount in his body on day 4 could be calculated in the following way:

$$Kd = \frac{0.693}{1.6 \text{ days}}$$

$$= 0.44 \text{ days}^{-1}$$

More simply, we could draw a line on semilog paper which represents the elimination of digoxin in this patient (see Fig. 1). After 1 day, 65% remains; after 4 days, only 18% remains. Therefore:

$$Ab = Ab \text{ max} \times 18\%$$
$$= 1.00 \text{ mg} \times 18\%$$
$$= 0.18 \text{ mg.}$$

The loading dose for this patient would then be the difference between Ab max and the amount in the body at 4 days.

$$1.00-0.18 \text{ mg} = 0.82 \text{ mg}$$

Two oral doses of 0.5 mg administered 6 hours apart, will approximate the calculated loading dose considering the fact that oral digoxin is not completely available. At the end of each six hour period, the patient should be evaluated for symptoms of digitalis toxicity. In six hours absorption and tissue distribution should be virtually complete so that one should be able to observe the full effects of the dose.

24. A 70-year-old, 70 kg male with a steady state serum creatinine of 1.5 mg% was admitted for management of moderate CHF which had not been previously controlled on digoxin 0.25 mg daily x 1 month. The object of therapy was to reach a level of 2.0

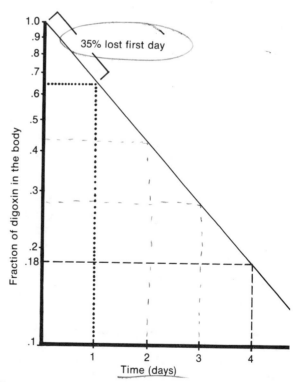

Figure 1: Graph representing the elimination of digoxin for a patient with normal renal function.

ng/ml. His hospital course was as follows:

| Hospital | | Digoxin | Digoxin |
Day	Time	Dose	Level
1	8A	—	1.12
1	9A	.25	
2	9A	.375	
3	9A	.375	
4	9A	.375	
5	8A	—	1.4 ng/ml
5	9A	.375	
6	9A	.375	
6	11A	—	3.4 ng/ml

A. Estimate this patient's creatinine clearance.

Jeliffe (39b) has derived a formula whereby the creatinine clearance (Ccr) may be estimated from the serum creatinine (Eq. 30 in the *Clinical Pharmacokinetics* chapter):

$$\text{Ccr (ml/min)} = \frac{98 - 0.8 \text{ (Age in years} - 20)}{\text{SrCr}}$$

The equation takes into consideration the decreased muscle mass which occurs with aging and estimates the Ccr for a 70 kg man. Therefore, values must be corrected for patients whose weights differ substantially from this standard. The value is also multiplied by a factor of 0.9 for women. The estimated Ccr for this patient is:

$$\text{Ccr} = \frac{98 - 0.8\,(70 - 20)}{1.5}$$

$$= 38.7 \text{ ml/min}$$

Also see Questions 60-65 in the *Clinical Pharmacokinetics* chapter.

B. Estimate this patient's half-life for digoxin. Assume no serum levels are available.

This patient's half-life may be estimated in two ways: graphically or by calculation. The graphical method first requires that one estimate the fraction of digoxin which the patient eliminates in one dosing interval (one day). This can be done using the Jeliffe formula discussed in Method I of Question 19:

% eliminated daily = 14 + Ccr/5
= 14 + 38.7/5
= 22%

If we know that 22% is lost in one day, then the line describing this patient's elimination of digoxin can be drawn on semilog graph paper using the following two points: (Time = 0, Amount = 1.0) and (Time = 1 day, Amount = 0.78). The half-life, then, is the time required for the amount to fall by 50%: 2.8 days. See Fig. 2.

The second method involves estimating the clearance and volume of distribution for digoxin in this pa-

tient. With these values, it is possible to estimate the t½ using Eq. 16 in the *Clinical Pharmacokinetics* chapter:

$$t\frac{1}{2} = \frac{Vd}{Cl} \times 0.693$$

The clearance can be estimated using a modified version of Koup et al's equation (see Method III, Question 19):

$$Cl_{digoxin} = 1.0 \times 38.7 \text{ ml/min} + 40 \text{ ml/min}$$
$$= 79 \text{ ml/min or } 114 \text{ L/day}$$

The volume of distribution and half-life of digoxin vary tremendously in patients with renal failure (Ccr less than 25 mls/min) (40, 48a, 70). Koup et al (48a) observed volumes of distribution ranging from 195-489 L/1.73 m² in seven renal failure patients; Reunig et al (7) calculated volumes of distribution for renal failure patients reported in the literature and found a range of 230 to 380 L/1.73 m², 30-50% less than that observed in

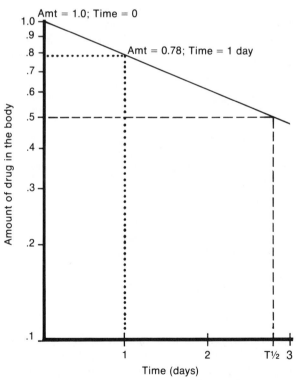

Figure 2: Estimation of half-life by the graphical method. See Question 24B.

subjects with normal renal function. It has been suggested by clinical pharmacokineticists at the University of California that an average value for Vd in renal failure patients (330 L/70 kg or 4.7 L/kg) be used. This patient's Ccr is above 25 ml/min which makes the Vd even more difficult to estimate. If it is assumed to be within normal limits (i.e. 7.3 L/kg), the Vd for digoxin in this patient would be 511 L. The estimated half-life using this patient's values would be:

$$t^{1/2} = \frac{511 \text{ L}}{114 \text{ L/day}} \times 0.693$$

$$= 3.1 \text{ days}$$

C. How long will it take for this patient to accumulate to plateau levels?

After four half-lives, the drug will have accumulated to 93% of its plateau levels. Therefore, approximately 12.0 days (4 x 2.8 days) will be required to reach steady state.

D. In view of the above calculations do you feel this patient was digitalized correctly?

Even though administration of the maintenance dose without a loading dose may appear to be a cautious approach, digitalizing a hospitalized patient or a patient with renal failure by the slow method of digitalization (see Question 20) is disadvantageous for several reasons (36):

(1) the time required to reach plateau levels is excessive and may be detrimental to the patient's health;

(2) if the patient's renal function fluctuates at all during the period of digitalization it will be difficult to estimate his body stores;

(3) if the patient fails to respond or develops toxicity during the period of accumulation, body stores will be difficult to estimate.

Jelliffe has stated that although the MD must be adjusted in patients with renal failure the loading dose remains the same (37). However, in view of the observation that the Vd in patients with severe renal failure may be decreased, this recommendation is no longer valid. A smaller estimate for the Vd should be used to calculate the loading dose for patients with a Ccr of 25 ml/min or less. A conservative estimate of Vd should be used for patients with moderate renal failure. After the loading dose has been administered and a serum level has been obtained, a more precise estimate of the patient's Vd can be made. At present, patients in renal failure should be digitalized with conservative doses of digoxin (e.g. 10 mcg/kg or less). Thereafter, dose adjustments should be based upon serum levels.

F. The objective of therapy is to achieve an average serum concentration (Cp_ave) of 2.0 ng/ml. How should

this patient be dosed to achieve this objective?

Since we know that the Cp_{min} produced by a daily dose of 0.25 mg is 1.12 ng/ml in *this* patient, we do not have to use literature estimates for Vd or F. From the formula for Cp_{min} it is possible to calculate the ratio of Vd/F for this patient. (Note: this formula for Cp_{min} was obtained by substituting Eq. 18 into Eq. 19 in the *Clinical Pharmacokinetics* chapter:

$$Cpss_{min} = \frac{F \times Dose \times Fraction\ remaining\ after\ \tau}{Vd \times Fraction\ eliminated\ in\ \tau}$$

$$Vd/F = \frac{250\ mcg \times 0.78}{1.12\ mcg/L \times 0.22}$$

$$= 791\ L$$

If the objective therapy is to achieve a $\overline{Cp}ss$ of 2.0 ng/ml, then the daily dose can be calculated by reorganizing Eq. 10 in the *Clinical Pharmacokinetics* chapter for the maintenance dose:

$$MD = \frac{Cl \times \overline{Cp}ss \times \tau}{F}$$

$$= \frac{Kd \times Vd \times \overline{Cp}ss \times \tau}{F}$$

$$= Vd/F \times \frac{0.693 \times \overline{Cp}ss \times \tau}{t^{1/2}}$$

$$= 791\ L \times \frac{0.693 \times 2.0\ mcg/L \times 1\ day}{2.8\ days}$$

$$= 391\ mcg\ or\ 0.391\ mg$$

To determine the loading dose, calculate Ab_{max} for a maintenance dose of 0.39 mg. See Eq. 18 in the *Clinical Pharmacokinetics* chapter:

$$Cpss_{max} = \frac{F}{Vd} \times \frac{Dose}{Fraction\ eliminated\ in\ \tau}$$

$$= \frac{1}{791\ L} \times \frac{391\ mcg}{0.22}$$

$$= 2.24\ mcg/L$$

$$Ab_{max} = Cpss_{max} \times \frac{Vd}{F}$$

$$= 2.24\ mcg/L \times 791\ L$$

$$= 1.77\ mg$$

However, the patient already has some digoxin in his body. The amount of drug in this patient's body at steady state just prior to the next dose of 0.25 mg can be calculated in the following way:

$$Ab_{min} = Cpss_{min} \times \frac{Vd}{F}$$

$$= 1.12 \text{ mcg/L} \times 791 \text{ L}$$

$$= 0.89 \text{ mg}$$

Therefore the loading dose for this patient should be the difference between these two values:

$$LD = 1.77 \text{ mg} - 0.89 \text{ mg}$$
$$= 0.88 \text{ mg}$$

This can be accomplished by administering 0.5 mg initially followed by 0.375 mg in six hours. It is assumed that this loading dose will be administered when plasma levels are at a minimum. This level can be maintained with a daily dose of 0.375 mg.

G. On hospital day five a serum level for digoxin was reported as 1.4 ng/ml. Based upon this observation, it was decided to increase the patient's dose to 0.375 mg daily. Was this a valid decision? Why or why not?

The decision was based upon the invalid assumption that 1.4 ng/ml was a reflection of the serum level which could be achieved by doses of 0.375 mg/day. As noted previously, without a loading dose digoxin will continue to accumulate and will not reach plateau levels for another 10 days.

H. A final digoxin level was drawn on the morning of hospital day seven. Clinically, the patient appeared much improved. The following day a level of 3.4 ng/ml was reported. How would you interpret this serum level?

This serum level was drawn only two hours after the dose was administered. Several investigators point out that complete equilibration between serum and tissue does not occur for 5-8 hours. Therefore serum levels taken within this period will not reflect tissue levels, nor will they correlate with any pharmacological or toxic effects of digoxin.

For further discussion of digoxin pharmacokinetics the reader is referred to the Clinical Pharmacokinetics chapter.

25. A 65-year-old alcoholic male is admitted to the hospital with a three day history of epigastric pain radiating to the back associated with nausea and vomiting. The patient also has cirrhosis of the liver and mild CHF well controlled on hydrochlorothiazide 50 mg bid and digoxin 0.25 mg daily. He also has a 3 year history of severe rheumatoid arthritis which is moderately relieved with hydrocortisone 50 mg tid. Since the initial impression was acute pancreatitis, the patient was placed on NG suction and 3 liters of D5 1/4 NS daily. The following evening the laboratory report disclosed the following:

K 3.3 mEq/L	HCO$_3$ 32mEq/L
Cl 90 mEq/L	Na 136 mEq/L
SGOT 8OU (40)	Alk phos 130 (80) U
C$_{cr}$ 60 cc/min	Mg 1.3 mEq/L
Digoxin 2.8 ng/ml	Amylase 1200U
Creat 1.2 mg%	

An ECG showed occasional PVC's and runs of bigeminy. What factors are predisposing this patient to digitalis toxicity?

This patient has a mild degree of **_hypokalemia_**. The association between digitalis toxicity and hypokalemia is well recognized. Jelliffe (36) has observed that twice as much digitalis is required to produce toxicity in patients with a serum potassium of 5 mEq/L than in those with a serum potassium of 3 mEq/l. Therefore, drugs, diseases and medical maneuvers which induce a hypokalemia or a drop in serum potassium from elevated to normal levels may unmask existing digitalis toxicity or allow toxicity to occur at lower doses. The mechanism of this potentiation is unclear; however, a low serum potassium has been observed to increase the uptake of digitalis by the myocardial tissue (68).

Hypokalemia may result when excessive amounts of potassium are lost via the kidney or gastrointestinal tract or when extracellular potassium redistributes to intracellular spaces. (See *Fluid and Electrolytes* chapter.)

Corticosteroids promote potassium excretion at the distal portion of the renal tubule. The degree of hypokalemia produced by the various glucocorticoids may be predicted on the basis of their mineralocorticoid potency. Hypokalemia is more frequently associated with hydrocortisone than with equivalent anti-inflammatory doses of prednisone. Similarly, dexamethasone which is devoid of mineralcorticoid activity would not be expected to produce hypokalemia. Diseases in which mineralocorticoid activity is high (e.g., Cushing's disease, hyperaldosteronism) also are associated with low serum potassium levels. (See *Glucocorticoid* chapter.)

All diuretics, with the exception of triamterene and spironolactone, may cause hypokalemia through kaliuresis. See the chapter on *Edema*.

Renal tubular acidoses is a disease characterized by an inability of the kidney to excrete acid and is associated with increased losses of urinary potassium. Although this patient does not have this disease it should be noted that drugs such as acetazolamide, amphotericin (63, 66) and outdated tetracycline cause a similar renal tubular defect resulting in increased urinary losses of potassium and hypokalemia.

Gastrointestinal secretions contain high concentrations of potassium (8-10 mEq/L). Therefore, nasogastric suction and vomiting may have contributed to this patient's hypokalemic state. Excessive loss of gastrointestinal potassium can also occur in patients with ileostomies, gastrointestinal fistulas, severe diarrhea or in those who take cathartics and other drugs which regularly produce diarrhea (e.g. neomycin, quinidine). Kayexelate, a non-absorbable cationic exchange resin which exchanges sodium for potassium in the gastrointestinal tract, results in decreased serum potassium.

The patient is in metabolic *alkalosis* as a result of the diuretic therapy, vomiting and nasogastric suctioning. Alkalosis results in the redistribution of potassium intracellularly and an increased renal excretion of potassium. In the former case, potassium moves into the cells to maintain electrical neutrality which has been altered by the presence of excess anion (HCO_3). Alkalosis in and of itself has been associated with an increased incidence of digitalis toxicity. Brater et al (82) attribute this to an intracellular depletion of potassium due to increased urinary excretion and a relative increase in the ratio of extracellular to intracellular potassium. This has the same effect on the membrane potential as digoxin.

Chronic alcoholism and the loss or removal of upper gastrointestinal fluids containing 1.0 mEq/L of magnesium are the major factors contributing to this patient's **hypomagnesemia.** The observation of hypomagnesemia in the absence of hypokalemia in four digitalis-toxic patients prompted an animal study to test the effect of this electrolyte imbalance on digitalis toxicity. The toxic dose of acetylstrophanthidin in dogs was reduced when the serum magnesium was reduced by hemodialysis (74). The prevalence of hypomagnesemia is higher in digitalis toxic patients (4), and $MgSO_4$ has been used successfully in the treatment of digitalis toxicity (65c, 77a). The long-term administration of magnesium free fluids (e.g. hyperalimentation), diuretics, amphotericin B, and hemodialysis have also been associated with hypomagnesemia (93).

A significant amount of digoxin is eliminated by the kidney as unchanged, active drug. It is therefore not surprising that the digoxin may accumulate to toxic levels in patients with **renal failure** (37). In contrast, digitoxin is primarily metabolized to inactive products by the liver so that the half life of this drug is only slightly altered, if at all (69), in patients with renal failure. Nevertheless, this author prefers the use of digoxin in patients with renal failure, since the elimination t½ of digoxin is always less than that of digitoxin regardless of the degree of renal function. Therefore, the time required for elimination in cases of toxicity will still be shorter for digoxin.

Very little digoxin is metabolized so that it is not surprising that its elimination was found to be unaltered in cirrhotic patients (61). Although never reported, diminished **liver function** may theoretically increase the half-life and serum levels of digitoxin because it is metabolized to a significant degree.

Age may be an important predisposing factor in the production of digitalis toxicity in this patient. The same intravenous dose of digoxin administered to elderly and young patients produced higher serum concentrations of digoxin in the elderly. Ewy et al (25) proposed that the higher levels and prolonged half life observed in these patients were due to diminished renal clearance of the drug and the smaller body size of this population. It is important to emphasize that although the serum creatinine of the elderly patients (average age 77 years) was within normal limits, the mean creatinine clearance (56 ml/min) was approximately half that observed in the younger patients. The response to digitalis may also be altered in the very young. Levine et al (52, 53) have recommended the use of lower doses in premature infants and neonates (less than one month of age). Toxic arrhythmias were observed when infants tested during the first 72 hours of life were given doses of digoxin comparable to those recommended for children and older infants. This may be due to the decreased renal function normally observed in newborns. Their studies demonstrate that the absorption, tissue fixation and/or excretion of digoxin in infants is similar to that of adults. They point out, however, that infants excrete a smaller percentage of digoxin metabolites than do adults.

Although not illustrated by this patient, it should be noted that **hypercalcemia** may theoretically predispose patients to digitalis toxicity. The electrical and contractile effects of calcium on the myocardium are similar to those of digitalis. For this reason, rapid intravenous infusions of calcium may facilitate the development of digitalis toxicity and normal or low doses of digitalis may induce toxicity in patients with hypercalcemia (e.g., hyperparathyroidism or metastatic cancer). The clinical significance of calcium-induced digitalis toxicity, however, has been questioned by Lown et al (58). There have been no reports of digitalis toxicity secondary to the oral administration calcium-containing products.

An increased prevalence of digoxin toxicity has also been observed in patients with advanced cardiac disease, chronic pulmonary disease, cor pulmonale, hypoxia and atrial fibrillation (5, 64). The concomitant administration of several drugs has been noted to decrease the myocardial threshold to digitalis toxicity. These include cyclopropane and large doses of reserpine (7).

Finally, **thyroid function** can alter a patient's sensitivity to digitalis. Hypothyroid patients respond to low doses whereas hyperthyroid patients frequently require higher doses (21). See chapters on *Cardiac Arrhythmias, Thyroid Disease* and *Clinical Phar-*

macokinetics.

26. Digoxin was prescribed for a 70-year-old male with mild congestive heart failure. The label on his prescription bottle instructed him to take one tablet (0.25 mg) twice daily for three days and one tablet daily thereafter. Ten days later the patient returned to clinic complaining of extreme fatigue, anorexia, nausea and a "funny" heart beat. Close questioning disclosed that the patient failed to decrease his digoxin to 0.25 mg daily. An ECG revealed multiple PVC's and second degree AV block. A "stat" digoxin serum level was 2.8 ng/ml. What are the signs and symptoms of digitalis toxicity?

Noncardiac symptoms of digitalis toxicity are related to the central nervous system (CNS), gastrointestinal tract and endocrine effects of the drug. Allergic reactions to digitalis are extremely rare. Thrombocytopenia secondary to digitoxin is also a rare phenomenon. Unilateral or bilateral gynecomastia is occasionally observed during digoxin administration and is reversible upon withdrawal of the drug.

Recent studies indicate that **CNS symptoms** of digitalis toxicity may be extremely common. Chronic digitalis intoxication resulting from misformulation was observed in 179 patients (51). Acute, extreme fatigue was a complaint in 95% of these patients. Approximately 80% experienced weakness of the arms and legs and 65% suffered from psychic disturbances occurring in the form of nightmares, agitation, listlessness and hallucinations. Visual disturbances were observed in 95% of these patients. Hazy vision, difficulty in reading and difficulty in red-green color perception were frequently present. Other complaints included glitterings, dark or moving spots, photophobia, and yellow-green vision. Disturbances in color vision returned to normal two to three weeks following discontinuation of digitalis.

Gastrointestinal symptoms including anorexia, nausea, vomiting, abdominal pain (65%) and less commonly diarrhea were present in 80% of the patients observed. Recent studies fail to support the old notion that gastrointestinal symptoms are related to impurities in digitalis products.

The clinical presentation of digitalis toxicity is highly unpredictable. Unfortunately, **cardiac symptoms** may precede non-cardiac symptoms of digitalis toxicity in up to 47% of cases. Frequently (26-66%), nonspecific cardiac arrhythmias may be the only manifestation of digitalis toxicity (51, 71). Vague gastrointestinal symptoms characteristic of digitalis toxicity may be difficult to evaluate since anorexia and nausea are also part of the clinical picture of congestive heart failure. Beller et al (5) observed an equal frequency of anorexia and nausea in both toxic and nontoxic patients. Even more frustrating is the fact that digitalis

toxicity may occasionally present as progressive congestive heart failure.

The **arrhythmogenic action** of digitalis is related to its complex effects on the electrophysiologic properties of the heart. Toxic doses of digitalis may simultaneously depress the automaticity of the normal pacemakers and increase the automaticity of subsidiary conduction tissues. Conduction velocity is diminished in all portions of the heart and there is an increased irritability of the ventricles. (82)

Digitalis-induced rhythm disturbances are nonspecific but are generally characterized by decreased conduction velocity manifested by atrioventricular (A-V) block or increased automaticity of the atrium, AV node or ventricles. It is estimated that rhythm disturbances occur in 80-90% of digitalis toxic patients (14). Ventricular arrhythmias (premature ventricular contractions [PVC's], bigeminy, multi-focal PVC's and tachycardia) and AV conduction disturbances (prolonged PR interval and second degree AV block) appear to be the most commonly encountered arrhythmias. Comprehensive reviews are available on the topic of digitalis induced arrhythmias (14, 15, 75).

Prospective studies show good correlation between serum digoxin levels and toxicity. Eighty-seven percent of digitalis toxic patients had levels greater than 2 ng/ml and 90% of the nontoxic patients had levels of less than 2 ng/ml. However, because a significant overlap between toxic and therapeutic levels exists, serum level determinations are currently most useful as an aid in confirming suspected digitalis toxicity and in individualizing dosing regimens so that toxicity is avoided (5, 81).

27. How should digitalis toxicity be managed?

If the cardiac arrhythmia is not life-threatening, simple withdrawal of digitalis may be the only treatment required. Potassium administration should be considered in patients with digitalis-induced ectopic beats who have low or normal serum potassium levels. The oral route of administration is generally adequate and should be used unless the patient cannot take medications by mouth. The following precautions should be considered when potassium is used to treat digitalis toxicity:

(a) potassium should be administered with caution in patients who have conduction disturbances characterized by second degree or complete atrioventricular (AV) block. Potassium also depresses conduction velocity in the AV node and its use may result in an augmentation of this cardiac arrhythmia,

(b) toxic doses of digitalis inhibit the uptake of potassium by myocardial, skeletal muscle and liver cells. For this reason, these patients may occasionally develop refractory hyperkalemia; large doses of potassium should be administered cautiously (8),

(c) because potassium is eliminated by the kidneys, excessive potassium loads should be avoided in patients with compromised renal function,

(d) cardiac arrhythmias have been observed following the rapid intravenous administration of concentrated potassium solutions.

If digitalis-induced arrhythmias are severe enough to warrant intravenously administered potassium, maximum recommended doses are 40 mEq (preferably 10 mEq/hr) at a concentration which does not exceed 80-100 mEq/L. The patient should be monitored for signs and symptoms of potassium toxicity with frequent ECG tracings (tall, peaked T waves; prolonged PR interval) and serum potassium determinations.

Virtually all of the antiarrhythmic agents have been used to treat digitalis-induced arrhythmias. Intravenous lidocaine, phenytoin and propranolol have been used with the greatest success (15). Lidocaine and phenytoin have a theoretical advantage over propranolol and quinidine-like agents in that they probably do not further depress AV conduction.

Although lidocaine has an elimination half-life of approximately two hours, an initial IV bolus may last only 10-20 minutes because of rapid tissue distribution. Generally, the drug is administered as a constant infusion (1-4 mg/min) following an initial bolus dose of 50-100 mg (1 mg/kg). Caution should be exercised in patients with congestive heart failure since it has been demonstrated that the volume of distribution and plasma clearance of lidocaine may be decreased in these patients (92). Elimination half-life and time to reach plateau are therefore prolonged and symptoms of lidocaine toxicity may not be evident for several hours (two-three half-lives). See chapters on *Cardiac Arrhythmias* and *Clinical Pharmacokinetics.*

Reports regarding the efficacy of phenytoin (DPH) as an antiarrhythmic agent have been variable; however, the drug appears to be particularly efficacious in the suppression of digitalis-induced tachyarrhythmias with or without first or second degree A-V block. A loading dose of up to one gram (in divided doses) may be required during the first 12 to 24 hours. Thereafter, the patient may be maintained at doses of 100 mg three to four times daily. The diluent for parenteral phenytoin contains 40% propylene glycol which is cardiotoxic (57); for this reason DPH should not be administered at a rate which exceeds 50 mg/min. Phenytoin is insoluble in aqueous solutions and should not be administered by intravenous infusion (see chapters on *Cardiac Arrhythmias* and *Clinical Pharmacokinetics*).

Intravenous propranolol has been useful in abolishing digitalis-induced atrial tachycardia with AV block and ventricular premature contractions. Quinidine-like actions of the drug may account for its efficacy as an antiarrhythmic agent. One to three mg should be given at a rate of one mg/min with careful ECG monitoring. A similar dose may be repeated after two minutes, but further doses should be withheld for four hours. Unlike phenytoin and lidocaine, propranolol depresses conduction velocity and may therefore augment AV and intraventricular block. It should not be used in asthmatic patients since it may induce bronchoconstriction and caution should be taken when it is used in diabetics since they may experience severe protracted hypoglycemia following its administration. (See *Diabetes* chapter). Should profound bradycardia occur, atropine may be used.

Procainamide and quinidine have been used less frequently because their intravenous administration is associated with hypotension and cardiotoxicity. Since conduction velocity is diminished by both of these drugs their use should be avoided when AV or intraventricular block is present. (See chapter on *Cardiac Arrhythmias*).

Other agents which are used less frequently because of unpredictable or toxic effects or limited availability include EDTA (a calcium chelating agent), magnesium (65c, 77a), cholestyramine (1b), and specific digoxin antibodies (84a).

28. LM, a 50-year-old man, is admitted with severe, progressive and debilitating symptoms of congestive heart failure. The patient's family history is significant in that his father and two brothers succumbed to heart attacks before the age of 40. The patient has had a 12 year history of CHF which has been symptomatic despite treatment with full therapeutic doses of digoxin and furosemide. He has no history of hypertension, but previous studies have suggested a diagnosis of cardiomyopathy. Over the past 8 months LM's DOE has become progressively worse, and for the past month he has been confined to bed because of extreme fatigue. He wakes up once or twice nightly with PND.

Physical examination revealed a dyspneic, cyanotic male in apparent distress, but with no complaints of chest pain. The blood pressure was 100/60 mm Hg and his pulse was 105/min. Marked jugular venous distension, bilateral rales, hepatomegaly and 3+ peripheral edema were also observed. Chest x-ray revealed marked cardiomegaly and pulmonary congestion. The patient was admitted to the coronary care unit where a Swan-Ganz catheter was passed from an antecubital vien to the pulmonary artery. Prior to therapy, the patient's pulmonary-capillary pressure was 27 mm Hg and his cardiac index was 1.4 L/min-m². Intravenous nitroprusside was initiated at a dose of 16 mcg/min and eventually increased to 200 mcg/min. At this dose, the patient's pulmonary-capillary pressure decreased to 15 mm Hg and his

cardiac index increased to 2.5 L/min-m². He was eventually discharged on digoxin 0.375 mg daily, furosemide 80 mg bid, spironolactone 50 mg bid, NTG ointment 2 inches q 4 h, and hydralazine 75 mg qid.

A. What was the importance of obtaining a pulmonary-capillary pressure and cardiac index in this patient? To what other hemodynamic measurements do these correspond?

Severe congestive heart failure which is resistant to conventional therapy occurs in association with intrinsic myocardial failure (e.g. myocardial infarction and cardiomyopathy). In its most severe form, this failure is characterized by an increased pulmonary-capillary pressure (PCP) and a decreased cardiac index as illustrated by this patient. The pulmonary-capillary pressure (or pulmonary wedge pressure-PWP) is the "hydrostatic pressure which forces fluids from the pulmonary vascular space into the interstitial or intraalveolar spaces" (25b). It is measured by inflating a balloon at the tip of the Swan-Ganz catheter and is a good index of left ventricular volume in the absence of mitral valvular disease. Other terms or measurements which generally correspond to this value are left ventricular filling pressure (LFP or LVFP), left ventricular end diastolic pressure (LVEDP), left atrial pressure and pulmonary vein pressure. These values reflect the preload on the heart and are primarily influenced by venous return, cardiac output, and less frequently mitral or aortic valve insufficiency. The normal PCP is 5 to 12 mm Hg. Clinically, the onset of pulmonary congestion occurs at 18 to 20 mm Hg; moderate pulmonary congestion is present at a level of 25 to 30 mm Hg and the onset of pulmonary edema occurs at values greater than 30 mm Hg (25b, 26a).

The cardiac index is cardiac output which has been corrected for body surface area and is measured by a thermodilution technique which is described elsewhere (25b). Symptoms of decreased perfusion to the kidneys, brain and skin are consequences of a diminished cardiac output. A normal value is 2.7 to 4.3 L/min-m²; subclinical hypoperfusion occurs at 2.2 to 2.7 L/min-m²; and cardiogenic shock is associated with a cardiac index of less than 1.8 L/min-m².

The objective of therapy is to decrease the PCP and increase the stroke volume or cardiac output in patients such as LM described above.

B. What was the rationale for nitroprusside therapy? What doses are used? What are the hazards of this type of therapy?

Nitroprusside dilates both the venous and arterial vessels. Thus, it increases venous capacitance and decreases the venous return or preload on the heart. A decrease in the PCP and pulmonary and systemic

venous resistance results. It also decreases peripheral vascular resistance (PVR) through its action on arterial vessels and in doing so decreases the afterload on the heart or impedance to left ventricular outflow. As a consequence of this effect, cardiac output is increased. An increase in the heart rate following nitroprusside therapy is infrequently observed in patients with congestive heart failure. This may be due to a decreased sensitivity of the baroreceptor in these patients or it may be related to the fact that an increased cardiac output may be achieved with minimal change in the arterial pressure. Since blood pressure is equal to the product of cardiac output and peripheral vascular resistance (BP = CO x PVR), only a minor change in blood pressure may be observed if the decreased PVR produced by nitroprusside is counterbalanced by a comparable increase in cardiac output (13a).

The major hazard associated with nitroprusside use is a sudden, profound hypotension which will decrease cardiac output. This occurred in 3 out of 43 patients in one study and was reversed in 5 to 10 minutes by discontinuing the nitroprusside and elevating the patient's feet (13a). Nitroprusside may also decrease cardiac output and increase heart rate in patients with cardiac failure associated with a normal or low pulmonary-capillary pressure (13a). Another concern with regard to all vasodilator therapy is that in decreasing the arterial pressure, coronary perfusion may also be decreased and the area of ischemia increased in patients with recent myocardial infarction. Chatergee and Parmley (13a) have reviewed this extensively and present evidence which argues to the contrary. However, since the effects of vasodilators on myocardial ischemia are not actually known, they suggest that the use of nitroprusside therapy be reserved for congestive heart failure patients with a pulmonary-capillary pressure greater than 18 mm Hg and with a mean arterial pressure (diastolic + ⅓ the pulse pressure) of greater than 60 mm Hg (13a). Other toxic effects of nitroprusside relating to cyanide and thiocyanate toxicity are discussed in the chapter on *Hypertension*.

Since severe hypotension is of major concern, these patients should be initiated on small doses of nitroprusside (16 mcg/min) which are increased slowly (3-6 mcg/min to a maximum of 430 mcg/min) until a decrease in the PCP or arterial pressure is observed. (13a)

C. Compare and contrast the other vasodilators which are used parenterally to treat refractory congestive heart failure.

Nitroprusside is the most frequently used agent for this purpose. However, intravenous phentolamine, trimethaphan and nitroglycerin have also been used with varying degrees of success.

Phentolamine is a short-acting alpha adrenergic blocking agent which predominantly affects the arterial vessels, but also increases venous capacitance. Like nitroprusside, it is most likely to increase the cardiac output in patients with elevated left ventricular filling pressures. Unlike nitroprusside 80% of patients with CHF developed an increased heart rate and increased myocardial oxygen consumption which is of major concern in patients with ischemic heart disease (15a, 25b). For this reason, nitroprusside is generally favored over phentolamine.

Nitroglycerin has been prepared extemporaneously for intravenous use (25b, 25d). The usual method is to dissolve sublingual NTG tablets in small volumes of sterile water for injection, 5% dextrose, or normal saline (400 mcg/ml or 500 mcg/30 ml) and pass it through a millipore filter (22 mm) into sterile vials (25a). Fung (25d) has recently discussed the problems associated with the quality control and stability of these products. Nitroglycerin primarily affects the venous capacitance vessels as opposed to the arterial bed. This activity accounts for the fact that the pulmonary-capillary pressure or left ventricular filling pressure (preload) is reduced in patients with a PCP greater than 18 mm Hg. However, because it may only slightly decrease or have no effect on afterload, cardiac output may remain unchanged or increase slightly. Nitroglycerin may actually decrease cardiac output in patients with low or elevated capillary wedge pressures by reducing the left ventricular filling pressure to less than 15 mm Hg (25b). For this reason nitroglycerin may be specifically useful in a patient whose primary problem is one of pulmonary congestion.

Trimethaphan, a ganglionic blocker, has been used infrequently due to the fact that it can produce profound postural hypotension. It apparently decreases pulmonary wedge pressure without increasing the heart rate, but produces no increase in cardiac output (13a).

D. Once LM was controlled with nitroprusside therapy, he was placed on NTG ointment and hydralazine. Why were both hydralazine and NTG used? What other vasodilating agents are available for ambulatory congestive heart failure patients unresponsive to conventional therapy?

Although nitroprusside has been used successfully in refractory congestive heart failure patients, its use is limited to an intensive care setting because it is short-acting and must be administered intravenously.

Various forms of the *nitrates* have been used. The *sublingual forms* are less than ideal for chronic use since they have such a short duration of action. The hemodynamic effects of sublingual NTG last only 20-30 minutes whereas those of isosorbide dinitrate (2.5-10 mg) may persist for 90-180 minutes (13a, 59a).

Preliminary studies indicate that relatively large doses of oral *isosorbide dinitrate* (20-80 mg) effectively decrease left ventricular filling pressure within 30 minutes and maintain a significantly lowered pressure for 4-5 hours (11a, 15a, 25c). Its effect on cardiac output is variable, but it appears to increase CO in patients with control LVFP's of greater than 20 mm Hg. This was attributed to a decrease in the afterload (11a). The effects on cardiac output were more short-lived (3 hours) than those on the LVFP. the heart rate remained constant whether initial LVFP's were less than or greater than 20 mm Hg. Although nitrates have a large first-pass effect, large oral doses may overwhelm the metabolic capacity of the liver or, the metabolites may be active.

More attention has been given to **NTG ointment** which appears to have prolonged hemodynamic effects (3-5 hours). Like the other nitrates, it decreases pulmonary and systemic venous pressures and LVFP, but has a variable effect on cardiac output. An apparent lack of response in some patients may be related to poor peripheral circulation and poor absorption of NTG from the ointment (25b, 65a). The dose may be titrated using 1-4 inches of 2% NTG applied to the skin of the chest, back, or back of the thigh. Effects should be observed within 15-30 minutes. If a response is not observed after 30 minutes, another application may be made. See the chapter on *Angina* for a more detailed discussion on the application of NTG ointment. (25b, 65a)

Vasodilators such as **hydralazine** and **minoxidil** (experimental) which primarily affect the arterial bed have also been used in the chronic therapy of CHF. Hydralazine (50-100 mg qid) decreases pulmonary and systemic resistance and produces relatively little change in the LVFP. It produces a sharp increase in the cardiac output by reducing arterial impedence. The tachycardia which is frequently observed in hypertensive patients is minor or absent in patients with CHF (15a).

It is apparent that the nitrates, which primarily affect preload or left ventricular filling pressure, and hydralazine, which primarily affects arterial impedence or cardiac output, will have complimentary effects in certain patients. In fact, the combination has been used successfully when one of the other agents has failed (13b).

Recently, the hemodynamic effects of a new vasodilator, **prazosin**, have been studied. Prazosin appears to be an ideal agent in that it affects both the venous and arterial beds and thus decreases the LVFP (preload) as well as arterial impedence (afterload). Additionally, it has a sympatholytic effect which prevents reflex tachycardia. Oral doses of 1-10 mg have an onset of action of 1 hour and the effects persist for

6 hours (65b). The first dose of prazosin should always be given under direct medical supervision since syncope following the initial dose has been reported.

It is not yet known what the effect of vasodilators will be on the long-term prognosis of CHF patients. This may depend, to a large degree on careful patient and agent selection. It is apparent, for example, that a certain population of patients defined on the basis of their hemodynamic parameters have a poor prognosis regardless of therapy (25b). However, it does appear that some patients may benefit, at least on the short term, from vasodilator therapy. The reported mortality rate for patients in cardiogenic shock following acute myocardial infarction has been close to 100% (13a). Chatergee et al have observed a decrease in mortality of 50% in patients receiving vasodilator therapy. However, the long-term prognosis for these patients treated in the hospital with vasodilators has been unfavorable. Studies will need to be performed to determine the value of this new therapeutic approach in the treatment of congestive heart failure.

REFERENCES

1. Armstrong PW et al: Nitroglycerin ointment in acute myocardial infarction. Am J Cardiol 38:474, 1976.
1a. Astwood EB: Chapter 70. Androgens and anabolic steroids, in The Pharmacological Basis of Therapeutics, 4th ed edited by LS goodman and A Gilman, Macmillan Co, NY, 1970.
1b. Banzano G et al: Digitalis intoxication. Treatment with a new steroid binding resin. JAMA 220:828, 1972.
2. Bartorelli C et al: Hypotensive and renal effects of diazoxide, a sodium-retaining benzothiadiazine compound. Circ 27:895, 1963.
3. Beaver WT: Mild analgesics, a review of their clinical pharmacology, Part I. Am J Med Sci 250:577, 1965.
4. Beller GA et al: Correlation of serum magnesium levels and cardiac digitalis intoxication. Am J Cardiol 33:225, 1974.
5. Beller GA et al: Digitalis intoxication. A prospective clinical study with serum level correlations. NEJM 284:989, 1971.
6. Bernard Jet al: Treatment of acute leukemias. Semin Hematol 9:181, 1972.
7. Bigger JT et al: Digitalis toxicity: drug interactions promoting toxicity and the management of toxicity. Semin in Drug Treat 2:147, 1972.
8. Braunwald E et al: Digitalis, Ann Rev Med 16:371, 1965.
8a. Brater C et al: Digoxin toxicity in patients with normokalemic potassium depletion. Clin Pharmacol Ther 22:21, 1977.
9. Brest AN et al: Clinical selection of diuretic drugs in the management of congestive heart failure. Am J Cardiol 22:168, 1968.
10. Brod J: Pathogenesis of cardiac edema. Brit Med J 1:222, 1972.
10a. Brown DD et al: Decreased bioavailability of digoxin due to antacids and kaolin-pection. NEJM 295:1035, 1976.
11. Brown DD et al: Plasma digoxin levels in normal human volunteers following chronic oral and intramuscular digoxin. J Lab Clin Med, 82:201, 1973.
11a. Bussmann W et al: Orally administered isosorbide dinitrate in patients with and without left ventricular failure due to acute myocardial infarction. Am J Cardiol 39:91, 1977.
12. Butler VP: Digoxin: immunologic approaches to measurement and reversal of toxicity. NEJM 283:1150, 1970.
13. Chamberlain TJ: Licorice poisoning, pseudoaldosteronism and heart failure. JAMA 213:1343, 1970.
13a. Chatergee K et al: The role of vasodilator therapy in heart failure. Prog Cardiovasc Dis 19:301, 1977.
13b. Chatergee K et al: Combination vasodilator therapy for severe chronic congestive heart failure. Ann Int Med 85:467, 1976.
14. Chung, EK: Digitalis induced cardiac arrhythmias. Am Heart J 79:845, 1970.
15. Chung, EK: The current status of digitalis therapy. Mod Treat 8:643, 1971.
15a. Cohn J et al: Vasodilator therapy of cardiac failure (2 parts). NEJM 297:27 and 254, 1977.
15b. Chopra D et al: Insensitivity to digoxin associated with hypocalcemia. NEJM 296:917, 1977.
16. Conn, HL, Merill, JP and Lauler DP: Modern Concepts in Congestive Heart Failure. Roche Therapeutic Series. Hoffman La-Roche Inc., NY, 1969.
16a. Crouthamel WG et al: The effect of congestive heart failure on quinidine pharmacokinetics. Am Heart J 90:335, 1975.

17. Demers R et al: Pretibial edema and sodium retention during lithium carbonate treatment. JAMA 214:1845, 1970.
18. Diet Committee of the San Francisco Heart Association in cooperation with the U.C. Hospital Pharmacy: Sodium in Medicinals. San Francisco Heart Association, San Francisco, 1973.
19. Doherty JE: The clinical pharmacology of digitalis glycosides: a review. Am J Med Sci 255:382, 1968.
20. Doherty JE: Digitalis glycosides: pharmacokinetics and their clinical implications. Ann Int Med 79:229, 1973.
21. Doherty, JE et al: Digoxin metabolism in hypo- and hyperthyroidism: studies with tritiated digoxin. Ann Int Med 64:489, 1966.
22. Doherty JE et al: Studies following intramuscular tritiated digoxin in human subjects. Am J Cardiol 15:170, 1965.
23. Early L: Diuretics. NEJM 276:966, 1967.
24. Early L: Diuretics (concluded). NEJM 276:1023, 1967.
25. Ewy GA et al: Digoxin metabolism in the elderly. Circ 39:449, 1969.
25a. Flaherty JT et al: Intravenous nitroglycerin in acute myocardial infarction. Circ 51:131, 1975.
25b. Forrester JS et al: Medical therapy of acute myocardial infarction by application of hemodynamic subsets (2 parts). NEJM 295:1356, 1976.
25c. Franciosa JA et al: Hemodynamic effects of orally administered isosorbide dinitrate in patients with congestive heart failure. Circ 50:1020, 1974.
25d. Fung H: Potency and stability of extemporaneously prepared nitroglycerin intravenous solutions. Am J Hosp Pharm 35:528, 1978.
25e. Flentie EH et al: Electrolyte effects of the sodium phosphate enema. Dis Colon Rectum 1:295, 1958.
26. Gantt CL: Diuretic therapy. Rational Drug Ther 6:1, 1972.
26a. Gorlin R: Practical cardiac hemodynamics. NEJM 296:203, 1977.
27. Greenblatt DJ et al: Pain and CPK elevation after intramuscular digoxin. NEJM 288:689, 1973.
28. Greenblatt DJ et al: Evaluation of digoxin bioavailability in single-dose studies. NEJM 289:651, 1973.
29. Halazan JF et al: Daunorubicin cardiac toxicity in children with ALL. Cancer 33:545, 1974.
29a. Halkin H et al: Determinants of the renal clearance of digoxin. Clin Pharmacol Ther 17:385, 1975.
30. Hall WH et al: Tritiated digoxin XXII. Absorption and excretion in malabsorption syndromes. Am J Med 56:437, 1974.
30a. Hall WH et al: Effect of cholestyramine of digoxin absorption and excretion in man. Am J Cardiol 39:213, 1977.
31. Heizer WD et al: Absorption of digoxin in patients with malabsorption syndromes. NEJM 285:257, 1971.
31a. Hendeles Le et al: Frequent toxicity from recommended intravenous aminophylline dosage regimens. Drug Intell Clin Pharm 11:12, 1977.
32. Hernandex A et al: Pharmacodynamics of 3H-Digoxin in infants. Pediat 44:418, 1969.
33. Hoffman BF et al: Effects of digitalis on electrical activity of cardiac fibers. Progr Cardiovas Dis 7:226, 1964.
34. Huffman DH: Absorption of orally given digoxin preparations. JAMA 222:957, 1972.
34a. Huffman DH et al: Absorption of digoxin from different oral preparations in normal subjects during steady state. Clin Pharmacol Ther 16:310, 1974.
35. Irons GV Jr et al: Digitalis induced arrhythmias and their man-

agement. Prog Cardiovas Dis 8:539, 1966.

36. Jelliffe RW: Factors to consider in planning digoxin therapy. J Chron Dis 24:407, 1971.

37. Jelliffe RW: An improved method of digoxin therapy. Ann Int Med 69:703, 1968.

38. Jelliffe RW et al: Reduction of digitalis toxicity by computer assisted glycosides dosage regimens. Ann Int Med 77:891, 1972.

39. Jelliffe RW et al: An improved method of digitoxin therapy. Ann Int Med 72:453, 1970.

39a. Jelliffe RW et al: A nomogram for digoxin therapy. Am J Med 57:63, 1974.

39b. Jelliffe RW: Creatinine clearance: Bedside estimate. Ann Int Med 70:604, 1973.

39c. Jenne JW et al: Apparent theophylline half-life fluctuations during treatment of acute left ventricular failure. Am J Hosp Pharm 34:408, 1977.

39d. Juhl RP et al: Effects of sulfasalazine on digoxin bioavailability. Clin Pharmacol Ther 20:387, 1976.

40. Jusko W et al: Pharmacokinetic design of digoxin dosage regimens in relation to renal function. J Clin Pharmacol 14:525, 1974.

41. Kannel WB et al: Role of blood pressure in the development of congestive heart failure. The Framingham study. NEJM 287:781, 1972.

42. Kessler KM et al: Quinidine elimination in patients with congestive heart failure or poor renal function. NEJM 290:706, 1974.

43. Klainer LM et al: The epidemiology of cardiac failure. J Chronic Dis 18:797, 1965.

44. Kleim M et al: Correlation of the electrical and mechanical changes in the dog heart during progressive digitalization. Circ Res 29:635, 1971.

45. Kleit SA et al: Diuretic therapy: current status. Am Heart J 79:700, 1970.

46. Koch-Weser J: Vasodilator drugs in the treatment of hypertension. Arch Int Med 133:1017, 1974.

47. Koch-Weser J: Mechanisms of digitalis action on the heart. NEJM 277:417, 1967.

48. Koch-Weser J: Mechanisms of digitalis action on the heart. NEJM 277:469, 1967.

48a. Koup JR et al: Digoxin pharmacokinetics: role of renal failure in dosage regimen design. Clin Pharmacol Ther 18:9, 1975.

48b. Koup JR et al: Pharmacokinetics of digoxin in normal subjects after intravenous bolus and infusion doses. J Pharmacokin Biopharm 3:181, 1975.

49. Kristensen M et al: Drug elimination ꞏnd renal function. J Clin Pharmacol 14:307, 1974.

49a. Sahiri K et al: Mechanism of diphenylhydantoin (DPH) induced decrease of serum digoxin levels, Clin Res 22:321A, 1974.

50. Langer G: The mechanism of action of digitalis. Hosp Pract 5:49, 1970.

50a. Lee G et al: Linear dose response and quantitative attenuation by potassium of the inotropic action of acetylstrophanthidin. Clin Pharmacol Ther 22:34, 1977.

51. Lely AH et al: Non-cardiac symptoms of digitalis intoxication. Am Heart J 83:149, 1972.

52. Levine OR et al: Digoxin dosage in premature infants. Pediat 29:18, 1972.

53. Levine OR et al: Digitalis intoxication in premature infants. J Pediat 61:70, 1962.

54. Lewis WS et al: Another disadvantage of intramuscular digoxin (Letter). NEJM 288:1077, 1973.

55. Lindenbaum J et al: Impairment of digoxin absorption by neomycin. Clin Res 20:410, 1970.

56. Lindenbaum J et al: Variation in biologic availability of digoxin from four preparations. NEJM 285: 1344, 1971.

57. Louis S et al: The cardiocirculatory changes caused by intravenous dilantin and its solvent. Am Heart J 74:523, 1967.

58. Lown B et al: Digitalis, electrolytes and the surgical patient. Am J Cardiol 6:309, 1960.

59. Luchi RJ et al: Unusually large digitalis requirements: a study of altered digoxin metabolism. Am J Med 45:322, 1968.

59a. Mantle JA et al: Isosorbide dinitrate for the relief of severe heart failure after myocardial infarction. Am J Cardiol 37:263, 1976.

60. Marcus FI et al: Administration of tritiated digoxin with and without a loading dose. A metabolic study. Circ 34:865, 1966.

61. Marcus RI et al: The metabolism of digoxin in cirrhotic patients. Gastroent 47:517, 1964.

62. Mason DT et al: Symposium on congestive heart failure II. Digitalis; new facts about an old drug. Am J Cardio 22:151, 1968.

63. McCurdy DK et al: Renal tubular acidosis due to amphotericin B. NEJM 278:124, 1968.

64. McIntosh HD et al: Problems in the use of digitalis in the management of congestive heart failure. Progr Cardiovasc Dis 7:360, 1965.

65. McKee PA et al: The natural history of congestive Heart failure: The Framingham Study. NEJM 285: 1441, 1971.

65a. Meister SG et al: Sustained haemodynamic action of nitroglycerin ointment. Brit Heart J 38:1031, 1976.

65b. Miller RR et al: Sustained reduction of cardiac impedence and preload in congestive heart failure with the antihypertensive vasodilator prazosin. NEJM 297:303, 1977.

65c. Mosely PK et al: Fluid and electrolyte disturbance as a complication of enema in Hirschprung's disease. Am J Dis Child 115:714, 1968.

65d. Neff MS et al: Magnesium sulfate in digitalis toxicity. Am J Cardiol 29:377, 1972.

66. Patterson RM et al: Renal tubular acidoses due to amphotericin B therapy. Arch Int Med 127:241, 1971.

67. Platman ST et al: Lithium retention and excretion. The effect of sodium and fluid intake. Arch Gen Psychiat 20:285, 1969.

68. Prindle KH Jr et al: Influence of extracellular potassium concentration on myocardial uptake and inotropic effect of tritiated digoxin. Circ Res 28:337, 1971.

69. Rasmussem K et al: Digitoxin kinetics in patients with impaired renal function. Clin Pharmacol Ther 13:6, 1972.

70. Reunig RH et al: Role of pharmacokinetics in drug dosage adjustment 1. Pharmacologic effect kinetics and apparent volume of distribution of digoxin. J Clin Pharmacol 13:4, 1973.

71. Rodensky PL et al: Observations on digitalis intoxication. Arch Int Med 108:61, 1961.

72. Sanchez N et al: Pharmacokinetics of digoxin: interpreting bioavailability. Brit Med J 4:132, 1973.

73. Schreiner GE & Lauler DP: *Edema and Diuretics*, Roche Therapeutic Series, Medcom, NY, 1969.

74. Seller RH et al: Digitalis toxicity and hypomagnesemia. Am Heart J 79:57, 1970.

75. Seltzer A et al: Production, recognition and treatment of digitalis toxicity. Calif Med 113:1, 1970.

76. Shaw TR: Clinical problems associated with the variable biologic availability of digoxin. Am Heart J 87:399, 1974.

77. Sheiner LB et al: Differences in serum digoxin concentrations between outpatients and inpatients: an effect of compliance? Clin Pharmacol Ther 15:239, 1974.

77a. Singh RB et al: Hypomagnesemia in relation to digoxin intoxication in children. Am Heart J 92:144, 1976.

78. Smith AJ: Clinical features of fluid retention complicating treatment with guanethidine. Circ 31:485, 1965.

78a. Smith HJ et al: Cardiomyopathy associated with amphetamine administration. Am Heart J 91:792, 1976.

79. Smith TW: Digitalis glycosides (first of two parts). NEJM 288:719, 1973.

80. Smith TW: Digitalis glycosides (second of two parts). NEJM 288:942, 1973.

81. Smith TW et al: Determination of therapeutic and toxic serum digoxin concentrations by radioimmunoassay. NEJM 281:1212, 1969.

82. Smith TW et al: Medical progress: digitalis (first of four parts). NEJM 289:945, 1973.

83. Smith TW et al: Digitalis (third of four parts). NEJM 289:1063, 1973.

84. Smith TW et al: Digoxin intoxication: the relationship of clinical presentation to serum digoxin concentration. J Clin Invest 49:2377, 1970.

84a. Smith TW et al: Reversal of advanced digoxin intoxication with Fab fragments of digoxin-specific antibodies. NEJM 294: 797, 1976.

85. Smith WO et al: Magnesium depletion induced by various diuretics. J Okla State Med Assoc 55:248, 1962.

86. Solomon HM et al: Interactions between digitoxin and other drugs in man. Am Heart J 83:277, 1972.

87. Sorby DL et al: On the evaluation of biologic availability of digoxin from tablets. Drug Intell Clin Pharm 7:79, 1973.

88. Stancer HC et al: Lithium carbonate and oedema (Letter). Lancet 2:985, 1971.

89. Steiness E et al: Bioavailability of digoxin tablets. Clin Pharmacol Ther 14:949, 1973.
90. Tainter ML and Ferris AJ: *Aspirin in Modern Therapy*. Bayer Co., N.Y., 1969.
91. Thomson AE et al: Clinical observations on an antihypertensive chlorothiazide analogue devoid of diuretic activity. Can Med Assoc J 78: 1306, 1962.
92. Thomson PD et al: Lidocaine pharmacokinetics in advanced heart failure, liver disease and renal failure. Ann Int Med 78:499, 1973.
92a. VonHoff DD et al: Daunomycin-induced cardiotoxicity in children and adults. A review of 110 cases. Am J Med 62:200, 1977.
93. Wacker WE et al: Magnesium metabolism (3 parts). NEJM 278:658, 712, 722, 1968.
94. WagnerJG: Appraisal of digoxin bioavailability and pharmacokinetics in relation to cardiac therapy. Am Heart J 88:133, 1974.
95. Wagner JG et al: Equivalence lack in digoxin plasma levels. JAMA 224:199, 1973.
95a. Walsh FM et al: Significance of non-steady-state serum digoxin concentrations. Am J Clin Path 65:446, 1975.
95b. Weinberger MW et al: Intravenous aminophylline dosage: Use of serum theophylline measurement for guidance. JAMA 235:2110, 1976.
96. Weintraub M et al: Compliance as a determinant of serum digoxin concentration. JAMA 224:481, 1973.
97. Well JV et al: Plasma volume expansion resulting from interference with adrenergic function in normal man. Circ 37:54, 1978.
98. White RJ et al: Plasma concentrations of digoxin after oral administration in the fasting and postprandial state. Brit Med J 1:380, 1971.
99. Williams JF et al: Studies on digitalis XIII. A comparison of the effects of potassium on the inotropic and arrhythmia producing actions of ouabain. J Clin Invest 45:346, 1966.
100. Zwillich CW et al: Theophylline-induced seizures in adults. Ann Int Med 82:784, 1975.
101. Zumhoff B et al: Rectal absorption of sodium from hypertonic sodium phosphate solutions. From the unpublished files of CB Fleet Co and the Clinical Biophysics Section, Sloan Kettering Institute for Cancer Research, New York.

Chapter 13

Edema

Richard J. Mangini
Lloyd Y. Young

Generalized edema represents an excessive accumulation of fluid in the interstitial spaces and is a clinical manifestation of many primary disorders. Initially, edema formation may be caused by an imbalance of local forces that determine the movement of fluids between the plasma and interstitial compartments: Intracapillary and interstitial hydrostatic and osmotic pressures.

Normally, the hydrostatic pressure at the arteriolar end of the capillaries greatly exceeds that in the surrounding tissues. As water and low molecular weight solutes move out of the vascular compartment, the oncotic pressure within the capillaries gradually increases. At the venous end of the capillaries, the hydrostatic pressure from the interstitium increases to the extent that interstitial fluid is driven back into the vascular tree with the assistance of the high oncotic pressure within the capillary. In this manner, tissue perfusion is maintained without altering the size of either the plasma or interstitial compartments. Edema forms when the balance of these forces shifts such that movement of fluid into the interstitial space is favored. Edema fluid will then accumulate until a new equilibrium occurs between the forces on the plasma and interstitial compartments. Therefore, manipulation of the oncotic pressure within the vasculature with osmotic agents, such as albumin or mannitol, and alterations of vascular hydrostatic pressure with diuretics can affect the removal of edema fluid. Since capillary hydrostatic pressure is primarily affected by sodium and water, the kidneys ultimately play the major role in the maintenance of the edematous state.

Edema may be localized as the result of a local inflammation, or its distribution may be generalized throughout the entire interstitial space. In the adult, interstitial fluid must increase by several liters (about 10 lbs) before edema becomes clinically apparent. Edema can be demonstrated by an indentation of skin and subcutaneous tissue following applied pressure. This sign, called *pitting edema,* is elicited by pressing the thumb into the skin of the patient against a bony surface, such as the ankle, tibia, fibula, or sacrum. The depth of the pit is then estimated and recorded in millimeters, although physicians often prefer the less precise terms of "2+" or "3+".

Characteristically, generalized edema first appears in the feet and ankles of the ambulatory patient in response to gravitational factors. If the patient is bedridden, the examiner searches for early edema by turning the patient over and indenting the posterior surfaces of the calves and the skin overlying the sacrum. If edema of the legs has been present for a long time in an ambulatory patient, the subcutaneous tissues and skin become fibrotic and pitting may not be elicited.

Should excess fluid accumulate in the peritoneal cavity, the term *ascites* is used. *Pleural effusion* or *hydrothorax* are terms used to denote fluid accumulation in the pleural cavity; *pericardial effusion* is a term which designates the accumulation of fluid in the pericardial cavity. The term *anasarca* is used to denote grossly generalized edematous conditions (67).

Edema is most commonly associated with congestive heart failure; alcoholic cirrhosis, nutritional deficiency, and nephrotic syndrome are next in order of frequency (249).

The pathogenesis of excessive sodium and water retention in congestive heart failure is adequately discussed in the chapter on *Congestive Heart Failure.* Basically, a decrease in cardiac output reduces the glomerular filtration rate which is perceived by the kidney as inadequate circulating blood volume. This initiates a series of events which increases sodium and water retention by the kidneys. Also, in uncompensated right-sided heart failure, venous and capillary hydrostatic pressures are increased resulting in edema formation.

Ascites and edema commonly occur in patients with alcoholic cirrhosis. The major factors which contribute to the excessive accumulation of fluids in these spaces are hypoalbuminemia, elevated intrahepatic and portal pressures, increased hepatic lymph flow, and increased sodium and water retention due to secondary hyperaldosteronism. The hypoalbuminemia, caused by decreased hepatic synthesis of albumin, poor nutrition, and loss of lymphatic protein into the ascitic fluid, results in a low capillary oncotic pressure. This, together with the elevated capillary hydrostatic pressure, elevated osmotic pressure of the ascitic fluid, and sodium retention, favors edema formation (248). Also see Question 34.

Edema associated with the nephrotic syndrome is primarily related to increased excretion of albumin by the kidney with the subsequent loss of oncotic pressure. The movement of water into the interstitium depletes intravascular volume and stimulates renal retention of sodium and water. This is discussed more thoroughly in the chapter on *Diseases of the Kidney.*

1. Since the increased sodium and water retention by the kidney plays a major role in the pathogenesis of edema, a complete understanding of the major sites for sodium and water reabsorption is essential. Review these and identify the major factors which affect sodium and water homeostasis.

A major function of the kidney is the maintenance of sodium and water balance. Normally, the kidney exerts its effect through conservation or enhanced excretion of sodium secondary to volume changes in the intravascular component of the extracellular fluid (ECF) compartment.

In general, the kidney serves as the only realistic route of sodium elimination. Renal glomerular filtration and tubular reabsorption are the major determinants of sodium content in the urine; under most circumstances, all but a very small fraction (i.e. approximately 1%) of the filtered sodium and water is reab-

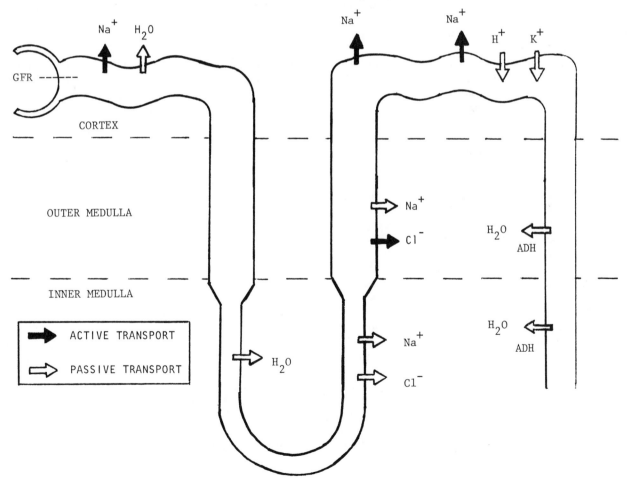

Figure 1: Probable sites of sodium reabsorption in the nephron

sorbed. All of the sodium present in the blood (25,000 mEq/24 hr) is filtered at the glomerulus. See Figure 1.

Under normal conditions, the **proximal tubule** reabsorbs 60-70% of the filtered sodium load. At this site, water is permeable and is passively and isotonically reabsorbed along an osmotic gradient created by active sodium reabsorption. Chloride is also passively reabsorbed down a negative electrochemical gradient formed secondary to sodium reabsorption. Therefore, no dilutional or concentrational changes occur in the proximal tubule with the filtrate remaining isotonic and isosmotic. However, a compositional change does occur here. As a result of the carbonic anhydrase-mediated secretion of hydrogen ion in exchange for sodium ions, approximately 90% of filtered bicarbonate will be reabsorbed as carbon dioxide along with sodium in this segment of the nephron.

Because of the large reabsorptive capacity of the proximal tubule, this site has a major role in regulating ECF volume. Proximal tubule reabsorption remains nearly constant despite moderate changes in glomerular filtration rate (GFR). However, if marked reductions in GFR occur, fractional sodium and water reabsorption by the proximal tubule increases. Thus, poor renal perfusion, which is often noted in cardiac failure, can lead to sodium retention.

In the **ascending limb of the loop of Henle,** 20 to 25% of the filtered sodium load is reabsorbed. Sodium and chloride are passively reabsorbed in the thin segment of the ascending loop. In the thick, "diluting" portion of this segment, (also called the cortical or distal portion of the ascending loop), chloride is actively reabsorbed and sodium passively follows the electrochemical gradient which is created. Because this portion of the tubule is relatively impermeable to water, the medullary interstitium becomes hypertonic and the filtrate becomes increasingly hypotonic as it approaches the distal tubule. The production of hypotonic filtrate in this portion of the segment is also referred to as the production of "free water."

In contrast, the **descending limb of the loop of Henle** is permeable to water. Therefore, in this portion of the nephron, equilibration with the hypertonic medullary interstitium reduces the filtrate volume and results in the production of an increasingly hypertonic filtrate toward the tip of the loop. This gradient of increasing medullary osmolality created by the countercurrent mechanism of the loop of Henle ultimately provides the driving force for the formation of concentrated urine in the presence of antidiuretic hormone (ADH). In the absence of ADH, the hypotonic filtrate generated by the ascending loop of Henle is passed through the collecting ducts and excreted as dilute urine. To summarize, this segment of the nephron contributes significantly to sodium homeostasis and provides a mechanism for urinary dilution or concentration.

At the **distal tubule,** the remaining 5 to 10% of the filtered sodium load is actively filtered in exchange for potassium and hydrogen ion. The efficiency of sodium reabsorption in the distal tubule is governed to a large extent by the mineralocorticoid, aldosterone.

The final reabsorptive site through which the filtrate must pass is the **collecting duct** where antidiuretic hormone (ADH) acts to increase water absorption without sodium. The susceptibility of this portion of the tubule to ADH is important in maintaining serum osmolality. Water reabsorption is enhanced via ADH stimulation in hypertonic states and excess water is eliminated in hypotonic states. The former situation produces a hypertonic urine, and the latter a hypotonic urine (8,37,65,94,99,122).

2. Identify the primary sites of action of the major diuretic classes. Relate this information to their relative diuretic potencies and effects on potassium.

Based on the knowledge of where a diuretic exerts its major effect along the kidney tubule, it is possible to predict the relative potency and electrolyte imbalances which are likely to result from their use.

The more proximal the site of action, the more potent will be the diuretic effect. Therefore, furosemide and ethacrynic acid which inhibit sodium reabsorption in the proximal portion of the ascending loop of Henle are the most potent diuretics. Fortunately, none of the diuretics exerts its major effect at the proximal tubule where a majority of the filtered sodium is absorbed. The thiazide diuretics inhibit sodium reabsorption at the distal portion of the ascending loop and are $1/6$ to $1/8$ as potent as the "loop" diuretics. Finally spironolactone and triamterene, which exert their effects at the distal tubule are the least potent diuretics. See Table 1. Also see Questions 5, 22, and 33 (79).

Table 1
RELATIVE POTENCY OF
THE DIURETICS

Furosemide	8
Ethacrynic acid	6
Thiazides	1
Triamterene	0.4
Spironolactone	0.4

Another generalization which can be made is that any diuretic which acts proximally to the distal tubule may potentially produce hypokalemia and alkalosis. This occurs because more sodium is presented to the distal tubule where sodium is exchanged for potassium and hydrogen ion. In contrast, spironolactone and triamterene, which inhibit sodium at the distal tubule, will produce potassium retention.

3. What are the major principles which should be observed in the treatment of edema?

Several principles should be considered in the treatment of any edematous condition. The first is that edema is a secondary clinical sign of an underlying disease and will persist until that disease is corrected. Therefore, treatment should always be directed towards correction of the primary disorder. Secondly, with the exception of cardiac disease, diuresis per se is frequently only a cosmetic maneuver. Hence, the mere presence of edema is not sufficient reason for the forced removal of excessive interstitial fluid. Third, once therapy directed at correcting the underlying disease has been initiated, several non-drug therapeutic maneuvers can be employed to alleviate edema (see Question 4). Finally, the mobilization of edema fluid into the intravascular compartment may occur more slowly than the rate of diuresis induced by drug therapy. Therefore, there is always the danger that intravascular volume depletion will result from overzealous diuretic therapy. For these reasons, clinicians should be willing to settle for less than complete correction of edema rather than risk the complications of overdiuresis which may considerably worsen the overall clinical condition of the patient (75,76,249).

4. Once edema is noted and therapy has been initiated for the underlying disease, what therapeutic maneuvers can be utilized before resorting to diuretic therapy?

Since sodium retention inherently causes fluid accumulation, *dietary restriction of salt* can have a major effect on the alleviation of some edematous conditions. *Dietary sodium restriction* alone frequently suffices for control of mild edema, and it is not unreasonable to place patients on a 2 to 4 gram per day salt (NaCl) diet. More severe restriction is unpalatable, meets with considerable patient lack of compliance, and in reality offers very little therapeutic advantage (249,284a). It should also be emphasized that vigorous sodium restriction in combination with diuretic therapy may cause profound volume depletion.

To provide a proper perspective, the daily average adult intake of salt is approximately 6 to 15 gm. By restricting a diet to no added salt (NAS), this value is reduced to 4 to 7 gm, and to 2 to 4 gm when salt is restricted during cooking. When suggesting or ordering low salt diets, clinicians should be clear as to whether they desire a 1 gm sodium diet or a 1 gm sodium chloride diet, since 1 gm of sodium represents approximately 2.5 gm of sodium chloride. The following conversions may be useful:

1 gm Na = 43 mEq
1 gm NaCl = 17 mEq of Na
1 mEq of Na = 23 mg

Mobilization of excess interstitial fluid into the vascular compartment by the use of *leg wraps* or *elastic hose* can also be useful adjuncts in the therapy of edema. *Bedrest* increases renal perfusion and is also an important adjunct to edema therapy; sodium excretion can be diminished by ten-fold by assumption of the standing position (249).

5. Describe the site and mechanism of action of the thiazide diuretics. What is the composition of urine produced by these agents?

Thiazide diuretics and the pharmacologically related quinazoline (quinethazone and metolazone) and phthalimidine (chlorthalidone) derivatives are moderately active diuretics which can induce excretion of approximately 5 to 10% of the filtered sodium load. They apparently inhibit sodium reabsorption in or somewhere between the thick diluting segment of the ascending loop of Henle and the distal tubule. These drugs impair free water clearance but do not affect urinary concentration.

Thiazide and thiazide-type diuretics also inhibit proximal tubular sodium and water reabsorption. This effect is partially related to the variable carbonic anhydrase inhibition that most of these agents display. However, factors other than carbonic anhydrase inhibition probably contribute to the overall proximal action. Some drugs, like metolazone, are practically devoid of carbonic anhydrase inhibitory activity and also inhibit proximal tubule sodium and water reabsorption. Although these agents have significant proximal activity, the major diuretic effect results from their more distal site of action.

The diuresis induced by thiazides is characterized by a urine rich in chloride, sodium, potassium, and to a lesser extent, bicarbonate (8, 12, 24, 37, 65, 94, 122, 242).

6. What is the thiazide of choice from a clinical standpoint?

Despite claims of superiority of different products by pharmaceutical companies, all thiazide and thiazide-type diuretics produce similar therapeutic effects under most clinical conditions, with the exception of metolazone (see Question 8). In addition, the incidence of major adverse reactions does not differ significantly between preparations, with the exception of ticrynafen (see Question 9). Products differ primarily in terms of dosage and duration of action (see Table 2). Except for patient convenience and possibly better patient compliance, prolongation of the pharmacologic action of a single dose of some of these analogs does not provide a distinct advantage (8, 9, 12, 65, 79, 94, 122).

Generic Name	Trade Name	Equivalent Dose	Duration of Action	Daily Dose
Chlorothiazide	Diuril	500 mg	6 to 12 hours	500 to 1000 mg
Hydrochlorothiazide	Hydrodiuril	50 mg	12 hours	50 to 100 mg
Bendroflumethiazide	Naturetin	5 mg	18 to 24 hours	5 mg
Trichlormethiazide	Naqua	2 mg	24 hours	1 to 4 mg
Polythiazide	Renese	2 mg	36 hours	1 to 4 mg
Chlorthalidone	Hygroton	50 mg	48 to 72 hours	50 to 100 mg
Quinethazone	Hydromox	50 mg	18 to 24 hours	50 to 100 mg
Metolazone	Zaroxolyn	5 mg	12 to 24 hours	5 to 10 mg

7. Discuss the absorption, metabolism, and distribution of the thiazides. What is the onset and duration of diuretic action?

The thiazides are rapidly absorbed, but the bioavailability varies among the different derivatives. Once absorbed, these agents are distributed in the ECF space, where they are variably protein bound. The thiazides cross the placental barrier and appear in the breast milk of nursing mothers.

These agents are primarily excreted unchanged in the urine by glomerular filtration and by active proximal tubular secretion, presumably by the same transport system that secretes p-aminohippurate and other weak organic acids.

A demonstrable diuretic effect is usually observed within two hours of oral administration. The duration of action varies with the rate of elimination. See Table 2 (12,65,94,122).

8. Discuss the efficacy, pharmacokinetics, and mechanism of action of metolazone. Does it have any advantage over currently available thiazide diuretics?

Metolazone is a new, long acting quinazoline sulfonamide diuretic which is effective in relieving edema of cardiac, hepatic, and renal origin in doses of 5 to 20 mg/day (21,58,61,129,171,180,235,259). It is also useful in the treatment of mild to moderate essential hypertension. The antihypertensive response to 2.5 to 5.0 mg of metolazone is equivalent to 50 mg of hydrochlorothiazide or 100 mg of chlorthalidone (42, 93, 213, 259).

Following oral administration, metolazone is rapidly but incompletely absorbed (271). Diuresis usually begins within the first hour and peaks between 1.5 to 3 hours. The diuretic and natriuretic effect generally persist for at least 24 hours in normal subjects (259). Metolazone, which is highly bound to plasma protein and to red blood cells, is primarily excreted unchanged in the urine. The drug also undergoes significant enterohepatic recycling (259,271).

Like the thiazides, metolazone is thought to inhibit sodium reabsorption in the cortical diluting segment of the ascending loop of Henle or in the early distal tubule. It may also block proximal tubular sodium reabsorption, even though it has little, if any, inhibitory effect on carbonic anhydrase (21a,218a,258a,259).

Because of its similar mode of action, the pharmacologic effects of metolazone are similar to those of thiazide diuretics in most cases (259). However, under certain circumstances there are some qualitative and quantitative differences between the effects of metolazone and thiazides on water and electrolyte excretion (21a,218a,258a,259).

Metolazone in large doses (up to 150 mg/day) can induce diuresis in patients with markedly reduced glomerular filtration rates (21,58,61,235), unlike thiazide diuretics which are ineffective when the GFR is less than 15 to 20 ml/min. In addition, the diuretic action of metolazone is reportedly synergistic with that of furosemide, an effect which is not uniformly seen with thiazides (85,116). This combination may be useful in treating edema refractory to single agents but can be associated with severe electrolyte disturbances (25,85,116). In normal volunteers, the natriuretic response to metolazone is associated with less kaliuresis than an equivalent natriuretic response to thiazides (21a,218a,258a). Nevertheless, hypokalemia frequently occurs during metolazone therapy and the overall incidence does not appear to differ significantly from that associated with the thiazide diuretics (93, 171, 218a, 259).

In conclusion, the above data suggest subtle differences in the mechanism of action of metolazone and the thiazide diuretics. However, except for the convenience of once-a-day dosing, metolazone does not offer any real advantage over currently available thiazide diuretics in most clinical situations. In patients with renal insufficiency, metolazone can produce diuresis when thiazides have failed (259), as can furosemide.

9. What advantages does the new diuretic, ticrynafen, have over presently available diuretics? What is its mechanism of action?

Ticrynafen is a new antihypertensive diuretic agent

undergoing clinical trials in the United States. Chemically, it resembles ethacrynic acid, but pharmacologically it works like the thiazides. Apparently, the natriuretic and antihypertensive effects of 500 mg of ticrynafen are equivalent to 50 mg of hydrochlorothiazide. The diuretic effect of 250 to 500 mg of ticrynafen is additive with that of 40 mg of furosemide.

Unlike thiazides, thiazide-type, and loop diuretics (all of which cause urate retention with chronic administration), ticrynafen possesses *uricosuric* activity. Ticrynafen apparently inhibits uric acid tubular reabsorption at both pre- and post-secretory sites. The uricosuric effect is maintained in patients receiving either thiazide or loop diuretics concomitantly. Therefore it appears that ticrynafen offers a significant advance in diuretic therapy by reducing the potential risks of elevated uric acid levels (204,262). The reader is also referred to the chapters on *Gout and Hyperuricemia* and *Essential Hypertension.*

10. A 54-year-old female with nephrotic syndrome was placed on hydrochlorothiazide 100 mg/day for peripheral edema. After some improvement, she noted some return of "swelling" after several weeks. An analysis of the urine electrolytes at that time revealed a low sodium content and relatively high potassium concentrations. Assess this situation. Does tolerance to the diuretic effects of thiazides occur?

This patient exemplifies some of the typical findings of diuretic tolerance or escape. Unlike the organomercurials or the carbonic anhydrase inhibitors, the diuretic actions of the thiazides are not influenced by acid-base balance. However, daily thiazide administration does not produce indefinite natriuresis in normal, hypertensive, or edematous subjects (75, 76, 77, 78, 79).

Earley and Orloff (74) describe the escape from the natriuretic effect of hydrochlorothiazide in a patient with nephrogenic diabetes insipidus. "Beginning on the first day of therapy, hydrochlorothiazide uniformly resulted in an increased excretion of sodium and, to a lesser extent, potassium. After the first day of therapy, the excretion of sodium decreased, and by the fourth to sixth day the output of sodium as well as potassium had returned to control levels." Although this involved a patient with diabetes insipidus, similar observations have been made in hypertensive patients whose extracellular fluid volume (ECFV) returns to normal despite continual thiazide therapy. (See the chapter on *Hypertension.*)

By enhancing sodium and water excretion, diuretics decrease the ECFV. If ECFV depletion occurs, aldosterone production increases resulting in greater distal sodium reabsorption in exchange for potassium. This explains the observation of low sodium and relatively

high potassium concentrations in the patient's urine. This phenomenon may occur in the presence of edema if the excess interstitial fluid has not had time to mobilize in the vascular compartment.

The reduced glomerular filtration rate associated with edematous conditions, as well as with ECFV contraction and diuresis increases the proximal tubular reabsorption of sodium. This effectively limits the amount of sodium which is delivered to the distal tubular sites where diuretics exert their major activity. Also, the diseases associated with edematous conditions are often intrinsically characterized by increased sodium reabsorption at the proximal tubule.

In summary, diuretic escape occurs as a result of enhanced aldosterone activity and the diminished delivery of sodium to the distal portion of the nephron. Spironolactone, an aldosterone antagonist may minimize and partially reverse this patient's tolerance to hydrochlorothiazide (75-79).

11. A 65-year-old white female is admitted to the emergency room of General Hospital in an obtunded state following a generalized seizure. The patient had developed progressive weakness, lethargy, anorexia, and dizzy spells in the week prior to admission and had become increasingly confused, disoriented, and agitated over the past two days. Medical problems include schizophrenia and psychogenic water drinking of three years duration and essential hypertension.

Current medications include chlorpromazine 100 mg three times daily, diazepam 10 mg every 8 hours as needed, and hydrochlorothiazide 25 mg twice daily which was begun ten days previously at her last clinic visit.

The patient did not appear dehydrated, and no edema was noted. Renal and adrenal functions were within normal limits. Laboratory data revealed the following: Na 110 mEq/L, Cl 68 mEq/L, K 2.9 mEq/L, HCO_3 38 mEq/L, BUN 9 mg%, blood glucose 125 mg%, plasma osmolality 255 mOsm/kg. The urinalysis showed the following: osmolality 536 mOsm/kg; Na 60 mEq/L; K 80 mEq/L. Can this clinical picture be explained on the basis of this patient's diuretic therapy?

True hyponatremia may be the result of an actual sodium deficiency or due to a dilutional effect. It is a rare side effect of diuretic therapy. Nevertheless, patients on severely restricted sodium diets can be over-diuresed and can develop hyponatremia, hypovolemia, and prerenal azotemia. This is probably more common with the more potent loop diuretics and treatment consists of fluid and electrolyte replacement (8,65).

Dilutional hyponatremia, resembling the **syndrome of inappropriate antidiuretic hormone** (SIADH) secretion, has been described following treatment with thiazide and loop diuretics (22, 66, 68, 74, 89, 95, 109, 110, 155, 185). Patients with congestive heart failure or hepatic cirrhosis are more likely to develop this diuretic-induced dilutional hyponatremia because of pre-existing defects in free water clearance. Strict low sodium diets and excessive fluid intake further enhance the risk. Additionally, impaired free water clearance can result in acute symptomatic hyponatremia in psychogenic water drinkers receiving thiazide diuretics (22,66,109,155).

Severe hyponatremia with serum sodiums ranging from 91 to 120 mEq/L was attributed to diuretics by Fichman (89). Twenty-five patients with diuretic-induced hyponatremia had a syndrome which was indistinguishable from SIADH except that alkalosis and hypokalemia were also present as seen in this patient. The diuretics implicated in this study included a variety of thiazide derivatives, furosemide (Lasix), and chlorthalidone (Hygroton) in conventional doses. Within 3 to 10 days after discontinuation of therapy, the hyponatremia disappeared and the ability to excrete a water load returned to normal. Repetitive episodes of hyponatremia occurred within 2 to 12 days after the reinstitution of these diuretics. An elevated ADH activity was noted in all 10 patients with diuretic related hyponatremia in whom ADH activity was measured. Treatment of dilutional hyponatremia includes fluid restriction and discontinuation of the offending diuretic agent (8,65). Also see chapter on *Diseases of the Kidney.*

12. This patient also has a diuretic-induced hypochloremic, hypokalemic alkalosis. How do diuretics induce these abnormalities? Which patients are most susceptible to clinically significant hypokalemia. How should this side effect be monitored and when should it be treated?

Hypokalemia and total body potassium depletion is a common side effect of the thiazides, thiazide-type, and loop diuretics (43,65,94,122). It is primarily caused by an exchange of sodium for potassium in the distal tubule. The urinary excretion of potassium is enhanced by: (a) an increased rate of delivery of sodium to the distal tubule; (b) diuretic related chloride loss and alkalosis; and (c) increased aldosterone secretion secondary to either the disease state or diuretic-induced volume depletion (151, 160, 161, 168, 199, 260). Also see the chapters on *Fluids and Electrolytes* and *Acid-Base Disorders.*

Most ambulatory, non-edematous, hypertensive patients who are chronically treated with thiazide diuretics or furosemide do not require prophylactic potassium supplementation despite small or moderate decreases in serum potassium (151,160,168,199,225). Also see the chapter on *Hypertension.*

Conversely, diuretic-treated patients with edema of hepatic and renal origin consistently demonstrate a significant reduction in total body potassium stores. Concurrent hypokalemia may be present, although total body potassium depletion commonly exists in these patients despite normal potassium levels. A number of factors appear to be involved in the development of potassium deficiency in this group of patients. These include high circulating aldosterone levels due to the patient's medical condition and/or secondary to diuretic-related volume depletion; cellular metabolic abnormalities associated with the disease state; poor nutritional status and muscle wasting; or diuretic-induced kaliuresis.

Similar potassium deficiencies have previously been reported in patients with edema due to congestive heart failure (151,160,168,199). However, recent clinical investigators have failed to find substantial decreases in potassium stores in these patients even when treated with diuretics (64,169,198). This discrepancy is probably due to improperly matched patients and controls in the earlier studies (198).

Patients should be monitored frequently in the first few months of diuretic therapy to determine their potassium requirements. Prophylactic or therapeutic potassium replacement should be given only when the therapeutic gains of treatment are balanced against its risks (167,168). Routine potassium supplementation should be avoided in non-edematous ambulatory hypertensive patients receiving kaliuretic diuretics as long as the serum potassium remains above 3.0 mEq/L and no symptoms related to potassium deficiency are apparent (151,160,168,199). On the other hand, potassium replacement is warranted in cirrhotic patients where hypokalemia and alkalosis may contribute to the development of hepatic coma, or in patients with congestive heart failure treated with digitalis in whom hypokalemia would increase the risk of digitalis arrhythmias (151,160,168,199). Also see the chapter entitled *Essential Hypertension.*

Hypochloremia: When sodium is reabsorbed, electroneutrality must be maintained by the concomitant reabsorption of an anion or the tubular secretion of a cation. Certain anions such as chloride or thiocyanate readily penetrate the tubular membrane, whereas others such as phosphate and bicarbonate are poorly permeable. Since chloride is readily reabsorbable and is abundant, considerable sodium reabsorption is accompanied by the concomitant reabsorption of chloride. Likewise, a sodium diuresis results in a chloride diuresis as well.

Under normal conditions urinary excretion of chloride is consistently greater than that of sodium, because the distal nephron allows for the reabsorption of sodium in "exchange" for the tubular secretion of potassium and hydrogen ions. Since there is no net change in electroneutrality, chloride does not accompany the reabsorbed sodium and is therefore excreted (150a,241a). It is also important to note that the chloride plasma concentration is only 75% that of sodium. Thus, the excretion of equimolar concentrations of sodium and chloride results in a relative plasma chloride loss that greatly exceeds that of sodium (154a).

Since diuretic therapy is aimed at an increased sodium excretion, concomitant chloruresis is unavoidable. Moreover, diuretic programs often include salt restriction which also decreases chloride intake. Also see the chapter on *Acid-Base Disorders.*

Metabolic Alkalosis: Diuretic induced alkalosis is generally associated with hypochloremia, although it need not be. Alkalosis can occur as the result of a shrinking extracellular fluid compartment along with normal renal bicarbonate reabsorption (241a).

13. What therapeutic measures are available to prevent, minimize, or correct hypokalemia? What doses should be prescribed?

Diuretic-induced hypokalemia sometimes can be prevented by increasing the dietary intake of potassium-containing foods. This may be useful in hypertensive patients being treated with low doses of diuretics; however, caloric restrictions in these patients may prevent adoption of such dietary measures (151,160,168). Also see Questions 16-17 in the *Essential Hypertension* chapter.

Oral potassium supplements are commonly used to replace diuretic-induced potassium losses. If potassium supplementation is indicated, either prophylactically or for replacement, the preparation of choice is *potassium chloride.* Since treatment with potassium-wasting diuretics may also produce a hypochloremic alkalosis, chloride ion must be replaced along with the potassium.

As long as hypochloremic alkalosis exists, hypokalemia cannot be corrected. In one study (241a), the administration of 80 mEq of potassium bicarbonate to a hypochloremic hypokalemic patient failed to correct the acid-base imbalance and only resulted in a modest retention of potassium. After discontinuation of the potassium bicarbonate supplement, about half of the potassium which had been retained during loading was excreted. In another study (150a), 120 to 140 mEq daily of potassium bicarbonate or phosphate did not correct the acid-base imbalance or the body potassium stores until the chloride deficiency was corrected. Although a slight, transient retention of potassium was noticed, all but one of the subjects were excreting as much potassium as they were ingesting by the second or third day. In contrast, a remarkable rise in serum potassium concentrations occurred when the chloride salt was administered.

Therefore, the use of potassium agents which are converted to bicarbonate *in vivo* (potassium gluconate [Kaon], potassium citrate [K-Lyte], or the combination of potassium acetate, potassium bicarbonate, and potassium citrate [Potassium Triplex]) will have very little effect on diuretic-induced hypokalemia if hypochloremic alkalosis is present. These more palatable preparations may be effectively used to replace potassium deficits only if hypochloremic alkalosis is not present (151,160,168,199,260,280).

Most patients, especially non-edematous hypertensive patients, requiring potassium supplementation can be adequately treated with 40 to 60 mEq/day or less of potassium. However, those patients with disease states associated with high circulating aldosterone levels may require doses of potassium in excess of 60 mEq/day (151,160,168,199,225,260).

Potassium sparing diuretics, spironolactone and triamterene, in conjunction with kaliuretic diuretics occasionally prevent potassium losses. Besides reducing potassium urinary losses, such combination treatment also minimizes alkalosis and may provide a more effective regimen for mobilizing edema fluid (151,160,260). These agents should not be used in conjunction with potassium supplements due to the risk of hyperkalemia. Also see the chapter on *Essential Hypertension* for additional information on potassium supplementation.

14. Potassium chloride elixir, 20 mEq tid, is prescribed for the above patient. One week later, the serum potassium is only 3.0 mEq/L. The patient confesses that she has not been taking the preparation because of its "awful taste." Are there any palatable potassium chloride preparations available? Are the KCl tablets acceptable to use?

One of the major problems of potassium supplementation is *patient non-compliance* due to the unpalatable taste of most potassium chloride preparations. Sometimes the problem can be alleviated by mixing solutions of potassium chloride in fruit juices or by trying somewhat more expensive potassium chloride effervescent tablets which partially alter the taste. Diluting potassium chloride solutions also reduces gastrointestinal upset.

Slow K, a slow release solid dosage form of potassium chloride crystals imbedded in a wax matrix, is equal to potassium chloride solutions in bioavailability and is associated with less gastrointestinal bleeding and ulceration than enteric-coated potassium tablets. Although *esophageal ulceration and stricture,* as well as *gastric and small bowel ulceration* have been reported with the wax-matrix slow release potassium preparations (86,133,170,188,191,226), the incidence is less than that associated with enteric coated tablets

(151). Slow release potassium tablets should be avoided in patients with impaired gastrointestinal mobility (151), and enteric-coated potassium tablets should be avoided at all times. Also see the chapter on *Peptic Ulcer Disease*. If these measures fail, one should consider discontinuing potassium supplementation and instituting potassium sparing diuretics.

15. A 52-year-old housewife is hospitalized with the complaint of increasing shortness of breath (SOB) and dyspnea on exertion (DOE) of two days duration. Past medical history includes a five year history of idiopathic osteoporosis treated with calciferol 4.0 mg/day and supplemental calcium lactate 1.0 gm/day. Admission laboratories were unremarkable except for a BUN of 47 mg% and a serum creatinine of 1.6 mg%. This patient's acute distress was treated with furosemide and aminophylline. Four days after her acute episode she was switched to hydrochlorothiazide 50 mg twice daily. On the seventh hospital day, the patient was noted to be lethargic and slightly confused. An elevated serum calcium level of 12.8 mg% was noted on the SMA-12 panel. The physician decided to discontinue hydrochlorothiazide, calcium lactate and calciferol. By the ninth hospital day the calcium level had fallen to 10.2 mg% at which time calciferol and calcium lactate were restarted. What effect do thiazide diuretics have on calcium homeostasis?

Thiazide diuretics have two major effects on calcium homeostasis: hypercalcemia and hypocalciuria. They *increase both total and ionized serum calcium* in normal subjects and in patients with various diseases during acute and chronic administration (31, 49, 73, 146, 159, 176, 194, 207-210, 243, 261, 300). Perhaps because of feedback inhibition on parathyroid hormone (PTH) secretion, these elevations of serum calcium are usually transient even with continued treatment, and they rarely reach levels of clinical significance. However, symptomatic hypercalcemia secondary to thiazides can occur, especially in patients with metabolic bone diseases associated with increased bone resorption as exemplified by this patient.

A rise in total serum calcium concentrations ranging from 11.3 to 12.0 mg% was observed on several separate occasions in a patient with essential hypertension being treated intermittently with hydrochlorothiazide (HCTZ) 50 mg twice daily (73). Calcium levels normalized when HCTZ was withdrawn. A subsequent trial of HCTZ 50 mg twice daily for 30 days in this patient produced a rise in total calcium levels from 10.0 mg% to 12.4 mg% by the ninth day which reverted to baseline by the fourteenth day. A case of symptomatic hypercalcemia (12.6 mg%) following three to four days of thiazide administration was noted in a patient with juvenile osteoporosis treated with calciferol; the

hypercalcemia subsided within five days of thiazide withdrawal. Thiazides also transiently increase calcium levels in hypoparathyroid subjects treated with vitamin D (209,210). This effect is temporary, self-limiting and unrelated to dose (31,176,194,261).

In contrast to the transient effects seen in most patients, thiazide administration commonly causes a sustained hypercalcemia in patients with primary hyperparathyroidism, probably because PTH secretion is not suppressed in response to increases in serum calcium (31,49,208,215,300).

Thiazide-induced hypercalcemia may be related to hemoconcentration and reduced calcium excretion (31,159,208); however, these mechanisms are not solely responsible. Hypercalcemia and the magnitude of fall in urinary calcium excretion correlate poorly (208). In 9 hemodialyzed patients who had little or no remaining renal function, elevated serum calcium concentrations were attributed to the thiazides and persisted for at least two weeks after the thiazide was withdrawn (159). Thus, thiazides may have provided strong extrarenal effects on calcium metabolism.

The increase in total and ionized plasma calcium may also be due to thiazide-induced release of calcium from bone into the extracellular fluid and may be caused by enhancement of the action of PTH or vitamin D (159,209,210,215,261). Hyperparathyroidism has been observed in six hypertensive patients undergoing chronic thiazide treatment (207). In addition, a high prevalence of hypercalcemia and primary hyperparathyroidism were found in patients receiving thiazide on routine medical health screening (49). Although these studies, as well as experimental investigations in animals (212), raise the possibility that thiazides may stimulate parathyroid gland hyperplasia (300), studies on PTH levels in thiazide-treated patients have shown either no change (261) or a decrease in PTH levels (51). Therefore, it is not clear whether thiazides may in fact induce hyperparathyroidism or only unmask underlying aberrations in parathyroid function.

The chronic administration of thiazides and thiazide-type diuretics can reduce urinary calcium excretion. The *hypocalciuric effect* of thiazides usually begins within two to three days following initiation of drug treatment and may occur in normal patients, patients with hypercalciuria, and in patients with hyperparathyroidism (31, 73, 82, 147, 164, 194, 202, 209, 210, 243, 298-300). This action of thiazides has been used successfully to prevent calcium nephrolithiasis and renal calculi formation (52, 82, 202, 298-300).

The mechanism by which thiazides reduce urinary calcium excretion remains an area of continuing investigation. Thiazide-induced hypocalciuria is due in part to diuretic-induced extracellular fluid volume (ECFV) depletion which enhances proximal tubular reabsorption of sodium, as well as calcium (31, 210, 264, 300). Since renal tubular reabsorption of calcium is closely related to that of sodium, it is reasonable to conclude that events, such as ECFV depletion, which affect sodium excretion will also affect calcium excretion. Moreover, the replacement of sodium losses reverses the hypocalciuric effect of thiazides (31,264).

There are other factors which contribute to this hypocalciuric effect. For example, the vast majority of hypoparathyroid patients have a blunted or absent hypocalciuric response to thiazide diuretics. This occurs despite extracellular fluid volume depletion and suggests that the presence of parathyroid hormone is essential for the hypocalciuric action of thiazides. Although thiazides enhance the hypocalciuric effect of circulating parathyroid hormone (PTH) on the renal tubules (31,73,194,208-210,300), a direct effect of thiazides on the renal tubule cannot be ruled out (57, 147, 300).

16. A 55-year-old obese male is seen in the outpatient clinic for evaluation of mild congestive heart failure and essential hypertension. The patient has been treated with chlorthalidone 50 mg/day and digoxin 0.25 mg/day for the last six months. Besides an increase in serum uric acid to 8.9 mg%, a modest increase in serum triglyceride levels and a mild elevation of serum cholesterol were noted. Can thiazide or thiazide-type diuretics affect either cholesterol or triglyceride serum levels?

An *increase in serum lipids* similar to that observed in the above case has been described in hypertensive patients undergoing treatment with thiazide and thiazide-type diuretics (5,6,124,141,236). The reported rise in lipid levels may become evident as soon as the first week of diuretic treatment and apparently persists (6). The mechanisms by which thiazides affect lipid metabolism are not known.

In a study of 63 patients with uncomplicated essential hypertension, 31 patients with diastolic blood pressures of 104 mm Hg or less received no drug therapy, and were maintained on a low sodium, lipid lowering, and calorie restricted diet (5). The remaining 32 patients with diastolic blood pressures greater than 104 mm Hg were treated with chlorthalidone and diet. Chlorthalidone doses ranged from 50 mg twice a week to 100 mg/day. In those patients treated with diet only, the serum triglyceride levels did not change; however, the serum cholesterol decreased slightly. Conversely, the chlorthalidone/diet treatment group had a 12 mg/dl (5.2%) and a 36 mg/dl (25.7%) increase in serum cholesterol and triglycerides respectively. Most of the changes in the chlorthalidone treatment group could be attributed to a subgroup of 15 patients. If analyzed separately, these patients had substantial elevations in serum lipids with increases in cholesterol and triglyc-

eride levels of 29 mg/dl (13.9%) and 66 mg/dl (51.9%) respectively. Lipid levels did not change significantly in the remaining 17 patients (5). Another study by the same investigator resulted in similar findings (6).

Of 300 hypertensives (124) who were evaluated for lipid changes for three years, no significant changes were noted in serum cholesterol or triglyceride levels in either the thiazide treated group or the control group which received no treatment. A subgroup within the treatment group however, was identified as having substantial increases in serum triglyceride and uric acid levels. Both of these changes were primarily limited to those patients who had gained weight during treatment. Equivalent weight gain in the control group did not produce similar results. Thus, weight gain should be avoided during thiazide treatment of essential hypertension. (Also see the *Essential Hypertension* chapter.)

17. Is the elevated uric acid in the above patient also due to diuretic treatment? Should urate-lowering treatment be initiated?

Diuretics have been implicated as a cause of **hyperuricemia** in over 20% of patients with this condition. In addition, more than 50% of diuretic-treated patients with essential hypertension are hyperuricemic. Increases of 1 to 2 mg% in uric acid levels are common during thiazide administration, although 4 to 5 mg% elevations have been reported.

Diuretic-induced hyperuricemia is due to decreased excretion of urates as well as extracellular fluid volume contraction. Replacement of urinary sodium and fluid losses abolishes the hyperuricemia caused by the diuretics.

The natural history of diuretic-induced hyperuricemia is not entirely clear. Although moderate elevations in plasma uric acid are common during chronic diuretic treatment, the development of acute gouty arthritis is relatively rare; however, it is not known whether these patients are at risk of developing gouty nephropathy.

Presently, the general consensus is that the majority of patients who develop elevated uric acid levels during treatment with diuretic agents will remain asymptomatic and need not be treated. Only those patients with uric acid levels persistently greater than 11.0 mg% (SMA 12/60 autoanalyzer), as well as those with a history of gout or a familial predisposition should be considered for treatment with urate lowering agents. Although treatment of asymptomatic hyperuricemia may be initiated to prevent the complications of elevated uric acid, there is no clearcut evidence that asymptomatic hyperuricemia alone is harmful (256, 296). Also see the chapter on *Gout and Hyperuricemia.*

18. A 63-year-old moderately obese woman was

referred to the diabetic clinic from the hypertension clinic at General Hospital for control of her adult onset diabetes mellitus of five years duration. The patient's chief complaint is polyuria and nocturia. She is presently spilling 3+ to 4+ glucose in her urine and her fasting blood sugars are running between 225 and 250 mg%. Although her physician from the diabetic clinic originally controlled her diabetes by diet alone, increasing complaints of polyuria and repeatedly elevated fasting blood glucose levels of greater than 190 mg% led to the institution of tolbutamide 500 mg three times a day one year prior to the present clinic visit. Following the initiation of tolbutamide, fasting blood glucose levels fluctuated between 130 to 150 mg% with only negative to trace glycosuria. Six months before the present clinic visit the patient was found to be mildly hypertensive and she was referred to the hypertension clinic where she was evaluated and begun on hydrochlorothiazide. After several visits to the hypertension clinic the patient was lost to follow-up for four months until her present visit to the hypertension clinic. The patient says she has maintained her diabetic diet and takes her medications regularly. Current medications include tolbutamide 500 mg three times a day; diazepam 5 mg every six hours as needed, and hydrochlorothiazide 50 mg twice daily for blood pressure control. Could the thiazide diuretic affect this patient's diabetic control?

Hyperglycemia and *glucose intolerance* have been reported to occur during treatment with thiazide diuretics (4,7,30,44,48,59,71,72,102,108,128,158,174, 190,230,234,245,253,294). Mild to moderate rises in fasting blood sugar (FBS) commonly occur within the first several weeks of thiazide administration in diabetic, as well as prediabetic patients. Occasionally, elevations in FBS may be more pronounced with increases as great as 350 mg%. In some patients, discontinuation of thiazides may be necessary, or alternatively, the addition or dosage adjustment of hypoglycemic agents may be required to control blood glucose levels.

Hyperosmolar nonketotic coma associated with marked hyperglycemia has also been reported as a serious sequela of thiazide's diabetogenic effects. Elderly, late onset diabetics appear to be at greatest risk. The incidence of hyperosmolar nonketotic coma is very low but the mortality rate ranges between 20 to 40% (59,102,174,253). Although diabetic and prediabetic patients are more prone to the diabetogenic effects of thiazides, significant carbohydrate disturbances may also become evident in nondiabetic patients after several years of chronic thiazide treatment (4, 30, 158, 174, 294).

The exact mechanism of diuretic-induced carbohydrate intolerance is unknown, but a number of possibilities exist. These include impaired pancreatic insulin release, extrapancreatic effects on glucose utilization, and thiazide-related changes in catecholamine release affecting carbohydrate metabolism. Impaired insulin release caused by thiazide-induced hypokalemia and decreased peripheral glucose utilization have also been suggested as mechanisms. Potassium replacement has reportedly reversed the hyperglycemic effect of thiazides, however, the association of hypokalemia and thiazide hyperglycemia has not been consistently demonstrated (4,48,72,128).

Furosemide (30,72,137,166,174, 201,270,273,281), as well as ethacrynic acid, and triamterene (7,87,128) have also been reported to affect carbohydrate metabolism. However, the effects of these drugs on blood sugar and glucose tolerance appear to be weaker and less consistent than those seen with thiazides. Nonetheless, in certain patients, the diabetogenic effect of these diuretic agents can be significant as evidenced by the fact that hyperosmolar nonketotic coma has been reported in patients treated with furosemide (72,166,270). (Also see the chapter on *Diabetes Mellitus.*)

19. A 67-year-old female is hospitalized with a 24-hour history of abdominal pain, nausea and vomiting. The patient has no history of alcohol abuse or hyperlipoproteinemias. Pertinent medical history includes congestive heart failure of six months duration treated with digoxin 0.25 mg/day, hydrochlorothiazide 100 mg/day, and KCl 40 mEq/day which were all discontinued on admission.

Physical examination on admission revealed a slightly obese female in apparent distress with moderate to severe epigastric pain. Admission laboratory values of significance were a serum amylase of 875 U/dl, and a BUN of 52 mg%. A subsequent 24-hour urinary amylase came back as 8450 U/24 hours.

The patient was treated for acute pancreatitis with nasogastric suction, intravenous fluids, and meperidine for pain. She rapidly improved over the next ten days with normalization of her serum amylase. At this time her previous medications for congestive heart failure were restarted. Within two days the patient again began to complain of abdominal tenderness. A repeat serum amylase revealed that the level had again risen to 315 U/dl. Can thiazide diuretics or any other diuretic agent cause pancreatitis?

Acute hemorrhagic necrotizing *pancreatitis* is a rare complication of thiazide diuretics (26, 69, 143, 195, 244, 286) and chlorthalidone (144). A number of fatalities have been reported (69,143,195,244,286), including two cases of fatal hemorrhagic pancreatitis in pregnant women receiving chlorothiazide (195). In another case, hyperglycemic, hyperosmolar coma and lactic acidosis secondary to thiazide-related pancreatitis appeared to contribute to the patient's death (69). Pancreatic atrophy was apparently the cause of death in a 9-year-old boy on long-term hydrochlorothiazide (244). The overall incidence of thiazide-induced pancreatitis appears to be low. However, 1.0 to 2.0 gm/day of chlorothiazide can cause a 1½- to 2-fold increase in serum amylase levels in 50% of patients (56).

Several case reports also implicate furosemide as a cause of acute pancreatitis (26,36,40,145,292). In two separate cases, drug rechallenge clearly identified furosemide as the causative agent (40,145).

In a recent study, drug histories were obtained from 100 patients with acute pancreatitis (26). These patients were cross-matched for sex and age with control patients who were admitted with abdominal pain but normal serum amylase levels. Diuretic intake was substantially more frequent in the patients with acute pancreatitis (26 versus 11%). Thiazides, particularly cyclopenthiazide, accounted for 58% of diuretic intake in patients with pancreatitis, furosemide accounted for 35%. Although the results of this study indicate that diuretics may induce acute pancreatitis, the clinical conditions in which diuretics were used could not be ruled out as possible etiologic factors.

20. A 64-year-old female who developed a purpuric rash three days prior to admission (PTA) was admitted with a diagnosis of thrombocytopenia purpura. The platelet count on admission was 14,000/mm³; the WBC and differential were unremarkable. Past medical history includes atrial flutter of two years duration treated with quinidine sulfate 200 mg every six hours and digitoxin 0.1 mg once daily; a six-month history of mild hypertension had been controlled on sodium restriction alone until three weeks PTA at which time chlorothiazide 0.5 gm twice daily was added for further blood pressure control. Routine hematological testing at this time was normal. All medications were discontinued on admission and within three days, the platelet levels began to rise and reached a level of 125,000/mm³ by the sixth hospital day. However, because of worsening atrial arrhythmias both quinidine and digitoxin were reinstituted at their previous dosage. Nevertheless, the platelet count continued to rise and the patient was discharged with a platelet count of 250,000/mm³ on the 15th hospital day. Can thiazide diuretics induce thrombocytopenia purpura?

The thiazide and thiazide-type diuretics can cause *thrombocytopenia* (17, 23, 83, 103, 138, 162, 192, 205, 255, 302). A low platelet count is usually the sole hematologic abnormality, but on occasion neutropenia or agranulocytosis may also be present (192, 255, 302). In most cases, thrombocytopenia is associated with purpura, although purpura in the absence of thrombocytopenia has been reported as well (92,132).

The time course from the initiation of thiazide treatment to the development of thrombocytopenia varies. Thrombocytopenia usually becomes clinically evident one week to several months after initiation of diuretic treatment, although as many as nine months may pass before thrombocytopenia is discovered. Platelet counts return to normal following withdrawal of thiazide diuretics. Although this patient is receiving other drugs which have been reported to cause thrombocytopenia, the temporal relationship of chlorothiazide makes it the most likely cause of thrombocytopenia.

In a retrospective study (162), 19 of 71 patients (26%) receiving diuretics (5 thiazides, 14 chlorthalidone) developed asymptomatic thrombocytopenia with platelet counts of less than 100,000/mm³ as compared to only 4 of 93 (<4%) cardiac patients not receiving diuretics. The thrombocytopenia may be related to dosage and duration of diuretic therapy. Further evidence for a toxic myelosuppression is the finding of a hypoplastic marrow with decreased megakaryocytes in several cases in which thrombocytopenia was associated with other blood dyscrasias (192,255). However, several other reports implicate an immunologic mechanism as the cause of thiazide-induced thrombocytopenia (23,83,103,138,205). Circulating IgM globulin was identified in one case (83). The possibility that there are two mechanisms by which thiazides cause thrombocytopenia cannot be ruled out.

Neutropenia (203,238,255,274,291), agranulocytosis (135,157,302), and immune hemolytic anemia (277) are other blood dyscrasias which have been associated with thiazide and thiazide-type diuretic treatment.

21. If a patient has experienced a mild rash to sulfisoxazole (Gantrisin), does this mean that the sulfonamide diuretics (furosemide, chlorthalidone, quinethazone and the thiazides) are contraindicated?

Some investigators believe that the metabolites of the antibacterial sulfonamides, rather than the parent compound, are responsible for skin lesions and hypersensitivity reactions (284). Since sulfonamides are acetylated and oxidized to varying extents it is possible for a patient to become allergic to one antibacterial sulfonamide and not another. One study showed that the cross-sensitivity between different antibacterial sulfonamides was approximately 17% (72a). Therefore, the cross sensitivity between chemically different sulfonamides such as the thiazide diuretics and sulfisoxazole should be practically nil. It would probably be safe to administer furosemide or a thiazide to a patient who had previously experienced a mild rash from an antibacterial sulfonamide, provided that the patient is closely monitored.

Ethacrynic acid does not contain a sulfa radical and may be used in a patient who proves to be cross-sensitive. (Also see the chapter entitled *Diabetes Mellitus*.)

22. How do furosemide (Lasix) and ethacrynic acid (Edecrin) affect sodium and water reabsorption in the renal tubule?

Furosemide and ethacrynic acid are the most potent diuretic agents currently available. Although their chemical structures are completely different, these agents are generally discussed in tandem because they are strikingly similar in their pharmacologic effects (8,24,37,65,94, 122,156,242,290a).

Furosemide and ethacrynic acid exert their major diuretic action by inhibiting active chloride transport (and thereby passive sodium reabsorption) in the thick diluting segment of the ascending loop of Henle (37,242,290a). Since 20 to 25% of the filtered sodium load is reabsorbed at this site, these agents can produce a substantial increase in the urinary excretion of sodium, chloride, and water. Potassium excretion is also increased. The maximal diuretic effect of furosemide and ethacrynic acid is much greater than that which can be achieved with thiazide diuretics (242, 290a).

These drugs may also inhibit the proximal tubular reabsorption of sodium. However, such proximal activity, if present, is relatively insignificant in terms of excreted sodium. Furthermore, the volume depletion or decreased glomerular filtration rate induced by these two diuretics leads to increased sodium reabsorption which more than cancels any inhibition of proximal tubule reabsorption these agents may have (37,242).

Additional data suggest that loop diuretics may enhance sodium excretion by shifting renal blood flow from the long juxtamedullary nephrons to shorter superficial cortical nephrons (65).

23. Is there any preference for the use of furosemide or ethacrynic acid?

Throughout this chapter, ethacrynic acid and furosemide are discussed in tandem because of their similarities. They share a common site of action in the renal tubule and induce a comparable diuresis. Both diuretics are equally potent; 40 mg of furosemide is essentially equivalent to 50 mg of ethacrynic acid. These drugs also share the same major side effects of electrolyte disturbances, hyperuricemia, and ototoxicity. Ethacrynic acid, however, is more disturbing to the gastrointestinal tract and the incidence of gastrointestinal bleeding may be significantly higher than with furosemide based on a prospective report (252). Blood dyscrasias have been reported with both drugs as well (62).

Ethacrynic acid has never been as popular as furosemide, although the reason for this is not clear. Perhaps the early reports of transient and permanent deafness associated with ethacrynic acid provide a partial explanation. The immediate availability of parenteral furosemide as opposed to ethacrynate sodium, which requires reconstitution, may be another reason for furosemide's popularity (8,9,65,122).

24. Characterize the clinical response to oral and parenteral furosemide.

Natriuresis usually begins 30 to 60 minutes after oral administration of furosemide. Diuresis peaks within the first or second hour and lasts for 6 to 8 hours. The diuresis following an intravenous injection begins within 5 minutes, peaks within the first 30 minutes, and is usually complete within 2 hours. Intramuscular administration has a somewhat slower onset of action than intravenous administration (24,65,94,122).

25. What is the bioavailability of furosemide? Are dose adjustments required when switching a patient from oral to parenteral furosemide?

Following oral administration, furosemide absorption is erratic and incomplete. As a consequence, plasma furosemide concentrations are significantly lower following oral as opposed to parenteral administration of the drug (134,153). Bioavailability data from several pharmacokinetic studies have shown that only 30 to 85% of an oral dose of furosemide reaches the systemic circulation (29,134,152,153). Branch et al (29) and Kelly et al (152,153) both report a mean bioavailability of approximately 50% in healthy subjects and in patients with renal failure. Huang et al (134) found a mean bioavailability of 76% in 12 patients with advanced renal insufficiency.

Although the bioavailability of oral furosemide is approximately half that of parenteral furosemide, most clinical investigations, with few exceptions (134), have demonstrated that the diuretic response from an oral dose of furosemide is similar to that of a comparable intravenous dose (3,20,29,63,152,153).

At present there is no strong evidence to indicate that dosage alterations of furosemide are required when switching from intravenous to oral administration. Except for a more rapid onset of diuretic activity, parenteral furosemide does not appear to offer any significant advantage over oral administration in treating fluid retention (29).

26. A 34-year-old woman is hospitalized for management of acute renal failure of unknown origin. Past medical history is non-contributory except for a history of mild hypertension and glucosuria during her last pregnancy five years ago. The patient is not currently taking any medications. Pertinent admis-

sion laboratory data include the following: BUN 85 mg%, serum creatinine 6.9 mg%, uric acid 8.9 mg%, sodium 131 mEq/L, and potassium 5.4 mEq/L. Urine output was less than 200 ml/24 hours. Because of excessive volume overload resulting in symptomatic congestive heart failure and pulmonary edema, it was decided to give furosemide 200 mg intravenously every 3 hours for 4 doses. Following the second injection, the patient became somewhat nauseated and complained of a full feeling in her ears. Immediately after the third dose the patient became moderately deaf, and was only able to hear loudly spoken words. No further furosemide was administered and the patient's hearing abnormalities disappeared within 3 hours. What patients are at risk of developing ototoxicity following administration of ethacrynic acid or furosemide? Is this toxicity always reversible?

Ototoxicity, primarily affecting the auditory component, is a serious complication of ethacrynic acid (28,54,121,186,187,193,214,221,237) and furosemide (54,177,220,221,227, 241,276,188) therapy. These sensorineuronal hearing losses may be transient (121, 193, 214, 237, 241, 276, 288), as demonstrated by this case, or permanent (177,186,214,220,227). With rare exception, diuretic-induced ototoxicity is limited to patients with renal insufficiency receiving rapid intravenous injections of moderate to large doses of either drug. Wigund et al (288) observed mild to severe transient hearing losses in 8 of 16 uremic patients receiving a furosemide infusion of 25 mg/min for 40 minutes and recommended slower infusions.

Deafness may occasionally occur following large oral doses of furosemide (227) or ethacrynic acid (214,237). Hearing impairment was also noted in two nonazotemic patients who received standard intravenous doses of ethacrynic acid; however, both of these patients were receiving therapeutic doses of aminoglycoside antibiotics concurrently (193). Other ototoxic drugs, especially the aminoglycoside antibiotics, can potentiate the ototoxic effects of the loop diuretics (140,186,187,193,221).

Bilateral hearing loss usually occurs within 5 to 30 minutes following intravenous administration of either loop diuretic (54,121,186,193,241,276). Concurrent complaints include vertigo, tinnitus, or a fullness in the ears similar to that experienced by this patient (214,220,227). In some cases, hearing impairment may not occur immediately (214,220,227). Insidious hearing losses that have gradually progressed for up to 6 months have been reported in six transplant patients (five children) following varying doses of oral and parenteral furosemide (220).

The etiology of this drug-induced ototoxicity is still debatable. Reproducible morphologic and functional changes in the stria vascularis which is responsible for the ionic concentrations of the endolymph can be produced by administering ethacrynic acid to animals (27,35,216,219). Cochlear damage in both laboratory animals and in humans has also been demonstrated (34,35,186,287).

Fortunately, the auditory complications of ethacrynic acid and furosemide are relatively rare. The Boston Collaborative Drug Surveillance Program noted that only 2 ot 165 patients (12 per 1,000) who received intravenous ethacrynic acid developed transient deafness (28), and no cases of ototoxicity occurred in over 2,300 hospitalized patients who received either oral or parenteral furosemide (113). However, a higher incidence of ototoxicity has been reported in patients with renal impairment. In a seven year prospective study of 602 hemodialysis and renal transplant patients, 107 (17.6%) demonstrated appreciable hearing losses during the observation period (221). In 71 patients the event which precipitated the hearing loss was identified. Furosemide and ethacrynic acid, alone (14 patients) or in combination with aminoglycoside antibiotics (8 patients) were the most frequent cause of hearing loss in these patients. Ototoxicity almost always occurred following rapid and repeated administration of these drugs. It was also evident from this and other studies (142) that in any given patient with renal disease, multiple factors may combine to produce a hearing deficit.

Clinicians should use large doses of loop diuretics cautiously especially if the patient is receiving aminoglycosides concurrently or is uremic. In these circumstances it would be advisable to order baseline audiograms. Rapid intravenous injections should be avoided (221,288).

27. What effect does furosemide have on calcium metabolism?

Although the calcium excretion usually parallels sodium excretion, not all natriuretic agents affect this ion in the same manner. As discussed in Question 15, the overall effect of thiazides is to decrease calcium excretion. Conversely, furosemide *increases renal calcium excretion* (97,265,267,272). The calciuric effect of furosemide can best be explained by the fact that a large percentage of the filtered sodium and calcium load is reabsorbed in the loop of Henle. By inhibiting active chloride transport in the loop of Henle, furosemide causes an increase in the excretion of both sodium and calcium. This calciuric action is usually transient, because shrinkage of the extracellular fluid volume following furosemide diuresis leads to enhanced proximal tubular reabsorption of sodium and water, as well as calcium.

Acute *hypocalcemia* does not occur in most patients receiving furosemide, probably because increased parathyroid hormone secretion secondary to furosemide-induced calciuria maintains serum calcium levels within normal limits (51,189). However, tetany has been reported following furosemide administration in patients with impaired parathyroid hormone function (97). Six hypoparathyroid patients were investigated to determine the effects of furosemide on total serum and ionized calcium levels. It was demonstrated that 80 mg/day of furosemide for four days caused a marked reduction in ionized calcium levels in all six patients, although total serum calcium remained essentially unchanged. The decrease in ionized calcium levels parallelled increased urinary calcium excretion in 5 of the 6 individuals. An increase in calcium excretion was not observed in one patient, suggesting that furosemide may affect calcium homeostasis by other mechanisms (97). Furosemide-induced hypercalcemia has also been reported (46). The clinical significance of this latter finding remains to be determined.

28. How is the hypercalciuric effect of furosemide utilized clinically?

Large parenteral doses of furosemide have been utilized clinically in the acute treatment of hypercalcemia (90,265). The calciuric action is only maintained if sodium and water losses are replaced simultaneously. In one study (265) eight hypercalcemic patients with serum calcium values ranging from 12.3 to 18.4 mg/100 ml were diuresed with furosemide, 80 to 100 mg every one to two hours. Urinary water, sodium, and potassium losses were monitored and replaced hourly. The furosemide diuresis was maintained for 6 to 7 hours with a mean calcium excretion of 82 mg per hour. The serum calcium levels fell to normal in three of the eight patients, and to near normal in another three patients. Minimal changes were observed in the remaining two patients.

This therapy was free of serious complications as long as fluid and electrolyte balance was maintained. However, because reduction in serum magnesium was consistently noted, the concomitant administration of 15 mg of magnesium per hour was recommended.

29. A 59-year-old female has been underoing biweekly hemodialysis for the past eight months. Present medications include ferrous sulfate 325 mg three times daily, folic acid 1 mg daily, aluminum hydroxide two capsules three times daily and furosemide 240 mg three times a day. During the patient's last visit she was noted to have numerous blisters which had appeared over the dorsal aspects of her hands and to a lesser extent her arms and feet. The patient first noticed these eruptions the day after she had worked in her yard gardening. Can furosemide be responsible for the skin lesions in this patient?

The high-dose furosemide treatment regimens which are commonly used in chronic renal failure patients have been implicated as a cause of *epidermolysis bullosa* (38,127,154). In one study, twelve of 56 patients with chronic renal failure who were treated with 0.5 to 2.0 grams/day of furosemide developed bullous dermatoses (127). Bullous pemphigoid lesions and erythema multiforme have also been reported after standard doses of furosemide (80,88,104).

The interval between the onset of furosemide treatment and the appearance of bullae is variable. Bullae may not become evident for as long as three years after the initiation of furosemide therapy. Clinically, the bullae vary in size and are easily ruptured; the intravesicular fluid is clear and the surrounding tissue is not involved. Bullous eruptions primarily occur in areas exposed to light, such as the dorsal aspect of the hands and feet, which may indicate that furosemide acts as a photosensitizing agent. This theory is also supported by the fact that a higher incidence of furosemide-induced bullae has been reported in the summer months (127). At present it is not clear whether a toxic or allergic mechanism is responsible for furosemide photosensitization. The bullae can persist for a few weeks to several months. They ultimately heal without scarring, and, in many cases, even with continued furosemide use (38,127,154).

Although the clinical presentation of the skin lesions described in these patients is similar to that of porphyria cutanea tarda, blood and urine screens for porphyria have been uniformly negative (38,127,154). Finally, bullous dermatosis resembling porphyria cutanea tarda has also occurred in patients undergoing hemodialysis who were not receiving furosemide (32,106). Therefore, the exact role of furosemide in the production of porphyria cutanea tarda-like syndrome in hemodialysis patients remains to be determined.

30. How does furosemide relieve pulmonary congestion?

The beneficial effect of furosemide in relieving acute pulmonary edema has traditionally been attributed to its potent diuretic activity. However, furosemide can induce hemodynamic changes and relieve pulmonary congestion prior to demonstrable diuretic effects (14,70,126,196). When furosemide 0.5-1.0 mg/kg was administered intravenously to 20 patients with left ventricular failure after acute myocardial infarctions, the left ventricular (LV) filling pressure was lowered by 6 mm Hg within 5 to 15 minutes. A marked increase (52%) in mean calf venous capacitance accompanied this drop in LV filling pressure. Since no significant increase in urine output occurred in the first five minutes and the mean increase in urine volume at the end of 15 minutes was only 20 ml, the authors concluded that furosemide's diuretic action was insufficient to account for its favorable hemodynamic changes.

31. What is bumetanide?

Bumetanide is an investigational loop diuretic whose diuretic action is comparable to that of furosemide, despite significant chemical differences. The urinary excretion pattern for the two drugs, with the exception of phosphate, is also similar. Clinical trials comparing the effectiveness of furosemide with bumetanide in patients with congestive heart failure, renal failure, and ascites, have demonstrated the effects of the two drugs to be indistinguishable.

The gastrointestinal absorption of bumetanide is rapid and nearly complete. Once absorbed bumetanide undergoes rapid oxidative metabolism and glucuronidation (half-life of 1.5 hours) with ultimate urinary and biliary excretion. The onset, peak, and duration of action of bumetanide is similar to that of furosemide. The overall diuretic response of oral and parenteral bumetanide appear to be equivalent under normal conditions (33,45,119). The diuretic response of 1.0 mg of bumetanide is equivalent to 40 mg of furosemide.

32. What are the indications for spironolactone?

Spironolactone is used primarily in combination with diuretics which have a more proximal site of action (e.g. thiazides and loop diuretics) to potentiate their natriuretic action and prevent kaliuresis. Spironolactone alone is also particularly useful in treating edema of diseases associated with high aldosterone levels. The diseases in which the anti-aldosterone effects of spironolactone may be desired include cirrhosis with ascites, nephrotic syndromes, some cases of cardiac failure, and idiopathic cyclical edema (24,65,94).

33. What is the mechanism of action of spironolactone (Aldactone)? How is the drug metabolized?

Spironolactone is a steroidal compound which antagonizes the renal tubular electrolyte effects of the mineralocorticoid, aldosterone. This agent acts at the distal convoluted renal tubule where it inhibits sodium and potassium cation exchange by competing with aldosterone for cellular receptor sites. By opposing aldosterone effects, spironolactone enhances sodium and water diuresis and promotes potassium retention. Its distal site of action, however, makes this agent a relatively mild diuretic (24,79,94,117,163).

The anti-aldosterone effect exerted by spironolactone is due primarily to its metabolites. Following oral administration, spironolactone is rapidly dethioacetylated (79%) to the principal active metabolite, canrenone (149,231,232), which is in equilibrium with canrenonate. In subjects receiving spironolactone chronically, approximately 72% of the drug's antimineral-

ocorticoid activity is due to canrenone (224). A number of sulfa containing metabolites of spironolactone also possess antimineralocorticoid activity and apparently contribute to the overall effect of spironolactone (223,224,232).

The liver is the major site of biotransformation of both spironolactone and canrenone. Five day urinary excretion data can account for only 14 to 31% of an administered dose of spironolactone (149,231). The elimination half-life of canrenone ranges from 13.5 to 24 hours in normal subjects (136,149,231,232) and is dose-related; it was 19.2 hours following a single daily spironolactone dose of 200 mg and 12.5 hours when the same amount was divided into four daily doses (150). Canrenone's half-life is prolonged in patients with chronic liver disease (59 hours, range 32 to 105 hours) or congestive heart failure (37 hours, range 19 to 48 hours) (136). However, the total daily dose requires no adjustment in these patients since plasma canrenone levels do not differ significantly from those in normal subjects, despite changes in the elimination half-life (136). No correlation has been made between plasma canrenone levels and liver function tests (232).

CASE A – ASCITES: A 57-year-old male with a two year history of hepatic cirrhosis secondary to long-term alcohol abuse was hospitalized for removal of excessive ascitic fluid. The patient has been treated in the past with sodium restriction and intermittent diuretic administration. His past medical history also includes congestive heart failure of six months duration presently controlled with digoxin 0.25 mg/day, which was continued on admission. Pertinent laboratory data were SGOT 175 IU, alkaline phosphatase 127 IU, and serum albumin of 2.1 gm%. Serum electrolytes were sodium 132 mEq/L, potassium 3.7 mEq/L, chloride 99 mEq/L and bicarbonate 29 mEq/L. Urinary electrolytes were sodium 10 mEq/L and potassium 15.0 mEq/L.

Following initial evaluation, the patient was placed on a strict 500 mg sodium diet. Diuretic therapy was initiated with furosemide 40 mg twice a day along with supplemental potassium chloride 20 mEq daily. The patient responded with a brisk diuresis. The 24 hour urine volume exceeded five liters. The patient lost over five kilograms during the first two days. However, on the night of the second day, he became slightly hypotensive and was lethargic. Therefore, the dose of furosemide was decreased to 40 mg/day; however, he remained hypotensive and lethargic. Over the next four days the 24-hour volume fell and by the sixth hospital day was less than 1.5 liters. At that time urine sodium and potassium were 3 mEq/L and 32 mEq/L respectively. Serum potassium had fallen to 2.8 mEq/L and the BUN was 52 mg%.

A 60 mEq infusion of potassium chloride was given because of the danger of digitalis-induced arrhythmias, and furosemide was discontinued. On the ninth hospital day it was decided to give spironolactone 50 mg four times daily. By the 11th hospital day, the 24-hour urine volume was 3 liters, and urinary sodium was 37 mEq/L and urinary potassium was 5 mEq/L. The patient was maintained on this regimen and lost 9 kg over two weeks. He was discharged on this treatment regimen. At a follow-up visit six weeks later, ascitic fluid had not reaccumulated, but the patient complained of swelling and soreness of his breasts.

34. What physiologic factors are involved in the formation of ascites?

Reduced plasma oncotic pressure secondary to defective albumin synthesis is generally considered to be a major cause of peripheral edema and ascites in patients with hepatic cirrhosis (248). The reduced plasma oncotic pressure decreases the extracellular fluid volume and renal sodium and water reabsorption increases as a result. Portal hypertension, which increases capillary hydrostatic pressure, does not appear to produce ascites by itself but tends to localize fluid accumulation to the intraperitoneal space in hypoalbuminemic patients (248). Obstruction of hepatic lymph outflow may also contribute to ascites formation (248). In patients with ascites, fluid accumulation will continue to occur at the expense of intravascular volume until equilibrium between capillary hydrostatic pressure and both plasma oncotic and tissue hydrostatic pressure is established.

As an alternative hypothesis, renal sodium retention itself, not hypoalbuminemia, actually initiates ascites (289). According to this theory, elevated intrahepatic pressure caused by structural abnormalities of the cirrhotic liver decreases the perfusion of the outer renal cortex. The renin-angiotensin aldosterone system is stimulated as a result, and sodium and water is retained. The hypoalbuminemia and portal hypertension serve only to dictate the site of fluid accumulation.

Regardless of whether the kidney initiates or secondarily causes ascites, it avidly reabsorbs sodium and water, in part due to the elevated aldosterone levels in cirrhotic patients. In some patients, the 24-hour urinary excretion of sodium can be less than 5 mEq/day. In patients with severe hepatic failure renal blood flow, glomerular filtration rate, and free water clearance may be markedly reduced. These patients are commonly resistant to medical treatment and have a poor prognosis (2,248).

35. How is ascites treated?

The goal of treatment of cirrhotic patients with ascites is to mobilize ascitic and edema fluid and to prevent its reaccumulation. Conservative therapy with sodium and fluid restriction and bedrest (2,98,248) is sometimes adequate. Patients with initially high urinary sodium excretion are most likely to respond to this type of treatment (2). Patients with low sodium excretion, but normal or near normal free water clearance and otherwise normal renal function, appear to benefit from the addition of diuretics (2). Spironolactone alone (13,81,115,248) or in combination with either furosemide or thiazide diuretics (2, 96, 98, 115, 248) can effectively mobilize ascitic fluid.

The 24-hour urinary sodium to potassium (Na:K) ratio, when used as an estimate of endogenous mineralocorticoid activity, may be of value in predicting diuretic response to spironolactone in cirrhotic patients with ascites (2,81). Patients with a low urinary baseline Na:K ratio (<1), which indicates high intrinsic mineralocorticoid activity respond well to 200 to 400 mg/day of spironolactone alone or in combination with furosemide (2,81). If spironolactone alone does not produce a response in these patients, the dose can be increased until the Na:K ratio reverses (81). If there is still no response following reversal of the Na:K ratio, then loop diuretics or thiazides should be added. Patients with a low Na:K ratio respond poorly to furosemide alone and the subsequent potassium losses can precipitate hepatic coma. Furosemide alone will usually be effective in patients with a high baseline Na:K ratio (>1), which suggests low aldosterone levels. Because of the low Na:K ratio in this patient, spironolactone, not furosemide, would have been a better choice to initiate treatment.

In general, the vast majority of cirrhotic patients have high circulating levels of aldosterone. The fluid loss into the peritoneal cavity with ascites causes a contraction of the effective extracellular fluid volume which decreases renal perfusion. The macula densa cells in the juxtaglomerular apparatus sense the decreased plasma volume and secrete renin which acts on angiotensin I. The angiotensin I is converted to angiotensin II in pulmonary tissues. Angiotensin II attempts to maintain plasma volume by constricting the vasculature and by stimulating the adrenals to produce aldosterone. The aldosterone then increases sodium and water retention. Hepatic shunting also serves to increase aldosterone production by similarly decreasing renal blood flow.

Approximately 90% of aldosterone is metabolized by a single pass through the liver. Hence hepatic dysfunction causes a decreased extraction of aldosterone. Additionally, aldosterone is highly bound to albumin which is in low concentrations because it is synthesized by the liver. Therefore, it is common to have high circulating levels of free aldosterone in cirrhotic patients with ascites. Since spironolactone is a competitive antagonist of aldosterone, it is reasonable to use relatively large doses (200 to 400 mg/day) in these patients, and clinicians commonly use spironolactone empirically in cirrhotics with excess interstitial fluid.

A major objective of diuretic therapy in cirrhotic patients with ascites is to produce a gradual and sustained diuresis. Patients with ascites can only mobilize about 300 cc of ascitic fluid daily; and patients with both edema and ascites can mobilize between 700 to 900 cc of fluid in a 24 hour period (246). Therefore, the maximal daily weight loss for these patients, ideally, should not exceed .5 to 1 kg depending on the presence of edema (98,248). Gradual diuresis avoids diuretic-induced depletion of the extracellular fluid volume by permitting ascitic fluid to equilibrate with the plasma volume. By using these guidelines, adverse effects from diuretic therapy, which may occur in as many as 75% diuretic-treated cirrhotics with ascites, can be minimized (247). Complications of diuretic therapy include electrolyte imbalance and metabolic alkalosis, both of which can contribute to the development of hepatic encephalopathy; hypovolemia; azotemia; and possible induction of the hepatorenal syndrome (247,248).

Although continuous diuretic treatment is usually required to maintain patients at a desired weight, intermittent diuretic administration can frequently be effective as well (96,98). Diuretic regimens must be individualized to produce maximum benefit with minimal side effects.

36. Comment on the swelling and soreness of this patient's breasts.

Spironolactone can cause gynecomastia, an estrogenic-like side effect which is characterized by the excessive development of male mammary glands. Clinically, there is bilateral and, on occasion, unilateral (290,301) breast enlargement. Underlying painful or tender masses or lumps, one to four centimeters in diameter, can be palpated (41, 50, 111, 114, 184, 254, 266, 290, 301).

The appearance of noticeable breast changes following the initiation of spironolactone ranges from several weeks to as long as two years. Disappearance of gynecomastia follows spironolactone withdrawal, usually within several weeks or months. However, complete remission can take more than a year in some cases (50).

The overall incidence of spironolactone-induced gynecomastia is not known. Although development of gynecomastia appears to be more common in patients receiving moderate to high doses of spironolactone chronically (41,50,111,184,266,290), this side effect has been reported in patients taking as little as 50 mg/day (50,301). Cirrhosis of the liver is also associated with hyperestrinism and gynecomastia since the liver is responsible for the metabolism of estrogen. Furthermore, this patient was also taking digoxin, and digoxin has also been associated with the develop-

ment of gynecomastia (114).

37. What other hormonal side effects have been attributed to spironolactone?

Besides gynecomastia, spironolactone has also been associated with decreased libido, impotence, and semen abnormalities in males (41, 111, 114, 254, 301). In females, breast soreness and enlargement, chloasma, as well as amenorrhea and other menstrual irregularities have been reported (173,254).

Spironolactone has also been associated with development of breast cancer in five women (179). However, data from the Boston Collaborative Drug Surveillance Program did not confirm this finding (139).

Amenorrhea and menstrual irregularities developed in 6 of 9 women with mild renal disease receiving standard (100 mg/day) doses of spironolactone (173). Amenorrhea occurred 1 to 9 months after therapy was initiated and in all cases, regular menstrual periods resumed within two months after discontinuation of spironolactone. In one case, resumption of spironolactone again induced amenorrhea. Spironolactone-induced amenorrhea and gynecomastia are also discussed in the chapter on *Essential Hypertension*.

38. A 40-year-old male with a four month history of arterial hypertension is treated with spironolactone (Aldactone) 50 mg tid. He presents with symptoms of weakness, weight gain, purplish striae on his abdomen and thighs, impaired glucose tolerance and truncal obesity. A plasma cortisol is elevated to 250 μg/100 ml (nl 4-10 μg/100 ml). Can spironolactone interfere with the measurement of plasma cortisol or other steroid hormones?

The Mattingly method for the estimation of free 11-hydroxycorticoids (11-OHCS), which includes cortisol, is based on a simple fluorometric analysis and is widely used in clinical practice. Very few pharmacologic agents have been known to interfere with this method for estimating plasma "cortisol" concentrations. Spironolactone, however, has been incriminated as an interfering fluorogen in plasma samples submitted for suspected adrenal disease (182, 295, 295a). Apparently, spironolactone spuriously elevates concentrations of plasma fluorogens that are read as 11-OHCS.

A standard regimen of spironolactone 75 to 100 mg daily can cause a four- to nine-fold increase in cortisol determinations. Higher dosages of spironolactone produce even higher cortisol levels. These falsely elevated values can occur after the first day of treatment and may persist several days after spironolactone is discontinued (182,295,295a). It is difficult to establish exactly how many days the spironolactone artifact continues to interfere with this test after therapy is discontinued. However, it appears that cortisol values return to normal within seven days. Therefore, in the case above, it would be prudent to wait seven days after the discontinuation of spironolactone before rescheduling the test. A single case has been reported in which plasma cortisol remained elevated one week after the discontinuation of spironolactone (251).

Since adrenal hyperfunction is sometimes considered in edematous disorders, clinicians should be aware of spironolactone's laboratory test interference with the Mattingly method of cortisol determinations. Urinary determinations of 17-hydroxycorticosteroids and 17-ketosteroids by the Peterson method and by the Norymberski method are not affected by spironolactone (181, 182, 206, 211, 269, 295a).

Spironolactone and its metabolite canrenone also spuriously elevate plasma 11-deoxycorticosterone (DOC) levels as measured by radioimmunoassay or competitive protein-binding radioassay (268). Furthermore, a metabolite of canrenone may interfere with an immunoassay for aldosterone (233).

39. Compare the mechanism of action and clinical effects of triamterene (Dryenium) and spironolactone (Aldactone).

In contrast to spironolactone, triamterene produces its diuretic effects by directly depressing renal tubular transport processes in the distal tubule even in the absence of aldosterone. Both of these potassium-sparing diuretics affect urine composition identically. Like spironolactone it is a weak diuretic when used alone and is most useful when used in combination with a more proximal acting diuretic agent (24, 65, 79, 94, 117).

Triamterene is incompletely absorbed from the gastrointestinal tract. The drug has a short half-life of 1.5 to 2.5 hours. Total body clearance is high because of rapid and extensive metabolism by the liver. Both the parent compound and the metabolite undergo biliary and renal excretion. As with spironolactone, the hepatic metabolism of triamterene may be altered in patients with cirrhosis (24,218). The diuretic effect of triamterene begins within two to three hours of its administration and its maximum duration is 12 to 16 hours.

Triamterene produces relatively few side effects. The most common are nausea, vomiting, leg cramps, and dizziness. The most serious and potentially fatal complication of triamterene therapy is hyperkalemia. Triamterene has also been reported to impart a faint blue coloring to the urine (65,94).

40. A 30-year-old alcoholic female with mitral insufficiency has been treated with digoxin 0.25 mg/day and triamterene 200 mg twice daily for 1 year. She now complains of a bright-red tongue, cracked corners of the mouth, and a burning, inflamed feeling in

her tongue. Could any of these symptoms be related to her drug therapy?

Triamterene is a diuretic with a structure similar to that of folic acid. The above symptoms of folate deficiency have occurred in alcoholic cirrhotics receiving triamterene (47,55,175). Megaloblastosis in these patients may be due to inhibition of dihydrofolate reductase (DHFR), an enzyme necessary for the formation of tetrahydrofolate. A case of megaloblastosis occurred in a cirrhotic patient with normal serum and red cell folate levels following two weeks of therapy with triamterene (55). Based on bone marrow aspirate examination, the conclusion was that triamterene in conventional doses produced significant in vivo inhibition in DHFR activity. In contrast, others (47) conclude that the in vivo effect of triamterene on DHFR inhibition is less apparent than that in vitro, and that triamterene has no effect on DNA synthesis in vivo.

Further investigation is needed to determine the role of triamterene in inducing megaloblastic anemia. Malnutrition may have contributed significantly to the folate deficiency.

41. A 48-year-old adult onset diabetic male with chronic renal failure (CrCl 47 ml/min) was recently diagnosed to be hypertensive (135/105 mm Hg). The patient was placed on a low sodium diet utilizing Co-Salt as a salt substitute in addition to his regular diabetic diet. Furosemide 40 mg bid, methyldopa 250 mg tid and triamterene 100 mg bid were prescribed. The patient also takes tolbutamide 0.5 gm bid.

Two days after initiation of the antihypertensive regimen the patient complained of shortness of breath, severe weakness, and dizziness. An EKG strip done in the emergency room showed cardiac arrhythmias typical of hyperkalemia. A serum potassium at this time was 6.9 mEq/L. Besides triamterene administration, what factors contributed to the development of hyperkalemia in this patient?

Hyperkalemia is a serious and potentially fatal complication of the potassium sparing diuretics, spironolactone and triamterene (53, 112, 120, 125, 148, 250, 278, 297). Hyperkalemia can occur even when these agents are given in combination with thiazide diuretics (53,120). Patients receiving potassium supplements including those from dietary sources and salt substitutes such as Co-Salt, and those with concomitant renal insufficiency are at particular risk of developing hyperkalemia (112,125,297). The Boston Collaborative Drug Surveillance Program (112) found that 8.6% of hospitalized patients receiving spironolactone developed hyperkalemia. However, the incidence of hyperkalemia was 20.3% in those patients with a BUN greater than 50 mg%; 15.8% in those receiving potassium supplements; and 42.1% in those with a BUN above 50 mg% who were also receiving potassium supplementation. Others have observed a 52% incidence of hyperkalemia in patients receiving a combination of spironolactone and potassium supplements (250). Diabetic patients, as illustrated in the case presentation, may be more prone to developing hyperkalemia with these agents (53,125,278). Also see the *Essential Hypertension* chapter.

42. Why are the diuretic effects of acetazolamide (Diamox) self-limiting?

The pharmacologic action of acetazolamide is dependent upon its ability to inhibit carbonic anhydrase, the enzyme which catalyzes the hydration of carbon dioxide to carbonic acid. After its formation, carbonic acid instantaneously dissociates into hydrogen and bicarbonate ions, independently of any enzymatic acceleration. Therefore, inhibition of carbonic anhydrase in the renal cells prevents the formation of carbonic acid and its subsequent breakdown to hydrogen and bicarbonate ions. Therefore fewer hydrogen ions are available to exchange with sodium in the proximal and distal tubules, and a sodium bicarbonate diuresis ensues.

Since the kidney is unable to effectively excrete hydrogen ions because of the carbonic anhydrase inhibition, metabolic acidosis follows after three to five days of continual administration. At this time, the excess hydrogen ions simply overwhelm the kidney, and hydrogen readily exchanges with sodium in spite of the continued carbonic anhydrase inhibition. In this manner, metabolic acidosis renders acetazolamide's diuretic action ineffective (200,249).

43. Since about 70% of sodium in the glomerular filtrate is reabsorbed in the proximal tubule, why is the proximally acting acetazolamide (Diamox) such a weak diuretic?

The carbonic anhydrase inhibitors exert their major pharmacologic actions in the proximal tubule where hydrogen secretion and bicarbonate reabsorption occur. However, sodium reabsorption is not dependent merely on hydrogen secretion, and many equally important factors influence sodium reabsorption in this segment of the nephron. Additionally, the ascending limb of the loop of Henle has the capacity to increase sodium reabsorption in direct proportion to the amount of sodium presented. Thus, the diuretic action of proximally acting agents is compromised to some extent (107,242).

Although acetazolamide is a weak diuretic, it affects a different nephron segment than many other diuretics. As a result, it will potentiate the natriuresis of these agents. Therefore, combination with furosemide or ethacrynic acid is sometimes quite useful in the therapy of resistant edema (43).

44. A 64-year-old man received one unit of mismatched blood during a surgical procedure. On his first post-op day his urine output was less than 25 ml/24 hours, and he was given 2,000 ml of a 10% solution of mannitol in normal saline. Is this a proper indication for the use of mannitol? What complications might be predicted from this dose?

Mannitol is a low molecular weight osmotic diuretic used in a number of clinical conditions including drug overdose, refractory edema, cerebral edema, and acute oliguric renal failure (101). The most important indication for its use is in the prophylaxis and early treatment of acute decreases in renal blood flow which can produce tubular necrosis and oliguria (200). Thus, mannitol has been used for the oliguria occurring after hemolytic transfusion reactions, severe traumatic injuries, and cardiovascular operations (11).

Mannitol is an ideal osmotic agent in that it is freely filterable at the renal glomerulus, is not metabolized, and does not undergo tubular reabsorption. Mannitol not only reduces isomotic sodium and water reabsorption in the proximal tubule but also impairs passive water and sodium transport in the ascending and descending loop of Henle (101).

The usual adult dose of mannitol ranges from 50 to 200 gm/24 hours, and in most instances 100 gm/24 hours suffices. The rate of administration depends upon the severity of the condition being treated, but as a general rule, the rate of administration should be adjusted to maintain a urine output of at least 40 to 50 ml/hr (11). Because crystallization of mannitol occasionally occurs, it should be administered through an in-line filter.

The dose of mannitol being administered to the patient (200 gms) is within the normal range. However, in oliguric patients a test dose of 12.5 gm of mannitol in 100 ml of solution should be infused over a period of 3 to 5 minutes. If no increase in urine output occurs in the ensuing 3 to 5 hours, mannitol probably would not be effective. Another test dose may be attempted if circulatory overload is not present.

The importance of the test dose in patients with renal insufficiency can be better appreciated upon recalling that mannitol is not metabolized and that its only route of excretion is by the kidneys. If large doses are administered to renal failure patients, it cannot be excreted and remains in the extracellular vascular compartment where it exerts alarming osmotic actions. A clinical picture of severe vascular overload occurs as evidenced by congestive heart failure, pulmonary edema, tissue and cellular dehydration, high plasma osmolality, and hyponatremia and hypochloremia. In a few cases, hemodialysis corrected the hyperosmolality and hyponatremia. However, peritoneal dialysis caused a further increase in plasma osmolality (15). Since fatalities have resulted from the inappropriate use of mannitol, this agent should be used cautiously with careful monitoring of urinary output and central venous pressure.

Alkalinization of the urine with acetazolamide and sodium bicarbonate have been recommended for the management of intravascular hemolysis resulting from mismatched blood transfusions; alkaline urine may prevent the renal precipitation of acid hematin which contributes to the development of renal failure (258). Prevention of the initial oliguria of acute renal failure can also be accomplished with the administration of furosemide or ethacrynic acid (197).

45. Organomercurial diuretics are highly effective diuretics. Why are they no longer used?

Under optimal conditions the organomercurials are about four times more effective than the thiazides in increasing sodium excretion. However, these agents have several disadvantages. They require repeated parenteral administration, are more toxic, and have self-limiting diuretic actions (75,76).

These agents were initially believed to act primarily on proximal tubular sodium reabsorption. However, the principal site of action is in the ascending limb of the loop of Henle. A small amount of mercuric ion is thought to combine intrarenally with cysteine and subsequently with renal tubular transport systems. The action of the mercurial diuretics may not be totally dependent on the mercuric ion. Acidifying agents enhance mercurial diuresis, while alkalinizing salts decrease diuresis. During mercurial diuresis, sodium and chloride are excreted in nearly equal amounts.

This results in a hypochloremic alkalosis with a subsequent diminution of diuretic effect. Mercurial diuretics also suppress the distal tubular secretion of potassium. Therefore, mercurial-induced potassium depletion is generally not profound.

Diuresis begins 1 to 2 hours after IM administration, peaks in 6 to 9 hours, and is essentially complete in 12 to 24 hours. Intravenous administration does not result in a quicker or more potent diuretic response and may be complicated by sudden fatal ventricular arrhythmias and thrombophlebitis. Other untoward reactions include a possible nephrotoxic effect and systemic mercury poisoning when used injudiciously in patients with poor renal function (8, 37, 39, 100, 200, 242, 249).

46. A 25-year-old comatose female is admitted to General Hospital following an acute ingestion of aspirin. In addition to standard therapeutic regimens, the intern initiates dexamethasone for its diuretic properties. Comment.

Glucocorticosteroids are sometimes used as adjuncts in the therapy of life-threatening "resistant" edema. The precise mechanism of this diuretic effect remains obscure. These agents are capable of markedly increasing the glomerular filtration rate and free water excretion without inducing a significant sodium diuresis. It has therefore been theorized that the steroids inhibit the action of antidiuretic hormone, or "third factor" activity. Glucocorticoid enhancement of diuretic therapy may not be apparent for 3 to 4 days (77,163,240,249).

REFERENCES

1. Ahmad S: Renal insensitivity to furosemide caused by chronic anticonvulsant therapy. Brit Med J 3:657, 1974.
2. Alexander WD et al: The urinary sodium: potassium ratio and response to diuretics in resistant oedema. Postgrad Med J 53:117, 1977.
3. Allison MEM et al: Diuretics in chronic renal disease: A study of high dosage frusemide. Clin Sci 41:171, 1971.
4. Amery A et al: Glucose intolerance during diuretic therapy. Lancet 1:681, 1978.
5. Ames RP et al: Increase in serum-lipids during treatment of hypertension with chlorthalidone. Lancet 1:721, 1976.
6. Ames RP et al: Elevation of serum lipid levels during diuretic therapy of hypertension. Amer J Med 61:748, 1976.
7. Anderson OO et al: Carbohydrate metabolism during treatment with chlorthalidone and ethacrynic acid. Brit Med J 2:798, 1968.
8. Anderton JL et al: Diuretics I: physiological and pharmacological considerations. Drugs 1:54, 1971.
9. Anderton JL et al: Diuretics II: clinical considerations. Drugs 1:141, 1971.
10. Andreasen F et al: Pharmacokinetics of furosemide in anephric patients and in normal subjects. Europ J Clin Pharmacol 13:41, 1978.
11. Anonymous: Mannitol — an osmotic diuretic. Med Letter 10:5, 1968.
12. Anonymous: Current drug therapy — thiazide diuretics. Amer J Hosp Pharm 32:473, 1975.
13. Arroyo V et al: A rational approach to the treatment of ascites. Postgrad Med J 51:558, 1975.
14. Austin SM et al: The acute hemodynamic effects of ethacrynic acid and furosemide in patients with chronic postcapillary pulmonary hypertension. Circ 53:364, 1976.
15. Aviram A et al: Hyperosmolality with hyponatremia caused by inappropriate administration of mannitol. Am J Med 42:648, 1967.
16. Baba S et al: Antiandrogenic effects of spironolactone: hormonal and ultrastructural studies in dogs and men. J Urol 119:375, 1978.
17. Ball P: Thrombocytopenia and purpura in patients receiving chlorothiazide and hydrochlorothiazide. JAMA 173:663, 1960.
18. Barilla DE et al: Selective effects of thiazide on intestinal absorption of calcium in absorptive and renal hypercalciurias. Metab 27:125, 1978.
19. Beaudry C et al: Severe allergic pneumonitis from hydrochlorothiazide. Ann Intern Med 78:251, 1973.
20. Beerman B et al: Elimination of furosemide in healthy subjects and in those with renal failure. Clin Pharmacol Ther 22:70, 1977.
21a. Bennett WB et al: Comparison of intravenous chlorothiazide and metolazone in normal man. Curr Ther Res 22:326, 1977.
21. Bennett WM et al: Efficacy and safety of metolazone in renal failure and the nephrotic syndrome. J Clin Pharmacol 13:357, 1973.
22. Beresford HR: Polydipsia, hydrochlorothiazide, and water intoxication. JAMA 214:879, 1970.
23. Bettman JW: Drug hypersensitivity purpuras. Arch Intern Med 112:840, 1963.
24. Beyer KH: The pharmacological basis for modern diuretic therapy. Ration Drug Ther 12:1, 1978 (Feb).
25. Black WD et al: Severe electrolyte disturbances associated with

metolazone and furosemide. South Med J 71:380, 1978.

26. Bourke JB et al: Drug-associated primary acute pancreatitis. Lancet 1:706, 1978.

27. Bosher SK et al: The effects of ethacrynic acid upon the cochlear endolymph and the stria vascularis. Acta Otolaryngol 75:184, 1973.

28. Boston Collaborative Drug Surveillance Program: Drug-induced deafness. JAMA 224:515, 1973.

29. Branch RA et al: Determinants of response to frusemide in normal subjects. Brit J Clin Pharmacol 4:121, 1977.

30. Breckenridge A et al: Glucose tolerance in hypertensive patients on long-term diuretic therapy. Lancet 1:61, 1967.

31. Brickman AS et al: Changes in serum and urinary calcium during treatment with hydrochlorothiazide: Studies on mechanisms. J Clin Invest 51:945, 1972.

32. Brivet F et al: Porphyria cutanea tarda-like syndrome in hemodialyzed patients. Nephron 20:258, 1978

33. Brogden RN et al: Bumetanide: A preliminary report of its pharmacological properties and therapeutic efficacy in oedema. Drugs 9:4, 1975.

34. Brummett RE et al: Cochlear damage resulting from kanamycin and furosemide. Acta Otolaryngol 80:86, 1975.

35. Brummett RE et al: The delayed effects of ethacrynic acid on the stria vascularis of the guinea pig. Acta Otolaryngol 83:98, 1977.

36. Buchanan N et al: Furosemide-induced pancreatitis. Brit Med J 2:1417, 1977.

37. Burg MB: Tubular chloride transport and the mode of action of some diuretics. Kid Internat 9:189, 1976.

38. Burry JN et al: Phototoxic blisters from high frusemide dosage. Brit J Dermatol 94:495, 1976.

39. Cafruny EJ: The site and mechanism of action of mercurial diuretics. Pharmacological Reviews 20:89, 1968.

40. Call T et al: Acute pancreatitis secondary to furosemide with associated hyperlipidemia. Am J Digest Dis 22:835, 1977.

41. Caminos-Torres R et al: Gynecomastia and semen abnormalities induced by spironolactone in normal men. J Clin Endocrinol Metab 45:255, 1977.

42. Cangiano JL: Effects of prolonged administration of metolazone in the treatment of essential hypertension. Curr Ther Res 20:745, 1976.

43. Cannon PJ et al: Ethacrynic acid and furosemide: renal pharmacology and clinical use. Progr Cardiovas Dis 12:99, 1969.

44. Carliner R et al: Thiazide and phthalimidine-induced hyperglycemia. JAMA 191:535, 1965.

45. Carriere S et al: Bumetanide, a new loop diuretic. Clin Pharmacol Ther 20:424, 1976.

46. Chandler PT et al: Increased serum calcium levels induced by furosemide. South Med J 70:571, 1977.

47. Chang JC et al: Effect of triamterene on nucleic acid synthesis. Clin Pharmacol Ther 13:372, 1972.

48. Chazan IA et al: Etiological factors in thiazide-induced or aggravated diabetes mellitus. Diabetes 14:132, 1965.

49. Christensson T et al: Hypercalcemia and primary hyperparathyroidism. Arch Intern Med 137:1138, 1977.

50. Clark E: Spironolactone therapy and gynecomastia. JAMA 193:157, 1965.

51. Coe FL et al: Evidence for secondary hyperparathyroidism in idiopathic hypercalciuria. J Clin Invest 52:134, 1973.

52. Coe FL: Treated and untreated recurrent calcium nephrolithiasis in patients with idiopathic hypercalciuria, hyperuricosuria, or no metabolic disorder. Ann Intern Med 87:404, 1977.

53. Cohen AB: Hyperkalemic effects of triamterene. Ann Intern Med 65:521, 1966.

54. Cooperman LB et al: Toxicity of ethacrynic acid and furosemide. Am Heart J 85:831, 1973.

55. Corcino J et al: Mechanism of triamterene-induced megaloblastosis. Ann Intern Med 73:419, 1970.

56. Cornish AL et al: Effects of chlorothiazide on the pancreas. NEJM 265:673, 1961.

57. Costanzo LS et al: On the hypocalciuric action of chlorothiazide. J Clin Invest 54:628, 1974.

58. Craswell PW et al: Use of metolazone, a new diuretic in patients with renal disease. Nephron 12:63, 1973.

59. Curtis J et al: Chlorthalidone-induced hyperosmolar hyperglycemic nonketotic coma. JAMA 220:1592, 1972.

60. Cutter RE et al: Pharmacokinetics of furosemide in normal subjects and functionally anephric patients. Clin Pharmacol Ther

61. Dargie HJ et al: High dosage metolazone in chronic renal failure. Brit Med J 4:196, 1972.

62. Dargie HJ et al: Adverse reactions to diuretic drugs. In Meyler's Side Effects of Drugs, Vol 8, edited by Dukes MNG, Ch 19, Excerpta Medica, Amsterdam-Oxford, 1975, p 483.

63. Davidov M et al: Intravenous administration of furosemide in heart failure. JAMA 200:824, 1967.

64. Davidson C et al: Effect of long-term diuretic treatment on body-potassium in heart disease. Lancet 2:1044, 1976.

65. Davies DL et al: Diuretics: Mechanism of action and clinical application. Drugs 9:178, 1975.

66. Day JO: Water intoxication in psychogenic water drinkers taking thiazide diuretics. South Med J 70:572, 1977.

67. DeGowin EL et al: Bedside Diagnostic Examination, Ed 2, Ch 7, The MacMillan Co., New York, 1971, p 323.

68. DeRubertis FR et al: Complications of diuretic therapy: severe alkalosis and syndrome resembling inappropriate secretion of antidiuretic hormone. Metab 19:709, 1970.

69. Diamond MT: Hyperglycemic hyperosmolar coma associated with hydrochlorothiazide and pancreatitis. NY State J Med 72:1741, 1972.

70. Dikshit K et al: Renal and extrarenal hemodynamic effects of furosemide in congestive heart failure after acute myocardial infarction. NEJM 288:1087, 1973.

71. Dollery CT et al: Drug-induced diabetes. Lancet 2:735, 1962.

72. Dollery CT: Diabetogenic effect of long-term diuretic therapy. In Modern Diuretic Therapy in the Treatment of Cardiovascular and Renal Disease, edited by Lant AF, Wilson GM, Excerpta Medica, Amsterdam, 1973, p 320.

72a. Dowling HF et al: Toxic reactions accompanying second courses of sulfonamides in patients developing toxic reactions during a previous course. Ann Intern Med 24:629, 1946.

73. Duarte CG et al: Thiazide-induced hypercalcemia. NEJM 284: 828, 1971.

74. Earley LE et al: The mechanism of anti diuresis associated with the administration of hydrochlorothiazide in patients with vasopressin resistant diabetes insipidus. J Clin Invest 41:1988, 1962.

75. Earley LE: Diuretics. NEJM 276:966, 1967.

76. Earley LE: Diuretics. NEJM 276:1023, 1967.

77. Earley LE: Salt and water transport in the kidney: mechanism of action of diuretics utilizing the thiazide diuretics as a model. In Diuretics and Clinical Medicine (Proceedings of the Peter Bent Brigham Symposium, Boston, Mass., May 16, 1967), Excerpta Medica Foundation, New York, 1968, p 22.

78. Earley LE et al: Sodium metabolism. NEJM 281:72, 1969.

79. Earley LE et al: Edema formation and the use of diuretics. Calif Med 114:56, 1971.

80. Ebringer A et al: Bullous haemorrhagic eruption associated with frusemide. Med J Aust 1:768, 1969.

81. Eggert RC: Spironolactone diuresis in patients with cirrhosis and ascites. Brit Med J 2:401, 1970.

82. Ehrig U et al: Effect of long-term thiazide therapy on intestinal calcium absorption in patients with recurrent renal calculi. Metabolism 23:139, 1974.

83. Eisner EV et al: Hydrochlorothiazide dependent thrombocytopenia due to IgM antibody. JAMA 215:480, 1971.

84. Elliott HC: Reduced adrenocortical steroid excretion rates in man following aspirin administration. Metab 11:1015, 1962.

85. Epstein M et al: Potentiation of furosemide by metolazone in refractory edema. Curr Ther Res 21:656, 1977.

86. Farquaharson-Roberts MA et al: Perforation of small bowel due to slow release potassium chloride (slow-K). Brit Med J 3:206, 1975.

87. Feldman E et al: Ethacrynic acid: a non-diabetogenic diuretic. Dis Chest 51:282, 1967.

88. Fellner MJ et al: Occurrence of bullous pemphigoid after furosemide therapy. Arch Dermatol 112:75, 1976.

89. Fichman MP et al: Diuretic-induced hyponatremia. Ann Intern Med 75:853, 1971.

90. Fillastre JP et al: Treatment of acute hypercalcemia with furosemide. Curr Ther Res 15:641, 1973.

91. Fine A et al: Malabsorption of furosemide caused by phenytoin. Brit Med J 2:1061, 1977.

92. Fitzgerald EW: Fatal glomerulonephritis complicating allergic purpura due to chlorothiazide. Arch Intern Med 105:305, 1960.

93. Fotiu S et al: Antihypertensive efficacy of metolazone. Clin

15:588, 1974.

Pharmacol Ther 16:318, 1974.

94. Frazier HD et al: The clinical use of diuretics — Parts 1 and 2. NEJM 288:246, 1973 and 288:455, 1973.

95. Fuisz RE et al: Diuretic-induced hyponatremia and sustained antidiuresis. Am J Med 33:783, 1962.

96. Fuller RK et al: An optimal diuretic regimen for cirrhotic ascites. A controlled trial evaluating safety and efficacy of spironolactone and furosemide. JAMA 237:972, 1977.

97. Gabow PA et al: Furosemide-induced reduction in ionized calcium in hypoparathyroid patients. Ann Intern Med 86:579, 1977.

98. Gabuzda GJ: Cirrhosis, ascites, and edema. Gastroent 58:546, 1970.

99. Ganong WF: Formation and excretion of urine. In Review of Medical Physiology, Ed 8, Ch 38, Lange Medical Publications, Los Altos, Calif, 1977, p 522.

100. Gantt CL: Diuretic therapy. Ration Drug Ther 6:1, 1972.

101. Gennari FJ et al: Osmotic diuresis. NEJM 291:714, 1974.

102. Gerich JE et al: Clinical and metabolic characteristics of hyperosmolar nonketotic coma. Diabetes 20:228, 1971.

103. Gesink MH et al: Thrombocytopenia purpura associated with hydrochlorothiazide therapy. JAMA 172:556, 1960.

104. Gibson TP et al: Erythema multiforme and furosemide therapy. JAMA 212:1709, 1970.

105. Gifford RW: A guide to the practical use of diuretics. JAMA 235:1890, 1976.

106. Gilchrest B et al: Bullous dermatosis of hemodialysis. Ann Intern Med 83:480, 1975.

107. Goldberg ME: The physiology, pharmacology and clinical uses of ethacrynic acid and furosemide. In Diuretics and Clinical Medicine (Proceedings of the Peter Bent Brigham Symposium, Boston, Mass., May 16, 1967), Excerpta Medica Foundation, New York, 1968, p 34.

108. Goldner MG et al: Hyperglycemia and glycosuria due to thiazide derivatives administered in diabetes mellitus. NEJM 262:403, 1960.

109. Gossain VV et al: Drug-induced hyponatremia in psychogenic polydipsia. Postgrad Med J 52:720, 1976.

110. Grantham JJ et al: Asymptomatic hyponatremia and bronchogenic carcinoma: the deleterious effects of diuretics. Am J Med Sci 249:273, 1965.

111. Greenblatt DJ et al: Gynecomastia and impotence complications of spironolactone therapy. JAMA 223:82, 1973.

112. Greenblatt DJ et al: Adverse reactions to spironolactone. JAMA 225:40, 1973.

113. Greenblatt DJ et al: Clinical toxicity of furosemide in hospitalized patients. Am Heart J 94:6, 1977.

114. Greenlaw C: Spironolactone induced gynecomastia. Drug Intell Clin Pharm 11:70, 1977.

115. Gregory PB et al: Complications of diuresis in the alcoholic patient with ascites: a controlled trial. Gastroent 73:534, 1977.

116. Gunstone RF et al: Clinical experience with metolazone in 52 African patients: synergy with frusemide. Postgrad Med J 47:789, 1971.

117. Gussin RZ: Potassium-sparing diuretics. J Clin Pharmacol 17:651, 1977.

118. Guyton AC: The body fluids and kidneys. In Textbook of Medical Physiology, Ed 4, Ch 33, 34, and 35. WB Saunders Co., Philadelphia, Pa., 1971.

119. Halladay SC et al: Diuretic effect and metabolism of bumetanide in man. Clin Pharmacol Ther 22:179, 1977.

120. Hansen KB et al: Changes in serum potassium levels occurring in patients treated with triamterene and a triamterene-hydrochlorothiazide combination. Clin Pharmacol Ther 8:393, 1967.

121. Hanzelik E et al: Deafness after ethacrynic acid. Lancet 1:416, 1969.

122. Harrington JT: Diuretics. Am J Hosp Pharm 32:316, 1975.

123. Harter HR: Fluid and electrolyte disturbances. In Manual of Medical Therapeutics, Ed 22, edited by Costrini NV, Ch 2, Little, Brown & Co., Boston, 1977, p 27.

124. Helgeland A et al: Serum triglycerides and serum uric acid in untreated and thiazide-treated patients with mild hypertension. Am J Med 64:34, 1978.

125. Herman E et al: Fatal hyperkalemic paralysis associated with spironolactone. Arch Neurol 15:74, 1966.

126. Hesse B et al: The early effects of intravenous furosemide on central haemodynamics, venous tone and plasma renin activity.

Clin Sci Mol Med 49:551, 1975.

127. Heydenreich G et al: Bullous dermatosis among patients with chronic renal failure on high dose frusemide. Acta Med Scand 202:61, 1974.

128. Hicks BH et al: A controlled study of clopamide, clorexolone, and hydrochlorothiazide in diabetes. Metab 22:101, 1973.

129. Hillenbrand P et al: Use of metolazone in the treatment of ascites due to liver disease. Brit Med J 4:266, 1971.

130. Hollifield JW: Failure of aspirin to antagonize the antihypertensive effect of spironolactone in low-renin hypertension. South Med J 69:1034, 1976.

131. Hook JB et al: Influence of probenecid and alterations in acid-base balance on the saluretic activity of furosemide. J Pharmacol Exp Therap 149:404, 1965.

131a. Homeida M et al: Influence of probenecid and spironolactone on furosemide kinetics and dynamics in man. Clin Pharmacol Ther 22:402, 1977.

131b. Honari J et al: Effects of probenecid on furosemide kinetics and natriuresis in man. Clin Pharmacol Ther 22:395, 1977.

132. Horowitz HI et al: Athrombocytopenia purpura caused by chlorothiazide. New York State J Med 59:1117, 1959.

133. Howie AD et al: Slow release potassium chloride treatment. Brit Med J 2:176, 1975.

134. Huang CM et al: Pharmacokinetics of furosemide in advanced renal failure. Clin Pharmacol Ther 16:659, 1974.

135. Ince WE: A case of agranulocytosis following chlorothiazide. Practitioner 189:74, 1962.

136. Jackson L et al: Elimination of canrenone in congestive heart failure and chronic liver disease. Europ J Clin Pharmacol 11:177, 1977.

137. Jackson WP et al: Effect of frusemide on carbohydrate metabolism, blood-pressure, and other modalities: a comparison with chlorothiazide. Brit Med J 2:333, 1966.

138. Jaffe MO et al: Purpura due to chlorothiazide (Diuril). JAMA 168:2264, 1958.

139. Jick H et al: Breast cancer and spironolactone. Lancet 2:368, 1975.

140. Johnson AH et al: Kanamycin ototoxicity — possible potentiation by other drugs. South Med J 63:511, 1970.

141. Johnson BF et al: The relation of antihypertensive treatment to plasma lipids and other vascular risk factors in hypertensives. J Clin Sci Mol Med 47:9P, 1974.

142. Johnson DW et al: Hearing function and chronic renal failure. Ann Otol 85:43, 1976.

143. Johnston DH et al: Acute pancreatitis. JAMA 170:2054, 1959.

144. Jones MF et al: Acute hemorrhagic pancreatitis associated with administration of chlorthalidone. NEJM 267:1029, 1962.

145. Jones PE et al: Frusemide-induced pancreatitis. Brit Med J 1:133, 1975.

146. Jorgensen FS et al: The effect of bendro flumethiazide on total, ultrafiltrable and ionized calcium in serum in normocalcaemic renal stone formers and in hyperparathyroidism. ·Acta Med Scand 194:323, 1973.

147. Jorgensen FS et al: The effect of bendroflumethiazide on the renal handling of calcium, magnesium and phosphate in normocalcaemic renal stone formers and in hyperparathyroidism. Acta Med Scand 194:327, 1973.

148. Kalbian VV: Iatrogenic hyperkalemic paralysis with electrocardiographic changes. South Med J 67:342, 1974.

149. Karim A et al: Spironolactone, I., Disposition and metabolism. Clin Pharmacol Ther 19:158, 1976.

150. Karim A et al: Spironolactone. III. Canrenone-maximum and minimum steady-state plasma levels. Clin Pharmacol Ther 19:177, 1976.

150a. Kassirer JP et al: The critical role of chloride in the correction of hypokalemic alkalosis in man. Am J Med 38:172, 1965.

151. Kassirer JP et al: Diuretics and potassium metabolism: A reassessment of the need, effectiveness and safety of potassium therapy. Kidney Internat 11:505, 1977.

152. Kelly MR: Pharmacokinetics of orally administered furosemide. Clin Pharmacol Ther 15:178, 1974.

153. Kelly MR et al: A comparison of the diuretic response to oral and intravenous furosemide in "diuretic-resistant" patients. Curr Ther Res 21:1, 1977.

154. Kennedy AC et al: Acquired epidermolysis bullosa due to high-dose frusemide. Brit Med J 1:1509, 1976.

154a. Kessler AH: The use of furosemide and ethacrynic acid in the treatment of edema. Pharmacol for Physicians 1:1, 1967.

155. Kennedy RM et al: Profound hyponatremia resulting from a thiazide-induced decrease in urinary diluting capacity in a patient with primary polydipsia. NEJM 282:1185, 1970.

156. Kim KE et al: Ethacrynic acid and furosemide. Diuretic and hemodynamic effects and clinical uses. Am J Cardiol 27:407, 1971.

157. Klein M: Agranulocytosis secondary to chlorthalidone therapy. JAMA 184:310, 1963.

158. Kohner EM et al: Effect of diuretic therapy on glucose tolerance in hypertensive patients. Lancet 1:986, 1971.

159. Koppel MH et al: Thiazide-induced rise in serum calcium and magnesium in patients on maintenance hemodialysis. Ann Intern Med 72:895, 1970.

160. Kosman ME: Management of potassium problems during long-term diuretic therapy. JAMA 230:743, 1974.

161. Kunau RT et al: Disorders of hypo- and hyperkalemia. Clin Nephrol 7:173, 1977.

162. Kutti J et al: The frequency of thrombocytopenia in patients with heart disease treated with oral diuretics. Acta Med Scand 183:245, 1968.

163. Laidlaw JC: The use of aldosterone antagonists in diuretic therapy and the use of diuretic agents in hypertension therapy. In *Diuretics and Clinical Medicine* (Proceedings of the Pet3r Bent Brigham Symposium, Boston, Mass., May 16, 1967), Excerpta Medica Foundation, New York, 1968, p 74.

164. Lamberg BA et al: Effect of chlorothiazide and hydrochlorothiazide on the excretion of calcium in urine. Scand J Clin Lab Invest 11:351, 1959.

165. Lauler DP: The role of renin and angiotensin in clinical medicine. In *Diuretics and Clinical Medicine.* (Proceedings of the Peter Bent Brigham Symposium, Boston, Mass., May 16, 1967), Excerpta Medica Foundation, New York, 1968, p 6.

166. Lavender S et al: Nonketotic hyperosmolar coma and furosemide therapy. Diabetes 23:247, 1974.

167. Lawson DH: Adverse reactions to potassium chloride. Q J Med 43:433, 1974.

168. Lawson DH: Clinical use of potassium supplements. Am J Hosp Pharm 32:708, 1975.

169. Lawson DH et al: Potassium supplements in patients receiving long-term diuretics for oedema. Q J Med 45:469, 1976.

170. Learmonth I et al: Potassium stricture of the upper alimentary tract. Lancet 1:251, 1976.

171. Levey BA et al: Biochemical and clinical effects of metolazone in congestive heart failure. Curr Ther Res 18:641, 1975.

172. Levinsky NG: Nonaldosterone influences on renal sodium transport. Ann NY Acad Sci 139:295, 1966.

173. Levitt JI: Spironolactone therapy and amenorrhea. JAMA 211:2014, 1970.

174. Lewis PJ et al: Deterioration of glucose tolerance in hypertensive patients on prolonged diuretic treatment. Lancet 1:564, 1976.

175. Lieherman FL et al: Megaloblastic anaemia possibly induced by triamterene in patients with alcoholic cirrhosis. Two case reports. Ann Intern Med 68:168, 1968.

176. Lindy S et al: Serum calcium and phosphorus in patients treated with thiazides and furosemide. Acta Med Scand 194:319, 1973.

177. Lloyd-Mostyn RH et al: Ototoxicity of intravenous frusemide. Lancet 2:1156, 1971.

178. Loriaux DL et al: Spironolactone and endocrine dysfunction. Ann Intern Med 85:630, 1976.

179. Loube SD et al: Breast cancer associated with administration of spironolactone. Lancet 1:1428, 1975.

180. Lowenthal DT et al: Use of a new diuretic agent (metolazone) in patients with edema and ascites. Arch Intern Med 132:38, 1973.

181. Lurie AO: Spironolactone and steroid assay. Lancet 2:326, 1969.

182. Lurie AO: Plasma cortisol assay: interference by spironolactone. JAMA 211:1851, 1970.

183. Maffly RH: How to avoid complications of potent diuretics. JAMA 235:2526, 1976.

184. Mann NM: Gynecomastia during therapy with spironolactone. JAMA 184:778, 1963.

185. Mataverde AQ et al: Hydrochlorothiazide induced water intoxication in myxedema. JAMA 230:1014, 1974.

186. Matz GJ et al: Ototoxicity of ethacrynic acid. Arch Otolaryng 90:60, 1969.

187. Mathog RH et al: Ototoxicity of ethacrynic acid and aminogly-

coside antibiotics in uremia. NEJM 280:1223, 1969.

188. McCall AJ: Slow-K ulcertaion of oesophagus with aneurysmal left atrium. Brit Med J 3:238, 1975.

189. McElligott M: Effect of frusemide on serum calcium. Ir J Med Sci 140:410, 1971.

190. McFarland KF et al: Changes in the fasting blood sugar after hydrochlorothiazide and potassium supplementation. J Clin Pharmacol 17:13, 1977.

191. McMahon FG et al: Gastric ulceration after "Slow-K". NEJM 295:733, 1976.

192. McMurdo R: Thrombocytopenia purpura due to chlorothiazide. Practitioner 192:403, 1964.

193. Meriwether WD et al: Deafness following standard intravenous dose of ethacrynic acid. JAMA 216:795, 1971.

194. Middler S et al: Thiazide diuretics and calcium metabolism. Metab 22:139, 1973.

195. Minkowitz S et al: Fatal hemorrhagic pancreatitis following chlorothiazide administration in pregnancy. Obstet Gynecol 24:332, 1964.

196. Mond H et al: Haemodynamic effects of furosemide in patients suspected of having myocardial infarction. Brit Heart J 36:44, 1974.

197. Montoreano R et al: Prevention of the initial oliguria of acute renal failure by the administration of furosemide. Postgrad Med J 47:7, 1971.

198. Morgan DB et al: Potassium depletion in heart failure and its relation to long-term treatment with diuretics: a review of the literature. Postgrad Med J 54:72, 1978.

199. Morgan TO: Clinical use of potassium supplements and potassium sparing diuretics. Drugs 6:222, 1973.

200. Mudge GH: Diuretics and other agents employed in the mobilization of edema fluid. In *The Pharmacological Basis of Therapeutics,* Ed 5, edited by Goodman LS and Gilman A. The MacMillan Co., New York, 1975.

201. Mustala O et al: Comparison of the diabetogenic effects of chlorothiazide and furosemide. Ann Med Fenn 54:75, 1965.

202. Nassim JR et al: Control of idiopathic hypercalciuria. Brit Med J 1:675, 1965.

203. Neaverson MA: Neutropenia due to chlorthalidone. Lancet 2:208, 1964.

204. Nemati M et al: Clinical study of ticrynafen: A new diuretic, antihypertensive, and uricosuric agent. JAMA 237:652, 1977.

205. Nordquist et al: Thrombocytopenia during chlorothiazide treatment. Lancet 1:271, 1959.

206. Norymberski JK et al: Assessment of adrenocorticol activity by assay of 17-ketogenic steroid in urine. Lancet 1:1276, 1953.

207. Paloyan E et al: Hyperparathyroidism coexisting with hypertension and prolonged thiazide administration. JAMA 210:1243, 1969.

208. Parfitt AM: Chlorothiazide-induced hypercalcemia in juvenile osteoporosis and hyperparathyroidism. NEJM 281:55; 1969.

209. Parfitt AM: The interactions of thiazide diuretics with parathyroid hormone and vitamin D. J Clin Invest 51:1879, 1972.

210. Parfitt AM: Thiazide-induced hypercalcemia in vitamin D-treated hypoparathyroidism. Ann Intern Med 77:557, 1972.

211. Peterson RE: Determination of urinary neutral 17-ketosteroids. Standard Methods of Clinical Chemistry 4:151, 1963.

212. Pickleman JR et al: Thiazide induced parathyroid stimulation. Metabolism 18:867, 1969.

213. Pilewski RM et al: Technique of controlled drug assay in hypertension. Comparison of hydrochlorothiazide with a new quinethazone diuretic, metolazone. Clin Pharmacol Ther 12:843, 1971.

214. Pillay VKG et al: Transient and permanent deafness following treatment with ethacrynic acid in renal failure. Lancet 1:77, 1969.

215. Popovtzer MM et al: The acute effect of chlorothiazide on serum-ionized calcium. J Clin Invest 55:1295, 1975.

216. Prazma J et al: Ototoxicity of ethacrynic acid. Arch Otolaryngol 95:448, 1972.

217. Prazma J et al: Ethacrynic acid ototoxicity potentiation by kanamycin. Ann Otol 83:111, 1974.

218. Pruitt AW et al: Variations in the fate of triamterene. Clin Pharmacol Ther 21:610, 1977.

218a.Puschett JB et al: Comparative study of the effects of metolazone and other diuretics on potassium excretion. Clin Pharmacol Ther 15:397, 1974.

219. Quick CA et al: Early changes in the cochlear duct from etha-

crynic acid: An electron microscopic evaluation. Larynogoscope 80:854, 1970.

220. Quick CA et al: Permanent deafness associated with furosemide administration. Ann Otol 84:94, 1975.

221. Quick CA: Hearing loss in patients with dialysis and renal transplants. Ann Otol 85:776, 1976.

222. Ramsey LE et al: Influence of acetylsalicyclic acid on the renal handling of a spironolactone metabolite in healthy subjects. Europ J Clin Pharmacol 10:43, 1976.

223. Ramsay LE et al: Spironolactone and potassium canrenoate in normal man. Clin Pharmacol Ther 20:167, 1976.

224. Ramsay LE et al: Spironolactone and canrenoate-K: Relative potency at steady state. Clin Pharmacol Ther 21:602, 1977.

225. Ramsay LE et al: Factors influencing serum potassium in treated hypertension. Q J Med 46:401, 1977.

226. Rider JA et al: Potassium chloride preparations and fecal blood loss. JAMA 231:836, 1975.

227. Rifkin SI et al: Deafness associated with oral furosemide. South Med J 71:86, 1978.

228. Rose HJ et al: Depression of renal clearance of furosemide in man by azotemia. Clin Pharmacol Ther 21:141, 1977.

229. Rose LI et al: Pathophysiology of diuretic-induced gynecomastia. Ann Intern Med 87:398, 1977.

230. Runyan JW: Influence of thiazide diuretics on carbohydrate metabolism in patients with mild diabetes. NEJM 267:541, 1962.

231. Sadee W et al: Pharmacokinetics of spironolactone, canrenone and conrenoate-K in humans. J Pharmacol Exp Ther 185:686, 1973.

232. Sadee W et al: Multiple dose kinetics of spironolactone and canrenoate-potassium in cardiac and hepatic failure. Europ J Clin Pharmacol 7:195, 1974.

233. Sadee W et al: Aldosterone plasma radioimmunoassay interference by a spironolactone metabolite. Steroids 25:301, 1975.

234. Samaan N et al: Diabetogenic action of benzothiadiazines. Lancet 2:1244, 1963.

235. Schoones R et al: Evaluation of metolazone: new diuretic in chronic renal disease. NY State Med J 71:566, 1971.

236. Schnaper H et al: Chlorthalidone and serum cholesterol. Lancet 2:295, 1977.

237. Schneider WJ et al: Acute transient hearing loss after ethacrynic acid therapy. Arch Intern Med 117:715, 1966.

238. Schotland MG et al: Neutropenia in a infant secondary to hydrochlorothiazide therapy. Pediat 31:754, 1963.

239. Schrier RW et al: Tubular reabsorption of sodium ion: influence of factors other than aldosterone and glomerular filtration rates (parts 1 and 2) NEJM 285:1231, 1971 and 285:1292, 1971.

240. Schrier RW et al: Nonosmolar factors affecting renal water excretion. NEJM 292:81, 1975.

241. Schwartz GH et al: Ototoxicity induced by furosemide. NEJM 282:1413, 1970.

241a. Schwartz WB: Pathogenesis and replacement of diuretic-induced potassium and chloride loss. Ann NY Acad Sci 139:506, 1966.

242. Seely JF et al: Site of action of diuretic drugs. Kid Internat 11:1, 1977.

243. Seitz H et al: Effect of hydrochlorothiazide on serum and urinary calcium and urinary citrate. Can Med Assoc J 90:414, 1964.

244. Shanklin DR: Pancreatic atrophy apparently secondary to hydrochlorothiazide. NEJM 266:1097, 1966.

245. Shapiro AP et al: Effect of thiazides on carbohydrate metabolism in patients with hypertension. NEJM 265:1028, 1961.

246. Shear L et al: Compartmentalization of ascites and edema in patients with hepatic cirrhosis. NEJM 282:1391, 1970.

247. Sherlock S et al: Complications of diuretic therapy in hepatic cirrhosis. Lancet 1:1049, 1966.

248. Sherlock S: Ascites, Chapter 8 in *Diseases of the Liver and Biliary System*, 5th ed, Blackwell Scientific Publications, London, 1975.

249. Shreiner GE et al: *Edema and Diuretics*, Medical Communications Inc., New York, 1969.

250. Simborg DW: Medication prescribing on a university medical service — the incidence of drug combinations with potential adverse interactions. John Hopkins Med J 139:23, 1976.

251. Simon NM: Plasma cortisol after spironolactone. NEJM 282:1214, 1970.

252. Slone D et al: Intravenously given ethacrynic acid and gastrointestinal bleeding. JAMA 209:1668, 1969.

253. Solvsteen P et al: Diabetic coma without ketoacidosis. Acta Med Scand 184:83, 1968.

254. Spark RF et al: Aldosteronism in hypertension. The spironolactone response test. Ann Intern Med 69:685, 1968.

255. Sprivastava G et al: Thiazide-induced bone-marrow aplasia. Indian J Pediat 34:407, 1967.

256. Steele TH: Diuretic-induced hyperuricemia. Clinics Rheumatic Dis 3:37, 1977.

257. Steinberg AD: Pulmonary edema following ingestion of hydrochlorothiazide. JAMA 204:825, 1968.

258. Steinmetz PR: Use of diuretics in renal disease. Mod Treat 7:401, 1970.

258a. Steinmuller SR et al: Effects of metolazone in man: Comparison with chlorothiazide. Kid Internat 1:169, 1972.

259. Stern A: Metolazone, a diuretic agent. Am Heart J 91:262, 1976.

260. Stockigt JR: Potassium homeostasis. Aust NZ J Med 7:66, 1977.

261. Stote RM et al: Hydrochlorothiazide effects on serum calcium and immunoreactive parathyroid hormone concentrations. Ann Intern Med 77:587, 1972.

262. Stote RM et al: Ticrynafen a uricosuric antihypertensive diuretic. Clin Pharmacol Ther 23:456, 1978.

263. Stripp B et al: Effect of spironolactone on sex hormones in man. J Clin Endocrinol Metab 41:777, 1975.

264. Suki WN et al: Mechanism of the effect of thiazide diuretics on calcium and uric acid. Clin Res 15:78, 1967.

265. Suki WN et al: Acute treatment of hypercalcemia with furosemide. NEJM 283:836, 1970.

266. Sussman RM: Spironolactone and gynecomastia. Lancet 1:58, 1963.

267. Tambyah JA et al: Effect of frusemide on calcium excretion. Brit Med J 1:751, 1969.

268. Tan SY et al: Interference of spironolactone in 11 deoxycorticosterone radioassays. J Clin Endocrinol Metab 41:791, 1975.

269. Tashima CK: Blood cortisol levels from spironolactone. JAMA 224:1188, 1973.

270. Tasker PRW et al: Nonketotic diabetic precoma associated with high-dose frusemide therapy. Brit Med J 1:626, 1976.

271. Tilstone WJ et al: Pharmacokinetics of metolazone in normal subjects and in patients with cardiac or renal failure. Clin Pharmacol Ther 16:322, 1974.

272. Toft H et al: Effect of frusemide administration on calcium excretion. Brit Med J 1:437, 1971.

273. Toivonen S et al: Diabetogenic action of frusemide. Brit Med J 1:920, 1966.

274. Turner NA et al: Neutropenia associated with chlorthalidone therapy. Med J Aust 1:361, 1964.

275. Tweeddale MG et al: Antagonism of spironolactone-induced natriuresis by aspirin in man. NEJM 289:198, 1973.

276. Venkateswaran PS: Transient deafness from high doses of frusemide. Brit Med J 4:113, 1971.

277. Vila JM et al: Thiazide-induced immune hemolytic anemia. JAMA 236:1723, 1976.

278. Walker BR et al: Hyperkalemia after triamterene in diabetic patients. Clin Pharmacol Ther 13:643, 1972.

279. Walker WG: Indications and contraindications for diuretic therapy. Ann NY Acad Sci 139:481, 1966.

280. Walker WG et al: Potassium homeostatis and diuretic therapy. In *Modern Diuretic Therapy in the Treatment of Cardiovascular and Renal Disease*, edited by Lant AF, Wilson GM, Excerpta Medica, Amsterdam, 1973, p 331.

281. Walsh CH et al: A study of the effect of frusemide on carbohydrate metabolism in diabetic subjects. J Irish Med Ass 67:187, 1974.

282. Walsh PC et al: Suppression of plasma androgens by spironolactone in castrated men with carcinoma of the prostate. J Urol 114:254, 1975.

283. Wedeen RP et al: Mechanisms of edema and the use of diuretics. Ped Clin N Amer 18:561, 1971.

284. Weinstein L: The sulfonamides. In *The Pharmacologic Basis of Therapeutics*, Ed 4, edited by Goodman LS and Gilman A, Ch 56. The MacMillan Co., New York, 1970, p 1177.

284a. Weiss ES et al: Congestive heart failure. In Manual of Medical Therapeutics, Ed 22, edited by Costrini NV, Ch 5, Little, Brown & Co., Boston, 1977, p 81.

285. Welt L: Edema. In *Harrison's Principles of Internal Medicine*, Ed 8, Ch 30, McGraw Hill, San Fransisco, 1977, p 176.

286. Wenger J et al: Acute pancreatitis related to hydrochlorothiazide

therapy. Gastroent 46:768, 1964.

287. West BA et al: Interaction of kanamycin and ethacrynic acid. Arch Otolarygol 98:32, 1973.

288. Wigand ME et al: Ototoxic side-effects of high doses of furosemide in patients with uremia. Postgrad Med J 47 (Apr Suppl):54, 1971.

289. Wilkinson SP et al: Renal retention of sodium in cirrhosis and fulminant hepatic failure. Postgrad Med J 51:527, 1975.

290. Williams E: Spironolactone and gynaecomastia. Lancet 2:1113, 1962.

290a. Williamson HE: Furosemide and ethacrynic acid. J Clin Pharmacol 17:663, 1977.

291. Williamson JM et al: Hypoplastic anemia and hydroflumethiazide. Scot Med J 11:9, 1966.

292. Wilson AE et al: Acute pancreatitis associated with furosemide therapy. Lancet 1:105, 1967.

293. Wilson DR et al: The effect of thiazide diuretics on carbohydrate-induced calciuria in patients with recurrent renal calculi. J Lab Clin Med 86:118, 1975.

294. Wolff FW et al: Drug-induced diabetes. JAMA 185:568, 1963.

295. Wood LC et al: Plasma cortisol after spironolactone. NEJM 282:1214, 1970.

295a. Wood LC et al: Interference in the measurement of plasma 11-hydroxycorticosteroids caused by spironolactone administration. NEJM 282:650, 1970.

296. Wyngaarden JB et al: Drug-induced hyperuricemia and gout. In *Gout and Hyperuricemia*, Grune and Stratton, New York, 1976, p 369.

297. Yap V et al: Hyperkalemia with cardiac arrhythmia. JAMA 236:2775, 1976.

298. Yendt ER et al: The effect of thiazides in idiopathic hypercalciuria. Am J Med Sci 251:449, 1966.

299. Yendt ER et al: The use of thiazides in the prevention of renal calculi. Can Med Assoc J 102:614, 1970.

300. Yendt ER et al: Prevention of calcium stones with thiazides. Kidney Internat 13:397, 1978.

301. Zarren HS et al: Unilateral gynecomastia and impotence during low-dose spironolactone administration in men. Milit Med 140:417, 1975.

302. Zuckerman AM et al: Agranulocytosis with thrombocytopenia following chlorothiazide therapy. Brit Med J 2:1338, 1958.

Chapter 14

Cardiac Arrhythmias

Mark A. Gill
Michael E. Winter

The pharmacist's involvement in the treatment of cardiac arrhythmias requires a synthesis of drug knowledge with electrophysiology and anatomy. Physical assessment techniques and their interpretation are important since disruption of the normal heart rhythm affects other organ systems. Pharmacists must develop clinical judgement to evaluate the efficacy of drug therapy for cardiac arrhythmias. Familiarity with the literature will be essential since the majority of therapeutic questions revolve around acute situations.

The *electrical system of the heart* consists of intrinsic pacemakers and conduction tissues. A diagram of the heart which depicts the pathways for conduction is provided in figure 1.

The rate of electrical firing of the heart is dependent upon the most rapid pacemaker. Spontaneous electrical firing or automaticity can occur anywhere in the heart under certain conditions; normally, however, the sino-atrial node (S-A node) which has the most rapid intrinsic rate (60-100 per minute) serves as the major pacemaker. Any electrical activity which is initiated by other automatic tissues is considered to be an arrhythmia. Most arrhythmias are labelled according to their anatomical locations and rates.

Firing of the S-A node initiates atrial contraction. The electrical impulse is conducted through the atria via internodal tracts to the atrioventricular node (A-V node) which is located near the coronary sinus between the left and right atria. The A-V node has pacemaker properties but normally serves to coordinate atrial and ventricular contraction.

The conduction system in the ventricles is more elaborate than the atria since the muscle mass is larger. Rapid and effective excitation is critical since ventricular contraction is the major determinant of cardiac output.

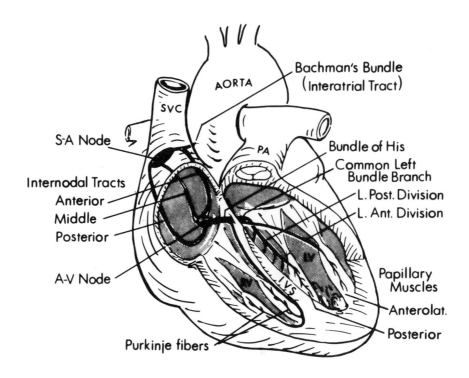

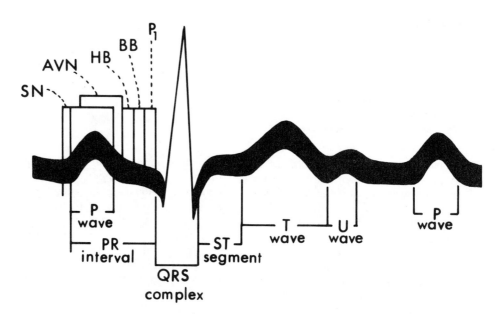

Figure 1: *Conduction system of the heart.* Above is an anatomical illustration of the location of pacemakers and conduction tissues. Below is an electrocardiogram. The P wave is atrial depolorization. Note that the P-R interval is formed from the following: S-A Node (SN), A-V Node (AVN), Bundle of His (HB), Bundle Branch (BB), and Purkinje fibers (P₁). The QRS complex is ventricular depolorization.

Figure 2

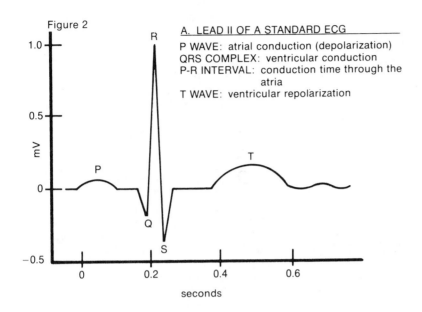

A. LEAD II OF A STANDARD ECG

P WAVE: atrial conduction (depolarization)
QRS COMPLEX: ventricular conduction
P-R INTERVAL: conduction time through the
    atria
T WAVE: ventricular repolarization

seconds

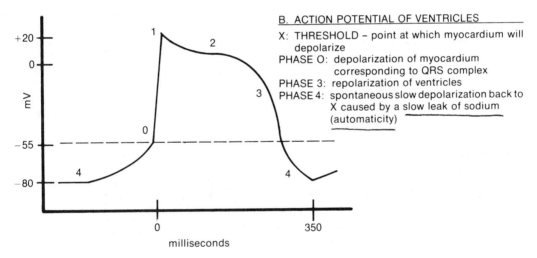

B. ACTION POTENTIAL OF VENTRICLES

X: THRESHOLD – point at which myocardium will
    depolarize
PHASE O: depolarization of myocardium
    corresponding to QRS complex
PHASE 3: repolarization of ventricles
PHASE 4: spontaneous slow depolarization back to
    X caused by a slow leak of sodium
    (automaticity)

milliseconds

C. CORRESPONDING IONIC FLUXES

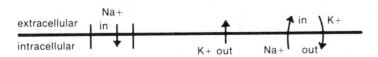

Figure 3:
EFFECT OF TYPE I ANTIARRHYTHMICS ON THE ECG
AND ACTION POTENTIAL

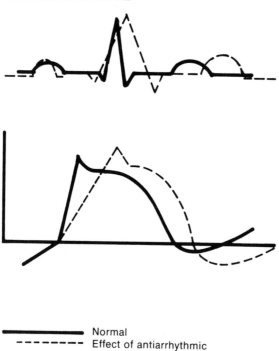

——————— Normal
- - - - - - - Effect of antiarrhythmic

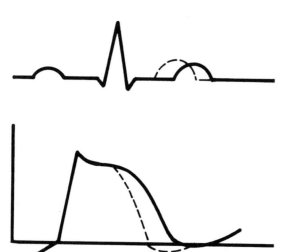

Figure 4: EFFECT OF TYPE II ANTIARRHYTHMICS ON
THE ECG AND ACTION POTENTIAL OF NORMAL
(UNDEPRESSED) CARDIAC TISSUE

Fibers leaving the A-V node are called the Bundle of His and separate into the bundle branches which traverse the septum between the ventricles. The final conducting components of the ventricles are the Purkinje fibers which emanate from the bundle branches to stimulate ventricular contraction.

Before studying the antiarrhythmic drugs individually, it is helpful if the direct pharmacologic properties are compared and contrasted. The antiarrhythmics are often divided into two or three basic classes of drugs:

ⓐ Type I antiarrhythmics: quinidine, procainamide, disopyramide

ⓑ Type II antiarrhythmics: phenytoin, lidocaine

ⓒ "Type III" antiarrhythmics: propranolol (this drug has properties in common with both Type I and Type II antiarrhythmics).

Figure 2 depicts a schematic diagram of an action potential with corresponding changes in the electrocardiogram. The ionic fluxes at the cell surface which occur with each phase of the action potential are provided as well.

The *Type I* antiarrhythmics decrease the slope of phase 4 (decrease automaticity); slow the rate of conduction (or the rate of rise of phase 0); and increase the time of recovery or repolarization (lengthening phases 1, 2, and 3 of the action potential). See figure 3. These are direct effects and do not involve the vagolytic properties of the Type I drugs. If vagal tone is decreased by these drugs, one may see an increase rather than a decrease in the conduction and repolarization of the atria and the atrioventricular node. This becomes important in rhythms characterized by rapid atrial rates, as such increases in conduction and repolarization may allow an increased number of electrical impulses to reach the ventricles resulting in a ventricular tachycardia. The vagal effects are not as important when the atrium has a normal rate (130).

Because the P-R and QRS intervals of the electrocardiogram (ECG) correspond to the rates of conduction in the atria, atrioventricular node and the ventricles respectively, the direct effects of a Type I antiarrhythmic would be to widen these intervals. The Q-T interval corresponds to the rate of ventricular repolarization (phases 1, 2 and 3) and would be widened by a Type I antiarrhythmic. See figure 3. Remember, however, that because of the vagolytic properties of the Type I antiarrhythmics, low doses can be expected to shorten the P-R interval and QRS complex.

The *Type II* antiarrhythmics, lidocaine and phenytoin, will slow the rate of spontaneous depolarization in Phase 4 (decrease automaticity). They usually will not change the slope of phase 0 (i.e., they do not change rate of conduction) and will shorten the time course of repolarization (phases 1, 2 and 3 of the action potential) (130). See figure 4. It is important to note that lidocaine can depress conduction in the myocardium in a manner similar to quinidine if the serum concentrations are sufficiently high, i.e., above the 2 to 7 mcg/ml level (126); phenytoin can actually increase the rate of conduction in depressed myocardial tissue (31). See figure 5.

Although the ECG changes of the Type II antiarrhythmics are not as dramatic as the Type I antiarrhythmics, one would expect a shortening of the Q-T interval as the repolarization process (phases 1, 2 and 3) of the action potential appear to be shortened. In the depressed myocardium, one might expect a shortening of the QRS interval with the administration of phenytoin because of its ability to increase conduction rate (phase 0) of a depressed action potential. See figure 5.

Propranolol is sometimes considered to be a Type I antiarrhythmic because it depresses phase 4 (automaticity) and also phase 0 (conduction) like quinidine. However, propranolol also appears to shorten the repolarization process (phases 1, 2 and 3) like the Type II antiarrhythmics. The exact classification type of propranolol is immaterial as long as the differences are appreciated. See figure 6.

Propranolol would be expected to have a direct effect of widening the QRS complex like the Type I antiarrhythmics and shortening the Q-T interval like the Type II antiarrhythmics. See figure 6. Although the beta-blocking properties of propranolol may be useful in treating certain types of arrhythmias, the antiarrhythmic effects are not solely dependent on beta-blockade (40).

1. How can knowledge of the effects of antiarrhythmics on the action potential and ECG be applied clinically?

Theoretically, one selects a drug which will reverse the underlying abnormality. For example, phenothiazines have been known to cause arrhythmias associated with typical ECG changes such as an alteration in the T-wave (corresponding to phases 1, 2 and 3 of the action potential) and notching or prolongation of the QT interval (an indication of a prolonged repolarization phase) (5). A reasonable choice of antiarrhythmics in this situation would be one of the Type II drugs (i.e., phenytoin or lidocaine) since they shorten phases 1, 2 and 3 of the action potential (6).

Another example is in the treatment of arrhythmias secondary to quinidine or procainamide toxicity. The type I drugs decrease phase 0 and prolong phases 1, 2 and 3; therefore, a Type II drug would be a logical choice since they increase phase 0 of the depressed myocardial tissue and increase the rate of repolarization (shorten phases 1, 2 and 3) (53).

2. A 59-year-old male was admitted to the CCU with

Figure 5:
EFFECT OF DIPHENYLHYDANTOIN ON ECG AND ACTION POTENTIAL OF DEPRESSED TISSUE

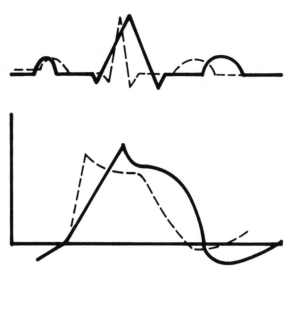

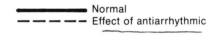
——————— Normal
— — — — — Effect of antiarrhythmic

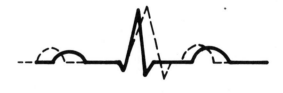

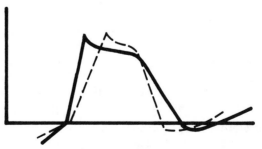

Figure 6: EFFECT OF PROPRANOLOL ON THE ECG AND ACTION POTENTIAL

a chief complaint of severe chest pain which was unrelieved by three nitroglycerin tablets. The pain radiated from the sternum up the neck and down his left arm and was associated with nausea, diaphoresis and shortness of breath. On admission the patient was in acute distress, obtunded and cyanotic. His blood pressure was 90/20. The ECG showed sinus bradycardia with ST segment depression and the presence of Q waves with a rate of 30 beats per minute. Does this patient require antiarrhythmic treatment? What drug would you recommend?

A logical first step in determining the need for, and type of antiarrhythmic therapy depends on the expected morbidity and mortality associated with the arrhythmia. Clearly the patient, not the electrocardiogram should be treated. **Sinus bradycardia** is a rhythm emanating from the S-A node with a rate of less than 60 beats per minute which is caused by a defect in impulse formation through a decrease in S-A node automaticity. This arrhythmia is seen in approximately 40% of patients with infarction of the right coronary artery (the artery that perfuses the S-A node) (95).

This patient deserves treatment since his cardiac output is not sufficient to maintain normal blood pressure and tissue perfusion. Maintenance of a normal rate alone may not be sufficient to improve cardiac output if significant cardiac damage has occurred. **Atropine** is the drug of choice and should be given intravenously in an initial dose of 0.6-1.0 mg. The goal of therapy is to maintain an adequate cardiac output (which may be monitored by blood pressure and urinary output) as well as a normal heart rate. Animal data indicate that atropine may increase ischemic changes if given in excessive doses (34). Generally, atropine may be repeated every three minutes until a maximum dose of 2 mg has been given (25,95). The appropriate dose may be repeated every three to four hours as needed (128).

If the patient is symptomatic and still has a rate of less than 45/min after adequate atropinization, a temporary transvenous artificial **cardiac pacemaker** should be inserted. In addition to maintaining a normal rate, artificial pacing suppresses ventricular ectopic beats that frequently appear when the automaticity of the S-A node falls below the intrinsic automaticity of the ventricles (25).

Isoproterenol may be used to treat bradycardia only if other measures have failed or are not available. It has several drawbacks in that excessive doses may increase ventricular irritability and induce ventricular tachyarrhythmias. In addition, isoproterenol increases myocardial oxygen consumption which may increase the infarct size (84). Isoproterenol should be administered as a constant infusion at a rate of 1-4 mcg/min.

3. A 24-year-old female is admitted with a chief complaint of shortness of breath. She has a ten-year history of asthma for which she takes oxtriphylline 400 mg qid and prednisone 10 mg daily. Physical examination reveals a patient in respiratory distress with a pulse of 90, a respiratory rate of 40/min, and a temperature of 102°F. Wheezes were heard on auscultation. The patient was given an intravenous bolus of aminophylline, 5.6 mg/kg, followed by an infusion of 0.9 mg/kg/hour. Within two hours after the loading dose had been administered, the nurses noted a pulse of 140. How should this patient's sinus tachycardia be managed?

Sinus tachycardia is a sinus rhythm except the rate is greater than 100 beats per minute. Its significance depends upon the etiology of the arrhythmia. Anxiety or stimulants such as caffeine, amphetamines or methylphenidate may produce a sinus tachycardia. This is generally benign and requires no treatment other than removal of the offending agent(s).

This patient could be exhibiting toxicity to aminophylline. Most young, otherwise healthy asthmatics, can tolerate this arrhythmia with careful observation. The aminophylline does not necessarily need to be stopped or decreased unless there is a potential for more dangerous complications. In addition, the fever may be indicative of an infection which may also contribute to this tachycardia.

Some patients may not tolerate an increase in heart rate such as this. For example, the tachycardia could increase myocardial oxygen consumption and exacerbate angina pectoris. Also, a rapid heart rate limits ventricular filling and thus reduces cardiac output. Therefore, in some patients, the risk of the arrhythmia may outweigh the benefits of aminophylline for bronchodilation. Propranolol is generally used to treat sinus tachycardia; however, it should be avoided in this patient since it may exacerbate the bronchospasm.

4. A 45-year-old female was admitted to the hospital with a chief complaint of palpitations. The prior medical history revealed that the patient had rheumatic fever at age 9. On physical examination the patient was noted to have an irregular pulse of about 130 beats per minute. The point of maximum impulse (PMI) was displaced to the mid-axillary line at the sixth intercostal space and the apical rate was 170 beats per minute. The lungs were clear but a murmur was noted. The ECG was read as atrial fibrillation. What is atrial fibrillation? Why is digitalis considered to be the drug of choice? What are the goals of therapy?

Atrial fibrillation is an irregularly irregular rhythm originating from ectopic atrial foci at a rate of 400-650 beats per minute. However, since the A-V node prevents the majority of these impulses from stimulating the ventricles, the ventricular rate (pulse) is significantly less. Atrial fibrillation is the second most common arrhythmia and is frequently associated with rheumatic heart disease (64).

Digitalis is considered to be the drug of choice for atrial fibrillation because it is the only drug that can reduce the ventricular rate and simultaneously reduce the major consequence of the arrhythmia, congestive heart failure (135).

Digitalis increases the force of myocardial contraction and decreases A-V conduction as reflected by a prolonged P-R interval. Intraventricular conduction is not affected; i.e., the QRS complex is not altered. Digitalis also prolongs the refractory period (repolarization) of the A-V node; this effect is most apparent when digitalis is used in the treatment of rapid atrial rates. There is an increase in the ectopic impulse formation which occurs in all areas of the heart except the S-A node; this effect is usually seen in the Purkinje fibers. Finally, digitalis decreases the rate of S-A node impulse formation. There are two mechanisms for this phenomenon. Vagal stimulation occurs with lower doses which can be reversed by atropine; however, there is also a direct effect that is not blocked by atropine.

Reflex vagal stimulation, depression of the S-A node, prolongation of the A-V nodal refractory period, and slowing of A-V conduction brought about by digitalis form the basis for the use of this drug in the treatment of supraventricular tachyarrhythmias — that is, arrhythmias originating in the S-A node or atria (17,89).

The primary goal of therapy is to slow the rate of ventricular contraction so that diastolic filling is increased and cardiac output is improved. Generally an arbitrary ventricular rate of 60-70/min is used as a therapeutic goal (119). This rate should be based upon a pulse obtained at the apex of the heart rather than at the radial artery since all of the ventricular beats may not be transmitted to the periphery. Clinicians should take care that objective and symptomatic relief and drug intoxication are not overlooked in their zeal to achieve a specific rate. Improved pulmonary, renal, and cerebral function will also give clues to increased cardiac output (19).

The second goal in the treatment of atrial fibrillation is to convert the arrhythmia to normal sinus rhythm (NSR) with electrocardioversion, **quinidine or procainamide**. It is important that patients who are to receive quinidine for atrial fibrillation be digitalized first to produce some degree of AV block. This is necessary because the vagolytic effects of quinidine may actually enhance AV conduction in these patients and increase the ventricular rate. The recent onset of the arrhythmia and the apparent absence of CHF would suggest that

this patient has a good chance of converting; however, the displaced PMI may indicate left ventricular hypertrophy which makes conversion less likely (55,66). (See chapters on *Congestive Heart Failure* and *Clinical Pharmacokinetics* for further discussion of digitalis.)

5. A 50-year-old male is admitted for fever and mental confusion. Vital signs include a pulse of 140, a temperature of 102°F, a respiratory rate of 35/min, and a blood pressure of 160/90. A chest x-ray (CXR) revealed an infiltrate in the right lower lobe and a normal sized heart. The ECG was read as atrial fibrillation. Two hours after digoxin 0.5 mg was given by intravenous push, the rate remained 130-140/min and an additional 0.5 mg was given intravenously. One hour later another 0.25 mg digoxin was given since the rate was 130/min. Two hours later the rate is still rapid at 125 beats per minute; should additional doses of digoxin be given?

Clinically, it appears that higher doses of digoxin are required for atrial fibrillation than for congestive heart failure (59). Several studies reveal that neither total dose or serum digoxin level are useful indicators of response in the treatment of atrial fibrillation (19,45,101). A modest, mean digoxin level of 1.4 ng/ml has been observed in patient with controlled atrial fibrillation (19). Goldman et al noted that in patients with acute illnesses (such as this patient's infection), doses of digoxin which produced toxicity did not control the ventricular response (45). An arterial blood gas would be helpful in this patient since hypoxia (secondary to the pulmonary infection) may predispose to digitalis toxicity (118,120).

It is still too early to conclude that digoxin is ineffective in this patient since at least four hours is required before digoxin is distributed into cardiac tissue (113). In fact, this may be delayed in some subjects for 12 hours (103).

Control of the infection and correction of any acid-base or electrolyte abnormality may allow digoxin to control the ventricular response without the risk of digoxin toxicity.

6. A 30-year-old male with a long history of hyperthyroidism controlled with methimazole, failed to refill his medications. He came to the emergency room complaining of nervousness, insomnia and a throbbing sensation in his chest. The ECG indicated atrial fibrillation. How should this patient be treated?

Atrial fibrillation attributed to hyperthyroidism has been reported to be refractory to digoxin (19). This resistance is due to the lower digoxin levels which occur in hyperthyroid subjects when equivalent doses of digoxin are administered to hyperthyroid and euthyroid individuals. Doherty et al suggested that a larger volume of distribution could account for the lower digoxin concentration since the elimination half-life was not altered in the hyperthyroid individuals (30). Croxson et al discounted this theory since they observed a shorter half-life in hyperthyroid patients and this was associated with an increased glomerular filtration rate (27).

Propranolol may be the drug of choice to treat atrial fibrillation induced by hyperthyroidism if there is no evidence of congestive heart failure. Propranolol slows A-V conduction but has little activity on atrial tissue to decrease the atrial rate (115). Although propranolol has antiarrhythmic properties, it rarely converts atrial fibrillation to normal sinus rhythm (NSR) when used alone. When used in conjunction with quinidine, 64.8% of patients will convert to NSR (135).

This patient may be treated with intravenous propranolol to rapidly reduce the ventricular rate and associated symptoms of hyperthyroidism. An intravenous (IV) dose of 0.5-0.75 mg propranolol may be repeated every two minutes up to a maximum of 0.1 mg/kg. Alternatively a total dose of 0.1 mg/kg may be diluted in 50-100cc D5W and infused over ten minutes (115). The patient should be monitored closely as these doses are given since decreased cardiac output is more likely to occur early in therapy (99). Others have administered propranolol to patients with arrhythmias and severe congestive heart failure and have observed improvement in cardiac output. Apparently in these cases the antiarrhythmic properties predominated and negative inotropic effects were minimal (78).

Once the ventricular rate is controlled with IV therapy, the drug may be given orally. Oral doses are larger than IV doses because of first pass metabolism after oral administration (35,97,112) (Also see chapter on *Clinical Pharmacokinetics.*) This extraction process varies significantly between patients as evidenced by a twenty-fold difference in peak serum levels observed after the administration of equivalent oral doses (111). This patient may be switched to an oral dose of 10 mg every four to six hours. This may be increased each day by 10 mg per dose until the ventricular rate is maintained at 60-80/min or the patient develops other evidence of propranolol toxicity (98).

The Boston Collaborative Drug Surveillance Program reported a 9.4% incidence of side effects associated with the use of propranolol (48). Reactions are most commonly related to the central nervous system and include fatigue, hallucinations, weakness, insomnia, and nightmares (57,115,124).

7. R.R., a 68-year-old female, was admitted with a chief complaint of shortness of breath. She was diagnosed as having atrial fibrillation and was digitalized. Although the apical rate is 80, she is still in atrial fibrillation. What are the possibilities of converting the atrial fibrillation to NSR? Describe the various approaches which may be used to make this conversion.

Digitalis alone very rarely converts atrial fibrillation to NSR (21); this probably relates to its inability to reduce atrial automaticity (47). The methods for conversion are neither completely effective nor totally without risk. The mortality rate for electrical conversion is reported to be 2% (79) while that associated with quinidine is 0.5-2.0% (82,129). In a patient without underlying cardiovascular disease these risks may not be justifiable. This patient does, however, present with complaints that require hospitalization and the potential for conversion now is greater than at some later date (79).

Electrical stimulation is a more rapid and effective method of conversion than is the use of antiarrhythmic drugs (50,100,102). Yet, electric shock may abruptly release catecholamines and induce arrhythmias, especially in the presence of digitalis (81). The rhythm is converted 80-90% of the time (50, 100,102); however, atrial fibrillation will recur in 72% of patients within one year (116).

Quinidine is an alternative to electric shock for cardioversion and has a variable response rate of 59% (26) to 82% (44).

8. The above patient responded to electrocardioversion without complications. Should she be placed on antiarrhythmic drugs chronically?

Chronic administration of quinidine prevents recurrences of atrial fibrillation in only 10-20% of patients (123) and there are some studies which indicate that quinidine may have no effect on the recurrence of atrial fibrillation at all (51,96,117). However, it is worthwhile to try to prevent recurrence since effective atrial contraction will improve cardiac output by 30% (94). There is some morbidity associated with the chronic use of quinidine since 30% of patients may develop side effects severe enough to require discontinuation of the medication (82).

Because this arrhythmia compromises the patient's limited cardiac reserve, arrhythmia suppression is probably indicated, but adverse drug reactions must be monitored carefully.

9. R.R. was placed on quinidine sulfate, 400 mg qid. Two weeks later she returned to the clinic complaining of diarrhea. The intern discontinued the quinidine sulfate and ordered quinidine polygalacturonate (Cardioquin) because of his understanding that this salt has fewer gastrointestinal side effects. Comment.

Nausea, vomiting, diarrhea, and anorexia are the most common side effects of quinidine and it is not clear whether they are caused by CNS effects or local gastrointestinal (GI) irritation.

A study by Gerstenbleth (38) indicated that the polygalacturonate (PG) salt did produce fewer GI side effects. The incidence of side effects was reduced from 56% to 13% when 270 mg of the PG salt was given in place of 200 mg of the sulfate. Both drugs had similar success rates in converting arrhythmias back to normal sinus rhythm. The amount of quinidine in the two dosage forms is approximately the same; however, the polygalacturonate salt is less soluble and releases free quinidine more slowly, producing fewer side effects.

Evidence that all of the quinidine from the polygalacturonate salt was completely absorbed from the GI tract is lacking since blood levels were not measured in this particular study and it was, therefore, not shown that comparable quinidine levels were achieved with both salt forms. Others have shown (43) that equivalent doses of the polygalacturonate salt produce much lower blood levels than the sulfate after seven days of a multiple dosing schedule. The substantial cost difference between the two drugs is also an important consideration, since patients can remain on this type of agent for a long period of time.

Even though many patients complain of diarrhea early in quinidine therapy, most become tolerant to this side effect. Should the symptoms become severe, the patient should be evaluated and treated for electrolyte and acid-base imbalance. If necessary, bothersome diarrhea may be controlled on a short term basis with small doses of opiates or diphenoxylate.

10. Mr. S.H. requests a refill on his recently prescribed quinidine prescription. As you are talking, you notice a bruise on his forehead and immediately think of quinidine-induced thrombocytopenia. You question him about it, but he says he passed out and hit his head as he fell. He says he has fainted on several occasions since he started taking his "new heart medicine." However, he was told not to worry because this drug can cause his "veins to dilate" and make his blood pressure go down. He was told that if he felt faint, he should just lie down and that he would be all right. Is this "quinidine syncope?" What is the mechanism by which syncope occurs? How is it treated? What are some other cardiovascular side effects of quinidine?

The patient's problem could be "quinidine syncope," but there is no way to ascertain this unless evidence of ventricular arrhythmias can be documented at the time of his syncopal episodes. Quinidine syncope is caused by drug-induced changes in ventricular rhythm (tachycardias and fibrillation) which decrease cardiac output and cause a loss of consciousness or "syncope." Pallor, muscular

twitching, seizures and apnea may also occur. The arrhythmias are often recurrent, apparently unrelated to dose, and can terminate spontaneously, as in the above case. The drugs of choice to treat this syndrome would include phenytoin or lidocaine which have an opposite electrophysiological effect. However, these are often not as effective as external cardiac massage, DC shock, or pacemakers. Of course, discontinuation of the quinidine is recommended. This is one of the most serious side effects of quinidine and can result in sudden death if left unrecognized (88,109). Quinidine may be hazardous in patients with compromised cardiac output since it also produces a dose-related hypotension by alpha adrenergic blockage (93) and has a direct negative inotropic effect (85).

11. Mr. J. was discharged from the hospital. A week before he was due to return to the clinic, he developed a fever with no associated infection. His only medication was quinidine. The physician is certain that it is not the quinidine that is causing the fever because he gave the patient a "test dose" of 200 mg of quinidine sulfate prior to discharge to determine if he was allergic or overly sensitive to the drug. Comment.

This is a typical reaction to quinidine. Fever most commonly occurs three to twenty days after the drug is started; however, the fever usually, but not always, is accompanied by other signs of an allergic reaction, such as a maculopapular or urticarial rash or thrombocytopenia (36,77).

12. How can ECG changes be used to monitor the toxic effects of quinidine? Do they correlate with serum levels?

Changes in the QRS complex (i.e., conducting velocity through the ventricles) correlate most closely with quinidine levels. Widening of the QRS complex begins when serum levels reach 2 mcg/ml (nonspecific assay) and there is progressive widening as the quinidine levels rise. The Q-T interval or refractory period also increase but do not correlate with the serum level as well as changes in the QRS (13,51).

A widening of the QRS of more than 25% (i.e., greater than 0.14 seconds) should be taken as a warning that toxic levels are being approached. Increases in the QRS complex of 50% or more are often followed by ventricular fibrillation. Most clinicians avoid QRS widening of more than 25% and few, if any, are willing to continue treatment if there is more than a 50% change in the QRS (51,52).

13. A 65-year-old white male, with a history of deep vein thrombophlebitis, has been going to the outpatient clinics for the past two months because he is on warfarin (Coumadin). On his last visit he was noted to

have a few PVC's, but there was no evidence of pulmonary embolism. He now comes to the pharmacy with a prescription for quinidine 200 mg qid #100 and an order to refill his Coumadin 10 mg qd. His next clinic appointment is in three weeks. Comment. What is the mechanism of the interaction between warfarin and quinidine?

The anticoagulant effect or depression of the prothrombin complex by quinidine or quinine is well known. Koch-Weser (69) reports that patients developed hematuria, conjunctival hemorrhages, guaiac positive stools, hematomas and epistaxis 6 to 10 days after the initiation of quinidine in doses of 200 mg qid when begun in combination with warfarin. Changes in the prothrombin time (PT) have been noted by the second or third day. This patient is obviously a candidate for such a reaction; therefore, his physician should be contacted by the pharmacist. An appropriate solution would be to check the prothrombin time in 2 or 3 days and caution the patient about symptoms of excessive anticoagulation (69).

The mechanism is possibly two-fold. Quinidine is highly protein bound so that drug-displacement or competition for binding sites is a postulated mechanism. However, quinidine is an organic base and warfarin is an organic acid so that they are most likely bound to different sites on the protein molecule; this would tend to negate the displacement theory. The second postulated mechanism is that quinidine may be a direct antagonist of vitamin K. The former mechanism may account for an initial change in the PT; however, this effect would be expected to be of relatively short duration. The latter mechanism would require a permanent reduction in the warfarin dosage (69,71).

14. K.C. is a 65-year-old 50 kg female who is admitted to the hospital for assessment and treatment of ileus. On physical examination her pulse is noted to be 130/minute and irregular. She has had a history of atrial fibrillation which was previously controlled with digoxin 0.25 mg and quinidine sulfate 200 mg qid. She has not taken either of these agents recently. It is also known that she has deteriorating renal function. The last creatinine clearance obtained was 15 cc/min. The medical staff plans to reinstitute digoxin and quinidine parenterally. They are aware of the effect of renal failure on digoxin elimination and will dose accordingly. However, they are unfamiliar with the parenteral administration and pharmacokinetics of quinidine. What would you recommend for this patient?

Since quinidine is usually well absorbed, one can assume that the parenteral dose is about equivalent to the oral dose; however, since different salt forms of the drug are used in the parenteral preparations, some adjustment is necessary. The usual oral form is quinidine sulfate, which is 87.4% quinidine. Quinidine gluconate, which is used parenterally, is only 62.3% quinidine. Therefore, 280 mg of quinidine gluconate contains the same amount of quinidine as 200 mg of quinidine sulfate (87).

The intramuscular injection of quinidine is painful and produces local muscle damage. Also, absorption is erratic and only 85-90% complete (49). Intravenous administration is more reliable, but has not been used routinely because of the cardiovascular toxicity which accompanies its use by this route. However, recent studies indicate that there are few adverse effects when the gluconate salt is administered slowly at a rate of 0.3-0.4 mg/kg/min (58). Since the volume of distribution for quinidine is 2.3 L/kg (49) and the therapeutic range is 2-5 mg/L (70), the loading dose may range from 4.6 to 11.5 mg/kg. The appropriate dose should be repeated at six to eight hour intervals since the reported elimination half time obtained using a specific assay is 7.3 hours (133).

Considerable controversy has been generated over the last few years regarding quinidine pharmacokinetics. Nonspecific assays measure quinidine metabolites and/or tablet contaminants (66) resulting in smaller estimates for the volume of distribution and clearance and larger estimates for therapeutic plasma levels than those which are derived from levels using a specific assay that measures only quinidine (See chapter on *Clinical Pharmacokinetics*). The literature reveals contradictory results in quinidine disposition in renal impairment. Bellet et al (9) reported higher serum levels with decreased renal function while Kessler et al (66) described similar half-times in normal and renal failure patients. More recently Ueda et al (133) found only 17% of quinidine excreted unchanged in the urine while Greenblatt et al (49) observed 35%. At this time most of the data indicate that the renal route of elimination for quinidine is minor and no dose adjustment would be expected in patients with decreased renal function (1). It would be appropriate, however, to follow such patients carefully for side effects or toxicities. If serum levels are to be used, the type of assay must be considered, as levels obtained from a nonspecific assay may be elevated due to the accumulation of quinidine metabolites.

15. K.C. received intravenous quinidine as ordered; however, because she became hypotensive, it was decided to switch her to procainamide. The plan is to administer procainamide parenterally until the ileus has resolved. Discuss the use of procainamide, its pharmacokinetic properties, and derive a parenteral and oral dosage regimen for this patient.

Therapeutic plasma levels for procainamide are reported to be 4 to 8 mg/L (72). The volume of distribution for procainamide is about 2 L/kg (68) indicating the loading dose necessary to achieve a plasma level of 8 mg/L would be 960 mg:

$$\text{Loading Dose} = \frac{\text{Volume of Distribution} \times \text{Desired Plasma Level}}{\text{Bioavailability}}$$

$$= \frac{2 \text{ L/kg} \times 60 \text{ kg} \times 8 \text{ mg/L}}{1.0 \text{ (for the intravenous route)}}$$

$$= 960 \text{ mg}$$

In order to avoid acute toxicities, the loading dose should be injected at a rate not exceeding 25 to 50 mg/min (42), 100 mg may be given over 2 minutes and repeated every 5 minutes. The small 100 mg doses should be repeated until sustained therapeutic control is achieved, the total loading dose has been administered or toxicity is encountered.

Procainamide toxicities include gastrointestinal distress, weakness, mild to serious hypotension, a wide QRS interval (10 to 30%), ventricular conduction disturbances and arrhythmias (59). The ECG changes are similar to those seen with quinidine. At levels below 12 mg/L cardiovascular toxicities are rare; however, these are quite common at levels above 16 mg/L (72). In order to maintain the procainamide level in the middle of the "therapeutic range" (6 mg/L) a maintenance dose needs to be administered. The usual maintenance infusion for procainamide is between 1.48 and 2.96 mg/kg/hr (68). A rational way to select a maintenance dose would be to adjust her procainamide clearance for the decrease in renal function. The normal procainamide clearance is about 540 ml/min (72); 50% (270 ml/min) is cleared metabolically and 50% (270 ml/min) is cleared renally. If one assumes that a normal creatinine clearance is 100 ml/minute, this patient has only 15% of her renal function remaining. Her total clearance could then be estimated to be 310 ml/minute (18.6 L/hour) if her metabolic clearance is unchanged. The maintenance dose would then be about 111 mg/hour (1.86 mg/kg/hr):

$$\text{Maintenance Dose (mg/hr)} = \frac{\text{Clearance (L/hr)} \times \text{Desired Steady State Plasma Level (mg/L)}}{\text{Bioavailability}}$$

$$= \frac{17.4 \text{ L/hr} \times 6 \text{ mg/L}}{1.0}$$

$$= 111.6 \text{ mg/hr}$$

The reported oral bioavailability of procainamide is 75 to 95%; however, an estimated 10% of the patients may absorb less than half of an oral dose (68). If a bioavailability of 85% (0.85) is assumed, the hourly oral dose of 130 mg can be estimated from the above formula. The hourly dose could then be accumulated and administered at each dosing interval. If no more than a 50% change in the plasma level is desired

within the dosing interval, the drug should be administered every half-life or less. In this case, the procainamide half-life would be about 5 hours.

$$\text{Half-Life (Hours)} = \frac{.693 \times \text{Volume of Distribution (L)}}{\text{Clearance (L/hr)}}$$

$$= \frac{.693 \times 140 \text{ L}}{18.6 \text{ L/hr}}$$

$$= 5.22 \text{ hours}$$

If a dosing interval of 4 hours is selected, a dose of 520 mg (130 mg/hr × 4 hr) should maintain procainamide levels in the therapeutic range of 4 to 8 mg/L. To most clinicians, the suggested dose would seem rather large considering the degree of renal impairment. There are two major factors that may account for the fact that adequate therapeutic control is maintained when lower doses are administered. The first is that patients with congestive heart failure appear to have a reduced procainamide clearance, resulting in higher than predicted plasma levels (72). The second is accumulation of the active metabolite, N-acetyl procainamide (NAPA). The amount of each procainamide dose which is converted to NAPA is between 11 and 60% and is controlled by the patients acetylation phenotype (fast vs slow) and the degree of renal impairment. Patients with renal failure that are also fast acetylators convert the largest percent of procainamide to NAPA (39,62,63,125). The half-life of NAPA is about 5 hours in patients with normal renal function and would be expected to increase to about 30 hours (39,62) in renal failure. This would allow for less frequent administration of procainamide (39). (See *Clinical Pharmacokinetics* chapter for a more detailed discussion.) At present NAPA is believed to be about equal to procainamide in antiarrhythmic activity, and it may be less toxic (33). There are patients in the literature with NAPA levels greater than 40 mg/L and the authors have observed NAPA levels greater than 55 mg/L without the usual signs of procainamide toxicity (4). At present it appears that while NAPA and procainamide levels may be useful in evaluating drug efficacy, only procainamide levels may currently be used to evaluate toxicity.

16. A.X. is a 54-year-old female with a long history of systemic lupus erythematosus (SLE) and recurrent debilitating PAT. What is the risk of administering procainamide to this patient? Characterize procainamide-induced SLE.

Twenty-nine percent of patients who take therapeutic doses of procainamide on a chronic basis will develop a reversible lupus-like syndrome characterized by arthralgias, myalgias, fevers, pleuritis, and pericarditis (54). Although the risk of developing this syndrome is minimal if procainamide is taken on a short-term basis (75), symptoms may occur as early as two weeks and as late as 2 years after therapy is initiated (114). The syndrome is believed to be caused by the parent compound since slow acetylators have a higher risk of developing the syndrome. The incidence of positive laboratory tests (e.g., anti-nuclear antibody (ANA), LE cells) without other symptoms is substantially higher (67,91,75). It has been estimated that 83% of patients will develop positive serologic tests. Since many of these may never become symptomatic, these findings are not particulary useful monitoring parameters and should not be used as the sole criterion to determine whether or not procainamide should be discontinued. These tests usually revert to normal within a few months when the drug is discontinued. The drug-induced syndrome also differs significantly from the idiopathic form in that there is not a higher incidence in females and it is rarely complicated by leukopenia, anemia, thrombocytopenia, hypergammaglobulinemia or renal failure (11,91,114).

No adverse effects were observed after 15 months of administration of procainamide to a patient with SLE (126), and it could be argued that since the syndromes differ substantially in their presentations, procainamide is not likely to exacerbate the pre-existing idiopathic form.

However, there are two reasons for avoiding the use of procainamide in this patient. First, her arrhythmia is recurrent and it is likely that she will need to take procainamide chronically; this will increase the risk of developing the syndrome. Secondly, the drug-induced complication is monitored on the basis of symptoms. Since arthralgias, myalgia, fever and pleuritis are all common symptoms of the idiopathic form, it would be virtually impossible to differentiate between the two forms without highly sophisticated, expensive serologic testing. Since quinidine has the same basic effects on the myocardium, it is a reasonable alternative to procainamide.

17. Quinidine was to be administered to a patient with atrial fibrillation by slow intravenous infusion. However, the mechanical infusion device delivered the entire dose over two minutes. The patient is no longer in atrial fibrillation but has a sinus rhythm with a rate of 80 and first degree AV block. What is AV block?

Atrioventricular block is divided into three major categories. First degree AV block is a delay in impulse conduction through the AV node and is characterized by a P-R interval greater than 0.21 seconds. All atrial impulses will be conducted as long as the AV node has completed the repolarization process from the previous impulse. Second degree AV block is characterized by a block of some of the atrial impulses so that a ventricular response is not elicited following every atrial beat. In this case some of the P waves produced by

atrial depolarization would not be followed by a QRS complex on the ECG. Second degree AV block is characterized as being either Mobitz Type I or Mobitz Type II. Mobitz Type I AV block is usually due to increased vagal tone or drug therapy such as digitalis and usually requires no treatment other than elimination of the precipitating factor. Mobitz Type II AV block may at times be difficult to distinguish from Type I; however, it is a more serious condition in that syncopal attacks associated with ventricular fibrillation are common. Most patients with Type II AV block will eventually develop complete or third degree AV block if they survive episodes of syncope and ventricular fibrillation. In third degree AV block, none of the atrial depolarizations are transmitted to the ventricles. Consequently, the ventricles are paced by ectopic foci or ventricular pacemakers. Although patients with third degree heart block can sustain an adequate cardiac output, they are subject to the risk of ventricular arrhythmias and cardiovascular collapse. The drugs most commonly used to treat AV block are the catecholamines, such as isoproterenol or possibly epinephrine (121,122). An artificial electrical pacemaker may also be appropriate. It should be noted that in patients with a high degree of AV blockade the administration of Type I or Type III antiarrhythmic agents as well as potassium or other myocardial depressants are contraindicated since they may increase the AV block and suppress the ventricular pacemakers resulting in cardiac standstill (121). If the patient is being paced electrically, the above mentioned agents may be useful if frequent PVC's are present. In patients with a high degree of AV block *no* cardiac depressants should be used unless electrical pacing is available.

In the case presented it appears that the patient has only first degree AV block (a direct effect of quinidine) and has sufficient cardiac output. In this situation it would probably be best to temporarily discontinue the quinidine and observe the patient; as the quinidine plasma levels decline the AV block should diminish. Of course, in the future it would seem reasonable to guard against rapid intravenous infusions of quinidine. Although routine intravenous administration is currently not recommended, it does appear that an infusion period of 22 to 45 minutes or 16 mg/minute (58,90) will minimize acute toxicities associated with quinidine administration.

18. A 56-year-old male is admitted with a chief complaint of palpitations which are not relieved by "rubbing the side of his neck". The rate was variable and the ECG was described as paroxysmal atrial tachycardia (PAT). What is PAT? How would rubbing the patient's neck affect the arrhythmia? How would you treat this patient?

PAT is an atrial arrhythmia with a rate of 140-220 beats per minute. It has a rapid onset and abrupt cessation. Rubbing the patient's neck just below the angle of the jaw stimulates baroreceptors located in the carotid sinus and produces vagal stimulation to the heart. Generally, this maneuver is sufficient to terminate the majority of attacks.

There are numerous approaches to the treatment of PAT. The rate can be reduced using digitalis, edrophonium or propranolol, or the arrhythmia can be suppressed with quinidine or procainamide. In an uncomplicated case such as this, either intravenous edrophonium (10 mg) (92) or propranolol are indicated. In a patient with congestive heart failure and PAT, digitalis is the drug of choice; however, the onset of rate reduction is usually delayed.

19. A 65-year-old female admitted in congestive heart failure was initially treated with 80 mg of IV furosemide and 1.0 mg digoxin. Approximately four hours later, after she had diuresed 2.5 liters, she developed a rapid pulse. An ECG showed an irregular rhythm with a rate from 120-200 which was interpreted as PAT with block. "Stat" laboratory data reported a serum potassium of 2.9 mEq/L, a serum creatinine of 3.2 mg%, and a plasma digoxin level of 2.8 ng/cc. Assess the etiology of this arrhythmia. How should it be treated?

Digitalis-induced PAT with block is a dangerous arrhythmia which has a mortality rate of 28-58% (14,20,21,83). Until proven otherwise, PAT with block should be considered a symptom of digitalis toxicity in patients taking digitalis. The presence of a high digoxin level, hypokalemia and an elevated serum creatinine in this patient all make digitalis toxicity quite likely. The digoxin and furosemide should be discontinued immediately. Potassium, the drug of choice for PAT due to digoxin, typically slows the atrial rate, improves AV conduction and converts the arrhythmia to NSR (83). However, it must be administered carefully since high levels of potassium may actually enhance AV block.

Since 60% of digoxin is excreted renally, the maintenance dose should be adjusted accordingly (22,59). (Also see chapters on *Congestive Heart Failure* and *Clinical Pharmacokinetics.*) Previously it was not recommended that the loading dose be altered (22,59); however, there is now data which indicates that patients with renal insufficiency have a decreased Vd for digoxin (3,30,60,65).

$$Vd = \frac{226 + 298 (C_{Cr})}{29 + C_{Cr}}$$

where Vd is the volume of distribution in liters for a 70 kg person (1.73 m^2) and C_{Cr} is the creatinine clearance per 1.73 m^2 (87). Therefore, the loading dose will have to be decreased in patients with significant renal failure. It should be remembered that the above equation is only an approximation, and the volume of distribution for digoxin in renal failure, though usually decreased, is highly variable. To complicate the situation further, autopsy data indicate that there is less myocardial binding of digoxin in patients with decreased renal function. This implies that these patients may actually require the higher digoxin serum concentrations which would occur as a result of the smaller volume of distribution (61). However, for this conclusion to be valid, the displacement of digoxin from the myocardial tissue would have to be from pharmacologically active receptor sites as well as non-specific binding sites. The major argument against this hypothesis is the lack of evidence indicating that patients with renal failure require higher serum digoxin concentration. (See chapter on *Clinical Pharmacokinetics.*)

20. R.P., a 23-year-old junior pharmacy student, noticed that he had a rapid pulse and sought help at the medical center emergency room (ER). He was found to have AV nodal tachycardia which responded to carotid sinus stimulation. Subsequently, R.P. read about his rhythm and learned that digitalis and electric shock were also used to treat it. Some time later, R.P. was asked how to treat a 73-year-old female with AV nodal tachycardia unresponsive to carotid massage. The student suggested digoxin. Comment.

R.P.'s arrhythmia was typical for the benign form of *nodal tachycardia,* a paroxysmal rhythm emanating from or around the AV node at a varying rate of 160-250 beats per minute. Carotid sinus massage is the therapy for very rapid rates, and digitalis or shock are alternative forms of therapy (12,21).

Unfortunately, the student did not obtain a full history before recommending digitalis for the elderly patient. This patient may have had a more serious form of nodal tachycardia. Non-paroxysmal nodal tachycardia has a slower rate (70-130 beats per minute) and is frequently (60%) caused by digitalis (21). There is no effective treatment for digitalis-induced nodal tachycardia other than discontinuation of the drug (14). Obviously, the student's recommendation would only worsen the arrhythmia if it were due to digitalis.

21. A patient is admitted to the CCU with a chief complaint of chest pain and an ECG consistent with an acute myocardial infarction (AMI). Except for S-T segment changes and U waves consistent with an AMI, the ECG is normal. Should this patient be given prophylactic antiarrhythmic treatment with lidocaine?

Since 40-80% of patients will develop arrhythmias

following an AMI, there is sound theoretical basis for the prophylactic administration of antiarrhythmic agents (15). Premature ventricular contractions (PVC's) occur most commonly and comprise 40-80% of all arrhythmias which occur following an AMI (21,86). Isolated PVC's are probably benign but may be the predecessors of the frequently fatal ventricular flutter or fibrillation. In fact, there may be inadequate warning of these dangerous arrhythmias in 40% of cases (29,73). Despite the apparent need for prophylaxis, studies performed with procainamide, quinidine, and lidocaine do not demonstrate a significant difference in the mortality rate of the treated group (73,74,98). In attempting to identify patients at risk for fatal arrhythmias in the setting of an AMI, Koch-Weser suggested that the following criteria be used to determine whether or not PVC's should be treated: PVC's that interrupt the T wave; PVC's which differ morphologically on the ECG or are multifocal in origin; PVC's which occur in a series of two or more, or exceed a frequency of five per minute should receive prophylactic treatment with antiarrhythmic drugs (73).

22. A patient with a well-documented MI develops unifocal PVC's at a rate of 25 per minute. What drug regimen should be instituted?

Although lidocaine and procainamide have different electrophysiological effects, they are comparable in their antiarrhythmic efficacy (11,107). Lidocaine is the drug of choice for PVC's following an acute myocardial infarction (135), because procainamide produces more depression of myocardial contractility, AV conduction and peripheral resistance (2,11).

Lidocaine should be administered to produce levels of 1-6 mcg/ml (41,131). This is usually accomplished by one or more bolus injections. Although an infusion can be initiated without loading doses, peak levels may not be reached for approximately six hours in normal patients since the elimination half-time is 100 minutes (131). Bolus doses should be based upon the relatively small central compartment of this two compartment drug, since the myocardium appears as though it were in the central compartment. A 1.5 mg/kg intravenous injection over one to two minutes should produce a level of 3 mcg/ml assuming an average central compartment volume of 0.5 L/kg (104). Two additional bolus doses of 0.8 mg/kg given at ten minute intervals should produce a therapeutic level of 3 mcg/ml in the steady state distribution volume of 1.32 L/kg (assuming an eight minute alpha phase half time with negligible loss of lidocaine between doses) (10). This may be followed by a maintenance infusion calculated on the assumption that each 10 mcg/kg/ minute produces a level of 1 mcg/ml. This also assumes that the MI has not compromised the patient's

cardiac output (130).

Cardiac output after myocardial infarction is frequently decreased necessitating a dosage reduction of lidocaine (130,131). It appears that both the clearance and volume of distribution of lidocaine are decreased to about 60% of the usual values indicating that both the loading and maintenance doses should be reduced (130,131). It is interesting to note that because both the volume of distribution and clearance are reduced by the same magnitude, the elimination half-life will remain unchanged (130). Many intensive care units are capable of measuring cardiac output which may be applied to published nomograms for estimating dosing requirements of lidocaine (130). In the absence of these sophisticated techniques, modest doses of lidocaine should be used with careful monitoring of side effects. It should be remembered that if side effects do occur during a maintenance infusion, it may require several hours for them to dissipate as the elimination half-life (100 minutes) rather than the distribution half-life (10 minutes) will be the primary factor in determining the rate with which the plasma level will be decreasing (130). Collinsworth et al suggest that two boluses of 0.75 mg/kg each, 15 minutes apart, followed by an infusion of 30 mg/kg/ min be given to AMI patients who do not have severe congestive heart failure (23).

23. A 50-year-old 70 kg male patient is admitted to the hospital from a nursing home because of mental confusion. He has a long history of alcoholism and is subsequently diagnosed as having developed hepato-renal syndrome. On the tenth hospital day, he developed multifocal PVC's associated with an acute upper GI bleed. The physician asks you to set up a lidocaine infusion at 4 mg/minute. Comment.

In patients with hepatic disease, it appears that lidocaine has an increased volume of distribution and decreased hepatic clearance which results in a prolonged elimination half-life of approximately 300 minutes (130). This would mean that unless a loading or bolus dose were administered therapeutic concentrations may not be achieved for several hours. Since the volume of distribution is probably increased it might be expected that more than the usual loading or bolus dose would be required. In most cases the "usual" size bolus (50 to 100 mg) would probably be given with additional injections administered (usually one-half of the original) if the arrhythmia reappeared within 10 to 30 minutes of the previous bolus dose. The maintenance infusion of 4 mg/min (57 mcg/kg/min) would be expected to achieve a steady state lidocaine level of 5.7 mcg/ml (see previous case) in a patient with normal cardiac and liver function. In this patient one would expect an even higher level secondary to the decreased hepatic clearance resulting from the alcoholic liver disease. Since there is no reliable method to quantify the degree of liver dysfunction, this patient should be started on an infusion of 30 mcg/kg/min or less and carefully monitored over the next 20 to 24 hours (three to five elimination half-lives of 300 minutes) for signs and symptoms of toxicity (130). Central nervous sytem and hemodynamic reactions are the most serious. Dizziness, drowsiness, paresthesias, visual disturbances and euphoria may be seen at the higher end of the therapeutic range, while confusion, dysarthria, psychoses, coma, respiratory failure and seizures may occur at levels above 6 mcg/ml (16,108). In this patient, lidocaine plasma levels would be helpful as many of the symptoms mentioned would be difficult to identify in a patient with hepato-renal syndrome and pre-existing mental confusion. Since less than 10% of lidocaine is excreted unchanged in the urine, and renal failure does not appear to affect either the volume of distribution or metabolic clearance of lidocaine, no additional adjustments would have to be made for the renal failure (108). (See chapter on *Clinical Pharmacokinetics* for additional information on lidocaine.)

24. What electrophysiological properties of phenytoin distinguish it from other antiarrhythmic drugs such as quinidine and procainamide?

Quinidine and procainamide depress both automaticity and conduction of electrical impulses in the myocardium. Phenytoin also depresses automaticity, but enhances conduction. This is significant because the suppression of automaticity is important in the abolition of many arrhythmias, whereas depression of conduction is sometimes detrimental to efficient cardiac function (31).

25. Which arrhythmias are amenable to treatment with phenytoin? What is the relative efficiency of the drug in each? A 67-year-old man enters the hospital with a recent diagnosis of atrial fibrillation due to rheumatic valve disease. The intern would like to use phenytoin. Comment.

Phenytoin is generally more effective in ventricular arrhythmias than in atrial ones. It has been shown to be of greatest use in digitalis-induced premature contractions, tachycardia, and bigeminy. It has some use in arrhythmias which are unresponsive to procainamide. Phenytoin is generally ineffective in the treatment of atrial fibrillation and flutter; it is sometimes effective in atrial and nodal tachycardias, atrial premature contractions, and wandering atrial pacemakers with tachycardia. It is sometimes useful in atrial arrhythmias unresponsive to other antiarrhythmic drugs. In the above case, digoxin and quinidine would probably be the drugs of choice (24,31,32,53).

26. The usual accepted plasma levels of phenytoin for anticonvulsant activity are 10 to 20 mcg/ml. How do these values compare with those required for antiarrhythmic activity?

Therapeutic response is generally not seen below 10 mcg/ml; however, a few patients may be responsive to phenytoin levels as low as 2 mcg/ml. The study by Bigger (13) indicates that over 70% of arrhythmias respond to levels of 10-18 mcg/ml, while 20% respond to levels of 2-10 mcg/ml. Only 10% require levels greater than 18 mcg/ml. In short, both the anticonvulsant and antiarrhythmic effects are seen with blood levels between 10 and 20 mcg/ml. Moreover, Bigger suggests that because the side effects almost always occur at levels above 20 mcg/ml, the appearance of side effects without a therapeutic response is an indication for discontinuation of phenytoin.

27. An intern asks that phenytoin 250 mg/10 cc be prepared in the pharmacy for IV use. What problems does this pose? How should these problems be handled?

In an animal study it was shown that 40% propylene glycol and the solvent supplied with phenytoin injectable had identical cardiac effects, the majority of which were antagonized by phenytoin. Large doses of propylene glycol caused a significant decrease in blood pressure, apnea, bradycardia, increased QRS amplitude, and amplification of the T wave. Larger doses depressed the S-A node and caused nodal or multifocal ventricular rhythms. Still larger doses produced asystole. It was also shown that the administration of phenytoin diluted with propylene glycol or its supplied diluent caused the same type of ECG and blood pressure changes, but these were only transient (80). Therefore phenytoin should be given in an appropriate ratio to its diluent.

Dilution of phenytoin in the usual IV solutions is not recommended because of rapid crystal formation (37,132). However, Bauman et al demonstrated insignificant (0.8%) phenytoin crystallization after eight hours in normal saline and Ringer's Lactate (7) at concentrations of 1 mg/ml. Unfortunately, the concentration is probably too low to be of use in the administration of a loading dose, but it may be suitable for maintenance dosing.

28. A 70-year-old male who has been on digoxin 0.25 mg qd for several years as well as hydrochlorothiazide 50 mg bid for the past two weeks enters with ventricular premature contractions. The resident orders phenytoin 200 mg IV. Is this rational? Why?

Phenytoin is considered by some to be the drug of choice for the treatment of digitalis intoxication. Fifty percent of reported episodes of digitalis toxicity were reversed with excellent results following phenytoin administration. It has also been shown that pretreatment with phenytoin may be useful in increasing the therapeutic ratio of digitalis in certain digitalis-sensitive patients. In the above case, it is likely that the patient is suffering from digitalis toxicity, especially in light of the recent diuretic therapy without supplemental potassium.

Before attempting to use phenytoin it would be more logical to evaluate his acid-base and electrolyte balance and correct any imbalances (17). If the arrhythmia continues and is compromising cardiac output, phenytoin may then be indicated. An additional advantage of using phenytoin in patients with congestive heart failure is that it will not further depress cardiac output (24,53). The prescribed dose of 200 mg would probably produce plasma levels of only 4 mcg/ml (volume of distribution of 50 L) which would be unlikely to result in a sustained therapeutic response. (See *Clinical Pharmacokinetics* chapter for further discussion.)

29. Phenytoin when used as an antiarrhythmic agent, is most commonly initiated via the parenteral route. Is the IM or IV route preferred, and how should it be administered?

The IV route is recommended because results are much more predictable; the IM route is not advised because the absorption, although complete, may be slow and erratic (110). When phenytoin is given by the IV route it should be infused at a maximum rate of 1 cc per minute (50 mg/min). The cardiovascular toxicities seen with IV administration are apparently due to the vehicle, propylene glycol, as they can be reproduced by infusions of propylene glycol without phenytoin.

It should also be noted that there may be a recurrence of the arrhythmia 20 to 30 minutes after the initial administration of phenytoin, because blood levels fall as the drug is distributed into body tissues. The total loading dose of phenytoin is about 1 gm. Usually 250 mg boluses are given at a maximum rate of 50 mg/min every hour for four doses. However, Bigger (13) recommends that 100 mg of phenytoin be given IV every 5 minutes until an antiarrhythmic effect is seen. As these boluses are administered, careful attention should be paid to the appearance of toxicities. In addition to the cardiovascular problems (see Question 27), the classical progression from nystagmus to ataxia and dysarthria to mental confusion usually correlate with phenytoin levels of 20, 30 and 40 mcg/ml respectively (76). If the arrhythmia recurs, treatment is repeated to a maximum dose of 1 gm. Some authors feel that side effects are fewer when the 100 mg bolus technique is used since any single injection produces an increase in the plasma phenytoin level of 3 to 4 mcg/ml (13,18,46,76,134).

Subsequent maintenance doses of 300 to 400 mg/day administered either orally or parenterally usually maintain therapeutic phenytoin plasma concentrations. (See the *Clinical Pharmacokinetics* chapter for further discussion of phenytoin pharmacokinetics.)

30. Ms. J.P., a 59-year-old 70 kg white female, is being seen in the cardiac clinic for frequent premature ventricular contractions (PVC's) which have been observed to occur in couplets. Quinidine has been tried but was discontinued secondary to diarrhea; she is presently on procainamide but has recently developed arthralgias. Laboratory tests for antinuclear antibodies and L.E. cells were both positive. She has normal renal and hepatic function. Would disopyramide be a reasonable choice? What would be an appropriate dosage regimen and what side effects might be anticipated?

Like quinidine and procainamide, disopyramide is a Type I antiarrhythmic agent and therefore should be a reasonable alternative. Effects are to decrease automaticity (phase 4) and conduction velocity (0 phase), and increase refractory period (phase 1, 2, and 3) of the AV node and His-purkinje system (8). Disopyramide has marked anticholinergic properties, which accounts for the most frequently observed side effects of dry mouth, urinary hesitancy, constipation and blurred vision (28). Presently disopyramide is only approved for ventricular arrhythmias, but it appears to be effective in atrial arrhythmias as are the other Type I antiarrhythmics. The usual adult dose is 400 to 800 mg/day in four divided doses. It appears to be well absorbed orally (83 to 90%) with peak levels being achieved one-half to three hours following oral administration. The decay half-life is about 5 to 6 hours but might be expected to increase if renal failure were present as 40 to 70% of the drug is excreted unchanged in the urine (56). Since the therapeutic plasma levels appear to be between 2 and 4 mg/L, the dosing interval of 6 hours is probably appropriate as the patient has normal renal function.

REFERENCES

1. Anderson RJ, Gambertoglio JG and Shrier RW: *Clinical Use of Drugs in Renal Failure.* C. Thomas, Springfield, Ill. 1976.
2. Anon: Lidocaine as an anti-arrhythmic agent. Medical Letter 13:1, 1971.
3. Aronson JK et al: Altered distribution of digoxin in renal failure — a cause of digoxin toxicity? Brit J Clin Pharmacol 3:1045, 1976.
4. Atkinson AJ et al: Dose-ranging trial of N-acetyl procainamide in patients with premature ventricular contraction. Clin Pharmacol Ther 21:575, 1977.
5. Ban TA et al: The effect of phenothiazines on the electrocardiogram. Canad Med Assoc J 91:537, 1964.
6. Barry D et al: Phenothiazine poisoning: a review of 48 cases. Calif Med 118:1, 1973

7. Bauman JL et al: Phenytoin crystallization in intravenous fluids. Drug Intell Clin Pharm 11:646, 1977.

8. Befeler B et al: Electrophysiologic effects of the antiarrhythmic agent disopyramide phosphate. Amer Cardiol 35:282, 1975.

9. Bellet S et al: Relation between serum quinidine levels and renal function. Amer J Cardiol 27:368, 1971.

10. Benowitz N: Clinical applications of the pharmacokinetics of lidocaine. Cardiovasc Drug Ther 6:77, 1974.

11. Bigger JT et al: The use of procainamide and lidocaine in the treatment of cardiac arrhythmias. Prog Cardiovasc Dis 1:515, 1969.

12. Bigger JT et al: Management of cardiac problems in intensive care units. Med Clin Amer 55:1183, 1971.

13. Bigger JT et al: Relationship between the plasma level of diphenylhydantoin sodium and its cardiac anti-arrhythmic effects. Circulation 38:363, 1968.

14. Bigger JT et al: Digitalis toxicity: Drug interactions promoting toxicity and the management of toxicity. Semin Drug Treat 2:147, 1972.

15. Bloomfield SS et al: Quinidine for prophylaxis of arrhythmias in acute myocardial infarction. NEJM 285:979, 1971.

16. Boston Collaborative Drug Surveillance Program: Drug induced convulsions. Lancet 2:677, 1972.

17. Brater et al: Digoxin toxicity in patients with normokalemic potassium depletion. Clin Pharmacol Ther 22:21, 1977.

18. Cantu RC et al: Comparison of blood levels with oral and intramuscular diphenylhydantoin. Neurol 18:782, 1968.

19. Chamberlain DA et al: Plasma digoxin concentrations in patients with atrial fibrillation. Br Med J 3:429, 1970.

20. Chung EK: Digitalis induced cardiac arrhythmias. Am Heart J 79:845, 1970.

21. Chung EK: Principles of Cardiac Arrththmias, Williams and Wilkins Co., Baltimore 1971.

22. Clayton BD: Reduction of digitalis glycoside intoxication by rational dosing procedures. Amer J Hosp Pharm 31:855, 1974.

23. Collinsworth KA et al: The clinical pharmacology of lidocaine as an anti-arrhythmic drug. Circulation 50:1217, 1974.

24. Conn RD: Newer drugs in the treatment of cardiac arrhythmia. Med Clin N Amer 51:1223, 1967.

25. Cooper JA et al: Atropine in the treatment of cardiac disease. Am Heart J 78:124, 1969.

26. Cramer G: Early and late results of conversion to atrial fibrillation with quinidine. Acta Med Scand S490:5, 1968.

27. Croxson MS et al: Serum digoxin in patients with thyroid disease. Brit Med J 236:566, 1975.

28. Deano D et al: The antiarrhythmic efficacy of intravenous therapy with disopyramide phosphate. Chest 71:597, 1977.

29. Dhurandhar RJ et al: Primary ventricular fibrillation complicating acute myocardial infarction. Amer J Cardiol 27:347, 1971.

30. Doherty JE et al: Digoxin metabolism in hypo- and hyperthyroidism, studies with tritiated digoxin. Ann Intern Med 64:489, 1966.

31. Dreifus LS et al: Current status of diphenylhydantoin. Am Heart J 30:709, 1970.

32. Eddy JD et al: Treatment of cardiac arrhythmias with phenytoin. Brit Med J 170:273, 1969.

33. Elson J et al: Antiarrhythmic potency of N-acetylprocainamide. Clin Pharm Ther 17:134, 1975.

34. Epstein S et al: The early phase of myocardial infarction: Pharmacologic aspects of therapy. Ann Intern Med 78:818, 1973.

35. Evans GH et al: Disposition of propranolol, V. drug accumulation and steady state concentrations during chronic oral administration in man. Clin Pharmacol Ther 14:487, 1973.

36. Foley RE et al: Drug fever of quinidine. Lahey Clin Found. Bull 15:49, 1966.

37. Frank JT: Letter. Drug Intell Clin Pharm 7:419, 1973.

38. Gerstenblith T et al: Quinidine utilization in cardiac arrththmias. NY State J Med 66:701, 1966.

39. Gibson TP et al: Acetylation of procainamide in man and its relationship to isonicotinic acid hydrazide acetylation phenotype. Clin Pharmacol Ther 19:395, 1976.

40. Gianelly RE et al: The antiarrhythmic properties of lidocaine and propranolol. A review. Geriat 25:120, 1970.

41. Gianelli R et al: Effect of lidocaine on ventricular arrhythmias in patients with coronary heart disease. NEJM 277:1215, 1967.

42. Giardina E et al: Intermittent intravenous procainamide to treat ventricular arrhythmias. Ann Intern Med 78:183, 1973.

43. Goldberg WM: The relationship of dosage schedules to blood level of quinidine using all available quinidine preparations. Canad Med Assoc J 91:991, 1964.

44. Goldman MJ: The management of chronic atrial fibrillation: Indications for and methods of conversion to sinus rhythm. Prog Cardiovasc Dis 2:465, 1960.

45. Goldman S et al: Inefficacy of "therapeutic" serum levels of digoxin controlling the ventricular rate in atrial fibrillation. Am J Cardiol 35:651, 1975.

46. Goldschlager AW et al: Ventricular standstill after intravenous diphenylhydantoin. Am Heart J 74:410, 1967.

47. Goodman LS and Gilman A (eds): The Pharmacological Basis of Therapeutics, 5th ed. MacMillan Co. NY, 1975.

48. Greenblatt DJ et al: Adverse reactions to beta adrenergic receptor blocking drugs: A report from the Boston Collaborative Drug Surveillance Program. Drugs 7:118, 1974.

49. Greenblatt DJ et al: Pharmacokinetics of quinidine in humans after intravenous, intramuscular and oral administration. J Pharm Exp Ther 202:365, 1977.

50. Hall JI et al: Factors affecting cardioversion of atrial arrhythmias with special reference to quinidine. Brit Heart J 30:84, 1968.

51. Halmos PB: Direct current conversion of atrial fibrillation. Brit Heart J 28:302, 1966.

52. Heisenbuktel RH et al: The effect of oral quinidine on intraventricular conduction in man: Correlation of plasma quinidine with changes in QRS duration. Am Heart J 80:453, 1970.

53. Helfant RH et al: The clinical use of diphenylhydantoin (Dilantin) in the treatment and prevention of cardiac arrhythmias. Am Heart J 77:315, 1969.

54. Henningsen NC et al: Effects of long term treatment with procainamide, a prospective study with special regard to ANA and SLE in fast and slow acetylators. Acta Med Scand 198:475, 1975.

55. Hillestad L et al: Quinidine in maintenance of sinus rhythm after electroconversion of chronic atrial fibrillation, a controlled clinical study. Brit Heart J 33:518, 1971.

56. Hinderling PH et al: Pharmacokinetics of the antiarrhythmic disopyramide in healthy humans. J Pharmacokin Biopharm 4:199, 1976.

57. Hinskelwood RD: Hallucinations and propranolol. Amer J Cardiol 18:463, 1966.

58. Hirschfeld DS et al: Clinical and electrophysiologic effects of intravenous quinidine in man. Circulation 50:S230, 1974.

59. Jelliffe RW: A mathematical analysis of digitalis kinetics in patients with normal and reduced renal function. Math Bio 1:305, 1967.

60. Jusko WJ et al: Pharmacokinetic design of digoxin dosage regimens in relation to renal function. J Clin Pharmacol 14:525, 1974.

61. Jusko WJ et al: Myocardial distribution of digoxin and renal function. Clin Pharmacol Ther 16:449, 1974.

62. Karlsson E et al: Acetylation of procainamide in man. A preliminary communication. Eur J Clin Pharmacol 8:79, 1975.

63. Karlsson E et al: Polymorphic acetylation of procainamide in healthy subjects. Acta Med Scand 197:299, 1975.

64. Katz L and Pick A: Clinical Electrocardiography. Lea and Febiger Co., Philadelphia, 1956.

65. Kern JW: The volume of distribution and dosing of digoxin in patients with reduced renal function. (In press) Drug Intell Clin Pharm, 1978.

66. Kessler KM et al: Quinidine elimination in patients with congestive heart failure or poor renal function. NEJM 290:706, 1974.

67. Klajman A et al: Occurrence, immunoglobulin pattern and specificity of antinuclear bodies in sera of procainamide treated patients. Clin Exp Immunol 7:641, 1970.

68. Koch-Weser J: Pharmacokinetics of procainamide in man. Ann NY Acad Sci 179:370, 1971.

69. Koch-Weser J: Quinidine induced hypoprothrombinemic hemorrhage in patients on chronic warfarin therapy. Ann Intern Med 68:511, 1968.

70. Koch-Weser J: Serum drug concentrations as therapeutic guides. NEJM 287:227, 1972.

71. Koch-Weser J et al: Drug interactions with coumarin anticoagulants, Part 1. NEJM 285:487, 1971.

72. Koch-Weser J et al: Procainamide dosage schedules, plasma concentrations and clinical effects. JAMA 215:1454, 1971.

73. Koch-Weser J et al: Anti-arrhythmic prophylaxis in acute

myocardial infarction. NEJM 285:1024, 1971.

74. Koch-Weser J et al: Anti-arrhythmic prophylaxis with pro-cainamide in acute myocardial infarction. NEJM 281:1253, 1969.

75. Kosowsky BD et al: Long term use of procainamide following acute myocardial infarction. Circulation 47:1204, 1973.

76. Kutt H et al: Diphenylhydantoin metabolism, blood levels and toxicity. Arch Neurol 11:642, 1964.

77. Larson RK: Mechanism of quinidine purpura. Blood 8:16, 1953.

78. Lemberg L et al: The use of propranolol in arrhythmias com-plicating acute myocardial infarction. Am Heart J 80:479, 1970.

79. Levi GF et al: Combined treatment of atrial fibrillation with quinidine and beta blockers. Brit Heart J 34:911, 1972.

80. Louis S et al: The cardiocirculatory changes caused by in-travenous dilantin and its solvent. Am Heart J 74:523, 1967.

81. Lown B: Electrical reversion of cardiac arrhythmias. Brit Heart J 29:469, 1967.

82. Lown B et al: Approaches to sudden death from coronary heart disease. Circulation 44:130, 1971.

83. Lown G et al: Paroxysmal atrial tachycardias with block. Circula-tion 21:129, 1960.

84. Marako PR et al: Factors influencing infarct size in experimental coronary artery occlusions. Circulation 43:67, 1971.

85. Mason DT et al: The clinical pharmacology and therapeutic ap-plications of the anti-arrhythmic drugs. Clin Pharmacol Ther 11:460, 1970.

86. Meltzer LE et al: The incidence of arrhythmias associated with acute myocardial infarction. Prog Cardiovasc Dis 9:50, 1966.

87. Meyers FH et al: A Review of Medical Pharmacology, 3rd ed. Lange Med. Pub. Los Altos, 1972, p. 139.

88. Miller DS et al: Quinidine induced recurrent ventricular fibrilla-tion (quinidine syncope). South Med J 64:597, 1971.

89. Moc GK et al: Digitalis and allied cardiac glycosides in Phar-macological Basis of Therapeutics, ed. LS Goodman and H Gil-man, 5th ed. Ch. 31, Macmillan Pub. Co., New York, 1975, p. 677.

90. Moc GK et al: Antiarrhythmic drugs in Pharmacological Basis of Therapeutics, ed. LS Goodman and H Gilman, 5th Ed., Ch. 32, Macmillan Pub. Co., New York, 1975, p. 692.

91. Molina J et al: Procainamide induced serologic changes in asymptomatic patients, arthritis and rheumatism. Arthr Rheum 12:608, 1969.

92. Moss AJ et al: Use of edrophonium in evaluation of supraven-tricular tachycardias. Am J Cardiol 17:58, 1966.

93. Moss AJ and Patton RD: Anti-arrhythmic Agents. Charles C. Thomas, Springfield, Ill. 1973.

94. McIntosh HD et al: The hemodynamic consequences of ar-rhythmias. Prog Cardiovasc Dis 8:330, 1966.

95. Nevins MA et al: The treatment of acute myocardial infarction. Med Clin N Am 38:435, 1974.

96. Oram S et al: Further experience of electrial conversion of atrial fibrillation to sinus rhythm: Analysis of one-hundred patients. Lancet 1:1294, 1964.

97. Patterson JW et al: The pharmacodynamics and metabolism of propranolol in man. Pharmacol Clinica. 2:127, 1970.

98. Pitt A et al: Lidocaine prophylaxis to patients with acute myocardial infarction. Lancet 1:612, 1971.

99. Prichard BN et al: Treatment of hypertension with propranolol. Brit Med J 1:7, 1969.

100. Radford MD et al: Long term results of D.C. reversion of atrial fibrillation. Brit Heart J 30:91, 1968.

101. Redfors A: Plasma digoxin concentration — its relation to digo-xin dosage and clinical effects in patients with atrial fibrillation. Brit Heart J 34:383, 1972.

102. Resnekov L: Electroversion of cardiac dysrhythmias. Am Heart J 79:581, 1970.

103. Reuning RH et al: Role of pharmacokinetics in drug dosage adjustment. I. Pharmacologic effect, kinetics and apparent vol-ume of distribution of digoxin. J Clin Pharmacol 13:127, 1973.

104. Rowland M et al: Disposition kinetics of lidocaine in normal subjects. Ann NY Acad Sci 179:383, 1971.

105. Russell M et al: Fatal results from diphenylhydantoin adminis-tered intravenously. JAMA 206:2118, 1968.

106. Rusy BF: Pharmacology of anti-arrhythmic drugs. Med Clin Amer 58:987, 1974.

107. Schwartz ML et al: Comparative anti-arrhythmic effects of in-travenously administered lidocaine and procainamide and orally administered quinidine. Amer J Cardiol 26:520, 1970.

108. Selden R et al: Central nervous system toxicity induced by lidocaine. JAMA 202:908, 1967.

109. Selzer A et al: Quinidine syncope: Paroxysmal ventricular fibril-lation occurring during treatment of chronic atrial arrhythmias. Ciculation 30:617, 1964.

110. Serrano EE et al: Plasma diphenylhydantoin values after oral and intramuscular administration of diphenylhydantoin. Neurol 23:311, 1973.

111. Shand DG: Pharmacokinetic properties of beta-adrenergic blocking drugs. Drugs 7:39, 1974.

112. Shand DG et al: The disposition of propranolol, I. Elimination during oral absorption in man. Pharmacol 7:159, 1972.

113. Shapiro W et al: Relationship of plasma digitoxin and digoxin to cardiac response following intravenous digitalization in man. Circulation 42:1065, 1970.

114. Sheldon JHS et al: Procainamide-induced systemic lupus erythematosus. Ann Rheum Dis 29:236, 1970.

115. Singh BN et al: Beta adrenergic receptor blocking drugs in car-diac arrhythmias. Drugs 7:426, 1974.

116. Sjelky P et al: Maintenance of sinus rhythm after atrial defibrilla-tion. Brit Heart J 32:741, 1970.

117. Skelky PS et al: Direct current shock therapy of cardiac ar-rhythmias. Brit Heart J 28:36, 1966.

118. Smith TW: Digitalis toxicity: epidemiology and clinical use of serum concentration measurements. Am J Med 58:470, 1975.

119. Smith TW: Drug therapy: digitalis glycosides. NEJM 288:719, 1973.

120. Smith TW et al: Digitalis. NEJM 289:945, 1010, 1063, 1125, 1973.

121. Sobel B et al: Cardiac dysrhymias in Harrison's Principles of Internal Medicine, ed. Thorn GW et al, eighth ed. Chapter 238 McGraw-Hill Book Company, New York, 1977, p. 1187.

122. Sokolow M et al: Conduction defect, in Clinical Cardiology, Lange Medical Publications. Los Altos, California, Ch. 14, p. 421.

123. Sokolow M et al: The clinical pharmacology and use of quinidine in heart disease. Prog Cardiovasc Dis 3:316, 1961.

124. Stephen SA: Unwanted effects of propranolol. Amer J Cardiol 18:463, 1966.

125. Strong JM: Pharmacokinetics in man of the N Acelylated metabolite of procainamide. Pharmacokin Biopharm 3:223, 1975.

126. Sugimoto T et al: Electrophysiologic effects of lidocaine in awake dogs. J Pharmacol Exper Ther 166:146, 1969.

127. Theilen EO et al: Beta-adrenergic receptor blocking drugs in the treatment of cardiac arrhythmias. Med Clin N Amer 52:1017, 1968.

128. Thomas M et al: Effect of atropine on bradycardia and hypoten-sion in acute myocardial infarction. Brit Heart J 28:409, 1966.

129. Thompson GW: Quinidine as a cause of sudden death. Circula-tion 14:757, 1956.

130. Thomson PD et al: Lidocaine pharmacokinetics in advanced heart failure, liver disease, and renal failure in humans. Ann Intern Med 78:499, 1973.

131. Thomson PD et al: The influence of heart failure, liver disease and renal failure on the disposition of lidocaine in man. Am Heart J 82:417, 1971.

132. Trissel LA: Handbook on injectable drugs. American Society of Hospital Pharmacists, Washington, D.C. 1977.

133. Ueda CT et al: Disposition kinetics of quinidine. Clin Phar-macacol Ther 19:30, 1976.

134. Unger AH et al: Fatalities following IV use of sodium diphenylhy-dantoin for cardiac arrhythmias. JAMA 200:159, 1967.

135. Warner H: Therapy of common arrhythmias. Med Clin N Amer 58:995, 1974.

Chapter 15

Angina

Moses S. Chow

A 57-year-old, 6 foot, 250 lb, hard-driving, hypertensive, male executive was hospitalized for evaluation. He was first seen in his private physician's office two days prior to admission, complaining of a dull, heavy, squeezing substernal chest pain that occasionally radiated to the left shoulder and arm and lasted only a few minutes. The chest pain was usually related to exertion and was frequently relieved by rest. There was no past history of cardiac problems. A family history revealed that his father died of a heart attack at the age of 60 and that his brother has had hypertension for 10 years. The patient has smoked one pack of cigarettes a day for 20 years. His electrocardiogram upon admission was essentially normal. His serum cholesterol and triglycerides were elevated. Other clinical laboratory tests were not unusual. During his graded exercise test (treadmill test) S-T segment depression of 1.0 mm, which lasted 0.1 seconds was demonstrated after 4 minutes at a speed of 3 miles per hour. His angina which occurred at that time responded well to nitroglycerin. During his angina attack, his heart rate was 150, his blood pressure was 160/100 and a fourth heart sound was slightly audible. (These findings are compatible with most anginal patients undergoing a stress exercise test.) This patient's diagnosis is stable angina pectoris, most likely secondary to coronary artery disease.

a. Define angina pectoris and identify the symptoms in this patient which are commonly associated with this syndrome.

Angina pectoris is generally considered to be a clinical syndrome caused by insufficient oxygenation of the heart and is characterized by **chest pain.** This patient's dull, heavy, squeezing substernal chest pain that radiated to his left shoulder and arm is typical, although the anginal pain may radiate to the back, neck or lower jaw. The patient with angina feels as though a weight is on his chest and often has difficulty in applying the word pain to this discomfort. Words such as gripping, heaviness, pressing, boring, choking, or squeezing are commonly used. This sensation results from an imbalance of myocardial oxygen supply and demand usually due to coronary artery obstruction by an atherosclerotic process. In a minority of cases, angina pectoris is associated with various disease states such as valvular heart disease, pulmonary hypertension, myocardial hypertrophy, coronary artery spasm, and diseases of the coronary micro-circulation (41,94).

Based on clinical features, several types of angina can be defined (41,102). **Stable angina** is the classical angina; it is precipitated by physical activity and is relieved by rest or nitroglycerin. **Unstable angina,** also referred to as crescendo angina, accelerated angina, acute coronary insufficiency, intermediate coronary syndrome, pre-infarction angina, and status anginosis, describes the condition in which angina becomes more severe in duration, intensity, or frequency, and is less responsive than usual to treatment (41). **Nocturnal angina** or angina decubitus refers to discomfort which occurs during recumbency. This is sometimes seen when congestive heart failure complicates coronary artery disease. Prinzmetal angina or **variant angina** refers to angina at rest and is associated with S-T segment elevation on the ECG. This type of angina is most likely related to spasm of a coronary artery (60).

b. Identify those factors which may have contributed to the progression of angina in this patient.

Studies of the natural history of angina indicate that progression of the disease is accelerated by advancing age, high serum cholesterol, high blood pressure, electrocardiographic abnormalities, cigarette smoking, and diabetes mellitus (16, 67, 84). In addition, anxiety, severe psychosocial problems, or Type A behavior pattern (hard-driving, competitive, ambitious) are also considered major risk factors (84,107). With the knowledge of these risk factors, it is possible to predict the probability that any given person will develop coronary artery disease (15,71). Successful modification of these risk factors over a long period may help to prevent the development of coronary heart disease and reduce mortality (18,109).

c. Discuss the prognosis of anginal patients and therapeutic interventions.

The prognosis of patients with angina pectoris is generally discouraging. In men (aged 50-69) with stable angina, the mortality rate is about 4 per cent per year, and within a period of 5 years, 25 per cent can expect to have a myocardial infarction. This is twice the average mortality rate in the general population (1.7 per cent per year in the 55-64 age group) (114). Women have a much lower incidence of angina; however, older women (aged 60 or over) with stable angina have a prognosis similar to men with the disease (68,132). Patients with unstable angina or variant angina have a higher rate of mortality (18,109,114).

The poor prognosis of patients with angina pectoris indicates that treatment of the underlying cause is most desirable. However, there are only a few situations where the underlying cause (e.g. pulmonary hypertension or valvular heart disease) can be treated. Therefore, most patients with angina are managed symptomatically.

Coronary artery surgery (aorto-coronary bypass, or sometimes internal mammary artery implant) is regarded as an important approach in the management of angina. The purpose of the surgery is to increase coronary circulation. Such surgery can decrease or relieve pain in 80-90 per cent of patients with angina (86). In low risk patients with good ventricular function, the surgical mortality is low, less than 1 per cent (109). Higher operative mortality occurs in patients with unstable angina (109). In patients with significant occlusive disease of the left main coronary artery, there is some evidence that the bypass surgery may prolong as well as improve the quality of life (83,98). In the great majority of patients with occlusive disease of other coronary arteries, significant differences in mortality have not been shown.

Medical management remains the therapy of first choice in most patients with angina pectoris. Even patients who have had coronary artery surgery require medical management (9). The patient with angina should avoid precipitating factors such as heavy meals, emotional upsets and exposure to extremes in temperature (46). Beverages containing caffeine, such as coffee, tea, or colas, may precipitate angina in some patients (9,46). Strenuous exercise should be avoided, but regular mild to moderate exercise should be encouraged. Control of risk factors and associated disease are also important in the medical management of angina. Smoking should be stopped, as it can increase heart rate and blood pressure and impair myocardial oxygen delivery (9,46). Hypertension, obesity, hyperlipidemia, anemia, hyperthyroidism, and arrhythmias should all be appropriately controlled.

The rest of the chapter will emphasize the drug treatment of angina pectoris. Practical situations illustrating the rational use of nitrates and beta-adrenergic blocking agents will be discussed.

1. What are the major determinants of myocardial oxygen consumption? How are they affected by nitroglycerin?

The most important determinant of myocardial oxygen consumption is the myocardial wall tension (product of ventricular systolic pressure times the radius of the ventricle divided by its wall thickness) (17,124). In simplistic terms, the left ventricular tension can be regarded as the product of systolic blood pressure and heart size (147). The other two major determinants of oxygen consumption are heart rate and contractility (17).

The primary action of nitroglycerin is to relax vascular smooth muscle (23,44,46,47,101,110). This reduces peripheral resistance and decreases venous return. Both of these effects favor decreased myocardial oxygen consumption by decreasing ventricular wall tension. Although the heart rate and contractile state are increased (52), most likely due to a reflex mechanism, the net effect of nitroglycerin is a decrease of myocardial oxygen consumption.

2. How does nitroglycerin affect the coronary circulation?

In normal man, sublingual nitroglycerin causes significant generalized coronary artery vasodilation. In patients with coronary artery disease, dilatation from the drug is insignificant in diseased segments. Nitroglycerin, however, may redistribute myocardial flow to the relatively ischemic subendocardial or endocardial region either by a direct vasodilation of the large intramural vessels or by decreasing the resistance in these regions as a result of reduction of heart size and wall tension (14,33,52,91,135,140).

3. Is there any relationship between the blood level of nitroglycerin or its metabolites and the observed cardiovascular effects?

There are no clinical data that correlate nitroglycerin's blood level to its cardiovascular effect. Nitroglycerin persists in the serum for only a short time after a dose, and the assays are not sufficiently sensitive to detect low levels. The vascular effects of the metabolites are insignificant. One metabolite, glycerol dinitrate, is only 2 to 5 per cent as potent as nitroglycerin in lowering blood pressure, and the other metabolite, glyceryl mononitrate, is inactive. (95).

4. How effective is nitroglycerin in the treatment of angina pectoris?

Nitroglycerin is generally recognized as a very effective agent in the treatment of angina pectoris. It relieves pain, increases work performance, and improves electrocardiographic patterns following standardized exercise stress testing in 90 per cent of patients with angina (111).

In a standardized interview, 76 per cent of patients

with coronary artery disease reported relief of chest pain from nitroglycerin in less than 3 minutes and 16 per cent reported relief after 3 or more minutes. Only 8 per cent failed to obtain relief (62).

A number of other studies indicate that nitroglycerin, when compared to placebo, significantly increases exercise tolerance or decreases the incidence of chest pain (4).

5. A new angina patient has a prescription which reads as follows: Nitroglycerin 1/100 grain, No. 100, Sig: one prn chest pain. Comment on the dose and the direction.

In individuals first starting nitroglycerin treatment , a low strength tablet, preferably 1/200 grain, is often sufficient to relieve anginal attacks. This dose is less likely to cause unpleasant side effects than larger doses. The patient should be instructed to dissolve the tablet under the tongue and to take not more than three tablets over a 15 minute period (8). As soon as the chest pain is relieved, the remaining tablet may be expelled from the mouth. Although nitroglycerin (NTG) effectively relieves anginal pain, it may also be used prophylactically 2 to 3 minutes prior to activities which trigger anginal attacks.

6. GT has been treated with nitroglycerin 1/150 grain for a year. One morning he experiences severe constant chest pain. He cannot contact his physician and has already taken 5 tablets of nitroglycerin in the past 40 minutes with no relief of the pain. How is angina distinguished from myocardial infarction?

Angina attacks are usually of short duration and respond well to rest or nitroglycerin. This patient's prolonged chest pain which is not relieved by nitroglycerin is perhaps an indication of an acute myocardial infarction or severe coronary insufficiency. The patient should be taken to an emergency room immediately. Patients who experience any change in the character of their pain should also see their physicians.

7. A 62-year-old angina patient was admitted to the CCU because of excruciating, persistent chest pain unrelieved by nitroglycerin. He was treated with morphine sulfate four hours after admission, and the pain gradually disappeared by the next morning. Leads II, III, and AVF on his admitting ECG showed elevated ST segments, and Q wave depths greater than 1/3 of the QRS height in lead III. CPK was 856 U/L, his SGOT was 90 U/L, and his LDH was 220 U/L. On the second day he experienced two brief episodes of chest pain lasting 8 minutes each. Discuss the use of nitrates in this patient.

It is apparent from this patient's history, ECG, and enzyme levels, that he had an acute inferior wall myocardial infarction on the day of admission. The

brief episodes of chest pain on the second hospital day represent recurring angina pectoris. Nitrates would be the drugs of choice in this situation.

The use of nitrates during acute MI was considered a contraindication a few years ago. At the present, this is no longer the case, and its use is even considered desirable because of possible beneficial effect on the myocardium. Hemodynamic improvement as well as reduction of S-T elevation have been well documented following nitrate administration in patients with acute MI (3,39,122). These patients, however, should receive careful hemodynamic monitoring, as severe hypotension and bradycardia can occur (26).

8. What is the stability of nitroglycerin? How does it lose its potency? Is there significant nitroglycerin loss when the bottle is opened during use?

The inactivation of nitroglycerin is increased by time, light, heat, air, and moisture (21). The drug should be stored in an amber glass container with a tight fitting screw cap.

At 201 days, nitroglycerin stored in amber and clear glass vials loses 5 per cent of its potency; in polystyrene vials, 14 to 29 per cent is lost; and in pill boxes, 72 per cent is lost. Strip-packaging has resulted in a 47 to 90 per cent loss of potency after 52 days (37). Storing nitroglycerin with large amounts of cotton filler or other tablets or capsules is undesirable. When nitroglycerin is stored in a glass vial with a large amount of cotton filler, only 33 per cent of its activity is retained after one week (119). Two aspirin tablets can absorb 400 micrograms of nitroglycerin when stored with this drug for a month (120). Recent stability studies of major brands of NTG (Lilly and Parke-Davis) indicate that with proper storage, i.e., in a light resistant container with tightly fitted screw cap, the drug is stable for at least 5 months, even if the tablets are repackaged or the original vial is opened 100 times for brief periods (35,57).

Nitroglycerin is a volatile liquid prepared in a tablet form. It has a significant vapor pressure at room temperature, and the vapor can escape if the container is not tightly sealed (120). Nitroglycerin can also escape from the surface of one tablet and absorb onto another. This inter-tablet migration of active ingredients may result in a potency 25 per cent above or below USP standards (120).

At 70° F, 400 mcg nitroglycerin would supply enough vapor for a 3 dram prescription vial over 10,000 times (120). Even if all the vapor escaped when the bottle was opened, the loss would not be significant. However, if the bottle is not closed tightly, the vapor can escape continuously and result in continued loss of potency.

9. What instructions should the patient receive regarding the proper storage and handling of nitroglycerin? How can a patient tell if the nitroglycerin tablet

is fresh?

Patients should be warned to keep the sublingual nitroglycerin tablets in the original container to prevent loss of potency. After each use, the cap should be tightly closed immediately. The cotton filler should be discarded after initial opening of the bottle. The drug should not be stored in the inside pocket of clothes, in the glove compartment of the car, near a fireplace or in other hot, humid locations. Some authors recommend storing the bottle in the refrigerator (21,82); however, the potency will most likely still be retained if it is stored at room temperature (21° C).

A fresh, potent NTG tablet should produce a burning sensation under the tongue when administered sublingually (27). Headache, if it occurs, is another indication of potency. If an individual dosage has been titrated, the presence or absence of the cardiovascular effects should provide information regarding potency as well as efficacy.

10. What are the most frequently encountered undesirable effects of nitroglycerin? How can they be minimized?

Headache is the most common side effect. One study demonstrated a 49 per cent incidence of headaches in angina patients with coronary artery disease and 81 per cent in patients without coronary disease (62). The headaches were usually of short duration (5 minutes) and seldom lasted for more than 20 minutes in those with coronary artery disease. Dizziness and syncopal episodes are the next most frequently experienced undesirable effects and occur in less than 10 per cent of patients (62). The incidence of adverse reactions differed in the Boston Collaborative Study (90) which reported a 2.7 per cent incidence of headache, and 0.7 per cent GI disturbance, and 0.5 per cent hypotension. The differences in the incidence of adverse reactions probably reflect the differences in the methodology of each study. While the Boston study utilized a general surveillance method to study the adverse reactions of NTG, an intense interview method was used in the other study. Since nitroglycerin is usually administered on a prn basis and the effects are often transient, a careful interview on each patient is needed to obtain all the information. Thus, the incidence reported in the Boston study is probably inaccurate. On the other hand, the other study's 49 per cent incidence of headaches in angina patients receiving nitroglycerin seems extraordinarily high. Clinically, the headaches generally are not a major problem.

If headache is a severe problem, reducing the dose (if possible) or the addition of salicylates may be helpful (59). Dizziness and syncopal episodes may occur more frequently in elderly patients and in those patients taking peripheral vasodilators (eg papaverine, isoxsuprine, etc.) or large amounts of alcohol. Such patients

should be instructed to sit down when taking nitroglycerin.

11. What is the onset and duration of action of sublingual isosorbide dinitrate (ISDN) as compared to nitroglycerin (NTG)?

If pain relief is evaluated subjectively, the onset of action of ISDN varies from 45 seconds to 5 minutes, whereas that of NTG varies from a few seconds to two minutes (20). Other studies also confirm that 5 mg of ISDN has an onset of action within 5 minutes and a duration of action one or two minutes longer than 0.4 mg nitroglycerin (111).

Comparative studies with fixed doses indicate that ISDN has a longer duration of action than nitroglycerin (20,72,111,128). The duration of action, as evidenced by increased exercise tolerance and ECG recordings, was less than 30 minutes for 0.4 mg sublingual nitroglycerin and 2 hours for 5 mg sublingual ISDN. However, data from fixed dose studies are less valid than data obtained from doses based on similar pharmacological effects. When duration of action was based upon hemodynamic changes, such as arterial pressure, ISDN activity lasted from 1 hour to 4 hours depending on dose. The hemodynamic changes induced by NTG (0.4 mg) did not last as long (128,139). It should be noted that the persistence of the hemodynamic changes induced by ISDN may not correspond to its beneficial action on exercise tolerance (47). When doses of ISDN and nitroglycerin that produced similar physiologic changes at rest were compared, the duration of the beneficial effects on exercise capacity for both was similar. Both drugs had a pharmacological half-time of 19 to 20 minutes (48).

12. CM is a 65 year old, 78 kg man who was hospitalized because of accelerating angina. He has a two year history of angina and during the last 3 months he has been taking isosorbide dinitrate 10 mg po qid, NTG 1/150 grain prn SL, propranolol 80 mg tid, and erythrityl tetranitrate 10 mg chewed tid. After admission, the intern maintained him on the same medications and added NTG ointment 2 inches q 4 hours. Are long acting nitrates effective in the treatment of angina pectoris?

The efficacy of the "long-acting" nitrates has been studied and reviewed by many investigators. The results of some studies indicate that oral nitrate preparations are ineffective or are less effective than the sublingual preparations in increasing exercise capacity, reducing the number of nitroglycerin tablets consumed, or reducing the number of anginal episodes (5,111,134). Others, however, demonstrate a long duration of beneficial effects based on clinical assessment or exercise testing (19, 24, 64, 105, 126, 137, 141), especially with high doses (118). Long lasting hemodynamic changes also have been observed following oral nitrates in patients with angina (45, 69, 104, 139, 141, 142).

Due to conflicting results from these studies, the efficacy of oral nitrates is still being debated. Although pharmacokinetic and bioavailability studies can help to resolve the controversy, such data, unfortunately, are far from complete. When 20 mg C[14] labeled pentaerythritol tetranitrate was administered to human subjects, the parent compound was found consistently in feces but not in the blood (32). Animal studies indicate that when nitrates are injected into the portal vein or given orally, little or none of the parent compound reaches the circulation (95). These studies tend to support the lack of efficacy of oral nitrates. On the other hand, in a bioavailability study of oral versus sublingual isosorbide dinitrate, the oral preparation was absorbed, but the peak level and area under the plasma concentration time curve of a 20 mg oral dose were half that of a 10 mg sublingual dose (22). Evidence of persistent hemodynamic changes after oral nitrates indicates the availability of either the parent drug or active metabolites. Unfortunately, the metabolites of oral nitrates are not well studied, though active as well as inactive products have been claimed (65,73,96).

In view of the present status of oral nitrates, these drugs should not be used indiscriminately. Only patients with unpredictable daily angina episodes who cannot be treated with propranolol deserve a trial of oral nitrates for sustained angina prophylaxis. (More definite findings regarding the efficacy of oral nitrates are forthcoming. A controlled trial using increasing doses of oral isosorbide dinitrate is being conducted at the present time.)

13. What are the acute as well as chronic undesirable effects of long-acting nitrates?

Quantitative information on the acute side effects of oral nitrate preparations is limited, but approximately 7 per cent of patients receiving nitroglycerin sustained release tablets or ISDN experience headaches according to the Boston Collaborative Program (87). However, this figure is based on data from a multicenter epidemiologic study; the possibility of undisclosed concomitant NTG use by some of these patients cannot be excluded.

Cross-tolerance to nitroglycerin following chronic administration of long-acting nitrates has been reported in both animals (15) and man (115,146). Schelling and Lasagna (115) reported that the changes in blood pressure and heart rate after sublingual nitroglycerin were significantly less following 4 weeks of oral pentaerythritol tetranitrate (PETN) as compared to the control period. The venodilating effect of nitroglycerin was also shown to be decreased after 120 mg oral ISDN per day for 6 weeks (146). Tolerance to nitrate-induced increase in exercise performance, however,

did not result from the prolonged use of sublingual ISDN or from nitroglycerin ointment (10,47).

The other possible undesirable effect of chronic nitrate therapy is physiologic drug dependence. Chronic (12 to 48 months) nitroglycerin exposure by industrial workers handling 37 per cent nitroglycerin-cellulose mixture resulted in a 5 per cent incidence of non-atheromatous ischemic heart disease after withdrawal from such exposure (75). The chronic nitroglycerin exposure supposedly resulted in a compensatory increase in vasomotor tone which led to excessive coronary vasoconstriction when the vasodilator effect of nitrates was suddenly removed (75).

14. Are ISDN *chewable* tablets effective for the treatment of angina?

ISDN chewable tablets have been reported to be as effective as nitroglycerin in patients not taking oral ISDN and more effective than nitroglycerin in those taking oral ISDN prophylactically (79). In the same study, sublingual nitroglycerin was found to be less effective than the placebo chewable preparation, though a statistical difference was not demonstrated. Thus, the validity of the result from this study is highly questionable. Others have reported that the onset of action of the chewable tablet is within 3 minutes and that 65 per cent of the patients studied are protected from pain for 30 minutes (117). In a comparative study of NTG and chewable ISDN in assessing anginal relief during treadmill exercise, the onset of action of 0.3-0.6 mg sublingual NTG was 75 seconds, whereas the onset of action of 0.5 mg chewable ISDN was 108 seconds (70). The maximum effect of NTG was observed at 193 seconds and at 315 seconds for ISDN. This study clearly demonstrates that sublingual NTG has a faster onset of action. As a whole, the clinical efficacy of chewable ISDN is not as well documented as sublingual NTG. Equivocal exercise benefit and long duration of hemodynamic effects have been reported with chewable ISDN (42,63).

15. Is nitroglycerin ointment useful as a long-acting nitrate preparation? How is it used? Can it be applied anywhere on the skin? What precautions should be taken in applying this preparation?

Although topical administration of nitroglycerin has been used for more than two decades for the treatment of angina, the efficacy of the ointment has been systematically investigated only recently. In a comparison of nitroglycerin ointment vs placebo in 14 angina patients, the ointment significantly increased the exercise capacity for as long as three hours (106). Concurrent reduction of electrocardiographic evidence of ischemia, decrease in systolic blood pressure, and increase in heart rate were also observed. In a recent double-blind crossover study, the ointment was also found to be more effective than placebo, with a duration of at least three hours (31).

The ointment contains 2 per cent nitroglycerin in a lanolin-petrolatum base. The onset of anginal relief is around 30 minutes, and the drug is absorbed continuously through the skin. The usual dose is 1 to 2 inches squeezed from the tube onto a Dose Measuring Applicator and then spread in a thin layer over any skin area without massaging or rubbing it in. Thirty minutes after the dose, the patient's blood pressure and heart rate should be measured. The effective dose is the one which will produce a 10 mm Hg fall in blood pressure and 10 beats per minute increase in heart rate when the patient is in a sitting position. If these effects are not achieved after the first dose, the amount can be increased ½ inch at a time until the desired effect or headache occurs. The largest dose which does not produce headache is the optimal dose. The ointment may be applied every 3 or 4 hours if needed. It is important to spread the drug over an area approximately equivalent to 6 inches by 6 inches; an application over the chest may provide additional psychological benefit. A plastic wrap covering the ointment assures increased utilization of the medication and decreases the absorption by clothing. Before the second application, the "old" ointment left on the skin should be removed. Nurses who apply the ointment should avoid contact with their own skin by using gloves or by careful use of an applicator. Chronic administration has not been observed to cause tolerance. However, gradual reduction of dose as well as frequency of use over a 4 to 6 week period is desirable when the drug is to be discontinued.

16. How does propranolol affect myocardial oxygen consumption?

Propranolol decreases heart rate, contractility, and left ventricular tension development (38,58,143). All of these actions tend to reduce myocardial oxygen consumption. On the other hand, propranolol frequently increases the ventricular ejection period and ventricular end diastolic pressure (38,58,143). These effects increase the myocardial oxygen consumption. The net effect of propranolol is a reduction of myocardial oxygen consumption (143,144). When 5 mg of propranolol was given intravenously to 20 patients at rest, the average myocardial oxygen consumption fell from 11.4 to 9.1 ml/100gm. In patients performing identical levels of exercise before and after propranolol, average myocardial oxygen consumption rose 7.1 ml/100gm before the drug dose, but only 4.9 ml/100gm after a 5 mg dose (143).

17. What are the effects of propranolol on coronary circulation?

In patients with coronary artery disease, propranolol decreases coronary flow, increases mean coronary vascular resistance, and increases oxygen extraction (38,41,143). These effects may be due to unopposed alpha-adrenergic activity in the coronary bed (38,46), or autoregulatory phenomena resulting from a decreased metabolic demand for blood flow (46,143). Coronary vasoconstriction following propranolol can be regarded as a benign effect rather than a potential hazard. In patients with chronic ischemic heart disease, vasoconstriction in the non-ischemic regions may divert blood flow into collateral channels, thereby augmenting the blood supply of ischemic regions (46).

18. How effective is propranolol in the treatment of various types of angina?

The effectiveness of propranolol in the treatment of stable angina is well documented. With adequate doses, the drug decreases the number of anginal episodes and nitroglycerin tablets consumed in most patients (13,89,105,112,144). It also enhances exercise performance (13,30,55,80,89,105,112). Long term therapy with propranolol has resulted in 32 per cent of patients per year being angina-free and 84 per cent per year having 50 per cent or more reduction in angina episodes (131). However, fixed dose controlled studies have failed to demonstrate beneficial effects from propranolol. The doses used in these studies may not have been adequate for many patients, thereby minimizing beneficial effects (46).

Patients with unstable angina (angina at rest) and variant angina also benefit from propranolol. With adequate doses, 38 per cent of the former and 73 per cent of the latter responded to propranolol as evidenced by reduction of number of pain episodes and electrocardiographic abnormalities (131). Antianginal response is dose related.

19. A 65-year-old male treated with nitroglycerin 1/150 grain prn for one year, is hospitalized for prolonged anginal episodes unrelieved by nitroglycerin. Propranolol therapy is being considered. What dose should be given and how should its effects be monitored?

Initially, propranolol should be given in a dose of 10 mg tid or qid. It should then be gradually increased in increments of 40 mg per day every 3 to 5 days until the desired clinical response is obtained, the pulse rate falls to 55-60 beats per minute, or until undesirable effects occur (38,78,81). The effective dose ranges from 80 to 1280 mg per day, depending on the patient (105).

20. Is there a relationship between dose, blood level, and the antianginal effect of propranolol?

Therapeutic benefit from propranolol may occur at an average dose of 144 mg per day and an average plasma concentration of 30 ng/ml (103). However, there is wide variation of the maximum effective dose and therapeutic plasma level among individuals (103,105). The plasma level to achieve the maximum therapeutic response was found to correspond to 64 to 98 per cent of total beta-blockade (103).

21. A day after propranolol therapy (10 mg qid) was initiated, a patient developed acute pulmonary edema requiring morphine and furosemide therapy. On that day his BUN was 50 mg per cent (normal: 10 to 20 mg per cent), and his serum creatinine was 3.5 mg per cent (normal: 0.7 to 1.2 mg per cent). Propranolol was discontinued, and the pulmonary edema gradually resolved. Seven days later propranolol 10 mg tid was reinstituted. Pulmonary edema immediately recurred. Is this a common reaction in this type of patient? What other adverse effects are frequently associated with the use of propranolol? Under what circumstances would its use be contraindicated?

The Boston Collaborative Drug Surveillance Program found that 25 (9 per cent) of 268 patients on propranolol experienced adverse reactions. Nearly one-third of these were life-threatening reactions: bradycardia, impaired A-V conduction, acute pulmonary edema, or hypotension. The rest of the reactions were less serious, mostly involving cardiac depression and neurologic disturbances. The frequency of the adverse reactions was not influenced by the dosage, but the reactions did occur more frequently in elderly or azotemic patients and after intravenous administration (53).

Zeft and associates (145) studied 65 patients and showed that the long term use of propranolol in doses of 160 to 400 mg resulted in a 9 per cent incidence of left ventricular failure; approximately 2 per cent developed asthma. Another long term study showed significant side effects in 8 per cent of patients (131). The side effects included gastrointestinal symptoms, hallucination, hypotension and asthma.

In an early report, nausea, tiredness, and lightheadedness were the most common side effects occurring in 1.0 to 1.5 per cent of 1500 patients on oral propranolol therapy. An additional 8 patients (approximately 0.5 per cent) developed dyspnea and wheezing; 13 (approximately 1 per cent) developed cardiac failure; 8 exhibited hypotension; and 2 patients developed bradycardia (127). The low incidence in this report probably reflects inadequate data collection.

Propranolol is contraindicated in patients with overt congestive heart failure (unless the failure is due to tachyarrhythmia), cardiogenic shock, heart block, significant aortic or mitral valve disease, bradycardia, chronic obstructive pulmonary disease, or acute asthma (6,58).

Propranolol-induced congestive heart failure may be treated with digitalis (78,113). However, the patient's heart rate should be monitored carefully because of the additive bradycardic effects of propranolol and digitalis.

22. Compare the properties of the various adrenergic blocking agents. Is there any advantage to using the newly developed adrenergic blocking agents for treatment of angina pectoris? How effective are these drugs in the treatment of angina pectoris?

Different adrenergic blocking agents have different pharmacologic properties (see Table I).

Table I

ADRENERGIC-BLOCKING AGENTS AND THEIR PROPERTIES*

Agent	Beta-blocking action	Membrane effect	Sympatho-mimetic effect
Propranolol	+	+	0
Sotalol	+	minimal	0
Practolol	+	minimal	+
Oxyprenolol	+	+	+
Alprenolol	+	+	+
Pindolol	+	minimal	+

* Modified from Sowton et al, 1975

Practolol is said to be more cardio-selective, because it has relatively little effect on the beta-receptors of the bronchial tree (36,108). It may, therefore, be useful in angina patients with asthma (15,43).

In controlled studies, comparable doses of propranolol, oxyprenolol and practolol increased the exercise tolerance, decreased the chest pain and reduced electrocardiographic evidence of myocardial ischemia to a similar degree in most patients (125,129). Despite the fact that only single doses were used, the results of these studies indicate that all beta-adrenergic agents have similar antianginal activity in patients with stable angina. In patients with variant angina, propranolol was much more effective than practolol (54). Presently, propranolol is the only beta-adrenergic blocker approved by the FDA for the treatment of angina.

23. JA is 66-year-old man whose stable angina has been controlled with NTG SL prn. Because of a recent increase in anginal episodes, propranolol was added to his therapeutic regimen. What is the rationale for using nitrates and beta-adrenergic blockers together? Is the combination clinically synergistic?

When nitrates and propranolol are used together certain cardiac effects are complementary. The increase in the heart rate induced by nitroglycerin is offset by the bradycardic effect of the beta-blockers; whereas the increase in the ejection time and the ventricular volume produced by beta blockers are opposed by NTG (38,46,113).

When sublingual nitrates are combined with propranolol, enhanced effects on exercise tolerance have been observed (112,133). Aronow and Kaplan (11) however, did not find any beneficial effect with the combination of propranolol and sublingual isosorbide dinitrate when compared to propranolol and placebo. In this study, the exercise performance test was done 90 minutes after drug administration. Thus, the results may be expected to be negative since the action of sublingual isosorbide dinitrate is usually quite short. (Also see Question 11).

Clinically, propranolol is used for the prophylactic treatment of angina pectoris. Sublingual nitrates can be used acutely or preferably just prior to anticipated exertion. Addition of propranolol to the nitrate therapy can reduce the need for sublingual nitrates in these patients.

24. What other drugs are used for the treatment of angina pectoris?

Digitalis and diuretics are useful in patients with angina secondary to congestive heart failure. These drugs are also used in the treatment of nocturnal angina. Nocturnal angina may be due to the shift of peripheral fluid and elevation of left ventricular end-diastolic volume which occurs in the recumbent position (7). Diuretics and digitalis decrease left ventricular volume and thus may be helpful in nocturnal angina associated with recumbency (7,46).

Coronary vasodilators such as dipyridamole, papaverine, ethaverine and prenylamine are advocated for the treatment of angina pectoris. To date, the efficacy of these agents has not been adequately demonstrated (7). Whether the long term use of these drugs has any beneficial effect on the development of coronary collateral vessels in humans has not been determined (129).

Verapamil, a drug introduced in 1962 as a coronary vasodilator, was found to decrease angina attacks and increase exercise tolerance in a double-blind crossover study in Europe. Previous studies had not adequately demonstrated its efficacy. This drug is not available in the United States, and its mechanism of antianginal action is controversial (2).

Sedatives are important adjuncts in the management of certain patients with angina. Benzodiazepines are helpful in those individuals whose emotional responses must be curbed to control their angina (81,113).

25. A 60-year-old man with vascular headaches complained of chest pain ten minutes after receiving 0.5 mg of ergotamine tartrate intramuscularly. An

ECG at that time showed S-T segment depression. Explain. What is the best therapy for this patient's chest pain?

All natural ergot alkaloids can increase blood pressure as a result of peripheral vasoconstriction. In patients with coronary artery disease, ergotamine and other ergot alkaloids can specifically produce coronary vasoconstriction which causes anginal pain and ischemic changes that are characterized by S-T segment depression (97). Ergotamine tartrate, ergonovine, and dihydroergotamine have actually been used to intentionally induce angina in some patients (136). The onset of angina usually occurs 5 to 10 minutes after parenteral administration of the ergot compounds and lasts 30 to 45 minutes. Sublingual nitroglycerin 0.6 mg usually relieves such chest pain in 5 minutes (136).

26. What other drugs can induce angina?

Methysergide, a serotonin antagonist and an ergot derivative, has been reported to induce or exacerbate angina-like symptoms at normal doses (4-6 mg per day) (49,50,61). The incidence of methysergide-induced angina is probably less than 1 per cent, and the anginal pain is usually reversible when the drug is discontinued (50). Electrocardiographic changes typical of myocardial infarction (MI) occurred in some patients while taking methysergide (61). Whether these were mere coincidences of an actual MI or drug induced changes was not established.

Hydralazine-induced angina pectoris is well documented (92,116). This drug increases cardiac output and heart rate which result in an increased oxygen demand which can precipitate or exacerbate angina pectoris. The anginal symptoms from hydralazine may be accompanied by electrocardiographic changes manifested by S-T segment depression and QRS and T wave alterations (92). These changes are more common in patients with coronary artery disease. The incidence of hydralazine-induced angina in hypertensive patients is about 7 per cent; it is much less if a cardiodepressive agent is also used concurrently (92).

Digitalis-induced angina has been reported in 15 out of 179 patients who suffered from digitoxin intoxication (77); however, in normal doses, digitalis usually does not induce angina. The overall hemodynamic effects of the drug may even result in a decrease in myocardial oxygen consumption in angina patients who are also in failure (121).

Diazoxide, an antihypertensive drug, causes an angina-like syndrome (66,74). As many as 50 per cent of patients receiving diazoxide have demonstrated ST-T changes (66,99), and as many as 43 per cent of these patients develop substernal discomfort (66). ST-T changes and substernal discomfort may be related to a sudden drop in blood pressure. Hypertensive crisis in patients with coronary artery disease should be treated with nitroprusside, since beneficial effects such as reduction of ischemic changes have been demonstrated from this drug (12,93).

Large doses of sympathomimetic agents (especially isoproterenol inhalers) and thyroid preparations can precipitate angina pectoris in some patients. Less frequently, insulin and fat emulsions for parenteral nutrition may induce angina (85).

27. The patient described at the beginning of this chapter is to be started on medical treatment. What would be a good drug regimen for him?

Sublingual nitroglycerin (NTG) would be the first drug of choice for this patient. With adequate instruction regarding the proper use of nitroglycerin, he may not need any further therapy. If the patient's angina interrupts his daily activity despite daily nitrate therapy, propranolol should be added provided there is no contraindication to its use. An additive effect is usually obtained when propranolol is combined with nitrates (78). If congestive heart failure is a complication of propranolol therapy, digitalis can be used (29,46,78). If a high dose of propranolol is contraindicated or is inadequate to control chest pain, nitroglycerin ointment or high doses of oral nitrates can be added to the regimen.

The appropriate use of nitrates, propranolol, and digitalis alleviates angina in about 80 per cent of patients (78). When the symptoms cannot be controlled by these drugs, surgical intervention should be considered.

28. MM is a glaucoma patient with recent onset of crescendo angina. The physician would like to use nitroglycerin ointment, propranolol, and sublingual NTG prn. Will any of these drugs have a deleterious effect on the existing glaucoma?

Although nitrates can increase intraocular pressure, they are not contraindicated in glaucoma. Any increase in intraocular pressure is probably transient (especially from sublingual NTG) and drainage from the anterior chamber is not impeded (138).

Propranolol will not adversely affect glaucoma and in some patients may actually reduce intraocular pressure (51).

29. A patient was hospitalized for a hypertensive work-up. All medications except nitroglycerin were discontinued and the patient was placed on a vanillymandelic acid (VMA) free diet. The patient experienced several anginal episodes and consumed a total of 12 nitroglycerin tablets during the day. The urinary VMA determination was 8 mg (normal 0-7 mg/24 hours) on that day. What might be the cause of the elevated VMA in this patient?

Besides possible underlying pathological conditions such as pheochromocytoma, nitroglycerin might also be the cause of such an elevation. Significant increases in 8-hour urinary VMA and catecholamine levels have been observed in patients taking large amounts (5.1 mg/day) of nitroglycerin (130). The mechanism of the drug interaction is not clear, and the possibility of interference with the determination for urinary VMA exists (56).

30. AC has been taking nitroglycerin and propranolol for two years. He is now taking propranolol 80 mg qid, applying nitroglycerin ointment 3 inches qid, and uses more than 10 tablets of nitroglycerin a day. Despite good compliance and appropriate use of these drugs, he still experiences chest pains. Cardiac catheterization and coronary angiogram revealed a fairly adequate functioning ventricle with 90 per cent occlusion of the right coronary artery and 75 per cent occlusion of the left circumflex artery. He is scheduled for aorto-coronary saphenous vein bypass surgery. How soon should the propranolol be discontinued before his surgery?

Due to difficulties often associated with decreased cardiac function following open heart surgery, propranolol should be discontinued prior to such surgery (1,34,88,100,123).

To determine the safe period for withdrawal of propranolol before open heart surgery, Faulkner et al studied propranolol levels after chronic therapy (40 to 240 mg per day). They found that the drug could not be detected in plasma or the left atrium 36 to 48 hours after withdrawal of propranolol. They recommended discontinuation of the drug 48 hours before coronary bypass surgery (40).

Coltart et al studied propranolol activity after oral and intravenous C^{14} propranolol. After the intravenous dose, half-life varied from 1.5 to 5 hours and very little propranolol was detected in the myocardial tissue 10 hours after the dose, although small amounts of inactive metabolites were present at that time. After oral propranolol, no radioactivity was found in the myocardial tissue, adipose tissue or skeletal muscle at the end of 24 hours. They recommended propranolol be discontinued 24 to 48 hours prior to surgery (25).

In pharmacokinetic studies, propranolol half-life varies from 3.4 to 6 hours after chronic oral doses of 80 mg every 6 hours (103). Since over 99 per cent of the drug is eliminated from the body after 43 hours (7 half-lives) and 93 per cent after 24 hours, it would be reasonable to discontinue propranolol 24 to 48 hours before the scheduled surgery in this patient.

There is some evidence that unnecessary early abrupt withdrawal may result in rebound infarction or crescendo angina (1,34,98,100,123). This seems to occur more frequently in patients with unstable angina. In view of the possible serious cardiovascular sequelae following sudden withdrawl of propranolol, some authors recommend tapering the dosage gradually prior to stopping the therapy. Whether this is the safest method for propranolol withdrawal remains to be established. It seems reasonable to stop the drug 24 to 48 hours prior to surgery or cardiac catheterization in the hospital setting. Any undesirable effect following the withdrawal of propranolol can be better handled in that setting.

CASE FOR STUDY I

TM is a 60-year-old, 160 lb man who presented in the emergency room with substernal pain unrelieved by 3 NTG 0.4 mg tablets. The patient has adult onset diabetes (for 8 years) and a long history of atherosclerotic heart disease. He has a 40-pack a year history of cigarette smoking and drinks socially. He also has hypertension and Type III hyperlipidemia. Pertinent past hospitalizations include open heart surgery (Vineberg procedure) 8 years ago, myocardial infarction in 1969, 1970, and 1974; CHF in 1970, 1973, and 1974. Angiogram in April 1974 revealed akinesis of inferior apical wall and bulging anteroseptal wall. The ejection fraction was 30 per cent (normal 65-70 per cent). Coronary vessels were small, and diffuse atherosclerosis was present in all coronary arteries. Right coronary artery was 99 per cent, LC 100 per cent, and LAD 95 per cent occluded. He was on the following medications prior to admission: digoxin 0.25 mg qd, furosemide 40 mg qd, KCl 20 mEq bid, ISDN 2.5 mg SL qid, NPH insulin 32 U q AM and 6 U regular insulin q AM, and methyldopa 250 mg tid. On admission, cardiac examination revealed a PMI outside the mcl and a II/VI systolic murmur. ECG showed occasional PVC's and ST depression in various leads. Other laboratory values including glucose were normal. Since this patient was not suitable for bypass surgery, he was treated medically with sublingual NTG prn, nitroglycerin ointment 1½ inches q6h, ISDN 5 mg sublingually q3h,

propranolol 20 mg qid, furosemide 80 mg qd, KCl 20 mEq bid, digoxin 0.375 mg qd and NPH Insulin 32 U qd. During the next few days, the patient's chest pain was poorly controlled and he required supplemental morphine sulfate on several occasions. Prapranolol was then increased to 30 mg qid and nitroglycerin ointment to 2 inches q4h. He was discharged 3 days later with good control of chest pain, blood pressure, heart rate (50 beats per minute), and glucose.

1) Is the combination of ISDN sublingual, nitroglycerin ointment, and NTG prn rational?
2) How could propranolol adversely affect this patient?
3) Should digitalis be used if the patient has a normal sized heart?
4) What is the effect of alcohol on cardiac function? Should this patient change his drinking habits?
5) If the patient's angina is not controlled by the present regimen, how much more nitrate or propranolol can be given? Is there any other therapeutic modality which can help this patient?

CASE FOR STUDY II

MB is a 77-year-old, 184 lb female who was admitted for evaluation of her chest pain. She has had angina for 2 years, hypertension for 15 years, and arthritis for 10 years. Her medications prior to admission include hydrochlorothiazide 100 mg qd, Rauwiloid 2 mg qd, ISDN 5 mg SL prn, ibuprofen 400 mg tid, and occasional antacid use. Physical examination and review of symptoms were consistent with her underlying disease, except the patient was lethargic and had dry skin. Admission laboratory results revealed BUN 29 mg%, resin sponge uptake 25.4 per cent, (normal 25 to 35 per cent), TT4 1.8 mcg% (normal 4.0 to 11 mcg%). The rest of the tests were normal. Chest x-ray showed slight cardiomegaly.

(1) What drug(s) should be given to control her increasing chest pain?
(2) How should her thyroid problem be treated and how would the treatment influence her cardiac problem?

REFERENCES

1. Alderman EL, et al: Coronary artery syndromes after sudden propranolol withdrawal. Ann Int Med 81: 625, 1974.
2. Andreasen F, et al: Assessment of verapamil in the treatment of angina pectoris. Europ J Cardiol 2/4: 443, 1975.
3. Armstrong PW, et al: Vasodilator therapy in acute myocardial infarction. A comparison of sodium nitroprusside and nitroglycerin. Circ 52: 1118, 1975.
4. Aronow WS: Medical treatment of angina pectoris. IV. Nitroglycerin as an antianginal drug. Am Heart J 84: 415, 1972.
5. Aronow WS: The treatment of angina pectoris. V. Long-acting nitrates as anti-anginal drugs. Am Heart J 84: 657, 1972.
6. Aronow WS: The medical treatment of angina pectoris. VI. Propranolol as an anti-anginal drug. Am Heart J 84: 706, 1972.
7. Aronow WS: The medical treatment of angina pectoris, VIII. Miscellaneous anti-anginal drugs. Am Heart J 85: 132, 1973.
8. Aronow WS: The medical treatment of angina pectoris. IX. The medical management of angina pectoris. Am Heart J 85: 275, 1973.
9. Aronow WS: Management of stable angina pectoris. Drug Therapy 3: 91, 1973.
10. Aronow WS, et al: Evaluation of nitroglycerin in angina in patients on isosorbide dinitrate. Circ 42: 61, 1970.
11. Aronow WS, et al: Evaluation of propranolol and of isosorbide dinitrate in angina pectoris. Curr Ther Res 11: 80, 1969.
12. Awan NA, et al: Reduction of S-T segment elevation with infusion of nitroprusside in patients with acute myocardial infarction. Am J Cardiol 38: 435, 1976.
13. Battock DJ, et al: Effects of propranolol and isosorbide dinitrate on exercise performance and adrenergic activity in patients with angina pectoris. Circ 39: 157, 1969.
14. Becker LC, et al: Effect of ischemia and antianginal drugs in the distribution of radioactive microspheres in the canine left ventricle. Circ Res 28: 263, 1971.
15. Bogaert MG: Organic nitrates in angina pectoris. Arch Internation de Pharmacodyn 197: 25, 1972.
16. Brand RJ et al: Multivariate prediction of coronary heart disease in the Western Collaborative Group Study compared to the findings of the Framingham Study. Circ 53: 348, 1976.
17. Braunwald E: Control of myocardial oxygen consumption. Physiologic and clinical considerations. Am J Cardiol 27: 416, 1971.
18. Browning RA, et al: Angina pectoris: Recent advances in understanding and implications for management. Miss Med 70: 235, 1973.
19. Brunner D, et al: Effectiveness of sustained-action isosorbide dinitrate on exercise-induced myocardial ischemia. Chest 66: 282, 1974.
20. Bunn WH, Jr., et al: Clinical evaluation of sublingual nitrates. Onset and duration of action of nitroglycerin and isosorbide dinitrate. Angiology 14: 48, 1963.

21. Burch EG, et al: Fresh nitroglycerin (glyceryl trinitrate). Am Heart J 72: 842, 1966.
22. Caron M, et al: Plasma concentrations of isosorbide dinitrate and metabolites in normal volunteers. Clin Res 23: 608A 1975.
23. Chiong MA, et al: Influence of nitroglycerin on myocardial metabolism and hemodynamics during angina induced by atrial pacing. Circ 45: 1044, 1972.
24. Cole SL, et al: Antianginal effects of oral, controlled-release nitroglycerin (NTG) in patients with coronary artery disease (CAD): Double-blind, randomized, multiple cross-over study. Clin Res 23: 177A 1975.
25. Coltart DJ, et al: Investigation of the safe withdrawal period for propranolol in patients scheduled for open heart surgery. Brit Heart J 37: 1228, 1975.
26. Come PC, et al: Nitroglycerin-induced severe hypotension and bradycardia in patients with acute myocardial infarction. Circ 54: 624, 1976.
27. Copelan HW: Burning sensation and potency of nitroglycerin sublingually. JAMA 219: 176, 1972.
28. Coronary Risk Handbook. Estimating risk of coronary heart disease in daily practice. New York: Amer Heart Assoc, 1973.
29. Crawford MH, et al: Combined propranolol and digoxin therapy in angina pectoris. Ann Int Med 83: 449, 1975.
30. Dagenais GR, et al: Exercise tolerance in patients with angina pectoris. Daily variation and effects of erythrityl tetranitrate, propranolol and alprenolol. Am J Cardiol 28: 10, 1971.
31. Davidov ME, et al: The effect of nitroglycerin ointment on the exercise capacity in patients with angina pectoris. Angiology 27: 205, 1976.
32. Davidson IWF, et al: Absorption, excretion and metabolism of pentaerythritol tetranitrate by humans. J Pharmacol Exper Ther 174: 42, 1970.
33. Dempsey PJ, et al: Pharmacology of the coronary circulation. Ann Rev Pharmacol 12: 99, 1972.
34. Diaz RG, et al: Withdrawal of propranolol and myocardial infarction. Lancet 1: 1068, 1973.
35. DiMatteo FP, et al: Stability of repackaged nitroglycerin for hospital inpatient distribution. Hosp Pharm 9: 299, 1974.
36. Dunlop D, et al: Selective blockade of adrenoceptive beta receptors in the heart. Brit J Pharmacol 32: 201, 1968.
37. Edelman BA, et al: The stability of hypodermic tablets of nitroglycerin packaged in dispensing containers. J Am Pharm Assoc NS11: 30, 1971.
38. Elliot WC, et al: Beta adrenergic blocking agents for the treatment of angina pectoris. Progr Cardiovasc Dis 12: 83, 1969.
39. Flaherty JT, et al: Intravenous nitroglycerin in acute myocardial infarction. Circ 51: 132, 1975.
40. Faulkner SL, et al: Time required for complete recovery from chronic propranolol therapy. NEJM 289: 607, 1973.
41. Fowler NO: Clinical diagnosis. Circ 46: 1079, 1972.
42. Franciosa JA, et al: Hemodynamic effects of orally administered isosorbide dinitrate in patients with congestive heart failure. Circ 50: 1020, 1974.
43. George CF, et al: Practolol in treatment of angina pectoris in a double-blind trial. Brit Med J 2: 402, 1970.
44. Gillis RA, et al: Effects of sublingual and intravenously administered nitroglycerin on the cardiovascular system of the dog. Am J Cardiol 28: 38, 1971.
45. Glancy DL, et al: Effects of swallowed isosorbide dinitrate on blood pressure, heart rate, and exercise tolerance in patients with coronary artery disease. Circ (Suppl. 2) 51 & 52: II-189,1975.
46. Goldstein RE, et al: Medical managements of patients with angina pectoris. Progr Cardiovasc Dis 14: 360, 1972.
47. Goldstein RE, et al: Nitrates in the prophylactic treatment of angina pectoris. (Editorial) Circ 48: 917, 1973.
48. Goldstein RE, et al: Clinical and circulatory effects of isosorbide dinitrate, comparison with nitroglycerin. Circ 43: 629, 1971.
49. Graham JR: Use of a new compound. UML-491 (1-methyl-D-lysergic acid butanolamide) in the prevention of various types of headache. NEJM 263, 1960.
50. Graham JR: Methysergide for prevention of headache. NEJM 270: 67, 1964.
51. Grant WM: Toxicology of the Eye. 2nd Ed. Charles C. Thomas, Springfield, IL, 1974, p. 861.
52. Greenberg H, et al: Effects of nitroglycerin on the major determinants of myocardial oxygen consumption. An angiographic and hemodynamic assessment. Am J Cardiol 36: 426, 1975.
53. Greenblatt DJ, et al: Adverse reactions to propranolol in hospitalized medical patients: A report from the Boston Collaborative Drug Surveillance Program. Am Heart J 86: 478, 1973.
54. Guazzi M, et al: Treatment of spontaneous angina pectoris with beta blocking agents. Brit Heart J 37: 1235, 1975.
55. Hamer J, et al: Effects of propranolol on exercise tolerance in angina pectoris. Am J Cardiol 18: 354, 1966.
56. Hansten PD: Drug Interactions. Lea and Febiger, Philadelphia. 1973, p. 447.
57. Hargrove W: Nitroglycerin facts today. Tile & Till 59: 65, 1973.
58. Harrison DC: Beta-adrenergic blockade, 1972, pharmacology and clinical uses. Am J Cardiol 19: 432, 1972.
59. Harrison TR, et al: Principles and problems of ischemic heart disease. Chicago Year Book Medical Publishers, Inc., 1968, p. 251.
60. Higgins CB, et al: Clinical and arteriographic features of Prinzmetal's variant angina: Documentation of etiologic factors. Am J Cardiol 37: 831, 1976.
61. Hudgson P, et al: Methysergide and coronary-artery disease. Lancet 1: 444, 1967.
62. Horwitz LD, et al: Clinical response to nitroglycerin as a diagnostic test for coronary artery disease. Am J Cardiol 19: 149, 1972.
63. Hurwitz L, et al: Isosorbide dinatrate and cardiovascular adaptation to exercise. Chest 69: 10, 1976.
64. Ikram H: A clinical trial of a new long-acting nitroglycerine preparation ("Nitrocontin") in angina pectoris. Curr Med Res & Opin 3: 719, 1976.
65. Jerie P: Efficacy of long-acting nitrates. II. Peroral isosorbide dinitrate. Am J Cardiol 38: 402, 1976.
66. Kanada SA, et al: Angina-like syndrome with diazoxide therapy for hypertensive crisis. Ann Int Med 84: 696, 1976.
67. Kannel WB, et al: Factors of risk in the development of coronary heart disease — Six-year follow-up experience. The Framingham Study. Ann Int Med 55: 33, 1961.
68. Kannel WB, et al: Natural history of angina pectoris in the Framingham Study. Prognosis and survival. Am J Cardiol 19: 154, 1972.
69. Kasparian H, et al: Comparative hemodynamic effects of placebo and oral isosorbide dinitrate in patients with significant coronary artery disease. Am Heart J 90: 68, 1975.
70. Kattus AA, et al: Effectiveness of isosorbide dinitrate and nitroglycerin in relieving angina pectoris during uninterrupted exercise. Chest 67: 640, 1975.
71. Keys A, et al: Probability of middle-aged men developing coronary heart disease in five years. Circ 45: 815,1972.
72. Klaus AP, et al: Comparative evaluation of sublingual long-acting nitrates. Circ 48: 519, 1973.
73. Krantz JJ, et al: Efficacy of long-acting nitrates. I. Sublingual versus oral administration. Am J Cardiol 38: 401, 1976.
74. Kumar GK, et al: Side effects of diazoxide. JAMA 235: 275, 1976.
75. Lange RL, et al: Non-atheromatous ischemic heart disease following withdrawal from chronic industrial nitroglycerin exposure. Circ 46: 666, 1972.
76. Lee G, et al: Improved exercise tolerance for six hours following isosorbide dinitrate capsules in patients with ischemic heart disease. Am J Cardiol 37: 150, 1976.
77. Lely AH, et al: Large scale digitoxin intoxication. Brit Med J 3: 737, 1970.
78. Lesch N, et al: Pharmacological therapy of angina pectoris. Mod Concepts Cardiovasc Dis 42: 5, 1973.
79. Leslie RE: A ten-year reevaluation. Nitroglycerin and isosorbide dinitrate in coronary insufficiency. Texas Med 67: 95, 1971.
80. Livesley B, et al: Double-blind evaluation of verapamil, propranolol and isosorbide dinitrate against a placebo in the treatment of angina pectoris. Brit Med J 1: 375, 1973.
81. Logue RB, et al: Medical management of angina pectoris. Circ 46:1132, 1972.
82. Mayer GA: Instability of nitroglycerin tablets. Canad Med Assoc J 110: 788, 1974.
83. McConahay DR, et al: Coronary artery bypass surgery for left main coronary artery disease. Am J Cardiol 37: 885, 1976.
84. Medalie JH, et al: Angina pectoris among 10,000 men. II. Psychosocial and other risk factors as evidenced by a multivariate analysis of a five year incidence study. Am J Med 60: 910, 1976.
85. Meyler L, Herxheimer A (Eds.): Side Effects of Drugs, Vol. VII. A survey of unwanted effects of drugs reported in 1968-71. Excerpta Medica, Amsterdam, 1972, p. 579.

86. Coronary arteriography and coronary artery surgery. Med Letter 18: 57, 1976.

87. Miller RR, Greenblatt DJ (Eds.): *Drug Effects in Hospitalized Patients.* John Wiley & Sons, New York, 1976, p. 56, 59.

88. Miller RR, et al: Propranolol withdrawal rebound phenomenon. Exacerbation of coronary events after abrupt cessation of antianginal therapy. NEJM 293: 416, 1975.

89. Miller RR, et al: Efficacy of beta adrenergic blockade in coronary heart disease: Propranolol in angina pectoris. Clin Pharm & Ther 18: 598, 1975.

90. Miller RR, Greenblatt DJ (Eds.): *Drug Effects in Hospitalized Patients.* John Wiley & Sons, New York, 1976, p. 57.

91. Moir TW: Brief reviews: Subendocardial distribution of coronary blood flow and the effects of antianginal drugs. Circ Res 30: 621, 1972.

92. Moyer JH, et al: Hydralazine in the treatment of hypertension. Med Clin N Amer 45: 375, 1961.

93. Mukherjee D, et al: Nitroprusside therapy. Treatment of hypertensive patients with recurrent resting chest pain, ST-segment elevation, and ventricular arrhythmias. JAMA 235: 2406, 1976.

94. Myerburg RJ: Diagnostic and therapeutic aspects of stable angina pectoris. Med Clin N Amer 55: 421, 1971.

95. Needleman P, et al: Organic nitrates: relationship between biotransformation and rational angina pectoris therapy. J Pharmacol Exp Ther 181: 189, 1972.

96. Needleman P: Efficacy of long-acting nitrates. I. Sublingual versus oral administration. Am J Cardiol 38: 400, 1976.

97. Nickerson M. Drugs inhibiting adrenergic nerves and structures innervated by them. Chapter 26 in *Pharmacological Basis of Therapeutics,* 4th Ed., edited by LS Goodman and A Gilman. The Macmillan Co, New York, 1971, p. 745.

98. Oberman A, et al: Surgical versus medical treatment in disease of the left main coronary artery. Lancet 2: 591, 1976.

99. O'Brien KP et al: Intravenous diazoxide in treatment of hypertension associated with recent myocardial infarction. Brit Med J 4: 74, 1975.

100. Olson HG, et al: The propranolol withdrawal rebound phenomenon: Acute and catastrophic exacerbation of symptoms and death following the abrupt cessation of large doses of propranolol in coronary disease. Brit Heart J 37: 1228, 1975.

101. Parker JO: The effect of nitroglycerin on coronary blood flow and the hemodynamic response to exercise in coronary artery disease. Am J Cardiol 27: 59, 1971.

102. Paul O: Angina pectoris. Rational Drug Ther 6: 1, 1972.

103. Pine M, et al: Correlation of plasma propranolol concentration with therapeutic response in patients with angina pectoris. Circ 52: 886, 1975.

104. Poliner L, et al: The comparative hemodynamic effects of oral and sublingual isosorbide dinitrate in patients with coronary insufficiency. Clin Res 24: 5A 1976.

105. Prichard BNC, et al: Assessment of propranolol in angina pectoris. Brit Heart J 33: 473, 1971.

106. Reichek N: Long-acting nitrates in the treatment of angina pectoris. JAMA 236: 1399, 1976.

107. Rosenman RH, et al: Multivariate prediction of coronary heart disease during 8.5 year follow-up in the Western Collaborative Group Study. Am J Cardiol 37: 903, 1976.

108. Ross G, et al: Effects of cardio selective beta-adrenergic blocking agent on the heart and coronary circulation. Cardiovasc Res 4: 148, 1970.

109. Ross RS: Ischemic heart disease: An overview. Am J Cardiol 36: 495, 1975.

110. Rossi GV: Antianginal drugs — A review. Am J Pharm 143: 153, 1971.

111. Russek HI: The therapeutic role of coronary vasodilators: glyceryl trinitrate, isosorbide dinitrate, and pentaerythritol tetranitrate. Am J Med Sci 252: 43, 1966.

112. Russek HI: Propranolol and isosorbide dinitrate synergism in angina pectoris. Am J Cardiol 21: 44, 1968.

113. Russek HI: Intractable angina pectoris. Med Clin N Amer 54: 333, 1970.

114. Scheidt S, et al: Unstable angina pectoris. Natural history, hemodynamics, uncertainties of treatment and the ethics of clinical study. Am J Med 60: 409, 1976.

115. Schelling JL: A study of cross-tolerance to circulatory effects of organic nitrates. Clin Pharmacol Ther 8: 256, 1967.

116. Schirger A, et al: Pharmacology and clinical use of hydralazine in the treatment of diastolic hypertension. Am J Cardiol 9: 854, 1962.

117. Semler HJ, et al: Angina prophylaxis by chewable isosorbide dinitrate. Curr Ther Res 13: 523, 1971.

118. Shane SJ: High-dose oral isosorbide dinitrate and ischemic heartpain. Canad Fam Phys 19: 61, 1973.

119. Shangraw RF: Unstable nitroglycerin tablets. (Letter) NEJM 286: 950, 1972.

120. Shangraw RF, et al: New developments in the manufacture and prepackaging of nitroglycerin in tablets. J Am Pharm Assoc NS12: 633, 1972.

121. Sharma B, et al: Clinical electrocardiographic and hemodynamic effects of digitalis (Ouabain) in angina pectoris. Brit Heart J 34: 631, 1972.

122. Shell WE, et al: Protection of jeopardized ischemic myocardium by reduction of ventricular afterload. NEJM 291: 481, 1974.

123. Slome R: Withdrawal of propranolol and myocardial infarction. Lancet 1: 156, 1973.

124. Sonnenblick EH, et al: Oxygen consumption or the heart. Physiological principles and clinical implications. Mod Concepts Cardiovasc Dis 49: 9, 1971.

125. Sowton E, et al: Comparative effects of beta-adrenergic blocking drugs. Thorax 30: 9, 1975.

126. Spier L: Uniform release nitroglycerin for prophylactic use. Clin Med 76: 23, 1969.

127. Stephen SA: Unwanted effects of propranolol. Am J Cardiol 18: 463, 1966.

128. Sweatman T, et al: The long-acting hemodynamic effects of isosorbide dinitrate. Am J Cardiol 29: 475, 1972.

129. Thadani U, et al: Comparison of adrenergic beta-receptor antagonists in angina pectoris. Brit Med J 1: 138, 1973.

130. Vigliani ED, et al: Biological effects of nitroglycal on the metabolism of catecholamines. Arch Environ Health 16: 477, 1968.

131. Warren SG, et al: Long-term propranolol therapy for angina pectoris. Am J Cardiol 37: 420, 1976.

132. Weinblatt AB, et al: Prognosis of women with newly diagnosed coronary heart disease — a comparison with course of disease among men. Am J Public Health 63: 577, 1973.

133. Weiner L, et al: Hemodynamic effects of nitroglycerin, propranolol and their combination in coronary heart disease. Circ 39: 623, 1969.

134. Weisse AB, et al: The current status of nitrites in the treatment of coronary artery disease. Progr Cardiovasc Dis 12: 72, 1969.

135. Weisse AB, et al: Effects of nitrate infusions on the systemic and coronary circulations following acute experimental myocardial infarction in the intact dog. Am J Cardiol 30: 362, 1972.

136. Wendkos MH: The anti-anginal effect of rapidly acting nitrates in subjects with ergot-induced angina. Am J Med Sci 253: 39, 1967.

137. Wendkos MH, et al: Comparative effect of placebo and sustained-release nitroglycerin in angina subjects. J Clin Pharmacol 13: 160, 1973.

138. Whitworth CG, et al: Use of nitrate and nitrate vasodilators by glaucomatous patients.Arch Ophthal 71: 492, 1964.

139. Willis WH, et al: Hemodynamic effects of isosorbide dinitrate vs. nitroglycerin in patients with unstable angina. Chest 69: 15, 1976.

140. Winbury MM: Redistribution of left ventricular blood flow produced by nitroglycerin. Circ Res 28 (Suppl. 1): 140, 1971.

141. Winsor T, et al: Hemodynamic response of oral long-acting nitrates: evidence of gastrointestinal absorption. Chest 62: 407, 1972.

142. Wolf R, et al: Hemodynamic investigations of the long-term action of nitrite in patients with coronary heart disease. Deutsche Med Wochenschr 100: 735, 1975.

143. Wolfson S, et al: Cardiovascular pharmacology of propranolol in man. Circ 40: 501, 1969.

144. Wolfson S, et al: Propranolol and angina pectoris. Am J cardiol 18: 345, 1966.

145. Zeft HJ, et al: The effect of propranolol in the long term treatment of angina pectoris. Arch Int Med 124: 588, 1969.

146. Zelis R, et al: Demonstration of nitrite tolerance: attenuation of the venodilator response to nitroglycerin by the chronic administration of isosorbide dinitrate. (Abstract) Circ 40 (Suppl. 111): 221, 1969.

147. Zelis R, et al: Angina pectoris. Diagnosis and treatment. Postgrad Med 59: 179, 1976.

Chapter 16

Thrombosis

Steven R. Kayser

Arterial and venous thromboemboli contribute to many of the leading causes of death in the U.S. today. In addition, adverse reactions to anticoagulants (especially warfarin) are among the most common causes of hospital admissions due to adverse drug reactions. It is important to consider the risk of adverse reactions whenever anticoagulant drugs are required to treat or prevent potentially life-threatening conditions. To minimize this risk, an understanding of the pharmacology of the anticoagulants as well as the physiologic and pathologic processes of blood coagulation and of the conditions being treated is essential.

Although there are many potential indications for anticoagulant therapy, beneficial effects have been established for only a few. These include pulmonary embolism, deep venous thrombosis, cerebral embolism, acute peripheral arterial embolism, atrial fibrillation with rheumatic heart disease, and prophylaxis of emboli from heart valve prostheses. The use of anticoagulants in the treatment of acute myocardial infarction and transient ischemic attacks is of questionable benefit.

When evaluating and managing anticoagulant therapy, it is essential that consideration be given to:

a) the indication for therapy, b) the anticipated duration of therapy, c) the therapeutic endpoint, d) other conditions present in the patient which may alter response to anticoagulants, e) the current drug history, and f) changes which may occur in any of these factors over time.

In this chapter some aspects of the general pharmacology of heparin, the oral anticoagulants, and drugs altering platelet behavior will be reviewed. Some of the more common drug interactions will also be discussed. The indanediones will not be considered, because it is the opinion of this author that the high incidence of toxicity associated with these drugs precludes their clinical use.

1. A thorough understanding of the normal clotting cascade is important to the understanding the pharmacology of both heparin and the oral anticoagulants. Discuss the normal clotting system and differentiate between the intrinsic and extrinsic system. Include a discussion of the role of platelets in the clotting cascade.

A complex series of events initiated by injury to the vascular endothelium results in the ultimate formation of a firm fibrin clot. When injury occurs, platelets adhere to collagen as well as to other exposed subendothelial tissue (52). After the initial adhesion of platelets to the site of injury, platelet aggregation is induced through platelet release of adenosine diphosphate (ADP) (207). (See Fig. 1)

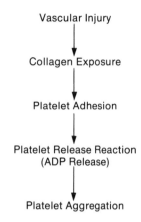

Vascular Injury

↓

Collagen Exposure

↓

Platelet Adhesion

↓

Platelet Release Reaction
(ADP Release)

↓

Platelet Aggregation

Figure 1
Formation of the Platelet Plug

The transformation of this temporary platelet plug to a permanent fibrin clot is achieved through activation of the extrinsic or intrinsic blood clotting system (81). (See fig. 2)

Each of the clotting factors exists in the blood in the inactive form and must be converted to an active (a) or enzymatic form before further clotting is stimulated (55). Exposure of subendothelial collagen initiates the *intrinsic* pathway by stimulating the activation of factor XII. Activated factor XII then stimulates the conversion of factor XI to its active form, which then stimulates the activation of factor IX. Activated factor IX, in the presence of calcium, phospholipids (platelet factor III), and factor VIII, stimulates the conversion of factor X to its active form. Activated factor X in the presence of Ca^{++}, phospholipid (platelet factor III), and factor V stimulate the conversion of prothrombin to thrombin (24).

The conversion of prothrombin to thrombin may also be achieved through the *extrinsic* clotting pathway. The release of material extrinsic to the blood, such as tissue extract or tissue thromboplastin, activates factor VII, which stimulates the activation of factor X. Factor X thus occupies a central position at the junction of the extrinsic and intrinsic systems.

Thrombin, which is generated by either pathway, stimulates the conversion of fibrinogen to fibrin in the presence of ionized calcium (189). The initial soluble fibrin clot is further converted to an insoluble fibrin polymer when factor XIII is activated by thrombin (72). In addition to stimulating the conversion of fibrinogen

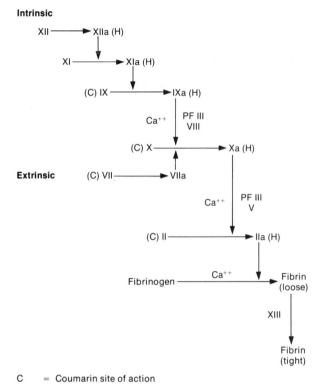

C   = Coumarin site of action
H   = Heparin site of action
PF III = Platelet Factor III (phospholipid)
a   = Activated

Figure 2
Soluble Clotting Cascade

to fibrin, thrombin stimulates further platelet aggregation and potentiates the activity of factor V, VIIa, VIII, and Xa (161).

Once thrombin is formed, it is partly removed by absorption into fibrin. This, plus other naturally occurring inhibitors of clotting factors, play a role in localizing fibrin formation to the sites of injury and in maintaining the fluidity of circulating blood. Agents have been identified in normal blood which inhibit the activated forms of factors II, X, XI and XII (23,222). The deposition of fibrin is also associated with activation of plasmin or fibrinolysin, a fibrinolytic enzyme which also prevents excessive coagulation. (See Fig. 3)

2. What is the etiology and the role of a "white thrombus" and a "red thrombus" in thromboembolic disease?

White thrombi, or arterial thrombi, are composed primarily of platelets, although they also contain fibrin and occasional leukocytes (55,203). They generally occur in areas of rapid blood flow and are formed in response to an injured or abnormal vessel wall.

Red thrombi, or stasis thrombi, are primarily found

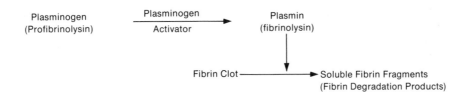

Figure 3   Mechanism of Action of Plasmin

in the venous circulation and are almost entirely composed of fibrin and erythrocytes. They have a small platelet head, and they form in areas of stasis when dilution of activated blood coagulation factors by blood flow is prevented (55).

Thus, the choice of an antithrombotic agent, may be influenced by the type of thrombus which is to be treated. Heparin and the coumarins are presently used to treat both white and red thrombi. Drugs affecting platelet function are now being investigated for their role in the prevention of certain thromboembolic disorders and are expected to be particularly useful in the treatment of white thrombi.

3. Discuss the common clotting tests used to evaluate the hemostatic mechanism.

The **bleeding time** is a measure of platelet aggregation and capillary contraction, and is of little value in monitoring anticoagulant therapy (93). Simple clotting factor deficiencies result in a normal bleeding time (125). The normal Ivy bleeding time is 2½-7 minutes (25).

The **whole blood clotting time,** (WBCT) or Lee-White clotting time, is infrequently used today because it lacks sensitivity. It is usually normal in the presence of factor VII deficiency (189). It is an insensitive measure of prothrombin deficiency and is only moderately sensitive in measuirng thromboplastin generation or fibrin formation (190). The clotting time by this method depends greatly on the size and types of tubes used, the temperature, degree of agitation, type of blood used (i.e. venous or capillary), and the skill of the laboratory technician. The normal clotting time is less than 15 minutes (34).

The **prothrombin time** (PT) of Quick (184) is prolonged by deficiencies of factors V, VII, X, and II; by low levels of fibrinogen; and by high levels of heparin (186,187). It thus reflects alterations in the extrinsic system and the common clotting pathway, but not the intrinsic system. The normal prothrombin time is 12±0.5 seconds (186). An individual patient's prothrombin time is compared to a control or standard curve determined by various dilutions of a commercially available thromboplastin. Therapeutic pro-

Table 1
TESTS USED TO MONITOR ANTICOAGULANT THERAPY

Tests	Factors Measured	Normal Value*	Drug Monitored
WBCT (Lee-White)	All except VII	9-14 min. (<15 min.)	Heparin
Prothrombin Time (PT)	II, V, VII, X	12 sec.	Warfarin
Partial Thromboplastin Time (PTT)	All except VII	60-85 sec.	Warfarin
Activated Partial Thromboplastin Time (APTT)	All except VII	24-36 sec.	Heparin
Activated Coagulation Time (ACT)	All except VII	80-130 sec.	Heparin

*University of California, San Francisco

thrombin times are in the range of 1½ to 2½ times the patient's control value. Prothrombin times have also been reported as percent activity (54,56). This should be avoided because of the risk of confusing a percentage activity with prothrombin time in seconds.

The **partial thromboplastin time** (PTT) reflects deficiencies of all the plasma coagulation factors except for factors VII and XIII (136), and thus measures deficiencies in the intrinsic and common clotting pathway but not the extrinsic pathway. Since the test is performed with platelet-poor plasma, it does not reflect the role of platelets in clotting. It has been used to measure the activity of oral anticoagulants (223), but it is not very sensitive to heparin (188). It is primarily used to screen for deficiencies in clotting factors of the intrinsic system in patients being considered for oral anticoagulant therapy. The normal PTT is 60 to 85 seconds. If platelets are present, or if the test is performed more than one hour after collection, values that are unexpectedly low may be observed (105).

The **activated partial thromboplastin time** (APTT) is sensitive to deficiencies of all the plasma coagulation factors except for factors VII and XIII. It is generally a more sensitive test than the PTT, and it is widely used to monitor heparin therapy (19,220,261). The APTT correlates well with the Lee-White clotting test but is more sensitive. Its advantage over the Lee-White method is that it can be performed within a few minutes. This test, like the PTT, is performed with platelet-poor plasma, thus it does not reflect the activity of platelets. Normal values for the APTT may vary but are usually between 24 to 36 seconds. Therapeutic values are one and one-half to two and one-half the patient's baseline APTT.

The *activated coagulation time* (ACT) of whole blood measures all of the factors except factor VII; its sensitivity to factors V and II has not been established (98). Since it is a whole blood test, it reflects the role of platelets in coagulation. The test is used to monitor heparin therapy (9,99) and can be performed at the bedside. Normal values are 80 to 130 seconds. (See Table 1)

4. How valid is it to use prolongation of coagulation tests to monitor the therapeutic and toxic effects of anticoagulation?

Most clinicians feel that it is necessary to monitor coagulation tests so that embolism and hemorrhage can be prevented (5,51,65,83,205,250). However, some clinicians do not agree and consider testing to be superfluous (20).

Most recent investigators have confirmed earlier observations that effective anticoagulant therapy will prolong coagulation tests 1½ to 2½ times the control value. Early studies indicated that maintenance of clotting times in excess of twice control provided optimal protection against experimentally-induced thrombi in dogs (33,249).

More recent studies indicate that a continuous infusion of heparin (in doses which maintain the APTT between 1½ to 2½ times the control level) safely and effectively prevents venous thromboembolism (19,102). This method of administration also decreases the incidence of hemorrhage (204).

Sevitt and Innes (209) studied patients who were being treated with oral anticoagulants to prevent thromboembolism. When they compared the prothrombin times of those patients who were treated successfully to those who were not, they found that prothrombin values which were less than two times the control correlated with treatment failure. Successful therapy correlated with prothrombin values greater than two times the control; however, no therapeutic advantage was observed when prothrombin times were greater than three times the control value.

Hemorrhage from anticoagulation is frequently, but not always, associated with excessive hypoprothrombinemia. A review of hemorrhagic complications secondary to anticoagulant therapy by Coon and Willis (40) revealed that more than two thirds of all hemorrhagic complications occurred when the PT was more than two times baseline activity. They concluded that while fewer thromboembolic complications occur when prothrombin times are maintained at twice normal or more, this is also the range associated with a greater incidence of hemorrhage. However, the morbidity and mortality associated with hemorrhage are far less than that associated with inadequately treated thromboembolic disease.

In conclusion, it is reasonable to control anticoagulant therapy with an appropriate laboratory test because the response to a given dose of heparin (176) or warfarin (171) can generally be correlated with a specific value. Maintenance of the selected clotting parameter between 1½ and 2½ times the control value appears to provide the greatest protection against embolization with minimal risk of hemorrhage. However, even in this range bleeding complications cannot always be avoided, especially in postoperative patients (19).

5. The oral anticoagulants, bishydroxycoumarin and warfarin have been called "vitamin K antagonists." What is meant by this?

Vitamin K is essential for the hepatic synthesis of four of the ten circulating proteins required for the formation of a clot. These factors are II, VII, IX and X (134,255). The ability of the coumarins to antagonize the hepatic synthesis of these factors has been known for years. The exact mechanism for this interaction is not known, but several have been proposed.

It was originally proposed that vitamin K and the coumarins act as simple competitive antagonists (39). This theory is supported by the observation that patients who are resistant to warfarin have a moderately decreased affinity at the receptor site for vitamin K and a markedly decreased affinity for the anticoagulant (166,167,173,226).

More complex mechanisms for the inhibition of hepatic synthesis of the vitamin K-dependent clotting factors have been proposed. The site of action of warfarin may be an enzyme that regulates the metabolism of vitamin K rather than a binding site for the vitamin (54). Animal studies have shown that in the presence of warfarin there is an accumulation of phylloquinone oxide (vitamin K_1 oxide), which is an antagonist of vitamin K (255).

It is apparent that the interaction between vitamin K and warfarin has not been clearly defined.

6. The pharmacokinetics of bishydroxycoumarin and warfarin differ. Discuss these differences.

Warfarin is completely absorbed in the upper gastrointestinal tract by passive diffusion (165,167). However, bishydroxycoumarin is poorly and variably absorbed; 15 to 30% is recovered in the stool as unchanged drug (167).

Peak absorption for both warfarin and bishydroxycoumarin occurs in 60 to 120 minutes (29,167). The volume of distribution (Vd) for warfarin and high doses of bishydroxycoumarin is about the same:

12.5% of body weight (165,167). This small volume of distribution is consistent with the extensive binding of warfarin to albumin, since it is equivalent to the Vd for albumin or 2.6 times the plasma volume (165).

The mean half-life of warfarin is independent of dose and is 42 hours (165). In contrast, the half-life of bishydroxycoumarin is 24 hours and is dependent upon the plasma concentration (263). Both warfarin and bishydroxycoumarin are highly protein bound; warfarin is bound on the order of 99.5% to serum albumin (263,251) and bishydroxycoumarin is 99% protein bound (263). However, the binding of coumarins is readily reversible and it is the free drug that is pharmacologically active. Recent work (251) indicates that no apparent relationship exists between the extent of protein binding of warfarin and the concentration of albumin or total protein in the serum. Furthermore, there appears to be no correlation between the prothrombin time and dose of warfarin, total warfarin concentration, or free warfarin concentration.

The coumarins are metabolized in the hepatic microsomes by mixed function oxidase enzymes. Warfarin is administered as a racemate which contains equal parts of the R and S isomer. The S-isomer is approximately five times more potent as an anticoagulant than is the R-isomer (132). S-warfarin is oxidized to 7-hydroxywarfarin and reduced to an alcohol 2 (SS alcohol), whereas R-warfarin is metabolized primarily by reduction to alcohol 1 (RS alcohol). Both racemates are metabolized to 6-hydroxywarfarin in small amounts. The warfarin alcohols have minimal anticoagulant activity and are excreted renally (36,100,129,130,131). The hydroxylated products are inactive (129) and are eliminated only by metabolism.

The reason why the R and S isomers differ in potency is unclear. The half-life of the R-isomer is 45 hours while the half-life of the S-isomer is 33 hours, and they both have the same volumes of distribution (100). It has been proposed that differences in permeability or affinity to the receptor site account for the differing potencies.

Knowledge of these two isomers is also important because drugs interact with warfarin stereoselectively. Phenylbutazone (132) and metronidazole (174) inhibit the S-isomer but have no effect on the R-isomer. Long-term warfarin therapy in thrombotic diseases may be made safer in the future by the administration of the R-isomer alone since it does not appear to interact with other drugs to the same extent as the racemic mixture and the S-isomer.

7. A 44-year-old white male accounting executive with a history of thromboembolic disease is considered a good candidate for anticoagulant therapy. The physician wants to begin his therapy on an out-

patient basis. How should this be done?

Whether warfarin therapy should be initiated with a loading dose, or more conservatively with maintenance doses, has been a subject of controversy (27,55,169,234). While clinicians in the U.S. have resolved the issue in their minds and use the maintenance-dose approach, the loading dose is still recommended by clinicians in Europe (58,59).

Since warfarin acts only on the synthesis of vitamin K-dependent clotting factors, its onset of activity is dependent, not only upon its own kinetics, but also upon the catabolic rate of the circulating clotting factors. The half-life of the four vitamin K-dependent clotting factors ranges from 5 hours for factor VII, to 60 hours for factor II (prothrombin); factors IX and X have intermediate half-lives of between 20 and 40 hours (54,117).

Some advocate the loading dose to achieve a more rapid therapeutic effect. Depression of any one of the clotting factors in the extrinsic pathway will prolong the prothrombin time, and this might be interpreted as therapeutic hypoprothrombinemia (54). However, even though factor VII from the extrinsic pathway disappears first because it has the shortest half-life of all the vitamin K-dependent factors, it has been shown that factors IX and X (intrinsic pathway) are more important in the pathogensis of thromboembolic disease (104,246).

Studies using a loading dose (1.5 mg/kg) versus a maintenance dose (10 or 15 mg daily) have shown that in the first 48 hours there is less factor VII activity when a loading dose is used; however, there are no significant differences between the methods with respect to the maximum suppression of any of the four factors (169).

In summary, even though a more rapid prolongation of the prothrombin time is achieved following a large loading dose, this method does not offer more rapid protection against thrombi formation. Furthermore, these large doses place the patient at risk for hemorrhage. The hemorrhagic potential in a patient unusually sensitive to the effects of warfarin (for example, if the patient should exhibit an alteration of metabolism or have an underlying hepatic abnormality) may be avoided by giving smaller doses.

This patient should be initiated on low maintenance doses, because he is to be treated on an outpatient basis, and because there is no evidence of an acute thrombotic episode. On a dose of 5 to 10 mg warfarin daily a therapeutic prothrombin time should be achieved in five to ten days. If an immediate effect is required, heparin would be the initial drug of choice.

8. The same patient has now taken warfarin for eight months, and he is believed to be free of his

thromboembolic disease. How should therapy be terminated?

Some investigators feel that if anticoagulant therapy is discontinued abruptly, a rebound hypercoagulable state will result. Therefore, they believe therapy should be withdrawn gradually (218). However, other studies indicate that abrupt discontinuation of oral anticoagulant therapy is not associated with a higher risk of thromboembolic complications (115,145,253). Since the half-lives of warfarin and the clotting factors responsible for emboli are long, one would expect that the elimination of warfarin and the build up of clotting factors to normal levels would be gradual, even if the anticoagulant were discontinued abruptly. Therefore, warfarin may be abruptly discontinued in this patient.

9. Seven days after a patient was started on a warfarin (Coumadin) dose of 15 mg daily, the dose is increased as a result of poor therapeutic control. After a subsequent increase in dosage you are consulted. The following information was found when this patient was monitored:

Day	15	16	17	18	19	20
Dosage of warfarin (mg)	17.5	10	20	22.5	22.5	25.0
Prothrombin time (control 11.8 sec)	17.8	18.0	18.0	18.5	19.0	18.5

What are the possible explanations for this patient's resistance to warfarin?

Many factors may be contributing to this patient's resistance or altered response to warfarin therapy.

Diet may be a potential source of resistance. Foods rich in vitamin K include cauliflower, beans, spinach, rice, pork, fish, and some cheeses (181). The role of increased dietary intake has not been clearly established, but this possibility should be considered. More frequently, a decreased absorption of vitamin K results in an increased sensitivity to warfarin.

Poor absorption may contribute to resistance since there have been cases of apparent resistance which resolved when warfarin was administered parenterally (171).

Altered metabolism of warfarin might also account for resistance. Patients in whom warfarin has a shorter half-life have shown a decreased hypoprothrombinemic response (165). For example, a patient who metabolizes warfarin to an enantiomer which is less active may require a higher dose. A patient with an increased clearance of both warfarin and phenindione has been reported (128).

The response of *myxedematous* patients to a single dose of warfarin is diminished (194). The response to chronic administration has not been studied, but the overall metabolic state of the patient must be consid-

ered as a possible reason for resistance to warfarin. In contrast, the rate of catabolism of vitamin K-dependent clotting factors is increased in hypermetabolic states such as fever and hyperthyroidism (133).

An increased rate of clearance of warfarin was observed in *alcoholics* who had a prothrombin content of 100% before warfarin was given. Since single doses were given, the significance of this report must be substantiated for chronic dosing (116).

Cigarette smokers metabolize certain drugs such as pentazocine and benzodiazepines in an altered manner. A retrospective analysis has shown no effect of cigarette smoking on warfarin metabolism (147).

A *hereditary* basis for resistance has been identified in animals and man (166,170,171). Findings consistent with an altered affinity of the receptor for the oral anticoagulants or for vitamin K have been reported. This is apparently mediated by a single autosomal gene. An altered affinity to bishydroxycoumarin has also been proposed (219).

Race apparently plays no role in the ability to metabolize warfarin. It was proposed that a greater response occurs in Japanese patients (73), but this has been refuted (11).

The mean coumarin anticoagulant requirement may be increased in patients with elevated serum cholesterol levels, perhaps due to an increased level of vitamin K in the plasma and liver (183). This has not been substantiated however. Serum triglyceride levels do not influence the warfarin dosage.

Drug interactions play a large role in altering the response to oral anticoagulants. Barbiturates, oral contraceptives, cholestyramine, glutethimide, griseofulvin, adrenocortical steroids and others reportedly inhibit coumarin action in man (263). A careful medication history is thus essential when an altered response to warfarin is interpreted. Also see Questions 10-12.

It is important to remember that if a patient appears to be unresponsive to warfarin, the dose should not be altered daily. Since the drug has a half-life of 42 hours, it takes longer than one or two days before a new steady state is reached. When changing a maintenance dose it takes six days to achieve 90% and 12 days to achieve 99% of the new steady state (263). Frequent dosing changes do not allow sufficient time to reach a new steady state, which makes evaluation of response difficult. Thus, many factors play a role in determining the response to warfarin. For other less well documented contributing factors the reader is referred to a review article by O'Reilly and Aggeler (171).

10. What is the incidence of drug interactions with warfarin? Discuss the interaction between warfarin and chloral hydrate.

One investigator reviewed the medication profiles of

363 patients who were on long-term anticoagulant therapy. Theoretically, 33% of prescription drugs and 30% of drugs taken as self-medication could have interacted with warfarin; however, the actual incidence of drug interactions in these patients was 9% (221). The potential for drug interactions is great, and the addition or withdrawal of any drug in the therapeutic regimen of patients receiving oral anticoagulants should be carefully monitored with appropriate laboratory tests (120). Numerous reviews are available which include extensive lists of drugs which potentially interact with warfarin (95,97,263,140,215). It is important to read the original literature carefully to assess the significance of a reported interaction with warfarin, since many of the drugs included in such lists may be of little clinical import.

Early reports indicated that chloral hydrate enhanced the metabolism of bishydroxycoumarin (46) and warfarin (137). However, since chloral hydrate is largely metabolized by alcohol dehydrogenase, a nonmicrosomal enzyme, it would not be expected to affect the metabolism of warfarin, which is metabolized by microsomal enzymes.

Trichloroacetic acid, a highly acidic, protein bound metabolite of chloral hydrate has been reported to displace warfarin from protein (26,30,263,208) and may potentiate therapeutic hypoprothrombinemia to a limited extent. This pharmacologic interaction of warfarin with chloral hydrate resulting in transient potentiation of anticoagulant activity does exist, but is clinically insignificant (30,89,195,231,236,237). Because a transient potentiation may occur and because patients frequently take sedative-hypnotics on an as-needed basis, a benzodiazepine would be more appropriate therapy since these drugs do not interact with warfarin (175).

11. J.B. is a 27-year-old male who has been referred for outpatient management of anticoagulant therapy. Pertinent past medical history includes epileptiform seizures secondary to injuries received during the Viet Nam war. He is presently managed on phenobarbital 30 mg tid and phenytoin 100 mg tid. Three weeks ago he was admitted to the hospital with symptoms of pleuritic chest pain, hemoptysis, dyspnea, and tachycardia. A lung scan confirmed the clinical diagnosis of pulmonary embolus. He was appropriately given heparin and begun on warfarin. On his first visit to clinic, his PT was noted to be 14.3 seconds (11.8 control) on 20 mg warfarin. What is the effect of phenobarbital and phenytoin on warfarin therapy?

All of the barbiturates in clinical use in the United States have been reported to induce warfarin metabolism. These include secobarbital (31,197), amobarbital (197), butabarbital (10), aprobarbital (110), heptabarbital (127), and phenobarbital (44,138,139,195).

The extent of enzyme induction in man, in part, may be genetically determined. It is also most likely dependent on the specific inducing drug, on its dosage, and the duration of exposure (263).

Barbiturates (e.g. phenobarbital in doses of 90-210 mg) may induce warfarin metabolizing enzymes after only one or two days of exposure and within one week in almost all cases. However, it may require longer (197). Recovery, after discontinuation of the barbiturate requires a corresponding duration of time (31).

The degree of induction, or the increase in warfarin dose required in J.B. cannot be predicted, and therapy will need to be adjusted based upon frequent laboratory and clinical assessment. The patient needs to be encouraged to take all of the medications on a regular schedule, since adjustment of the barbiturate dose may change his response to warfarin.

Since phenytoin and warfarin are both metabolized by hydroxylation in the liver, the potential for interaction must be considered. Although some investigators have hypothesized an interaction between warfarin and phenytoin, there are no documented cases (122,202). To further confuse the issue, one of these reports suggests an increased anticoagulant effect by phenytoin while the other suggests an increased phenytoin effect by warfarin. Thus, J.G. should be followed closely for signs of altered anticoagulant response as well as phenytoin toxicity.

12. F.P.A. is a 64-year-old white female who has been treated with ASA 600 mg qid for rheumatoid arthritis. Because of the development of left leg thrombophlebitis, she was started on warfarin (5 mg) which produced a protime of 24.6 sec (11.8 control). Since there are potential problems associated with the concomitant administration of ASA and warfarin, which anti-inflammatory agent would you recommend?

The selection of an anti-inflammatory agent for the patient receiving warfarin poses significant problems. All of the anti-inflammatory agents in current clinical use, including salicylates, phenylbutazone, indomethacin, ibuprofen, and glucocorticoids, potentially interact with warfarin. Some of the other problems encountered are not directly related to an interaction with warfarin, but rather to other pharmacologic properties of these agents.

Aspirin is a gastric irritant and can cause gastric bleeding. This property provides a potential site of hemorrhage for the patient on anticoagulant therapy. Other salicylate preparations, including sodium salicylate and choline salicylate are also gastric irritants.

As little as 300 mg of ASA will irreversibly acetylate platelets and thus inhibit their aggregation. The effect of a single dose may last four to seven days, or roughly for the duration of the platelet life span (245). Sodium salicylate does not affect platelet function (244). Likewise, choline salicylate would not be expected to interfere with platelet function.

In addition, large doses (3-8 gm/day) of salicylates intrinsically prolong the prothrombin time (185). Evidence for clinically significant protein displacement of warfarin by salicylates is lacking, although this has been proposed (144).

Phenylbutazone is a gastric irritant and thus may produce hemorrhagic foci. This drug also displaces warfarin from protein so that unbound or active warfarin levels are increased early in therapy. Another characteristic of phenylbutazone is that it selectively inhibits the metabolism of the more active S-isomer (132,206). These observations explain the early and sustained potentiation of warfarin by phenylbutazone (7,172). Phenylbutazone may also inhibit platelet function (35).

Indomethacin, like salicylates and phenylbutazone, has gastric irritant properties, but it has been shown not to interact in a clinically significant fashion with warfarin (239). Like ASA and phenylbutazone, indomethacin has been shown to alter platelet function (262).

Despite early claims that **ibuprofen** would not cause gastric irritation, it is now believed that it does. However, it is felt that there is less irritation with ibuprofen than with other nonsteroidal anti-inflammatory agents. Ibuprofen does not interact with warfarin when administered in doses from 1,200-2,400 mg per day for up to 14 days (178). This agent has been shown to inhibit collagen, ADP, and adrenaline-induced platelet aggregation, but not to the same extent as ASA or indomethacin (163).

Glucocorticoids may cause gastric irritation and may even induce ulceration. (For discussion about this effect, see the chapter on Glucocorticoids.) Corticosteroids have been reported to antagonize the hypoprothrombinemic effect of oral anticoagulants by inducing a hypercoagulable state (241); however, this interaction requires further substantiation. Corticosteroids may cause increased bruising by decreasing the vascular integrity which may predispose a patient to hemorrhage. Corticosteroids do not inhibit platelet function.

It can be concluded that there is no ideal anti-inflammatory agent for the patient on warfarin. Of the agents available for clinical use, ibuprofen is the most attractive because of its relative lack of interfering properties. Corticosteroids are not used except in more severe forms of rheumatoid disease because of other long-term adverse effects. After ibuprofen, choline salicylate or indomethacin may be tried.

13. A 26-year-old woman is taking warfarin for a thromboembolic episode thought to be secondary to oral contraceptives. She is concerned about the effect of warfarin on her menstrual flow. What would you reply?

Menstrual flow may be increased and prolonged in patients on anticoagulants. However, unless there is some underlying pathology of the reproductive tract which would make this condition a great risk by comparison, it is of little significance (8). The patient should be advised to have her prothrombin times checked monthly and she should watch for an unusual increase in flow or blood loss.

The contribution of oral contraceptives to thromboembolic disease is discussed in the chapter, Oral Contraception, in this book as well as in other literature (61,62).

14. A 30-year-old woman has been taking warfarin for continuing therapy of a resolved pulmonary embolus. She has just learned she is pregnant. What would you recommend?

Since the coumarin anticoagulants cross the placental barrier, the fetus is at risk for the direct adverse effects as well as the possible teratogenic effects of the drug (71,101). Nasal bone deformities have been attributed to maternal consumption of warfarin during the first trimester (118); also, stippling of the bones (chondrodysplasia punctata) has more recently been reported in mothers taking warfarin throughout pregnancy (21,179,212,242). However, other factors such as other drugs and diseases cannot be ruled out as teratogens in these cases. Additional risks arise from possible maternal and fetal hemorrhage. Experience has shown that the risk of hemorrhage is lowered if the coumarin therapy is closely monitored and oral therapy is discontinued and replaced with heparin prior to delivery. Heparin does not cross the placenta and is a possible alternative to coumarins.

In the case of this patient, it would be appropriate to determine first if continued anticoagulant therapy is indicated. If it is, then warfarin should not be administered during the first trimester or during delivery and may be replaced by heparin during these periods. If exposure to the drug has already occurred, then appropriate counseling should be arranged.

15. Anticoagulant-induced hemorrhage is one of the most difficult adverse reactions to predict. What are the most common sites of bleeding, and of these, which are most frequently associated with mortality?

Hemorrhage occurred in 8% of over 2400 courses of anticoagulant therapy in a recent survey (39). In these patients, hemorrhage was of sufficient magnitude to require termination of therapy in 2.5%. The remaining episodes of bleeding (5.5%) were considered minor and required alteration of dose, but not discontinuation of therapy. The most common site of major hemorrhage in this series was the gastrointestinal tract. This was followed by vaginal bleeding, wound bleeding, and severe epistaxis. The most common site of minor bleeding was the genitourinary tract. This was followed by epistaxis, then gastrointestinal bleeding.

During long-term anticoagulant therapy, serious hemorrhagic complications most commonly occur intracranially and in the gastrointestinal tract (13,14). In fact, 90% of the serious hemorrhagic episodes that are crippling or fatal are caused by bleeding in these sites. Although hypertension does not appear to increase the risk of hemorrhage in a patient on anticoagulants, the presence of the condition does make hemorrhage worse if it occurs. Gastrointestinal hemorrhage occurs more frequently and is more severe in patients on anticoagulants; it is frequently associated with underlying lesions (e.g. ulcers) and can occur within the therapeutic range of laboratory control (14).

Minor hemorrhage is usually due to capillary breaks and includes purpura, hematomas, episcleral hemorrhage, epistaxis, and hematuria (15,16,17). There seems to be no correlation between minor bleeding and serious bleeding.

Unusual sites of bleeding have included intrapulmonary hemorrhage (192), hemorrhage into the pericardial space (146), intestinal hemorrhage resulting in obstruction (45), adrenal hemorrhage, hemarthroses, and retroperitoneal hemorrhage (141).

Although this list is by no means complete, and there are other reports and figures for incidence of hemorrhage (152), generalizations can be made. Major hemorrhage appears to occur in 2-3% of all courses of anticoagulant therapy, while minor hemorrhage occurs in approximately 4.5%. Bleeding can occur even when laboratory parameters are within the therapeutically accepted range (19).

16. A patient has been receiving warfarin for six months with good laboratory control. He now notes that his urine has a slightly pink color. In the emergency room a prothrombin time of 30 seconds is reported. Upon careful questioning, it is discovered that he took two tablets yesterday, instead of one tablet. The intern wants to administer vitamin K, 20 mg IM. What do you recommend?

No official minimum daily requirement for vitamin K has been established. It has been found experimentally, however, that it is on the order of 0.03 mcg/kg body weight for an adult male (75). Besides dietary sources, some vitamin K is produced by colonic bacteria (235). However, this souce is of little significance since vitamin K instilled into the cecum is reportedly not absorbed (235).

The presence of a pink urine suggests the presence of red cells in the urine. (One should of course rule out the ingestion of interfering drugs such as phenolphthalein.) Microscopic hematuria has been said to occur in approximately one-third of patients on anticoagulant therapy; however, this case represents more than just microscopic bleeding.

Hematuria may be an early sign of more serious bleeding, but in most cases this condition is associated with minor bleeding episodes. In a reliable patient, discontinuing the warfarin until the prothrombin time returns to a therapeutic level usually suffices, although a more rapid return to normal can be accomplished if vitamin K is administered. Administration of 10 mg phytonadione (vitamin K) orally or intravenously will return the prothrombin time to normal within 4 to 24 hours in a case of minor hemorrhage (55,80,214,234). Intramuscular administration provides a site for bleeding and should be avoided. Intravenous administration should be slow, at a rate not exceeding 5 mg per minute to avoid flushing of the face, constriction of the chest, and vascular collapse.

Phytonadione is the only vitamin K that should be used because of its more specific and more rapid effect (232). This is due to the presence of the phytol side chain which is lacking in the menadione derivatives. However, the administration of phytonadione in a situation of minor bleeding can complicate further warfarin therapy since vitamin K may make the patient refractory to warfarin for 7 to 14 days (39,55,181,257).

It would be wise to counsel the patient about the importance of taking his medication properly. Discontinuing the warfarin until the prothrombin time returns to a therapeutic range would be the proper therapy for this patient.

17. A patient has ingested 100 mg of warfarin and now presents with hematemesis and bright red blood per rectum. How would you recommend treating him?

The surreptitious ingestion of warfarin has been well documented either in suicide attempts or in attempts to produce factitious disease (123,168). The presence of a major gastrointestinal hemorrhage indicates that this patient is in much more serious condition than the previous one. In this case, volume replacement as well as replacement of clotting factors is required. This can best be accomplished by the administration of fresh frozen plasma or fresh whole blood (39,181). Vitamin K may also be administered. Larger doses (10-25 mg) are usually given intravenously.

The possibility of a vitamin K-induced hypercoagulable state has been discussed, but this has not been documented in the literature (181).

18. Discuss how heparin acts as an anticoagulant,

its half-life, and route of elimination. By what route should it be administered and what is the therapeutic endpoint?

In contrast to the slow, indirect acting oral anticoagulants, heparin is a rapid acting anticoagulant that is effective only when administered parenterally (53,59).

Heparin prevents clot formation by dramatically accelerating the action of a naturally occurring inhibitor of thrombin, antithrombin III. Heparin induces a conformational change in antithrombin III which results in rapid inhibition of thrombin (200,201). Antithrombin also neutralizes the activated forms of factors XII, XI, IX, X and probably VII, and this effect is also accelerated by heparin. The effect that heparin has on platelets may vary. It has been claimed that platelets in normal subjects given heparin obtained from beef lung showed slower aggregation than subjects who had been given heparin obtained from hog mucosa (160). However, this has been disputed (217). While the effect of heparin *in vivo* on platelets is debatable (164,200), there does not appear to be conclusive evidence indicating a therapeutic advantage for one source over another.

The plasma half-life of heparin is one and one-half hours (66,67) and does not change with dose; however, the pharmacologic half-life is dose-dependent and increases with increasing dose (159). After injection of 100, 200, and 400 units/kg, the pharmacologic half-lives are 56, 96, and 152 minutes respectively.

Following intravenous administration of heparin, an anticoagulant effect is noted immediately. Heparin, in doses less than 5000 units, is primarily metabolized in the liver. With larger doses, approximately 20% is excreted unchanged in the urine (63). It has been proposed that heparin is metabolized in the liver by an enzyme, heparinase, and then excreted as uro-heparin (107).

Heparin may be administered intravenously, subcutaneously, or intramuscularly. Intramuscular administration should be avoided because of the potential for hematoma formation (53,87,111). Subcutaneous and intravenous administration will be discussed in more detail in following questions.

Heparin therapy is aimed at achieving a clotting time which is 1½-2½ the control value (i.e. the pre-heparin clotting time). Several tests may be used, but the APTT or ACT tests offer the best correlation for control for heparin therapy (19,98).

19. What other pharmacological actions besides prolongation of the blood clotting time does heparin have? Are these clinically useful?

Other pharmacologic actions of heparin include a lipemia clearing action (64); blockade of the local and generalized Schwartzman and Arthrus phenomena;

inactivation of serotonin and certain snake venoms; and an increase in the I^{131} triiodothyronine uptake of red blood cells (3). This drug has also been recommended for the treatment of asthma, weeping exzema, and hay fever (57).

Despite all of these proposed uses for heparin, it is used clinically only for the treatment of thrombotic conditions.

20. Heparin is the anticoagulant that is used to initiate anticoagulant therapy when an immediate effect is desired. Discuss the advantages and disadvantages of intermittent versus continuous intravenous infusion of heparin.

Traditionally, heparin has been administered intravenously on an intermittent basis. Usually 5000 to 15,000 units are administered every four to six hours (91,247). This method provides supratherapeutic levels of heparin immediately after injection and subtherapeutic levels just prior to the next dose.

Continuous intravenous infusion is designed to prevent this and has been suggested by many studies (51,58,87,94,143,176,224). Such an infusion is much easier to control if a constant infusion pump is used (94,224). Laboratory control of continuous infusion is best done using the APTT (19,51) or the ACT tests (224) since these require a minimum of time to perform and can be used to immediately determine if any alteration in dosage is necessary. The therapeutic clotting time should be in the range of 1½-2½ times a patient's control.

There are numerous disadvantages for the use of intermittent administration. There is a requirement for large doses and frequent injections; the clotting tests must be done at certain times (just prior to the next scheduled dose); and there is difficulty in maintaining the clotting time in the therapeutic range (224). The advantage is that the method requires less sophisticated administration equipment.

Continuous infusion offers numerous advantages. There is flexibility in dosage adjustment; less heparin is required; clotting times can be done at any time; and the clotting time can be maintained continuously in the therapeutic range (224).

Salzman (204) has demonstrated that continuous infusion of heparin, to 1½ to 2½ times the control APTT, is associated with less bleeding than is intermittent infusion of heparin, with or without laboratory control.

21. A.T. has just been admitted to the hospital with symptoms of a pulmonary embolus. It is decided to give him heparin therapy intravenously. You have suggested continuous therapy and are asked to determine the proper dosage. A.T. weighs 70 kg. Describe the proper dosage regimen for this patient.

Heparin should be administered immediately when

there is a high suspicion that a pulmonary embolism has occurred (229). Intravenous doses of 5,000 to 15,000 units of heparin are administered after baseline clotting tests are obtained (79). An initial heparin resistance exists that is partially due to the release of platelet factor 4, a protein within platelets that neutralizes heparin and is released during thrombotic events (156). Larger doses of the drug may also be necessary to overcome the enhanced platelet-thrombin interaction (227).

Once this initial bolus dose is administered, continuous infusion of heparin may be started. A minimum heparin dose of 35-50 units/kg is required to anticoagulate blood to a clinically desirable level (66). Since this patient weighs 70 kg, it will be necessary to maintain a level of from 2,450 to 3,500 units in the body at all times. Because the half-life of heparin is 1½ hours, the infusion can be started at the rate of 1,225 to 1,750 units every 1½ hours or 900-1,200 units every hour. If no loading dose or bolus dose was administered, then therapy should include an initial dose of 2,450-3,500 units. This amount is usually exceeded by the initial dose recommendation of 5,000-15,000 units; thus, the continuous infusion can be started 1½ hours after the bolus has been given. Therapy should be monitored closely; any deviation in laboratory control can be adjusted by altering the rate of infusion. The heparin solution should be administered through a constant infusion pump, not by gravity flow, because the flow-rate can be altered if the patient changes position and nursing error is more likely to occur in "speeding-up" or "slowing-down" the intravenous solution.

Because there is an initial insensitivity to heparin (53,91) a return to normal sensitivity and a decrease in dose requirement should be anticipated over time. Frequent laboratory assessment of clotting tests will enable detection of these changes.

22. A 60-year-old male is entering the hospital for an elective cholecystectomy. He has a history of thromboembolism secondary to varicose veins and venous stasis. The surgeons have heard of a new regimen of low-dose subcutaneous anticoagulant therapy. Describe the indications for and proper administration of this therapy.

Clinical evidence indicates that patients are at a higher risk for deep venous thrombosis during the postoperative period; this phenomenon persists until at least the seventh postoperative day. The period of reactivation following postoperative immobilization is another critical time for thrombus formation (210). Studies using ^{125}I fibrinogen have shown that approximately 20-30% of all surgical patients, 40-50% of elderly surgical patients, and more than 50% of patients who undergo hip-nailing procedures or prostatec-

tomies develop postoperative venous thrombosis (106,157).

Some researches have postulated that if the hypercoagulable state that occurs in the operative period can be prevented, embolism can be prevented (210). This theory serves as the basis for the administration of low-dose subcutaneous heparin to prevent venous thrombosis. Both encouraging (4, 76, 77, 113, 114, 124, 158, 211, 248, 253) and discouraging (12, 68, 77, 95, 199) results have been reported; however, the International Multicenter Trial published in 1975 is strong evidence for the efficacy of this procedure (114). While the design of the trial may be criticized (213), the results do show clinically significant benefits in reduction of venous thrombosis and pulmonary embolism with low doses of subcutaneous heparin. Furthermore, this form of heparin therapy is associated with a small, generally insignificant risk of bleeding (77).

Low-dose heparin is most effective for elective gynecological or abdominothoracic surgery (37,76,77,86,113,124,158,211,253). However, prevention of venous thromboembolism is less effective after hip fracture (76,112), elective hip surgery (92,150), or prostatic surgery (158). Low-dose heparin may also be useful in prophylaxis of venous thromboembolism in certain high-risk medical patients (76).

The use of heparin in low subcutaneous doses augments the activity of an inhibitor of activated factor X (113,248). This inhibitor of factor Xa, or anti-Xa, is probably the same as antithrombin III (259), and thus may share the previously mentioned activities of antithrombin III.

The protocols for low-dose heparin generally recommend that 5000 units of heparin be administered subcutaneously from 2 (76,113,158) to 12 hours (211,253) preoperatively and that this dose be continued every 8 to 12 hours for 5 to 7 days postoperatively, or until the patient is fully mobile. APTT values indicate that the clotting time is moderately elevated for approximately five hours after 5,000 units of heparin has been administered subcutaneously (76).

It is important when heparin is administered subcutaneously (usually in the fat of the abdomen) that the area of injection is not traumatized because of the risk for bleeding. Heparin should not be administered intramuscularly because of the risk of hematoma formation (87).

23. A patient who has been treated with heparin is to be discharged from the hospital because his pulmonary embolus has resolved. The medical staff would like to continue him on anticoagulant therapy and have decided to switch him to warfarin. What is the best method for switching from heparin to warfarin? Will heparin prolong the prothrombin time?

Heparin therapy should be continued for 7 to 10 days following a pulmonary embolus. Since the onset of warfarin's anticoagulant effect is delayed, both heparin and warfarin may be given simultaneously from the first day, or alternatively warfarin may be started on the third to the fifth day of heparin therapy (55,82). Occasionally, heparin and warfarin are begun simultaneously and the heparin is discontinued in 48 hours. This is usually done when a loading dose of warfarin is administered and is based on the incorrect supposition that the therapeutic effects of warfarin have been achieved (2,181). As discussed earlier, the early prolongation of the prothrombin time only reflects the depletion of factor VII, and it should be re-emphasized that depletion of this factor does not afford protection from thromboembolism (54). See Question 7.

Heparin and maintenance doses of warfarin are administered concurrently until a therapeutic prothrombin time is reached. However, care must be taken to measure the prothrombin time when heparin's effect is at a minimum, since heparin will interfere with determination of the one-stage prothrombin time (151). When heparin is administered on an intermittent basis, the prothrombin time should be measured just before the next dose of heparin. With continuous-infusion heparin, the prothrombin time may be monitored at any time during the infusion. There may be a prolongation of one or two seconds in the prothrombin time during continuous infusion (204). Low-dose subcutaneous heparin may cause transient prolongation in the PT, but only immediately after administration.

24. Are female patients at a higher risk for complications of heparin therapy?

Some evidence indicates that elderly females over the age of 60 are at a greater risk for bleeding complications secondary to heparin (109,240). These authors report a statistically significant difference between age and sex in the risk of bleeding. Other drugs which affect platelet function, such as aspirin or phenylbutazone were not specifically eliminated as a contributing cause of bleeding in either study. The failure of these investigators to express the doses of heparin in terms of body weight tends to invalidate their studies (240). A subsequent prospective study did not confirm an increased incidence of bleeding in elderly females (19). Nevertheless, until there is substantial evidence to the contrary, it seems reasonable to use extra care in monitoring these patients for signs of bleeding.

25. Mrs. Brown has been receiving heparin 5,000 units (5cc of 1,000 units/cc) every 6 hours for 5 days for treatment of a pulmonary embolism. Her ACTs

have been 2 minutes 50 seconds on this regimen. On the 6th day she inadvertently was given 50,000 units (5cc of 10,000 units/cc). Within one-half hour she was noted to be diaphoretic and hypotensive. Bright red blood was noted upon rectal examination and a large retroperitoneal mass was noted. How should this patient be managed?

Mrs. Brown has definite signs of hemorrhage from the gastrointestinal tract, a site associated with considerable mortality. The drug should be discontinued immediately, and in this case specific treatment should include maintenance of fluid volume and replacement of clotting factors. Unlike albumin, fresh whole blood or fresh frozen plasma provide clotting factors (252). If hemorrhage is not present and the only manifestation of the overdose is a prolonged clotting time, administration of the drug can simply be discontinued and the effects will clear in a few hours.

Since heparin is highly negatively charged, agents with a positive charge have been used to antagonize its effects. Protamine sulfate is most useful immediately after the administration of heparin. It is infused intravenously as a 1% solution in a dose of 1 mg per 100 units of heparin. However, if a significant period of time has elapsed, the dose of protamine must be reduced. Protamine itself acts as an anticoagulant in high doses (82).

26. A 41-year-old male with a history of angina pectoris was treated with daily subcutaneous injections of heparin (20,000 units). After one year of therapy, the patient fell and fractured his ribs. Generalized demineralization of the skeleton was observed in the patient's X-rays. Can this condition have been caused by the heparin injections? What other side effects may be caused by heparin?

The development of *osteoporosis* has been associated with the administration of more than 10,000 units of heparin for six months or longer (88,108). The size of the dose appears to be more important than the duration of therapy. Symptoms resolve upon discontinuation of therapy. The incidence of osteoporosis as a result of anticoagulant therapy is low, and this condition may reflect the more common use of oral coumarin anticoagulants in the long-term treatment of thromboembolic disease, rather than heparin.

Other problems of heparin therapy include generalized *hypersensitivity* reactions such as rhinitis, urticaria, conjunctivitis, and a reversible temporal alopecia (260).

Heparin may interfere with aldosterone secretion and cause *hypoaldosteronism* (254). This can occur in healthy and edematous salt-restricted patients who receive 30,000-40,000 units of heparin per day (142). It usually takes four to five days for this rare side effect to become apparent and a corresponding time for aldosterone levels to return to normal. These patients should be monitored for elevated potassium levels.

Thrombocytopenia secondary to heparin administration was first recognized in the early 1960s (85,155). Recently it has been reported with increased frequency (18,22,74,193). Despite extensive investigation, the exact mechanism for the thrombocytopenia has not been established. It characteristically occurs after 3 to 12 days of heparin therapy, is unrelated to dose, and resolves 3 to 5 days after heparin is discontinued. Since thrombocytopenia increases the risk for bleeding in patients already on an anticoagulant, it is important to carefully look for its occurrence with frequent platelet counts and smears.

27. A 46-year-old sales executive with rapidly progressive angina is unresponsive to nitroglycerin, weight reduction, and propranolol. Is this patient a candidate for anticoagulant therapy?

Anticoagulants are usually not indicated for the treatment of angina. When deciding whether to use anticoagulants for any condition, the risks must be weighed against the potential advantages. Some health professionals have suggested that anticoagulants "benefit" these patients if they are given within two years of the onset of symptoms. However, most clinicians do not feel that anticoagulants play a role in the treatment of angina (135).

28. A 65-year-old female with atrial fibrillation that is unresponsive to antiarrhythmic agents is admitted to the hospital for elective DC electrocardioversion. Should she be placed on anticoagulants prior to this procedure?

Anticoagulation is recommended for patients prior to electrocardioversion therapy if they have chronic coronary heart disease, mitral valvular disease, cardiomyopathy, prosthetic heart valves, or have recently suffered a myocardial infarction. Because the risk of reversion to the original rhythm disturbance is greater within the first month, it is recommended by some health professionals that anticoagulation be continued for four weeks after this procedure (191).

29. A patient has just suffered his first acute myocardial infarction. In addition to the usual protocol, it is decided that he will be treated with heparin and then warfarin. Do you concur?

Since the early 1960s various clinical trials have been conducted in attempts to define whether anticoagulants are beneficial in the treatment of myocardial infarction. There is still no agreement on this controversy (38,149,198).

Many studies have failed to meet the criteria required for a good clinical trial (70,84a,90). Although some of the studies that have met the criteria have

reported a decreased mortality in treated patients (41,42,148,228), it is now generally accepted that mortality is not altered by anticoagulant therapy. It has been shown in some studies that morbidity (strokes and non-fatal systemic emboli) may be decreased with anticoagulant therapy (43,60,256). One review indicated that anticoagulants reduced the morbidity of patients who had an admitting serum glutamic oxaloacetic transaminase greater than 150, a white blood count of greater than 15,000/mm³, congestive heart failure, a history of previous infarction, and who were older than 60 (60).

If it is decided that a patient is to be treated with anticoagulants, a careful history of previous bleeding must be obtained so that a patient is not exposed to additional risk.

In summary, anticoagulants may be useful in the high-risk patient during hospital recuperation from a myocardial infarction, but anticoagulant therapy is not acceptable at present for all myocardial infarction patients. Early mobilization or treatment with low-dose subcutaneous heparin (76,243) may be more useful in preventing thrombosis.

30. A 26-year-old airline pilot is admitted to the hospital with a chief complaint of severe precordial chest pain of two days duration. Two weeks before admission he noted the onset of pain and tenderness in his left calf with mild left-sided ankle edema. A lung scan showed a perfusion defect of the right upper lobe and left lower lobe.

A pulmonary arteriogram revealed the same defect. His activated clotting time was 1 minute 25 seconds. It was felt that the patient had multiple pulmonary emboli, probably secondary to left leg thrombophlebitis and venous stasis. How should anticoagulant therapy be initiated? How long should it be maintained?

Anticoagulants are the treatment of choice for pulmonary emboli. The actual incidence of pulmonary embolism has not changed much, but because more sophisticated diagnostic procedures are available, more cases are diagnosed (47,225).

When anticoagulant therapy is indicated, heparin is the drug of choice because of its immediate onset of action. However, heparin therapy is only prophylactic. It prevents the development and propagation of a thrombus from the area of the embolus into the pulmonary artery and further prevents thrombus formation at original thrombus site (216). Although lysis of the embolus begins in 24 hours, three weeks or more are required for complete resolution (50). The body's own fibrinolytic system is responsible for lysis of the embolus since heparin is devoid of any fibrinolytic activity.

Because each patient responds differently to heparin, initial dosages used in treating pulmonary embolism vary. Early in the course of massive pulmonary embolism, large doses may have little effect on clotting parameters (53). As the acute episode clears, normal sensitivity returns and lower dosages are needed. Intravenous dosages range from 5,000 to 10,000 units every 4 to 6 hours. Because resolution of an embolus may take several weeks, oral anticoagulants are frequently given. Since warfarin has a delayed onset of action, it should be initiated simultaneously with heparin. After seven to ten days the therapeutic response to warfarin should have been achieved and heparin can be discontinued (180,182,216).

Little agreement exists regarding the duration of anticoagulant therapy in the treatment of pulmonary embolism. Unless there is a past history of venous thromboembolism, a recurrent thrombotic tendency, or a continuing predisposing cause, it is unnecessary to continue treatment beyond six weeks (48,49,176).

31. Drugs that affect platelet behavior have been suggested as possible alternatives to anticoagulants in the treatment of both arterial and venous thromboembolism. What is the present clinical status of these agents?

Several comprehensive reviews have appeared in the recent literature which discuss the clinical use of antiplatelet drugs (84,244,245) and describe the various mechanisms of action of these drugs (78,103,153,154).

The possible indications for antiplatelet agents in the treatment of arterial thromboembolism include patients with prosthetic heart valves, cerebrovascular disorders, coronary heart disease, peripheral vascular disease, and renal allograft rejection. Antiplatelet drugs have also been proposed to be of value in the treatment of venous thromboembolism.

Many drugs have been reported to affect platelet behavior (153,154), but only a few have been shown to have potential value in the treatment of thromboembolic disease. Those drugs with the greatest promise include aspirin, clofibrate, dextran, dipyridamole, hydroxychloroquine, and sulfinpyrazone. Other agents which may affect platelet behavior are listed in Table 2.

Aspirin, by acetylation of platelets and possibly by inhibition of prostaglandins, inhibits collagen-induced ADP release and epinephrine-induced platelet aggregation. As little as 300 mg will accomplish this effect for the lifetime of the platelets (245).

Studies of the use of aspirin in the treatment of transient ischemic attacks (TIAs) and ischemic heart disease are promising but inconclusive in that there are some major weaknesses in study design. Some well designed cooperative clinical trials of aspirin in both of these conditions are currently underway, and

it is hoped that these studies will provide more conclusive evidence of the effect or lack of effect of aspirin in these conditions.

The trials of aspirin in venous thromboembolism are also inconclusive, and no benefit has been shown with their use. Aspirin may be useful in the treatment of peripheral ischemia in patients with thrombocytosis and spontaneous platelet aggregation.

Clofibrate has been shown to reduce platelet adhesion and to prolong platelet survival in some patients with coronary artery disease. However, these studies suffer from poor trial design and clofibrate cannot be recommended for this use. This drug has no clinical antithrombotic effect in the prevention of cerebrovascular or coronary artery disease.

Dextran suppresses platelet function by a mechanism which is unclear. It may alter platelet membranes, interfere with platelet procoagulant (factor 3) availability, or inhibit the spreading capability of platelets. The effects are dose-related and are more pronounced with the high molecular weight dextran.

Dextran is most useful in the prevention of venous thromboembolism. The results have been conflicting, however, in that there are an equal number of reports which document the efficacy and the lack of efficacy of this drug. At present, it cannot be recommended to replace anticoagulants.

Although in pharmacological doses (400 mg qd), *dipyridamole* does not affect platelet behavior, higher concentrations *in vitro* inhibit platelet aggregation. Clinically, the combination of dipyridamole and warfarin is more effective than warfarin alone in preventing embolization from prosthetic valves. Its usefulness has not been demonstrated in venous thromboembolism, cerebrovascular disease, or coronary heart disease.

Hydroxychloroquine in doses of 500 mg per day appears promising in the prevention of venous thromboembolism. It weakly inhibits platelet aggregation induced by ADP. Its use in other conditions has not been documented.

Table 2

DRUGS AFFECTING PLATELET BEHAVIOR THAT ARE NOT USED CLINICALLY FOR THIS PURPOSE

Alcohol	Indomethacin
Carbenicillin	Lidocaine
Chlorpromazine	Nitrofurantoin
Colchicine	Penicillin
Cyproheptadine	Phenformin
Ethacrynic acid	Phenylbutazone
Furosemide	Promethazine
Guaifenesin	Prostaglandin E
Heparin	Theophylline
Ibuprofen	Tricyclic antidepressants

Sulfinpyrazone inhibits platelet release and pro-longs platelet survival. The best evidence for an antithrombotic effect of sulfinpyrazone comes from its ability to reduce the incidence of shunt thrombosis in patients with arteriovenous shunts used for chronic hemodialysis. Its use in coronary artery disease or in the treatment of cerebral ischemia must be substantiated by further clinical trials.

CASE HISTORY FOR STUDY

M.J. is a 48-year-old white male with a past history of intravenous drug abuse. Three years ago he developed staphylococcal and candida endocarditis requiring treatment with methicillin and amphotericin B. Upon resolution of his endocarditis, a Bjork-Shiley (tilting disc) mitral valve prosthesis was implanted because of mitral stenosis and recurrent heart failure. Other significant past medical history included hepatitis in 1965.

Medications have included warfarin 5 mg daily, methadone (dose managed by methadone maintenance clinic), digoxin 0.25 mg daily, ferrous sulfate 0.325 tid, and diazepam 10 mg tid. He admitted to occasional alcohol ingestion. He denied over-the-counter drug use.

His anticoagulant therapy has been complicated by several episodes of hemorrhage which required hospitalization. These have included a major gastrointestinal hemorrhage which resulted in bowel necrosis, requiring resection; a major uroligic bleeding episode; and several soft tissue bleeding episodes. His prothrombin times during these episodes ranged from 18.0 to 71.8 seconds.

Throughout these episodes, which required vitamin K administration as well as fresh-frozen plasma and whole blood, he denied taking his medications other than as directed. He denied changes in his diet. He denied any acute illnesses such as fevers, chills, GI disorders or symptoms consistent with any other metabolic disorder. With the exception of prothrombin times, laboratory data including plasma warfarin levels were not unusual.

Because of frequent hemorrhagic events and questionable reliability of the patient, warfarin was discontinued and aspirin 0.650 gm qd, and dipyridamole 100 mg qid were begun. He has remained free of thromboembolic and hemorrhagic reactions to date.

REFERENCES

1. Anticoagulants in myocardial infarction. Med Lett 16:17, 1974
2. Anticoagulants in thromboembolism. Med J Aust 2:1097, 1972.
3. Heparin, NEJM 279:320, 1968.
4. Low dose heparin prophylaxis of deep vein thrombosis. Med Lett 15:35, 1973.
5. Clinical uses of heparin. Med Lett 6:21, 1964.
6. Aagard GN: Drug spotlight on anticoagulants. Postgrad Med 55:212, 1974.
7. Aggeler PM et al: Potentiation of anticoagulant effect of warfarin by phenylbutazone. NEJM 276:496, 1967.
8. Alexander B et al: A guide to anticoagulant therapy. Circ. 34:123, 1961.
9. Allison, SB et al: The activated clotting time in the control of heparin therapy. Bull Geisinger Med Ctr 21:199, 1969.
10. Antlitz AM et al: Effect of butabarbital on orally administered anticoagulants. Curr Ther Res 10:70, 1968.
11. Aoki N: Japanese not hypersensitive to warfarin. NEJM 285:1327, 1971.
12. Arden GP et al: Subcutaneous heparin treatment. Brit Med J 2:486, 1972.
13. Askey JM: Hemorrhage during long-term anticoagulant drug therapy, Part I: Intracranial hemorrhage. Calif Med 104:6, 1966.
14. Askey JM: Hemorrhage during long-term anticoagulant drug therapy, Part II: Gastrointestinal hemorrhage. Calif Med 104:88, 1966.
15. Askey, JM: Hemorrhage during long-term anticoagulant drug therapy, Part III: The relationship of minor to serious bleeding. Calif Med 104:175, 1966.
16. Askey JM: Hemorrhage during long-term anticoagulant drug therapy, Part IV: Selection and management of patients. Calif Med 104:284, 1966.
17. Askey JM: Hemorrhage during long-term anticoagulant drug therapy, Part V: Unusual bleeding episodes. Calif Med 104:377, 1966.
18. Babcock RB et al: Heparin-induced immune thrombocytopenia. NEJM 295:237, 1976.
19. Basu, D et al: A prospective study of the value of monitoring heparin treatment with the activated partial thromboplastin time. NEJM 287:324, 1972.
20. Bauer G: Clinical experiences of a surgeon in the use of heparin. Amer J Card 14:29, 1964.
21. Becker MH et al: Chondrodysplasia punctata. Is maternal warfarin therapy a factor? Amer J Dis Child 129:356, 1975.
22. Bell WR et al: Thrombocytopenia occurring during the administration of heparin. A prospective study in 52 patients. Ann Int Med 85:155, 1976.
23. Bennett B et al: Blood coagulation mechanism. Clin Hematol 2:3, 1973.
24. Bennett B et al: The normal coagulation mechanism. Med Clin N Amer 56:95, 1972.
25. Biggs R (editor): *Human Blood Coagulation, Haemostasis and Thrombosis.* Blackwell Scientific Publications, London, 1972, p 607.
26. Bostom Collaborative Drug Surveillance Program: Interaction between chloral hydrate and warfarin. NEJM 286:53, 1972.
27. Bove, LG: No load warfarin therapy — long overdue. J Maine Med Assoc 63:159, 1972.
28. Bowie, EJW et al: Evaluation of the hemostatic mechanism. Med Clin N Amer 54:889, 1970.
29. Breckenridge A et al: Kinetics of warfarin absorption in man. Clin Pharmacol Ther 14:955, 1973.
30. Breckenridge A et al: Drug interactions with dichloral-phenazone, chloral hydrate, and phenazone (antipyrine). Clin Sci 40:351, 1971.
31. Breckenridge A et al: Dose-dependent enzyme induction. Clin Pharmacol Ther 14:514, 1973.
32. Brogden RN et al: Streptokinase: a review of its clinical pharmacology, mechanism of action and therapeutic uses. Drugs 5:357, 1973.
33. Carey LC et al: Comparative effects of dicumarol, tranexan, and heparin on thrombus propogation. Ann Surg 152:919, 1960.
34. Castleman B (editor): Normal laboratory values. Case records of the Massachusetts General Hospital. NEJM 290:39, 1974.
35. Cazenave JP: Inhibition of platelet adherence to a collagen coated surface by non-steroidal antiinflammatory drugs, pyrimido-pyrimidine and tricyclic compounds and lidocaine. J Lab Clin Med 83:797, 1974.
36. Chan KK et al: Absolute configuration of the four warfarin alcohols. J Med Chem 15:1265, 1972.
37. Clagett GP et al: Prevention of venous thromboembolism in surgical patients. NEJM 290:93, 1974.
38. Controversy in Internal Medicine. Edited by FJ Ingelfinger, AS Relman, M Finland. Philadelphia, WB Saunders Company, 1974.
39. Coon WW et al: Some aspects of the pharmacology of oral anticoagulants. Clin Pharmacol Ther 11:312, 1970.
40. Coon WW et al: Hemorrhagic Complications of Anticoagulant Therapy. Arch Int Med 133:386, 1976.
41. Cooperative Study: Long-term anticoagulant therapy after myocardial infarction. JAMA 193:929, 1965.
42. Cooperative Study: Long-term anticoagulant therapy after myocardial infarction. Final report of the veterans administra-

tion cooperative study. JAMA 207:2263, 1969.

43. Cooperative Clinical Trial: Anticoagulants in acute myocardial infarction. JAMA 225:724, 1973.

44. Corn M: Effect of phenobarbital and glutethimide on biological half-life of warfarin. Thromb Diath Haemorrh 16:606, 1966.

45. Crisler C et al: Intestinal obstruction in patients receiving anticoagulants. Med Clin N Amer 50:1009, 1970.

46. Cucinell SA et al: The effect of chloral hydrate on bishydroxycoumarin metabolism, a fatal outcome. JAMA 197:366, 1966.

47. Cugel DW et al: The limitations of laboratory methods in the diagnosis of pulmonary embolism. Med Clin N Amer 51:175, 1967.

48. Dalen JE et al: Resolution rate of actue pulmonary embolism. Med Clin N Amer 51:175, 1967.

49. Dalen JE et al: Resolution rate of acute pulmonary embolism in man. NEJM 280:1194, 1969.

50. Dalen JE et al: Diagnosis and management of massive pulmonary embolism. Dis Month (Aug) 1967.

51. Davies EW: The laboratory control of intravenous heparin therapy. Med J Aust 2:1001, 1971.

52. Deykin D: Emerging concepts of platelet function. NEJM 290:144, 1974.

53. Deykin D: The use of heparin. NEJM 280:937, 1969.

54. Deykin D: Warfarin therapy. NEJM 283:691 & 801, 1970.

55. Deykin D: Local and systemic factors in the pathogenesis of thrombosis. Calif Med 112:31, 1970.

56. Didisheim R: Tests of blood coagulation and hemostasis I. The prothrombin time. JAMA 196:33, 1966.

57. Dougherty TF et al: Physiologic actions of heparin not related to blood clotting. Am J Cardiol 14:18, 1964.

58. Douglas AS: Management of thrombotic diseases. Semin Hematol 8:95, 1971.

59. Douglas AS et al: Anticoagulant and thrombolytic therapy. Clin Hematol 2:175, 1973.

60. Drapkin A et al: Anticoagulant therapy after acute myocardial infarction. Relation of therapeutic benefit to patient's age, sex, and severity of infarction. JAMA 222:541, 1972.

61. Drill JA et al: Oral contraceptives and thromboembolic disease II: Estrogen content of oral contraceptives. JAMA 219:593, 1974.

62. Drill JA: Oral contraceptives and thromboembolic disease, I. Prospective and retrospective studies. JAMA 219:583, 1972.

63. Eiker HB et al: Studies with radioactive heparin in humans. Angiology 11:40, 1960.

64. Engelberg H: Heparin and the removal of triglyceride from the blood stream. Am J Cardiol 14:8, 1964.

65. Engelberg H: The clinical use of heparin. Curr Ther Res 18:34, 1975 (supp).

66. Estes JW: Kinetics of the anticoagulant effect of heparin. JAMA 212:1492, 1970.

67. Estes JW et al: A retrospective study of the pharmacokinetics of heparin. Clin Pharm Ther 10:329, 1970.

68. Evarts CM et al: Thromboembolism after total hip reconstruction. Failure of low doses of heparin in prevention. JAMA 225:515, 1973.

69. Fearnside ML et al: Long-term anticoagulation in venous thromboembolism disease by subcutaneous calcium heparin injection. Med J Aust 2:891, 1971.

70. Feinstein AR: More blood for the anticoagulant battle. NEJM 292:1400, 1975.

71. Fillmore SJ et al: Effect of coumarin compounds on the fetus. Ann Int Med 73:731, 1970.

72. Finlayson JS: Crosslinking of fibrin. Sem Thromb Hemostasis 1:33, 1974.

73. Flannery, EP et al: Japanese restaurant syndrome. NEJM 285:412, 1971.

74. Fratantoni JC et al: Heparin-induced thrombocytopenia: confirmation of diagnosis with in vitro methods. Blood 45:395, 1975.

75. Frick PG et al: Dose response and minimal daily requirement for vitamin K in man. J Appl Physiol 23:387, 1967.

76. Gallus AS et al: Small subcutaneous doses of heparin in prevention of venous thrombosis. NEJM 288:11, 1973.

77. Gallus AS et al: Prevention of venous thrombosis with small, subcutaneous doses of heparin. JAMA 235:1980, 1976.

78. Gallus AS et al: Antithrombotic drugs. Part II. Drugs 12:132, 1976.

79. Gallus AS et al: Antithrombotic drugs. Part I. Drugs 12:41, 1976.

80. Gamble JR et al: Clinical comparison of vitamin K_1 and water soluble vitamin K. Arch Int Med, 95:52, 1955.

81. Gaston LW: The blood-clotting factors. NEJM 270:236 & 290, 1964.

82. Genton E: Guidelines for heparin therapy. Ann Int Med 80:77, 1974.

83. Genton E et al: Observations in anticoagulant and thrombolytic therapy in pulmonary embolism. Prog Cardiovas Dis 17:335, 1975.

84. Genton et al: Platelet-inhibiting drugs in the prevention of clinical thrombotic disease. NEJM 293:1174, 1236, 1296; 1975.

84a. Gifford RH et al: A critique of methodology in studies of anticoagulant therapy for acute myocardial infarction. NEJM 280:351, 1969.

85. Godlub S et al: Heparin induced thrombocytopenia in man. J Lab Clin Med 59:430, 1962.

86. Gordon-Smith IC et al: Controlled trial of two regimens of subcutaneous heparin prevention of postoperative deep-vein thrombosis. Lancet 1:1133, 1972.

87. Griffith GC et al: The clinical usage of heparin. Amer J Cardiol 14:39, 1964.

88. Griffith GC et al: Heparin osteoporosis. JAMA 193.85, 1965.

89. Griner PF et al: Chloral hydrate and warfarin interaction: clinical significance? Ann Int Med 74:540, 1971.

90. Gross H et al: Anticoagulant therapy in myocardial infarction, an overview of methodology. Am J Med 52:421, 1972.

91. Gurewich V et al: Some guidelines for heparin therapy of venous thromboembolic disease. JAMA 199:116, 1967.

92. Hampson WGJ: Failure of low-dose heparin to prevent deep-vein thrombosis after hip replacement arthroplasty. Lancet 4:1, 1974.

93. Handley AJ: Heparin administration by constant infusion pump. Brit Med J 2:482, 1967.

94. Handley AJ: Low-dose heparin after myocardial infarction. Lancet 11:623, 1972.

95. Hansten PD: Drug Interactions, 2nd ed. Lea & Febiger, Phila., 1973.

96. Harker LA et al: Studies of platelet and fibrinogen kinetics in patients with prosthetic heart valves. NEJM 283:1302, 1970.

97. Hartshorn EA: Handbook of Drug Interactions. Drug Intelligence Publ., Hamilton, Ill., 1970.

98. Hattersly PG: Activated coagulation time of whole blood. JAMA 196:436, 1966.

99. Hattersly PG: The activated coagulation time of whole blood as a routine pre-operative screening test. Calif Med 114:15, 1971.

100. Hewick DS et al: Plasma half-lives, plasma metabolites and anticoagulant efficacies of the enantiomers of warfarin in man. J Pharm Pharmacol 25:458, 1973.

101. Hirsh J et al: Anticoagulants in pregnancy. A review of indications and complications. Am Heart J 83:301, 1972.

102. Hirsh J: The value of monitoring heparin therapy in the prevention of occurrence in patients with venous thromboembolic disease. Thromb Diath Haemorrh 56:181, 1973 Suppl.

103. Hirsh J et al: The current status of platelet suppressive drugs in the treatment of thrombosis. Thromb Diath Haemorrh 33:406, 1975.

104. Hoak, JC et al: The antithrombotic properties of coumarin drugs. Ann Int Med 54:73, 1961.

105. Hougie C: Recalcification time test and its modifications (PTT, APTT and expanded PTT) in Hematology, Williams WJ et al (Ed) McGraw Hill, New York 1972 pp 1400-1403.

106. Hume M et al: 1^{125} fibrinogen and the prevention of venous thrombosis. Arch Surg 107:803, 1973.

107. Jaques, LB et al: The disappearance of heparin activity with liver globulins and determinations of heparinase. Thromb Diath Hemorrh 10:71, 1963.

108. Jaffe MD et al: Multiple fractures associated with long-term sodium heparin therapy. JAMA 193:158, 1965.

109. Jick H et al: Efficacy and toxicity of heparin in relation to age and sex. NEJM 279:284, 1968.

110. Johansson SA: Apparent resistance to oral anticoagulant therapy and influence of hypnotics on some coagulation factors. Act Med Scand 184:297, 1968.

111. Jorpes JE: Heparin, its chemistry, pharmacology, and clincial use. Am J Med 33:692, 1962.

112. Kakker VV et al: Lancet 11:101, 1972.

113. Kakkar VV et al: Low doses of heparin in prevention of deep-vein thrombosis. Lancet 11:669, 1971.

114. Kakkar VV et al: Prevention of fatal postoperative pulmonary embolism by low doses of heparin. An international multicentre trial. Lancet 3:45, 1975.

115. Kamath VR et al: Ischemic heart disease and withdrawal of anticoagulant therapy. Lancet 1:1025, 1969.

116. Kates, RMH et al: Increased rate of clearance of drugs from the circulation of alcoholics. J Med Sci 258:35, 1969.

117. Kazmier FJ et al: Effect of oral anticoagulants on factors VII, IX, X, and II. Arch Int Med 115:667, 1965.

118. Kerber JJ et al: Pregnancy in a patient with a prosthetic mitral valve associated with a fetal anomaly attributed to warfarin sodium. JAMA 203:223, 1968.

120. Kleinman, PD et al: Studies of the epidemiology of anticoagulant drug interactions. Arch Int Med 126:522, 1970.

121. Koch-Weser J et al: Hemorrhagic diathesis induced by surreptitious ingestion of coumarin drugs. Med Clin N Amer 56:263, 1972.

122. Koch-Weser J: Hemorrhagic reactions and drug interactions in 500 warfarin-treated patients (Abstract). Clin Pharmacol Ther 14:139, 1974.

123. Kawwn, HD et al: Hemorrhagic diathesis induced by surreptitious ingestion of coumarin drugs. Med Clin N Amer 56:263, 1972.

124. Lahnborg G et al: Effect of low-dose heparin on incidence of postoperative pulmonary embolism detected by photoscanning. Lancet 1:329, 1974.

125. Leslie J et al: The diagnosis of long-standing bleeding disorders, in *Disorders of Hemostasis,* Miescher, PA et al (eds.) Grune and Stratton, Inc., NY, 1971 p 140.

126. Levine WG: Anticoagulants in *Pharmacological Basis of Therapeutics.* Goodman, S et al (eds.) 4th ed, The Macmillan Co., New York, 1970, p 1445.

127. Levy G: Pharmacokinetic analysis of the effect of barbiturate on the anticoagulant action of warfarin in man. Clin Pharmacol Ther 11:372, 1970.

128. Lewis, RJ et al: Warfarin resistance. Am J Med 42:620, 1967.

129. Lewis, RJ et al: Warfarin metabolism in man: identification of metabolites in urine. J. Clin Invest 49:907, 1970.

130. Lewis, RJ et al: The metabolic fate of warfarin studies on the metabolites in plasma. Ann NY Acad Sci 179:205, 1971.

131. Lewis RJ et al: Warfarin metabolites: the anticoagulant activity and pharmacology of warfarin alcohols. J Lab Clin Med 81:915, 1973.

132. Lewis RJ et al: Warfarin. Stereochemical aspects of its metabolism and the interaction with phenylbutazone. J Clin Invest 53:1607, 1974.

133. Loeliger EA et al: The biological disappearance rate of prothrombin factors VII, IX, and X from plasma in hypothyroidism, hyperthyroidism, and during fever. Thromb Diath Haemorrh 10:267, 1964.

134. Lowenthal J et al: The nature of the antagonism between vitamin K and indirect anticoagulants. J Pharmacol Exp Therap 143:273, 1964.

135. Lyon AF et al: Indications for anticoagulant therapy. Am Heart J 77:132, 1969.

136. MacAuley MA et al: Relationship of the partial thromboplastin time to the Lee-White coagulation time. Am J Clin Path 50:403, 1968.

137. MacDonald MG et al: The effects of phenobarbital, chloral betaine, and gluthethimide administration on warfarin plasma levels and hypoprothrombinemic responses in man. Clin Pharmacol Ther 10:80, 1969.

138. MacDonald MG et al: Clinical observations of possible barbiturate interference with anticoagulation. JAMA 204:97, 1968.

139. MacDonald MG et al: The effects of phenobarbital, chloral betaine, and glutethimide administration on warfarin plasma levels and hypoprothrombinemic responses in man. Clin Pharmacol Ther 10:80, 1969.

140. MacLeaod SM et al: Pharmacodynamic and pharmacokinetic drug interactions with coumarin anticoagulants. Drugs 11:461, 1976.

141. Macon WL et al: Significant complications of anticoagulant therapy. Surg 68:571, 1970.

142. Majoor CLH: Aldosterone suppression by heparin, NEJM 279:1172, 1968.

143. Martyn DT et al: Continuous intravenous administration of heparin. Mayo Clin Proc 46:347, 1971.

144. Medical News. Possible interaction occurs with aspirin and two drugs. JAMA 214:39, 1970.

145. Michaels L: Incidence of thromboembolism after stopping anticoagulant therapy relationship of hemorrhage at the time of termination. JAMA 215:595, 1971.

146. Miller RL: Hemopericardium with use of oral anticoagulant therapy. JAMA 209:1362, 1969.

147. Mitchell AA: SMoking and warfarin dosage. NEJM 287:1153, 1972.

148. Modan B et al: Reduction of hospital mortality from acute myocardial infarction by anticoagulant therapy. NEJM 292:1359, 1975.

149. Modan B et al: The case for anticoagulants in acute myocardial infarction. Arch Int Med 136:1230, 1976.

150. Morris GK: Prevention of deep-vein thrombosis by low-dose heparin in patients undergoing total hip replacement. Lancet 2:797, 1974.

151. Moser KM et al: Effect of heparin on the one-stage prothrombin time. Ann Int Med 66:1207, 1967.

152. Mosley DH et al: Long-term anticoagulant therapy, JAMA 186:914, 1963.

153. Mustard JF et al: Factors influencing platelet function, adhesion, release and aggregation. Pharmacol Rev 22:97, 1970.

154. Mustard JF et al: Platelets, thrombosis and drugs. Drugs 9:19, 1975.

155. Natelson EA et al: Heparin-induced thrombocytopenia. An unexpected response to treatment of consumption coagulopathy. Ann Int Med 71:1121, 1969.

156. Nath H et al: Platelet factor 4 — antiheparin protein releasable from platelets. Purification and properties. J Lab Clin Med 82:754, 1973.

157. Neuschatz J et al: The prevention of postoperative thrombosis — a simple safe approach. JAMA 130:966, 1972.

158. Nicolaides AN et al: Small doses of subcutaneous sodium heparin in preventing deep venous thrombosis after major surgery. Lancet 11:890, 1972.

159. Nies DS: Pulmonary embolism in clinical pharmocology, in *Basic Principles in Therapeutics.* Melmon K et al (eds), The Macmillan Co., New York, 1972, p 230.

160. Novak E et al: A comparative study of the effect of lung and gut heparins on platelet aggregation and protamine neutralization in man. Clin Med 79:22, 1972.

161. Nussbaum M et al: Anticoagulants and anticoagulation. Med Clin NA 60:855, 1971.

162. O'Brien JR: The effect of heparin on the early stages of blood coagulation. J Clin Pathol 13:93, 1960.

163. O'Brien JR: Effect of anti-inflammatory agents on platelets. Lancet 1:894, 1968.

164. O'Brien JR: Heparin and platelets. Curr Ther Res 18:79, 1975.

165. O'Reilly RA et al: Studies on the coumarin anticoagulant drugs: the pharmacodynamics of warfarin in man. J Clin Invest 42:1542, 1963.

166. O'Reilly RA et al: Hereditary transmission of exceptional resistance to coumarin anticoagulant drugs. First reported kindred. NEJM 271:809, 1964.

167. O'Reilly RA et al: Studies on the coumarin anticoagulant drugs: a comparison of the pharmacodynamics of dicoumarol and warfarin in man. Thromb Diath Hemorrh 11:1, 1964.

168. O'Reilly RA et al: Surreptitious ingestion of coumarin anticoagulant drugs. Ann Int Med 64:1034, 1966.

169. O'Reilly RA et al: Studies on coumarin anticoagulant drugs. Initiation of warfarin therapy without a loading dose. Circ 38:169, 1968.

170. O'Reilly RA: Hereditary resistance to oral anticoagulant drugs: a second reported kindred. Clin Res 17:317, 1969.

171. O'Reilly RA et al: Determinants of the response to oral anticoagulant drugs in man. Pharmacol Rev 22:35, 1970.

172. O'Reilly RA et al: Pharmacokinetic analysis of potentiating effect of phenylbutazone on anticoagulant action of warfarin in man. J Pharm Sci 59:1258, 1970.

173. O'Reilly RA: Vitamin K and oral anticoagulant drugs as competitive antagonists in man. Pharmacol 7:149, 1972.

174. O'Reilly RA: The stereoselective interaction of warfarin and metronidazole in man. NEJM 295:354, 1976.

175. Orme M et al: Interactions of benzodiazepines with warfarin. Brit Med J 2:611, 1972.

176. O'Sullivan EF et al: Heparin in the treatment of venous throm-

boembolic disease: administration, control, and results. Med J Aust 2:153, 1968.

177. O'Sullivan EF: Duration of anticoagulant therapy in venous thromboembolism. Med J Aust. 2:1104, 1972.

178. Penner JA et al: Lack of interaction between ibuprofen and warfarin. Curr Ther Res 18:862, 1975.

179. Pettifor JM et al: Congenital malformations associated with the administration of oral anticoagulants during pregnancy. J Ped 86:459, 1975.

180. Phelps MD: Thrombophlebitis and pulmonary embolism. Med Clin N Amer 53:341, 1969.

181. Pitney WR: Mechanisms of Thrombosis in Clinical Aspects of Thromboembolism, 1st ed. p. 85. Williams and Wilkins, Baltimore 1972.

182. Pollak EW et al: Pulmonary embolism, an appraisal of therapy in 516 cases. Arch Surg 107:66, 1973.

183. Pyorala K: Coumarin anticoagulant requirement in relation to serum cholesterol and triglyceride level. Acta Med Scand 183:437, 1968.

184. Quick AJ: Clinical interpreation of the one-stage prothrombin time. Circ 24:1422, 1961.

185. Quick AJ et al: Influence of acetylsalicylic acid and salicylamide on the coagulation of blood. J Pharmacol Exp Ther 128:95, 1960.

186. Quick AJ: Detection and diagnosis of hemorrhagic states. JAMA 197:418, 1966.

187. Quick AJ: Quick on Quick's test. NEJM 288:1079, 1973.

188. Rapaport SL et al: Clotting factor assays on plasma from patients receiving intramuscular or subcutaneous heparin. Am J Med Sci 234:678, 1957.

189. Ratnoff OD: The blood clotting mechanism and its disorders. Dis. Month (Nov.) 1965.

190. Ravel R: Blood Coagulation in Clinical Laboratory Medicine, Application of Laboratory Data, 2nd ed. Year Book Medical Publishers, Inc. 1973, p 80.

191. Resnekov L: Present status of electroversion in the management of cardiac dysrhythmias. Circ 47:1356, 1973.

192. Reussi, C et al: Unusual complications in the course of anticoagulant therapy. Am J Med 46:460, 1969.

193. Rhodes GR et al: Heparin-induced thrombocytopenia with thrombotic and hemorrhagic manifestations. Surg Gynec Obstet 136:409, 1973.

194. Rice AJ et al: Decreased sensitivity to warfarin in patients with myxedema. Am J Med Sci 262:211, 1971.

195. Rickles, FR et al: Chloral hydrate and warfarin. NEJM 286:611, 1972.

196. Robinson DS et al: The effect of phenobarbital administration on the control of coagulation achieved during warfarin therapy in man. J Pharmacol Exp Ther 153:250, 1966.

197. Robinson DS et al: Interaction of commonly prescribed drugs and warfarin. Ann Int Med 72:853, 1970.

198. Rogel S et al: Anticoagulants in ischemic heart disease. Arch Int Med 136:1229, 1976.

199. Roos J et al: Subcutaneous heparin and postoperative deep-vein thrombosis. Lancet 11:932, 1972.

200. Rosenberg RD: Heparin action. Circ 49:603, 1974.

201. Rosenberg RD: Actions and interactions of antithrombin and heparin. NEJM 292:146, 1975.

202. Rothermich NO: Diphenylhydantoin intoxication (Letter) Lancet 2:640, 1966.

203. Salzman EW et al: Reduction in venous thromboembolism by agents affecting platelet function. NEJM 284:1287, 1971.

204. Salzman EW et al: Management of heparin therapy. Controlled prospective trial. NEJM 292:1046, 1975.

205. Sassahara AA: Therapy for pulmonary embolism. JAMA 229:1795, 1974.

206. Schary WL et al: Warfarin-phenylbutazone interaction in man: A long term multiple dose study. Res Comm Chem Path Pharmacol 10:663, 1975.

207. Schnetzer TW: Platelets and thrombogenesis — current concepts. Am Heart J 83:552, 1972.

208. Sellers EM et al: Kinetics and clinical importance of displacement of warfarin from albumin by acidic drugs. Ann NY Acad Sci 179:213, 1971.

209. Sevitt S et al: Prothrombin time and thrombotest in inured patients on prophylactic anticoagulant therapy. Lancet 1:124, 1964.

210. Sharnoff JG: Results in the prophylaxis of postoperative thromboembolism. Surg Gynecol Obstet 123:303, 1966.

211. Sharnoff JG et al: Prevention of fatal postoperative thromboembolism by heparin prophylaxis. Lancet 11:1006, 1970.

212. Shaul WL et al: Chondrodysplasia punctata and maternal warfarin use during pregnancy. Amer J Dis Child 129:360, 1975.

213. Sherry S: Low-dose heparin prophylaxis for postoperative venous thromboembolism. NEJM 293:300, 1975.

214. Shoshkes M et al: Vitamin K_1 in treatment of bishydroxycoumarin-induced hypoprothrombinemia, comparison of intravenous and intramuscular administration. JAMA 161:1145, 1956.

215. Sigell LT et al: Drug interactions with anticoagulants. JAMA 214:2035, 1970.

216. Silver D et al: Management of pulmonary embolism. Med Clin N Amer 54:361, 1970.

217. Silverglade A: Biological equivalence of beef lung and hog mucosal heparins. Curr Ther Res 18:91, 1975.

218. Sise HS et al: The risk of interrupting long-term anticoagulant treatment. A rebound hypercoagulable stage following hemorrhage. Circ 24:1137, 1961.

219. Solomon HM et al: The anticoagulant response to bishydroxycoumarin I. The role of individual variation. Circ 24:1137, 1961.

220. Spector I et al: Control of heparin therapy with activated partial thromboplastin times. JAMA 201:157, 1967.

221. Starr KJ et al: Drug interactions in patients on long-term dual anticoagulant and antihypertensive adrenergic neuron-blocking drugs. Brit Med J 4:133, 1972.

222. Stormorken H et al: Physiopathology of hemostasis in Disorders of Hemostasis, Miescher, PA et al (eds), Grune and Stratton, Inc., New York, 1971, p 3.

223. Struver GD et al: The partial thromboplastin time (cephalin time) in anticoagulant therapy. Am J Clin Path 38:473, 1962.

224. Swanson M et al: Heparin therapy by continuous intravenous infusion. Am J Hosp Pharm 28:792, 1971.

225. Szucs MM Jr Et al: Diagnostic sensitivity of laboratory findings in acute pulmonary embolism. Ann Int Med 74:161, 1971.

226. Thierry, MJ et al: Vitamin K and warfarin distribution and metabolism in the warfarin resistant rat. Am J Physiol 219:854, 1970.

227. Thomas DP: Therapeutic role of heparin in acute pulmonary embolism Curr Ther Res 18:21, 1975.

228. Tonascia J: Retrospective evidence favoring use of anticoagulants for myocardial infarction. NEJM 292:1362, 1975.

229. Tibbutt DA et al: Pulmonary embolism: Current therapeutic concepts. Drugs 11:161, 1976.

230. Tozer TN:Peronal communication, re: research by M Rowland, University of California School of Pharmacy, San Francisco, 1973.

231. Udall JA: Chloral hydrate and warfarin therapy. Ann Int Med 75:141, 1971.

232. Udall JA: Don't use the wrong vitamin K. Calif Med 112:65, 1966.

233. Udall JA: Human sources and absorption of vitamin K in relation to anticoagulant.

234. Udall JA: Drug interference with warfarin therapy. Clin Med 77:20, 1970.

235. Udall JA: Human sources and absorption of vitamin K in relation to anticoagulant stability. JAMA 194:107, 1965.

236. Udall JA: Warfarin-chloral hydrate interaction. Pharmacological activity and clinical significance. Ann Int Med 81:341, 1974.

237. Udall JA: Clinical implications of warfarin interactions with five sedatives. Amer J Card 35:67, 1975.

238. Van Cleve RB: Letting go of the bear's tail. Experience with discontinuation of long-term anticoagulant therapy. JAMA 196:1156, 1966.

239. Vessell ES: Failure of indomethacin and warfarin to interact in normal human volunteers. J Clin Pharmacol 15:486, 1975.

240. Viewig WVR et al: Complications of intravenous administration of heparin in elderly women. JAMA 213:1303, 1970.

241. Wadman B: Thromboembolic complications during corticosteroid treatment of temporal arteritis (Letter). Lancet 1:907, 1972.

242. Warkany J: A warfarin embryopathy. Marginal comment. Amer J Dis Child 129:287, 1975.

243. Warlow C et al: A double-blind trial of low doses subcutaneous heparin in the prevention of deep-venous thrombosis after myocardial infarction. Lancet 2:934, 1973.

244. Weiss HJ: Platelet physiology and abnormalities of platelet func-

tion. NEJM 293:580, 1975.

245. Weiss HJ: Antiplatelet drugs — A new pharmacologic approach to the prevention of thrombosis. Amer Heart J 92:86, 1976.

246. Wessler S: Thrombosis in the presence of vascular stasis. Am J Med 33:648, 1962.

247. Wessler S et al: *A Guide to Anticoagulant Therapy*. American Heart Association, New York, 1970.

248. Wessler S et al: Theory and practice of minidose heparin in surgical patients. A status report. Circ 47:4, 1973.

249. Wessler S et al: Studies in intravascular coagulation IV. The effect of heparin and dicumarol on serum-induced venous thrombous. Circ 12:553, 1955.

250. Wessler S: Anticoagulant therapy — 1974. JAMA 8:757, 1974.

251. Yacobi A et al: Serum protein binding as a determinant of warfarin body clearance and anticoagulant effect. Clin Pharmacol Ther 19:552, 1976.

252. Westphal RG: Rational alternatives to the use of whole blood. Ann Int Med 76:987, 1972.

253. Williams HT: Prevention of postoperative deep-vein thrombosis with peri-operative subcutaneous heparin. Lancet 11:950, 1971.

254. Wilson ID et al: Selective hypoaldosteronism after prolonged heparin administration. Am J Med 36:635, 1964.

255. Woolf IL et al: Vitamin K and warfarin metabolism, function, and interaction. Am J Med 53:261, 1972.

256. Working Party Report: Assessment of short-term anticoagulant administration after cardiac infarction. Brit Med J 1:335, 1969.

257. Wright IS: Anticoagulant therapy-practical management. Am Heart J 77:280, 1969.

258. Wright IS: Recent developments in antithrombotic therapy. Ann Int Med 71:823, 1969.

259. Yin ET et al: Identity of plasma-activated Factor X inhibitor with antithrombin III and heparin co-factor. J Biol Chem 216:3712, 1971.

260. Zinn WJ: Side reactions of heparin in clinical practice. Am J Cardiol 14:36, 1964.

261. Zucker S et al: Control of heparin therapy. Sensitivity of the activated partial thromboplastin time for monitoring the antithrombotic effects of heparin. J Lab Clin Med 73:320, 1969.

262. Zucker MB: Effect of acetylsalicylic acid, other nonsteroidal antiinflammatory agents, and dipyridamole on human blood platelets. J Lab Clin Med 76:66, 1970.

263. Koch-Weser J et al: Drug interactions with coumarin anticoagulants. NEJM 285:487,547, 1971.

Chapter 17

Asthma, Chronic Bronchitis, and Emphysema
J. Robert Powell

Asthma, chronic bronchitis, and emphysema are diseases which may or may not be related, are caused or exacerbated by similar or different sources, and may or may not be effectively treated in the same manner. Because of their similarities the three disease classifications are being presented together as a matter of convenience. However, the inconsistencies between and within disease classifications are emphasized in order to assist in the development of a therapeutic regimen for the individual patient. The use of umbrella-like classifications such as "Chronic Obstructive Lung Disease" are discouraged since it creates the illusion that all three diseases may be treated as one — an approach which is definitely wrong. Objective methods for assessing the degree of severity are stressed so that an assessment of drug therapy efficacy can be performed.

The diagnosis and treatment of asthma, bronchitis, emphysema and respiratory failure is based on an understanding of normal and abnormal lung physiology. Pulmonary function testing and analysis of arterial blood gases and pH initially assist in defining the disease process and severity, and will later provide objective, baseline information for determining change in the disease and efficacy of therapy. While a brief overview of pulmonary physiology is presented here, more comprehensive reviews are recommended. (46, 196, 274).

1. What are the principal functions of the lung? Describe the utility of spirometry in assessing pulmonary function.

The primary function of the lung is respiration, which is defined in man as the transport of oxygen (O_2) from the environment to the cells and the transport of carbon dioxide (CO_2) from the cells to the environment. The lung also acts as an organ which filters blood, metabolizes biochemical compounds, protects the body from inhaled microorganisms and toxins, and acts as a reservoir for the left ventricle. Gas exchange can be divided into three major stages: *ventilation* or how air gets to and from the alveoli; *diffusion* or how oxygen and carbon dioxide cross the alveolar walls; and *circulation* or how oxygen and carbon dioxide are transported from and to the lung.

The diagnosis and continued assessment of asthma, chronic bronchitis, and emphysema are based upon clinical and laboratory evaluation. The principal laboratory tests are spirometry for determining lung volumes and flow rates, carbon monoxide diffusing capacity for measuring the gas diffusion properties of the lung, and determination of arterial blood gases and pH.

The spirometer (Fig. 1) can be used to measure many lung volumes and flow rates. As the person exhales a bell goes up and a pen on the rotating recording paper goes down. The ***tidal volume*** is the volume of gas inspired and expired during normal breathing. When the subject makes a maximal inspiration and expiration, the ***vital capacity (VC)*** is measured. The volume of gas remaining in the lung after maximal expiration is the ***residual volume (RV)***. ***Total lung capacity (TLC)*** is the sum of the vital capacity and the residual volume. During an exacerbation of asthma the vital capacity is decreased, the residual volume is increased, and the total lung capacity may be normal or increased. Once the patient recovers, the lung volumes may markedly change toward normal. Patients with symptomatic chronic bronchitis may have a markedly decreased VC and slightly increased RV with a near normal TLC. Pure emphysemics tend to have a markedly increased TLC and RV with a slight increase in VC. Although the above information is useful, patients frequently do not have pure asthma, chronic bronchitis, or emphysema, but suffer from a combination of diseases (e.g., asthmatic bronchitis). Lung volumes vary with height, body build, gender, age, and disease.

Measurement of timed forced expiratory volume by a spirometer is performed by having the subject inspire maximally and then expire as hard and completely as possible. The volume expired in the first second is called the forced expiratory volume at one second, **FEV$_{1.0}$**, and the total volume expired is the vital capacity (VC). Normally the FEV$_{1.0}$ is 80 percent of the VC. When there is airway resistance, obstructive disease such as asthma, chronic bronchitis, or emphysema, the FEV$_{1.0}$ is reduced more than the VC, producing a FEV$_{1.0}$/VC ratio which is less than 80 percent. In restrictive diseases such as pulmonary fibrosis both FEV$_{1.0}$ and VC are reduced so that the FEV$_{1.0}$/VC ratio is normal or increased (274).

The **_maximal midexpiratory flow rate (MMFR)_** is the flow rate measured over the middle half of expiration or is the slope of the line connecting the first and last quarter of the forced vital capacity. Usually the MMFR is closely related to the FEV$_{1.0}$. However, the FEV$_{1.0}$ mainly reflects resistance in the large airways while the MMFR is sensitive to the airflow resistance in the large and small airways (bronchioles). When there is constriction of these smaller airways the MMFR is reduced while the FEV$_{1.0}$ may be normal.

2. Why is there a different pattern of forced expiratory volumes in restrictive versus obstructive disease?

In restrictive disease inspiration is limited by decreased compliance of the lung or by weakness of inspiratory muscles. The total lung capacity may be increased in obstructive disease; however, expiration ends prematurely. This is caused by increased bronchial smooth muscle tone in asthma, loss of radial traction in the parenchyma in emphysema, and edema or thick mucoid secretions in the airway lumen of chronic bronchitis. An increase in airway resistance (asthma) or a decrease in the elastic recoil properties of the lung (emphysema) may decrease the FEV$_{1.0}$.

3. What criteria can be used to determine bronchodilatability?

The degree the patient can be bronchodilated is frequently used as a basis for diagnosis and treatment. The following procedure is used. The FEV$_{1.0}$ and/or VC are measured before and after administration of a

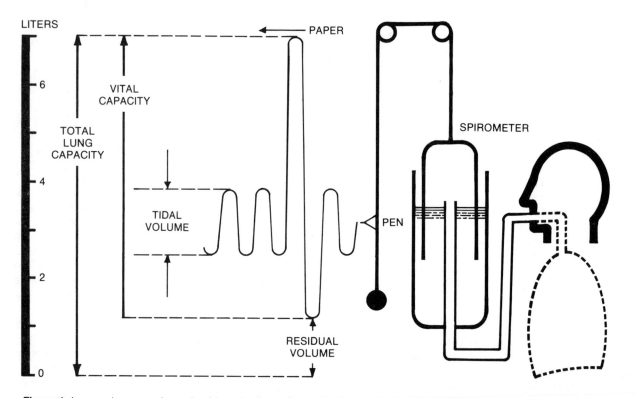

Figure 1. Lung volumes as determined by spirometry. Determination of the residual volume requires the use of a body plethysmograph.

rapid-acting, potent bronchodilator, e.g., isoproterenol inhalation (117). The pulmonary function measurement after the drug is administered should be at the time the bronchodilator has reached the maximal bronchodilator effect. If there has been at least a 15 to 25% increase in $FEV_{1.0}$ or VC following drug administration, the patient is said to be bronchodilatable and will possibly benefit from bronchodilator drug therapy. However, if this response is not found, it does not rule out bronchospasm since the ability of the airways to dilate is dependent upon the degree of bronchospasm which is present (117). When the initial $FEV_{1.0}$ is very low, as in a patient with severe asthma, the response to bronchodilators may not be detectable. As the patient recovers, the initial $FEV_{1.0}$ increases and the response to a bronchodilator will be maximal. Then, as the initial $FEV_{1.0}$ approaches the ideal for that patient, the response to a bronchodilator will diminish because the patient should not have pulmonary function which is greater than that of a similar nondiseased person.

Patients with severe asthma may receive symptomatic relief from isoproterenol inhalation, although there is no change in $FEV_{1.0}$ pre- and post-drug administration. An explanation for this apparent paradox is the finding that patients with severe asthma may have elevated TLC and RV (278). After isoproterenol inhalation the air trapped in the lung may decrease without significantly affecting the $FEV_{1.0}$.

4. What are major limitations in the use of $FEV_{1.0}$, and VC in monitoring patients with obstructive airways disease?

The $FEV_{1.0}$, VC, and MMFR are effort-dependent tests. That is, if the person is not exerting a maximal forced expiration, the data will be spurious. Another restriction is the sensitivity of the $FEV_{1.0}$ in reflecting bronchospasm in the small peripheral airways. When a patient who has had a severe exacerbation of asthma is subjectively feeling much better, the $FEV_{1.0}$ may be approaching normality and yet there is residual peripheral bronchospasm in the smaller bronchioles which is only reflected by the MMFR (179,180). The situation may occur when a patient is discharged from the emergency room after several hours of treatment because he is feeling much better and the $FEV_{1.0}$ has markedly increased. If peripheral constriction of the small bronchioles is still present, it could form the basis for developing an attack soon after leaving the hospital, which could make readmission necessary.

5. The principal problem in emphysema is destruction of alveolar and capillary walls resulting in a decrease in the alveolar surface area available for diffusion. How can this abnormality be detected?

The diagnosis of emphysema is most easily made at autopsy. However, measuring the diffusing capacity of carbon monoxide (D_{CO}) in the lung also is useful in diagnosing emphysema. The simplest technique for measuring D_{CO} is to have the patient inspire a gas mixture containing a low concentration of carbon monoxide (CO) and hold his breath for 10 seconds during which CO leaves the alveolar space and enters the blood. The larger the D_{CO}, the more CO enters the blood during the 10 second period. Diffusing capacity is decreased in emphysema, sarcoidosis, pulmonary edema, asbestosis, and berylliosis and is normal in bronchial asthma. Diffusing capacity is low in patients with anemia and high in polycythemia, making a correction for hemoglobin concentration necessary.

6. A patient who comes to the emergency room for treatment of an acute asthmatic attack has the following arterial blood gases and forced volumes: P_aO_2 55 mm Hg, P_aCO_2 35 mm Hg, $FEV_{1.0}$ 0.5 L, and FVC 0.9 L. Fifteen minutes after being given isoproterenol inhalation and intravenous aminophylline the tests were repeated: P_aO_2 45 mm Hg, P_{CO2} 37 mm Hg, $FEV_{1.0}$ 0.8 L, and FVC 1.3 L. How can you explain the decrease in P_aO_2 with bronchodilation (increased $FEV_{1.0}$, increased FVC)?

In the normal lung, the ventilation (V) of all areas is matched to an appropriate blood flow (perfusion, Q) so that an efficient gas exchange of O_2 and CO_2 takes place. The ventilation and blood flow in the lungs of a normal, upright person increases from the apex to the base. When there is obstruction in the airways, those areas of the lung which are less obstructed than others will be ventilated more. At this time, it is felt that areas of the lung which are poorly ventilated will be perfused less than areas which are ventilated more (106). In effect, the body is trying to maintain matched ventilation and perfusion. As the patient recovers from an acute exacerbation of bronchial asthma and obstruction is relieved, the distribution of ventilation and perfusion approach normality (277).

During an asthmatic attack bronchodilator drugs may alter the compensated ventilation-perfusion (V/Q) relationship and produce a V/Q abnormality resulting in a decrease in the P_aO_2. Isoproterenol (142,258), terbutaline (143), salbutamol (222), theophylline (258), and atropine (69) have all been associated with ventilation-perfusion inequality and may subsequently cause the P_aO_2 to transiently decrease in obstructed patients.

The following hypothesis may explain this effect of bronchodilators. Beta_2 adrenergic stimulation causes dilation of the pulmonary blood vessels as well as bronchial smooth muscle. Drugs which are beta_2 stimulants may produce a larger decrease in vascular resistance in those areas which are strongly vasoconstricted by hypoxia. This may cause shunting of blood away from areas of higher ventilation increasing perfusion of poorly ventilated lung, and cause the arterial P_aO_2 to decrease. If drugs were found which produced selective beta$_2$ stimulation of bronchial smooth muscle, ventilation-perfusion inequalities might be avoided. Salbutamol (201), metaproterenol (182), and terbutaline (154), appear to have less of an effect in this regard than isoproterenol and may even increase P_aO_2.

The decrease in P_aO_2 is usually small when it occurs; however, a decrease of 10 to 15 mm Hg may occur in some patients. There is no way of predicting which patients will experience this effect, although it is felt that some patients are more susceptible to the vasodilator effect of these drugs. Because of the unpredictable nature of this effect, all patients receiving bronchodilators who are hypoxemic and either hypocapneic or normocapneic should receive supplemental oxygen to prevent further falling down the steep portion of the hemoglobin-oxygen dissociation curve.

7. Describe the use of arterial blood gas determinations in the treatment of asthma.

The ultimate test which reflects the efficacy of ventilation, diffusion, and circulation in lung disease is the measurement of the partial pressure of oxygen and carbon dioxide (P_aO_2, P_aCO_2) and pH in arterial blood. Several general principles should be considered when using arterial blood gases and pH in patient monitoring. The duration and degree of bronchial obstruction correlates well with the extent of P_aO_2 reduction. McFadden and Lyons (181) found that when the mean predicted $FEV_{1.0}$ percentage was 59, 35 and 18%, the mean P_aO_2 was 83, 71, and 63 mm Hg. The use of serial determinations of arterial blood gases and pH have become a routine method for assessing the severity of obstructive lung disease and for determining the need for more intensive therapy. Without measuring these parameters, there is no reliable method for monitoring respiration in patients who are severely ill. Frequent determinations of arterial blood gases and pH are especially critical in the following situation. A patient with very severe asthma with a P_aO_2 47 mm Hg, P_aCO_2 43 mm Hg, and pH 7.38 (stage IV, table 7), may regress to a potentially fatal point where P_aO_2 is 46 mm Hg, P_aCO_2 is 55 mm Hg, and the arterial pH is 7.30 (stage V) within several hours. Knowing the clinical, respiratory, and acid-base status of severely ill patients will enable the clinician to institute lifesaving therapy.

8. What are the proposed mechanisms of action for the diverse group of chemicals known as bronchodilators?

Within the last ten years there has been a virtual explosion in the number of new drugs used to treat asthma. Many of these drugs are a direct result of research on the physiology, immunopharmacology, and pharmacology of the lung. A schematic representation of the mechanisms by which drugs can produce bronchodilation or bronchoconstriction is shown in Fig. 2 (7,92). This scheme has changed many times in the past and will certainly change in the future. It will be helpful to use Fig. 2 as a map with the following discussion.

Antigen is introduced into the body and stimulates the release of IgE from peripheral lymphoid tissue in atopic individuals. The IgE becomes fixed to mast cells (sensitized mast cell) which on re-exposure to the antigen will cause the formation and release of histamine, eosinophil chemotactic factor of anaphylaxis (ECF-A) and slow reacting substance of anaphylaxis (SRS-A). These mediators either directly cause bronchoconstriction or, possibly during an acute response to antigen, they may also stimulate the afferent vagus nerve which initiates a parasympathetic reflex resulting in the release of acetylcholine from the efferent vagus. Acetylcholine may directly cause smooth muscle contraction and further release of mediators. Within the mast cell are the beta$_2$ adrenergic, alpha adrenergic, and cholinergic pathways which modulate bronchial smooth muscle tone possibly by regulating mediator release. In general, bronchodilation is associated with increased intracellular concentration of cyclic AMP and a decreased level of cyclic GMP, while bronchoconstriction is associated with a decrease in cyclic AMP and an increase in cyclic GMP. The relationship between cyclic AMP and GMP may be thought of as a push-pull mechanism. Bronchodilators usually lead to an increase in cyclic AMP or a decrease in cyclic GMP and drugs which cause bronchoconstriction usually have the opposite effect.

Beta$_2$ adrenergic stimulation increases cyclic AMP in bronchial smooth muscle and produces bronchodilation. Drugs which stimulate the beta$_2$ adrenergic receptor are: isoproterenol, epinephrine, isoetharine, terbutaline, metaproterenol, and salbutamol. Propranolol will block the beta$_2$ adrenergic receptor and will produce bronchospasm in asthmatics. The use of propranolol in even mild asthmatics is contraindicated because of the importance of this effect (284). Selective beta$_1$ adrenergic blocking agents, such as metaprolol can be used with caution in asthma patients who require a beta blocker for treating cardiac arrhythmias or hypertension (242). Prostaglandins E$_1$ and E$_2$ appear to bypass the beta$_2$ receptor producing an increase in cyclic AMP and bronchodilation. The duration of action of PGE$_1$ and E$_2$ inhalation is about the same as that of isoproterenol inhalation (53). A major limitation to prostaglandins when given by inhalation is the pharyngeal and tracheal irritation resulting in protracted coughing and expectoration (133). Prostaglan-

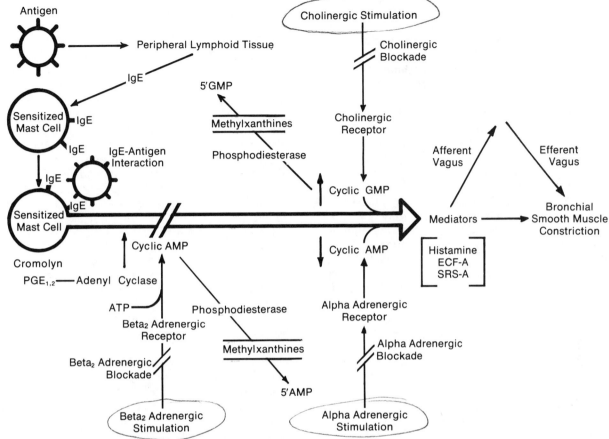

Figure 2. Schematic presentation of the immunopharmocologic and pharmocologic factors influencing bronchial smooth muscle tone. (Adapted from refs 7,92).

din F2α is a potent bronchoconstrictor. It has been postulated that an imbalance of prostaglandins with opposite activity may be involved in the pathogenesis of asthma (1). Aspirin and indomethacin inhibit prostaglandin synthesis and the effects of PGF2α on bronchial smooth muscle. Although these drugs have been suggested for the treatment of asthma, some patients have suffered severe attacks of asthma after taking aspirin or indomethacin (177). (See *Rheumatoid Arthritis* chapter).

Phosphodiesterase is the enzyme which converts cyclic AMP to 5'AMP. By inhibiting phosphodiesterase, the methylxanthines (theophylline, caffeine, theobromine) increase intracellular cyclic AMP and produce bronchodilation. The metabolism of cyclic GMP to 5'GMP is also mediated by phosphodiesterase and inhibited by theophylline. Although the action of theophylline on the metabolism of cyclic AMP and GMP appears to be antagonistic, theophylline is only known to be a bronchodilator. This could suggest lesser importance of the effect on cyclic GMP or, possibly, another mechanism of action for theophylline such as a direct effect on bronchial muscle.

Alpha-adrenergic stimulation (phenylephrine) is associated with decreasing intracellular cyclic AMP concentration, which enhances the ability of the IgE-antigen interaction to cause release of histamine and SRS-A from the lung (132). Alpha-adrenergic blocking agents (phentolamine, thymoxamine) have been shown to be bronchodilators in a limited number of subjects (81,98).

Cholinergic stimulation (acetylcholine) enhances the immunological release of mediators from human lung, and is associated with increased intracellular cyclic GMP concentration. This effect can be blocked by use of a muscarinic blocking agent (atropine) (132).

Drugs which increase intracellular cyclic AMP may reduce the immunological release of mediators, decrease discharges across the parasympathetic ganglia, and directly dilate bronchial smooth muscle. Anticholinergic drugs may prevent the muscarinic effects of acetylcholine on smooth muscle and on the mast cell. Some investigators feel that further describing the intracellular biochemical processes may lead to the establishment of several classes of asthmatic individuals who have different defects in control mechanisms of mediator release.

9. Discuss the development of beta₂ sympathomimetic drugs. How do they differ from isoproterenol and epinephrine? What is the sympathomimetic drug of choice in the treatment of bronchospasm?

Epinephrine, isoproterenol, and ephedrine are the adrenergic stimulant drugs that have been available many years for the treatment of acute or chronic bronchospasm. In the mid-1960's Lands and coworkers suggested the presence of two types of beta adrenergic receptors, beta₁ and beta₂, in addition to the alpha receptor (150,151) (Table 1). Since that time a large number of chemicals have been investigated with the hope of finding a selective beta₂ adrenergic bronchodilator which does not have either the alpha or beta₁ side effects of epinephrine, ephedrine, or isoproterenol. Now, with the availability of selective beta₂ agonists (even more should be marketed in the near future), there is a great deal of confusion concerning the properties of these new drugs compared to the standards, epinephrine and isoproterenol. Sympathomimetic bronchodilator drugs are classified in three groups according to *in vitro* receptor activity: drugs with alpha, beta₁, and beta₂ activity (epinephrine); beta₁ and beta₂ activity (isoproterenol); and only beta₂ activity (salbutamol) (Table 2).

The major differences between epinephrine or isoproterenol and the new selective beta₂ sympathomimetic drugs metaproterenol (37, 75, 112, 174, 183, 186, 205), terbutaline (73, 74, 76, 105, 153, 154, 232), salbutamol (2, 39, 18, 102, 186, 195, 218, 222, 259, 268), rimiterol (9, 48, 238, 253), fenoterol (9), salmefamol (135), carbuterol, hexoprenaline (264), and trimetoquinol (280), are that the more selective beta₂ agonists: (a) generally do not directly stimulate the myocardium unless administered in high doses or intravenously; (b) are active when swallowed; (c) have a slower onset of action; (d) and some have a much longer duration of action. It is not claimed that the beta₂ stimulants produce more bronchodilation than

isoproterenol, but it has been shown that when isoproterenol and salbutamol produce an equivalent degree of bronchodilation, the cardiac stimulation secondary to salbutamol can be much less than from isoproterenol. It is difficult to estimate the beta₁ effect of these drugs when given intravenously by simultaneously measuring the changes in FEV₁.₀ and heart rate because there may be a reflex tachycardia in response to the beta₂-induced vasodilation. However, Gibson and Coltart (87) reported that although isoproterenol and salbutamol produced the same degree of tachycardia, only isoproterenol had a positive inotropic cardiac effect (beta₁). Other workers have found that intravenous isoproterenol and salbutamol were equipotent as bronchodilators, but salbutamol was approximately one-sixth as potent as isoproterenol in chronotropic effect (204,254). The selectivity of the newer drugs may be most important during an exacerbation of asthma when tachycardia is common. If a beta₂ drug would produce bronchodilation without increasing the heart rate further, and if epinephrine produced bronchodilation and further increased the heart rate, then it would be reasonable to choose the beta₂ drug. Smith and associates (246) made this comparison in a double-blind study of subcutaneously injected terbutaline or epinephrine in treating 49 adults with acute bronchial asthma. When both drugs were given in doses which produced a similar change in FEV₁.₀ and FVC, terbutaline caused a significantly greater increase in heart rate. Neither drug produced a significant change in blood pressure and the incidence of side effects was similar. Based on the results of this study, one must question if terbutaline is a selective beta₂ agonist. Since hypotension was not found, one might suspect terbutaline has a direct beta₁ cardiac effect. Is there a significant advantage of terbutaline over epinephrine in treating acute bronchial asthma? If either drug has an advantage, the results of this study would indicate it is epinephrine. However, to conclusively answer this question a range of doses should be studied in the various types of pa-

Table 1
EFFECTS OF ADRENERGIC RECEPTOR STIMULATION

Alpha	Beta₁	Beta₂
Bronchoconstriction	Cardiac stimulation (inotropic and chronotropic)	Bronchodilation
Vasoconstriction		Vasodilation
Sphincter constriction in GI tract and bladder	Increased lipolysis	Skeletal muscle tremor Increased muscle glycogenolysis
Contraction of pilomotor muscles		
Increased hepatic glycogenolysis		

Table 2
CHARACTERISTICS OF SYMPATHOMIMETIC BRONCHODILATORS

Drug	Alpha	Beta$_1$	Beta$_2$	Duration of action of aerosol (hr)	Route of Administration
Epinephrine	+3	+3	+3	1-2	IM,SQ, Aerosol, Nebulizer Solution
Isoproterenol	**	+3	+3	1-2	IV,SL, Aerosol
Ephedrine	+1	+2	+2	4	Oral
Isoetharine	**	+1	+3	1-2	Aerosol, Nebulizer Solution, Oral*
Metaproterenol (Orciprenaline)		+1	+3	3-4	IV, IM, Aerosol, Nebulizer Solution, Oral
Terbutaline	±		+3	4-6	IV*, SQ, Aerosol, Oral
Salbutamol* (Albuterol)	±		+3	4-6	IV, Aerosol, Nebulizer Solution, Oral
Rimiterol*	±		+3	1-2	Aerosol
Fenoterol*			+3	8-10	Aerosol
Salmefamol*			+3	8-10	Aerosol

*Not available in USA
**Alpha effect possible due to combination with phenylephrine

tients with bronchoconstriction of various degrees of severity.

When the selective beta$_2$ sympathomimetic drugs are given in therapeutic doses by inhalation or the oral route, tachycardia does not usually occur. However, when these drugs are given by subcutaneous injection or by mouth, tremors may occur in 20 to 35% of cases (261). The skeletal muscle tremor appears to originate peripherally and is due to an increase in the amplitude of normal physiologic tremor (168). There is evidence that the tremor is caused by stimulation of a beta$_2$ type receptor in skeletal muscle (152). In order to decrease the incidence or degree of tremor from metaproterenol, terbutaline, or salbutamol; it is safest to start with a low dosage and then slowly increase the dose to achieve the desired effect. When tremor occurs, it may add to the patient's anxiety and result in an effective drug being discontinued.

Isoproterenol aerosol can usually be effectively used without causing alarming cardiac effects. However, if one is treating a patient known to be sensitive to the cardiac effects of isoproterenol or when an aerosolized bronchodilator with a prolonged duration of action is desirable, then it may be appropriate to choose one of the newer agents. In comparing orally effective sympathomimetics, ephedrine probably causes more nausea and CNS stimulation, while beta$_2$ drugs produce more tremors. The milligram potency is not a basis for selection. The ideal drug is yet to be developed. The choice of a sympathomimetic bronchodilator should be based primarily on the needs of the patient and consideration of the characteristics of the various drugs.

10. How should an aerosol delivered bronchodilator be used? What precautions should be taken when an aerosol bronchodilator is used? Is there

any advantage to giving bronchodilator drugs by aerosol versus an intermittent positive pressure breathing (IPPB) apparatus?

Many patients squirt a bronchodilator aerosol into the mouth five to six times within several seconds as if they were using a breath deodorant spray. All patients should be clearly instructed on the correct procedure for using an aerosol and be given an explanation of the serious risk of toxicity which accompanies overuse of this medication. The following recommendations are for an isoproterenol, handheld, freon propellant aerosol which delivers a metered dose between 75-125 mcg. The patient exhales to near residual volume and as he is inhaling to near vital capacity, he expresses one dose from the aerosol into his mouth, drawing it into the lungs. After the inhalation is completed, the patient will hold his breath for several seconds and then repeat the entire procedure. The aerosol may dispense the spray in a tight shotgun-like pattern which takes several inches to expand. Because of this, one should avoid placing the spray too far distally in the oral cavity which causes more of the dose to be deposited on the pharynx than usual. Patients should not use the spray more than 4 to 6 times in the above manner in a 24-hour period. The need for more frequent use may be taken as an indication for prompt medication evaluation in order to abort an exacerbation.

Even when the aerosol is administered in a proper manner to patients with airway obstruction, there is no assurance that the drug will be delivered to the constricted airways (54). In this situation, oral or intravenous routes of administration may be more efficacious. Administration of isoproterenol may contribute to bronchospasm, infrequently, by direct action on smooth muscle or from beta blockade produced by an isoproterenol metabolite, 3-0-methylisoproterenol

(134,203,247). When isoproterenol is given to hypoxic patients, oxygen should be given concurrently to prevent worsening hypoxia due to ventilation-perfusion abnormalities. The association of adrenergic aerosol overuse with death could be discussed with the patient to impress the seriousness of aerosol abuse.

The use of IPPB machines to deliver bronchodilator aerosols has not been shown to be of more therapeutic benefit than giving the drug by a portable, hand-held nebulizer or a freon-propelled aerosol dispenser (42,52,71,93,184). However, IPPB machines have the distinct disadvantage of costing hundreds of dollars more than a nebulizer. When a patient is fatigued or has difficulty in coordinating the use of a nebulizer or propellant-powered dispenser, IPPB may be a useful means for drug delivery.

11. Continuous intravenous isoproterenol infusion has been recommended in the treatment of patients in status asthmaticus who have not responded adequately to standard therapy and may require assisted ventilation. Discuss how this therapy is initiated and monitored.

The use of continuous intravenous isoproterenol should only be considered when standard therapeutic measures are inadequate and when facilities are present for maintaining a constant infusion rate and for monitoring blood pressure, ECG, and arterial blood gases. Klaustermeyer and coworkers (139), studied isoproterenol infusions in seven adult patients who were moderately severe to severe asthmatics, but were not in status asthmaticus. They found graded isoproterenol infusion rates from 0.0375 to 0.225 mcg/kg/min to be effective and safe with the maximum bronchodilation effect occurring within 2-5 minutes of starting the infusion. Cardiac effects were noted in all, but were not serious. Two patients complained of pain at the site of infusion which may be caused by the acidity of the solution. Wood and coworkers (276) studied isoproterenol continuous infusions in 19 children with status asthmaticus and respiratory failure. Seventeen children responded within 10 hours of receiving 0.08-2.7 mcg/kg/min isoproterenol continuous I.V. infusion. Intravenous salbutamol appears to have a bronchodilating effect similar to isoproterenol, but much less of an effect on heart rate (204).

12. Why do sympathomimetics appear to have less cardiac effects when given orally or by inhalation than by I.V. injection?

When isoproterenol is administered intravenously, the major urinary fraction is free isoproterenol (52%) and no conjugated isoproterenol is found (47). However, when given orally or inhaled, about three-fourths of the material collected in the urine is conjugated isoproterenol with a small amount of 3-0-methyliso-proterenol and a very small quantity of free isoproterenol. Significant O-methylation of isoproterenol occurs in the lung during absorption (15). Approximately 90% of the inhaled dose is swallowed and absorbed in the gastrointestinal tract (213). Isoproterenol is conjugated in the gut wall during absorption and enters the circulation mostly as inactive drug (85).

The observation that inhaled sympathomimetics have less cardiac effect than when given intravenously may be due to a large proportion of the dose being swallowed and not absorbed in an active form and secondly, because there may be metabolism of some sympathomimetics within the lung. Although beta$_2$ drugs are effective when given orally, a significant portion of the dose may be metabolized or not absorbed (56,64,199,266,275). When a beta$_2$ drug is used as an aerosol, of the 90% or so which is swallowed, some may be absorbed in an active form.

13. Other than sympathomimetics and theophylline, which drugs are effective bronchodilators?

Within the last 15 years, cigarettes containing the anticholinergic drug stramonium were used as a bronchodilator in treating asthma and chronic bronchitis. Atropine is an effective bronchodilator when given intravenously or by aerosol (282). However, the drug has not been routinely used because the required dose may have serious extrapulmonary effects (tachycardia, failure of accommodation) and there is fear of mucus inspissation. Recent evidence indicates that atropine aerosol is an effective bronchodilator which is well tolerated and has no adverse effect on sputum (141). The recently recognized importance of the parasympathetic nervous system in asthma and chronic bronchitis has stimulated the development of several anticholinergic drugs which are currently under investigation: ipratropium bromide (SCH 1000), deptropine, and atropine methonitrate. The majority of research has been an ipratropium bromide administered by aerosol (256). Preliminary studies indicate the drug may be most useful in chronic bronchitis or intrinsic asthma.

Alpha-adrenergic blocking agents have been shown to be bronchodilators in a limited number of reports. Alston and coworkers (3) found that the adenylcyclase activity in leucocytes (corresponding to the beta receptor) of patients with acute asthma shows a diminished response to isoproterenol stimulation. However, when an alpha-adrenergic blocking drug (phentolamine, thymoxamine) is combined with isoproterenol, the adenyl-cyclase response approaches normal. A study in 10 patients with reversible airway obstruction indicated that the combination of an alpha blocker produced more bronchodilation than isoproterenol alone (202). Although the use of alpha-adrenergic blocking agents could conceptually benefit the patient who does not respond to beta stimulation, subsequent *in vitro* studies have clouded the issue by showing alpha blockade to increase intracellular cyclic GMP in lymphocytes (100). Both alpha-adrenergic blocking agents and anticholinergic drugs should remain investigational until more information is available.

14. Knowing that G.S. took her last dose of aminophylline two hours before coming to the emergency room, the physician in the emergency room started a continuous aminophylline intravenous infusion at a rate of 63 mg/hr (0.9 mg/kg/hr). Theophylline plasma concentrations determined 12 and 24 hours after the infusion was initiated were 5.5 and 5.0 mcg/ml, respectively. Knowing that there is a log-linear improvement in FEV$_1$ and FVC as the theophylline plasma concentration increases from 5 to 20 mcg/ml (189), the intern wanted to increase the infusion rate to achieve a plasma theophylline concentration of 20 mcg/ml. What is the optimum theophylline plasma concentration to be achieved in status asthmaticus and in chronic asthma in outpatients?

The therapeutic theophylline plasma concentration range is generally stated to be either 5 to 20 mcg/ml or 10 to 20 mcg/ml. This range is commonly applied to the use of theophylline in the treatment of adults or children with acute or chronic asthma or bronchitis. One would assume that a theophylline plasma concentration-bronchodilation response relationship has been described for children and adults with acute and chronic asthma or bronchitis. However, it has not. Virtually all dose-response studies of theophylline have been performed in adults or children with asthma which was stable and not severe at the time of the study (123,128,156, 172,189,262, 272). People with severe asthma or status asthmaticus are frequently characterized by their inability to bronchodilate on exposure to isoproterenol inhalation or subcutaneous injection of epinephrine. In a series of 58 patients with severe asthma, patients did not show signs of bronchodilatability for 3.7 days after hospital admission (range 1 to 18 days) (221).

As with most biologic characteristics, the therapeutic range of a theophylline plasma concentration-response relationship is subject to inter- and intrapatient variability. Patients with severe asthma or those in status asthmaticus may show no response or a relatively poor response to high plasma levels of theophylline. However, in mild asthmatics who are very sensitive to bronchodilators, the theophylline plasma concentration-response relationship might start at 3 mcg/ml and be maximal at 8 mcg/ml. Patients with chronic asthma who are not acutely ill will demonstrate a plasma concentration-response which is in-

termediate to these two extremes.

For most drugs the upper limit of the therapeutic drug plasma concentration range is set at the point above which the toxicity incidence is unacceptable. The incidence of minor theophylline toxicity incidence is acceptable below 20 mcg/ml and grand mal seizures have only been reported above 20 mcg/ml.

Thus, the optimum theophylline plasma concentration is variable and not a fixed number for all patients in all situations. However, it may be useful to think in terms of target concentrations. For example, the target theophylline plasma concentration in severe airway obstruction requiring a continuous intravenous aminophylline infusion may be 15 to 20 mcg/ml. The initial target for the outpatient taking oral theophylline may be to achieve a peak theophylline plasma concentration between 10 to 15 mcg/ml. If this does not produce satisfactory results, the target can be raised to 15 to 20 mcg/ml. It is possible some patients may tolerate and benefit from concentrations exceeding 20 mcg/ml. Alternatively, patients with a pre-existing seizure disorder may not tolerate a theophylline plasma concentration as high as 20 mcg/ml.

15. After several days of receiving a continuous aminophylline infusion of 126 mg/hr which produced a steady-state theophylline plasma concentration (Cpss) of 10 mcg/ml, it was clear that G.S. was not getting much better. The intern wanted to achieve a new Cpss of 18 mcg/ml, whereas the pharmacy student recommended increasing the dose until minor toxicity was encountered and then slightly decreasing the dose until toxicity subsided. The pharmacy student argued that this is a well accepted method for achieving the maximum tolerable dose which is based on the fact that minor theophylline toxicity always precedes severe toxicity. Discuss minor and severe theophylline toxicity and the use of minor toxic symptoms as a prodrome for severe toxicity.

Theophylline toxicity is closely associated with the theophylline plasma concentration and can often be relieved by reducing the dose and plasma concentration. Historically, nausea and vomiting were thought to be the result of a local irritant effect of theophylline on the gastric mucosa. It was primarily this concept which led to the development of the highly soluble theophylline salts and complexes (e.g., oxtriphylline, theophylline sodium glycinate). Recent studies have shown nausea and vomiting may occur while the patient is receiving intravenous aminophylline and that these side effects are most common at theophylline plasma concentrations above 18 to 20 mcg/ml (107, 124, 128, 285). Jenne et al (128) did not find theophylline toxicity at theophylline plasma concentrations below 13 mcg/ml. Hypotension is a potentially lethal side effect of theophylline and is usually caused by administering the intravenous dose too rapidly. There is very little information available on the ability of theophylline to cause cardiac arrhythmias. Tachycardia is most frequent above theophylline plasma concentrations of 20 mcg/ml. When the drug is given by "I.V. push" or through a central venous pressure catheter the heart can be exposed to extremely high theophylline concentrations prior to distribution equilibrium (32). Both of these procedures should be avoided.

Table 3
THEOPHYLLINE SEIZURES:
CHARACTERISTICS OF 21 CASES REPORTED
SINCE 1972 (125,128,235,281,285)

Characteristic	Percent of Cases Where Information Was Available
Mortality	48
Age >61 years	68
Alcoholic/cirrhotic	24
Congestive heart failure	19
Severe illness as signified by the intravenous route of theophylline administration	90
Theophylline plasma concentration at time of seizure >40 mcg/ml	85
Prodromal symptoms (nausea) experienced prior to seizure	33
Therapeutic response to anticonvulsants	13

Until several years ago grand mal convulsions were thought to occur mainly in children who had received a theophylline overdosage. Since 1972 there have been at least 21 cases of convulsions reported in adults (125,128,235,281,285). The common characteristics of these 21 cases are summarized in Table 3. Although the incidence of mortality appears to be very high, many of the people were in respiratory failure and had other complications at the time of the seizure which may have contributed to the death. The seizure usually occurred at least 24 hours after aminophylline therapy was started and at a theophylline plasma concentration above 40 mcg/ml. This suggests drug accumulation as a result of an overestimate of the patient's theophylline clearance resulting in an overdose. The patient characteristics are consistent with this explanation in that many were elderly, had liver damage or potential damage, had congestive heart failure, or were severely ill. Theophylline clearance is decreased in cirrhosis and congestive heart failure. Although theophylline clearance is not well described in severely ill patients or people over 60 years of age, both factors alter the clearance of other drugs. Many of the seizures could not be controlled by diazepam,

phenytoin, or phenobarbital. Because some patients required a bronchodilator at the time of seizure, theophylline was not immediately discontinued in all patients and the seizure was treated with anticonvulsants. In these patients the seizures stopped only after theophylline was discontinued. When treating theophylline-associated seizures, theophylline must be discontinued and a rapid-acting anticonvulsant drug should be used.

Many clinicians will choose a standard dose of theophylline for treating all patients. When this dose does not produce the desired effect, the dosage is increased until the desired effect is attained or the patient complains of nausea or vomiting. Then, the dose is decreased slightly until this minor toxicity subsides. This reasoning is based on the assumption that minor theophylline toxicity will precede major toxicity. Zwillich and coworkers (285) looked for prodromal minor toxicity in eight seizure cases and found only one patient in eight had complained of minor toxicity prior to the seizure. To avoid seizures in patients, it appears the safest method would be to prevent the theophylline plasma concentration from exceeding 20 mcg/ml.

16. Discuss theophylline disposition and factors which may affect theophylline disposition.

Theophylline is eliminated primarily by hepatic metabolism with only 10% of the dose eliminated unchanged in the urine (20,49,126). Based on studies in the rat, a proposed scheme for theophylline metabolism is presented in Fig. 3 (162).

In man there are three theophylline metabolites found in the urine: 3-methylxanthine; 1,3-dimethyluric acid; and 1-methyluric acid from 1-methylxanthine. 1-Methylxanthine is not found in human urine and is not found in rat urine in the absence of allopurinol. It is possible that allopurinol could inhibit this metabolic step in man. The conversion of theophylline to 1,3 dimethyluric acid and 1-methylxanthine in the rat is mediated by hepatic microsomal enzymes which are inducible by phenobarbital and to a greater degree by 3-methylcholanthrene. The induction of theophylline metabolism in the rat by 3-methylcholanthrene has been offered as an explanation for the increased theophylline clearance in cigarette smokers. The conversion of theophylline to 3-methylxanthine may be a saturable step in the metabolism of theophylline at higher plasma concentrations (126). The metabolite 3-methylxanthine has been found in the plasma of several patients taking theophylline routinely. Nothing is known of the activity of 3-methylxanthine or the other metabolites. This information may be of importance in renal failure.

The parameters of theophylline disposition in man which are of importance clinically are total body clearance (L/hr/kg), the elimination rate constant (hr^{-1}) or half-life (hr), and the volume of distribution (L/kg). Theophylline disposition is influenced by age, disease, and smoking habit (Table 4).

There appear to be at least three age populations with respect to theophylline clearance: premature infants (5,86), children (60,163), and adults (128,188). Theophylline disposition has not been described in full-term infants from birth to one year or in adults over 60 years of age. Hepatic cirrhosis (207), congestive heart failure (127,146,208,217,270), and severe airway obstruction (217) decrease theophylline clearance.

The influence of status asthmaticus or severe bronchitis in adults on theophylline clearance remains a question. Neither the study by Weinberger and associates (270), or Koup and associates (146), have differentiated the strong effect of smoking from asthma or bronchitis in their patient samples. The theophylline clearance which Weinberger found in a heterogeneous group of adults with asthma, bronchitis, emphysema with complications of congestive heart failure, cancer, and acute myocardial infarction was the same as the clearance in healthy nonsmokers (118, 216). If all Weinberger's patients were nonsmokers one might assume that none of the disease characteristics in their sample influenced theophylline clearance. With the exception of premature infants, the differences in theophylline clearance between the groups are due to differences in the rate of metabolism as reflected in the half-life and not from changes in the volume of distribution.

Eventually the clinician should be able to better predict the theophylline dose which will produce the desired theophylline plasma concentration by knowing those characteristics of the patient which will influence theophylline disposition. Presently, one must use the disposition parameters outlined in Table 4. Since there is no information on the interaction of effects, i.e., a patient with cirrhosis, congestive heart failure, and severe asthma who is a heavy smoker; the clinician should make an educated, conservative guess as to the patient's clearance and base the initial theophylline regimen on that guess. A theophylline plasma determination can then be used to estimate the individual patient's clearance and a dosage adjustment can be made if necessary.

17. M.B. is a 100 kg, 25-year-old male admitted to the emergency room for acute asthma which has progressively worsened over the last week. He has been taking one 200 mg aminophylline uncoated tablet four times a day for the last several months in addition to use of his isoproterenol inhaler. His last aminophylline dose was two hours ago. It is noted that he smokes heavily and chews Mailpouch to-

bacco. The decision is made to give M.B. an aminophylline loading dose and continuous I.V. infusion which should keep his theophylline plasma concentration around 10 mcg/ml. Calculate dosage regimen recommendation.

The first consideration is to estimate the theophylline plasma concentration before giving the loading dose. Assuming that M.B. has a theophylline half-life of an average smoker (4 hours) and that he takes a tablet every 6 hours, little drug accumulation would be expected to occur. After taking an aminophylline uncoated tablet the peak plasma concentration is usually reached within 1 to 2 hours after the dose. Assuming a one-compartment model, instantaneous absorption, and no accumulation, the plasma concentration is estimated:

$$\text{Volume of distribution} = 0.45 \text{ L/kg} \times 100 \text{ kg} = 45\text{L}$$

$$C_p = \frac{\text{Dose}}{V_d} = \frac{160 \text{ mg theophylline}}{45 \text{ L}} = 3.6 \text{ mcg/ml or mg/L}$$

This estimation can be more accurately described and verified as follows:

$$C_{p\ max} = \frac{\text{Dose}}{V_d} \times \frac{1}{1-e^{-k_d\tau}}$$

$$\text{where } k_d = \frac{0.693}{t\frac{1}{2}} = \frac{0.693}{4.3\text{hr}} = 0.161 \text{ hr}^{-1}$$

where τ is the time interval between doses

$$= \frac{160 \text{ mg}}{45 \text{ L}} \times \frac{1}{1-e^{-(0.161 \text{ hr}^{-1}) (6 \text{ hr})}}$$

$$= 5.7 \text{ mcg/ml}$$

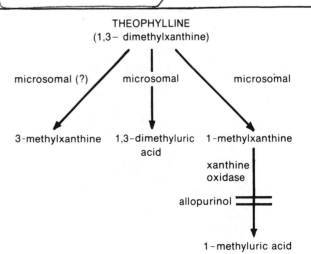

THEOPHYLLINE
(1,3– dimethylxanthine)

Figure 3. Potential Route of Theophylline Metabolism in Man

If M.B.'s plasma concentration is now about 4 mcg/ml and the desired plasma concentration is 10 mcg/ml, a theophylline dose must be given which will increase the theophylline plasma concentration 6 mcg/ml (10−4 = 6). The loading dose will be

LD = 6 mg/L × 45L = 270 mg theophylline

Since theophylline can be given I.V. only as amino-phylline (80 percent theophylline) the correct aminophylline loading dose is:

270 mg theophylline × 1.25 = 337.5 mg aminophylline

Giving a 340 mg aminophylline loading dose over 20 to 30 minutes should result in a plasma concentration near to 10 mcg/ml for M.B. The continuous theophylline infusion rate is calculated using the following steady-state equation:

Theophylline infusion rate
(mg/hr/kg)

= Theophylline Clearance × Steady-state theophylline
(L/hr/kg)   plasma concentration
                (mg/L)

The desired theophylline plasma concentration is known to be 10 mg/L, and now one must guess the theophylline clearance. There is no clearance estimate for severe asthmatics who smoke, but there is for healthy smokers (0.081 L/hr/kg) and severe asthmatics (0.038 L/hr/kg) although there may be an error in this estimation as noted above. When assuming a theophylline clearance it is probably best to err on the conservative side since the dose can always be increased once the initial dose is known to be safe. Choosing a theophylline clearance of 0.055 L/hr/kg the infusion rate would be:

Table 4
THE EFFECT OF AGE AND DISEASE ON THEOPHYLLINE DISPOSITION

	No. Subjects	Clearance (L/hr/kg)±SD	Half-Life (hrs)	Volume of distribution (L/kg)±SD
Age				
Premature infants with apnea:				
a. Aranda et al (5)	6	0.018(±0.002)	30.2	0.69(±0.10)
b. Giacoia et al (86)	8	0.039(±0.015)	19.9	1.15(±0.73)
Children-Asthma (nonacute):				
1-4 years — Loughnan et al (163)	10	0.100(±0.036)	3.4	0.45(±0.13)
6-17 years — Ellis et al (60)	30	0.087(±0.035)	3.7	0.42(±0.06)
4-15 years — Maselli et al (172)	38	0.093	3.2	0.40
Adults:				
a. healthy 19-31 years — Mitendo et al (188)	9	0.075(±0.019)	4.4	0.49(±0.08)
b. healthy 22-27 years — Ellis et al (60)	6	0.057(±0.018)	5.8	0.45(±0.09)
Disease				
Adults:				
Pulmonary edema — Piafsky et al (208)	9	0.041(±0.047)	22.9	0.60(±0.24)
Hepatic cirrhosis — Piafsky et al (207)	4	0.023(±0.009)	30.0	
Asthma (unknown severity) 34 to 53 years — Mitenko et al (188)	7	0.068(±0.016)	4.3	0.42(±0.06)
Acute, severe COPD plus some patients with pneumonia, cirrhosis, CHF — Weinberger et al (270)	15	0.038(±0.023)	—	—
Children:				
Status asthmaticus (no complications) 4-10 years — Weinberger et al (270)	6	0.073(±0.019)	—	—
Smoking habit (Adults)				
Nonsmokers:				
a. Powell et al (216)	15	0.040(±0.008)	8.3	0.47(±0.08)
b. Hunt et al (118)	8	0.038	7.0	0.38(±0.04)
Smokers:				
a. Powell et al (216)	7	0.063(±0.019)	5.4	0.50(±0.06)
b. Hunt et al (118)	8	0.081	4.3	0.50(±0.12)

Theophylline infusion rate	= 0.055 L/hr/kg × 10 mg/L
	= 0.55 mg/hr/kg
Aminophylline infusion rate	= 0.55 mg/hr/kg × 1.25
	= 0.69 mg/hr/kg
M.B.'s aminophylline	
infusion rate	= 0.69 mg/hr/kg × 100 kg
	= 69 mg/hr

18. Twenty-four hours after the theophylline infusion was begun M.B.'s asthma was no better; the theophylline plasma concentration was 9 mcg/ml at that time. The decision was made to increase his plasma concentration to 18 mcg/ml. How would you do this?

The theophylline clearance which was initially estimated is probably close to M.B.'s actual clearance based on the predicted steady-state concentration and that found at 24 hours. When making clearance estimations based on an assumed steady-state plasma concentration, it is imperative that the accuracy of the infusion rate be checked. That is, if M.B. was to receive 100 mg/hr (630 mg aminophylline/Liter D_5W) for 24 hours (2400 ml) and he only received 1200 ml, then the true infusion rate would be 31.5 mg/hr. In this case M.B.'s clearance would be:

Theophylline infusion rate	= 31.5 mg/hr × 0.8
	= 25.2 mg/hr
Theophylline clearance	= 25.2 mg/hr ÷ 9 mg/L
	= 2.8 L/hr

However, the I.V. infusion was accurate and his clearance is close to the initial estimation (0.055 L/hr/kg · 100 kg = 5.5 L/hr). To achieve the new steady-state theophylline concentration, a loading dose should be given with the new infusion rate. Otherwise, it may take a day or more to go from 9 to 18 mcg/ml by only increasing the infusion rate.

Theophylline loading dose	= (18−9 mcg/ml) × 45L
	= 405 mg or 506 mg
	aminophylline
Theophylline infusion rate	= 5.5 L/hr × 18 mg/L
	= 99 mg/hr
	or 124 mg/hr aminophylline

19. About 30 hours after this new aminophylline infusion rate (124 mg/hr) was initiated, M.B. had a grand mal seizure. The aminophylline infusion was immediately stopped, a blood sample drawn, and anticonvulsants administered. No sign of seizure activity was noted 20 minutes after the aminophylline was discontinued. The cause of the seizure was probably due to a medication error since he had received 4 times the intended dose over the last 30 hours. Instead of giving 124 mg/hr (1240 mg aminophylline/ Liter D-5-W at 100 ml/hr), he had received 496 mg/hr (1240 mg aminophylline/500 ml D-5-W at 200 ml/hr). His plasma theophylline concentration at the time of

the seizure was 85 mcg/ml. How should this patient be treated? How can theophylline-induced seizures be prevented?

After stopping the theophylline, the patient must be evaluated for other causes of seizures, e.g., falling out of bed and striking his head, previous neurologic damage, extremely high doses of corticosteroids or penicillin, rapid change in arterial pH or hypoxia. It may be necessary to treat residual bronchospasm in patients experiencing theophylline associated seizures. Although there is no information on the safety of sympathomimetic bronchodilators in this situation, CNS stimulation or seizures from the newer sympathomimetics is rare. Neither terbutaline nor its metabolites penetrate the blood-brain barrier in mice (18). Based on this information, low doses of terbutaline could be used and carefully evaluated. The terbutaline dose could be increased when the previous dose is felt to be safe.

Theophylline should be stopped until it is estimated that the theophylline plasma concentration is within the 5 to 20 mcg/ml range. The infusion which will maintain the theophylline plasma concentration within this range can then be started. Serial theophylline plasma determinations following the seizure provide the safest means for determining the correct time to start dosing theophylline and make it possible to estimate the elimination rate constant (k_d). Then, by assuming the volume of distribution to be 0.45 L/kg, a reasonably accurate estimation of theophylline clearance ($k_d V_d$) is made which can be used for estimating a new infusion rate. When the drug assay is not available, the theophylline half-life should be estimated and theophylline should be not given for 3 to 4 half-lives following the seizures. Any estimate of theophylline half-life should be an overestimation since it should be assured that the plasma concentration is below 20 to 25 mcg/ml before theophylline is re-started.

In the above case, the overdosage should have resulted in a plasma concentration of 72 mcg/ml instead of the intended 18 mcg/ml assuming first order elimination. Theophylline pharmacokinetics at this high plasma concentration have not been described and may not be first order. However, assuming the half-life is still 4 hours, in three half-lives the theophylline plasma concentration should decay to 10.6 mcg/ml.

$$C_{p(t)} = C_{p(o)}e^{-(k_d)(t)}$$
$$= 85 \text{ mcg/ml} \times e^{-(0.173hr^{-1})(12 \text{ hr})}$$
$$= 10.6 \text{ mcg/ml}$$

A theophylline plasma assay could be rapidly performed at 12 hours and when it is in the above region, the correct aminophylline infusion rate can be used (124 mg/hr).

Theophylline seizures are generally caused by overdosing the patient. This may be caused either by an overestimate of the theophylline clearance or by a medication error. Helpful precautions which can be employed to avoid theophylline seizures or toxicity include:

(a) Dose theophylline on a milligram per kilogram body weight basis using the characteristics of the patient to estimate theophylline clearance.

(b) Utilize theophylline plasma concentration determinations.

(c) Place one-fourth of the 24-hour theophylline dose into an I.V. bottle to run over 6 hours. In this way, if all the contents of the bottle inadvertently are infused in 10 or 20 minutes, the patient will not be in serious danger. One should avoid giving the 24-hour dose in a single I.V. bottle.

(d) Use an intravenous infusion set which delivers 60 drops per milliliter.

(e) Use an intravenous infusion pump.

The problem of dosing theophylline in patients with a history of seizures has not been studied. We encountered a patient who had asthma and epilepsy treated with anticonvulsants. On several hospital admissions for the treatment of severe asthma the patient experienced a grand mal seizure. On each occasion the theophylline plasma concentration was around 20 mcg/ml when the seizure occurred. When the theophylline dose was decreased so that the plasma concentration would not exceed 15 mcg/ml, the patient was seizure-free. This is certainly not proof that theophylline caused the seizures or that lowering the dose had a beneficial effect. However, it may suggest that some patients with epilepsy may be sensitive to theophylline and may require close observation or the use of other bronchodilators.

Table 5
THEOPHYLLINE CONTENT OF THEOPHYLLINE PHARMACEUTICAL ALTERNATIVES

	Percent Pure Theophylline
Theophylline NF	100
Theophylline monohydrate NF	91
Aminophylline USP	80
Oxtriphylline (choline theophyllinate)	65
Theophylline monoethanolamine	75
Theophylline calcium salicylate	48
Theophylline sodium glycinate	50

20. M.B. is now well enough to start taking oral medications. Discuss those factors influencing theophylline product selection and dosage. How are theophylline plasma concentration determinations used in outpatients?

The choice of a theophylline product for chronic use is dependent on patient convenience, bioavailability,

and cost. Theophylline dosage forms used in outpatients include: aqueous or hydro-alcoholic solutions, suspensions, uncoated tablets, soft gelatin capsules, enteric coated tablets, sustained-release tablets and capsules, suppositories, and retention enemas.

The development of many theophylline dosage forms and salts was based on the feeling that the gastrointestinal side effects of theophylline are caused by a local effect of the drug on the gastric mucosa. Although this may in part be true, the association of nausea and vomiting with high theophylline plasma concentrations seems to indicate a centrally mediated mechanism.

Based on a series of recent studies, it appears that theophylline is completely absorbed from the gastrointestinal tract if the dosage form has not been designed to slow or delay absorption, and if the dosage form remains in the body. Solutions and uncoated tablets of theophylline, aminophylline, and oxtriphylline are completely and rapidly absorbed reaching a peak plasma concentration in 1 to 2 hours when given on an empty stomach (61,94,107,215,225,273). When a meal high in fat, protein and carbohydrate precedes a solution of uncoated tablet, absorption may be delayed but absorption is still complete (215,225,273). When aminophylline suppositories are retained in the body for 6 hours or longer, theophylline absorption is nearly complete (231). The absorption of enteric coated or sustained-release theophylline dosage forms may be incomplete and erratic (187,223,224), although some sustained-release dosage forms are quite reliable (128).

Based on bioavailability, convenience, and cost, an uncoated tablet of theophylline or its salts is the recommended dosage form to use in adults and children who can swallow tablets. There can be a ten-fold difference in cost between products. For example, based on the 1976 Red Book average wholesale cost, the cost of giving a patient 200 mg theophylline four times a day for one year would be $402.96 for Elixophyllin versus $46.72 for the most expensive generic aminophylline uncoated tablet.

For patients being converted from intravenous to oral theophylline therapy, the oral theophylline dose will be the same as the intravenous dose if similar plasma concentrations and effect are desired. In other words, the hourly intravenous dose is multiplied times the number of dosage interval hours to obtain the oral theophylline dose. When converting a patient from intravenous aminophylline to oral theophylline, oxtriphylline or another salt, a dosage adjustment must be made because of differences in the actual theophylline content (Table 5). Although outpatients are often given theophylline on a qid regimen (9 AM, 1 PM, 5 PM, 9 PM), many patients may only require a dose every 8 hours or less if they have a relatively low theophylline clearance or long half-life, e.g., non-smokers.

Assuming that M.B.'s 124 mg/hour intravenous aminophylline dose was satisfactory, his oral dose would be 600 mg aminophylline as uncoated tablets every 6 hours (6 hr × 124 mg/hr = 744 mg). The 600 mg dose is slightly less than the 6-hour infusion rate, 744 mg/6 hours, to allow for peak plasma concentrations which would be higher than was produced by the constant infusion.

When prescribing theophylline for an outpatient who has never taken the drug before, an initial estimation of the dose should be made according to the patient's weight and smoking history. This estimation should be conservative to prevent toxicity from occurring at home and should be re-evaluated within a week or so. Theophylline plasma concentration determinations and an objective and subjective analysis may be used in following outpatients. The time the blood sample should be drawn is determined by the question being asked. If toxicity is suspected, a blood sample can be drawn while symptoms are present or when a peak plasma concentration is suspected. A blood sample drawn at the midpoint of the dosage interval or just before the next dose may be more useful in evaluating therapy than obtaining a sample just after the dose is given and absorption is occurring. Saliva has been recommended as a sampling medium for estimating the theophylline plasma concentration (147). Although the saliva theophylline concentration is about 50% of the plasma concentration in most patients, there is significant inter- and intrasubject variation in this percentage (215,225). If a patient has had his saliva to plasma theophylline ratio determined, then future theophylline saliva determinations may be a rough estimation of the plasma concentration. Otherwise, a theophylline saliva concentration may only indicate whether the patient is taking the drug.

Sustained-release preparations may be of use in patients with a high theophylline clearance. Asthma patients frequently complain of dyspnea in the middle of the night or early in the morning. It is conceivable that some of these patients have a subtherapeutic theophylline plasma concentration at this time due to the long dosage interval from 10 PM to 7 AM. One could try using a sustained release product alone or substitute a sustained-release preparation or suppository for the usual night time dose of a solution or uncoated tablet in order to prolong absorption and raise the early morning plasma concentration.

21. C.M. is a 20 kg, 8-year-old girl who has just been diagnosed in the clinic as having asthma. Using the above recommendations, what theophylline dosage form and dose would you recommend?

The dosage can be calculated using the clearance estimation of Ellis and Associates (60):

Theophylline dose/6 hrs
$$= \text{Theophylline clearance for 6 hrs} \times C_{pss}$$
$$= (0.087 \text{ L/hr/kg} \times 6 \text{ hr} \times 20 \text{ kg}) \times 10 \text{ mg/L}$$
$$= 104 \text{ mg}$$
Aminophylline dose/6 hours = 130 mg

Since an 8-year-old child can usually take tablets, C.M. could try taking 1½ 100 mg (150 mg) aminophylline uncoated tablets every 6 hours. One could make the regimen more conservative by using the clearance estimate for the population (0.087 L/hr/kg) minus one standard deviation (0.035 L/hr/kg) which is 0.052 L/hr/kg. The same procedure can be used for the initial estimation of theophylline dosage in adults.

22. What is the indication for dosage forms which contain theophylline and other drugs?

The more than 30 drugs which are available in combination with theophylline include sympathomimetics, sedatives, antacids, expectorants, antihistamines, anesthetics, a narcotic, diuretic and an anticholinergic drug. Of all the combination ingredients, sympathomimetics appear to be most rational. Combination products which contain theophylline and ephedrine do produce bronchodilation. However, there is reason to believe that the use of such products will result in less than optimal therapy. Weinberger and Bronsky (271,272) have shown that theophylline produces more bronchodilation than ephedrine in children. When ephedrine was given to children who had an average theophylline plasma concentration of 10 mcg/ml, ephedrine did not increase the therapetuic effect, but did increase the incidence of toxicity. If the theophylline dose is to be titrated to a plasma concentration between 5 to 20 mcg/ml, toxicity may occur at a relatively low theophylline plasma concentration when a combination product is used because of the inherent inflexibility of these products. Theophylline-ephedrine products frequently contain phenobarbital which may increase corticosteroid clearance (22) and could increase theophylline clearance (162).

Since there is even less indication for the other drugs in combination theophylline products, the use of such products should be discouraged.

23. Dihydroxypropyltheophylline (dyphylline) and hydroxypropyltheophylline (proxyphylline) are theophylline analogues which are used in the U.S. and Europe, respectively. How do they compare to theophylline as bronchodilators?

Neither drug is metabolized to theophylline in man. There is no basis for recommending the use of either drug since the relative potencies and toxicities are not known. Compared to theophylline, dyphylline may be eliminated more rapidly (241).

24. What is the mechanism of action of corticosteroids in asthma? In which patients are corticosteroids indicated?

Since corticosteroids were first used to treat asthma in the early 1950's (34,233), multiple mechanisms of action have been proposed (8) even though objective documentation of the clinical efficacy in acute asthma has been difficult (178,211). Actions of corticosteroids which would benefit the asthmatic patient include: inhibit the formation of antibody and the formation and release of chemicals mediating the allergic reaction, decrease the threshold of beta$_2$ stimulation in bronchial smooth muscle, enhance the endogenous synthesis of epinephrine and inhibit its degradation, decrease mucosal edema, and induce bronchodilator effectiveness in patients who were previously unresponsive. Corticosteroids are indicated in the treatment of acute and chronic patients with severe asthma where maximal bronchodilator usage has not provided an adequate effect.

25. Present an approach to the use of systemic corticosteroids in acute and chronic asthma based on current knowledge of adrenal function in the disease and corticosteroid pharmacokinetics. Also indicate the therapeutic goals which should be applied to these drugs in asthma.

Although corticosteroids are toxic, these drugs may be underused in the treatment of some asthma patients because the toxicity is often emphasized over the therapeutic effect. Either under- or overuse may result in unnecessary morbidity and mortality. The proper dosage which should be used is not well defined. Monitoring serial pulmonary function tests, total eosinophil count, and plasma 11-hydroxycorticosteroids may be useful in arriving at the individual steroid dosage. It has been suggested that an adequate corticosteroid dose will maintain the total eosinophil count less than 80–100/mm^3 (115). When the total eosinophil count is greater than this value, it may be an indication that the corticosteroid dose should be increased.

Another approach to corticosteroid use is based on adrenal function in asthma and the application of pharmacokinetic principles. The normal plasma concentration of cortisol (hydrocortisone) varies between 10 and 30 mcg/100ml, with diurnal changes (57). Approximately 80 to 95% of plasma cortisol is bound to the gamma globulin, transcortin, leaving only a small fraction of cortisol free and active (55). During a stressful situation the adrenals may produce more cortisol. Asthma patients who are asymptomatic or acutely ill and not receiving corticosteroids may have a normal adrenocortical response and in some cases it can be decreased (17,138). Patients on continuous corticosteroid therapy have a reduced plasma cortisol concentration, a decreased response to ACTH, and an increased cortisol metabolic clearance rate (35, 57, 214, 234). Patients taking alternate day corticosteroids have normal plasma cortisol and normal response to ACTH (67,214). It has been suggested that to achieve a therapeutic response from corticosteroids in severe asthma, the plasma cortisol concentration should be between 100 and 150 mcg/ml (45). It is felt that this concentration is necessary to produce an appreciable amount of unbound cortisol which can diffuse to the sites of action and produce the therapeutic effect. To achieve and maintain the above cortisol plasma concentration range, a hydrocortisone hemisuccinate loading dose of 4 mg/kg body weight and continuous infusion of 3 mg/kg every 6 hours has been recommended (44). Since cortisol clearance varies between individuals (57), and cortisol clearance is increased in patients on continuous corticosteroid therapy or patients taking phenobarbital (22), the continuous hydrocortisone dosage would have to be adjusted for the patient's cortisol concentration if the above approach is used. Alternatively, 30 mg/kg/day of methylprednisolone in 4 to 6 divided I.V. doses has been recommended. There is no indication that these large steroid doses are more efficacious than giving 4 to 10 mg/kg/day doses of methylprednisolone.

Tapering the corticosteroid dosage in acutely ill patients can be initiated when the patient has sustained improvement by decreasing the dosage 25 to 50% every two days until a daily oral prednisone dose of about 20 mg is reached. This dosage is further tapered over the next week or two until it is stopped. Patients on chronic corticosteroid therapy can be tapered to their pre-hospitalization dosage usually within a week after the attack has subsided. A major goal when using chronic corticosteroid therapy is to arrive at the smallest daily corticosteroid dosage possible by tapering the dose until mild asthma symptoms are evident and then, slightly increase the dose until the patient is relieved.

When long-term corticosteroid therapy is used in asthma, the most common side effects which occur are growth retardation in children, gastritis or peptic ulcer, weight gain, hypertension, osteoporosis, increase in intraocular pressure, easy bruisability and electrolyte disturbances. However, all corticosteroid side effects can be encountered. Many of the side effects are dose related (159,175). Growth retardation in asthmatic children given a daily prednisolone dosage of 3 mg/meter^2 for 6 months is less than that with 4 mg/meter^2/day (136). Maunsell and coworkers (175) found the incidence of corticosteroid side effects in a series of 170 asthma patients to be 4% when receiving a daily prednisone dose of 2 to 5 mg for at least 6 months, 14% receiving 6 to 10 mg, and 16% at 11 to 20 mg prednisone per day. Patients who are elderly (159) or who have low serum albumin concentration (157) appear to be more susceptible to side effects. Although the primary protein which binds cortisol is globulin (high affinity, low capacity), at high corticosteroid doses the binding capacity of globulin may be exceeded and binding to albumin (low affinity, high capacity) may become more important. Patients receiving large corticosteroid doses who have low serum albumin may receive a greater pharmacologic effect since a higher concentration of free drug would be expected.

Before a patient is begun on a chronic corticosteroid regimen, every effort should be made to optimize therapy with less toxic drugs and possibly avert the use of corticosteroids. When a patient must take corticosteroids chronically, the goal should be to use the smallest dose which is necessary to keep the patient symptom-free or nearly so, while giving the drug in a manner which will most limit side effects. Side effects may be limited by choosing a corticosteroid with minimal mineralocorticoid activity, giving the daily dose early in the morning, using an alternate day dosing regimen, and using either beclomethasone or cromolyn with systemic corticosteroids. (Also see *Glucocorticoid* chapter.)

26. Beclomethasone dipropionate has recently been introduced as a corticosteroid aerosol for treating chronic asthma in children and adults. Discuss the pharmacologic and pharmacokinetic characteristics of beclomethasone which make it significantly different from previously used corticosteroids.

Beclomethasone dipropionate has very potent topical anti-inflammatory activity which is far greater than beclomethasone alone or either dexamethasone or betamethasone (104). The inhalation dose is 400 mcg per day and is usually not greater than 800 mcg per day in severe cases. Adrenal function tests are at most minimally affected by inhalation of 1000 mcg beclomethasone dipropionate per day, whereas daily doses of 2000 mcg or more appear to suppress adrenal function (24,38,50,80,89,104,166). The reason beclomethasone dipropionate is an effective corticosteroid in asthma, while producing little or no systemic corticosteroid side effects or adrenal suppression at usual doses, is the drug has a local effect in the lung and most of that which is absorbed systemically appears to be inactive. An intravenous dose of 1000 mcg will produce complete suppression of plasma cortisol, indicating the drug has the ability to produce adrenal suppression at usual doses but must be inactivated prior to systemic distribution following inhalation. Results of pharmacokinetic studies of beclomethasone dipropionate are difficult to evaluate because of the analytic techniques used (169,170). Eighty to ninety percent of the inhaled dose is swallowed and absorbed from the gut. Although a large proportion of an oral dose is absorbed, it is felt that most of the dose is converted to inactive metabolites by first pass metabolism in the liver.

27. When should beclomethasone aerosol be used? What are the goals ot therapy? Which factors will influence the response to beclomethasone dipropionate?

Beclomethasone dipropionate aerosol has been studied in controlled trials in corticosteroid-dependent patients and patients who were being considered for corticosteroid therapy because they had not been adequately controlled by other drugs. In general, these are the two types of asthma patients in whom the drug is indicated. The goal in the first group is to reduce or eliminate the need for systemic corticosteroids in patients taking them chronically, thereby limiting side effects. In the second group, the goal is to preclude the use of chronic systemic corticosteroids in patients who have not used them chronically.

Blinded, controlled trials of beclomethasone dipropionate aerosol in adults (19, 33, 77, 79, 111, 113, 171, 244, 265) and children (90,164) of the above two groups clearly indicate the drug is superior to placebo in maintaining or improving clinical and pulmonary function status. Generally, decreasing the maintenance dose of oral corticosteroid in patients treated with beclomethasone dipropionate is easier in patients receiving less than 10 mg prednisone per day or an equivalent dose of other corticosteroids (19, 99, 111, 113). The finding that many patients who receive less than 10 mg prednisone per day can be completely transferred to beclomethasone dipropionate aerosol may be partially explained by the relative potency of the two drugs. Beclomethasone dipropionate 300 mcg aerosol is approximately equivalent to 7.5 mg prednisone per day in objective and subjective response (149), and the usual dose of beclomethasone is 400 mcg/day. In uncontrolled studies where corticosteroid-dependent patients were followed for at least one year, oral corticosteroids or corticotropin could be withdrawn in one-third to three-fourths of patients (23,63,95,99). Since some studies have not determined the minimum effective corticosteroid dose before starting beclomethasone, the percentage of patients in whom corticosteroids can be withdrawn may actually be less. Some patients may require periodic short term oral corticosteroid dosing during an exacerbation of asthma. If the oral corticosteroid dosage reduction is performed too quickly, the result may be an episode of adrenal insufficiency or an acute asthma attack. When use of beclomethasone dipropionate aerosol unsuccessfully reduces or replaces systemic corticosteroids, Cushingoid side effects may regress or disappear. Beclomethasone dipropionate aerosol may be more effective in patients with (a) extrinsic asthma, (b) less impaired pulmonary function, (c) a large degree of reversible airway obstruction, and (d) patients without impaired adrenal function. This is not surprising since almost any drug used in asthma will be more effective in the above situations.

28. How should beclomethasone dipropionate aerosol be used in treating asthma? Discuss the dosage, method of administration, and a scheme for replacing systemic corticosteroids with beclomethasone.

The dosage of beclomethasone dipropionate aerosol which has been effective in children and adults is 400 mcg per day given as two puffs four times a day. Although increasing the dosage is not beneficial in most patients (80), selected patients who respond poorly to the 400 mcg per day dose and who are taking large systemic corticosteroid doses (>15 mg prednisone per day) may show significant improvement in pulmonary function at daily beclomethasone doses of 800 to 1000 mcg (21,50). Daily dosages less than 400 mcg may be effective in some patients.

The method of using the aerosol is the same as was previously described for aerosolized sympathomimetics. Since beclomethasone has a local effect in the lung, it would be expected to be less effective or ineffective when significant bronchial obstruction exists. If the patient is obstructed but bronchodilatable, beclomethasone dipropionate aerosol may be more effective if a fast-acting sympathomimetic aerosol is used prior to steroid aerosol administration. The patient must understand that he is not to expect an acute effect from either beclomethasone or cromolyn and for this reason should not dose himself with more than has been prescribed.

In studies where beclomethasone has been used to reduce or replace systemic corticosteroids, the rate of systemic corticosteroid dose reduction has varied from complete withdrawal in several days to decreasing the daily prednisone dose in 1 mg increments at monthly intervals (24,33). Because the risks of rapid systemic corticosteroid withdrawal far outweigh the potential benefits in most cases, a conservative approach is recommended with frequent evaluation for signs or symptoms of adrenal insufficiency or disease exacerbation. Patients must be advised that when Addisonian symptoms occur (nausea, vomiting, muscle and joint pain, depression, fatigue, anorexia, etc.) or asthma worsens, they must inform their physician. Adrenal function tests should be performed initially and at intervals during the withdrawal phase in order to indicate whether further systemic corticosteroid is indicated at that time. Corticosteroid-dependent patients undergoing dosage reduction should be informed to increase the systemic corticosteroid dosage

should the above problems arise. Patients who have been completely withdrawn from systemic corticosteroids can be given a supply of oral corticosteroid which they can use during periodic asthma exacerbations.

29. What side effects of corticosteroid aerosols, other than adrenal, are of concern? Discuss how they can be treated and prevented.

Candida albicans infection of the mouth, pharynx, and larynx is the most common side effect associated with continuous use of beclomethasone dipropionate aerosol. The incidence appears to be dose related occurring in 71% of cases at 800 mcg per day and in 33 to 41% of cases at 400 mcg per day, versus 9 to 27% when corticosteroids were not given (21,176,185). There have been no reports of fungal pulmonary infections to date. The infection may spontaneously resolve, or may clear with dosage reduction with or without combined treatment with topical nystatin or amphotericin B. There are currently no conclusive data on the influence of steroid aerosols on the actual infection rate, i.e., fungal, bacterial, and viral. Some investigators believe it may be higher than initially estimated (99,111).

Betamethasone valerate and triamcinolone acetonide aerosols appear to have similar efficacy and side effects as beclomethasone dipropionate.

A more detailed review of corticosteroid therapy may be found in the *Glucocorticoid* chapter.

30. Cromolyn (cromolyn sodium, disodium chromoglycate) is used as aprophylactic drug in the treatment of asthma. Discuss the pharmacologic and pharmaceutical properties of this anti-asthmatic drug.

Cromolyn blocks the release of mediators (histamine, serotonin, SRS-A) from the mast cell in the lung caused by the interaction of antigen with a sensitized mast cell (Fig. 2). It is felt that cromolyn stabilizes the membrane of the sensitized mast cell, thereby preventing the release of mediators of anaphylaxis. By presenting the release of mediators of anaphylaxis, cromolyn has the ability to prevent the occurrence of an allergic or asthmatic reaction when it normally would occur. Cromolyn is ineffective when given after the host is exposed to the antigen. Cromolyn is not a bronchodilator and should not be used as one (51).

Cromolyn is available for clinical use in 20 mg gelatin capsules with lactose as an inert adjuvant. The capsule is placed in a special turboinhaler (Spinhaler) which punctures the capsule. When the patient places the turboinhaler in his mouth and inhales, the capsule spins and vibrates, causing the micronized powder to be inhaled. Of the 1 to 2 mg cromolyn which is inhaled into the lung, only about 9% is absorbed systemically. Ninety percent of the dose which is inhaled into the lungs plus the 18 to 19 mg which is deposited in the oropharynx and trachea is eventually swallowed and eliminated by way of the gastrointestinal tract. Neither the drug nor lactose is felt to accumulate in the lung.

31. What conclusions can be drawn from the cromolyn efficacy studies in adults and children with chronic asthma?

Many of the early controlled clinical studies of cromolyn were conducted in England using a product which contained 0.1 mg isoproterenol in addition to 20 mg cromolyn. These studies have been criticized because of the inability to dissociate the effect of cromolyn from isoproterenol. The discussion presented here will be based on those studies where only cromolyn was used. Both short (11,59,82,116,121,173,192,239) and long term (62,72,119,261) (one year or more) studies have reported cromolyn to be superior to placebo in preventing or suppressing asthma symptoms. The response to cromolyn was usually measured by a change in asthma symptoms (wheeze, tightness of chest, cough), incidence of acute attacks, requirement for bronchodilators or corticosteroids, and a subjective charge in patient preference for cromolyn compared to placebo. Although the effect of cromolyn was marked in many patients, there was either a minimal effect or no benefit noted in some patients. Forced expiratory volume at one second and peak expiratory flow rate (PEFR) may either increase or show no improvement following cromolyn therapy (36, 121, 228, 240). The observation that some patients show symptomatic improvement without a change in $FEV_{1.0}$ or PEFR may result from a reduction in hyperinflation caused by the drug. Chronic bronchial infection appears to be an important factor which limits the therapeutic response (27). When cromolyn is given for more than one year most patients who had a favorable response initially continue to benefit from the drug (194,240). Unexpectedly, cromolyn has been shown to be effective in exercise-induced asthma (59, 91, 243).

32. What type of asthma patient can be expected to benefit most from cromolyn?

Cromolyn appears to be most effective when used prophylactically to treat the extrinsic type of asthma patient. The cromolyn responsive patient is frequently young, has seasonal symptoms which are related to a specific allergen, and does not have permanent lung damage from bronchitis or emphysema. Although extrinsic asthmatics benefit most from cromolyn, some extrinsic types do not respond while many intrinsic types are well-controlled on the drug (240,261). Because of the inability to predict therapeutic response

to cromolyn, any patient who does not respond adequately to bronchodilators may be treated with 20 mg cromolyn inhaled four times a day for four weeks. If there is no subjective or objective change in the patient at that time, cromolyn may be discontinued.

33. How significant is the steroid-sparing effect of cromolyn? Outline a safe method for steroid withdrawal in patients receivng cromolyn.

The percentage of patients in clinical studies receiving cromolyn in whom the corticosteroid dose can be reduced and the degree of reduction is dependent upon patient selection. Extrinsic asthmatics respond better to cromolyn than patients diagnosed as having intrinsic asthma, bronchitis, or emphysema. In studies evaluating a steroid-sparing effect of cromolyn, prior to starting the study it is critical all patients receive the lowest possible oral corticosteroid dose. With these factors in mind, the use of cromolyn may permit the corticosteroid dose to be decreased about 25 to 50% in 50 to 75% of patients (6,62,119,121,173,194,220). Some patients can be completely weaned from corticosteroids while a few patients may actually worsen after cromolyn is administered.

The method for reducing the corticosteroid dose is similar to that described earlier for beclomethasone. The risk of causing an exacerbation of asthma or Addisonian effects from too rapid steroid withdrawal is clearly avoidable in most cases by conservative dosage reduction and frequent patient evaluation. Patient education and participation in the therapeutic plan should be stressed. When the patient encounters symptoms of asthma or steroid withdrawal, he should have a supply of oral corticosteroid to self-administer. After cromolyn therapy is started and before an attempt is made to reduce the corticosteroid dosage, it may be advantageous to first switch to an alternate day corticosteroid regimen.

Hambleton and associates (101) compared a fixed cromolyn dose to an individualized theophylline regimen in controlling symptoms of children with chronic asthma and found the two treatments had similar efficacy. Although the patients in this study were not steroid-dependent asthmatics, the possibility of a steroid-sparing effect for theophylline was raised. Indeed, it is reasonable to expect that any treatment which significantly alleviates the symptoms of chronic severe asthma may have a steroid-sparing effect.

34. What are some clinically useful guidelines for using cromolyn?

One of the main causes for therapeutic failure from cromolyn is thought to be poor patient compliance with the prescribed regimen. An attempt should be made to have the patient inhale 20 mg cromolyn four times a day. Since cromolyn exerts a direct, local effect in the lung, it may be desirable to give the patient a rapid-acting sympathomimetic aerosol prior to cromolyn inhalation. This may improve the distribution of cromolyn in the lung and prevent bronchospasm following inhalation of the powder. Cromolyn should be started when the patient is stable and not for at least a week or two following an acute asthma attack. When a severe attack does occur, cromolyn should be withheld because the powder may provoke bronchospasm of the sensitive airways. If the drug is to be effective, the patient must understand and demonstrate the correct use of the Spinhaler. Some patients, particularly those with seasonal asthma, may be able to adjust the cromolyn dose to fit their requirements (261). The drug may be used seasonally prior to antigen exposure or may be tapered to less than four capsules a day. Although it has been suggested that some patients not responding to four capsules a day may benefit from an increased dosage, there is little evidence to support this contention.

35. Describe the side effects of cromolyn.

The most remarkable characteristic of cromolyn is its very low incidence of serious side effects. The most bothersome side effect is the cough which probably results from inhaling a dry powder. Other than a few cases of allergy, the drug has shown little evidence of toxicity.

36. Many patients with bronchitis or asthma, particularly during an exacerbation, have thick tenacious sputum which is difficult to eliminate. Inspissation contributes to airway obstruction, and removal of mucous plugs, if present, is an important treatment goal. Discuss the pharmacologic treatments which are currently available: hydration, expectorants, and mucolytics.

The chemical composition of bronchial secretions is predominantly sodium, chloride, calcium, carbohydrate, protein, lipid, and nucleic acid. These secretions from goblet cells and bronchial glands cover the bronchial mucosa. The constant, synchronized action of cilia propels mucous containing foreign particles toward the upper region of the respiratory tract. This process is partially responsible for keeping the respiratory tract sterile. Thickened, tenacious mucous which forms plugs within the bronchi is a characteristic feature of status asthmaticus and is thought to limit the response to bronchodilator drugs.

It would be expected that water would be the best expectorant available. Dehydration occurs in some patients with status asthmaticus and has been suggested to be a cause of death (251). Adequate hydration in severely ill patients is insured by giving intravenous fluids. Although water requirements are greater for the dehydrated patients, care must be taken to prevent overhydration in all patients. The clinician must frequently evaluate the state of hydration based on history (thirst), physical examination (skin turgor, edema), and laboratory tests (hemoglobin, hematocrit, BUN, Cr, serum and urine electrolytes, and urine volume and specific gravity).

Expectorant drugs such as potassium or sodium iodide (68) or guaifenesin (110) are supposed to stimulate production of a watery, less viscous sputum which is easier to expectorate. Iodides are thought to have a proteolytic effect. Mucolytic and proteolytic drugs (N-acetylcysteine, pancreatic dornase, streptokinase, bromhexine) decrease sputum viscosity by acting on disulfide bonds of mucoproteins or by depolymerizing the high content of DNA in purulent sputum (158). A prerequisite to using these drugs is to insure that the patient is hydrated. Guaifenesin is not more efficacious than placebo (110). Although there is evidence to suggest that iodides are effective expectorants, the clinical utility of iodides is limited by hypersensitivity, acute intoxication, and mild, but unpleasant, side effects. Both N-acetylcysteine and pancreatic dornase have the unfortunate side effect of bronchospasm (12,219) which, combined with poorly documented efficacy, restricts the usefulness of both drugs.

When oxygen is given, care must be taken to insure proper humidification which may aid expectoration and prevent further dessication of secretions from dry tank oxygen. Air humidification may be particularly important when the patient is intubated and the upper airway is bypassed.

37. The treatment of hypoxia is facilitated by the use of conventional drugs, but often requires supplemental oxygen. As with other drugs, the safe and effective use of oxygen requires a thorough understanding of the pathophysiology of the problem being treated, factors influencing the dose and method of administration, and toxicity. Discuss these topics concerning the use of oxygen in the treatment of hypoxia caused by asthma or chronic bronchitis.

The oxygen concentration in arterial blood is determined by the hemoglobin concentration, factors influencing the oxygen-hemoglobin dissociation curve such as pH, and the ventilation-perfusion relationship in the lung. Oxygen delivery to the tissues is a function of the available arterial oxygen concentration, cardiac output, distribution of blood to tissues, and the ability of the tissues to extract oxygen from blood. Supplemental oxygen can correct hypoxemia while leaving the tissues hypoxic due to extrapulmonary factors influencing oxygen delivery and utilization.

The limitations of oxygen administration are direct and indirect toxicity. When oxygen is given in high concentrations approaching 100 percent of inspired gas over several days, permanent damage to the alveoli may occur which may further aggravate the transfer of gas by the lungs. Indirect oxygen toxicity occurs principally in chronic bronchitics who have chronic elevation of the $PaCO_2$ and depend on hypoxia as the main stimulus to breathe. When supplemental oxygen is given to these patients, the PaO_2 will increase, the hypoxic drive to breathe can be depressed causing hypoventilation and ultimately result in increasing hypercapnea and acidosis (267). The goal in this situation may be to use an oxygen dose (flow rate) which alleviates hypoxia while producing an acceptable rise in $PaCO_2$ and decline in ventilation. When too much oxygen is administered, somnolence may increase over a period of hours to days. If this process continues without a reduction in the oxygen dose, the patient may not awaken.

The indications for oxygen therapy are difficult to rigidly define (198). Short-term supplemental oxygen is indicated in acute respiratory failure and during an exacerbation of asthma, bronchitis, or emphysema when the patient is hypoxemic ($PaO_2 < 55$ mm Hg). Long-term, low-dose oxygen may be useful in patients with chronic bronchitis and/or emphysema with hypoxemia ($PaO_2 < 55$ mm Hg) and cor pulmonale and/or secondary polycythemia; and in patients with hypoxemia and exercise intolerance which is improved with supplemental oxygen (16, 137, 190, 229, 248).

The correct dose of oxygen must be tailored to each patient's requirement. Many chronic bronchitics adjust well to chronic hypoxia by compensatory changes in red blood cell production, oxygen-hemoglobin dissociation, and oxygen transport and utilization in tissues. Alternatively, a patient with heart failure and anemia may not tolerate chronic hypoxia nearly as well. In assessing the need and efficacy of supplemental oxygen, arterial blood gas measurements are essential and must be used in conjunction with a clinical evaluation. In the above situations, the arterial blood gases may be the same, but the person who has compensated for chronic hypoxia would not need supplemental oxygen, whereas the uncompensated patient may require oxygen. When using long-term supplemental oxygen in chronic bronchitics with cor pulmonale or exercise intolerance, one should document a decrease in pulmonary hypertension and decrease in signs and symptoms of cor pulmonale or an increase in exercise tolerance. Patients with chronic bronchitis and cor pulmonale may receive oxygen up to 15 hours per day. The toxicity from long-term, low-dose oxygen administration is yet to be determined. (40,206). In patients with exercise intolerance, oxygen is used prior to and during exercise.

High oxygen concentrations (50-100%) are used in respiratory arrest and serious respiratory failure. To achieve this oxygen concentration in the inspired air, one uses a tight fitting mask with a non-return valve or an endotracheal tube as an artificial airway. When oxygen concentrations between 20 to 40% are desired, one may use nasal prongs, nasal catheters, or various face masks. The Venturi mask (Ventimask) is available in models which deliver 24, 28, or 35% oxygen. Oxygen supplementation is usually beneficial when the PaO_2 is below 45 mm Hg and may not be of value when the PaO_2 is greater than 60 mm Hg. During an exacerbation of chronic bronchitis in a patient who retains carbon dioxide, a loose guide to follow would be to keep the PaO_2 above 45 to 50 mm Hg and not exceed 70 mm Hg. This can frequently be achieved by using 24 to 28 percent oxygen. The correct dose is always determined by measurement of arterial blood gases and clinical evaluation.

38. Doxapram, ethamivan, nikethamide, and picrotoxin have been used most commonly in the past as respiratory stimulants in the treatment of respiratory depression caused by sedative-hypnotic drug intoxication or oxygen therapy in patients with respiratory failure due to obstructive pulmonary disease. These drugs also have been used to hasten the recovery from anesthesia following surgery. Comment on the current usefulness of these drugs in the above situations.

Although these drugs have been advocated as selective respiratory stimulants working by a central or peripheral mechanism, clinical experience indicates that they are nonspecific central nervous system stimulants which have questionable selectivity for respiratory stimulation. That is, in order to produce respiratory stimulation, the required dosage will frequently cause side effects resulting from nonspecific CNS stimulation including seizures, vomiting, arrythmias, tremors, hypertension, flushing, sweating, and hyperpyrexia. The margin of safety for these drugs is very slight.

Respiratory stimulants are not indicated in treating respiratory depression from acute sedative-hypnotic intoxication or in hastening the recovery of patients from anesthisia (167,209). When assisted ventilation is required in either situation, mechanical ventilation is more safe, reliable, and effective than using a respiratory stimulant drug.

The major controversy in the use of respiratory stimulants is in the treatment of acute respiratory failure in patients with chronic bronchitis and/or emphysema. Since there is an indication that doxapram may be more effective (58) and less toxic (155) than the other respiratory stimulants, most recent efficacy studies have used doxapram for the above indication. Patients in respiratory failure due to chronic bronchitis and/or emphysema require oxygen either by using a graded oxygen dose, which is high enough to meet the patient's requirement without causing more severe hypercarbia, or by using controlled mechanical ventilation. The conservative approach would favor the use of controlled oxygen administration and when this fails (e.g. severe hypercarbia and respiratory depression occur before adequate oxygenation is achieved) respiration is totally controlled by a mechanical ventilator. An effort is made to give the patient maximal treatment prior to using mechanical ventilation because of the attendant hazards of mechanical ventilation (e.g. dependance on the ventilator, hemodynamic changes). Timing in the initiation of mechanical ventilation is critical. If intubation and ventilation are delayed until severe hypoxemia or acidosis, and complications exist, it may be too late; whereas, if used too early, the patient may be exposed to an unnecessary risk. Respiratory stimulants have been advocated in combination with controlled oxygen therapy to prevent hypercarbia and respiratory depression from occurring and possibly avoiding the use of intubation and mechanical ventilation. Herein is the controversy (14,279). A continuous intravenous doxapram infusion of 2 to 3 milligrams per minute clearly prevents carbon dioxide retention associated with controlled oxygen therapy for a 2 to 3 hour period (193,226). However, neither study showed the eventual need for mechanical ventilation to be decreased. In the study by Moser and associates (193) approximately 40% of patients in both the placebo and doxapram groups eventually required intubation/ventilation, even though doxapram was continued from 6 to 48 hours in more than 60% of the doxapram group. The controversy is yet to be settled; however, the eventual efficacy of respiratory stimulants in this situation should be viewed with skepticism because of toxicity and the possibility that these drugs may disproportionately increase oxygen consumption.

39. Theophylline, caffeine, salicylate, and progesterone are also known to be drugs with respiratory stimulant activity. Describe the situation(s) in which some of these drugs are used as respiratory stimulants.

The Pickwickian Syndrome is the eponym used to describe the syndrome of alveolar hypoventilation associated with obesity (30). Features of this syndrome include extreme obesity, somnolence, cyanosis, secondary polycythemia, and right ventricular heart failure. The syndrome gains its name from the somnolent fat boy, Joe, described in the *Pickwick Papers* by Charles Dickens. As a result of hypoventilation, these patients are chronically dyspneic, somnolent, and usually have a reduced PaO_2 with or without an elevated $PaCO_2$. Although weight reduction is the treatment of choice, this is rarely successful. In a series of outpatients, long-term use of progesterone (sublin-

gual medroxyprogesterone acetate 20 mg every 8 hours) has been shown to increase PaO_2, decrease $PaCO_2$, and result in clinical improvement (252).

Apnea occurs frequently during the neonatal period, especially in premature infants. Although the sequelae of apnea and hypoxia in neonates are not definitely established, apnea has been suggested to be the cause of central nervous system damage in surviving infants. The management of apnea includes tactile stimulation, adjustment of the ambient temperature, continuous airway distending pressure, and assisted ventilation. Recent studies suggest that both theophylline and caffeine significantly decrease the frequency of apneic spells (4,148,237,263). Although a target drug concentration range of 5 to 20 mcg/ml has been suggested for both theophylline and caffeine, it must be emphasized that this is based on data obtained with theophylline in treating adult asthmatics. The concentration range where therapeutic and toxic effects are to be expected must be established for the respective drugs in treating neonates with apnea.

40. Define asthma, chronic bronchitis, and emphysema and describe the inter-relationships of these diseases.

Asthma and chronic bronchitis are defined by clinical characteristics while emphysema is defined by pathological findings at autopsy. Asthma is characterized by episodic increased airways responsiveness (obstruction) to a variety of stimuli which results in decreased bronchial caliber and increased airflow resistance. Reversibility of expiratory airflow resistance by bronchodilator drugs is frequently used to confirm the diagnosis. An asthma attack may occur after exposure to pollens, animal dander, house dust, foods, chemicals (drugs, dyes, industrial chemicals), or as the result of respiratory infection, physical exercise, or psychologic factors. Asthma associated with allergy is called extrinsic and when allergy is not thought to be the cause, the term intrinsic asthma is used. Characteristics of intrinsic and extrinsic asthma, chronic bronchitis, and emphysema are summarized in Table 6. From a therapeutic viewpoint, extrinsic asthma is usually more responsive to treatment. Children with extrinsic asthma may outgrow the disease manifestations and be virtually symptom-free by the time they reach adulthood. When the onset of asthma occurs in middle age, it is usually intrinsic in nature, more severe and perennial. There is considerable overlap in this classification.

Chronic bronchitis is a disease of insidious onset which has been arbitrarily characterized by excessive mucous production in the tracheobronchial tree, resulting in a cough producing mucous on most days for at least three months of the year and for a minimum of two consecutive years. Chronic bronchitis is almost

Table 6
CHARACTERISTICS OF ASTHMA (INTRINSIC AND EXTRINSIC),
CHRONIC BRONCHITIS, AND EMPHYSEMA

Characteristic	Asthma		Chronic Bronchitis	Emphysema
	Extrinsic	Intrinsic		
Age group	Children, young adults	Middle age	Middle age and older	Usually ≥ 50 years
Atopic history	+	0	0	0
Allergen skin test	+	0	0	0
Blood eosinophil count	↑	↑	Normal	Normal
Serum IgE	↑	Normal	Normal	Normal
Cigarette smoking	0	0	+	+
Pulmonary function				
Forced expiratory volume at 1 sec	↓	↓	↓	↓
Forced vital capacity	↓	↓	↓	↓
Residual volume	↑	↑	↑	↑↑
Total lung capacity	Normal, ↑	Normal, ↑	Normal, ↓	↑↑
Diffusing capacity	Normal	Normal	Normal	↓
Response to bronchodilators	↑↑	↑	0, ↑	0
Response to cromolyn	↑↑	0, ↑	0	0
Aspirin sensitivity	0	0, ↑	0	0

+ = present
0 = absent
↑ = increased
↓ = decreased

always associated with cigarette smoking or air pollution. It often occurs in combination with emphysema and less frequently with asthma. Airflow obstruction is the result of mucosal thickening and accumulation of secretions. An acute exacerbation is frequently caused by upper respiratory infection or exposure to smog.

Emphysema is defined as a permanent enlargement of the respiratory air space as a result of destruction of the alveolar septa. The major cause of airway obstruction in emphysema is loss of elastic recoil within the airways resulting from destruction of lung parenchyma. Cigarette smoking is also a major etiologic factor. When emphysema occurs in younger adults who do not smoke, it is frequently associated with an alpha₁ antitrypsin deficiency.

There does not appear to be any relationship between asthma and emphysema. Even long-standing, severe asthma is not associated with emphysema. In some adults, the distinction between asthma and chronic bronchitis may be less clear. Asthma attacks may become less frequent and severe; however, the degree of recovery between attacks may be less complete. In effect, the patient appears to be in transition between asthma and chronic bronchitis. The airway obstruction becomes more sustained and chronic cough with sputum develops. Emphysema is more common in patients with chronic bronchitis than in patients without chronic bronchitis, although it does occur in the pure form. Many believe that chronic bronchitis precedes emphysema.

41. K.K. is a 21-year-old female with a 15 year history of asthma. Upon admission to the emergency room she was noted to have intense dyspnea at rest which limited her speech, anxiety, wheezing, and a cough with tenacious sputum. The asthma attack started 72 hours ago and has been worsening despite the fact she has been conscientiously taking her medications. Physical examination revealed inspiratory wheezes, use of the sternocleidomastoid and other accessory muscles for breathing, tachypnea, heart rate 120 beats per minute, and pulsus paradoxicus. Pulmonary function tests were $FEV_{1.0}$ 0.5L observed/4.5L predicted (11%), FVC 0.9L observed/5.5L predicted (16%), peak expiratory flow rate <60L/min. observed, PaO_2 55 mm Hg, $PaCO_2$ 35 mm Hg on room air and arterial blood pH 7.45. Other significant findings include hyperinflation of the lungs on x-ray, leukocytosis, and a total peripheral blood eosinophil count of 1000 cells per cubic millimeter. No apparent improvement was noted after she was given three 0.3 ml subcutaneous injections of epinephrine (1:1000) over a 90 minute period.

What is the significance of the above signs, symptoms, and laboratory data with regard to the present severity and prognosis? Which of these characteristics are most important to follow in both acute and chronic asthma?

This patient has status asthmaticus based upon the severe nature of her clinical presentation and the inability to respond to several doses of a rapidly-acting parenteral bronchodilator. All of the above signs, symptoms, and laboratory data are consistent with the diagnosis of severe asthma. The primary goal during this early danger phase of acute asthma is to prevent the patient from dying from asphyxia. During the acute attack the most important parameters to monitor are the arterial blood gases and pH. Arterial blood gas measurements are made frequently during acute, severe attacks of asthma, bronchitis, and emphysema. Blood gases are useful in assessing the current respiratory state and are a guide for therapy. Useful indicators of severity are disturbances of consciousness, an elevated or rising $PaCO_2$, $PaO_2 < 50$ mm Hg, pulsus paradoxicus (change in systolic blood pressure between inspiration and expiration), lung hyperinflation on roentgenogram, pneumothorax, and a low $FEV_{1.0}$ which is not responsive to bronchodilators (221).

Rebuck and Reed (221) present an excellent description of severe asthma based on their observations in a large series of patients. They found the recovery pattern to be highly variable between individuals and, therefore, recommend using an $FEV_{1.0}$-bronchodilation response curve as a tool for following the course of severe asthma (Fig. 4). The procedure requires the $FEV_{1.0}$ to be measured daily before and after inhalation of a rapid-acting sympathomimetic drug. The change in $FEV_{1.0}$ taken before and after isoproterenol, for example, is plotted on the ordinate versus the initial $FEV_{1.0}$ taken before isoproterenol on the abscissa. The successive daily points are connected to make an $FEV_{1.0}$-response curve. They noted two portions of the curve which were designated as corresponding to the "nonresponsive" and "responsive" phases of severe asthma. The horizontal portion of the curve, nonresponsive phase, reflects a daily improvement in initial $FEV_{1.0}$, but no bronchodilator response. During the vertical responsive phase of the graph, the initial $FEV_{1.0}$ may decrease, however the improvement in $FEV_{1.0}$ following bronchodilator is close to the predicted or ideal $FEV_{1.0}$ for that patient. The mean time to reach the responsive phase was 3.7 days (range 1-18 days) in 63 patients. Once the danger phase has passed the $FEV_{1.0}$-response curve may be useful in assessing the efficacy of drug therapy and determining the duration of hospitalization. Achieving the responsive phase may be a goal to be achieved prior to discharging the patient from the hospital. A common avoidable mistake is allowing the patient to leave the hospital too early, only to have the patient return for treatment of severe asthma which may be more severe than it was initially.

Airway resistance may also be measured by the peak expiratory flow rate (PEFR), which is similar to the $FEV_{1.0}$ but may be more easily and conveniently obtained by means of a small hand-held device (Wright Peak Flow Meter). Because of the portability and ease-of-use of a peak flow meter, the patient may

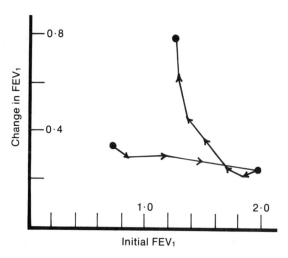

Figure 4. $FEV_{1.0}$ response curve. Change in $FEV_{1.0}$ following inhaled bronchodilator is plotted against initial $FEV_{1.0}$ on successive days. The direction of the arrowheads shows the sequence of the readings. (Modified from ref. 221.)

make routine daily measurements at home. Several measurements should be made during the day because of the normal lability in asthma. By measuring pulmonary function daily in the "real" environment of the patient, a response to treatment can be documented when adding or substituting a new drug. The clinician may be interested to see if PEFR increases during the day or perhaps only at night when many patients become symptomatic. Alternatively, when cromolyn or beclomethasone are being used and systemic corticosteroids are being withdrawn, the clinician may have the patient be alert to any decrease in PEFR.

As the patient recovers from an acute exacerbation, monitoring pulmonary function tests may be more indicative of the patient's status than arterial blood gas measurements. Care must be taken, however, not to place too much emphasis on any one test or sign. The overall pattern of the disease process which is derived from signs, symptoms, and laboratory data is much more important than any single measurement.

Recently, the total blood eosinophil count has been advocated as a tool in the diagnosis and management of asthma, particularly corticosteroid-dependent asthma (115,165). The range in nonatopic, nonasthmatic, healthy individuals is 50 to 250 eosinophils per cubic millimeter. In asthma, the count frequently approaches or exceeds 1000 and is not usually below 350 to 400 eisinophils per cubic millimeter of blood. In corticosteroid-dependent asthmatics there appears to be a positive correlation between airway resistance and total eosinophil count. Horn and coworkers (115) have suggested that a therapeutic guide for dosing corticosteroids in steroid-dependent patients would be to use a corticosteroid dosage sufficient to lower the total eosinophil count to 85 per cubic millimeter or less. It should be noted that epinephrine (144), isoproterenol (200), and theophylline also have an eosinopenic effect, while beta adrenergic blockade with propranolol (144) produces eosinophilia. Cromolyn exerts an indirect effect on the eosinophil by inhibiting the release of eosinophil chemotactic factor of anaphylaxis and other mediators from the mast cell. In one study, patients with eosinophilia initially showed a greater response to bronchodilators and corticosteroids than those who did not have eosinophilia. Many patients with a total eosinophil count exceeding 1200 per cubic millimeter required corticosteroids in addition to bronchodilators to achieve an adequate response (114). Since the total eosinophil count increases with airway resistance and beta adrenergic blockade, and is decreased by drugs which favorably effect asthma, this parameter may gain increasing usefulness as a guide to the treatment of acute and chronic asthma. However, it must be remembered that many other pulmonary and nonpulmonary diseases also effect the eosinophil count, e.g. helminth infections, Hodgkin's disease, sarcoidosis, granulomatous infections, and drug hypersensitivities.

Physical examination, pulmonary function, and laboratory tests should be performed frequently enough to describe the patient when the disease is in remission and during exacerbations. This information may enable the clinician to abort an exacerbation by starting early treatment. When the patient does experience an acute attack, the clinician will know the degree of improvement which should be expected from previous evaluations. A summary of spirometric and arterial blood gases which could be expected in the different stages of severity of asthma is presented in Table 7.

42. The treatment of chronic asthma has become confusing because of the plethora of drugs and dosage forms available. What are the therapeutic goals in treating chronic asthma? Discuss the design of drug regimens.

The therapeutic goals for chronic asthma include: (a) prevent acute, severe illness requiring hospitalization, (b) maintain the patient's routine daily activity, (c) avoid or limit drug toxicity, and (d) educate and encourage the patient to participate in the formulation and revision of drug therapy.

When an allergen is the cause of asthma, the most effective treatment can be having the patient avoid exposure to the antigen. When this is not possible hyposensitization may be tried by injecting small graded doses of the antigen giving rise to "blocking antibodies." Although hyposensitization is effective in some patients, the treatments are time consuming and often provide only transient relief. Perhaps it is for these reasons that hyposensitization is not more popular.

In selecting drugs or dosage forms for the treatment of chronic asthma one should consider the characteristics of the patient, the disease, the drug, and the dosage form. With the possible exception of cromolyn, drug selection is not based on the type of asthma, but selection is made on the severity of the disease. Generally, the simplest single drug regimen is tried initially and when adequate relief is not achieved, a second drug is added. There is no one drug of choice to use initially. A sympathomimetic aerosol or tablet, a theophylline oral preparation, or cromolyn can be tried initially. However, usually only one drug should be added at a time and a two to four week evaluation period be set before another drug is added. Most patients have mild, periodic bronchoconstriction which

Table 7
STAGES OF SEVERITY OF ASTHMA

Stage	Description	$FEV_{1.0}$ FVC (% predicted)	Pa O_2[+] mm Hg	Pa CO_2 mm Hg	pH
	Normal values	100, 100	80-100	35-45	7.38-7.43
I	*Asymptomatic* to *mild*	60, 75*		35-45	7.38-7.43
II	*Moderate:* mild hypoxia, hypocapnea and respiratory alkalosis due to hyperventilation	45, 65*	70-80	35-42	$\geq$7.40
III	*Severe* obstruction with tachypnea and dyspnea. Greater hypoxia, hyperventilation and hypocapnea, and respiratory alkalosis.	20, 35*	50-70*	<35	>7.43
IV	*Very severe:* marked hypoxia, hypoventilation causing paradoxically normal pH and Pa CO_2	not possible	<50*	35-45*	7.40*
V	*Potentially fatal:* hypoxia, hypercapnea, respiratory acidosis. Exhaustion and narcosis.	not possible	<50*	>45-50*	<7.38*

*Key tests for monitoring patient in different asthma stages.

[+]In the absence of supplemental oxygen

Adapted from Franklin W: Treatment of severe asthma. N Engl J Med 290:1469, 1974.

may only require intermittent use of a sympathomimetic drug aerosol. When asthma is seasonal, drug therapy should start just prior to the season and can often be discontinued after the season has passed. Patients with perennial asthma usually require a fixed round-the-clock oral bronchodilator regimen with either fixed or intermittent doses of an aerosolized bronchodilator. To this regimen one can add cromolyn, beclomethasone and, last of all, a systemic corticosteroid.

When a fixed regimen is required, an oral bronchodilator (sympathomimetic or theophylline) is the corner-stone of therapy to which other drugs are added. This is because oral bronchodilators usually have a longer duration of action than aerosols and these drugs are much less expensive than cromolyn or beclomethasone aerosol. Cromolyn may be the drug of first choice in some patients with extrinsic or exercise induced asthma. Which oral bronchodilator is the drug of first choice — ephedrine, terbutaline, metaproterenol, salbutamol, or theophylline? As with many good questions, there is no good answer. There are few well designed comparative studies. Theophylline is an excellent candidate for the oral bronchodilator of choice because: (a) theophylline may be more efficacious and less toxic than ephedrine in children, (b) tremors are probably not as common with theophylline as with the beta$_2$ sympathomimetic drugs, and (c) theophylline is by far the least expensive oral bronchodilator available. There is no indication that using an oral sympathomimetic drug with theophylline is any more efficacious than using maximal, tolerable doses of either drug alone.

When the patient has been receiving an oral bronchodilator and an aerosol resulting in an inadequate response, either cromolyn or beclomethasone aerosol can be added. After these drugs have failed to alleviate severe chronic asthma, oral corticosteroids are indicated. Care must be taken to use the lowest oral corticosteroid dose required to control asthma and which produces minimal toxicity.

The design of an optimal drug therapy regimen for the individual patient may require many months of evaluation and re-evaluation. The process of evaluating the patient and changing the regimen is continuous due to changes in the disease with season, age, environment, and unknown variables. Most patients only require an aerosol, oral bronchodilator, cromolyn, or beclomethasone; whereas, a few may need all these drugs in addition to oral corticosteroids for effective management.

43. When several doses of a parenteral bronchodilator do not alleviate an acute asthmatic attack, hospitalization is indicated for more intensive therapy and evaluation. Discuss the treatment of status asthmaticus.

Patients in status asthmaticus are given supplemental oxygen and intravenous aminophylline as soon as possible. The rational use of supplemental oxygen requires serial arterial blood gas determinations. An inspired oxygen concentration of 20 to 50% is adequate for treating most patients. Care must be taken to avoid oxygen toxicity from direct cellular damage or hypoventilation resulting from removal of the hypoxic stimulus to breath.

The intravenous aminophylline loading dose should be adjusted for the estimated theophylline plasma concentration at that time. The initial aminophylline maintenance dose should be regulated according to weight, age, presence of congestive heart failure, cirrhosis, smoking history and possibly disease severity. This initial dosage should be re-evaluated within 18 to 30 hours if theophylline plasma concentrations are available and when toxicity occurs. When the theophylline assay is not available, the dosage should not be increased before 30-48 hours, i.e. when the plasma concentrations are approaching steady-state, in order to insure the safety of the initial dose.

Intravenous corticosteroids should be used in patients who are corticosteroid dependent or who do not respond to aminophylline. Some clinicians advocate the use of intravenous pharmacologic corticosteroid doses in all patients requiring hospitalization for asthma. One reason for this is that the beneficial effect of corticosteroids may not be seen for at least 6 hours after receiving the drug (178) and a delay in using corticosteroids will further retard the onset. Another justification seems to be that many clinicians believe the toxicity associated with short-term, high dose corticosteroids (e.g. psychosis and gastrointestinal hemorrhage) is rare and is an acceptable hazard compared to the benefit received. Perhaps intravenous pharmacologic corticosteroid doses should be used in all asthmatics requiring hospitalization, however the toxicity is significant when it occurs and the benefit from this therapy is difficult to demonstrate. When corticosteroids are used, they can be carefully tapered to the previous maintenance dose over several weeks or completely withdrawn over 7 to 14 days in patients not requiring chronic corticosteroid therapy.

Intravenous fluids should be used with caution to insure hydration and not overhydration. A sympathomimetic drug is often administered on a fixed regimen by an IPPB device. Usually after 10 to 15 minutes of inhalation therapy and then postural drainage and percussion, the patient will be able to cough up thick mucous which may contain plugs. The role of intravenous isoproterenol infusion in treating patients who have not responded to conventional therapy is uncertain due to limited information available.

When upper respiratory infection is a complication

of an acute asthma exacerbation, the infecting organism is frequently a virus in children and a bacteria in older adults with intrinsic asthma. If bacterial infection is suspected, prompt treatment should be initiated with ampicillin or another broad spectrum antibiotic which is effective against the most commonly cultured organisms, Hemophilus influenzae and Diplococcus pneumonia. Antibiotic therapy should be re-evaluated when the results of culture and sensitivity studies are known.

If the patient's clinical condition deteriorates to the point of imminent respiratory failure, intubation and continuous mechanical ventilation must be considered. Artificial ventilation is usually instituted after all of the above forms of therapy have been used and the PaCO2 is rising to 50 mm Hg with respiratory acidosis.

44. Which drugs can either induce an asthmatic attack in susceptible individuals or are dangerous to use in patients experiencing an acute attack?

Drug-induced bronchospasm may be caused by a direct pharmacologic effect, allergic reaction, idiosyncratic reactions, and local irritation (145). Beta adrenergic blocking drugs can produce an increase in airway resistance and bronchospasm in patients with asthma and in some with allergic rhinitis (284). The incidence and severity of this effect may be directly related to the activity at the beta2 adrenergic receptor in the lung. Drugs which produce a more selective blockade on the beta1 receptor in the heart (practolol, metaprolol) may be safer than propranolol in treating asthma patients with arrythmias or hypertension (13,96,97,129). Cholinergic stimulants (acetylcholine, bethanechol) can also induce bronchospasm in asthma.

Aspirin has been shown to cause asthma symptoms resulting from bronchospasm in many patients with nasal polyps. Although the basis for this action has been suggested to be immunologic, pharmacologic, or genetic, the true cause is unknown (65, 66, 88, 161, 230). Most patients are adults with nonallergic rhinitis and nasal polyps (236), although the syndrome has been reported in children (283). Asthma symptoms appear within minutes to several hours after aspirin ingestion. Even though aspirin is avoided, patients with this triad may develop an intrinsic-type asthma which is perennial and difficult to treat. These patients may also be sensitive to indomethacin, phenylbutazone, tartrazine dye, various other anti-inflammatory drugs, and approved dyes which may be used to color drug dosage forms (43,131). Indeed, it is ironic that some medications used to treat asthma contain dyes which may cause the asthma to worsen (31). Many other drugs in isolated reports have been associated with bronchospasm (145).

When drug-induced bronchospasm occurs, the severity ranges from mild wheezing to death if untreated. The treatment is to stop taking the offending chemical and treat the patient according to the severity of the attack.

Patients in status asthmaticus are exhausted and anxious because of a fear of suffocation. The use of sedatives or narcotics to alleviate the patient's anxiety is felt to be a definite contraindication in severe asthma, chronic bronchitis or emphysema because the result may be oversedation and respiratory depression, particularly in the presence of hypercarbia (26, 41, 197). A decrease in wheezing following sedative administration may be misinterpreted as clinical improvement when it is probably due to a reduction in airflow velocity from respiratory depression. The most effective way to alleviate anxiety is to effectively treat the asthma. Time should be taken to explain to the patient his treatment and prognosis, and to impart a feeling of confidence in the patient. Once a patient has been placed on artificial ventilation, sedatives can be used to help the patient relax and prevent "fighting" the forced ventilation.

45. In 1968, epidemiological studies in England indicated an increased mortality of asthmatics between 5 to 39 years old which was attributed to excessive use of sympathomimetic aerosols (247). Discuss this finding.

Although asthma can be fatal, the mortality is relatively low compared to the morbidity. The cause of death for many patients appears to be either undertreatment or overtreatment. That is, these patients do not receive treatment as early as they should or drugs which should be used are either not used or not given in adequate doses. Alternatively, almost all medications used to treat asthma have the potential to cause or contribute to death. The increased incidence of death has been attributed to overuse of the isoproterenol aerosol. The toxicity was thought to be caused either by the patient using the aerosol too frequently and/or due to the fact that the aerosol used in England delivered twice the isoproterenol dose per puff as comparable products available in the United States (120,249). The aerosol propellant has been investigated for cardiac arrythmogenic potential. Studies conducted more recently in Australia have found an increase in the number of deaths in patients 5 to 54 years old which was not associated with sympathomimetic aerosol use (83,84). It is possible that the primary cause of death in the original study was severe asthma which was not treated appropriately. Aerosol overuse may have reflected the severity of asthma. Whether the aerosol was responsible or not, a point which can be drawn from these studies is that patients must be educated in the proper procedure to follow when the disease worsens and in the correct use of medications.

46. What is the prognosis and what are the therapeutic goals in treating chronic bronchitis and emphysema?

Chronic bronchitis and emphysema frequently progressively worsen and can lead to respiratory failure and death. Thus, the prognosis of these diseases is distinctly different from that of asthma since death due to asthma is unusual. The medical treatments of chronic bronchitis and emphysema are discussed together since it is common for patients to have both diseases concomitantly.

The most important goal in treating patients with chronic bronchitis and emphysema is to avoid further exposure of the patient to cigarette or pipe smoke or significant air pollution. A prospective study of the preclinical stages of "chronic obstructive lung disease" in 792 working men followed for eight years indicates smoking causes an obstructive and hypersecretory disorder which often coexist, but which are distinct (70). The obstructive disorder is due to intrinsic airways disease and emphysema. In those people affected with this disorder there is a rapid decline in FEV with advancing age which is not reversible. However, smokers who stop smoking may revert to a normal rate of FEV decline with aging which may delay or prevent disability. The hypersecretory disorder caused by smoking or air pollution predisposes the individual to bronchial infection and is similar, if not identical, to what is generally termed chronic bronchitis. The hypersecretory disorder will usually remit when exposure to smoke or air pollution is stopped. The results of this study appear to be in direct opposition to earlier studies which indicated there is a progressive decline in pulmonary function in patients with chronic obstructive pulmonary disease (chronic bronchitis and/or emphysema) which is not influenced by discontinuance of smoking or treatment (29,130). A possible explanation is that those people who stopped smoking in the later two studies had advanced to a terminal disease stage which will continue to decline regardless of the intervention. Prevention of lung disability from chronic bronchitis is dependent upon early disease detection and having the patient stop smoking. In the patient who does not stop smoking, therapy will probably have no influence on the long-term course of either disease.

Other therapeutic goals are to alleviate symptoms, prevent death from respiratory failure, and prevent overmedication. Unfortunately, the clinician frequently encounters patients with chronic bronchitis or emphysema very late in the disease course when little can be done. Overmedication is common in this situation due to the clinician's desire to help the patient and the patient's desire to breathe again. These patients may be taking homeopathic doses of many drugs, high doses associated with toxicity, several drugs having nearly identical pharmacologic actions, oral or inhalation corticosteroids, or long-term oral antibiotic treatment with inappropriate drugs such as chloramphenicol or cephalexin. When any of these situations are noted, the patient may benefit by a reevaluation of the regimen and setting appropriate therapeutic goals.

The treatments used for chronic bronchitis and emphysema include bronchodilators when bronchospasm is present, antibiotics for intermittent infections, low flow oxygen, respiratory and exercise therapy, and the management of cor pulmonale.

47. R.F. is a thin 55-year-old night watchman who has recently noted that breathlessness markedly limits his ability to work. He has been a heavy smoker for many years and acknowledges that he has several respiratory infections a year and has had a productive cough for many years. Physical examination reveals slightly labored breathing at rest through pursed lips, slight tachypnea at rest, wheezing, over-inflated chest, and low flat diaphragms. Inspiration is achieved by retraction of the intercostal and supraclavicular muscles while expiration is noted to be prolonged. Pulmonary function tests show a decreased $FEV_{1.0}$ and FVC which increases only 10% following isoproterenol aerosol, slightly depressed PaO_2 with normal $PaCO_2$ and pH, and a slightly decreased carbon monoxide diffusing capacity. The final diagnosis is chronic bronchitis and emphysema with a questionable degree of bronchospasm.

Should R.F. be treated with a bronchodilator and, if so, how?

Bronchospasm may be difficult to document in a patient with chronic bronchitis and/or emphysema. Although wheezing is generally associated with bronchospasm, it may also be caused by obstruction of the airways from excess secretions and edema, tumors, or most any other fixed obstruction. Pulmonary function tests give an indication as to the bronchodilatability of the patient; however, when these objective guidelines give equivocal results, the clinician is forced to base the decision of drug efficacy on changes in physical signs and symptoms before and after the drug and, most importantly, on the patient's opinion of efficacy. In R.F.'s case, a clinician could prescribe an oral or aerosol bronchodilator on a fixed regimen and reevaluate pulmonary function tests, physical signs, and the patient's self-assessment several weeks later. If there is no response, the bronchodilator should be discontinued.

Most patients with chronic bronchitis and emphysema have some degree of bronchospasm which is highly variable between and within individuals (122,160). Ventilation-perfusion abnormalities due to bronchodilators are common in this group of patients (269). The same bronchodilators used to treat asthma are used to treat chronic bronchitis and emphysema. The principles for using these drugs in treating acute, severe and chronic disease are also the same. However, the efficacy of bronchodilators in treating the individual with chronic bronchitis and emphysema must be judiciously considered.

48. What role do corticosteroids have in the treatment of chronic bronchitis and/or emphysema?

Corticosteroids produce little or no improvement in objective pulmonary function indices in most patients with chronic bronchitis and/or emphysema (10, 140, 191). However, a few patients have shown marked improvement in objective and subjective measures (10). In patients where reversible airway obstruction is suspected and when an adequate response has not been achieved from maximal conventional therapy, a short-term corticosteroid efficacy trial can be initiated using objective measures of pulmonary function (forced expiratory volumes, diffusing capacity) as criteria for assessing improvement. Subjective assessment of corticosteroid efficacy may be misleading due to the sense of well-being many patients experience. Less judicious use of corticosteroids in treating chronic bronchitis and/or emphysema should be discouraged (191).

49. R.F.'s physician is concerned about the frequency of his upper respiratory infections. What is the relationship between respiratory infection to the pathogenesis and symptomatology of chronic bronchitis? Should he prescribe a long-term prophylactic antibiotic regimen or should he use antibiotics only for treating acute exacerbations?

A prominent feature of chronic bronchitis is the acute exacerbation which is characterized by an increase in sputum production and viscosity, a change in sputum color from colorless or gray to yellow or green, cough, wheezing, dyspnea, and malaise. Exacerbations have been associated with acute respiratory infections due most commonly to *Hemophilus influenzae* or *Diplococcus pneumoniae*, although *Mycoplasma pneumoniae* and various viruses are also implicated. However, a critical review of the role of infection in chronic bronchitis by Tager and Speizer (257) was unable to show a clear etiologic role for infection. Sputum cultures during an exacerbation frequently exhibit mixed flora with no predominant pathogen. There may be little difference in the sputum bacterial flora during periods of exacerbation or remission (250). Bacterial and viral respiratory infections appear to contribute to chronic bronchitis exacerba-

tions in about 45% of all episodes. However, the effect of the combination or interaction of respiratory infections with air pollution or cigarette smoking is not well investigated (257).

The antibiotics chosen for prophylaxis of chronic bronchitis are tetracycline, ampicillin, or erythromycin given orally as 0.5 to 1.0 gram daily. Antibiotic prophylaxis of acute exacerbations has been recommended and condemned. The difference of opinion is due to the conflicting results of clinical studies, the potential for selection of resistant bacteria, and monetary cost (257). Prophylactic antibiotics are used in one of two ways. The first method is to give the patient a seven day supply of one of the above antibiotics with instructions to start taking the drug at the first sign of an exacerbation, which is usually a change in sputum color to yellow or green. The rationale for this method lies in the hope that the exacerbation will be aborted because a small bacterial population is being treated. A second approach is to treat the patient year-round or during the season when exacerbations are experienced which is usually during the winter. The use of prophylactic antibiotics by either method may offer benefit to highly selected patients such as those with many exacerbations during the winter, but will probably have little effect on alleviating symptoms in most patients.

Although the use of antibiotics to treat acute exacerbations of chronic bronchitis is generally accepted, the efficacy of this treatment is also yet to be proven (257). The choice of drug, dosage, and treatment duration is based on clinical experience and not scientific investigation. Although many regard microbiologic culture and sensitivity studies of the sputum to be of little value, this information may prove useful in antibiotic selection if the patient does not respond within 24 to 48 hours of empiric antibiotic treatment (25,28).

The fact that antibiotic efficacy in chronic bronchitis is not proven does not mean that these drugs should not be used. However, it does mean that antibiotics should be used judiciously until more discriminating information is available. Viral respiratory infections in patients with chronic bronchitis are associated with increased colonization of potentially pathogenic bacteria and may predispose the patient to infection by *Hemophilus influenzae* (245). Perhaps this observation may help explain the widely accepted empiric use of tetracycline or ampicillin for treatment of all exacerbations regardless of the etiology.

REFERENCES

1. Alanko K et al: Anticholinergic blocking of prostaglandin induced bronchoconstriction. Brit Med J 1:294, 1973.
2. Alliott RJ et al: Effects of salbutamol and isoprenaline/phenylephrine in reversible airways obstruction. Brit Med J 1:539, 1972.

3. Alston WC et al: Response of leucocyte adenyl cyclase to iso-prenaline and effect of alpha-blocking drugs in extrinsic bronchial asthma. Brit Med J 1:90, 1974.

4. Aranda JV et al: Efficacy of caffeine in treatment of apnea in the low-birth-weight infant. J Peds 90:467, 1977.

5. Aranda JV et al: Pharmacokinetic aspects of theophylline in premature newborns NEJM 295:413, 1976.

6. Arner B et al: Steroid sparing effect of disodium cromoglycate in chronic bronchial asthma. Acta Allergol 26:383, 1971.

7. Austen KF: A review of immunological, biochemical, and pharmacological factors in the release of chemical mediators from human lung. In *Asthma,* edited by Austen, K.F. and Lichtenstein, L.M., Ch. 8, Academic Press, New York. 1973.

8. Aviado DM et al: Antiasthmatic action of corticosteroids: A review of the literature on their mechanism of action. J Clin Pharmacol 10:3, 1970.

9. Beardshaw J et al: Comparison of the bronchodilator and cardiac effects of hydroxy phenylorciprenaline and orciprenaline. Chest 65:507, 1974.

10. Beerel FR et al: Prednisone treatment for stable pulmonary emphysema. Amer Rev Resp Dis 104:264, 1971.

11. Bernstein IL et al: A controlled study of cromolyn sodium sponsored by the American Academy of Allergy. J Allergy Clin Immunol 50:235, 1972.

12. Bernstein IL et al: Iatrogenic bronchospasm occurring during clinical trials of a new mucolytic agent. Dis Chest 46:469, 1964.

13. Beumer HM: Adverse effects of β-adrenergic receptor blocking drugs on respiratory function. Drugs 7:130, 1974.

14. Bickerman HA et al: The case against the use of respiratory stimulants. Chest 58:53, 1970.

15. Blackwell EW: Metabolism of isoprenaline after aerosol or direct intrabronchial administration in man and dog. Brit J Pharmacol 50:581, 1974.

16. Block AJ: Low flow oxygen therapy: treatment of the ambulant outpatient. Amer Rev Resp Dis 110 (part 2):71, 1974.

17. Blumenthal MN et al: Adrenal-pituitary function in bronchial asthma. Arch Intern Med 117:34, 1966.

18. Bodin NO et al: The tissue distribution of H³-terbutaline (Bricanyl) in mice. Acta Physiol Scand 84:40, 1972.

19. British Thoracic and Tuberculosis Association: Inhaled corticosteroids compared with oral prednisone in patients starting long-term corticosteroid therapy for asthma. Lancet 2:469, 1975.

20. Brodie BB et al: Metabolism of theophylline (1,3-dimethylxanthine) in man. J Biol Chem 194:215, 1952.

21. Brompton Hospital/Medical Research Council Collaborative Trial: Double-blind trial comparing two dosage schedules of beclomethasone dipropionate aerosol in the treatment of chronic bronchial asthma. Lancet 2:303, 1974.

22. Brooks SM et al: Adverse effects of phenobarbital on corticosteroid metabolism in patients with bronchial asthma. NEJM 286:1125, 1972.

23. Brown HM et al: Treatment of allergy of the respiratory tract with beclomethasone dipropionate steroid aerosol. Postgrad Med J 51 (Suppl. 4):59, 1975.

24. Brown HM et al: Beclomethasone dipropionate: A new steroid aerosol for the treatment of allergic asthma. Brit Med J 1:585, 1972.

25. Brummer DL et al: Chemoprophylaxis of chronic bronchitis. Amer Rev Resp Dis 104:776, 1971.

26. Buranakul B et al: Causes of death during acute asthma in children. Amer J Dis Child 128:343, 1974.

27. Burgher LW et al: A perspective on the role of cromolyn sodium as an antiasthmatic agent. Chest 60:210, 1971.

28. Burrows B et al: Antibiotic management in patients with chronic bronchitis and emphysema. Ann Intern Med 77:993, 1972.

29. Burrows B et al: Course and prognosis of chronic obstructive lung disease. A prospective study of 200 patients. NEJM 280:397, 1969.

30. Burwell CS et al: Extreme obesity associated with alveolar hypoventilation — a pickwickian syndrome. Amer J Med 21:811, 1956.

31. Buswell RS et al: Oral bronchodilator containing tartrazine. JAMA 235:1111, 1976.

32. Camarata SJ et al: Cardiac arrest in the critically ill. I. A study of predisposing causes in 132 patients. Circ 44:688, 1971.

33. Cameron SJ et al: Substitution of beclomethasone aerosol for oral prednisolone in the treatment of chronic asthma. Brit Med J 4:205, 1973.

34. Carryer HM et al: Effect of cortisone on bronchial asthma and hay fever occurring in subjects sensitive to ragweed pollen. Proc Mayo Clinic 25:482, 1950.

35. Cayton RM et al: Plasma cortisol and the use of hydrocortisone in the treatment of status asthmatics. Thorax 28:567, 1973.

36. Chai H et al: Therapeutic and investigational evaluation of asthmatic children. J Allergy 41:23, 1968.

37. Chervinsky P et al: Comparison of metaproterenol and isoproterenol aerosols: spirometric evaluation after two months therapy. Ann Allergy 27:611, 1969.

38. Choo-Kang YFJ et al: Beclomethasone by inhalation in the treatment of airways obstruction. Brit J Dis Chest 66:101, 1972.

39. Choo-Kang YFJ et al: Controlled comparison of bronchodilator effects of three beta-adrenergic stimulating drugs administered by inhalation to patients with asthma. Brit Med J 2:287, 1969.

40. Clark JM: The toxicity of oxygen. Amer Rev Resp Dis 110 (part 2):40, 1974.

41. Cochrane GM et al: A survey of asthma mortality between ages 35 and 64 in greater London hospitals in 1971. Thorax 30:300, 1975.

42. Cohen AA et al: Comparative effects of isoproterenol aerosols on airways resistance in obstructive pulmonary diseases. Am J Med Sci 249:309, 1965.

43. Cohon MS: Tartrazine revisited. Drug Intell Clin Pharmacy 9:198, 1975.

44. Collins JV et al: The use of corticosteroids in the treatment of acute asthma. Quart J Med 174:259, 1975.

45. Collins JV et al: Intravenous corticosteroids in treatment of acute bronchial asthma. Lancet 2:1047, 1970.

46. Comroe JH: *Physiology of Respiration.* 2nd edition, Year Book Medical Publishers Inc., Chicago, 1974.

47. Conolly ME et al: Metabolism of isoprenaline in dog and man. Brit J Pharmacol 46:458, 1972.

48. Cooke NJ et al: Response to rimiterol and salbutamol aerosols administered by intermittent positive pressure ventilation. Brit Med J 2:250, 1974.

49. Cornish HH et al: A study of the metabolism of theobromine, theophylline, and caffeine in man. J Biol Chem 228:315, 1957.

50. Costello JF et al: Response of patients receiving high dose beclomethasone dipropionate. Thorax 29:571, 1974.

51. Cox JSG: Disodium cromoglycate. Mode of action and possible relevance to the clinical use of the drug. Brit J Dis Chest 65:189, 1971.

52. Curtis JK et al: IPPB therapy in chronic obstructive pulmonary disease. An evaluation of long-term home treatment. JAMA 206:1037, 1968.

53. Cuthbert MF: Effect on airway resistance of prostaglandis E₁ given by aerosol to healthy and asthmatic volunteers. Brit Med J 4:723, 1969.

54. Dashe CK et al: The distribution of nebulized isoproterenol and its effect on regional ventilation and perfusion. Amer Rev Resp Dis 110:293, 1974.

55. Daughday WH: Binding of corticosteroids by plasma proteins. J Clin Invest 37:519, 1958.

56. Davies DS et al: Metabolism of terbutaline in man and dog. Brit J Pharmacol 1:129, 1974.

57. Dwyer J et al: A study of cortisol metabolism in patients with chronic asthma. Aust Ann Med 16:297, 1967.

58. Edwards G et al: A double-blind trial of five respiratory stimulants in patients in acute respiratory failure. Lancet 2:226, 1967.

59. Eggleston PA et al: A double-blind trial of the effect of cromolyn sodium on exercise-induced bronchospasm. J Allergy Clin Immunol 50:57, 1972.

60. Ellis EF et al: Pharmacokinetics of theophylline in children with asthma. Pediat 58:542, 1976.

61. Ellis EF: Bioavailability of theophylline. Abstract J Allergy Clin Immunol 55:94, 1975.

62. Engström I et al: The corticosteroid-sparing effect of disodium cromoglycate in children and adolescents with bronchial asthma. Acta Allergol 26:90, 1971.

63. Eriksson NE et al: Long-term treatment of steroid dependent asthmatic patients with beclomethasone dipropionate. Allergologia et Immunopathologia 3:77, 1975.

64. Evans ME et al: The metabolism of salbutamol in man. Exenobiotica 3:113, 1973.

65. Falliers CJ: Familial coincidence of asthma, aspirin intolerance,

and nasal polyposis. Ann Allergy 32:65, 1974.

66. Falliers CJ: Aspirin and subtypes of asthma: risk factor analysis. J Allergy Clin Immunol 52:141, 1973.

67. Falliers CJ et al: Pulmonary and adrenal effects of alternate day corticosteroid therapy. J Allergy Clin Immunol 49:156, 1972.

68. Falliers CJ et al: Controlled study of iodotherapy for childhood asthma. J Allergy 38:183, 1966.

69. Field GB: The effect of posture, oxygen, isoproterenol, and atropine on ventilation perfusion relationships in the lung in asthma. Clin Sci 32:279, 1967.

70. Fletcher C et al: *The Natural History of Chronic Bronchitis and Emphysema.* Oxford University Press, New York, 1976.

71. Fowler WS et al: Treatment of pulmonary emphysema with aerosolized bronchodilator drugs and intermittent positive-pressure breathing. Mayo Clin Staff Proc 28:743, 1953.

72. Fox ZR et al: Response to disodium cromoglycate in children with chronic asthma. Can Med Assoc J 106:975, 1972.

73. Freedman BJ: Trial of a terbutaline aerosol in the treatment of asthma and a comparison of its effects with those of a salbutamol aerosol. Brit J Dis Chest 66:222, 1972.

74. Freedman BJ: Trial of a new bronchodilator, terbutaline, in asthma. Brit Med J 1:633, 1971.

75. Freedman BJ et al: A comparison of the actions of different bronchodilators in asthma. Thorax 23:590, 1968.

76. Fromgren H: A clinical comparison of the effect of oral terbutaline and orciprenaline. Scand J Resp Dis 51:195, 1970.

77. Gaddie J et al: Beclomethasone dipropionate aerosol: studies in chronic bronchial asthma. Postgrad Med J 51 (Suppl. 4):50, 1975.

78. Gaddie J et al: Aerosols of salbutamol, terbutaline, and isoprenaline/phenylephrine in asthma. Brit J Dis Chest 67:215, 1973.

79. Gaddie J et al: Aerosol beclomethasone dipropionate in chronic bronchial asthma. Lancet 1:691, 1973.

80. Gaddie J et al: Aerosol beclomethasone dipropionate: a dose response study in chronic bronchial asthma. Lancet 2:280, 1973.

81. Gaddie J et al: The effect of an α-adrenergic receptor blocking drug on histamine sensitivity in bronchial asthma. Brit J Dis Chest 66:141, 1972.

82. Gaddie J et al: The effect of disodium cromoglycate on pulmonary function in asthma. Brit J Dis Chest 66:254, 1972.

83. Gandevia B: Pressurized sympathomimetic aerosols and their lack of relationship to asthma mortality in Australia. Ann Allergy 31:30, 1973.

84. Gandevia B: The changing pattern of mortality from asthma in Australia. Med J Aust. 1:747, 1968.

85. George CF et al: Metabolism of isoprenaline in the intestine. J Pharm Pharmacol 26:265, 1974.

86. Giacoia G et al: Theophylline pharmacokinetics in premature infants with apnea. J Pediat 89:829, 1976.

87. Gibson DG et al: Haemodynamic effects of intravenous salbutamol in patients with mitral valve disease: comparison with isoprenaline and atropine. Postgrad Med J 47:40, 1971.

88. Giraldo B et al: Aspirin intolerance and asthma: A clinical and immunologic study. Ann Intern Med 71:479, 1973.

89. Godfrey B et al: Treatment of childhood asthma for 13 months and longer with beclomethasone dipropionate aerosol. Arch Dis Child 49:591, 1974.

90. Godfrey S et al: Beclomethasone aerosol in childhood asthma. Arch Dis Child 48:665, 1973.

91. Godfrey S: The physiologic assessment of the effect of DSCG in the asthmatic child. Respiration 27 (Suppl.):353, 1970.

92. Gold WM: Cholinergic pharmacology in asthma. In *Asthma*, edited by Austen, K.F. and Lichtenstein, L.M., Ch. 11, Academic Press, New York, 1973.

93. Goldberg I et al: The effect of nebulized bronchodilator delivered with and without IPPB on ventilatory function in chronic obstructive emphysema. Amer Rev Resp Dis 91:13, 1965.

94. Graham G et al: Rapidly dissolving tablets of theophylline. Aust J Pharm Sci NS 3:66, 1974.

95. Grant IWB: Experience with beclomethasone dipropionate aerosol in the treatment of chronic asthma. Postgrad Med J 51 (Suppl. 4):58, 1975.

96. Greenblatt DJ et al: Adverse reactions to β-adrenergic receptor blocking drugs: a report from the Boston Collaborative Drug Surveillance Program. Drugs 7:118, 1974.

97. Greico MH et al: Mechanism of bronchoconstriction due to beta adrenergic blockade. Studies with practolol, propranolol, and atropine,. J Allergy Clin Immunol 48:143, 1971.

98. Gross GN et al: The long-term treatment of an asthmatic patient using phentolamine. Chest 66:397, 1974.

99. Gwynn CM et al: A 1 year follow-up of children and adolescents receiving regular beclomethasone dipropionate. Clin Allergy 4:325, 1974.

100. Haddock AM et al: Response of lymphocyte guanyl cyclase to propranolol, noradrenaline, thymoxamine, and acetylcholine in extrinsic bronchial asthma. Brit Med J 2:357, 1975.

101. Hambleton G et al: Comparison of cromoglycate (cromolyn) and theophylline in controlling symptoms of chronic asthma. Lancet 1:381, 1977.

102. Hambleton G et al: Evaluation of the effects of isoprenaline and salbutamol aerosols on airways obstruction and pulse rates of children with asthma. Arch Dis Child 45:766, 1970.

103. Hargrave SA et al: Effect of bromhexine on the incidence of postoperative bronchopneumonia after upper abdominal surgery. Brit J Dis Chest 69:195, 1975.

104. Harris DM: Some properties of beclomethasone dipropionate and related steroids in man. Postgrad Med J 51(Suppl. 4):20, 1975.

105. Harris L: Comparison of cardiorespiratory effects of terbutaline and salbutamol aerosols in patients with reversible airways obstruction. Thorax 28:592, 1973.

106. Heckscher T et al: Regional lung function in patients with bronchial asthma. J Clin Invest 47:1063, 1968.

107. Hendeles L et al: Absolute bioavailability of oral theophylline. Amer J Hosp Pharm 34:525, 1977.

108. Hendeles L et al: Frequent toxicity from IV infusions in critically ill patients. Drug Intell Clin Pharm 11:12, 1977.

109. Hermann G et al: Successful treatment of persistent extreme dyspnea "status asthmaticus". J Lab Clin Med 23:135, 1937.

110. Hirsh SR et al: The expectorant effects of glyceryl guaiacolate in patients with chronic bronchitis. Chest 63:9, 1973.

111. Hodson ME et al: Beclomethasone dipropionate aerosol in asthma. Transfer of steroid-dependent asthmatic patients from oral prednisone to beclomethasone dipropionate aerosol. Amer Rev Resp Dis 110:403, 1974.

112. Hollbrand BI et al: Trial of bronchodilating drugs given by metered aerosol with a comparison of two bedside methods of estimating airway resistance. Brit Med J 1:1014, 1966.

113. Holst PE et al: A controlled trial of beclomethasone dipropionate in asthma. N Zeal Med J 79:769, 1974.

114. Honsinger RW et al: The eosinophil and allergy: why? Allergy Clin Immunol 49:142, 1974.

115. Horn BR et al: Total eosinophil count in obstructive pulmonary disease. NEJM 292:1152, 1975.

116. Howell JBL et al: A double blind trial of disodium cromoglycate in the treatment of allergic bronchial asthma. Lancet 2:539, 1967.

117. Hume KM et al: Forced expiratory volume before and after isoprenaline. Thorax 12:296, 1957.

118. Hunt SN et al: Effect of smoking on theophylline disposition. Clin Pharmacol Ther 19:546, 1976.

119. Hyde JS et al: Long-term prophylaxis of childhood asthma using cromolyn sodium. Ann Allergy 29:483, 1971.

120. Inman WH et al: Rise and fall of asthma mortality in England and Wales in relation to use of pressurized aerosols. Lancet 2:279, 1969.

121. Irani FA et al: Evaluation of disodium cromoglycate in intrinsic and extrinsic asthma. Amer Rev Resp Dis 106:179, 1972.

122. Ishikawa S et al: The effect of nebulized bronchodilators on air flow resistance in chronic airways obstruction. Amer Rev Resp Dis 99:703, 1969.

123. Jackson RH et al: Clinical evaluation of elixophyllin with correlation of pulmonary function studies and theophylline serum levels in acute and chronic asthma patients. Dis Chest 45:75, 1964.

124. Jacobs MH et al: Clinical experience with theophylline: relationships between dosage, serum concentration, and toxicity. J. Amer Med Assoc 235:1983, 1976.

125. Jacobs MH et al: Theophylline toxicity due to impaired degradation. Amer Rev Resp Dis 110:342, 1976.

126. Jenne JW et al: Relationship of urinary metabolites of theophylline to serum theophylline levels, Clin Pharmacol Ther 19:375, 1976.

127. Jenne JW et al: Effect of congestive heart failure on the elimination of theophylline. J Allergy Clin Immunol 53:80, 1974.

128. Jenne JW et al: Pharmacokinetics of theophylline: application to adjustment of the clinical dose of aminophylline. Clin Pharmacol Ther 13:349, 1973.

129. Johnsson G et al: Effects of intravenous propranolol and metaprolol and their interaction with isoprenaline on pulmonary function, heart rate, and blood pressure in asthmatics. Europ J Clin Pharmacol 8:175, 1975.

130. Jones NL et al: Serial studies of 100 patients with chronic airways obstruction in London and Chicago. Thorax 22:327, 1967.

131. Juhlin L et al: Urticaria and asthma induced by food and drug additives in patients with aspirin hypersensitivity. J Allergy Clin Immunol 50:92, 1972.

132. Kaliner M et al: Immunologic release of histamine and slow reacting substance of anaphylaxis from human lung: IV. Enhancement of cholinergic and alpha adrenergic stimulation. J Exp Med 136:556, 1972.

133. Kawakami Y et al: Evaluation of aerosols of prostaglandins E1 and E2 as bronchodilators. Europ J Clin Pharmacol 6:127, 1973.

134. Keighley JF: Iatrogenic asthma associated with adrenergic aerosols. Ann Intern Med 65:985, 1966.

135. Kennedy MCS et al: The bronchodilator effect of a new adrenergic aerosol-salmefamol. Acta Allergy 27:22, 1972.

136. Kerrebijn KF et al: Effect on height of corticosteroid therapy in asthmatic children. Arch Dis Child 48:556, 1968.

137. Kettel L et al: Recommendations for continuous O_2 therapy in chronic obstructive lung disease. Chest 64:505, 1973.

138. Kilborn JR et al: Studies of adrenocortical function in continuous asthma. Thorax 20:93, 1965.

139. Klaustermeyer WB et al: Intravenous isoproterenol: rationale for bronchial asthma. J Allergy Clin Immunol 55:325, 1975.

140. Klein RC et al: The response of patients with "idiopathic" obstructive pulmonary disease and "allergic" obstructive bronchitis to prednisone. Ann Intern Med 71:711, 1969.

141. Klock LE et al: A comparison study of atropine sulfate and isoproterenol hydrochloride in chronic bronchitis. Amer Rev Resp Dis 112:371, 1975.

142. Knudson RJ et al: An effect of isoproterenol on ventilation perfusion in asthmatic versus normal subjects. J Appl Physiol 22:402, 1967.

143. Koch G: Terbutaline in bronchial asthma effect on lung volumes, ventilatory performance, pulmonary gas exchange and circulation at rest and during exercise. Scand J Resp Dis 53:187, 1972.

144. Koch-Weser J: Beta adrenergic blockade and circulating eosinophils. Arch Intern Med 121:255, 1968.

145. Kounis NG: A review: Drug-induced bronchospasm. Ann Allergy 37:285, 1976.

146. Koup JR et al: System for clinical pharmacokinetic monitoring of theophylline therapy. Amer J Hosp Pharm 33:949, 1976.

147. Koysooko R et al: Relationship between theophylline concentration in plasma and saliva in man. Clin Pharmacol Ther 15:454, 1974.

148. Kuzemko JA et al: Apneic attacks in the newborn treated with aminophylline. Arch Dis Child 48:404, 1973.

149. Lal S et al: Comparison of beclomethasone dipropionate aerosol and prednisolone in reversible airways obstruction. Brit Med J 3:314, 1972.

150. Lands AM et al: Differentiation of receptor systems activated by sympathomimetic amines. Nature 214:597, 1967.

151. Lands, AM et al: A comparison of the cardiac stimulating and bronchodilator actions of selected sympathomimetic amines. Proc Soc Exp Biol Med 116:331, 1964.

152. Larsson S et al: Studies of muscle tremor induced by beta-adrenergic stimulating drugs. Scand J Resp Dis 88:51, 1974.

153. Leegaard J et al: Terbutaline in children with asthma. Arch Dis Child 48:229, 1973.

154. Legge JS et al: Comparison of two oral selection $beta_2$ adrenergic stimulant drugs in bronchial asthma. Brit Med J 1:637, 1971.

155. Leszczynski SO et al: The toxicity of five respiratory stimulants: A comparative study. Clin Trials J 7:320, 1970.

156. Levy G et al: Pharmacokinetic analysis of the effect of theophylline on pulmonary function in asthmatic children. J Pediatr 86:789, 1975.

157. Lewis GP et al: Prednisone side effects and serum protein levels. Lancet 2:781, 1971.

158. Lieberman J: The appropriate use of mucolytic agents. Am J Med 49:1, 1970.

159. Lieberman P et al: Complications of long-term steroid therapy for asthma. J Allergy Clin Immunol 49:329, 1972.

160. Light RW et al: Response of patients with chronic obstructive lung disease to the regular administration of nebulized isoproterenol. Chest 67:634, 1975.

161. Lockley RF et al: Familial occurrence of asthma, nasal polyps, and aspirin intolerance. Ann Intern Med 78:57, 1973.

162. Lohman SM et al: Theophylline metabolism by the rat liver, microsomal system. J Pharmacol Exp Ther 196:213, 1976.

163. Loughnan PM et al: Pharmacokinetic analysis of the disposition of intravenous theophylline in young children. J Pediatr 88:874, 1976.

164. Lovera J et al: Beclomethasone dipropionate by aerosol in the treatment of asthmatic children. Postgrad Med J 51 (suppl. 4):96, 1975.

165. Lowell FC: The total eosinophil count in obstructive pulmonary disease. NEJM 292:1182, 1975.

166. Maberly DJ et al: Recovery of adrenal function after substitution of beclomethasone dipropionate for oral corticosteroids. Brit Med J 1:778, 1973.

167. Mark LC: Analeptics: changing concepts, declining status. Am J Med Sci 254:296, 1967.

168. Mardsen CD et al: Peripheral beta adrenergic receptors concerned with tremor. Clin Sci 33:53, 1967.

169. Martin LE et al: Metabolism of beclomethasone dipropionate by animals and man. Postgrad Med J 51 (suppl. 4):11, 1975.

170. Martin LE et al: Absorption and metabolism of orally administered beclomethasone dipropionate. Clin Pharmacol Ther 15:267, 1974.

171. Martin PD et al: A controlled trial of beclomethasone dipropionate by aerosol in chronic asthmatics. N Zeal Med J 79:773, 1974.

172. Maselli R et al: Pharmacoligic effects of intravenously administered aminophylline in asthmatic children. J Pediatr 76:777, 1970.

173. Mathison DA et al: Cromolyn treatment of asthma: Trials in corticosteroid dependent asthmatics. JAMA 216:1454, 1971.

174. Mattila MJ et al: The effect of bronchodilator aerosols on the PEFR in asthmatic patients. Acta Med Scand 180:421, 1966.

175. Maunsell K et al: Long-term corticosteroid treatment of asthma. Brit Med J 1:661, 1968.

176. McAllen MK et al: Steroid aerosols in asthma. An assessment of betamethasone valerate and a 12-month study of patients on maintenance. Brit Med J 1:171, 1974.

177. McDonald JR et al: Aspirin intolerance in asthma: Detection by oral challenge. J Allergy Clin Immunol 50:198, 1972.

178. McFadden ER Jr et al: A controlled study of the effects of single doses of hydrocortisone on the resolution of actue attacks of asthma. Am J Med 60:52, 1976.

179. McFadden ER et al: Acute bronchial asthma: relations between clinical and physiologic manifestations. NEJM 288:221, 1974.

180. McFadden ER Jr. et al: A reduction in maximum mid-expiratory flow rate. A spirographic manifestation of small airway disease. Am J Med 52:725, 1972.

181. McFadden ER Jr. et al: Arterial blood gas tension in asthma. NEJM 278:1027, 1968.

182. Meissner P et al: Pulmonary function in bronchial asthma. Brit Med J 1:470, 1968.

183. Miller J: A comprehensive evaluation of metaproterenol, a new bronchodilator. J Clin Pharmacol 7:34, 1967.

184. Miller RD et al: The treatment of pulmonary emphysema and diffuse pulmonary fibrosis with nebulized bronchodilators and intermittent positive pressure breathing. Dis Chest 28:309, 1955.

185. Milne LJR et al: Beclomethasone dipropionate and oropharyngeal candidasis. Brit Med J 3:397, 1974.

186. Milner AD et al: Bronchodilator and cardiac effects of isoprenaline, orlprenaline and salbutamol aerosols in asthma. Arch Dis Child 46:502, 1971.

187. Mitenko PA et al: Bioavailability and efficacy of a sustained release theophylline tablet. Clin Pharmacol Ther 16:720, 1974.

188. Mitenko PA et al: Pharmacokinetics of intravenous theophylline. Clin Pharmacol Ther 14:509, 1973.

189. Mitenko PA et al: Rational intravenous doses of theophylline. NEJM 289:600, 1973.

190. Mithoefer JC: Indications for oxygen therapy in chronic obstructive pulmonary disease. Amer Rev Resp Dis 110 (part 2):35, 1974.

191. Morgan WKC et al: A controlled trial of steroids in obstructive

airway disease. Ann Intern Med 61:248, 1964.

192. Morrison-Smith J et al: A clinical trial of disodium cromogylcate (Intal) in the treatment of asthma in children. Brit Med J 2:340, 1968.

193. Moser KM et al: Respiratory stimulation with intravenous doxapram in respiratory failure. NEJM 288:427, 1973.

194. Munro-Ford R: Treatment of various types of asthma with disodium cromoglycate (Intal): A two year appraisal. Ann Allergy 29:8, 1971.

195. Murray AB et al: The effects of pressurized isoproterenol and salbutamol in asthmatic children. Pediat 54:746, 1974.

196. Murray JF: The Normal Lung – The Basis for Diagnosis and Treatment of Pulmonary Disease. W. B. Sanders Co., Philadelphia, Pa, 1976.

197. Neder GA et al: Death in status asthmaticus. Chest 44:263, 1963.

198. Neff TA: Selection of patients for oxygen therapy. Chest 68:481, 1975.

199. Nilsson HT et al: The metabolism of terbutaline in man. Xenobiotica 2:363, 1972.

200. Ohman JL Jr. et al: Effect of propranolol on the eosinopenic responses of cortisol, isoproterenol, and aminophylline. J Allergy Clin Immunol 50:151, 1972.

201. Palmer KNV et al: Comparison of effect of salbutamol and isoprenaline on spirometry and blood gas tensions in bronchial asthma. Brit Med J 2:23, 1970.

202. Patel KR et al: Alpha-receptor-blocking drugs in bronchial asthma. Lancet 1:348, 1975.

203. Paterson JW et al: Isoprenaline resistance and use of pressurized aerosols in asthma. Lancet 2:426, 1968.

204. Paterson JW et al: Selectivity of bronchodilator action of salbutamol in asthmatic patients. Brit J Dis Chest 65:23, 1971.

205. Pelz HH: Metaproterenol, a new bronchodilator: comparison with isoproterenol. Amer J Med Sci 253:321, 1967.

206. Petty TL et al: Continuous oxygen therapy in chronic airway obstruction. OBservation on possible oxygen toxicity and survival. Ann Intern Med 75:361, 1971.

207. Piafsky KM et al: Disposition of theophylline in chronic liver disease. Clin Pharmacol Ther 17:241, 1975.

208. Piafsky KM et al: Disposition of theophylline in pulmonary edema. Clin Res 22:726A, 1974.

209. Picchioni AL: Clinical status and toxicology of analeptic drugs. Amer J Hosp Pharm 28:201, 1971.

210. Pierce AK: Acute respiratory failure. In Pulmonary Medicine, edited by Guenter CA and Welch MH Ch. 5, J. B. Lippincott Co., Philadelphia, 1977.

211. Pierson WE et al: A double-blind trial of corticosteroid therapy in status asthmaticus. Pediat 54:282, 1974.

212. Pontoppidan H et al: Acute respiratory failure in the adult. NEJM 287:690, 743, 799, 1972.

213. Portman GA et al: Absorption and elimination profile of isoproterenol (I). J Pharm Sci 54:973, 1965.

214. Portner MM et al: Successful initiation of alternate day prednisone in chronic steroid dependent asthmatic patients. J Allergy Clin Immunol 49:16, 1972.

215. Powell JR et al: Bioavailability of theophylline administered orally in solution. Parts I and II. Abstract from the 19th Academy of Pharmaceutical Sciences Meeting. November 1975, Atlanta, Georgia.

216. Powell JR et al: The influence of cigarette smoking and sex on theophylline disposition in adults. (Abstract). Amer Rev Resp Dis 115 (part 2):152, 1977.

217. Powell JR et al: Theophylline clearance in acutely ill patients with asthma and chronic obstructive pulmonary disease with and without congestive heart failure and pneumonia. (Abstract) Amer Rev Resp Dis 115 (part 2):

218. Radwan L et al: Arterial oxygen tension following salbutamol inhalation. Scand J Resp Dis 54:23, 1973.

219. Raskin P: Bronchospasm after inhalation of pancreatic dornase. Amer Rev Resp Dis 98:697, 1968.

220. Read J et al: Steroid-sparing effect of disodium cromoglycate (Intal) in chronic asthma. Med J Aust 1:566, 1969.

221. Rebuck AS et al: Assessment and management of severe asthma. Am J Med 51:788, 1971.

222. Riding WD et al: A comparison of the cardiorespiratory effects of salbutamol and isoproterenol-phenylephrine aerosols in asthma. Amer Rev Resp Dis 104:688, 1971.

223. Riegelman S et al: Bioavailability of enteric coated aminophylline tablets. Progress Report to the Bureau of Drugs, FDA, Washington, DC 1976.

224. Riegelman S et al: Bioavailability of three types of aminophylline oral sustained release dosage forms. Progress report to the Bureau of Drugs, FDA, Washington, D.C. 1976.

225. Riegelman S et al: Bioavailability of uncoated aminophylline tablets. Progress report to the Bureau of Drugs, FDA, Washington, D.C. 1976.

226. Riordan JF et al: A controlled trial of doxapram in acute respiratory failure. Brit J Dis Chest 69:67, 1975.

227. Ritchie JM: Central nervous system stimulants II. The xanthines, The Pharmacological Basis of Therapeutics, Fifth Edition. Edited by LS Goodman, A. Gilman, New York, The Macmillan Co, 1975. p367.

228. Robertson DG et al: Trial of disodium cromoglycate in bronchial asthma. Brit Med J 1:552, 1969.

229. Sackner MA: A history of oxygen usage in chronic obstructive pulmonary disease. Amer Rev Resp Dis 110 (part 2):25, 1974.

230. Samter M et al: Concerning the nature of intolerance to aspirin. J Allergy 40:281, 1967.

231. Sansom LN et al: Bioavailability of aminophylline suppositories. Abstract from the 21st Academy of Pharmaceutical Sciences Meeting, November 1976, Orlando, Florida.

232. Santa Cruz R et al: Tracheal mucous velocity in normal man and patients with obstructive lung disease: effects of terbutaline. Amer Rev Resp Dis 109:458, 1974.

233. Schwartz E: Oral hydrocortisone therapy in bronchial asthma and hayfever. J Allergy 25:112, 1954.

234. Schwartz HJ et al: Steroid resistance in bronchial asthma. Ann Intern Med 69:493, 1968.

235. Schwartz MS et al: Aminophylline-induced seizures. Epilepsia 15:501, 1974.

236. Settipane GA et al: Aspirin intolerance: A prospective study in an atopic and normal population. J Allergy Clin Immunol 53:200, 1974.

237. Shannon DC et al: Prevention of apnea and bradycardia in low birthweight infants. Pediatr 55:589, 1975.

238. Shenfield GM et al: Clinical assessment of bronchodilator drugs delivered by aerosol. Thorax 28:124, 1973.

239. Shioda H et al: Disodium cromoglycate (Intal) in the treatment of bronchial asthma in children. Acta Allergol 25:221, 1970.

240. Silverman M et al: Long term trial of disodium cromoglycate and isoprenaline in children with asthma. Brit Med J 3:378, 1972.

241. Simons FER et al: The pharmacokinetics of dihydroxypropyltheophylline: a basis for rational therapy. J Allergy Clin Immunol 56:347, 1975.

242. Skinner C et al: Comparison of effects of metoprolol and propranolol on asthmatic airway obstruction. Brit Med J 1:504, 1976.

243. Sly RM Effect of cromolyn sodium on exercise-induced airway obstruction in asthmatic children. Ann Allergy 29:362, 1971.

244. Smith AP et al: A controlled trial of beclomethasone dipropionate for asthma. Brit J Dis Chest 67:208, 1973.

245. Smith CB et al: Interactions between viruses and bacteria in patients with chronic bronchitis. J Infect Dis 134:552, 1976.

246. Smith PR et al: A comparative study of subcutaneously administered terbutaline and epinephrine in the treatment of acute bronchial asthma. Chest 71:129, 1977.

247. Speizer FE et al: Observations on recent increase in mortality from asthma. Brit Med J 1:335, 1968.

248. Stark RD et al: Daily requirement of oxygen to reverse pulmonary hypertension in patients with chronic bronchitis. Brit Med J 3:724, 1972.

249. Stolley PD: Asthma mortality. Why the United States was spared an epidemic of deaths due to asthma. Amer Rev Resp Dis 105:883, 1972.

250. Storey PB et al: Chronic obstructive airway disease: Bacterial and cellular content of sputum. Amer Rev Resp Dis 90:730, 1964.

251. Straub PW et al: Hypovolemia in status asthmaticus. Lancet 2:923, 1969.

252. Sutton FD et al: Progesterone for outpatient treatment of Pickwickian Syndrome. Ann Intern Med 83:476, 1975.

253. Svedmyr N et al: The effect of a new adrenergic beta-2 receptor stimulating agent (Rimiterol, R798) in patients wich chronic obstructive lung disease. Scand J Resp Dis 53:302, 1972.

254. Svedmyr N et al: The effects of salbutamol and isoprenaline on beta receptors in patients with chronic obstructive lung disease. Postgrad Med J 47:44, 1971.

255. Sykes MK et al: *Respiratory Failure*, 2nd Ed. Blackwell Scientific Publications—OXFORD, England, 1976.

256. Sumposium: The place of parasympatholytic drugs in the management of chronic obstructive airways disease. Postgrad Med J (Supplement 51 (7), 1975.

257. Tager I et al: Role of infection in chronic bronchitis. NEJM 292:563, 1975.

258. Tai E et al: Response of blood gas tensions to aminophylline and isoprenaline in patients with asthma. Thorax 22:543, 1967.

259. Tattersfield AE et al: Salbutamol and isoproterenol: A double blind trial to compare bronchodilator and cardiovascular activity. NEJM 281:1323, 1969.

260. Thiringer G et al: Evaluation of skeletal muscle tremor due to bronchodilator agents. Scand J Resp Dis 56:93, 1975.

261. Turner-Warwick M et al: Long term study of disodium cromoglycate in treatment of severe extrinsic or intrinsic bronchial asthma. Brit Med J 4:383, 1972.

262. Turner-Warwick M: Study of theophylline plasma levels after oral administration of new theophylline compounds. Brit Med J 2:67, 1957.

263. Uauy R et al: Effect of theophylline on severe primary apnea of prematurity. A preliminary report. Pediatr 55:595, 1975.

264. Van As A et al: A new bronchodilator hexoprenaline in obstructive pulmonary disease. Scand J Resp Dis 54:28, 1973.

265. Vilsvik JS et al: Beclomethasone dipropionate aerosol in adult steroid-dependent obstructive lung disease. Scand J Resp Dis 55:169, 1974.

266. Walker SR et al: The clinical pharmacology of oral and inhaled salbutamol. Clin Pharmacol Ther 13:861, 1972.

267. Warrell DA et al: Effect of controlled oxygen therapy on arterial blood gases in acute respiratory failure. Brit Med J 2:452, 1970.

268. Warrell DA et al: Comparison of cardiorespiratory effects of isoprenaline and salbutamol in patients with bronchial asthma. Brit Med J 1:65, 1970.

269. Watanabe S et al: Bronchodilator and corticosteroid effects on regional and total airway resistance in patients with asthma, chronic bronchitis and chronic pulmonary emphysema. Amer Rev Resp Dis 106:392, 1972.

270. Weinberger MM et al: Intravenous aminophylline dosage: use of serum theophylline measurements for guidance. JAMA 235:2110, 1976.

271. Weinberger MM et al: Interaction of ephedrine and theophylline. Clin Pharmacol Ther 17:585, 1975.

272. Weinberger MM et al: Evaluation of oral bronchodilator therapy in asthmatic children. J Pediatr 84:421, 1974.

273. Welling PG et al: Influence of diet and fluid on bioavailability of theophylline. Clin Pharmacol Ther 17:475, 1975.

274. West JB: *Respiratory Physiology – The Essentials.* The Williams and Wilkins Co., Baltimore, 1974.

275. Williams FM et al: The influence of the route of administration on the urinary metabolites of isoetharine. Xenobiotica 4:345, 1974.

276. Woods DW et al: Intravenous isoproterenol in the management of respiratory failure in childhood status asthmaticus. J Allergy Clin Immunol 50:75, 1972.

277. Woolcock AJ et al: Abnormal pulmonary blood flow distribution in bronchial asthma. Aust Ann Med 15:196, 1966.

278. Woolcock AJ et al: Improvement in bronchial asthma not reflected in forced expiratory volume. Lancet 1:1323, 1965.

279. Woof CR: The use of "respiratory stimulant" drugs. Chest 58:59, 1970.

280. Yamamura Y et al: Clinical effectiveness of a new bronchodilator, Inolin, on bronchial asthma. Ann Allergy 26:504, 1968.

281. Yarnell PR et al: Focal seizures and aminophylline. Neurology 25:819, 1975.

282. Yu DYC et al: Inhibition of antigen-induced bronchoconstriction by atropine in asthmatic patients. J Appl Physiol 32:823, 1972.

283. Yunginger JW et al: Aspirin induced asthma in children. J Pediatr 82:218, 1973.

284. Zaid G et al: Bronchial response to β-adrenergic blockade. NEJM 275:580, 1966.

285. Zwillich CW et al: Theophylline-induced seizures in adults: correlation with serum concentrations. Ann Intern Med 82:784, 1975.

Chapter 18

Peptic Ulcer Disease

Robert K. Maudlin

To have a basic understanding of gastrointestinal (GI) physiology, the following references may be helpful: Sleisenger and Fordtran: *Gastrointestinal Disease: Pathology, Diagnosis, Management,* W.B. Saunders Company, Philadelphia 1975, or Frohlich: *Pathophysiology: Altered Regulatory Mechanisms in Disease,* J.B. Lippincott Company, Philadelphia 1976, pages 461-498; however, a brief discussion is in order.

The stomach stores and mixes food with acid, mucus, and pepsin prior to controlled release into the duodenum. The cells of the gastric mucosa secrete mucus, pepsinogen, and hydrochloric acid along with miscellaneous enzymes and ions. This mixture constitutes 1-3% of the gastric juice, the remainder being water. Approximately 2000-3000 ml is secreted daily. The pH may be as low as 0.87 but is generally higher (pH 2-3) due to neutralization by food, saliva, and alkaline intestinal contents.

Mucus is a mixture of polysaccharides and mucoproteins which functions mainly as a viscous, protective that absorbs pepsin, neutralizes and buffers acid, and physically hinders digestion of the gastric mucosal lining.

Hydrochloric acid (HCl) is secreted by parietal cells located in the body of the stomach and its secretion is controlled primarily by a balance between stimulators (acetylcholine, histamine, and gastrin) and inhibitors (secretin and cholecystokinin). Some authorities are of the opinion that acid secretion is mediated by three separate receptors (acetylcholine, histamine, and gastrin) on the parietal cell (63). Others think that histamine is the final common mediator (30). The main function of HCl is to maintain the pH of the stomach in the optimal range to convert pepsinogen to pepsin (pH 1.8-2.5).

Pepsinogen is secreted by the chief cells and its release is vagally mediated. At the appropriate pH, pepsinogen is converted to pepsin which is capable of digesting proteins in the diet.

Although all ulcerating lesions of the gastroduodenal area have traditionally been labelled as peptic ulcers, these lesions differ in anatomical location, etiology, clinical presentation and genetic relationships.

Peptic ulcer disease (PUD) is characteristic to man and occurs in 10%-15% of the population. Prior to 1900,

gastric ulcers occurred more commonly than duodenal ulcers and both were more common in women. Today, both trends have reversed throughout the world except in Japan where gastric ulcer is still more common. Gastric ulcers are two to three and a half times more prevalent in males, and males have up to ten times more duodenal ulcers than females. The incidence of gastric ulcers seems to increase with age. Ulcers occur most commonly between the ages of 20 to 50 years; however, it is estimated that 2% of adults with PUD have had symptoms dating from childhood. A good discussion of childhood peptic ulcer and its treatment is presented by Nuss and Lynn (114).

The traditional acid-peptic theory remains valid for the **duodenal ulcer.** Patients with these ulcers have higher ''average'' outputs of hydrochloric acid than do ulcer-free persons. The word average is important since nearly half of the persons with duodenal ulcer have normal acid secretion. While some persons with duodenal ulcers may secrete more acid, their ulcers will heal spontaneously with little or no therapeutic intervention, and this healing is not accompanied by a decrease in gastric acid output. Several theories have been proposed to explain the complex interrelationship between acid secretion and duodenal ulcer. For example, the person with duodenal ulcer may have an abnormally high ''vagal tone'' (44); excessive humoral (gastrin) stimulation of acid (21, 154); impaired inhibition of gastric secretion (108); or a greater capacity to secrete acid (35, 159, 131). Unfortunately, all of these theories evolve entirely around acid secretion, and it is important to realize that peptic activity may have an equally important role in duodenal ulcer pathogenesis.

Although some patients with **gastric ulcer** are hypersecretors of acid, most secrete either normal or less than normal amounts. Therefore, it is probably reasonable to focus more attention on mucosal resistance than on acid and pepsin in this type of ulcer. One can postulate that gastric ulcer is the result of gastric stasis due to poor emptying (45). This is followed by gastritis which lowers mucosal resistance to minimal amounts of acid and pepsin (125, 96). The gastric mucosa has the capacity to prevent the penetration of normal concentrations of acid; however, when acid concentrations are increased, the mucosal barrier is broken and hydrogen ions penetrate the stomach wall resulting in mucosal damage (37, 38, 117, 28). Pyloric sphincter dysfunction may also contribute to the pathogenesis of gastric ulcers by allowing reflux of duodenal contents into the stomach (53). The resultant bile, bile salts, and urea reaching the stomach will cause a break in the gastric mucosa even at low concentrations of acid, permitting the back-diffusion of hydrogen ions (107). The acid damage to mucosa and acid-pepsin leads to ulceration (43). However, these sequence of events are only theoretical and the true cause of gastric ulcer is still to be established.

1. What is the Zollinger-Ellison syndrome?

This syndrome is characterized by single or multiple non-beta islet cell adenomas of the pancreas which release large quantities of gastrin into the plasma. This results in a 10-20 fold increase in the amount of acid secreted and a high incidence of ulcers. Diagnosis is based on elevated serum gastrin levels and on an enormously elevated "basal" secretion of HCl that is minimally stimulated following the administration of histamine (less than 60%). The clinical picture and treatment may be reviewed elsewhere (91, 116).

2. What are stress ulcers?

The cause of stress ulcers (acute peptic ulcers, Curling's ulcer, or Cushing's ulcer) remains unknown, but there appears to be a disruption in mucosal resistance to normal levels of acid-pepsin (35b). This may result from a quantitative and qualitative change in gastric mucus and/or a reduced rate of gastric mucosal cell renewal (99). Multiple gastric ulcers occur in 0.4-11% of patients following central nervous system disease, myocardial infarction, sepsis, burns, various types of surgery, and fractures (47). Pain may be absent and acute hemorrhage is the presenting sign in most patients. Perforation occurs in 8-18% of these patients and the mortality rate is approximately 60-65% despite treatment. A conservative therapeutic approach (antacids and fluid replacement) may be employed; however, surgical intervention is necessary in more severe or unresponsive cases. It has been proposed that postoperative acute peptic ulcers may be caused by thrombosis and that premedication with heparin may be of prophylactic value (136).

3. Is there any correlation between the incidence of peptic ulcer disease and other pathological conditions?

Apparently, extragastric factors influence the stomach in unexplained ways. The results of studies originating nearly 50 years ago established that people with peptic ulcer disease have lower systolic blood pressure (70-100 mm Hg) than normals. This curious relationship carries forward to the present (58, 103, 157). Patients with chronic renal failure have high basal serum gastrin levels, possibly because of an inability to eliminate gastrin. High basal gastric acid levels and the presence of duodenal ulcers have been reported in 53% of such patients on renal dialysis (137). In patients with hyperparathyroid disease there is an increased incidence of peptic ulcer. This may result from hypercalcemia which enhances the release of gastrin. The association between diabetes mellitus and peptic ulcer disease is related to insulin-induced hypoglycemia which causes a profound basal stimulation of acid (133). Duodenal ulcer is at least three times more common in emphysemics, and emphysema occurs three to four times more commonly in people with peptic ulcer disease. Hypoxia may lower mucosal resistance to acid.

4. What is the clinical picture of a person with peptic ulcer disease?

The typical "lay" description of an ulcer personality is that of a hard-driving, highly charged, aggressive businessman who rarely relaxes and who ends up winning the presidency of the company and a peptic ulcer. Such a description may be apropos for some, but not all patients. Clinically, ulcer patients complain of recurrent episodes of abdominal pain over a period of several years. The pain may be nonspecific but is usually described as a gnawing or burning in the epigastric region reaching maximum intensity just prior to meals. The pain is readily relieved by food, antacid, or vomiting. Although the pain may awaken the patient from his sleep, it is unusual to experience pain on awakening in the morning. About 10% of persons with PUD will present with complications: hematemesis, GI bleeding, perforation, or obstruction. Peptic ulcer is a chronic disease and is characterized by remission and exacerbation of symptoms over 20-30 years.

5. What are some of the diagnostic tests performed in persons with suspected peptic ulcer disease?

The most readily available diagnostic tool in peptic ulcer disease is the upper GI (UGI) series. Some 70-85% of gastric and duodenal ulcers can be detected by the radiologist. Marginal and postsurgical ulcers are more difficult to diagnose radiologically. Because of the development of the forward and side viewing flexible fibroscope (gastroscope) a correct diagnosis can be achieved in greater than 95% of the cases. Biopsy and brush cytology through the gastroscope may be used to differentiate benign and malignant ulcers (5-10% of gastric ulcers are malignant).

Since the day "no acid, no ulcer" was first uttered, interest has centered around analyzing the quality and quantity of acid secretion. Reliability and reproducibility of these data were lacking until the maximal acid output test with basal controls was defined. Today these tests probably have only two indications: to determine the presence or absence of achlorhydria in patients with gastric ulcer and to demonstrate basal hypersecretion in patients suspected of Zollinger-Ellison syndrome (134). In the former, achlorhydria might indicate that the ulcer is a carcinoma; however, since achlorhydria is found in only 20% of carcinomatous ulcers, it is difficult to justify its use even in this instance. The two-hour test is most reliable. The initial hour measures basal acid secretion (at 15 minute intervals). Following the last "basal" collection, histamine acid phosphate (0.04 mg/kg SC), beta-imidazole (Histalog) (1.7 mg/kg IM) or pentagastrin (Peptavlon) (6 mcg/kg SC) is administered. Gastric contents are again collected; the volume, pH, and titratable acidity are measured; and the maximal acid output in milliequivalents is calculated.

In general, duodenal ulcer patients are hypersecretors, while gastric ulcer patients are normal or low secretors. Patients with Zollinger-Ellison syndrome have enormous basal secretion rates which are usually greater than 60% of their post histamine stimulation rate. The drug of choice for this procedure is pentagastrin, as it has fewer and less severe adverse effects than the other agents. It is currently available only from Ayerst. If histamine acid phosphate is used, an antihistamine (e.g. diphenhydramine (Benadryl) or chlorpheniramine (Chlortrimeton) should be administered 30 minutes before the basal collection is completed.

6. Is the dictum "no acid — no ulcer" absolute, or is it possible to have a benign peptic ulcer in the absence of gastric acid?

There are reports of ulcer disease without the presence of acid in the older literature (62), prior to the use of maximal acid stimulation tests. Since the introduction of such tests the dictum has stood firmly.

There is good evidence that for unexplained reasons, some patients will have transitory refractoriness of parietal cells and resultant achlorhydria. Yet, repeated stimulation testing will show acid secretion (118).

7. B.A., a 42-year-old male, has been bothered with joint pain in his fingers and wrists, especially in the morning. On the basis of preliminary diagnosis of rheumatoid arthritis, B.A. was instructed to begin therapy with aspirin 1.0 gram four times daily. His medication profile indicates that he has recurrent peptic ulcer disease, a prescription for propantheline (Propanthine) is still filled regularly, and he has taken no antacids for six months. B.A. states that he has had no problems with the ulcer for 6-8 months and only takes the propantheline as a precautionary measure. He failed to mention the ulcer problem to his rheumatologist. What is the relationship between aspirin ingestion and gastrointestinal bleeding?

There is an increased fecal blood loss in patients

ingesting aspirin. The loss is usually 5 ml more than that occurring in control subjects and occurs in 70% of the people ingesting normal doses (approximately 3 grams per day). Gastroscopy reveals that this occult blood loss originates primarily from the lesser curvature of the stomach.

The degree of topical irritation, erosion, and subsequent blood loss is related to both the concentration of aspirin and its duration of contact with the gastric mucosa. When the drug is administered orally in a solid dosage form, a saturated solution of non-ionized molecules is achieved around the aspirin particles. This serves as a reservoir for additional absorption.

The pKa of aspirin is 3.5, implying that 50% of the drug is in the non-ionized, lipid soluble, readily absorbable form at a pH of 3.5. At the GI pH of 2.5, 91% of the drug is in this form. Therefore, the acid environment of the stomach promotes aspirin absorption. Once aspirin is absorbed into the gastric mucosal cell (pH of 7) ionization occurs. Since a high concentration gradient of non-ionized drug exists on the mucosal surface, aspirin accumulates in the cell. This apparently disrupts the mucosal membrane barrier, allowing hydrogen ions to back-diffuse into the mucosa. Electronmicroscopy studies show that a single 600 mg dose of aspirin will produce mucosal damage with early karyolysis, cytoplasmic edema, and mucous granule loss from disrupted apical cell membranes (18). The result is cell damage, erosion, exfoliation (36) and bleeding (34). Support for the concept that acid is essential for aspirin-induced bleeding is based on comparisons of fecal blood loss before and after aspirin administration to normal subjects and those with achlorhydria. Fecal blood loss in the control subjects increased from a basal level of 0.47 ml/day to 4.7 ml/day following aspirin, while the loss in the achlorhydric subjects increased from 0.29 ml to 1.2 ml. Also, direct gastroscopic studies following the ingestion of 600 mg of aspirin with 10 mEq of acid demonstrated visible gastric lesions in 50% of subjects (152), but the same dose without acid caused gastric lesions in only 17% of the subjects examined (155).

The above studies imply that the bleeding induced by aspirin is a local effect of the drug and that acid is necessary; however, other studies (both in animals and man) suggest a central mechanism of action. The implication arises as a result of GI bleeding following intravenous administration of aspirin. Animal studies using normal or large doses have demonstrated the occurrence of gastric irritation. There seems to be some species specificity in these studies in that all the erosions and bleeding occurred in rats and not in guinea pigs, rabbits, or dogs. Studies in man have failed to show that the intravenous administration of aspirin in normal doses causes gastrointestinal blood loss above the normal levels of 0.17 to 1.7 ml/day (33,

54, 86).

Aspirin interference with adenosine diphosphate (ADP) induced platelet aggregation, occurs within a few hours and lasts the entire life span of the platelet (2-6 days) following doses as low as 150 mg. A single dose of 650 mg approximately doubles the mean bleeding time in normal persons. Whether platelet dysfunction plays a role in gastrointestinal bleeding secondary to aspirin is only speculative, but it may contribute to continued or prolonged hemorrhage once "local" erosion has occurred. Individuals with defective platelet function are more susceptible to hemorrhage following mucosal erosion, and some individuals may have platelets that are intrinsically more sensitive to aspirin (109). The hypoprothrombinemic effect of aspirin occurs only with very large doses (over six grams per day).

8. Is there an association between aspirin ingestion and subsequent development of peptic ulcer disease (PUD)?

Although aspirin ingestion is clearly associated with gastric mucosal erosion and increased GI blood loss, its association with gastric ulcers is less clear. Data from retrospective studies show an association between gastric ulcers and recent aspirin ingestion. In an Australian study, 57% of patients with gastric ulcer ingested aspirin at least once daily compared with only 22% of controls. There was no correlation between aspirin ingestion and the development of duodenal ulcer (57). The Boston Collaborative Drug Surveillance Program reported that 19.2% of patients hospitalized with newly diagnosed uncomplicated benign gastric ulcer used aspirin at least four times weekly compared with 6.9% of controls. No association was found between aspirin use 1-3 days a week and gastric ulcer. Also, no association between aspirin use and duodenal ulcer was established (97). In another study, 52% of 61 patients with gastric ulcer ingested 15 or more aspirin tablets per week compared to 10% of matched controls (23).

The results of these studies imply that heavy, regular aspirin use is more common among hospital admissions for benign gastric ulcer and major upper GI bleeding than other admission diagnoses among such aspirin users. No convincing data exist suggesting an association between aspirin ingestion and duodenal ulcer. This author feels that this knowledge should not prevent clinicians from using aspirin in persons without a hisory of PUD. The estimated attributable incidence rate of hospital admission is 15 for major bleeding and 10 for gastric ulcer per 100,000 heavy, regular aspirin users per year (97). A cautious approach would be to use aspirin with antacids, if at all, in persons with a past history of documented PUD or "aspirin gastritis." In a patient with active PUD, aspirin should be avoided. The alternatives depend on the indication for aspirin, but can be selected from acetaminophen (analgesia or antipyresis); or ibuprofen, fenoprofen, naproxen, tolmetin (anti-inflammatory).

9. How can aspirin-induced gastric irritation and bleeding be minimized?

The addition of sodium bicarbonate, calcium carbonate, magnesium oxide, and magnesium carbonate to aspirin tablets and the formulation of similarly buffered aspirin solutions have shown promise in reducing blood loss caused by aspirin. The oral administration of aspirin and acid will cause more mucosal erosions and bleeding than the administration of acid alone. Replacement of the acid with sodium bicarbonate significantly reduces the erosions and bleeding (152.) The degree to which aspirin-induced blood loss is reduced is directly related to the buffer capacity of the formulation (85). Apparently, buffering reduces the concentration of acid available for damaging the mucosa and also maintains more of the aspirin is in the ionic nonabsorbable form so that it may pass out of the stomach without being absorbed into the mucosal cell. Commercially available buffered aspirin formulations, with the exception of Alka Seltzer, are not significantly "safer" than aspirin alone. Alka Seltzer, unfortunately, is high in sodium content (521mg/tablet) and costly. Ascriptin A/D (Maalox 300mg/aspirin 325mg) is better than Ascriptin in that it contains twice as much Maalox per dose. One must remember that tablet antacids are not equivalent mg for mg with liquid formulations. The dose of Maalox liquid to provide 40-80mEq of neutralizing capacity is 1200-2400mg (15-30 ml). The crushing of aspirin tablets and the addition of 15-20 ml of water with a full therapeutic dose of a non-aluminum-containing antacid, is most efficacious in decreasing aspirin's ulcerogenic effect. A non-aluminum antacid is recommended because aluminum can complex with aspirin and reduce its bioavailability. Hourly administration of aluminum and magnesium hydroxides can increase the urinary pH and thereby reduce serum levels of aspirin by 30-70% (92). Therefore, co-administration of aspirin and antacids requires regular monitoring of serum salicylate concentrations and assessment of the patient's clinical response.

10. Do products such as ibuprofen (Motrin), fenoprofen (Nalfon), Naproxen (Naprosyn) and tolmetin (Tolectin) cause less gastrointestinal (GI) bleeding than aspirin?

Early studies and manufacturers' promotional data compared less than anti-inflammatory doses of ibuprofen with aspirin (e.g. ibuprofen 900 mg/day versus aspirin 4 grams/day). However, the results of later studies demonstrated that doses of 1600-2400mg of ibuprofen, 1600-3200 mg of fenoprofen, 500 mg of naproxen, or 1275-1500 mg of tolmetin caused GI distress in about

10% of subjects (half that of aspirin). Actual bleeding and ulceration has been reported with all of these agents (10, 84, 128). (Also see chapter on **Rheumatoid Arthritis).**

11. K.G., a 35-year-old male, was hospitalized one year ago for work-up and treatment of a duodenal ulcer. His ulcer is currently asymptomatic requiring no medications. K.G. has just returned from a fishing trip and has a severe, extensive case of poison ivy dermatitis. His family physician wants to use a tapering regimen of oral prednisone to treat him and is concerned about using corticosteroids in a patient with a past history of PUD. What is the relationship between corticosteroids and PUD?

A convincing association between corticosteroids and PUD is difficult to substantiate in the medical literature.

Some evidence implies that steroids induce ulcers by altering the protective composition of mucus and/or by interfering with the gastric mucosa's ability to secrete mucus (149, 106). Steroids also reduce the rate of shedding of gastric mucosal cells by decreasing the rate of cell renewal (99). Reports that steroids potentiate the development of ulcers from other causes (e.g. aspirin ingestion) also imply that they impair normal defense mechanisms (50).

Many studies have shown that steroids do not affect basal acid secretion; however, such data are not easily reproducible. Reproducible data can be obtained by using maximal stimulation tests; studies utilizing this technique have shown that steroid treated patients do have an increase in acid secretion that is primarily related to an increase in concentration rather than volume (146).

Because corticosteroids decrease the mucosal barrier and increase acidity, a relationship with peptic ulcer disease seems reasonable. However, the available literature does not support the association. A review of 42 double-blind studies involving 5331 patients reported peptic ulcers in 0.8% of 2346 controls and 1.3% of 2985 steroid treated patients. This difference is not statistically significant (32). Those treated with steroids for more than 30 days had a greater incidence of peptic ulcers than those treated for less than 30 days. However, long-term placebo usage was associated with peptic ulcers more often than short-term placebo use, and the ulcers did not occur significantly more often with long-term steroid therapy than with long-term placebo therapy (1.7% versus 1.2%) (32). Patients taking more than 20 mg of prednisone (or its equivalent) did not develop significantly more ulcers than those taking a low daily dose (1.6% versus 1.3%) (32). This lack of correlation with dose confirms an earlier contention of the Boston Collaborative Drug Surveillance Program (14). The only correlation between

steroids and PUD seems to be in patients receiving a total dose of more than 1000 mg of prednisone. More than 5% of such patients developed ulcers while they occurred in 0.1% of those receiving less than 1000 mg (32). Although an association between corticosteroids and peptic ulcer is unprovable at present, most clinicians feel that such an association does exist. Therefore, for K.G., who is to receive a short course of steroids for poison ivy dermatitis, it seems reasonable to proceed with the steroids, but to administer them with a full therapeutic dose of an antacid.

12. E.C., is a 47-year-old female who has been treated with thiazide diuretics for 5 years. Approximately one year ago, it was noted that her serum potassium level was 2.7 mEq/liter. She was started on a potassium chloride (KCl) liquid 60mEq daily. Over the next 8 months she tried virtually every KCl liquid formulation available and was unable to tolerate their taste. Lack of potassium supplementation resulted in a recurrence of hypokalemia. Out of frustration her local physician started her on potassium chloride enteric-coated tablets one gram daily, 2 months ago. For the past few days E.C. has been experiencing moderate epigastric pain. Last night she passed an abundant tarry stool and on arrival at the emergency room, she was vomiting blood. Radiography revealed a large ulcer on the posterior wall of the antrum surrounded by edematous swelling. Her physician is cognizant of small bowel ulcerations attributable to enteric-coated potassium chloride tablets, but wants to know the likelihood of gastric ulceration induced by this medication.

Reports of small-bowel ulceration secondary to the administration of enteric-coated KCl or enteric-coated KCl plus thiazide diuretic preparations began to appear in the mid 1960's. These small-bowel lesions were described as circumferential ulcers which led to intestinal stenosis, obstruction, and occasionally perforation. In general, the patients had been taking the KCl for weeks or months; however, in a few cases ulceration occurred after only 1 or 2 doses (6, 16, 111). It was determined that the enteric-coated form of KCl was the causative agent (13), and that variable sensitivity to potassium chloride's ulcerogenic properties existed. The enteric-coating, which was intended to prevent inactivation of the KCl by digestive juices and gastric irritation, allowed for rapid dissolution and absorption over a short portion of the intestine. The resultant high concentration of potassium chloride in the absorbing segment caused venous spasm or paralysis, venous stasis, and submucosal edema, with subsequent ulceration and stenosis.

Gastric ulcers have been produced in animals following administration of KCl in solution, from a rapidly-disintegrating tablet, or as an enteric-coated tablet, but until recently, no reports in man existed. Five cases of gastric ulcer, during treatment with enteric-coated KCl tablets, have now been reported. Studies of the tablets show they are capable of rapidly releasing the salt even in an acid medium. There was no defect noted in the manufacture of these tablets (78).

Therefore, in this case, it must be concluded that enteric-coated KCl tablets are capable of dissolving in the acid medium of the stomach. This is a situation not unlike that occurring in the small bowel. Considering all of the available evidence against the use of enteric-coated KCl tablets, it is surprising that drug companies continue to manufacture such dosage forms.

13. The occurrence of ulceration following the use of potassium chloride seems to require that the salt be rapidly released in the gastrointestinal tract. Would a preparation that slowly releases potassium chloride prevent such side effects and yet be efficacious?

Slow release products (Slow-K and Kaon-Cl) are effective in correcting hypokalemia. When these "slow-release" products were compared with a 10% KCl solution, the solution produced quicker and higher initial excretion levels; however, after four days both dosage forms were equivalent. The slow-release products circumvented the palatability problem of the solution without increasing untoward effects. Fecal occult blood was noted only in one patient receiving the KCl solution (11). Cases of ulceration and stricture have been reported from lodgement of these slow-release potassium tablets in a Meckel's diverticulum, in an esophageal compression associated with enlarged left atrium, and in previously normal adults (101, 157a). *Medical Letter* consultants consider these products to be dangerous and feel that they should not be used (150). Nevertheless, the incidence of these side effects is low and the European experience is quite favorable. Therefore, slow-release potassium chloride should be considered as an expensive alternative when other forms of oral potassium therapy prove unsatisfactory. The enteric-coated tablets should not be used under any circumstance.

14. What other drugs are capable of inducing peptic ulcer disease?

Since its introduction (1963) as a potent anti-inflammatory agent, *indomethacin* has attracted much publicity and controversy regarding its true role in therapy. It took two years for the first reports of peptic ulceration to reach the literature (140); however, there has been a steady stream of reports since that time (130, 147). Gastrointestinal upset, bleeding, or ulceration are now considered to be the most common side effects of indomethacin and occur in 15% of patients (22, 140). Apparently, indomethacin causes changes in gastric mucus secretion similar to that caused by corticosteroids, and it allows a back-diffusion of hydrogen ions similar to that caused by aspirin (106, 143). Although most ulcers induced by indomethacin occur following the ingestion of large doses (150-300 mg/day) over a long period of time (1½ to 3 years), they have also occurred with much lower doses and after short term therapy (151a). GI upset may be reduced by administering indomethacin with food or antacids. Nonetheless, it should be withheld from patients with a history of PUD.

Phenylbutazone (Butazolidin and Azolid) and Oxyphenbutazone (Tandearil and Oxalid) are anti-inflammatory agents causing frequent gastrointestinal problems. The incidence of peptic ulceration with phenylbutazone is estimated to be 1-2%. The liability is increased by continuous therapy with doses greater than 400 mg/day. The likelihood of peptic ulcers from oxyphenbutazone is reported to be less; however, occult blood loss occurs with both of these agents, and they are contraindicated in patients with existing peptic ulcer disease. A combination product of 100 mg phenylbutazone, 100 mg aluminum hydroxide, and 150 mg magnesium trisilicate (Butazolodin Alka and Azolid A) is also available. The combination is intended to reduce gastrointestinal irritation; however, the quantity of antacids present per capsule is equivalent to less than 2 ml of Gelusil. It is difficult to believe that the antacids in this product are of any prophylactic benefit. The mechanism of the ulcerogenic properties of these drugs is supposedly similar to that of indomethacin.

Reserpine (Serpasil and Reserpoid) in large doses increases gastric acid secretion. Acute duodenal ulcers have been reported in people taking this drug; however, the incidence must be very low considering the number of patients who have ingested this drug over a period of years.

Although the incidence of peptic ulceration following **methotrexate** is not known, 15 deaths have been reported "usually as a result of gastrointestinal ulceration and hemorrhage, hematopoietic suppression, or overwhelming infection" in patients being treated for psoriasis alone (46). Methotrexate should be withheld from patients with both psoriasis and peptic ulcer disease since the benefits do not outweigh the hazards in such patients. In general, methotrexate and other antineoplastics should be used with caution in patients with peptic ulcer disease.

Caffeine, a long-acting stimulator of acid secretion, was previously used as an aid to diagnose peptic ulcers. It has largely been replaced by pentagastrin for this purpose. Though not considered to be ulcerogenic itself, it enhances the secretion of hydrochloric acid and this effect may be more pronounced in people with peptic ulcers than in normals (94a). Caffeine containing beverages such as coffee, tea, cocoa and cola-drinks should be avoided by peptic ulcer patients whenever possible.

Alcoholic beverages in concentrations of about 10%, stimulate gastric secretions which are rich in acid but poor in pepsin. As the concentration of alcohol increases, gastric secretion is inhibited. Concentrations of greater than 40% are directly irritating to the mucosa and cause chronic gastritis on prolonged ingestion (128a). The amount of alcohol in a strong cocktail is, like aspirin, capable of significantly increasing gastric mucosal permeability to hydrogen ions (139). Therefore, people with peptic ulcer disease should restrict their intake of alcoholic beverages and avoid medications containing high concentrations of alcohol.

Tetracycline and doxycycline have been implicated in four cases of esophageal ulceration (12a, 35a). All four cases were young women ingesting their medicine just before going to sleep. Tetracycline 500 mg dissolved in 2 ml of water has a pH of 2.3; doxycycline 100 mg forms a thick gel with a pH of 3.0 after three hours of 2 ml of water. It is possible that these cases represent reflux of the antibiotic into the esophagus, and with their high degree of acidity, the antibiotics caused an ulcer. Tetracyclines should be used cautiously, if at all, in patients with esophageal obstruction or reflux. Importantly, they should be given with a full glass of water and not ingested within one hour of going to sleep. Antacids should not be used with the tetracyclines.

Epigastric pain has been reported in 7-20% of patients on *iron therapy* (142a). This pain is directly related to the total amount of absorbable iron per dose and can be reduced or eliminated by decreasing the dose or by taking the dose after meals. Esophageal ulceration has been reported following the ingestion of a single 525 mg ferrous sulfate tablet which became lodged in the hypopharynx. Iron salts should be taken with a full glass of water and not within an hour of going to sleep.

15. What is the relationship between cigarette smoking and peptic ulcer disease?

Virtually all studies indicate that cigarette smokers have more duodenal ulcers than a comparable non-smoking population (110). People who smoke more than one pack per day for more than three years have a chronic reduction in pancreatic output of bicarbonates while those who smoke less have a similar reduction only while smoking. This reduction in bicarbonate decreases the endogenous neutralization of acid within the duodenum and is offered as a theory in duodenal ulcer production (142). Cigarette smokers with pre-existing gastric ulcers have larger ulcers than nonsmokers. In contrast to earlier reports (42), the cessation of smoking has not been shown to increase the healing rate (68).

16. What therapeutic measures are currently advo-

cated in the management of peptic ulcer disease?

Although the literature is replete with changing concepts and new therapeutic modalities, actual therapy of peptic ulcer disease has changed little over the years. Patients are still managed with some or all of the following: rest, diet, sedatives, anticholinergics and antacids. Histamine H2-receptor antagonists are also likely to be widely used.

17. It was recognized during the first century A.D. by Celsus that the diet should sooth and not irritate the stomach. Since then, this concept has repeatedly been reinforced in the minds of the medical community and the lay public (26). Is this supported by scientific assessment?

The Council on Foods and Nutrition of the American Medical Association has stated: "all the elaborate food lists used today for treating gastrointestinal disorders must be regarded as based on unverified impressions and traditional lore". This statement, though not fully accepted by the medical community, has been supported by controlled studies (17, 18). It must be concluded that individualization of the dietary program with small frequent feedings best meet the patients' needs (2).

18. M.X., a 32-year-old male, has been "troubled" with gastrointestinal pain of 12 weeks duration. He self-diagnosed an ulcer and began drinking a quart of milk with each meal, between meals, and at bedtime. What is the place of milk in the therapy of peptic ulcer?

Amino acids derived from the hydrolysis of the milk protein, casein, stimulate acid secretion in man (156). Additionally, the calcium in milk increases the secretion of acid in both normal subjects and those with duodenal ulcer (89). Whole, low-fat, and nonfat milk (240 ml) produce a significant increase in mean gastric acid secretion in both normal and ulcer subjects and can approximate 20-35% of the maximal acid output stimulated by betazole or pentagastrin. While milk has some acid buffering capabilities, it is mild with 1 ml of whole, low-fat and nonfat milk buffering 4.6, 4.3, and 4.7 ml of 0.1N HCl respectively *in vitro* (75). *In vivo* experiments have shown that continuous intragastric milk drips only slightly affect the pH of stomach contents in patients with duodenal ulcer (41, 120). Frequent ingestion of whole milk in the treatment of peptic ulcer is associated with an accelerated mortality from arteriosclerotic heart disease (132). Milk taken at bedtime, as in the case of M.X., will stimulate acid secretion during the night while the patient is sleeping (134).

19. What is the role of rest and sedation in the management of peptic ulcer disease?

Certainly no unanimity exists in assessing the value

of these modes of treatment. Possibly more tradition than fact associates anxiety and tension with ulcers. Psychotherapy does not promote or prevent the recurrence of peptic ulcers. Although patients with severe symptoms respond better with hospitalization, this may only be due to improved compliance with prescribed regimens in this environment. Sedatives should be considered as adjunctive therapy and prescribed only for selected patients.

20. Clinical observations and scientific studies often differ markedly in their conclusions. Such seems to be the case with anticholinergic drug therapy. What is the consensus on the efficacy and indications for anticholinergic therapy in duodenal ulcer disease?

Since radiologists are unable to differentiate between active and healed ulcers, and since a firm relationship has never been established between symptomatic relief and ulcer healing, it is not surprising that there are relatively few controlled clinical trials evaluating anticholinergic therapy. Studies in the early 1960's showed that synthetic anticholinergic drugs relieved symptoms better than either atropine or placebo. In an often quoted study, the recurrence rate following glycopyrrolate (Robinul) therapy was only 15% after 18 months compared with 71% for placebo. Ulcer complications developed in only 5% of the glycopyrrolate-treated patients compared with 59% of the placebo-treated patients (148). Although this study appears impressive, there were no data supporting the comparability of the two groups; the follow-up period (18 months) was short, and assessment was based on "ulcer-like symptoms, deformity, irritability of duodenum, or painless bleeding", which are all difficult to evaluate. Later, glycopyrrolate was shown not to reduce relapse (153). Doses of 1-11 mg (average of 5.1 mg) per day did not reduce the frequency and severity of symptoms or antacid consumption when compared to placebo (113). These data support the contention that there is no consistent evidence from controlled trials that in commonly recommended doses, anticholinergic drugs favorably alter the acute or long-term course of peptic ulcer disease (61, 76a). Some clinicians advocate dosages which cause dry mouth, blurred vision, urinary retention and tachycardia in an attempt to decrease gastric secretory response, prolong gastric emptying, and enhance therapeutic response. It is difficult to conceive of a patient who would tolerate such side effects.

Daytime administration of anticholinergics to prolong the action of antacids has been advocated; however, glycopyrrolate administered one hour before meals does not facilitate the action of four grams of calcium carbonate given one hour after meals (54a).

Anticholinergics given in large doses (e.g. propan-theline 30-45 mg) at bedtime in conjunction with antacids may afford relief to patients with nocturnal pain.

21. Z.E., a 35 year-old-male, has a five year history of recurrent duodenal ulcer. His family physician reports Z.E. has not responded well to chronic Pro-Banthine therapy and would like to prescribe equivalent doses of Robinul. Do any of the anticholinergic agents on the market have therapeutic advantages over one another?

All available anticholinergic agents can be classified into two categories: quaternary ammonium compounds and tertiary ammonium compounds. Uncontrolled studies have generated much confusion concerning their organ specificity and side effects. In general, *equivalent therapeutic doses* of all of these agents affect the same organs and cause the same side effects. Some authorities advocate the quaternary ammonium compounds because these agents do not cross the blood-brain barrier and therefore, lack annoying central effects. Although these agents are promoted as lacking central effects, there are reports of restlessness, fatigue, euphoria, and psychotic episodes, which must be considered to be CNS manifestations.

Since quaternary ammonium anticholinergics are poorly and unreliably absorbed, valid comparisons with belladonna alkaloids can only be made on parenteral administration. While tertiary ammonium compounds like atropine are 100% absorbed, the quaternary ammonium compounds like propantheline and methscopolamine are only 15-20% absorbed orally (9). Inadequately controlled studies often compare medications based on a lack of side effects rather than on a valid therapeutic response. The absence of side effects may simply reflect a subtherapeutic dose.

Therapy initiated with a belladonna alkaloid is equally efficacious, less expensive, and as well absorbed orally as any other available anticholinergic.

22. What are some of the contraindications to anticholinergic therapy?

Anticholinergics should be used with caution in patients with pyloric or intestinal obstruction, gastric hypomotility, gastric retention, and prostatic hypertrophy (104). In addition, people with hiatal hernia should avoid anticholinergic agents especially at bedtime, because gastric reflux into the esophagus with secondary inflammation and pain can result from paralysis of the sphincter between the esophagus and stomach. Elevation of the head may minimize such reflux during the night.

There is no contraindication to the use of systemic anticholinergics in patients with open-angle glaucoma (69).

23. Is there any value to combination products con-

taining anticholinergics and a sedative (e.g. Donnatal, Librax, etc.)?

Although these combination products accounted for 44.3% of the $97.7 million anticholinergic business in 1973, such products administered in maximal recommended doses do not reduce basal or histamine stimulated acid secretion (144). This is not surprising when one considers the amount of each ingredient contained in the product as well as their onset and duration of action. A therapeutic dose of the anticholinergic often results in excessive amounts of the sedative (4).

24. What is the mechanism of action and goal of antacid therapy in PUD?

Initially, it was proposed that antacids decreased the corrosiveness of gastric acid or prevented peptic digestion (15). Although four grams of calcium carbonate *in vitro* is capable of neutralizing all the gastric acid secreted by an average person with duodenal ulcer for 27 hours, *in vivo* antacids seldom raise the gastric pH above 4.0. At this pH greater than 99% of the acid has been eliminated; however, the gastric contents remain "corrosive." Though antacids may raise the gastric pH to greater than 1.8-2.5 (where pepsinogen is optimally converted to pepsin) inherent "antipeptic" activity has not been found (40,82). Claims of coating, demulcent, protective, absorbent or amphoteric properties of antacids also remain unsupported. Considering these points and the realization that there is no convincing evidence that antacids enhance the healing, decrease the frequency, or prevent the recurrence or complications of ulcer disease (119), the goal of antacid therapy remains that of relieving the pain.

25. It is reported that 15 ml of magnesium hydroxide will raise the pH of 150 ml of 0.1N HCl to 8.3 *in vitro* (71). Such studies also tabulate the pH that 15 ml of other antacids will raise the same solution. Conclusions are drawn that certain antacids are superior to others. Does such *in vitro* data imply *in vivo* superiority?

Such laboratory models do not mimic an antacid in the stomach of a patient with PUD. Therefore, 15 ml of magnesium hydroxide will not raise the stomach pH anywhere near 8.3. Such studies do provide a rough comparison of the potency of various antacids. However, using a different model, *in vitro* testing shows that if 1 ml of various liquid antacids is titrated to pH 3.0 with 0.1N HCl, assessments can be made that correlate well with *in vivo* neutralizing capacity. The endpoint of pH 3.0 has no physiological or pathological implication, it is simply the *in vitro* point that empirically correlates best with *in vivo* potency. Using this technique, a quantitative comparison of the *in vivo* activity of various liquid antacid preparations can be made (see Table 1). Obviously, other factors such as cost, taste, sodium content, bowel effect, patient's renal function and other pathology influence the selection of an antacid for a particular patient.

26. On morning rounds, a newly admitted patient with radiologically and clinically confirmed duodenal ulcer is discussed. Antacid therapy is deemed necessary for relief of severe epigastric pain. What is an effective antacid dose for patients with PUD?

Half the acid in the stomach is neutralized when the intragastric pH is raised from 1.3 to 1.6. As much as 99% of acid can be neutralized by raising the gastric pH from 1.3 to 3.3-3.5. Reduction of the acid content of gastric juice decreases the amount of acid available for back diffusion through the gastric mucosa, and peptic activity is diminished as the pH is raised above 1.8 to 2.5. Maintaining the intragastric pH in this arbitrary range throughout the day seems reasonable. Although the absolute amount of antacid must be individualized, duodenal ulcer patients require large amounts of antacids to achieve adequate buffering. Effective doses are 75 to 150 mEq of buffer which requires 30-60 ml of antacids such as Maalox or Mylanta (see Table 1). Gastric ulcer patients usually require lower doses providing 40-80 mEq of buffer (76). Other authorities recommend dosages of 40-80 mEq for all PUD patients (94, 112). This author recommends that 40-80 mEq doses be

Table 1

NEUTRALIZING CAPACITY OF VARIOUS ANTACIDS (55,9⋅

Antacid	Capacity (mEq/ml)	Volume (ml) required to neutralize 80 mEq
Delcid	7.1	11.3
Ducon	7.0	11.4
Mylanta II	4.1	19.3
Titralac	3.9	20.5
Camalox	3.6	22.3
Aludrox	2.8	28.5
Maalox	2.6	31.0
Creamalin	2.6	31.1
Di-Gel	2.5	32.7
Mylanta	2.4	33.6
Silain-Gel	2.3	34.6
Marblen	2.3	35.1
Wingel	2.2	35.6
Gelusil M	2.2	35.9
Riopan	2.2	36.2
Amphojel	1.9	41.4
A-M-T	1.8	44.7
Kolantyl Gel	1.7	47.3
Trisogel	1.6	48.5
Malcogel	1.6	48.5
Gelusil	1.3	60.1
Robolate	1.1	70.8
Phosphaljel	0.4	190.5

tried initially because gastrointestinal side effects are usually encountered with larger doses. Additionally, the ingestion of as much as 60 ml an hour (nearly 1.5 quarts/day) is expensive and patient compliance is poor, especially in view of the palatability of large amounts of these products.

27. It is decided to give the patient 80 mEq neutralizing capacity of an antacid per dose. You are asked to comment on the frequency of administration and the duration of therapy.

Antacid regimens usually are as follows: take as needed for pain, take every hour between meals, or take one hour after meals and at bedtime. The first regimen is less than optimal for the above patient with active disease and severe pain. If all antacids do is relieve pain, they should be administered at intervals to keep the patient pain free. The second regimen is widely used, especially in "refractory" patients, because the stomach usually empties every 30-45 minutes when no food is present. Patients are generally afforded prompt and complete relief if they comply to this demanding program. The third regimen is gaining popularity and its efficacy is supported in the literature. Ducon and Maalox in 15 ml doses administered one hour after a test meal and at bedtime to patients eating normal meals can completely relieve pain in 30%-55% of ulcer patients (124). The duration of action of antacids administered in this manner is prolonged to three or four hours depending on the antacid. In this hospitalized patient with acute duodenal ulcer, although frequent administration of antacid may not be absolutely necessary, most authorities still recommend hourly doses during waking hours for a minimum of two months (112). Others recommend hourly antacid regimens until the pain is alleviated, to be followed by doses after meals and bedtime for an additional six to eight weeks (76). Finally, others recommend that antacids be ingested immediately after meals and at bedtime for six to eight weeks. The agreement on six to eight weeks of therapy is in accordance with the concept that 50% of duodenal ulcers heal completely in six weeks.

28. C.S., a 68-year-old woman, has noted increasing epigastric pain, which she feels is an "old ulcer acting up." She relates that bicarbonate of soda has always worked better than antacids. Her medication profile notes she is currently taking: Digoxin, 0.125 mg per day and furosemide, 80 mg per day for congestive heart failure and Diasal salt substitute (potassium chloride with a trace of glutamic acid). She has mild chronic renal failure and a past history of PUD. How should she be advised?

Sodium bicarbonate is a rapid acting, highly effective, absorbable antacid that is short acting and capa-

ble of causing systemic alkalosis. The latter two properties limit its usefulness in the management of peptic ulcer disease. The maximum daily intake of bicarbonate should be limited to 200 mEq in people under 60-years-old and to 100 mEq in people over 60, although up to 24 mEq/kg/day for 3 weeks will not increase plasma pH in persons with normal renal function (40). In renal disease, however, a decrease in bicarbonate excretion may lead to alkalosis. It is assumed that people over the age of 60 have some degree of renal impairment. Therefore, frequent administration, as required in peptic ulcer disease, is undesirable in the elderly. In addition, sodium bicarbonate should be withheld from a patient with CHF, renal failure, and on a sodium restricted diet due to its sodium content (each gram of sodium bicarbonate contains 12 mEq of sodium). Suggesting an alternative low-sodium antacid is reasonable. Her GI complaints, however, may represent toxicity to digoxin or furosemide. She should be referred to her physician for further evaluation.

29. The most widely prescribed antacids are aluminum and magnesium hydroxides, either alone or in combination with each other. What are the relative advantages and disadvantages of each of these antacids?

Aluminum hydroxide (Amphojel) has poor neutralizing capacity, is short acting and predictably causes constipation. Claims for demulcent, protective, adsorbent, and amphoteric properties have been disproved. Aluminum hydroxide formulations are mixtures of hydrated aluminum hydroxide and anhydrous aluminum oxide. Excessive amounts of the anhydrous compound render formulations virtually useless. Tablet formulations are largely nonreactive, ineffective, and should not be prescribed. If the gel form of the aluminum hydroxide dries out, all of its activity is lost despite reconstitution with water. Tremendous variability between the products of different manufacturers and even between lots of the same manufacturer still exist. No doubt, factors such as these have contributed to the variable reports on the efficacy of aluminum hydroxide.

Aluminum hydroxide is a relatively non-toxic agent with constipation being the most troublesome side effect. In man, less than 1 mg of aluminum appears in the urine when normal doses are used; animal studies reveal no toxicity following huge doses. However, patients on dialysis may accumulate aluminum (see Question 32). In some individuals, a syndrome of phosphate depletion (hypophosphatemia, hypophosphaturia, increased GI absorption of calcium, hypercalciuria, increased resorption of skeletal calcium and phosphorus, debility, and bone pain) can be produced with aluminum antacids. Doses of 60 ml of aluminum-magnesium hydroxide or 30 of aluminum hydroxide administered four times daily can increase the fecal excretion of phosphorus and decrease the urinary excretion to undetectable levels after six days of therapy. As early as the 20th day of therapy, negative phosphorus balance can result (95). This is a problem only with patients on a very low phosphate diet or in those with chronic diarrhea.

Magnesium hydroxide (oxide and carbonate) is an effective antacid preparation with good neutralizing capacity *in vitro*. The same cannot be said for the trisilicate form found in Gelusil and A.M.T. Magnesium trisilicate has a slow onset, and a 2 gram dose given hourly will raise the pH of the stomach to just above 2.5 (15). All magnesium salts are poorly absorbed (15-30% of an oral dose) and are unlikely to cause toxicity in patients with normal renal function. If the maximum daily dose exceeds 50 mEq of magnesium, then caution should be observed in patients with kidney disease (40). Magnesium hydroxide's most bothersome effect is an osmotic diarrhea. This property is advantageous when magnesium hydroxide (milk of magnesia) is used as a laxative.

30. Aluminum and magnesium are usually prescribed in combination with each other (Maalox, Aludrox, Mylanta, WinGel, Creamalin, Maalox Plus, Di-Gel and others) to minimize gastrointestinal side effects and to increase activity. Are these mixtures more potent than either agent alone?

While aluminum and magnesium hydroxide mixtures are popular and effective antacids, the neutralizing capacity of the magnesium salt is reduced by the addition of aluminum hydroxide. Magnesium hydroxide has an initial pH of 9, and 600 mg can maintain a pH above 8 even in the presence of 200 mEq of hydrochloric acid. In contrast, if 600 mg of aluminum hydroxide is added to 600 mg of magnesium hydroxide, the mixture has a pH of 8 and the pH will fall to 4 after adding only 5 mEq of hydrochloric acid. The pH will remain at 4, however, in spite of the addition of 30 mEq more acid. (112)

31. K.E.G., a 57-year-old male, is hospitalized for acute epigastric pain. His history is compatible with PUD and gastroscopy confirms a rather marked duodenal ulcer of the mid-portion of the duodenal cap. Antacid therapy is initiated with 60 ml of Mylanta II liquid hourly. The second morning after admission, the patient complains that he has had severe diarrhea (six loose stools) throughout the night. Could this be secondary to the antacid and what can be done?

Although the above mixture is formulated, at least in part, to minimize possible diarrhea secondary to the magnesium salt or constipation secondary to the aluminum salt, individual patients commonly experience GI side effects. Diarrhea seems to appear more commonly. In the case of K.E.G., a large dose equivalent to approximately 240 mEq of neutralizing capacity (See Table 1) has been prescribed. Even aggressive clinicians seldom advocate more than 150-160 mEq per dose. Also, the 60 ml dose contains 4.8 grams of magnesium hydroxide, which is about twice the laxative dose of the drug. Therefore, it is not surprising that K.E.G. was experiencing diarrhea. The dose of Mylanta II should be reduced to 80 mEq of neutralizing capacity (approximately 20 ml). If diarrhea continues, then some doses can be replaced with an equivalent amount of aluminum hydroxide. Likewise, a patient experiencing constipation from such a mixture should replace sufficient dosages with an equivalent amount of magnesium hydroxide.

32. D.L., a 42-year-old male, has been on hemodialysis three times weekly for four years. Aluminum hydroxide, 60 ml, four times daily to increase fecal excretion of phosphates is part of his drug regimen. Over the past several months, his family has noted a progressive mental deterioration and the loss of recent memory, involuntary muscle twitching, and personality changes. This neurologic syndrome was attributed to renal failure and the dialysis by the family. Can antacids cause such a syndrome?

Only minimal amounts of aluminum are absorbed from antacid therapy. The normal human intake of aluminum is 10 to 100 mg daily, with an average blood concentration of 11 mcg/100 ml and minute tissue concentrations (23a, 112a). No biologic function for aluminum has been documented. It is felt that epithelial barriers to aluminum absorption exist in the lung, GI tract and skin. However, a syndrome such as that described above, which also includes speech abnormalities, a disordered EEG, and psychosis progressing to death within six to seven months has been noted in persons on dialysis for three or more years. It is now believed that this syndrome is secondary to high concentrations of aluminum in brain gray matter (1b), though confirmation is necessary.

33. A patient is confused concerning his antacid therapy. Calcium carbonate was prescribed by a physician as the best antacid available. A recent visit to a second physician brought comments that calcium carbonate was not good, dangerous, and should not be taken. The patient realizes that people have differing opinions but he is surprised at such divergent opinions. What is your comment?

Calcium carbonate is found in liquid antacid combination products such as Ducon 375 mg/5ml, Camalox 250 mg/5ml, Marblen (quantity not listed), Eugel 325 mg/ml, Glycogel 325 mg/5ml, and Titralac 1000 mg/5ml. Certain antacid tablets also contain calcium carbonate, i.e. Amitone 420 mg, Alkets 800 mg, and Tums 489 mg per tablet; however, they are not as effective mg-for-mg as liquids. Hourly administration of 4.0 grams of calcium carbonate maintains an intragastric pH in the range of 3.7 to 5.8 in fasting patients (81a). Recent data continue to support the fact that calcium carbonate has the greatest neutralizing capacity of the available antacids (54a, 71, 143). The most bothersome problems with this antacid are its poor taste and its predictable constipating action.

However, calcium carbonate has some potentially serious adverse effects which may override its advantages. About 8-24% of calcium is absorbed from a given oral dose of the carbonate salt. With the 4-5 gram per hour doses that are required to maintain an elevated pH in fasting patients, there is a 30% chance of developing hypercalcemia (145). Hypercalcemia and subsequent renal calculi are serious problems in patients with decreased renal function; when this antacid is used, the calcium intake should be kept below 160 mEq (8 grams of calcium carbonate) per day. In contrast to sodium bicarbonate, aluminum hydroxide, and magnesium hydroxide, calcium carbonate stimulates rebound acid secretion (see Question 34). Also, prolonged calcium carbonate therapy, together with foods containing vitamin D or calcium, may cause the milk-alkali syndrome (Question 35). Weighing all of these factors (effective, inexpensive, rapid acting versus its bad taste and ability to cause constipation, hypercalcemia, renal calculi, rebound hyperacidity and milk-alkali syndrome) against the efficacy of other available antacid mixtures prompts the controversy. It is doubtful that the therapeutic benefits of calcium carbonate outweigh the risks in this author's opinion.

34. At Grand Rounds the subject is peptic ulcer disease. Following a discussion of the pathology and presentation of the patient, the discussion turns to antacid-induced acid-rebound. Why don't all antacids cause rebound activity?

Study of the ability of various antacid formulations to induce gastric hypersecretion when administered one hour after a test meal has shown that calcium carbonate stimulates rebound-secretion while aluminum hydroxide-magnesium hydroxide formulations (Maalox and Riopan) and sodium bicarbonate do not (54, 89). Neither 30 nor 60 ml of the mixed hydroxides stimulated acid secretion, nor did 2, 4, and 8 gram doses of sodium bicarbonate. In contrast, a 4 gram dose of calcium carbonate raised the mean acid secretion to 6.9 mEq/hour as compared to a mean control value of 4.3 mEq/hour in 10 of 14 patients with chronic duodenal ulcer. Eight grams of the calcium salt raised the mean secretion to 6.9 mEq/hour compared to a control value of 4.1 mEq/hour in 11 of 11 patients. This hypersecretion could not be attributed to hypercalcemia and alkalinization of the antrum. Fordtran (54) concluded that acid-rebound due to calcium carbonate

is at least in part due to contact of the calcium ion in the small bowel. Levant and co-workers' (89) study of fasting subjects attributed the hypersecretion to an increase in gastrin release.

35. J.K. is a 49-year-old shoe salesman who three years prior to admission reported dull abdominal pain which occurred daily 30-60 minutes after meals and after retiring. At that time, he sought medical attention, and radiographic examination revealed a large gastric ulcer. He was treated with Maalox and belladonna and phenobarbital tablets without complete relief. Two weeks ago, he returned to his local physician complaining of additional abdominal pain. He was treated as an out-patient with a bland diet, six ounces of milk every two hours, and four grams of calcium carbonate every two hours between milk feedings while awake. He is now admitted to General Hospital with the following history: About four days ago he became dizzy on standing. This was followed by nausea and vomiting, anorexia, weakness, lethargy, abdominal pain and diarrhea. On admission, his serum calcium is 16.4 mg/100ml (9.0 - 11.0 mg/100ml), serum phosphorus 4.8 mg/100ml (3.0 - 4.5 mg/100ml), serum carbon dioxide content 38 mEq/liter (24 - 30 mEq/liter), and serum creatinine 2.1 mg/100ml (0.7 - 1.2 mg/ml). A diagnosis of "milk alkali" syndrome secondary to the calcium carbonate and milk regimen was made. His ulcer regimen was changed to aluminum hydroxide gel 30 ml hourly and a regular diet. Nine days later all laboratory values were within normal range and the symptoms had resolved. At that time, an upper GI series revealed a large persistent gastric ulcer. The patient underwent surgery, and the post-operative course was uneventful. J.K. was discharged five weeks after admission. Explain the pathogenesis of milk alkali syndrome secondary to calcium carbonate and milk.

Although 88% of ingested calcium carbonate appears in the stool (73), when large amounts of alkaline calcium salts and milk are ingested, hypercalcemia may occur. A regimen such as J.K.'s can result in serum calcium levels greater than 12 mg/100ml in 25% of patients. Hypercalcemia suppresses parathyroid hormone production. Such suppression reduces phosphorus excretion and elevates serum phosphorus. Hypercalcemia and elevated serum phosphorus levels can cause renal damage and reduce glomerular filtration in animals. Reduced glomerular filtration rate can lead to further accummulation of calcium and phosphorus and more kidney damage (102).

36. In peptic ulcer disease, as in any disease treated with medications, clinicians must be aware that patient non-compliance is one of the major causes of therapeutic failure. Is there evidence that

non-compliance is a problem in antacid therapy?

Non-compliance is a major problem not only with ambulatory patients, but also with hospitalized ulcer patients. Unlike other hospitalized patients, people with ulcer disease are often allowed to medicate themselves. A bottle of antacid is left at the patient's bedside and the patient is instructed to take doses in the prescribed manner. "Bottle counts" demonstrate that only 42-43% of ulcer patients take their medication as directed (129). Interestingly, this poor compliance occurred in spite of specific instructions by the patient's physician and the nurse who brought the antacid to the patient. Specific instructions also appeared on the label of each bottle. No correlation to compliance could be established between the quantity of antacid prescribed, the severity of ulcer pain, or the age of the patient. In another study, physicians felt that 70% of their patients were complying with prescribed regimens based on clinical response and confidence in the patient. On bottle-count, only 46% actually complied. Twenty-two of the 28 physicians overestimated their patients' reliability (25).

37. Commercially available antacids often contain other ingredients. What benefits can be obtained from these other "active" ingredients?

Simethicone (contained in Mylanta, Di-Gel, Silain-Gel, and Maalox Plus) is a surfactant claimed to cause small gas bubbles to coalesce and form larger ones, thereby facilitating elimination of gas. No controlled trials have shown whether such a change is clinically important in disorders that require antacid therapy. Manufacturers claim that it is useful in reducing postoperative gas pain and in reducing radiologically visualized gaseous accumulation. However, this does not imply improved efficacy, and the rationale for its inclusion in an antacid to be used in peptic ulcer disease is still unclear (40).

Alginic acid is said to produce a layer of antacid material which floats on top of gastric contents; however, there is no evidence demonstrating that this characteristic provides any beneficial effects in ulcer disease. Products such as Gaviscon do not increase the pH of the gastric contents as a whole. Reports supporting the efficacy of these products lack controls and are generally testimonial in nature.

Other additives such as activated charcoal, kaolin, pectin, methylcellulose, and gastric mucin also lack evidence supporting their efficacy for inclusion in antacid formulations.

38. Dr. W.W. is concerned with the proper selection of an antacid preparation for his hypertensive patients with PUD. What is the best antacid preparation for these patients?

It has been claimed that the maximum safe daily intake of sodium is 200 mEq for persons under 60 years of age and 100 mEq for those over 60 years. Doubling the average sodium intake (2400-6000 mg of sodium or 6-15 grams of salt) may cause a 10 mm Hg rise in blood pressure (65). Antacid formulations vary considerably in their sodium content. During the acute phase when antacids are administered every hour (possibly around the clock) large quantities of sodium may be ingested. See Table 2 for a list of commonly prescribed antacids and their sodium, potassium, and magnesium contents. In patients on sodium restricted diets, a product low in sodium should be selected. However, once the acute phase has passed and antacids are administered after meals and at bedtime, the problem of excess sodium ingestion from antacids is not significant. In the near future, all antacid formulations containing greater than 0.2 mEq (5 mg) of sodium per dosage unit will show on the label the sodium content per tablet or per unit volume. This will greatly facilitate the selection of antacids for sodium restricted patients.

39. D.F., a 24-year-old belly-dancer, has been bothered by chronic urinary tract infections for six years. Eight days ago a urologist placed her on tetracycline hydrochloride 250 mg every six hours for her most recent infection. D.F. has documented allergies to penicillins and sulfonamides and is now experiencing nausea and diarrhea from the tetracycline. (Apparently, D.F. started taking "soda" along with her tetracycline two days ago and has noted a decrease in the nausea.) Her physician is aware that di- and tri-valent cations (aluminum, calcium, and magnesium) will decrease the effectiveness of tetracycline but wonders about sodium bicarbonate. Should she continue with the bicarbonate and tetracycline together?

Shortly after the introduction of the tetracycline, aluminum hydroxide gel was noted to interfere with absorption, resulting in markedly reduced serum levels. Other divalent and trivalent cations, including iron, also markedly depress blood levels achieved with oral tetracycline (151). These polyvalent cations form insoluble chelates with the tetracyclines and thereby reduce absorption (80). Decreased tetracycline absorption has also been reported in the absence of chelation. A 50% decrease in tetracycline absorption occurred in patients receiving sodium bicarbonate (2.0 grams). Apparently, elevation in gastric pH decreases the dissolution rate of tetracycline (7). This latter study suggests that decreased tetracycline absorption might be expected with any agent which increases gastric pH. Tetracyclines should not be administered within one to two hours of antacids. If D.F. cannot tolerate the drug without the antacid, alternative antibiotics should be considered.

40. What other drug interactions may occur with

Table 2
ELECTROLYTE CONCENTRATIONS OF VARIOUS ANTACIDS

Liquid	Sodium Content	Potassium Content	Magnesium Content
Aludrox	1.17 mEq/30ml		3.0-3.7 mEq/5ml
Amphojel	2.13 mEq/30ml	0.5 mg/30ml	
A-M-T	2.21 mEq/30ml	6.8 mg/30ml	7.4 mEq/5ml
Basaljel	2.34 mEq/30ml	0.6 mg/30ml	
Camalox	0.67 mEq/30ml		
Creamalin	0.78 mEq/30ml		25.7 mEq/5ml
Delcid	3.00 mEq/30ml		
Ducon	4.66 mEq/30ml		
Gelusil	1.69 mEq/30ml		5.7 mEq/5ml
Gelusil M	1.49 mEq/30ml		12.6 mEq/5ml
Maalox	0.65 mEq/30ml	1.2 mg/30ml	
Milk of Magnesia	0.18 mEq/30ml		2.9 mEq/5ml
Mylanta	1.01 mEq/30ml		6.85 mEq/5ml
Mylanta II	2.09 mEq/30ml		
Oxaine	1.57 mEq/30ml		
Phosphaljel	3.39 mEq/30ml	0.6 mg/30ml	
Riopan	0.18 mEq/30ml	0.12 mg/30ml	6.51 mEq/5ml
Robalate	2.43 mEq/30ml		
Silain-Gel	0.06 mEq/30ml		2.91 mEq/5ml
Tricreamalate	10.61 mEq/30ml	78.0 mg/30ml	6.8 mEq/5ml
Trisogel	2.35 mEq/30ml		
Titralac	3.21 mEq/30ml		
Wingel	1.41 mEq/30ml		5.48 mEq/5ml

antacid therapy?

It has been suggested that antacids will decrease the absorption of weakly acidic drugs (e.g. nalidixic acid, nitrofurantoin, and the sulfonamides) by increasing the portion of ionized drug. However, since all of these agents are given in multiple doses, a delay in absorption does not necessarily mean a decrease in total absorption. The clinical significance of these interactions has not been adequately assessed.

Antacids would also increase the amount of ionized penicillin G; however, they might also protect the drug from acid degradation. This interaction may be of more theoretical than clinical importance.

The finding that bishydroxycoumarin forms insoluble chelates with magnesium and aluminum (100) implies that antacids might reduce the absorption of weakly acidic anticoagulants. However in vivo investigation of 15 ml magnesium hydroxide with 300 mg of bishydroxycoumarin (BHC) resulted in a 75% increase in mean peak plasma levels of BHC and a 50% increase in the area under the plasma level curve compared to controls. A 30 ml dose of aluminum hydroxide administered in the same manner did not alter BHC plasma levels. It was suggested that chelate formation may be involved in the increased BHC absorption when administered with magnesium hydroxide. In identical studies with warfarin, antacids did not affect absorption (1).

The coadministration of aluminum-magnesium hydroxides (Maalox) 120 ml/day and sodium polystyrene sulfonate (Kayexalate) 10 gm four times daily in fruit juice resulted in systemic alkalosis in 10 patients. Both antacids are considered "nonsystemic" and incapable of inducing systemic alkalosis. The resin evidently binds magnesium ion in exchange for sodium; therefore, no insoluble magnesium carbonate is formed in the colon and accumulation of bicarbonate results (51, 135). Antacids, particularly magnesium trisilicate, have been reported to impair the absorption of orally administered iron salts by forming poorly soluble substances (66a). If this combination of drugs must be given, their administration times should be widely spaced. Reports of decreased chlorpromazine blood levels and a 10-45% decrease in urinary excretion implies antacids reduce the absorption of phenothiazines (48, 49). Aluminum hydroxide and Riopan reportedly reduce the rate and amount of isoniazid that is absorbed (74). Administration of these agents should be at widely spaced intervals to avoid this interaction.

It is not generally realized that certain "nonsystemic" antacids increase urinary pH. The increase in urinary pH depends on the kind of antacid, the dose, and the pH before antacid administration. Subjects who have a relatively low baseline urine pH show the most pronounced antacid effect. The effect of seven days antacid therapy on the urinary pH of 11 healthy volunteers was (56b):

ANTACID	pH EFFECT
Aluminum hydroxide 10 ml QID	none
Calcium carbonate and glycine 5 ml QID	increased 0.4
Magnesium hydroxide 5 ml QID	increased 0.5
Aluminum/magnesium hydroxide (Maalox) 15 ml QID	increased 0.9

Since these are relatively low doses, larger therapeutic doses of antacids are likely to influence the elimination kinetics of drugs such as salicylates, certain sulfonamides, amphetamine and quinidine. A significant increase in serum quinidine levels and QT intervals have been attributed to concomitant antacid therapy (56a). Aluminum and magnesium hydroxide can reduce serum salicylate concentrations by 30 to 70% (92, 92a).

41. The histamine H_2-receptor antagonists offer a new therapeutic approach to acid-peptic disease. Discuss these various compounds and their mechanism of action.

Conventional antihistamines, termed H_1-receptor antagonists, inhibit histamine stimulated contraction of the bronchi and gut, but do not block the stimulatory effect of histamine on gastric acid secretion. In 1972, a new class of antihistamines was discovered that blocked gastric acid and pepsin secretion in response to not only histamine, but also gastrin, food, distention, caffeine, vagal and other cholinergic agonists. This implies that histamine may be involved in all modes of acid stimulation (12). To date, three agents have been studied extensively in man. The first was **buramide**, which was very effective but could only be given intravenously because of poor oral absorption. **Metiamide** is effective orally and doses of 200-300 mg inhibit both basal and meal stimulated acid secretion by about 80% in duodenal ulcer patients (97). In contrast, oral anticholinergics in maximally tolerated doses only reduce meal stimulated acid secretion by 23% over 3 hours (126). In Zollinger-Ellison syndrome, metiamide inhibits acid secretion by 85-100% (127). Healing of duodenal ulcers reportedly occurs in 62% and 73% of patients depending on dosage (1 gram and 1.3 grams respectively) as opposed to 25% of placebo treated patients (27). Metiamide does not alter serum gastrin release nor does it affect gastric emptying. Unfortunately, agranulocytosis occurred in four patients (one fatal) after a few weeks of metiamide therapy (56). This adverse reaction has been attributed to metiamide's thiourea chemical structure (propylthiouracil is a thiourea compound). The recently released **cimetidine** (Tagamet) is not a thiourea. Doses of 300 mg and 800 to 1600 mg per day reduce gastric acid secretion by 55% and 67% respectively in duodenal ulcer patients (67,123). Studies in normal subjects have noted a 70% reduction in acidity over 24 hours when cimetidine was taken before meals and a 72% reduction when taken after meals. When given after meals the peak blood levels occurred at the time when the buffer capacity of food was waning. Therefore, cimetidine administration after meals seems most appropriate (123). Cimetidine reduces meal stimulated acid output by 50% at blood levels which are achieved over 6 hours by oral doses of 2.5 and 3.5 mg/kg. Cimetidine is readily absorbed orally and the bioavailability is the same as by the IV route. About 70% is excreted unchanged in the urine within 6 hours and dosages should be reduced in renal failure. It appears to have a high margin of safety. With doses above 1000 mg/day, serum creatinine increases by up to 0.4 mg/dl in 60% of patients. In 11% the serum creatinine rises above the normal range but appears to be transient and returns to normal on stopping therapy. Rarely gynecomastia has been noted in males (66a).

42. What are the current indications for cimetidine?

Generally, cimetidine is felt to be an alternative or as a supplement to antacid therapy in unresponsive **duodenal ulcer** patients. This is based on the newness of the drug and the fact that intensive antacid therapy has been effective. A minimum of 3 weeks and up to 6 weeks of cimetidine therapy is necessary to heal 65-70% of active duodenal ulcers. Longer therapy or additional therapeutic agents may be necessary to maintain healing. Recurrences of ulcers within a month of stopping therapy at 2, 4 or 6 weeks ranged from 53-67%. Maintenance therapy using 400 mg twice daily has reduced relapses in 6 to 18 months from greater than 50% to 10%. Further studies assessing the efficacy and safety of long-term cimetidine are necessary before maintenance regimens become routine. Cimetidine is becoming the treatment of choice over total gastrectomy for *Zollinger-Ellison Syndrome*. Usual doses of 1.0-1.6 grams/day result in ulcer healing and reduction in pain and diarrhea in most cases. Occasionally, doses up to 2.4 grams/day are necessary along with antacids and/or anticholinergics. There are no controlled studies using cimetidine in *acute gastric ulcers*. Its use in over 300 patients with *gastric ulcer* and in *reflux esophagitis* has been disappointing.(67,123)

43. Elsewhere in the world other therapeutic modalities for the treatment of PUD such as inhibition of acid secretion, direct inactivation of pepsin, increase in gastric mucus production, and inhibition of gastrin release are also employed. What investigational products for the treatment of peptic ulcer disease are likely to become available?

Orally effective **prostaglandins** (16, 16 dimethyl prostaglandin E_2) also inhibit all forms of acid secretion (volume, concentration, and total output). A dose of 1 mcg/kg inhibited 80% of pentagastrin-stimulated secretion (115), while a 127 mcg capsule caused a 37% reduction in volume, 39% reduction in concentration, and a 60% reduction in output (158). Diarrhea seems to be the most common adverse effect.

Sulfated Amylopectin (Depepsen) inhibits gastric peptic activity without changing acidity. It does not inhibit trypsin, chymotrypsin, or pancreatic lipase, but weakly alters salivary amylase activity. Studies have shown a 50% decrease in luminal peptic activity for 30 minutes after a 500 mg oral dose. Considerable antipeptic activity was present after one hour. After 17 to 34 days, ten Depepsen-treated patients showed an $81.5 \pm 19.4\%$ reduction in gastric ulcer size (patients treated for 19 to 37 days with a placebo showed a $37.1 \pm 44.9\%$ reduction in ulcer size) (160). Amylopectin has also been studied for prophylactic use in patients recently recovered from duodenal ulcer. Recurrence rates were significantly less in patients treated with amylopectin (16%) in comparison with placebo-treated patients (75%) after 1 year of follow-up (150). These findings need confirmation.

Gefarnate (Gefarnil) is related to an anti-ulcer substance found in cabbage. Apprently, it has been used to protect against the gastric lesions induced by reserpine, phenylbutazone and prednisone (20). Additional investigation of this agent is needed.

Carbenoxolone is a licorice derivative that has received extensive investigation in the treatment of gastric ulcers. Its effectiveness appears related to enhanced mucus secretion, increased life span of gastric epithelium, inhibition of back-diffusion of hydrogen ions induced by bile, and, possibly, inhibition of peptic activity. The usual dosage regimen is 50 to 100 mg three times daily. The higher dose causes a high incidence of side effects but considerably better therapeutic response. The major side effects are sodium and water retention leading to edema, alkalosis, hypertension, and hyperkalemia. Some authorities advocate administration of a thiazide diuretic if edema occurs. A potassium supplement may also be necessary. The concomitant administration of spironolactone blocks carbenoxolone's healing action. Since most of the side effects of carbenoxolone may be attributable to the glycyrrhizinic acid present in the product, a formulation with all but 3% of the acid removed has been prepared (Caved-S). Though studies to date are few, the therapeutic benefits of carbenoxolone are apparently retained without the side effects (83). Prolonged therapy with carbenoxolone is not justified if healing has not occurred within the first 12 weeks. Also, there is no evidence to support the use of maintenance therapy with small doses to prevent relapse. Special capsules of carbenoxolone formulated to release the drug in the duodenum (Duogastrone) were not effective in duodenal ulcer disease; it may be too much to ask of pharmaceutical science to design a dosage form that will consistently release the active ingredient at a particular spot in a diseased bowel. Carbenoxolone will undoubtedly be released in the U.S. in the future, but it is questionable what impact it will make on the history of ulcer disease.

44. Once a peptic ulcer has healed, what is the prognosis for the patient?

Once the ulcer has healed, therapy should not stop. The goal of therapy is to prevent recurrence of another ulcer. Antacid therapy should continue on a moderate basis (after meals and at bedtime) when needed; foods known to cause gastrointestinal upset should be avoided; secretagogues such as caffeine and alcohol should be used in moderation; and ulcerogenic drugs should be avoided whenever possible. Such a regimen is difficult to adhere to even during active disease. Yet, it is necessary to educate patients to treat their disease even during remission. The available statistics show that 50 - 75% of duodenal ulcer patients will have a recurrence within 2 years and 20 - 30% of those with gastric ulcer will have a recurrence within one year. Such statistics could undoubtedly be favorably improved by better patient education about his disease and the more rational utilization of our current therapeutic tools.

45. When is surgery indicated for the treatment of peptic ulcer disease, and what are the procedures of choice?

In general, three factors dictate whether surgery is indicated for therapy of peptic ulcer disease: 1) high recurrence rate, 2) frequent complications, and 3) the possibility of underlying malignancy. Since malignancy is associated with gastric ulcers, failure to heal at an acceptable rate (e.g. 50% within 3 weeks and 90% within 6 weeks) in the face of a good medical regimen, is an indication for surgery. Complications of PUD such as perforation, pyloric obstruction, or continued hemorrhage also require surgical intervention. Most patients become surgical candidates only after they have had a long history of exacerbation and remission of their ulcer disease.

Most of the available surgical techniques produce almost identical results, and the success of surgery depends more on patient selection than on the procedure (60). Operative techniques are judged on the basis of associated mortality, recurrent ulcer rates, and post-operative nutritional disturbances (39). A vagotomy is performed to reduce the neural component of gastric secretion, a pyloroplasty to facilitate drainage when gastric emptying is delayed, an antrectomy to eliminate gastrin release, and a gastrectomy to remove parietal cell mass.

46. What is the "dumping" syndrome?

Clinically, this syndrome is reported as a sensation of epigastric fullness or churning, warmth, sweating, tachycardia, weakness, and syncope which occurs 5 to 30 minutes after meals and lasts 20 to 60 minutes. Intestinal cramping and diarrhea also occur. This symptom complex occurs in up to 80% of post-surgical ulcer patients, but rapidly improves over a few months. About 20 to 35% of patients will have chronic symptoms and 5 to 10% will have severe disabling symptoms. It occurs most commonly following a gastrojejunostomy.

This syndrome is caused by the rapid entry of hypertonic solution in the upper intestine, resulting in an osmotic accumulation of fluid in the bowel lumen. The splanchnic blood flow increases and plasma volume falls; peripheral vasodilation ensues with an increase in peripheral blood flow. Ultimately, there is a decrease in blood flow to the heart and brain. It is most likely that the symptomatology of "dumping" is due to this unfavorable distribution of blood.

Treatment consists of small, frequent low carbohydrate feedings to reduce the volume and number of calories per meal. Drug therapy which is designed to slow the intestinal transit time includes anticholinergics, ganglionic blocking agents, antihistamines, and sedatives; these agents do not consistently relieve the symptoms. The serotonin antagonist, cyproheptadine (Periactin), has been prescribed on the basis that an excess of serotonin will cause a syndrome complex indistinguishable from that of "dumping." However, the role of serotonin in dumping is unknown and cyproheptadine use has not produced impressive results. Additional surgery has been advocated in a few patients to further slow intestinal transit (138) or to increase intestinal absorption (52).

A pre-operative technique is now available which enables the clinician to predict the likelihood that a patient will develop "dumping" symdrome. Hypertonic glucose solutions are rapidly injected into the jejunum via an intestinal tube, and observations of clinical response, plasma volume decrease, peripheral blood flow changes, and skin temperature are made. Such a test may prove useful in matching patients with the surgical procedure that affords them the least morbidity (70).

CASE FOR STUDY

O.R.C., a 30-year-old white male, 74" tall and weighing 240 pounds, is a married father of five children ranging from 4 to 11 years of age. He was first seen by his family physician in July 1976, complaining of anterior chest discomfort, "heartburn," and burning epigastric pain, of 6-7 months duration. The epigastric pain sometimes lasted 1-3 hours and was severe enough to "double him over." Its onset was not associated with any foods and was occasionally relieved by antacids. On several occasions he was awakened from sleep with severe pain. Food seemed to relieve the pain and as a consequence of this he gained 20 pounds over the past several months. He smokes one package of cigarettes a day, drinks 10-15 cups of coffee a day, and "rarely" drinks alcoholic beverages. His past medical history was unremarkable except for long-standing back pain dating back to a farming accident at age 16. Since then he has had chronic low back pain. Six years ago a laminectomy was performed, and three years ago he had a fusion. Apparently he got good initial results from each procedure, only to have a recurrence. Initially, aspirin 650-1000 mg as needed helped, but he began to associate aspirin with increasing stomach pain and discontinued this medication. At the time of his initial office visit his current medications were: carisoprodol 350 mg three times daily and acetaminophen with codeine 60 mg three tablets a day. He has no drug allergies. The family history was noncontributory.

A review of systems was noncontributory. The physical examination revealed normal vital signs with a blood pressure of 122/70, pulse 70, and respirations 14. The general physical examination was essentially normal except for obesity. There was no abdominal tenderness. Laboratory studies were unremarkable with a hemoglobin of 14.4 gm%, hematocrit of 42%, white cell count of 9,650 and sedimentation rate of 13 mm/hr. The SMA 12/60 and urinalysis were within normal limits, and the stool was negative for occult blood.

A preliminary diagnosis of peptic ulcer disease was made, belladonna with phenobarbital 15 mg tablets one or two before meals and at bedtime were prescribed, and the patient was scheduled for an upper gastrointestinal (UGI) study. The UGI study revealed a prepyloric superficial gastric ulcer and some degree of chronic duodenal ulcer disease. These findings were discussed with the patient, and a regimen consisting of rest, bland diet (avoiding alcohol, tobacco, caffeine, pepper, spices, etc.), hourly milk or snack, calcium carbonate 1 gram as needed, and belladonna-phenobarbital tablets was prescribed. He was to return for X-ray follow-up in two to three months.

O.R.C. returned for re-evaluation of his peptic ulcer disease in September 1976, stating he had been relatively free of epigastric pain and was complying with the prescribed regimen. Two months later he returned with complaints of increasing epigastric pain which he associated with significant family problems and lack of adherence to his diet. A repeat UGI study revealed a rather marked duodenal ulcer deformity of the midportion of the duodenal cap. The changes were consistent with chronic duodenal ulcer disease and had increased in their prominence since the previous study. He had gained 10 pounds which he attributed to the diet and milk. The additional weight gain aggravated his back pain, and a local rheumatologist added ibuprofen 1600 mg/day to his regimen. The patient found this aggravated his stomach pain and stopped taking it after a week. The management and complications of peptic ulcer disease were discussed with him, and it was decided to cut down on the milk and intensify the antacid regimen to calcium carbonate 1 gram, one hour after meals and at bedtime.

O.R.C. was not seen until February 1977, when he returned to the office complaining of burning epigastric pain which occurred approximately 1 to 2 hours after meals and awakened him at night. Because the pain subsided shortly after his last visit, he discontinued the antacids after 2 or 3 weeks of therapy. An esophagogastroscopy revealed deformity of the duodenal bulb with marked narrowing of the midportion, the presence of two small superficial erosions, and a large ulcer crater. The pylorus, stomach, and esophagus were normal. After consultation between O.R.C.'s family physician and pharmacist, it was decided that surgery was not indicated because there was no assurance that a rigorous medical regimen had failed.

During an office visit, the family physician and pharmacist discussed with O.R.C. his peptic ulcer disease, his particular clinical course to date, and its apparent prognosis, its cost, and the patient's responsibility in successful managment.

His pharmacist outlined the following treatment regimen:

1. A diet as tolerated was offered with no food to be taken after the small evening meal.
2. Discontinuance of alcohol consumption during this acute phase and minimal usage therafter.
3. Personal re-evaluation of the importance of cigarette smoking.
4. Aluminum and magnesium hydroxide combination (Delcid-10 ml, Maalox, Mylanta, Creamalin, etc. - 30 ml) to be taken hourly between meals while awake and doubling the dosage at bedtime. When necessary, replacement of a dose or two each day with aluminum hydroxide (in the case of diarrhea) or magnesium hydroxide (in the case of constipation).
5. An anticholinergic (propantheline 30-45 mg) was prescribed for use at bedtime if night pain was unresponsive to antacids alone.

O.R.C. was followed at monthly intervals for three months. His pain stopped after 2 to 3 days of this intensive therapy and he no longer complained of night pain. His weight stabilized at 235 pounds. Although UGI studies or endoscopic examination have not been repeated, it is assumed that O.R.C. has had a positive response to therapy and that his ulcer has healed. He has been advised to take no medications, either prescription or non prescription, without consulting his pharmacist.

PEPTIC ULCER DISEASE CASE QUESTIONS

1. Speculate why O.R.C.'s antacid therapy had not relieved his espigastric pain prior to his first physician visit in July, 1976.
2. Why does food relieve ulcer pain?
3. What is the relationship between O.R.C.'s past history of a pack of cigarettes per day, 10 to 15 cups of coffee per day and "rarely" drinking alcoholic beverages with his epigastric pain? Should these points be considered in the treatment program?
4. Initially, aspirin helped control O.R.C.'s back pain; however, it caused increasing stomach pain. What is the association between aspirin ingestion and epigastric pain and bleeding?
5. Comment on the initial treatment regimen of belladonna with phenobarbital 15 mg prior to O.R.C.'s upper GI study.
6. Comment on each component of the regimen of rest, bland diet, hourly milk or snack and calcium carbonate as needed and the belladonna/phenobarbital tablets prescribed after confirmation of peptic ulcer disease.
7. Weight gain, possibly secondary to the "ulcer diet" and milk aggravated O.R.C.'s back pain for which ibuprofen was prescribed. Is ibuprofen a good choice for a patient with O.R.C.'s history? Could the ibuprofen be contributing to the exacerbation of epigastric pain?
8. Comment of the intensified ulcer regimen of cutting down on the milk and taking calcium carbonate after meals and bedtime.
9. Comment on each component of treatment regimen outlined by O.R.C.'s pharmacist.

REFERENCES

1a. Abbarath TR et al: Ulceration by oral ferrous sulfate. JAMA 236:2320, 1976.

1b. Alfrey AC et al: Syndrome of dyspraxia and multifocal seizures associated with chronic hemodialysis. Trans Am Soc Art Intern Organs 18:257, 1972.

1. Ambre J et al: Effect of coadministration of aluminum and magnesium hydroxides on absorption of anticoagulants in man. Clin Pharmacol Ther 14:231, 1973.

2. American Dietetic Assoc: Position paper on bland diet in the treatment of chronic duodenal ulcer disease. J Amer Diet Assoc 59:244, 1971.

3. Arky R: Diphenylhydantoin and the beta cell. NEJM. 286: 371, 1972.

4. Asher LM: The choice of anticholinergic drugs in the treatment of functional digestive disease. Amer J Dig Dis 4:260, 1959.

5. Aspinall R: Differential effect of spironolactone on the ulcerogenic and anti-inflammatory activities of indomethacin. Proc Soc Exp Biol Med 135:561, 1970.

6. Baker D: Small bowel ulceration apparently associated with thiazides and potassium therapy. JAMA 190:586, 1964.

7. Barr W et al: Decrease of tetracycline absorption in man by sodium bicarbonate. Clin Pharmacol Ther 12:779, 1971.

8. Baskin WN et al: Aspirin-induced ultrastructural changes in human gastric mucosa. Ann Int Med 85:299, 1976.

9. Beerman B et al: Gastrointestinal absorption of certain anticholinergic drugs. Eur J Clin Pharmacol 5:87, 1972.

10. Beirne JA: Gastrointestinal blood loss caused by tolmetin, aspirin and indomethacin. Clin Pharmacol Ther 16:821, 1974.

11. Ben Ishay D et al: Bioavailability of potassium from a slow-release tablet. Clin Pharmacol Ther 14:250, 1973.

12. Black JW et al: Definition and antagonism of histamine H-2-receptors. Nature 236:385, 1972.

12a. Bokey L et al: Oesophageal ulceration associated with doxcycline. Med J Aust 1:236, 1975.

13. Boley S: Experimental evaluation of thiazides and potassium as a cause of small-bowel ulcer. JAMA 192:93, 1965.

14. Boston Collaborative Drug Surveillance Program: Acute adverse reactions to prednisone in relation to dosage. Clin Pharmacol Ther 13:694, 1972.

15. Brody M et al: Antacids — comparative biochemical and economic considerations. Amer J Dig Dis 4:435, 1959.

16. Buchan D et al: Small bowel ulceration associated with enteric coated potassium chloride and hydrochlorothiazide. Canad Med Assoc J 19:176, 1965

17. Buchman E et al: Unrestricted diet in the treatment of duodenal ulcer. Gastroent 56:1016, 1969.

18. Buchman E et al: dietary treatment in duodenal ulcer Amer J Clin Nutr 22:1536, 1969.

19. Buckley R: Diphenylhydantoin in the treatment of duodenal ulcer. JAMA 219:511, 1972.
20. Butler DE et al: Developments in non anticholinergic anti-ulcer agents. Amer J Dig Dis 15:157, 1970.
21. Byrnes DJ et al: Serum gastrin in patients with peptic ulceration. Brit Med J 2:626, 1970.
22. Calabro JJ: Indomethacin: a current view of its use in rheumatic disorders. Drug Ther 1:34, 1971.
23. Cameron AJ: Aspirin and gastric ulcer. Mayo Clin Proc 50:565, 1975.
23a. Campbell IR et al: Aluminum in the environment of man. AMA Arch Indust Health 15:359, 1957.
24. Caron H et al: Patients cooperation with a medical regimen, JAMA 203:120, 1968.
25. Caron H et al: Objective assessment of cooperation with an ulcer diet: relation to antacid intake and to assigned physician. Amer J Med Sci 216:61, 1971.
26. Caron H et al: Popular beliefs about the peptic ulcer diet. J Amer Diet Assoc 60:306, 1972.
27. Celestin: Treatment of duodenal ulcer by metiamide. Lancet 2:779, 1975.
28. Chapman ML et al: Pentagastrin infusion glycine instillation as a measure of acid absorption in the human stomach: comparison to an instilled acid load. Gastroent 63:962n 1972.
29. Cline MJ: Cancer Chemotherapy, W.B. Saunders Company, Philadelphia, 1971, pp. 22-23.
30. Code CF: New antagonists excite an old histamine prespector. NEJM 290:738, 1974.
31. Cole P et al: Drug consultation — its significance to the discharged hospital patient and its relevance as a role for the pharmacist. Amer J Hosp Pharm 28:954, 1971.
32. Conn HO et al: Nonassociation of adrenocorticosteroid therapy and peptic ulcer. NEJM 294:473, 1976.
33. Cooke AR, et al: Failure of intravenous aspirin to increase gastrointestinal blood loss. Brit Med J 3:330, 1969.
34. Cooke AR: The role of acid in the pathogenesis of aspirin — induced gastrointestinal erosions and hemorrhage. Amer J Dig Dis 18:225, 1973.
35. Cox AJ: Stomach size and its relation to chronic peptic ulcer. Arch Pathol 54:407, 1952.
35a. Crowson TD et al: Esophageal ulcers associated with tetracycline therapy. JAMA 235, 1976.
35b. Crawford FA et al: The stress ulcer syndrome. Am J Surg 121:644, 1971.
36. Davenport HW: Damage to the gastric mucosa: effects of salicylates and stimulation. Gastroent 49:189, 1965.
37. Davenport HW: Back diffusion of acid through the gastric mucosa and its physiological consequences. Prog Gastroent 2:42, 1970.
38. Davenport HW: Why the stomach does not digest itself. Sci Amer 226:86, 1972.
39. Dawson JL: Peptic ulcer — surgical treatment. Brit Med J 4:102, 1969.
40. Department of Health, Education and Welfare, Food and Drug Administration: Over the counter drugs — antacids. Fed Register 38:8714, 1973.
41. Doll R et al: Continuous intragastric milk drip in treatment of uncomplicated gastric ulcer. Lancet 1:70, 1956.
42. Doll R et al: Effect of smoking on the production and maintenance of gastric and duodenal ulcers. Lancet 1:657, 1958.
43. Donaldson RM: Breakdown of barriers in gastric ulcer. NEJM 288:316, 1973.
44. Dragstedt LR: Peptic Ulcer: an abnormality in gastric secretion. Amer J Surg 117:143, 1969.
45. Dragstedt LR et al: Gastric stasis; a cause of gastric ulcer. Scand J Gastroent (suppl) 6:243, 1970.
46. Editorial: Psoriasis, methotrexate, and cirrhosis. JAMA 212:314, 1970.
47. Eiseman B et al: Stress ulcers — a continuing challenge. NEJM 282:372, 1970.
48. Fann WE et al: The effects of antacids on the blood levels of chlorpromazine. Clin. Pharmacol Ther 14:135, 1973.
49. Fann WE: Chlorpromazine — Effects of antacids on its gastrointestinal absorption. J Clin Pharmacol 2:388, 1973.
50. Fenster LF: The ulcerogenic potential of glucocorticoids and possible prophylactic measures. Med Clin N Amer 57:1289, 1973.
51. Fernandez PC et al: Metabolic acidosis reversed by the combina-

tion of magnesium hydroxide and a cation exchange resin. NEJM 286:23, 1972.
52. Fineberg C et al: The correction of postgastrectomy malabsorption by jejunal interposition. Surg Clin N Amer 53:581, 1973.
53. Fisher RS et al: Pyloric-sphincter dysfunction in patients with gastric ulcer. NEJM 288:273, 1973.
54. Fordtran JS: Acid rebound NEJM 279:900, 1968.
54a. Fordtran JS et al: Antacid pharmacology in duodenal ulcer. NEJM 274:921, 1966.
55. Fordtran JS et al: In vivo and in vitro evaluation of liquid antacids. NEJM 288:923, 1973.
56. Forrest JAH et al: Neutropenia associated with metiamide. Lancet 1:392, 1975.
56a. Gerhardt RE et al: Quinidine excretion in aciduria and alkalinuria. Ann Int Med 71:927, 1969.
56b. Gibaldi M et al: Effect of antacids on pH of urine. Clin Pharmacol Ther 16:520, 1974.
57. Gillies M et al: Gastric ulcer, duodenal ulcer and gastric carcinoma a case-control study of certain social and environmental factors. Med. J Aust 2:1132, 1968.
58. Glass G: Blood pressure and peptic ulcer. Lancet 1:864, 1971.
59. Goligher J et al: Five to eight year results of Leeds/York controlled trial of elective surgery for duodenal ulcer. Brit Med J 2:781, 1968.
60. Goligher J et al: Clinical comparison of vagotomy and pyloroplasty with other forms of elective surgery for duodenal ulcer. Brit Med J 2:787, 1968.
61. Greenblatt DJ et al: Anticholinergics. NEJM. 288:1215, 1973.
62. Greenspan R, et al: Gastric ulcer with true anacidity and pain relief with alkali. Gastroent 17:420, 1951.
63. Grossman MI et al: Inhibition of acid in dog by metiamide, a histamine antagonist acting on H-2 receptors. Gastroent 66:517, 1974.
64. Grossman MI et al: Fecal blood loss produced by oral and intravenous administration of various salicylates. Gastroent 40:383, 1961.
65. Guyton A et al: Physiologic control of arterial pressure. Bull N Y acad Med 45:811, 1969.
66. Hall GJ et al: Inhibition of iron absorption with magnesium trisilicate. Med J Aust 2:95, 1969.
66a. Hall WH: Breast changes in males on cimetidine. NEJM 295:841, 1976.
67. Henn RM et al: Inhibition of gastric acid secretion by cimetidine in patients with duodenal ulcer. NEJM 293:371, 1975.
68. Herrman R et al: Factors influencing the healing rate of chronic gastric ulcer. Amer J Dig Dis 18:1, 1973.
69. Hiatt RL et al: Systemically administered anticholinergic drugs and intraocular pressure. Arch Ophthal 84:735, 1970.
70. Hinshaw D: Pre- and postoperative "dumping studies" in patients with peptic ulcer. Amer J Surg 122:269, 1971.
71. Hirschman JL et al: Peptic ulcer disease. J Amer Pharm Assoc NS11:445, 1971.
72. Hune JN et al: Progress in patients with peptic ulceration treated for more than five years with Poldine, including a double-blind study. Brit Med J 2:13, 1966.
73. Hurst PE et al: The effect of oral anion exchange resins on fecal anions-comparison with calcium salts and aluminum hydroxide. Clin Sci 24:187, 1963.
74. Hurwitz A et al: Effects of antacids on gastrointestinal absorption of isoniazid in rat and man. Amer Rev Resp Dis 109:41, 1974.
75. Ippoliti AF et al: The effect of various forms of milk on gastric acid secretion. Ann Int Med 84:286, 1976.
76. Isenberg JI: Therapy of peptic ulcer. JAMA 233:540, 1975.
76a. Ivy KJ: Anticholinergics — do they work in peptic ulcer? Gastroent 68:154, 1975.
77. Jabbari M et al: Role of acid secretion in aspirin-induced gastric mucosal injury. Can Med Assoc J 102:178, 1970.
78. Jacobs E et al: Gastric ulcers due to the intake of potassium chloride. Amer J Dig Dis 18:289, 1973.
79. Janowitz HD: Jejunal ulcer in the presence of gastric ancylia — a case report. Gastroent 17:425, 1951.
80. Kabins SA: Interactions among antibiotics and other drugs. JAMA 219:206, 1972.
81. Kaye MD et al: A controlled trial of glycopyrronium and l-hyoscyamine in the long-term treatment of duodenal ulcer. Gut 11:559, 1970.
81a. Kirner JB et al: The effect of various antacids upon hydrogen ion concentration of the gastric contents. Amer J Dig Dis 7:85, 1940.

82. Kuruvilla JT: Antipeptic activity of antacids. Gut 12:897, 1971.

83. Langman MJS: Peptic ulcer — medical treatment. Brit Med J 4:100, 1969.

84. Lee P: Adverse reactions in patients with rheumatoid diseases: retrospective analysis of causes of admission and outpatient attendance in a specialist center. Ann Rheum Dis 32:565, 1973.

85. Leonards JR et al: reduction or prevention of aspirin-induced occult gastrointestinal blood loss in man. Clin Pharmacol Ther 10:571, 1969.

86. Leonards JR et al: Aspirin induced occult gastrointestinal loss: local vs. systemic effects. J Pharm Sci 59:1511, 1970.

87. Leonards JR et al: Safe and effective therapy with aspirin. Drug Ther 2:78, 1972.

88. Leonards JR et al: Gastrointestinal blood loss from aspirin and sodium salicylate tablets in man. Clin Pharmacol Ther 14:62, 1973.

89. Levant JA et al: Stimulation of gastric secretion and gastrin release by single oral doses of calcium carbonate in man. NEJM 289:555, 1973.

90. Levin E: Peptic Ulcer in the aged. Geriatrics 27:83, 1972.

91. Levin ME: Endocrine syndromes associated with pancreatic islet cell tumors. Med Clin N Amer 52:295, 1968.

92. Levy G et al: Decreased serum salicylate concentration in children with rheumatic fever treated with antacid. NEJM 293:323, 1975.

92a.Levy G et al: Urine pH and salicylate therapy. JAMA 217:81, 1971.

93. Levy G: Aspirin use in patients with major gastrointestinal bleeding and peptic ulcer disease. NEJM 290:1158, 1974.

94. Littman A et al: Antacid and anticholinergic drugs. Ann Int Med 82:544, 1975.

94a.Littman A: A single aspiration gastric analysis in duodenal ulcer and control patients. Gastroent 28:958, 1955.

95. Lotz M et al: Phosphorus-depletion syndrome in man. NEJM 278:409, 1968.

96. MacDonald WC: Correlation of mucosal histology and aspirin intake in chronic gastric ulcer. Gastroent 65:381, 1973.

97. Mainardi M et al: Metiamide an H-2-receptor blocker, as inhibitor of basal and meal stimulated gastric acid secretion in patients with duodenal ulcer. NEJM 291:373, 1974.

98. Malherbe C et al: Effect of diphenylhydantoin in insulin secretion in man. NEJM 286: 339, 1972.

99. Max M et al: Influence of adrenocorticotropin, cortisone, aspirin, and phenylbutazone on the rate of exfoliation and the rate of renewal of gastric mucosal cells. Gastroent 58:329, 1970.

100. McCallister J et al: Diffuse reflectance studies of solid-solid interactions IV. Interaction of bishydroxycoumarin, furosemide, and other medical agents with various adjuvants. J Pharm Sci 59:1286, 1970.

101. McMahon FG et al: Gastric ulcer after Slow-K. NEJM 295:733, 1976.

102. McMillan DE et al: The milk alkali syndrome: a study of the acute disorder with comments on the development of the chronic condition. Medicine 44:485, 1965.

103. Medalie J et al: Association between blood pressure and peptic ulcer incidence. Lancet 2:1225, 1970.

104. Medical Letter: Medical treatment of peptic ulcer. 11:105, 1969.

105. Medical Letter: Who needs slow-release potassium tablets? 17:73, 1975.

106. Menguy R et al: Effect of cortisone on mucoprotein secretion by gastric antrum of dogs: pathogenesis of steroid ulcer. Surgery 54:19, 1963.

107. Menguy R et al: Influence of bile on the canine gastric antral mucosa. Amer J Surg 119:177, 1970.

108. Menguy R: Pathophysiology of peptic ulcer. Amer J Surg 120:282, 1970.

109. Mills DG et al: Effect of in vitro aspirin on blood platelets of gastrointestinal bleeders. Clin Pharmacol Ther 15:187, 1973.

110. Monson R: Cigarette smoking and body form in peptic ulcer. Gastroent 8:337, 1970.

111. Morgenstern L: The cirumferential small-bowel ulcer. JAMA 191:101, 1965.

112. Morrissey JF et al: Antacid therapy. NEJM 290:550, 1974.

112a.Niedermeier W et al: Emission spectrometric determination of trace elements in biologic fluids. Appl Spectroscopy 25:53, 1971.

113. Norgaard RP et al: Effect of long-term anticholinergic therapy on gastric acid secretion with observations on the serial measurement of peak histalog response. Gastroent 58:750, 1970.

114. Nuss D et al: Peptic ulceration in childhood. Surg Clin N Amer 51:945, 1971.

115. Nylander B et al: Gastric secretory inhibition induced by three methyl analogs of prostaglandin E-2 administered intragastrically to man. Scand J Gastroent 9:751, 1974.

116. O'Brien TK et al: Alimentary hypoglycemia associated with the Zollinger-Ellison syndrome. Amer J Med 54:637, 1973.

117. Overholt BF et al: Acid diffusion into the human gastric mucosa. Gastroent 54:182, 1968.

118. Palmer WL: Achlorhydria and ulcer. NEJM 285:1487, 1971.

119. Piper DW: Antacid and anticholinergic drug therapy of peptic ulcer. Gastroent 58:750, 1967.

120. Piper DW: Milk in the treatment of gastric disease. Amer J Clin Nutr 22:191, 1969.

121. Pounder RE et al: 24-hr control of intragastric acidity by ametidine in duodenal-ulcer patients. Lancet 2:1069, 1975.

122. Pounder RD et al: Healing of gastric ulcer during treatment with cimetidine. Lancet 1:337, 1976.

123. Pounder RE: Effect of cimetidine on 24-hour intragastric acidity in normal subjects. Gut 17:133, 1976.

124. Powell RL et al: A clinical evaluation of a new concentrated antacid. J Clin Pharmacol 11:296, 1971.

125. Rhodes J: Etiology of gastric ulcer. Gastroent 63:171, 1972.

126. Richardson CT et al: The effect of an H-2-receptor antagonist on food stimulated acid secretion, serum gastrin, and gastric emptying in patients with duodenal ulcer. J Clin Invest 55:536, 1975.

127. Richardson CT et al: The value of a histamine H-2-receptor antagonist in the management of patients with the Zollinger-Ellison Syndrome. NEJM 294:133, 1976.

128. Ridolfo AS: Effects of fenoprofen and aspirin on gastrointestinal microbleeding in man. Clin Pharmacol Ther 14:226, 1973.

128a.Ritchie JM: The aliphatic alcohols. The Pharmacological Basis of Therapeutics, 5th ed, Goodman and Gilman editors, MacMillan Co, New York 1975.

129. Roth H et al: Studies on patient cooperation in ulcer treatment. Gastroent 38;630, 1960.

130. Rothermich NO: An extended study of indomethacin. JAMA 195:531, 1966.

131. Samloff IM et al: Serum group I pepsinogens by radioimmunoassay in control subjects and patients with peptic ulcer. Gastroent 69:83, 1975.

132. Sandweiss DJ: The sippy treatment for peptic ulcer — fifty years later. Amer J Dig Dis 6:929, 1961.

133. Sapp OL: Treatment of duodenal ulcer. Amer Fam Physician 7:129, 1973.

134. Schiff ER: Treatment of uncomplicated peptic ulcer disease. Med Clin N Amer 55:305, 1971.

135. Shroeder ET: Alkalosis resulting from combined administration of a non-systemic antacid and a cation-exchange resin. Gastroent 56:868, 1969.

136. Sharnoff J et al: Stress ulcers and heparin prophylaxis. Brit Med J 1:444, 1972.

137. Shepherd A et al: Peptic ulceration in chronic renal failure. Lancet 1:1357, 1973.

138. Silver D et al: The mechanism of the dumping syndrome. Surg Clin N Amer 46:425, 1966.

139. Smith BM et al: Permeability of the human gastric mucosa: alteration by ASA and ethanol. NEJM 285:176, 1971.

140. Smyth CJ: Indomethacin in rheumatoid arthritis. A comparative objective evaluation with adrenocorticosteroids. Arthr Rheum 8:921, 1965.

141. Smyth CJ: Indomethacin — its rightful place in treatment. Ann Int Med 72:430, 1970.

142. Solomon TE et al: Cigarette smoking and duodenal-ulcer disease. NEJM 286:1212, 1972.

142a.Sovell: Iron Deficiency Symposium, Academic Press, New York 1970.

143. Sparberg M: The therapy of peptic ulcer disease. Ration Drug Ther 7:1, 1973.

144. Steigmann L et al: Belladonna alkaloid sedative mixture, effects on gastric acidity and motility. Amer J Dig Dis 1:174, 1956.

145. Stiel J et al: Hypercalcemia in patients with peptic ulceration receiving large doses of calcium carbonate. Gastroent 53:900, 1967.

146. Strickland R et al: Effect of prednisolone on gastric function and structure in man. Gastroent 56:675, 1969.

147. Sturges HF et al: Ulceration and stricture of the jejunum in a patient on a long-term indomethacin therapy. Amer J Gastroent 59:162, 1973.
148. Sun D: Long-term anticholinergic therapy for prevention of recurrences in duodenal ulcer. Amer J Dig Dis 7:706, 1964.
149. Sun D: Effect of corticotropin on gastric acid, pepsin, and mucus secretion in dogs with fistulas. Amer J Dig Dis 14:107, 1969.
150. Sun et al: A controlled study on the use of propantheline and amylopectin sulfate (SN-263) for recurrences in duodenal ulcer. Gastroent 58:756, 1970.
151. Sweeney WM et al: Absorption of tetracycline in human beings as affected by certain excipients. Antibiot Med Clin Therap 4:642, 1957.
151a. Taylor Rt et al: Gastric ulceration occurring during indomethacin therapy. Brit Med J 4:734, 1968.
152. Thorsen WB et al: Aspirin injury to the gastric mucosa. Arch. Int. Med 121:499, 1968.
153. Trevino H et al: The effect of glycopyrrolate on the course of symptomatic duodenal ulcer. Amer J Dig Dis 12:983, 1967.
154. Trudeau WL et al: Relations between serum gastrin levels and rates of gastric hydrochloric acid secretion. NEJM 284:408, 1971.
155. Vickers NF: Mucosal effects of aspirin and acetaminophen: report of a controlled gastroscopic study. Gastrointest Endon 14:94, 1967.
156. Walsh JH et al: pH dependence of acid secretion and gastrin release in normal and ulcer subjects. J Clin Invest 55:462, 1975.
157. Westlund K: Blood pressure and peptic ulcer. Lancet 1:86, January 1971.
157a. Weiss SM: Gut lesions due to slow release KCl tablets. NEJM 296:111, 1977.
158. Wilson DE et al: Inhibition of stimulated gastric secretion by an orally administered prostagla capsule. Ann Int Med 84:688, 1976.
159. Wormsley KG et al: Maximal histalog test in control subjects and patients with peptic ulcer. Gut 6:427, 1965.
160. Zimon D et al: Specific inhibition of gastric pepsin in the treatment of gastric ulcer. Gastroent 56:19, 1969.

Chapter 19

Diseases of the Liver

Richard Grant Closson
Lloyd Y. Young

Hepatitis, or inflammation of the liver, is a complex collection of clinical abnormalities. Hepatitis may be active or chronic, acute or subclinical. It can be divided into five categories based upon the etiology and/or clinical course as follows:

  a. Typical acute viral hepatitis
  b. Atypical viral hepatitis
  c. Active chronic (lupoid) hepatitis
  d. Toxic hepatitis
  e. Drug-induced hepatitis

Hepatitis may also be a manifestation of infectious diseases. The liver may be infected by bacteria, mycobacteria, fungi, protozoa, Rickettsiae, and other agents. Although hepatitis frequently has a viral etiology, it can also be caused by other pathogens and chemical agents.

CASE A: VIRAL HEPATITIS.

M.S. is a 31-year-old unmarried merchant seaman with a chief complaint of headache, nausea, vomiting and general malaise for four days. Six weeks ago aboard ship he was involved in an industrial accident, sustaining multiple internal abdominal injuries. He was hospitalized in a large Asian city where his treatment required an emergency exploratory laparotomy, splenectomy and transfusion of six units of whole blood. He recovered sufficiently to be returned to the United States in two weeks, but not before he had visited a busy tattoo parlor and had become decorated with a bicentennial eagle. On his return to this country he continued to convalesce at the house he shares with eight other people. Shortly after his return, three other people in the household developed similar mild symptoms.

1. The history, symptoms and admitting signs of dark urine and scleral icterus point to a diagnosis of typical viral hepatitis. Discuss the major differences between Type A and Type B viral hepatitis with regard to incubation period and mode of transmission.

Typical acute viral hepatitis is an infection in which the eventual necrosis of the liver cells is responsible for most of the symptomatology. Currently it is felt that two major forms of viral hepatitis exist: viral hepatitis — Type A and viral hepatitis — Type B. Viral hepatitis Type A (also known as infectious hepatitis or IH) has a short incubation period and is caused by hepatitis virus A. Viral hepatitis — Type B (also known as serum hepatitis or SH) has a long incubation period and is caused by hepatitis virus B. There may also be a third non-A, non-B hepatitis, but its significance is not yet clear (166a).

Viral Hepatitis – Type A is most commonly transmitted by the fecal-oral route, or by ingestion of contaminated water, shellfish or meat. The incubation period (time between infection and development of symptoms) ranges between one-half and two months. The patient's feces and blood become infectious two to three weeks prior to the onset of jaundice (this is based on an average incubation period of 25 days). The infective stage probably lasts only a few days after the onset of jaundice; however, chronic excretion of virus has been reported (240). The urine or nasopharyngeal secretions of patients may contain viral particles but appear to be poorly infective.

Viral Hepatitis – Type B is usually transmitted parenterally. The incubation period ranges from two to six months, but may be as brief as 28 days. Infective viremia has been demonstrated up to 87 days before the onset of clinical symptoms (169) and chronic viremia of greater than five years duration has been observed (240). The most common etiology of viral hepatitis B is the transfusion of blood products. The infection rate increases almost linearly with the number of units transfused. The amount of contaminated blood necessary for disease transmission is microscopic, as evidenced by the report of infection in 5 of 10 volunteers injected with 0.00004 ml of whole blood (59).

Viral hepatitis type B may also be transmitted by hemodialysis, organ transplantation, use of contaminated needles, syringes, dental tools, tattooing equipment, or skin puncture by outdoor elements such as twigs, branches and rocks. Confirmation of the infectivity of hepatitis-associated antigen found in saliva, urine and feces would complete the evolution of thought regarding the pathogenesis of viral hepatitis type B (see below).

2. Which blood products are associated with a high risk of hepatitis. Which products have a low risk of hepatitis?

The risk of infection from the transfusion of blood or a blood derivative is determined by the number of donors per unit of transfusate, and the use of effective sterilization procedures. Examples of "High Risk" products (from multiple donors, unsterilized) include pooled plasma and clotting factor concentrates. "No Risk" or "Safe" products (adequately sterilized) include human serum albumin, plasma protein fraction, hyperimmune globulins and gamma globulin.

3. Describe the typical time course for development of symptoms of acute viral hepatitis. Can M.S.'s diagnosis be made more specific from his history and this information?

Typical acute viral hepatitis usually first becomes apparent with the onset of vague symptoms, often referable to the gastrointestinal tract. When transmitted orally, abrupt fatigue, headache, anorexia, nausea, and vomiting may be the first manifestations of the disease. Right upper quadrant abdominal fullness or pain may be described by the patient as well as a flu-like syndrome, including fever, myalgia, pharyngitis and coryza. When the disease is acquired parenterally, the onset is more insidious and many of these symptoms, particularly the fever, may not occur. From 2 to 14 days after the onset of symptoms, jaundice will appear. Dark urine (bilirubinuria) and light stools precede jaundice by 1 to 4 days.

Jaundice marks the end of the prodromal phase and the beginning of the icteric phase. From this stage on, the clinical features of viral hepatitis A and B are identical. Fever subsides, the gastrointestinal symptoms diminish, jaundice peaks in 1½ weeks and then begins to decrease. Jaundice usually lasts for 6 to 8 weeks and by the time it resolves, the patient should feel well with the exception of residual fatigue. The posticteric recovery phase may last for 2 to 6 more weeks. Complete recovery requires 3 to 4 months in most cases.

A more specific diagnosis of viral hepatitis type A or type B could be based upon history of exposure to a likely source and an appropriate time course for development of symptoms. The history of M.S.'s disease contains several exposures to possible disease sources which prevent exclusion of either form of viral hepatitis. Likewise, other pathogens and chemical agents, in this case, cannot be excluded.

4. As part of the attempt to confirm the diagnosis of viral hepatitis in M.S., determination of Hepatitis-Associated (Australia) Antigen is ordered. What is Hepatitis-Associated Antigen (HAA)? How may it be used in the diagnosis and prevention of viral hepatitis?

Hepatitis-Associated Antigen (HAA) is also called Australia antigen, serum hepatitis antigen (SH-antigen) and hepatitis-B antigen (HB-Ag). For a complete description of the current knowledge of the agent of hepatitis B, the reader is referred to a recent review (213). The antigen appears to be a small virus or virus-like agent which can be found in the serum, bile, urine, feces and saliva of patients with viral hepatitis B (227,245,249,257). Apparent discrepancies between patient history and the presence of HAA are probably the result of unconfirmed nonparenteral transmission of the disease and/or low HAA test sensitivity. Because there is considerable overlap between the transmission routes and incubation periods, previous distinctions that were made between hepatitis A and B based upon these criteria are probably invalid (132,263). As tests for HAA become more sensitive, a diagnosis of type A or B hepatitis may be made based upon the presence or absence of HAA.

Testing for the presence of HAA has had a great impact in the area of blood banking and blood component therapy. The American Association of Blood Banks now requires that all blood be screened for the presence of HAA, because it is well established that hepatitis does occur following the administration of HAA-positive blood products (87,159). Screening for and elimination of HAA-positive blood products at Philadelphia General Hospital decreased the incidence of post-transfusion hepatitis from 17.9% to 5.9% (245). As more sensitive testing procedures become available, this incidence should decrease even further.

5. Does the presence of HAA in this patient confirm a diagnosis of viral hepatitis B?

The presence of HAA in M.S.'s serum is evidence that he has had viral hepatitis B at some time. The argument that the current antigenemia is due to his current infection is strong but not ironclad.

The fact that antigenemia associated with viral hepatitis B is usually transient supports a diagnosis of hepatitis B in M.S. However, persistent antigenemia occurs in some patients with chronic hepatitis, Down's syndrome, chronic renal disease (on hemodialysis), acute and chronic lymphocytic leukemia, and Hodgkin's disease. There is also a fairly large group of apparently normal patients (approximately 0.1% in the United States) who have persistent HAA without signs or symptoms of clinical disease. Sutnick has discussed the theoretical basis for this phenomenon in an excellent review (245). Therefore, it is possible that M.S. has viral hepatitis A and that his antigenemia is due to some other condition. If these can be ruled out, the antigenemia strongly suggests a diagnosis of acute viral hepatitis B.

6. Assume that a diagnosis of acute viral hepatitis (A or B) has been confirmed. Outline a rational plan for treatment.

The management of viral hepatitis is nonspecific and is based upon manipulation of activity, diet, and medication. Most studies of therapy are uncontrolled. Initial hospitalization may be necessary if symptoms are severe or to diagnose atypical variants that carry high morbidity.

Recommendations for *bedrest* vary greatly depending upon author and era. Most patients with severe disease will feel like staying in bed; patients who feel well and have good appetites may be allowed to walk as their strength permits. Prolonged bedrest beyond the duration of clinical disease is unnecessary. Despite the fact that hepatic blood flow decreases dramatically in the upright position (at rest or during exercise) (44,217), there is no evidence that excessive rest enhances recovery. In addition to the subjective improvement of symptoms, serum transaminase levels may be used as a guide to ambulation. Some patients may show a secondary rise in these enzymes after two or three weeks of illness that may occur in the presence of continued clinical improvement. This does not necessarily mean progression of the disease and does not require additional bedrest.

During the acute illness, the patient should receive a *high carbohydrate diet* (one source suggests 16 carbohydrate calories per kilogram body weight per day); however, severe nausea and vomiting may necessitate intravenous feeding. Hyperalimentation with concentrated dextrose-protein solutions can be used, but is unnecessarily expensive and unwarranted in a well-nourished adult. Should prehepatic coma develop, protein intake should be discontinued. When appetite returns, oral feeding may be begun and advanced as tolerated. Small, frequent feedings (5 to 6 per day) are usually more palatable to the patient. Carbohydrates have a protein "sparing" effect in that when they are provided in sufficient quantities to meet the patient's caloric requirements, all available protein may be used for tissue regeneration.

Phenothiazines may be used to treat nausea and vomiting associated with viral hepatitis but these symptoms are usually self-limited and improve in a few days and phenothiazines themselves rarely cause cholestatic jaundice. Serum transaminase levels may be used to monitor this side effect because the transient elevations associated with viral hepatitis occur well into the convalescent period when phenothiazines would no longer be needed.

There is no basis for the use of water-soluble vitamin supplementation in patients with acute hepatitis who are well-nourished. In chronic liver disease, however, the degradation of pyridoxine may be increased. Supplemental vitamin B-6 does not correct the deficiency as well as pyridoxine-5'-phosphate (133a). Fat-soluble vitamin supplementation may be reasonable because the absorption of fat (and, perhaps, fat-soluble vitamins) is impaired in viral hepatitis (36). In chronic liver disease, 25-hydroxyvitamin D serum levels are abnormally low (146a), apparently due to diminished absorption of vitamin D (37a), impaired 25-hydroxylation (233a) and decreased absorption of enterohepatically circulated 25-hydroxyvitamin D (37a). Normal serum levels of the vitamin can be maintained with adequate supplementation which is greater than for normal persons (233a). In acute hepatitis, vitamin K body stores are usually adequate to maintain clotting factor levels in spite of possible vitamin K malabsorption. Nevertheless, in chronic liver disease, supplemental phytonadione injections or clotting factor concentrations may often be warranted.

There is no specific drug therapy for typical acute viral hepatitis. Corticosteroids have been used to decrease inflammation, but recent evidence suggests that this action may not be separable from immunosuppression which carries considerable risk in patients with severe disease. Other studies (96,197) fail to demonstrate that corticosteroids alter the morbidity or mortality of severe viral hepatitis and even suggest that they may be deleterious. These dismal results should not be confused with the use of corticosteroids in the treatment of chronic active hepatitis where immunosuppression appears to be of value.

7. Is alcohol contraindicated in a patient with acute viral hepatitis?

Although ethanol restriction is usually placed upon viral hepatitis patients, there is little direct experimental evidence to support this practice. The common acknowledgement of ethanol's hepatotoxic effects and its association with portal (Laennec's) cirrhosis have probably led to the recommended avoidance of alcohol by hepatitis patients. Alcohol is known to cause striking metabolic imbalances within the liver: it promotes fatty acid synthesis, favors triglyceride accumulation and decreases fatty acid oxidation (142). Patients with and without active viral hepatitis have been given 0.5 ml or 1.0 ml ethanol per kilogram, intravenously to study the effect on hepatic enzymes (83). The ethanol had no significant effect on the mean levels of SGOT, SGPT, LDH, or sorbitol dehydrogenase. Other studies have shown that moderate alcohol consumption does not interfere with convalescence nor the incidence of residua.

8. Are antibiotics and antiviral agents useful for the treatment of uncomplicated viral hepatitis in M.S.?

Presently there is no justification for the use of systemic antibiotics to treat viral hepatitis. The inability to isolate the hepatitis viruses has hampered the development of effective antiviral agents. There is some evidence that an investigational agent, ribavirin (Virazole — ICN Pharmaceuticals), produces clinical improvement in patients with viral hepatitis type A. The drug seems to have little effect on the course of hepatitis type B but may hasten the disappearance of HB-Ag from the blood of chronic carriers (155). Clinical trials are under way but it will be several years before the drug is available for general use if the results are favorable. Human leukocyte interferon, a naturally-occurring antiviral substance, appears to depress the immunological markers of hepatitis B infection but has not been observed to affect the disease course (54a,93). There are no current antibiotic or antiviral agents that would be useful in the treatment of M.S.'s uncomplicated hepatitis.

9. What role would serum immune (gamma) globulin administration have in the management of this patient's viral hepatitis? What dose should be used and how should it be administered?

It has been apparent for more than 30 years that the administration of gamma globulin can greatly attenuate some cases of viral hepatitis. Recently it has become apparent that most of the antibody in pooled gamma globulin is specific for hepatitis virus A which accounts for its poor ability to prevent hepatitis B. If it is given after suspected contact, it can minimize hepatitis A. Its prophylactic value is greatest when administered early in the incubation period and decreases with time after exposure. Immune serum globulin is not effective if it is given more than six weeks after exposure. Nor is it useful in the treatment of active clinical disease (192).

Whether gamma globulin will effectively attenuate viral hepatitis A is based upon several factors: (a) the dose administered, (b) the concentration of hepatitis virus antibody in the dose, (c) the amount of virus in the infecting dose, and (d) the time interval between infection and administration of immune serum globulin. Official preparations of immune serum globulin contain 16 percent globulin. The recommended dose has ranged between 0.02 ml/kg and 0.2 ml/kg of body weight. Under most conditions, protection is afforded by intramuscular injection of 0.01 ml of immune serum globulin per pound of body weight or approximately 0.02 ml/kg. While larger doses do not generally provide greater protection for a single exposure, the duration of protection is increased to four to six months if this dose is doubled; this has important implications for travelers to foreign countries. Pregnancy is not a contraindication to the use of immune serum globulin (192).

Due to the possibility of severe hypersensitivity reactions, the intravenous route should not be used. Discomfort may occur at the site of intramuscular injection.

Globulin with a high titer of hepatitis B antibody has been experimentally produced in small quantities (244). It appears that this product ("Hepatitis B Immune Globulin" or HBIG) can minimize symptoms or prevent infection entirely if given soon after exposure to the hepatitis B virus (92,97a,191,198). The protection lasts four months, but longer follow-up shows a rapid rise in the incidence of infection. The incidence of disease at 9 months post exposure in HBIG treated subjects is not different from that in subjects who did not receive HBIG (92). It is suggested that this may be due to a delayed onset of the disease, a second exposure to hepatitis B virus, or an interference with the development of long-lasting immunity.

The value of gamma globulin in preventing posttransfusion hepatitis (PTH), which can be caused by both hepatitis virus A and B, is being studied. In a well-controlled study, patients receiving blood transfusions were concomitantly given a 6% preparation of gamma globulin which had been specially made for intravenous use (122). There was a significant reduction in the incidence of PTH in the patients receiving the combination of blood and gamma globulin as compared to the controls who received blood without gamma globulin. Despite these promising results, currently available immune serum globulin is only effective for prophylactic use against viral hepatitis A.

CASE B: PRIMARY BILIARY CIRRHOSIS

J.K., a 50-year-old housewife, entered General Hospital complaining of severe and persistent itching, intractable insomnia, jaundice, pale stools and dark urine. Two years prior to admission she consulted a physician for a yellow growth on her upper eyelid, at which time a serum cholesterol of 505 mg/ 100 ml was noted. Physical examination disclosed a well nourished, jaundiced woman with extensive scratch marks, bruises, and scabs on her arms and back. Her liver was enlarged to four finger breadths below the right costal margin and the tip of her spleen was palpable. Laboratory evaluation disclosed an elevated serum bilirubin, alkaline phosphatase, cholesterol, and gamma globulin, and a liver biopsy was compatible with primary biliary cirrhosis. A two year history of pruritus has been unresponsive to hydrocortisone, antihistamines, sedatives, and topical antipruritic agents. Despite a happy family and social life the patient has considered suicide for relief of her itching.

10. What causes the pruritus associated with jaundice? What agents can be used to treat this symptom? Discuss their mechanisms of action, dose, administration and side effects.

The exact cause of the pruritus which accompanies obstructive liver disease is unknown, but it is currently believed to be due to high levels of bile acids in blood and tissues. Bile acids are the final products of cholesterol degradation. In man, the liver synthesizes only about 800 mg of bile acids per day; however, almost all the 25 grams of bile acids that are secreted each day into the biliary tree are reabsorbed from the small bowel (256).

Cholestyramine (Cuemid, Questran) is an insoluble quarternary ammonium anion exchange resin that disrupts biliary enterohepatic recycling by firmly binding bile acids in the bowel and holding them in an insoluble complex that is eliminated in the feces. Cholestyramine, therefore, relieves pruritus by reducing bile acid in the serum and ultimately, that deposited in dermal tissues. The resin is ineffective in patients with complete biliary obstruction because no bile reaches the intestines to be bound.

Cholestyramine is administered orally. The recommended adult dosage is one teaspoonful (about 4 grams) three or four times daily with meals. It should be mixed with fruit juices, soups, or applesauce because of its offensive pungent odor and should be allowed to stand in the selected vehicle for one or two minutes prior to stirring so that it will absorb moisture and disperse evenly. With these doses, the pruritus dramatically improves within one to three weeks (220,256); however, relief of itching has also occurred as early as 4-11 days (49).

Toxicity is negligible, although large doses may induce steatorrhea and hypoprothrombinemia. By increasing the fecal excretion of bile salts, cholestyramine interferes with fat absorption and, therefore, with the absorption of fat-soluble vitamins. Patients receiving long term resin therapy should receive water-soluble formulations of vitamin A, D, or K or IM injections of these vitamins. Gastrointestinal side effects including nausea, abdominal cramping, diarrhea or constipation are more common and occur in about 20% of treated patients. However, most patients are more than willing to tolerate these side effects which are minor when compared to the incessant pruritus.

Since cholestyramine is a binding resin, no oral medications should be given within one to two hours of cholestyramine administration to assure adequate absorption. Cholestyramine has been demonstrated to decrease serum levels of digitoxin and thyroid hormones significantly. Hansten (99) reports that at least six hours are necessary between doses of cholestyramine and warfarin to prevent decreased warfarin absorption.

Phenobarbital increases the liver's capacity to conjugate bilirubin. Originally, it was used to stimulate glucuronyl transferase in patients with Crigler-Najjar syndrome but it also effectively reduces high levels of unconjugated bilirubin due to Gilbert's syndrome, intrahepatic cholestasis (chronic obstructive jaundice), intrahepatic biliary atresia, benign recurrent cholestasis, primary biliary cirrhosis and hemolysis (250).

In addition to inducing the production of glucuronyl transferase, phenobarbital also increases the excretion and flow of bile salts (239) if the biliary ductal system is patent. Phenobarbital administration has been uniformly ineffective in reducing serum bilirubin levels in patients with extrahepatic biliary atresia (45,239).

The usual dose of phenobarbital is 100-200 mg per day. For hyperbilirubinemia of the newborn, the dose is 5-10 mg/kg of body weight. The drug does not cure the underlying disease but only alleviates a manifestation of that disease. Serum bilirubin can be decreased to 20-50% of pretreatment levels by phenobarbital and relief from pruritus occurs within 7 days (239).

Corticosteroids seem effective in lowering serum bilirubin levels in certain types of liver disease. Williams and Billing (264a) observed some benefit when prednisolone was administered to jaundiced patients with infectious hepatitis, obstructive jaundice, and decompensated cirrhosis. They were unable to define prednisolone's mechanism of action; however, they ruled out increased biliary excretion, increased renal excretion, and decreased red cell breakdown as the mechanism of the decreased hyperbilirubinemia. Glucocorticoids are not effective in lowering elevated serum bilirubins secondary to complete extrahepatic biliary obstruction.

11. What is chronic active hepatitis? Describe its course and prognosis.

Although the terminology is confusing and ambiguous, *chronic active hepatitis* is currently the most widely accepted term for a disease that has been variously called chronic liver disease in young women, plasma cell hepatitis, active juvenile cirrhosis, chronic liver disease in young people, progressive hepatitis, lupoid hepatitis, autoimmune hepatitis, and liver disease in young women with hyperglobulinemia.

This is a progressively chronic disease with sporadic flares of active disease which primarily affects the liver but also affects other organs and systems. It may occur at any age and in either sex; however, half of the patients are between the ages of ten and thirty and 70-80% are women. About one-third develop the disease in an abrupt fashion with clinical and laboratory features indistinguishable from acute infectious hepatitis; however, unlike acute infectious hepatitis it continues over several months until manifestations of chronic active hepatitis become apparent. In the remainder, the symptoms slowly develop over two to six months.

The clinical features of chronic active hepatitis are extremely variable and usually consist of some combination of the following: intermittent fatigue, weakness, weight loss, anorexia, fever of unknown origin, vague abdominal pains, arthralgias, and skin rashes. Hepatomegaly and splenomegaly are common, as are endocrine abnormalities such as amenorrhea, cushingoid facies, abdominal striae, and acne (164). Aspiration liver biopsy is the only reliable means of establishing this diagnosis.

Laboratory abnormalities observed in this disease include the following (71):

Laboratory Test	Value
Albumin	1-3.5 gm%
Anemia, thrombocytopenia, leukopenia	40-60% occurrence
Bilirubin	1-30 mg%
Gamma-globulin	1-4 gm%
Glutamic oxalacetic transaminase (SGOT)	40-500 Sigma units
Glutamic pyruvic transaminase (SGPT)	40-500 Sigma units
Hepatitis-associated antigen (HAA)	25% positive
LE cell test	10-20% positive
Smooth muscle antibody	65-85% positive
Antinuclear antibody (ANA)	often positive
Erythrocyte Sedimentation Rate (ESR)	often elevated

12. Are there any drugs which will alter the course and prognosis of chronic active hepatitis?

This form of hepatitis is exceptional in that its course and prognosis may be influenced favorably by drug treatment. Morbidity and mortality are decreased by corticosteroids and azathioprine. The six-year survival for untreated disease is about 55% (164). Treatment with azathioprine for six months decreases the mortality to 40%. However, the addition of prednisone or the use of prednisone alone produces an 80 percent remission after two years of treatment (234). Treatment is recommended for at least 18 months due to the high relapse rate.

Most often treatment begins with 60-100 mg/day of prednisolone or its equivalent (138). However, Cook and associates (40) reported that as little as 15 mg/day of prednisone impressively increased albumin synthesis, decreased bilirubin, decreased gamma globulin, and reduced mortality from 51.2% in the control group to 15.2% in the treated group. When combined with azathioprine, the maintenance dose of prednisone may be as low as 10 mg/day after initial doses of 30 mg/day are slowly tapered (243a). The dosage of azathioprine is 50-75 mg/day. Recently, human leukocyte interferon (93) and transfer-factor (248) have been tried in chronic active hepatitis without observable effect on the disease course.

13. Women with chronic active hepatitis occasionally become pregnant. What modifications and considerations should be made in treating a pregnant patient with this disease?

Whelton and Sherlock (261) reviewed the literature and described eight pregnant patients with chronic active hepatitis that progressed to cirrhosis. They concluded that the mother's welfare was of primary concern and consequently recommended treatment which differs very little from that recommended for non-pregnant individuals. The prognosis for the pregnant patient is the same as that for a non-pregnant woman with comparable disease. Fluid retention is treated with salt restriction, diuretics, and potassium supplementation and the need for folate supplementation is emphasized. The treatment of bleeding esophageal varices is generally unaltered; however, if vasopressin is considered, the drug's oxytocic activity should be kept in mind.

Many patients are receiving corticosteroids when pregnancy is diagnosed. This is usually well into the first trimester, the most dangerous time for the fetus with respect to corticosteroid teratogenesis. The benefits of therapy for the mother probably outweigh the low risk of congenital abnormality associated with corticosteroids. Since corticosteroid requirements increase in stress, parenteral supplementation should be given at the time of delivery if the mother has been taking chronic suppressive doses. The use of immunosuppressant drugs is reserved for patients with disease that is refractory to corticosteroids. Since the risks to the developing fetus are high, the decision to use these agents must be made on an individual basis.

14. A patient taking several drugs develops signs of liver dysfunction. What drugs can cause hepatic abnormalities? How can one establish the contribution of drugs to liver disease?

This question arises frequently. Although it can be answered superficially by consulting lists or tables, an adequate answer can be provided only by researching primary references which describe the hepatic disorder caused by each drug. When the type and time course of drug injury are characterized, an assessment can be made with regard to the drug's contribution to the case in question.

Table 1 lists drugs that have been reported to cause liver injury or dysfunction. For each entry there is at least one reference to a reported case. Whenever possible, the cited report is (a) the most recent description containing references to significant previous reports, or (b) comprehensive and representative of earlier and later briefer reports. Combination drugs are listed by constituents.

15. Characterize the signs, symptoms and course of drug-induced hepatitis. What is the most common mechanism by which drugs induce hepatitis?

Whenever a patient presents with hepatitis, a drug-induced etiology must be considered. Although a few drugs such as tetracycline or acetaminophen produce "toxic" reactions that are dose related and predictable, the most common mechanism of drug induced hepatitis is hypersensitivity. These drugs produce syndromes that are similar in six respects:

(1) They are not reproducible in animals.

(2) Only very few patients exposed to the drug will exhibit this syndrome.

(3) The lesions are not dose-related.

(4) The interval between exposure and onset of symptoms is variable and may range from one day to many months, with the most common interval being two to five weeks.

(5) Histologically, the hepatic lesions usually fall into categories of either hepatocellular injury or cholestasis, although strict differentiation is difficult.

(6) The lesions may be accompanied by extrahepatic signs of drug hypersensitivity (125).

The first clinical manifestations may be general signs of hypersensitivity, like fever, rash and pruritus which are often accompanied by the more common symptoms of hepatitis such as anorexia and nausea. Jaundice and bilirubinuria follow within a few days. Discontinuance of the offending drug will result in a

TABLE 1
DRUGS REPORTED TO CAUSE LIVER DYSFUNCTION

Acetaminophen (34)	Methimazole (80)
Acetohexamide (91)	Methotrexate (47)
Adriamycin (238)	Methoxyflurane (119)
Alcohol (143)	Methyldopa (30)
Allopurinol (232)	Methyltestosterone (54)
Aminosalicylic acid (233)	Mithramycin (196)
Amitriptyline (267)	Mitomycin (165)
Ampicillin (158)	Naproxen (135)
Aspirin (84,271)	Nicotinic acid (67)
Azathioprine (236)	Nitrofurantoin (90)
BCNU (55)	Norethandrolone (168)
Busulfan (253)	Norethindrone (179)
Cannabis (123)	Norethisterone (134,235)
Carbamazepine (194)	Norethynodrel (19)
Carbasone (193)	Novobiocin (43)
Carbenicillin (265)	Oral contraceptives (172)
Carbimazole (148)	Oxacillin (56)
Carisoprodol (125)	Oxymetholone (13)
Cephalexin (158)	Oxyphenbutazone (16)
Chlorambucil (130)	Oxytetracycline (58)
Chloramphenicol (100)	Papaverine (215)
Chlordiazepoxide (145)	Penicillin (255)
Chlorothiazide (113)	Perphenazine (41)
Chlorpromazine (20)	Phenacemide (140)
Chlorpropamide (200,207)	Phenazopyridine (89)
Chlortetracycline (58)	Phenelzine (108)
Chlorthalidone (125)	Phenindione (180)
Clindamycin (70)	Phenobarbital (176)
Conjugated estrogens (168)	Phenylbutazone (65)
Cyclophosphamide (8)	Phenytoin (182)
Dantrolene (173)	Probenecid (203)
Dapsone (163)	Procainamide (124)
Desipramine (188)	Prochlorperazine (160)
Diazepam (125)	Propoxyphene (48)
Disulfiram (68)	Propylthiouracil (74)
Ergotamine (262)	Pyrazinamide (166)
Erythromycin estolate (149)	Quinacrine (4)
Estradiol (254)	Quinethazone (114)
Ethionamide (39)	Quinidine (33)
Ferrous sulfate (150)	Rifampin (222)
Fluoxymesterone (168)	Sodium salicylate (61)
Fluroxene (204)	Sulfamethoxazole (62)
Guanoxan (82)	Sulfisoxazole (62)
Halothane (31)	Tetracycline (209)
Hycanthone (72)	Thioridazine (201)
Hydralazine (118)	Thiouracil (110)
Hydrochlorthiazide (260)	Tolbutamide (95)
Idoxuridine (52)	Tranylcypromine (24)
Imipramine (229)	Trifluoperazine (129)
Indomethacin (76)	Trimethadione (136)
Isoniazid (17)	Trimethobenzamide (21)
Meprobamate (125)	Tripelennamine (16)
Mercaptopurine (66)	Tromethamine (88)
Mestranol (19)	Vitamin A (167)

clearing of the general symptoms of hypersensitivity within a few days; however, hepatic dysfunction usually takes two to three weeks to resolve. Signs of hypersensitivity should encourage the search for a sensitizing agent. Although the reported incidence of hypersensitivity to individual drugs is usually very low, this etiology in suspected cases should not be ruled out casually.

When drugs produce hepatocellular damage, the results of liver function tests will usually mimic those seen in acute viral hepatitis. When cholestasis is present, the disease appears as if extrahepatic biliary obstruction is present, except for early elevations in serum transaminases. White blood cell counts are usually normal or only slightly elevated. Eosinophilia occurs but is not seen consistently. In cases where it may be important to establish a histologic diagnosis, liver biopsy is being used increasingly. Guidelines for interpretation of results from this procedure have been suggested (223).

16. How should a case of drug-induced hepatitis be treated?

Discontinuation of the suspected drug and appropriate supportive therapy as described in Question 6 may be all that is required. However, in severe cases the use of corticosteroids may be justified since death has occurred and some cases have been treated with apparent success (46,237).

Occasionally, the overall welfare of the patient dictates continued administration of the offending drug and in these instances the concomitant administration of corticosteroids may be warranted (125). It should be noted, however, that drug-induced hepatitis may resolve spontaneously despite continued use of the etiologic agent (224).

CASE C: DRUG-INDUCED HEPATITIS.

A 69-year-old man is hospitalized with complaints of malaise and fever of 102°F for two days, nausea, vomiting, jaundice, and a morbilliform pruritic rash over his entire body. His urine is dark yellow to brown and contains bile and urobilinogen. His stools are light and clay-colored. Four weeks prior to admission, he had a prostatectomy under halothane anesthesia and required two units of whole blood. No other complications occurred during the procedure. Three weeks prior to admission he was discharged with sulfamethoxazole (1 gm qid). Laboratory results include WBC 11,900 (Eos 28%), SGOT 85 IU/L, Bili T/D=12.7 mg%/8.5 mg%, Alk Phos 200 U.

17. What signs and/or symptoms are suggestive of hepatitis in this patient? Discuss how the etiology of this patient's hepatitis can be determined.

Malaise, fever, nausea, vomiting, jaundice, dark urine, light stools, hyperbilirubinemia suggest hepatitis.

There are three possible causes for this patient's hepatitis (halothane, blood transfusions and sulfamethoxazole), and steps must be taken to differentiate the role of each. Because the exposure to halothane occurred one month prior to the onset of symptoms, it can probably be excluded as a cause of

the hepatitis (see Question 18). The time between blood transfusion and onset of symptoms (30 days) most likely excludes viral hepatitis type B; however, viral hepatitis type A must still be considered. The generalized rash and eosinophilia suggest hypersensitivity, which is a common cause of drug-induced hepatitis. Sulfamethoxazole could be the offending agent and should be discontinued. Follow up: Within one week the patient was asymptomatic and abnormal liver and blood tests were also much improved (151).

CASE D: HALOTHANE HEPATITIS.

A 45-year-old woman underwent halothane anesthesia for a radical mastectomy. Three weeks later halothane was used during another surgery for a retinal detachment. Four days after the second surgery she became icteric and a diagnosis of halothane hepatitis was made.

18. Characterize halothane hepatitis. What is a reasonable exposure-free period between doses?

Halothane is a non-explosive inhalation anesthetic that is very useful when electrocauterizing must be done. It has been considered an extremely safe agent that provides precise, controllable, predictable, and uncomplicated anesthesia. The National Halothane Study representing 42 medical centers and 856,000 patients reported that on the basis of careful statistical analysis, the death rate following halothane anesthesia was lower than the death rate for all anesthetic practices combined. Thus, this agent continues to be widely used in spite of sporadic reports of halothane-induced hepatotoxicity (42).

The precise mechanism by which halothane produces hepatotoxicity is not known. Since halothane is a halogenated hydrocarbon, it may act as a true hepatotoxin, i.e., given in sufficient dose it will consistently produce human hepatotoxicity that can be reproduced in animals. Investigators have not confirmed this mechanism, although Hughes and Lang (112) have recently induced hepatic necrosis for the first time in a species other than man following repetitive halothane anesthesia. A second unsubstantiated hypothesis is that halothane unmasks or facilitates the development of viral hepatitis.

The most widely accepted postulate is that halothane hepatotoxicity represents a hypersensitivity phenomenon. It is difficult to determine whether halothane is a hepatotoxin or a sensitizing agent since there is nothing pathognomonic about the two types of hepatitis. Nevertheless, most authorities believe that halothane toxicity only occurs in sensitized individuals (1,29,32). The circumstantial evidence for sensitization lies in the postoperative findings of fever, myalgia, arthralgia, eosinophilia, rash, and jaundice in most halothane-affected patients. The increased risk of a second halothane exposure further suggests the probability of sensitization. In one study, one-half of 22 patients who had a second exposure to halothane developed signs and symptoms of hepatic damage (6).

Although there is a greater risk if the interval between exposures is brief, hepatitis has also occurred following re-exposure to halothane after an interval of several years. Because of medical-legal implications, some hospitals now insist on a three month period between repeated exposures to halothane (146). However, this arbitrary interval has been challenged by others (29).

To decrease the risk of halothane hepatotoxicity, a careful history should be obtained and past medical records reviewed to avoid administering halothane to patients with possible prior sensitization. Although an unexplained fever commonly occurs postoperatively (63), halothane should not be readministered to such patients if this fever was accompanied by eosinophilia, rash, arthralgia, abnormal liver function tests, or jaundice. Thus, a clinician's responsibility is to follow such parameters postoperatively in every surgical patient who receives halothane and to obtain the necessary base-line information (e.g. WBC count with differentials, liver function studies, and temperatures).

19. A patient taking erythromycin has developed abdominal distress of a more severe nature than is usually associated with the use of this antibiotic. How should this be interpreted?

Erythromycin base appears to be free of hepatotoxicity; however, the propionyl ester of erythromycin lauryl sulfate ("estolate") causes a rare allergic cholestatic hepatitis and jaundice. Although erythromycin is marketed as several salts in addition to the base, only the "estolate" has been associated with this hypersensitivity reaction. The first reports of this reaction appeared three years after the introduction of the drug (128,210); more cases were reported shortly thereafter (57,86,117,152,199,208,212). This activity continued until the existence of this hypersensitivity reaction was well established (28,73,97,162).

Gilbert (86) examined the molecular structure of erythromycin estolate and compared it to triacetyloleandomycin which also has caused cholestatic hepatitis (although oleandomycin phosphate does not). On the basis of the observation that the only compounds in the macrolide antibiotic group that have been reported to cause allergic cholestatic hepatitis have a specific analogous hydroxyl group replaced by an ester, he postulated that esterification at this molecular position may confer the properties of a hapten on the macrolide antibiotic.

Because this reaction is one of allergic hypersensitivity, any number of symptoms could appear. Nevertheless, epigastric or right upper quadrant tenderness and pain, fever, vomiting, anorexia, pruritus, dark urine, and light-colored stools are common. Other reported symptoms include dyspnea, heartburn, disturbances in color vision, vertigo, continuous headache, generalized myalgia, erythematous rash on the trunk and constipation.

The reaction is usually accompanied by other indicators of hepatic dysfunction: an elevated transaminase, alkaline phosphatase, bilirubin (particularly the direct fraction) and erythrocyte sedimentation rate. Eosinophilia may be absent, moderate, or marked and the prothrombin time may be slightly increased.

Other laboratory tests may aid the differential diagnosis by their normal values. The serum amylase should be within normal limits, thus tentatively excluding pancreatitis and cholecystogram should be normal, ruling out cholecystitis. However, in two cases the gall bladder was reported not to have been visualized on x-ray examination and this was attributed to the failure of the liver to excrete the contrast material (78).

A history of hypersensitivity to drugs and other allergens has been associated with several of the reported cases. The most valuable test for final diagnosis is rechallenge of the patient with the suspected agent and this has been done, purposely or inadvertently, in many reports (211).

As with any drug hypersensitivity reaction, immediate treatment begins with the discontinuance of the drug. Analgesics may be given for severe pain. Of the narcotic analgesics, meperidine is a common choice due to the unsupported theory that it causes less severe spasms of the sphincter of Oddi than do other narcotic analgesics. Corticosteroids have been used for their anti-inflammatory action; however, there are no controlled studies which establish their value.

Abnormalities of liver function generally disappear shortly after the drug is discontinued. However, one patient still showed evidence of hepatic dysfunction and hepatomegaly six months after the onset of the reaction (101).

A more detailed review of the literature regarding this entire subject has been provided by Braun (25).

Recently, interest in this specific drug hypersensitivity has been revived by reports of erythromycin estolate-induced abdominal pain occurring both with and without jaundice. The authors suggest the incidence of this reaction is greater than previously suspected (121,174,214). Since other erythromycin products do not cause such problems, the estolate salt of erythromycin (Ilosone) should be avoided.

20. If a patient experiences hepatotoxic reaction to a drug, must all chemically related drugs be avoided

in that patient for fear of cross-reaction with the hepatotoxin?

The administration of a drug to a patient who has a history of a hepatotoxic reaction to a drug with similar chemical structure is a thorny problem since there has been little investigation in this area. However, there are a few reports of such instances.

Several case reports indicate that there may be no cross-sensitivity among *penicillins* with regard to their hepatotoxic effect. Liver enzyme elevations in four patients receiving carbenicillin decreased when carbenicillin was replaced with penicillin G, ampicillin, methicillin, nafcillin, or cloxacillin. Only one of the above patients exhibited generalized signs of hypersensitivity to carbenicillin and these signs continued during therapy with penicillin G and nafcillin in spite of improving liver function tests. Rechallenge with lower doses of carbenicillin resulted in signs of hepatic dysfunction (265). One case of oxacillin hepatitis resolved during continued penicillin G therapy; another case showed no hepatic cross-sensitivity between oxacillin and cephalothin (56).

Sulfamethoxazole is a commonly used sulfonamide with a history of causing hepatotoxic reactions (62). In one instance of drug-induced hepatitis, inadvertent treatment with sulfisoxazole (81) resulted in a return of hepatitic symptoms and signs within 30 hours.

Two patients with *chlorpropamide* hepatotoxicity did well when switched to *tolbutamide* (98). Interestingly, the patients had no adverse reaction when later switched back to chlorpropamide. Another patient had no adverse reaction when switched to tolbutamide, but nausea and vomiting recurred when another trial of chlorpropamide was begun (98). One case of chlorpropamide jaundice occurred in a patient who previously used tolbutamide without this problem and who later reacted to chlorpropamide rechallenge (200). While tolbutamide seems to cause liver damage less frequently than other sulfonylureas, its substitution in the chlorpropamide-sensitive patient is not without risk. One patient who developed jaundice from chlorpropamide again became jaundiced when he was subsequently given tolbutamide (35).

Phenothiazines have long been considered to be cross-reactive with chemically-related drugs. Chlorpromazine induced jaundice recurred in two patients switched to thioridazine (201); however, only one of five chlorpromazine sensitive patients reacted to promazine challenge (109). Reports of antipsychotic drug-induced jaundice rarely specify how the psychosis was subsequently managed. It is, therefore, difficult to determine the incidence of hepatic cross-reactivity for these drugs.

Two *tricyclic antidepressants* appeared to cross-react in a patient. When desipramine was substituted for imipramine in a patient who was allergic to the latter drug, the rash worsened and terminated in hepatic necrosis (188). This is not surprising considering that desipramine is a metabolic product of imipramine.

Phenindione is an indandione-derived *anticoagulant* used primarily in Europe. Two cases of "phenindione hepatitis" have been reported in which signs of hepatic dysfunction and systemic hypersensitivity persisted for weeks after the drug was replaced by nicoumalone, another anticoagulant (185). The time courses of administration of these two drugs is unclear so that it is impossible to determine whether the patients' adverse reactions to phenindione were sustained by the presence of nicoumalone. If this could be documented, it would be an example of cross-sensitivity between chemically-unrelated compounds; nicoumalone is a derivative of hydroxycoumarin. In another case, phenindione-induced fever, rash and jaundice persisted for five days after ethyl biscoumacetate therapy was substituted. The latter drug was discontinued and the symptoms subsided six days later (64). Cross-reactivity between drugs of different anticoagulant classes has not been observed for non-hepatic sensitivity reactions (14).

Halothane hepatitis has been discussed in Question 18. Methoxyflurane is a similar halogenated hydrocarbon that also causes hepatitis and there appears to be both clinical and laboratory evidence for cross-reactivity between these *anesthetics* in patients sensitive to one of them. Two patients with a history of halothane hepatitis developed hepatitis after receiving methoxyflurane (120,144). Lymphocytes from two of three patients with a history of halothane hepatitis were stimulated in the presence of methoxyflurane (178). This is also evidence for cross-sensitivity between these two agents. Fluroxene is also a halogenated volatile anesthetic; however, it is theorized that this agent will cross-react in patients sensitive to halothane or methoxyflurane because it is chemically stable (31).

When *oral contraceptives* cause hepatic dysfunction, alternative contraceptive methods should be used. Due to their effectiveness and convenience, however, the patient may still prefer to use these agents. Both the presence and absence of cross-reactivity between these agents have been reported. A patient who developed jaundice twice on a combination containing norethindrone 2 mg and mestranol 0.1 mg (Ortho-Novum 2 mg) tolerated a pill containing chlormadinone 2 mg and mestranol 0.08 mg (C-Quens) without ill effects (219). A similar patient who was jaundiced during three pregnancies and two trials of Ortho-Novum 2 mg, was symptom free while taking chlormadinone acetate 0.5 mg daily (247). Adlercreutz and Ikonen described a woman who suffered pruritus during pregnancy and jaundice during norethynodrel 5 mg and mestranol 0.075 mg (Conovid, Enovid) therapy. Two years later the same patient started taking lynestrenol 2.5 mg and mestranol 0.075 mg (Lyndiol 2.5) and developed migraine, vomiting and right costal margin pain. She received lynestrenol alone for 60 days without symptoms; however, when she was again given Lyndiol 2.5, the pain and vomiting returned (3). Another patient who became jaundiced while taking norethynodrel 5 mg and mestranol 0.75 mg (Enovid), developed no symptoms when rechallenged with norethynodrel 10 mg alone. When she was given mestranol 0.16 mg, she developed pruritus and an increased BSP retention; estradiol 0.16 mg produced only the latter (254). In summary, while the progestins contained in the oral contraceptives have occasionally caused hepatic symptoms when used alone (134,179), estrogens appear to be more potent hepatotoxins (60). In a patient whose liver is seriously affected by combination oral contraceptives, progestin-only contraception may be the solution. (See also chapter on Oral Contraception.)

21. What is toxic hepatitis? Describe the usual clinical picture and differentiate this entity from drug-induced hepatitis due to hypersensitivity.

Toxic hepatitis may be caused by any of several mechanisms including altered protein synthesis and cellular energy production, impaired hepatic blood flow, or altered lipid metabolism. Agents that are toxic to liver cells may also damage other organ tissue, and the latter may be more important in the overall clinical picture. Symptoms are similar to those of viral hepatitis without the preicteric fever. Anorexia, nausea, and vomiting are seen most often; jaundice and hepatomegaly are usually apparent. The convalescent period is generally shorter for toxic hepatitis.

Certain features distinguish toxic hepatitis from drug-induced hepatitis due to hypersensitivity. The lesions can be reproduced in experimental animals; they occur in *all subjects* administered the chemical; the liver damage is *related to dose;* the appearance of the syndrome usually occurs in a predictable length of time after exposure; and each hepatotoxin causes a characteristic, reproducible histologic lesion (125).

CASE E: ASPIRIN HEPATOTOXICITY.

J.H., a 25-year-old white woman with a history of systemic lupus erythematosus (SLE) was admitted to General Hospital for evaluation of increasing fatigue, weight loss, anorexia, vague abdominal discomfort, and tinnitus. One month prior to admission a diagnosis of SLE was made when she developed diffuse migratory polyarthritis, fever, prostration, generalized lymphadenopathy and a symmetrical malar erythema. Laboratory workup at that time included a positive LE cell test, ANA, and Coomb's test without the presence of hemolytic anemia, a hypergammaglobulinemia and decreased serum complements. Other laboratory results were within normal limits and no organ involvement was noted. The patient had given birth to her first child six weeks prior to the onset of symptoms. Substantial clinical improvement occurred when she was treated with aspirin 4.8 grams daily.

Physical examination was unremarkable except for marked tenderness in her right upper quadrant. Laboratory tests disclosed SGOT and SGPT levels of 540 and 465 units respectively; thymol turbidity was elevated and BSP retention was 32%. Creatine phosphokinase (CPK), alkaline phosphatase, bilirubin and prothrombin times were WNL, and the serum salicylate level was 40 mg/100ml. A diagnosis of chronic active (lupoid) hepatitis is being considered. The medical staff are awaiting the results of the smooth muscle antibody test and the pathology report on the liver biopsy. Aspirin is discontinued because of her tinnitus and prednisone 20 mg/day is instituted.

22. Whenever a patient presents with abnormal liver function tests, drug-induced hepatic disease must always be considered. The only drug J.H. was taking at the onset of symptoms was aspirin. Has aspirin been implicated as a hepatotoxic agent? Assess the possible etiologies of this patient's hepatitis.

In a case such as this, clinicians might attribute the liver dysfunction to a progressive disease process since mild hepatomegaly has been associated with SLE. In actual clinical practice, however, SLE-induced hepatic dysfunction is extremely uncommon (251).

A hepatitis associated antigen test (HAA) should be ordered, because J.H. might have had a blood transfusion during her pregnancy approximately 2½ months ago. This time span falls within the usual 60-180 day incubation period for viral hepatitis, type B. Should this test be negative, there still exists the possibility of coincidental viral hepatitis, type A. J.H.'s clinical and laboratory evaluations are also compatible with chronic active hepatitis, because extrahepatic manifestations commonly occur before the actual appearance of liver dysfunction. The liver biopsy and the smooth muscle antibody test may be able to confirm this later diagnosis. It should be noted, however, that Seaman and associates (225) documented a case of aspirin-induced hepatoxicity in an SLE patient with a liver biopsy compatible with chronic active hepatitis. Other hepatic diseases should also be ruled out.

Recent reports demonstrate unequivocally that hepatocellular injury occurs in patients with high salicylate blood levels. Thirteen of 23 children convalescing from rheumatic fever demonstrated elevations of SGOT and SGPT when treated with high doses of aspirin or sodium salicylate (153). Also, salicylates induced hepatoxicity in six patients with juvenile rheumatoid arthritis when salicylate serum levels exceeded 25 mg/100ml. All six of these patients had elevated SGOT and SGPT and four of these six had other evidence of liver dysfunction. In two patients, liver biopsies revealed mononuclear cell infiltration of the portal triads, and in one patient scattered single cell parenchymal necrosis was observed (205).

Russell and associates (218) noted transient SGOT elevations in 8 of their 32 juvenile rheumatoid arthritic patients treated with salicylates.

In two separate reports involving four SLE patients, aspirin apparently induced hepatocellular injury that was clearly dose related (225,266). When aspirin therapy was discontinued, liver function tests (LFT's) returned to normal within five to ten days. Subsequent rechallenge with aspirin resulted in liver function abnormalities when serum salicylate levels higher than 25 mg/100ml were achieved. In all cases, salicylate hepatotoxicity occurred in patients with salicylate serum levels ranging from 18-45 mg/100ml. The fact that this effect is dose related and may occur in 50% of such patients implies that the salicylates are true hepatotoxins. Moreover, similar hepatocellular injury has been reproduced in rabbits given high doses of salicylates (270).

The hepatic injury is clearly hepatocellular in nature. Liver biopsies have demonstrated parenchymal injury, including necrosis, extra- and intracellular acidophilic bodies, ballooning of hepatocytes, and degenerative changes.

In conclusion, aspirin-induced hepatotoxicity is dose related, reversible, reproducible in animals, and requires a certain duration of administration (acute aspirin poisonings generally do not cause hepatocellular injury). This duration of therapy, however, need not be prolonged. Rich and Johnson (205) noted serum transaminase elevations within 6 to 32 days after initiation of therapy. The 50% incidence of ASA-hepatoxicity (270) seems somewhat unrealistic considering the large number of patients who are treated with doses of salicylates which produce serum levels of 20 mg% or more. Clearly more studies are needed to place this drug-induced disease into proper perspective.

In this particular case, liver function tests (LFT's) should be followed. Once they have returned to normal, it may be important from both a diagnostic and treatment point of view, to rechallenge her with aspirin, while continually monitoring both serum salicylate levels and LFT's. Since J.H. responded so well to aspirin therapy in the past, another trial should be considered if the aspirin challenge test is negative. This is also rational because aspirin is a safer drug than corticosteroids and because the liver dysfunction it produces is rapidly reversible. It should be noted, however, that Athreya and co-workers (7) reported a single case of aspirin-induced liver dysfunction that persisted for more than 60 days after aspirin therapy was discontinued in a ten-year-old black girl with rheumatoid arthritis and sickle thalassemia.

23. A 38-year-old woman with a history of chronic alcoholism is admitted to General Hospital with a three day history of anorexia, nausea, vomiting, weakness, weight loss, abdominal pain, diarrhea, and fever. Physical examination reveals hepatosplenomegaly, ascites, and spider angiomas. Clinically, she appears severely ill and presents with some signs of hepatic precoma. How should alcoholic liver disease be managed? Should corticosteroids be used in a patient with suspected alcohol-induced toxic hepatitis?

Alcoholic hepatitis is considered a "toxic hepatitis" because it is preceded by chronic toxin exposure and subclinical liver changes. Its pathogenesis, clinical features, prognosis, and therapy are controversial.

The therapy of severe alcoholic hepatitis is similar to that recommended for viral hepatitis: a high protein (except where coma is an immediate risk) high carbohydrate caloric diet, and bedrest followed by advancement of physical activity as tolerated. Patients should definitely abstain from ethanol. Because malnutrition due to dietary neglect is often seen in alcoholism, vitamin supplementation is recommended for many of these patients.

While corticosteroids have been widely used in such patients, only three controlled trials have been completed, and results are conflicting (37,105,186). Helman and associates (105) studied 37 patients with alcoholic hepatitis. The clinical course of those treated with prednisone was not significantly different from that of a placebo group. Prednisolone treated patients with severe disease (see citation for criteria), however, had a higher survival rate than placebo-treated patients. In no case could any effect of prednisolone be demonstrated histologically. It appears from this study that corticosteroid therapy is of value to the patient in pre-coma or early hepatic coma; however, its use carries an unjustifiable risk in the moderately or mildly ill alcoholic hepatitis patient whose prognosis is generally good.

Porter and co-workers (186) reached somewhat different conclusions even though their 20 patients were more severely ill than those studied by Helman et al (105). Although the group receiving parenteral 6-methylprednisolone 40 mg/day exhibited a two-fold increase in survival rate as compared to the untreated group, the differences were not statistically significant. This may have been due to the small number of patients evaluated.

Twenty of 45 severe acute alcoholic hepatitis patients received prednisone 0.5 mg/kg/day for three weeks, then 0.25 mg/kg/day for three additional weeks; twenty-five served as untreated controls. Nine of 25 (36%) controls and 7 of 20 (35%) prednisone-treated persons died. No differences were found between the treated and control groups with respect to the duration of hospitalization, rate of improvement in serum bilirubin, SGOT, and prothrombin time; or clinical presentation (37). In conclusion, the effectiveness of corticosteroids in the treatment of alcoholic hepatitis still needs further evaluation. A national cooperative study has been called for in editorials (50,137).

24. How may liver dysfunction alter a patient's response to drugs?

Metabolism by the liver is the major route of elimination for many drugs. However, unlike renal function, it is difficult to quantitate liver failure in that the degree of functional impairment may not proportionally affect drug disposition. Moreover, many attendant diseases may accentuate or compensate for a diseased liver's metabolic restriction. A simple example will illustrate the complexity of this problem. In a patient with acute viral hepatitis, liver enzyme blood levels may indicate substantial hepatic damage, and maximum functional capacity may actually be depressed. However, an increase in hepatic blood flow, sometimes seen in hepatitis (147), may compensate for decreased function producing no net change in the absolute amount of drug metabolized or the serum half-life for the drug. The other extreme of this example is the situation of far advanced liver disease when hepatic enzyme blood levels may be normal or even low. The diminished hepatic function combined with shunting of hepatic blood flow may severely compromise drug metabolism. The decreased rate of metabolism could be partially offset by decreased albumin production by the liver since hypoalbuminemia may increase the fraction of free drug in the blood. Many of the pathologic factors involved and the difficulties in collecting useful data have recently been reviewed (264).

25. In spite of methodological and interpretative problems, results from studies of drug pharmacokinetics in liver disease may be useful if employed cautiously. However, the serum half-lives are only of importance for drugs extensively eliminated by the liver. List and discuss those drugs which have been studied.

ANALGESICS

In patients with chronic liver diseases, the half-life of oral *acetaminophen* is increased from 2 hours to an average of 3.3 hours. There is a correlation between half-life and serum albumin levels and prothrombin ratios. There is no correlation between half-life and transaminase, alkaline phosphatase or bilirubin levels (77). In the hepatic necrosis resulting from acetaminophen overdosage, the half-life is also prolonged (190).

The half-life of *meperidine* is doubled in patients with acute viral hepatitis (6.99 hours vs. 3.37 hours) (161) and cirrhosis (7.04 hours vs. 3.21 hours) (127). No correlation between plasma half-life and liver function tests could be established in either of these studies.

ANTIBIOTICS

The elimination half-life of intravenous carbenicillin is doubled (1.9 hours vs. 1.0 hour) in patients with varying degrees of hepatic dysfunction (107). Renal impairment and the reduced creatinine clearance that can accompany hepatic disease contributed to the prolongation of carbenicillin half-life observed in four patients (107).

The calculated biologic half-life of *nafcillin* in a cirrhotic patient was 1.4 hours; a similar patient without hepatic disease had a nafcillin half-life of 1.0 hours (171).

The elimination of intravenous *chloramphenicol* has been reported to be decreased (10,133) and unchanged (104) in the presence of hepatic impairment. A prolonged half-life appears to correlate with hypoalbuminemia and hyperbilirubinemia (10). Diminished drug metabolism and low serum albumin levels elevate serum levels of free chloramphenicol thereby increasing the risk of bone marrow depression (242,243).

Clindamycin pharmacokinetics are moderately altered in patients with stable alcoholic cirrhosis. A 31% prolongation of the half-life (from 3.42 hrs. to 4.46 hrs.) correlated well with serum bilirubin and SGOT concentrations (9). In patients with severe liver disease, the prolongation of clindamycin's half-life may be more dramatic. An average half-life of 6.4 hours was observed in ten patients with acute hepatitis or cirrhosis (23). However, in a conflicting report, patients with acute and chronic hepatitis and cirrhosis given single and multiple intravenous doses of clindamycin, showed only a slight increase in half-life, but no dramatic accumulation of drug or exacerbation of hepatitis (106).

Antitubercular drug kinetics may be altered by liver disease. The half-life of isoniazid is prolonged in patients with chronic liver disease (2,139). *Rifampin,* too, has an extended half-life in patients with liver disease (2,189), but its combination with isoniazid does not appear to further prolong the half-life of either drug (2). *Aminosalicylic acid* may not be affected by liver disease (104). See Tuberculosis chapter regarding the hepatotoxicity of these agents.

The antibiotic combination of *trimethoprim-sulfamethoxazole* has been studied in patients with both minor and severe hepatic damage (206). There was a wide variation in trimethoprim half-lives in the patients with severe liver disease, but the average trimethoprim half-life was not significantly different from normals or patients with mild liver disease. Sulfamethoxazole seemed to be handled normally in all patients.

ANTIINFLAMMATORY AGENTS

Despite the fact that the liver is a major site of conversion of cortisone to hydrocortisone, the half-life of *cortisone* was normal in three patients with hepatic cirrhosis; however, the half-life of *hydrocortisone* was three times normal (320 minutes v. 98 minutes) (181).

A knowledge of *prednisone* and *prednisolone* kinetics in liver disease is important because these drugs may be used to treat chronic active liver disease. Active liver disease seems to impair the metabolism of prednisone to active prednisolone and slows the elimination of prednisolone (187). In addition, low serum albumin levels correlate with high levels of unbound or free prednisolone. While this may increase drug activity in patients with liver disease, it may also increase the incidence of side effects (141). Other groups have observed a delay in the conversion of prednisone to prednisolone (51) and insignificant alterations in the kinetics of these drugs (221) in patients with liver diseases.

The elimination half-life of *phenylbutazone* does not appear to be affected by liver disease (115,259). However, other investigators point out that concurrent or pre-treatment with other drugs may stimulate phenylbutazone metabolism and obscure the effects of liver disease (139). Levi and associates only observed a prolonged half-life in these patients when no other drugs were given (139). *Oxyphenbutazone* kinetics may not be affected by liver disease (115).

In patients with halothane jaundice, chronic hepatitis, and hepatic cirrhosis, an increase in the peak plasma concentrations and a decrease in the half-life of intravenous *colchicine* were observed (258). The high peak level was attributed to a diminished apparent volume of distribution. As a result, it was suggested that more free colchicine was presented to the kidney for excretion thereby decreasing the half-life of the drug.

ANTICONVULSANTS

Since the plasma binding of *phenytoin* decreases in patients with liver disease (111), more free drug should be available for elimination. However, the half-life and clearance of phenytoin appear to be unchanged in patients with acute hepatitis (18). A possible explanation is that the increased amount of drug available for extraction is offset by a diminished extraction capacity of the liver. (See phenobarbital discussion below).

CARDIAC AGENTS

The elimination of a single intravenous dose of *digitoxin* in patients with chronic active hepatitis, was enhanced when compared to normal subjects (241); the half-life of digitoxin was about one-half (4.4 days) of that seen in normals (8.1 days). Changes in hepatic metabolism, biliary secretion and enterohepatic circulation were suggested as possible explanations. There was no evidence of impaired clearance when a single intravenous dose of *digoxin* was given to patients with alcoholic cirrhosis (one patient in hepatic precoma) (154). Multiple intravenous doses of digoxin produced normal plasma digoxin levels without toxic accumulation in patients with acute hepatitis (269). *Methyldigoxin,* on the other hand, accumulates in patients with hepatitis, suggesting that hepatic demethylation pathways are impaired (269). It should be emphasized that some patients with severe liver disease may still be predisposed to the toxic effects of digitalis because of decreased serum potassium levels and other physiologic changes.

The half-life of *lidocaine* is prolonged (77,246) and the urinary excretion is increased (77) in patients with liver disease. Half-life has (77) and has not been (246) correlated with serum albumin and prothrombin ratios.

Propranolol is very efficiently metabolized by the liver, and hepatic dysfunction increases the half-life and volume of distribution and decreases the clearance of this drug (22). This effect is in addition to the decreased clearance caused by the drug's beta-adrenergic blocking effect on hepatic blood flow.

SEDATIVE-HYPNOTICS

Barbiturate derivatives are often avoided in patients with liver disease because it is assumed that their kinetics are altered. Intravenous *amobarbital* was handled abnormally by patients with various forms of chronic liver disease whose serum albumin levels were less than 3.5 gm% (156). The average half-life was 39.4 hours in these patients compared with 21.1 hours in the controls and 17.7 hours in patients with liver disease and serum albumin levels above 3.5 gm%. The rate of amobarbital metabolism correlated with the patients' degree of Bromsulphalein retention, but not with other liver function tests. The clinical effect of the single intravenous dose of amobarbital was similar in patients with impaired and normal drug metabolism.

Intravenous *hexobarbital* given to patients with acute hepatitis (27) resulted in almost double the control half-life (490 minutes v. 261 minutes). After recovery from hepatitis, as judged by normalization of laboratory data, the hexobarbital half-life decreased, but was still elevated with respect to the normal values.

Pentobarbital kinetics were shown in early studies not to change with liver disease (104,226), but a recent report suggests that pentobarbital metabolism is decreased in patients with cirrhosis (175).

Phenobarbital plasma half-life is prolonged in patients with hepatitis, and even more so in patients with cirrhosis. This effect may be partially modified by an increased renal excretion of unchanged phenobarbital (5).

Diazepam and related benzodiazepines have been considered safe for use in patients with liver disease until recently. Klotz and co-workers found that the half-life of diazepam was doubled in patients with alcoholic cirrhosis, acute viral hepatitis, and chronic active hepatitis, probably as a result of impairment of hepatic demethylation (126). They found no correlation between diazepam half-life and any liver function tests. (See also chapter on General Care: Anxiety and Insomnia.)

Oxazepam is an active metabolite of diazepam and is glucuronidated before excretion. Since oxazepam elimination is normal in patients with acute viral hepatitis and cirrhosis (230), it may be a safer drug to use in patients with hepatic disease.

The plasma half-life of *meprobamate* is prolonged in patients with cirrhosis and chronic hepatitis to 24.3 hours (normal 12.6 hours) (102). Pre-treatment with phenobarbital for ten days did not alter these results.

MISCELLANEOUS DRUGS

The pharmacokinetics of *doxorubicin* are significantly altered by liver disease. Plasma levels of the drug and its metabolites are several times that of normal in patients with hepatic impairment. Toxicity and drug-related death are more frequent in liver diseased patients who receive normal doses. When the dose is reduced by 50-75% in these patients, the plasma Adriamycin levels are similar to those seen in patients without liver disease taking normal doses (11).

Chlorpromazine metabolism is normal in cirrhotic patients, and the clinical effects of the drug are comparable in normal and diseased patients (157). An earlier report had shown normal chlorpromazine plasma clearance, but greater than normal electroencephalographic changes and patient drowsiness in patients with hepatic cirrhosis (195).

Disulfiram is used to treat ethanol abusers, who may often have liver dysfunction. Recovery of excreted radioactive disulfiram from the breath, urine and feces is about the same in patients with alcoholic hepatitis or mild cirrhosis as from normal subjects. Thus it was concluded that the absorption and rate of metabolism are normal in patients with liver disease (228).

When *theophylline* (as aminophylline) was infused into four patients with cirrhosis (183), the biologic half-life increased from 9.19 hours to 30.0 hours. Theophylline doses should be decreased in cirrhotics to avoid toxic theophylline accumulation. For further discussion, see chapter on Asthma.

The results of studies on the influence of liver disease on *tolbutamide* kinetics are confusing and conflicting. The half-life of this drug in patients with liver disease has been reported to be unchanged (170), decreased (103) and prolonged (104,252).

CASE F: HEPATIC ENCEPHALOPATHY.

R.H., a 25-year-old female was admitted with a one month history of easy fatigability, anorexia, forgetfulness, and confusion. On physical examination the patient was markedly jaundiced and cachetic. Mild palmar erythema and several telangiectasias on the chest and face were observed; there were spider angiomas on the upper chest. The lungs were clear. The heart was enlarged and there was a harsh grade 3 systolic murmur along the lower left sternal border. The abdomen was markedly distended with a palpable fluid wave. Neurological examination was negative.

The urine was dark brown in color and gave a 3+ test for bile; the sediment contained a few bile-stained white cells. The hematocrit was 40.7%, WBC count was 7500, with 74% neutrophils, 7% bands, 9% monocytes, and 1% basophils. The prothrombin time was 44.2 seconds with a control of 13 seconds; the partial thromboplastin time (PTT) was greater than 80 seconds. A stool specimen produced a 4+ guiac test. The BUN was 6 mg%, glucose 56 mg%, conjugated bilirubin was 5.2 mg%, the total bilirubin was 9.9 mg% and the protein was 6.0 gm%. The serum sodium was 138 mEq/L, and the potassium 3.5 mEq/L. The SGOT was 3900 IU, alkaline phosphatase 200 U, serum creatinine 1.8 mg% and urine cultures were negative. A test for hepatitis-associated antigen (HAA) was positive by counter electrophoresis and by radioimmunoassay. A liver biopsy was advised, but the patient refused to grant permission.

On the fourth hospital day, a gastric aspirate was 3+ for occult blood, the arterial ammonia was 110 mg/100 ml, the hematocrit was 39.5%, and the SGOT was 2400 units. The 24 hour urinary volume was 2500 ml while on furosemide (Lasix) 120 mg/day and spironolactone (Aldactone) 100 mg/day. As the day progressed, the patient became increasingly somnolent, exhibited impaired intellectual function, asterixis, and continued marked ascites despite a 15 lb (7Kg.) weight loss since the day of admission.

26. This patient exhibits palmar erythema, spider angiomas, and asterixis. What do these signs indicate?

Palmar erythema involves an intense diffuse flushing of the skin over the hypothenar eminence (the "meaty" part of the palm opposite from the thumb) and is usually less intense on the thenar prominence (the "meaty" part of the palm at the base of the thumb) and the distal digits of the fingers. Palmar erythema is usually seen in diseases involving the liver, but it may also appear in pregnancy.

Spider angiomas are fiery red vascular figures in the skin consisting of a central point from which superficial arterioles radiate, giving the total appearance of a spider's legs. When pressure is applied to that central point (e.g. with a pencil tip) the radicles blanch and fill centrifugally when the pressure is released. The cause of arterial spiders is not known. While spiders may occur in a variety of diseases they are most commonly associated with pregnancy and diseases of the liver. In both of these conditions spiders are commonly accompanied by palmar erythema.

Asterixis (flapping tremor of the hands) describes the phenomenon of jerky alternations of extension and flexion at the wrists and joints of fingers when patients extend their arms 90° from their body with the hands open and palms upright as if pushing against a wall. This flapping tremor is most commonly seen in impending hepatic coma, uremia, or cerebral vascular disease (53).

27. Why is this patient's blood glucose level decreased?

Hypoglycemia may be the consequence of the severe liver damage. Felig and associates (75) noted that plasma glucose levels below 60 mg/100 ml occurred in 8 of 15 consecutive patients with acute viral hepatitis. Apparently these patients have reduced liver glycogen stores and have a decreased capacity for hepatic gluconeogenesis since the plasma glucose response to glucagon was only one-third that of normal controls.

On the other hand, it should be noted that potassium depletion in cirrhotic patients, whether caused by diuretics used to treat the ascites, vomiting, diarrhea, or secondary hyperaldosteronism, can be associated with a diabetic-like glucose tolerance curve. Hypokalemia in these patients decreases the output of insulin and growth hormone. These abnormalities reverse with potassium repletion. Thus, cirrhotics may also exhibit hyperglycemia (184).

28. What might account for the falling SGOT at a time when the patient appears to be more clinically ill? What other laboratory findings are worth noting at this time?

Since this patient appears more ill clinically, one would have to postulate that the decreasing SGOT most likely represents a depletion of liver transaminase rather than an improvement in her disease state (32).

The finding of occult blood in the gastric aspirate indicates mild bleeding into the gastrointestinal tract. This is especially ominous since blood liberates much more ammonia and induces a greater toxicity per gram of protein than does meat or milk (38).

In a bleeding patient one would expect to see a rise in BUN. But in this patient, the liver damage has progressed to the point that it is unable to convert ammonia to urea adequately. Thus, the BUN is low despite a creatinine of 1.8%.

The patient was wise to refuse the liver biopsy considering that her prothrombin time is 44.2 seconds.

29. What is the pathogenesis of hepatic coma?

Hepatic encephalopathy or coma is defined as a disorder of consciousness occurring in patients with advanced liver disease or portal systemic shunting. It is characterized by intellectual deterioration, mental confusion, disturbances of awareness, fluctuating neurological signs and distinctive electroencephalographic changes. The manifestations of this metabolic disorder vary in intensity and are entirely reversible. The brain does not show pathological changes that would account for these symptoms (268).

Rational therapy of hepatic encephalopathy requires an understanding of its pathogenesis. Undoubtedly, toxic substances other than ammonia are involved in the genesis of hepatic coma; however, in the large majority of cases the symptoms are, in fact, related directly or indirectly to ammonia intoxication (38).

30. What is the standard therapy of hepatic coma? How should this particular patient be handled?

Although this patient represents a classical case of hepatic encephalopathy, other complications common to patients with advanced hepatic disease should be ruled out. These include a subdural hematoma, central nervous system trauma, hypoglycemia, sepsis, drug intoxication, or electrolyte imbalance. Treatment of hepatic coma should be prompt because once profound coma appears, patients generally respond less well to therapeutic maneuvers.

Attempts should be made to stop the gastric bleeding since the absorption of blood from the gastrointestinal tract is a major source of ammonia. Gastric cooling by ice water lavage may temporarily decrease her gastric oozing. Balloon tamponade or vasopressin are not indicated since her bleeding is not yet severe enough to warrant those measures. Vitamin K₁ (phytonadione) should be administered in a parenteral dose of approximately 30 mg in an attempt to generate hepatic clotting factors; however, this patient's liver may be unable to respond. A few units of fresh frozen plasma or clotting factor concentrates may also be desirable.

Since protein is a major source of ammonia, it must be completely eliminated from the diet until the patient becomes more alert. As soon as the patient emerges out of coma, protein intake should be gradually reinstituted to enable the liver to regenerate. In the meantime, one should provide a caloric intake of 2000-3000 calories per day either by nasogastric tube or by IV administration to minimize protein breakdown.

Ammoniagenic material must be removed from the bowel since the gastrointestinal tract serves as the major port of entry for ammonia. *Laxatives* such as magnesium sulfate or magnesium citrate (2-3 ounces orally) serve as excellent cathartics in these patients and have the added advantage of repleting low body magnesium stores (116). Magnesium may accumulate in patients with impaired renal function and confuse the clinical picture because of its central nervous system depressant effects. R.H.'s renal status is not yet severely impaired, as evidenced by her serum creatinine of 1.8 mg%. Prolonged magnesium administration should not be necessary.

The bowel continues to serve as a source of ammonia even when patients are NPO because of bacterial enzymatic hydrolysis of urea and deamination of amino acids. Thus, *non-absorbable oral antibiotics* such as neomycin should be administered in doses of 4-8 grams daily to minimize bacterial growth and hence, the production of ammonia. Neomycin rectal enemas can also be administered as 1-2 gram doses in 100-200 ml of normal saline twice a day.

For this particular patient one approach to therapy would be one gram of neomycin four times daily orally, a magnesium citrate laxative, and a one gram neomycin retention enema at bedtime along with the previously mentioned therapeutic maneuvers. Renal function should be monitored if neomycin must be used for more than a few days since 0.5-5% is absorbed, and in the presence of renal impairment, neomycin will accumulate in the serum (26). Since neomycin is both nephrotoxic and ototoxic (202), this accumulation may lead to further renal damage and produce additional problems in this already seriously ill patient. It must be emphasized that renal impairment is not a prerequisite for ototoxicity. Low serum levels of neomycin, when present for a long period of time, may have a toxic effect on the hair cells of the cochlea causing irreversible sensorineural hearing loss (12,85,94,202).

31. Chronic therapy with neomycin may induce staphylococcus enterocolitis, malabsorption, ototoxicity and nephrotoxicity even in the absence of anuria. Thus, this product is less than ideal for chronic use. For these reasons, the non-absorbable sulfonamides such as phthalylsulfathiazole (Sulfathalidine) and succinylsulfathiazole (Sulfasuxidine) are sometimes preferred for prolonged cases of hepatic encephalopathy; however, sulfas are also absorbed to a small extent and may present problems in anuric patients. Lactulose now seems to be preferable to these agents for chronic therapy. What is lactulose and what is its mechanism of action?

Lactulose (Cephulac) is a synthetic disaccharide which reaches the colon largely unhydrolyzed in man because the small intestine has no disaccharidase. Of the ingested dose, 0.4-2% is absorbed and excreted upsplit into the urine. In the colon lactulose is metabolized by normally occurring bacteria to lactic acid, acetic acid and gas; an osmotic and fermentative diarrhea ensues (15,69). Originally, the effect of lactulose in chronic hepatic coma was thought to be related to its ability to replace urease proteolytic bacteria such as *E. coli, Proteus* and *Bacteroides,* with *lactobacilli* that do not possess urease activity; however, this theory has not been confirmed. Presently, it is thought that the therapeutic action of lactulose is related to a reduction in fecal pH which facilitates the transfer of ammonia from the blood into the colonic lumen. In addition, lactulose converts unionized bowel ammonia to the poorly absorbed ammonium ion (116,216,231). While this certainly is a reasonable explanation, it should also be recalled that ammonia by itself may not be entirely responsible for the cerebral symptoms of hepatic encephalopathy. The acidification of colonic contents might also affect the reabsorption of other nitrogenous materials. (131)

Therapy with lactulose syrup (67 gm/100 ml) is usually initiated in 30-45 ml doses three times daily with meals. These doses are then adjusted individually in each patient to promote two to three soft bowel movements daily (69,216,231). Bircher and associates (15) further recommend titrating patients to a sustained acidic colonic environment of pH 5.5 or less as measured by pHydrion indicator paper, because an occasional patient may demonstrate diarrhea without a lowered fecal pH. Doses range from 20-200 ml/day and an overall success rate of approximately 83% can be obtained in properly titrated patients.

Clinically significant benefits do not occur immediately. Simmons and associates (231) noted that at least five days of therapy are required and Rorsman and Sulg (216) reported that the optimal effects of lactulose therapy are not observed for 10-14 days. This delay in clinical effects is probably due to the gradual decrease of toxic compounds already absorbed. This does not explain why neomycin has a more rapid onset of action. In some patients neomycin is more beneficial than lactulose. In others, lactulose has been effective when neomycin has failed.

To date, lactulose has not been associated with any significant side effects other than occasional flatulence, mild abdominal cramping, and the expected diarrhea. Rarely, patients will complain of the sweet taste of the lactulose syrup, but this can easily be overcome by adding it to fruit juices or desserts.

32. M.K. is a 23-year-old woman with a history of acute hepatic necrosis following halothane anesthesia. Despite standard therapeutic maneuvers she has remained in a deep coma for the past five days. A trial of levodopa is being considered. What is the rationale for the use of this drug? What are its proposed mechanisms of action?

Parkes and associates (177) reported that *levodopa* remarkably improved abnormal EEG tracings and dramatically aroused three of five patients suffering from acute hepatic coma. Five grams of levodopa were administered in 100 ml of fluid by a nasogastric tube in two of the patients while the third received this dose by rectal enema. Arousal began 15 minutes after the drug was administered. The previously comatose patients were able to sit up, open their eyes, and maintain a simple conversation. These effects were maximal at 30 minutes and no longer detectable after one hour. Similar results were obtained by Fischer and James (79) in four additional patients when levodopa 50mg/Kg body weight was administered in six divided doses per day.

It is proposed that certain manifestations of hepatic encephalopathy reflect the abnormal accumulation of false neurotransmitters which act by replacing norepinephrine at nerve endings in the peripheral and central nervous system. False neurotransmitters such as phenylalanine, tyrosine, and their derivatives are produced from protein in the gut by bacterial enzymatic breakdown. Under normal circumstances, these substances are removed from the circulation by the liver. Thus, impaired hepatic function results in the flooding of the central and peripheral nervous system with these false neurotransmitters which then replace the normal endogenous neurotransmitters. Consistent with this hypothesis is that (a) the high arterial ammonia levels commonly seen in hepatic coma merely reflect the presence of increased amino acids and amines, (b) neomycin gut sterilization decreases production of amines other than ammonia, and (c) asterixis is a sign of disordered extrapyramidal movement, and like Parkinsonism, may reflect the lack of dopamine in the basal ganglia. Since levodopa is able to penetrate the central nervous system it should re-

plenish the depleted central nervous system stores of norepinephrine and dopamine and thereby (theoretically) result in prompt awakening (79).

Levodopa's notorious tendency to cause gastritis and gastrointestinal bleeding severely limits its usefulness in a condition where gastrointestinal bleeding may already be a complication of hepatic failure. Clearly controlled studies must be done to evaluate any real benefits obtained from levodopa before this agent is widely used.

33. Discuss those drugs which should be avoided in this patient because they may exacerbate hepatic coma.

All central nervous system depressant medications such as sedatives and analgesics should be discontinued because they may worsen the underlying central nervous sytem disorder in patients with impending hepatic coma.

The diuretics, especially the furosemide given to this patient, should be discontinued because electrolyte abnormalities as well as acid-base balance alterations will affect the compartmental distribution of ammonia. Extracellular fluid losses of potassium are replenished by intracellular potassium. In order to maintain cellular electroneutrality, hydrogen and sodium ions move intracellularly to compensate for the potassium exodus. This exchange results in an increase in the pH of the extracellular fluid and this pH gradient favors the conversion of the ammonium ion to the unionized ammonia which more readily penetrates cells and the blood brain barrier (38,268).

CASES FOR STUDY

CASE G: J. B. is a 35-year-old woman with several complaints, not the least of which is her present syndrome which resembles incipient viral hepatitis: nausea, vomiting, and anorexia for more than a week. She has been markedly tired for almost that long and has had a fever for the last four days. Her medical history includes adult-onset diabetes mellitus (onset — 29 years) which is controlled with tolbutamide 1.5 gm/day; mild hypertension (BP 140/95) treated with hydrochlorothiazide 100 mg/day; and chronic urinary tract infections currently minimized by maintenance doses of nitrofurantoin. For the past two months, she has been bothered by an infection of her fingertips. This was originally treated with penicillin and probenecid; however, when a fungal infection was diagnosed, she was given griseofulvin 500 mg/day. Other pertinent drug use included the following:

OrthoNovum 1-80 for 4 years.
Chlordiazepoxide 10 mg as needed.
Indomethacin as needed for arthritic hand pain.
Dialose Plus as needed for constipation (she got these from her mother-in-law several years ago and hasn't used many).

CASE H: W. D., a 23-year-old man in previously good health, now complains of anorexia, nausea, vomiting, and tenderness in the right upper quadrant. His temperature is 38.3° C. He was admitted to the hospital ten days ago because of a painful left elbow of four days duration. One week prior to admission, the patient used his left arm to inject some unidentifiable drugs intravenously. Arthrocentesis on the day of admission confirmed the diagnosis of infection, showing clusters of Gram-Positive cocci. Culture yielded *Staphylococcus aureus* sensitive to penicillin, methicillin, cephalothin, chloramphenicol, erythromycin, and tetracycline.

On the second hospital day, intravenous oxacillin was begun at a dose of 8 gm/day and surgical drainage of the left elbow was performed the next day using thiamylal sodium as the anesthetic. The patient received propoxyphene hydrochloride for pain until the fifth hospital day and acetaminophen thereafter.

On the eleventh hospital day, the patient's SGOT value is 500 IU/ml (normal, 10-40) and his serum alkaline phosphatase value is 7.9 Bodansky units (normal, 2-5). The patient's total serum bilirubin value is normal. The patient gives no history of blood transfusions (56).

1. What signs and/or symptoms are suggestive of hepatitis in these patients?
2. What possible etiologies come to your mind from each case?
3. How would you attempt to differentiate the true cause from other possibilities?
4. How would you treat these patients?

REFERENCES

1. Aach R et al: Halothane and liver failure. JAMA 211:2145, 1970.
2. Acocella G et al: Kinetics of rifampicin and isoniazid administered alone and in combination to normal subjects and patients with liver disease. Gut 13:47, 1972.
3. Adlercreutz H et al: Oral contraceptives and liver damage. Brit Med J 2:1133, 1964.
4. Agress CM: Atabrine as a cause of fatal exfoliative dermatitis and hepatitis. JAMA 131:14, 1946.
5. Alvin J et al: The effect of liver disease in man on the disposition of phenobarbital. J Pharmacol Exp Ther 192:224, 1975.
6. Anon: Halothane hepatitis. Medical Letter 14:43, 1972.
7. Athreya BH et al: Aspirin induced abnormalities of liver function. Amer Dis Child 126:638, 1973.
8. Aubrey DA: Massive hepatic necrosis after cyclophosphamide. Brit Med J 3:588, 1970.
9. Avant GR et al: The effect of cirrhosis on the disposition and elimination of clindamycin. Amer J Dig Dis 20:223, 1975.
10. Azzollini F et al: Elimination of chloramphenicol and thiamphenicol in subjects with cirrhosis of the liver. Int J Clin Pharmacol 6:130, 1972.
11. Benjamin RS et al: Adriamycin chemotherapy — efficacy, safety, and pharmacologic basis of an intermittent single high-dosage schedule. Cancer 33:19, 1974.
12. Berk DP et al: Deafness complicating antibiotic therapy of hepatic encephalopathy. Ann Int Med 73:393, 1970.
13. Bernstein MS et al: Hepatoma and peliosis hepatis developing in a patient with Fanconi's anemia. NEJM 284:1135, 1971.
14. Bingle J et al: Phenindione sensitivity. Lancet 2:377, 1959.
15. Bircher J et al: Treatment of chronic portal-systemic encephalopathy with lactulose. Amer J Med 51:148, 1971.
16. Bjorneboe M et al: Infective hepatitis and toxic jaundice in a municipal hospital during a five-year period. Acta Med Scand 182:491, 1967.
17. Black M et al: Isoniazid-associated hepatitis in 114 patients. Gastroent 69:289, 1975.
18. Blaschke TF et al: Influence on acute viral hepatitis on phenytoin kinetics and protein binding. Clin Pharmacol Ther 17:685, 1975.
19. Boake WC et al: Intrahepatic cholestatic jaundice of pregnancy followed by Enovid-induced cholestatic jaundice. Ann Int Med 63:302, 1965.
20. Bolton BH: Prolonged chlorpromazine jaundice. Amer J Gastroent 48:497, 1967.
21. Borda I et al: Hepatitis following the administration of trimethobenzamide hydrochloride. Arch Int Med 120:371, 1967.
22. Branch RA et al: The pharmacokinetics of (+) - propranolol in normal subjects and patients with chronic liver disease. Brit J Clin Pharm 2:183P, 1975.
23. Brandl R et al: Zur pharmakokinetik von clindamycin bei gestorter leber — und nierenfunktion. Dtsch Med Wschr 97:1057, 1972.
24. Brandt C et al: Liver injury associated with tranylcypromine therapy. JAMA 188:752, 1964.
25. Braun P: Hepatotoxicity of erythromycin. J Inf Dis 119:300, 1969.
26. Breen KJ et al: Neomycin absorption in man: Studies of oral and enema administration and effect of intestinal ulceration. Ann Int Med 76:211, 1972.
27. Breimer DD et al: Pharmacokinetics of hexobarbital in acute hepatitis and after apparent recovery. Clin Pharmacol Ther 18:433, 1975.
28. Brown AR: Two cases of untoward reaction after "Ilosone." Brit Med J 2:913, 1963.
29. Bruce DL: What is a "safe" interval between halothane exposures. JAMA 221:1140, 1972.
30. Cacace LG et al: Alpha-methyldopa hepatitis. Drug Intel Clin Pharm 10:144, 1976.
31. Carney FMT et al: Halothane hepatitis: a critical review. Anesth Analg 51:135, 1972.
32. Castleman B et al: Case records of the Massachusetts General Hospital, case 10-1970, NEJM 282:558, 1970.
33. Chajek T et al: Quinidine-induced granulomatous hepatitis. Ann Int Med 81:774, 1974.
34. Clark R et al: Hepatic damage and death from overdose of paracetamol. Lancet 1:66, 1973.
35. Collens WS et al: Cholestatic jaundice following use of sulfonylurea drugs. NY State J Med 65:907, 1965.
36. Colwell AR: Fecal fat excretion in patients with jaundice due to viral hepatitis. Gastroent 33:591, 1957.
37. Compra JL et al: Prednisone therapy of acute alcoholic hepatitis — report of a controlled trial. Ann Int Med 79:625, 1973.
37a. Compston JE et al: Intestinal absorption of 25-hydroxyvitamin D and osteomalacia in primary biliary cirrhosis. Lancet 1:721, 1977.
38. Conn HO: A rational program for the management of hepatic coma. Gastroent 57:715, 1969.
39. Conn HO et al: Ethionamide-induced hepatitis. Amer Rev Resp Dis 90:542, 1964.
40. Cook GC et al: Controlled prospective trial of corticosteroid therapy in active chronic hepatitis. Quart J Med 40:159, 1971.
41. Cook GC et al: Jaundice and its relation to therapeutic agents. Lancet 1:175, 1965.
42. Cooperative Study: Subcommittee on the National Halothane Study of the Committee on Anesthesia, NAS-NRC, Summary of the national halothane study JAMA 197:775, 1966.
43. Cox RP et al: Novobiocin jaundice. NEJM 261:139, 1959.
44. Culbertson JW et al: The effect of the upright position upon the hepatic blood flow in normotensive and hypertensive subjects. J Clin Invest 30:305, 1951.
45. Cunningham MD et al: Phenobarbitone in cholestasis. Lancet 1:1089, 1968.
46. Cutts M: Chlorpromazine hepatitis treated with cortisone. Ann Int Med 46:1160, 1957.
47. Dahl MGC et al: Methotrexate hepatotoxicity in psoriasis — comparison of different dose regimens. Brit Med J 1:654, 1972.
48. Daikos GK et al: Propoxyphene jaundice. JAMA 232:835, 1975.
49. Datta DV et al: Treatment of pruritus of obstructive jaundice with cholestyramine. Brit Med J 1:216, 1963.
50. Davidson CS: Alcoholic hepatitis. NEJM 284:1378, 1971.
51. Davis M et al: Plasma pharmacokinetics of prednisone and prednisolone in normal subjects and patients with liver disease. Digestion 12:264, 1975.
52. Dayan AD et al: Idoxuridine and jaundice. Lancet 2:1073, 1969.
53. DeGowin EL et al: *Bedside Diagnostic Examination*, 2nd ed, Macmillan and Company, New York, 1969, pp442, 444, 754.
54. deLorimier AA et al: Methyltestosterone, related steroids, and liver function. Arch Int Med 116:289, 1965.

54a. Desmyter J et al: Administration of human fibroblast interferon in chronic hepatitis-B infection. Lancet 2:645, 1976.

55. DeVita VT et al: Clinical trials with 1,3-bis(2-chloroethyl)-1-nitrosourea, NSC-409962. Cancer Res 25:1876, 1965.

56. Dismukes, WE: Oxacillin-induced hepatic dysfunction. JAMA 226:861, 1973.

57. Dittler EL: Upper abdominal pain and intrahepatic cholestasis as manifestations of sensitivity to Ilosone. Amer J Gastroent 38:691, 1962.

58. Dowling HF et al: Hepatic reactions to tetracycline. JAMA 188:307, 1964.

59. Drake ME et al: The effect of nitrogen mustard on virus of serum hepatitis in whole blood. Proc Soc Expt Biol Med 80:310, 1952.

60. Drill VA: Benign cholestatic jaundice of pregnancy and benign cholestatic jaundice from oral contraceptives. Amer J Ob Gyn 119:165, 1974.

61. Drivsholm AA et al: The influence of treatment with sodium salicylate on the serum glutamic oxalacetic transaminase activity. Scand J Clin Lab Invest 13:442, 1961.

62. Dujovne CA et al: Sulfonamide hepatic injury. NEJM 277:785, 1967.

63. Dykes MHM: Unexplained postoperative fever: its value as a sign of halothane sensitization. JAMA 216:641, 1971.

64. East EN et al: Severe sensitivity reaction (hepatitis, dermatitis and pyrexia) attributable to phenylindanedione. Can Med Assoc J 77:1028, 1957.

65. Ecker JA: Phenylbutazone hepatitis. Amer J Gastroent 43:23, 1965.

66. Einhorn M et al: Hepatotoxicity of mercaptopurine. JAMA 188:802, 1964.

67. Einstein N et al: Jaundice due to nicotinic acid therapy. Amer J Dig Dis 20:282, 1975.

68. Eisen HJ et al: Disulfiram hepatotoxicity. Ann Int Med 83:673, 1975.

69. Elkington SG et al: Lactulose in the treatment of chronic portal-systemic encephalopathy. NEJM 281:408, 1969.

70. Elmore M et al: Clindamycin-associated hepatotoxicity. Amer J Med 57:627, 1974.

71. Fallon H et al: Chronic active hepatitis. JAMA 221:888, 1972.

72. Farid Z et al: Hepatotoxicity after treatment of schistosomiasis with hycanthone. Brit Med J 2:88, 1972.

73. Farmer CD et al: Intrahepatic cholestasis associated with the ingestion of erythromycin estolate (Ilosone). Gastroent 45:157, 1963.

74. Fedotin MS et al: Liver disease caused by propylthiouracil. Arch Int Med 135:319, 1975.

75. Felig P et al: Glucose homeostasis in viral hepatitis. NEJM 283:1436, 1970.

76. Fenech FF et al: Hepatitis with biliverdinaemia in association with indomethacin therapy. Brit Med J 3:155, 1967.

77. Finlayson NDC et al: Antipyrine, lidocaine, and paracetamol metabolism in chronic liver disease. Gastroent 67:790, 1974.

78. Fischer HW et al: Mimicry of acute cholecystitis by erythromycin estolate reactions, reports of 2 cases. Amer J Med Sci 247:283, 1964.

79. Fischer JE et al: Treatment of hepatic coma and hepatorenal syndrome: mechanism of action of L-Dopa and Aramine. Amer J Surg 123:222, 1972.

80. Fischer MG et al: Methimazole-induced jaundice. JAMA 223:1028, 1973.

81. Fries J, and Siraganian R: Sulfonamide hepatitis. NEJM 274:95, 1966.

82. Frohlich ED et al: Some clinical effects of guanoxan. Clin Pharmacol Ther 7:599, 1966.

83. Galambos JT et al: The effect of intravenous ethanol on serum enzymes in patients with normal or diseased liver. Gastroent 44:267, 1963.

84. Garber E et al: Aspirin hepatotoxicity. Ann Int Med 82:592, 1975.

85. Gibson WS: Deafness to orally administered neomycin. Arch Otolaryng 86:163, 1967.

86. Gilbert FJ: Cholestatic hepatitis caused by esters of erythromycin and oleandomycin. JAMA 182:1048, 1962.

87. Gocke DJ: A prospective study of post-transfusion hepatitis: the role of Australia antigen. JAMA 219:1165, 1972.

88. Goldenberg VE et al: Hepatic injury associated with tromethamine. JAMA 205:81, 1968.

89. Goldfinger SE et al: Hypersensitivity hepatitis due to phe-nazopyridine hydrochloride. NEJM 286:1090, 1972.

90. Goldstein LI et al: Hepatic injury associated with nitrofurantoin therapy. Amer J Dig Dis 19:987, 1974.

91. Goldstein MJ et al: Jaundice in a patient receiving aceto-hexamide. NEJM 275:97, 1966.

92. Grady GF et al: Hepatitis B immune globulin — prevention of hepatitis from accidental exposure among medical personnel. NEJM 293:1067, 1975.

93. Greenberg HB et al: Effect of human leukocyte interferon on hepatitis B virus infection in patients with chronic active hepatitis. NEJM 295:517, 1976.

94. Greenberg LH et al: Audiotoxicity and nephrotoxicity due to or-ally administered neomycin JAMA 194:827, 1965.

95. Gregory DH et al: Chronic cholestasis following prolonged tol-butamide administration. Arch Path 84:194, 1967.

96. Gregory PB et al: Steroid therapy in severe viral hepatitis: a double-blind, randomized trial of methyl-prednisolone versus placebo. NEJM 294:681, 1976.

97. Grieco MH: Hypersensitivity abdominal pain induced by eryth-romycin propionate estolate. Med Times 97:149, 1969.

97a. Gunby P: Hepatitis B vaccines show promise in early human trials. JAMA 237:2022, 1977.

98. Hamff LH et al: The effects of tolbutamide and chlorpropamide on patients exhibiting jaundice as a result of previous chlor-propamide therapy. Ann NY Acad Sci 74:820, 1959.

99. Hansten PD: Drug Interactions, 3rd ed Lea & Febiger, Philadel-phia, 1975, p 31.

100. Hargraves MM et al: Aplastic anemia associated with administra-tion of chloramphenicol, (case 2). JAMA 149:1293, 1952.

101. Havens WP: Cholestatic jaundice in patients treated with eryth-romycin estolate. JAMA 180:30, 1962.

102. Held H et al: Zur pharmakokinetik von meprobamat bei chronis-chen hepatopathien und arzneimittelsucht. Klin Wochenschr 47:78, 1969.

103. Held VH et al: Pharmakokinetik von glymidine (glycodiazin) und tolbutamid bei akuten und chronischen leberschaden. Arzneim Forsch 23:1801, 1973.

104. Held H et al: Drug metabolism in actue and chronic liver disease. Digestion 4:151, 1971.

105. Helman RA et al: Alcoholic hepatitis: Natural history and evalua-tion of prednisolone therapy. Ann Int Med 74:311, 1971.

106. Hinthorn DR et al: Use of clindamycin in patients with liver dis-ease. Antimicrob Ag Chem 9:498, 1976.

107. Hoffman TA et al: Pharmacodynamics of carbenicillin in hepatic and renal failure. Ann Int Med 73:173, 1970.

108. Holdsworth CD et al: Hepatitis caused by the newer amine-oxidase-inhibiting drugs. Lancet 2:1459, 1961.

109. Hollister LE: Allergic reactions to tranquilizing drugs. Ann Int Med 49:17, 1958.

110. Holoubek JE et al: Thiouracil hepatitis. Amer J Med 5:138, 1948.

111. Hooper WD et al: Plasma protein binding of diphenylhydantoin. Effects of sex hormones, renal and hepatic disease. Clin Phar-macol Ther 15:276, 1974.

112. Hughes HC et al: Hepatic necrosis produced by repeated admin-istration of halothane to guinea pigs. Anesthes 36:466, 1972.

113. Husebye KO: Jaundice with persisting pericholangiolitic in-flammation in a patient treated with chlorothiazide. Amer J Dig Dis 9:439, 1964.

114. Hutchison JC et al: Cholestatic jaundice following administra-tion of quinethazone. Curr Ther Res 6:199, 1964.

115. Hvidberg EF et al: Plasma half-life of phenylbutazone in patients with impaired liver function. Clin Pharmacol Ther 15:171, 1974.

116. Jacobson S et al: Recognition and management of acute and chronic hepatic encephalopathy. Med Clin N Amer 57:1569, 1973.

117. Johnson DF et al: Allergic hepatitis caused by propionyl eryth-romycin ester of lauryl sulfate. NEJM 265:1200, 1961.

118. Jori GP et al: Hydralazine disease associated with transient granulomas in the liver. Gastroent 64:1163, 1973.

119. Joshi PH et al: The syndrome of methoxyflurane-associated hepatitis. Ann Int Med 80:395, 1974.

120. Judson JA et al: Possible cross-sensitivity between halothane and methoxyflurane. Anesthes 35:527, 1971.

121. Karachalios GN: Abdominal pain and erythromycin estolate. Lancet 1:199, 1973.

122. Katz R et al: Post-transfusion hepatitis — effect of modified gamma globulin added to blood in vitro. NEJM 285:925, 1971.

123. Kew MC et al: Possible hepatotoxicity of cannabis. Lancet 1:578, 1969.
124. King JA et al: An unexpected reaction to procainamide. JAMA 186:603, 1963.
125. Klatskin G: Toxic and drug-induced hepatitis; in Schiff L, Ed.: Diseases of the Liver, 4th ed. J. B. Lippincott, Philadelphia, 1975.
126. Klotz U et al: The effects of age and liver disease on the disposition and elimination of diazepam in adult man. J Clin Invest 55:347, 1975.
127. Klotz U et al: The effect of cirrhosis on the disposition and elimination of meperidine in man. Clin Pharmacol Ther 16:667, 1974.
128. Kohlstaedt KG: Propionyl erythromycin ester lauryl sulfate and jaundice. JAMA 178:89, 1961.
129. Kohn N et al: Cholestatic hepatitis associated with trifluoperazine. NEJM 264:549, 1961.
130. Koler RD et al: Hepatotoxicity due to chlorambucil. JAMA 167:316, 1958.
131. Kosman ME: Lactulose (Cephulac) in portosystemic encephalopathy. JAMA 236:2444, 1976.
132. Krugman S et al: Infectious hepatitis: evidence for two distinctive clinical epidemiological and immunological types of infection. JAMA 200:365, 1967.
133. Kunin CM et al: Persistence of antibiotics in blood of patients with acute renal failure. II. Chloramphenicol and its metabolic products in the blood of patients with severe renal disease or hepatic cirrhosis. J Clin Invest 38:1498, 1959.
133a. Labadarios, D, et al: Vitamin B6 deficiency in chronic liver disease — evidence for increased degradation of pyridoxal-5'-phosphate. Gut 18:23, 1977.
134. Langlands AO et al: Jaundice associated with norethisterone-acetate treatment of breast cancer. Lancet 1:584, 1975.
135. Law IP et al: Jaundice associated with naproxen. NEJM 295:1201, 1976.
136. Leard SE et al: Hepatitis, exfoliative dermatitis and abnormal bone marrow occurring during tridione therapy. NEJM 240:962, 1949.
137. Leevy CM et al: Alcoholic hepatitis and corticosteroids. Med Clin N Amer 57:1191, 1973.
138. Lesesne HR et al: Treatment of liver disease with corticosteroids. Med Clin N Amer 57:1191, 1973.
139. Levi AJ et al: Phenylbutazone and isoniazid metabolism in patients with liver disease in relation to previous drug therapy. Lancet 1:1275, 1968.
140. Levy RW et al: Fatal hepatorenal syndrome associated with phenurone therapy. NEJM 242:933, 1950.
141. Lewis GP et al: Prednisone side-effects and serum-protein levels. Lancet 2:778, 1971.
142. Lieber CS: Liver adaptation and injury in alcoholism. NEJM 288:356, 1973.
143. Lieber CS: Hepatic and metabolic effects of alcohol. Gastroent 65:821, 1973.
144. Lindenbaum J et al: Hepatic necrosis associated with halothane anesthesia. NEJM 268:525, 1963.
145. Lo KJ et al: Cholestatic jaundice associated with chlordiazepoxide (Librium) therapy. Amer J Dig Dis 12:845, 1967.
146. Lomanto C et al: Problems in diagnosing halothane hepatitis. JAMA 214:1257, 1970.
146a. Long RG et al: Serum-25-hydroxy-vitamin-D in untreated parenchymal and cholestatic liver disease. Lancet 2:650, 1976.
147. Lundbergh P et al: Changes in hepatic circulation at rest, during and after exercise in young males with infectious hepatitis compared with controls. Acta Med Scand 196:315, 1974.
148. Lunzer M et al: Jaundice due to carbimazole. Gut 16:913, 1975.
149. Lunzer MR et al: Jaundice due to erythromycin estolate. Gastroent 68:1284, 1975.
150. Luongo MA et al: The liver in ferrous sulfate poisoning. NEJM 251:995, 1954.
151. Macoul KL: Hepatitis attributed to sulfamethoxazole. NEJM 275:39, 1966.
152. Masel MA: Erythromycin hepato-sensitivity: a preliminary report of two cases. Med J Aust 1:560, 1962.
153. Manso C et al: Effect of aspirin administration on serum glutamic oxaloacetic and glutamic pyruvic transaminases in children. Proc Soc Expt Biol Med 93:84, 1956.
154. Marcus FI et al: The metabolism of tritiated digoxin in cirrhotic patients. Gastroent 47:517, 1964.
155. Maugh TH: Chemotherapy: antiviral agents come of age. Science 192:128, 1976.
156. Mawer GE et al: Metabolism of amylobarbitone in patients with chronic liver disease. Brit J Pharmacol 44:549, 1972.
157. Maxwell JD et al: Plasma disappearance and cerebral effects of chlorpromazine in cirrhotics. Clin Sci 43:143, 1972.
158. McArthur JE et al: Stevens-Johnson syndrome with hepatitis following therapy with ampicillin and cephalexin. NZ Med J 81:390, 1975.
159. McCollum RW: Report of a conference: serum antigens in viral hepatitis. J Inf Dis 120:641, 1969.
160. McFarland RB: Fatal drug reaction associated with prochlorperazine (compazine). Amer J Clin Path 40:284, 1963.
161. McHorse TS et al: Effect of acute viral hepatitis in man on the disposition and elimination of meperidine. Gastroent 68:775, 1975.
162. McKenzie I et al: Two cases of jaundice following "Ilosone." Med J Aust 1:349, 1966.
163. Millikan LE et al: Drug reactions to sulfones. Arch Derm 102:220, 1970.
164. Mistilis SP et al: Active chronic hepatitis. Amer J Med 48:484, 1970.
165. Moertel CG et al: Mitomycin c therapy in advanced gastrointestinal cancer. JAMA 204:1045, 1968.
166. Morrissey JF et al: The detection of pyrazinamide-induced liver damage by serum enzyme determinations. Amer Rev Resp Dis 80:855, 1959.
166a. Mosley JW et al: Multiple hepatitis viruses in multiple attacks of acute viral hepatitis. NEJM 296:75, 1977.
167. Muenter MD et al: Chronic vitamin A intoxication in adults. Amer J Med 50:129, 1971.
168. Naeim F et al: Peliosis hepatis. Arch Pathol 95:284, 1973.
169. Neefe JR et al: Hepatitis due to the injection of homologous blood products in human volunteers. J Clin Invest 23:836, 1944.
170. Nelson E: Rate of metabolism of tolbutamide in test subjects with liver disease or with impaired renal function. Amer J Med Sci 248:657, 1964.
171. Nunes HL et al: Turnover and distribution of nafcillin in tissues and body fluids of surgical patients. Antimicrob Ag Chem 1964:237, 1965.
172. Ockner RK, and Davidson CS: Hepatic effects or oral contraceptives. NEJM 276:331, 1967.
173. Ogburn RM et al: Hepatitis associated with dantrolene sodium. Ann Int Med 84:53, 1976.
174. Oliver LE et al: "Biliary colic" and Ilosone. Med J Aust 1:1148, 1973.
175. Ossenberg FW et al: Pentobarbital pharmacokinetics in cirrhosis. Digestion 8:448, 1973.
176. Pagliaro L et al: Barbiturate jaundice. Gastroent 56:938, 1969.
177. Parkes JD et al: Levodopa in hepatic coma. Lancet 2:1341, 1970.
178. Paronetto F et al: Lymphocyte stimulation induced by halothane in patients with hepatitis following exposure to halothane. NEJM 283:277, 1970.
179. Perez-Mera RA et al: Jaundice associated with norethindrone acetate therapy. NEJM 267:1137, 1962.
180. Perkins J: Phenindione jaundice. Lancet 1:125, 1962.
181. Peterson RE et al: The physiological disposition and metabolic fate of cortisone in man. J Clin Invest 36:1301, 1957.
182. Pezzimenti JF et al: Anicteric hepatitis induced by diphenylhydantoin. Arch Int Med 125:118, 1970.
183. Piafsky KM et al: Disposition of theophylline in chronic liver disease. Clin Pharmacol Ther 17:241, 1975.
184. Podolsky S et al: Potassium depletion in hepatic cirrhosis: a reversible cause of impaired growth hormone and insulin response to stimulation. NEJM 288:644, 1973.
185. Portal RW, and Emanuel RW: Phenindione hepatitis complicating anticoagulant therapy. Brit Med J 2:1318, 1961.
186. Porter HP et al: Corticosteroid therapy in severe alcoholic hepatitis. NEJM 284:1350, 1971.
187. Powell LW et al: Corticosteroids in liver disease: Studies on the biological conversion of prednisone to prednisolone and plasma protein binding. Gut 13:690, 1972.
188. Powell WJ et al: Lethal hepatic necrosis after therapy with imipramine and desipramine. JAMA 206:642, 1968.
189. Pozzi E et al: Blood levels of rifampicin in liver diseases. Intn'l J Clin Pharmacol 10:44, 1974.
190. Prescott LF et al: Plasma-paracetamol half-life and hepatic necrosis in patients with paracetamol overdosage. Lancet 1:519, 1971.

191. Prince AM et al: Hepatitis B "immune" globulin: effectiveness in prevention of dialysis-associated hepatitis. NEJM 293:1063, 1975.

192. Public Health Service Advisory Committee on Immunization Practices: Immune serum globulin for protection against viral hepatitis. Ann Int Med 77:427, 1972.

193. Radke RA et al: Carbasone toxicity. Ann Int Med 47:418, 1957.

194. Ramsay ID: Carbamazepine-induced jaundice. Brit Med J 4:155, 1967.

195. Read AE et al: Effects of chlorpromazine in patients with hepatic disease. Brit Med J 3:497, 1969.

196. Ream NW et al: Mithramycin therapy in disseminated germinal testicular cancer. JAMA 204:1030, 1968.

197. Redeker AG et al: Randomization of corticosteroid therapy in fulminant hepatitis. NEJM 294:728, 1976.

198. Redeker AG et al: Hepatitis B immune globulin as a prophylactic measure for spouses exposed to acute type B hepatitis. NEJM 293:1055, 1975.

199. Reed C et al: Toxic jaundice due to propionyl erythromycin ester lauryl sulphate ("Ilosone"). Med J Aust 1:810, 1962.

200. Reichel J et al: Intrahepatic cholestasis following administration of chlorpropamide. Amer J Med 28:654, 1960.

201. Reinhart MJ et al: Suggestive evidence of hepatotoxicity concomitant with thioridazine hydrochloride use. JAMA 197:767, 1966.

202. Reuben RJ et al: Neomycin ototoxicity and nephrotoxicity — a case report following oral administration. Laryng 78:1734, 1968.

203. Reynolds ES et al: Fatal massive necrosis of the liver as a manifestation of hypersensitivity to probenecid. NEJM 256:592, 1957.

204. Reynolds ES et al: Massive hepatic necrosis after fluroxene anesthesia — a case of drug interaction? NEJM 286:530, 1972.

205. Rich RR et al: Salicylate hepatotoxicity in patients with juvenile rheumatoid arthritis. Arthr Rheum 16:1, 1973.

206. Rieder VJ et al: Pharmakokinetik der wirkstoffkombination trimethoprim + sulfamethoxazol bei leberkranken im vergleich zu gesunden. Arzneim. Forsch. 25:656, 1975.

207. Rigberg LA et al: Chlorpropamide-induced granulomas. JAMA 235:409, 1976.

208. Riley WA: Hepatitis following administration of Ilosone. N Carolina Med J 23:361, 1962.

209. Robinson MJ et al: Tetracycline-associated fatty liver in the male. Amer J Dig Dis 15:857, 1970.

210. Robinson MM: Antibiotics increase incidence of hepatitis. JAMA 178:89, 1961.

211. Robinson MM: Demonstration by "challenge" of hepatic dysfunction associated with propionyl erythromycin ester lauryl sulfate. Antibiot Chemother 12:147, 1962.

212. Robinson MM: Hepatic dysfunction associated with triacetyloleandomycin and propionyl erythromycin ester lauryl sulfate. Amer J Med Sci 243:502, 1962.

213. Robinson WS et al: The virus of hepatitis, type B·(in two parts). NEJM 295:1168,1232, 1976.

214. Rogers RS: Abdominal distress and erythromycin estolate. Lancet 2:1198, 1972.

215. Ronnov-Jessen V et al: Hepatotoxicity due to treatment with papaverine. NEJM 281:1333, 1969.

216. Rorsman G et al: Lactulose treatment of chronic hepatoportal encephalopathy. Acta Med Scand 187:337, 1970.

217. Rowell LB et al: Indocyanine green clearance and estimated hepatic blood flow during mild to maximal exercise in upright man. J Clin Invest 43:1677, 1964.

218. Russell AS et al: Serum transaminase during salicylate therapy. Brit Med J 2:428, 1971.

219. Sabel GH et al: Biliary stasis after mestranolnorethindrone ingestion. Ob Gyn 31:375, 1968.

220. Schaffner F: Cholestyramine, a boon to some who itch. Gastroent 46:67, 1964.

221. Schalm SW et al: Pharmacokinetics of prednisone and prednisolone in chronic active liver disease (CALD). Gastroent 69:863, 1975.

222. Scheuer PJ et al: Rifampicin hepatitis. Lancet 1:421, 1974.

223. Scheuer PJ et al: Guidelines for diagnosis of therapeutic drug-induced liver injury in liver biopsies. Lancet 1:854, 1974.

224. Schneider EM et al: Chlorpromazine jaundice: the effect of continued chlorpromazine ingestion in the presence of chlorpromazine jaundice. South Med J 51:287, 1958.

225. Seaman WE et al: Aspirin-induced hepatotoxicity in patients with systemic lupus erythematosus. Ann Int Med 80:1, 1974.

226. Sessions JT et al: The effect of barbiturates in patients with liver disease. J Clin Invest 33:1116, 1954.

227. Serpeau D et al: Hepatitis-associated antigen in human bile. Lancet 2:1266, 1971.

228. Shamszad M et al: Metabolism of ^{35}S-disulfiram in normals and in patients with liver disease. Gastroent 68:983, 1975.

229. Short MH et al: Cholestatic jaundice during imipramine therapy. JAMA 206:1791, 1968.

230. Shull HJ et al: Normal disposition of oxazepam in acute viral hepatitis and cirrhosis. Ann Int Med 84:420, 1976.

231. Simmons F et al: A controlled clinical trial of lactulose in hepatic encephalopathy. Gastroent 59:827, 1970.

232. Simmons F et al: Granulomatous hepatitis in a patient receiving allopurinol. Gastroent 62:101, 1972.

233. Simpson DG et al: Hypersensitivity to para-aminosalicylic acid. Amer J Med 29:297, 1960.

233a. Skinner RK et al: 25-Hydroxylation of vitamin-D in primary biliary cirrhosis. Lancet 1:720, 1977.

234. Soloway RD et al: Chronic active liver disease: classification and treatment. Postgrad Med 53:88, 1973.

235. Somayaji BN et al: Norethisterone jaundice in two sisters. Brit Med J 2:281, 1968.

236. Sparberg M et al: Intrahepatic cholestasis due to azathioprine. Gastroent 57:439, 1969.

237. Stein AA et al: Hepatic pathology in jaundice due to chlorpromazine. JAMA 161:508, 1956.

238. Stern MH et al: Hepatotoxicity in patients treated with adriamycin and 6-mercaptopurine for refractory leukemia. Amer J Clin Path 63:758, 1975.

239. Stiehl A et al: The effects of phenobarbital on bile salts and bilirubin in patients with intrahepatic and extrahepatic cholestasis. NEJM 286:858, 1972.

240. Stokes J et al: The carrier state in viral hepatitis. JAMA 154:1059, 1954.

241. Storstein L et al: Digitoxin pharmacokinetics in chronic active hepatitis. Digestion 12:353, 1975.

242. Suhrland LG et al: Delayed clearance of chloramphenicol from serum in patients with hematologic toxicity. Blood 34:466, 1969.

243. Suhrland LG et al: Chloramphenicol toxicity in liver and renal disease. Arch Int Med 112:747, 1963.

243a. Summerskill WHJ et al: Prednisone for chronic active liver disease: dose titration, standard dose, and combination with azathioprine compared. Gut 16:876, 1975.

244. Surgenor DM et al: Clinical trials of hepatitis B immune globulin. NEJM 293:1060, 1975.

245. Sutnick AL: Australia antigen: progress report. Med Clin N Amer 57:1029, 1973.

246. Thompson PD et al: Lidocaine pharmacokinetics in advanced heart failure, liver disease, and renal failure in humans. Ann Int Med 78:499, 1973.

247. Thompson RPH et al: Contraception with chlormadinone acetate in woman with previous contraceptive jaundice. Brit Med J 1:152, 1970.

248. Tong MJ et al: Failure of transfer-factor therapy in chronic active type B hepatitis. NEJM 295:209, 1976.

249. Tripatzis I: Australia antigen in urine and feces. Amer J Dis Child 123:401, 1972.

250. Trolle D: Decrease of total serum-bilirubin concentration in newborn infants after phenobarbitone treatment. Lancet 2:705, 1968.

251. Tumulty PA: Systemic lupus erythematosus. In Harrison's Principles of Internal Medicine, 6th ed, McGraw Hill Book Co., New York, 1970, p 1962.

252. Ueda H et al: Disappearance rate of tolbutamide in normal subjects and in diabetes mellitus, liver cirrhosis, and renal disease. Diabetes 12:414, 1963.

253. Underwood JCE et al: Jaundice after treatment of leukemia with busulfan. Brit Med J 1:556, 1971.

254. Urban E et al: Liver dysfunction with mestranol but not with norethynodrel in a patient with enovid-induced jaundice. Ann Int Med 68:598, 1968.

255. Valdivia-Barriga V et al: Generalized hypersensitivity with hepatitis and jaundice after the use of penicillin and streptomycin. Gastroent 45:114, 1963.

256. Van Itallie TB et al: The treatment of pruritus and hypercholesteremia of primary biliary cirrhosis with cholestyramine. NEJM 265:469, 1961.

257. Villarejos VM et al: Role of saliva, urine and feces in the transmission of type B hepatitis. NEJM 291:1375, 1974.

258. Wallace SL et al: Colchicine plasma levels. Amer J Med 48:443, 1970.

259. Weiner M et al: Observations on the metabolic transformation and effects of phenylbutazone in subjects with hepatic disease. Amer J Med Sci 228:36, 1954.

260. Weisburst M et al: Jaundice and rash associated with the use of phenobarbital and hydrochlorothiazide. S Med J 69:126, 1976.

261. Whelton MJ et al: Pregnancy in patients with hepatic cirrhosis: Management and outcome. Lancet 2:995, 1968.

262. Whelton MJ et al: Ergot poisoning in acute hepatic necrosis. Gut 9:287, 1968.

263. Widman FK: The Australia antigen: where do we stand? Parts I and II. Postgrad Med 50:167, 1971 and 51:257, 1972.

264. Wilkinson GR et al: Drug disposition and liver disease. Drug Metab Rev 4:139, 1975.

264a. Williams R et al: Action of steroid therapy in jaundice. Lancet 2:392, 1961.

265. Wilson FM et al: Anicteric carbenicillin hepatitis: eight episodes in four patients. JAMA 232:818, 1975.

266. Wolfe JD et al: Aspirin hepatitis. Ann Int Med 80:74, 1974.

267. Yon J et al: Hepatitis caused by amitriptyline therapy. JAMA 232:833, 1975.

268. Zieve L: Pathogenesis of hepatic coma. Arch Int Med 118:211, 1966.

269. Zilly W et al: Pharmacokinetics and metabolism of digoxin and b-methyl-digoxin-12a-^{3}H in patients with acute hepatitis. Clin Pharmacol Ther 17:302, 1975.

270. Zimmerman HJ: Aspirin-induced hepatic injury (editorial) Ann Int Med 80:103, 1974.

271. Zucker P et al: Aspirin Hepatitis. Amer J Dis Child 129:1433, 1975.

Chapter 20

Diseases of the Kidney

John G. Gambertoglio
Richard J. Mangini

An increasingly large number of persons have developed irreversible loss of renal function. Between 50 and 75 per million people per year have kidney disease of such severity that they require chronic dialysis, renal transplantation or die from end-stage renal failure. The five-year survival rate for patients on chronic hemodialysis is 55 to 85%; two-year graft survival rates in patients receiving live related or cadaver donor kidneys are approximately 70% and 46% respectively (1). Thus, although life certainly can be prolonged by dialysis and transplantation, these means of therapy are far from perfect.

The clinical presentation, pathogenesis, and treatment of the more commonly encountered forms of renal disease will be described in this chapter. These are acute and chronic renal failure, and glomerular diseases such as nephrotic syndrome and lupus nephritis. Diabetes insipidus and the syndrome of inappropriate secretion of antidiuretic hormone will be discussed briefly. Commonly used drugs which have been associated with nephrotoxic effects will also be reviewed in the following chapter.

The dosing of drugs in renal failure and their removal by hemodialysis will not be presented here;

however, this information may be found in other sources (2).

It is necessary to have a basic understanding of the disease process in order to assess therapy, and excellent texts have recently become available describing renal disease in detail (3,4). However, in this chapter emphasis is placed on drugs and drug therapy in association with the various renal diseases.

ACUTE RENAL FAILURE:

B.M. is a 38-year-old male, admitted to the hospital because of persistent nausea, vomiting, and diarrhea that is thought to be due to a viral infection. He has a history of hypertension and has been treated with sodium restriction and methyldopa. Initial diagnostic studies were performed which prevented him from obtaining an adequate oral intake. At this time his blood pressure was noted to be elevated, and he was started on 80 mg of furosemide once a day. Three days later the patient's blood pressure was 70/30 with a rapid pulse and his urine volume was only 100 ml per 24 hours. The patient complained of a dry mouth and decreased skin turgor was noticeable on physical examination. Serum electrolytes revealed a sodium of 130 mEq/L, potassium of 7.0 mEq/L, chloride of 110 mEq/L and bicarbonate of 19 mEq/L. The serum creatinine was 4.0 mg% and the blood urea nitrogen (BUN) was 60 mg%. Plasma osmolality was 290 mOsm/kg. Examination of the urine revealed the following: sodium 7 mEq/L; potassium 25 mEq/L; urea 900 mg%; creatinine 70 mg% and osmolality 800 mOsm/kg.

The patient was immediately given intravenous fluid therapy and a dose of mannitol. Within the next few hours urine volume exceeded 80 ml/hour and over the next few days, serum electrolytes, creatinine and BUN returned to normal.

1. What is the definition of acute renal failure?

Acute renal failure (ARF) can be defined as a sudden decline in renal function, accompanied by an accumulation of nitrogenous waste products normally excreted by the kidney. It is caused by a process within the kidney itself and is not reversed by correction of extrarenal factors, i.e. pre-renal and post-renal causes of azotemia (see Questions 2 and 3). Urine volume may vary over a wide range in ARF. In general, if the urine volume is less than 400 ml per day, the term oliguric ARF is used. However, the urine volume may be much higher than this, exceeding one liter or more. This latter type is referred to as nonoliguric or high-output acute renal failure. Thus, a patient with acute renal failure who is accumulating metabolic wastes may have a small or relatively large daily urine output. Commonly, the term acute tubular necrosis (ATN),

which describes a histopathological change within the kidney is used; however, patients with ARF frequently do not exhibit evidence of tubular necrosis. In fact, histological changes within the kidney do not correlate very well with the functional capacity of the kidney. Therefore, the terms acute tubular necrosis and acute renal failure are not synonymous (7, 9, 11, 12, 14, 15).

2. What is pre-renal azotemia?

Pre-renal azotemia may be defined as a decline in creatinine clearance or glomerular filtration rate (GFR) caused by an event which decreases renal perfusion pressure or causes severe renal vasoconstriction. The most common etiology is hypovolemia which decreases renal blood flow and produces renal ischemia. The hypovolemia may be secondary to blood loss or excessive fluid losses from the gastrointestinal tract or from severe burns. The overuse of diuretics, as exemplified in the above case, can also cause pre-renal azotemia, especially if patients are on sodium restricted diets. Vasodilatation of peripheral blood vessels secondary to antihypertensive drugs or septicemia can decrease renal perfusion. Other causes of pre-renal azotemia include decreased cardiac output secondary to impaired cardiac function, e.g. myocardial infarction, congestive heart failure; obstruction of the renal vasculature by emboli; and increased renal vascular resistance due to surgery and anesthesia. In most instances pre-renal failure is readily reversible when the extra-renal factors are corrected. However, should the pre-renal cause be prolonged for an extended period, irreversible damage to the kidneys could result (7,14).

3. What is post-renal azotemia?

Post-renal azotemia is simply an accumulation of waste products which is caused by an obstruction along the urinary tract. Obstruction of the ureters may be caused by stones, blood clots, uric acid and sulfonamide crystals, and papillary necrosis from analgesic abuse. Tumors and retroperitoneal fibrosis (methysergide therapy) may also cause obstruction by impinging on or surrounding the ureters. Carcinoma, infection of the bladder, prostatic hypertrophy and ganglionic blockers may lead to bladder neck obstruction. Finally, there may even be obstruction along the urethra. The finding of anuria (no urine excretion) or alternating anuria and polyuria (large urine volume) in a patient with decreased renal function is very suggestive of obstruction. Removal of the obstruction, when possible, will reverse the renal failure (7,14).

4. When a patient such as B.M. suddenly develops oliguria and a rising BUN and creatinine, how is it determined whether it is pre-renal azotemia, post-

renal azotemia, or acute renal failure?

Since pre-renal and post-renal azotemia are usually readily reversible, precipitating causes must first be considered. Once these are excluded as an explanation of the patient's renal failure, then the diagnosis of acute renal failure must be considered.

A *history and physical examination* of the patient and specific serum and urine laboratory tests must be performed to elicit the cause of the azotemia. The physical examination should include percussion of the abdomen for an enlarged bladder, palpation for kidney enlargement, and a pelvic examination in females for cervical malignancy or a rectal examination in males for an enlarged prostate in order to rule out obstruction. In addition, excretion urography and bladder catheterization may be needed. To evaluate the presence of pre-renal azotemia, the clinician should be alert for signs of volume depletion such as dry mucous membranes, decreased skin turgor, and orthostatic hypotension with an increased pulse rate. B.M. exhibited many of the characteristic physical findings of pre-renal azotemia.

Specific *laboratory tests* are very helpful in distinguishing the cause of azotemia. In general, one can differentiate pre-renal failure from acute renal failure by examination of the urine. In pre-renal azotemia (in an otherwise normal patient) tubular function is intact and the kidney responds normally to a decrease in renal perfusion or volume depletion. Therefore, if oliguria is due to pre-renal factors, the urine should be highly concentrated; the urinary sodium concentration should be decreased, and the urine urea and creatinine concentrations should be increased. Generally, patients in acute or intra-renal failure do not have intact tubular function and will not be able to

conserve sodium and water normally.

Table 1, from Schrier (7,14) compares the usual urinary findings in pre-renal azotemia and acute renal failure. The urinary findings of the patient B.M. further substantiate a diagnosis of pre-renal azotemia as opposed to acute renal failure.

In addition to these findings, the plasma urea to creatinine ratio is greater than 10 to 1 in pre-renal azotemia.

Diuretic agents administered prior to the collection of urine for the above tests will decrease urine osmolality and increase urinary sodium concentration. Thus, interpretation of these urinary findings in a patient with pre-renal azotemia may seem to be more consistent with acute renal failure. Therefore, the urine must be obtained prior to diuretic administration.

Urine composition is not very useful in distinguishing post-renal failure from ARF, since in certain types of obstruction it may be similar to that of pre-renal azotemia or acute renal failure.

Some investigators utilize the response to a volume load or to diuretic agents (furosemide, mannitol) to distinguish pre-renal azotemia from acute renal failure. If the kidneys fail to increase the urine volume substantially, then the cause may be acute renal failure. Before administering fluids or mannitol, obstruction should be ruled out, since a fluid or diuretic challenge could lead to volume overload and congestive heart failure or pulmonary edema (7,9,14).

5. What are some of the general causes of acute renal failure?

There are a number of causes of acute renal failure. These may be classified into three major categories. The first are diseases affecting the glomerulus and small blood vessels of the kidney. Examples of this include: systemic lupus erythematosus, subacute bacterial endocarditis, acute post streptococcal glomerulonephritis, malignant hypertension, pregnancy and drug-induced vasculitis. The second category includes disorders that result in ischemia to the kidney: severe trauma, major hemorrhage, crush injuries, post-operative and blood transfusion reactions, and sepsis. The last major category is nephrotoxins. Included in this are the following chemicals or drugs: heavy metals (mercury), ethylene glycol, carbon tetrachloride, pesticides, radiocontrast media, and antibiotics. Finally, approximately 20% of the cases of ARF are termed idiopathic because no identifiable cause exists (7,9,14).

6. What are some of the complications of acute renal failure and how are they treated?

The major cause of death in patients with acute

TABLE 1
URINARY FINDINGS IN PRE-RENAL AZOTEMIA AND ACUTE RENAL FAILURE

	Pre-renal Azotemia	Acute Renal Failure
Urine sodium concentration	<10 mEq/L	>20 mEq/L
Urine to plasma urea ratio	>14 to 1	<14 to 1
Urine to plasma creatinine ratio	>14 to 1	<14 to 1
Urine osmolality	>100 mOsm/kg above plasma osmolality	≤plasma osmolality
Renal failure index $\left(\dfrac{U(Na)}{U/P\ Cr}\right)$	<1	>3
Urine sediment	Normal	cellular debris, casts, protein.

Adapted from Schrier, R. W. and Conger, J. D., 1976 (14).

renal failure is *infection.* Unfortunately, dialysis does not reduce this complication. Proper and careful use of intravenous and urinary catheters is mandatory, as is the correct dosage regimen of antibiotics used to treat the infection.

Maintaining proper *fluid and electrolyte balance* is a significant problem in acute renal failure. Since the renal failure may be either oliguric or nonoliguric, fluid and electrolyte losses may be either large or small. *Hyponatremia* may occur in nonoliguric acute renal failure if the sodium loss in the urine exceeds its replacement in intravenous fluids. *Hyperkalemia* may result from the diminished excretion of potassium as well as the acidosis and general catabolic state of the patient. Other complications that can take place in acute renal failure are hypocalcemia, hypercalcemia, hyperphosphatemia, hyperuricemia, hypermagnesemia, and metabolic acidosis. Treatment of some of these complications is discussed under chronic renal failure. Proper fluid balance is essential in these patients in order to avoid either volume depletion or volume overload. The latter may lead to hypertension, congestive heart failure or pulmonary edema. Hemodialysis is important in controlling fluid and electrolyte problems.

The *central nervous system* is affected in acute renal failure and may result in lethargy, confusion, agitation, hyperreflexia, asterixis, coma, and even seizures. In addition, *gastrointestinal disturbances* such as stomatitis, anorexia, nausea, vomiting and diarrhea may occur. Gastrointestinal hemorrhage may develop due to acute ulcerations in the stomach and colon. The bleeding diathesis of uremia and heparin administration during dialysis may further contribute to the GI bleeding. Finally, there may be acute *uremic pericarditis,* although this is infrequent. All of these complications are an indication for dialysis which is the primary treatment modality. In fact, prophylactic dialysis may be performed in order to prevent the development of uremic symptoms.

Additional complications seen in acute renal failure include anemia, leukocytosis and inadequate wound healing.

In conclusion, treatment of acute renal failure includes proper maintenance of fluid and electrolyte balance and an adequate caloric intake to prevent protein catabolism and a negative nitrogen balance. Both hemodialysis and peritoneal dialysis are major treatment modalities which have significantly reduced the morbidity and mortality from acute renal failure (7,9,14).

7. What is the rationale for the use of mannitol and furosemide in acute renal failure? How should they be used? What are the complications which may accompany their use?

Mannitol or potent diuretics such as furosemide or ethacrynic acid are commonly used in patients with acute renal failure (ARF). However, their exact role and clinical usefulness has not been established. In general, the sooner these agents are used after the acute episode begins, the greater the response will be. Early diuretic use may prevent acute pre-renal failure from progressing to irreversible parenchymal damage. In addition, diuretics may convert an oliguric ARF to the nonoliguric type. There is insufficient evidence that mannitol or furosemide will reverse ARF once it is established. Furthermore, their use in the prevention of acute renal failure is controversial.

Mannitol is a nondiffusable hexahydric sugar. Following intravenous administration, it distributes within the plasma and interstitial spaces, but does not enter cells (5,17). Dosage recommendations are quite variable, but, in general, 10 to 25 grams of mannitol are infused intravenously over approximately 5 to 10 minutes. Urine output is then measured, and if it is not greater than 40 ml/hour over a one to three hour period, a repeat dose may be given. Should the patient fail to respond to a second challenge, no further mannitol should be administered. If there is an adequate response (greater than 40 ml/hr), then mannitol should be continued, either by a continuous infusion or by repeated injections, in order to maintain a high rate of urinary flow (approximately 100 ml/hr). This is continued until the patient is able to sustain a sufficient urine output on his own. Within a 24-hour period, no more than 100 grams of mannitol should be administered unless the urinary flow rate exceeds 100 ml/hour.

Complications in the use of mannitol include excessive intravascular volume expansion, hyponatremia, fluid overload, pulmonary edema, congestive heart failure, and hypertension. Since mannitol is entirely excreted unchanged in the urine, patients with pre-existing renal failure can potentially accumulate the drug. Another consideration is that mannitol is available as a 25% super-saturated solution which commonly crystallizes. This can be avoided by heating the solution or using a less concentrated solution, e.g. 20%. (Also see chapter on Edema).

In patients with congestive heart failure, excessive hydration, or chronic renal failure, *furosemide* or *ethacrynic acid* may be used as alternatives. Furosemide is used more frequently since it is less ototoxic than ethacrynic acid (10,13). In terms of diuretic potency, however, they are essentially equivalent. In a number of studies, doses of 200 to 3200 mg of furosemide have been administered to obtain an adequate diuretic response (6,8,18). Initially an intravenous (bolus or infusion) dose of 80 mg is administered, which is then doubled every few hours until a high urine flow is achieved. Often, rather than using high dose furosemide, the patient is started on dialysis.

Side effects associated with the use of large parenteral doses of furosemide in renal failure include tinnitus and transient deafness (16,19). The hearing loss appears related to both the dose and rate of infusion of furosemide. Hyperuricemia, diarrhea and leg cramps may also be observed.

8. What is the recovery phase and prognosis of acute renal failure?

Following an episode of acute renal failure, urine volume progressively increases. This *diuretic phase* signals the return of renal function and usually begins two days to six weeks after oliguria. Again, it is important that attention be given to proper fluid and electrolyte balance during this phase, which may last from a few days to several weeks. Over the next several months, renal function will progressively improve and in most cases complete clinical recovery results. However, creatinine clearance does not completely return to normal in the majority of patients, especially the elderly. Thus, many are left with a mild reduction in glomerular filtration rate and maximum concentrating ability, but this decreased function is often not clinically important. Rarely, this mild renal impairment may progress after recovery from the initial episode of acute renal failure (7,9,14).

CHRONIC RENAL FAILURE:

M.S. is a 49-year-old female with chronic renal failure secondary to a long history of diabetes and hypertension. She presently has been admitted to the hospital with a chief complaint of severe abdominal pain, nausea, and vomiting. An upper gastrointestinal series has revealed a small peptic ulcer. She also complains of arthritic type pain in her knees and hands, for which she has been treating herself with aspirin. Because the aspirin frequently caused her gastrointestinal irritation, she has been taking Maalox with each dose. On physical examination she appears pale and in moderate distress from her abdominal pain. Her blood pressure was 170/100 mm Hg; her heart rate was 70/minute and her respiratory rate was 14/minute. Her eye grounds revealed arteriolar narrowing without exudates. Heart and chest examination were within normal limits. Her extremities revealed characteristic arthritic changes. No spleen or liver enlargement were noted. X-ray showed bony deformities secondary to arthritis. Laboratory data included the following:

Sodium 143 mEq/L
Potassium 5.8 mEq/L
Chloride 110 mEq/L
Bicarbonate 18 mEq/L

Calcium 7.5 mg%
Phosphate 5.4 mg%
Uric acid 12 mg%
Hemoglobin 8 gm%
Hematocrit 24%
Platelet count 74,000/mm³
Glucose fasting 200 mg%
Serum creatinine 6.0 mg%
Blood urea nitrogen 80 mg%
Creatinine clearance 20 ml/min
Her present medications include:
Hydrochlorothiazide 50 mg bid
Aldomet 500 mg qid
Maalox 30 cc prn
ASA 600 mg prn
Regular insulin 10 units q AM

9. What is the definition of chronic renal failure? What are the causes of chronic renal failure?

Chronic renal failure may be defined as a progressive deterioration in renal function as evidenced by a rise in BUN and serum creatinine, a decline in creatinine clearance, and the development of uremic symptoms. The term *uremia* refers to the symptom complex associated with severe renal functional impairment. It may take months, or even years, to reach what is termed end-stage renal failure. The downhill progression of renal function depends on the primary cause of the renal failure, the frequency of relapsing episodes of acute renal failure, and on the occurrence of complications which accompany renal failure (1,20-28).

The causes of chronic renal failure are multiple; some of them are: prolonged acute renal failure, chronic pyelonephritis, idiopathic glomerulonephritis, poststreptococcal glomerulonephritis and polycystic kidney disease. Some systemic diseases leading to chronic renal failure are diabetes, amyloidosis, systemic lupus erythematosus (SLE), and hypertension. Nephrotoxic compounds such as analgesics, antibiotics, and heavy metals can also cause chronic renal failure. The degree of renal failure and the rapidity with which the end stage is reached depend upon the type and severity of disease state involved. For example, a patient with diffuse proliferative nephritis secondary to lupus has a poorer prognosis than a lupus patient with a focal proliferative renal lesion (1,20-28).

10. Is chronic renal failure reversible?

In general, kidney damage which leads to chronic renal failure is irreversible. However, there are cases in which renal function that is already compromised may become further reduced over a period of days to months because of reversible pre-renal or post-renal factors. These reversible factors must be sought and corrected to prevent further deterioration of the patient's renal function and to restore it to pre-existing levels. These factors include obstructive uropathy, urinary tract infection, or any cause of acute renal failure which diminishes renal perfusion. (See Questions 2 and 3.) Drugs can also cause reversible renal toxicity. Examples include diuretic-induced hypovolemia; decreased renal perfusion secondary to antihypertensives; and nephrotoxic compounds such as methicillin, amphotericin, cephaloridine and the aminoglycosides. Obstruction can also occur secondary to crystalluria induced by sulfonamides, uricosurics, or radiocontrast dyes (1,20-28).

11. What are the major complications of chronic renal failure?

The major complications of chronic renal failure include the following:

Hematological	anemia
Hemostatic defects	bleeding
Metabolic	carbohydrate intolerance
	hyperuricemia
Endocrine	abnormalities in calcium and phosphorus
	hyperparathyroidism
	renal osteodystrophy
	sexual dysfunction
	infertility
Cardiovascular	hypertension
	congestive heart failure
	pericarditis
	atherosclerosis
Gastrointestinal	anorexia
	nausea
	vomiting
	G.I. bleeding
	ulcers
Neurological	headache
	lethargy
	muscular irritability and cramps
	asterixis
	paresthesias
	motor weakness
	seizures
	coma
Dermatological	pallor
	hyperpigmentation
	ecchymosis
	pruritus
	uremic frost
	calcium deposition
Fluid/Electrolyte	sodium and potassium imbalance
	acidosis
	extracellular fluid imbalance
Psychological	depression
	anxiety
	psychosis
Infection	increased susceptibility
	hepatitis

Some of these complications of chronic renal failure are discussed in more detail in the following sections (1,20-28).

12. What are the characteristics of the anemia of chronic renal failure? What is its etiology and how is it treated?

Patients with chronic renal failure inevitably develop anemia, and the occurrence of pallor and fatigue are the earliest clinical signs. The anemia usually becomes evident when the creatinine clearance falls to approximately 25 to 50 ml/min (24,34,45). Although there is no absolute correlation between the BUN and hematocrit or hemoglobin, as uremia becomes progressively severe, the anemia worsens. It has been demonstrated that patients with chronic glomerulonephritis with BUN values over 100 mg% had, as a group, significantly lower hemoglobin values than patients with BUN values of less than 100 mg%.

The anemia of chronic renal failure, will usually stabilize at a hematocrit value of approximately 20 to 25% in the absence of other associated anemias. The anemia is characteristically normochromic and normocytic in nature unless a concomitant iron or folate deficiency exists. Uremic anemia is generally well-tolerated except in elderly patients, or those with angina pectoris, cerebral ischemia or congestive heart failure.

A number of factors have been demonstrated to contribute to the anemia of chronic renal failure. *Reduced erythrocyte production* appears to be the most significant etiologic factor. Due to progressive damage to kidney tissue, erythropoietin production, an endocrine product of the kidney, is diminished (33,34). As a result, red blood cell formation in the marrow is reduced and anemia occurs. However, the fact that anephric patients can respond, (though inefficiently) to hemorrhage or hypoxia with a reticulocytosis demonstrates that total hormonal control of erythropoiesis may not lie within the kidney. In fact, extrarenal production, through a hepatic erythropoietin globulin has been described (42). However, this non-renal source is minimal, since anephric patients usually cannot stimulate erythropoiesis as well as patients with remnant kidneys (34).

Inhibitors of erythropoiesis may also exist in the plasma of patients with chronic renal failure. These substances may inhibit the production of erythropoietin, the bone marrow response to erythropoietin and/or the synthesis of heme (34). The existence of these substances is confirmed by the observation that dialyzed patients who have no increase in blood erythropoietin levels display improvement in erythropoiesis. This, as well as other evidence, indicates that there may be a dialyzable erythroid depressant factor in renal failure (34,42,47).

The red blood cell lifespan is reduced to 30 to 60% of normal values in chronic renal failure patients. The *hemolysis* is generally mild, and is due to the abnormal chemical environment of uremia. The exact nature of these hemolytic factors in uremic plasma is unknown, and the hemolysis is not uniformly reversed with dialysis. Other causes contributing to or aggravating the hemolysis are malignant hypertension, hypersplenism, and dialysis fluid that has been contaminated with copper, nitrates, or chloramine. In addition use of a hypotonic dialysate may lead to a fatal hemolytic episode (34). Yawata et al (51) found that 50% of uremic patients have a uremic plasma factor which inhibits the RBC hexose monophosphate shunt's ability to generate NADPH, thereby reducing the RBC's ability to handle oxidative stress. Hence, survival is reduced. Some patients may need to be screened for red-cell hexose monophosphate shunt deficiency since drugs known to cause glucose-6-phosphate dehydrogenase hemolytic anemia may produce the same reaction in these patients.

Blood loss is a frequent contributing factor to the anemia of chronic renal disease (34). Because of the impaired hemostasis of uremia, gastrointestinal tract and intradermal bleeding are frequent. More often than not, these patients have positive guaiac stools. In addition, dialysis patients have an obligate blood loss that is related to the techniques and complications inherent in dialysis. Patients on hemodialysis are always given heparin during the procedure and occasionally they may be receiving warfarin or antiplatelet drugs to prevent clotting. Thus, bleeding may occur from the administration of these drugs.

Iron deficiency may develop, especially in dialysis patients, secondary to the blood loss. Some studies have shown that iron absorption from the gastrointestinal tract in uremic patients is reduced compared to controls. However, other studies have demonstrated no difference, or even greater absorption in uremics (36,44).

Folic acid deficiency as evidenced by low folate levels and macrocytosis is not uncommon in renal failure (39,41,43,50). However, a recent study by Paine et al (46) noted subnormal serum folate levels in only 10% of chronic renal failure patients not on dialysis, and none had a megaloblastic anemia. Nevertheless, folate deficiency occurs most frequently in patients on dialysis since folic acid is readily removed by dialysis (49).

The treatment of the anemia of chronic renal failure includes a variety of approaches. Initially it is important to correct any iron deficiency, and the patient is usually treated with oral *iron,* such as ferrous sulfate 300 mg three times a day, or parenteral iron if the patient shows evidence of malabsorption. Iron is not significantly removed by dialysis. *Folic acid* is usually administered by oral supplementation at a dose of 1 mg per day. Thus, patients on dialysis frequently receive iron, folic acid, and a multivitamin. In addition, adequate nutrition from the diet is important (43).

At the initiation of *hemodialysis,* the hematocrit frequently falls and then progressively increases over the next 6 to 12 months. The effect of dialysis on erythropoiesis rarely restores hematocrit to normal but can raise it up to the low thirties in some patients (34). Although it does not fully correct the defect, regular dialysis has been shown to improve erythrokinetics and is essential in the management of uremic anemia (30,42).

Blood transfusions are avoided, if possible, in patients with chronic renal failure because there is risk of hepatitis, iron overload, and further suppression of erythropoiesis. There is also the risk of sensitizing a potential kidney transplant recipient to HLA antigens on the anticipated renal allograft (37). However, this issue is controversial (27) and transfusions are given periodically in order to restore the oxygen carrying capacity of the blood and to alleviate patient's symptoms.

Androgens can increase erythropoiesis in many chronic renal failure patients. They act by directly or indirectly raising erythropoietin levels, thereby increasing RBC production. Various clinical trials have been conducted using a number of androgenic compounds at different dosages. The interpretation of many of these studies is complicated because most are not controlled and patients were sometimes iron and vitamin deficient, given blood transfusion, or not treated for sufficient periods of time. Thus, direct comparison of the data to determine which androgen is the most suitable or the most potent is extremely difficult.

The different androgens used include the orally administered 17-alpha-alkylated androgens such as oxymetholone and methyltestosterone; testosterone esters such as testosterone enanthate; and 19-nortestosterone derivatives such as nandrolone decanoate, both of which are given intramuscularly. Male patients usually require larger amounts of a given androgen than females to elicit a similar hematologic response. Furthermore, anephric patients generally do not respond as well to androgen therapy as do patients with intact kidneys. The reason for this difference is not readily explainable, but may be related to the doses of the individual androgens. In addition, kidney remnants appear to be essential for androgen-induced rises in erythropoietin. Nephrectomized patients may require a higher dose of androgen. Finally, the maximum response from androgen therapy may not occur until three months or more after treatment has been initiated.

Side effects reported from the use of androgens in chronic renal failure patients on dialysis include: virilization, weight gain, muscle soreness, abnormal hair growth, priapism, acne, as well as swelling and hematoma at injection sites. Some of these effects are particularly disturbing to female patients who sometimes refuse androgen therapy. Hepatic dysfunction with hepatomegaly and abnormal liver function tests may occur. The orally administered 17-alpha-alkylated compounds are generally considered more hepatotoxic than the others and have been associated with the development of hepatocellular carcinoma.

However, despite these effects, androgens are useful to dialysis patients in improving their anemia and in reducing symptoms. In addition, the androgens may reduce the number of blood transfusions required. Nandrolone decanoate (Decadurabolin) 100-200mg is commonly administered intramuscularly at weekly intervals. Alternative therapy includes oral administration of fluoxymesterone (Halotestin) in doses of 30 mg/day for males and 10 mg/day for females. At least three to six months should be allowed for evaluation of an adequate response, and monitoring for adverse effects is essential (29,31,32,35,37,38,40,42,48).

Other methods that have been used in treating the anemia of chronic renal failure include splenectomy, histidine supplementation and even exogenous erythropoietin (24,34).

13. Describe the hemostatic defects in uremia. How are they managed?

Uremia is frequently complicated by excessive bleeding as evidenced by ecchymosis, purpura, low-grade gastrointestinal bleeding, epistaxis, and, less commonly, profuse gastrointestinal hemorrhage.

The estimates of moderate to severe hemorrhage vary from 12 to 63% of patients depending on the study (55). Capillary fragility and a decrease in plasma coagulation factors have been excluded by most as major causes of uremic bleeding. A quantitative deficiency of platelets in uremics has been suggested as a cause for the bleeding tendency in uremics since thrombocytopenia (less than 150,000/mm³) has been reported in up to 53% of renal failure patients. However, values of less than 50,000/mm³ are rarely seen (55), and it is generally agreed that thrombocytopenia is not a significant causative factor of uremic bleeding. Platelet lifespan has also been shown to be normal. A functional platelet defect in uremic platelets has been demonstrated although its exact nature is unknown. Earlier reports suggested an inhibition or deficiency of platelet factor 3 (52,54,56); however, the prolonged bleeding times observed in uremics cannot

totally be accounted for on this basis. The possibility of defects in platelet adhesion and ADP-induced aggregation have also been considered. Apparently, abnormalities of several platelet functions lead to the overall platelet defect (54,56).

A specific uremic toxin responsible for defective platelet function has not been identified. However, guanidinosuccinic acid, phenol, and phenolic acids, toxins that are known to accululate in uremia, have been shown to produce qualitative platelet defects. Whatever the specific toxin, the platelet abnormalities of uremia can be corrected and normal hemostasis maintained with frequent hemodialysis or peritoneal dialysis. Whenever bleeding occurs, thorough dialysis is the treatment of choice (54).

A regular dialysis program and avoidance of antiplatelet drugs can substantially reduce the occurrence of uremic bleeding. A list of drugs which have clinically important antiplatelet activity is provided below:

acetylsalicylic acid	indomethacin
carbenicillin	oxyphenbutazone
dextran	penicillin G
dipyridamole	phenylbutazone
hydroxychloroquine	sulfinpyrazone
(53,57).	

14. What effect does renal failure have on calcium metabolism?

Hypocalcemia associated with hyperphosphatemia and vitamin D resistance are frequent problems of chronic renal failure which may lead to the secondary complication of renal osteodystrophy. The low serum calcium is usually well tolerated because of concomitant parathyroid stimulation and acidosis which maintain free ionized calcium at near normal levels. Rapid fluctuation in the pH, especially toward alkalosis, should be avoided since tetany can be precipitated.

Hyperphosphatemia is one of the earliest causes of low calcium levels in renal failure. As the creatinine clearance begins to fall, the amount of filtered phosphate also begins to fall. However, a secondary elevation in parathyroid hormone (PTH), stimulated by a slight phosphate-induced hypocalcemia, maintains normal phosphate and calcium levels. PTH enhances phosphate excretion by inhibiting tubular reabsorption of phosphate, mobilizing bone calcium, and increasing gastrointestinal absorption of calcium. However, as creatinine clearance falls below 25 cc/min, parathyroid hormone inhibition of phosphate reabsorption can no longer maintain phosphate excretion because of the small amount of phosphate which is filtered. Phosphate levels begin to rise, which in turn causes calcium levels to fall, the latter stimulating further parathyroid hormone secretion. The parathyroid attempts to maintain normal calcium levels, despite the concomitant hyperphosphatemia, by increasing bone resorption and increasing gastrointestinal absorption of calcium. This secondary hyperparathyroidism results in an elevated calcium-phosphate solubility product (Ca x PO₄) which predisposes the patient to deposition of calcium salts in the kidney, blood vessels, heart and other vital organs. The secondary hyperparathyroidism also leads to bone resorption and fibrosis which is evidenced radiologically as osteitis fibrosa cystica.

Furthermore, vitamin D resistance also plays an important role in uremic hypocalcemia. This resistance, which can occur in mild degrees of renal insufficiency, is due to an inability of the kidney to convert 25-hydroxycholecalciferol to the active hormonal form of vitamin D, 1,25-dihydroxycholecalciferol. An elevated renal intracellular concentration of phosphate also inhibits vitamin D activation and may be a causative factor of vitamin D resistance in renal failure.

Vitamin D resistance decreases gastrointestinal absorption of dietary calcium and phosphate, reduces sensitivity of bone to parathyroid hormone, and enhances the development of defective bone mineralization (osteomalacia). Despite high circulating levels of parathyroid hormone, calcium levels are reduced because of parathyroid hormone insensitivity. This results in a low calcium-phosphate solubility product.

Invariably, most patients will demonstrate biochemical and pathological features of both vitamin D resistance and hyperparathyroidism. Bony lesions vary, with most patients exhibiting both osteomalacia and osteitis fibrosa cystica, known collectively as renal osteodystrophy. Calcium-phosphate solubility products also vary depending upon the predominance of vitamin D resistance or hyperparathyroidism. Below is a diagram summarizing the calcium abnormalities of renal failure (Fig. 1) (58,59,75,76,91).

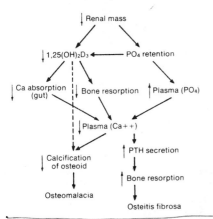

Figure 1: Pathogenisis of secondary hyperparathyroidism and osteodystrophy (osteitis fibrosa plus osteomalacia) in chronic renal insufficiency. Adapted from Kidney International (reference 78) with permission.

15. How should the calcium abnormalities and bone disease of renal failure be managed?

Due to the improved survival of patients with renal failure associated with the advent of hemodialysis, the occurrence of symptomatic renal osteodystrophy has increased (59). Since multiple factors are involved in the development of renal osteodystrophy, the therapeutic approach for each patient must be individualized.

Specific treatment of calcium abnormalities and bone disease in renal failure is based primarily on: serum calcium, phosphate, and PTH levels; histologic/radiologic appraisal of renal osteodystrophy; and the degree of clinical disability (59).

Initial therapeutic management of these patients includes replacement of *water soluble vitamins* (especially ascorbic acid and pyridoxine) which are essential for normal bone metabolism (59).

Early in the course of renal failure, efforts are made to lower serum phosphate and reverse secondary hyperparathyroidism. Hyperphosphatemia is commonly treated by *dietary phosphate restriction* and by administering 15 to 30 cc of *aluminum carbonate* (Basaljel) or *aluminum hydroxide* (Amphojel) with or immediately following each meal and at bedtime. Aluminum hydroxide capsules may also be useful in this regard. Aluminum binds dietary phosphate as well as gastrointestinal secretions of phosphate and as a result lowers the serum phosphate level. Aluminum antacid therapy, by its effective control of serum phosphate, can reverse metastatic calcification and osteitis fibrosa cystica (59,90,94). (Also see Question 16.) Hypophosphatemia should be avoided to prevent a reciprocal hypercalcemia and bony demineralization. Control of phosphate levels with phosphate binding antacids may also partially or completely reverse vitamin D resistance, because intracellular phosphate levels within the renal tubular cells may regulate 1,25-dihydroxycholecalciferol production. High phosphate levels can inhibit activation of vitamin D and form 24,25-dihydroxycholecalciferol instead, which is believed to be an inactive product in man (76).

Calcium salts and vitamin D or both must be instituted cautiously, and only after phosphate levels have been lowered in order to prevent metastatic calcifications.

Calcium salts are indicated in uremic patients, since both vitamin D dependent and independent calcium absorptive processes are impaired when creatinine clearances approach 25 ml/min (59). Low protein diets also compound the problem, since dietary calcium is also reduced (70,71,77). Large supplements of calcium can overcome malabsorption defects because they are probably absorbed by passive ionic diffusion which is independent of vitamin D (59,71). In this manner, patients can maintain their calcium levels without vitamin D therapy. Supplemental calcium should be given in a minimum dose of 1.5 mEq/kg/day (approximately 2 gm of elemental calcium for a 70 kg man) (59,70). Larger doses of 4 to 10 gm/day can be given if necessary (59,66,71). Although calcium absorption from the carbonate salt is not maximal (71), this salt is commonly recommended because it aids in the reduction of acidosis (83,85,95). In dialyzed patients, the use of a high calcium concentration in the renal dialysate is another method of improving calcium balance (59).

Prophylactic *vitamin D* is only indicated for those patients with symptomatic and radiologically evident bone demineralization (rickets or osteomalacia) secondary to vitamin D resistance. Large doses of vitamin D (cholecalciferol or ergocalciferol) are usually required because of the decreased conversion in renal failure of vitamin D to an active form. Vitamin D therapy should be initiated carefully because the long half-life of the drug could lead to the development of sustained hypercalcemia and nephrocalcinosis (73). In addition, the degree of vitamin D resistance is not known for the individual patient. An initial dose of 10,000 to 20,000 units per day of vitamin D should be used and slowly increased as needed (59,61,95). Some patients may require 10 to 50 times the normal therapeutic dose of vitamin D.

Because of the relative inactivity of vitamin D in renal failure, the use of *dihydrotachysterol (DHT)*, which does not require renal activation (59,80,93), has been suggested. This drug also has the advantage of a short duration of action (79,81). Doses of 0.25 to 0.375 mg/day (up to 1 mg in some patients) of DHT have been used successfully in dialyzed patients to reverse calcium absorption defects and to clinically and radiologically improve renal bone disease (72, 80, 81, 93). Equivalent doses of cholecalciferol were ineffective. Doses of DHT that are effective in dialyzed patients are not effective in non-dialyzed patients, suggesting that additional non-specific dialyzable factors may reduce this drug's effectiveness (80); thus, greater doses of DHT may be necessary for non-dialyzed patients.

There has been extensive research on the possible usefulness of the active vitamin D metabolites in reversing calcium abnormalities in renal failure. Brickman et al (61,62,63,64) administered *1,25-dihydroxycholecalciferol*, the active form of vitamin D, in molar equivalents of up to 100 units of cholecalciferol per day to renal failure patients. A rapid increase in calcium absorption and a rise in serum calcium was observed. Doses of up to 40,000 units of cholecalciferol produced no significant change in calcium levels and absorption. The data indicate the possible benefits of using active vitamin D metabolites in treating renal osteodystrophy (59,76).

Since the production of 1,25-dihydroxycholecal-ciferol is costly, less expensive and highly active congeners which also do not require renal activation are presently being investigated. At this time, *1-alpha-hydroxycholecalciferol*, a vitamin D_3 analog which requires hepatic activation to 1,25-dihydroxycholecalciferol is undergoing extensive clinical trials. Initial results are promising (65, 66, 67, 68, 69, 74, 75, 82, 84, 86, 87). A majority of patients with renal osteodystrophy treated with 1-alpha-hydroxycholecalciferol orally in doses of 1 to 4 mcg/day have shown increased calcium absorption, a reduction in circulating parathyroid hormone levels, and enhanced bone mineralization with histologic, roentgenographic and symptomatic improvement of renal bone disease. Calcium levels should be closely monitored since hypercalcemia is a possible side effect (66,82,86). Elevated calcium levels decrease rapidly within 24 to 48 hours following withdrawal of 1-alpha-hydroxycholecalciferol (66,82,84,86), which is an advantage of this drug over other vitamin D analogs. Additionally, coadministration of anticonvulsant agents may blunt the response to this drug (88,89).

Pharmacologic doses (100 to 500 mcg/day) of *25-hydroxycholecalciferol* given orally are also effective in improving calcium absorption and in reversing renal bone disease in dialyzed patients (59,92). These results indicate that 25-hydroxycholecalciferol, even in anephric patients where activation to 1,25-dihydroxycholecalciferol does not occur, may have some therapeutic value.

In the rare patient with resistant secondary hyperthyroidism, parathyroidectomy may be indicated (59).

16. What are the uses and complications of antacid therapy in renal failure patients?

Antacids are commonly employed in renal failure patients for a variety of reasons. These patients may have significant gastrointestinal (GI) upset and ulceration caused by local irritation from ammonia or other uremic toxins on the GI tract. In addition, many of them receive concomitant corticosteriod therapy or other GI irritating drugs. Finally, they take antacids to bind dietary phosphate for reasons discussed previously. (See Question 15.)

Therapy to decrease phosphate levels is usually initiated with 30 ml of an aluminum-containing antacid, administered with, or immediately following meals. The aluminum binds with dietary phosphate forming an insoluble complex which is unabsorbable and excreted in the stool. The chemical reaction occurring within the gastrointestinal tract is demonstrated by the following equation (101):

$$Al(OH)_3 + 3HCl \longrightarrow AlCl_3 + 3H_2O$$
$$AlCl_3 + PO_4 \longrightarrow AlPO_4 + 3Cl$$
$$(insoluble)$$

Phosphate binding capacity varies directly with the

quantitative amount of aluminum contained in the antacid preparation. Of the aluminum containing antacids, aluminum carbonate gel (Basaljel) appears to demonstrate the greatest phosphate binding capacity, whereas the magaldrate (Riopan) shows the least ability to bind phosphate. (See Table 2.)

TABLE 2
PHOSPHATE BINDING CAPACITY OF SELECTED ANTACIDS

Product	Contents	Phosphate Binding Capacity	Elemental Aluminum Content (gm/30 ml)
Amphojel	Aluminum hydroxide	+2	0.636
Basaljel	Aluminum carbonate	+4	0.87
Phosphaljel	Aluminum phosphate	0	
Gelusil	Aluminum & magnesium hydroxide	+3	
Maalox	Aluminum & magnesium hydroxide	+3	0.716
Mylanta	Aluminum & magnesium hydroxide & simethicone	+2	
Riopan	Aluminum-magnesium Hydroxide complex	+1	0.276
Titralac	Calcium carbonate & glycine	0	0

*Adapted from Bailey (101).

Aluminum antacid therapy is not without hazard, however. *Excessive phosphate depletion,* secondary to aluminum antacid therapy and dialysis can result in multiple complications (96,104,105,107,109,111,112). These include hypercalcemia, hypercalciuria, osteomalacia and fracture caused by enhanced resorption of skeletal calcium and phosphorus, as well as defects in erythrocyte, leukocyte, and platelet function related to decreased adenosine triphosphate levels. The symptoms of phosphate depletion include generalized muscle weakness, malaise, tremors, absence of deep tendon reflexes, bone pain, mental depression, convulsions, and even coma. The complications of hypophosphatemia are generally reversible upon phosphate replacement.

Long-term administration of aluminum may not in itself be without toxicity. Aluminum antacids are supposedly nonabsorbable, and aluminum does not appear to accumulate in normal subjects after repeated doses of aluminum compounds (114). Nevertheless, significant *elevations in serum* and *tissue aluminum* have been noted in renal failure patients receiving aluminum hydroxide. Berlyne et al (102,103) have described a syndrome of aluminum toxicity in uremic rats consisting of periorbital bleeding, lethargy, anorexia, and death. Elevated plasma levels of aluminum as well as deposition of aluminum in numerous organs including the brain, liver, heart, muscle, and

especially bone was found. Berlyne et al recommend that the use of aluminum salts in renal failure patients be curtailed because of the possibility of aluminum toxicity. However, their failure to measure phosphate levels as well as their administration of parenteral and soluble oral salts of aluminum make their conclusions difficult to evaluate (100). In fact, Thurston et al (117) found that even though small amounts of aluminum are absorbed and deposited in bone, no toxicity related to aluminum itself could be demonstrated in uremic rats. They did show, however, that in normal rats growth-stunting, secondary to aluminum antacid therapy, was related to phosphate depletion. It is thought that some of the toxicity related to aluminum antacid treatment is related to phosphate depletion and can be prevented by avoidance of hypophosphatemia.

Alfrey et al (97) also demonstrated elevated levels of aluminum in muscle, bone, and brain tissue in dialyzed patients who were receiving aluminum antacid therapy. They suggest a relationship between the excess aluminum levels and the development of a fatal neurologic syndrome referred to as the dialysis encephalopathy syndrome. Additional studies are needed to further define this complication.

Magnesium-containing products should be used cautiously, if at all, in renal failure patients. Significant amounts of magnesium from antacids and cathartics can be absorbed from the gastrointestinal tract. Since magnesium levels within the body are controlled by glomerular filtration and distal tubular reabsorption, a lowering of the glomerular filtration rate below 20 ml/min results in a reduced clearance of magnesium (98,99,116,119,120). If a patient with this degree of renal failure or worse is presented with a magnesium load, *magnesium intoxication* may develop. The occurrence of magnesium toxicity in renal failure patients, secondary to antacid or cathartic therapy, is well documented (98,108,113). Ingestion of 150 to 300 ml per day of magnesium-containing products can result in rapid intoxication in these patients (101). Moderate amounts of magnesium-containing antacids can be used if the patient is on regular dialysis (e.g. hemodialysis for six hours, three times a week) and avoids ingestion of large quantities of magnesium. However, if the patient has severe renal dysfunction that does not yet require dialysis or is on irregular maintenance dialysis, magnesium compounds should be avoided.

Hypermagnesemia is evidenced clinically by central nervous system signs of lethargy, weakness, hyporeflexia, and hypotension. Electrocardiographic abnormalities can be noted at serum concentrations of 8 mEq/L, while complete heart block, coma, and respiratory depression usually occur at higher blood levels. Treatment for hypermagnesemia consists of administration of parenteral calcium salts (5 to 10 mEq) if severe symptoms of intoxication such as respiratory depression or cardiac arrhythmias are present. Unfortunately, calcium injections are not uniformly effective (98,99). If kidney function is adequate, intravenous furosemide and saline administration can be used to enhance renal magnesium excreation. Dialysis against a bath containing little (1.5 mEq/L) or no magnesium can substantially reduce magnesium levels within four to six hours (98). In addition, all magnesium-containing preparations should be discontinued.

Calcium-containing antacids should also be used with caution because of the possibility of developing the milk alkali syndrome, hypercalcemia, nephrocalcinosis, and/or worsening renal function (106,115). Calcium carbonate also has been associated with a rebound increase in gastric acid secretion (110). The significance of this in patients with renal failure is not yet determined. However, this problem is of concern since calcium preparations seem to be effective acid-neutralizing agents, and patients with renal failure frequently receive calcium salts for calcium replacement therapy. (Also see chapter on Peptic Ulcer Disease.)

Constipation and fecal impaction are also associated with calcium and aluminum antacids. In fact, intestinal obstruction may even result due to the development of solid concretions of antacid in the intestine, especially in patients with renal failure (118). Such obstructions have resulted in rectal-vaginal fistula formation and may require surgical intervention and removal.

17. How is potassium balance affected by chronic renal failure?

Most of the daily load of potassium, approximately 100 mEq, is removed from the body by the kidney. Gastrointestinal losses account for only minimal amounts of potassium elimination.

Potassium is normally filtered at the glomerulus and undergoes nearly complete reabsorption throughout the renal tubule. The potassium excreted in the urine is chiefly the result of distal tubular secretion. A variety of factors affect this distal secretion of potassium including: aldosterone, sodium load presented to the distal reabsorptive site, hydrogen ion secretion, the amount of unreabsorbable anions, urinary flow-rate, diuretics, and potassium intake (125,133,138).

Serum potassium levels are relatively well-maintained within normal limits in patients with chronic renal failure. With a creatinine clearance greater than 5 ml per minute, the development of hyperkalemia is rare without an endogenous or exogenous load of potassium. This balance is maintained despite a decreasing nephron population and an overall drop in glomerular filtration. The remaining nephron population undergoes adaptive hypertrophy to enhance the distal tubular secretion of potassium per nephron, which is mediated by elevated levels of aldosterone. Increased gastrointestinal secretion and fecal losses may account for up to 50% of the daily potassium losses in patients with severe renal insufficiency (1,125). The gut secretion of potassium is controlled in part by aldosterone and can be inhibited by spironolactone (135).

Episodic *hyperkalemia* can develop in a patient with chronic renal failure under several conditions. Excess potassium loads may result from exogenous sources such as increased dietary intake or drugs. (See Table 3.)

TABLE 3
POTASSIUM CONTENT OF SELECTED DRUGS (129)

Drug	Potassium Content (mg/dose)
Bromo-Seltzer	53.2/80 grains
Co-Salt	390/gm
Effersyllium Powder	293/teaspoon
Ex Lax	27.5/tablet
Potassium Penicillin G	66/million units
Quadrinal Tablets	76/tablet
Sumycin Syrup	26.5/5cc
Viokase Powder	1020/100 gm

Endogenous sources of potassium include cellular destruction, as for example in the hemolysis of red blood cells, rhabdomyolysis, and catabolic states. Metabolic or respiratory acidosis may cause a redistribution of intracellular potassium to the extracellular space. For each 0.1 unit change in blood pH, there is a corresponding opposite change of 0.6 mEq/L in the serum potassium level (1). Potassium-sparing diuretics such as spironolactone or triamterene should be avoided in the presence of renal failure since they decrease tubular secretion of potassium, and their use has been associated with fatal hyperkalemia (124,126). Diabetic patients with normal renal function may develop hyperkalemia from the administration of these diuretics (125). Some diabetic patients with only mild degrees of renal failure may also develop hyperkalemia as a result of low plasma renin levels and subsequently lowered aldosterone levels (1,125).

Paradoxically, *hypokalemia* can occur in chronic renal failure patients. The potassium deficiency can be due to inadequate dietary intake or excessive gastrointestinal (GI) losses. This is related to the anorexia, nausea, vomiting, and diarrhea which accompanies the GI irritation that occurs in the uremic patient. Protracted vomiting may lead to hypokalemia through induction of a hypochloremic alkalosis and through loss of potassium rich fluids. Furthermore, hypovolemia and other conditions may induce hyperaldosteronism which will enhance urinary losses of potassium (1,125).

Other causes of hypokalemia include glucocorticoid therapy, Cushing's syndrome, licorice abuse, laxative abuse, excessive diuretic therapy, and renal tubular acidosis (125). Also see chapters on Fluids and Electrolytes and Congestive Heart Failure.

18. How should hyperkalemia be treated?

Treatment of hyperkalemia depends upon the serum level of potassium as well as the presence or absence of symptoms and electrocardiographic (ECG) changes. Manifestations of hyperkalemia include weakness, confusion, and muscular or respiratory paralysis. Early ECG changes include peaked T waves, followed by a decreased R wave amplitude, widened QRS complex, and a prolonged P-R interval. This may progress to complete heart block with absent P waves and finally a sine wave occurs. Ventricular arrhythmias or cardiac arrest may ensue if no effort to lower serum potassium is initiated. Hyperkalemic ECG changes are uncommon at potassium levels of less than 7 mEq/L but occur regularly at levels above 8 mEq/L.

Usually no specific treatment is required if hyperkalemia is mild (less than 6.5 mEq/L), and if there are no ECG changes or only peaked T waves. If potassium levels rise above 6.5 mEq/L, especially with neuromuscular symptoms or changes in the ECG, treatment should be instituted.

Treatment of hyperkalemia consists of three basic modalities. The first is calcium administration to counteract the effects of excess potassium on the heart. Second, glucose or alkali therapy lowers serum potassium by shifting it from extracellular to intracellular fluid compartments. Thirdly, exchange resins or dialysis are used to remove potassium from the body.

In the presence of life-threatening arrhythmias, five to ten ml of a 10% calcium gluconate solution may be given intravenously over 2 minutes to antagonize the cardiac toxicity of hyperkalemia. The injection may be repeated in five minutes and continous monitoring of the ECG is mandatory. The cardiac response to an injection of calcium begins within 5 minutes and lasts from 1 to 2 hours. Since administration of calcium does not lower the serum potassium, other modes of treatment must also be instituted. Patients receiving digitalis should be given calcium cautiously.

Additional emergency treatment consists of sodium bicarbonate 50 mEq injected intravenously over 5 minutes. This may be repeated every 10 to 15 minutes as needed to reverse ECG abnormalities. Sodium bicarbonate is used since the alkaline systemic pH it produces favors the shift of potassium intracellularly, and because the sodium load enhances distal tubular potassium secretion. It should be used cautiously in patients with congestive heart failure.

Glucose plus insulin infusions also shift potassium intracellularly. One unit of insulin for every 2 grams of glucose is administered. Two to three hundred ml of a 20% glucose solution containing 20 to 30 units of regular insulin are infused over 30 to 60 minutes. This should produce a 1 to 2 mEq/L reduction of serum potassium for approximately 12 to 24 hours. The glucose-insulin infusion can then be continued at a slower rate and titrated against the serum potassium level. Sodium bicarbonate may be added to the solution containing glucose and insulin. The onset of effect is less than 30 minutes with either alkali or glucose-insulin therapy. The volume of fluid administered is a consideration in oliguric patients or those with heart failure or hypertension.

Cation exchange resins also lower serum potassium and maintain low potassium levels. Rectal retention enemas containing 50 gm of sodium polystyrene sulfonate (Kayexalate) suspended in 50 ml of 70% sorbitol and 100 ml of tap water can reduce serum potassium levels by 0.5 to 2.0 mEq/L, 30 to 90 minutes following a single dose. The enema should be retained for at least 30 to 60 minutes and may be repeated as needed thereafter. The sorbitol is used in order to prevent fecal impactions.

On a chronic basis, oral Kayexalate may be given in a dose of 15 to 20 grams three to four times daily. The dose should be suspended in 20 ml of 70% sorbitol with water added if necessary. The onset of action when given orally ranges from 2 to 12 hours, somewhat longer than when given rectally. The oral route of administration may be preferred by some patients despite some nausea. Semi-diarrhea should be induced with sorbitol before the administration of oral Kayexalate to prevent constipation and fecal impaction. Since this resin exchanges sodium for potassium, consideration must be given to patients with heart failure or elevated blood pressure. Although the oral administration of Kayexalate is often considered unpalatable, it should not be mixed with high potassium containing solutions or citrus juices as this will render the resin ineffective.

Hemodialysis and peritoneal dialysis are also effective means of lowering serum potassium, but the results take several hours, making these methods relatively slow. Thus, they should not be used as the primary mode of treatment in emergency situations (1,121-123, 125, 127, 128, 130-132, 134-138).

19. How does renal failure affect uric acid metabolism? How is it managed?

Chronic renal failure is associated with hyperuricemia that is due to reduced excretion of uric acid by the kidneys. Uric acid is normally freely filtered at the glomerulus; only a small fraction of protein-bound urate is not filtered. Up to 98% of the filtered urate load is reabsorbed by the proximal tubules, then secreted distal to the site of reabsorption. It is now believed that uric acid undergoes another reabsorptive process in the latter portion of the proximal tubule after it is secreted. The small fraction of filtered uric acid (6-10%) which finally appears in the urine results from the secreted uric acid that escapes proximal tubular reabsorption. The final reabsorption process is believed to protect the nephron from excessive concentrations of uric acid, and therefore from uric acid stones (141).

As kidney function decreases and the nephron population is reduced the fractional excretion of filtered urate increases. This means that as the tubular reabsorptive and secretory capacity diminishes with renal failure, there is an increase in the fractional amount of glomerularly filtered urate which escapes reabsorption. Therefore, as renal function decreases, glomerular filtration takes over a greater proportion of the renal excretion of uric acid. In the anuric patient gastrointestinal secretion provides the only means of urate excretion from the body (141,142,148).

The degree of hyperuricemia correlates with the severity of renal dysfunction. Serum urate levels are usually maintained within normal limits until the creatinine clearance drops below 30 ml/min, at which point serum urate levels begin to rise. Urate levels may rise well above 20 mg% with severe renal failure (142,148).

Excessive urate levels may give rise to three complications: gouty attacks and arthritis; uric acid stones; and urate deposition nephropathy. For unknown reasons gouty attacks and arthritis are not likely to occur in renal failure despite the presence of excessive urate levels. Only if a patient has had a previous gouty history should gouty attacks be expected. Rarely is urate-lowering therapy begun to prevent gouty attacks in these patients (140). Instead, treatment is initiated in the hope of preventing further renal dysfunction caused by the latter two complications of hyperuricemia. Post renal obstruction caused by uric acid stones or interstitial nephritis secondary to renal urate deposition can possibly be prevented by allopurinol therapy. If sufficient renal function remains, fluids and alkalinization of the urine alone may be adequate. Uricosuric drugs are ineffective in lowering urate levels if the creatinine clearance is less than 30 ml/min, since tubular function is diminished (142, 143, 148). There is also the possibility that uricosurics could give rise to a greater incidence of stone formation because of the increased excretion of uric acid.

Allopurinol can be started at 200 to 300 mg per day as a divided or single dose (143,144,147). Since allopurinol and oxypurinol (a major active metabolite) are both cleared renally, accumulation occurs with decreased renal function (139). Therefore it is necessary to titrate the dose in renal failure. A fair number of patients may be adequately controlled on a smaller dose. Since gouty attacks are uncommon in these pa-

tients, prophylactic colchicine is not necessary. Its toxicity which may be greater in renal failure (145,146) is thereby avoided.

In patients with chronic, irreversible renal failure who have creatinine clearances less than 5 to 10 ml/min, urate-lowering therapy should be questioned as there is essentially no renal function left to save. Invariably most of these patients will come to dialysis which may obviate the need for drug therapy since uric acid is dialyzable.

20. What are the carbohydrate abnormalities seen in chronic renal failure?

Approximately 70% of uremic patients have varying degrees of "uremic diabetes" manifested by an abnormal glucose tolerance test, elevated fasting insulin levels, and normal fasting blood sugars. Peripheral insensitivity to circulating insulin is a well-established mechanism of carbohydrate intolerance in uremic patients (149,151,152,155,156,158). This insensitivity has been attributed to several physiologic conditions and chemical substances present in renal failure, including: acidosis, elevated growth hormone, excessive urea and guanidinosuccinic acid levels, and total body potassium deficiency (149,151,152,155,158). However, no one factor has been proven to be conclusively responsible.

Although peripheral insulin antagonism is the major apparent cause of uremic diabetes, defects in insulin secretion and metabolism may also play a role (151,152). Uremic diabetes rarely requires treatment since marked symptomatic hyperglycemia and ketoacidosis are rare. However, abnormalities of carbohydrate metabolism in uremics can be partially normalized within several weeks following initiation of hemodialysis (151,156). The exact mechanism by which this is accomplished is unknown.

It is well known that the kidney, as well as the liver, is important in the degradation of insulin within the body (150,152,158,159). Thirty to 40% of the insulin reaching the kidneys is cleared by this organ. Insulin is normally filtered by the glomerulus; it then undergoes nearly complete proximal tubular reabsorption and catabolism, with less than 2% of the filtered load appearing in the urine. Renal metabolism accounts for removal of approximately 6 to 8 units of insulin per day, or 18% of the daily production (156,159). Patients with mild-to-moderate renal failure have reduced renal degradation of insulin, but they still manage to catabolize a significant amount of insulin (150,153). However, in patients with severe renal disease, the insulin half-life is prolonged and the amount of insulin renally degraded is substantially reduced with less than 0.17 units/day of insulin being removed by the kidneys (150,152,156,157,158). Insulin requirements of diabetic patients may be decreased in severe renal failure because of altered insulin kinetics. Marked insulin sensitivity with fatal hypoglycemia has been reported in these patients (152,154,159). (See the Diabetes chapter for further discussion of this problem.)

21. What is the relationship between hypertension and chronic renal disease, and how should it be treated?

※The kidney plays a major role in the control of blood pressure by regulating extracellular fluid volume and through the renin-angiotensin system (164,167,182). Hypertension is known to induce renal failure by damaging the renal vasculature. As a consequence, the impaired renal perfusion leads to increased renin secretion which further aggravates the hypertension and worsens the renal failure. A vicious cycle is thus established, and in many cases it is unclear which came first, the hypertension or the renal failure (172). In an individual with chronic renal failure, it is often difficult to establish if the hypertension is associated predominantly with volume expansion or high renin levels. However, the primary cause of the hypertension in most of these patients is extracellular volume expansion. This volume overload exists because the kidney is no longer able to excrete fluids efficiently (163,172,181).

※Since elevated blood pressure results in kidney damage, aggressive antihypertensive therapy can improve renal function and long-term survival (174, 183, 184). Therefore, the aim of antihypertensive treatment in chronic renal failure patients is to prevent further renal damage. When treating hypertensive patients with renal failure, drugs which cause excessive venous pooling and thus have a substantial orthostatic component (e.g. guanethidine) should be avoided. An acute drop in blood pressure can further reduce or even eliminate any remaining renal function. The treatment of hypertension in patients with renal failure is thus complicated by the fact that either too high or too low a blood pressure may have a detrimental effect on residual kidney function. Hence, antihypertensive drugs which minimally reduce or have no effect on renal blood flow are commonly used (e.g. methyldopa, hydralazine). Despite the use of these drugs, patients may still develop an elevated BUN and serum creatinine at the initiation of therapy. This is caused by the reduced renal perfusion secondary to lowered blood pressure. Therapy should be continued, as the elevation is transient and should not be taken as a sign of worsening renal function unless severe hypotension is present (183).

Diuretics are relatively mild antihypertensive agents and act primarily by reducing extracellular fluid volume. In patients with renal failure which does not yet require dialysis, diuretics are the most common treatment modality. Because the effectiveness of thiazides,

as diuretics, is reduced when the creatinine clearance is less than 20-30 ml/min, furosemide is usually the preferred agent. The ability of furosemide to maintain urine flow in patients with renal failure has been adequately demonstrated (18,170,173,178,179). Because diuretics increase renin release, a better response is observed in patients classified as low-renin hypertensives. Less diuretic-induced renin stimulation occurs in these patients compared to normal or high renin producers (180).

If adequate blood pressure control is not achieved by appropriate extracellular fluid reduction, the addition of *methyldopa* or *hydralazine* is usually considered. Neither drug adversely affects renal blood flow. Because a reflex tachycardia can develop from hydralazine, a beta-blocker such as *propranolol* is commonly added (185). Occasionally, methyldopa may be able to control the reflex sympathetic effect from hydralazine. In some patients, all three drugs may be necessary to control blood pressure (172,177). An additional agent, with which we have had little experience thus far, is *clonidine*. It is very similar to methyldopa in that it has a central mode of action and maintains renal blood flow. Its antihypertensive effects are additive to the vasodilator and beta-blocker combination (175). In patients unable to tolerate methyldopa, this may be a reasonable alternative. Propranolol, methyldopa, and clonidine all cause suppression of renin release (161,172).

Minoxidil in combination with propranolol and furosemide is effective in the control of hypertension in chronic renal failure patients refractory to other therapy (176). Early comparative studies show that minoxidil may be of greater therapeutic benefit than hydralazine (165). Minoxidil seems to be a promising agent in the treatment of hypertension.

In patients with severe acute hypertension and renal failure, the direct-acting vasodilators *diazoxide* (171) or *nitroprusside* (160) are frequently used. The control of hypertension by diazoxide has been shown to be a critical factor in improving renal function in patients with chronic renal failure (171). The continued administration of nitroprusside to patients with renal failure can lead to accumulation of the toxic metabolite thiocyanate (162,168). Neither diazoxide, nitroprusside, minoxidil, nor hydralazine adversely affect renal blood flow, and all are potent stimulators of renin release (172).

Reserpine and guanethidine are rarely used in the patient with renal failure because of frequent side effects. Additionally, guanethidine adversely affects renal blood flow.

Hemodialysis is extremely effective in reducing extracellular fluid volume and lowering blood pressure (166,170,172). Since volume expansion is the major cause of hypertension in chronic renal failure patients, hemodialysis is effective in controlling blood pressure in the majority of cases (164,170). When hemodialysis is initiated, the dosage of antihypertensive medications may be lowered, or even discontinued in some patients. However, in a minority of patients whose hypertension is primarily related to elevated renin levels, the response to dialysis is usually not significant (172).

Bilateral nephrectomy has been used to control blood pressure when antihypertensive drug treatment and dialysis have failed. This procedure eliminates the source of the excessive renin production and hopefully controls the patient's hypertension (169).

In summary, aggressive antihypertensive therapy should be initiated in renal failure patients with hypertension. The aim of such therapy is to improve the patient's renal function if possible, and to prevent further organ damage and complications of hypertension. Antihypertensive drug administration is clearly the most important therapeutic approach. However, dialysis or nephrectomy may also be necessary.

GLOMERULONEPHRITIS:

22. What is glomerulonephritis?

Glomerulonephritis is a broad term, used in referring to diseases which predominately damage the filtering unit of the kidney, the glomerulus. Glomerulonephritis can be further classified on the basis of histologic changes present within the glomerulus. (See Table 4.) Histologic classification is important in determining the patient's prognosis and aggressiveness of treatment.

TABLE 4
GENERAL HISTOLOGIC CLASSIFICATION
OF GLOMERULONEPHRITIS

Histologic Classification	Example
Minimal Change	Idiopathic nephrotic syndrome.
Membraneous Nephropathy	Renal vein thrombosis, malaria, mercury nephropathy, gold nephropathy, lupus nephritis.
Focal Glomerulosclerosis	Idiopathic nephrotic syndrome.
Proliferative Glomerulonephritis. Includes sub-classifications; exudative, mesangial, mesangio-capillary, focal, with extensive crescents, etc.	Lupus nephritis, Henoch-Schonlein purpura, polyarteritis, post-infectious glomerulonephritis nephritis secondary to subacute bacterial endocarditis.

Glomerular disease can appear as an acute or chronic syndrome or as a rapidly progressing one. Primary glomerular disease is manifested by varying degrees of proteinuria, hematuria, red blood cell casts, and pyuria. Elevation of the blood urea nitrogen (BUN) and creatinine also frequently occur.

The pathologic causes of glomerular lesions are primarily two-fold: circulating immune complex deposition and anti-glomerular basement membrane antibody disease.

Immune complex deposition is believed to be associated with a number of disease states, including lupus nephritis, acute serum sickness, and acute post-infectious glomerulonephritis. Circulating immune complexes deposit in the glomerular capillary bed and activate the complement system. This brings about release of vaso-active peptides, leukocytosis, and an inflammatory reaction. The inflammatory reaction bares the vascular endothelium exposing collagen thereby activating the coagulation process. Platelet aggregation and Hageman factor activation result in fibrin formation and deposition. The overall degree and pattern of glomerular damage depends on the amount and size of the complexes, the rate of formation, the antigen-antibody ratio, and the degree of participation of the inflammatory reaction. Although immune complex deposition is believed to be the most common cause of glomerulonephritis, the inciting antigen is rarely identified.

Circulating antibodies to glomerular basement membrane (GBM), such as that associated with Goodpasture's syndrome, occurs infrequently, accounting for less than 5% of all cases of glomerulonephritis. Anti-GBM disease is generally rapidly progressive and has a poor prognosis.

A complete discussion of the prognosis and treatment of all classifications and causes of glomerulonephritis are beyond the scope of this chapter. However, the following sections will encompass pathogenesis, histologic classification and treatment of the glomerular lesions caused by systemic lupus erythematosus (SLE), and the nephrotic syndrome which develops secondary to glomerular disease (186-193).

LUPUS NEPHRITIS:

E.P. is a 17-year-old Oriental female who was in good health until 6 months prior to admission when she saw her physician because of a two to three week history of headaches. She complained of stiffening of the knee joints and was anemic, but was not treated at this time for these conditions. The patient's headaches were controlled with ergonovine, acetominophen, and Darvon, and her birth control pills (Demulen) were discontinued because they were a possible cause of her headaches.

She remained well until 5 days prior to admission when she noted general malaise. Two days prior to admission she developed fever and vomiting. This continued until the patient was seen in the emergency room, at which time a urinalysis showed 5 to 10 RBC/hpf and 10 to 25 WBC/hpf and a few bacteria. She was sent home with a week's supply of ampicillin only to return the next day with a total body maculopapular rash that had a butterfly distribution on her face. Physical examination showed a normal blood pressure, slight ankle and facial edema, and mild alopecia. Urinary laboratory data of importance included the following: 10 to 25 RBC/hpf, 10 to 25 WBC/hpf in the urine, BUN 51 mg%, creatinine 2.5 mg% and 6 gm/24 hours of protein in the urine. Additional laboratory data include: positive SLE preparation, positive antinuclear antibody (ANA), elevated erythrocyte sedimentation rate (ESR) of 34, hemoglobin of 9.9 gm%, and a hematocrit of 29.6%. Previous urinary cultures showed no growth. The diagnoses were systemic lupus (SLE) with renal involvement; ampicillin allergy; and possible drug-induced exacerbation of SLE.

Following admission, a renal biopsy was performed which showed a diffuse proliferative glomerular lesion. The patient had a low serum complement, low fibrinogen, and high fibrin-split products at this time. She was treated with 90 mg of prednisone a day for 7 days in divided doses and had a moderate response as evidenced by a drop in the serum creatinine to 1.6 and urinary protein output to 1.5 gm/day. The patient was discharged on 60 mg of prednisone a day.

23. What is systemic lupus erythematosus (SLE)?

Systemic lupus erythematosus (SLE) is a chronic polysystemic autoimmune disease of connective tissue. This disease has a genetic predisposition and occurs predominantly in young females and in blacks. Presenting complaints include malaise, lethargy, low-grade fever, headache, and arthritic-like joint pain. Patients are frequently anemic as well. Dermatologic abnormalities are common. As many as 85% of patients are found to have an erythematous rash having a butterfly-malar distribution on the face as found in our patient E.P. There may also be cardiac and pulmonary involvement as evidenced by pericarditis, pericardial or pleural effusions, and cardiac murmurs. In addition, both the central nervous system (CNS) and the kidney may be damaged. CNS involvement is manifested by psychotic reactions, palsies, convulsions, and strokes, while abnormalities of the kidney are evident by proteinuria, hematuria, and azotemia. Uremia and CNS damage constitute the major causes of death in lupus patients.

Useful laboratory tests that would diagnose SLE include a positive ANA test (>95%), positive SLE preparation (76-100%), and an elevated ESR.

24. How is SLE treated?

Treatment is primarily suppressive. The aggressiveness of the therapy depends on the degree of organ involvement. Bed rest and avoidance of emotional stress are helpful. Salicylates or other nonsteroidal anti-inflammatory drugs usually help to relieve arthritic-like joint pain. Antimalarial therapy is useful for generalized skin rashes, while topical steroids can be used for localized skin involvement. Prednisone or other glucocorticosteroids are generally required in varying doses to control other systemic manifestations of lupus. High, divided-dose therapy is usually necessary for treatment of exacerbations of the disease, while once-a-day or every-other-day therapy with steroids can be used in the interim for maintenance, if required. In the absence of renal involvement, cytotoxic drugs are rarely indicated (200, 201, 207, 214).

25. How serious is the renal involvement of SLE?

Renal involvement in lupus is of major concern, since renal failure is one of the leading causes of death in lupus patients. A large portion of patients with lupus (35 to 90%) develop some degree of renal damage. This damage is believed to be secondary to the glomerular deposition of DNA- anti-DNA-immune complexes with activation of complement which, in turn, results in a destructive inflammatory reaction. Therapy of lupus patients with renal involvement is more aggressive because of the poor prognosis of the untreated disease (222,230).

26. What are the types of renal lesions found in lupus?

Lupus nephritis has three major histologic and pathologic variants, each with its own typical clinical features and prognosis (197,217,222,231).

1. *Focal Proliferative Lupus Nephritis* is found in up to a third of the patients in whom biopsies are performed. It is characterized by incomplete glomerular damage in less than 50% of the glomeruli. Other structural damage is minimal. Histologic evidence shows focal mesangial and endothelial cell proliferation with cellular infiltrates in the affected glomeruli. Immunoglobins are believed to be responsible for the glomerular damage (197,222,230,239). Renal involvement is characterized clinically by microscopic hematuria, pyuria, and mild proteinuria. However, patients with this type of lupus rarely develop the nephrotic syndrome, hypertension, or end-stage renal insufficiency (197,222).

2. *Diffuse Proliferative Lupus Nephritis* occurs in 45 to 90% of patients with lupus nephritis. This condition is characterized histologically by involvement of most of the glomeruli. Although the glomerulus is the major site of renal damage, the renal tubules and interstitium also show evidence of damage. The

glomerular pathologic features include irregular mesangial-endothelial cellular proliferation; local basement-membrane thickening, subendothelial deposits of immunocomplexes (electron dense particles), and generalized inflammation and fibrosis (222,230,239).

Unlike the focal proliferative lesion, the nephrotic syndrome, hypertension, and renal insufficiency (which may progress rapidly) are frequent complications of the diffuse proliferative lesion. Clinical activity of the disease and the overall prognosis of patients with this lesion have been correlated with the presence of subendothelial deposits of immunocomplexes, as well as the graded histologic severity of the diffuse proliferative lesion (222,230,239).

3. **Membranous Lupus Nephritis** is not common and occurs in only 15% of lupus nephritis patients. As with other lesions, this condition is characterized by hematuria, pyuria, and proteinuria. However, the latter is especially marked and most patients develop the nephrotic syndrome at some time during the course of this disease. Despite the fact that renal failure may develop in a large portion of patients after a number of years, the long-term prognosis of these patients is good (222).

Glomerular basement-membrane thickening without cellular proliferative changes is the chief histologic finding. In addition, immuno-complexes appear chiefly on the epithelial site of the glomerular basement membrane (197,222,230,239).

Although transformation from one type of lesion to another was thought to be rare (197), it is becoming apparent that such transformation may occur frequently (222). It has been suggested that these histologic lesions represent a continuum where the membranous changes may actually represent a resolution stage of the disease (225).

27. How is lupus nephritis treated?

Glucocorticoids form the basis for the treatment of lupus nephritis. Because of the good prognosis for patients with focal proliferative nephritis (197, 222, 239), aggressive therapy is usually not indicated. The usual dose of steroid to control systemic manifestations of the disease will more than suffice, although higher doses are occasionally required (239). Alternate-day steroids have been observed to have their best success in this form of lupus nephritis (194). Patients may also enjoy drug-free periods. Prolonged high-dose steroids or the addition of immunosuppressive agents, although effective (222), are rarely necessary for this form of the disease, and may, in fact, expose the patient to undue risk of drug toxicity (230). The question as to whether drug therapy is necessary at all has also been raised (197). Deaths in these patients usually are related to extrarenal causes (197, 217, 232).

Approximately one-third of the patients with membranous lupus nephritis on steroid therapy will experience a partial or complete clinical remission of renal disease. The remaining patients have a persistent proteinuria, despite steroid therapy. A gradual downhill course of renal failure develops in about 50% of the patients (197). The severity and duration of proteinuria may indicate the prognosis of impending renal failure. High-dose steroids are frequently continued in these patients in the hope of inducing a remission. However, excessive doses should be avoided since a large portion of deaths reported in this group of patients has been attributed to complications of aggressive immunosuppressive therapy, not renal failure (239).

Because of the serious nature of diffuse proliferative lupus nephritis, aggressive therapy is indicated in patients with this glomerular lesion. Treatment consists of 60 to 100 mg/day or 1 mg/kg/day of prednisone during periods of disease activity. Doses as high as 2 mg/kg/day may be required to control these acute exacerbations. The dose required will depend primarily on the severity of the initial renal lesion (230,239,242). More than 50% of the patients treated will show partial or complete remission of clinically evident renal abnormalities. The patients are then continued on maintenance steroids, usually indefinitely. Generally, maintenance doses are higher than those required to control the other systemic manifestations of lupus (except CNS lupus). Alternate-day steroids are invariably ineffective in this form of lupus nephritis (194, 213).

Regardless of the fact that patients are maintained on corticosteroids, the relapse rate is extremely high (greater than 50%). Therefore, increased doses of steroids or the addition of cytotoxic agents, or both, are necessary to try to control renal flare-ups. (See Question 28).

Despite aggressive steroid therapy, diffuse proliferative lupus nephritis has a grave prognosis. Five-year survival rates for steroid-treated patients have been reported from uncontrolled studies to be 20 to 25% (197,217,222,231,232). A majority of deaths in these patients are related to renal disease. Overall, patients treated with high-dose steroids appear to do better than those patients treated with low-dose steroids or no steroids at all (231). However, steroids apparently exert little beneficial effect in those patients with severe renal disease with extensive glomerular involvement (222). Because of inadequate response to steroids in many of these patients, and due to the fact that prolonged steroid therapy is associated with numerous severe side effects, other treatment regimens for diffuse proliferative lupus nephritis have been investigated.

28. Are cytotoxic agents useful in treating diffuse proliferative lupus nephritis?

The usefulness of cytotoxic agents in the treatment of lupus nephritis has been debated and investigated at length. Differences in study design, patient selection criteria, treatment regimens, length of follow-up and monitoring parameters make evaluation of the data extremely difficult. The following is a brief overview of the current literature.

Uncontrolled clinical studies suggest a possible therapeutic benefit of *azathioprine* when used alone, or when added to steroids in patients with lupus nephritis (195,196,199,212,223-227,229,230,234). In one such study (229), 16 pediatric and adult patients primarily with diffuse proliferative lupus nephritis were treated with a combination of 2 to 3 mg/kg/day of azathioprine and 20 mg/day or less of prednisone. Proteinuria improved in 14 patients and complete remission was achieved in six. Glomerular filtration returned to normal in three patients and remained normal in twelve. One patient, who had severe renal dysfunction at the start of the study, died as the result of renal disease. Decreased cellular proliferation, inflammation, and electron dense particle depostion was demonstrated in 10 of 11 biopsied patients. Additionally, a subendothelial to subepithelial shift of electron dense particles was noted in six patients after 24 to 36 months. A subsequent uncontrolled study by these investigators (225a) indicates that dissolution of subendothelial deposits, with or without a shift of electron dense particles, correlates with clinical improvement in renal function. The authors conclude that the presence or absence of subendothelial deposits of electron-dense material, regardless of light microscopic classification, offers the best long-term prognostic indicator of renal function in patients with lupus nephritis and that azathioprine has a favorable effect in resolving these deposits.

The results of controlled clinical investigations concerning the usefulness of azathioprine in lupus nephritis are equivocal, but encouraging data have been reported (202,221,240). In one study (240), the addition of azathioprine, 2.5 mg/kg/day, to prednisone therapy in 16 lupus patients markedly improved morbidity, mortality, and renal function parameters when compared to 19 control patients receiving prednisone alone. Additionally, patients receiving the combination required smaller quantities of steroid. However, this study has been criticized for lack of renal biopsy information, making comparison between the treatment groups difficult.

In a retrospective study of 110 lupus patients (221), 68 were classified as patients with a poor prognosis (CNS lupus or severe lupus renal disease); these patients were divided into two groups, those who received azathioprine and those who did not. Azathio-

prine was found not to be useful in treating acute exacerbations of renal disease, nor did it affect one-year survival rates. However, after one year, a significant reduction in mortality was noted in the azathioprine group. Although this study indicates the possible advantages of azathioprine in these patients, the study suffers from a lack of steroid dosage information in the two groups and from a preponderance of patients with membranous lupus nephritis in the azathioprine-treated group, a factor which favors this group.

In an impressive well-designed controlled study, 50 patients with moderate to severe diffuse proliferative lupus nephritis were allocated to four treatment groups: high-dose steroids, azathioprine alone, azathioprine plus steroids, or azathioprine plus heparin. All regimens containing azathioprine were significantly more effective than regimens of high-dose steroids alone in terms of improvement of renal function and survival (202).

A number of other controlled studies (205,209, 210,224,238) however, failed to show that the addition of azathioprine to steroid therapy has a significant beneficial effect on the overall prognosis of lupus nephritis patients. In controlled 6- and 36-month studies of 16 patients with mild to moderate renal disease (209,210) the addition of azathioprine to tapering doses of prednisone did not reduce the incidence of renal flare-ups. No deaths were reported in either treatment group. More recently, a ten-week double-blind controlled study of 38 patients with mild to moderate renal disease caused by diffuse proliferative lupus glomerulonephritis assessed the potential benefits of adding cyclophosphamide, azathioprine, or placebo to patients already receiving low doses of steroids used to suppress extrarenal manifestations of lupus (238). In any score of lupus activity improvement, including three measures of renal function, the addition of azathioprine to prednisone was no more effective than prednisone alone. A 28-month follow-up of these patients (206) indicated that azathioprine plus prednisone had no overall effect on unfavorable outcomes (death or dialysis). However, deterioration of renal function was apparently more common in the group being treated with steroids only. A prospective, controlled evaluation of 24 patients with varying lupus glomerular lesions (including focal proliferative and membraneous glomerulonephritis) failed to demonstrate any improvement in survival or renal function at a mean follow-up period of 18 to 24 months when azathioprine 2 to 4 mg/kg/day was added to prednisone (224). A steroid-sparing effect, which has been noted in other controlled studies, could not be found (205,209,238).

To summarize, the exact role of azathioprine in the treatment of lupus nephritis is still unclear. Azathioprine alone, or in combination with steroids, does not appear to be useful in treating acute renal flare-ups nor in improving short-term survival, and it remains to be demonstrated whether the addition of azathioprine to the treatment regimen of patients with severe renal disease from diffuse proliferative lupus nephritis will be of any long-term benefit.

The possible therapeutic usefulness of *cyclophosphamide* in treating lupus nephritis, as with azathioprine, has been studied in uncontrolled clinical trials (203,204,218). A subsequent controlled study (220) indicated that cyclophosphamide at a mean dose of 125 mg/kg/day alone was ineffective in inducing remissions of lupus nephritis when compared to prednisone alone. However, controlled investigations utilizing cyclophosphamide plus steroids have produced promising, but inconclusive, results (198,206,211,237,238). Ten-week double-blind controlled studies in patients with diffuse proliferative lupus nephritis (237,238) have indicated that cyclophosphamide (3 to 4 mg/kg/day) in combination with prednisone produced greater improvement of immunologic indicators of lupus activity and urinary sediment when compared to prednisone plus azathioprine or prednisone plus placebo. However, renal function was not favorably affected by any treatment regimen. A subsequent long-term follow-up (206) of 38 of these patients showed similar findings, although the incidence of an unfavorable outcome (death/dialysis) was lowest in the cyclophosphamide group. No steroid-sparing effect could be demonstrated. A prospective randomized study of 39 lupus patients with proliferative glomerulonephritis (211) showed no difference between high-dose steroid therapy and cyclophosphamide plus moderate-dose steroids following six months of treatment. However, after an average of 24 months, the frequency of progression of renal disease was lower in the cyclophosphamide group. In addition, the cyclophosphamide group required smaller doses of steroids.

Chlorambucil has also been used in the treatment of lupus nephritis. In uncontrolled studies (216,223,235, 236), patients with lupus nephritis have shown improvement in parameters of renal function following treatment with chlorambucil. Chlorambucil was used in these studies because the patients were steroid toxic and because chlorambucil is relatively non-toxic compared with the other cytotoxic agents discussed above.

Epstein and Grausz (216) demonstrated that by utilizing appropriate immunologic laboratory tests as a guide to drug therapy (see below), a 77.7% five-year survival rate could be achieved in patients with diffuse proliferative lupus nephritis. Patients received varying doses of steroids and/or chlorambucil depending upon laboratory test results. The authors attributed the improved survival to early, aggressive use of drug therapy based on laboratory data, not on clinical signs and symptoms.

High-dose steroid therapy, combined with a single dose of nitrogen mustard, does not improve the prognosis of the diffuse lesion when compared to high-dose steroid treatment alone in an uncontrolled study (208).

In conclusion, although impressive improvements in five-year survival (75 to 80%) have been demonstrated in uncontrolled clinical trials utilizing cytotoxic agents (222), the use of these drugs should still be considered investigational and reserved for steroid-resistant cases of diffuse proliferative lupus nephritis. The possible benefits from these agents must be balanced against the severity of drug toxicity. Complications of cytotoxic therapy include bone-marrow suppression, increased incidence of infection, and the possible induction of malignancies. Severe exacerbations of renal lupus that is frequently resistant to treatment have been reported following withdrawal of both azathioprine and cyclophosphamide (233,241) therapy. In addition, azathioprine is hepatotoxic, while alopecia, hemorrhagic cystitis, and suppression of gonadal function are frequent complications of cyclophosphamide treatment (241). Suppression of gonadal function has also been reported following the use of chlorambucil.

Drug monitoring parameters required to adjust drug doses are numerous and too complicated to discuss in entirety; however, by following the clinical and laboratory parameters listed in Table 5, exacerbations of lupus nephritis can be detected and appropriate adjustment in drug dosage instituted.

TABLE 5
MONITORING PARAMETERS FOR LUPUS NEPHRITIS

Laboratory Test	Trend	Explanation
ANA (Antinuclear antibody)	+	Indication of autoimmune disease.
CH$_{50}$ total hemolytic complement	←	Immune complex binds complement. Indicates glomerular damage.
Urinary light chains	←	Good early indicator of oncoming exacerbation. Indicates tubular damage.
Anti-DNA antibody (double-stranded)	←	Antibody to native DNA antigen. Good indicator of active disease.
Urinary FSP (fibrin-split products)	←	Demonstrates ongoing fibrin utilization and deposition. Good indicator of active disease.
Serum fibrinogen	←	Demonstrates ongoing fibrin utilization and deposition. Good indicator of active disease.
Proteinuria/Hematuria/ Pyuria	←	Demonstrated glomerular damage. Clinical evidence of active disease.
Creatinine/BUN	←	Demonstrates renal damage. Clinical evidence of active disease/permanent damage.
(215,216,222,228)		

Recently it has been suggested that patients with end-stage renal failure secondary to lupus should have their steroid and cytotoxic drug doses reduced to levels which can control systemic manifestations of the disease. At this stage, drug treatment appears ineffective in reversing renal damage and only increases the risk of infection. Dialysis and transplantation may provide the most beneficial results in these patients (205,219).

NEPHROTIC SYNDROME:

C.H. is a 12-year-old male who was admitted to the hospital because of increasing peripheral edema. The physical examination at entrance demonstrated no physical abnormalities except a 4+ pitting edema on both legs. Blood pressure and renal function were normal. SMA-12 panel was unremarkable except for a serum cholesterol of 387 mg% and a serum albumin of 1.8 gm%. Urinalysis at this time revealed a 4+ proteinuria as well as oval fat bodies. No red or white blood cells were seen. The patient excreted 9.5 gm of protein in a 24-hour period. A renal biopsy showed lipoid nephrosis. Systemic causes of the nephrotic syndrome were ruled out. Prednisone was begun at a dose of 40 mg/day. The patient was discharged with the diagnosis of idiopathic nephrotic syndrome.

29. What is the nephrotic syndrome?

Lesions of the glomerulus which enhance permeability of the glomerular apparatus to circulating proteins lead to a group of clinical abnormalities collectively known as the nephrotic syndrome. Virtually any glomerulopathy can result in the nephrotic syndrome. The clinical entities which characterize this syndrome, as illustrated in the patient above, have been well defined by Schreiner (305). They include: proteinuria of greater than 3.5 grams per day; hypoalbuminemia of less than 3.0 gram%; hypercholesterolemia of greater than 300 mg%; lipiduria; and edema.

The initial glomerular lesion leading to the syndrome can be idiopathic, induced by systemic disease, or caused by other exogenous factors such as drugs. These include the following (263,268,305,308):

a. Lupus nephritis and other collagen vascular diseases

b. Diabetic nephrosclerosis

c. Various other glomerular diseases

d. Primary/secondary amyloidosis

e. Infection (i.e. malaria, syphilis, staph/streptococcal infections)

f. Drugs (i.e. gold, probenecid, penicillamine, trimethadone, mercurial diuretics)

g. Allergens (poison oak, bee sting)

h. Severe right-sided heart failure

Protein loss primarily consists of albumin and other lower molecular weight proteins. The presence of higher molecular weight proteins in the urine signals poor selectivity and is indicative of a more severe glomerular lesion with a poorer prognosis (268,308). Hypoproteinemia causes a loss of oncotic pressure and a shift of intravascular fluid into the interstitial spaces. Intravascular hypovolemia results. Then, in an effort to replenish the intravascular deficit, sodium and water reabsorption are stimulated by aldosterone and a decreased hydrostatic pressure. At steady-state there is an interstitial edema and a near normal intravascular volume (268). Hyperlipidemia and lipiduria as evidenced by fatty casts and oval fat bodies in the urine are also characteristic of the nephrotic syndrome. Hyperlipidemia may be a major factor in the early cardiovascular deaths observed in these patients (268). Nephrotic patients also display an enhanced susceptibility to infections, especially pneumococcal, and an increased tendency toward thromboembolic episodes (268). Additional symptoms include anorexia, fatigue, and headache. The syndrome may or may not advance to renal failure, depending upon the severity of the glomerular lesion. [Classification of glomerular lesions varies from author to author, making true evaluation of the present literature difficult. Classifications will be based on the work by MacDonald (285), Darly et al. (263), and Glassock et al (268).]

30. What is lipoid or minimal-change nephrosis? How is it treated?

Lipoid or minimal-change nephrosis (also known as "nil lesion") has the best prognosis of all the glomerular lesions of idiopathic nephrotic syndrome. It is usually associated with childhood nephrotic syndrome, but sometimes it occurs in adults. Minimal alterations of glomerular structure are evident on light microscopy. However, electron microscopy demonstrates fusion of foot processes with little or no cellular proliferation (285,308). The lesion has not, for the most part, been associated with immune complex deposition.

Steroid therapy is the basis of treatment for minimal change nephrotic syndrome, and its effectiveness is well documented (252,268,275,276,277,292,296,301, 321). Varying remission rates have been reported in different studies. These may be attributed to differences in patient selection or treatment regimens as well as to the remitting and relapsing nature of the disease. Nonetheless, an estimated 90% or more of patients will respond to steroids initially (268).

A variety of steroid-dosing schedules have been suggested (263,268,305,308). Generally, high doses of prednisone (1 to 2 mg/kg/day) are administered initially. This is tapered, as complete remission or marked improvement in proteinuria occur, which usually takes two to eight weeks or longer. Patients are then maintained on lower doses of steroids or every-other-day steroids for varying periods of time (several weeks) following remission. They are eventually taken off medication if the remission is maintained during the follow-up period. It is important to reduce proteinuria to a level of 2 grams per day or less as this is associated with a marked improvement in life expectancy (292).

Patients who respond initially are still prone to relapses when steroids are reduced or withdrawn. Up to two-thirds of these patients may suffer a relapse (268), which can be treated with a full course of steroid therapy. Certain patients, however, fail to maintain remission without repeated courses of steroids and become steroid-dependent. These patients, as well as a small percentage of lipoid nephrotic patients who are initially resistant to steroid therapy, pose a treatment problem.

31. Can cytotoxic agents be used to treat lipoid nephrosis if patients are steroid dependent or resistant?

Because of the development of steroid toxicity in patients with frequently relapsing, steroid dependent lipoid nephrosis, the possible therapeutic benefit of several cytotoxic drugs has been investigated in this disease (309).

In early uncontrolled studies, persons with lipoid nephrosis who were steroid dependent or resistant and who were treated with varying doses of cyclophosphamide, had immediate and usually prolonged remissions (262,266,293). More recently, a number of clinical trials (250,257,259,287,296,298, 307,312,314) and controlled studies (249,258,303,313) have clearly confirmed the usefulness of adding cyclophosphamide to steroids in the treatment of lipoid nephrosis. Beneficial responses are seen primarily in those patients who are steroid sensitive initially. In a controlled study, Barratt et al (249) demonstrated a significant reduction in relapses from steroid-induced remissions when an eight-week course of cyclophosphamide was added to the steroid regimen. At 60 weeks, nine of ten patients with steroid treatment alone had relapsed, while only two of ten patients with steroids plus cyclophosphamide had relapsed. Tsao and Yeung (313) conducted a paired trial comparing cyclophosphamide with prednisone. They found that although prednisone induced a more rapid remission, patients treated with cyclophosphamide (3 to 5 mg/kg/day) were much less likely to relapse. Chui et al (258), in a controlled study comparing steroid treatment versus steroid plus cyclophosphamide, showed a relapse rate of 90.9% and 16.7% respectively at 25-months follow-up. A prospective controlled study from the International Study of Kidney Diseases in Children has further documented the effectiveness of cyclophosphamide in the treatment of these patients (303).

Acute and long-term assessment of cyclophosphamide indicates that the remissions induced in lipoid nephrotic patients by cyclophosphamide alone or in combination with steroids are longer and relatively more stable than those produced by steroids alone.

In early reports it was believed that leukopenia was essential for effectiveness of cyclophosphamide (266,272,293). However, more recent information indicates no correlation between the degree of leukopenia and the therapeutic response to the drug (250,258, 283,286,303). In fact, those patients subjected to higher doses of cyclophosphamide showed a higher incidence of toxicity without additional therapeutic benefit. It now appears that the major determinant of response to cyclophosphamide is the duration of treatment (248,250,257,287,298). Moreover, the beneficial effects of cyclophosphamide are not diminished by repeated courses (250,259). Furthermore, cyclophosphamide may also restore steroid responsiveness in patients who may become steroid insensitive during the disease course (251,307,312).

The usefulness of cyclophosphamide in inducing remissions in steroid-dependent patients with lipoid nephrosis is well documented. Its usefulness in treating patients with steroid "resistant" nephrosis remains to be clarified. Patients with steroid "resistant" lipoid nephrosis may in fact have undetectable focal glomerular sclerosis (see Question 32). At present, it appears that cyclophosphamide is the cytotoxic agent of choice for inducing remissions in lipoid nephrotic patients who are steroid dependent. However, its use must be balanced against its long list of toxicities (319) including hemorrhogic cystitis, alopecia, bone marrow suppression, and impaired systemic immunity to infections. A side effect of major concern in these patients, many of whom are children, is the drug's *effects on gonadal function.* Oligo/azoospermia, menstrual disturbances, and amenorrhea have been reported following cyclophosphamide therapy in adults and adolescents (254, 267, 268, 269, 281, 297, 299, 302, 314, 315, 317). Children treated in the pre-pubertal period may also develop subsequent gonadal dysfunction. Spermatogenesis and ovarian function may be permanently impaired or return spontaneously after a period of time (254). Both the duration (297) and the total dose (267) of cyclophosphamide have been correlated with gonadal toxicity. It has been recommended (268, 287, 303) that cyclophosphamide therapy be limited to eight to ten weeks with the dose not to exceed 2.5 to 3.0 mg/kg/day so as to derive maximum benefit with the least amount of toxicity.

Chlorambucil has been shown to be effective in both the treatment of steroid-dependent and steroid-resistant nephrotic syndrome in a limited number of studies (272-274). In an uncontrolled study, Grupe

(273) used a combination of prednisone and chlorambucil in 23 children with steroid-dependent nephrotic syndrome. Chlorambucil was used at a dose of 0.1 to 0.2 mg/kg/day for 2½ to 12 weeks until leukopenia was induced. Complete remissions occurred in all cases and only 13% had relapsed in 26.6 months. A more recent controlled study by this same group (274) has confirmed earlier, impressive observations. In this study they treated 21 children who had frequently relapsing nephrotic syndrome with either prednisone alone (6 weeks), or with prednisone (6 weeks) plus chlorambucil (6 to 12 weeks) in a dose of 0.26 to 0.41 mg/kg/day. All 11 control (steroid alone) patients relapsed within seven months while none of the 10 patients receiving the combination relapsed at an average follow-up of 19.6 months. Evidence indicates that chlorambucil-induced remissions in these patients may be more stable than those induced by either steroids or cyclophosphamide. Further controlled studies comparing both agents are required to document this possibility. Chlorambucil, like cyclophosphamide, may affect gonadal function (291,304).

Although there are early reports of *azathioprine*-induced remissions in the treatment of lipoid nephrosis (244,272), more recent studies do not confirm the usefulness of this drug in these patients. Michael et al (289) found that a group of patients with idiopathic nephrotic syndrome did not benefit from a combination of prednisone and azathioprine. Abramowicz et al (243) treated 5 patients who did not respond to steroids and 35 steroid-dependent lipoid-nephrotic patients with either prednisone plus azathioprine or prednisone plus placebo. The azathioprine-treated patients did not show a statistically different response from those patients in the placebo group.

In summary, treatment of lipoid nephrosis should always be initiated with an adequate trial of steroids, because a majority of patients will respond initially to this therapy. Cytotoxic agents such as cyclophosphamide or chlorambucil can be utilized in patients with lipoid nephrosis who are steroid-dependent, especially those patients with frequent relapses, or those who develop late steroid unresponsiveness.

32. What is the prognosis of nephrotic syndrome associated with focal glomerular sclerosis?

Focal glomerular sclerosis may be present in 10 to 20% of adults with the nephrotic syndrome (268). It may be a variant of lipoid or minimal-change lesion or, as has been argued, a separate clinical entity (268,295). Juxtamedullary focal segmental glomerular sclerosis is the typical histologic lesion and is invariably associated with immunoglobulin (IgM) deposits (268,271,278,294). Clinically, the course of these patients is characterized by recurrent hematuria, steroid-resistant proteinuria, and progressive renal

failure in a variable number of patients. In general, these patients are usually older and have a poorer prognosis when compared to patients with lipoid nephrosis (271,278,294). However, children with focal glomerular sclerosis fare better than adults (294).

Response to steroids is usually poor (243,256,268, 271,277,278,283,294,316,318). Only a minority of patients experience a partial or complete remission with steroid treatment and a majority of these patients subsequently have a relapse (271,295). Response to cytotoxic agents such as cyclophosphamide or azathioprine has been equally disappointing (256, 283, 294, 295, 316).

Because of the difference in response to treatment and the overall poorer prognosis of these patients with focal sclerosis, it is imperative to differentiate between lipoid nephrosis and focal segmental glomerulosclerosis.

33. Are there any other glomerular lesions associated with idiopathic nephrotic syndrome?

Idiopathic membranous glomerulopathy is another cause of nephrotic syndrome (255,260,268,270,300). This lesion can be demonstrated in a large portion of adults with idiopathic nephrotic syndrome, but in only a small percentage of children (268,300). Histologically, the glomeruli are characterized by diffuse thickening of the basement membrane with little or no hypercellularity. The lesion is associated with subepithelial or intramembraneous deposits of IgG immune complexes of unknown origin (263,268,285). The disease usually follows an indolent course, with renal failure progressing over a number of years. Usually, only those patients who demonstrate heavy, persistent proteinuria go on to develop renal insufficiency. Spontaneous clinical remissions and relapses may occur (268,275). Although steroid and immunosuppressive therapy do not appear to significantly affect the course of the disease, the prognosis for this lesion is good and the mortality is relatively low (268,300). Five-year survival is reported to be between 85 and 100% (268,300). However, complete agreement on the long-term survival is lacking (255).

Proliferative glomerulonephritis (and its subcategories) is another histologic type of glomerular lesion which can lead to idiopathic nephrotic syndrome (268). The lesion is chiefly characterized by variable mesangial proliferation, as well as by varying amounts of epithelial and endothelial electron dense deposits on electron microscopic examination (263,285). Complement consumption can frequently be demonstrated. These patients usually display a steady downhill progression of renal function, depending upon the type of proliferative changes (263). Clearer definition of subcategories of proliferative nephritis, as well as better-controlled studies, are needed to determine the actual prognosis of this group of patients.

34. What is the treatment of idiopathic nephrotic syndrome secondary to proliferative or membranous glomerular lesions?

Steroid immunosuppression in patients with these more severe glomerular lesions has been somewhat disappointing. Although possible beneficial effects have been reported (264,268) especially in cases of mild proliferative changes (274), the majority of clinical trials fail to demonstrate a significant effect of steroids in these patients. Steroids have little or no beneficial effect on proteinuria or on the long-term prognosis of both idiopathic membraneous glomerulopathy (252,255,265,268,275,277,282,292,301,321) or proliferative glomerulonephritis (252,255,265,268, 277,282,321).

Because of the poor response to steroids, the cytotoxic agents azathioprine and cyclophosphamide have been extensively investigated in these patients. Despite the fact that therapeutic responses from these agents, either alone or in combination with steroids, have been reported in uncontrolled clinical trials (247,284,289,320), it is generally agreed that the therapeutic benefit derived from these agents is minimal at best and that there are substantial risks associated with the therapy involved (243,255,265,268, 288,306,311).

Available controlled studies have not demonstrated the effectiveness of *azathioprine,* either alone or in combination with steroids, in altering the course of the disease. Sharpstone et al (306) found in 20 adults with proliferative glomerulonephritis that a steroid-azathioprine combination was no more effective than prednisone alone. Abramowicz et al (243) conducted a controlled trial of 17 steroid-dependent nephrotic patients with proliferative and other glomerular lesions. These investigators showed that azathioprine (60 mg/m²/day) was no more effective than a placebo in reducing proteinuria in these patients. The Medical Research Council Working Party (288) reported similar findings in 72 children and adult patients with idiopathic nephrotic syndrome due to proliferative or membraneous lesions. No beneficial effect was found by combining azathioprine with steroids.

The response to *cyclophosphamide* has been equally discouraging. Booth and Aber (253), in a controlled clinical study conducted in 28 adults with idiopathic nephrotic syndrome with proliferative glomerular lesions, found no advantage of cyclophosphamide or azathioprine over placebo in treating these patients. In a prospective controlled study of 22 adult patients with idiopathic membranous nephropathy (261), cyclophosphamide did not favorably affect the progression of the disease after one year of daily treatment.

Immunosuppressive therapy continues to be used to treat these glomerular lesions with the hope of preventing or reversing immunologically mediated glomerular damage, despite the fact that controlled studies have failed to show that the prognosis of the disease is favorably altered by such treatment. The general ineffectiveness of steroid and cytotoxic agents cannot be fully explained. It may be related to the fact that although immune complexes initiate the disease process, other factors such as platelet aggregation and fibrin deposition sustain the disease (245). The recent success of investigators using antiplatelet drugs such as dipyridamole (280) and indomethacin (290), anticoagulants, or hemostatic-altering drugs plus immunosuppressive agents (279,282) lends support to this concept. In addition, reduced protein excretion, improved protein selectivity, and the ultimate improvement in glomerular filtration rate following initiation of indomethacin therapy may be related to inhibition in renal prostaglandin synthesis (246, 290). More controlled studies are required to determine the true effectiveness of this type of treatment.

35. How is the edema of nephrotic syndrome treated?

Unless the edema is a threat to health, vigorous treatment should be avoided. For mild edema, bed rest and sodium restriction will usually suffice. A high protein diet, unless contraindicated by coexisting azotemia, is also indicated to promote maximal albumin synthesis and restoration of oncotic pressure. If these measures are not successful, cautious diuresis may be indicated. Diuresis should be carried out slowly since these patients can rapidly develop hypovolemia due to poor oncotic pressure. A slow weight loss of no more than 0.5 to 0.8 kg per day can be carried out using spironolactone 100-200 mg/day, if the patient is not in renal failure. Thiazide-type diuretics (especially metazolone) and low doses of loop diuretics, such as furosemide are also effective: a combination of spironolactone with either thiazides or a loop diuretic may be particularly useful (268).

DIABETES INSIPIDUS:

J. J. is a 14-year-old male who had a partial hypophysectomy 48 hours ago to reduce an expanding pituitary tumor. However, over the last 24 hours he has put out 7.8 liters of dilute urine (specific gravity 1.001) with a urine osmolality of 225 mOsm/kg and a serum osmolality of 332 mOsm/kg. Intake during this period was 4.9 liters. The patient complains of intense thirst and shows signs of mild dehydration. Post-traumatic diabetes insipidus is the diagnosis.

36. What is diabetes insipidus?

Diabetes insipidus is a syndrome that is characterized by the excretion of large volumes of dilute urine and polydipsia and is caused by a relative deficiency of antidiuretic hormone (ADH), also known as vasopressin.

ADH, in combination with the thirst mechanism, is essential for the maintenance of normal extracellular fluid osmolality and water balance. ADH is manufactured in the supraoptic nucleus of the hypothalamus and is stored in the posterior pituitary. The major physiologic factor which controls day-to-day ADH production and release is serum osmolality. Elevations in serum osmolality, sensed by hypothalamic osmoreceptors, result in an increased ADH production and secretion. A decrease in serum osmolality has the opposite effect. ADH generation is secondarily controlled by volume depletion, which is mediated through vagal nerve impulses from arterial and venous baroceptors, as well as through cardiopulmonary stretch receptors. Pain, emotion, stress, temperature, and drugs can also influence the synthesis and secretion of ADH. Once in the circulation, ADH is transported to the kidney where it binds to renal tubular cell membranes and activates adenyl cyclase, which generates cyclic-AMP. The overall result of this biochemical reaction is an increase in the permeability of the renal collecting tubules to water, thereby increasing water reabsorption and lowering serum osmolality.

Usually, ADH deficiency results from damage to the neurohypophysis. The deficiency is generally transient if the damage is traumatic, but it may be permanent if, for example, it is due to congenital malformation. There is also a congenital nephrogenic origin of diabetes insipidus. That is, the pituitary gland produces a sufficient amount of ADH. However, the renal tubules are resistant to the action of the hormone, resulting in polyuria and polydipsia.

Diagnosis of diabetes insipidus is based on the presence of polyuria, polydipsia, a urine specific gravity of less than 1.010, and a urine osmolality which is less than that of the plasma. These are exhibited in the case history above. Differentiation between pituitary and nephrogenic diabetes insipidus is made by establishing the patient's responsiveness to aqueous vasopressin. Diabetes insipidus must also be differentiated from psychogenic water drinking by a water deprivation test.

Diabetes insipidus is generally not an emergency situation. In fact, as long as patients have an intact thirst mechanism and an adequate fluid supply, they are not in immediate danger of fluid and electrolyte imbalance. Treatment is initiated nonetheless, not only to relieve the inconvenience of polydipsia and polyuria, but also to avoid rapid dehydration in a situation of involuntary water deprivation (e.g. head injury,

unconsciousness). Treatment consists of vasopressin, thiazide diuretics, and a variety of drugs which produce the syndrome of inappropriate anti-diuretic hormone secretion (SIADH) (326,334,337,344,347). (See Question 41.)

37. Are there drugs that cause diabetes insipidus?

A number of drugs may increase water clearance, which in some instances, leads to clinically evident diabetes insipidus.

Lithium carbonate commonly produces a reversible nephrogenic diabetes insipidus, probably by blocking the activation of ADH-sensitive adenyl cyclase, resulting in ADH insensitivity. Impaired activation of cyclic-AMP dependent protein kinase has also been suggested. Additionally, lithium impairs free-water clearance by decreasing proximal tubular reabsorption of sodium and water. The possibility of a central mode of action has also been raised. The syndrome usually appears a few weeks following the initiation of drug treatment, but can take months to develop. This may be related to lithium accumulation within the renal tissue. The syndrome reverses within three to four weeks after drug discontinuation, which is the recommended treatment if electrolyte balance is a problem. It is possible that lowering the dose reduces the polyuria, therefore, this should be tried first. Thiazides may also be tried, but diminution of lithium's antimanic action is possible secondary to a sodium/lithium diuresis.

Other drugs have been associated with a reversible syndrome of nephrogenic diabetes insipidus. Singer et al report that 8 of 24 patients treated with *demethylchlortetracycline* (DMCT, demeclocycline) for acne developed renal concentrating defects. This drug-induced diabetes insipidus is caused by an unresponsiveness to ADH and is dose-related. Polydipsia and polyuria occur uniformly in patients receiving 1200 mg/day or more. It reverses with a reduction in dose or drug discontinuation. DMCT reduces cyclic-AMP levels in the renal medulla by inhibiting ADH-stimulated adenyl cyclase. The activity of cyclic-AMP-dependent protein kinase may also be impaired. While tetracycline and chlortetracycline have the same, but weaker, *in vitro* effects, they have not been reported to cause clinical diabetes insipidus. Other cases of diabetes insipidus secondary to DMCT have been reported.

Several *oral hypoglycemics,* acetohexamide, tolazamide, and glyburide, possess diuretic properties unlike chlorpropamide. This effect is not related to inhibition of ADH release or activity. These agents increase free water clearance by increasing proximal tubular reabsorption of sodium and water.

Vasopressin-resistant polyuria, with or without oliguria, may frequently follow *methoxyflurane* anesthesia. The polyuria may be related to the elevated fluoride concentrations found in these patients; however, the exact biochemical abnormality induced by methoxyflurane or the fluoride metabolite has not been clearly elucidated. Several cases of nephrogenic diabetes insipidus have also occurred during *propoxyphene* poisoning (344,345,352).

38. What forms of vasopressin are available? How are they dosed?

Three forms of vasopressin are commonly available for general use:

(a) Pitressin injection aqueous 20 units/cc.
(b) Pitressin tannate in oil 5 units/cc.
(c) Lysine vasopressin (Diapid) 2 units/spray.

Pitressin or vasopressin injections are used only in cases of diabetes insipidus secondary to a pituitary deficit, since they are ineffective in the nephrogenic variant. Initial treatment with *aqueous pitressin* provides short amelioration of polyuria. Aqueous pitressin requires repeated doses approximately every 3 to 4 hours, as indicated by a urine output of greater than 150-200 ml/hour. The initial dose is approximately 5 units IM or SC; however, smaller amounts may be used. The dose may be increased to 20 units or higher if control is inadequate with lower doses. The short duration of action of aqueous pitressin is advantageous because water intoxication is uncommon, and titration is easier in initial therapy where the severity and duration of the problem are not yet determined.

If it appears that the diabetes insipidus will be chronic, *pitressin tannate in oil suspension* is used because of its 24 to 72 hour duration of action. Following a test dose of 1.5 to 2.5 units, a maintenance dose of 2.5 to 5.0 units IM as determined by urine output is administered (preferably at night). In administering the tannate in oil preparation, it is important to remember that it is a suspension requiring thorough agitation before use. The ignorance of this fact has been the cause of a number of "vasopressin-resistant" cases of diabetes insipidus. Despite the fact that water intoxication is most likely to occur with this preparation, it is recommended over the aqueous solution for maintenance therapy (331,333).

Lysine vasopressin (Diapid), available as a nasal spray, is more acceptable for many patients than the tannate in oil vasopressin (322). This preparation is dosed every 3 to 6 hours as required to control polyuria. It is conveniently administered, and water intoxication is rare. The local, systemic, and pulmonary allergic reactions commonly associated with the older, still available, posterior pituitary snuff powder have practically been eliminated (322,332,342). The dose is one to two sprays in one or both nostrils (to a total of four sprays), four times a day initially. If polyuria is not controlled, it is recommended that the

dosing frequency be decreased rather than increasing the amount of drug per dose, since excessive amounts will be lost by swallowing. Overnight control may be difficult due to this preparation's short duration of action.

A new synthetic vasopressin analog, *1-desamino-8D arginine vasopressin (DDAVP)* is currently undergoing clinical trials in the United States. This agent will probably become the agent of choice in treating pituitary deficient diabetes insipidus. DDAVP, like lysine vasopressin, offers the convenience of intranasal administration. However, DDAVP's longer duration of action (average 12 hours), allows more satisfactory control of symptoms with usually one or two inhalations a day of 2.5 to 20 mcg. No significant hypersensitivity reactions have been reported (336, 338,351,354).

Patients should be monitored for electrolyte changes caused by excessive or insufficient vasopressin. Intake of hypertonic fluids should be avoided because the increased sodium load increases urine volume. On the other hand, excessive intake of water without electrolytes will cause a dilutional hyponatremia. Urine output, urine osmolality, serum osmolality, and specific gravity must be monitored while the patient is in the hospital. While at home, the patient must follow his symptoms of polyuria and polydipsia. Vasopressin resistance can also be induced by hypokalemia, hypercalcemia, and hypercalciuria (331,333). These electrolyte abnormalities should be avoided.

39. How is chlorpropamide used in diabetes insipidus? Are any other drugs useful?

As with vasopressin, *chlorpropamide* is effective only in the treatment of diabetes insipidus of pituitary origin. It cannot be used in nephrogenic diabetes insipidus. (See Question 42 for mechanisms.) Chlorpropamide's effectiveness depends on residual pituitary function. As residual pituitary function increases, so does chlorpropamide's effectiveness. Dosage is also important for drug effect. The greater the dose, the more effective will be the control of polyuria. A low dose of 125 mg/day is used initially. The patient remains on this dose for three to four days, at the end of which time maximal antidiuresis should be achieved. If polyuria is not controlled at this time, the dose is increased to 250 mg a day for an additional three to four days, then to 375 mg a day if needed. A dose of 500 mg a day may be tried, but is not recommended since hypoglycemia will usually occur at this dose. Instead of a 500-mg dose, the addition of a thiazide diuretic such as hydrochlorothiazide 50 to 100 mg twice daily with 375 mg of chlorpropamide is useful and effective. The addition of a thiazide potentiates the effectiveness of chlorpropamide through its ability to decrease free water clearance and reduce urine volume by 30 to 50%. Its ability to inhibit insulin release may also blunt the hypoglycemia induced by chlorpropamide. Because of its effectiveness and ease of administration, chlorpropamide has become a popular choice for the treatment of mild to moderate diabetes insipidus in patients with partial posterior pituitary deficiency (324, 327, 330, 339, 340, 344, 346, 347, 349, 352, 355).

Prompt reversal of clinical signs and symptoms of vasopressin-sensitive diabetes insipidus has also been reported in a majority of patients treated with 600 mg/day of *carbamazepine*. The effects of carbamazepine as with chlorpropamide appear to be dose-related. Additionally, the combination of carbamazepine and chlorpropamide has been used to treat diabetes insipidus. This combination offers equal effectiveness, while allowing dosage reduction and a decrease in the toxicity of each agent (325, 328, 344, 347, 350).

The antidiuretic effect of *clofibrate* (Atromid-S), a lipid-lowering agent, has been successfully utilized to treat patients with diabetes insipidus. Clofibrate in doses of 1.5 to 2.25 gm/day strikingly decreases urine volume within 24 hours in a number of patients with pituitary-deficient diabetes insipidus. Response depends on residual pituitary function and dose. The mechanism appears to be one of enhanced release of pituitary ADH. Clofibrate's effects appear to be weaker than those of chlorpropamide or carbamazepine at usual therapeutic doses, and its long-term efficacy has not been established (329, 343, 344, 347).

Acetaminophen has also been reported to improve polyuria and water balance in pituitary diabetes insipidus (348).

40. How do thiazides decrease urine volume in patients with diabetes insipidus?

Thiazides decrease urine volume by decreasing free water clearance. Thiazide diuretics induce volume depletion, resulting in increased proximal tubular reabsorption of sodium and water. This decreases the solute load to the distal tubule and reduces free water clearance. A low sodium diet enhances, while a high sodium diet blunts thiazide antidiuresis. Additionally, thiazides act in the cortical loop of Henle where sodium is reabsorbed without water in an effort to dilute urine or increase free water clearance. If thiazides block the action of this diluting segment, the kidneys are unable to generate free water and are not able to excrete a water load since maximal dilution cannot occur. Hence, urine volume is less than would be expected for a particular water load.

The overall effect of the above mechanisms is a drop in the urine volume by 30 to 50% in patients with both pituitary and nephrogenic diabetes insipidus.

Thiazides are rarely used alone because of their limited action, except in nephrogenic diabetes insipidus where they are the only drug treatment available. The usual dose is 50 to 100 mg twice a day of hydrochlorothiazide or an equivalent dose of other thiazides. Furosemide has also been successfully used to reduce urine volume (333, 347).

SYNDROME OF INAPPROPRIATE ANTIDIURETIC HORMONE SECRETION

E.T. is a 52-year-old woman who has been admitted to the hospital with a chief complaint of dizziness and chronic fatigue. The patient is in good health except for a five-year history of diabetes mellitus, treated at present with 250 mg/day of chlorpropamide which was recently added to dietary control. On admission, the patient's laboratory values were normal, except for a hematocrit of 34% and serum sodium of 120 mEq/L. On the day after admission, the serum osmolality was noted to be 268 mOsm/kg; the urine osmolality was 384 mOsm/kg. A syndrome of chlorpropamide-induced inappropriate secretion of ADH (SIADH) was suggested. Hyponatremia responded to fluid restriction and discontinuation of chlorpropamide.

41. What is the syndrome of inappropriate secretion of antidiuretic hormone (SIADH)?

The syndrome of inappropriate secretion of antidiuretic hormone is one in which hyponatremia is associated with adequate circulation and an expanded extracellular fluid volume. The symptoms are related to body fluid hypotonicity and water intoxication; neurologic symptoms predominate. The initial symptoms include progressive mental confusion, drowsiness, and lethargy. Overt psychotic behavior, coma, and grand mal convulsions will ensue if the hyponatremia persists, especially if the serum sodium is less than 110 mEq/L. Ultimately, irreversible neurologic damage and death can occur.

The diagnosis of the syndrome can be made on the basis of five criteria. First, hyponatremia and hypoosmolality of the serum caused by excessive water retention secondary to SIADH. Second, renal sodium wasting, relative to sodium intake despite hyponatremia. This phenomenon is related to volume expansion which causes: an increase in GFR, and sodium diuresis; a decrease in the proximal tubular reabsorption of sodium via third factor or naturetic hormone; and a decrease in aldosterone secretion which increases distal sodium excretion. Then, a third criteria of the syndrome is the formation of a less than maximally dilute urine in the face of serum hypotonicity. Fourth, the absence of evidence for dehydration; and finally, the fifth criteria, normal renal and adrenal function. In fact, these patients tend to have a low blood urea nitrogen (BUN).

SIADH is becoming well known as the cause of hyponatremia in "oat cell" carcinoma of the lung and other pulmonary diseases, as well as certain cerebral diseases (e.g. meningitis, aneurysm). Inappropriate secretion of antidiuretic hormone may also play a partial role in the development of hyponatremia in certain clinical disorders such as congestive heart failure, cirrhosis, hypothyroidism, and Addison's disease (323, 335, 344).

42. Can drugs induce the syndrome of inappropriate secretion of antidiuretic hormone?

A syndrome resembling SIADH has been associated with a number of drugs. These are listed below:

Chlorpropamide	Amitriptyline
Tolbutamide	Thiothixene
Carbamazepine	Flupenazine
Clofibrate	Thioridazine
Cyclophosphamide	Anesthestics
Vincristine	Barbiturates (pre-operative)
Diuretics	Narcotics
Oxytocin	Diazoxide
Phenformin	Acetaminophen

Of these drugs, *chlorpropamide* is probably the best known offender. The antidiuretic effect of chlorpropamide has occurred in patients with diabetes mellitus, diabetes insipidus, and in normal water-loaded patients. *Tolbutamide* has also been associated with this syndrome of drug-induced SIADH, but it does not appear to be a substantial problem. (See chapter on Diabetes Mellitus.)

Clofibrate (Atromid-S), a hypolipidemic agent, has been reported to have significant SIADH-like activity which is useful in the treatment of pituitary diabetes insipidus (see Question 39). Normal subjects also demonstrate an inability to excrete a water load while receiving clofibrate. However, dilutional hyponatremia, secondary to clofibrate, has not been reported in Atromid-treated hyperlipidemic patients, but it has been seen in a psychogenic water drinker receiving 6 to 8 gm/day of clofibrate.

The European literature has shown *carbamazepine* (Tegretol) to be effective in reducing polyuria in experimental subjects with diabetes insipidus (see Question 39). The SIADH has been reported in a psychogenic water drinker while on 1,200 to 1,800 mg/day of carbamazepine. The antidiuretic effect of carbamazepine was also found to be dose-related. Recently the combination of carbamazepine and chlorpropamide was shown to have additive dose-related antidiuretic effects. Carbamazepine has no intrinsic ADH activity, but apparently induces water retention by increasing ADH release.

Impaired water excretion secondary to *cyclophosphamide* has been documented. Impaired water load

excretion has been reported in 17 of 19 cancer patients receiving 50 mg/kg of cyclophosphamide. Signs of hyponatremia, hypo-osmolality, and inappropriately concentrated urine appeared within 4 to 12 hours following the dose. The effect lasted up to 20 hours. The course of events can be related in time to the excretion of active metabolites in the urine. There were no signs of SIADH when patients did not receive the drug nor could the hyponatremia be related to the type of cancer the patient exhibited. A single case of transient hyponatremia following a 3-gram parenteral dose of cyclophosphamide has been reported in a patient with oat cell carcinoma. Hyponatremia persisted for 10 days. Drug-induced SIADH or the release of an ADH substance following drug kill were suggested as the cause of the hyponatremia. This complication of cyclophosphamide may be important during initial treatment, since patients are required to increase fluid intake during cyclophosphamide therapy to prevent the hemorrhagic cystitis. Therefore patients must be watched during drug administration for signs of water intoxication; once the drug is stopped, water intoxication is no longer a problem since the "SIADH" activity dissipates over 20 hours following the last injection.

SIADH secretion has been associated with *vincristine* (Oncovin) treatment in both adults and children. Inappropriate antidiuretic hormone secretion manifested by the signs and symptoms of hyponatremia have occurred following repeated doses as well as single injections of vincristine (Oncovin). Severe water intoxication as evidenced by seizures and/or coma have occurred in some cases. Other manifestions of vincristine neurotoxicity are invariably associated with vincristine-induced SIADH secretion. Discontinuation of vincristine results in correction of hyponatremia, usually within two weeks. An abnormal secretion of ADH from the neurohypophysis has been suggested as a possible mechanism. Enhanced neurohypophyseal secretion of ADH may be related to a disruptive effect of vincristine on the microtubules of the neurohypophysis. Although the exact frequency of vincristine SIADH is not known, there is evidence which indicates that this is a dose-dependent effect.

Diuretic-induced hyponatremia may be caused by excessive saluresis or by inhibition of urinary dilution. The latter prevents maximal urinary dilution during a water load (such as excessive fluid intake) which results in a dilutional hyponatremia and hypo-osmolality in the presence of less than maximally dilute urine. This syndrome is indistinguishable from SIADH except that hypokalemia and alkalosis are usually present. It has been postulated that a low potassium level causes sodium to move intracellularly, resulting in hyponatremia and that the secondary extracellular volume depletion stimulates ADH release. However, this mechanism is disputed, since volume depletion is only a minor force in ADH release. The syndrome is reversible if the drug is discontinued.

Oxytocin, a hormone used to induce labor, has weak ADH-like activity and produces hyponatremia especially in patients whose volume overloaded. Symptomatic SIADH has also been reported in patients receiving *amitriptyline, thiothixene, fluphenazine,* and *phenformin* (323,335,341,344,345).

43. How is SIADH treated?

The treatment of SIADH depends upon the signs and symptoms of water intoxication. First, the underlying cause should be removed or corrected. Patients with drug-induced water intoxication usually respond to discontinuation of the offending agent, and all patients, regardless of the etiology of intoxication, respond to fluid restriction. Administration of less than 1000 cc/day of fluid encourages proximal tubular sodium reabsorption and enhances aldosterone secretion. If there is danger of permanent central nervous sytem damage, hypertonic saline (3 or 5%) should be infused slowly for transient but rapid correction of the hyponatremia.

Neurologic signs of hyponatremia may be reversed by rapid infusion of 1 mg/kg of *furosemide* to initiate a diuresis and by hourly replacement of urinary sodium losses with a concentrated saline solution. Potassium as well as other electrolyte losses induced by furosemide must be replaced.

Lithium carbonate and *demethylchlortetracycline,* because of their ability to inhibit the renal action of ADH, have been used successfully in the treatment of SIADH. These drugs may be particularly useful in ambulatory patients whose underlying cause of SIADH cannot be corrected and when other treatment modalities are ineffective or are not feasible. Demethylchlortetracycline is preferred over lithium because it is associated with less serious side effects. Phenytoin, which inhibits the central release of ADH acutely, does not appear to be clinically effective in the chronic treatment of SIADH (323,335,341,344).

INTRODUCTION

1. Alfrey AC: Chronic renal failure: Manifestations and pathogenesis. Chapt 11, in *Renal and Electrolyte Disorders,* Ed. by RW Schrier, Little, Brown, Co., Boston, 1976, p 319.
2. Anderson RJ et al: *Clinical Use of Drugs in Renal Failure,* Charles C. Thomas, III, 1976.
3. Brenner BM and Rector FC: *The Kidney,* WB Saunders, Phil, 1976.
4. Schrier RW (Ed): *Renal and Electrolyte Disorders.* Little, Brown Co, Boston, 1976.

ACUTE RENAL FAILURE

5. Barry KG et al: Oliguric renal failure: evaluation and therapy by the intravenous infusion of mannitol. JAMA 179:510, 1962.
6. Cantarovich F et al: Furosemide in high doses in the treatment of acute renal failure. Postgrad Med J 47 (suppl): 13, 1971.

7. Cronin RE and Schrier RW, Acute renal failure: diagnosis, pathogenesis, and management. Hosp Med 12:26, 1976.
8. Fries D et al: The use of large doses of furosemide in acute renal failure. Postgrad Med J 47 (suppl): 18, 1971.
9. Levinsky NG and Alexander EA: Acute Renal Failure, Chapt 21, in *The Kidney,* Ed. by BM Brenner and FC Rector, WB Saunders Company, Philadelphia, 1976, p 806.
10. Meriwether WD et al: Deafness following a standard intravenous dose of ethacrynic acid. JAMA 216:795, 1971.
11. Merrill JP: Acute renal failure, Chapt 17, *Diseases of the Kidney,* 2nd Ed., Ed. by MB Strauss and LG Welt, Little Brown and Co., Boston, 1971, p 637.
12. Muehreke RC: *Acute renal failure: Diagnosis and Management,* CV Mosby Co., St. Louis, 1969.
13. Pillay VKG et al: Transient and permanent deafness following treatment with ehtacrynic acid in renal failure. Lancet 1:77, 1969.
14. Schrier RW and Conger JD: Acute renal failure: Pathogenesis, diagnosis, and management, chapt 21, in *Renal and Electrolyte Disorders,* Ed. by RW Schrier, Little, Brown and Company, Boston, 1976, p 289.
15. Schrier RW: Acute renal failure: diagnosis, management and pathogenesis. Calif Med 115:28, 1971.
16. Schwartz, GH et al: Ototoxicity induced by furosemide. NEJM 282:1413, 1970.
17. Silverberg DS et al: The use of mannitol in oliguric renal failure, Med Clin N Amer 50:1159, 1966.
18. Sulliven JF et al: Use of furosemide in the oliguria of acute and chronic renal failure. Postgrad Med J 47 (suppl): 26, 1971.
19. Wigand ME et al: Ototoxic side-effects of high doses of furosemide in patients with uraemia. Postgrad Med J 47 (suppl): 54, 1971.

CHRONIC RENAL FAILURE

20. Crowe LR and Hatch FE: Diagnosis and management of chronic renal insufficiency. Hosp Med 12:6, 1976.
21. Merrill JP et al: Uremia (Part 1) NEJM 282:953, 1970.
22. Merrill JP et al: Uremia (Part 2) NEJM 282:1014, 1970.
23. Pullman TN et al: Chronic renal failure. Clin Symposia 25:2, 1973.
24. Schonfeld PY and Humphreys MH: A general description of the uremic state. Chap 33, in *The Kidney,* Ed. by BM Brenner and FC Rector, WB Saunders, Phil, 1976, p 1423.
25. Schrier RW: Medical management of chronic renal disease. Calif Med 114:44, 1971.
26. Schwartz WB et al: Medical management of chronic renal failure. Am J Med 44:786, 1968.
27. Walser M: The conservative management of the uremic patient. Chapt 39, *The Kidney,* Ed. by BM Brenner and FC Rector, WB Saunders, Phil, 1976, p 1613.
28. Wang F: Conservative management of chronic renal failure. Med Clin N Amer 55:137, 1971.

ANEMIA AND CHRONIC RENAL FAILURE

29. Alexander MR: Use of androgens in chronic renal failure patients on maintenance hemodialysis. Am J Hosp Pharm 33:242, 1976.
30. Bailey GL: *Hemodialysis, Principles and Practice.* Academic Press, New York, 1972.
31. DeGowin RL et al: Erythropoiesis and erythropoietin in patients with chronic renal failure treated with hemodialysis and testosterone. Ann Int Med 72:913, 1970.
32. Doane BD et al: Response of uremic patients to nandrolone decanoate, Arch Int Med 135:972, 1975.
33. Erslev AJ: Renal biogenesis of erythropoietin, Am J Med 58:25, 1975.
34. Eschbach JW et al: The hematological consequences of renal failure. Chapt 36, in *The Kidney.* Ed. by BM Brenner and FC Rector, WB Saunders, Phil, 1976, p 1522.
35. Eschbach JW et al: Improvement in the anemia of chronic renal failure with fluoxymesterone. Ann Int Med 78:527, 1973.
36. Fam AG et al: Iron absorption in chronic renal failure. Proc Eur Dial Trans Assoc 7:81, 1970.
37. Fried W et al: The hematologic effect of androgen in uremic

patients: study of packed cells volume and erythropoietin responses. Ann Int Med 79:823, 1973.

38. Goodman J and Bessman AN: Effect of nortestosterone decanoate on red cell 2, 3 diphosphoglycerate and hematocrit in hemodialysis patients. Clin Pharmacol Ther 17: 167, 1974.

39. Hampers CL et al: Megaloblastic hematopoiesis in uremia and in patients on long-term hemodialysis. NEJM 276:551, 1967.

40. Hendler ED et al: Controlled study of androgen therapy in anemia of patients on hemodialysis. NEJM 291:1046, 1974.

41. Hines JD et al: Abnormal folate binding proteins in azotemic patients. Blood 42:997, 1973.

42. Koch, KM et al: Anemia of the regular hemodialysis patient and its treatment. Nephron 12:405, 1974.

43. Kopple JD et al: Vitamin nutrition in patients undergoing maintenance hemodialysis. Kidney Intn'l 7:S-79, 1975.

44. Milman N and Larsen L: Iron absorption in patients with chronic uremia undergoing regular hemodialysis. Acta Med Scand 199:113, 1976.

45. Naets JP: Hematologic disorders in renal failure. Nephron 14:181, 1975.

46. Paine CJ et al: Folic acid binding proteins and folate balance in uremia. Arch Int Med 136:756, 1976.

47. Shahidi NT: Androgens and erythropoiesis. NEJM 289:72, 1973.

48. Shaldon S et al: Testosterone therapy for anemia in maintenance dialysis. Brit Med J 3:212, 1971.

49. Skoutakis VA et al: Folic acid dosage for chronic hemodialysis patients. Clin Pharmacol Ther 18:200, 1975.

50. Whitehead VM: Homeostatis of folic acid in patients undergoing maintenance hemodialysis. NEJM 279:970, 1968.

51. Yawata Y et al: Abnormal red cell metabolism causing hemolysis in uremia: a defect potentiated by tap water hemodialysis. Ann Int Med 79:362, 1973.

HEMOSTATIC DEFECTS IN CHRONIC RENAL FAILURE

52. Hutton RA: Hemostatic mechanism in uremia. Am J Clin Path 21:406, 1968.

53. Mustard JF et al: Platelets, thrombosis, and drugs. Drugs 9:19, 1975.

54. Merrill JP: Uremia, NEJM 282:953, 1970.

55. Rabiner SF: Bleeding in uremia. Med Clin N Am 56:221, 1972.

56. Weiss HJ: Bleeding disorders due to abnormal platelet function. Med Clin N Am 57:517, 1973.

57. Weiss HJ: Platelet physiology and abnormalities of platelet function (second ot two parts). NEJM 293:580, 1975.

CALCIUM METABOLISM IN CHRONIC RENAL FAILURE

58. Arnaud CD: Hyperparathyroidism and renal failure. Kidney Intn'l 4:89, 1973.

59. Avioli LV and Teitelbaum SL: Renal Osteodystrophies, Chapt 37, in The Kidney, Ed by BM Brenner and F Rector, WB Saunders Co, Phil, 1976, p 1542.

60. Beale MG et al: Vitamin D: The discovery of its metabolites and their therapeutic applications. Pediat 57:729, 1976.

61. Brickman AS et al: Treatment of renal osteodystrophy with calciferol (vitamin D) and related steroids, Kidney Intn'l 4:161, 1973.

62. Brickman AS et al: 1,25 Dihydroxy-vitamin D3 in normal man and patients with renal failure. Ann Int Med 80:161, 1974.

63. Brickman AS et al: Action of 1,25-dihydroxy-cholecalciferol, a potent, kidney-produced metabolite of vitamin D, in uremic man. NEJM 287:891, 1972.

64. Brickman AS et al: 1,25-dihydroxycholecalciferol. Arch Int Med 134:883, 1974.

65. Castells S et al: Metabolic effects of 1-α-hydroxycholecalciferol on renal osteodystrophy. Curr Ther Res 19:410, 1976.

66. Catto GRD et al: The investigation and treatment of renal bone disease. Am J Med 61:64, 1976.

67. Catto GRD et al: 1-α-hydroxycholecalciferol: A treatment for renal bone disease. Brit Med J 1:12, 1975.

68. Chalmers TM et al: 1-alpha-hydroxycholecalciferol as a substitute for the kidney hormone 1,25-dihydroxycholecalciferol in chronic renal failure. Lancet 2:696, 1973.

69. Chan JCM et al: 1-α-hydroxyvitamin D3 in chronic renal failure. JAMA 234:47, 1975.

70. Clarkson EM et al: Net intestinal absorption of calcium in patients with chronic renal failure. Kidney Intn'l 3:258, 1973.

71. Coburn JW et al: Intestinal absorption of calcium and the effect of renal insufficiency. Kidney Intn'l 4:96, 1973.

72. Corby PE: Treatment of bone disease in patients on chronic hemodialysis with dihydrotachysterol, Trans Amer Soc Artif Int Organs 22:60, 1976.

73. David DS: Vitamin D intoxication post renal transplantation. Ann Surg 171:455, 1970.

74. Davie MWJ et al: 1-alphahydroxycholecalciferol in chronic renal failure. Ann Int Med 84:281, 1976.

75. DeLuca HF: The kidney as an endocrine organ involved in the function of vitamin D. Am J Med 58:39, 1975.

76. DeLuca HF: Recent advances in our understanding of vitamin D endocrine system. J Lab Clin Med 87:7, 1976.

77. Eastwood JB et al: Some biochemical, histological, radiological and clinical features of renal osteodystrophy. Kidney Intn'l 4:128, 1973.

78. Goldsmith RS et al: Effects of calcium and phosphorus on patients maintained on dialysis. Kidney Intn'l 7:S118, 1975.

79. Harrison HE et al: Comparison between crystalline dihydrotachysterol and calciferol in patients requiring pharmacologic vitamin D therapy. NEJM 276:894, 1967.

80. Kaye M et al: Effect of dihydrotachysterol on calcium absorption in uremia. Metab 21:815, 1972.

81. Kaye M et al: Arrest of hyperparathyroid bone disease with dihydrotachysterol in patients undergoing chronic hemodialysis. Ann Int Med 73:225, 1970.

82. Madsen S et al: 1-alpha-hydroxycholecalciferol treatment of adults with chronic renal failure. Acta Med Scand 200:1, 1976.

83. Makoff DL et al: Chronic calcium carbonate therapy in uremia. Arch Int Med 123:15, 1969.

84. Mawer EB et al: Metabolic fate of administered 1,25-dihydroxycholecalciferol in controls and in patients with hypoparathyroidism. Lancet 1:1203, 1976.

85. Meyrier A et al: The influence of a high calcium carbonate intake on bone disease in patients undergoing hemodialysis. Kidney Intn'l 4:146, 1973.

86. Nielsen SP et al: 1-α-hydroxycholecalciferol. Long term treatment of patients with uremic osteodystrophy. Nephron 16:359, 1976.

87. Pierides Am et al: Variable response to long term 1-α-hydroxycholecalciferol in haemodialsys osteodystrophy. Lancet 1:1092, 1976.

88. Pierides Am et al: Barbiturate and anticonvulsant treatment in relation to osteomalacia with haemodialysis and renal transplantation. Brit Med J 1:190, 1976.

89. Pierides Am et al: 1-α-hydroxycholecalciferol in hemodialysis renal osteodystrophy. Adverse effects of anticonvulsant therapy. Clin Nephrol 5:189, 1976.

90. Pinggera WF et al: Uremic osteodystrophy: the therapeutic consequences of effective control of serum phosphorus. JAMA 222:1640, 1972.

91. Rasmussen H et al: The cellular basis of metabolic bone disease. NEJM 289:25, 1973.

92. Rutherford WE et al: Effect of 25-hydroxycholecalciferol on calcium absorption in chronic renal disease. Kidney Intn'l 8:320, 1975.

93. Sagar S et al: Dihydotachysterol and vitamin D resistance in renal failure. Arch Int Med 130:768, 1972.

94. Verberckmoes R et al: Disappearance of vascular calcifications during treatment of renal osteodystrophy. Ann Int Med 82:529, 1975.

95. Wang F: Conservative management of chronic renal failure. Med Clin N Amer 55:137, 1971.

ANTACIDS IN CHRONIC RENAL FAILURE

96. Abrams EE et al: Case reports: antacid induction of phosphate depletion syndrome in renal failure. West J Med 120:157, 1974.

97. Alfrey AC et al: The dialysis encephalopathy syndrome. Possible aluminum intoxication. NEJM 294:184, 1976.

98. Alfrey AC: Disorders of magnesium metabolism. Chapt 7, in Renal and Electrolyte Disorders Ed. by RW Schrier, Little, Brown & Co., 1976, p 223.

99. Alfrey AC et al: Hypermagnesemia after renal homotransplantation. Ann Int Med 73:367, 1970.
100. Bailey RR: Aluminum toxicity in rats and man. Lancet 2:276, 1972.
101. Bailey GL and Vona JP: Pharmacodynamics in renal failure. Chapt 4 in *Hemodialysis: Principles & Practice* Ed: GL Bailey, Academic Press, New York, 1972, p 117.
102. Berlyne GM et al: Aluminum toxicity in rats. Lancet 1:564, 1972.
103. Berlyne GM: Aluminum toxicity. Lancet 2:47, 1972.
104. Bloom WL and Flinchum D: Osteomalacia with pseudofractures caused by the ingestion of aluminum hydroxide. JAMA 174:181, 1960.
105. Boelens PA et al: Hypophosphatemia with muscle weakness due to antacids and hemodialysis. Am J Dis Child 120:350, 1970.
106. David DS et al: Hypercalcemia after renal transplantation. NEJM 289:398, 1973.
107. Dent CE et al: Medical memoranda: Osteomalacia due to phosphate depletion from excessive aluminum hydroxide ingestion. Brit Med J 1:551, 1974.
108. Ditzler JW: Epsom-salts poisoning and a review of magnesium-ion physiology. Anesth 32:378, 1970.
109. Fitzgerald FT: Hypophosphatemia-Medical Staff Conference. West J Med 122:482, 1975.
110. Levant JA et al: Stimulation of gastric secretion and gastrin release by single oral doses of calcium carbonate in man. NEJM 289:555, 1973.
111. Lichtman MA et al: Erythrocyte adenosine triphosphate depletion during hypophosphatemia in a uremic subject. NEJM 280:240, 1969.
112. Lotz M et al: Evidence for a phosphorus-depletion syndrome in man. NEJM 278:409, 1968.
113. Mansouri K et al: Zinc, copper, magnesium and calcium in dialyzed and nondialyzed uremic patients. Arch Int Med 125:88, 1970.
114. Poole JW et al: Investigation of aluminum blood levels in man after oral administration of an aluminum-containing complex, potassium glucaldrate. J Pharm Sci 54:651, 1965.
115. Randall RE et al: The milk-alkali syndrome. Arch Int Med 107:63, 1961.
116. Randall RE Jr. et al: Hypermagnesemia in renal failure: etiology and toxic manifestations. Ann Int Med 61:73, 1964.
117. Thurston H et al: Aluminum retention and toxicity in chronic renal failure. Lancet 1:881, 1972.
118. Townsend CM Jr et al: Intestinal obstruction from medication bezoar in patients with renal failure. NEJM 288:1058, 1973.
119. Wacker WEC and Parisi AF: Magnesium metabolism. NEJM 278:712, 1968.
120. Wacker WEC and Parisi AF: Magnesium Metabolism. NEJM 278:772, 1968.

POTASSIUM BALANCE IN CHRONIC RENAL FAILURE

121. Berlyne GM: Dangers of kayexalate in the treatment of hyperkalemia in renal failure. Lancet 1:167, 1966.
122. Cacioppo PL and Hollander L: Orange juice treated with exchange resin. NEJM 287:361, 1972.
123. Chamberlain MJ: Emergency treatment of hyperkalemia. Lancet 1:464, 1964.
124. Cohen AB: Hyperkalemic effects of triamterene. Ann Intern Med 65:521, 1966.
125. Gabow P: Disorders of potassium metabolism, Chapt 5 in *Renal and Electrolyte Disorders* Ed. by RW Schrier, Little, Brown and Co., Boston, 1976, p 143.
126. Herman E et al: Fatal hyperkalemic paralysis associated with spironolactone. Arch Neurol 15:74, 1966.
127. Levinsky NG and Alexander EA: *Acute renal failure*, Chapt 21 in *The Kidney*, Ed. by BM Brenner and FC Rector, WB Saunders Co., Phil, 1976, p 806.
128. Levy N et al: Citrus juice treated with exchange resins. NEJM 289:753, 1973.
129. Pearson RE et al: Potassium content of selected medicines, foods and salt substitutes. Hosp Pharm 6:6, 1971.
130. Pullman TN et al: Chronic renal failure. Clinical Symposia 25:2, 1973.
131. Rovner DR: Use of pharmacologic agents in the treatment of hypokalemia and hyperkalemia. Rational Drug Therapy 6:1, 1972.
132. Schrier RW: Medical Management of chronic renal disease, Calif Med 114:44, 1971.
133. Schwartz WB: Potassium and the Kidney. NEJM 253:601, 1955.
134. Schwartz WB et al: Medical management of chronic renal failure. Am J Med 44:786, 1968.
135. Thorn GW, Ed: Clinician: Potassium in Clinical Medicine. Searle and Co., San Juan, Puerto Rico, 1973.
136. Townsend CM et al: Intestinal obstruction from medication bezoar in patients with renal failure. NEJM 288:1058, 1973.
137. Wang F: Conservative management of chronic renal failure. Med Clin N Am 55:137, 1971.
138. Whang R Hyperkalemia: diagnosis and treatment. Am J Med Sci 272:19, 1976.

URIC ACID AND CHRONIC RENAL FAILURE

139. Elion GB et al: Renal clearance of oxypurinol, the chief metabolite of allopurinol. Am J Med 45:69, 1968.
140. Fessel WF et al: Correlates and consequences of asymptomatic hyperuricemia. Arch Int Med 132:44, 1973.
141. Rieselbach RE et al: Influence of the kidney upon urate homeostasis in health and disease. Am J Med 56:665, 1974.
142. Smyth CJ: Ch 59, Diagnosis and treatment of gout, in *Arthritis and Allied Conditions*, Ed. 9, Ed. by Hot5$nder JL. Lea & Febiger, Phila., 1972, p 112.
143. Symposium: Gout with renal complicatons. Ann Rheum Dis. 25:668, 1966.
144. Yu TF: Milestones in the treatment of gout. Am J Med 56:676, 1974.
145. Wallace SL et al: Plasma levels of colchicine after oral administration of a single dose. Metab 22:749, 1973.
146. Wallace SL et al: Colchicine plasma levels: implications as to pharmacology and mechanism of action. Am J Med 48:443, 1970.
147. Wilson JD et al: Allopurinol in the treatment of uremic patients with gout. Ann Rheum Dis 26:136, 1967.
148. Wyngaarden JB: Ch 58, The etiology and pathogenesis of gout, in *Arthritis and Allied Conditions*, Ed. 8. Ed by Holland, JL. Lea & Febiger, Phila., 1972, p 1072.

CARBOHYDRATE ANBORMALITIES IN CHRONIC RENAL FAILURE

149. Bagdade JD: Disorders of carbohydrate and lipid metabolism in uremia. Nephron 14:153, 1975.
150. Corvilain J et al: Labeled insulin catabolism in chronic renal failure and in the anephric state: Diabetes 20:467, 1971.
151. DeFronzo RA et al: Carbohydrate metabolism in uremia, a review. Medicine 52:469, 1973.
152. Feldman HA et al: Endocrinology and metabolism in uremia and dialysis: A clinical review. Medicine 54:345, 1975.
153. Fuss M et al: I^{125}-insulin metabolism in chronic renal failure treated by renal transplantation. Kidney Intn'l 5:372, 1974.
154. Greenblatt DJ: Insulin sensitivity in renal failure. NY State J Med 74:1040, 1974.
155. Horton DS et al: Carbohydrate metabolism in uremia. Ann Int Med 68:63, 1968.
156. Knochel JP et al: The pathophysiology of uremia, in *The Kidney*, by Brenner BM and Rector F, WB Saunders Comp, Philadel, 1976, pg 1448.
157. Navalesi R et al: Insulin metabolism in chronic uremia and in the anephric state: effect of the dialytic treatment. J Clin Endocrinol Metab 40:70, 1975.
158. Rabkin R et al: Effect of renal disease on renal uptake and excretion of insulin in man. NEJM 282:182, 1970.
159. Rubinstein AH et al: Role of the kidney in insulin metabolism and excretion. Diabetes 17:161, 1968.

HYPERTENSION IN CHRONIC RENAL FAILURE

160. Ahearn DJ et al: Treatment of malignant hypertension with sodium nitroprusside. Arch Int Med 133:187, 1974.
161. Buhler FR et al: Propranolol inhibition of renin secretion: a spe-

cific approach to diagnosis and treatment of renin-dependent hypertensive diseases. NEJM 287:1209, 1972.

162. Cacace L et al: Treatment of hypertensive emergencies with sodium nitroprusside. Drug Intell Clin Pharm 4:187, 1970.

163. Davies DL et al: Abnormal relation between exchangeable sodium and the renin-angiotensin system in malignant hypertension and in hypertension with chronic renal failure. Lancet 1:683, 1973.

164. Del Greco F et al: Hypertension of chronic renal failure: role of sodium and the renal pressor system. Kidney Intn'l 7:S176, 1975.

165. Gottlieb TB et al: Combined therapy with vasodilator drugs and beta-adrenergic blockade in hypertension: a comparative study of minoxidil and hydralazine. Circ. XLV:571, 1972.

166. Hull AR et al: The control of hypertension in patients undergoing regular maintenance hemodialysis. Kidney Intn'l 7:S184, 1975.

167. Kincaid-Smith P et al: Hypertension and the kidney. Kidney Intn'l 8:S151, 1975.

168. Koch-Weser J: Hypertensive emergencies. NEJM 290:211, 1974.

169. Lazarus JM et al: Urgent bilateral nephrectomy for severe hypertension. Ann Int Med 76:733, 1972.

170. Lazarus JM et al: Hypertension in chronic renal failure: treatment with hemodialysis and nephrectomy. Arch Int Med 133:1059, 1974.

171. Mathew TH et al: The use of diazoxide in hypertensive crises. Drugs 2:73, 1971.

172. McDonald KM: The kidney in hypertension. Chapt. 9, in Renal and Electrolyte Disorders, Ed. by RW Schrier, Little, Brown Co., Boston, 1976, p 263.

173. Muth RG: Diuretic properties of furosemide in renal disease. Ann Int Med 69:249, 1968.

174. Mroczek WJ et al: The value of aggressive therapy in the hypertensive patient with azotemia. Circ. XL:893, 1969.

175. Pettinger WA: Clonidine, a new antihypertensive drug. NEJM 293:1179, 1975.

176. Pettinger WA et al: Minoxidil — an alternative to nephrectomy for refractory hypertension. NEJM 289:167, 1973.

177. Pettinger WA: Treatment of hypertension in the patient with renal disease. Chapt 47 in The Kidney, Ed. by BM Brenner and FC Rector, WB Saunders Co., Phil, 1976, p 1879.

178. Rastogi SP et al: High dose furosemide in the treatment of hypertension in chronic renal insufficiency and of terminal renal failure. Postgrad Med J 47 (April Suppl):45, 1971.

179. Ulvila JM et al: Blood pressure in chronic renal failure: effect of sodium intake and furosemide. JAMA 220:233, 1972.

180. Vaughan ED Jr et al: The volume factor in low and normal renin essential hypertension. Its treatment with either spironolactone or chlorthalidone. In Hypertension Manual, Ed by JH Laragh, New York, Yorke Medical Books, 1973, p 851.

181. Vertes V et al: Hypertension in end-stage renal disease. NEJM 280:978, 1969.

182. Weidmann P et al: Hypertension in terminal renal failure. Kidney Intn'l 9:294, 1976.

183. Woods JW et al: Management of malignant hypertension complicated by renal insufficiency. NEJM 277:57, 1967.

184. Woods JW et al: Management of malignant hypertension complicated by renal insufficiency, a follow up study. NEJM 291:10, 1974.

185. Zacest R et al: Treatment of essential hypertension with combined vasodilation and betaadrenergic blockage. NEJM 286:617, 1972.

GLOMERULONEPHRITIS

186. Cameron JS: A clinician's view of the classification of glomerulonephritis, in Glomerulonephritis, Proc Intn'l Symp, Royal Melbourne Hospital, Part II, ed by P. Kincaid-Smith, et al, John Wiley & Sons, New York, 1973, p 63.

187. Churg J et al: Classification of glomerulonephritis based on morphology, in Glomeruloonephritis, Proc Intn'l Symp, Royal Melbourne Hospital, Part II, ed. by P. Kincaid-Smith et al, John Wiley & Sons, New York, 1973, p 43.

188. MacDonald M: Electron microscopy in the classification of glomerulonephritis, in Glomerulonephritis, Proc Intn'l Symp, Royal Melbourne Hospital, Part II, ed by P. Kincaid-Smith, et al: John Wiley & Sons, New York, 1973, p 111.

189. Medical Staff Conference: Immunological mechanisms of glomerulonephritis. West J Med 116:47, 1972.

190. Merrill JP: Glomerulonephritis, Part I, NEJM 290:257, 1974.

191. Merrill JP: Glomerulonephritis, Part II, NEJM 290:313, 1974.

192. Merrill JP: Glomerulonephritis, Part III, NEJM 290:374, 1974.

193. Wilson CB et al: Glomerulonephritis, Disease-a-month 22:4, 1976 (June).

LUPUS NEPHRITIS

194. Ackerman GL: Alternate-day steroid therapy in lupus nephritis. Ann Int Med 72:511, 1970.

195. Adams DA et al: Azathioprine treatment of immunological renal disease. JAMA 199:119, 1967.

196. Alwall N et al: On corticosteroid and azathioprine treatment of glomerular renal diseases. Acta Med Scand 192:455, 1972.

197. Baldwin DS et al: The clinical course of the proliferative and membranous forms of lupus nephritis. Ann Int Med 73:929, 1970.

198. Balslov JT et al: Cytostatic treatment of glomerular diseases. Acta Med Scand 200:31, 1976.

199. Bardana EJ Jr et al: Azathioprine in steroid-insensitive nephropathy. Am J Med 49:789, 1970.

200. Bardana EJ Jr et al: Recent advances in the immunopathogenesis of systemic lupus erythematosus. West J Med 122:130, 1975.

201. Barnett EV et al: Systemic lupus erythematosus. Calif Med 111:467, 1969.

202. Cade R et al: Comparison of azathioprine, prednisone, and heparin alone or combined in treating lupus nephritis. Nephron 10:37, 1973.

203. Cameron JS et al: Lupus nephritis: long-term follow-up in Glomerulonephritis, Proc Intn'l Symp, Royal Melbourne Hospital, Part II, ed by P. Kincaid-Smith et al: John Wiley & Sons, New York, 1973, p 1187.

204. Cameron JS et al: Treatment of lupus nephritis with cyclophosphamide. Lancet 2:846, 1970.

205. Coplon N et al: Hemodialysis in end-stage lupus nephritis. Trans Amer Soc Artif Int Organs 19:302, 1973.

206. Decker JL et al: Cyclophosphamide or azathioprine in lupus glomerulonephritis, a controlled trial; results at 28 months. Ann Intern Med 83:605, 1975.

207. Decker JL et al: Systemic lupus erythematosus contrast and comparisons. Ann Intern Med 82:391, 1975.

208. Dillard MG et al: The effect of treatment with prednisone and nitrogen mustard on the renal lesions and life span of patients with lupus glomerulonephritis. Nephron 10:273, 1973.

209. Donadio JV Jr et al: Treatment of lupus nephritis with prednisone and combined prednisone and azathioprine. Ann Int Med 77:829, 1972.

210. Donadio JV Jr et al: Further observations on the treatment of lupus nephritis with prednisone and combined prednisone and azathioprine. Arthr Rheum 17:573, 1974.

211. Donadio JV Jr et al: Progressive lupus glomerulonephritis. Treatment with prednisone and combined prednisone and cyclophosphamide. Mayo Clin Proc 51:484, 1976.

212. Drinkard et al: Azathioprine and prednisone in the treatment of adults with lupus nephritis. Clinical, histological, and immunological changes with therapy. Medicine, 49:411, 1970.

213. Dubois EL: Management of systemic lupus erythematosus. Mod Treat 3:1245, 1966.

214. Ehrlich GE: Systemic lupus erythematosus. JAMA 232:1361, 1975.

215. Epstein WV: Immunologic events preceding clinical exacerbation of systemic lupus erythematosus. Am J Med 54:631, 1973.

216. Epstein WV et al: Favorable outcome in diffuse proliferative glomerulonephritis of systemic lupus erythematosus. Arth Rheum 17:129, 1974.

217. Estes D et al: The natural history of systemic lupus erythematosus by prospective analysis. Medicine 50:85, 1971.

218. Feng, PH et al: Cyclophosphamide in treatment of systemic lupus erythematosus: 7 years' experience. Br Med J, 2:450, 1973.

219. Fries JF et al: Late-stage lupus nephropathy. J Rheum 1:166, 1974.

220. Fries JF et al: Cyclophosphamide therapy in systemic lupus erythematosus and polymyositis. Arth Rheum 16:154, 1973.

221. Ginzler E et al: Long term maintenance therapy with azathioprine in systemic lupus erythematosus. Arth Rheum 18:27, 1975.

222. Glassock RJ et al: The glomerulopathies, in *The Kidney*. Ed. by Brenner BM and Rector F, WB Saunders Comp, Philadel, 1976, pg 941.

223. Grupe WE et al: Cytotoxic drugs in steroid-resistant renal disease. Am J Dis Child 112:448, 1966.

224. Hann BH et al: Azathioprine plus prednisone compared with prednisone alone in the treatment of systemic lupus erythematosus, Ann Intern Med 83:597, 1975.

225. Hayslett JP et al: The effect of azathioprine on lupus glomerulonephritis. Medicine 51:393, 1972.

225a. Hecht B et al: Prognostic indices in lupus nephritis. Medicine 55:163, 1976.

226. Lindeman RD et al: Long-term azathioprine-corticosteroid therapy in lupus nephritis and idiopathic nephrotic syndrome. J Chron Dis 29:189, 1976.

227. Maher JF et al: Treatment of lupus nephritis with azathioprine. Arch Int Med 125:293, 1970.

228. Martin EW Jr et al: The nephritis of systemic lupus erythematosus. Calif Med 117:49, 1972.

229. Michael AF et al: Immunosuppressive therapy of chronic renal disease. NEJM 276:817, 1967.

230. Nanra RS et al: Lupus nephritis clinical course in relation to treatment, in *Glomerulonephritis,* Proc Intn'l Symp, Royal Melbourne Hospital, Part II, ed. by P. Kincaid-Smith et al, John Wiley & Sons, New York, 1973, p 1193.

231. Pollak VE et al: The clinical course of lupus nephritis relationship to the renal histologic findings in *Glomerulonephritis,* Proc Intn'l Symp, Royal Melbourne Hospital, Part II, ed. by P. Kincaid-Smith et al, John Wiley & Sons, New York, 1973, p 1167.

232. Pollack VE et al: Clinical and experimental natural history of the renal manifestations of systemic lupus erythematosus. J Lab Clin Med 63:537, 1964.

233. Sharon E et al: Exacerbation of systemic lupus erythematosis after withdrawal of azathioprine therapy. NEJM 288:122, 1973.

234. Shelp WD et al: Effect of azathioprine on renal histology and function in lupus nephritis. Arch Int Med 128:566, 1971.

235. Snaith ML et al: Treatment of patients with systemic lupus erythematosus including nephritis with chlorambucil. Brit Med J 2:197, 1973.

236. Snaith ML et al: Chlorambucil in the treatment of systemic lupus erythematosus. Am Heart J 87:533, 1974.

237. Steinberg AD et al: Cyclophosphamide in lupus nephritis: a controlled trial, Ann Int Med 75:165, 1971.

238. Steinberg AD et al: A double-blind controlled trial comparing cyclophosphamide, azathioprine, and placebo in the treatment of lupus glomerulonephritis. Arth Rheum 17:923, 1974.

239. Striker GE et al: The course of lupus nephritis: a clinical-pathological correlation of fifty patients in *Glomerulopnephritis.* Proc Intn'l Symp Royal Melbourne Hospital Part II ed by P. Kincaid-Smith et al John Wiley & Sons New York 1973 p 1143.

240. Sztejnbok M et al: Azathioprine in the treatment of systemic lupus erythematosus. Arthr Rheum 14:639, 1971.

241. Wagner L: Immunosuppressive agents in lupus nephritis: a critical analysis. Medicine 55:239, 1976.

242. Yount WJ et al: Corticosteroid therapy of the collagen vascular disorders. Med Clin N Amer 57:1343, 1973.

NEPHROTIC SYNDROME

243. Abramowicz M et al: Controlled trial of azathioprine in children with nephrotic syndrome; a report for the international study of kidney disease in children. Lancet 1:959, 1970.

244. Adams DA et al: Azathioprine treatment of immunological renal disease, JAMA 199:119, 1967.

245. Ardlie NG: Mechanism of platelet aggregation and release; their possible role in vascular injury, in *Glomerulonephritis,* Proc. Intn'l Symp, Royal Melbourne Hospital, Part II, ed by P. Kincaid-Smith, et al, John Wiley & Sons, New York, 1973, p 891.

246. Arisz L et al: The effect of indomethacin on proteninuria and kidney function in the nephrotic syndrome. Acta Med Scand 199:121, 1976.

247. Bardana EJ Jr et al: Azathioprine in steriod-insensitive nephropathy. Am J Med 49:789, 1970.

248. Barratt TM et al: Comparative trial of 2 week and 8 weeks cyclophosphamide in steroid-sensitive relapsing nephrotic syndrome of childhood. Arch Dis Child 48:286, 1973.

249. Barratt TM et al: Controlled trial of cyclophosphamide in steroid-sensitive relapsing nephrotic syndrome of childhood. Lancet 2:479, 1970.

250. Barratt TM et al: Cyclophosphamide treatment in steroid-sensitive nephrotic syndrome of childhood. Lancet 1:55, 1975.

251. Bergstrand A et al: Idiopathic nephrotic syndrome of childhood cyclophosphamide induced conversion from steroid refractory to highly steroid sensitive disease. Clin Nephrol 1:302, 1973.

252. Black DAK et al: Controlled trial of prednisone in adult patients with the nephrotic syndrome. Brit Med J 3:421, 1970.

253. Booth LJ et al: Immunosuppressive therapy in adults with proliferative glomerulonephritis. Lancet 2:1010, 1970.

254. Buchanan JD et al: Return of spermatogenesis after stopping cyclophosphamide therapy. Lancet 2:156, 1975.

255. Cameron JS et al: Memranous nephropathy, in *Glomerulonephritis,* Proc. Intn'l Symp, Royal Melbourne Hospital, Part II, ed by P. Kincaid-Smith, et al, John Wiley & Sons, New York, 1973, p 473.

256. Cameron JS et al: Observations on the "minimal change" lesion: adult onset patients and results of cyclophosphamide treatment in children, op cit, p 211.

257. Cameron JS et al: Long-term stability of remission in nephrotic syndrome after treatment with cyclophosphamide. Brit Med J 4:7, 1971.

258. Chiu J et al: A controlled prospective study of cyclophosphamide in relapsing, corticosteroid-responsive minimal-lesion nephrotic syndrome in childhood. J Pediat 82:607, 1973.

259. Chiu J et al: Long-term follow-up of cyclophosphamide therapy in frequent relapsing minimal lesion nephrotic syndrome. J Pediat 84:825, 1974.

260. Churg J et al: Membranous nephropathy in *Glomerulonephritis,* Proc. Intn'l Symp. Royal Melbourne Hospital, Part II, edited by P. Kincaid-Smith, et al, John Wiley & Sons, New York, 1973, p 443.

261. Donadio JV Jr et al: Controlled trial of cyclophosphamide in idiopathic membranous nephropathy. Kid Intn'l 6:431, 1974.

262. Drummond KN et al: Cyclophosphamide in the nephrotic syndrome of childhood: its use in two groups of patients defined by clinical, light microscopic and immunopathologic findings. Canad Med Assoc J 98:524, 1968.

263. Earley, LE et al: Nephrotic syndrome. West J Med 115:23, 1971.

264. Ehrenreich T et al: Treatment of idiopathic membranous nephropathy. NEJM 295:741, 1976.

265. Erwin DT et al: The clinical course of idiopathic membranous nephropathy. Mayo Clin Proc 48:697, 1973.

266. Etteldorf JN et al: Cyclophosphamide in the treatment of idiopathic lipoid nephrosis. J Pediat 70:758, 1967.

267. Etteldorf JN et al: Gonadal function, testicular histology, and meiosis following cyclophosphamide therapy in patients with nephrotic syndrome. J Pediat 88:206, 1976.

268. Glassock RJ et al: The glomerulopathies, in *The Kidney,* by Brenner BM and Rector F, WB Saunders Comp, Philadel, 1976, pg 941.

269. Fairley KF et al: Sterility and testicular atrophy related to cyclophosphamide therapy. Lancet 1:568, 1972.

270. Gluck, MC et al: Membranous glomerulonephritis; evolution of clinical and pathologic features. Ann Int Med 78:1, 1973.

271. Grishman E et al: Pathology of nephrotic syndrome with minimal or minor glomerular changes, in *Glomerulonephritis,* Proc. Intn'l Symp, Royal Melbourne Hospital, Part II, ed by P. Kincaid-Smith, et al. John Wiley & Sons, New York, 1973, p 165.

272. Grupe WE et al: Cytotoxic drugs in steroid-resistant renal disease. Am J Dis Child 112:448, 1966.

273. Grupe WE: Chlorambucil in steroid-dependent nephrotic syndrome. J Pediat 82:598, 1973.

274. Grupe WE et al: Chlorambucil treatment of frequently relapsing nephrotic syndrome. NEJM 295:746, 1976.

275. Hayslett JP et al: Clinicopathological correlations in the nephrotic syndrome due to primary renal disease. Medicine 52:93, 1973.

276. Hopper J Jr et al: Lipoid nephrosis in 31 adult patients, renal biopsy study by light, electron, and fluorescence microscopy with experience in treatment. Medicine 49:321, 1970.

277. Jao W et al: Lipoid nephrosis: An approach to the clinicopathologic analysis and dismemberment of idiopathic nephrotic syndrome with minimal changes. Medicine 52:445, 1973.

278. Jenis EH et al: Focal segmental glomerulosclerosis. Amer J Med 57:695, 1974.

279. Kincaid-Smith P: The natural history and treatment of mesangio-capillary glomerulonephritis, in *Glomerulonephritis,* Proc. Int'l Symp, Royal Melbourne Hospital, Part II, ed. by P. Kincaid-Smith, et al, John Wiley & Sons, New York, 1973, p 591.

280. Kincaid-Smith P et al: Dipyridamole and anticoagulants in renal disease due to glomerular and vascular lesions; a new approach to therapy. Med J Aust 1:145, 1970.

281. Kumar R et al: Cyclophosphamide and reproductive function. Lancet 1:1212, 1972.

282. Laver MC et al: The natural history and treatment of membranous glomerulonephritis, in *Glomerulonephritis,* Proc. Intn'l Symp., Royal Melbourne Hospital, Part II, ed. by P. Kincaid-Smith, et al, John Wiley & Sons, New York, 1973, p 461.

283. Lim VS et al: Adult lipoid nephrosis: Clinicopathological correlations, Ann Int Med 81:314, 1974.

284. Lindeman RD et al: Long-term azathioprine-corticosteroid therapy in lupus nephritis and idiopathic nephrotic syndrome. J Chron Dis 29:189, 1976.

285. MacDonald MK: Electron microscopy in the classification of glomerulonephritis, in *Glomerulonephritis,* Proc. Intn'l Symp. Royal Melbourne Hospital, Part II, ed by P. Kincaid-Smith et al. John Wiley & Sons, New York, 1973, p 111.

286. McCrory WW et al: Therapeutic and toxic effects observed with different dosage programs of cyclophosphamide in treatment of steroid-responsive but frequently relapsing nephrotic syndrome. J Pediat 82:614, 1973.

287. McDonald J et al: Long-term assessment of cyclophosphamide therapy for nephrosis in children. Lancet 2:980, 1974.

288. Medical Research Council Working Party: Controlled trial of azathioprine and prednisone in chronic renal disease. Brit Med J 2:239, 1971.

289. Michael AF et al: Immunosuppressive therapy of chronic renal disease. NEJM 276:817, 1967.

290. Michielsen P et al: Indomethacin treatment of membrano-proliferative and lobular glomerulonephritis, in *Glomerulonephritis,* Proc. Intn'l Symp., Royal Melbourne Hospital, Part II, ed by P. Kincaid-Smith et al, John Wiley & Sons, New York, 1973, p 611.

291. Miller DG: Alkylating agents and human spermatogenesis. JAMA 217:1662, 1971.

292. Miller RB et al: Long-term results of steroid therapy in adults with idiopathic nephrotic syndrome. Am J Med 46:919, 1969.

293. Moncrieff MW et al: Cyclophosphamide therapy in the nephrotic syndrome in childhood. Brit Med J 1:666, 1969.

294. Nash MA et al: The significance of focal sclerotic lesions of glomeruli in children. J Pediat 88:806, 1976.

295. Newman WJ et al: Focal glomerular sclerosis: Contrasting clinical patterns in children and adults. Medicine 55:, 1976.

296. Ooi BS et al: Longitudinal studies of lipoid nephrosis. Arch Intern Med 130:883, 1972.

297. Pennisi AJ et al: Gonadal function in children with nephrosis treated with cyclophosphamide. Am J Dis Child 129:315, 1975.

298. Pennisi AJ et al: Cyclophosphamide in the treatment of idiopathic nephrotic syndrome. Pediat 57:948, 1976.

299. Penso J et al: Testicular function in prepubertal and pubertal male patients treated with cyclophosphamide for nephrotic syndrome. J Pediat 84:831, 1974.

300. Pollak VE et al: The natural history of membranous glomerulonephropathy, in *Glomerulonephritis,* Proc. Intn'l. Symp., Royal Melbourne Hospital, Part II, ed. by P. Kincaid-Smith, et al, John Wiley & Sons, New York, 1973, p 429.

301. Pollak VE et al: Natural history of lipoid nephrosis and of membranous glomerulonephritis. Ann Int Med 69:1171, 1968.

302. Qureshi MSA et al: Cyclophosphamide therapy and sterility. Lancet 2:1290, 1972.

303. Report of the international study of kidney diseases in children, Prospective, controlled trial of cyclophosphamide therapy in children with nephrotic syndrome. Lancet 2:423, 1974.

304. Richter P et al: Effect of chlorambucil on spermatogenesis in the human with malignant lymphoma. Cancer 25:1026, 1970.

305. Schreiner GE, ed: *Clinician: The Nephrotic Syndrome.* Searle & Co., San Juan Puerto Rico, 1972.

306. Sharpstone P et al: Nephrotic syndrome due to primary renal disease in adults: II. A controlled trial of prednisolone and azathioprine. Brit Med J 2:535, 1969.

307. Siegel NJ et al: Minimal-lesion nephrotic syndrome with early resistance to steroid therapy. J Pediat 87:377, 1975.

308. Smith RG et al: The nephrotic syndrome: current concepts. Ann Int Med 76:463, 1972.

309. Steinberg AD et al: Cytotoxic drugs in treatment of nonmalignant diseases. Ann Int Med 76:619, 1972.

310. Suc JM et al: Treatment of glomerulonephritis with indomethacin and heparin, in *Glomerulonephritis,* Proc. Intn'l Symp., Royal Melbourne Hospital, Part II, ed. by P. Kincaid-Smith et al, John Wiley & Sons, New York, 1973, p 927.

311. Teehan BP et al: Steroid-resistant idiopathic nephrotic syndrome. Arch Int Med 130:877, 1972.

312. Trainin EB et al: Late responsiveness to steroids in children with the nephrotic syndrome. J Pediat 87:519, 1975.

313. Tsao YC et al: Paired trial of cyclophosphamide and prednisone in children with nephrosis. Arch Dis Child 46:327, 1971.

314. Uldall PR et al: Cyclophosphamide therapy in adults with minimal-change nephrotic syndrome. Lancet 1:1250, 1972.

315. Uldall, PR et al: Sterility and cyclophosphamide. Lancet 1:1212, 1972.

316. Velosa JA et al: Focal sclerosing glomerulonephropathy: a clinicopathologic study. Mayo Clin Proc 50:121, 1975.

317. Warne GL et al: Cyclophosphamide-induced ovarian failure. NEJM 289:1159, 1973.

318. Wellington J et al: Lipoid nephrosis. A reassessment, in *Glomerulonephritis,* Proc. Intn'l Symp., Royal Melbourne Hospital, Part II, ed. by P. Kincaid-Smith, et al, John Wiley & Sons, New York, 1973, p 183.

319. West CD: Alkylating agents in the treatment of nephrotic syndrome, in *Glomerulonephritis,* Proc. Intn'l Symp., Royal Melbourne Hospital, Part II, ed. by P. Kincaid-Smith, et al, John Wiley & Sons, New York, 1973, p 199.

320. White RHR et al: Immunosuppressive therapy in steroid-resistant proliferative glomerulonephritis accompanied by the nephrotic syndrome. Brit Med J 2:853, 1966.

321. White RHR et al: Clinicopathological study of nephrotic syndrome in childhood. Lancet 1:1353, 1970.

DIABETES INSIPIDUS AND SYNDROME OF INAPPROPRIATE ANTIDIURETIC HORMONE SECRETION

322. Anon: Lypressin (Diapid) and other drugs for diabetes insipidus. Medical Letter 14:97, Dec. 22, 1972.

323. Bartter RC et al: The syndrome of inappropriate secretion of antidiuretic hormone. Am J Med 42:790, 1967.

324. Bode HH et al: Restoration of normal drinking behavior by chlorpropamide in patients with hypodypsia and diabetes insipidus. Am J Med 51:304, 1971.

325. Bonnici F: Antidiuretic effects of clofibrate and carbamazepine in diabetes insipidus: studies on free water clearance and response to a water load. Clin Endocrinol 2:265-275, 1973.

326. Coggins CH et al: Diabetes insipidus. Am J Med 42:807, 1967.

327. Cushard WG Jr et al: Oral therapy of diabetes insipidus with chlorpropamide. Calif Med 115:1, 1971.

328. Czako, L and Laszlo FA: Antidiuretic effect of carbamazepine in diabetes insipidus. Intn'l J Clin Pharmacol 11:58, 1975.

329. DeGennes JL et al: Antidiuretic effect of clofibrate in therapy of diabetes insipidus. Horm Metab Res 5:461, 1973.

330. Froyshov I, Haugen HN: Chlorpropamide treatment in diabetes insipidus. Acta Med Scan 183:397-400, 1968.

331. Goodman LS and Gilman A: The Pharmacological Basis of Therapeutics, 4th ed., MacMillan Co. London, 1970, pp 874-885.

332. Harper LO et al: Allergic alveolitis due to pituitary snuff. Ann Int Med 73:581, 1970.

333. Harrison TR: Principles of Internal Medicine, 7th ed, McGraw-Hill Book Co., NY, 1974, pp 465.

334. Hayes RM: Antidiuretic hormone. NEJM 295:659, 1976.

335. Ivy HK: The syndrome of inappropriate secretion of antidiuretic hormone. Med Clin N Am 52:817, 1968.

336. Kauli R, Laron Z: A vasopressin analogue in treatment of diabetes insipidus. Arch Dis Child 49:482-485, 1974.

337. Kurtzman NA et al: Physiology of antidiuretic hormone and the interrelationship between hormone and the kidney. Nephron 15:167, 1975.

338. Lee WN et al: Vasopressin analog DDAUP in the treatment of diabetes insipidus. Am J Dis Child 130:166, 1976.

339. Mahoney JH et al: Hypernatremia due to hypodipsia and elevated threshold for vasopressin release effects of treatment with

hydrochlorothiazide, chlorpropamide and tolbutamide. NEJM 279; 1191, 1968.

340. Miller M, Moses AM: Mechamism of chlorpropamide action in diabetes insipidus. J Clin Endocrinol Metab 30:488-496, 1970.

341. Miller M et al: Drug-induced states of impaired water excretion. Kidney Intn'l 10:96, 1976.

342. Mimica N et al: Lypressin nasal spray: usefulness in patients who manifest allergies to other antidiuretic hormone preparations. JAMA 203:802, 1968.

343. Moses AM et al: Clofibrate-induced antidiuresis. J Clin Invest 52:535, 1973.

344. Moses AM et al: Pathophysiologic and pharmacologic alterations in the release and action of ADH. Metabolism 25:697, 1976.

345. Moses AM et al: Drug-induced dilutional hyponatremia. NEJM 291:1234, 1974.

346. Murase T, Yoshida S: Mechanism of chlorpropamide action in patients with diabetes insipidus. J Clin Endocrinol Metab 36:174 — 177, 1973.

347. Nawar T et al: Non-hormonal drugs for the treatment of diabetes insipidus. Cand Med Assoc J 107:1225, 1972.

348. Nusynowitz ML, Forsham PH: The antidiuretic action of acetaminophen. Am J Med Sci 252:429-435, 1966.

349. Rado JP, Szende L, Borbely L, Tako J: Clinical value and mode of action of chlorpropamide in diabetes insipidus. Am J Med Sci 260:359 — 372, 1970.

350. Rado JP: Combination of carbamazepine and chlorpropamide in the treatment of "hyporesponder" pituitary diabetes insipidus. Clin Endocrin Metab 38:1, 1974.

351. Robinson, A.G.: DDAVP in the treatment of central diabetes insipidus. NEJM 294:507, 1976.

352. Singer I et al: Drug induced states of nephrogenic diabetes insipidus. Kidney Intn'l 10:82, 1976.

353. Wales JK, Fraser TR: The clinical use of chlorpropamide in diabetes insipidus. Acta Endocrinol 68:725-736, 1971.

354. Ward MK, Fraser TR: DDAVP in treatment of vasopressin-sensitive diabetes insipidus. Br Med J 3:86-89, 1974.

355. Webster B, Bain J: Antidiuretic effect and complications of chlorpropamide therapy in diabetes insipidus. J Clin Endocrinol Metab 30:215-227, 1970.

Chapter 21

Adverse Effects of Drugs on the Kidney

Richard J. Mangini
John G. Gambertoglio

Many drugs used in the treatment of a wide variety of medical conditions can induce significant adverse effects upon the kidney. Nephropathy due to some agents is suggested by isolated case reports, while that due to others is clearly documented by laboratory investigations and clinical studies. The potential for and frequency of renal damage due to a particular drug depends primarily upon the drug's mechanism and site of nephrotoxicity. However, the exact incidence of nephrotoxicity of any drug is difficult to pre-

renal damage may develop. First, a parent drug or metabolite may exert a direct toxic effect on renal cells (protoplasmic toxin). Tubular cell damage and necrosis are usually the primary consequences of direct nephrotoxicity of drugs. In addition, a drug can indirectly cause kidney damage by creating a condition within the patient which can potentially lead to deterioration in renal function (e.g. hypertension induced by oral contraceptives). A drug may also act as an immunogen and elicit an immune reaction whereby

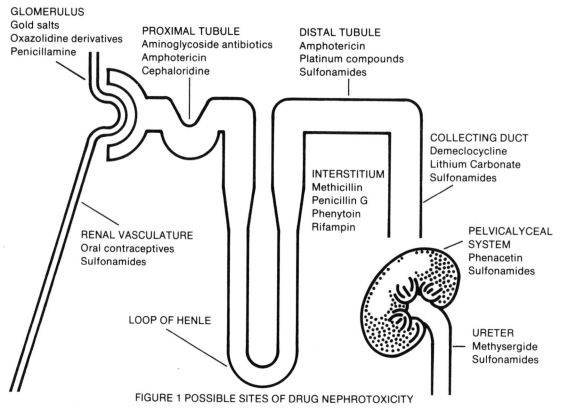

GLOMERULUS
Gold salts
Oxazolidine derivatives
Penicillamine

PROXIMAL TUBULE
Aminoglycoside antibiotics
Amphotericin
Cephaloridine

DISTAL TUBULE
Amphotericin
Platinum compounds
Sulfonamides

COLLECTING DUCT
Demeclocycline
Lithium Carbonate
Sulfonamides

INTERSTITIUM
Methicillin
Penicillin G
Phenytoin
Rifampin

RENAL VASCULATURE
Oral contraceptives
Sulfonamides

PELVICALYCEAL
SYSTEM
Phenacetin
Sulfonamides

LOOP OF HENLE

URETER
Methysergide
Sulfonamides

FIGURE 1 POSSIBLE SITES OF DRUG NEPHROTOXICITY

dict and can be influenced by a number of factors including concurrent administration of other nephrotoxic agents, preexisting renal disease, or the underlying disease state for which the drug is being used.

Drug nephrotoxicity may occur at a number of sites (See Figure 1). These include the renal vasculature, the glomerulus, the renal tubule (both proximal and distal), the collecting ducts, the interstitium, the pelvicalyceal system, and ureters.

Several mechanisms exist whereby drug-induced

the renal vasculature (vasculitis), glomerulus (glomerulonephritis), or tubules and interstitium (tubulointerstitial disease) may be damaged. The immune reaction to a drug is due to antibody formation in response to either a drug antigen or a drug hapten-protein which combine to form a complete antigen. The formed antigen-antibody complex, either circulating or tissue bound, can elicit an inflammatory response with resultant renal tissue damage. An additional mechanism by which drugs can cause kidney damage is mechanical obstruction of the tubules, collecting ducts, or ureters (obstructive nephropathy). This may result from 1) a parent compound or metabolite exceeding its solubility in the urine and precipitating out of solution forming crystals and stones, 2) a drug increasing the excretion of a poorly soluble or insoluble material, or 3) creating a condition in which the ureters may be impinged upon (e.g. retroperitoneal fibrosis). A further mechanism whereby renal function may be reduced is by a drug-induced decrease in renal blood flow (pre-renal azotemia). Finally, for some drugs the mechanism of their nephrotoxicity is unknown.

Because the number of drugs that induce nephrotoxicity is so great, they have been placed in table format to facilitate their discussion. In the table these drugs are listed and followed by a number which gives a subjective rating of the frequency of nephrotoxicity. The numbers denoting the frequency of this occurrence are:

1. *Invariable*
2. *Frequent*
3. *Uncommon*
4. *Rare*

Discussion of the histopathologic findings and mechanism of toxicity for each drug follows. In the "clinical remarks" section, salient clinical features such as pertinent laboratory data, clinical presentation, prognosis, as well as the dose and duration of therapy associated with the adverse effect are discussed. References are listed so that the reader may obtain more detailed information if desired. It is hoped that this table will provide a useful reference source for the nephrotoxic effects of drugs in man.

DRUG INDUCED NEPHROTOXICITY

Drug; Rate of Occurrence; Histopathology; Mechanism	Clinical Remarks
Acetazolamide	
A. Acute oliguric renal failure — **3**.	A. See benzothiadiazides A.
B. Tubular dysfunction secondary to diuretic-induced hypokalemia — **4**.	B. See benzothiadiazides B.
C. Obstructive nephropathy secondary to one of two mechanisms: acetazolamide crystalluria (obstructive tubular damage) or calcium phosphate stones (hydronephrosis/nephrocalcinosis) — **4**. (46,96,120,204,207,248,326,358,397,401,407,411, 440,521,552)	C. Patients may develop obstructive nephropathy secondary to acetazolamide (a sulfonamide derivative). Acutely, acetazolamide crystals are more likely to precipitate causing obstructive renal tubular damage. Chronically, however, calcium phosphate stone formation appears to be a greater problem. Reduced citrate excretion is the primary factor involved in calcium stone formation. In addition, the alkaline urine produced by acetazolamide-induced carbonic anhydrase inhibition can further potentiate precipitation of calcium phosphate stones. Patients with previous hypercalciuria are at a greater risk. Both types of obstruction present similarly with dysuria, renal colic, and/or hematuria; however, renal failure is more common following acetazolamide crystalluria. Treatment with bicarbonate and fluids is recommended in this group of patients. Alkalinization of the urine should be avoided in patients with calcium phosphate stones; instead they should be treated by restricting dietary calcium and increasing fluid intake.
Acetaminophen	
See phenacetin. Occurs with a frequency of **3-4**.	
Acetylsalicylic acid	
A. Altered renal function secondary to inhibition of renal prostaglandin. Not a direct nephrotoxic effect — **3-4**. It has also been suggested that aspirin may interfere with the tubular secretion of creatinine. (40,74,75,278,462)	A. Aspirin administration may decrease creatinine clearance and increase serum creatinine levels. The BUN may or may not be elevated. This effect is dose-related and is more pronounced in patients with pre-existing renal impairment. Acute aspirin-induced alterations in kidney function are readily reversible.
B. Chronic tubulointerstitial toxicity with papillary necrosis — **3-4**.	B. See phenacetin.
Allopurinol	
A. Obstructive nephropathy secondary to xanthine or oxypurinol crystals and stone formation — **4**. Hydronephrotic changes may be present in the kidney. (11,24,163,194,218,296,464,465)	A. Allopurinol and its active metabolite oxypurinol increase the excretion of xanthine which is poorly soluble as is oxypurinol. Under rare conditions excessive xanthine or oxypurinol urinary concentrations, which exceed solubility, may occur. These substances may then precipitate, leading to obstructive tubular damage that is clinically evident by renal colic and hematuria. Acute oliguric renal failure may subsequently develop.

Drug; Rate of Occurrence;
Histopathology; Mechanism   **Clinical Remarks**

B. Renal toxicity secondary to a hypersensitivity reaction — **4.** Although biopsy data is scarce, interstitial nephritis, renal vasculitis and glomerulonephritis have all been reported as the primary renal lesion.
(151,261,269,350,361,553)

B. A generalized hypersensitivity reaction may develop several weeks after initiation of allopurinol therapy. Fever, maculopapular pruritic rash (which may progress to exfoliative dermatitis), eosinophilia, hepatomegaly, and gastro-intestinal bleeding may all be present. Azotemia and oliguric renal failure can rapidly develop. When these conditions are noted, discontinuation of allopurinol is imperative. Although steroids appear to be beneficial, the disease course may be prolonged. Several deaths have been reported. Co-administration of thiazide diuretics and pre-existing renal impairment may increase the possibility of a hypersensitivity reaction.

Amikacin

Tubular toxicity. A direct nephrotoxic effect — **2-3.**
(240,272a,356,377,485,505)

As many as 16% of patients treated with amikacin have been reported to develop elevations in BUN and serum creatinine during treatment. The true incidence, as with other aminoglycoside antibiotics, is difficult to determine because of the severe nature of the infections for which it is used. In addition, a complex metabolic disorder associated with renal dysfunction has been reported. See Gentamicin.

Amphotericin

Tubular toxicity. A direct nephrotoxic effect — **1.** Proximal/distal tubular damage. Flattened tubular epithelial cells, tubular dilatation, and necrosis, as well as intratubular and interstitial calcification, are prominent biopsy findings. Tubular basement membrane thickening may also be noted. Renal vasoconstriction resulting in decreased glomerular filtration rate and renal plasma flow, apparently contribute to the development of amphotericin nephrotoxicity as well.
(68,71,137,210,231,316,328,344,345,358,359,378, 393,406,433,453,475,517)

Nephrotoxicity is the major dose-limiting factor of amphotericin treatment. More than 80% of all patients receiving amphotericin therapy will develop varying degrees of renal insufficiency. Cylindruria is frequently the initial sign of tubular damage as are other abnormalities ·in the urinalysis. Additional clinical evidence of tubular dysfunction may develop including decreased concentrating ability, polyuria, distal renal tubular acidosis, hypokalemia, hypomagnesemia, and defective citrate excretion. Elevations of BUN and creatinine occur in the majority of patients.

The correlation between the degree and persistence of renal insufficiency as related to the total dose of amphotericin is disputed. However, total doses of greater than 5 grams should be used with caution since there is evidence to suggest a greater incidence of permanent renal damage at this dose level. At lower total doses of amphotericin, renal insufficiency and other signs of tubular dysfunction are usually reversible if the dose is adjusted or the drug is discontinued. Possible methods of reducing amphotericin nephrotoxicity have been suggested in uncontrolled trials. These include alternate day therapy, alkali administration, or mannitol infusions. However, in a recent controlled trial, mannitol infusion did not prove useful. The success of other treatment modalities in decreasing nephrotoxicity require further evaluation. At present, primary treatment is temporary reduction or discontinuation of the drug, especially if BUN values are greater than 50 mg% and creatinine levels are above 3 mg%.

Ampicillin

Acute tubulointerstitial toxicity. A hypersensitivity reaction — **4.**
Interstitial infiltration with lymphocytes, plasma cells, and eosinophils associated with tubular necrosis has been demonstrated in patients receiving ampicillin.
(37,138,200,337,441,506,547).

The clinical findings of ampicillin-induced nephrotoxicity are similar to those associated with methicillin interstitial nephritis (See methicillin); however, these may, in some cases, develop more rapidly than with methicillin. Renal function usually returns to normal on drug discontinuation. If renal toxicity due to ampicillin occurs, patients should not receive other penicillin analogs. Cephalosporin derivatives may also cross-react.

Azathioprine

Acute tubulointerstitial toxicity. A hypersensitivity reaction — **4.** Acute and chronic tubular damage associated with interstitial leukocyte and eosinophil infiltration. (483)

Oliguria and renal dysfunction secondary to azathioprine has been reported in a single patient. Renal failure was associated with systemic reactions of fever, rash, muscular pain, headache, and gastrointestinal symptoms.

Bacitracin

Tubular toxicity. A direct nephrotoxic effect — **2.** Proximal tubular necrosis is the principal pathohistologic finding.
(197,290,328,453).

Acute tubular necrosis and renal failure is a common complication of parenteral bacitracin therapy limiting this drug to primarily topical use. After several days of treatment, renal damage may become apparent as mild proteinuria, hematuria, cylindruria, and azotemia. Acute renal failure may subsequently develop. Urinary abnormalities and azotemia are reversible, although renal insufficiency may persist and eventually contribute to death. Patients being irrigated with triple antibiotic solutions containing bacitracin have also developed renal failure.

Drug; Rate of Occurrence; Histopathology; Mechanism	Clinical Remarks

Benzothiadiazides (Thiazide diuretics)

A. Pre-renal azotemia caused by volume depletion from excessive diuretic therapy. Not a direct nephrotoxic effect — **3.**
(87,358,371)

A. Hypotension, secondary to diuretic-induced volume depletion results in poor renal perfusion, reduced glomerular filtration and impaired tubular function. Acute oliguric renal failure can result. Excessive sodium restriction can potentiate hypovolemia. Severe volume contraction is more common with the potent loop diuretics.

B. Tubular toxicity. An indirect nephrotoxic effect — **4.**
Prolonged hypokalemia can produce proximal tubular hydropic degeneration and atrophy as well as interstitial cellular infiltration and fibrosis. Various glomerular lesions including arterio/glomerulosclerosis may also be demonstrated.
(116a,180,243a,358,427,456,457,458,544a)

B. Hypokalemic nephropathy occurs primarily in patients who abuse diuretics. Frequently, these patients have psychiatric problems and commonly abuse other agents including laxatives. Metabolic alkalosis and other electrolyte disturbances are usually present as well. Inability to concentrate urine is the primary renal defect initially identified, while chronic renal failure develops slowly. There is evidence that the severity of renal damage is related to the duration of hypokalemia. Renal damage secondary to infectious pyelonephritis may be superimposed and can further compromise renal function in these patients. Early tubular cell damage and functional defects appear to be reversible with potassium repletion; however, the extent of reversibility of more severe lesions is not clear.

C. Acute tubulointerstitial toxicity. Hypersensitivity reaction — **4.**
Light microscopy from available cases invariably show a diffuse interstitial mononuclear cell infiltrate. Interstitial edema and some fibrosis may also be present. Tubular degenerative changes and atrophy are demonstrated as well.
(170,183,321,350,541)

C. Diuretic-induced allergic interstitial nephritis has been rarely reported and occurs primarily in patients with preexisting glomerular disease. The consistent presence of a peripheral eosinophilia and frequent appearance of a rash suggest a hypersensitivity reaction. Impaired renal function with severe oliguria may ensue. Renal function usually improves when the drug is discontinued with or without steroids. Loop diuretics can also cause interstitial nephritis.

D. Renal toxicity associated with various pathological lesions — **4.**
(2,49,173,195,281,371)

D. There are several documented cases of acute renal failure due to thiazide-related necrotizing vasculitis with associated vasculitic skin lesions. In addition, single cases of fatal glomerulonephritis with purpura, renal colic, and acute tubular necrosis have been reported.

Calcium Salts

Nephrocalcinosis — **4.**
Renal biopsies, although scarce, have shown tubular and interstitial calcifications as well as variable degrees of interstitial inflammation and fibrosis.
(14,17,73,351,426,430,530)

The milk-alkali syndrome is a well documented clinical entity. Prolonged intake of milk (as well as calcium salts) and absorbable alkali can lead to a systemic alkalosis and a positive calcium balance with hypercalcemia. A generalized calcinosis may result including nephrocalcinosis with subsequent development of renal insufficiency.

Capreomycin

Tubular toxicity. A direct nephrotoxic effect — **2.**
Although biopsy information is scarce, proximal tubular dilatation and cellular flattening have been shown. Although not specifically demonstrated, toxicity to glomerular vasculature has also been postulated.
(189,290,328,358,378,542,557)

Mild azotemia, as well as proteinuria, hematuria, pyuria, and cylindruria, are frequent complications of capreomycin therapy. As many as 36% of treated patients have BUN elevations of 20 mg% or more, and 10% have elevations above 30 mg%. Toxicity has not been related to dose or duration of therapy. Dosage should be reduced if the BUN rises above 30 mg%. Severe electrolyte disturbances (hypokalemia, hypomagnesemia, and hypocalcemia) apparently related to tubular dysfunction may also occur infrequently. Renal abnormalities are generally reversible, although one fatality has been reported.

Carbamazepine

Suspected tubular toxicity. A direct nephrotoxic effect — **4.**
(388)

A single case of nonoliguric renal failure secondary to carbamazepine has been reported. The patient recovered rapidly upon withdrawal of the drug.

Cefazolin

Tubular toxicity. A direct nephrotoxic effect — **4.**
(48,114,290,303,376,476)

Cefazolin has caused subtle histologic changes in rat and rabbit kidneys following prolonged high-dose injections. Lesions are much less extensive and less frequent than those caused by equivalent doses of cephaloridine. The frequency and severity of nephrotoxicity with cefazolin in humans, if any, has yet to be determined.

Drug; Rate of Occurrence;
Histopathology; Mechanism   **Clinical Remarks**

Caphalexin

Mechanism is unknown. No biopsies available in the cases reported — **4.**
(185,376,519)

Hematuria associated with eosinophilia has been reported in two patients receiving 20 to 24 grams/day of cephalexin in combination with probenecid. Each patient had a history of hypersensitivity reactions to penicillin analogs prior to the cephalexin reaction (one had nephritis from methicillin). Nonoliguric acute renal failure and hepatotoxicity secondary to cephalexin has also been reported. All reactions cleared when the drug was withdrawn. The exact role of cephalexin as a nephrotoxin is unclear.

Cephaloridine

Tubular toxicity. A direct nephrotoxic effect — **3.** Damage is confined to the proximal tubules. Disappearance of the tubular cell brush border is an early sign of toxicity. Tubules are usually dilated with flattened, vacuolated epithelial cells. The presence of tubular necrosis is variable. Tubular basement membranes are intact while glomeruli are normal.
(37,79,130,132,160,174,175,270,298,309,328,331, 343,376,391,409,474,475,476,479,543)

Animal data and clinical experience indicate that cephaloridine is the most nephrotoxic cephalosporin. This is because toxic concentrations accumulate in proximal tubular cells due to cephaloridine's inability to readily diffuse across the luminal membrane. Nephrotoxicity has primarily been associated with doses greater than the recommended daily dose of 4 grams or doses that are excessive for the patient's renal function. Serum levels of greater than 100 mcg/ml correlate with the appearance of renal toxicity. Patients with preexisting renal failure are more susceptible to the development of nephrotoxicity at lower doses, as are patients receiving other nephrotoxic antibiotics or potent loop diuretics. Cephaloridine-induced renal impairment is uncommon in the absence of excessive dosing and/or existence of predisposing factors. Toxicity is characterized by mild proteinuria (evidence of tubular dysfunction), granular casts, rising BUN and serum creatinine, and acute oliguric renal failure. Tubular epithelial cell shedding is frequently noted and has been suggested as an early indicator of tubular cell irritation. Nephrotoxicity is usually reversible upon drug withdrawal.

Cephalothin

A. Tubular toxicity. A direct nephrotoxic effect — **3-4.**
   Proximal tubular cell damage and necrosis is the primary renal lesion.
   (31,37,50,82,88,126,127,162,171,175,202,223, 226,282,283,284,309,317,328,376,389,404,409, 414,417,455,475,476,479,538)

A. In laboratory animals, it requires two to six times the amount of cephalothin compared to cephaloridine to produce equivalent proximal tubular necrosis. In humans, nephrotoxicity as evidenced by mild proteinuria, elevation of BUN and/or creatinine has been reported in patients with normal renal function as well as those with preexisting renal impairment. Cephalothin nephrotoxicity occurs much less frequently than that due to cephaloridine and follows the use of excessive doses or drug accumulation. Nephrotoxicity may be enhanced by co-administration of loop diuretics, colistin, and gentamicin.

B. Acute tubulointerstitial toxicity. A hypersensitivity reaction — **4.**
   (13,77,91,103,140,157,376)

B. Several cases of acute interstitial nephritis have been reported during cephalothin therapy. Cephalothin has also been reported to cause exacerbation of methicillin-induced nephritis. Because of the possibility of cross sensitivity, cephalothin should be administered with caution, if at all, to patients who develop methicillin interstitial nephritis (for the characteristic clinical course of interstitial nephritis see Methicillin).

Clindamycin

(See Gentamicin) — **4.**
(80)

Clofibrate

Mechanism unknown — **4.**
(59,136,415)

The pharmacokinetics of clofibrate are altered in patients with renal disease and the incidence of clofibrate-induced acute muscular syndrome appears to be substantially greater in these patients. Patients developing this syndrome may also undergo further decompensation of renal function, which may or may not return to baseline upon drug discontinuation.

Colistimethate/Colistin

Tubular toxicity. A direct nephrotoxic effect—**2-3.** Tubular dilatation with epithelial cell degeneration and necrosis is a frequent finding. Tubular lumens are usually filled with cellular debris and casts.
(5,65,83,153,165,205,206,223,241,242,286,325, 328,377,390,422,453,504,545)

Colistimethate is less toxic, but possesses less antibacterial activity than polymixin B. Renal toxicity, as evidenced by hematuria, proteinuria, cylindruria, and mild azotemia occur frequently (in as many as 20% of treated patients), usually within the first three to four days of therapy. Severe renal insufficiency is a less common occurrence with proper doses, although there is disagreement about this. Doses should not exceed 5 mg/kg/day. The drug should be discontinued or the dose should be reduced if an elevation in the BUN is noted. Renal abnormalities are generally reversible, but may progress for one to two weeks following drug discontinuation. Irreversible renal failure and death have been reported in a number of cases. Patients with renal insufficiency accumulate the drug and are more susceptible to renal toxicity as are those who are taking cephalothin concurrently.

Drug; Rate of Occurrence;
Histopathology; Mechanism   **Clinical Remarks**

Co-Trimoxazole

Tubular toxicity. A direct nephrotoxic effect — **4.** Available light microscopy has revealed acute tubular necrosis, with some interstitial inflammatory changes. Impaired tubular secretion of creatinine has also been suggested as a possible cause of elevated creatinine levels in some patients. (20,42,268,437,507)

Deterioration of renal function, evident by a rising serum creatinine and BUN, as well as by reduced creatinine clearances, has been attributed to co-trimoxazole treatment. All patients who developed worsening renal function while receiving co-trimoxazole had pre-existing renal disease. Drug-related renal dysfunction usually reverses rapidly on withdrawal of co-trimoxazole. However, permanent renal impairment has been reported. In normal patients and with proper dosage adjustment in renal failure, co-trimoxazole nephrotoxicity does not appear to be a substantial problem.

Dextran

A. Obstructive nephropathy secondary to intratubular dextran precipitation — **4.**
Proximal/distal intratubular dextran precipitates have been demonstrated. However, osmotic intratubular nephrosis in the absence of these deposits has also been reported, suggesting tubular cell swelling as an alternative cause of obstructive nephropathy in some patients. (41,98,163b,329,366,510)

A. Dextran infusions rarely cause acute renal failure. High urinary concentrations of dextran in the presence of dehydration and/or reduced renal perfusion may result in tubular stasis, intralumenal precipitation of dextran, and tubular plugging. Oliguric/anuric acute renal failure can subsequently develop. Maintenance of urine flow by the use of mannitol injections or loop diuretics reportedly prevents obstructive nephropathy. Dextrans should be withdrawn at the first indication of renal dysfunction.

B. Glomerular toxicity. A hypersensitivity glomerulonephritis — **4.**
(371)

B. This is not a well documented complication of dextran.

Doxorubicin (Adriamycin)

Mechanism unknown — **4.**
Light microscopy shows non-specific changes. Mild glomerular proliferation with occasional crescent formation as well as severe interstitial fibrosis and tubular atrophy has been found. Electron microscopy shows fusion of foot processes. (72)

Acute renal failure has been reported in a single 78-year-old patient while undergoing treatment with doxorubicin (180 mg total dose) for squamous cell carcinoma. Temporal relationships suggest that doxorubicin was the cause of renal failure. Renal function gradually returned to normal following doxorubicin withdrawal.

Enflurane

Tubular toxicity. A direct nephrotoxic effect due to the production of a toxic metabolite, fluoride — **4.**
(113,148,216,225,314,342)

High-output renal failure may develop shortly after enflurane anesthesia. As with methoxyflurane, toxicity is related to the production of inorganic fluoride. However, the amount of enflurane metabolized to inorganic fluoride is far less than that of methoxyflurane. Because of this difference in metabolism, the incidence of nonoliguric renal failure due to enflurane is low. Renal toxicity may be a problem only in those patients with an impaired ability to excrete fluoride ion.

Epsilon Aminocaproic Acid (EACA)

A. Obstructive nephropathy secondary to intraureteral clot formation — **4.**
(488)

A. EACA-induced intrarenal fibrin deposition may lead to obstruction with renal colic and post-renal azotemia when used to treat hematuria.

B. Glomerular-tubular damage — **4.**
(97,349)

B. Glomerular capillary thrombosis associated with acute tubular necrosis and renal failure has been reported.

C. Pre-renal azotemia caused by drug-induced hypotension. Not a direct nephrotoxic effect — **4.**
(500)

C. EACA can cause substantial drops in blood pressure, which can result in poor renal perfusion.

Ergot Alkaloids

See Methysergide.

Ethacrynic Acid

See Benzothiadiazides A, B and C.

Drug; Rate of Occurrence; Histopathology; Mechanism	Clinical Remarks

Ethambutol

Acute tubulointerstitial toxicity. An apparent hypersensitivity reaction, although direct nephrotoxicity has been proposed as a possible mechanism as well — **4**.
(104,378,497)

There are case reports which suggest that ethambutol and/or isoniazid may be nephrotoxic. An abnormal urinalysis (hematuria, pyuria, mild proteinuria, granular casts, glycosuria), elevated serum creatinine, and BUN are the principal clinical and laboratory findings. Eosinophilia and drug rash suggestive of an immune process have been noted as well. Renal toxicity appears reversible although persistent renal dysfunction has been reported in some patients. It is difficult, however, to clearly implicate ethambutol or isoniazid as nephrotoxic agents because of the multiple drug regimens (including rifampin) patients with tuberculosis receive.

Furosemide

See Benzothiadiazines A, B, and C.

Gentamicin

Tubular toxicity. A direct nephrotoxic effect — **2-3**. Renal damage is confined primarily to the proximal tubules which show dilatation as well as epithelial cell vacuolization, flattening, and regeneration. Lysosomes with myeloid bodies are a prominent finding in proximal epithelial tubular cells. The presence of tubular epithelial cell necrosis is variable. Tubular basement membranes are generally intact. Glomeruli are normal.
(25,28,50,80,81,82,118,126,127,161,162,171,190, 223,226,234,243,247,249,267,272a,283,284,289,317, 318,328,362,377,389,405,417,455,475,529,538)

The incidence of gentamicin nephrotoxicity varies from 2 to 16% of patients treated. However, the true incidence is difficult to determine because of the severe and complicated nature of the infectious illnesses for which gentamicin is used. Kidney toxicity, clinically evident by cylindruria, proteinuria, elevations of BUN, and creatinine, is usually mild, although acute nonoliguric or oliguric renal failure may develop. Gentamicin-induced renal dysfunction is generally reversible upon discontinuation of the drug, but complete resolution may take several weeks to months. Enzymuria may be a useful early warning indicator of gentamicin tubular damage. Toxicity is dose-related in rats and probably in humans. Patient age, preexisting renal disease, duration of treatment, high serum trough levels (2 mcg/ml or more) and coadministration of furosemide or other nephrotoxic drugs may all increase the incidence of gentamicin renal toxicity. Cephalothin is reported to enhance the nephrotoxic potential of gentamicin. Although controlled animal studies have not confirmed this effect, and in fact, some animal studies suggest a protective effect, this combination should be given with caution. Recently it has been suggested that the concurrent administration of clindamycin may also potentiate gentamicin nephrotoxicity. Renal function should be monitored in patients receiving gentamicin. Elevations of BUN and/or creatinine during therapy require appropriate dosage reduction or drug discontinuation.

In addition, a complex metabolic disorder apparently due to renal tubular dysfunction and hypoparathyroidism has been reported as a consequence of aminoglycoside therapy. This syndrome is characterized by hypomagnesmia and hypocalcemia secondary to inappropriate magnesium wasting. Excessive urinary loss of potassium, phosphate, sodium, and uric acid may also be seen. Circulating parathyroid hormone levels have been noted to be low despite hypocalcemia. Electrolyte wasting, requiring replacement in most cases, may persist for two to eight weeks even after withdrawal. Some patients with this syndrome may develop progressive renal impairment There appears to be a higher incidence of this disorder in patients with malignant disease especially those receiving adriamycin chemotherapy.

Gold Salts

Glomerular toxicity. Immune-complex membranous glomerulonephritis — **3**.
Subepithelial deposition of an unidentified immunogen apparently leads to progressive and irregular accumulation of a membranous-like material around the deposits. Focal fusion of foot processes also occurs. Deposits of gold which suggest an additional direct nephrotoxic effect, are commonly demonstrated in tubular epithelial cells and infrequently in the interstitium and glomeruli. The exact contribution of tubular lesions caused by gold deposits to the overall process of gold nephropathy is unclear.
(208,272,473,498,513,514,518,527,551)

Gold therapy can, on occasion, result in clinically evident kidney damage. Renal dysfunction is initially noted by the onset of proteinuria, the severity of which may lead to the nephrotic syndrome. Azotemia may eventually develop as well. Kidney impairment is generally reversible on withdrawal of gold therapy, with or without steroids, but can persist for an extended length of time. Chronic renal failure and death have been reported. The drug should not be readministered. Gold nephropathy cannot consistently be related to dose, duration of therapy, or blood levels of gold.

Griseofulvin

Pathology unknown — **4**.
(470,501)

Transient proteinuria has been associated with griseofulvin therapy.

Drug; Rate of Occurrence; Histopathology; Mechanism	Clinical Remarks

Halothane

Tubular toxicity. A direct nephrotoxic effect due to toxic metabolites — **4.**
Dense deposits of intratubular and interstitial oxalate crystals as well as patchy interstitial fibrosis and tubular atrophy have been demonstrated.
(110,342,355,511)

Renal failure developing after exposure to halothane anesthesia has been reported. The clinical and pathologic findings are similar to those found in patients with oliguric renal failure due to methoxyflurane (see methoxyflurane); thereby suggesting halothane as a possible cause of renal failure. Although up to 43% of patients receiving halothane have urinary oxalate crystals postoperatively, serum fluoride levels do not rise appreciably since only a small amount of halothane is biotransformed to inorganic fluoride. Compared to methoxyflurane, halothane nephrotoxicity appears to occur rarely.

Hydralazine

A. Glomerular toxicity, probably autoimmune glomerulonephritis — **4.**
   Definitive renal biopsy material is not available.
   (9,220,410)

A. Glomerulonephritis has been associated with hydralazine therapy. Nephritis is a rare sequela of hydralazine-induced lupus syndrome. Hematuria, proteinuria, urinary casts and an elevated BUN are indicators of renal involvement. Renal impairment is not dose-related and generally clears on drug discontinuation.

B. Post-renal obstructive nephropathy secondary to retroperitoneal fibrosis — **4.**
   Fibrotic processes in the retroperitoneal area encompass ureters unilaterally or bilaterally, and possibly major blood vessels. Compression and deviation of the ureters, as well as hydronephrosis, are evident radiologically.
   (93,213)

B. Retroperitoneal fibrosis has rarely been associated with hydralazine therapy. Patients present clinically with abdominal, back, or loin pain. Edema of the lower extremities, secondary to venous and lymphatic obstruction, may also be present. Erythrocyte sedimentation rate (ESR) is usually elevated. Uremia is the main indicator of renal abnormalities.

Indomethacin

A. Vascular-glomerular toxicity. An apparent hypersensitivity vasculitic reaction — **4.**
   Proliferative glomerulonephritis with epithelial crescents and fibrinoid necrosis has been shown.
   (333)

A. Glomerulonephritis, associated with nonthrombocytopenic purpura has been reported in two patients during and shortly following indomethacin therapy. Both patients developed renal failure, which was the cause of death in one patient. Although indomethacin cannot be conclusively implicated, the evidence is suggestive.

B. Altered renal function secondary to inhibition of renal prostaglandins by indomethacin. Not a direct nephrotoxic effect — **4.**
   (16a,133,181,201,235)

B. Indomethacin has been reported to decrease urinary sodium, reduce urinary volume, and occasionally, substantially decrease creatinine clearance. Indomethacin-induced changes in renal function appear to be dose-dependent and are readily reversible.

Isoniazid

See Ethambutol.

Kanamycin

Tubular toxicity. A direct nephrotoxic effect — **2-3.**
Proximal tubular cell swelling, degeneration, and necrosis. Distal tubules may also be affected. Glomeruli are normal.
(45,69,161,172,297,328,377,453,475)

Proteinuria, microscopic hematuria, cylindruria, and mild azotemia are the usual signs of renal toxicity. Acute oliguric renal failure, though infrequent, may result from kanamycin therapy, especially in high doses. Prolonged therapy at any dose appears to increase the incidence of toxicity as does preexisting renal insufficiency. Previous or concurrent administration of other nephrotoxic drugs, especially streptomycin or viomycin, may also enhance nephrotoxicity. Renal damage is slowly reversible when the dose is adjusted or the drug is discontinued. A high incidence of renal abnormalities due to kanamycin was reported in early clinical trials when doses of 25 to 50 mg/kg/day were used. The incidence of renal insufficiency is lower when kanamycin is given at the recommended dose of 15 mg/kg/day.

Laxatives

Tubular toxicity. An indirect nephrotoxic effect — **4.**
Prolonged hypokalemia can result in proximal tubular hydropic degeneration and atrophy as well as interstitial cellular infiltration and fibrosis. Various glomerular lesions including arterio/glomerulosclerosis may also be demonstrated.
(116a,124a,243a,427,456,459a,544a)

Hypokalemic nephropathy may occur in chronic laxative abusers. These patients frequently have psychiatric problems and commonly abuse other agents including diuretics. Metabolic alkalosis and other electrolyte disturbances are usually present as well. Inability to concentrate urine is the primary renal defect that is initially identified in these patients. Chronic renal failure develops slowly. There is evidence which indicates that the severity of renal damage is related to the duration of hypokalemia. Renal damage secondary to infectious pyelonephritis may be superimposed and can further compromise renal function in these patients. Early tubular cell damage and functional defects appear to be reversible with potassium repletion; however, the extent of reversibility of more severe lesions is not clear.

**Drug; Rate of Occurrence;
Histopathology; Mechanism**

Clinical Remarks

Lithium carbonate

A. Nephrogenic diabetes insipidus. A direct tubular toxicity — **2.**
Lithium most likely blocks the activation of ADH-sensitive adenyl cyclase in the renal medulla, resulting in ADH insensitivity. Impaired activation of cyclic-AMP dependent protein kinase has also been suggested. Additionally, lithium impairs free-water clearance by decreasing proximal tubular reabsorption of sodium and water. The possibility of a CNS mode of action has also been raised.
(368a,479a)

A. Lithium carbonate appears to be the drug most commonly associated with diabetes insipidus. Polyuria occurs frequently in lithium-treated patients. The syndrome, which presents as a reversible nephrogenic diabetes insipidus, usually appears a few weeks following the initiation of drug treatment, but can take months to develop. This may be related to lithium accumulation within the renal tissue. The syndrome reverses within three to four weeks after drug discontinuation, which is the recommended treatment if electrolyte balance is a problem. Thiazide diuretics are useful in decreasing urine volume and may additionally allow lithium dosage reduction by decreasing lithium renal clearance. (see B)

B. Renal toxicity. An apparent direct nephrotoxic effect — **4.**
Focal and diffuse interstitial fibrosis with tubular atrophy and glomerulorsclerosis have been found in patients on chronic lithium therapy.
(232a,306a,352a)

B. Recent evidence indicates that patients receiving long-term lithium treatment who have a history of lithium-induced nephrogenic diabetes insipidus and/or have had episodes of lithium intoxication may develop varying degrees of chronic renal failure as indicated by a falling creatinine clearance. In addition, there is a single case of marked proteinuria that was temporally related to lithium therapy.

Mephenytoin

Glomerular toxicity. A hypersensitivity reaction. Diffuse proliferative glomerulonephritis, possibly auto-immune — **4.**
Glomeruli show diffuse proliferative changes with mesangial and subendothelial electron dense deposits.
(307,487)

Proteinuria with the nephrotic syndrome is a rarely reported side effect of mephenytoin. Nephrotoxicity has only been reported in association with other systemic-immune reactions such as lymphadenopathy and drug-induced lupus syndrome.

Mercurial diuretics

A. Tubular toxicity. A direct nephrotoxic effect — **3.**
(177,328,358,453)
B. Glomerular toxicity. Immune-complex membranous glomerulonephritis — **4.**
(70,76,84,358,429,453)

A. Tubular degeneration and necrosis sometimes occurs especially in the presence of renal insufficiency because of the abnormal retention of mercury. Proteinuria, hematuria, cylindruria, as well as apparent resistance to diuresis are early signs of toxicity. Acute renal failure is reversible and may require dialysis and/or dimercaprol treatment.

B. Proteinuria severe enough to cause the nephrotic syndrome has been reported.

Mercury containing ointments

Glomerular toxicity. Immune complex glomerulonephritis — **3-4.**
Membranous as well as minimal proliferative glomerular changes have been found in renal biopsies. In addition, varying degrees of tubular damage have been shown.
(30,34,276,463)

The nephrotic syndrome has been reported following chronic use of topically applied mercury containing ointments and cosmetic creams. Renal abnormalities are apparently reversible upon discontinuation of these preparations.

Methicillin

Acute tubulointerstitial toxicity. A hypersensitivity reaction — **3.**
Light microscopy examination of renal biopsy material invariably demonstrates interstitial infiltration of mononuclear cells, primarily lymphocytes, as well as eosinophils. Tubular damage is primarily adjacent to cellular infiltrates. Antitubular basement antibodies have been recently demonstrated, although immunofluorescent studies have been equivocal. Whether a tubular or interstitial lesion initiates methicillin nephrotoxicity has not been determined. Methicillin-elicited involvement of humoral and/or cellular components of the immune system have been suggested as being responsible for renal toxicity. (13, 13a, 23, 54, 58, 103, 107,131a, 139, 163a, 164, 188, 188a, 200, 215, 233, 240a, 264, 268a, 315a, 337a, 352, 376, 388a, 394, 395, 396, 444, 454, 478, 498a, 546, 555).

The clinical onset of renal damage due to methicillin is evident by abnormalities in the urinary sediment. Hematuria, sterile pyuria, and mild to moderate proteinuria usually appear one to four weeks following the initiation of methicillin. Signs and symptoms of an immune reaction, including eosinophilia, drug fever, and rash, invariably precede or occur concurrently with the development of urinary/renal abnormalities. Eosinophiluria is an additional diagnostic finding. Renal impairment, which may be severe, commonly develops. Clinical evidence of drug toxicity is usually rapidly reversible on drug discontinuation with complete resolution taking several weeks. However, prolonged courses of renal dysfunction are not uncommon and rarely permanent renal impairment may occur. Steroids may be beneficial in some cases. Other penicillin analogs should be avoided because of the possibility of a cross-reaction. Cephalosporin derivatives as an alternative antibiotic may also exacerbate methicillin nephritis. Duration but not the dose of methicillin treatment appears to affect the incidence of nephrotoxicity.

Drug; Rate of Occurrence; Histopathology; Mechanism	Clinical Remarks

Methotrexate

Obstructive nephropathy secondary to methotrexate crystal formation — **3.**
Intraluminal precipitation of methotrexate results in tubular dilatation and damage. Direct tubular toxicity has also been suggested.
(108,178,256,259,260,420,496)

Methotrexate, which has limited solubility in acidic urine, may precipitate and lead to reversible obstructive renal tubular damage when used in high doses. Alkalinization of the urine and maintenance of an adequate urine flow are essential in preventing methotrexate crystalluria. Renal failure secondary to methotrexate also decreases methotrexate clearance and may lead to other systemic toxicities of methotrexate.

Methoxyflurane

Tubular toxicity. A direct nephrotoxic effect due to toxic metabolites — **3.**
Segmental degeneration and necrosis of proximal tubular epithelial cells with interstitial edema is a predominent finding. Calcium oxalate crystals are characteristically present in the tubular lumen and frequently in the interstitium. Increased interstitial connective tissue and interstitial fibrosis may also be found, especially in patients with prolonged or permanent renal dysfunction. Glomeruli are normal.
(10,29,67,99,100,106,111,112,116,141,150,176,221, 244,277,288,294,328,338,339,340,341,348,355, 400,424,435,508,511,516)

Nephrotoxicity resulting from methoxyflurane therapy is a dose-duration-related phenomenon caused by the production of toxic metabolites, inorganic fluoride and oxalic acid. Excessive serum levels of inorganic fluoride are associated with a vasopressin-resistant diabetes insipidus and high output renal failure which usually occurs shortly after methoxyflurane administration. Inability to concentrate urine usually lasts 10 to 20 days, but may persist for three months or longer. In a small number of patients oliguric renal failure and death may also result. Intratubular and interstitial calcium oxalate crystal deposition with progressive interstitial fibrosis probably contributes significantly to the development of chronic renal failure. Methoxyflurane nephrotoxicity is reportedly enhanced by concurrent administration of tetracyclines (see Tetracycline, D) and aminoglycoside antibiotics. It has been shown that enzyme induction caused by pre-treatment with barbiturates enhances the production of nephrotoxic metabolites. Patient age and weight have also been suggested as contributing factors in nephrotoxicity.

Methyldopa

A. Obstructive nephropathy secondary to retroperitoneal fibrosis — **4.**
Fibrotic processes in the retroperitoneal areas encompass ureters unilaterally or bilaterally and possibly major blood vessels. Compression and deviation of the ureters, as well as hydronephrosis can be seen radiologically. An autoimmune process has been suggested as a cause of retroperitoneal fibrosis.
(93,252)

A. Retroperitoneal fibrosis is a rare complication of methyldopa therapy. Patients present clinically with abdominal, back, or loin pain, edema of the lower extremities secondary to venous and lymphatic obstruction may also be present. Erythrocyte sedimentation rate (ESR) is usually elevated. Uremia is the main indication of renal damage.

B. Obstructive nephropathy secondary to stone formation — **4.**
Bilateral renal calculi have been found associated with hydronephrotic changes. Renal stones are black in color.
(375)

B. Methyldopa is poorly soluble and may rarely precipitate in the urine, possibly providing a nidus for calcium stone formation.

C. Acute tubulointerstitial toxicity. A hypersensitivity reaction — **4.**
(350,541)

C. Weak evidence suggests that methyldopa either alone or in combination with a thiazide diuretic may cause acute renal failure. Systemic evidence of a hypersensitivity reaction is usually present as well.

Methysergide

Postrenal obstructive nephropathy secondary to retroperitoneal fibrosis — **3-4.**
Fibrotic processes in the retroperitoneal area encompass ureters unilaterally or bilaterally and possibly major blood vessels. Compression and deviations of the ureters as well as hydronephrosis are evident radiologically.
(47,92,149,213,484,489)

Long-term therapy with ergot alkaloids, primarily methysergide, may result in retroperitoneal fibrosis. Methysergide-induced retroperitoneal fibrosis may lead to ureteral obstruction, hydronephrosis, and chronic renal failure. Onset of flank or loin pain and oliguria are signs of retroperitoneal fibrosis with obstruction. Treatment is discontinuation of the drug, glucocorticosteroids, and surgery if necessary. Patients should not receive methysergide for more than six months without a four- to eight-week drug-free period.

Mithramycin

Tubular toxicity. A direct nephrotoxic effect — **2-3.**
Proximal tubular cell swelling, necrosis, and atrophy. Distal tubules may also be involved. Glomeruli are normal.
(275)

Patients receiving 10 to 50 mg/kg/day of mithramycin for varying periods of time frequently demonstrate evidence of mild renal tubular damage (mild proteinuria). Elevation of creatinine and BUN secondary to severe renal tubular damage occurs less frequently. Renal toxicity appears to be cumulative since the creatinine clearance decreases with subsequent courses. Abnormalities in renal function are generally reversible, but they have persisted in some cases.

Drug; Rate of Occurrence; Histopathology; Mechanism	Clinical Remarks

Nafcillin

Acute tubulointerstitial toxicity. A hypersensitivity reaction — **4.**
(268a,308,403)

Evidence of an allergic interstitial nephritis secondary to nafcillin has been reported in one patient who previously developed methicillin nephritis. (See Methicillin.) However, the occurrence of nafcillin-induced renal toxicity appears to be far less than that of methicillin. Pseudoproteinuria has also recently been reported during nafcillin therapy.

Neomycin

Tubular toxicity. A direct nephrotoxic effect — **2.**
Focal proximal tubular epithelial cell vacuolization with variable degenerative and necrotic changes are prominent findings. Tubular basement membranes are generally intact but may be thickened. Glomeruli are normal.
(44,119,123,155,156,161,217,274,293,327,328,334, 377,439,453)

Neomycin is considered to be the most nephrotoxic of the aminoglycosides. Abnormal urinalysis (hematuria, proteinuria, cylindruria), azotemia, and oliguric renal failure commonly occur during parenteral neomycin administration. The high incidence of neomycin nephrotoxicity prohibits its use as a parenteral agent. Although poorly absorbed, several cases of acute renal failure have been reported following oral ingestion and following the use of neomycin-containing irrigation solutions. Preexisting renal insufficiency, as well as concomitant use of other nephrotoxic drugs, appear to enhance neomycin's nephrotoxic potential. Renal damage is generally reversible if neomycin is withdrawn at the first evidence of tubular damage.

Nitrofurantoin

A. Obstructive nephropathy secondary to stone formation — **4.**
Small irregular bright purple crystals.
(323)

A. Three cases of nitrofurantoin crystalluria have been reported. All occurred in geriatric patients with urinary catheters receiving chronic nitrofurantoin prophylaxis. Although none of these patients developed acute renal failure, the possibility of obstructive nephropathy exists.

B. Acute tubulointerstitial toxicity. A hypersensitivity reaction — **4.**
(371)

B. This is a poorly documented, reversible complication of nitrofurantoin therapy.

Oral Contraceptives

A. Vascular-glomerular toxicity. Renal failure secondary to hypertensive arteriolar nephrosclerosis — **4.**
Fibrinoid necrosis and other structural changes of the afferent arterioles and interlobular arteries are present. Thrombotic microangiopathy may also be present in the glomerular capillary loops. Glomeruli may also show ischemic and necrotic changes. Other nonspecific changes have been noted.
(26,52,64,125,145,203,253,452,512,558,559)

A. Development of malignant hypertension, secondary to estrogen containing oral contraceptives, can lead to azotemia and acute oliguric renal failure, as well as irreversible end-stage renal failure and death. Hemolytic anemia may also be present, secondary to microangiopathy. Malignant hypertensive kidney disease usually appears after prolonged therapy with oral contraceptives. Additionally, nephrosclerotic changes and renal failure have been reported in a patient with only minor elevations in blood pressure. Blood pressure should be monitored during oral contraceptive administration and the drug should be discontinued if hypertension occurs.

B. Vascular-glomerular toxicity. Renal failure secondary to renal vein thrombosis — **4.**
Thromboemboli may be demonstrated within a renal vein. The kidneys may demonstrate membranous or ischemic glomerular changes, as well as nephrosclerotic lesions associated with any secondary hypertension.
(222,363,482)

B. This is a rare complication of oral contraceptive therapy. The severity and rapidity of onset of renal impairment depends primarily on the location of the thrombus and the degree of occlusion. The patient may present acutely with the sudden onset of lower back pain. Evidence of renal damage may range from an abnormal urinalysis (hematuria/proteinuria) to severe azotemic renal failure or nephrotic syndrome (chronic). Renovascular hypertension may also develop.

Oxacillin

Acute tubulointerstitial toxicity. A hypersensitivity reaction — **4.**
(78,376)

A biopsy-documented interstitial nephritis, presumably due to oxacillin has been reported. The clinical findings with regard to oxacillin-induced interstitial nephritis are similar to those that occur with methicillin-induced interstitial nephritis. (See Methicillin.) However, the incidence of oxacillin-induced renal toxicity appears to be far less than that of methicillin.

Oxazolidine Derivatives
(Trimethadione, Paramethadione)

Glomerular toxicity. Membranous glomerulonephritis probably by an immune complex mechanism — **3.**
Focal glomerular basement membrane thickening and splitting is a prominent finding on light and

The nephrotic syndrome is a well-documented complication of therapy with oxazolidine derivatives. The onset of clinically evident renal damage is variable, reportedly occurring anywhere from 4 to 65 months after the initiation of treatment. Heavy proteinuria, hypoalbuminemia, and edema are the hallmarks of renal toxicity. Elevations in BUN and creatinine are less common. Toxicity is apparently not related to dose or duration. Although several

Drug; Rate of Occurrence; Histopathology; Mechanism	Clinical Remarks

electron microscopy. Partial fusion of foot processes may also be found as granular deposits and membranous-bound structures. Intracapillary eosinophils have been recently observed suggesting a hypersensitivity reaction. (27,28,43,60,121,228,236,358,360,382,392,436,481, 502,534,549)

deaths have been reported, prognosis is good with abnormalities in renal function generally clearing completely within four to six weeks following drug discontinuation alone. Steroids and alkylating agents have been used to treat resistant cases. Oxazolidine derivatives should be withdrawn if evidence of renal toxicity appears.

Para-Aminosalicylic Acid

Probably acute tubulointerstitial toxicity. A hypersensitivity reaction — **4.** (101,117,263,313,332,368,378,398,477)

Generalized systemic hypersensitivity reaction (fever, rash, eosinophilia, lymphadenopathy) may occur with para-aminosalicylic acid alone or in combination with other antitubercular agents. The kidney (hematuria, proteinuria, sterile pyuria) as well as other organ systems may be involved. Acute oliguric renal failure may develop.

Penicillamine

Glomerular toxicity. Immune-complex membranous glomerulonephritis — **2-3.** Irregular glomerular membrane thickening, foot process fusion, and subepithelial deposition of electron dense particles are prominent electron microscopic findings. Focal and diffuse proliferative changes may also be found, especially in rare cases of rapidly progressing glomerulonephritis due to penicillamine. Immunofluorescent studies have demonstrated granular staining and the presence of IgG immune-complex deposition. (3,18,122,152,167,168,229,239,257,258,295,319,320 358,385,434,466,490,491,492,522)

Renal toxicity is associated with both the DL and D form of penicillamine. Kidney abnormalities usually develop only after several months or more of drug administration. Proteinuria is the main indicator of renal toxicity, although hematuria and sterile pyuria are also frequent findings. Ultimately, the nephrotic syndrome may develop. Significantly impaired renal function (elevated serum creatinine) is uncommon, although persistant proteinuria and progressive renal failure and death have been reported. Renal abnormalities are normally reversible, requiring several weeks to months to clear completely following penicillamine withdrawal. The benefit of short-term steroid therapy is equivocal. Rarely, a rapidly progressive glomerulonephritis associated with pulmonary hemorrhages (a condition resembling Goodpasture's syndrome) occurs. Antinuclear antibodies are usually positive and the prognosis of these patients is poor.

Penicillin

A. Acute tubulointerstitial toxicity. A hypersensitivity reaction — **4.** See Methicillin for biopsy details. (23,105,138,196,200,376,395,396,454,478,523)

Renal failure, secondary to penicillin-induced interstitial nephritis, is well documented, although the incidence is less than that of methicillin. The clinical findings are identical to those associated with methicillin nephritis. (See Methicillin.) Renal impairment usually reverses when the drug is discontinued; however, if the drug is continued, impairment can progress to fatal renal failure. If nephritis develops, patients should not receive other penicillin analogs because of the possibility of a cross-reaction. Cephalosporin derivatives may also exacerbate penicillin nephritis.

B. Glomerular toxicity. A hypersensitivity reaction — **4.** Proliferative/exudative glomerulonephritis with crescent formation has been reported. It is commonly associated with a generalized vasculitis. (290,453,454)

Rapidly developing renal insufficiency, associated with clinical evidence of a systemic allergic reaction may occur following small doses of penicillin administered for a short period of time. When this condition becomes known, penicillin should be withdrawn immediately.

Pentamidine Isothionate

Tubular toxicity. A direct nephrotoxic effect — **2.** Although renal histopathological material is scarce, proximal tubular epithelial degeneration and necrosis have been shown. (128,154,279,524,525,533)

Renal dysfunction is the most common serious adverse effect of pentamidine. As many as 24% of patients treated with pentamidine show evidence of renal impairment. Proteinuria, pyuria, and cylindruria are frequent abnormalities found on urinalysis. Azotemia is usually mild and reversible on drug withdrawal. However, more severe renal impairment which may directly contribute to death has been reported, especially in patients with prior renal damage and those who receive other nephrotoxic drugs concomitantly.

Phenacetin

Chronic tubulointerstitial toxicity with papillary necrosis. A direct nephrotoxic effect — **3.** The main insult to the kidney appears to be located in the inner renal medulla where high concentrations of different analgesics have been identified. Roentgenographic changes in the pelvicalyceal system are commonly demonstrated. Papillary necrosis

Analgesic nephropathy and its associated syndrome of abuse is well documented. Patients who chronically abuse analgesics are predominantly middle-aged women who usually present clinically with a history of headaches, malaise, weakness, and a variety of psychiatric complaints. They may also have a refractory normochromic microcytic anemia, peptic ulcer disease, and mild renal impairment. Ischemic heart disease and premature aging may also be prominent findings. Denial of analgesic use may make diagnosis difficult.

**Drug; Rate of Occurrence;
Histopathology; Mechanism**   **Clinical Remarks**

is a frequent finding, while papillary calcification is less common. Kidney size may be significantly reduced, especially late in the course of the disease. Histologically, medullary interstitial fibrosis with minimal cellular proliferation, tubular degeneration, and atrophy, as well as tubular basement membrane thickening, are usually present, even before clinical evidence of renal disease. Worsening of renal function correlates with progression of medullary changes as well as the development of cortical and glomerular involvement. Papillary necrosis is invariably present in patients with severe renal dysfunction. Whether papillary necrosis or medullary interstitial damage is the initial lesion is debatable. (1,4,16,191,192,193,310,328,378a,379,383,384,412, 421,469,494,537,540)

Although conclusive evidence is lacking, phenacetin is apparently the common denominator of analgesic nephropathy in humans. A number of epidemiologic and environmental factors appear to control the incidence of this drug-induced disease. Renal impairment is usually insidious in onset. A reduced concentrating capacity is frequently the earliest sign of renal damage. Mild proteinuria, microscopic hematuria, sterile pyuria, renal tubular acidosis, and azotemia also present at various times in the course of the disease. Renal involvement may progress to end-stage renal failure. Sloughed papillary tissue can additionally cause obstructive uropathy with ureteral colic and macroscopic hematuria. Infectious pyelonephritis is commonly superimposed and may further compromise renal function. Toxicity is felt to be related to the amount of drug consumed. Although different criteria exist, analgesic nephropathy should be suspected in anyone ingesting in excess of two kilograms of phenacetin over a five-year period. Reversibility and prognosis are related to the severity of renal damage and whether or not the patient refrains from further analgesic use. A significant increase in renal pelvis carcinoma has been documented in patients with analgesic-induced papillary necrosis. Tumors may develop years after withdrawal of phenacetin.

Aspirin is a more potent inducer of papillary necrosis in laboratory animals than phenacetin. In addition, in animals and humans, aspirin has a decided effect on tubular epithelium, as evidenced by cyclindruria and renal tubular epithelial cell shedding during aspirin therapy. However, renal papillary necrosis has only rarely been shown to occur following aspirin therapy alone. Likewise pyrazolone derivatives (including phenylbutazone) and acetaminophen cannot be implicated, despite the fact that high concentrations of the latter are found in the renal medulla. Experimental data strongly suggest that the use of combination analgesics potentiates nephrotoxicity.

Phenazopyridine

Obstructive nephropathy secondary to phenazopyridine crystal and stone formation — **4.**
Highly pigmented tubular casts and crystals have been demonstrated in the renal tubules. Degenerative or regenerative changes in the tubular epithelial cells primarily in the collecting ducts, secondary to phenazopyridine crystal and stone formation, have been found.
(8,159,373)

Transient oliguria and impaired renal function have been reported as a complication of phenazopyridine. In most cases patients had preexisting renal disease and usually had received large doses of this drug. Urinalysis showed pigmented urine, casts, and crystals. Patients also showed peripheral skin pigmentation. Urinary phenazopyridine stones have also been seen that did not reduce renal function. Since this drug undergoes extensive renal clearance, it should be avoided in patients with renal insufficiency.

Phenindione

Acute tubulointerstitial toxicity. A hypersensitivity reaction — **4.**
Evidence of tubulointerstitial disease is invariably present. Mononuclear cell infiltration of interstitial tissue and tubular damage can be demonstrated in a majority of biopsy specimens. Although glomeruli are usually normal, nonspecific alterations in glomerular morphology have been seen.
(21,63,187,245,300,350,486)

Clinically, patients present with fever and rash (which may progress to exfoliative dermatitis) usually two to four weeks after drug initiation. Hepatic abnormalities may also be present. The development of renal toxicity as evidenced by an abnormal urinalysis (proteinuria, hematuria, sterile pyuria) and azotemia may be delayed and may occur after drug discontinuation. Impaired kidney function may or may not revert to normal. A number of cases of anuric renal failure and death have been reported and steroids may be beneficial for this condition. The drug should be withdrawn at the first sign of hypersensitivity or renal damage.

Phenylbutazone

A. Tubular toxicity — **4.**
   Tubular damage is the major pathological finding, although various glomerular lesions including capillary thrombi have been demonstrated. The exact mechanism is unknown, although hypersensitivity appears likely.
   (312,322,347)

A. Acute renal failure, secondary to a possible hypersensitivity reaction to phenylbutazone has been reported. Although complete recovery usually follows drug withdrawal, several deaths have occurred.

B. Obstructive nephropathy secondary to uric acid crystals — **4.**
   Uric acid crystals, stone deposition in ureters, renal calculi and hydronephrosis have been observed.
   (490a,528)

B. Bilateral ureteral obstruction leading to anuria has been reported in a patient receiving phenylbutazone. Renal colic without anuria has also been reported.

C. Chronic tubulointerstitial toxicity with papillary necrosis — **4.**

C. See phenacetin.

Drug; Rate of Occurrence; Histopathology; Mechanism	Clinical Remarks

D. Vascular-glomerular toxicity. A hypersensitivity reaction — **4.**
Renal biopsy consistent with thrombotic thrombocytopenic purpura.
(144)

D. Thrombotic thrombocytopenic purpura, apparently induced by phenylbutazone, leading to acute anuric renal failure has been reported in one patient. Despite steroid therapy, the patient died.

Phenytoin (Diphenylhydantoin)

A. Acute tubulointerstitial toxicity. A hypersensitivity reaction — **4.**
Peritubular and interstitial infiltrates of lymphocytes, plasma cells, and eosinophils as well as tubular atrophy have been demonstrated. Anti-tubular basement membrane antibodies have also been found in one patient.
(7,250,357,396,470a,539)

A. Reversible oliguric renal failure has been reported as part of a multi-system immune reaction to phenytoin. Besides abnormalities in the urinalysis (proteinuria, hematuria) and renal function (elevated BUN and serum creatinine), fever, skin rash (maculopapular to exfoliative dermatitis), lymphadenopathy, leukocytosis with eosinophilia, and abnormal liver function tests are prominent findings. The immune reaction usually occurs within several days to several weeks following initiation of phenytoin. Phenytoin should be withdrawn at the first indication of a drug reaction and steroids should be instituted if necessary.

B. Glomerular toxicity. Autoimmune glomerulonephritis — **4.**
Definitive biopsy material lacking.
(254,255,480,539)

B. Varying degrees of proteinuria have been occasionally reported in patients with phenytoin-induced lupus. The exact relationship of renal damage to phenytoin therapy in these reported cases is difficult to determine since the patients were frequently on more than one anticonvulsant medication.

Platinum Compounds (Cis Diamine Dichloroplatinum)

Tubular toxicity. A direct nephrotoxic effect — **1-2.**
Light microscopy reveals distal tubular damage ranging from epithelial cell flattening and tubular dilatation to severe tubular cell degeneration and necrosis. The proximal tubules may be affected as well but to a much lesser degree. Focal necrosis of the collecting duct epithelium has been shown as well as the presence of granular and hyaline casts within the collecting ducts. Other nonspecific changes have been noted.
(124,204a,224,228a,237,238,311,503,526,550)

Platinum (cis diamine dichloroplatinum) nephrotoxicity during chemotherapy is the primary factor limiting treatment. An elevated BUN and serum creatinine are frequent findings, especially with the higher dosage regimens, and usually appear within one to two weeks following initiation of platinum treatment. Platinum chemotherapy should be withheld if the creatinine clearance falls below 50 ml/min. Following discontinuation, renal dysfunction reverses within two weeks, but frequently the course of recovery may be prolonged. Cases of irreversible anuric renal failure due to platinum which contributed to death have also been reported, especially in patients receiving high dose and/or repeated courses of platinum. Evidence suggests prehydration and treatment with diuretics, especially mannitol, may reduce the incidence of platinum renal toxicity, while concurrent administration of other nephrotoxic drugs such as gentamicin and cephalothin may increase the incidence.

Polymixin B

Tubular toxicity. A direct nephrotoxic effect — **2.**
Proximal tubular epithelial cells are affected primarily with resultant tubular degeneration and necrosis.
(241,242,246,262,290,328,377,390,402,453,554)

Polymixin B possesses more antibacterial activity than colistimethate but is more toxic. Adverse renal tubular toxicity, as evidenced by light-to-moderate proteinuria, cylindruria, defective concentrating ability, and mild azotemia are common. These abnormalities usually appear within three to four days after therapy with this drug begins.

Severe renal insufficiency occurs less frequently if proper doses are used. Toxicity is apparently dose-related; thus, it is recommended that the dose should not exceed 2.5 mg/kg/day. Renal abnormalities are generally reversible following prompt discontinuation of the drug or dosage reduction following creatinine elevations. Patients with previous renal insufficiency are more susceptible to nephrotoxicity because of drug accumulation.

Probenecid

A. Obstructive nephropathy secondary to uric acid crystals — **4.**
(53,328)

A. Patients receiving probenecid may develop hematuria and renal colic as a consequence of excessive drug-induced uricosuria and uric acid crystal formation.

B. Glomerular toxicity? A hypersensitivity reaction — **4.**
(53,169,232,460)

B. Proteinuria is a rare complication of probenecid therapy. The development of the nephrotic syndrome has been reported in a patient following repeated challenges with probenecid. With each episode, renal abnormalities cleared following discontinuation of the drug.

Procainamide

Glomerular toxicity. Autoimmune glomerulonephritis — **4.**
Subendothelial deposits of electron-dense material have been demonstrated in several cases of procainamide-induced lupus.
(32,90,304,442,535,536)

Symptomatic immune glomerulonephritis is a rare complication of procainamide-induced lupus. It has been suggested that histological evidence of kidney damage may be present without clinical evidence of renal dysfunction.

Drug; Rate of Occurrence; Histopathology; Mechanism	Clinical Remarks

Pyrazolone Derivatives (Antipyrine, Phenazone)

See phenacetin.

Quinidine

Mechanism unknown. Autoimmune glomerulonephritis suspected — **4**. (556)

Lupus nephritis, secondary to quinidine has been suggested. Although nephritis is a rare complication of drug-induced lupus, the presence of antinuclear antibodies, reduced serum complement levels, abnormal urinary sediment, and a slight reduction in creatinine clearance support the possibility of quinidine-induced lupus nephritis.

Radiocontrast Media

A. Tubular toxicity. A direct nephrotoxic effect — **3**. Both proximal and distal tubular necrosis have been demonstrated; cortical and medullary necrosis have been reported as well. Varying degrees of interstitial inflammation and nonspecific glomerular changes may also be present. Contrast-induced alterations of renal plasma flow and glomerular filtration have been proposed as additional mechanisms of renal toxicity. (6,15,33,55,86,129,135,142,143,166,209,214,227, 328,330,358,365,416,438,459,461,467,472,509, 527a,531)

A. Acute oliguric renal failure, secondary to a number of radiocontrast media have been reported following various radiologic procedures. Renal insufficiency usually occurs within 12 to 48 hours following these procedures and reaches its nadir by the seventh day. Renal function generally returns to normal over several weeks; however, on occasion prolonged or irreversible nephrotoxicity and death may occur. The overall incidence does not appear to be high, but does depend on the agent used and its iodine content. A number of predisposing factors have also been identified: excessive dosing, dehydration, preexisting renal disease, and diabetes.

B. Obstructive nephropathy, secondary to uric acid crystal and stone formation or intratubular precipitation of proteins — **4**. (15,39,328,358,365,370,381,419)

B. A significant uricosuric effect of certain radiocontrast media has been documented. Iopanoic acid and calcium ipodate demonstrate the greatest uricosuric potential. Hypertonic urographic contrast agents have also been shown to cause intratubular precipitation of mucoproteins. Acute renal failure in patients with myelomatosis has been reported following intravenous urography. This has been associated with a radiocontrast media with a high protein binding capacity such as the now rarely used acetrizoates. Patients with preexisting hyperuricemia, proteinuria and dehydration may be predisposed to acute obstructive renal failure.

Rifampin

Acute tubulointerstitial toxicity. Probably a hypersensitivity reaction — **3**.
Light microscopy consistently demonstrates tubular cell damage and necrosis that is frequently associated with interstitial inflammation. However, tubular necrosis alone has been reported. Glomeruli usually appear normal, but mild proliferative changes sometimes have been noted. Circulating anti-rifampin antibodies have been found. Although renal immunofluorescent studies are generally negative, evidence suggesting antitubular basement membrane antibodies have recently been demonstrated. Even though a hypersensitivity reaction seems likely, a toxic mechanism has not been ruled out. (85,94,102,109,186,211,212,285,291,335,378,386, 418,425,431,468,497,560)

Rifampin nephrotoxicity has been associated primarily with irregular or intermittent drug intake. Patients may develop flu-like and abdominal symptoms one-half to two hours following any reintroduction of rifampin, which usually lasts 24 hours. Acute renal failure may subsequently develop at variable intervals of time in a small number of these patients as may hepatotoxicity, hemolysis, and other hematologic abnormalities. Renal insufficiency improves within two to six weeks, although chronic renal failure has been reported. Rifampin-induced hemolysis may itself result in acute obstructive renal failure secondary to precipitation of hemoglobin. Light-chain proteinuria and acute renal failure have also been noted in patients receiving continuous rifampin treatment. Patients on rifampin therapy should be warned not to discontinue and restart the drug without consulting their physician.

Spironolactone

Mechanism unknown — **4**. (19,384a)

Further deterioration of renal function which could not be attributed to salt or water depletion has been reported in six patients with previous renal impairment.

Streptomycin

Tubular toxicity. A direct nephrotoxic effect — **4**. Proximal tubular necrosis has been found. (51,161,230,328,346,377,453)

Compared to the other aminoglycoside derivatives, streptomycin is the least nephrotoxic. Early investigators noted a high incidence of cylindruria and proteinuria, although azotemia was not common with daily doses of 1 to 1.5 grams. However, the frequency of BUN elevations increases with higher doses and in patients with preexisting renal insufficiency. Renal toxicity is reversible. Since the drug has been purified streptomycin nephrotoxicity has become uncommon.

Drug; Rate of Occurrence;
Histopathology; Mechanism   **Clinical Remarks**

Streptozotocin

Tubular toxicity. A direct nephrotoxic effect — **1.**
Proximal tubular damage evidenced on light microscopy by cellular degeneration and necrosis of proximal tubular epithelium. Patchy interstitial cellular infiltrates may also be found. Glomeruli are generally normal. Immunofluorescent studies are negative.
(61,146,266,315,336,380,443,447,448,449,495)

Nephrotoxicity following streptozotocin treatment is common, occurs in up to 65% of patients treated, and is a primary limiting factor in streptozotocin therapy. It has been suggested, but not established, that nephrotoxicity is dose-dependent and possibly route-dependent as well. Mild to moderate proteinuria is usually the initial clinical sign of tubular damage and frequently develops after the second or third dose of streptozotocin. Other signs of more severe tubular toxicity including Fanconi syndrome (hypophosphatemia, glycosuria, renal tubular acidosis, etc) and nephrogenic diabetes insipidus may develop as well as azotemia, and, less commonly, anuria. Treatment should be withheld at the first sign of proteinuria and should not be reinstituted until this has returned to normal unless therapy demands otherwise. Proteinuria alone is generally transient, while severe tubular dysfunction and renal failure may persist for several weeks following drug discontinuation. However, irreversible renal failure contributing to death has been reported.

Streptozotocin has also been documented to induce kidney tumors in rats, while in humans abnormal glomerular nodules have been reported.

Sulfinpyrazone

A. Obstructive nephropathy secondary to uric acid crystals — **4.**
(328,464)

A. Patients receiving sulfinpyrazone may develop hematuria and renal colic secondary to excessive drug-induced uricosuria and uric acid crystal formation.

B. Renal toxicity. An apparent hypersensitivity reaction; pathology unknown — **4.**
(57)

B. A single case of sterile pyuria and amorphous urinary debris, with associated elevation of BUN and creatinine has been reported. Abnormalities cleared on drug discontinuation, reappeared on rechallenge, and subsequently disappeared when sulfinpyrazone was again stopped.

Sulfonamides

A. Obstructive nephropathy secondary to sulfonamide crystalluria — **3-4.**
Sulfonamide crystals can be found in urinary specimens. They may also be demonstrated in the calyces, pelvis, ureters as well as distal tubule lumens where they are associated with tubular epithelial cell flattening, tubular dilatation and necrosis. Retrograde pyelogram may also show dilatation of the ureters and pelvis.
(66,115,134,299,302,328,358,378,453,475,544)

A. Obstructive nephropathy is the most common nephrotoxic effect reported. Toxicity has been documented primarily with the older, less soluble sulfa preparations (sulfapyridine, sulfathiazole, sulfadiazine) and their acetyl metabolites when given in high doses to patients with acidic urine. Crystalluria associated with hematuria and dysuria indicates renal tubular damage which may progress to renal colic and acute oliguric/anuric renal failure. A number of fatalities were reported in early cases. Treatment and preventive measures include adequate fluid intake and alkalinization of the urine. For established cases of anuric renal failure, ureteral catheterization and alkaline irrigation as well as dialysis may be required. The newer, more soluble sulfonamides, such as sulfisoxazole, rarely cause crystalluria. There does not appear to be any substantial risk of anuria secondary to crystalluria with these agents.

B. Renal toxicity. A hypersensitivity reaction — **4.**
A variety of pathologic lesions (tubulointerstitial disease, glomerulonephritis, vasculitis) have been associated with sulfonamide administration.
(22,158,179,299,302,328,353,354,364,374,378,399,432,453,475)

B. Nephrotoxicity due to a hypersensitivity reaction is not common but may be serious. Acute renal failure is usually associated with evidence of a generalized allergic reaction. Nephrotic syndrome following topically applied sulfadiazine silver has been reported as well.

Tetracyclines

A. Prerenal azotemia secondary to an antianabolic effect — **2-3.**
(12,56,89,131,147,198,199,271,273,287,301,367,377,408,413,428,445,471,493,548)

A. An elevated BUN occurs frequently. Patients with preexisting renal impairment are more susceptible to tetracycline-induced azotemia because of drug accumulation. In addition, concomitant administration of diuretics with tetracycline may enhance the incidence of azotemia. Drug-related azotemia can be severe enough to cause nausea, vomiting, and diarrhea. If fluids and electrolytes are not replaced, dehydration with further worsening of renal function will occur. Tetracyclines should be withdrawn immediately. Doxycycline appears to have minimal antianabolic effect since it does not accumulate in renal failure. With the possible exception of doxycycline, tetracycline derivatives should be avoided in patients with impaired renal function.

B. Tubular toxicity. A direct nephrotoxic effect — **3.**
Fatty vacuolization of proximal tubular epithelial cells, as well as fatty metamorphosis of the liver are characteristic pathological findings. Focal ischemic tubular necrosis may also be found.
(265,292,305,324,328,423)

B. Hepatorenal failure may develop following intravenous tetracycline administration. Patients present clinically with nausea, abdominal pain, lethargy, jaundice (scleral icterus, dark urine) and renal failure (usually nonoliguric). Pregnant or postpartum women appear to be at greatest risk, especially when treated with large doses (more than 2 gm/day) and when there is a preexisting renal impairment. For these patients prognosis is poor and recovery is prolonged in those who survive. Avoid parenteral tetracyclines in pregnant or postpartum women.

Drug; Rate of Occurrence; Histopathology; Mechanism	Clinical Remarks
C. Tubular toxicity. A direct nephrotoxic effect of degradation products — **4**. Proximal and distal tubular damage has been shown. (36,182,184,219,328,377,499)	C. Ingestion of outdated tetracycline has resulted in a reversible Fanconi-like syndrome. Clinical evidence of tubular damage usually appears within three to four days following ingestion of the degraded tetracycline. The characteristic clinical signs and symptoms include nausea, polydypsia, polyuria, glycosuria, aminoaciduria, hyperphosphaturia, proteinuria, and proximal renal tubular acidosis. Usually this condition is reversed when the drug is discontinued; however, prolonged defects in urinary acidification have been reported. Although improved manufacturing techniques have all but eliminated degradation of this drug as a problem, do not use outdated tetracycline.
D. Synergistic renal toxicity. Mechanism unknown — **4**. Calcium oxalate stones were demonstrated in one study. (10,294,424,435)	D. The incidence of acute renal failure following methoxyflurane anesthesia is increased by the administration of parenteral tetracycline immediately before or following methoxyflurane.
E. Nephrogenic diabetes insipidus. Direct tubular toxicity — **2-3**. Tetracyclines reduce cyclic-AMP levels in the renal medulla by inhibiting ADH-stimulated adenyl cyclase. The activity of cyclic-AMP dependent protein kinase may also be impaired. (368a,479a)	E. Demeclocycline-induced diabetes insipidus is ADH-unresponsive and dose-related. Polydipsia and polyuria occur uniformly in patients receiving 1200 mg/day or more and reverse with dosage reduction or drug discontinuation. While tetracycline and chlortetracycline have the same, but weaker, *in vitro* effects, they have not been reported to cause clinical diabetes insipidus.

Thiotepa

Obstructive nephropathy secondary to bladder/ureter inflammation and fibrosis — **4**. The kidneys show hydronephrotic changes. A possible direct toxic effect on renal tubular cells is postulated as well. (450,515)	One case of renal failure that followed bladder instillation of thiotepa has been reported. The primary complaints included dysuria, urgency, frequency of urination, and hematuria. Two instances of renal shutdown following parenteral thiotepa have also been reported.

Tobramycin

Tubular toxicity. A direct nephrotoxic effect — **2-3**. (35,62,202,272a,282,377,387)	As with gentamicin, the incidence of tobramycin nephrotoxicity is difficult to evaluate because of the severe nature of the infections for which it is used. The incidence of azotemia during tobramycin therapy has been reported to be between 1.5 to 20%. Toxicity appears to be dose- and duration-related. As with gentamicin, evidence exists to suggest that cephalothin may also enhance the nephrotoxic potential of tobramycin. In addition, a complex metabolic disorder associated with renal tubular dysfunction has been reported. See Gentamicin.

Tolbutamide

Mechanism unknown — **4**. (451)	One case of the nephrotic syndrome attributed to tolbutamide has been reported. This appears to be a rare complication.

Vancomycin

Mechanism unknown — **4**. (280,290,306,328,377,453,520)	Proteinuria, hematuria, and elevations of the BUN have been reported. However, purification of the drug has resulted in disappearance of additional reports of nephrotoxicity. Renal toxicity is no longer considered a significant complication of vancomycin therapy.

Viomycin

Renal toxicity. A direct nephrotoxic effect — **2-3**. Both glomerular and tubular damage have been found. (358,369,378,532)	A large number of patients on prolonged therapy eventually develop renal toxicity. Evidence of nephrotoxicity includes proteinuria, hematuria, pyuria, and cylindruria which commonly appear within the first two weeks of treatment. Azotemia and severe electrolyte disturbances (hypocalcemia, hypokalemia) may also develop. Nephrotoxicity is readily reversible.

Vitamin D

Nephrocalcinosis — **4**. Tubular calcification is the principle finding. (14,95,251,372,446)	Excessive amounts of vitamin D can cause a marked elevation in serum calcium which may lead to metastatic calcifications, including nephrocalcinosis. Renal insufficiency may subsequently develop.

REFERENCES

1. Abel JA: Analgesic nephropathy — a review of the literature, 1967-1970. Clin Pharmacol Ther 12:583, 1971.
2. Abry J et al: Fatal tubular necrosis during chlorothiazide administration. NY State J Med 60:1638, 1960.
3. Adams DA et al: Nephrotic syndrome associated with penicillamine therapy of Wilson's disease. Am J Med 36:330, 1964.
4. Adams PG et al: The radiological diagnosis of analgesic nephropathy. Clin Radio 26:417, 1975.
5. Adler S et al: Nonoliguric renal failure secondary to sodium colistimethate: a report of four cases. Am J Med Sci 262:109, 1971.
6. Adornato B et al: Acute renal failure. A complication of cerebral angiography. Arch Neurol 33:687, 1976.
7. Agarwal BN et al: Diphenylhydantoin-induced acute renal failure. Nephron 18:249, 1977.
8. Alano FA et al: Acute renal failure and pigmentation due to phenazopyridine (Pyridium). Ann Int Med 72:89, 1970.
9. Alarcon-Sebovia SD et al: Clinical and experimental studies on the hydralazine syndrome and its relationship to systemic lupus erythematosus. Medicine 46:1, 1967.
10. Albers DD et al: Renal failure following prostato vesiculectomy related to methoxyflurane anesthesia and tetracycline complicated by candida infection. J Urol 106:348, 1971.
11. Albin A et al: Nephropathy, xanthinuria, and orotic aciduria complicating Burkitt's lymphoma treated with chemotherapy and allopurinol. Metab 21:771, 1972.
12. Alestig K: Studies on doxycycline during intravenous and oral treatment with reference to renal function. Scand J Infect Dis 5:193, 1973.
13. Alexander MR et al: Methicillin nephritis. Drug Intell Clin Pharm 8:115, 1974.
13a. Allen JD et al: Staphylococcal septicemia treated with methicillin. NEJM 266:111, 1962.
14. Anning ST et al: The toxic effect of calciferol. QJ Med 17:203, 1948.
15. Ansari Z et al: Acute renal failure due to radiocontrast agents. Nephton 17:28, 1976.
16. Arger PH et al: Analgesic abuse nephropathy. Urol 7:123, 1976.
16a. Arisz L et al: The effect of indomethacin on proteinuria and kidney function in the nephrotic syndrome. Acta Med Scand 199:121, 1976.
17. Aufderheide AC: Renal tubular calcium oxalate crystal deposition. Arch Path 92:162, 1971.
18. Bacon PA et al: Penicillamine nephropathy in rheumatoid arthritis. Quart J Med 45:661, 1976.
19. Bailey RR: The kidney and antihypertensive therapy. Drugs 11(suppl 1):70, 1976.
20. Bailey RR et al: Deterioration in renal function in association with co-trimoxazole therapy. Med J Aust 1:914, 1976.
21. Baker SB et al: Acute interstitial nephritis due to drug sensitivity. Brit Med J 1:1655, 1963.
22. Bakken K: The allergic reaction of the kidney to sulfonamide medication. J Path Bacteriol 59:501, 1947.
23. Baldwin DS et al: Renal-failure and interstitial nephritis due to penicillin and methicillin. NEJM 279:1245, 1968.
24. Band PR et al: Xanthine nephropathy in a patient with lymphosarcoma treated with allopurinol. NEJM 283:354, 1970.
25. Baar RS et al: Hypomagnesemic hypocalcemia secondary to renal magnesium wasting. A possible consequence of high-dose gentamicin therapy. Ann Int Med 82:646, 1975.
26. Barcenas CG et al: Recovery from malignant hypertension with anuria after prolonged hemodialysis. South Med J 69:1230, 1976.
27. Bar-Khayim Y et al: Trimethadione (Tridione)-induced nephrotic syndrome. A report of a case with unique ultrastructural renal pathology. Am J Med 54:272, 1973.
28. Barnett ML et al: Nephrotic syndrome occurring during tridione therapy. Am J Med 4:760, 1948.
29. Barr GA et al: An animal model for combined methoxyflurane and gentamicin nephrotoxicity. Brit J Anaesth 45:306, 1973.
30. Barr RD et al: Nephrotic syndrome in adult Africans in Nairobi. Brit Med J 2:131, 1972.
31. Barrientos A et al: Renal failure and cephalothin. Ann Int Med 84:612, 1976.
32. Barry KG: Post-traumatic renal shutdown in humans. Milit Med 128:224, 1963.
33. Barshay ME et al: Acute renal failure in diabetic patients after intravenous infusion pyelography. Clin Nephrol 1:35, 1973.
34. Becker CG et al: Nephrotic syndrome after contact with mercury. Arch Int Med 110:82, 1962.
35. Bendush CL et al: Tobramycin sulfate: A summary of worldwide experience from clinical studies. J Infect Dis 134:S219, 1976.
36. Benitz KF et al: Renal toxicity of tetracycline degradation products. Proc Soc Exp Biol 115:930, 1964.
37. Benner EJ: Renal damage associated with prolonged administration of ampicillin, cephaloridine, and cephalothin. Antimicrob Agents Chemother 417, 1969.
38. Bennett WM et al: Gentamicin nephrotoxicity — morphologic and pharmacologic features. West J Med 126:65, 1977.
39. Berdon WE et al: Tamm-Horsfall proteinuria. Radiology 92:714, 1969.
40. Berg KJ: Acute effect of acetylsalicylic acid in patients with chronic renal insufficiency. Europ J Clin Pharmacol 11:111, 1977.
41. Bergentz SE et al: Diuresis and viscosity in dehydrated patients: influence of dextran 40,000 with and without mannitol. Ann Surg 161:582, 1965.
42. Berglund F et al: Effect of trimethoprim-sulfamethoxazole on the renal excretion of creatinine in man. J Urol 114:802, 1975.
43. Bergstrand A et al: Renal histology during treatment with oxazolidine-diones (trimethadione, ethadione, and paramethadione). Pediat 30:601, 1962.
44. Berk DP et al: Deafness complicating antibiotic therapy of hepatic encephalopathy. Ann Int Med 73:393, 1970.
45. Berman LB et al: Kanamycin nephrotoxicity. Ann NY Acad Sci 76:149, 1958.
46. Bertino JR: Thrombocytopenia and renal lesions associated with acetazoleamide (Diamox) therapy. Arch Int Med 99:1006, 1957.
47. Bilde T et al: Idiopathic retroperitoneal fibrosis. Acta Chir Scand 137:573, 1971.
48. Birkhead HA et al: Toxicology of cefazolin in animals. J Infect Dis 128:S379, 1973.
49. Bjornberg A et al: Thiazides: a cause of necrotising vasculitis. Lancet 2:982, 1965.
50. Bobrow SN et al: Anuria and acute tubular necrosis associated with gentamicin and cephalothin. JAMA 222:1546, 1972.
51. Bobrowitz ID: Ethambutol compared to streptomycin in original treatment of advanced pulmonary tuberculosis. Chest 60:14, 1971.
52. Bock KD et al: Peracute primary malignant nephrosclerosis with irreversible renal failure and malignant hypertension after taking oral contraceptives. Dtsch Med Wschr 98:757, 1973.
53. Boger WP et al: Probenecid (Benemid). Its uses and side effects in 2,502 patients. Arch Int Med 95:83, 1955.
54. Border WA et al: Antitubular basement membrane antibodies in methicillin-associated interstitial nephritis. NEJM 291:381, 1974.
55. Borges FJ: Acute renal failure after oral cholecystography. Lancet 2:340, 1964.
56. Boston Collaborative Drug Surveillance Program: Tetracycline and drug-attributed rises in blood urea nitrogen. JAMA 220:377, 1972.
57. Brown J: Abnormalities of urinary sediment and renal failure following sulfinpyrazone therapy. Arch Int Med 136:1060, 1976.
58. Brauninger GE et al: Nephropathy associated with methicillin therapy. JAMA 203:125, 1968.
59. Bridgman JF et al: Complications during clofibrate treatment of nephrotic-syndrome hyperlipoproteinemia. Lancet 2:506, 1972.
60. Briggs JN et al: Toxic effects of tridione. Lancet 1:59, 1949.
61. Broder LE et al: Pancreatic islet cell carcinoma. Results of therapy with streptozotocin in 52 patients. Ann Int Med 79:108, 1973.
62. Brogden RN et al: Tobramycin: A review of its antibacterial and pharmacokinetic properties and therapeutic use. Drugs 12:166, 1976.
63. Brooks RH et al: Dermatitis, hepatitis and nephritis due to pheindione. Ann Int Med 52:706, 1960.
64. Brown CB et al: Haemolytic uraemic syndrome in women taking oral contraceptives. Lancet 1:1479, 1973.
65. Brumfitt W et al: Colistin in pseudomonas pyocyanea infections and its effect on renal function. Brit J Urol 38:495, 1966.
66. Bull GM et al: Acute renal failure due to poisons and drugs. Lancet 1:134, 1958.

67. Bullock JD et al: Flecked retina. Appearance secondary to oxalate crystals from methoxyflurane anesthesia. Arch Ophth 93:26, 1975.
68. Bullock WE et al: Can mannitol reduce amphotericin B nephrotoxicity? Antimicrob Agents Chemother 10:555, 1976.
69. Bunn PA: Kanamycin. Med Clin N Am 54:1245, 1970.
70. Burack WR et al: A reversible nephrotic syndrome associated with congestive heart failure. Circ 18:562, 1958.
71. Burgess JL et al: Nephrotoxicity of amphotericin B with emphasis on changes in tubular function. Am J Med 53:77, 1972.
72. Burke, JF et al: Doxorubicin hydrochloride-associated renal failure. Arch Int Med 137:385, 1977.
73. Burnett CH et al: Hypercalcemia without hypercalciuria or hypophosphatemia, calcinosis, and renal insufficiency: A syndrome following prolonged intake of milk and alkali. NEJM 240:787, 1949.
74. Burry HC et al: Salicylates and renal function in rheumatoid arthritis. Brit Med J 1:613, 1976.
75. Burry HC et al: Apparent reduction of endogenous creatinine clearance by salicylate treatment. Brit Med J 2:16, 1976.
76. Bursion J et al: Nephrosis due to mercurial diuretics. Brit Med J 1:1277, 1958.
77. Burton JR et al: Acute renal failure during cephalothin therapy. JAMA 229:679, 1974.
78. Burton JR et al: Acute interstitial nephritis from oxacillin. Johns Hopkins Med J 134:58, 1974.
79. Busutill AA et al: Possible cephaloridine nephrotoxicity in a neonate. Lancet 1:264, 1975.
80. Butkus DE et al: Renal failure following gentamicin in combination with clindamycin. Nephron 17:307, 1976.
81. Bygbjerg IC et al: Gentamicin-induced nephrotoxicity. Scand J Infect Dis 8:203, 1976.
82. Cabanillas F et al: Nephrotoxicity of combined cephalothin-gentamicin regimen. Arch Int Med 135:850, 1975.
83. Caldwell ADS et al: Comparative study of the effect of three antibiotics on renal function. Brit J Pharmacol 37:283, 1969.
84. Cameron JS et al: Membranous glomerulonephritis and the nephrotic syndrome appearing during mersalyl therapy. Guy's Hosp Rep 114:101, 1965.
85. Campese VM et al: Acute renal failure during intermittent rifampicin therapy. Nephron 10:256, 1973.
86. Canales CO et al: Acute renal failure after the administration of iopanoic acid as an oral cholecystographic agent. NEJM 281:89, 1969.
87. Cannon PJ et al: Ethacrynic acid and furosemide: Renal pharmacology and clinical use. Progr Cardiovas Dis 12:99, 1969.
88. Carling PC et al: Nephrotoxicity associated with cephalothin administration. Arch Int Med 135:797, 1975.
89. Carney S et al: Minocycline excretion and distribution in relation to renal function in man. Clin Exp Pharmacol Physiol 1:299, 1974.
90. Case records of the Massachusetts General Hospital (case no. 21-1968). NEJM 278:1167, 1968.
91. Case records of the Massachusetts General Hospital (case 49-1975). NEJM 293:1308, 1975.
92. Case records of the Massachusetts General Hospital (case 5-1973). NEJM 288:254, 1973.
93. Case records of the Massachusetts General Hospital (case 13-1976). NEJM 294:712, 1976.
94. Chan WC et al: Renal failure during intermittent rifampicin therapy. Tubercle 56:191, 1975.
95. Chaplin H et al: Vitamin D intoxication. Am J Med Sci 221:369, 1951.
96. Charron RC et al: Acetazolamide therapy with renal complications. Conad J Ophthal 9:282, 1974.
97. Charytan C et al: Glomerular capillary thrombosis and acute renal failure after epsilon aminocaproic acid therapy. NEJM 280:1102, 1969.
98. Chinitz JL et al: Pathophysiology and prevention of dextran-40-induced anuria. J Lab Clin Med 77:76, 1971.
99. Churchill D et al: Persisting renal insufficiency after methoxyflurane anesthesia. Am J Med 56:575, 1974.
100. Churchill D et al: Toxic nephropathy after low dose methoxyflurane anesthesia: drug interaction with secobarbital? CMAJ 114:326, 1976.
101. Climie H: Acquired idiosyncrasy to sodium p-aminosalicylate. Lancet 2:308, 1950.

102. Cochran M et al: Permanent renal damage with rifampicin. Lancet 1:1428, 1975.
103. Cohen SN et al: Drug-induced nephropathy. JAMA 227:325, 1974.
104. Collier J et al: Two cases of ethambutol nephrotoxicity. Brit Med J 2:1105, 1976.
105. Colvin RB et al: Penicillin-associated interstitial nephritis. Ann Int Med 81:404, 1974.
106. Committee on Anesthesia NAS-NRC: Statement regarding the role of methoxyflurane in the production of renal dysfunction. Anesth 34:505, 1971.
107. Compton AB et al: Nephropathy caused by methicillin therapy for staphylococcal septicemia. South Med J 69:872, 1976.
108. Condit P et al: Renal toxicity of methotrexate. Cancer 23:126, 1969.
109. Cordonnier D et al: Acute renal failure after rifampicin. Lancet 2:1364, 1972.
110. Cotton JR et al: Acute renal failure following halothane anesthesia. Arch Pathol Lab Med 100:628, 1976.
111. Cousins MJ et al: Methoxyflurane nephrotoxicity. A study of dose response in man. JAMA 225:1611, 1973.
112. Cousins MJ et al: The etiology of methoxyflurane nephrotoxicity. J Pharm Exper Ther 190:530, 1974.
113. Cousins MJ et al: Metabolism and renal effects of enflurane in man. Anesth 44:44, 1976.
114. Craig WA et al: Pharmacology of cefazolin and other cephalosporins in patients with renal insufficiency. J Infect Dis 128:S347, 1973.
115. Craft AW et al: Acute renal failure and hypoglycaemia due to sulphadiazine poisoning. Postgrad Med J 53:103, 1977.
116. Crandell WB et al: Nephrotoxicity associated with methoxyflurane anesthesia. Anesth 27:591, 1966.
116a. Cremer W et al: Symptoms and course of chronic hypokalemic nephropathy in man. Clin Nephrol 8:112, 1977.
117. Cuthbert J: Acquired idiosyncrasy to sodium p-aminosalicylate. Lancet 2:209, 1950.
118. Dahlgren JG et al: Gentamicin blood levels: a guide to nephrotoxicity. Antimicrob Agents Chemother 8:58, 1975.
119. Davia JE et al: Uremia, deafness, and paralysis due to irrigating antibiotic solutions. Arch Int Med 125:135, 1970.
120. Davies DW: Acetazolamide therapy with renal complications. Brit Med J 1:214, 1959.
121. Davis JP et al: A comparison of paradione and tridione in the treatment of epilepsy. J Pediat 34:273, 1949.
122. Day AT et al: Hazards of penicillamine therapy in the treatment of rheumatoid arthritis. Postgrad Med J 50 (suppl 2):71, 1974.
123. DeBeukelaer MM et al: Deafness and acute tubular necrosis following parenteral administration of neomycin. Am J Dis Child 122:250, 1971.
124. DeConti RC et al: Clinical and pharmacological studies with cis-diammine dichloroplatinum (II). Cancer Res 33:1310, 1975.
124a. DeGraff J et al: Severe potassium depletion caused by the abuse of laxatives. Acta Scand Med 166:407, 1960.
125. Delin K et al: Multiple arterial occlusions and hypertension probably caused by an oral contraceptive: a patient in whom the development of renovascular hypertension has been followed. Clin Nephrol 6:453, 1976.
126. Dellinger P et al: Effect of cephalothin on renal cortical concentrations of gentamicin in rats. Antimicrob Agents Chemother 9:587, 1976.
127. Dellinger P et al: Protective effect of cephalothin against gentamicin-induced nephrotoxicity in rats. Antimicrob Agents Chemother 9:172, 1976.
128. DeVita VT et al: Pneumocystis carinii pneumonia. NEJM 280:287, 1969.
129. Diaz-Buxo JA et al: Acute renal failure after excretory urography in diabetic patients. Ann Int Med 83:155, 1975.
130. Dillon ML et al: Cephaloridine in patients with impaired renal function. JAMA 218:250, 1971.
131. Dijkhuis HJPM et al: Tetracycline and BUN level. JAMA 223:441, 1973.
131a. Ditlove J et al: Methicillin nephritis. Medicine 56:483, 1977.
132. Dodds MG et al: Enhancement by potent diuretics of renal tubular necrosis induced by cephaloridine. Brit J Pharmacol 40:227, 1970.
133. Donker AJM et al: The effect of indomethacin on kidney function and plasma renin activity in man. Nephron 17:288, 1976.

134. Dorfman LF et al: Sulfonamide crystalluria: a forgotten disease. J Urol 104:482, 1970.

135. Dormandy KM et al: A case of renal failure following renal angiography. Lancet 2:18, 1957.

136. Dosa S et al: Acute-on-chronic renal failure precipitated by clofibrate. Lancet 1:250, 1976.

137. Douglas JB et al: Nephrotoxic effects of amphotericin B, including renal tubular acidosis. Am J Med 46:154, 1969.

138. Down PF et al: Postpartum renal failure associated with eclampsia and penicillin hypersensitivity. Brit J Obstet Gyn 82:831, 1975.

139. Doyle WF et al: Interstitial nephritis associated with methicillin therapy: case reported. Milit Med 139:384, 1974.

140. Drago JR et al: Acute interstitial nephritis. J Urol 115:105, 1976.

141. Dryden GE: Incidence of tubular degeneration with microlithiasis following methoxyflurane compared with other anesthetic agents. Anesth Analg 53:383, 1974.

142. Dudzinski PG et al: Acute renal failure following high dose excretory urography in dehydrated patients. J Urol 106:619, 1971.

143. Duggan FJ et al: Acute renal insufficiency following oral cholecystography. J Urol 109:156, 1973.

144. Dunea JG et al: Thrombotic thrombocytopenia purpura with acute anuric renal failure. Am J Med 41:1000, 1966.

145. Dunn FG et al: Malignant hypertension associated with use of oral contraceptives. Brit Heart J 37:336, 1975.

146. DuPriest RW et al: Streptozotocin therapy in 22 cancer patients. Cancer 35:358, 1975.

147. Edwards OM: Azotemia aggravated by tetracycline. Brit Med J 1:26, 1970.

148. Eichhorn JH et al: Renal failure following enflurane anesthesia. Anesth 45:557, 1976.

149. Elkind AM et al: Silent retroperitoneal fibrosis associated with methysergide therapy. JAMA 206:1041, 1968.

150. Elkington SG et al: Renal and hepatic injury associated with methoxyflurane anesthesia. Ann Int Med 69:1229, 1968.

151. Ellman MH et al: Toxic epidermal necrolysis associated with allopurinol administration. Arch Dermatol 111:986, 1975.

152. Elsas LJ: Wilson's disease with reversible renal tubular dysfunction. Correlation with proximal tubular ultrastructure. Ann Int Med 75:427, 1971.

153. Elwood CM et al: Acute renal failure associated with sodium colistimethate treatment. Arch Int Med 118:326, 1966.

154. Emmer M et al: Pneumocystis carinii pneumonia and pentamidine isethionate toxicity. Ann Int Med 69:637, 1968.

155. Emmerson BT et al: Studies on the nephrotoxic effect of neomycin. Aust Ann Med 13:149, 1964.

156. Emspruch BC et al: Clinical and experimental nephropathy resulting from use of neomycin sulfate. JAMA 173:809, 1960.

157. Engle JE et al: Reversible acute renal failure after cephalothin. Ann Int Med 83:232, 1975.

158. Evans WE et al: Acute renal failure in a multisystem allergic reaction to sulfamethoxazole. Drug Intell Clin Pharm 9:660, 1975.

159. Eybel CE et al: Skin pigmentation and acute renal failure in a patient receiving phenazopyridine therapy. JAMA 228:1027, 1974.

160. Fair WR: The effect of cephaloridine on normal renal function. J Urol 107:2, 1972.

161. Falco FG et al: Nephrotoxicity of aminoglycosides and gentamicin. J Infect Dis 119:406, 1969.

162. Fanning WL et al: Gentamicin and cephalothin associated rises in blood urea nitrogen. Antimicrob Agents Chemother 10:80, 1976.

163. Farebrother DA et al: Experimental crystal nephropathy (one year study in the pig). Clin Nephrol 4:243, 1975.

163a. Federman MJ et al: Occurrence of nephritis with prolonged administration of methicillin. Clin Res 17:539, 1969.

163b. Feest TG et al: Low molecular weight dextran: a continuing cause of acute renal failure. Brit Med J 2:1300, 1976.

164. Feigen RD et al: Hematuria and proteinuria associated with methicillin administration. NEJM 272:903, 1965.

165. Fekety FR et al: The treatment of gram-negative bacillary infections with colistin. Ann Int Med 57:214, 1962.

166. Feldman HA: Recurrent radiographic dye-induced acute renal failure. JAMA 229-72, 1974.

167. Fellers FX et al: Nephrotic syndrome induced by penicillamine therapy. Am J Dis Child 98:659, 1959.

168. Felts JH et al: Nephrotic syndrome induced by penicillamine therapy. Lancet 1:53, 1968.

169. Ferris TF et al: Nephrotic syndrome caused by probenecid. NEJM 265:381, 1961.

170. Fialk MA et al: Allergic interstitial nephritis with diuretics. Ann Int Med 81:403, 1974.

171. Fillastre P et al: Acute renal failure associated with combined gentamicin and cephalothin therapy. Brit Med J 2:396, 1973.

172. Finland M: Symposium on kanamycin. Ann NY Acad Sci 132:1089, 1966.

173. Fitzgerald EW Jr.: Fatal glomerulonephritis complicating allergic purpura due to chlorothiazide. Arch Int Med 105:153, 1960.

174. Foord RD: Cephaloridine and the kidney, in Progress in Antimicrobial and Anticancer Chemotherapy, Proc. 6th Intn'l Congress Chemother, University of Tokyo Press, 1970, p 597.

175. Ford RD: Cephaloridine, cephalothin and the kidney. J Antimicrob Chemother 1 (suppl):119, 1975.

176. Frascino JA et al: Renal oxalosis and azotemia after methoxyflurane anesthesia. NEJM 283:676, 1970.

177. Freeland RB et al: Renal tubular necrosis due to nephrotoxicity of organic mercurial diuretics. Ann Int Med 57:34, 1962.

178. Frei E et al: New approaches to cancer chemotherapy with methotrexate. NEJM 292:846, 1975.

179. French AJ: Hypersensitivity in the pathogenesis of the histopathologic changes associated with sulfonamide chemotherapy. Am J Path 22:679, 1946.

180. Friedman IS et al: Chlorothiazide and electrolyte depletion in chronic glomerulonephritis. Arch Int Med 105:31, 1960.

181. Friedman WF et al: Pharmacologic closure of patent arteriosus in the premature infant. NEJM 295:526, 1976.

182. Frimpter GW et al: Reversible fanconi Syndrome caused by degraded tetracycline. JAMA 184:111, 1963.

183. Fuller TJ et al: Diuretic-induced interstitial nephritis. Occurrence in a patient with membranous glomerulonephritis. JAMA 235:1998, 1976.

184. Fulop M et al: Potassium-depletion syndrome to nephropathy apparently caused by "outdated tetracycline." NEJM 272:986, 1965.

185. Fung-Herrera CG et al: Cephalexin nephrotoxicity. JAMA 229:318, 1974.

186. Gabow PA et al: Tubulointerstitial and glomerular nephritis associated with rifampicin. JAMA 235:2517, 1976.

187. Galea EG et al: Fatal nephropathy due to phenindione sensitivity. Lancet 1:920, 1963.

188. Gallagher PJ et al: Haematuria during methicillin therapy. Postgrad Med J 47:511, 1972.

188a. Galpin JE et al: Acute interstitial nephritis due to methicillin and similar drugs. Kid Intn'l 8:411, 1975.

189. Garfield JW et al: The auditory vestibular and renal effects of capreomycin in humans. Ann NY Acad Sci 135:1039, 1966.

190. Gary NE et al: Gentamicin-associated acute renal failure. Arch Int Med 136:1101, 1976.

191. Gault MH: Evidence for the nephrotoxicity of analgesics. CMAJ 107:756, 1972.

192. Gault MH: Analgesic nephropathy. Am J Med 57:740, 1971.

193. Gault MH et al: Syndrome associated with the abuse of analgesics. Ann Int Med 65:906, 1968.

194. Gelbart DR et al: Allopurinol-induced interstitial nephritis. Ann Int Med 86:196, 1977.

195. Gelfand ML: Renal colic associated with chlorothiazide and hydrochlorothiazide therapy. NEJM 265:129, 1961.

196. Geller M et al: Penicillin-associated pulmonary hypersensitivity reaction and interstitial nephritis. Ann Allergy 37:183, 1976.

197. Genkins G et al: Bacitracin nephropathy. JAMA 155:894, 1954.

198. George CRP et al: Tetracycline toxicity in renal failure. Med J Aust 1:1271, 1971.

199. George CRP et al: Minocycline toxicity in renal failure. Med J Aust 1:640, 1973.

200. Gilbert DN et al: Interstitial nephritis due to methicillin, penicillin and ampicillin. Ann Allerg 28:378, 1970.

201. Gill JR et al: Bartter's syndrome: a disorder characterized by high urinary prostaglandins and a dependence of hyperreninemia on prostaglandin synthesis. Am J Med 61:43, 1976.

202. Gillett P et al: Tobramycin/cephalothin nephrotoxicity. Lancet 1:547, 1976.

203. Girndt J et al: Severe hypertension with cardiac failure and nephrosclerosis after oral contraceptives. Dtsch Med Wschr 99:404, 1974.

204. Glushien AS et al: Renal lesions of sulfonamide type treatment with acetazolamide (Diamox). JAMA 160:204, 1956.

204a.Gonzalez-Vitale JC, et al: The renal pathology in clincial trials of cis-platinum (II) diamminedichloride. Cancer 39:1362, 1977.

205. Goodwin NJ: Colistin sulfate versus sodium colistimethate. Ann Int Med 70:232, 1968.

206. Goodwin NJ: Colistin and sodium colistimethate. Med Clin N Amer 54:1267, 1970.

207. Gordon EE et al: The effects of acetazolamide on citrate excretion and formation of renal calculi. NEJM 256:1215, 1957.

208. Gottlieb NL et al: Pharmacodynamics of Au and Au labeled aurothiomalate in blood: correlation with courses of rheumatoid arthritis, gold toxicity and gold excretion. Arthr Rheum 17:170, 1974.

209. Gottlieb A et al: Fatal renal insufficiency after oral cholecystography. NEJM 267:389, 1962.

210. Gouge TH et al: An experimental model of amphotericin B nephrotoxicity with renal tubular acidosis. J Lab Clin Med 78:713, 1971.

211. Graber CD et al: Light chain proteinuria and humoral immunoincompetence in tuberculous patients treated with rifampin. Am Rev Resp Dis 107:713, 1973.

212. Graber CD et al: Light chain proteinuria and cellular mediated immunity in rifampin treated patients with tuberculosis. Chest 67:408, 1975.

213. Graham JR et al: Fibrotic disorders associated with methysergide therapy for headache. NEJM 274:359, 1966.

214. Grainger RG: Renal toxicity of radiological contrast media. Brit Med Bull 28:191, 1972.

215. Gratton WA: Hematuria and azotemia associated with administration of methicillin. J Pediat 64:285, 1964.

216. Graves CL et al: Cardiovascular and renal effects of enflurane in surgical patients. Anesth Analg 53:898, 1974.

217. Greenberg LH et al: Audiotoxicity and nephrotoxicity due to orally administered neomycin. JAMA 194:237, 1965.

218. Greene ML et al: Urinary xanthine stones — a rare complication of allopurinol therapy. NEJM 280:426, 1969.

219. Gross JM: Fanconi syndrome developing secondary to the ingestion of outdated tetracycline. Ann Int Med 58:523, 1963.

220. Hahn BH et al: Immune responses to hydralazine-induced lupus erythematosus. Ann Int Med 76:365, 1972.

221. Halpren BA et al: Interstitial fibrosis and chronic renal failure following methoxyflurane anesthesia. JAMA 223:1239, 1973.

222. Hamilton CR et al: Renal vein thrombosis and pulmonary thromboembolism. Hopkins Med J 124:331, 1969.

223. Hansten PD: Cephalothin, gentamicin, colistin hazards. JAMA 223:1158, 1973.

224. Hardaker WT: Platinum nephrotoxicity. Cancer 34:1030, 1974.

225. Harnett MN et al: Nonoliguric renal failure and enflurane. Ann Int Med 81:560, 1974.

226. Harrison WO et al: Gentamicin nephrotoxicity: failure of three cephalosporins to potentiate injury to rats. Antimicrob Agents Chemother 8:209, 1975.

227. Harrow BR et al: Acute renal failure following oral cholecystography. Am J Med Sci 249:52, 1965.

228. Haugen HN: Tridione nephropathy. Acta Med Scand 159:375, 1957.

228a.Hayes DM et al: High dose cis-platinum diamminedichloride. Cancer 39:1372, 1977.

229. Hayslett JP et al: Focal glomerulitis due to penicillamine. Lab Invest 19:376, 1968.

230. Heilman DH et al: Streptomycin absorption, diffusion, excretion and toxicity. Am J Med Sci 210:576, 1945.

231. Hellesbusch AA et al: The use of mannitol to reduce the nephrotoxicity of amphotericin B. Surg Gyn Obst 134:241, 1972.

232. Hertz P: Probenecid-induced nephrotic syndrome. Arch Pathol 94:241, 1972.

232a.Hestbech J et al: Chronic lesions following long-term treatment with lithium. Kidney Intn'l 12:205, 1977.

233. Hewitt WL et al: Untoward side effect associated with methicillin therapy. Antimicrob Agents Chemother 765, 1961.

234. Hewitt WL: Gentamicin: toxicity in perspective. Postgrad Med J 50 (suppl 7):55, 1974.

235. Heymann MA et al: Closure of the ductus arteriosus in premature infants by inhibition of prostaglandin synthesis. NEJM 295:530, 1976.

236. Heymann W: Nephrotic syndrome after the use of trimethadione and paramethadione in petit mal. JAMA 202:893, 1967.

237. Higby DJ et al: Diaminodichoroplatinum. A phase I study showing responses in testicular and other tumors. Cancer 33:1219, 1974.

238. Hill JM et al: Clinical studies of platinum coordination compounds in the treatment of various malignant diseases. Cancer Chemother Rep 59:647, 1975.

239. Hirschman SZ et al: The nephrotic syndrome as a complication of penicillamine therapy for hepatolenticular degeneration. Ann Int Med 62:1297, 1965.

240. Hirth RS: Nephrotoxicity of amikacin (BB-K8), an aminoglycoside antibiotic. Vet Path 12:68, 1975.

240a.Hodgin UG: Renal insufficiency during administration of methicillin. Rocky Mount Med J 63:43, (Sept) 1966.

241. Hoeprich PD et al: Toxicity of colistin and polymyxin B. NEJM 270:633, 1964.

242. Hoeprich PD: The polymyxins. Med Clin N Am 54:1257, 1970.

243. Hoffman RP et al: Impaired renal function secondary to gentamicin — identifying the special risk patient. Drug Intell Clin Pharm 11:135, 1977.

243a.Hollander W et al: Nephropathy of potassium depletion, in Diseases of the Kidney, 2nd ed., Ed by Strauss MB and Welt LG, Little, Brown and Company, 1971, p 933.

244. Hollenberg NK et al: Irreversible acute oliguric renal failure. A complication of methoxyflurane anesthesia. NEJM 286:877, 1972.

245. Hollman A et al: Phenindione sensitivity. Brit Med J 2:730, 1964.

246. Hopper J: Polymyxin B in chronic pyelonephritis observations on the safety of the drug and its influence on renal function. Am J Med Sci 225:402, 1953.

247. Houghton DC et al: A light and electron microscopic analysis of gentamicin nephrotoxicity in rats. Am J Path 82:589, 1976.

248. Howlett SA: Renal failure associated with acetazolamide therapy for glaucoma. South Med J 68:504, 1975.

249. Hsu CH et al: Potentiation of gentamicin nephrotoxicity by metabolic acidosis. Proc Soc Exp Biol Med 146:894, 1974.

250. Hyman LR et al: Diphenylhydantoin nephropathy. Evidence for an autoimmune pathogenesis. Kid Intn'l 8:450, 1975.

251. Irnell L: Metastatic calcification of soft tissue in overdosage of vitamin D. Acta Med Scand 185:107, 1969.

252. Iversen BM et al: Retroperitoneal fibrosis during treatment with methyldopa. Lancet 2:302, 1971.

253. Jackson B et al: The haemolytic uraemic syndrome and oral contraceptives. Aust N Z J Med 6:580, 1976.

254. Jacobs JC: Systemic lupus erythematosus in childhood. Pediat 32:257, 1963.

255. Jacobs JC: Systemic lupus erythematosus in childhood. Report of thirty-five cases, with discussion of seven apparently induced by anticonvulsant medication, and of prognosis and treatment. Pediat 32:257, 1963.

256. Jacobs SA et al: Pharmacokinetics of high dose methotrexate. Clin Res 23:425a, 1975.

257. Jaffe JA: Effects of penicillamine on the kidney and on taste. Postgrad Med J 44(Suppl):15, 1968.

258. Jaffe JA et al: Nephropathy induced by D-penicillamine. Ann Int Med 69:549, 1968.

259. Jaffe N et al: Adjuvant methotrexate and citrovorum factor treatment of osteogenic sarcoma. NEJM 291:994, 1974.

260. Jaffe N et al: Toxicity of high-dose methotrexate (NSC-740) and citrovorum factor (NSC-3590) in osteogenic sarcoma. Cancer Chemother Rep Part 3, 6:31, 1975.

261. Jarzobski J et al: Vasculitis with allopurinol therapy. Am Heart J 79:116, 1970.

262. Jawetz E: Laboratory and clinical observations on polymyxin B and E. Am J Med 10:111, 1957.

263. Jeffery B et al: Acquired hypersensitivity to sodium PAS, streptomycin, and penicillin. Brit Med J 2:647, 1952.

264. Jensen AH et al: Permanent inpairment of renal function after methicillin nephropathy. Brit Med J 4:406, 1971.

265. Kahn CB et al: Hypoglycemia secondary to tetracycline-induced hepatorenal failure. Milit Med 140:185, 1975.

266. Kahn CR et al: Pancreatic cholera: beneficial effects of treatment with streptozotocin. NEJM 292:941, 1975.

267. Kahn T et al: Gentamicin and renal failure. Lancet 1:498, 1972.

268. Kalowski S et al: Deterioration in renal function in association with co-trimoxazole therapy. Lancet 1:394, 1973.

268a. Kancair LM et al: Comparison of methicillin and nafcillin in the treatment of staphylococcal endocarditis. Clin Res 24:25A, 1976.

269. Kantor GL: Toxic epidermal necrolysis, azotemia, and death after allopurinol therapy. JAMA 212:478, 1970.

270. Kaplan K et al: Cephaloridine: studies of therapeutic activity and untoward effects. Arch Int Med 121:17, 1968.

271. Kasanen A et al: Doxycycline in renal insufficiency. Curr Ther Res 16:243, 1974.

272. Katz A et al: Gold nephropathy: an immunopathologic study. Arch Pathol 96:133, 1973.

272a. Keating MJ et al: Hypocalcemia with hypoparathyroidism and renal tubular dysfunction associated with aminoglycoside therapy. Cancer 39:1410, 1977.

273. Keenan TD et al: Aggravation of renal functional impairment by tetracycline. NZ Med J 78:164, 1973.

274. Kelly DR et al: Deafness after topical neomycin wound irrigation. NEJM 280:1338, 1969.

275. Kennedy BJ: Metabolic and toxic effects of mithramycin during tumor therapy. Am J Med 49:494, 1970.

276. Kibukamusoke JW et al: Membranous nephropathy due to skin lightening cream. Brit Med J 2:646, 1974.

277. Kiefer L et al: Partial recovery from renal failure following methoxyflurane anesthesia. JAMA 227:201, 1974.

278. Kimberly RP et al: Aspirin-induced depression of renal function. NEJM 296:418, 1977.

279. Kirby HB et al: Pneumocystis carinii pneumonia treated with pyrimethamine and sulfadiazine. Ann Int Med 75:505, 1971.

280. Kirby WM et al: Vancomycin: Clinical and laboratory studies. Antibiotics Annual 109, 1956-1957.

281. Kjellbo H et al: Possibly thiazide-induced renal necrotising vasculitis. Lancet 1:1034, 1965.

282. Klastersky J: Empiric therapy for cancer patients: comparative study of ticarcillin-tobramycin, ticarcillin-cephalothin, and cephalothin-tobramycin. Antimicrob Agents Chemother 7:640, 1975.

283. Klastersky J: Gram-negative infections in cancer: Study of empiric therapy comparing carbenicillin-cephalothin with and without gentamicin. JAMA 227:45, 1974.

284. Kleinknect D et al: Acute renal failure after high doses of gentamicin and cephalothin. Lancet 1:1129, 1973.

285. Kleinknect D et al: Acute renal failure after rifampicin. Lancet 1:1238, 1972.

286. Koch-Weser J et al: Adverse effects of sodium colistimethate. Manifestations and specific reaction rates during 317 courses of therapy. Ann Int Med 72:857, 1970.

287. Korkeila J: Antianabolic effect of tetracyclines. Lancet 1:974, 1971.

288. Kosek JC et al: Morphology and pathogenesis of nephrotoxicity following methoxyflurane (penthrane) anesthesia. Lab Invest 27:575, 1972.

289. Kosek JC et al: Nephrotoxicity of gentamicin. Lab Invest 30:48, 1974.

290. Kucers A and McK Bennett N: The Use of Antibiotics, 2nd ed., William Heinemann Medical Books Ltd, 1976, p 167,341,420,546.

291. Kumar S et al: Light-chain proteinuria and reversible renal failure in rifampin-treated patients with tuberculosis. Chest 70:564, 1976.

292. Kunelis CT et al: Fatty liver of pregnancy and its relationship to tetracycline therapy. Am J Med 38:359, 1965.

293. Kunin CM: Absorption or orally amdinistered neomycin and kanamycin. NEJM 262:380, 1960.

294. Kuzuci EY: Methoxyflurane, tetracycline and renal failure. JAMA 211:1162, 1970.

295. Lachmann PG: Nephrotic syndrome from penicillamine. Postgrad Med J 44 (Suppl):23, 1968.

296. Landgrebe AR et al: Urinary-tract stones resulting from the excretion of oxypurinol. NEJM 292:626, 1975.

297. Lawson DH et al: Effect of furosemide on antibiotic-induced renal damage in rats. J Infect Dis 126:593, 1972.

298. Lawson DH et al: The nephrotoxicity of cephaloridine. Postgrad Med J 46 (Suppl):36, 1970.

299. Lederer M et al: Death during sulfathiazole therapy. JAMA 119:8, 1942.

300. Lee HA: Phenindione nephropathy with recovery: studies of morphology and renal function. Postgrad Med J 40:326, 1964.

301. Lee P et al: Doxycycline: studies in normal subjects and patients with renal failure. NZ Med J 75:355, 1972.

302. Lehr D: Clinical toxicity of sulfonamides. Ann NY Acad Sci 69:417, 1957.

303. Levison ME et al: Pharmacology of cefazolin in patients with normal and abnormal renal function. J Infect Dis 128:S354, 1973.

304. Levo Y et al: Clinicopathological study of a patient with procainamide-induced systemic lupus erythematosus. Ann Rheum Dis 35:181, 1976.

305. Lew HT et al: Tetracycline nephrotoxicity and non-oliguric acute renal failure. Arch Int Med 118:123, 1966.

306. Lindholm DD et al: Persistence of vancomycin in the blood during renal failure and its treatment by hemodialysis. NEJM 274:1047, 1966.

306a. Lindop GBM et al: The renal pathology in a case of lithium-induced diabetes insipidus. J Clin Path 28:472, 1975.

307. Lindquist T: Lupus erythematosus disseminatus after administration of mesantoin. Acta Med Scand 158:131, 1957.

308. Line DE et al: Massive pseudoproteinuria caused by nafcillin. JAMA 235:1259, 1976.

309. Linton AL et al: Relative nephrotoxicity of cephalosporin antibiotics in an animal model. CMAJ 107:414, 1972.

310. Linton AL: Renal disease due to analgesics. Recognition of the problem of analgesic nephropathy. CMAJ 107:749, 1972.

311. Lippman AJ et al: Clinical trials of cis-diamminedichloro-platinum (NSC-119875). Cancer Chemother Rep 57:191, 1973.

312. Lipsett MB et al: Phenylbutazone toxicity: report of a case of acute renal failure. Ann Int Med 41:1075, 1954.

313. Livingstone R et al: Acquired idiosyncrasy to sodium p-aminosalicylate. Lancet 2:308, 1950.

314. Loehning RW et al: Possible nephrotoxicity from enflurane in a patient with severe renal disease. Anesth 40:203, 1974.

315. Loftus L et al: Clinical and pathological effects of streptozotocin. J Lab Clin Med 84:407, 1974.

315a. London RD: Hematuria associated with methicillin therapy. J Pediat 70:285, 1967.

316. Lovine G et al: Nephrotoxicity of amphotericin B a clinical-pathologic study. Arch Int Med 112:853, 1963.

317. Luft FC et al: Nephrotoxicity of cephalosporin-gentamicin combination in rats. Antimicrob Agents Chemother 9:831, 1976.

318. Luft FC et al: Experimental aminoglycoside nephrotoxicity. J Lab Clin Med 86:213, 1976.

319. Luke RG et al: Proteinuria associated with D-penicillamine therapy of cystinuria. J Urol 99:207, 1968.

320. Luke RG: Porteinuria associated with D-penicillamine therapy of cystinuria. J Urol 99:207, 1968.

321. Lyons H et al: Allergic interstitial nephritis causing reversible renal failure in four patients with idiopathic nephrotic syndrome. NEJM 288:124, 1973.

322. MacCarthy JM et al: Hepatic necrosis and other visceral lesions associated with phenylbutazone therapy. Brit Med J 2:240, 1955.

323. MacDonald JB et al: Nitrofurantoin crystalluria. Brit Med J 2:1044, 1976.

324. MacFarlane MD et al: Fatty metamorphosis of the liver after IV tetracycline. Drug Intell Clin Pharm 6:310, 1972.

325. MacKay DN et al: Serum concentrations of colistin in patients with normal and impaired renal function. NEJM 270:394, 1964.

326. MacKenzie AR: Acetazolamide-induced renal stone. J Urol 84:453, 1960.

327. MacLean LD: Renal failure following the administration of intra-peritoneal neomycin. Minn Med 40:557, 1957.

328. Maher JF: Toxic Nephropathy, in The Kidney Ed 1 by BM Brenner and F Rector, WB Saunders Company 1976 pg 1355.

329. Mailloux L et al: Acute renal failure after administration of low-molecular-weight dextran. NEJM 277:1114, 1967.

330. Malt RA et al: Renal tubular necrosis after oral cholecystography. Arch Surg 87:743, 1963.

331. Mandell GL: Cephaloridine. Ann Int Med 79:561, 1973.

332. Mann B: An unusual case of PAS allergy. Tubercle 34:23, 1953.

333. Marsh FP et al: Non-thrombocytopenia purpura and acute glomerulonephritis after indomethacin therapy. Ann Rheum Dis 30:501, 1971.

334. Masur H et al: Neomycin toxicity revisited. Arch Surg 111:822, 1976.

335. Mattson K et al: Acute renal failure following rifampicin administration. Scand J Resp Dis 55:291, 1974.
336. Mauer SM et al: Induction of malignant kidney tumors in rats with streptozotocin. Cancer Res 34:158, 1974.
337. Maxwell D et al: Ampicillin nephropathy. JAMA 230:586, 1974.
337a. Maynaud C et al: Interstitial nephritis after methicillin. NEJM 292:1132, 1975.
338. Mazze RI et al: Renal dysfunction associated with methoxyflurane anesthesia. JAMA 216:278, 1971.
339. Mazze RI et al: Methoxyflurane metabolism and renal dysfunction: clinical correlation in man. Anesth 35:247, 1971.
340. Mazze RI et al: Dose-related methoxyflurane nephrotoxicity in rats: a biochemical and pathological correlation. Anesth 36:571, 1972.
341. Mazze RI et al: Combined nephrotoxicity of gentamicin and methoxyflurane anesthesia in man. Brit J Anaesth 45:394, 1973.
342. Mazze RI et al: Inorganic fluoride nephrotoxicity: prolonged enflurane and halothane anesthesia in volunteer. Anesth 46:265, 1977.
343. McAllister TA: Absence of nephrotoxicity during cephaloridine therapy. Lancet 2:710, 1972.
344. McChesney JA et al: Hypokalemic paralysis induced by amphotericin B. JAMA 189:1029, 1964.
345. McCurdy DK et al: Renal tubular acidosis due to amphotericin B. NEJM 278:124, 1968.
346. McDermott W: Toxicity of streptomycin. Am J Med 2:491, 1947.
347. McDonald FD et al: Phenylbutazone anuria. South Med J 60:1318, 1967.
348. McIntyre JWR et al: Oxalemia following methoxyflurane anesthesia in man. Anesth Analg 52:946, 1973.
349. McKay DG et al: Therapeutic implications of disseminated intravascular coagulation. Am J Cardiol 20:392, 1967.
350. McMenamin RA et al: Drug induced interstitial nephritis, hepatitis and exfoliative dermatitis. Aust NZ J Med 6:583, 1976.
351. McMillan DE et al: The milk alkali syndrome: a study of the acute disorder with comments on the development of the chronic condition. Medicine 44:485, 1965.
352. Medical Staff Conference: Methicillin induced interstitial nephritis. West J Med 123:380, 1975.
352a. Medlock TR et al: Lithium induced nephrotic syndrome. Kidney Intn'l 11:547, 1976.
353. Melnick PJ: Acute interstitial nephritis with uremia. Arch Path 36:499, 1943.
354. Merkel WC et al: Pathologic lesions produced by sulfathiazole. JAMA 119:770, 1942.
355. Merkle RB et al: Human renal function following methoxyflurane anesthesia. JAMA 218:841, 1971.
356. Meyer RD et al: Amikacin therapy for serious gram-negative bacillary infections. Ann Int Med 83:790, 1975.
357. Michael JR et al: Reversible renal failure and myositis caused by phenytoin hypersensitivity. JAMA 236:2773, 1976.
358. Michielsen P et al: Renal diseases due to drugs in Drug Induced Diseases, Vol 4, Ed. by L Meyler and HM Peck, Excerpta Medica, 1972, p 261.
359. Miller RP et al: Amphotericin B toxicity: a followup report of 53 patients. Ann Int Med 71:1089, 1969.
360. Millichap JG et al: Nephrotoxic effects of drugs used in treatment of petit mal. Lancet 1:1074, 1953.
361. Mills RM: Severe hypersensitivity reactions associated with allopurinol. JAMA 216:799, 1971.
362. Milman N: Renal failure associated with gentamicin therapy. Acta Med Scand 196:87, 1974.
363. Moffat NA et al: Renal vein thrombosis treated by thrombectomy: a case report. J Urol 106:635, 1971.
364. More RH et al: The pathology of sulfonamide allergy in man. Am J Path 22:703, 1946.
365. Morgan C Jr et al: Intravenous urography in multiple myeloma. NEJM 275:77, 1966.
366. Morgan T et al: Renal failure associated with low-molecular-weight dextran infusion. Brit Med J 2:737, 1966.
367. Morgan T et al: The effect of oxytetracycline and doxycycline on protein metabolism. Med J Aust 1:55, 1972.
368. Morrison JB: Acquired idiosyncrasy to sodium p-amino-salicylate. Lancet 2:308, 1950.
368a. Moses AM et al: Pathophysiologic and pharmacologic alterations in the release and action of ADH. Metab 25:697, 1976.
369. Moyer JH et al: The effects of an intermittent dosage schedule of viomycin on renal function and on plasma electrolytes. Am Rev Resp Med 68:541, 1953.
370. Mudge GH: Uricosuric action of cholecystographic agents. NEJM 284:929, 1971.
371. Muehrcke RD: Chart of the etiology and pathogenesis of acute tubular necrosis, in Acute Renal Failure: Diagnosis and Management, 1st ed., CV Mosley Co, St. Louis, 1964, p 167.
372. Mulligan RM: Metastatic calcification. Arch Pathol 43:177, 1947.
373. Mulvaney WP et al: Urinary phenazopyridine stones. A complication of therapy. JAMA 221:1511, 1972.
374. Murphy F et al: Clinicopathologic studies of renal damage due to sulfonamide compounds. Arch Int Med 73:433, 1944.
375. Murphy KJ et al: Bilateral renal calculi in patients receiving methyldopa. Med J Aust 2:20, 1976.
376. Murple GB et al: The nephrotoxicity of antimicrobial agents. NEJM 296:663, 1977.
377. Murple GB et al: The nephrotoxicity of antimicrobial agents. NEJM 296:722, 1977.
378. Murple GB et al: The nephrotoxicity of antimicrobial agents. NEJM 296:784, 1977.
378a. Murray T et al: Chronic interstitial nephritis: etiological factors. Ann Int Med 82:453, 1975.
379. Murray T et al: Analgesic abuse and renal disease. Ann Rev Med 26:537, 1975.
380. Myerowitz RL et al: Nephrotoxic and cytoproliferative effects of streptozotocin. Cancer 38:1550, 1976.
381. Myers GH Jr et al: Acute renal failure after excretory urography in multiple myeloma. Am J Roent 113:583, 1971.
382. Nabarro JDN et al: Nephrotic syndrome complicating tridione (troxidone) therapy. Lancet 1:1091, 1952.
383. Nanra RS: Pathology, aetiology and pathogenesis of analgesic nephropathy. Aust NZ J Med (Suppl 1) 6:33, 1976.
384. Nanra RS: Analgesic nephropathy. Med J Aust 1:745, 1976.
384a. Neale TJ et al: Spironolactone-associated aggravation of renal functional impairment. NZ Med J 83:147, 1976.
385. Neild GH et al: D-penicillamine-induced membranous glomerulonephritis. Lancet 1:1201, 1975.
386. Nessi R et al: Acute renal failure after rifampicin: a case report and survey of literature. Nephron 16:148, 1976.
387. Neu HC: Tobramycin: An overview. J Infect Dis 134:S3, 1976.
388. Nicholls DP et al: Acute renal failure from carbamazepine. Brit Med J 4:490, 1972.
388a. Nolan CM et al: Nephropathy associated with methicillin therapy: Prevalence and determinants in patients with staphylococcal bacteremia. Arch Int Med 137:997, 1977.
389. Noone P et al: Acute renal failure after high doses of gentamicin and cephalothin. Lancet 1:1387, 1973.
390. Nord NM et al: Polymyxin B and colistin: a critical comparison. NEJM 270:1030, 1964.
391. Norrby R et al: Interaction between cephaloridine and furosemide in man. Scand J Infect Dis 8:209, 1976.
392. Northway JD et al: Successful therapy of trimethadione nephrosis with prednisone and cyclophosphamide. J Pediat 71:259, 1967.
393. Olivero JJ et al: Mitigation of amphotericin B nephrotoxicity by mannitol. Brit Med J 1:550, 1975.
394. Olsen S et al: Interstitial nephritis and acute renal failure following cardiac surgery and treatment with methicillin. Acta Med Scand 199:305, 1976.
395. Ooi BS et al: IgE levels in interstitial nephritis. Lancet 1:1254, 1974.
396. Ooi BS et al: Acute interstitial nephritis. Am J Med 59:614, 1975.
397. Orchard RT et al: Sulphonamide crystalluria with acetazolamide. Brit Med J 3:646, 1972.
398. Owen D: Renal failure due to para-aminosalicylic acid. Brit Med J 2:483, 1958.
399. Owens CJ et al: Nephrotic syndrome following topically applied sulfadiazine silver therapy. Arch Int Med 134:332, 1974.
400. Panner BJ et al: Toxicity following methoxyflurane anesthesia. JAMA 214:86, 1970.
401. Parfitt AM: Acetazolamide and sodium bicarbonate induced nephrocalcinosis and nephrolithiasis. Relationship to citrate and calcium excretion. Arch Int Med 124:736, 1969.
402. Parker RH et al: Toxicity associated with intravenous and intramuscular polymyxin B sulfate. Clin Res 12:244, 1964.

403. Parry MF et al: Nafcillin nephritis. JAMA 225:178, 1973.
404. Pasternak DP et al: Reversible nephrotoxicity associated with cephalothin therapy. Arch Int Med 135:599, 1975.
405. Patel V et al: Enzymuria in gentamicin-induced kidney damage. Antimicrob Agents Chemother 7:364, 1975.
406. Patterson RM et al: Renal tubular acidosis due to amphotericin B nephrotoxicity. Arch Int Med 127:241, 1971.
407. Pepys MB: Acetazolamide and renal stone formation. Lancet 1:837, 1970.
408. Perkash I et al: Possible tetracycline toxicity in azotemia. J Urol 102:102, 1969.
409. Perkins RL: Cephaloridine and cephalothin: Comparative studies of potential nephrotoxicity. J Lab Clin Med 71:75, 1968.
410. Perry HM: Late toxicity to hydralazine resembling systemic lupus erythematosus or rheumatoid arthritis. Am J Med 54:58, 1973.
411. Persky L et al: Calculus formation and ureteral colic following acetazolamide (Diamox) therapy. JAMA 161:1625, 1956.
412. Phillips BM et al: Does aspirin play a role in analgesic nephropathy? Aust NZ J Med (Suppl 1) 6:48, 1976.
413. Phillips ME et al: Tetracycline poisoning in renal failure. Brit Med J 2:149, 1974.
414. Pickering JM et al: Declining renal function associated with administration of cephalothin. South Med J 63:426, 1970.
415. Pierides AM et al: Clofibrate-induced muscle damage in patients with chronic renal failure. Lancet 2:1279, 1975.
416. Pillay VKG et al: Acute renal failure following intravenous urography in patients with long-standing diabetes mellitus and azotemia. Radiol 95:633, 1970.
417. Plager JE et al: Association of renal injury with combined cephalothin-gentamicin therapy among severely ill patients with malignant disease. Cancer 37:1937, 1976.
418. Poole G et al: Potentially serious side effects of high-dose twice-weekly rifampicin. Brit Med J 3:343, 1971.
419. Postlethwaite AE et al: Uricosuric effect of radiocontrast agents. Ann Int Med 74:845, 1971.
420. Pratt CB et al: Clinical trials and pharmacokinetics of intermittent high-dose methotrexate — "leucovorin rescue" for children with malignant tumors. Cancer Res 34:3326, 1974.
421. Prescott LF: Analgesic nephropathy — the international experience. Aust NZ J Med (Suppl 1) 6:44, 1976.
422. Price DJE et al: Effects of large doses of colistin sulphomethate sodium on renal function. Brit Med J 4:525, 1970.
423. Pride GL et al: Disseminated intravascular coagulation associated with tetracycline-induced hepatorenal failure during pregnancy. Am J Obstet Gynecol 115:585, 1973.
424. Proctor EA et al: Polyuric acute renal failure after methoxyflurane and tetracycline. Brit Med J 4:661, 1971.
425. Ramgopal et al: Acute renal failure associated with rifampicin. Lancet 1:1195, 1973.
426. Randall RE et al: The milk-alkali syndrome. Arch Int Med 107:163, 1971.
427. Relman AS et al: Kidney in potassium depletion. Am J Med 24:764, 1958.
428. Ribush N et al: Tetracyclines and renal failure. Med J Aust 1:53, 1972.
429. Riddle M et al: The nephrotic syndrome complicating mercurial diuretic therapy. Brit Med J 1:1274, 1958.
430. Rifkind BM et al: Chronic milk-alkali syndrome with generalized osteosclerosis after prolonged excessive intake of "Rennie's" tablet. Brit Med J 1:317, 1960.
431. Riska N et al: Adverse reactions during rifampicin treatment. Scand J Resp Dis 53:87, 1972.
432. Robson M et al: Acute tubulo-interstitial nephritis following sulfadiazine therapy. Israel J Med Sci 6:561, 1970.
433. Rosch JM et al: Reduction of amphotericin B nephrotoxicity with mannitol. JAMA 235:1995, 1976.
434. Rosenberg LE et al: Nephrotoxic effects of penicillamine in cystinuria. JAMA 201:698, 1967.
435. Rosenberg H et al: Renal and hepatic toxicity of methoxyflurane in combination with tetracycline or oxytetracycline treatment in rats. Acta Pharmacol 34:46, 1974.
436. Rosenblum J et al: Trimethadione (Tridione) nephrosis. Am J Dis Child 97:790, 1959.
437. Rosenfeld JB et al: Effect of long-term co-trimoxazole therapy on renal function. Med J Aust 2:546, 1975.
438. Roy AD: Acute renal failure after aortography. Lancet 2:16, 1957.
439. Ruben RJ et al: Neomycin ototoxicity and nephrotoxicity. Laryngoscope 78:1734, 1968.
440. Rubenstein MA et al: Acetazolamide-induced renal calculi. J Urol 114:610, 1975.
441. Ruley EJ et al: Interstitial nephritis and renal failure due to ampicillin. J Pediat 84:878, 1974.
442. Rutherford BD: Procainamide-induced systemic lupus erythematosus. NZ Med J 68:235, 1968.
443. Sadoff L: Nephrotoxicity of streptozotocin (NSC-85998). Cancer Chemother Rep 54:457, 1970.
444. Sanjad SA et al: Nephropathy, an underestimated complication of methicillin therapy. J Pediat 84:873, 1974.
445. Sasse L: BUN levels and tetracycline. JAMA 224:530, 1973.
446. Scarpelli DG et al: A comparative cytochemical and cytologic study of vitamin D induced nephrocalcinosis. Am J Path 36:331, 1960.
447. Schein PS et al: Islet cell tumors: current concepts and management. Ann Int Med 79:239, 1973.
448. Schein PS et al: Streptozotocin for malignant insulinomas and carcinoid tumor. Arch Int Med 132:555, 1973.
449. Schein PS et al: Clinical antitumor activity and toxicity of streptozotocin (NSC-85998). Cancer 34:993, 1974.
450. Schellhammer PF: Renal failure associated with the use of thiotepa. J Urol 110:498, 1970.
451. Schnall C et al: Nephrosis occurring during tolbutamide administration. JAMA 167:214, 1958.
452. Schoolwerth AC et al: Nephrosclerosis postpartum and in women taking oral contraceptives. Arch Int Med 136:178, 1976.
453. Schreiner GE et al: Toxic nephropathy. Am J Med 38:409, 1965.
454. Schrier RW et al: Nephropathy associated with penicillin and homologues. Ann Int Med 64:116, 1966.
455. Schultze RG et al: Possible nephrotoxicity of gentamicin. J Infect Dis 124:S145, 1971.
456. Schwartz WB: Pathogenesis and replacement of diuretic-induced potassium and chloride loss. Ann NY Acad Sci 139:506, 1966.
457. Schwartz WB et al: Effects of electrolyte disorders on renal structure and function. NEJM 276:383, 1967.
458. Ibid: p 452.
459. Schwartz WB et al: Intravenous urography in the patient with renal insufficiency. NEJM 269:277, 1963.
459a. Schwartz WB et al: Metabolic and renal studies in chronic potassium depletion resulting from overuse of laxatives. J Clin Invest 32:258, 1953.
460. Scott JT: Probenecid nephrotic syndrome and renal failure. Ann Rheum Dis 27:249, 1968.
461. Seaman WB et al: Renal insufficiency following cholecystography. Am J Roent 90:859, 1963.
462. Seaman WE et al: Effect of aspirin on liver function tests in patients with RA or SLE and in normal volunteers. Arth Rheum 19:155, 1976.
463. Seedat YK et al: Nephrotic syndrome due to cosmetics containing mercury. S Afr Med J 47:506, 1973.
464. Seegmiller JE et al: Use of the newer uricosuric agents in the management of gout. JAMA 173:1076, 1966.
465. Seegmiller JE: Management and treatment. Fed Proc 27:1097, 1968.
466. Seelig MS: Penicillamine and the nephrotic syndrome. JAMA 199:767, 1967.
467. Setter JG et al: Acute renal failure following cholecystography. JAMA 184:102, 1963.
468. Seufert CD: Acute renal failure after rifampicin therapy. Scand J Resp Dis Supple 84:174, 1973.
469. Shelley JH: Phenacetin, through the looking glass. Clin Pharmacol Ther 8:427, 1967.
470. Shenilukht LA: Side effects during griseofulvin treatment and methods of their preventions. Vest Derm Vener 10:39, 1965.
470a. Sheth KJ et al: Interstitial nephritis due to phenytoin hypersensitivity. J Pediat 91:438, 1977.
471. Shils ME: Renal disease and the metabolic effects of tetracycline. Ann Int Med 58:389, 1963.
472. Sidd JJ et al: Unilateral renal damage due to massive contrast dye injection with recovery. J Urol 97:30, 1967.
473. Silverberg DS et al: Gold nephropathy. A clinical and pathologic study. Arthr Rheum 13:812, 1970.

474. Silverblatt F et al: Nephrotoxicity due to cephaloridine: a light and electron-microscopic study in rabbits. J Infect Dis 122:33, 1970.

475. Silverblatt F: Antibiotic nephrotoxicity. A review of pathogenesis and prevention. Urol Clin N Am 2:557, 1975.

476. Silverblatt F et al: Nephrotoxicity of cephalosporin antibiotics in experimental animals. J Infect Dis 128:S367, 1973.

477. Silverman JD: Stimultaneous hypersensitivity to streptomycin and para-aminosalicyic acid. Dis Chest 30:103, 1956.

478. Simenhoff MB et al: Acute diffuse interstitial nephritis. Am J Med 44:618, 1968.

479. Simpson IJ et al: Nephrotoxicity and acute renal failure associated with cephalothin and cephaloridine. NZ Med J 74:312, 1971.

479a. Singer I et al: Drug induced states of nephrotoxic diabetes insipidus. Kid Intn'l 10:82, 1976.

480. Singsen BH et al: Antinuclear antibodies and lupus-like syndromes in children receiving anticonvulsants. Pediat 57:529, 1976.

481. Sinks LF et al: Trimethadione nephrosis. Am J Dis Child 105:196, 1963.

482. Slick GL et al: Hypertension, renal vein thrombosis and renal failure (occurring in a patient on an oral contraceptive agent). Clin Nephrol 3:70, 1974.

483. Sloth K et al: Acute renal insufficiency during treatment with azathioprine. Acta Med Scand 189:145, 1971.

484. Slugg PH et al: Complications of methysergide therapy. JAMA 213:297, 1970.

485. Smith CR et al: Controlled comparison of amikacin and gentamicin. NEJM 296:349, 1977.

486. Smith K: Acute renal failure in phenindione sensitivity. Brit Med J 2:24, 1965.

487. Snead C et al: Generalized lymphadenopathy and nephrotic syndrome as a manifestation of mephenytoin (mesantoin) toxicity. Pediat 57:98, 1976.

488. Stark SN et al: Epsilon aminocaproic acid therapy as a cause of intrarenal obstruction in hematuria of hemophiliacs. Scand J Hemat 2:99, 1965.

489. Stecker JF et al: Retroperitoneal fibrosis and ergot derivatives. J Urol 112:30, 1974.

490. Stein J et al: Nephrotic syndrome induced by penicillamine. CMAJ 98:505, 1968.

490a. Steinbrocker O et al: Butazolidin in the treatment of gout. Med Clin N Am 611, 1954.

491. Steinlieb I: Penicillamine and the nephrotic syndrome. JAMA 198:1311, 1966.

492. Steinlieb I et al: D-penicillamine induced Goodpasture's Syndrome in Wilson's Disease. Ann Int Med 82:673, 1975.

493. Stenbaek O et al: The effect of doxycycline on renal function in patients with advanced renal insufficiency. Scand J Infect Dis 5:199, 1973.

494. Stewart JH et al: Analgesic abuse and kidney disease. Aust NZ J Med 6:498, 1976.

495. Stolinsky DC et al: Streptozotocin in the treatment of cancer: phase II study. Cancer 30:61, 1972.

496. Stoller RG et al: Pharmacokinetics of high-dose methotrexate (NSC-740). Cancer Chemother Rep Part 36:19, 1975.

497. Stone WJ et al: Acute diffuse interstitial nephritis related to chemotherapy of tuberculosis. Antimicrob Agents Chemother 10:164, 1976.

498. Strunk SW et al: Ultrastructural studies of the passage of gold thiomalate across the renal glomerular capillary wall. Arthr Rheum 13:39, 1970.

498a. Sudhir SV et al: Focal glomerulonephritis and interstitial nephritis in methicillin treated, heroin-related infective endocarditis. South Med J 70:1132, 1977.

499. Sulkowski SR et al: Simulated systemic lupus erythematosus from degraded tetracycline. JAMA 189:152, 1964.

500. Swartz C et al: Cardiac and renal hemodynamic effects of the antifibrinolytic agent, epsilon aminocaproic acid. Curr Ther Res 8:336, 1966.

501. Swartz JM: Infections caused dermatophytes. NEJM 267:1359, 1963.

502. Talmo RC et al: Trimethadione nephrosis treated with cortisone and nitrogen mustard. NEJM 269:15, 1963.

503. Talley RW et al: Clinical evaluation of toxic effects of cis-diamminedichloroplatinum (NSC-119875) — phase 1 clinical study. Cancer Chemother Rep 57:465, 1973.

504. Tallgren LG et al: The therapeutic success and nephrotoxicity of colistin in acute and chronic nephropathies with impaired renal function. Acta Med Scand 177:717, 1965.

505. Tally FP et al: Amikacin therapy for severe gram-negative sepsis. Ann Int Med 83:484, 1975.

506. Tannenberg AM et al: Ampicillin nephropathy. JAMA 218:449, 1971.

507. Tasker PR et al: Use of co-trimoxazole in chronic renal failure. Lancet 1:1216, 1975.

508. Taves DR et al: Toxicity following methoxyflurane anesthesia. JAMA 214:91, 1970.

509. Teal JS et al: Acute renal failure following spinal angiography with methylglucamine iolthalamate. Radiology 104:561, 1972.

510. Thomas JM et al: Dextran 40 in the treatment of peripheral vascular diseases. Arch Surg 106:138, 1973.

511. Tobey RE et al: Renal function after methoxyflurane and halothane anesthesia. JAMA 223:649, 1973.

512. Tobon H: Malignant hypertension, uremia and hemolytic anemia in a patient on oral contraceptives. Obstet Gynec 40:681, 1972.

513. Tornroth T et al: Gold nephropathy prototype of membranous glomerulonephritis. Am J Pathol 75:573, 1974.

514. Tornroth T et al: The development and resolution of glomerular basement membrane changes associated with subepithelial immune deposits. Am J Pathol 79:219, 1975.

515. Ultmann JE et al: Triethylenethiophosphoramide (thio-tepa) in the treatment of neoplastic disease. Cancer 10:902, 1957.

516. Urgena RB et al: Nephrotoxicity from methoxyflurane anesthesia: a 6 year retrospective study. Brit J Anaesth 45:358, 1973.

517. Utz JP et al: Amphotericin B toxicity: combined clinical staff conference at the National Institutes of Health. Ann Int Med 61:334, 1964.

518. Vaamonde CA et al: The nephrotic syndrome as a complication of gold therapy. Arthr Rheum 13:826, 1970.

519. Verma S et al: Cephalexin-related nephropathy. JAMA 234:618, 1975.

520. Waisbren BA et al: Comparative clinical effectiveness and toxicity of vancomycin, ristocetin, and kanamycin. Arch Int Med 106:179, 1960.

521. Wallace MR et al: Exacerbation of nephrolithiasis by a carbonic anhydrase inhibitor. NZ Med J 79:687, 1974.

522. Walshe JM: Management of penicillamine nephropathy in Wilson's disease: a new chelating agent. Lancet 2:1401, 1969.

523. Walter L et al: Allergic interstitial nephritis: Report of a case with activation of complement by the alternate pathway. Clin Nephrol 3:153, 1974.

524. Walzer PD et al: Pneumocystis carinii pneumonia in the United States: epidemiologic, diagnostic and clinical features. Ann Int Med 80:83, 1974.

525. Wang JJ et al: Unusual complications of pentamidine in the treatment of pneumocystis carinii pneumonia. J Pediat 77:311, 1970.

526. Ward JM et al: Prevention of renal failure in rats receiving cis-diamminedichloroplatinum (II) by administration of furosemide. Cancer Res 37:1238, 1977.

527. Watanabe I et al: Gold nephropathy: ultrastructural, fluorescence, and microanalytic studies of two patients. Arch Pathol Lab Med 100:632, 1976.

527a. Weinrauch LA et al: Coronary angiography and acute renal failure in diabetic azotemic nephropathy. Ann Int Med 86:56, 1977.

528. Weisman JI et al: Anuria following phenylbutazone therapy. NEJM 252:1086, 1955.

529. Wellwood JM et al: Evidence of gentamicin nephrotoxicity in patients with renal allografts. Brit Med J 3:278, 1975.

530. Wenger J et al: The milk-alkali syndrome: Hypercalcemia, alkalosis, and azotemia following calcium carbonate and milk therapy of peptic ulcer. Gastroent 33:745, 1957.

531. Wennberg JE et al: Renal toxicity of oral cholecystographic media. Bunamiodyl sodium and iopanoic acid. JAMA 186:461, 1963.

532. Werner CA et al: The toxicity of viomycin in humans. Am Rev Resp Med 63:49, 1951.

533. Western KA et al: Pentamidine isothionate in the treatment of pneumocystis carinii pneumonia. Ann Int Med 73:695, 1970.

534. White JC: Nephrosis occurring during trimethadione therapy. JAMA 139:376, 1949.

535. Whittingham S et al: Systemic lupus erythematosus induced by procaine amide. Aust Ann Med 4:358, 1970.

536. Whittle TS et al: Procainamide-induced systemic lupus erythematosus. Renal involvement with deposition of immune complexes. Arch Pathol Lab Med 100:469, 1976.

537. Wigley RAD: The New Zealand experience. Aust NZ J Med Suppl 1, 6:37, 1976.

538. Wilfert JN et al: Renal insufficiency associated with gentamicin therapy. J Infect Dis 124:S148, 1971.

539. Wilske KR et al: Findings suggestive of systemic lupus erythematosus in subjects on chronic anticonvulsant therapy. Arthr Rheum 8:260, 1965.

540. Wilson DR: Analgesic nephropathy in Canada: A retrospective study of 351 cases. CMAJ 107:752, 1972.

541. Wilson M et al: Renal failure from methyldopa therapy. Aust NZ J Med 4:415, 1974.

542. Wilson TM: Capreomycin, ethambutol and rifampin. Clinical experience in Manchester. Scand J Resp Dis Suppl 69:3, 1969.

543. Winchester JF et al: Absence of nephrotoxicity during cephaloridine therapy for urinary-tract infection. Lancet 2:514, 1972.

544. Winterborn MH et al: Anuria due to sulphadiazine. Arch Dis Childhood 48:915, 1973.

544a. Wolff HP et al: Psychiatric disturbance leading to potassium depletion, sodium depletion, raised plasma-renin concentration, and secondary hyperaldosteronism. Lancet 1:258, 1968.

545. Wolinsky E et al: Neurotoxic and nephrotoxic effects of colistin in patients with renal disease. NEJM 266:759, 1962.

546. Woodroffe AJ et al: Nephropathy associated with methicillin administration. Aust NZ J Med 4:256, 1974.

547. Woodroffe AJ et al: Acute interstitial nephritis following ampicillin hypersensitivity. Med J Aust 1:65, 1975.

548. Wray SH et al: The effects of tetracycline on blood urea. Postgrad Med J 41:18, 1965.

549. Wren JC et al: Nephrotic syndrome occurring during paramethadone therapy. JAMA 153:918, 1953.

550. Yagoda A et al: Cis-dichlorodiammineplatinum (II) in advanced bladder cancer. Cancer Chemother Rep 60:917, 1976.

551. Yarom R et al: Nephrotoxic effect of parenteral and intraarticular gold. Arch Pathol 99:36, 1975.

552. Yates-Bell JG: Renal colic and anuria from acetazolamide. Brit Med J 2:1392, 1958.

553. Young JL et al: Severe allopurinol hypersensitivity. Association with thiazides and prior renal compromise. Arch Int Med 134:553, 1974.

554. Yow EM et al: Toxicity of polymyxin. Arch Int Med 92:248, 1953.

555. Yow MD et al: A ten-year assessment of methicillin-associated side effects. Pediat 58:329, 1976.

556. Yudis M et al: Quinidine-induced lupus nephritis. JAMA 235:2000, 1976.

557. Yue WY et al: Toxic nephritis with acute renal insufficiency caused by administration of capreomycin. Dis Chest 49:549, 1966.

558. Zacherle BJ et al: Irreversible renal failure secondary to hypertension induced by oral contraceptives. Ann Int Med 77:83, 1972.

559. Zech P et al: Malignant hypertension with irreversible renal failure due to oral contraceptives. Brit Med J 2:1655, 1975.

560. Zierski M: Clinical aspects of side effects on intermittent rifampicin regimen. Scand J Resp Dis Suppl 84:166, 1973.

Chapter 22

Gout and Hyperuricemia

Lloyd Y. Young

Primary gout is considered to be an inborn error of uric acid metabolism. It is manifested by hyperuricemia, acute or chronic recurrent arthritis, and deposits of monosodium urates. *Gout* should be considered as a clinical diagnosis and *hyperuricemia* as a biochemical one. These two terms are not synonymous as each can occur without the other.

Clinically, early gout is characterized by highly variable recurrent episodic attacks of acute gouty arthritis. During the early phase of gout, attacks are predominately monoarticular, but as many as 39% of all patients may experience polyarticular gout as their first manifestation (35). In more advanced gout, monosodium urate crystals deposit in tissues and joints, but surprisingly, tophi do not predispose the affected joint to attacks.

Urate tophi are classically located in the cartilage of the ear pinna and in the great toe. However, urate crystals can deposit almost anywhere and involve not only cartilagenous areas and peripheral joints, but also bursae, tendons, skin, and kidneys. Although rare, urate deposits have even been reported in the eyelids, tongue, vocal cords, penis, and aorta. If underlying hyperuricemia is left untreated, approximately 50% to 60% of gouty patients will develop monosodium urate tophi.

CASE A (QUESTIONS 1-9, 19-22): WS, a 44-year-old male, was admitted to the Emergency Room with severe pain in his left great toe. About 2:00 a.m. he was awakened by the pain which he likened to the pain which he felt when he dislocated his shoulder. Yet his toe felt as if icy cold water was poured over it. He had a low grade fever initially followed by chills. The pain, which was at first moderate, became more intense. It felt like a violent stretching and tearing of the toe, then it developed into a gnawing pain, then a pressure and a tightening. His toe was so exquisitely painful that he could not tolerate the weight of the bedcovers, nor even the jar of a person walking into the room.

After a small dose of narcotic analgesic, additional history was obtained from the patient. Three days prior to this admission he strained his leg by jumping off a scaffold onto sand. At that time he thought that he had wrenched his knees. By that evening, he began to notice pain in the dorsum of his left foot and at the anterior portion of the ankle. By the next morn-

ing he was unable to bear weight and visited a physician who gave him a shot of hydrocortisone. He noticed slight improvement from this shot, however the pain became more severe later. His left foot, knee, posterior calf, and thigh have been involved, although the dorsum of his left foot has been the major area of complaint.

For the past several weeks he has noted intermittent pains around the heel of his foot, some leg cramps, and occasional pain in the inner aspect of both elbows. Recently, both knees have been somewhat stiff, and he has had some paresthesias in his left leg. His other medical problems include hypertension, obesity, ulcer-type stomach distress, and deep venous thromboembolism.

1. The diagnosis of acute gout is made by the physician. What are the manifestations of gout in this patient?

This patient's description of the exquisitely severe pain in his left great toe is remarkably similar to the classic description of the acute gouty attack which was so well described by Thomas Sydenham in the 17th century — pain so severe that the patient cannot bear the weight of the bedcovers on his affected toe and cannot even bear the jar of a person walking into his room.

An acute attack of gout commonly occurs at night (47) and may be preceded by prodromal symptoms such as mood changes, diuresis, local pruritus or discomfort in the to-be-affected joint. It is interesting that this patient noted intermittent pains around the heel of his foot, some leg cramps, paresthesias in his left leg, and occasional pain in the elbows for several weeks prior to this acute gouty attack. It is also said that an acute attack can sometimes be precipitated by a stressful event such as trauma, surgery, or uricosuric agents (47), and this patient stressed his leg by jumping off a scaffold onto sand.

The classic description of gouty arthritis also includes male predominance, persistent hyperuricemia, onset in middle age, and a high incidence of podagra (gouty pain in the great toe) as the initial event (35,36). WS is a 45-year-old male who presents with podagra as his first gouty manifestation. While the big toe is the most commonly affected joint (47), the ankle, knee, and, less commonly, the wrist and the elbow can be affected. In one study of acute gout, 83% of the involved joints were those in the lower extremity. However, the foot was spared in about a third of the patients. Furthermore, polyarthritis was the first manifestation of gout in as many as 39% of these patients (35).

Crystals of monosodium urate and large numbers of polymorphonuclear leukocytes can usually be aspirated from involved joints of patients with acute gouty arthritis (82). However, urate crystals may not be found in an occasional patient with gouty arthritis (1). Therefore, the diagnosis of acute gouty arthritis cannot be ruled out if urate crystals are not present in the first search of joint fluid. Repeated search of other involved joints (1), or even of the same joint five hours later (82) may demonstrate the diagnostic monosodium urate crystals.

Acute painful attacks of gout are often accompanied by severe inflammation of the joint as well as of periarticular tissues and skin. This patient not only experienced pain in his great toe, but also experienced discomfort in the dorsal area of his left foot, his left knee, and posterior calf. Other signs of systemic inflammation include febrile reactions, mild leukocytosis, and elevation of the erythrocyte sedimentation rate. Fever is common and maximum temperatures usually range from 101° F to 103° F. The leukocytosis is generally moderate and is usually about 10,000/mm^3 (35).

2. At the onset of this patient's attack (i.e. three days prior to admission), he received a shot of hydrocortisone in a physician's office. Are corticosteroids effective in the treatment of symptomatic gout?

A very brief course of ACTH or corticosteroids is sometimes effective in relieving an attack of severe gout (31). However, the consensus of opinion is that steroids should only be used in cases refractory to colchicine, indomethacin, or phenylbutazone. Such refractory cases are often fulminating, prolonged and polyarticular, and can occur in as many as 5 to 10% of patients (111). Upon cessation of corticosteroid antiinflammatory effects, a rebound attack of gout can occur within three to five days and be more severe than the original gouty attack (47). Therefore, intramuscular injections of ACTH or corticosteroids should be gradually discontinued over two to three days and should be administered in conjunction with 0.5 to 1.5 mg of daily colchicine (111).

Interestingly, this patient's attack did progressively increase in severity for about three days after his cortisone shot.

3. Colchicine is ordered by the hospital physician for WS. How effective is it and how should it be administered?

Colchicine is not a general anti-inflammatory drug and unlike indomethacin, phenylbutazone, fenoprofen, or naproxen, is relatively specific for relieving the symptoms of acute gout. The malaise of familial Mediterranean fever (30) and the arthritis associated with sarcoidosis (31) are the only other diseases with a rheumatological component which are relieved by colchicine. Therefore, the response to colchicine can be considered diagnostic and is of importance when synovial fluid cannot be obtained from small joints for inspection of urate crystals. As a result, colchicine continues to be the agent of choice for an acute attack of gout as it provides relief to greater than 95% of patients when administered early in the course of an attack.

For the fully developed acute attack, the traditional dose of colchicine has been one or two 0.5 to 0.6 mg tablets initially, following by 0.5 to 0.6 mg hourly until there is relief of joint pain or development of gastrointestinal side effects such as diarrhea, nausea, or vomiting. Colchicine is administered hourly to minimize gastrointestinal toxicity because patients vary considerably with respect to the amount of colchicine they can tolerate. However, even with hourly colchicine, titration of dose to a maximal therapeutic response without gastrointestinal toxicity is difficult. Therefore, some (111) no longer advise hourly colchicine, but instead recommend that 0.5 mg be administered every two or three hours following an initial 1.0 mg dose. When given in this manner, gastrointestinal problems with colchicine are rare, and the therapeutic response is not compromised. If, through past experience, the approximate therapeutic or toxic dose of colchicine is known for a particular patient, one-half to two-thirds of this dose can be administered at once with the remainder given as 0.5 to 0.6 mg every other hour. This method of administration saves the patient much suffering since delays in treatment may result in greater failure rates as well as increased severity and duration of attacks (99).

4. Since colchicine is the only medication for acute gout with specific diagnostic value, does its mechanism of action provide insights as to the pathophysiology of the acute attack?

The specific mechanism of action of colchicine remains unproven, and it will probably remain so until there is complete understanding of the pathogenesis of acute gouty inflammation. Nevertheless, experimental evidence has resulted in some reasonable theories. Currently it is felt that the following cycle of events takes place during an acute gouty attack. Precipitation of monosodium urate crystals elicits an inflammatory reaction with infiltration of granulocytes. These granulocytes then phagocytize the urate crystals resulting in the release of vasoactive polypeptides which are thought to be mediators of pain and inflammation (49). The subsequent biochemical changes in the local environment, such as the increased production of lactic acid during phagocytosis, produce a fall in synovial fluid pH leading to a decrease in urate solubility and precipitation of more urate crystals (12,85). Colchicine is thought to interfere with the role that granulocytes appear to play in perpetuating the acute attack.

Colchicine interferes with leukocyte locomotion, mobilization, chemotaxis, and adhesiveness; lysosomal degranulation in the granulocyte cell; and kinin release from plasma under the influence of leukocytes (101). The range of colchicine concentrations necessary to produce these changes *in vivo* is broad. Wallace, in consideration of the plasma and intracellular concentrations which are attainable with normal colchicine dosing, concludes that colchicine's mechanism of action is based upon interference with leukocyte chemotaxis or with the random motility of the leukocyte (100,101). Malawista claims that colchicine's mechanism of action in the treatment of acute gout probably depends upon interference with microtubular subunit protein aggregation (50,54). This latter mechanism is a result of colchicine's ability to arrest cellular mitosis at metaphase and could explain the interference with the mobilization of the leukocytes (107). However, there are objections (100) to this latter theory, and a point-counterpoint continues in the literature as to the true interaction between colchicine and polymorphonuclear granulocytes. Other work suggests that synovial cells may also have a vital role in both the production of gouty arthritis and the mechanism of action of colchicine (68).

5. WS has a history of an ulcer-like stomach distress; will intravenous colchicine be less toxic to the gastrointestinal tract than the oral form?

Although colchicine causes gastrointestinal (GI) distress by both oral and intravenous administration, clinicians generally recommend the latter route for patients unable to tolerate oral colchicine (46,99,115). However, a review of the literature did not uncover any well-controlled studies that compared the gastrointestinal problems caused by these two routes of administration.

Intestinal mucosal cells have a very rapid rate of turnover, and colchicine is known to inhibit the mitosis of cells. Therefore, it is postulated that colchicine induces nausea, vomiting, diarrhea, and abdominal pain by having a direct local toxic effect on cells lining the gastrointestinal tract. Since intravenous administration avoids the initial passage of colchicine through the gastrointestinal tract, it would be expected to cause less irritation than oral administration. Nevertheless, gastrointestinal toxicity from intravenous colchicine does occur, probably because large amounts of the drug enter the gastrointestinal

tract by biliary excretion and by back-diffusion from blood (101,107). Additionally, other mechanisms may be responsible for the GI toxicity of colchicine. The fact that the GI effects are eliminated by anesthesia in animals, suggests a neurogenic component (66). Furthermore, less apparent GI toxicity from intravenous administration may simply be a result of the smaller doses which are used by this route of administration. If the more moderate approach to dosing oral colchicine is used (see Question 3), the GI toxicity by both routes of administration may well be comparable.

6. If intravenous colchicine is to be used for WS, how should it be administered?

The entire dose of colchicine 2-3 mg should be diluted to 30cc with normal saline and administered slowly over a period of five minutes. This dose may be repeated in 6 to 8 hours if needed (31). Small, repeated intravenous doses of colchicine are not necessary and greatly enhance the probability of the development of phlebitis (99). Clinicians should be aware that colchicine solutions are extremely irritating. Care must be taken to prevent extravasation during intravenous administration because ulnar nerve damage has been reported (101). The needle used to draw up the colchicine solution into the syringe should be discarded, and a new needle used for the actual venopuncture.

7. WS is in excruciating pain and requests an analgesic. Should he receive a narcotic analgesic considering that colchicine therapy has already been initiated? What other therapeutic endeavors should be utilized?

Benefits from colchicine usually occur within 12 hours, although relief may begin as early as six to eight hours after the first oral dose. Pain, redness, and swelling are completely gone within 48 to 72 hours (107). Since relief from colchicine is not immediate, appropriate analgesics should be used for relief of pain until colchicine has had a chance to work. Salicylates must be avoided because they decrease urate tubular secretion (112), decrease urate solubility (49), and displace urate from binding sites on albumin (17). The narcotic analgesics are effective and have the added advantage of decreasing the troublesome diarrhea which accompanies colchicine use.

A cradle should be placed over this patient's foot to keep the weight of the bedsheets off his affected toe. Rest of his gouty foot and elevation also are of benefit. Cold applications to the foot are sometimes helpful, but heat should not be applied to the affected foot as it may intensify the inflammation (47).

8. WS's colchicine order was "1.0 mg initially followed by 0.5 mg hourly until there is relief of joint

pain or onset of gastrointestinal side effects." During work rounds the following morning, the medical house staff discovers that WS has not had relief from his colchicine, and has continued to receive it hourly. Apparently, the student nurse team leader did not consider his diarrhea or abdominal pains to be severe enough to discontinue the colchicine. What toxicities may be expected?

The colchicine order should have stated the maximum number of doses which this patient was to receive. A maximum of 10 to 15 tablets is generally recommended (46,107) because as little as 7 mg of colchicine can be fatal (107). However, the lethal dose has been estimated to be about 65 mg (69).

Toxic effects from colchicine are usually reversible and consist most commonly of nausea, diarrhea, abdominal pain, and vomiting. More severe toxic effects from therapeutic doses of colchicine affect the hepatic, hematopoietic, and nervous systems, but usually occur only in elderly patients (107) or those with prior cardiac, hepatic, or renal disease (66). Reports of a toxic effect of colchicine on sperm production (59,72) have been refuted (13).

Acute poisonings or large overdosages of colchicine cause life-threatening multiple system disturbances. *Nervous system* dysfunctions have been manifested as persistent mental confusion, loss of deep tendon reflexes, ascending paralysis, and respiratory failure. *Gastrointestinal system* toxicities result in abdominal pain, vomiting, severe watery diarrhea, and a hemorrhagic gastritis which has led to dehydration and shock. Hepatotoxicity and pancreatitis may also be associated with colchicine's effects on the gastrointestinal system. *Musculoskeletal problems* such as myopathy, myoglobinuria, and large increases in muscle enzymes have been reported. *Hematologic* abnormalities include severe leukopenia followed by recovery leukocytosis and complete bone marrow aplasia. *Renal* complications present as reversible azotemia with a urinalysis showing proteinuria, myoglobinuria, hematuria, and many hyaline casts. *Respiratory* system dysfunction may be the result of neurological failure as well as of chest wall weakening and pulmonary edema with hypoxemia (66).

9. Since this patient's acute gouty attack does not seem to be relieved with colchicine, how should other medications be used?

Phenylbutazone and indomethacin are comparable to colchicine in effectiveness in relieving acute gouty attacks. Both of these agents are popular because severe gastrointestinal toxicity is not a predicted consequence of vigorous oral therapy, and patients need not be awakened hourly for their medication. These drugs may also be more predictable than colchicine in relieving acute gouty attacks of more than several

days duration (31). Therefore, either indomethacin or phenylbutazone can be used to treat this patient's fulminating attack.

Indomethacin has become the drug most frequently prescribed for the treatment of acute attacks of gouty arthritis (47), and now Medical Letter consultants (4) even consider it to be the drug of choice. When used in doses of 50 mg three times daily for two to three days followed by gradually tapering doses, this nonsteroidal anti-inflammatory agent is very effective. Side effects are minimal when used in this manner, but gastrointestinal disturbances, headaches, rash, and leukopenia have been reported. Although the earlier use of indomethacin also resulted in dramatic therapeutic responses, the drug was associated with a high incidence of dose-related side effects because large doses of 100 to 200 mg four times daily were recommended at that time.

Phenylbutazone (Butazolidin) and its metabolite, *oxyphenbutazone* (Tandearil) are excellent alternative drugs for use in acute gouty arthritis. Either of these two drugs can control 85 to 95% of acute attacks within 24 to 36 hours. Therefore, phenylbutazone and oxyphenbutazone were the drugs of choice for patients unable to tolerate colchicine, prior to the recommendation that lower doses of indomethacin be used (47). Indeed, Gutman (33) at one time suggested that the time had come for oxyphenbutazone (or phenylbutazone) to replace colchicine as the drug of choice for acute gout. However, he continued to recommend oral colchicine up to his death (32).

Recommended phenylbutazone doses are 200 mg four times daily for the first day, followed by 200 mg three times daily for two additional days. Doses are then rapidly tapered and discontinued over the next two days. For the best therapeutic results with infrequent gastrointestinal side effects, Yu (111) recommends administering 200 mg of phenylbutazone four times daily together with colchicine 1.0 to 2.0 mg daily. After the phenylbutazone is discontinued, she continues the colchicine in prophylactic doses of 1.0 mg per day.

The potential hematological toxicities of phenylbutazone are well documented (see chapter on *Rheumatoid Arthritis*) but are rare with short term therapy. Nevertheless, these adverse reactions do occur and are severe enough to warrant the use of colchicine or indomethacin as the first agents of choice. Seegmiller (87) reported a case of thrombocytopenia which occurred after a single day of phenylbutazone therapy, and acute massive gastrointestinal hemorrhages have also occurred after only one day of phenylbutazone (60,77). Other common phenylbutazone side effects include sodium and fluid retention, mild uricosuria, peptic ulceration, nausea, vomiting, and skin rashes.

Ibuprofen (29), *fenopren* (103), and **naproxen** (95,105) are new anti-inflammatory and analgesic medications widely used in the treatment of rheumatoid arthritis because they are effective and have minimal gastrointestinal toxicities. Early clinical trials indicate that these agents are also effective alternatives for the treatment of acute gouty arthritis. In a multicenter trial of 41 patients, naproxen (750 mg initially followed by 250 mg three times daily) was as effective as phenylbutazone (200 mg four times daily for 48 hours followed by 200 mg three times daily) in aborting the acute gouty attack (95). Other studies with naproxen (105), fenoprofen (103), and ibuprofen (29) also substantiate the findings of efficacy and minimal toxicity. Until more clinical experience accumulates, these new propionic acid anti-inflammatory agents should be considered as alternatives to colchicine, indomethacin, or phenylbutazone.

CASE B (Questions 10-15): A 54-year-old male with a history of congestive heart failure is admitted to General Hospital with a diagnosis of acute myelogenous leukemia. On admission the BUN was 49 mg/100 ml, serum creatinine was 2.1 mg/100 ml, and the uric acid was 16.2 mg/100 ml. On the following hospital day chemotherapy was begun with thioguanine, cytosine arabinoside, and allopurinol. His white blood cell count decreased within a week from 90,000/mm³ on admission to 7,500/mm³ as a result of the cytotoxic treatment. On the 7th day he complained of nausea, and his urine volume decreased to 35 ml/24 hours. At this time, the BUN increased to 115 mg/100 ml, serum creatinine increased to 10.6 mg/100 ml, and his serum uric acid increased to 22.6 mg/100 ml. Intravenous furosemide and urine alkalinization had no effect on his clinical condition, and hemodialysis was started because of continued clinical deterioration. During the ensuing two days, the urine output increased and then gradually returned to normal. His renal function continued to improve, and 16 days after hemodialysis was initiated, the serum creatinine was again 2.1 mg/100 ml.

10. What are some physiological causes of hyperuricemia?

An early genetic mutation error during the evolution of man resulted in the loss of uricase, an enzyme necessary to degrade uric acid into more soluble products. As a consequence, uric acid is not metabolized in man. It serves no biological function and is merely the end product of purine metabolism. Since there is no established mechanism for the breakdown of uric acid, the uric acid which is formed must be eliminated renally to prevent accumulation. Therefore, elevated serum uric acid levels can result from an increase in the production in uric acid; a decrease in the renal excretion; or a combination of these two mechanisms.

Overproduction of uric acid may result from excessive de novo purine synthesis, excessive nucleoprotein turnover, or excessive dietary purines (25). The **excessive de novo purine synthesis** is primarily associated with enzyme mutation defects. For example, a deficiency of hypoxanthine-guanine-phosphoribosyl-transferase (HG PRTase) is associated not only with hyperuricemia and gout, but also with mental retardation, choreoathetosis, and self-mutilation by biting. This phenomenon has been named the Lesch-Nyhan syndrome (51,84). Increased phosphoribosyl-pyrophosphate synthetase (PRPP) initiates the acceleration of amidotransferase in de novo purine biosynthesis (91). Likewise, the deficiency of glucose-phosphatase in glycogen storage disease Type I (von Gierke) is associated with gout and hyperuricemia through excessive purine biosynthesis, as is the hereditary possession of a mutant glutathione reductase (91). Excessive dietary purines in, for example, yeast or liver can also cause hyperuricemia.

Excessive nucleoprotein turnover from neoplastic diseases such as multiple myeloma, leukemias, lymphomas, and Hodgkin's disease as well as from myeloproliferative disorders such as myeloid metaplasia or polycythemia vera, have all been associated with gout and hyperuricemia.

Underexcretion of uric acid is the result of decreased renal function. Uric acid concentrations are the same in plasma and in the glomerular filtrate. Thus, uric acid is considered to be completely filtered by the renal glomerulus. Nearly all the filtered urate, even when augmented by hyperuricemia, is reabsorbed in the proximal tubule. Of the uric acid appearing in the urine, approximately 80-86% of the uric acid in the urine is a result of active tubular secretion in the distal end of the proximal tubule (23,46,93). The filtered urate which escaped reabsorption constitutes only about 14 to 20% of the excreted uric acid load (32). Therefore, excreted uric acid is almost entirely attributable to the tubular secretory process. Reabsorption of filtered urate follows first-order kinetics because more urate is reabsorbed when large urate loads are filtered (49). Accordingly, despite the large filtered urate loads in man during hyperuricemia, urate is eliminated into the urine at a slow steady pace which discourages uric acid precipitation in the urinary tract (32). While high plasma urate levels stimulate renal tubular secretion to some extent, the above mechanisms prevent massive dumping of sparingly soluble uric acid into the urine in response to small fluctuations in plasma concentration (93). The renal excretion of uric acid is actually more complex and another postsecretory distal tubular reabsorptive site for urate probably exists (75,94).

11. What was the probable cause for the elevated serum uric acid level noted upon this patient's admission?

Upon superficial review, it would appear that the hyperuricemia in this patient is a result of both overproduction and underexcretion of uric acid. However, the major cause of hyperuricemia in this case is probably due to the increased turnover of nucleic acids because of the leukemia. Mild to moderate renal failure is not usually a cause of hyperuricemia as long as the creatinine clearance is greater than 15 ml/minute. Apparently, renal urate secretory mechanisms remain functional and do not become defective until the glomerular filtration rate falls below 10 ml/minute. At this level of renal function, the defective secretory mechanism is unable to entirely compensate for the decrease in urate reabsorption, and hyperuricemia occurs (75).

12. Efforts are made to lower the serum uric acid. Should this patient also receive prophylactic colchicine to prevent an acute attack of gouty arthritis?

Major texts and review articles claim that colchicine is generally effective in reducing recurrences of acute attacks, and various dosage schedules for this purpose are recommended (69,97,115). Usually, the prophylactic dose is about 0.5 to 2.0 mg every night or every other night (107). However, it is sometimes difficult to attribute benefits to colchicine, or for that matter to any drug or procedure, because gout is a highly variable disease without a predictable pattern. Nevertheless, considerable clinical experience indicates that prophylactic colchicine clearly decreases the frequency and severity of acute gouty attacks.

Gutman and Yu (110,111,115) reported that the periodicity of acute gouty attacks continued or increased in frequency and severity in 80% of 208 patients who did not receive preventive colchicine. This trend was reversed in about 75% of these patients by prophylactic colchicine, with or without uricosurics. Prior to colchicine preventive therapy, 39% of 260 gouty patients followed for an average of 6.4 years, were categorized as having severe attacks with an additional 61% as having moderately severe attacks. Symptom-free patients or those with mild gouty arthritis were excluded from this study. After prophylaxis was instituted with colchicine in doses of 0.5 mg to 2.0 mg per day, only 2% of these patients suffered severe attacks; 12% had moderately severe attacks; 32% had mild attacks; and 53% reported virtually no attacks. According to Yu (111) more than 500 of their patients have now been studied and some have been followed for more than 20 years. She concludes "the agony of acute gouty arthritis is long forgotten, and the chronic stiffness and aching likewise are no more remembered. The use of colchicine for the pre-

vention of recurrent acute gouty arthritis is now well accepted."

One aspect of Gutman's (110) prophylactic program which contributed much to its success, was the instruction to his patients to take abortive doses of colchicine (2 to 3 mg for a day or two) at the first sign of an attack and to proceed with full doses if the attack progressed. Additionally, extra doses of colchicine were to be taken when patients anticipated excessive stress.

Although prophylactic colchicine is successful in minimizing recurrences of acute gouty arthritis, it does not correct the hyperuricemia of gout, nor does it prevent the formation of tophi. Approximately 30% of Gutman's patients who were treated with colchicine alone began to show evidence of tophi over a period of 5.4 years.

Prophylactic colchicine would be unnecessary in this patient. He does not have a history of recurrent gouty arthritis and is not at high risk of developing an acute attack of gout. While high serum urate values are common in patients with renal insufficiency, gouty arthritis rarely occurs. In one study of 496 patients with chronic renal failure, only six developed gout (91). This absence of gouty attacks has been attributed to either a decreased lifespan or to a decreased ability to respond to an inflammatory stimulus. If acute recurrent attacks should occur, colchicine therapy can be initiated at that time. (Also see Question 31.)

13. How does colchicine prevent acute gouty attacks?

The mechanisms for acute gouty attacks are still speculative, as are the mechanisms for colchicine prophylaxis. There is some thought that small daily doses of colchicine prevent acute gouty attacks by interfering with synoviocyte participation in the inflammatory process of gout. The reasoning for this theory is based upon the fact that normal joint fluid contains only about four polymorphonuclear leukocytes per cubic millimeter. Since so few leukocytes are present, it seems rather unrealistic to expect that these leukocytes could mediate an acute attack. Because synovial membrane leukocytes can either act in lieu of, or complement the polymorphonuclear leukocytes in promoting the acute gouty attack (68), it would seem reasonable that colchicine's prophylactic activity is exerted on these synovial membrane phagocytes (50,102).

14. Why was urine alkalinization tried in this patient; what agents are available?

Urine alkalinization should be instituted when severe hyperuricemia is present as it was in this case. Uric acid is poorly soluble in water, but a pKa of 5.75 allows for greater solubility of the ionized form in alkaline environments (115). At a urine pH of 5, only six to eight milligrams of uric acid are soluble per 100 ml of urine. However, when urine is alkalinized to pH 7, the solubility of uric acid increases twenty-fold to 120-160 mg per 100 ml (89). Since the prevalence of uric acid urolithiasis in patients with gout is 1,000 times that of the non-gouty individuals and since urinary calculi occur in 10% to 20% of gouty patients (114,115), the importance of urine alkalinization can be appreciated.

Urine can be alkalinized using **sodium** or **potassium bicarbonate** in an initial oral dose of four grams followed by one to two grams every four hours (3). Intravenous sodium bicarbonate can also be used, as it was in this patient. The urine pH should be tested (e.g. nitrazine paper) at intervals throughout the day and the dose of bicarbonate should be adjusted accordingly. **Potassium** or **sodium citrate** can also be used in doses of one gram three to six times daily (16). The citrates have the same urine alkalinizing properties of sodium bicarbonate without neutralizing gastric secretions (55) and without promoting a dumping syndrome. The bicarbonate and citrate doses should be evenly divided throughout the day and night. During the night, the urine becomes the most concentrated and acidic; thus it may be necessary to add an intravenous dose to the IV solution during the night in hospitalized patients. **Acetazolamide** (Diamox) is also capable of alkalinizing urine, but it can produce a mild metabolic acidosis which is undesirable in a patient with renal decompensation.

Although an alkaline urine is desirable to increase the solubility of uric acid, it is often difficult to achieve clinically without affecting other organ systems. In this patient with congestive heart failure, sodium intake must be considered. The ability of the kidneys to excrete potassium may also be of critical importance. The cation content of various alkalinizing agents is listed as follows:

Product	mEq/gram
$Na\,HCO_3$	11.9
Na Citrate · $2H_2O$	8.4
$K\,HCO_3$	9.9
K Citrate · H_2O	9.3

15. Hemodialysis was initiated in this patient. Is uric acid dialyzable, and is there a preference for hemodialysis as compared to peritoneal dialysis?

Uric acid is readily dialyzable despite the finding that uric acid is bound to plasma proteins (17,93). Apparently, this urate-albumin bond is weak and influenced by many factors. In fact, hemodialysis is so efficient in removing uric acid that each six-hour dialysis can reduce the uric acid level by 50%. In 16 patients with hyperuricemic renal failure, each six-hour dialysis removed between 1.5 grams to 13.4 grams of uric acid. The amounts of uric acid removed by hemodialysis are much more than that reported with peritoneal dialysis. Although 3.4 to 4.8 grams of uric acid have been removed by peritoneal dialysis, hemodialysis is estimated to be between 10 to 20 times more efficient in eliminating uric acid (45). Disequilibrium does not occur even with rapid hemodialysis.

CASE C (Questions 16-22): One month after suffering an acute myocardial infarction, a 56-year-old man maintains his scheduled appointment at his physician's office for routine evaluation. His physical examination is unremarkable and his laboratory evaluations are all within normal limits except for a uric acid value of 12.0 mg/100 ml noted on an SMA-12 panel.

16. Is this hyperuricemia clinically significant?

There are several methods for the analysis of uric acid and each method and laboratory has different standard normal values for the same sample. The phosphotungstate or colorimetric method, commonly utilized in automated laboratory screening panels, is not as specific as the uricase method of uric acid analysis and generally provides values that are approximately 1 mg/100 ml higher (27).

In normal subjects, plasma becomes saturated with sodium urate at a concentration of 7 mg/100 ml. However, supersaturated solutions of sodium urate form readily, and serum urate concentrations as high as 40 to 60 mg/100 ml are not uncommon in untreated nongouty patients with myeloproliferative disorders (91). It is not clear how uric acid can stay in a supersaturated solution and then, suddenly under certain conditions begin to precipitate out. However, it is known that plasma urate-binding protein deficiency, urate affinity for chondroitin sulfate, local pH changes, cold, trauma, and stress can cause seeding of urate crystals (31).

When maximum serum uric acid values from the Framingham Heart Study (36) were analyzed, gouty arthritis was noted to occur in 1.8% of those patients with levels between 6.0 to 6.9 mg/100 ml, and in 11.8% of those with levels between 7.0 to 7.9 mg/100 ml. On the other hand, 15% of the men who had actually developed gouty arthritis did not have a serum uric acid value above 6.9 mg/100 ml and 81% of subjects with serum uric acid values of greater than 7.0 mg/100 ml did not develop gouty arthritis. Thus, although the risk of developing gouty arthritis generally increases with increasing serum uric acid levels, it is impossible to define a specific serum uric acid level above which treatment would be definitely indicated. The clinical significance of each level must be interpreted in the context of the patient history.

17. Should asymptomatic hyperuricemia, such as noted in this patient, be treated?

Individuals with high serum uric acid levels are more likely to develop acute gouty arthritis than normouricemic individuals, and the magnitude of the risk increases with increasing degrees of hyperuricemia. However, it would be excessive to treat all hyperuricemic individuals with uric acid lowering medications for life solely for the prevention of acute attacks of *gouty arthritis.* A large percentage of hyperuricemic patients may never experience an acute attack of gout. If an attack should occur, it can easily be treated within 48-72 hours, and after the acute episode has subsided, uric acid lowering medications can then be started.

The key issue in the treatment of hyperuricemia concerns the effect of uric acid on renal function. *Renal disease* is the most common complication of gout except for the arthritis, and renal failure is the eventual cause of death in as many as 25% of gouty patients (47). The renal damage may occur as a result of uric acid crystal deposition in the collecting tubules, followed by an inflammatory reaction, and perhaps fibrosis. More recent work seems to imply that an increased filtered urate load per se may be nephrotoxic (48). Even more alarming is the finding that the onset of uric acid nephrolithiasis preceded acute gouty arthritis by more than five years in 40% of 305 patients (114). Actual kidney damage in gout, however, usually occurs in a setting that includes either hypertension, diabetes, renal vascular disease, glomerulonephritis, pyelonephritis, renal calculi, or some other cause of primary nephropathy independent of gout. Furthermore, hyperuricemia alone had no adverse effect on renal function in an analysis of 524 gouty subjects who were followed for more than 12 years (7). In view of the contradictory data, it is abundantly clear that additional data are needed to determine the precise role of uric acid in renal dysfunction (86). Currently, there are no rational guidelines for the treatment of asymptomatic hyperuricemic patients, because there are no definitive studies to show the fate of untreated patients with hyperuricemia.

Consequently, an indisputable decision to treat this patient cannot be made in spite of his rather high serum uric acid of 12.0 mg/100 ml and the potential risk of renal disease. However, he probably should be treated with sulfinpyrazone for the reasons described in Question 18.

18. Why would uricosuric treatment with sulfinpyrazone be appropriate for this patient?

Sulfinpyrazone (Anturane) is a phenylbutazone analogue that is also a very effective uricosuric agent. Like all uricosurics, it inhibits tubular secretion of uric acid at low doses; but at normal therapeutic doses, it inhibits the tubular reabsorption of uric acid. Therapy should be initiated slowly, at a dose of 50 mg twice daily and raised gradually by increments of 100 mg weekly to the daily maintenance dosage range of 200 to 400 mg in divided doses. Untoward reactions and precautions are similar to those of probenecid with gastrointestinal distress and hypersensitivity skin rashes being the most common. Hematological reactions have rarely been associated with the administration of sulfinpyrazone, but there is a potential for blood dyscrasias since this drug is a congener of phenylbutazone.

Superficially, sulfinpyrazone appears to be merely another uricosuric agent similar to probenecid. However, this drug possesses antithrombotic properties which are speculated to be mediated by inhibition of platelet activation and inhibition of prostaglandin synthesis (76).

Antiplatelet drugs are currently being investigated as to whether usage prevents arterial thrombotic phenomena in all risk patients. Therefore, the Anturane Reinfarction Trial Research Group conducted a prospective double-blind study of sulfinpyrazone in patients recently recovered from a myocardial infarction in 26 hospitals in the United States and Canada. Sulfinpyrazone 200 mg four times daily or a placebo was administered to 1475 selected patients who had suffered a myocardial infarction 25 to 35 days previous to inclusion into this study. Sulfinpyrazone did not prevent recurrences of myocardial infarction, but surprisingly reduced the incidence of total mortality, cardiac mortality, and sudden cardiac death by about 50% (5). Since cardiac arrhythmias are the major cause of death after a myocardial infarction, the assumed conclusion is that sulfinpyrazone in some unexplained manner prevented fatal arrhythmias.

This patient with a uric acid of 12.0 mg/100 ml is at increased risk of developing acute gouty arthritis and perhaps of developing a gouty nephropathy because uric acid saturates plasma at a concentration of about 7.0 mg/100 ml. Furthermore, he is at risk of developing a fatal arrhythmia as a result of his myocardial infarction one month ago. In view of both problems it would seem reasonable to initiate sulfinpyrazone 50 mg twice daily for one week in this patient. This dosage should be increased gradually in 100 mg weekly increments until he is receiving 200 mg four times daily. (Also see Question 20.)

19. WS, who suffered the acute gouty attack described in Case A, has returned to his physician's office for routine evaluation. Since he suffers from gouty arthritis, the decision has been made to treat him with probenecid (Benemid). What is the mechanism of action of probenecid and when should serum uric acid levels begin to decrease?

It is entirely appropriate that WS be treated with a

uric acid lowering drug now that his acute attack has subsided. Such medications are indicated for all patients who have documented urate deposition disease. The goal of therapy should be to dissolve all existing tophaceous deposits and to maintain the serum urate level at less than 7.0 mg/100 ml. Lifetime treatment with either uricosurics or allopurinol may be necessary.

Uricosuric drugs such as probenecid (Benemid) and sulfinpyrazone (Anturane) increase uric acid excretion by inhibiting the renal tubular reabsorption of uric acid. Although low doses of these agents can theoretically inhibit tubular uric acid secretion, so predominant is the inhibition of tubular reabsorption that paradoxical urate retention with low doses is not observed clinically (34). When these drugs are used regularly in effective daily doses, they not only decrease the plasma level of uric acid, but also prevent the formation of tophi and mobilize already existing tophaceous deposits. However, these agents must be used consistently as plasma urate levels will rise to their initially high levels within a day or two after cessation of these drugs (34).

When therapy is begun, a prompt fall in plasma urate concentrations is usually seen and is accompanied by rapid urinary excretion of uric acid (107). After the first day or two, the urinary uric acid excess disappears in normal man, but in hyperuricemic individuals, the excess uric acid is continually mobilized until the body pool of urate is reduced to normal levels (34).

20. How should uricosuric therapy be initiated and what are the most commonly reported side effects?

Probenecid is well absorbed orally, and peak plasma concentrations occur within two to four hours. Its biological half-life is six to twelve hours and its active metabolites help to prolong the uricosuria. The dose of probenecid should be 250 mg twice daily for the first week of therapy; thereafter 500 mg may be given twice a day. If necessary, the dose may be increased to 2.0 grams daily. Initiation of uricosuric therapy must begin slowly because excretion of large amounts of uric acid increases the risk of urate stone formation in the kidney. This may be followed by connective tissue reaction with subsequent renal damage. This risk can be minimized by starting with small doses of uricosurics so that the kidney is not overwhelmed with a flood of uric acid. Alkalinization of the urine in order to increase uric acid solubility, and maintenance of a high fluid intake to maintain urine flow of at least two liters per day also minimizes renal stone formation. With few exceptions, it is not necessary to alkalinize the urine provided a high fluid intake is assured. Since probenecid is a weak acid, an alkaline urine would enhance its tubular secretion; and

an acid urine would stimulate probenecid reabsorption (111).

Probenecid is safe and generally well tolerated. The most common complaints are gastrointestinal distress and drug induced dermatitis. Gastrointestinal irritation occurs in at least 2% of patients and this percentage increases when larger doses are administered (12). In two series of 169 gouty patients, gastrointestinal distress occurred in 8%, drug hypersensitivity with fever and rash in 5%, and precipitation of acute gouty attacks in 10% (34). These percentages are in general accord with those of other investigators.

21. When should the use of uricosuric therapy be avoided?

The fact that uricosuric drugs do not affect the production of uric acid but merely increase its excretion places limitations on their use. Probenecid cannot be used in patients with a glomerular filtration rate (GFR) less than 20 to 30 ml/min (111) or a BUN greater than 40 mg/100 ml (31). If the GFR is 40 to 50 ml/min, the dose of probenecid needs to be increased (111). Patients with a history of frequent renal stones and patients who are gross over-excretors (more than 1000 mg/day) of uric acid should not be treated with uricosurics (111). Additionally, these agents should not be used in patients suffering an acute attack of gout.

22. Explain why aspirin can either lower or raise the serum uric acid.

This paradoxical action of salicylates on uric acid excretion is simply dose-dependent. At low oral doses of one to two grams per day, salicylates decrease urate secretion and elevate plasma urate. Larger doses of five to six grams per day decrease tubular reabsorption causing marked uricosuria and lower serum urate levels (110). Intermediate doses have little or no effect. When the high doses of salicylate sufficiently suppress tubular reabsorption, the net response is a uricosuric one because the amount of urate normally reabsorbed is greater than that secreted. With intermediate doses of two to three grams per day, tubular secretion and inhibition of tubular reabsorption more or less negate each other resulting in little or no net change in the urinary excretion of uric acid. Clinically, however, this balancing effect is highly unpredictable and it is best to avoid aspirin in critical gouty patients.

Actually, all the uricosuric agents, including probenecid and sulfinpyrazone, share this dose-dependent handling of uric acid (12). Investigations also indicate that all uricosuric drugs significantly decrease urate binding to plasma proteins; however, the physiological significance of these findings are as yet unknown. Speculations are that impaired urate binding significantly decreases urate solubility (17,49).

CASE D (Questions 23-24): A 50-year-old obese female is admitted to General Hospital with complaints of nausea, vomiting, and right upper quadrant pain which began three months ago during the Thanksgiving holiday. Since then the pain has been intermittent in nature and has generally been associated with anorexia and a dark urine. Physical examination showed a well-developed, well-nourished, obese, slightly jaundiced female. Her liver was not palpable but was enlarged to percussion. Laboratory findings were within normal limits except for a total serum bilirubin of 1.8 mg%, and an elevated serum uric acid of 10.5 mg%. Renal function tests were normal.

Approximately five years ago she suffered an acute attack of gout which was treated with colchicine followed by a short course of probenecid. After a few months she discontinued both medications on her own because of gastrointestinal distress. She was started on isoniazid and ethambutol approximately two months ago for tuberculosis. In addition she has been receiving levodopa for her parkinsonism for the past three years.

23. Could her problems be drug-related?

Both isoniazid and ethambutol have been associated with liver dysfunction which is compatible with many aspects of her present symptomatology. Liver function tests should be performed and her hepatic status should be re-evaluated in view of her jaundice, hepatomegaly, anorexia, dark urine, and elevated bilirubin.

Her hyperuricemia is probably drug-induced. There are several isolated reports of hyperuricemia associated with levodopa (2,41,70), and at least two cases of gout which have occurred during levodopa therapy for parkinsonism (39). It should be noted, however, that levodopa can also produce false rises with colorimetric determinations for serum uric acid (19). It is not yet clear whether hyperuricemia is the result of levodopa therapy or simply associated with parkinsonism itself. Nevertheless, hyperuricemia associated with levodopa is being reported and cases should be verified with the more specific uricase spectrophotometric method of laboratory determination for uric acid. (Also see *Parkinsonism* chapter.)

Prolonged use of ethambutol is also associated with hyperuricemia. Approximately 50% of 15 patients receiving standard therapeutic doses of this antituberculous agent experienced a rise in serum urate as early as 24 hours after the administration of a single dose of ethambutol or as late as 90 days after starting continuous ethambutol therapy. However, most patients who ultimately showed a significant rise in

serum uric acid did so within the first three weeks of therapy. During the first five days of therapy a mean elevation in serum uric acid of 1 mg/100 ml was noted. Eight of nine randomly selected patients studied prospectively exhibited a rise in the serum urate concentration of 2.4 mg per 100 ml or greater 9 to 90 days after initiating ethambutol therapy. The exact mechanism responsible for this effect of ethambutol remains undefined but appears to be associated with a reduced renal clearance of uric acid (74).

24. This patient is female, obese, fifty years of age, and complains of right upper quadrant pain which began during the last gluttonous Thanksgiving holiday. Her symptoms and physical findings are probably more compatible with gallbladder disease than liver disease; therefore an oral Telepaque (iopanoic acid) cholecystogram is scheduled for the following morning. Considering the pharmacology of Telepaque, what special precautions should be initiated?

Gallbladder agents such as iopanoic acid (Telepaque) are usually administered as a single dose in the evening prior to the scheduled morning cholecystogram. Food is restricted from the patient until after the examination and it is likely that many patients limit fluid intake as well. In fact, directions for two of the currently used agents call for no fluid intake except small amounts of water for one, and nothing by mouth except ordinary amounts of water for the other (65). Furthermore, patients probably restrict fluids because of the gastrointestinal symptoms which accompany gallbladder disease or because of the nauseating side effects of the oral cholecystographic agents themselves. Since the gallbladder dyes are now known to be potent uricosuric agents (65,73), it is essential that the standard precautions taken with all uricosurics be instituted. This is particularly important because the peak uricosuric activity of iopanoic acid occurs at night when urines are acidic and concentrated.

A standard three gram dose of iopanoic acid (Telepaque) is a potent uricosuric comparable to two grams of probenecid. At these doses, Telepaque increases twenty-four hour urate excretion by 68% which is similar to the 60% obtainable with probenecid. Further comparisons show that Telepaque has a plasma half-life of 12-20 hours and increases the excretion of uric acid for 5-6 days (73). Probenecid has a plasma half-life of approximately 6-12 hours and has a duration of activity of approximately two days (62). The peak uricosuric activity of both drugs usually appears within three to seven hours (34,73).

This potent uricosuric activity of iopanoic acid (Telepaque) has several important clinical ramifications. Uricosuric agents can precipitate acute attacks of gout (47). Intrarenal precipitation of uric acid may result from the increased uricosuria. Usually these problems can be averted by merely increasing urine volume, alkalinizing the urine, and gradually increasing the dosage of the uricosuric agent. Increasing fluid intake does not affect absorption of the dye, nor does it affect its concentrations within the gallbladder.

As a further precaution, renal function tests should be monitored because nephrotoxicity has been reported after the administration of oral cholecystographic agents (18,88). Whether this renal failure is related to the uricosuric property of these agents is not yet known. Switching from Telepaque to another radiocontrast agent is not a reliable alternative because calcium ipodate (Orograffin), meglumine iodipamide (Cholografin), and sodium diatrizoate (Hypaque) also cause uricosuria (73).

25. A large number of diverse pharmacological agents other than probenecid and sulfinpyrazone possess varying degrees of uricosuric properties. Although most of these drugs are organic acids, they do not seem to share any other similarities either in chemical structure or in pharmacological properties. What are some of these medications?

Acetohexamide	Halofenate
Azauridine	Iopanoic acid
Benzbromarone	Meglumine
Calcium ipodate	iodipamide
Chlorprothixene	Out-dated
Citrate	tetracyclines
Clofibrate	Phenolsulfophthalein
Dicoumarol	Phenylbutazone
Estrogens	Phenindione
Ethylbiscoumacetate	Probenecid
Glycine	Salicylates
Glycopyrrolate	Sodium
Guaiphenesin	diatrizoate
	Sulfinpyrazone
	Tridihexethyl
	chloride
	Zoxazolamine

26. A 50-year-old white male with a long history of congestive heart failure is currently being treated with digoxin 0.25 mg/day, furosemide 40 mg/day, and KCl 20 mEq/day. A review of his laboratory data summary sheet shows a temporal relationship between the elevation of his serum urate values (from 5.2 to 8.8 mg/100 ml) and the initiation of furosemide therapy. Can ethacrynic acid or another diuretic be used instead?

Hyperuricemia is a commonly encountered side effect of thiazide diuretics but other diuretic agents including furosemide, ethacrynic acid, chlorthalidone, acetazolamide, and mercurial diuretics have been implicated (22,64,92,108). Hansten (37) reports that 40 to

50% of patients treated with thiazides ultimately have serum uric acid levels greater than 7 mg/100 ml. The precise mechanism of action of diuretics on urate transport is not yet known, but they seem to have a dual dose-dependent action much like that of the salicylates and phenylbutazone. The oral administration of thiazides over a long period of time is associated with uric acid retention; but rapid intravenous administration of chlorothiazide 500 mg results in uricosuria and 1.5 grams in divided doses results in urate retention (22).

Steele and Oppenheimer (92) demonstrated that diuretics do not affect urate transport directly but rather affect uric acid levels indirectly by inducing extracellular fluid volume contraction. Their studies with furosemide and ethacrynic acid substantiated the conclusions of other investigators working with thiazides that diuretic-induced hyperuricemia could be prevented if urinary salt and water losses were replaced. Their saline-replenished group, in contrast to the control group, did not exhibit diuretic-induced uric acid retention. They conclude that the mechanism for urate retention during diuretic-induced volume depletion may well be due to a redistribution of renal blood flow or to an action of intrarenally generated angiotensin (54a). Diuretic-induced hyperuricemia could also be due to a generalized increase in solute reabsorption secondary to volume contraction (109).

Although all the mechanisms of diuretic-induced hyperuricemia have not been fully elucidated, it is known that one mechanism involves extracellular fluid volume depletion. Therefore, any diuretic able to produce sufficient volume contraction has the potential to produce hyperuricemia. An exception is ticrynafen, a newly synthesized phenoxyacetic acid diuretic which is currently being studied (66a).

27. A 48-year-old post-menopausal waitress is seen in comprehensive clinic with mild complaints of headache, urinary urgency, dysuria, and pyuria. Her past medical history shows that she has mild hypertension and has had two acute attacks of gout in the past three years. Both her hypertension and gout are well controlled with allopurinol 100 mg tid, probenecid 500 mg tid, sodium bicarbonate 2 grams qid, and hydrochlorothiazide 50 mg bid. Urine cultures report moderate E. coli sensitive to all antibacterial agents tested. Her diagnosis is that of a mild recurrent urinary tract infection and her physician prescribes, in addition to her current medications, methenamine mandelate (Mandelamine) 1 gram qid, flurazepam (Dalmane) 30 mg hs prn sleep and propoxyphene 65 mg with APC (Darvon Compound-65) q 4 h prn headache. What are some of the problems presented by these new medications?

Methenamine mandelate has a fairly wide antibacterial spectrum which includes *E. coli*. However, methenamine's urinary antiseptic action depends on the liberation of formaldehyde which is formed from methenamine in an acid urine. It is of no value in cases where the urine is alkaline. Since she is ingesting eight grams of sodium bicarbonate daily to alkalinize her urine, the methenamine will be inactivated. Discontinuation of the sodium bicarbonate and acidifying the urine is not indicated since this action could precipitate the formation of renal uric acid stones.

In the choice of an alternate urinary antibacterial, ampicillin should not be considered. The Boston Collaborative Drug Surveillance Group (9) has reported that drug rashes were observed in 22.4% of 67 patients receiving the combination of ampicillin and allopurinol as compared to 7.5% of 1257 patients receiving only ampicillin and 2.1% of patients receiving only allopurinol. They suggested that the allergenicity of ampicillin may either be enhanced by allopurinol or perhaps the underlying hyperuricemia. The choice of a sulfonamide such as sulfisoxazole would be good and no significant drug interaction should result although probenecid has been reported to raise the plasma level of conjugated sulfa drugs (58). At the same time the alkalinization of the urine will decrease sulfonamide and probenecid plasma levels by promoting renal excretion. Therefore, a higher urinary concentration will be achieved (104). Probenecid also does not affect the elimination or blood levels of streptomycin, chloramphenicol, or the tetracyclines (34).

Flurazepam should not cause any problems but Darvon Compound-65 contains aspirin and should not be used. Pascale (63) has reported that two 300 mg tablets of aspirin every six hours can completely antagonize the uricosuric effects of two grams of probenecid. An explanation of this drug interaction is not yet available, but it probably involves several mechanisms. Renal tubular transport competition is probably the most logical explanation (113). Doses of salicylate which do not produce serum salicylate levels above 5 mg/100 ml do not appear to significantly affect probenecid uricosuria (37). Interestingly, salicylates do not affect the ability of probenecid to inhibit the tubular secretion of penicillin (12). Acetaminophen (Tylenol) does not interfere with probenecid and is a reliable alternative for antipyresis and mild analgesia in these patients (46).

28. Considering the mechanism of action of allopurinol, what are the indications for its use?

Xanthine oxidase is an essential enzyme that converts the more soluble acid precursors, hypoxanthine and xanthine, to uric acid. Allopurinol (Zyloprim) and its metabolite, oxypurinol, prevent the formation of uric acid by nature of their potent xanthine oxidase inhibiting properties.

Thus, allopurinol is especially useful in:

a. Patients with severe tophaceous gout.

b. Patients who are allergic or exhibit an intolerance to both uricosuric agents.

c. Gouty patients not controlled by uricosurics.

d. Patients who already have kidney stones or who show a marked predisposition to renal calculi formation.

e. Patients with advanced renal failure.

f. Patients with myeloproliferative disorders whose nucleic acid turnover is very high. This is particularly true when cytotoxic therapy is initiated.

g. Patients with high rates of urate excretion (greater than 1250 mg/24 hours), because uricosuric therapy can lead to renal lithiasis in these individuals.

29. What is the proper dose of allopurinol, and when should one start to see an effect?

The ability of allopurinol to lower serum uric acid is a dose-related phenomenon. The higher the dose of allopurinol, the greater the fall in serum uric acid levels. Generally, the dose required to normalize hyperuricemia in patients with mild disease is 200 to 300 mg/day and 400 to 600 mg/day in those with moderate or severe disease (79). Higher doses may be used, but most clinicians prefer to add a uricosuric to the allopurinol. Gutman and Yu (112), in testing the effectiveness of allopurinol in patients unable to use uricosurics, demonstrated that 300 mg of daily allopurinol adequately reduced the serum urate below 7 mg% in approximately 70% of patients and generally halved urinary uric acid. In the other 30% of their patients 400 to 600 mg/day was necessary; in some instances 200 mg/day sufficed. Actually, uric acid formation can be decreased as much as desired simply by adjusting the dosage of allopurinol. More than 1200 mg of allopurinol per day is not used because of the availability of uricosuric therapy and because there is no clinical advantage in maintaining the uric acid at zero.

Serum uric acid levels usually begin to fall within one to two days after initiation of allopurinol therapy; maximal uric acid suppression usually requires seven to ten days (79,113). Clinical improvement takes longer. After approximately six months one should observe a gradual decrease in size of established tophi and the absence of new tophaceous deposits.

30. Must allopurinol be given in divided doses?

Approximately 80% of an oral dose of allopurinol is rapidly absorbed when administered by the oral route. Once absorbed (30 minutes to two hours), allopurinol is rapidly cleared from plasma with a probable plasma half-life of less than two hours (24). A small portion of allopurinol is excreted in the urine unchanged but the remainder is rapidly oxidized to alloxanthine (oxypurinol). Oxypurinol is slowly eliminated from the blood by renal excretion, and has a prolonged plasma half-life of 18 to 44 hours in man (38). Neither oxypurinol or allopurinol is bound to plasma proteins and both are filtered at the glomerulus. However, oxypurinol, unlike allopurinol, then undergoes proximal tubular reabsorption.

Oxypurinol, too, is a potent inhibitor of xanthine oxidase, but is one-fifth to one-tenth as potent as allopurinol *in vitro. In vivo,* however, it accounts for much of allopurinol's xanthine oxidase inhibitory effects because of its prolonged half-life. Although it is probably less than 50% absorbed, oxypurinol is comparable to allopurinol in effectiveness when doses are adjusted (24). Nevertheless allopurinol is more consistent in its effects and lower doses are required than with oxypurinol probably because oxypurinol is erratically absorbed (38).

Due to oxypurinol's long half-life and its acknowledged xanthine oxidase inhibitory effects, allopurinol can be administered on a once daily basis. In fact, dosing with allopurinol on any dosing schedule results in the same steady effect within a few days (38). The daily administration of a single 300 mg tablet of allopurinol gives results identical in all parameters to 100 mg three times daily (78). Smaller doses should be used in patients with renal failure.

31. Several clinicians state that there is an increase in the number of acute gouty attacks during the early stages of allopurinol administration and have recommended that prophylactic colchicine be administered concomitantly. In addition, the manufacturer has suggested that allopurinol therapy be initiated with low doses and that it be gradually increased at weekly intervals. Is this adverse effect of allopurinol clinically significant?

Since allopurinol merely suppresses uric acid formation, it is hard to understand how it can cause an acute attack of gout. In fact, there is no substantial evidence that this phenomenon occurs. However, if one accepts the fact that there is a greater incidence of acute gouty attacks after starting uricosuric therapy, then one can speculate that any agent which lowers serum urate has the potential to precipitate an acute attack. Scott (83) hypothesizes that the solid urate tophus is in equilibrium with its surrounding tissue environment; as the urate concentration of the surrounding tissue environment falls, the solid urate crystals slowly dissolve. Since serum uric acid levels are not constant but fluctuate, the equilibrium can shift in the other direction and cause the formation of crystalline tophi. In this circumstance an acute attack can occur. However, it would seem that this equilibrium could shift at any time, not just during the early phases of allopurinol therapy.

While some clinicians feel that there is a slight tendency for exacerbation of symptoms during the first six weeks of allopurinol administration (44), others (79) are not at all convinced that the use of allopurinol increases the incidence of acute attacks. Allopurinol therapy should be initiated slowly, simply because nothing is lost by so doing. Patients generally have been gouty or hyperuricemic for a good many years before the diagnosis is first made. The extra week or two required to reach usual therapeutic doses of allopurinol should not make a difference. Furthermore, sudden changes in treatment should be avoided; if a patient is already on colchicine or a uricosuric, allopurinol should be added to the current drugs. If desired, the other medications can be tapered off after two to six weeks. Generally, colchicine prophylaxis is unnecessary when initiating allopurinol or uricosuric therapy, except in a few instances. Preventive colchicine should be used in patients with a history of frequent acute gouty attacks, in patients recovering from a recent gouty attack; and perhaps in patients started on a single 300 mg tablet of allopurinol. The decision to use colchicine prophylaxis should be based on the clinical circumstances of the individual patient.

31. A semi-comatose leukemic patient is to be started on chemotherapy. His physician wishes to know how to handle the increased uric acid load, considering the patient cannot swallow prophylactic medications.

There is at present no injectable preparation commercially available which effectively lowers urinary uric acid. Thus, alkalinization of urine with adequate fluid intake via the intravenous route is the only available alternative if a nasogastric tube is contraindicated. Recently, Burroughs Wellcome and Company in Tuckahoe, New York has been investigating an intravenous allopurinol monosodium salt with very good success. By following established hospital procedures for the use of new investigational drugs and by contacting Burroughs Wellcome, arrangements might be made for the intravenous use of allopurinol in this case.

Brown (14) in a limited study of sixteen patients reported that intravenous allopurinol can be administered with apparent safety and definite therapeutic effectiveness. The recommended dose for patients unable to take oral medications is 200 to 400 mg/M^2/24 hours. The total daily dose can be administered as divided doses or as a continuous twenty-four hour infusion. It is important to initiate allopurinol therapy before antileukemic therapy is begun. As noted previously, serum uric acid levels are generally not affected for 1 to 2 days and maximal uric acid suppression generally requires 7 to 10 days (79,113). In one series of 16 patients, allopurinol therapy that was started concomitantly with chemotherapy was not effective in preventing either further increases in uric acid levels or acute renal failure (45).

If mercaptopurine (Purinethol) or azathioprine (Imuran) are used, clinicians should be aware that these drugs are also metabolized by xanthine oxidase. Thus the dosage of these drugs should be decreased to as little as one-third or one-fourth the usual dosage when allopurinol is administered concomitantly (81).

33. Mrs. L.N. is a 70-year-old black female with a ten-day history of fever, chills and non-productive cough. A rash, described as a generalized erythematous, pruritic, maculopapular dermatitis with desquamation, began on her lower extremities about two weeks prior to admission. She denies any previous history of asthma, hay fever, or other allergies. Her past medical history included a 15-year history of hypertension. She has been treated with hydrocholorothiazide for three years and has been on digoxin 0.125 mg/day for the past year because of dyspnea on exertion and rales. Allopurinol 100 mg tid was started six weeks ago for uric acid levels of 9-11mg%. Significant laboratory findings upon admission include the following: SGOT 250 U; alkaline phosphatase 195 U; serum creatinine 2.8 mg/100 ml, BUN 50 mg/100 ml, and an eosinophilia of 15%. Drug-induced disease is to be ruled out. Allopurinol is the only medication recently started; describe the nature and characteristics of allopurinol hypersensitivity reactions.

Allopurinol is exceptionally well tolerated with no severe dose-related adverse reactions of any major magnitude (81). Doses up to 1200 mg have been administered without untoward effects (80). Of the adverse drug reactions that are sometimes encountered with allopurinol, hypersensitivity-type reactions have been the most notorious. These generally present as mildly erythematous, purpuric, or maculopapular skin rashes which subside within a few days after the medication is discontinued (107). The rash most commonly occurs in patients with impaired renal function and is generally accompanied by fever, malaise, and aching. It often appears within one to five weeks of therapy and is frequently preceded by pruritus. However, the rash has appeared as part of a delayed hypersensitivity reaction as late as three months in one case and twenty-five months in another (80).

More severe hypersensitivity reactions have also been associated with allopurinol. One fatal case of generalized maculopapular exfoliative dermatitis with severe systemic allergic vasculitis has been reported (40). Another allopurinol-induced fatality has been attributed to toxic epidermal necrolysis with oliguria, sepsis and pneumonia (42). Two non-fatal cases of allopurinol hypersensitivity angiitis were characterized by pruritic dermatitis and renal failure three to five weeks after initiation of therapy (63). Five additional cases (10,109a) have been reported, making a total of nine reported cases of severe hypersensitivity reactions to allopurinol.

All nine cases shared similar characteristics. The onset of illness occurred about four weeks after initiation of therapy, and began with fever and pruritus or dermatitis. Variable hepatic impairment was present in all cases, although the predominant features were exfoliating dermatitis and renal failure. The dermatitis and renal failure were attributed to a systemic vasculitis and the non-fatal cases did not improve until large steroid doses were instituted despite immediate discontinuation of allopurinol. Furthermore, it has been hypothesized that the variable nature of the liver toxicity may indicate that it is not part of the picture of systemic vasculitis, but may well represent a separate immunological reaction to allopurinol (10). Seven of the above nine cases of allopurinol vasculitis were accompanied by eosinophilia and all exhibited fever, dermatitis, and renal impairment. Severe hypersensitivity reactions to allopurinol may also occur more commonly in patients with renal impairment, although in the majority of cases, renal dysfunction is the result of, rather than the cause of these reactions.

34. S.R. is a 50-year-old male who enters General Hospital with complaints of malaise, anorexia, low grade fever and right upper quadrant pain. Physical examination revealed a jaundiced male with an enlarged tender liver and spider angiomas. Significant laboratory abnormalities include the following: SGOT 345 U; SGPT 80 U; bilirubin (total) 4.0 mg/100 ml; BUN 40 mg/100 ml. His only medication is allopurinol. Has allopurinol-induced hepatotoxicity been reported?

A thorough literature survey indicates that unexplained abnormal liver function tests and hepatomegaly have been associated with allopurinol therapy. Blechman and co-workers (8) reported a case of marked hepatomegaly, documented by a liver scan and irregularity in the uptake of radioactive gold, in a 36-year-old male treated with 200 mg of allopurinol per day. This patient developed a localized rash, which later subsided without discontinuing therapy. Alkaline phosphatase, bilirubin, SGOT, thymol turbidity and cephalin flocculation tests were within normal limits. Ogryzlo and co-workers (67), in a study of the metabolic and clinical effects of allopurinol in 80 subjects, noted small transitory elevations of SGOT and SGPT and occasional traces of urinary urobilinogen. These liver enzymes were not persistently elevated and were noted to coincide with alcohol intake in the patients concerned. Mikkelsen (61) reported transient elevations of SGOT in four patients and a persistent SGOT elevation of 86-144 units in one patient without any other abnormal liver function tests. Scott (83) reported a slight rise in alkaline phosphatase and an abnormal retention of BSP in 14 of the 20 patients he studied; however, a high incidence of abnormal liver function tests was also noted in his control group. Other investigators (33,106,113) have reported similar transient abnormalities in liver function tests in patients receiving allopurinol therapy.

Lidsky and Sharp (52) observed intrahepatic obstructive jaundice in two patients receiving 600 and 900 mg of allopurinol daily for three weeks. Both of these patients had renal impairment with creatinine clearances of 32 and 51 ml/min respectively. A liver biopsy of one of these patients disclosed "periportal inflammatory infiltrates containing eosinophils." The liver abnormalities disappeared after the allopurinol was discontinued. Readministration of allopurinol at one-half the dose to one of these patients two years

after the episode of jaundice did not produce evidence of liver dysfunction. In three other patients with renal disease, Lidsky and Sharp (52) reported abnormal liver enzymes without evidence of jaundice. They concluded that there is an increased susceptibility to the hepatotoxic effects of allopurinol in patients with renal insufficiency. In the reports of allopurinol allergic vasculitis by Jarzobski (40), Kantor (42), and Mills (63), liver dysfunction was noted as part of the generalized multiple systems degeneration. Liver biopsies in those instances showed fibrinoid necrosis and pleomorphic infiltrates with eosinophilia. Thus, hepatoxicity can result from allopurinol therapy.

More recently, Butler and associates describe a case of massive hepatic necrosis in a patient receiving allopurinol (15). Additionally, Chawla reports yet another case and reviews the literature as well (20).

Addendum: Excellent new guidelines for the management of asymptomatic hyperuricemia became available after this chapter had been typeset. (Ann Intern Med 88:666, 1978.)

REFERENCES

1. Abeles M et al: Acute gouty arthritis — the diagnostic importance of aspirating more than one involved joint. JAMA 238:2526, 1977.
2. Al-Hujal M et al: Hyperuricemia and levodopa. NEJM 285-859, 1971.
3. American Hospital Formulary Service: Monograph on sodium bicarbonate, Section 40:08. American Society of Hospital Pharmacists, Washington, D.C., 1973.
4. Anon: Drugs for gout. Med Lett 18:49, 1976.
5. Anturane Reinfarction Trial Research Group: Sulfinpyrazone in the prevention of cardiac death after myocardial infarction. NEJM 298:289, 1978.
6. Band PR et al: Xanthine nephropathy in a patient with lymphosarcoma treated with allopurinol. NEJM 283:354, 1970.
7. Berger L et al: Renal function in gout. Am J Med 59:605, 1975.
8. Blechman WJ et al: Use of allopurinol in gout, hyperuricemia, and uric acid lithiasis. South Med J 60:215, 1967.
9. Boston Collaborative Drug Surveillance Program: Excess of ampicillin rashes associated with allopurinol or hyperuricemia. NEJM 286:505, 1972.
10. Boyer TD et al: Allopurinol — hypersensitivity vasculitis and liver damage. West J Med 126:143, 1977.
11. Boyett JD et al: Allopurinol and iron metabolism in man. Blood 32:460, 1968.
12. Brazeau P: Inhibitors of tubular transport of organic compounds. Chap. 41 in *The Pharmacological Basis of Therapeutics*, 5th ed., edited by LS Goodman and A Gilman. Macmillan Co. N.Y., 1975, pp.860-866.
13. Bremner WF et al: Colchicine and testicular function in man. NEJM 294:1384, 1976.
14. Brown CH et al: Clinical efficacy and lack of toxicity of allopurinol given intravenously. Ca Chemother Rep 54:125, 1970.
15. Butler RC et al: Massive hepatic necrosis in a patient receiving allopurinol. JAMA 237:473, 1977.
16. Calkins E: The treatment of gout. Rational Drug Ther 5:1, 1971.
17. Campion DS et al: Binding of urate by serum proteins. Arthr Rheum 18(Suppl): 747, 1975.
18. Canales CO et al: Acute renal failure after the administration of iopanoic acid as a cholecystographic agent. NEJM 281:89, 1969.
19. Cawein MJ et al: False rise in serum uric acid after L-dopa. NEJM 281:1489, 1969.
20. Chawla CK et al: Allopurinol hepatoxicity — case report and literature review. Arthr Rheum 20:1546, 1977.
21. Davis PS et al: Effect of a xanthine oxidase inhibitor (allopurinol) on radioiron absorption in man. Lancet 2:470, 1966.
22. Demartini FE: Hyperuricemia induced by drugs. Arthritis Rheum 8:823, 1965.
23. Diamond HS et al: Effect of urine flow rate on uric acid excretion in man. Arthr Rheum 15:338, 1972.
24. Elion GB: Enzymatic and metabolic studies with allopurinol. Ann Rheum Dis 25:608, 1966.
25. Emmerson BT: Hyperuricemia — To treat or not? Drugs 9:141, 1975.
26. Emmerson BT et al: Haemosiderosis associated with xanthine oxidase inhibition. Lancet 1:239, 1966.
27. Fessel WJ: Asymptomatic hyperuricemia in gout: A clinical comprehensive. Ed. by AB Gutman. Prepared by MEDCOM for Burroughs Wellcome Co, Research Triangle Park, North Carolina, 1971.
28. Fox IH et al: Depletion of erythrocyte phosphoribosylpyrophosphate in man. NEJM 283:1177, 1970.
29. Franck WA et al: Ibuprofen in acute polyarticular gout. Arthr Rheum 19:269, 1976.
30. Goldfinger SE: Colchicine for familial Mediterranean fever. NEJM 287:1302, 1972.
31. Goldfinger SE: Drug therapy: treatment of gout. NEJM 285:1303, 1971.
32. Gutman AB: The past four decades of progress in the knowledge of gout, with an assessment of the present status. Arthr Rheum 16:431, 1973.
33. Gutman AB: Treatment of primary gout: the present status. Arthr Rheum 8:911, 1965.
34. Gutman AB: Uricosuric drugs with special reference to probenecid and sulfinpyrazone. Adv Pharmacol 4:91, 1966.
35. Hadler NM et al: Acute polyarticular gout. Am J Med 56:715, 1974.
36. Hall AP et al: Epidemiology of gout and hyperuricemia. Am J Med 42:27, 1967.
37. Hansten PD: *Drug Interactions*. 3rd ed. Philadelphia, Lea and Febiger, 1975, p. 315, and p. 380.
38. Hitchings GH: Pharmacology of allopurinol. Arthr Rheum 18(Suppl):863, 1975.
39. Honda H et al: Gout while receiving levodopa for parkinsonism. JAMA 219:55, 1972.
40. Jarzobski J et al: Vasculitis with allopurinol therapy. Am Heart J 79:116, 1970.
41. Jonas S: Hyperuricemia and levodopa. NEJM 285:1488, 1971.
42. Kantor GL: Toxic epidermal necrolysis, azotemia, and death

after allopurinol therapy. JAMA 212:478, 1970.

43. Kelley WN: Hypouricemia. Arthr Rheum 18(Suppl):731, 1975.

44. Kersley GD: Treatment of gout. Ann Rheum Dis 25:353, 1966.

45. Kjellstrand CM et al: Hyperuricemic acute renal failure. Arch Intern Med 133:349, 1974.

46. Klinenberg JR: Current concepts of hyperuricemia and gout. Calif Med 110:231, 1969.

47. Klinenberg JR: Hyperuricemia and gout. Med Clin N Amer 61:299, 1977.

48. Klinenberg JR et al: Renal function abnormalities in patients with asymptomatic hyperuricemia. Arthr Rheum 18(Suppl):725, 1975.

49. Klinenberg JR et al: Urate deposition disease. Ann Intern Med 78:99, 1973.

50. Kowal CD: Gouty arthritis and colchicine. NEJM 291:681, 1974.

51. Lesch M et al: Familial disorder or uric acid metabolism and central nervous system function. Am J Med 36:561, 1964.

52. Lidsky MD et al: Jaundice with the use of 4-hydroxy-pyrazalo (3,4-d) pyrimidine (4-HPP). From Proceedings of the Annual Meeting of the American Rheumatism Association, June 15-16, 1967, New York (Abstract) as published in Arthritis Rheum 10:294, 1967.

53. Loebl WY et al: Withdrawal of allopurinol in patients with gout. Ann Rheum Dis 33:304, 1974.

54. Malawista SE: The action of colchicine in acute gouty arthritis. Arthr Rheum 18(Suppl):835, 1975.

54a. Manuel MA et al: Changes in urate handling after prolonged thiazide treatment. Am J Med 57:741, 1974.

55. Martindale W: *Extra Pharmacopoeia* (ed by RG Todd). 25th ed. The Pharmaceutical Press, London, 1967, p. 1142.

56. Mazur A et al: Relation of uric acid metabolism to release of iron from hepatic ferritin. J Biol Chem 227:653, 1957.

57. McCoombs RP: Systemic allergic vasculitis. JAMA 194:157, 1965.

58. Merck, Sharp and Dohme: Benemid — Manufacturer's Product Information, West Point, PA, 1972.

59. Merlin HE: Azoospermia caused by colchicine: a case report. Fertil Steril 23:180, 1972.

60. Meyler L et al: *Side Effects of Drugs.* Vol 6, Williams and Wilkins, Baltimore, 1968, p. 116, 449, 500.

61. Mikkelsen WM et al: The effects of allopurinol on serum and urinary uric acid. Arch Intern Med 118:224, 1966.

62. Mikkelsen WM et al: Physiological and biochemical basis for the treatment of gout and hyperuricemia. Med Clin N Amer 53:1331, 1969.

63. Mills RM: Severe hypersensitivity reactions associated with allopurinol. JAMA 216:799, 1971.

64. Moser RH: *Diseases of Medical Progress:* A Study of Iatrogenic Disease. 3rd ed. Charles C. Thomas, Springfield, IL, 1969, p. 123.

65. Mudge GH: Uricosuric action of cholecystographic agents. NEJM 284:931, 1971.

66. Naidus RM et al: Colchicine toxicity. Arch Intern Med 137-394, 1977.

66a. Nemati M et al: Clinical study of ticrynafen. JAMA 237:652, 1977.

67. Ogryzlo MA et al: The treatment of gout and disorders of uric acid metabolism with allopurinol. Can Med Assoc J 95:1120, 1966.

68. Ortel RW et al: Acute gouty arthritis and response to colchicine in the virtual absence of synovial fluid leukocytes. NEJM 290:1363, 1974.

69. Osol A et al: *The United States Dispensatory.* 27th ed. JB Lippincott Co, Philadelphia, 1973, p. 333.

70. Paladine WJ: Gout and levodopa. NEJM 286:376, 1972.

71. Pascale LR et al: Therapeutic value of probenecid in gout. JAMA 149:1188, 1952.

72. Poffenbarger PL et al: Colchicine for familial Mediterranean fever: possible adverse effects. NEJM 290:56, 1974.

73. Postlewaite AE et al: Uricosuric effect of radiocontrast agents. Ann Intern Med 74:845, 1971.

74. Postlewaite AE et al: Studies on the mechanism of ethambutol-induced hyperuricemia. Arthr Rheum 15:403, 1972.

75. Rastegar A et al: The physiologic approach to hyperuricemia. NEJM 286:470, 1972.

76. Relman AS: New job for an old drug. NEJM 298:333, 1978.

77. Robinson WD et al: The present status of colchicine and uricosuric agents in management of primary gout: and discussion. Arthr Rheum 8:865, 1965.

78. Rodnan GP et al: Allopurinol and gouty hyperuricemia. JAMA 231:1143, 1975.

79. Rundles RW et al: Allopurinol in the treatment of gout. Ann Intern Med 64:229, 1966.

80. Rundels RW: Metabolic effects of allopurinol and alloxanthine. Ann Rheum Dis 25:615, 1966.

81. Rundles RW et al: Drugs and uric acid. Ann Rev Pharmacol 9:345, 1969.

82. Schumacher R et al: Acute gouty arthritis without crystals identified on initial examination of synovial fluid. Arthr Rheum 18(Suppl):603, 1975. .

83. Scott JT et al: Allopurinol in the treatment of gout: a comparative trial of allopurinol against uricosuric treatment. Br Med J 2:321, 1966.

84. Seegmiller JE et al: An enzyme defect associated with the sex-linked human neurological disorder and excessive purine synthesis. Science 155:1682, 1967.

85. Seegmiller JE et al: Biochemistry of uric acid and its relation to gout. NEJM 268:712, 1963.

86. Seegmiller JE: Directions and prospects for future research on gout. Arthr Rheum 18(Suppl):883, 1975.

87. Seegmiller JE: The acute attack of gouty arthritis. Arthr Rheum 8:714, 1965.

88. Setter JC et al: Acute renal failure following cholecystography. JAMA 184:102, 1963.

89. Smith LH jr: Disorders of purine metabolism. In Cecil-Loeb *Textbook of Medicine,* ed by PB Beeson and W McDermott, 14th ed. WB Saunders, Philadelphia, 1975, p. 1647-1660.

90. Smith MJV: Placebo versus allopurinol for renal calculi. J Urology 117:690, 1977.

91. Smyth CJ: Disorders associated with hyperuricemia. Arthr Rheum 18(Suppl):713, 1975.

92. Steele TH et al: Factors affecting urate excretion following diuretic administration in man. Am J Med 47:564, 1969.

93. Steele TH: Control of uric acid excretion. NEJM 284:1193, 1971.

94. Steele TH: Renal excretion of uric acid. Arthr Rheum 18(Suppl):793, 1975.

95. Sturge RA et al: Multicentre trial of naproxen and phenylbutazone in acute gout. Ann Rheum Dis 36:80, 1977.

96. Talbott JH: Clinical experiences. Arthr Rheum 18(Suppl):663, 1975.

97. Talbott JH: *Gout.* 3rd ed. Grune and Stratton, New York, 1967, pp. 216, 256.

98. Vesell ES et al: Impairment of drug metabolism in man by allopurinol and nortriptyline. NEJM 283:1484, 1970.

99. Wallace S: Colchicine: clinical pharmacology in acute gouty arthritis. Am J Med 30:439, 1961.

100. Wallace SL: Colchicine and new anti-inflammatory drugs for the treatment of acute gout. Arthr Rheum 18(Suppl):847, 1975.

101. Wallace S et al: Colchicine plasma levels: implications as to pharmacology and mechanism of action. Am J Med 48:443, 1970.

102. Wallace SL: Gouty arthritis and colchicine. NEJM 291:681, 1974.

103. Wanasukapunt S et al: Effect of fenoprofen calcium on acute gouty arthritis. Arthr Rheum 19:933, 1976.

104. Weinstein L: The sulfonamides, Ch 56 in *The Pharmacological Basis of Therapeutics,* ed by LS Goodman and A Gilman, 5th ed, Macmillan, New York, 1975, p. 1113-1179.

105. Wilkens RF et al: The treatment of acute gout with naproxen. J Clin Pharmacol 15(Part 2):363, 1975.

106. Wilson JD et al: Allopurinol in the treatment of uremic patients with gout. Ann Rheum Dis 26:136, 1967.

107. Woodbury DM et al: Analgesics — antipyretics, anti-inflammatory agents, and drugs employed in the therapy of gout. In *The Pharmacological Basis of Therapeutics,* ed by LS Goodman and A Gilman, 5th ed. Macmillan, New York, 1975.

108. Wyngaarden JB: Gout and other disorders of uric acid metabolism. In *Harrison's Principles of Internal Medicine,* ed by MM Wintrobe et al, 8th ed, McGraw Hill, New York, 1977, pp. 642-651.

109. Wyngaarden JB: Diuretics and hyperuricemia. NEJM 283:1170, 1970.

109a. Young JL jr et al: Severe allopurinol hypersensitivity. Arch Intern Med 134:553, 1974.

110. Yu TF et al: Efficacy of colchicine prophylaxis in gout. Ann Intern Med 55:179, 1961.

111. Yu TF: Milestones in the treatment of gout. Am J Med 56:676, 1974.
112. Yu TF et al: Mutual suppression of the uricosuric effects of sulfinpyrazone and salicylate: a study in interactions between drugs. J Clin Invest 42:1330, 1963.
113. Yu TF et al: Effect of allopurinol (4-hydroxypyrazolo-(3,4-d) pyrimidine) on serum and urinary uric acid in primary and secondary gout. Am J Med 37:885, 1964.
114. Yu TF et al: Uric acid nephrolithiasis. Ann Intern Med 67:1133, 1967.
115. Yu TF et al: Principles of current management of primary gout. Am J Med Sci 144:893, 1967.

Chapter 23

Rheumatoid Arthritis

Brian S. Katcher

In the United States, arthritis affects about 20 million persons, and one in four families is affected. Although rheumatoid arthritis occurs less frequently than osteoarthritis, which is primarily a disease of age, it is more serious because it is potentially crippling. About one-fourth of those with arthritis have rheumatoid arthritis. Women are affected about three times more often than men. Although the disease most often occurs after the third decade of life, it can occur at any age and children are frequently affected (5,127).

Rheumatoid arthritis is a chronic systemic disease of unknown etiology which primarily affects the joints. Exacerbations and remissions occur throughout the course of this disease, which tends to be progressive. Aspirin and other drugs are employed to reduce inflammation and hence reduce the risk of joint damage. In some cases, the course of the disease is so rapidly progressive that more toxic drugs such as gold are employed in an attempt to arrest its progress. However, rheumatoid arthritis is generally not a life-threatening disease, and the potential for drug toxicity must always be considered in this light. Nevertheless, early treatment can prevent the crippling which might otherwise occur.

CASE A – EARLY ACUTE RHEUMATOID ARTHRITIS: T.W. is a previously healthy 42-year-old, 55 kg, woman who has been suffering increasingly from morning stiffness which persists for several hours, generalized muscle and joint pain, anorexia, and fatigue during the past four months. Her symptoms have been much worse during the past month and a half. Both hands are swollen and she no longer is able to wear her wedding ring. Pain in both hands and feet, as well as extreme general fatigue, have forced her to limit her activities. Physical examination revealed symmetrical swelling, tenderness, and heat of the metacarpophalangeal, proximal interphalangeal, and the metatarsalphalangeal joints. Pertinent laboratory findings included: erythrocyte sedimentation rate by Westergren method 52 mm/hr (normal less than 15 mm/hr); hemoglobin 10.6 gm% (normal 12 to 16 gm%); hematocrit 34% (normal 36 to 47%); albumin 3.8 gm/100 ml (normal 4.3 to 5.6 gm/100 ml); serum uric acid 3.0 mg% (normal 2-8 mg%); and latex fixation for rheumatoid factor was positive in a dilution of 1:320. Tests for lupus erythematosus (LE), antinuclear antibodies (ANA), and tuberculin sensitivity were negative. X-ray films of the hands and feet showed soft tissue swelling with no evidence of tophi or calcification. Other routine laboratory data and physical findings were normal.

1. What signs and symptoms of rheumatoid arthritis are manifested by this patient?

The presentation of rheumatoid arthritis is quite variable making it difficult to differentiate between it and a variety of other rheumatoid diseases (106,127). However, all of the signs and symptoms noted in T.W. are prominent features of rheumatoid arthritis (5,127). Symptoms of fatigue, anorexia, and morning stiffness usually precede localized joint involvement. About half of the patients with rheumatoid arthritis initially experience fatigue which later in the disease serves as a reliable index of disease activity (238). Morning stiffness usually lasts more than an hour before the patient "limbers up" and may last most of the day. Stiffness may also occur after any prolonged period of inactivity such as sitting in a chair (127). Duration of morning stiffness is also a reliable index of disease activity. Additionally, generalized muscle weakness and pain are prominent; grip strength is usually substantially weakened.

Bilateral swelling and pain of the small joints of the hands and feet most commonly occur, although wrists, knees, shoulders, hips, ankles, and the cervical spine are also frequently affected. Significant deformities may be present. This is a disease of the joints, but extra-articular manifestations are frequently seen. These range from harmless but characteristic subcutaneous rheumatoid nodules, which appear below the elbows in 25% of patients, to involvement of virtually any organ system. Rarely, these extra-articular manifestations can be life-threatening, as in rheumatoid vasculitis (5,127).

The laboratory findings in rheumatoid arthritis are those of a chronic inflammatory disease. There is no truly specific test for the disease. T.W.'s elevated erythrocyte sedimentation rate (ESR) is a nonspecific indication of inflammation. Her mild anemia is typical of chronic disease. Serum iron concentrations are decreased, but iron binding capacity is normal; binding capacity will be increased if she should subsequently develop a blood-loss iron deficiency anemia due to aspirin or other drug therapy. The degree of anemia correlates with the activity of the disease; it is refractory to iron therapy and is thought to be due to failure of iron release from reticuloendothelial tissues and excessive uptake by the liver (5,127,273).

Serum albumin is often low as illustrated by this patient. Although low serum albumin could theoretically result in decreased protein binding of salicylates and result in higher free (and therefore active) drug serum levels (176), this does not usually occur (80,90), because the degree of hypoalbuminemia is generally mild. However, this potential disease-drug interaction should be considered; it may be even more important with drugs like phenylbutazone, indomethacin, fenoprofen, or naproxen which are more highly protein bound than salicylate (131).

Rheumatoid factor, a macroglobulin which reacts with IgG to form an immune complex, is found in the sera of 80% of patients with rheumatoid arthritis. However, the presence of rheumatoid factor is not pathognomonic, because it does not appear in some patients with rheumatoid arthritis, high titers may occur in other disease states, and healthy individuals may have rheumatoid factor in their sera. Rheumatoid factor does not parallel disease activity, but high titers early in the course of the disease indicate a graver prognosis (65,127,172,209,235,273). The LE preparation and test for antinuclear antibodies were performed to rule out systemic lupus erythematosus, but it should be noted that both these tests may be positive in as many as 15% of patients with rheumatoid arthritis (127).

Many of these clinical and laboratory features of rheumatoid arthritis are useful parameters for monitoring disease activity and its response to therapy. These and others are listed in Table 1.

2. A diagnosis of rheumatoid arthritis is made. How should T.W. be treated?

The primary treatment objectives are reduction of inflammation and pain, preservation of function, and prevention of deformity. A conservative approach of aspirin, rest, and physical therapy is the safest and most effective means of achieving these objectives (62,63).

Aspirin given in large doses, as discussed in sub-

Table 1

USEFUL PARAMETERS FOR ASSESSING DISEASE ACTIVITY AND DRUG RESPONSE IN RHEUMATOID ARTHRITIS

Digital joint swelling (measured with a ring sizer)
Duration of morning stiffness (hours)
Erythrocyte sedimentation rate
Grip strength (in mm Hg as determined by squeezing a folded sphygmomanometer)
Number of painful joints
Number of tender joints
Number of swollen joints
Time until onset of fatigue (hours)
Time to walk 50 feet (seconds)

sequent questions, is one of the mainstays of therapy, but nondrug means should be employed concurrently. Systemic rest reduces inflammation, and articular rest achieved by splinting the affected joints may produce dramatic results (238). A comparison of complete bed confinement with ad lib activity in hospitalized patients demonstrated that absolute bed rest is unnecessary. However, most of the patients in this study benefited from hospitalization, probably due to a reduction of physical and emotional stresses and regular physical and salicylate therapy (177). Therefore, a liberal rest program should be prescribed for T.W. If an adequate rest program cannot be carried out at home, several weeks of hospitalization should be considered.

Since active exercise increases inflammation, passive exercises should be utilized for T.W. until her acute inflammation subsides; this will prevent muscle atrophy and flexion contractures. The inflammatory process requires higher than normal temperatures within the joint space. The external application of heat, which might be achieved by soaking her hands and feet in warm water, increases blood flow to the joint and cools it, thereby reducing inflammation and pain. Several heat applications per day of approximately 15 minutes each are more effective than a single longer treatment. An effective approach would be to prescribe heat and exercise treatments three times a day after meals and at bedtime after taking the prescribed doses of aspirin tablets (76).

Finally, emotional support in the form of open communication should take place. As many as 50% of patients experience their first symptoms after a severe emotional stress such as death of a loved one, sickness in the family, divorce, or change in jobs (127). Disability from the disease may cause further emotional problems (272). Therefore, it is important that some time be spent with the patient and her family to insure that treatment has an optimal effect.

3. T.W., who weighs 55 kg, is to begin taking aspirin 5 grains, three tablets four times a day (3.6 gm daily)

with heat applications and sufficient rest. Is this an appropriate dose of aspirin?

Although a large number of aspirin tablets must be ingested each day in order to achieve an anti-inflammatory effect, the required dose varies considerably among individuals. Individual differences in metabolic capacity seem to account for these differences (55,74,90,92). Serum concentrations of salicylate of 15 to 30 mg/100 ml are considered therapeutic.

A wide range of plateau serum levels is achieved with 65 mg/kg/day, the dose that has been prescribed for T.W. Plasma salicylate levels ranging from 5 to 28 mg/100 ml were observed among nine patients with rheumatoid arthritis who received this dose for three days (194). Similarly, a range of 12 to 35 mg/100 ml was observed among 26 healthy individuals after three days of this regimen (74). When a mixed group of patients with backache and rheumatoid arthritis were given this dosage, a similar range, from 13 to 29 mg/100 ml, was reported. The disease state did not appear to affect the final salicylate level achieved, despite differences in albumin concentrations (80). Therefore, T.W. will be taking an aspirin dose which is likely to result in anti-inflammatory blood levels. However, a serum salicylate determination at her next visit is necessary to confirm this, and further dosage adjustment will probably be required.

A reasonable initial dose of aspirin can also be based upon doses that have been proven effective in clinical trials of aspirin in patients with rheumatoid arthritis. Two studies demonstrated a daily aspirin dose of 5.2 gm to be more effective than either 2.6 gm or placebo in reduction of the duration of morning stiffness, delay in the onset of fatigue, increase in grip strength, decrease in ESR, decrease in joint swelling or tenderness, and patient preference. The 2.6 gm per day dose and the placebo preparation were not significantly different from one another (21a,27). However, a daily aspirin dose of 3.6 gm is more effective than placebo as judged by similar criteria for anti-inflammatory effect (185). Therefore, this beginning dose of aspirin may be effective for T.W. After several days, serum salicylate will reach a plateau, and improvement should be noted at that time (also, see Question 5).

4. What instructions should accompany this patient's aspirin prescription?

First, this patient should appreciate the important role that large regularly taken doses of aspirin play in the treatment of rheumatoid arthritis. In addition to providing substantial analgesia, large doses of aspirin are anti-inflammatory. When anti-inflammatory doses of aspirin are replaced with large oral doses of meperidine, codeine, or propoxyphene, patients experience a marked increase in symptoms. Fatigue and

stiffness become severe, finger joint size is increased, range of motion is decreased, and grip strength is decreased (70). The daily ingestion of large amounts of aspirin is commonly approached with considerable skepticism unless the patient receives some explanation and encouragement.

Gastric intolerance is the major limitation to the successful use of large doses of aspirin (16) and may take the form of epigastric distress or painless bleeding (270). Small amounts of blood loss occur with each aspirin dose, but individuals vary as to the amount of blood which is lost (140). Although continual aspirin use may eventually lead to a blood-loss anemia in some patients, major gastrointestinal bleeding from aspirin is a rare occurrence (114a, 114b, 133a, 148a). The gastric effects of aspirin can be minimized by concurrent ingestion of food; a full glass of water, or better, a cup of warm nonirritating beverage; and/or with antacids. Food seems to prevent the epigastric discomfort and sour eructations sometimes caused by aspirin (106). Adequate liquid and antacids facilitate the dissolution of aspirin; undissolved aspirin particles on the gastric mucosa are responsible for gastric blood loss (139) and gastric upset. If repeated therapeutic doses of antacids are required, their effect on urinary pH must be considered (see Question 7). The gastrointestinal effects of aspirin are discussed in the chapters on *Peptic Ulcer Disease* and *General Care: Pain*.

Aspirin is hydrolyzed to salicylic and acetic acids in the presence of moisture, so the container should be closed tightly and not be stored in the bathroom. Although childproof safety closures are required on aspirin containers and are effective in reducing accidental ingestion (232), many arthritic patients are unable to cope with these safety closures. Tight grasp and pressure on the lateral sides of the fingers encourages ulnar deviation, a deformity in which the fingers are shifted toward the little finger side of the hand. Excessive thumb pressure contributes to dislocation of thumb joints in patients with rheumatoid arthritis. Also, it is likely that this patient's grip strength is diminished. The greater the diameter of the bottle top, the easier it will be to open and close. To prevent deformities, she should be encouraged to use the palm of her hand in performing this task (7). If aspirin is dispensed in a conventional closure container, it is necessary to explain the hazards of accidental ingestion by children and to obtain a signed release form. (Also see the chapter on *Poisonings*.)

5. Four days later T.W.'s serum salicylate level was 17 mg/100 ml and her symptoms were marginally improved. How rapidly can the aspirin dose be increased? Discuss high-dose salicylate kinetics.

In the smaller doses used for analgesia, salicylate has a half-life of about 2½ hours (216). However, when aspirin is taken in the large daily doses used for anti-inflammatory effect, two of the five major pathways of elimination become saturated, and serum salicylate levels accumulate over several days to plateau levels far in excess of those achieved with smaller doses (75,143,144). Presently, T.W.'s salicylate levels have approached steady state, but another three or four days will be required until a new plateau is reached with an increased dose. Consequently, dosage changes should be made only after waiting periods of several days.

After ingestion, aspirin is rapidly hydrolyzed to salicylate. Salicylate is eliminated from the body by direct renal excretion and by biotransformation to salicyluric acid (capacity limited), salicyl phenolic glucuronide (capacity limited), salicyl acyl glucuronide, and gentistic acid with subsequent renal excretion (144). This is depicted in Fig. 1. The pharmacokinetics of anti-inflammatory doses of salicylate are therefore complex. Salicylate kinetics follow parallel first order and Michaelis-Mentin elimination processes. These processes have been characterized in computer simulations and appear to demonstrate a nonlinear relationship between dose and steady state levels (143,144). Accordingly, an increase in the daily dose would be expected to result in a more than proportionate increase in the plateau level of salicylate (144). However, even the original report of these accumulation effects alludes to the fact that increases in the apparent volume of distribution with increasing doses may compensate for the accumulation kinetics described by these computer simulations (144). Subsequent work eventually confirmed this dose-dependent change in the volume of distribution (145). More recently, it was demonstrated that total salicylate clearance remains constant throughout the therapeutic range of 15 to 30 mg/100 ml, because not only metabolism, but also plasma protein binding becomes saturated, and with increasing dose an increasing fraction of unbound drug compensates for decreasing unbound clearance by presenting more free drug to the liver and kidneys. This apparently stable total clearance allows prediction of appropriate dose increments with reference to steady state levels attained with initial doses (75). Therefore, if T.W.'s dose is increased from three tablets four times a day (3.6 gm or 65 mg/kg daily) to four tablets four times a day (4.8 gm or 87 mg/kg daily), the steady state level will be increased proportionately, and a level of approximately 23 mg/100 ml can be anticipated. Although dosage increments can be calculated, it is important that blood levels be used to monitor dosing and that the patient be cautioned to reduce the dosage at signs of tinnitus, because these recommendations are based on results obtained from a limited number of subjects.

These recommendations differ from some texts which describe salicylate accumulation kinetics without adequate consideration of the dose-dependent effects of changes in the volume of distribution. These texts warn that huge increases in serum concentrations may be attained with small increases in daily dose. A report of two patients who experienced a 300% increase in salicylate levels three days after their daily dose was increased from 65 mg/kg to 100 mg/kg is often cited in support of this point (194). However, both of these patients had initial serum concentrations below 15 mg/100 ml; therefore, they may not have achieved sufficient levels for enzyme saturation and the subsequent two- or three-fold decrease in clearance which occurs in higher dose salicylate kinetics. Also, urinary pH may have shifted in these patients, and this is an important determinant of serum salicylate level (see Question 7). Others have observed what seemed initially to be capacity-limited kinetics, only to later find that they were seeing the effects of antacids on urinary pH (269). Furthermore, a more recent comparison of these two doses demonstrated serum level increases roughly proportionate to the dose increase in four patients whose initial levels were within the therapeutic range of 15 to 30 mg/100 ml (80). These and other reports (74,75,145), suggest that after an initial decrease in clearance due to saturable metabolism, the combined effects of dose-dependent volume of distribution and dose-dependent metabolism offset one another so that total clearance remains relatively constant within the therapeutic anti-inflammatory range. Therefore, dosage increments result in linearly proportional increases in serum salicylate levels.

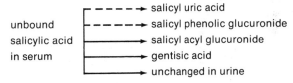

Fig. 1. Changes in salicylate kinetics with increased dose. The dotted lines indicate processes that become saturated. Protein binding is also dose-dependent; therefore, a more than proportionate increase in unbound drug in the serum occurs with any increase in dose. With anti-inflammatory doses, urinary excretion becomes relatively more important as a route of elimination.

6. Could tinnitus, rather than blood levels, be used as an endpoint for salicylate dosing for T.W.? Discuss the relative merits of each approach.

Gradually increasing the daily dose of aspirin to the point of tinnitus, a ringing or high-pitched buzzing sensation in the head, and then cutting back slightly by a couple of tablets a day is a time-honored technique which clinically results in maximal anti-inflammatory activity (16,70). A study of salicylate-induced tinnitus in 67 patients and 7 healthy volunteers demonstrated this symptom to be a useful therapeutic endpoint in those with normal hearing (180). As might be expected (see Question 3), the number of tablets required per day varied widely, but those who noted tinnitus did so at an average serum salicylate level of 29.5 mg/100 ml, and no patient experienced tinnitus at a serum level less than 19.6 mg/100 ml. Thus, when tinnitus occurs one can be confident that therapeutic serum levels are present. However, the 15 subjects in this study who had pre-existing hearing loss failed to experience tinnitus even though their serum levels ranged from 31 to 68 mg/100 ml. Thus, patients with known pre-existing hearing loss, and older subjects who may have undetected hearing loss, should have serum salicylate levels determined as a guide to therapy (180).

Tinnitus is followed by bilateral hearing loss as serum levels approach 30 mg/100 ml, and this hearing loss becomes progressively greater with higher levels until it plateaus at serum levels of about 50 mg/100 ml (180,186). Both symptoms are completely reversible (186).

Therefore, if T.W. has good hearing, tinnitus can be used as a therapeutic endpoint. However, serum salicylate levels are preferred over tinnitus as guides to dosing. First, noncompliance as well as factors other than dosing (see Question 7) may affect blood levels, and serum salicylate levels provide a precise way of monitoring for these effects. The results of an undetected fall in serum salicylate levels might otherwise be attributed to worsening of the disease state and taken as an indication of the need for treatment with more toxic drugs (115). Furthermore, salicylate-induced hepatotoxicity, which fortunately occurs infrequently, is apparently dose-related; if the patient can be successfully maintained at serum levels less than 25 mg/100 ml, the risk of hepatotoxicity is reduced (123). (Also see the chapter on *Diseases of the Liver.*)

7. After several weeks of treatment with excellent results, T.W. experienced tinnitus on the day of a scheduled clinic visit. A serum salicylate was ordered and reported as 32 mg/100 ml. Previously, her serum salicylate levels were about 25 mg/100 ml. The only change in her treatment had been a recent discontinuation of the antacid (Maalox) she was taking with each aspirin dose. Explain this increase in her serum salicylate. How can this problem be avoided in the future?

When aspirin is used in anti-inflammatory doses, the renal excretion of unchanged salicylate becomes an important elimination pathway (see Question 5 and Fig. 1), and the renal excretion of salicylate is highly pH-dependent (142,143). Both sodium bicarbonate and the supposedly "nonsystemic" antacids are ca-

pable of increasing urinary pH and thereby increasing salicylate excretion. When sodium bicarbonate 4 gm daily was administered to 13 subjects, urinary pH increased from a range of 5.6 to 6.1 to a range of 6.2 to 6.9 and the average serum salicylate level fell from 27 mg/100 ml to 15 mg/100 ml (142). Similarly, regular therapeutic doses of magnesium and aluminum hydroxides (Maalox) resulted in appreciable increases in urinary pH and decreases in serum salicylate concentrations ranging from 30 to 70% in a group of pediatric patients. In this study, aspirin absorption was not impaired by the antacid (146). Daily administration of Maalox 15 ml qid increases the average urinary pH approximately 0.7 to 0.9 units after several days of therapy; an equivalent fall in urinary pH is noted within two days after discontinuation of the antacid (14, 78, 79). Levy and Leonards point out that a decrease in urinary pH from 6.5 to 5.5 in a patient whose serum salicylate is within the therapeutic range of 20 to 30 mg/100 ml would cause a doubling of the serum salicylate with resulting toxicity (142). Consequently, T.W.'s discontinuation of her Maalox may have resulted in a more acidic urine which would explain her current tinnitus and high salicylate level. This illustrates the importance of not altering regular treatment with therapeutic doses of antacid without simultaneous adjustment of aspirin dosage.

If she is able to tolerate aspirin without an antacid, the aspirin dose can be lowered. Serum salicylate levels should then be obtained to ensure adequacy of therapy. She should take her aspirin with plenty of fluid to promote its dissolution, and thereby decrease irritation and reduce gastrointestinal blood loss. Occasional large doses of Maalox will not substantially alter urinary pH (14), nor will smaller doses such as a teaspoonful qid (79). Other antacids such as calcium carbonate (Titralac) may also raise urinary pH, although to a lesser degree (78).

Because urinary pH is such an important determinant of salicylate blood levels, it has been suggested that these patients monitor their urine with pH paper (142). Urinary pH follows a circadian pattern which is not changed by antacids but is shifted to a more basic range. Because of this circadian pattern, pH determinations should be compared with those made at the same time of day (14).

8. T.W. is scheduled to have an impacted wisdom tooth removed. Will her aspirin therapy interfere with this procedure?

Aspirin prolongs bleeding time and should therefore be discontinued about a week before the procedure (270). Several mechanisms may be responsible. First, low doses of aspirin impair platelet aggregation by irreversible acetylation; this accounts for prolonged bleeding times for several days after a single dose

(270). Second, both aspirin and sodium salicylate appear to increase blood fibrinolytic activity (181,182). Finally, near-toxic doses of salicylates induce a hypoprothrombinemia which is reversible by vitamin K (270). Salicylate-induced hypoprothrombinemia is usually not clinically significant, but on rare occasions it can be the cause of bleeding when associated with severe liver dysfunction or malnutrition (82).

A study comparing the effects of aspirin and acetaminophen on the post-operative course after extraction of impacted wisdom teeth demonstrated significantly more bleeding with aspirin. This study involved 32 subjects, each of whom had bilaterally impacted wisdom teeth that were removed separately so each patient received aspirin once and acetaminophen once (236). Furthermore, bleeding that could not be completely arrested after dental surgery has been attributed to aspirin (47). T.W. should not resume taking aspirin until her gums have begun to heal. Since sodium salicylate has no effect on platelets, and this is probably the major cause of increased bleeding time, it would be a good alternative drug during this period of time.

9. Aspirin is ordered for a patient who was recently hospitalized for evaluation and treatment of his rheumatoid arthritis. The medication profile in the pharmacy indicates that this patient is allergic to aspirin. What should be done?

The patient should be asked to describe his reaction to aspirin. Most patients who claim to be allergic to aspirin merely suffer from *gastrointestinal distress,* which is not an allergic reaction. In these patients, aspirin can be safely administered with plenty of fluid, with food, or if necessary, with an antacid.

On the other hand, *aspirin intolerance in association with asthma* is cause for serious concern. Challenge with aspirin in these patients may initiate an explosive asthmatic reaction which can be fatal (223). Asthma, rhinorrhea, and nasal polyps usually accompany this type of aspirin intolerance. About 2 to 4% of asthmatics will exhibit aspirin intolerance (1,271). These patients experience a high degree of cross-reactivity to other chemicals, including indomethacin (Indocin), naproxen (Naprosyn), ibuprofen (Motrin), fenoprofen (Nalfon), mefenamic acid (Ponstel), sodium benzoate (a widely used preservative), tartrazine (a dye, FD&C No. 5, which is widely used in foods and drugs), and other substances (1, 208, 223, 246, 250, 251, 261). However, sodium and choline salicylate have been administered to aspirin-sensitive patients without untoward reactions (223). It appears that any drug which is an effective inhibitor of prostaglandin synthesis will elicit this reaction (250, 251, 261).

Some patients develop *urticaria* upon exposure to aspirin. This reaction is apparently different from the one described above because there is no cross-reactivity with other analgesics or chemicals. However, there is cross-reactivity with sodium salicylate, indicating that the salicylate radical is responsible (1).

10. The patient with the alleged aspirin-allergy described above avoids aspirin because it has upset his stomach in the past. However, he often uses Excedrin, a proprietary aspirin-containing combination product, for analgesia. Should his rheumatoid arthritis be treated with aspirin or a less irritating form of salicylate? Briefly describe these other forms of salicylate.

The treatment of rheumatoid arthritis should be initiated with aspirin. Each dose of aspirin should be taken with a full glass of water to promote dissolution of the tablets and thereby reduce or prevent irritation. If needed, antacids may be added, although their effect on urinary pH and therefore on blood levels must be considered (see Question 7).

Aspirin is more potent than other salicylates as an anti-inflammatory agent (35). Although aspirin is rapidly hydrolyzed to salicylate (216,270), and salicylate is responsible for a substantial portion of the overall anti-inflammatory effect, aspirin levels persist for a somewhat longer period of time in the joint fluid than in the blood (242,243). The salicylates exert their anti-inflammatory effect by a number of mechanisms, but inhibition of prostaglandin synthesis, perhaps by acetylation of the enzyme prostaglandin synthetase, may be the most important factor in their action (176). Acetylation of prostaglandin synthetase is accomplished by aspirin but not salicylate. In animal studies, aspirin is a more potent inhibitor of prostaglandin synthesis than sodium salicylate (260). Therefore, it is not surprising that patients frequently find that their morning stiffness is decreased by taking aspirin an hour or so before arising, even though their blood salicylate is at therapeutic levels when they take this dose. Moreover, nearly all of the clinical research demonstrating the effectiveness of salicylates has been done with aspirin; therefore, other forms of salicylate cannot be assumed to be equal in effectiveness without further clinical trials. Finally, aspirin is more readily available and less expensive than other forms of salicylate.

Choline salicylate (Arthropan Liquid) may be tried in those who cannot tolerate the gastrointestinal effects of aspirin. It is less irritating, but consultants to the Medical Letter point out that there is little evidence that it is as effective as aspirin (9).

Buffered aspirin solutions such as Alka-Seltzer cause minimal gastrointestinal upset, but they are unsuitable for the treatment of rheumatoid arthritis since their buffering will result in an appreciable rise in urinary pH. Furthermore, Alka-Seltzer contains more than a gram of sodium for each 10 grains of aspirin (8,9).

Buffered aspirin tablets dissolve more rapidly than conventional aspirin tablets and thereby cause less gastrointestinal blood loss and perhaps less upset (139). However, the amount of buffering agent in commercially available tablets is small and the advantage is not great. (Also see chapter on *Peptic Ulcer Disease.*)

Tablets of **aspirin in combination with other drugs** should not be used in the treatment of rheumatoid arthritis. APC is a widely used analgesic combination which contains aspirin, phenacetin, and caffeine. Phenacetin lacks anti-inflammatory effect and repeated doses may cause papillary necrosis (see chapter on *Adverse Effects of Drugs on the Kidney*); caffeine is of no therapeutic benefit (270). This man has been taking Excedrin (aspirin, caffeine, salicylamide, and acetaminophen) for analgesia. Salicylamide is ineffective, and acetaminophen lacks anti-inflammatory activity (270).

Most **enteric coated aspirin** tablets are unreliably absorbed (107,134,138,141), although a Canadian preparation with reliable absorption characteristics has been described (29,30).

11. A 28-year-old woman with rheumatoid arthritis has recently become pregnant and is concerned about the possible effects of aspirin on her baby. Has her uninterrupted consumption of aspirin since conception placed the fetus at risk? How should her rheumatoid arthritis be managed during her pregnancy? Comment on the effects of aspirin late in pregnancy.

A prospective study of more than 50,000 pregnancies revealed similar malformation rates among children whose mothers had been intermediately or heavily exposed to aspirin and those whose mothers had not been exposed to aspirin during the first four months of pregnancy (237). Lack of teratogenicity was also noted in the babies of 144 mothers who had used salicylates heavily throughout pregnancy (256). Therefore, it appears unlikely that aspirin is teratogenic.

About three-quarters of women with rheumatoid arthritis undergo a temporary remission during pregnancy. Relief generally occurs during the first trimester and persists more than a month into the postpartum period (198). If this woman does not experience relief, she may safely continue taking aspirin during the first and second trimesters, but aspirin may have adverse effects later in pregnancy as discussed below. The effects of other anti-inflammatory drugs on the fetus are either unknown or adverse. (Also see the chapter on *Glucocorticoids.*)

Although a prospective study of 41,000 pregnancies did not detect any effect of maternal aspirin consumption on perinatal mortality or birthweight (229), others have noted an increase in perinatal mortality and decreased birthweight associated with maternal consumption of aspirin (256). The association noted in the latter study was probably due to its more careful patient selection involving maternal urine screens for salicylate and also the fact that all the women in this study continued to take aspirin every week until delivery (37).

The exact mechanism by which aspirin apparently causes a greater incidence of stillbirths is unknown, but it may be related to its anti-prostaglandin effect which could cause **closure of the ductus of arteriosus in utero.** The ductus arteriosus is normally open in utero and closes at birth. It allows run-off into the aorta of most of the fetal right ventricular stroke volume, allowing the high resistance pulmonary vascular bed to be bypassed. Closure in utero results in pulmonary hypertension with poor perfusion to the brain, liver, kidney, and other areas. The detrimental effects of aspirin-induced closure of the ductus arteriosus in utero have been produced experimentally in lambs (101) and have been implicated in at least one human birth (11). This effect has been used to therapeutic advantage in premature infants who required closure of the ductus arteriosus (100). It should be noted that all of the nonsterioidal anti-inflammatory drugs are prostaglandin inhibitors (261); therefore, all of them are probably capable of causing closure of the ductus arteriosus in utero. Furthermore, aspirin-induced **coagulation defects** may also contribute to the higher stillbirth rate and clearly place the mother at greater risk of hemmorhage (36,37). (Also see Question 8.) Finally, **fetal and neonatal salicylate pharmacokinetics** should be considered. Because of greater protein binding in the fetus, neonatal salicylate concentrations are about 1.5 times higher than those in the mother (77,147), and newborns eliminate salicylates more slowly than adults (77). Consequently, aspirin should be avoided during the final stages of pregnancy.

12. A 58-year-old man with rheumatoid arthritis has been taking aspirin 4.6 gm (14 tablets) daily for 18 months with good control of his symptoms. He recently read about a relatively new group of drugs, the proprionic acid derivatives, which are supposedly as effective as aspirin, less irritating to the stomach than aspirin, and more convenient in that fewer tablets are needed. Comment.

Naproxen (Naprosyn), fenoprofen (Nalfon), and ibuprofen (Motrin) are proprionic acid derivatives that have recently been marketed in the U.S. They are representative of a larger series of compounds, others of which are available abroad; fenbufen and ketoprofen are currently undergoing extensive investigation in this country. Tolmetin (Tolectin) is another new drug which is more closely related to indomethacin but shares many properties with the proprionic acid derivatives (41,150). Double-blind controlled clinical trials comparing naproxen, fenoprofen, or ibuprofen with aspirin in rheumatoid arthritis have shown these drugs to be as effective or nearly as effective as aspirin while causing fewer side effects (2, 19, 22, 54, 72, 103, 104, 112, 113). However, these studies generally lack good regulation of aspirin dosage. For example, after completion of a multi-center double-blind study comparing aspirin and naproxen in 80 patients, it was concluded that naproxen was as effective as aspirin, but significantly fewer side effects were observed with naproxen (22). However, it was later observed that many of the side effects observed with aspirin were signs of salicylism; salicylate levels were not monitored because titration of aspirin dosage on the basis of salicylate levels would have unblinded the study (23). Other studies have used a fixed dosage of aspirin that was probably too low for some patients. All anti-inflammatory drugs have ulcerogenic properties (270), but these drugs cause significantly less microbleeding than does aspirin (44, 94, 154, 160, 164, 211, 218). Furthermore, they cause less gastritis, so compliance is more likely. In summary, the proprionic acid derivatives approach aspirin in effectiveness, but none of them is superior to aspirin. The incidence of gastritis and degree of microbleeding is less, but as with aspirin, there is a small but real risk of gastric hemorrhage.

Thus, these drugs should be viewed as effective alternatives to aspirin. However, in patients such as this man who is asking about them, aspirin remains the drug of choice. He is apparently able to tolerate aspirin, and it has produced the desired results. For others, who are unable to tolerate aspirin, these drugs are the next best choice. Several double-blind crossover trials comparing indomethacin, which is sometimes tried in those who cannot or will not take aspirin, with naproxen demonstrated that naproxen is equal in efficacy to indomethacin, but naproxen causes substantially fewer side effects (32,132,249).

13. The patient in the previous question would like to try one of the proprionic acid derivatives in place of aspirin, and his physician agrees to such a trial. Which one should be used?

Only two cross-over trials have compared these drugs with each other (113,210). In both studies naproxen was most effective and ibuprofen was least effective. Fenoprofen was second most effective in both studies and was more effective than ketoprofen. Naproxen also caused the least number of side effects in both studies. Thus, on the basis of efficacy and side effects, naproxen must be regarded as the first choice among these drugs. It has the additional advantage of

a long half-life which allows bid dosing rather than the tid or qid dosing which is required with its congeners. In fact, it was recently demonstrated that naproxen can be administered in a single daily dose of 500 mg at bedtime (32). However, individuals appear to vary in their response to these drugs; thus, naproxen can only tentatively be suggested as the best choice (113,150).

14. Naproxen was ordered for the patient who was described above. His symptoms were well controlled for about eight months until he had a relapse (generalized synovitis) and was restarted on aspirin. At that time he observed that although his inflammation had returned, he was not experiencing a great deal of pain. Comment.

The proprionic acid derivatives are potent analgesics. When naproxen 400 mg was compared with a combination of aspirin 323 mg plus codeine 30 mg in a double-blind crossover study of 62 patients with pain after dental surgery, naproxen was slightly more effective (221). Other trials have also demonstrated the effectiveness and prolonged duration of analgesia provided by naproxen (20,165,220). Like aspirin, these drugs have analgesic properties at lower doses and anti-inflammatory properties at higher doses. For example, ibuprofen has anti-inflammatory activity at 2400 mg/day, but at 1200 mg/day it provides analgesia without anti-inflammatory activity (81). In this case, the anti-inflammatory effect of full doses of naproxen was not adequate; therefore, aspirin therapy was resumed. If needed, both drugs can be given together (268).

15. Because of its hematological toxicity, most clinicians limit their use of phenylbutazone to brief courses of medication for acute arthritic flares. How does phenylbutazone affect blood elements?

Blood dyscrasias are the most frequently reported serious adverse reactions among patients receiving phenylbutazone or oxyphenbutazone (45). Of 1,276 reports of adverse reactions to phenylbutazone reported to the United Kingdom Committee on Safety of Medicines, 398 were blood disorders and 205 of these were fatal (45). Leukopenia, agranulocytosis, thrombocytopenia, and aplastic anemia have been observed, and many fatalities, most often from aplastic anemia or agranulocytosis, have been reported (45,108,170,171,207). One literature review of 3934 patients at risk determined that 32 of these patients (0.15%) developed agranulocytosis (170). Therefore, because of hematological complications, as well as severe gastrointestinal effects, edema, toxic hepatitis and other side effects, it is recommended that phenylbutazone be limited to short-term therapy of not more than a week during any one treatment period (270).

16. A patient with congestive heart failure treated with digitoxin 0.2 mg/day, furosemide 40 mg/day and

supplemental potassium recently experienced a flare of her arthritic pain after a fall. She now presents with a prescription for one week of treatment with phenylbutazone. Comment.

Phenylbutazone should be used only with the greatest of caution in this patient since cardiac decompensation and pulmonary edema are recognized adverse reactions to phenylbutazone therapy (270). Despite warnings in the manufacturer's package insert and several published cases, many clinicians do not appreciate the sodium and fluid retaining properties of this drug. Nevertheless, frank edema may occur during the first two weeks of therapy in 10% of patients, and this is generally more apparent in those with pre-existing cardiac disease (176). In some cases, plasma volume may increase by as much as 50% (227). The exact mechanism of this edema formation is unknown, but it appears to involve an increased renal tubular reabsorption of sodium and may be mediated by the hypothalamus.

An additional factor to consider is that phenylbutazone is a potent inducer of hepatic microsomal enzymes. The limited data available suggest that a dramatic fall in digitoxin blood levels may occur with concomitant administration of phenylbutazone (242). Although not established, the possibility of this drug interaction should be considered. Therefore, this patient should be observed closely for signs of underdigitalization or phenylbutazone-induced fluid retention.

CASE B – PROGRESSIVE RHEUMATOID ARTHRITIS: A 52-year-old woman with rheumatoid arthritis has been treated with rest, heat, and anti-inflammatory doses of aspirin for eight months, but her disease has continued to progress as evidenced by more extensive joint involvement and worsening of her constitutional symptoms. Increasing ankle pain is forcing her to consider seeking employment which would require her to spend less time on her feet; inflammation and pain in her hands is particularly severe and is approaching the same level experienced before treatment. Additionally, she is suffering from dry eyes and mouth.

X-ray examination revealed soft tissue swelling of the feet and hands, narrowing of joint spaces, and erosions of the second and third metacarpophalangeal joints bilaterally. Abnormal laboratory data included rheumatoid factor in a dilution of 1:1280, an ESR of 65 mm/hr, a hemoglobin of 9.8 gm%, a hematocrit of 31%, and a serum albumin of 3.8 gm/100 ml. Her serum salicylate level was 22 mg/100 ml.

At this point, it is decided to begin her on gold while continuing her basic conservative treatment.

17. Comment on the choice of gold for this woman. Compare gold with other drugs which might have been used to arrest the progress of her disease. What sort of response can be expected?

The majority of patients with rheumatoid arthritis can be managed with conservative therapy; however, some will continue to have progressive disease which will require more aggressive treatment with more toxic drugs. In spite of their potency, glucocorticoids do not seem to alter the natural history of rheumatoid arthritis (58). However, in addition to suppressing joint inflammation (49,59,60,69), gold favorably alters the natural history of the disease. Radiologic examinations in controlled studies demonstrate that progression of the disease is significantly slowed or halted (161,162,233). Therefore, most rheumatologists would consider using gold in a situation like the one described above.

Possible alternatives to gold might include an antimalarial, which is less likely to be effective in inducing a remission (56), or penicillamine, cyclophosphamide, or azathioprine. Although the use of the latter three drugs in rheumatoid arthritis is still experimental at the time of this writing, they are currently being used by many rheumatologists. Recent comparisons of gold with these drugs confirm its major role in the treatment of early progressive rheumatoid arthritis (43,56,91,111).

Dwosh et al (56) compared the efficacy of weekly injections of gold 50 mg with chloroquine 250 mg po hs and azathioprine 1 to 2 mg/kg/day po; treatments were randomly assigned among 33 patients. After 24 weeks all treatments were equally effective, but there was marginally less improvement with chloroquine. Because of the long-term risks of azathioprine, particularly the increased risks of malignancy and opportunistic infection, the authors concluded that gold was the treatment of first choice in progressive disease unresponsive to salicylates alone (56). In a six month comparison of gold and penicillamine in 86 patients, both drugs produced a similar response, but more side effects were caused by penicillamine (111). Also, 12 of 14 gold withdrawals in this trial were due to rash; more recent experience suggests that patients with gold-induced rash can resume gold therapy after resolution of their rash (Question 23). In a less detailed report summarizing several years experience with gold, penicillamine, and cyclophosphamide in 171 patients, it was concluded that the highest number of complete remissions was obtained with gold (91). Although excellent response was obtained with cyclophosphamide, these clinicians disapproved of its use because of fears of malignancy. Therefore, they used a more aggressive approach toward the employment of gold which was restarted in patients with rash and the dose increased in unresponsive patients. Currey et al

(43) compared gold 50 mg per week with azathioprine 2.5 mg/kg/day and cyclophosphamide 1.5 mg/kg/day in early progressive rheumatoid arthritis. Although results with all three drugs were similar, cyclophosphamide being marginally the most effective, concern for the long-term hazards of immunosuppressant drugs led to their conclusion that azathioprine and cyclophosphamide should be considered as useful alternatives to gold in early progressive rheumatoid arthritis if risks prove acceptable (also see Question 28). In summary, gold is more effective than anitmalarials, equal to penicillamine and azathioprine, and slightly less effective than cyclophosphamide.

Because of its potential for toxicity, gold should not be employed in mild disease (87). However, it is most likely to be effective when it is employed early in the course of progressive disease (40,71,87,162). In one series of 57 gold-treated patients who were followed over five to six years, there was a clear correlation between an early start of gold therapy and the arrest of joint erosions. The greatest success in halting the progression of the disease was obtained in those in whom gold was initiated within 10 months after the onset of rheumatoid arthritis (162).

Age, sex, or the presence or absence of rheumatoid factor or antinuclear antibodies do not significantly alter the response to gold (87). Gold should be added to, rather than replace, basic conservative management (63,70). It has been demonstrated that gold adds substantially to the response obtained from aspirin or fenoprofen (46). Response to gold generally requires several months (56,60,71). Improvement in such parameters as joint count, duration of morning stiffness, time to walk 50 feet, grip strength, hemoglobin, hematocrit, ESR, albumin, and rheumatoid factor can be expected, although toxicity may supervene or the patient may remain unresponsive.

18. Comment on this woman's complaint of dry eyes and dry mouth. Will this alter her response to gold?

These symptoms are suggestive of Sjögren's syndrome, a chronic inflammatory disease of the salivary, lacrimal and other glands. It is associated with a variety of connective tissue diseases and occurs in about 10 to 15% of those with rheumatoid arthritis. The treatment is generally symptomatic (127). It is significant in this case because it has been listed in textbooks (71) and in the manufacturers' literature as a contraindication to gold therapy. Evidently, this proscription is based on a widely quoted but poorly controlled study which demonstrated a high incidence of gold toxicity in a small number of patients with Sjögren's syndrome. However, a review of 101 gold-treated patients, 41 of whom had Sjögren's syndrome, revealed that no such predilection exists. In fact, patients with Sjögren's syndrome appeared to tolerate gold treatment better than those without the syndrome (83). This finding is important, because Sjögren's syndrome is not an infrequent occurrence, and these patients constitute a population who are likely to benefit from treatment with gold.

19. Which gold preparation should be used for this woman?

There are two gold preparations in wide use: gold sodium thiomalate (Myochrysine) and aurothioglucose (Solganol). Gold sodium thiomalate is an aqueous solution, while aurothioglucose is an oil suspension. Each contains approximately 50% gold; dosages are expressed as milligrams of the salt.

It has been generally held that both gold compounds are equally effective and equally toxic (87). However, several recent reports provide justification for choosing aurothioglucose in preference to gold sodium thiomalate (86,93,135,215). First, **vasomotor reactions** which usually manifest as nausea, weakness, flushing, or fainting occur in as many as 5% of patients receiving gold sodium thiomalate solution; the reactions are generally mild and transient, but two cases of myocardial infarction caused by this vasomotor reaction have been reported (86,96). The etiology is unknown but may involve the vehicle or preservative. It does not occur with aurothioglucose. Although myocardial injury secondary to this vasomotor reaction is extremely rare, it has been suggested that elderly patients with concomitant cardiovascular disease receive only aurothioglucose when gold is indicated (86). Secondly, nonvasomotor reactions consisting of **transient stiffness, arthralgias, and myalgias** were reported in 15 of 100 patients after injections of gold sodium thiomalate; these reactions decreased in severity or disappeared when aurothioglucose was substituted (93). Thirdly, in another series of 125 patients receiving either aqueous solution or oil suspension of gold salts, there was a significantly higher incidence of **skin eruptions, stomatitis, and albuminuria** among those receiving the aqueous solution (135). This finding of fewer side effects with aurothioglucose suspension has also been observed by others (215). Finally, two groups of investigators have observed a significantly **higher percentage of improvement** with aurothioglucose (135,215). Therefore, the slow release of aurothioglucose from its oil suspension appears to confer upon it the advantages of less toxicity and greater efficacy. An oral gold compound is currently under investigation (67).

20. What dosage schedule should be employed for the initiation of this woman's gold therapy? Should serum gold levels be used as a guide to therapy?

The standard treatment schedule consists of 50 mg

weekly, after initial 10 and 25 mg test doses. Injections are given into the gluteal muscles each week until either the total dose reaches one gram, or toxicity or major clinical improvement supervenes. After one gram, if the response has been satisfactory, maintenance doses of 50 mg every other week for two to 20 weeks are advised, advancing subsequently to every third week and then every fourth week for an indefinite period of time (71,87).

Variations of this standard treatment regimen have recently been subjected to controlled clinical trials. Increasing the weekly dose by 250% (33) or increasing it to 1 mg/kg (215) appears to offer no advantage. Brief reports of other studies employing larger than standard doses also describe no therapeutic advantage, and toxicity is generally more frequent (87,88). A preliminary report on a double-blind trial comparing a 10 mg weekly dose with the usual 50 mg dose suggests that this smaller dose may be equally effective (173). In another trial, a 25 mg weekly dose was compared with more than twice as much gold in a flexible dosage schedule aimed at producing serum levels between 300 and 400 mcg%; there was no difference in response or toxicity (230). Further evidence is needed to confirm the efficacy of these lower doses of gold.

Although atomic absorption spectroscopy can be applied for the clinical evaluation of serum gold levels (51,156), results have been generally discouraging. Some have claimed that response is related to optimal levels which require higher than conventional doses in some patients (133,157); however, this has not been confirmed by retrospective (121,219) and prospective (230) studies. Furthermore, the presence or absence of toxicity cannot be correlated with serum gold levels (121,169,219).

Thus, the standard treatment schedule described above should be used for this woman.

21. How should gold therapy be monitored for toxicity?

Patients receiving weekly gold injections should have a weekly urinalysis and frequent complete blood counts — at least every other week. In addition, the patient should be interviewed each week prior to the injection to detect the occurrence of pruritis, skin eruption, purpura, sore throat, metallic taste, indigestion, or other symptoms of possible toxicity (71,120).

(a) *Cutaneous reactions:* Dermatological reactions are by far the most common forms of gold toxicity. Pruritis is usually the first symptom. A metallic taste may precede or accompany painful ulcers in the mouth (120). Erythema or a fine morbiliform rash on the neck or extremities may occur after the first few injections. This reaction usually disappears within several days, and subsequent injections may be tolerated. Dermatitis often occurs after 300 mg of gold has

been given. A common form is a highly pruritic localized eruption resembling pityriasis rosea. However, gold dermatitis may assume many different forms, so any eruption, especially if it is pruritic, should be considered suspect. Exposure to sunlight may worsen the dermatitis. Exfoliative dermatitis from gold toxicity occurs very rarely, but the risk must be considered (71,87). Therapy should be stopped if dermatitis occurs, but it can eventually be reintroduced in a reduced dosage schedule when the rash has cleared (see Question 23).

(b) *Urinalysis:* Mild and transient albuminuria may occur during gold treatment, but therapy can be continued without serious problems (71,102,120). However, any increase indicates a possible gold nephropathy; in such cases gold should be discontinued. Although transient proteinuria occurs in 3 to 10% of the patients treated, the nephrotic syndrome is infrequent (87). (Also see the chapter on *Adverse Effects of Drugs on the Kidney*.)

(c) *Blood count:* Leukopenia below 4000 WBC/mm^3, a rapid reduction of hemoglobin, decrease in platelets below 75,000/mm^3, or eosinophilia may be considered indications of potential toxicity (71). However, patients with Felty's syndrome, a complex of rheumatoid arthritis, splenomegaly, and leukopenia, can be started on gold therapy in spite of their initially low white blood count; their blood picture can revert to normal with successful treatment (58,89). Eosinophilia greater than 800/mm^3 often precedes or accompanies dermatological reactions (87,120). It should be noted, however, that eosinophilia can also be a manifestation of rheumatoid arthritis (71).

Thrombocytopenia is a life-threatening reaction to gold. It is difficult to treat because of the long half-life of gold and because gold deposits in many areas of the body. A number of cases of gold-induced thrombocytopenia have responded successfully to treatment with steroids, dimercaprol (BAL), and transfusion of platelets (28,61). Other cases have responded to splenectomy and immunosuppressants (28). Penicillamine is an inefficient chelator of gold and should therefore not be used in the treatment of gold toxicity (48). Substantial removal of gold by peritoneal dialysis has been reported; more study of this technique is needed (38).

Careful monitoring of gold therapy and appropriate management of toxicity have substantially reduced the risks inherent in this mode of therapy. The estimated mortality rate from gold toxicity is less than 0.4% (71,87).

22. When it is explained to the woman described in case B that it will probably take several months before any effect can be expected from her gold shots, she asks for additional medication to control her

pain and inflammation. Which of the many anti-inflammatory and analgesic drugs available would be most appropriate?

First, she should continue taking *aspirin* since she is apparently able to tolerate it well and she currently has anti-inflammatory salicylate levels. Other medication should be added to her current regimen. None of the anti-inflammatory drugs which might be added is superior to aspirin. Their addition to aspirin may provide the immediate relief which is desired, but the chance of gastrointestinal toxicity from combined oral anti-inflammatory drug therapy is probably increased.

Corticosteroids would probably not be a good choice in this situation, because it has been suggested that they may dampen the efficacy of gold treatment (58,87). Furthermore, corticosteroids appear to decrease salicylate levels, although this combination is frequently used (90,95). This interaction was previously attributed to increased renal excretion; however, subsequent work suggests that corticosteroids induce the metabolism of salicylate (58). More importantly, less toxic drugs are available.

Likewise, *phenylbutazone* is also too toxic to be considered in this situation which may require treatment for several months. Furthermore, phenylbutazone should not be administered with gold since the risks of hematological disorders are additive. Also, rash is a frequent side effect of phenylbutazone (153), and should rash or blood dyscrasia occur while both gold and phenylbutazone are being administered, it would be difficult to identify the offending agent (87).

Indomethacin can be given with gold, but its interaction with aspirin should receive careful consideration. A number of years ago, the Cooperating Clinics Committee of the American Rheumatism Association conducted an excellent three month, eleven clinic, double-blind trial in which neither patients nor physicians could differentiate between placebo or indomethacin; all patients were allowed liberal access to aspirin (166). Because of this surprising finding, a number of investigators have attempted to document a drug interaction between aspirin and indomethacin. Some have found that aspirin impairs the absorption of indomethacin (118,217), while others have been unable to confirm this effect (24,34,122). Response to salicylate does not appear to be affected by indomethacin (15,122). In light of the poor results obtained in the Cooperating Clinics study, one might argue that aspirin does impair the action of indomethacin, because it has been adequately demonstrated that indomethacin is effective in rheumatoid arthritis (32,53,132,199,203,249), albeit less so than aspirin (190). Moreover, when indomethacin and placebo, indomethacin and aspirin, and aspirin and placebo were compared in a double-blind crossover trial, each treatment produced similar results; thus,

there is no clinical advantage to using indomethacin and aspirin together (24).

Naproxen, fenoprofen, ibuprofen, and tolectin are less likely to enhance the gastrointestinal toxicity of aspirin than the drugs described above. However, they are all highly protein bound, so some interaction with aspirin is likely (124,131). Concomitant aspirin administration lowers the average blood levels of fenoprofen (217) and naproxen (226); however, as with indomethacin, the question of clinical significance must be answered. In an eight-week double-blind crossover study of 36 patients with rheumatoid arthritis (268), aspirin plus placebo was compared with aspirin plus naproxen. The aspirin-naproxen combination was more effective, was preferred by patients, and was as well tolerated as aspirin alone. Therefore, the additive effect of these two drugs appears to override any drug interaction. Thus, it would be appropriate to add naproxen to this woman's therapy.

23. After 10 weeks of treatment with aurothioglucose (total 435 mg) the woman described in case B developed pruritus and a rash on her abdomen. Gold was withheld, and she was given a prescription for triamcinolone cream. Comment on this reaction. Should gold therapy be abandoned?

Dermatological reactions to gold occur in 15 to 20% of those treated (130). The mechanism is unknown. It is unlikely that they are hypersensitivity reactions, because they usually occur after a cumulative dose of 400 to 800 mg, patch and intradermal skin tests are negative, and gold therapy can usually be reinstituted at a later date (88).

Because of fears of subsequent exfoliative dermatitis, many clinicians have abandoned gold therapy after the appearance of dermatitis or stomatitis. However, Klinefelter (130) has described successful reinstitution of gold in 28 of 30 patients who developed dermatological reactions. Interestingly, one of these patients presented initially with severe exfoliative dermatitis; many years elapsed before she was again treated with gold, but it ultimately brought her arthritis under fairly good control. The approach that was used for reinstitution of gold after dermatological reactions was as follows: After waiting at least six weeks after the lesions had healed completely, a 1 mg test dose was given intramuscularly. At intervals of two to four weeks the dose was increased from 1 to 2 mg, then from 2 to 5 mg, then to 10 mg, and thereafter 5 mg increments were added until a dose of 50 mg was attained. There was no further gold toxicity in any of the 28 patients whose gold was reinstituted in this manner (130). Others have also successfully restarted gold after disappearance of rashes (91). Because of the potential benefit of subsequent treatment, gold should not be abandoned in this woman.

24. The patient described in case B responded well to gold therapy, and now, one year later her rheumatoid arthritis is in remission. She is currently receiving monthly gold shots. How long should treatment be continued?

Treatment should continue indefinitely in order to sustain the remission. When successfully treated patients from an early multi-center trial of gold were compared to their controls two years after therapy had ended, there was no difference between the two groups (59). Conversely, a more recent double-blind controlled study which included maintenance dosing demonstrated that slowed progression of the disease was sustained during 28 months of treatment (233). Other patients have been maintained in remission for many years with continued injections (161, 162, 168, 241).

25. A 60-year-old man with rheumatoid arthritis of three years duration has been receiving weekly gold injections for 20 weeks with neither toxicity nor therapeutic benefit. He has now received a cumulative dose of 1 gm. Comment.

According to conventional wisdom, this would be considered a therapeutic failure, and gold would be abandoned. However, a different point of view has emerged as a result of a large prospective study which was designed to re-examine old beliefs and test new approaches to chrysotherapy (215). As part of this study, patients who failed to improve after 20 weeks of treatment were given weekly injections of 150% of the initial dose for eight additional weeks; if no response was noted, the dose was then increased to twice the original dose for four additional weeks. Nearly half of the nonresponders thereby attained a satisfactory clinical response without any increase in toxicity. Others (91) have reported good results from 100 mg weekly injections in patients who failed to respond after 20 weeks of 50 mg injections. More study is needed, but these results are promising. It should be noted, however, that increased dosages during the first 20 weeks of gold therapy have not produced better response (see Question 20).

26. A middle aged woman who has been taking aspirin for her rheumatoid arthritis for approximately three years presents a prescription for hydroxychloroquine 200 mg, 20 tablets, 1 hs. What sort of response can be expected? What instructions should she receive?

This is the correct dose, but four to six weeks may be required before any results are noted, and maximal benefits may not be apparent for at least three months (5,58,153). Reviews of a number of controlled double-blind studies carried out over five to twelve month periods provide clear evidence that antimala-

rials slow the rate of deterioration of functional capacity, induce a decline in rheumatoid factor, and lower serum globulin levels (163,205). Progression of bone lesions is not affected. About two-thirds of those treated with antimalarials will respond favorably (58,163). These drugs should not be used in patients with psoriasis, because antimalarials may exacerbate proriasis (153). They should not be used concurrently with gold; should rash or other toxicity develop, it would be difficult to identify the offending drug (87). Salicylate treatment should be continued (5,70).

The major hazard with antimalarials is the risk of retinopathy. Therefore, this woman should be examined by an ophthalmologist every three to six months (58a,153,224). Also, she should be advised to wear dark glasses when in sunlight or bright light (see Question 27). She should be warned of the potential hazard of ingestion by children; as little as a gram can be fatal in a three-year-old child (31,167).

27. What is the risk of retinopathy from antimalarials when used for the treatment of rheumatoid arthritis?

All of the 4-amino-quinolines are capable of causing permanent and sometimes progressive loss of vision from retinopathy. Hydroxychloroquine, which became available after chloroquine had been in wide use, appears no safer than chloroquine in this regard (10). Hydroxychloroquine 200 mg is approximately equivalent to chloroquine 250 mg.

The incidence of retinopathy is higher with chloroquine doses of 500 mg or more per day than with 250 mg per day (191,224). Hinkind and Rothfield (99) found retinal lesions in 8 of 45 patients who had been taking 250 to 750 mg of chloroquine daily for one or more years. However, Scherbel and co-workers (224) found only two cases of retinal changes in 408 patients taking antimalarials for one to nine years. The ceiling doses were 250 mg of chloroquine and 400 mg of hydroxychloroquine daily. Neither case had visual impairment. Elman and co-workers (58a) found one case of chloroquine-induced retinopathy among 270 consecutive patients treated with 250 mg per day, 10 months annually for periods up to 15 years. MacKenzie (163) has summarized his experience with 2000 patients receiving chloroquine in doses of 250 mg per day for many years. Six patients had retinal changes without scotoma or vision loss. Sixty-five of his patients have consumed more than a kilogram of chloroquine, but none of his 2000 patients have had any loss of vision because of the drug. He attributes his success to conservative daily dosage and regular ophthalmologic examinations including measurement of red light thresholds. He also recommends that his patients use dark glasses in bright sunlight, since the deposits of drug in the eye seem to impair the normal retinal defense mechanisms against light.

The retinopathy caused by these drugs is alarming because it can be progressive even after stopping the drug, since large amounts of the drug are stored in the body. In two instances (25), visual disturbances from chloroquine retinopathy did not occur until several years after therapy had been discontinued. It has been suggested that the risk of retinopathy makes these drugs too dangerous to use in rheumatoid arthritis (214). However the risk is small, and it must be weighed against the satisfactory, although not spectacular, benefits obtained in this sometimes crippling disease (105). Furthermore, there are effective techniques for monitoring for a pre-retinopathy which is reversible on discontinuation of the drug (196,197). With ophthalmologic exams every three to six months and conservative daily dosage (chloroquine 250 mg or hydroxychloroquine 200 mg) the risk is minimized.

It should be noted that benign corneal deposits of antimalarial drug occur in about 10% of patients (224). If this keratopathy is not annoying, therapy may be continued (191). This is a harmless side effect which can be reversed by withdrawal of the drug for a few months. It is not related to the more serious, and infrequent, retinopathy. Both corneal deposits and retinopathy can occur with or without visual disturbance (10,25,191,224). Therefore, an ophthalmologist must be consulted to monitor for signs of retinopathy (58a,153,224).

28. M.M. is a 55-year-old man with progressive rheumatoid arthritis which has been unresponsive to gold. He developed a rash during a course of treatment with hydroxychloroquine, requiring its discontinuation. Salicylates and other nonsteroidal antiinflammatory drugs do not provide adequate relief. What treatment alternatives are available?

Glucocorticoids might be considered at this point, but the smallest possible dose should be used and the dose should not exceed 10 mg of prednisone daily (5,127). Except for vasculitis and other serious systemic manifestations of rheumatoid arthritis where glucocorticoids may be life-saving, rheumatoid arthritis is not a life-threatening disease. Therefore, the predictable toxicity that would occur with prolonged glucocorticoid treatment must be weighed against the potential benefits. Nevertheless, the use of small doses is sometimes necessary. These drugs are discussed in detail in a separate chapter of this text.

Penicillamine is becoming recognized as an effective mode of treatment for rheumatoid arthritis, and it may be a reasonable alternative for this man. A number of controlled trials have demonstrated the efficacy of penicillamine in rheumatoid arthritis (52, 174, 184, 231), and in one uncontrolled trial pertinent to this patient, 14 of 17 patients who failed to respond to gold therapy improved with penicillamine (255).

Like gold, penicillamine causes rashes, blood dyscrasias, and renal toxicity. However, patients who have developed a given toxic manifestation from gold do not necessarily manifest the same toxicity with penicillamine (255). Loss of taste and gastrointestinal upset are frequent (111). In an effort to reduce toxicity, many investigators employ the "go slow-go low" regimen described by Jaffe (116): Patients are begun on 250 mg/day and the dose is increased by 250 mg increments after four to eight week intervals in an attempt to find the lowest possible effective maintenance dose. The Multicentre Trial Group used a dose of 1.5 gm/day in their successful trial of penicillamine (184). It was subsequently demonstrated that doses of 0.5 to 0.6 gm/day are nearly as effective as 1.0 to 1.2 gm/day, but with less toxicity (52,174). Dosage must be titrated for each patient. Lower dosage does not eliminate the risk of severe toxicity; this drug requires stringent monitoring procedures similar to those applied to gold (116).

There is no doubt that the immunosuppressant drugs such as *azathioprine* or *cyclophosphamide* are effective in severe progressive cases of rheumatoid arthritis (17,39,56,109,201,254,258). Because an early successful trial of cyclophosphamide was associated with a high degree of toxicity from average daily doses of 1.7 mg/kg (39), others attempted using lower doses, but 0.8 to 1 mg/kg/day was shown to be ineffective (151). Subsequently, it was demonstrated that cyclophosphamide 1.1 mg/kg/day in conjunction with low doses of prednisone is more effective than prednisone alone (239). Azathioprine is usually administered in doses of 2 to 3 mg/kg/day (58), but 1 to 2 mg/kg/day appears to be effective (56). The acute toxicities of these drugs are discussed in the chapter on *Cancer Chemotherapy.*

The potential dangers of malignancy as a result of therapy with immunosuppressive drugs has been a source of considerable concern (3). The relatively high incidence of malignancy among immunosuppressed renal transplant patients is well documented, although some have attributed this to the oncogenic effects of a foreign tissue graft or of uremia (201). However, a review of the causes of death among 28 patients with rheumatoid arthritis treated with cytotoxic drugs, 141 patients whose rheumatoid arthritis was treated conventionally, and data obtained from local, state, and national vital statistics, determined that neoplasia, particularly lymphoproliferative disease, was substantially more frequent in those treated with cytotoxic drugs (193). Therefore, until more definitive data become available, it must be assumed that treatment with these drugs increases the risk of malignancy. Nevertheless, these agents have a definite place in the management of severe systemic manifestations of rheumatoid arthritis.

Among the newer experimental drugs, *levamisole* appears to be quite promising. Unlike most drugs which are effective in rheumatoid arthritis by depressing the immune response, levamisole has immunostimulant qualities. Uncontrolled (213,262) and controlled (222) trials have demonstrated improvement in such parameters as grip strength, morning stiffness, ESR, joint tenderness, and walking time. Further study is needed.

In summary, of the various agents available, penicillamine appears to be the best choice for this patient. Although penicillamine is readily available, its use is still investigational in the U.S. at the time of this writing.

REFERENCES

1. Abrishami MA et al: Aspirin intolerance — a review. Ann Allergy 39:28, 1977.
2. Alexander SJ: Clinical experience with naproxen in rheumatoid arthritis. Arch Intern Med 135:1429, 1975.
3. Alexson E et al: Acute leukemia after azathioprine treatment of connective tissue disease. Amer J Med Sci 273:335, 1977.
4. Almeyda J et al: Cutaneous reactions to antirheumatic drugs. Brit J Dermatol 83:707, 1970.
5. American Rheumatism Association: Primer on the rheumatic diseases. JAMA 224:687 (suppl), 1973. Also available for a modest charge as a 152 page reprint from The Arthritis Foundation, 3400 Peachtree Road, N.E., Atlanta, Georgia 30326.
6. Anon: *Arthritis: The Basic Facts,* The Arthritis Foundation, New York.
7. Anon: Methods to protect the hands in the presence of rheumatoid arthritis. Circ Lett 19, Nov 25 1975, Northern Calif Chapt of The Arthritis Foundation, San Francisco.
8. Anon: Is all aspirin alike? Med Lett 16:57, 1974.
9. Anon: Arthropan liquid and other salicylates for arthritis. Med Lett 18:119, 1976.
10. Anon: Chloroquine retinopathy. NEJM 275:730, 1966.
11. Arcilla RA et al: Congestive heart failure from suspected ductal closure in utero. J Pediat 75:74, 1969.
12. Arden GB et al: Antimalarial therapy and early retinal changes in patients with rheumatoid arthritis. Brit Med J 1:270. 1966.
13. Arendt-Racine EC et al: Drug trial in rheumatoid arthritis: a new design. Clin Pharmacol Ther 23:233, 1978.
14. Ayers JW et al: Circadian rhythm of urinary pH in man with and without chronic antacid administration. Eur J Clin Pharmacol 12:415, 1977.
15. Barraclough DRE et al: Salicylate therapy and drug interaction in rheumatoid arthritis. Aust NZ J Med 5:518, 1975.
16. Bayles TB: Salicylate therapy for rheumatoid arthritis. In *Arthritis and Allied Conditions,* 8th ed, edited by JL Hollander and DJ McCarty, Lea & Febiger, Philadelphia, 1972, p 448.
17. Berry H et al: Trial comparing azathioprine and penicillamine in treatment of rheumatoid arthritis. Ann Rheum Dis 35:542, 1976.
18. Bick RL: Bleeding times, platelet adhesion, and aspirin. Am J Clin Path 65:69, 1976.
19. Blechman WJ et al: Ibuprofen or aspirin in rheumatoid arthritis therapy. JAMA 233:336, 1975.
20. Bloomfield SS et al: Naproxen, aspirin, and codeine in postpartum uterine pain. Clin Pharmacol Ther 21:414, 1977.
21. Boardman PL et al: Ibuprofen in the treatment of rheumatoid arthritis and osteo-arthritis. Ann Rheum Dis 26:560, 1967.
21a. Boardman PL et al: Clinical measurement of the anti-inflammatory effects of salicylates in rheumatoid arthritis. Brit Med J 4:264, 1967.
22. Bowers DE et al: Naproxen in rheumatoid arthritis: a controlled trial. Ann Intern Med 83:470, 1975.
23. Bowers DE et al: Naproxen in rheumatoid arthritis (letter). Ann Intern Med 85:400, 1976.
24. Brooks PM et al: Indomethacin-aspirin interactions: a clinical appraisal. Brit Med J 3:69, 1975.
25. Burns RP: Delayed onset of chloroquine retinopathy. NEJM 275:693, 1966.
26. Calabro JJ et al: Fever associated with juvenile rheumatoid arthritis. NEJM 276:11, 1967.
27. Calabro JJ et al: Anti-inflammatory effect of acetylsalicylic acid in rheumatoid arthritis. Clin Orth Rel Res 71:124, 1970.
28. Canada AT: Gold induced thrombocytopenia. Amer J Hosp Pharm 30:340, 1973.
29. Canada AT et al: The bioavailability of enteric-coated acetylsalicylic acid: a comparative study in rheumatoid arthritis, I. Curr Ther Res 18:727, 1975.
30. Canada AT et al: The bioavailability of enteric-coated acetylsalicylic acid: a comparison with buffered ASA in rheumatoid arthritis, II. Curr Ther Res 19:554, 1976.
31. Cann HM et al: Fatal acute chloroquine poisoning in children. Pediat 27:95, 1961.
32. Castles JJ et al: Multicenter comparison of naproxen and indomethacin in rheumatoid arthritis. Arch Intern Med 138:362, 1978.
33. Cats AL: Multicenter controlled trial of the effects of different dosage of gold therapy followed by a maintenance dosage. Agents Actions 6:355, 1976.
34. Champion DG et al: The effect of aspirin on serum indomethacin. Clin Pharmacol Ther 13:239, 1972.
35. Collier HOJ: A pharmacological analysis of aspirin. Adv Pharmacol Chemother 7:333, 1969.
36. Collins E et al: Maternal effects of regular salicylate ingestion in pregnancy. Lancet 2:335, 1975.
37. Collins E et al: Aspirin during pregnancy (letter). Lancet 2:797, 1976.
38. Combs RJ et al: Gold toxicity and peritoneal dialysis. Arthr Rheum 19:936, 1976.
39. Cooperating Clinics Committee of the American Rheumatism Assoc: A controlled trial of cyclophosphamide in rheumatoid arthritis. NEJM 283:883, 1970.
40. Cooperating Clinics Committee of the American Rheumatism Assoc: A controlled trial of gold salt therapy in rheumatoid arthritis. Arthr Rheum 16:353, 1973.
41. Cordrey LJ: Tolmetin sodium, a new anti-arthritis drug: double-blind and long-term studies. J Amer Geriat Soc 24:440, 1976.
42. Cotty VF et al: Augmentation of human blood acetylsalicylate concentrations by the simultaneous administration of acetaminophen and aspirin. Toxicol Appl Pharmacol 41:7, 1977.
43. Currey HLF et al: Comparison of azathioprine, cyclophosphamide, and gold in treatment of rheumatoid arthritis. Brit Med J 3:763, 1974.
44. Curtarelli G et al: Gastro-intestinal bleeding under treatment with naproxen. Scand J Rheumatol suppl 2:48, 1973.
45. Cuthbert MF: Adverse reactions to non-steroidal antirheumatic drugs. Curr Med Res Opin 2:600, 1974.
46. Davis JD: Fenoprofen, aspirin, and gold induction in rheumatoid arthritis. Clin Pharmacol Ther 21:52, 1977.
47. Davis MJ: Aspirin-induced prolonged bleeding: report of case. J Dent Child 43:350, 1976.
48. Davis P et al: Interaction of D-penicillamine with gold salts. Arthr Rheum 20:1413, 1977.
49. DeBlecourt JJ: Gold treatment in rheumatoid arthritis. In *Rheumatoid Arthritis,* edited by Fehr, Muller and Harwerth, Academic Press, NY, 1971, p 631.
50. Deodhar SD et al: Measurement of clinical response to anti-inflammatory drug therapy in rheumatoid arthritis. Quart J Med 42:387, 1973.
51. Dietz AA et al: Serum gold: I. estimation by atomic absorption spectroscopy. Ann Rheum Dis 32:124, 1973.
52. Dixon A et al: Synthetic D(−)penicillamine in rheumatoid arthritis. Ann Rheum Dis 34:416, 1975.
53. Donnelly P et al: Indomethacin in rheumatoid arthritis. Brit Med J 1:69, 1967.
54. Dornan J et al: Comparison of ibuprofen and acetylsalicylic acid in the treatment of rheumatoid arthritis. Canad Med Assoc J 110:1370, 1974.
55. Dromgoole SH et al: Correlation of plateau serum salicylate with

rate of salicylate metabolism. Clin Pharmacol Ther 20:120, 1976.

56. Dwosh IL et al: Azathioprine in early rheumatoid arthritis. Arthr Rheum 20:685, 1977.
57. Ebringer A: Chloroquine myopathy. Brit Med J 2:770, 1971.
58. Ehrlich GE: Remittive pharmaceutical agents. In *Rheumatic Diseases: Diagnosis and Management,* edited by WA Katz, JB Lippincott Co, Philadelphia, 1977, p 897.
58a. Elman A et al: Chloroquine retinopathy in patients with rheumatoid arthritis. Scand J Rheumatol 5:161, 1976.
59. Empire Rheumatism Council: Gold therapy in rheumatoid arthritis: report of a multi-center controlled trial. Ann Rheum Dis 19:95, 1960.
60. Empire Rheumatism Council: Gold therapy in rheumatoid arthritis: final report of a multi-center controlled trial. Ann Rheum Dis 20:315, 1961.
61. England JM et al: Gold induced thrombocytopenia and response to dimercaprol. Brit Med J 2:748, 1972.
62. Engleman EP: Conservative management of rheumatoid arthritis. Med Clin N Amer 52:669, 1968.
63. Engleman EP: Conservative management of rheumatoid arthritis. In *Arthritis and Allied Conditions,* 8th ed, edited by JL Hollander and DJ McCarty, Lea & Febiger, Philadelphia, 1972, p 441.
64. Englund DW: Long term large scale clinical evaluation of indomethacin. Arthr Rheum 9:502, 1966.
65. Epstein WV: Laboratory tests in rheumatic diseases. Med Clin N Amer 61:377, 1977.
66. Faidi AR: Aspirin intolerance in asthmatic patients: case histories. Ann Allergy 38:268, 1977.
67. Finkelstein AE et al: Auranofin: new oral gold compound for treatment of rheumatoid arthritis. Ann Rheum Dis 35:251, 1976.
68. Fosdick WM et al: Long term cyclophosphamide therapy in rheumatoid arthritis. Arthr Rheum 11:151, 1968.
69. Fraser NF: Gold treatment in rheumatoid arthritis. Ann Rheum Dis 4:71, 1945.
70. Fremont-Smith K et al: Salicylate therapy in rheumatoid arthritis. JAMA 192:1133, 1965.
71. Freyberg RH et al: Gold therapy for rheumatoid arthritis. In *Arthritis and Allied Conditions,* 8th ed, edited by JL Hollander and DJ McCarty, Lea & Febiger, Philadelphia, 1972, p 455.
72. Fries JF et al: Fenoprofen calcium in rheumatoid arthritis: a controlled double-blind crossover evaluation. Arthr Rheum 16:629, 1973.
73. Furst DE et al: A double-blind trial of high versus conventional dosages of gold salts for rheumatoid arthritis. Arthr Rheum 20:1473, 1977.
74. Furst DE et al: Salicylate metabolism in twins: evidence suggesting a genetic influence and induction of salicylurate formation. J Clin Invest 60:32, 1977.
75. Furst DE et al: Salicylate clearance: the consequence of saturability in plasma protein binding and metabolism (abstract). Clin Pharmacol Ther 23:113, 1978.
76. Fye KH: Rheumatoid arthritis. Medical Staff Conference Presentation, Univ Calif San Francisco, March 15, 1978.
77. Garrettson LK et al: Fetal acquisition and neonatal elimination of a large amount of salicylate. Clin Pharmacol Ther 17:98, 1975.
78. Gibaldi M et al: Effect of antacids on pH of urine. Clin Pharmacol Ther 16:520, 1974.
79. Gibaldi M et al: Time course and dose dependence of antacid effect on urine pH. J Pharm Sci 64:2003, 1975.
80. Gibson T et al: Kinetics of salicylate metabolism. Brit J Clin Pharmacol 2:233, 1975.
81. Godfrey RG et al: Effect of ibuprofen dosage on patient response in rheumatoid arthritis. Arthr Rheum 18:135, 1975.
82. Goldsweig HG et al: Bleeding, salicylates and prolonged prothrombin time: three case reports and a review of the literature. J Rheumatol 3:37, 1976.
83. Gordon MH et al: Gold reactions are *not* more common in Sjogren's syndrome. Ann Intern Med 82:47, 1975.
84. Gordon RA et al: D-penicillamine-induced myasthenia gravis in rheumatoid arthritis. Ann Intern Med 87:578, 1977.
85. Gottlieb NL et al: Gold excretion correlated with clinical course in rheumatoid arthritis. Arthr Rheum 15:582, 1972.
86. Gottlieb NL et al: Acute myocardial infarction following gold sodium thiomalate induced vasomotor (nitroid) reaction. Arthr Rheum 20:1026, 1977.
87. Gottlieb NL: Chrysotherapy. Bull Rheum Dis 27:912, 1977.

88. Gottlieb NL et al: Gold compounds in rheumatoid arthritis. Scand J Rheumatol 6:225, 1977.
89. Gowan JDC et al: Response of rheumatoid arthritis with leukopenia to gold salts. NEJM 288:1007, 1973.
90. Graham GG et al: Patterns of plasma concentrations and urinary excretion of salicylate in rheumatoid arthritis. Clin Pharmacol Ther 22:410, 1977.
91. Gumpel JM: Cyclophosphamide, gold and penicillamine — disease modifying drugs in rheumatoid arthritis — taylored dosage and ultimate success. Rheumatol Rehab 15:217, 1976.
92. Gupta N et al: Correlation of plateau serum salicylate level with rate of salicylate metabolism. Clin Pharmacol Ther 18:350, 1975.
93. Halla JT et al: Postinjection nonvasomotor reactions during chrysotherapy. Arthr Rheum 20:1188, 1977.
94. Halvorsen L et al: Comparative effects of aspirin and naproxen on gastric mucosa. Scand J Rheumatol, suppl 2:43, 1973.
95. Hansten PD: *Drug Interactions,* 3rd ed, Lea & Febiger, Philadelphia, 1975.
96. Harris BK: Myocardial infarction after a gold-induced nitroid reaction (letter). Arthr Rheum 20:1561, 1977.
97. Hart FD: Presentation of rheumatoid arthritis and its relation to prognosis. Brit Med J 2:621, 1977.
98. Helby-Petersen P et al: A double-blind crossover comparison of naproxen and placebo in rheumatoid arthritis. Scand J Rheumatol, suppl 2:145, 1973.
99. Henkind P et al: Ocular abnormalities in patients treated with synthetic antimalarial drugs. NEJM 269:433, 1963.
100. Heyman MA et al: Closure of the ductus arteriosus in premature infants by inhibition of prostaglandin synthesis. NEJM 295:530, 1976.
101. Heyman MA et al: Effects of acetylsalicylic acid on the ductus arteriosus and circulation in fetal lambs in utero. Circ Res 38:418, 1976.
102. Hill DF: Gold therapy for rheumatoid arthritis. Med Clin N Amer 52:733, 1968.
103. Hill HFH et al: Multi-centre double-blind cross-over trial comparing naproxen and aspirin in rheumatoid arthritis. Scand J Rheumatol, suppl 2:176, 1973.
104. Hill HFH et al: Naproxen. A new non-hormonal anti-inflammatory agent. Ann Rheum Dis 33:12, 1974.
105. Hollander JL: The calculated risk of arthritis treatment. Ann Intern Med 62:1062, 1965.
106. Hollander JL: *The Arthritis Handbook,* Merck Sharpe and Dohme, West Point, Pa, 1974.
107. Hollister LE et al: Studies of delayed-action medication — IV salicylates. Clin Pharmacol Ther 6:5, 1965.
108. Huguley CM: Hematological reactions. JAMA 196:408, 1966.
109. Hunter T et al: Azathioprine in rheumatoid arthritis: a long-term follow-up study. Arthr Rheum 18:15, 1975.
110. Huskisson EC: Long-term use of fenoprofen in rheumatoid arthritis: the therapeutic ratio. Curr Med Res Opin 2:545, 1974.
111. Huskisson EC et al: Trial comparing D-penicillamine and gold in rheumatoid arthritis. Ann Rheum Dis 33:532, 1974.
112. Huskisson EC et al: Treatment of rheumatoid arthritis with fenoprofen: comparison with aspirin. Brit Med J 1:176, 1974.
113. Huskisson EC et al: Four new anti-inflammatory drugs: responses and variations. Brit Med J 1:1048, 1976.
114. Huskisson EC: Anti-inflammatory drugs. Semin Arthr Rheum 7:1, 1977.
114a. Ingelfinger FJ: Aspirin and the stomach. In *Controversy in Internal Medicine II,* edited by FJ Ingelfinger, RV Ebert, M Finland, and AS Relman, WB Saunders Co, Philadelphia 1974, p 509.
114b. Ingelfinger FJ: The side effects of aspirin. NEJM 290:1196, 1974.
115. Jacobs JC et al: Micromeasurement of plasma salicylate in arthritic children. Arthr Rheum 21:129, 1978.
116. Jaffe JA: The technique of penicillamine administration in rheumatoid arthritis. Arthr Rheum 18:513, 1976.
117. Jayson MIV: Report of symposium: Penicillamine. Ann Rheum Dis 34:273, 1975.
118. Jeremy R et al: Interaction between aspirin and indomethacin in the treatment of rheumatoid arthritis. Med J Aust 2:127, 1970.
119. Jessar RA: Medical management. In *Total Management of the Arthritis Patient,* edited by GE Ehrlich, JB Lippincott Co, Philadelphia, 1973, p 15.
120. Jessop JD: The present status of chrysotherapy. Pract 208:28, 1972.
121. Jessop JD et al: Serum gold determinations in patients with

rheumatoid arthritis receiving sodium aurothiomalate. Ann Rheum Dis 32:228, 2973.

122. Kaldestad E et al: Interactions of indomethacin and acetyl salicylic acid as shown by the serum concentrations of indomethacin and salicylate. Europ J Clin Pharmacol 9:199, 1975.

123. Kanada SA et al: Aspirin hepatotoxicity. Am J Hosp Pharm 35:330, 1978.

124. Kantor TG: Anti-inflammatory and analgesic drugs. In *Rheumatic Diseases: Diagnosis and Management,* edited by WA Katz, JB Lippincott Co, Philadelphia, 1977, p 876.

125. Katona G: Four years of clinical experience with naproxen — and objective methods of evaluation. Scand J Rheumatol, suppl 2:101, 1973.

126. Katz A et al: Gold nephropathy. An immunopathologic study. Arch Path 96:133, 1973.

127. Katz WA: Rheumatoid arthritis. In *Rheumatic Diseases: Diagnosis and Management,* edited by WA Katz, JB Lippincott Co, Philadelphia, 1977.

128. Kaye RL et al: Treatment of rheumatoid arthritis: a review including newer and experimental anti-inflammatory agents. Arch Intern Med L36:1023, 1976.

129. Kirsner JB: Drug induced peptic ulcer. Ann Intern Med 47:666, 1957.

130. Klinefleter HF: Reinstitution of gold therapy in rheumatoid arthritis after mucocutaneous reactions. J Rheumatol 2:21, 1975.

131. Koch-Weser J et al: Binding of drugs to serum albumin. NEJM 294:311 and 294:526, 1976.

132. Kogstad O: A double-blind cross-over study of naproxen and indomethacin in patients with rheumatoid arthritis. Scand J Rheumatol, suppl 2:159, 1973.

133. Krusius FE et al: Plasma levels and urinary excretion of gold during routine treatment of rheumatoid arthritis. Ann Rheum Dis 29:232, 1970.

133a. Langman MJS: Aspirin is not a major cause of acute gastrointestinal bleeding. In *Controversy in Internal Medicine II,* edited by FJ Ingelfinger, RV Ebert, M Finland, and AS Relman, WB Saunders Co, Philadelphia, 1974, p 493.

134. Lasagna L et al: How reliable are enteric-coated aspirin preparations. Clin Pharmacol Ther 6:568, 1965.

135. Lawrence JS: Comparative toxicity of gold preparations in treatment of rheumatoid arthritis. Ann Rheum Dis 35:171, 1976.

136. Lawwill T et al: Chloroquine accumulation in human eyes. Amer J Ophth 65:530, 1968.

137. Lee P et al: Assessment of disease activity and drug evaluation. In *Recent Advances in Rheumatology, Part II,* edited by WW Buchanand and WC Dick, Churchill Livingstone, New York, 1976, p 1.

138. Leonards JR et al: Absorption and metabolism of aspirin administered in enteric coated tablets. JAMA 193:99, 1965.

139. Leonards JR et al: Effect of pharmaceutical formulation on gastrointestinal bleeding from aspirin tablets. Arch Intern Med 129:457, 1972.

140. Leonards JR et al: Gastrointestinal blood loss during prolonged aspirin administration. NEJM 289:1020, 1973.

141. Levy G et al: Failure of USP disintegration test to assess physiological availability of enteric coated tablets. NY State J Med 64:3002, 1964.

142. Levy G et al: Urine pH and salicylate therapy (letter). JAMA 217:81, 1971.

143. Levy G et al: Limited capacity for salicyl phenolic glucuronide formation and its effect on the kinetics of salicylate elimination in man. Clin Pharmacol Ther 13:258, 1972.

144. Levy G et al: Salicylate accumulation kinetics in man. NEJM 287:430, 1972.

145. Levy G et al: Relationship between dose and apparent volume of distribution of salicylate in children. Pediat 54:713, 1974.

146. Levy G et al: Decreased serum salicylate concentrations in children with rheumatic fever treated with antacid. NEJM 293:323, 1975.

147. Levy G et al: Distribution of salicylate between neonatal and maternal serum at diffusion equilibrium. Clin Pharmacol Ther 18:210, 1975.

148. Levy G et al: Commentary: rational aspirin dosage regimens. Clin Pharmacol Ther 23:247, 1978.

148a. Levy M: Aspirin use in patients with major upper gastrointestinal bleeding and peptic-ulcer disease. NEJM 290:1158, 1974.

149. Lewis JR: Evaluation of inbuprofen (Motrin): a new antirheumatic

agent. JAMA 233:364, 1975.

150. Lewis JR: New antirheumatic agents: fenoprofen calcium (Nalfon), naproxen (Naprosyn), and tolmetin sodium (Tolectin). JAMA 237:1260, 1977.

151. Lidsky MD et al: Double-blind study of cyclophosphamide in rheumatoid arthritis. Arthr Rheum 16:148, 1973.

152. Lloyd LA et al: Ocular complications of chloroquine therapy. Canad Med Assoc J 92:508, 1965.

153. Lockie LM: Phenylbutazone, indomethacin and chloroquines in therapy of rheumatoid arthritis. In *Arthritis and Allied Conditions,* 8th ed, edited by JL Hollander and DJ McCarty, Lea & Febiger, Philadelphia, 1972, p 483.

154. Loebl DH et al: Gastrointestinal blood loss: effect of aspirin, fenoprofen, and acetaminophen in rheumatoid arthritis as determined by sequential gastroscopy and radioactive fecal markers. JAMA 237:976, 1977.

155. Loew D et al: Dose-dependent influence of acetylsalicylic acid on platelet functions and plasmatic coagulation factors. Haemostasis 5:239, 1976.

156. Lorber A et al: Gold determination in biological fluids by atomic absorption spectroscopy: application to chrysotherapy in rheumatoid arthritis patients. Arthr Rheum 11:170, 1968.

157. Lorber A et al: Monitoring serum gold values to improve chrysotherapy in rheumatoid arthritis. Ann Rheum Dis 32:133, 1973.

158. Lussier A et al: Long term study of naproxen challenged by short-term double blind cross-over study with placebo in rheumatoid patients. Scand J Rheumatol, suppl 2:113, 1973.

159. Lussier A et al: Naproxen: a novel approach to dose-finding efficacy trials in rheumatoid arthritis. Clin Pharmacol Ther 14:434, 1973.

160. Lussier A et al: Gastrointestinal microbleeding after aspirin and naproxen. Clin Pharmacol Ther 23:402, 1978.

161. Luukkainen R et al: Effect of gold treatment on the progression of erosions in RA patients. Scand J Rheumatol 6:123, 1977.

162. Luukkainen R et al: Effect of gold on progression of erosions in rheumatoid arthritis: better results with earlier treatment. Scand J Rheumatol 6:189, 1977.

163. MacKenzie AH: An appraisal of chloroquine. Arthr Rheum 13:280, 1970.

164. Magnusson B et al: A comparative study of gastrointestinal bleeding during administration of ketoprofen and naproxen. Scand J Rheumatol 6:62, 1977.

165. Mahler DL et al: Assay of aspirin and naproxen analgesia. Clin Pharmacol Ther 19:18, 1976.

166. Mainland DM and the Cooperating Clinics Committee of the American Rheumatism Association: A three month trial of indomethacin in rheumatoid arthritis, with special reference to analysis inference. Clin Pharmacol Ther 8:11, 1967.

167. Markowitz JA et al: Chloroquine poisoning in a girl. JAMA 189:950, 1964.

168. Marshall CM: Gold therapy in rheumatoid arthritis: a review of ten years' treatment. Med J Aust 2:239, 1965.

169. Mascarenhas BR et al: Gold metabolism in patients with rheumatoid arthritis treated with gold compounds — reinvestigated. Arthr Rheum 15:391, 1972.

170. Maurer EF: The toxic effects of phenylbutazone. NEJM 253:404, 1955.

171. McCarthy DD et al: Hematological complications of phenylbutazone therapy. Canad Med Assoc J 90:1061, 1964.

172. McDuffie FC et al: Immunologic tests in the diagnosis of rheumatic diseases. Bull Rheum Dis 27:900 and 27:906, 1977.

173. McKenzie JMM: An initial report on a double-blind trial comparing small and large doses of gold in the treatment of rheumatoid disease. Rheumatol Rehab 16:78, 1977.

174. Mery C et al: Controlled trial of D-penicillamine in rheumatoid arthritis: dose effect and the role of zinc. Scand J Rheumatol 5:241, 1976.

175. Meyer W: Clinical observations on gold therapy in rheumatoid arthritis. In *Rheumatoid Arthritis,* edited by Fehr, Muller and Harworth, Academic Press, NY, 1971, p 631.

176. Miller RL et al: Inflammatory disorders. In *Clinical Pharmacology,* 2nd ed, edited by K Melmon and H Morrelli, Macmillan, New York, 1978, p 678.

177. Mills JA et al: Value of bed rest in patients with rheumatoid arthritis. NEJM 284:453, 1971.

178. Mills JA: Nonsteroidal anti-inflammatory drugs. NEJM 290:781

and 290:1002, 1974.

179. Mohammed I et al: Effect of penicillamine therapy on circulating immune complexes in rheumatoid arthritis. Ann Rheum Dis 35:458, 1976.

180. Mongan E et al: Tinnitus as an indication of therapeutic serum salicylate levels. JAMA 226:142, 1973.

181. Moroz LA: Increased blood fibrinolytic activity after aspirin ingestion. NEJM 296:525, 1977.

182. Moroz LA: Aspirin, fibrinolysis and menstruation (letter). NEJM 296:1299, 1977.

183. Mowat AG et al: Naproxen in rheumatoid arthritis: extended trial. Ann Rheum Dis 35:498, 1976.

184. Multicentre Trial Group: Controlled trial of D(-)penicillamine in severe rheumatoid arthritis. Lancet 1:275, 1973.

185. Multz CV et al: A comparison of intermediate-dose aspirin and placebo in rheumatoid arthritis. Clin Pharmacol Ther 15:310, 1974.

186. Myers EN et al: Salicylate ototoxicity: a clinical study. NEJM 273:587, 1965

187. Nevins M et al: Phenylbutazone and pulmonary oedema. Lancet 2:1358, 1969.

188. Northcross BM: Clinical effects of indomethacin in rheumatic diseases. J New Drugs 5:259, 1965.

189. Nozik RA et al: Ocular complications of chloroquine. A series and case presentation with a simple method for early detection of retinopathy. Amer J Ophth 58:744, 1964.

190. O'Brien WM: Indomethacin: a survey of clinical trials. Clin Pharmacol Ther 9:94, 1968.

191. Okun E et al: Chloroquine retinopathy. Arch Ophth 69:51, 1963.

192. O'Sullivan JB et al: The prevalence of rheumatoid arthritis: follow-up evaluation of the effect of criteria on rates in Sudbury, Massachusetts. Ann Intern Med 76:573, 1972.

193. Parsons JL et al: The causes of death in patients with rheumatoid arthritis treated with cytotoxic agents (abstract). J Rheumatol 1:suppl 1:75, 1974.

194. Paulus HE et al: Variations of serum concentrations and half-life of salicylate in patients with rheumatoid arthritis. Arthr Rheum 14:527, 1971.

195. Payne RW: Treatment of rheumatoid arthritis with indomethacin. J Okla Med Assoc 58:533, 1965.

196. Percival SP et al: Chloroquine: ophthalmological safety and clinical assessment in rheumatoid arthritis. Brit Med J 3:579, 1968.

197. Percival SP et al: Ophthalmological safety of chloroquine. Brit J Ophth 53:101, 1969.

198. Persellin RH: The effect of pregnancy on rheumatoid arthritis. Bull Rheum Dis 27:922, 1977.

199. Pinals RS et al: Relative efficacy of indomethacin and acetylsalicylic acid in rheumatoid arthritis. NEJM 276:512, 1967.

200. Pinckard RN et al: The influence of acetylsalicylic acid on the binding of acetrizoate to human albumin. Ann NY Acad Sci 226:341, 1973.

201. Pirofsky B et al: Immunosuppressive therapy in rheumatic disease. Med Clin N Amer 61:419, 1977.

202. Pisciotta AV: Drug-induced leukopenia and aplastic anemia. Clin Pharmacol Ther 12:13, 1971.

203. Pitkeathly DA et al: Indomethacin in inpatient treatment of rheumatoid arthritis. Ann Rheum Dis 25:334, 1966.

204. Pollock BH et al: Neoplasia and cyclophosphamide. Arthr Rheum 16:524, 1973.

205. Popert AJ: Chloroquine: a review. Rheumatol Rehab 15:235, 1976.

206. Popert AJ et al: Chloroquine diphosphate in rheumatoid arthritis. Ann Rheum Dis 20:18, 1961.

207. Pretty HM et al: Agranulocytosis: a report of 30 cases. Canad Med Assoc J 93:1058, 1965.

208. Prince HE: Aspirin and cross reactivity (editorial). Ann Allergy 39:47, 1977.

209. Ragan C et al: The clinical features of rheumatoid arthritis: prognostic indices. JAMA 181:663, 1962.

210. Reynolds PMG et al: A single-blind crossover comparison of fenoprofen, ibuprofen and naproxen in rheumatoid arthritis. Curr Med Res Opin 2:461, 1974.

211. Ridolfo AS et al: Effects of fenoprofen and aspirin on gastrointestinal microbleeding in man. Clin Pharmacol Ther 14:226, 1973.

212. Roe RL: Drug therapy in rheumatic diseases. Med Clin N Amer 61:405, 1977.

213. Rosenthal M et al: Immunotherapy with levamisole in rheumatic diseases. Scand J Rheumatol 5:216, 1976.

214. Rothermich NO: Coming catastrophies with chloroquine? Ann Intern Med 61:1203, 1964.

215. Rothermich NO et al: Chrysotherapy. A prospective study. Arthr Rheum 19:1321, 1976.

216. Rowland M et al: The clinical pharmacology of salicylates. Calif Med 110:410, 1969.

217. Rubin A et al: Interactions of aspirin with nonsteroidal anti-inflammatory drugs in man. Arthr Rheum 16:635, 1973.

218. Rubin A et al: A profile of the physiological disposition and gastrointestinal effects of fenoprofen in man. Curr Med Res Opin 2:529, 1974.

219. Rubinstein HM et al: Serum gold II. levels in rheumatoid arthritis. Ann Rheum Dis 32:128, 1973.

220. Ruedy J et al: A comparison of the analgesic efficacy of naproxen and propoxyphene in patients with pain after orthopedic surgery. Scand J Rheumatol, suppl 2:56, 1973.

221. Ruedy J: A comparison of the analgesic efficacy of naproxen and acetylsalicylic acid-codeine in patients with pain after dental surgery. Scand J Rheumatol, suppl 2:60, 1973.

222. Runge LA et al: Treatment of rheumatoid arthritis with levamisole. Arthr Rheum 20:1445, 1977.

223. Samter M et al: Intolerance to aspirin: clinical studies and consideration of its pathogenesis. Ann Intern Med 68:975, 1968.

224. Scherbel AL et al: Ocular lesions in rheumatoid arthritis and related disorders with particular reference to retinopathy. NEJM 273:360, 1965.

225. Seaman WE et al: Effect of aspirin on liver tests in patients with RA or SLE and in normal volunteers. Arthr Rheum 19:155, 1976.

226. Segre E et al: Interaction of naproxen and aspirin in the rat and in man. Scand J Rheumatol, suppl 2:37, 1973.

227. Shafar J: Phenylbutazone-induced pericarditis. Brit Med J 2:795, 1965.

228. Shafii M: Psychotherapeutic treatment for rheumatoid arthritis: one thousand years ago. Arch Gen Psychiat 29:85, 1973.

229. Shapiro S et al: Perinatal mortality and birth-weight in relation to aspirin taken during pregnancy. Lancet 1:1375, 1976.

230. Sharp JT et al: Comparison of two dosage schedules of gold salts in the treatment of rheumatoid arthritis. Arthr Rheum 20:1179, 1977.

231. Shiokawa Y et al: Clinical evaluation of D-penicillamine by multicentric double-blind comparative study in chronic rheumatoid arthritis. Arthr Rheum 20:1464, 1977.

232. Sibert JR: Child-resistant packaging and accidental child poisoning. Lancet 2:289, 1977.

233. Sigler JW et al: Gold salts in the treatment of rheumatoid arthritis: a double-blind study. Ann Intern Med 80:21, 1974.

234. Silverberg DS et al: Gold nephropathy. A clinical and pathologic study. Arthr Rheum 13:812, 1970.

235. Silverberg J et al: Rheumatoid factors in Graves' disease. Ann Intern Med 88:216, 1978.

236. Skjelbred P et al: Acetylsalicylic acid vs paracetamol: effects on post-operative course. Eur J Clin Pharmacol 12:257, 1977.

237. Slone D et al: Aspirin and congenital malformations. Lancet 1:1373, 1976.

238. Smith RD et al: Rest therapy for rheumatoid arthritis. Mayo Clin Proc 53:141, 1978.

239. Smyth CJ et al: Cyclophosphamide therapy for rheumatoid arthritis. Arch Intern Med 135:789, 1975.

240. Smuthe H: Nonsteroidal therapy in inflammatory joint disease. Hosp Pract 10:51, 1975.

241. Soler-Bechara J et al: Maintenance gold therapy for rheumatoid arthritis — analysis in 167 patients. Arthr Rheum 8:469, 1965.

242. Solomon HM et al: Interactions between digitoxin and other drugs in man. Amer Heart J 83:277, 1972.

243. Soren A: Transport of salicylates from blood to joint fluid. Arch Intern Med 132:668, 1973.

244. Soren A: Dissociation of acetylsalicylic acid in blood and joint fluid. Scand J Rheumatol 6:17, 1977.

245. Sperling IL: Adverse reactions with long-term use of phenylbutazone and oxyphenbutazone. Lancet 2:535, 1969.

246. Stenius BSM et al: Hypersensitivity to acetylsalicylic acid (ASA) and tartrazine in patients with asthma. Clin Allergy 6:119, 1976.

247. Stevem P et al: Immunological studies in a case of gold salt induced thrombocytopenia. Scand J Haem 5:271, 1968.

248. Steinberg AD et al: Cytotoxic drugs in treatment of non-malignant diseases. Ann Intern Med 76:619, 1972.

249. Szanto E: A double-blind comparison of naproxen and indomethacin in rheumatoid arthritis. Scand J Rheumatol 3:118, 1974.

250. Szczeklik A et al: Aspirin-induced asthma. J Aller Clin Immunol 58:10, 1976.

251. Szczeklik A et al: Asthmatic attacks induced in aspirin-sensitive patients by diclofenac and naproxen. Brit Med J 2:231, 1977.

252. Tamler E: Ocular complications of chloroquine therapy. Calif Med 103:30, 1965.

253. Thompson HE et al: Evaluation of indomethacin, a non-steroid agent in rheumatic disease. Ariz Med 2:289, 1965.

254. Townes AS et al: Controlled trial of cyclophosphamide in rheumatoid arthritis. Arthr Rheum 19:563, 1976.

255. Tsang IK et al: D-penicillamine in the treatment of rheumatoid arthritis. Arthr Rheum 20:666, 1977.

256. Turner G et al: Fetal effects of regular salicylate ingestion in pregnancy. Lancet 2:338, 1975.

257. Turner R: Aspirin and newer anti-inflammatory agents in rheumatoid arthritis. Amer Fam Phys 16:111, 1977.

258. Urowitz MB et al: Azathioprine in rheumatoid arthritis: a double-blind, cross-over study. Arthr Rheum 16:411, 1973.

259. Vaamonde CA et al: The nephrotic syndrome as a complication of gold therapy. Arthr Rheum 13:826, 1970.

260. Vane JR: Inhibition of prostaglandin synthesis as a mechanism of action for aspirin-like drugs. Nature New Biol 231:232, 1971.

261. Vane JR: The mode of action of aspirin and similar compounds. J Aller Clin Immunol 58:691, 1976.

262. Veys EM et al: Longterm evaluation of intermittent levamisole treatment in rheumatoid arthritis. J Rheumatol 4:27, 1977.

263. Walzer R et al: Gold dermatitis. Arch Dermatol 104:107, 1971.

264. Walzer RA et al; Severe hypersensitivity reaction to gold. Arch Dermatol 106:231, 1972.

265. Weinreb MS: Electro-oculograms in the early diagnosis of chloroquine retinopathy. Calif Med 106:183, 1967.

266. Willkens RF: Drug letter. Arthr Rheum 15:229, 1972.

267. Willkens RF: Double-blind crossover trial of naproxen and placebo in patients with rheumatoid arthritis. Scand J Rheumatol, suppl 2:132, 1973.

268. Willkens RF et al: Combination therapy with naproxen and aspirin in rheumatoid arthritis. Arthr Rheum 19:677, 1976.

269. Winter ME: Personal communication. Clinical Pharmacokinetics Laboratory, Univ Calif San Francisco 1978.

270. Woodbury DM et al: Analgesic-antipyretics, anti-inflammatory agents, and drugs employed in the therapy of gout. In The Pharmacological Basis of Therapeutics, 5th ed, edited by L Goodman and A Gilman, Macmillan Co, New York, 1975, p 325.

271. Zeiss CR et al: Refractory period to aspirin in a patient with aspirin-induced asthma. J Aller Clin Immunol 57:440, 1976.

272. Zeitlin DJ: Psychological issues in the management of rheumatoid arthritis. Psychosomatics 18:7, 1977.

273. Ziff M et al: Laboratory findings in rheumatoid arthritis. In Arthritis and Allied Conditions, 8th ed, edited by JL Hollander and DJ McCarty, Lea & Febiger, Philadelphia, 1972, p 367.

274. Zvaifler NJ: Anti-malarial treatment of rheumatoid arthritis. Med Clin N Amer 52:759, 1968.

Chapter 24

Diabetes Mellitus

Mary Anne Koda-Kimble

Although an estimated four million Americans have diabetes, only half of them are diagnosed. There is still no cure for diabetes, but insulin and the oral hypoglycemics have improved the quality and prolonged the duration of the diabetic's life.

Education of the patient with respect to his diabetes, medication, urine testing and diet is a major component of diabetic management. Compliance studies have shown time and again that poor control is often the result of medication error, misinterpretation of urine test results and ignorance of the disease (271). The pharmacist can play a major contributory role in this area.

Before beginning the chapter, the student is encouraged to review the pathophysiology of diabetes mellitus and the pharmacology of the drugs used in its treatment. In this chapter, the practical application of basic pharmacology is emphasized through case study questions. The major areas covered include (1) urine testing, (2) insulin in the treatment of juvenile diabetes, (3) the use of oral hypoglycemics in the treatment of adult onset diabetes, (4) drug-induced diabetes, and (5) drug-induced hypoglycemia.

CASE A – ADULT ONSET DIABETES: JS is a 48-year-old obese female with adult onset diabetes. Nine years ago the patient noted the onset of recurrent episodes of moniliasis and upper respiratory tract infections. At that time she was noted to have a fasting blood glucose of 295 mg/dl and was placed on a 1200 calorie ADA (American Diabetic Association) diet. Eight months later she complained of extreme thirstiness, urinary frequency (every one and one-half hours), and nocturia three times nightly. She was noted to have a 4+ glycosuria and a fasting blood glucose of 400 mg/dl at that time and was placed on phenformin (DBI-TD) 100 mg bid and acetohexamide (Dymelor) 500 mg bid. One month later the dose of phenformin was decreased to 100 mg daily because the patient complained of diarrhea. On this regimen, her urine glucose, as measured by Tes-Tape, has been trace to negative and random fasting blood glucose levels have been 130-170 mg/dl.

Concurrent problems include: (a) Hypertension which is currently treated with hydrochlorothiazide (HydroDiuril) 50 mg bid and methyldopa (Aldomet) 500 mg bid; (b) Premenopausal symptoms (hot flashes and depression) treated with conjugated estrogens (Premarin) 1.25 mg daily; (c) Obesity treated with diet and phenmetrazine (Preludin Endurets) one daily; (d) Bilateral cataracts; and (e) Mild renal failure as evidenced by proteinuria and a serum creatinine of 1.9.

1. What is diabetes? What are the two recognized clinical presentations of this disease?

Diabetes is a disorder of carbohydrate, fat and protein metabolism which is due to an absolute or relative lack of insulin and is primarily manifested as hyperglycemia and glycosuria. Almost all cases are caused by genetically determined pancreatic insufficiency; however, it may also be caused by destruction of the pancreas secondary to pancreatitis or hemachromatosis and by a variety of diabetogenic drugs (see Question 4) and endocrine disorders. The long-term vascular complications of diabetes often constitute the most devastating aspects of this disease and include retinopathy, nephropathy, and neuropathy. They may or may not be related to the carbohydrate intolerance per se and there is considerable debate as to whether these can be minimized or prevented by rigid control of blood glucose levels (see Question 17) (240e,268).

There are two major clinical presentations of diabetes. Eighty percent of all diabetics are diagnosed after the age of 35 and are of the obese, *adult-onset* type as illustrated by the patient above. This group retains some pancreatic function and is relatively easily controlled on diet alone or diet plus oral hypoglycemic agents. Twenty to thirty percent may eventually require insulin although they rarely develop ketoacidosis. Many of these individuals may have normal or even high levels of insulin (insulinplethoric) and it is thought that their symptoms may be related to sluggish insulin secretion in response to glucose and a relative tissue resistance to insulin which is observed in obese subjects (57a,240e). Apparently, the number of receptors per surface cell area is diminished which results in a decreased responsiveness to a given amount of insulin. Another 10% of the diabetics are stable, non-obese, adult-onset types, and another 5% have brittle, adult-onset diabetes which more closely resembles the juvenile-onset presentation.

Only 5% of the diabetic population has juvenile-onset diabetes. These patients have no pancreatic reserve (insulinopenic) and always require insulin for the management of their symptoms. Their blood glucose levels may fluctuate widely despite treatment ("brittle") and they are more prone to ketosis than are the adult onset diabetics. It is important to emphasize that the clinical course of some juvenile-onset diabetics is quite stable and is characterized by infrequent hypoglycemic and ketoacidotic episodes (240e,268).

2. Compare carbohydrate homeostasis in a diabetic and non-diabetic individual in the fasting and postprandial state. Relate the acute symptoms of diabetes to the altered metabolism which occurs in these patients.

To understand the symptomatology of diabetes, it is necessary to compare carbohydrate homeostasis of the normal and diabetic individual in the postprandial and fasting state (90,240d). Despite the fact that most symptoms may be related to hyperglycemia, the action of insulin is quite complex and its deficiency will result in disturbances of fat and protein as well as carbohydrate metabolism.

The homeostatic mechanisms in the body are aimed at maintaining a blood glucose level within a range of 40-160 mg/100 ml at all times. A minimum level of 40 mg/100 ml is required to provide adequate fuel for the brain which is only able to use glucose as fuel and is not dependent upon the presence of insulin for its utilization. Glucose spills into the urine resulting in energy and water loss when blood glucose levels exceed the reabsorptive capacity of the kidneys (180 mg/100 ml). Muscle and fat also use glucose as a major source of energy but require the presence of insulin. If glucose is not available, these tissues are able to use other substrates such as amino acids and fatty acids for fuel. It is only necessary to focus on what happens to glucose in the liver, fat, muscle and brain to obtain a basic understanding of glucose metabolism in the normal, fed individual (see Fig. A).

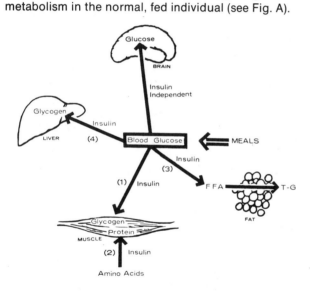

Figure A: Normal Carbohydrate Metabolism — Postprandial

Following the ingestion of food, blood glucose concentrations rise thus stimulating the release of insulin. Insulin promotes the uptake of glucose, fatty acids and amino acids and their conversion to storage forms in most tissues. It also decreases the blood sugar so that none will be unnecessarily wasted in the urine. In muscle, insulin promotes the uptake of glucose and the conversion to its storage form, glycogen (A-1). It also stimulates the uptake of amino acids and their conversion to protein (A-2). In adipose tissue, glucose is converted to free fatty acids (FFA) and stored as triglycerides (TG) (A-3). The presence of insulin also prevents the breakdown of these triglycerides to free

fatty acids, a form which may be transported to other tissues for utilization. The liver does not require insulin for glucose transport but the presence of insulin does facilitate the conversion of glucose to glycogen (A-4). Glycogenolysis (the breakdown of liver glycogen) is the major source of glucose during the fasting state.

In the fasting individual (Fig. B), hypoglycemia inhibits the release of insulin. Additionally, a number of hormones (e.g. glucocorticoids, epinephrine, growth hormone, and glucagon) are released which oppose the effect of insulin and promote an increase in blood sugar. As a result of this lack of insulin, several processes occur which maintain and conserve a minimum blood glucose level for the central nervous system. Glycogen in the liver is broken down to glucose (B-1); amino acids are converted to glucose by a process called gluconeogenesis (B-2); there is a diminished uptake of glucose by insulin-dependent tissues to conserve as much as possible for the brain; and finally, triglycerides are broken down to free fatty acids which are used as fuel by those tissues (primarily muscle and fat) which are unable to use glucose in the absence of insulin (B-3).

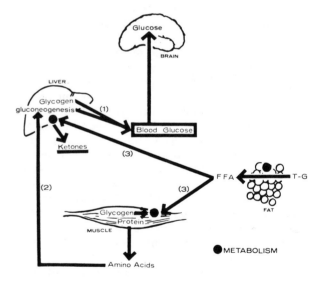

Figure B: Normal Carbohydrate Metabolism — Fasting

It follows that when hyperglycemia secondary to a meal occurs in a diabetic, the absence of insulin prevents the utilization of glucose by fat and muscle and the blood glucose level remains high (see Fig. C-1). Glucose spills into the urine taking excess water with it by the process of osmosis, thus explaining the symptoms of polyuria and polydipsia (C-2). Excessive sugar provides an excellent medium for bacterial growth, predisposing the patient to urinary tract infections, upper respiratory tract infections and vaginal moniliasis as illustrated by the above case. Although there is a large amount of glucose in the bloodstream, it is not accessible to the cells. This lack of intracellular glucose is interpreted by the body as starvation and fasting metabolism is initiated to provide fuel for the cells. Free fatty acids are mobilized and metabolized to ketones (C-3); protein breaks down to amino acids to provide substrate for gluconeogenesis (C-4); and liver glycogen is broken down to glucose (C-5). All of these processes result in symptoms of ketoacidosis, muscle wasting and the perpetually elevated blood glucose level which is observed in diabetics.

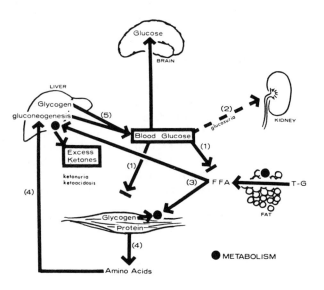

Figure C: Carbohydrate Metabolism — Diabetes

3. Discuss the bihormonal theory in the pathogenesis of diabetes mellitus. What are the therapeutic implications of this theory with regard to somatostatin?

Two major developments in the field of diabetology have enabled investigators to explore the role of glucagon in the pathogenesis of diabetes. The first has been the ability to measure plasma glucagon levels by radioimmunoassay, and the second was the discovery of somatostatin. The latter is a peptide isolated from the hypothalamus which inhibits the release of growth hormone, glucagon, insulin and many other hormones.

Unger and others (108a,108b,240d,267a,267b) have proposed that *glucagon* plays an essential role in the pathogenesis of the hyperglycemia and ketoacidosis observed in diabetics. Unlike non-diabetic individuals, diabetics have elevated glucagon levels postprandially. It has been proposed that excess glucagon contributes to the hyperglycemia by stimulating the release of glucose by the liver (glycogenolysis). In support of this theory is the observation that somatostatin diminishes postprandial hyperglycemia in insulin-dependent diabetics which parallels a suppression of glucagon levels (108a,108d,270). Of importance is the fact that the effect of somatostatin on insulin secretion is unimportant in individuals who lack pancreatic function. Since a decrease in the fasting blood glucose is observed in non-diabetic as well as diabetic patients, glucagon is apparently an important determinant of fasting blood glucose levels.

Felig and others (91a,246a) have disputed the essential role of glucagon in the pathogenesis of diabetes. They point to evidence which indicates that the administration of supraphysiologic doses of glucagon fails to produce a deterioration of the glucose tolerance test in normal individuals or diabetics treated with appropriate doses of insulin. Also, the effect of glucagon in hepatic glycogenolysis is short-lived and cannot account for the sustained hyperglycemia observed in diabetics. It is the contention of these diabetologists that absolute or relative insulin deficiency is the primary cause of diabetes. They propose that the excessive levels of glucagon observed in diabetics is a direct consequence of the lack of insulin in that there is evidence that insulin as well as glucose suppresses the release of glucagon. They agree that glucagon may modify the severity of diabetes, but only when there is a concomitant deficiency of insulin. Clearly, the issue of whether or not diabetes is a bihormonal disease is not resolved.

There are several therapeutic implications which can be extrapolated from the bihormonal theory. If glucagon is a major determinant of the fasting and postprandial hyperglycemia observed in diabetics, then inhibition of glucagon secretion with **somatostatin** should enhance the hypoglycemic effects of insulin. Gerich and others (108c,108d,270a) have shown that somatostatin does lower the postprandial blood glucose in insulin-dependent diabetics and abolishes or minimizes the immediate hyperglycemia which follows a standard meal in a diabetic who has been pretreated with subcutaneous insulin. The response of adult-onset type diabetics is not as predictable (108d, 270a). This may be related to the fact that a majority of these patients retain some pancreatic function so that the action of somatostatin in suppressing insulin secretion becomes relatively more important. Felig and others (91a,257a) have observed an initial hypoglycemia followed by hyperglycemia in fasting maturity-onset diabetics and non-diabetics following prolonged infusion of somatostatin. This effect may be averted with concomitant insulin therapy; however, they warn of the possibility that somatostatin may worsen diabetes in individuals who still have residual pancreatic function.

Somatostatin may also be useful in preventing or attenuating ketoacidosis in juvenile onset diabetics (108b). It has been postulated that the presence of glucagon, which converts the liver to a ketogenic state, as well as insulin deficiency is required to produce ketoacidosis.

Currently, there are several drawbacks to the use of somatostatin by ambulatory patients. It is not active orally, is extremely short-acting (t ½ = 2 minutes) and must, therefore, be administered by intravenous infusion (108a,108d); the effects of subcutaneous administration last for only 2 hours (108a). It is a substance that has innumerable physiologic and pharmacologic actions, many of which would be undesirable if it were administered chronically (108d). For example, it inhibits the secretion of growth hormone, thyrotrophic hormone, gastrin and renin in addition to insulin and glucagon. The inhibition of growth hormone would be extremely undesirable in a pediatric patient. Therefore, it will be necessary to develop a long-acting analogue which has greater pharmacologic specificity before routine or chronic use can be considered.

4. Are there any drugs taken by JS in Case A above which could cause or exacerbate her diabetes? Which drugs are most commonly implicated in iatrogenically induced diabetes? What is the significance of their diabetogenic effect?

JS is taking three drugs which could potentially affect her diabetic control: Hydrochlorothiazide, Preludin (a sympathomimetic), and Premarin (an estrogen). Although the author knows of no reports implicating Preludin or Premarin per se in the exacerbation of diabetes, the risk versus benefits of their use should be reassessed in this patient.

Other drugs which may compromise diabetic control include the following:

Alcohol. Glucose intolerance has been observed in association with chronic alcoholism (175a,219a,107b); however, it is not clear whether this is a direct effect of alcohol or secondary to the liver or pancreatic dysfunction present in many of these individuals. Nikkila et al (194a) challenged non-obese, non-diabetic males with alcohol in doses which equalled 25% of the total caloric intake for 7 days. A deterioration in both oral and intravenous glucose tolerance tests was observed following this period. Since the plasma insulin response to glucose was unchanged, these investigators postulate that this effect was related to an increased tissue resistance to insulin. These findings are in contrast with another study in which four

healthy young adults with no history of diabetes were also challenged with alcohol (206). The only subject who developed a diminished glucose tolerance had a strong family history of diabetes. In all cases the diabetogenic effect was reversible. The latter study was provoked by the observation of two patients who developed brief episodes of diabetes apparently related to the ingestion of alcohol. Subsequent rechallenge with large doses of alcohol (266-513 ml administered over 1-3 days) induced glucose intolerance and an augmented response of insulin to glucose in both of these patients. It is important to emphasize that no change in glucose tolerance was observed the morning following a single challenge with alcohol the evening prior to testing in amounts which produced levels of 1 mg/ml. In fact, single doses of ethanol *increased* the peripheral utilization of intravenous glucose and increased the response of insulin to both intravenous and oral glucose during the time alcohol levels were elevated which is consistent with the more commonly observed alcohol-induced hypoglycemia (194a) (see Question 61).

The mechanism of this effect is unknown; but it is not related to the caloric value of alcohol, suppression of insulin release, or stimulation of glucocorticoid release. Alcohol augments hepatic glycogenolysis and may decrease the peripheral utilization of glucose. In well-nourished individuals alcohol may increase blood glucose levels by 10%. It should be re-emphasized that alcohol-induced hypoglycemia is more commonly observed (27).

Arginine HCl. 30 gm of arginine hydrochloride infused intravenously over a period of 30 minutes produces maximal increases in the blood glucose of 16-29 mg/100 ml 20-30 minutes after the infusion is begun. The glycemic response in diabetic patients is greater. Arginine also stimulates the release of insulin, glucagon and growth hormone. Elevations of blood glucose are not due to gluconeogenesis from this amino acid. A more likely explanation is glucagon stimulation of hepatic glycogenolysis (91).

(L) Asparaginase can cause clinically significant hyperglycemia and glucosuria 2-4 days following a single therapeutic dose. Abnormal release of insulin in response to glucose lasts from days to months but generally is reversible. Hyperglycemia occurred in 5/39 patients in one series and in 3/5 patients in another. It is proposed that asparaginase inhibits insulin synthesis or destroys pancreatic tissue (104).

Birth Control Pills. See chapter on *Oral Contraception.*

Clonidine. Insulin secretion is inhibited by alpha-adrenergic stimulation. Since clonidine markedly suppresses norepinephrine levels, it was predicted that its administration would increase basal insulin levels and produce a fall in plasma blood glucose levels. Unexpectedly, a single 0.5 mg dose of clonidine decreased basal insulin levels and increased the plasma glucose by 12 mg/dl in non-diabetic subjects. Multiple doses of clonidine for four days also increased the plasma glucose by a similar magnitude but did not decrease basal insulin levels. However, the acute release of insulin in response to intravenous glucose was diminished under these circumstances. Since these effects were prevented by pretreatment with the alpha adrenergic blocker, phentolamine, Metz et al propose that clonidine selectively stimulates alpha adrenergic receptors affecting metabolic functions. Although the significance of this effect in diabetic patients has not been studied, it would seem reasonable to follow diabetics for deterioration of control if clonidine is prescribed for hypertension (185a).

Dextrothyroxine. Eighteen diabetics received 4-8 mg of dextrothyroxine for varying periods of time. Fasting blood sugars were significantly increased after two weeks. Continual treatment resulted in further deterioration in 8 of the 18 patients. One developed acidosis and several required readjustment of their medications. Hypoglycemia occurred in two patients after discontinuation of the drug (294).

Diazoxide. See Question 5.

Diphenylhydantoin (phenytoin). See Question 6.

Diuretics. See Question 7.

Glucagon. Glucagon is a hormone elaborated from the alpha cells of the human pancreas. Injection of 1-2 mg results in increased blood sugar within 5 to 20 minutes. The hormone promotes the breakdown of glycogen to glucose by increasing the activity of phosphorylase, an enzyme which acts at the first step of glycogenolysis. It works poorly in debilitated patients who may not have adequate glycogen stores. Its action is brief and must be supplemented with oral glucose as soon as the patient is responsive (268). See Question 3.

Glucocorticoids. See chapter on *Clinical Use and Toxicity of the Glucocorticoids* (59,110,182,246).

Glucose. Normal persons receiving 3 to 4 liters of 15% glucose/day for 5 to 7 days should be able to maintain a blood glucose of 100 mg% or less. If higher levels are observed, the patient may be diabetic and proper diagnostic tests should be performed (52).

Glycerin. Hyperglycemia was reported in a 68-year-old patient who had ingested large amounts (2.3 gm/kg) of glycerin over three days for the treatment of acute glaucoma. Since glycerin is metabolized to glucose, it should be used cautiously in elderly, dehydrated diabetics. The usual dose is 1-1.5 gm/kg and the high doses used in this patient may have been a factor in the development of hyperglycemia (67).

Levodopa. A single 0.5-1 gm dose of levodopa (L-dopa) significantly increases plasma levels of immunoreactive glucagon above basal levels in diabetic and non-diabetic subjects. This parallels an increase in plasma glucose levels and precedes elevated levels of growth hormone (155a,218a). The concomitant administration of 100 gm of oral glucose will suppress the effect of L-dopa on glucagon secretion in non-diabetics but not in diabetics. The mechanism by which L-dopa enhances the secretion of glucagon is not known, but the various theories are discussed by Klimes et al (155a). It is probable that this effect accounts for the deterioration in glucose tolerance which was observed in 14/19 parkinsonian patients following 12 months of chronic L-dopa therapy (240c).

Marijuana. It has been postulated that "when the stress of marijuana ingestion is greater than the adaptive capacity of the glucose regulating system, diabetic ketoacidosis might evolve."

It should be noted that the single patient under study was also taking chlorpromazine, which has also been reported to decrease glucose tolerance. If the author's postulate is true, chlorpromazine may have compromised the patient's glucose regulating system. The pharmacology of marijuana is poorly understood at this time; future studies are needed to validate or negate this report (137).

Nicotinic Acid. Doses of 1.5-3.0 grams used in the treatment of hypercholesterolemia or psychiatric disorders have been reported to cause hyperglycemia, glucosuria, ketonuria and increased insulin requirements (19 units in one case). The effect is reversible and its mechanism is unknown (6,144,189).

Phenothiazines. A retrospective study published in 1968 (261) suggested the incidence of elevated blood glucose levels in psychiatric patients increased after the introduction to chlorpromazine (17.2% as opposed to 4.2% prior to chlorpromazine). The increased levels occurred most often in women over 50 years of age who had a family history of diabetes and who had been treated for more than one year with 100 mg of chlorpromazine or more daily. There was a 25% remission rate after discontinuation of the drug or a decrease in its dose. Several isolated reports have been published (109,133,147,261).

A more recent study (269) suggests that the incidence of impaired glucose tolerance after long and short term therapy with chlorpromazine is not significantly different from that of the control population (16% vs. 10%).

Potassium Depletion. Hypokalemia and/or total body depletion of potassium has been associated with hyperglycemia, glucose intolerance, and a reduced output of insulin and growth hormone (119). These abnormalities have been observed in patients with cirrhosis and hyperaldosteronism. Administration of 180 mEq of KCl daily for a period of 2 weeks or more reversed the diabetic glucose tolerance to normal in cirrhotic patients (208).

Propranolol. Two episodes of hyperosmolar non-ketotic coma (HNC) were reported in a 46-year-old hypertensive male who had been taking Apresoline 200 mg and propranolol 240 mg daily for one year. Hyperglycemia with ketosis developed when the patient was taken off propranolol. In this patient, propranolol blunted the rise in free fatty acids in response to hyperglycemia and diminished the insulin response to tolbutamide. It is postulated that large doses may potentially precipitate HNC in untreated diabetics by inhibiting lipolysis and impairing insulin response to glucose (208).

Sympathomimetics. Epinephrine 0.5 mg SQ stimulates glycogenolysis which results in an increased blood glucose. The effect occurs only if there are adequate stores of liver glycogen. Other sympathomimetics do not have as potent an effect on blood sugar as does epinephrine.

Hyperglycemia, acetonuria and glucosuria were reported in three nondiabetic children who received therapeutic oral doses of phenylephrine. A 19-month-old child received 1.25 mg every 4 hours; a 2½-year-old child received 10 mg every 4 hours (21,139,210).

Theophylline, a phosphodiesterase inhibitor, increases intracellular levels of c-AMP and thereby increases insulin secretion in response to glucose in prediabetics and hypocalcemic individuals, but not in diabetics. Despite this action, *hyperglycemia* which is resistant to insulin therapy is observed following theophylline infusion because its glycogenolytic and gluconeogenic effects predominate (47,107a,202a).

5. A 54-year-old male is admitted for medical management of hypertension and progressive renal failure. He has been treated with a variety of medications, most recently alphamethyldopa 2 gm/day; furosemide 80 mg bid, and guanethidine 200 mg daily. His blood pressure on admission is 220/180. Current medications were continued on a prn basis; however, intravenous diazoxide 300 mg was also initiated. On the fifth hospital day the patient became confused and disoriented. Serum chemistries drawn at this time revealed the following:

Blood glucose 1800 mg%; serum ketones negative; Na 126 mEq/L; K 3.7 mEq/L; serum osmolality 360 mOsm/L; creatinine 5.0 mg/100 ml.

The patient recovered following treatment with insulin and hypotonic intravenous fluids. Discuss the etiology of this patient's symptomatology.

The patient described above has developed hyperosmolar non-ketotic coma secondary to the administration of **diazoxide.** The occurrence of this syndrome supposedly results from the presence of levels of insulin which are sufficient to prevent lipolysis but insufficient to promote the utilization of glucose. It

occurs most frequently in adult onset diabetics.

Although diazoxide has a predictable hyperglycemic effect in therapeutic doses following oral or intravenous administration, severe complications similar to the case described above are relatively rare. Almost all reported cases of hyperglycemic coma have been of the hyperosmolar non-ketotic type. Patients with uremia may be predisposed to the development of this complication (25,50). Ketotic coma has been reported in a ketosis prone diabetic following the administration of diazoxide.

Finnerty (98) treated 700 hypertensive patients with intravenous diazoxide and noted transient (1-4 hours) increases in blood sugar in 40% of nondiabetics and 75% of diabetics. He noted that in some diabetics hyperglycemia may persist from 24-48 hours. Thiazide diuretics (83) and furosemide may enhance but apparently do not increase the frequency with which this effect occurs. Pretreatment with tolbutamide will abolish or attenuate the hyperglycemia but will not interfere with the antihypertensive action of diazoxide (193,289).

Fajans (83) studied and summarized the theoretical mechanism of diazoxide's hyperglycemic effect. He concluded that diazoxide blocks the secretion of insulin and diminishes fasting and postprandial plasma insulin levels in diabetics, nondiabetics and in patients with insulinomas. It may also have an extrapancreatic mechanism through inhibition of phosphodiesterase which elevates levels of 3'5' cyclic AMP. Cyclic AMP then enhances enzymes which promote glycogenolysis and increase gluconeogenesis. Decreased peripheral utilization of glucose by diazoxide has also been proposed as a mechanism for the hyperglycemia. Since glucagon secretion is decreased by diazoxide, stimulation of this hormone cannot account for its effect (17a). The potency and consistency of this action of diazoxide is demonstrated by its value in the management of hyperglycemia of several etiologies (120,281).

6. A 53-year-old male with a family history of diabetes mellitus develops *grand mal* seizures following trauma to his head. He is to be treated with phenytoin (DPH). What is the effect of DPH on blood glucose and plasma insulin levels? Is the use of DPH contraindicated in this patient?

Several reports of DPH-induced glucosuria, hyperglycemia, diminished glucose tolerance tests (66, 85,203,264) and hyperosmolar non-ketotic coma (43,155) have appeared in the literature. With the exception of a single case (85) all were associated with toxic amounts of **phenytoin** (as judged by neurologic symptomatology) or the presence of other diabetogenic factors (stress, corticosteroids, dialysis). With the exception of two critically ill patients who developed hyperosmolar non-ketotic coma (113), all of these abnormalities were reversible following discontinuation of the drug. In most cases a family history of diabetes was absent or unspecified.

Malherbe, et al (178) and Fariss, et al (85) have demonstrated that pretreatment with therapeutic doses of phenytoin for as little as 3 days diminishes insulin release in response to glucose in non-diabetic patients.

Fariss, et al (85) demonstrated a dose relationship of this effect in a single patient. Doses of 200-300 mg/day reduced plasma insulin response but did not diminish glucose tolerance. The latter could not be demonstrated until doses of 400 mg were administered.

The clinical value of this pharmacologic effect in the diagnosis of early diabetes (172) and the treatment of insulinomas (158) is currently under investigation. It should be noted that DPH obscured the diagnosis of insulin secreting adenoma in one case (158).

Clinically, hyperglycemia does not appear to be a significant problem in patients who are taking chronic, non-toxic doses of DPH (63,188). Nevertheless, close monitoring is warranted in those patients who are (a) receiving high doses of DPH; (b) taking other diabetogenic medications; or (c) diabetic risks (178). The use of DPH is not contraindicated in this patient.

7. A 45-year-old male with a family history of diabetes mellitus and mild hypertension is to be initiated on hydrochlorothiazide 50 mg twice daily. Discuss the diabetogenic effect of hydrochlorothiazide and other diuretics.

That thiazide *diuretics* have a diabetogenic effect is well recognized and accepted. The phenomenon was first observed in 1959. Despite the appearance of numerous case reports and short term studies thereafter, the paucity of long term prospective studies which would clarify the significance and incidence of this effect is astounding. In reviewing the literature, one is able to make very few definitive conclusions:

(a) The diabetogenic effect may be observed following therapeutic doses of diuretics as soon as 3-5 days after the onset of therapy (51,114,288).

(b) Diuretics may aggravate existing diabetes (93,134,229,254). They may also precipitate clinical diabetes in patients with chemical diabetes (114).

(c) There have been a few case reports implicating diuretics as a cause of diabetic coma. Six of these have been associated with chlorthalidone (61, 64, 74, 190, 254); two with thiazides. It has also been suggested that diuretics may be an etiologic factor in the production of hyperosmolar non-ketotic coma (64, 70, 108).

(d) Case reports or studies of diuretic-induced hyperglycemia *in man* exist for the following diuretics:

(1) Thiazides (34,45,51,114,230).

(2) Chlorthalidone (15,45,61,64).

(3) Ethacrynic Acid (71).

(4) Furosemide (34,142,277).

(5) Triamterene (121).

Thiazide diuretics and chlorthalidone are most frequently implicated.

(e) Patients with existing diabetes mellitus or a family history of the disease appear to be predisposed to this effect (45,114). However, diuretic-induced hyperglycemia and/or decreased glucose tolerance has also been reported in non-diabetic patients (288).

(f) Diminished glucose tolerance resulting from diuretic therapy is in most cases reversible following withdrawal of the drug (45,114).

(g) Hypokalemia has been associated with the diabetogenic effects of diuretics; and, in some cases, potassium supplements have reversed an abnormal glucose tolerance induced by these agents (218,288). Although potassium deficiency per se is associated with a diminished glucose tolerance (119), hypokalemia is not a consistent finding in patients with diuretic-induced hyperglycemia (45,51,114). It should also be noted that in some studies, maintenance of a normal serum potassium failed to prevent the occurrence of diuretic-induced hyperglycemia.

(h) The mechanism of diuretic-induced hyperglycemia has not been elucidated. Most investigators have theorized that it may share a mechanism of action similar to that of diazoxide (see Question 5). (Also see chapter on *Edema.*)

8. Briefly describe the tests that are used to diagnose diabetes.

Several tests are currently used to diagnose diabetes, all of which measure an individual's ability to handle a glucose load (82).

The *oral glucose tolerance test (OGTT)* measures an individual's ability to handle a glucose load over a period of time and is the most reliable diagnostic test for diabetes. Following an overnight fast, a morning fasting blood sugar is drawn and a 100 gram glucose load is then ingested by the patient. Thereafter, blood samples are drawn at half hour intervals for 2 hours and again at 3 hours following the ingestion of this glucose load. Urine samples are often taken simultaneously and tested for glucose to estimate the individual's renal threshold for glucose. In non-diabetics the blood glucose returns to normal (less than 110 mg/100 ml) in less than two hours. In the diabetic, the glucose peak is higher and occurs much later than in the normal curve; levels also decline at a slower rate. Siperstein has recently criticized the criterion used to diagnose diabetes by the GTT (240a).

Other tests which are used as diagnostic or screening tests for diabetes include the following:

(a) *Fasting Blood Glucose (FBG).* This blood sample is taken in the morning prior to breakfast. A normal value for venous blood is 60-100 mg/100 ml. Although a high value is fairly diagnostic of diabetes, a normal value is meaningless since a delay in glucose metabolism may be the only defect in early diabetes. It is therefore conceivable that a mild diabetic could handle the glucose provided by the dinner meal within 9½ hours, the required fasting time. Many laboratories now measure *serum* glucose values which are normally 15 mg% higher than those of blood glucose (268).

(b) The *two hour postprandial (2HPP)* blood glucose is used as a screening test for diabetes. A blood glucose level is drawn 2 hours following a 100 gram glucose load. In non-diabetics, blood glucose levels return to normal in less than 2 hours following a glucose challenge whereas hyperglycemia persists in a diabetic. Values for this test are generally higher than the two hour oral glucose tolerance test values due to less stringent diet preparation and the inconsistent use of the standard glucose dose.

(c) *Glucosuria (Urine Glucose Tests).* A positive test for glucose in the urine is not diagnostic for diabetes but is an indication for more definitive testing. It is important to realize that glucosuria occurs in many other conditions (e.g. pregnancy or faulty renal function), and that it is not a persistent finding in diabetes. Glucosuria generally occurs when the mean blood glucose level is 180 mg/100 ml or more and rarely occurs when this level is less than 130 mg/100 ml. There is an exception to this rule in that the renal threshold for glucose may increase with age so that older diabetics may "spill" no glucose at all despite a high blood glucose level.

9. What are the two basic types of tests available to determine the presence of glucose in the urine? Discuss the principal differences between the two.

The two methods of testing for urine glucose are (a) the glucose oxidase method (Clinistix, Diastix, Tes-Tape) which is specific for glucose, and (b) the copper reduction method (Clinitest, Benedict's Solution) which may detect the presence of other reducing substances in the urine as well as glucose.

Even though the glucose oxidase method is specific for glucose and the simplest to perform, it is not the test of choice for monitoring insulin therapy because of its *qualitative* nature. Despite the fact that "quantitative" figures appear on many of the product labels, it appears that glucose oxidase tests are quantitative only when the amount of glucose in the urine is less than 0.25%. Larger amounts (2, 3 and 4%) were interpreted as 0.5% or less in 502 out of 804 urines tested with Tes-Tape (171). This high rate of interpretation error cannot be tolerated when hyperglycemia must be controlled to prevent ketoacidosis.

Glucose oxidase tests are, however, superior to the copper reduction methods in the screening of patients for diabetes because of their simplicity, specificity and ability to detect such minute amounts of sugar in the urine. They are also the tests of choice for monitoring adult onset diabetics who rarely "spill" glucose into the urine if properly controlled (171).

Although copper reduction methods (Clinitest, Benedict's Solution) are not as specific for glucose or as convenient to perform, they are more reliable in quantitating large amounts of sugar in the urine. For this reason, the copper reduction is the test of choice for insulin-dependent diabetics, many of whom adjust their insulin dosage in accordance with urinary glucose levels.

Recently, a glucose oxidase test which makes use of another colorimetric system (Diastix) has been marketed. It is the *only* glucose oxidase method which makes quantitative claims. Preliminary studies (143, 262) indicate that at low and intermediate levels of glucosuria (<1.5%) Diastix is comparable to Clinitest. However, false low readings are observed in the presence of high concentrations of glucose (>1.5%) or moderate to large amounts of ketones. This is also the author's experience. Another difficulty with the test is that it is frequently difficult to discriminate between the 1% and 2% readings because the color reaction is frequently speckled rather than uniform. This is definitely an undesirable feature for use by a brittle, difficult-to-control diabetic. If future studies confirm the manufacturer's "quantitative" claim, Diastix may become the test of choice for the juvenile diabetic because it is simple to use. Also, when quantitation is not critical for a particular patient and compliance in testing is of greater importance, Diastix is definitely the method of choice.

10. What is the chemical basis for each of the tests used to detect sugar in the urine? How do drugs interfere with the correct interpretation of these tests? Can misleading interpretations be avoided?

Glucose Oxidase Tests:

The following series of reactions form the basis of the glucose oxidase tests (89):

(a) β D-glucose in urine + Oxygen in air $\xrightarrow{\text{glucose oxidase}}$ Gluconic Acid + H_2O_2

(b) $H_2O_2 \xrightarrow{\text{peroxidase}}$ nascent oxygen

(c) $\uparrow$ nascent oxygen + reduced O-tolidine (pink) $\xrightarrow{\quad * \quad}$ oxidized O-tolidine (blue)

*site of drug inhibition

Strong reducing substances prevent the oxidation of O-tolidine, the indicator for glucose oxidase tests and may thereby produce a false negative reaction. Substances strong enough to prevent this oxidation generally cause a false positive Clinitest reaction as well. Weaker reducing substances such as the glucuronide metabolites of many drugs are capable of reacting with the Clinitest tablets but will not inhibit the enzyme test.

Feldman et al (89) attempted to estimate the potential incidence of error in reading urine glucose tests. They found a 23% incidence of false low readings by the Diastix or Clinistix method when urine was fortified with glucose. Approximately 50% of these false low readings could be accounted for by the presence of ascorbic or gentisic acid in the urine. Tes-Tape appeared to be less sensitive to the presence of these reducing substances.

Feldman et al (88) attempted to identify substances responsible for false negative glucose oxidase reactions and came to the following conclusions:

(a) *Gentisic acid,* a strong reducing metabolite of salicylates, may inhibit the glucose oxidase test and cause a false positive Clinitest reaction. Fifty percent (5/10) of the urine specimens from patients ingesting 2.4 to 2.7 gm of aspirin daily caused false negative glucose oxidase readings whereas 5/7 readings were false negative in patients ingesting 3.6 to 5.6 gm of aspirin daily. In most cases those urines which inhibited the glucose oxidase also caused a false positive copper reduction test. Patients with alcaptonuria excrete large amounts of homogentisic acid which reacts similarly to gentisic acid (88).

(b) An unknown reducing *metabolite of L-dopa* is capable of inhibiting the glucose oxidase test. Six of 25 urine specimens caused false positive Clinitest reactions and false negative Clinistix reactions in patients ingesting 0.75 to 3.0 gm of L-dopa. The ratio of false readings increased (13/17 samples) in patients taking 3.5 to 5.0 gm of L-dopa.

(c) A single urine from a patient ingesting 2 gm of *methyldopa (Aldomet)* caused a false positive Clinitest but did not inhibit the glucose oxidase reaction. Five urine samples from patients taking 1-2 gms of methyldopa did not cause false readings in either of the tests.

(d) The urine of patients with carcinoid syndrome who excrete large amounts of *5HIAA* may be expected to react similarly (88,89).

Gifford et al (111) noted that the urine of two patients receiving *ascorbic acid* (250 mg IM and 500 mg po) gave false negative Tes-Tape and Clinistix results. *In vitro* ascorbic acid must be present in concentrations of 0.08 mg/ml to cause a false negative reaction. Ascorbic acid is frequently added in large amounts to tetracycline parenteral products as an antioxidant. Gifford also noted similar results in the urines of patients taking therapeutic doses of dipyrone and mercuhydrin (111).

Drugs which do *not* influence the glucose oxidase test *in vitro* include the following:

xanthine 2 mg/ml
caffeine 10 mg/ml
glucuronic acid <20 mg/ml
reducing sugars 10 mg/ml (galactose, lactose, fructose)

penicillin 10,000 u/ml	+ Clinitest
streptomycin 5 mg/ml	+ Clinitest
cephaloridine 5 mg/ml	+ Clinitest
cephalothin 5 mg/ml	+ Clinitest
INH 5 mg/ml	+ Clinitest

Even in the presence of strong reducing substances, glucosuria can be detected on the Tes-Tape if the reading is taken in the area wet by diffusion or at the margin of wet and dry tape. The tape apparently acts as a mini ascending chromatography system in which the glucose is separated from the interfering substance. The same principle may be used with the Clinistix if care is taken to dip only a portion of the test patch (88,111).

Copper Reduction Method:

The following reaction represents the basis for the copper reduction test for glucose (Clinitest, Benedict's Solution):

$$Cu^{++}SO_4^{=} \xrightarrow[\substack{\text{reducing} \\ \text{substance}}]{\text{Glucose or any} *} Cu^{+++}O_3^{=}$$

cupric sulfate   cuprous oxide (reduced)

*Drug interference

Although lists of drugs which may potentially cause false positive reactions with copper reduction tests are available, there is very little documentation for the significance of these reactions. Should a patient be taking one of these drugs, it is suggested that the urine be double checked with Tes-Tape and be interpreted in the manner described above (See Table 1). Also see discussion of specific drugs under glucose oxidase tests.

Table 1
SUBSTANCES WHICH MAY CAUSE A FALSE POSITIVE GLUCOSURIA BY THE COPPER REDUCTION METHOD (14,88,157,161)

Ascorbic acid (large quantities)	Methyldopa (88)
	Nalidixic acid (157)
BAL	Para-aminosalicylic acid (14)
Cephalothin (161)	Penicillin (massive doses)(88)
Cephaloridine (88)	Probenecid (14)
Chloral hydrate	Salicylates (88)
Isoniazid (88)	Streptomycin (88)
L-dopa (88)	Sugars (galactose, lactose,
Metaxalone (14)	fructose) (14)

11. What is the 2 Drop Clinitest method of testing for urine glucose?

The 2 Drop Clinitest method uses 2 drops rather

than 5 drops of urine and is useful in quantitating very high levels (2%, 3% and 5%) of glucosuria. It is not as accurate as Diastix, Tes-Tape or the 5 drop Clinitest, however, in quantitating small amounts of glucose (<376 mg/100 ml) in the urine. Because the urine is more dilute, the "pass-through" phenomenon does not occur as frequently (see Question 18). Color charts are available from the Ames Company for interpretation of the 2 drop Clinitest (143,194).

12. All urine glucose tests require visual acuity for their interpretation. Is there any way a blind diabetic can test for glucosuria?

Free (101) recently suggested a method which could be used by the blind to test his urine for the presence of glucose. A test tube containing ¼ teaspoonful of dry baker's yeast is filled with urine, covered with a rubber finger cot and agitated. If as little as ¼% of glucose is present the finger cot will be inflated in 20-30 minutes because carbon dioxide is released as the glucose is fermented.

13. AG is a 13½-year-old female who is admitted to the hospital with symptoms of polydipsia, polyuria, weight loss, easy fatigability, and a recent history of multiple upper respiratory tract infections. Her temperature was 39°C and her chest was congested. A urinalysis revealed 4+ glucose by the Clinitest method with no ketones. Her blood glucose at this time was 400 mg/dl. A diagnosis of juvenile-onset diabetes and pneumonia was made. The physician ordered appropriate fluids, intravenous cephalothin (Keflin), and insulin "to be given according to the rainbow schedule." What is meant by the "rainbow" or "sliding scale" method for insulin dosing?

These terms refer to a method of adjusting dosages of subcutaneous *regular insulin* according to urine glucose readings obtained by the *copper reduction method.* The presence of acetone also influences the dose. Because there is no standard schedule, the physician must specifically indicate the number of units (s)he desires for each reading. Generally, insulin doses are in the range of 5 units for each "plus" sign. For example:

0-1+	0-5 U
2+	5-10U
3+	10-15U
4+	15-20U
Mod. acetone	An additional 5U

Such a schedule is used for the hospitalized diabetic whose insulin requirements may vary with stress (e.g., infections, surgery or any acute illness) or to determine the initial insulin requirements of a newly diagnosed diabetic. Generally the urine is tested every four hours and insulin administered accordingly. However,

Bressler (35) recently recommended that this interval be increased to six hours since all diabetics who have been treated with insulin eventually develop antibodies which may delay the onset and prolong the action of regular insulin beyond that which is seen in nondiabetics.

14. The nurse caring for AG obtained a 3+ result on the Tes-Tape and a 1+ result by the Clinitest method. She does not know which value to use to determine the insulin dose. She had been instructed to use both methods because the physician was aware of the fact that Keflin might interfere with the test results of Clinitest. What is your response?

Many health professionals do not realize that a 3+ (1/2%) result from a Tes-Tape is not equivalent to a 3+ (1%) on the Clinitest. As a result, many even set up the Rainbow Schedule using the Tes-Tape. In this case, the results of the two tests are equivalent and the nurse should use the Clinitest result to determine her insulin dose. The fact that the Clinitest reading was the same as the Tes-Tape indicates that the Clinitest reading is true for glucose and not a false positive secondary to the Keflin.

It is important to note that each method for testing urine glucose uses a different colorimetric system and that the "+" values for each correspond to different glucose concentrations. (See Table 2.)

Table 2
CORRESPONDING URINE GLUCOSE PERCENTAGES FOR THE "PLUS" SYSTEMS OF VARIOUS URINE GLUCOSE TESTS

Test	Negative	Trace	+	++	+++	++++
Clinitest	0%	¼%	½%	¾%	1%	2%
Diastix	0%	1/10%	¼%	½%	1%	2%
Tes-Tape	0%	*	1/10%	¼%	½%	2% or more

*No such reading

15. How should AG's insulin requirements be ascertained?

Severely ill and ketotic diabetics are generally hospitalized to determine their insulin requirements on the basis of frequent urine and blood glucose measurements. This process involves two basic steps. The first is to determine the total amount of insulin required in a 24-hour period. This is done by testing for urine glucose using the copper reduction method (Clinitest) every four hours (before meals and at bedtime) and administering 4-5 units of regular insulin ½-1 hour before meals for each "plus" which is measured. Additional doses may be given throughout the night if necessary (also refer to the earlier discussion on "rainbow schedule" — Question 13) (268).

In addition it is possible to draw serial blood glucoses to determine the accuracy of the doses. The latter procedure also gives some indication of the patient's renal threshold for glucose. Adjusting the insulin dose according to the degree of glycosuria is unsatisfactory in those patients (usually geriatrics) who have high renal thresholds. Their insulin requirements must be determined on the basis of blood sugars. It is also possible to approximate the initial insulin requirement by the quantitative determination of glucose in a 24-hour urine collection. One unit of insulin is said to "cover" each gram of glucose spilled in the urine.

Once the 24-hour requirements of regular insulin are ascertained and the patient is under control, multiple injections of regular insulin may be replaced by a single injection of intermediate acting insulin (NPH or lente). The dose of NPH is ⅔ to ¾ of the 24-hour requirement and should be supplemented with regular insulin as indicated by the urine sugars. If the total requirement exceeds 40 units, the insulin may be given in two doses, generally ⅔ in the morning and ⅓ in the evening. When the patient has been switched to an intermediate acting insulin, many physicians will order a blood sugar at 4 p.m., the time at which insulin exerts its peak activity. This is done to ascertain that there is no midafternoon hypoglycemia. The urine test taken before the evening meal most closely reflects the activity of the morning dose of NPH and the morning fasting urine test reflects the activity of the evening dose of NPH. Upon discharge, the dose is decreased by 4-6 units to compensate for increased activity which also has an insulin-like effect (76,180,268).

16. If AG had presented with a milder form of the disease (e.g., FBG 230 mg/dl, 2+ glucose in the urine, urine and serum negative for ketones, recurrent vaginitis), how could her insulin requirements be determined on an outpatient basis?

Dosing a mild, nonketotic diabetic on an outpatient basis is accomplished by giving an arbitrarily small dose of intermediate acting insulin and adjusting this dose on the basis of frequent (before meals and at bedtime) urine testing. The patient is given an initial dose of 10-20 units of NPH or lente insulin, instructed to test her urine four to five times daily and to increase or decrease her insulin dose according to a prescribed schedule. For example, if she spills 3+ to 4+ (i.e., 1-2% glucose) in her urine all day, she is to increase her insulin dose the following morning by four units. If she spills 1+ to 2+ (0-¼% glucose) in her urine for the entire day, there is no change in the dose; and if she spills 0 to 1+ (0-¼% glucose), the insulin dose is decreased by four units. The patient returns weekly for a fasting blood glucose test and for re-evaluation of her therapy (76,268).

17. What are the long-term goals of insulin therapy for AG? What are the arguments for and against

"tight" vs. "loose" control?

The degree to which diabetics should be controlled is a major area of controversy among diabetologists. For years there have been proponents for both "loose" and "tight" diabetic control. Those who favor "tight" (also described as "good," "rigid," and "chemical") control base their mode of therapy on the belief that late complications of diabetes can be minimized, prevented, or delayed by the normalization of the blood glucose concentration (40a,145a,225a). The evidence for this is adequately reviewed by Job et al (145a), Cahill (40a), Engerman et al (80a), and Rossini (225a). Briefly, there are several retrospective studies which suggest that the prevalence and progression of retinopathy is related to the degree of diabetic control (80a,145a). In addition, there are several animal studies which show that diabetic-like lesions in the eye, kidney, and nerve are decreased or prevented if blood glucose concentrations are normalized (40a,80a,145a,225a). There is also evidence that when blood glucose levels are elevated, an enzyme (aldose reductase) converts glucose to sorbitol (a sugar alcohol) in the Schwann cell of the spinal roots and peripheral nerves and in the lens of the eye. Sorbitol is metabolized very slowly and does not readily diffuse into extracellular spaces. The osmotic gradient which results causes swelling, and if this process persists, it is postulated that other biochemical changes will ultimately produce neuropathy and cataract formation (103a,225a). Finally, a small prospective study performed by Job et al (145a) which compared patients on single injections of insulin with those on two to three injections of insulin showed there was less retinopathy in the multiple injection group over a four-year follow-up period. The criticisms of this study as outlined by Siperstein et al (240b) point to the difficulties in gathering this type of prospective data. Rossini (225a) also advocates close control on the grounds that poor control may result in several short term complications: ketoacidosis and hyperosmolar coma, poor wound healing, impaired phagocytosis, and hyperlipemia.

Proponents of "loose" control strive to achieve a blood glucose level which maintains the patient in an asymptomatic state. Thus, they are likely to accept a blood glucose level which is clearly in the hyperglycemic range, but generally below the renal threshold for that patient. They are more concerned about the hazards of hypoglycemia and may prefer to see small amounts of glucose in the urine (trace to 1%) in patients who are particularly susceptible to insulin reactions. The argument for loose control is primarily based upon the premise that the late complications occur independently of hyperglycemia and that the morbidity associated with hypoglycemia outweighs the benefits that may accrue from tight control. Siperstein et al (240b) argue that animal studies cannot be extrapolated to humans and that the observation that sorbitol accumulates in certain tissues cannot be consistently shown to be causally related to long-term diabetic complications. They also note that muscle capillary membrane thickening (generally considered to be a long term complication of diabetes) has been observed at the time of diagnosis or very early in the course of diabetes and hold that the evidence for the prevention of microangiopathy by strict regulation of the blood glucose level is inconclusive.

What then, is a reasonable and realistic approach to the management of a diabetic patient? Ingelfinger pointedly criticizes diabetologists from both camps (138a). Those who advocate "good" control have failed to define what this constitutes, and the evidence cited by the advocates of loose control for the dangers of hypoglycemia is weak. There are other difficulties. Our current methods for monitoring "control" rely heavily on patient-performed urine glucose testing. It has been clearly demonstrated that these are inaccurate 50% of the time (179a) and that they correlate poorly with the blood glucose. Also, it is impossible to predict the degree of blood glucose fluctuation throughout the day from either a fasting or a random blood glucose level or from a quantitative 24-hour urine glucose sample. Gabbay (103b) has suggested that in the future, **Hemoglobin A_{IC}** (HbA$_{IC}$) levels may be used as an index of long term diabetic control. Hb A$_{IC}$ is a minor hemoglobin component which is identical to Hb A except that a glucose group is linked to the terminal amino acid. It is elevated in diabetics and is apparently formed by a relatively irreversible, non-enzymatic process. There is evidence which suggests that it accumulates in red blood cells during their 120-day life span and that the levels reflect the average blood glucose level for the preceding few weeks.

Until diabetologists can come to some agreement on the degree of control, Drash (77a) has proposed some therapeutic goals:

a. Control the symptoms of diabetes (polyuria, polyphagia, polydipsia, infection) and avoid hypoglycemia.

b. Maintain normal growth and maturation in the child with diabetes.

c. Maintain normal blood lipid levels.

d. Minimize urinary glucose loss. This may be defined as aglycosuria in patients who are not prone to hypoglycemic reactions. For those who are, attempt to minimize urine glucose spillage to less than 1%. An occasional 24-hour urinary glucose should be less than 7% of the total carbohydrate dietary intake which is 25 gm for the average teenager.

e. Drash (77a) believes that the attainment of normal blood glucose concentrations is an unreasonable goal in the insulin-dependent diabetic population because

of the high degree of variability which exists. In actuality, euglycemia (60-100 mg% in the fasting state and no greater than 150 mg% postprandially) may be almost impossible to achieve even with multiple injections of insulin. In the study of Job et al (145a), the fasting blood glucose concentrations and 24-hour urinary glucose results for patients on multiple insulin injections were not significantly different from those on single insulin injections. In an editorial, Strauss (253a) refers to data which would indicate that 60-80% of the diabetic population is in "poor" control by anyone's criteria. Even the criteria used by most investigators for "good" control (179a) do not meet the definition of euglycemia.

It is the author's opinion that the clinician should attempt to achieve a fasting blood glucose level which is as close to normal as possible and which simultaneously achieves goals "a" through "d" above. In reality, all of the goals will have to be tailored to the individual patient's life-style, diabetic presentation, ability to comprehend the complexities of this disease and ability to adhere to a carefully controlled regimen. It is the author's experience that the ideal goals presented above are rarely achieved.

18. After two weeks of hospitalization, the patient was discharged on U-100 NPH insulin, 20 units subcutaneously each morning. She was instructed to test her urine with Clinitest tablets four times daily, to keep a record of her results, and return to the clinic for re-evaluation in one week. Review all the instructions which should be discussed with the patient with regard to the use of Clinitest (e.g. procedure, interpretation, storage, drug interference).

Because of its importance, this urine test must be performed and interpreted correctly. A number of surveys (179a,271) have shown that the diabetic's lack of understanding of his disease and the errors he makes in treating himself account for a good number of the "labile" or difficult-to-control diabetics. For this reason, some discussion of the basic points regarding the use of Clinitest should be pursued with each patient. The following should be considered in such discussions (5,30):

(a) The **frequency** of testing varies with the degree of control. If the patient is labile, she may be requested to test her urine 3-4 times daily, usually before meals and at bedtime. In addition, the physician may wish the patient to test her urine at an hour when the insulin is exerting its maximum and/or minimum effect. If her diabetes has been controlled on one dose of insulin for some time, she may test her urine once daily or 2-3 times weekly. The urine should be tested more frequently at the first sign of infection or with the occurrence of any change in activity, diet, or emotional stress (154).

(b) The patient should be reminded to test a **double voided speciman.** That is, the patient should void one-half hour prior to testing time (to eliminate the glucose that has accumulated since her previous voiding), drink a glass of water, and test a freshly voided specimen. The second voiding should more accurately reflect the amount of sugar in the blood at the time of testing. This procedure is particularly important for the early morning test (196). Interestingly, dilute or second voided samples of urine have been associated with false high readings by Clinitest (88). This does not negate the need for double voiding; however, testing of both the first and second voided specimens may be required in difficult-to-control cases.

(c) **Procedure.** A Clinitest tablet is dropped into a test tube containing 10 drops of water and 5 drops of urine. The tablet generates its own heat and anaerobic environment with the production of foam. For this reason the tube should not be agitated during the reaction (5).

(d) The patient should observe the reaction while it is occurring since a very high glucose content results in the so-called **"pass through" phenomenon.** This is demonstrated by a fleeting, bright orange color which occurs during the "boiling" and which fades to a greenish brown when the reaction ceases. The latter color may be misinterpreted as 0.75-1%, when there is actually *more than* 2% glucose in the urine (30).

(e) Because the color may fade with time, it must be read precisely **15 seconds** after the "boiling" has ceased. The time dependence of this color reaction should be stressed upon persons who might leave to do other chores while the reaction is taking place.

(f) A patient who spills 4+ (2%) or more glucose into her urine should also test her urine for acetone. Persistence of large amounts of glucose in the urine should be called to the physician's attention.

(g) Several drugs may interfere with the test and cause a false positive reaction (See Table 1). There is very little quantitative documentation in the literature with respect to these laboratory/drug interferences, but patients who take large amounts of salicylates or ascorbic acid should be warned of the possible effects. If unexpected positive readings occur, the patient may double check her urine by the glucose oxidase method to see if glucose was the reducing substance actually measured. See Question 10.

(h) Because Clinitest tablets disintegrate rapidly in the presence of moisture and light, they should not be stored in the bathroom medicine cabinet (the most logical location from the patient's viewpoint). The disintegration is easily detected since the appearance of the tablet changes from the normal speckled robin's egg blue to white with splotches of dark blue (5).

(i) The tablets are poisonous and caustic. They should be manipulated with the lid of the container and kept out of the reach of small children. Should ingestion occur, do not induce vomiting.

19. The patient returned to clinic and her urine glucose results for the past week were as follows:

7 am	1+
11 am	4+
4 pm	tr–1+
9 pm	1–2+

Interpret the results and discuss other patterns of response which might be anticipated in a patient taking a single dose of intermediate-acting insulin. How would each of these responses be managed?

After the patient has left the hospital, changes in diet and activity make further adjustment of dose on an out-patient basis almost inevitable. Several problems may arise: The patient may experience midmorning hyperglycemia secondary to the slow onset of NPH as illustrated in this case. Supplementation of the morning dose of NPH with small amounts of regular insulin (4-6 units) will generally correct this problem. The urine tested before the mid-day meal most closely corresponds to the activity of the morning dose of regular insulin. If a patient experiences mid-afternoon hypoglycemia but nighttime and early morning hyperglycemia, the morning dose of NPH should be cut down and an additional dose added in the evening. This pattern occurs in patients who have a transient response to NPH. In other patients the activity of NPH may be delayed in onset so that hyperglycemia is experienced throughout the day and hypoglycemia at night. Because increasing the morning NPH would result in severe nighttime hypoglycemia, this problem is managed by the addition of regular insulin to a lower dose of morning NPH. An evening snack may also help to alleviate the nighttime hypoglycemia (35,268).

20. On the basis of the urine test results, the physician instructed the patient to add 10 units of regular insulin to the 20 units of NPH insulin. How should the patient be instructed to mix and withdraw the insulins into a syringe?

(a) Both regular and NPH insulins should be provided in the same concentrations. Never attempt to mix and measure insulins of different concentrations.

(b) The calibration of the syringe should correspond to the concentration of the insulins used. Calibrations are color coded with the labels on the vial: U-100 Black; U-80 Green; U-40 Red.

(c) Gently roll the vial of NPH between the palms so that the suspension is uniformly dispersed. Vigorous agitation results in foaming and therefore inaccurate measurement of the insulin. All insulins are suspensions with the exception of regular and globin insulin.

(d) Inject 20 units of air into the NPH vial and withdraw the needle.

(e) Inject 10 units of air into the regular vial and withdraw 10 units of insulin. Eliminate bubbles.

(f) Insert the needle into the NPH vial making certain that the needle is submerged in fluid and withdraw 20 units of insulin. Patients are instructed to withdraw regular insulin first, because contamination of the second vial with small amounts of insulin already withdrawn into the syringe almost always occurs. Thus, if NPH, a suspension, is withdrawn *first,* the vial of regular, clear insulin becomes clouded with small amounts of NPH. Although this is probably clinically insignificant, patients become concerned that the regular insulin has "spoiled."

(g) The elimination of bubbles within the barrel of the syringe and at the hub of the needle should be stressed. Although some disposable syringes with permanently attached needles have eliminated this dead space, it may be equivalent to 0.1 cc in those with detachable needles. This may introduce an error of 10 units for U-100, 8 units for U-80 and 4 units for U-40 insulin.

(h) If the patient is using a low-dose U-100 syringe, determine whether each calibration is equivalent to 1 unit or 2 units. If each calibration is equal to 2 units make absolutely certain the patient understands how to correctly measure the insulin dose.

(i) Observe the patient mixing and withdrawing her insulins to determine if she understands your instructions.

21. Eight weeks later, AG began to note symptoms of hypoglycemia (irritable and sweaty) in the late afternoon. Her insulin dose was gradually decreased until she was taking only 3 to 4 units daily. What has happened? Is it advisable to discontinue the insulin? How can such small doses be accurately measured?

Hypoglycemia commonly occurs in juvenile diabetics within days or weeks following the diagnosis of their disease. This is due to an apparent remission and is often referred to as the "honeymoon period." Even though insulin requirements during this phase of the disease may be minute (as little as 1-2U), it is best to maintain the patient on insulin because she will invariably become insulin-dependent. Discontinuation may result in resistance to the hormone at a later date and will only give the patient false hopes (123,215,268). Also see Question 35.

It will be necessary to dilute standard concentrations of insulin in order to measure accurate amounts of such small doses.

Although saline has been used to dilute insulin for desensitization procedures, it is recommended that such insulin be used within 2-3 hours of dilution. Insulin diluting fluid (available from the manufacturer on request) is recommended for the dilution of insulin which will be used over a longer period of time (268).

22. At the age of 23, AG's renal function began to deteriorate secondary to diabetic nephropathy. How will her insulin dose be affected? She currently requires 50 units of insulin daily.

Severe renal disease in which a patient is anuric can "improve" the diabetic state and decrease the requirements for insulin tremendously. Although the liver degrades 50% of insulin, the kidney is the most important site of extrahepatic breakdown. Therefore, diminished kidney function leads to retention of active insulin. Other proposed mechanisms of hypoglycemia in diabetics with renal failure include anorexia and impaired glycogenolysis and gluconeogenesis by the liver.

It should also be noted that uremic patients may also require increased amounts of insulin. The diabetogenic factor has not yet been isolated, but it is suspected that there is diminished tissue responsiveness to insulin (32,173,197,216,227).(Also see chapter on *Diseases of the Kidney.*)

23. Compare the various insulins with respect to their onset, peak effect and duration of action, pH, appearance, and container description.

The figures for onset, peak effect, and duration of action for the various insulins listed in Table 3 are average figures for the newly diagnosed, uncomplicated diabetic (232). In actuality these figures may be altered by innumerable factors, only some of which are mentioned below:

(a) Route. The onset, peak and duration of activity are usually delayed and prolonged following subcutaneous versus intravenous and intramuscular administration (30a,106).

(b) The vascularity of the site of injection may alter the rate of absorption (see Question 28 and 30).

(c) Any temperature resultant physical changes of insulin may alter the time-response curve (see Question 27).

(d) Individuals vary in their response to insulin. Bressler (35) discusses the transient, normal and delayed responses of various patients to NPH insulin. He notes that over a period of time patients may alter their response to insulin. As antibodies to insulin develop, the time response curve changes.

(e) As the dose of insulin increases, the duration of action also increases (106).

24. Several new forms of insulin are currently available. Describe the following insulins and their potential advantages: Single Peak Insulin, Mono Component Insulin, Neutral Regular Insulin, U-100 Insulin.

U-100 Insulin. U-100 insulin (100U/cc) was introduced in an effort to standardize the concentration of insulin available to all diabetics. Eventually, it is hoped

Table 3
COMPARISON OF VARIOUS INSULIN PREPARATIONS

Insulin	Onset (min)	Peak (hrs)	Duration (hrs)	pH	Appearance	Container Description
Acid Regular Insulin	20-30	3-5	5-8	2.8-3.5	clear	round
Neutral Regular Insulin	20-30	3-5	5-8	7.4	clear	round
Semilente	30-45	4-6	12-16	neutral	cloudy	hexagonal
Globin	4 hrs	6-8	12-18	acid	clear	round
NPH	60-90	8-12	24-28	neutral	cloudy	square
Lente	60-90	8-12	24-28	neutral	cloudy	hexagonal
PZI	60-90	14-20	36+	neutral	cloudy	round
Ultralente	5-8 hrs	16-18	36+	neutral	cloudy	hexagonal

that the use of U-40 and U-80 insulin will be discontinued and that all patients will use U-100 insulin. Other advantages include compatability with the emerging decimal system and elimination of errors resulting from the use of an incorrectly calibrated syringe.

Neutral Regular Insulin (NRI). It has recently been found that modern manufacturing techniques yield an unmodified insulin that is more stable at a neutral (7.4) than an acid (2.8) pH. Acid regular insulin loses 20% of its activity after one year at room temperature whereas NRI maintains its potency over the same period of time. Preliminary studies indicate that the pharmacologic activity of NRI is comparable to ARI whether used alone or in combination with other insulins (106,107).

Single Peak and Single (Mono) Component Insulin. If USP insulin is separated chromatographically, three peaks ("a", "b", and "c") are produced. The "a" and "b" peaks are large molecular weight pro-insulin-like substances and insulin aggregates which make up 8% of USP insulin. Thus, USP insulin contains 92% pure insulin and insulin-like materials (peak "c").

Recently, efforts have been made to improve the purity of commercially available insulins through chromatographic techniques. Currently, all Lilly insulins are "single peak" (SP) insulins. The "c" peak is composed of 90% pure insulin and 9% insulin-like materials which have a similar molecular weight (desamido insulin, arginine insulin, esterified insulins, etc.).

Single component (SC) insulin made by Eli Lilly and monocomponent (MC) insulin made by a European manufacturer, Novo, are products of further purification processes and are composed of more than 99% pure insulin. The process is complex, expensive and yields are low in that 40% of the insulin is lost. Since there is a world shortage of insulin, it is unlikely that this product will be commercially available in the near future (107,225).

It has been presumed that many of the complications related to insulin were caused by immunologic reactions to the impurities of USP insulin rather than to the insulin molecule itself. Therefore, the impetus for purifying insulin was that such a product would be less antigenic, and immunologically mediated problems such as allergy and resistance would be minimized. Yue et al (293a) recently reviewed the data from human investigations and made the following conclusions:

a. Purified insulins *are* antigenic although apparently less so than conventional insulin products. Treatment with monocomponent pork insulin did not produce a drop in insulin antibody levels in patients who had previously been treated with commercial insulin. Furthermore, insulin antibodies could be detected in 10/14 patients treated with MC pork only, after 20 months of therapy. The antibody levels were lower than a control population receiving conventional insulins (46% of control). Root et al (226) have also shown that SC pork insulin is less immunogenic than USP pork insulin. Similar results have been reported for single peak beef-pork insulin (258). Since antibodies to the "a" and "b" components of insulin can still be detected in patients receiving the purified insulin, these lower antibody levels may simply reflect insufficient purification to prevent antibody formation. However, antigenicity of the insulin molecule itself cannot be ruled out at this time.

b. Switching a patient from USP insulin to the more purified insulins may decrease insulin requirements, but this change is modest and gradual and may not be significant.

c. Purified insulins are not consistently successful in the therapy of insulin resistance. This may be related to the fact that SP insulin is a mixture of beef and pork insulin rather than pure pork insulin which is less antigenic than beef. See Question 31. It may also reflect the fact that insulin resistance is not always caused by increased insulin antibody formation. In any case, Yue, et al do recommend that purified insulins be tried if high levels of insulin antibody can be demonstrated

(258,293a).

d. The incidence of local reactions and lipoatrophy are decreased by purified insulins. See Question 29.

e. Systemic insulin allergy responds variably to therapy with purified insulin. Since systemic allergy has also been reported in patients treated with purified insulin, this effect may represent an immunologic reaction to the insulin molecule rather than to the contaminants.

25. You receive a prescription with instructions to premix 5 cc PZI U-40 with 5cc regular insulin U-40 for a seven-year-old child who will be going to summer camp and cannot be trusted to mix his own insulin. Would you mix it? What are the alternatives?

This mixture has no rational basis since PZI contains an excess of protamine which would bind the regular insulin. A 1:1 mixture of Regular:PZI would essentially be equivalent to PZI only. Some effects of the regular insulin might be maintained if the two insulins are mixed just prior to injection, but these effects will be lost if the two insulins are premixed for any length of time. The child should be taught to draw the insulin himself. It is important to withdraw the regular insulin prior to the PZI so that the vial of regular will not be contaminated with excess protamine. Alternatively, a mixture of ultra and semi-lentes insulins may be used as they are compatible with each other and have time characteristics which are similar to PZI and regular insulin. A recent letter to the editor concerned a patient who was using a PZI/regular mixture. It was suspected the patient had a hypoglycemic reaction because the two insulins had been mixed improperly (179,268).

26. What are the stability characteristics of various insulin mixtures?

Whenever a patient is using a mixture of two insulins, compatibility should be considered (see Table 4). When using a mixture of modified and regular insulin, instructions should always be given to withdraw the regular first. Regular insulin often becomes cloudy as a result of contamination with modified insulin suspensions.

Generally, all insulin mixtures are stable and will retain the qualities of the individual preparations if they are mixed just prior to injection. The stability of many insulin mixtures, hitherto unstable on the basis of pH

Table 4
STABILITY OF VARIOUS INSULIN MIXTURES

Mixture	Proportion	Incompatability	Stability
Neutral or Acid Regular: PZI	1:1 = PZI 2:1 = NPH 3:1 = NPH + Reg	Excess protamine in PZI combines with regular, prolonging its action. No advantages to any of these combinations.	Mix just prior to injection.
Acid Regular*: NPH	May be mixed in any proportion.	Even though there is no excess protamine, physical changes may occur with time, presumably due to pH differences.	Mix just prior to injection.
Neutral Regular*: NPH	May be mixed in any proportion.	No incompatibilities	May be mixed 2-3 months prior to injection.
Acid Regular*: Lente	Should not be mixed in a proportion greater than 1:1	Presumably physico-chemical changes may occur with the change in pH, resulting in an unpredictable time action curve.	Mix just prior to injection.
Neutral Regular*: Lente	May be mixed in any proportion.	No incompatibilities.	May be mixed 2-3 months prior to injection.
Lentes	May be mixed in any proportion.	No imcompatibilities.	Stable indefinitely. May be premixed.
Regular: Normal Saline	May be mixed in any proportion.	pH change; dilution of buffer; exact incompatability unknown.	Use within 2-3 hours of mixing.
Regular: Insulin Diluting Fluid	May be mixed any proportion.	No incompatibilities.	Stable indefinitely. May be premixed.

*(1) Acid Regular Insulin (ARI) = Squibb's U-40 and U-80 Regular Insulin.
 (2) Neutral Regular Insulin (NRI) = Squibb's U-100 Regular Insulin; Lilly's U-40, U-80 & U-100 Insulin.

differences, has been increased by the introduction of neutral regular insulin. Problems may occasionally arise when insulins are mixed far in advance of the injection time, as they may be in a unit-dose area. This situation may also occur when two insulins are pre-mixed for a child, or for geriatric or blind patients who are incapable of withdrawing accurate doses. Because the adsorption of insulin onto plastic syringes has not been studied, it is recommended that insulin be predrawn within 24 hours of the injection time and that the patient agitate the syringe prior to injection.

27. A diabetic patient plans to spend her summer vacation in the mountains. She would like to know if the insulin will deteriorate if it is placed in a cold mountain stream. Discuss the effects of temperature on insulin stability.

The insulin should remain quite stable under the conditions mentioned above. At temperatures of 68-75°F the decrease in potency is clinically insignificant for a duration of a vial's use. Modified insulins appear to be more stable at room temperature than acid regular insulins (106,249). Lente insulins, NPH, and PZI maintain their potency for a period of at least 24 months at room temperature. During this time the fine precipitates *may* aggregate, making withdrawal of a uniform dose difficult. Color changes may be associated with a denaturation of protein and should be interpreted as consistent with loss of potency (249). Neutral regular insulin is stable for 18 months at room temperature. Acid regular insulin, on the other hand, may lose up to 25% of its potency at room temperature over the same period of time (41). No one has studied the stability of insulins at temperatures of 75-100°F. At 100°F all insulins lose a significant amount of potency within 1-2 months. Deterioration occurs extremely rapidly at temperatures of 122°F (249). Lilly states that a "brief" exposure of NPH and PZI to 100°F may not result in significant loss of potency (269); however, aggregation of particles may occur at a much more rapid rate and insulins should be checked for this if they are delivered under improper storage conditions. Diabetics and pharmacists living in regions where the summers are hot report a greater difficulty in controlling the disease during this time of year. They attribute this to physical changes in the insulin caused by exposure to high temperatures. All insulins maintain their potency and physical properties for 36 months if stored in the refrigerator (249). Freezing apparently does not affect the potency of insulin but may cause aggregation of the precipitate (268).

These data have several implications. Many patients prefer injecting insulin which has been warmed to room temperature. This may be more than a comfort measure since the injection of cold insulin has been considered a contributing factor in the formation of lipodystrophies. See Question 29. The patient may keep the vials of insulin currently in use out of the refrigerator; nevertheless, they should be stored in a cool area, not near the radiator or on a sunny window-sill. Insulin dispensed within a hospital need not be refrigerated. Finally, unless the weather is unusually warm, patients who are traveling generally do not have to purchase special paraphernalia to keep their insulin refrigerated. Insulation of the insulin between several layers of clothing should be sufficient.

28. A 40-year-old woman with insulin-dependent diabetes comes to clinic with a chief complaint of episodes of hunger, irritability, sweaty palms and difficulty concentrating. One and one-half weeks ago, her morning and evening doses of NPH insulin were increased by 5 units (10 units total) because her fasting blood glucose levels had been greater than 250 mg/100 ml for the past three clinic visits. What is this patient's problem? What factors should be considered in assessing this woman's complaint? How should she be managed?

The patient is exhibiting signs and symptoms of hypoglycemia, the most common and dangerous complication of insulin therapy. Symptoms of hypoglycemia occur when the blood sugar falls below 50 mg/100 ml or when there is a rapid fall in blood glucose and include (in order of appearance) a parasympathetic response (nausea, hunger, eructation); diminished cerebral function (confusion, agitation, lethargy, personality changes); a sympathetic response (tachycardia, sweating, tremor); coma and convulsions. Ataxia and blurred vision also occur commonly (256), and nightmares and drenching bedclothes are common complaints of patients who develop insulin reactions at night. It occurs most frequently in newly diagnosed diabetics who have not yet learned to maintain the delicate balance between insulin dose, exercise and food intake. Unlike the non-diabetic whose insulin levels vacillate in accordance with blood glucose levels, the diabetic must match food intake and exercise with fixed levels of exogenous insulin.

At first glance, it would seem reasonable to decrease the dose of insulin. However, since the dose adjustment appears to have had good justifications, it is necessary to further characterize the reactions keeping in mind that *exercise* and *diet* are also major determinants of the blood glucose. First, it is important to determine the time of day that the reactions occurred and whether or not there were any extenuating circumstances which may have precipitated them. The first episode occurred on Friday mid-afternoon, and the second occurred early Saturday afternoon. A more detailed history revealed that on the weekend following the increment in the insulin dose, the patient had unexpected house guests. She spent all day Friday cleaning her home and took her guests out for a shopping spree on Saturday. Lunch was delayed and she developed symptoms of nausea, lightheadedness and sweatiness which were promptly relieved by a glass of orange juice. The patient's unusual spurt of activity and irregular eating probably contributed to her reactions. Even though the first reaction occurred at a time when NPH insulin generally has its peak activity, thus suggesting that the dose may be excessive, the patient's increased exercise was probably the greater contributing factor.

Other factors which may enhance the hypoglycemic activity of insulin must be ruled out. Is the patient taking any drugs which decrease the blood glucose? (See Question 61.) Is the patient developing a different onset and duration of action to the NPH insulin? See Question 23. How and where was the patient injecting her insulin? It has been demonstrated that the onset of insulin action is much faster and more predictable after intramuscular than after subcutaneous injection (30a,258a) and that absorption of insulin from the leg is much more rapid than from the arm (195). More recently it has become clear that injection of insulin into the leg followed by exercise results in a more rapid absorption of insulin from this site as well as a more profound hypoglycemic effect. Exercise does not affect the absorption of insulin from the arm or the degree of hypoglycemia produced when insulin is injected at this site. This indicates that injection of insulin into the arm actually reduces exercise-induced hypoglycemia. Finally, exercise reduces insulin absorption from the abdomen during the post-exercise period, thereby delaying and/or diminishing the hypoglycemic effect of insulin administered at this site (160a). Finally, one should actually observe the patient measuring and injecting her insulin. Some of the U-100 syringes are calibrated such that one calibration is equal to two, rather than one unit. This can be a source of measurement error for patients who are accustomed to the one-for-one calibration system.

If all of the above factors have been ruled out, the patient should be instructed to maintain her insulin dose, to moderate her exercise, and to take her meals at regular intervals. If the reactions continue, her dose of insulin should be re-evaluated.

29. A diabetic child has developed indentations on her thigh at the sites of insulin injection. Can this be due to the insulin? How can it be treated?

The patient has developed a lipodystrophy caused in insulin. Lipodystrophy may present as atrophy (subcutaneous concavities caused by a wasting of the lipid tissue) or, less commonly, as hypertrophy (the occurrence of tumorous-like fat pads at the site of injection).

Lipoatrophies have been noted to occur in 0.66-54.8% of patients using insulin. They occur predominantly in women and children. Subcutaneous atrophy appears 2 months to 2 years following initiation of therapy but has been observed as soon as one month (20,81). Early cases were predominantly associated with the use of protamine zinc insulin; however, atrophy has since been reported with the use of lente, NPH, globin and soluble (regular) insulins (272). The mechanism of this reaction is still unknown. It has been attributed to injection of refrigerated insulin, failure to rotate the injection site and insulin impurities. For this reason patients have been routinely advised to avoid injecting one site (2 cm) more frequently than once every 3-4 weeks. Spontaneous regression of lipoatrophy is rare (20) but may occur slowly after many months or years (81). Recently, investigators have had gratifying results by injecting single peak or monocomponent insulin directly into the atrophic areas (259a,279). 89/103 patients (85%) noted dramatic improvement or complete disappearance of the atrophy within one year of treatment (279). Watson et al (272) injected neutral (Actrapid by Novo) or biphasic (Rapitard by Novo) insulin into atrophic areas of 7 patients. They observed complete recovery, usually within 6 months of therapy (272). Small amounts of dexamethasone added to insulin (4 mcg/unit) produced significant improvement of lipoatrophic areas in 6/9 patients after 6 months of therapy (166a).

Lipohypertrophies occur after many months or years of repeated injections into the same site of any type of insulin. It is said to occur more frequently (up to 36.5%) in young patients than in adults (3%) (20,81,263). This type of lipodystrophy tends to be self-perpetuating because the site of injection becomes anesthetic. Rotation of injection sites may result in spontaneous regression of these lipomas (20,21). Injections of purified insulin into these sites does not appear to improve this form of lipodystrophy (293a).

30. Lipodystrophy has been said to have only cosmetic significance. Is this true?

On the contrary, the absorption of insulin from such areas can be quite variable and unpredictable. Absorption of insulin is significantly delayed from areas of hypertrophy presumably due to the decreased vascularity of fatty tissue. For the same reason the disappearance half-life from the thigh and arm differ considerably (310 vs. 232 minutes). This can be an important consideration in a young diabetic whose symptoms are difficult to control (124,195).

31. What factors determine the relative antigenicity of the various types of insulin?

At least two types of antibodies to insulin are formed. One is a blocking antibody (usually IgG) which occurs in the serum of all diabetics six weeks to three months after treatment is initiated. These antibodies may combine with and neutralize the activity of exogenous insulin, but in normal diabetics their binding capacity is fairly low (10-20 U) (57,291). Insulin derived from various animal species differs in its affinity for these antibodies. Another antibody (IgE) is responsible for the mediation of allergic reactions (75).

One of the claims made for the lente insulins is that they contain no foreign protein, that is, protamine or globin, and are therefore less antigenic than other modified insulins. Actually, there is little difference in the incidence of sensitivity between lente and NPH (76). More local reactions are recorded with the use of modified insulins, but it is questionable whether this is due to their inherent antigenicity or their longer retention at the site, leading to greater antigenicity.

The relative antigenicity between insulins from various species generally correlates with their structural similarity to human insulin. For example, pork insulin, which differs in one amino acid, is less antigenic than beef insulin, which differs by three amino acids. Dealanated and sulfated insulins (174a) are experimental modifications which are said to be less antigenic and less neutralizable than other insulins. Occasionally, a patient who is resistant to all mammalian sources of insulin will respond favorably to fish insulin (268a,291).

The antigenicity of the highly purified form of insulin is discussed in Question 24.

32. A diabetic patient notices that the clerk has given him the correct insulin but that its origin is pork rather than pork and beef. Should the animal source make a difference? Will a change in insulin brands make a difference?

The animal source of insulin can make a difference. Because the patient has been able to tolerate the mixture, it is unlikely that allergic problems will arise. Theoretically, pork insulin will not substitute for beef unit for unit. Often much less insulin is needed (presumably because it is less antigenic), and for this reason a change in insulin source should be avoided (69,292).

Diabetics frequently change brands of insulin depending upon which is the least expensive. Although Lilly insulin is more purified than Squibb insulin, any change in dose which might result from differences in their antigenicity is not significant. See Question 24.

33. A 12-year-old diabetic has just started insulin therapy and has noticed a red, itchy spot at the site of injection. Should his insulin be changed? What other factors would you consider if the area was not

pruritic? Would your response be the same if a rash occurred all over his body?

This is probably a *local reaction* to insulin. Erythema, pain, swelling and itching may occur at the site of injection in more than 50% of patients initiated on insulin. It generally occurs 20-40 minutes after injection and lasts 2-6 hours. However, such reactions may occur up to 12 hours after injection, reach their maximum intensity in 6 to 12 hours and subside in 1 to 7 days (25,81,200). Paley (200) could not relate the reaction to the type of insulin, pH or preservatives. Fabrykant (81) attributed the reaction to shallow subcutaneous injection and observed a lower incidence in patients who thrust the needle into the skin perpendicularly rather than at an angle. Paley (200) noted an indolent reaction with superficial necrosis and scabbing following *intradermal* injection of insulin. The reaction may also be due to a non-insulin protein (107), and this is supported by evidence that the incidence is decreased with the use of more purified forms of insulin (293a). Galloway et al (107) noted that in maturity onset diabetics allergy was associated with obesity and discontinuous use of insulin. They suggest that many of these reactions may have been prevented with either loss of weight or the uninterrupted use of insulin.

Frequently, spontaneous desensitization to insulin occurs by the time the first vial is completed (3 weeks to 3 months) and the local reaction subsides. If the reaction persists (as observed by Fabrykant [81]), one should check the patient's injection technique.

Alcohol which has been used to sterilize the syringe may also cause local irritation. This may be avoided by boiling the syringes, or by using plastic disposable syringes. Alternatively one may switch the patient ot a more purified form of insulin (see Question 24) or to another animal source of insulin.

Widespread urticaria and anaphylaxis secondary to insulin is, fortunately, rare, but has been reported (20,174,293a). The acute reaction should be treated with antihistamines, epinephrine and glucocorticoids as indicated. The animal source of the patient's insulin should be changed. Alternatively, the patient may be desensitized with very dilute amounts of insulin over a three day period and protected with antihistamines during the procedure (174,180a,286a).

34. A 54-year-old obese maturity onset diabetic whose disease was poorly controlled on a combination of chlorpropamide and phenformin was finally switched to insulin. Although her disease was initially well controlled on 20 units of insulin daily, requirements gradually increased to 100 units daily. Other medical problems included hypertension which was well controlled with hydrochlorothiazide and recurrent urinary tract infections. She made no

attempt to control her weight. **Why does this patient require such high doses of insulin?**

This patient demonstrates many factors which are associated with **insulin insensitivity.** This relatively common condition is defined as an acute or chronic insulin requirement of 60-200 units daily. The presence of diabetogenic factors plays an important role in the pathogenesis of high insulin requirements in these patients, whereas, insulin antibodies are relatively unimportant etiologic factors. Diabetogenic factors present in this patient include obesity, diuretic therapy, and infection. Other factors which may increase insulin requirements include diabetogenic drugs (see Question 4) and hormones (growth hormone, glucagon, catacholamines, glucocorticoids, thyroxine); pregnancy; ketoacidosis; mild liver diseases and emotional stress. Treatment consists of strict dieting, and elimination of diabetogenic factors.

35. In the years that followed, the patient was placed on a strict diet. Insulin was discontinued and chlorpropamide in combination with phenformin was resumed. Her diabetes was in fair control until six years later when she was admitted with ketoacidosis. Despite correction of her acidotic state and treatment of her urinary tract infection she continued to require 300 units of insulin per day. At this time her blood sugars averaged 300 mg%. Why does this patient require such high doses of insulin?

True **insulin resistance** is strictly defined as a requirement of 200 units or more per day for at least one week in the absence of acidosis, coma or infection. This phenomenon is rare and is primarily due to the presence of high titers of insulin blocking antibody. It occurs most frequently in adult onset diabetics over 40 years of age who have been treated with insulin intermittently. Frequently, insulin insensitivity occurs simultaneously (96). There are several modes of treatment all of which are aimed at minimizing antigen-antibody reaction. This may be done by decreasing antibody levels or administering *less antigenic insulin.* Resistance may regress spontaneously if high requirements are maintained for a period of time. Such patients have been successfully treated with insulins which more closely resemble human insulin. These include pork insulin and sulfated insulin (33,116,174a,286a). When insulin from other animal sources is used, the dose should be decreased by 50% in order to avoid hypoglycemic reactions which can occur if the two insulins are not cross sensitive. Single peak and/or monocomponent pork insulin have been used in an attempt to eliminate administration of the large, more antigenic pro-insulin molecules; however, results have been variable (258,293a). Fish insulin, whose structure differs significantly from mammalian insulin may be useful in the treatment of insulin resistance (286a,291).

Sulfonylureas have been administered on the theory that antibodies are not active against endogenous insulin. Beneficial effects at maximum doses may not occur for months but insulin requirements are often decreased by 25% (26). A dramatic fall in insulin requirement may be observed as soon as 3 days after 30-60 mg *prednisone* daily is initiated. The mechanism of its effect is unknown. Finally, insulin resistance has been treated by *withdrawing exogenous insulin,* thus allowing antibody titers to decline (149).

CASE B – DIABETIC KETOACIDOSIS: This is the sixth admission for RC, a 25-year-old female with insulin-dependent diabetes diagnosed at the age of 10. Three days prior to admission the patient developed flu-like symptoms with nausea, vomiting and anorexia and discontinued her insulin therapy despite the fact that she had 4+ glucose in her urine. Because she was becoming progressively weak and lethargic she came to the emergency room for evaluation.

The patient was a lean female who appeared ill and dehydrated. Her supine blood pressure was 120/80 and her sitting blood pressure was 90/60. Her respiratory rate was 30/minute but not Kussmaul in character. Her temperature was 39°C. Her lips and tongue were dry and she had poor skin turgor. Other physical findings were non-contributory.

Admission laboratory values were as follows: WBC 15,000 mm³; Hematocrit 46%; Na 129 mEq/L; K 5.7 mEq/L; Cl 92 mEq/L; HCO₃ 12 mEq/L; Serum glucose 800 mg/dl. Serum ketones were present in a 1:2 dilution (Acetest). Arterial blood gases included a pH of 7.2. Urinalysis showed 4+ glucosuria, moderate ketones and a specific gravity of 1.025.

On the night of admission (10 p.m.) the patient was rehydrated with normal saline. She was given an intravenous bolus of insulin in a dose of 0.1 U/kg and an infusion of insulin at a rate of 5 U/hr. By 4 a.m. the following morning, her serum glucose was 275 mg/dl, but her bicarbonate levels remained low (13 mEq/L). The insulin infusion was continued and 5% dextrose, and 40 mEq of potassium phosphate per liter were added to her replacement fluids. By 10 a.m., her serum bicarbonate was 20 mEq/L. The insulin infusion was discontinued and she was placed on 0.1 U/kg regular insulin SC every 6 hours.

36. Briefly describe the overall approach to the management of a patient with diabetic ketoacidosis.

Therapy of diabetic ketoacidosis includes replacement of fluid and electrolyte losses, administration of insulin to correct the underlying metabolic abnormalities and identification and correction of precipitating factors (54a,91b,150a,174b).

The average patient has lost 10% of his body weight in fluids at the time of diagnosis (6 to 10 liters). The initial goal of *fluid therapy* is to restore intravascular volume and establish urine flow. Since the fluid losses are hypotonic and the patient is generally in a hyperosmolar state, hypotonic half-normal saline (0.45%) has been advocated as a replacement fluid (91b,154c). Recently, some have recommended replacement with normal saline since a substantial amount of water in hypotonic saline is available to move into the intracellular compartment. Normalization of the blood glucose will cause a shift of extracellular water into intracellular spaces; this may further compromise the intravascular volume and place the patient in shock. Furthermore, it has been postulated that increased levels of sorbitol in the central nervous system may pull available water into the cells leading to cerebral edema (12a,54a). Thus, it is recommended that water be administered as isotonic saline so that it remains in the intravascular space (54a).

Although total body potassium is generally depleted secondary to gastrointestinal and urinary losses, serum potassium levels may be high, low, or normal because of shifts of potassium from intracellular to extracellular spaces which may occur in an acid environment. As acidosis and hyperglycemia are corrected, potassium redistributes into intracellular spaces and hypokalemia may result. Most authors suggest that *potassium* be added to replacement fluids (40 mEq/L) when levels fall to less than 5 mEq/l and/or serum glucose levels begin to fall. This should be done only if urine flow has been established. Hypokalemia should be treated more vigorously by adding 60 mEq of potassium to each liter of replacement fluid (91b,154c). Potassium chloride is the salt which is used most frequently; however, some use potassium phosphate to replace the phosphate depletion which is observed in these patients (54a, 150a, 174b).

The administration of *bicarbonate* to patients in ketoacidosis is controversial for several reasons. As insulin corrects the metabolic abnormalities, the ketones which are generally readily metabolized will be eliminated and the pH will return to normal. Administration of bicarbonate may produce a relative CNS acidosis and cause further deterioration of coma. Theoretically, as peripheral acidosis is corrected, the respiratory rate diminishes and carbon dioxide is retained. Since carbon dioxide crosses the blood brain barrier relatively more easily than bicarbonate, a central nervous system acidosis is produced (211a). More importantly, correction of acidosis may increase hemoglobin affinity for oxygen and produce tissue anoxia. This occurs because patients with diabetic ketoacidosis (DKA) have low levels of red cell 2,3-DPG (2,3 diphosphoglyceric acid) which shifts the oxyhemoglobin dissociation curve to the left (decreased hemoglobin affinity for oxygen). Since acidosis shifts the curve to the right, patients with DKA generally have normal oxygen dissociation from hemoglobin. Correction of the acidosis, therefore, eliminates the compensatory effect and the patient becomes compromised. Finally, rapid correction of the acidosis may produce a hypokalemia. Most authors do not administer bicarbonate unless the pH is less than 7.1 or the HCO_3 is less than 10 mEq/L because cardiovascular function may be compromised at this level. Then, conservative doses (88 mEq) are administered and doses are not repeated until the patient is re-evaluated in four hours (12a,54a,91b,1454c).

Insulin should be administered until the venous pH is greater than 7.3 or the HCO_3 is greater than 14 mEq/L. Since correction of the acidosis may lag behind correction of the blood glucose, these parameters are used to determine the duration of insulin therapy. When the blood glucose reaches 250 mg/dl, 5% glucose should be added to the replacement fluids to prevent precipitous hypoglycemia (91b,154a,174b). The presence of ketones in the urine and serum as measured by Acetest are not useful monitoring parameters because total body serum ketones as measured enzymatically do not correlate with the greatest serum dilution that gives a positive test using the nitroprusside reagent. This is not surprising since this reagent only measures acetoacetate and acetone, and the major ketone released from the liver is betahydroxybutyrate. Also see Question 37. The fall in acetoacetate concentration lags behind that of betahydroxybutyrate and acetone is eliminated so slowly that it may be detected in the urine up to 48 hours after acidosis has been corrected (54a,174b). Once this goal has been achieved the patient may be switched to subcutaneous insulin every four to six hours. Also see Question 38.

37. Which ketones do the Acetest tablet and Ketostix measure? How should positive and negative results be interpreted? Do any drugs or chemicals cause ketonuria?

All tests for ketones detect acetone and acetoacetic acid, not betahydroxybutyric acid, the major ketone responsible for ketoacidosis. For this reason, a negative test for ketones does not rule out ketoacidosis in a patient who has suggestive signs and symptoms. Ketonuria in the absence of glucosuria is generally indicative of insufficient carbohydrate in the diet or starvation. No insulin is indicated in this instance. Acetest tablets are more sensitive to the presence of acetoacetic acid than are Ketostix (143).

False positive reactions may be caused by bromsulfophthalein and large quantities of phenylketones. Additionally, levodopa has been noted to cause a false positive test for ketones in the urine by the Ketostix and Labstix method. Positive Acetests were inconsistently noted (46,287).

Phenformin may cause a ketonuria by unknown mechanisms especially when administered to juvenile, ketoacidotic prone patients. In a study of 109 patients it was found that ketonuria was present in all diabetics in the presence of normal or slightly increased blood levels of glucose when phenformin was administered. When phenformin is being used in a labile diabetic, the blood sugars should be checked prior to adjustment of the insulin dose since ketonuria may occur in the presence or absence of an increased blood glucose (270).

38. Evaluate the insulin therapy prescribed for this patient.

There is little or no consensus among diabetologists with regard to the appropriate dose or route of administration of insulin in a patient with diabetic ketoacidosis. However, large doses (50-200 units every 2 to 4 hours) have been traditionally advocated on the basis of in vitro data and retrospective studies which suggest that there may be some degree of insulin resistance in the acidotic state (12a, 12b, 91b, 154c, 159a, 245a). A portion of this dose is generally given intravenously to obtain an immediate effect and the remainder is administered subcutaneously or intramuscularly for a sustained effect.

In the early and mid seventies several reports of successful treatment of ketoacidosis with low doses of insulin were published (12c,154b,199a,234a), and the requirement of large doses of insulin was challenged. Since that time, several more reports of success have been published. In general, the doses used in adults range from 4 to 8 units per hour (0.1 U/kg/hr) by intravenous infusion. An initial loading dose of 0.1 U/kg/hr is administered by some, but not by others. These doses produce a serum insulin concentration of 20 to 200 μU/ml (199a,239a). This falls within the physiologic range of insulin concentration observed in patients undergoing glucose tolerance testing and is a level which produces the maximum rate of fall in the blood glucose concentration (12a, 12b, 150a). Within this concentration range, the blood glucose concentration falls at a rate of 75-100 mg/dl/hour (12c,150a,154b,174b,239a). Alberti et al (12a) have suggested that each 1 U/hr increment in the insulin dose increases the insulin concentration by approximately 20 μU/ml. Hourly intramuscular injections of low doses of insulin in similar doses produce comparable results (12c,154a). Low-dose intravenous infusions of insulin (0.1 U/kg loading dose followed by 0.1 U/kg/hr intravenous infusion) have also been used successfully in the treatment of pediatric patients with ketoacidosis (150a,174b).

The proponents of low-dose insulin therapy claim that it is more rational than high dose therapy for the following reasons:

a. Insulin has a very short half-life (4-5 minutes). Therefore intermittent intravenous boluses every 2-4 hours will produce "peaks" and "valleys" and may leave gaps in insulin coverage, whereas constant infusions maintain "physiologic" levels throughout the treatment period (199a).

b. The onset and duration of action of insulin administered subcutaneously is variable and unpredictable in a hypovolemic patient. Poor or delayed absorption in such patients may predispose them to late hypoglycemic reactions. In contrast, the onset of action of constant intravenous infusions is immediate, and the pharmacologic action can be terminated almost immediately after the infusion is discontinued (12a,12b,199a).

c. The time required to reduce blood glucose levels to 250 mg/dl is the same for patients treated with high-dose and low-dose insulin regimens (107c, 129a, 154a, 199b), but the incidence of complications related to overtreatment may be greater following high-dose therapy. See "e" and "f" below.

d. The low-dose method offers a simpler approach to the dosing of insulin in a patient with diabetic ketoacidosis. Recommendations for administering high doses of insulin are almost always complex and vary from author to author. Doses vary with the degree of ketoacidosis and/or blood glucose level and the frequency of administration is always a dilemma when the onset and duration of action of insulin administered subcutaneously and intramuscularly is so unpredictable. Using the low-dose method, the initial dose is established on a unit/kg basis and the rate is simply increased if an adequate response is not observed within the hour. All of the factors which determine the rate of fall of glucose during insulin infusions have not been identified. It does not appear to be affected by the presence of insulin antibodies, the degree of ketoacidosis, or the initial blood glucose level. The rate of fall can be substantially less in patients who have concurrent infections (199a) and there have been instances reported of requirements of insulin which are higher than those usually recommended (239d,272a).

e. Since the rate of fall of blood glucose concentrations is predictable and because discontinuation of the infusion results in negligible blood levels of insulin with 20 minutes, late hypoglycemic reactions can be averted through the use of low-dose therapy. This is upheld by the findings of Kitabchi et al who noted hypoglycemia in 25% of patients treated with high-dose insulin and the absence of hypoglycemia in patients treated with low-dose insulin (154a). Another theoretical advantage in avoiding a rapid fall in blood glucose concentrations is that cerebral edema may be avoided (54a).

f. Hypokalemia associated with high-dose insulin therapy also appears to occur less frequently (12c, 154a).

It is important to emphasize that the concept of low-dose insulin therapy is not uniformly embraced by all diabetologists (91c,177a,159a,239d). The strongest statement against its widespread use is made by Madison (199a) who recommends that it only be used as a research tool until a large, prospective, randomized trial comparing the two methods of administration has confirmed the theoretical claims made by proponents of low-dose therapy. Currently there are only two small prospective studies which compare high-dose and low-dose insulin regimens. Both favor low-dose therapy (129a,154a).

In summary, if the low-dose method is used, it is recommended that the patient be given an intravenous loading dose of 0.1 U/kg of insulin followed by an infusion at the rate of 0.1 U/kg/hr. Fifty units of insulin in 250 or 500 ml of normal saline will deliver 1 unit/5 ml and 1 unit/10 ml respectively if adsorption of insulin onto the infusion system is not considered. The advantages and disadvantages of adding 1 to 2% salt-poor albumin to the mixture to minimize adsorption are considered in Question 39. The goals of therapy are discussed in Question 36. Initially, blood glucose should be measured hourly to assure that the patient is responding to therapy. If a predicted drop is not observed, the infusion rate should be increased or the patient should be switched to high dose therapy.

39. Is the adsorption of insulin onto intravenous bottles and infusion sets significant?

Weisenfeld et al (273) studied this problem and found that a significant percentage of dilute solutions of insulin (2-40 units/1500 ml normal saline) could be lost through adsorption onto the glass containers and polyvinylchloride (PVC) infusion sets. The percent lost to one infusion system decreased as the concentration of insulin increased but was still significant (4-16%) at a concentration of 40 U/500 ml. There was a 20% loss at concentrations of 20 U/500 ml, 25% loss at 10 U/500 ml and 30% loss at 5 U/100 ml. The same investigators found that the addition of 3.5 mg/ml of human serum albumin diminished the loss to approximately 5%. The activity of the insulin bound to serum albumin was not tested.

These results have been confirmed by other investigators, and adsorption onto polyvinylchloride (PVC) containers has been documented as well (133a, 163a, 203a, 205a). Practically, the addition of small amounts of albumin (1-2%) is costly. Since insulin is clearly available from these systems as evidenced by elevated insulin levels and hypoglycemic responses in patients receiving insulin from systems without added albumin (12a,129a,174b,199a), it would seem reasonable to simply be aware of the potential decrease in bioavailability and to monitor the patient's response to therapy accordingly. The preparation of more concentrated solutions of insulin, as suggested in Question 38 above should also minimize significant insulin loss.

40. What is the University Group Diabetic Program (UGDP) study? Discuss the objectives, conclusions and criticisms of the study and its impact on the current use of oral hypoglycemic agents.

The UGDP (267c,d,e) was a prospective study initiated in 1961 to evaluate the effectiveness of antidiabetic therapy in preventing vascular and late complications of diabetes. Eight hundred patients from 12 different diabetic clinics were included. All of these patients were recently diagnosed maturity onset diabetics of the nonketotic type who had a life expectancy of five years or more and who could be maintained free of symptoms on diet alone. The patients were then randomly assigned to one of five treatment programs: (a) tolbutamide in a fixed dose of 1.5 grams, (b) placebo or diet alone, (c) insulin in a fixed dose, (d) insulin in variable doses, and (e) phenformin in fixed doses. An unexpected finding of a higher incidence of cardiovascular deaths in the tolbutamide and phenformin treated groups resulted in early termination of the study. After eight years, 26 cardiovascular deaths occurred in the tolbutamide group as opposed to 10-13 similar deaths in each of the other groups. Similar results were reported for the phenformin group (267c).

The conclusions of this controversial study have given the medical profession cause for radical reappraisal of therapy. The conclusions of the study and recommendations from various groups which followed its publication are summarized below. UGDP investigators made the following statements:

"The findings of this study indicate that the combination of diet and tolbutamide therapy is no more effective than diet alone in prolonging life. Moreover, the findings suggest that tolbutamide and diet may be less effective than diet alone or than diet and insulin at least insofar as cardiovascular mortality is concerned" (4).

"The results . . . have [also] given little hope thus far that degenerative complications of diabetes are preventable by simple control of blood glucose level" (267b).

The FDA reviewed the study with the AMA Council on Drugs and the American Diabetes Association, agreed with the findings of the study, and made the following prescribing recommendations to physicians:

"Pending results of [further] studies, the FDA recommends that Orinase . . . and other sulfonylurea type agents . . . should be used only in patients with symptomatic adult onset diabetes mellitus who cannot be adequately controlled by diet alone and who are not insulin dependent . . . Diabetic patients currently taking tolbutamide or other chemically related sulfonylurea agents who are under adequate medical supervision should continue on their current regimens until advised by their physicians" (4,80).

In 1975, the FDA published proposed labeling for the sulfonylreas. Although this is still not official, it is useful to be apprised of the current FDA position. The *indications* section would be addended to read as follows (7f):

"(Drug) is indicated to control symptoms due to hyperglycemia in patients with maturity-onset, non-ketotic diabetes mellitus whose symptoms cannot be controlled by diet alone and in whom insulin cannot be used because of patient unwillingness, erratic adherence to the injection regimen, poor vision, physical or mental handicap, insulin allergy, employment requirements, or similar factors."

"(Drug) may be used to lower blood glucose in asymptomatic patients whose blood glucose elevation cannot be controlled by diet alone and in whom insulin cannot be used for any of the above reasons. In considering the use of (drug) in asymptomatic patients, it should be recognized that whether or not controlling the blood glucose is effective in preventing the long term cardiovascular or neural complications of diabetes is an unanswered question."

"The use of (drug) may be associated with an increased risk of cardiovascular mortality as compared to diet alone or diet plus insulin; see WARNINGS. For this reason, it should be used only when the advantages in the individual patient justify the potential risk. The patient should be informed of the advantages and potential risks of (drug) and of alternative modes of therapy and should participate in the decision to use the drug."

"Use of (drug) must be considered by both the physician and the patient as treatment in addition to diet and not as a substitute for diet or as a convenient mechanism for avoiding dietary restraint."

"(Drug) should be given only to patients demonstrated to be responsive to it."

The *warnings* section would include a statement regarding the increased risk of cardiovascular mortality and require that the patient participate in the decision to take the drug. Finally, the *dosage and administration* section would require that patients be tested for secondary failure on a yearly basis.

The American Diabetes Association issued the following recommendations with respect to the study:

"Tolbutamide, as well as other oral hypoglycemic agents, has no place in the routine treatment of chem-ical or latent diabetes, suspected diabetes, or pre-diabetes. Such therapy has never had a place in diabetic ketoacidosis or in those prone to it. The clearest indication for oral agents is diabetes of mild or moderate severity in a patient who proves to be poorly controlled with diet and who is unable or unwilling to take insulin.

"In adult-onset diabetes with hyperglycemia and glycosuria, symptomatic or not, and in the absence of ketosis, a trial with an appropriate diet should come first. If this does not establish satisfactory control, insulin is to be preferred to other therapeutic agents because it is more uniformly effective in controlling hyperglycemia and the UGDP study indicates that it may be safer" (223).

The controversial study has been highly criticized with respect to its design and interpretation (87, 87a, 235, 239).

(a) It is said that the tolbutamide-treated patients had more cardiovascular risks. They were older, more obese, more had angina, higher blood cholesterols and more were on digitalis.

(b) There was some evidence that the death rate in the tolbutamide group was slacking off in the final period while the placebo death rate was rising.

(c) The dose of tolbutamide was fixed. This could not be expected to maintain proper control in all patients, and with improper control, one could expect a greater incidence of complications.

(d) The majority of deaths occurred in two or three treatment centers.

(e) There are studies with results contrary to those of the UGDP (153,199,266).

For further detail the reader is referred to an article written by Seltzer (239) who summarized criticisms of the UGDP study. Prout et al (214) wrote an article in the following issue of Diabetes which summarized the response of UGDP investigators to these criticisms.

In an effort to resolve the controversy, the National Institutes of Health requested the Biometric Society to assess the scientific quality of the UGDP study and other controlled trials of oral hypoglycemic agents. The committee of biostatisticians made the following conclusions (7d):

"On the question of cardiovascular mortality due to tolbutamide and phenformin, we consider that the UGDP trial has raised suspicions that cannot be dismissed on the basis of other evidence presently available."

"We find most of the criticisms levelled against the UGDP findings on this point unpersuasive. The possibility that deaths may have been allocated to cardiovascular causes preferentially in the groups receiving oral therapy exists and, in view of the 'nonsignificance' of differences in total mortality, some reservations about the conclusion that the oral hyperglycemics are toxic must remain. Nonetheless, we consider the evidence of harmfulness moderately strong. The risk is clearly seen in the group of older women . . .''

Unfortunately, the findings of the Biometric Society rekindled the controversy (see criticism of the Biometric study by Feinstein — 87a) and the issue remains unresolved. The clinician, however, is still left with the practicalities of managing the patient and this issue is considered in Question 41.

41. A 58-year-old, 60 kg female with a 7 year history of diabetes which was well controlled on diet until 6 months ago, began developing recurrent monilial infections and nocturia. Her fasting blood glucose at the time was 300 mg%. Her diabetes has since been well-controlled (2 HPP <140 mg%) on 15 units NPH daily. Although she feels much better subjectively, she insists on switching to an oral agent. Characterize the patient who will respond successfully to oral hypoglycemics. How efficacious are the sulfonylureas in controlling blood glucose? What criteria must be met before oral hypoglycemic agents are initiated? How should the patient on oral hypoglycemic agents be monitored?

This patient is very likely to have a successful response to the oral agents. She is greater than 30-40 years of age (i.e. adult onset); she has had diabetes for less than 10 years with no history of ketosis; her fasting blood sugar is currently less than 200 mg%; she is not obese; and her insulin requirements are less than 30 units (i.e., she has some pancreatic reserve) (255).

A review of several studies indicates that there is no significant difference in the initial success rate among the various sulfonylureas available. Approximately ⅔ to ¾ of those patients who meet those criteria specified above will achieve satisfactory control with these agents initially. The primary failure rate for these agents varies between 10-20%. Two to four percent develop secondary failure (see Question 43). As the duration of therapy increases to 7-10 years, the final overall success rate may drop to 10-30% (22, 23, 24, 48, 284, 212, 239a).

Prior to the UGDP study, most physicians would have used oral therapy in adult onset diabetics with or without a trial of diet. Now many would use insulin. On the basis of the proposed FDA labeling (7f) and a recent review of the topic by Dunphy (78a), the following recommendations for the clinical use of oral hypoglycemic agents are made:

a. First, there must be documentation of the diagnosis of diabetes as indicated by an abnormal glucose tolerance test, an elevated fasting blood glucose and/or the presence of symptoms. Glucosuria and elevated random blood glucose levels constitute only presumptive evidence for diabetes. Also see Question 8.

b. A documented trial of diet therapy alone must be attempted before oral agents are initiated. If this is not possible, the reasons must be clearly delineated.

c. The patient should participate in the decision to use the drug. This involves explaining as clearly as possible, the state of the controversy concerning the efficacy and toxicity of these agents and the other modes of therapy available (i.e. insulin).

d. Document the fact that insulin cannot be used for one of the reasons listed by the FDA (see Question 40).

e. If the patient consents, establish the baseline cardiac and diabetic status. Clearly document the patient's responsiveness to therapy in terms of general well-being, alleviation of symptoms, diminished glucosuria and improved fasting blood glucose levels.

f. Every one to two years document the continued effectiveness of the oral agent by giving the patient a trial off medications with very close monitoring.

g. Finally, continually monitor the patient for deterioration of cardiovascular status, and make consistent attempts to control the patient's weight through appropriate dietary therapy.

42. C.L. is a 50-year-old non-obese female with a 3 month history of diabetes mellitus which has not been well controlled on diet alone. Two weeks prior to her clinic visit tolbutamide 0.5 gm bid was prescribed. Although nocturia has improved somewhat, she still complains of having to urinate 2 to 3 times nightly. Her fasting blood glucose is now 200 mg%; it was 220 mg% two weeks ago. Does this patient represent a "primary" treatment failure to the sulfonylureas?

Although this patient is certainly not responding to the dose of tolbutamide prescribed, she should not be considered a *primary failure* until she has been given a one-month trial on maximum doses of the sulfonylurea in question. Maximum doses of the various sulfonylureas (listed below) have been determined clinically, and are those doses above which the occurrence and severity of toxic effects far exceed therapeutic benefits gained. For example, Canesa et al (44) noted that the incidence of adverse reactions with daily doses of 2 gm chlorpropramide (CPA) was 38.4%. These declined to 21% and 0% following daily doses of 1 gm and 0.5 gm respectively. As noted in Question 41, 10-20% of those patients placed on sulfonylureas will not respond to treatment.

Maximum doses for the sulfonylureas vary among clinics and according to individual preferences of practitioners. Those most frequently recommended in the literature are listed below:

Tolbutamide	2.0-3.0 gm
Acetohexamide	1.5 gm
Tolazamide	1.0 gm
Chlorpropamide	0.5 gm

43. C.L.'s tolbutamide doses were gradually increased to 1 gm tid, and the diabetes was successfully controlled (fasting blood glucose (FBG) 120 mg% and no nocturia) for some time. Although she had been extremely meticulous about her diabetic therapy she gradually began to slip out of control in her second year of therapy. What has happened? How should this patient be managed?

The patient described represents a **secondary treatment failure** to the sulfonylureas. This is defined as a failure of these agents to control blood glucose levels following a month of more of successful treatment. Presumed causes include natural progression of the disease, tolerance to the drug, poor initial selection of patients, inadequate dose, dietary noncompliance or metabolic stress. True secondary failure to the drug (i.e. no identifiable underlying diabetogenic factors) is relatively rare 2-4% (see Question 41).

There are several treatment alternatives for this patient.

(a) She can be switched to another oral agent. Acetohexamide and tolazamide may be used successfully in approximately 25-33% of those patients who have failed to respond (primarily or secondarily) to other sulfonylureas (23,24). There is some evidence that chlorpropamide may control 60% of tolbutamide secondary failures (48). The figures for phenformin are not known but may approach or equal that of the sulfonylureas (276).

(b) Prior to its withdrawal from the market (see Question 56), phenformin was used to treat cases of secondary failure. The addition of phenformin to the sulfonylurea satisfactorily controlled 50-60% of those patients who failed to respond to single agents (23, 24, 25, 48, 163). Fifty milligrams of phenformin were initially added to low doses of the sulfonylurea and then increased gradually (e.g. 50 mg/week) until control was achieved. Typical dose regimens included 100 mg of phenformin/day administered in divided doses in combination with a sulfonylurea in approximately one-half the maximum dose (163). A definitive effect should have been observed within 7-14 days. If there was no effect at maximum doses, it was necessary to switch the patient to insulin.

(c) If control is very poor and symptoms are severe, the patient should be switched to insulin until control is achieved. Fifty percent of the patients can usually be returned with success to oral therapy following control with insulin. The reason for this is that a plasma factor present during uncontrolled diabetes makes the disease relatively resistant to any type of therapy. This resistance usually subsides in one to two weeks (268).

44. Compare the half-lives, duration of action, metabolism, and route of elimination of the four commercially available sulfonylureas: tolbutamide, tolazamide, acetohexamide and chlorpropamide. (See Table 5.)

Tolbutamide is the sulfonylurea with the shortest duration of action (6-12 hours). It is essentially totally metabolized in the liver to inactive compounds (carboxytolbutamide and hydroxytolbutamide) which are excreted in the urine (260). Approximately 85% of the drug administered as a fine powder is recovered in the urine; 9% is recovered in the feces. The latter may be due to incomplete absorption or biliary excretion. Of that excreted in the urine, 66% occurs as the carboxy metabolite and 33% as the hydroxy metabolite. The average half-life of tolbutamide in diabetic subjects is 4.3 ± 0.9 hrs (205) and its volume of distribution is approximately 15 liters (252).

Chlorpropamide (CPA), the longest acting (duration 24-72 hours) sulfonylurea, was previously thought to be excreted unchanged in the urine (145). More recent studies using more sophisticated analytical techniques indicate that as much as 80% may be metabolized in diabetic subjects. At least 3 metabolites have been identified, and it is suspected that there are others; their activity is unknown. Approximately 20% (range 20-61%) is excreted in the urine as unchanged drug. Brotherton et al (38) pointed out that half-lives previously reported for this drug may have been facticiously prolonged as a result of poor methodology. However, Taylor (259), using the modified assays, reconfirmed that the average half-life for CPA is approximately 36 hours. It must be emphasized that these are average values and that the half-life of chlorpropamide varies widely from subject to subject (25-70 hours).

Tolazamide is the newest of the sulfonylureas and shares an intermediate duration of action (10-16 hours) with acetohexamide. Unlike the other sulfonylureas, its onset of action is delayed (4-6 hours vs. 1-2 hours) as a result of delayed absorption. Tolinase has six metabolites. Three of these are active but less so than the parent compound. Eighty-five percent of the administered dose may be recovered from the urine implying biliary excretion or incomplete absorption (Upjohn Research Files).

Acetohexamide (AH) is an intermediate acting (10-16 hours) sulfonylurea which is principally metabolized and eliminated as L-hydroxyhexamide (HH), a compound with equal or greater hypoglycemic activity than AH (278). Galloway et al (105) studied the disposition of AH in 5 patients with maturity onset diabetes and in 2 non-diabetic patients. They found that the half-life of AH conversion to HH was 1.6 hours (range 0.8-2.4 hours) and that the t½ for hydroxyhexamide was 5.3 hrs (range 3.7-6.4). The combined half-life of drug and metabolites was 5.3 hours (range 3.7-11). Three other minor metabolites of unknown activity were recovered from the urine. Intravenous studies and fecal collections indicate that approximately 15% of the drug is eliminated through biliary excretion. Acetohexamide is presumably metabolized in the liver; however, an enzyme has been isolated from rabbit kidney which is capable of reducing acetohexamide to hydroxyhexamide (62). Confirming studies in man could not be found.

Although the half-life is similar to that of tolbutamide, limited blood glucose data and clinical experience seem to indicate that the duration of activity

for this agent is unrelated to its serum levels. A major advantage of this drug, as well as tolazamide therefore, would be the ability to administer it on a once daily basis thereby improving the chances of compliance.

45. A 78-year-old adult onset diabetic has been well-controlled on diet and acetohexamide 500 mg daily. Over a period of months she is noted to develop mild-moderate renal failure. She lives alone, her cataracts impair her eyesight and she has severe arthritic deformities of her fingers and wrist joints. Oral hypoglycemics are to be continued. What is the agent of choice?

Any drug which depends on the kidney for its elimination as unchanged drug or active metabolite will accumulate in patients with renal failure.

Table 5
BASIC BIOPHARMACEUTICS AND PHARMACOKINETICS OF THE ORAL HYPOGLYCEMICS

Drug	Recommended Dose (gm)	Maximum Dose (gm)	Half-life	Onset and Duration	Metabolism and Excretion	Comments
Tolbutamide (Orinase)	0.5-3.0 divided doses	2-3	5.6 hours	Onset — 1 hour 6-12 hours	Totally metabolized to inactive form. Inactive metabolite excreted in kidney.	Generally first drug of choice; most benign; least potent; short half-life. Especially useful in kidney disease.
Acetohexamide (Dymelor)	0.25-1.5 single or divided doses	1.5	5 hours	Onset — 1 hour 10-14 hours	Metabolite's activity equal to, or greater than parent compound. Metabolite excreted via kidney	Essentially no advantage over tolbutamide although few patients who fail on tolbutamide are controlled. Significant uricosuric effects.
Tolazamide (Tolinase)	0.1-1.0 Single or divided	0.75-1.0	7 hours	Onset — 4-6 hours 10-14 hours	Absorbed slowly. Metabolite active but less potent than parent compound. Excreted via kidney.	Essentially no advantage over tolbutamide except that many patients are controlled on single daily doses and compliance may be improved. Said to be equipotent with less severe side effects.
Chlorpropamide (Diabinese)	0.1-0.5 single dose	0.5	35 hours	Onset — 1 hour 72 hours	Previously thought not to be metabolized but recently found that metabolism may be quite extensive. Activity of these unknown. Significant percent excreted unchanged.	More potent than tolbutamide. Caution in elderly patients and those with kidney disease.
*Phenformin (DBI)	0.05-0.1 in single or divided doses	Usually 200 mg (dose limited by GI effects)	3 hours	Initially onset 3-4 days; then onset is rapid. Duration 12 hours for TD form.	Metabolized but activity of metabolite unknown. 90 percent excreted via kidney in 24 hours	Additive with sulfonylureas and insulin. Drug of choice for obese diabetics. Used to treat secondary failures and to stabilize brittle juvenile diabetics.

*See Questions 56 and 60.

Although chlorpropamide may be metabolized to great extent (see Question 44), a significant portion may still be excreted into the urine unchanged, so that it should be avoided in such patients. Furthermore, the activity of its metabolites is not yet known. Petit-pierre et al (204) have studied the disposition of chlorpropamide in patients with renal failure. Chlorpropamide is primarily secreted by the tubules so that there is no apparent relationship between its half-life and the glomerular filtration rate (GFR). Five of 11 patients with GFR's less than 40 cc/min had normal half-lives. When patients with renal failure were grouped into types of nephropathies, it was found that 8/10 with chronic pyelonephritis which involved the tubules had half-lives which exceeded 50 hours (average 86 hours). Average serum creatinine levels and GFR's for both groups were approximately the same. It was further noted that as the half-life increased, measurable serum metabolites of CPA also increased from 2% to 8%. CPA should definitely be avoided in patients with tubular nephropathies.

It would appear that tolbutamide, a drug which is completely metabolized to inactive product, would be the drug of choice. Ueda et al (267) studied the disposition of tolbutamide in patients with severe renal failure. He noted that the half-life was prolonged in these patients and correlated well with GFR and serum levels of non-protein nitrogen (NPN). In those patients whose GFR was less than 10 cc/min and whose NPN was greater than 100 mg%, the half-life was increased to 16-26 hours. It should be emphasized, however, that he noted no prolongation of hypoglycemia in these patients. He postulates that his assay measured inactive metabolite as well as unchanged drug. However, since protracted hypoglycemia has been reported in elderly patients with renal failure who are taking tolbutamide (see Question 48), close follow-up of these patients is mandatory. The significant renal metabolism of insulin may also account for prolonged hypoglycemia occasionally observed in patients of this type. See Question 22.

Both tolazamide and acetohexamide (13,55,168) have produced prolonged hypoglycemia in patients with renal insufficiency. Because both are metabolized to active products that are excreted in the urine, their use should be avoided in these patients (see Question 44).

Any degree of renal failure is an absolute contraindication to the use of phenformin because of its association with lactic acidosis. See Question 60.

46. A 60-year-old male with cirrhosis of the liver is found to have diabetes mellitus. Tolbutamide 0.5 gm tid is initiated. How will the patient's liver function affect the disposition of tolbutamide and the patient's response to tolbutamide?

Since metabolism by the liver is the primary route of tolbutamide elimination, patients with hepatic disease might be expected to have an exaggerated response to this drug. Ueda et al (267) studied the disposition of tolbutamide in cirrhotic patients and found that the half life was prolonged to 7.8-11.2 hours (normal: 4.3 hours) in 5/10 patients. Moreover, the hypoglycemic response in many of these patients was both delayed and prolonged. However, because this exaggerated response in cirrhotics was not necessarily observed in those with prolonged tolbutamide half-lives, the authors concluded that it could not be attributed to delayed disappearance of the drug. It was postulated that this unusual response was a result of impaired uptake and release of glucose by the liver. It should be noted that the degree to which tolbutamide elimination was delayed could not be predicted by the severity of liver function tests.

Because liver disease may be a predisposing factor to severe, prolonged hypoglycemia induced by the sulfonylureas, these drugs should be used with caution in cirrhotic patients. The rare incidence of cholestatic jaundice secondary to the use of these agents may confuse the diagnostic picture in these patients and should be considered if signs and symptoms of obstruction progress (see Question 52).

47. Compare the individual sulfonylureas with respect to the incidence and severity of their side effects.

Adverse reactions attributed to the sulfonylureas are infrequent (approximately 5%) and mild. Allergic skin manifestations and gastrointestinal reactions (nausea, fullness, heartburn), account for the majority of complaints. In general, the incidence and severity of reported side effects are directly related to the half-life of the sulfonylurea:

Tolbutamide 1-3% (22,124,198)
Acetohexamide 5% (23)
Tolazamide 5% (24)
Chlorpropamide 5-8% (48,212,284).

The breakdown of adverse effects varies little among the sulfonylureas. For example, in one prospective study involving 9,168 patients (198), 292 reactions resulting from tolbutamide were reported. Withdrawal of the drug was necessary in 1.5% (140) of these patients. Allergic skin manifestations (0.5%) and gastrointestinal disturbances — nausea, fullness, heartburn (0.25-0.7%) — were the most common complaints. Hypoglycemia, hematologic reactions (0.12%) jaundice and purpura were rare complications.

The most frequent reported adverse effects for the sulfonylureas include the following:

(a) Hypoglycemia — Question No. 48.
(b) Alcohol intolerance — Question No. 50.
(c) Skin reactions — Question No. 51.

(d) Gastrointestinal reactions.

(e) Hepatotoxicity — Question No. 52.

(f) Hypothyroidism — Question No. 53.

(g) Blood dyscrasias — Question No. 54.

(h) Inappropriate ADH — Question No. 55.

48. C.A. is a 68-year-old female who has had a 10 year history of adult onset diabetes mellitus and a 5 year history of advanced renal failure. Over the past several months her diabetes has been well controlled on tolazamide 700 mg/day. Three days prior to admission she developed anorexia and vomiting. She was admitted to the hospital in coma with a blood glucose of 40 mg%, a creatinine of 10 mg% and a BUN of 200 mg%. What is this woman's diagnosis? Were there any predisposing factors? How should she be treated (55,228)?

C.A. has developed a case of severe hypoglycemia secondary to a sulfonylurea. In 1967, Cohen et al (55) reviewed the literature for cases of protracted hypoglycemia secondary to the sulfonylureas. Of the 102 published reports 40% were due to tolbutamide, the most widely used agent. The remaining 60% were attributed to chlorpropamide and acetohexamide. Tolazamide has been infrequently implicated, presumably because it is the newest of the sulfonylureas (228).

It is the exceptional case which is not surrounded by predisposing factors. Among these are old age, hepatic or renal dysfunction, irregular eating habits, unexpected starvation following the ingestion of the usual dose and the initiation of high doses in elderly patients. Drug interaction must also be considered (see Question 49).

This case demonstrates many of these factors. She is an elderly woman with renal impairment who is on relatively high doses of sulfonylurea. Additionally, she continued to take her usual dose in the face of poor dietary intake. Her vomiting and subsequent dehydration resulted in an acute worsening of her renal function.

As noted above, prolonged hypoglycemia has been reported in patients taking tolbutamide (55,244) despite the fact that it is totally metabolized to an inactive product. Therefore, although one would expect that those products which depend on the kidney for their metabolism or elimination of active products would certainly be most dangerous in patients with diminished renal function, it is apparent that other factors are important as well.

Cohen (55) demonstrated that the absorption and excretion of acetohexamide was diminished in a uremic patient. However, this was compensated to a great extent by its increased metabolism to an inactive product. Although the half-life of acetohexamide was clearly prolonged in 3/7 uremic patients who had developed hypoglycemia, prolongation was equivocal in

4. The lowering of blood sugar in all of these patients in response to intravenous tolbutamide or acetohexamide was delayed and exaggerated. Prolonged hypoglycemia in uremic patients may in part be explained by the fact that the kidney is the most important site of extrahepatic breakdown of insulin (227). Also see Question 22. Inadequate stores of hepatic glycogen to correct the hypoglycemia is also a contributing factor.

These patients respond within minutes to intravenous glucose. Although the sulfonylurea is discontinued it is important to remember that severe hypoglycemia may recur for 3 to 7 days. This patient was sent home in 24 hours only to return the next day in coma despite adequate feedings and the discontinuation of her medication.

49. Several drugs are known to potentiate the sulfonylureas. Discuss the significance of these drug interactions.

Hansen et al (127a) recently reviewed sulfonylurea drug interactions. Only those associated with hypoglycemic reactions in humans are discussed below. Other drugs reported to interact with the sulfonylureas include alcohol, allopurinol, novobiocin, and oxyphenbutazone (127a).

Chloramphenicol. A recent report indicates that chloramphenicol decreases the metabolism of tolbutamide. A patient who had been taking 2.0 grams of chloramphenicol daily took 1.5 grams of tolbutamide for 3 days. The combination resulted in a severe hypoglycemic reaction which lasted for four days. Blood levels of tolbutamide doubled in 8 days while the half-life tripled (54,127a).

Clofibrate. An increased hypoglycemic response to tolbutamide and severe hypoglycemia in a patient taking this combination may be due to an inhibition of tolbutamide metabolism by clofibrate (127a). Others have suggested that clofibrate has intrinsic hypoglycemic properties of its own (25a).

Dicumarol. When given in conjunction with the sulfonylureas, dicumarol may induce a significant prolongation of the half-life.

Tolbutamide — The half-life of tolbutamide was increased from 4.9 to 17 hours. The increase began on the third day of anticoagulant therapy and declined one week after therapy was stopped. It is significant that phenindione did not have this effect. It is proposed that dicumarol decreases the metabolism of tolbutamide (127a,166).

Chlorpropamide — Dicumarol more than doubled the half-life of chlorpropamide (from 36 hours to 80-90 hours). The prolonged half-life returned to normal 6 weeks after the drug was discontinued. Because it was thought that chlorpropamide was not metabolized at the time the study was done, the proposed mechanism of the interaction was a decreased renal clearance of the drug. Since that time, however, it has been shown that chlorpropamide *is* metabolized although the activity of the metabolites is unknown (127a,165,245).

Phenylbutazone. 100 mg 5 times daily initiated a profound hypoglycemic reaction (9 mg%) in a patient taking acetohexamide. Later experiments indicate that half-life was increased by decreasing renal excretion. The potentiation of tolbutamide may be due to its decreased metabolism. 100 mg qid x 7 days resulted in a prolongation of the action of acetohexamide from 5 to 24 hours (95).

Phenyramidol. 400 milligrams 3 times daily for 4 days increased the half-life of tolbutamide from 6 hours to 18 hours. It is suggested that phenyramidol inhibits the metabolism of tolbutamide. This interaction is of particular importance because profound and fatal hypoglycemic reactions have been reported (127a,245).

Probenecid. The effect of probenecid on the half-life of tolbutamide is controversial. An earlier report indicated that probenecid prolonged the half-life of tolbutamide, but a more recent report indicates there is no effect (37,251).

Salicylates. Large doses of aspirin (2.0 gm tid) increased chlorpropamide serum levels by 50% in one day and doubled it in four days. The mechanism may be a delay in the excretion of the drug or its displacement from protein (202,251,286).

Sulfonamides. Hypoglycemia may be induced by sulfaphenazole and sulfisoxazole in patients taking tolbutamide. The hypoglycemic reactions reportedly induced by sulfisoxazole occurred in two elderly patients who were given the usual dose of 2.0 gm daily. The onset was immediate in one case and gradual in the other. Both had decreased renal function. The proposed mechanism was competition for excretion, although displacement from protein is certainly another possibility (53,127a,244).

50. A 58-year-old male with adult onset diabetes, asthma and asymptomatic hyperuricemia (9.0 mg%) complains of frequent episodes of flushing, nausea, headache and tachycardia. His current medications include chlorpropamide 500 mg daily, theophylline elixir (Elixophylline) 45 cc qid, and aspirin 600 mg qid for headaches. Could any of his drugs be contributing to his current complaints? How can these episodes be avoided?

Nausea and tachycardia are frequent complications of high doses of theophylline. However, the concomitant occurrence of flushing and headache should alert the clinician to the possibility of a disulfiram-type reaction secondary to chlorpropamide.

Alcohol intolerance may occur in up to 30% of those patients who take normal doses (250-500 mg) of chlorpropamide (99) following the ingestion of very small amounts of alcohol (e.g. a single glass of beer) (156). For this reason, it is entirely plausible that the ingestion of large volumes of elixirs with high alcoholic contents may precipitate such a reaction. Examples of such products include Elixophylline (20%) and Nyquil (25%), an over-the-counter sleep preparation.

The typical reaction occurs within 2 to 3 minutes after the ingestion of alcohol and peaks in 15 to 20 minutes. It generally subsides within one hour but may last as long as 3 to 4 hours (2,99).

The most outstanding feature is intense facial flushing accompanied by a pounding headache and a feeling of breathlessness. Conjunctival injection, nausea, tachycardia and truncal flushing may occur (2,199).

The underlying mechanism of the reaction is still in debate but may be secondary to noncompetitive inhibition of aldehyde dehydrogenase by the sulfonylureas (207). Inhibition of this enzyme, which is responsible for the metabolism of both alcohol and serotonin, may result in the accumulation of acetaldehyde and serotonin. It should be noted that the elevation of these latter two substances has not been demonstrated in patients suffering from this syndrome (99).

Chlorpropamide is most often implicated, although alcohol intolerance has infrequently been reported following the ingestion of acetohexamide, tolazamide and tolbutamide. Switching the patient from chlorpropamide to one of the other sulfonylureas may alleviate his problem. Alternatively, theophylline may be administered as a tablet. It is interesting to note that in one physician's experience, the reaction was avoided by the prior ingestion of antihistamine. This is not recommended, however, in view of the additive sedative effects of antihistamines and alcohol.

The patient's asymptomatic hyperuricemia may be secondary to low doses of aspirin which block the secretion of uric acid into the urine, or a false positive reading induced by the theophylline if the colorimetric assay was used. If true hyperuricemia exists, a trial of acetohexamide may be justified in this patient. Yu et al (293) demonstrated that a significant degree of uricosuria may be attained following the ingestion of usual antidiabetic doses of acetohexamide.

51. An adult-onset diabetic who gives a history of allergy to sulfisoxazole develops a mild pruritic, maculopapular rash 3 weeks following the initiation of tolbutamide. What kinds of skin reactions have been attributed to the sulfonylureas? Was the use of a sulfonylurea contraindicated in this patient? Can she be treated with another sulfonylurea?

Pruritis and/or rash are among the most commonly reported side effects attributed to the sulfonylureas.

The majority are minor and reversible (within 2 to 14 days (241) if the offending drug is discontinued. Although there have been occasional reports of spontaneous clearing despite continuation of therapy, the rash has also been noted to increase in severity following discontinuation of the drug (20,241).

The rash, which usually is maculopapular, erythematous and discrete in nature, generally involves the face, neck, upper trunk and proximal portion of the arms. It may or may not be preceded or accompanied by pruritis (241). Baker reviewed the literature for cutaneous reactions to the sulfonylureas (20). Infrequently, patients may develop erythema multiforme, exfoliative dermatitis, photosensitivity reactions and lichenoid eruptions.

Because sulfonylureas have a sulfa-like structure, many authors have suggested that their use be avoided in those patients who are allergic to sulfonamides. Unless a severe reaction is documented, this author does not feel that there is a contraindication to the use of sulfonylureas in this situation. Dowling et al (77) demonstrated that the incidence of cross-sensitivity among various sulonamides was 17%. One would expect that the incidence between two classes of drugs with sulfa-like structures would be considerably less. Some patients who have developed rash to one sulfonylurea may be managed successfully with another sulfonylurea (20,36,126). However, cross-sensitivity among the sulfonylureas has also been documented (20,212) and is said to be common.

Because this patient's reaction is mild, one may consider a trial of another sulfonylurea.

52. Four weeks following the initiation of chlorpropamide therapy, a 56-year-old male develops a fever and complains of nausea, vomiting and a pruritic rash. His urine has turned dark and his stools are clay colored. He seeks medical advice at the urging of friends who have noted his yellowed complexion. Initial laboratory tests indicate that he has an elevated serum bilirubin, alkaline phosphatase and eosinophil count. Could the patient's signs and symptoms be related to his CPA therapy? If so, could they be alleviated by decreasing the dose or changing to another sulfonylurea?

Mildly elevated liver function tests (alkaline phosphatase, cephalin flocculation, SGPT) have been associated with the ingestion of all the sulfonylureas (19, 23, 24, 42, 129). Clinical jaundice, however, is relatively rare. Chlorpropamide has been most frequently implicated (129,220), but few cases have been reported since 1960 when the doses routinely used were lowered considerably from 1-3 gm to 250-500 mg. Jaundice has also been reported following therapeutic doses of tolbutamide (19,122) and acetohexamide

(78,117). No reports of tolazamide jaundice were documented; however, it is the most recently marketed sulfonylurea and its literature is not extensive.

Early reports of CPA-induced cholestatic jaundice would seem to indicate that this is a hypersensitivity type reaction in that many of the cases were associated with a rash and eosinophilia (126). Liver biopsies generally reveal intrahepatic cholestasis with minimal cellular damage (focal necrosis). Most cases are reversible in one to two months if the drug is discontinued soon after the onset of symptoms. In most cases symptoms developed within 6 weeks (126) although a latent period of up to 24 months (122) has been reported. In a single report, 3 patients who developed jaundice following high doses of chlorpropamide did not experience recurrent symptoms when placed on 3.0 gms of tolbutamide or low doses (250 mg) of chlorpropamide (126). Another patient who was treated similarly developed recurrent jaundice within 5 weeks (58).

A two month trial without CPA is warranted in this patient and an attempt should be made to control his diabetes with insulin.

53. A 55-year-old female with a 5 year history of diabetes mellitus which has been well controlled with tolbutamide 0.5 gm tid, complains of weight gain, cold intolerance and fatigue. She is found to have a T3 resin uptake of 15.5% (25-35%), a low basal metabolic rate, and depressed tendon reflexes. A diagnosis of hypothyroidism is made. Could tolbutamide have induced these symptoms?

Although the antithyroid effects of carbutamide (a sulfonylurea which has been removed from the market) have been well documented in man and animals (181), it remains unclear whether any of the sulfonylureas currently used share these effects.

Hanno and Awwad (128) demonstrated that tolbutamide reversibly inhibits the organic binding of I^{131} in man following a minimum of six months of therapy. The degree of this inhibition may be correlated with the total dose and duration of therapy. None of those patients in which inhibition was significant exhibited clinical signs or symptoms of hypothyroidism.

Portioli et al (211), and Hunton et al (138) screened patients who had been taking sulfonylureas for coexisting hypothyroidism. Both found that the incidence of hypothyroidism (based on diminished T3 resin uptake and/or PBI) was higher in these patients than in those diabetics treated with diet and/or insulin or in non-diabetics. Hunton et al (138), who used a low PBI as the basis of their diagnosis, stated that 20% of those patients taking sulfonylureas would develop hypothyroidism. One should also consider that tolbutamide and chlorpropamide *may* decrease the binding of T3 and T4 to thyroid binding globulin (131) and may thereby induce a false low PBI. None of the patients in these two studies exhibited overt signs and symptoms of hypothyroidism.

Burke et al (40) attempted, but were unable to confirm the findings of Hunton et al (138). They found no evidence of hypothyroidism in patients who had been on long-term sulfonylurea therapy.

Only four cases of symptomatic hypothyroidism, which clearly improved following discontinuation of sulfonylurea, have been reported. Tolbutamide 0.5 gm daily for a period of 6 weeks to 5 years was responsible for all of these (39,224,231,234). Until a well-controlled prospective study is done, it must be concluded that although sulfonylureas may occasionally induce mild abnormalities of thyroid function (decreased I[131] uptake, decreased PBI, decreased T3 resin uptake) (127,241), clinically significant hypothyroidism is very rare. Since in all of these cases, symptomatic improvement and normalization of laboratory tests was noted as soon as four weeks following discontinuation of the medication, a trial withdrawal of tolbutamide may be warranted in this patient.

54. Blood dyscrasias secondary to the sulfonylureas are extremely rare. What types of hematologic abnormalities have been reported?

A review of the literature revealed rare cases of sulfonylurea induced blood dyscrasias. See Table 6.

55. A 65-year-old female has been receiving chlorothiazide, digoxin and chlorpropamide 500 mg daily. On examination, her blood sugar is found to be higher than usual, so her chlorpropamide is increased to 750 mg/day. Her renal function is within normal limits. Three months later she complains of progressive weakness, anorexia, nausea and dizzy spells. Laboratory examination reveals a serum sodium of 120 mEq/L, a serum osmolality of 320 mOsm/L and a urine osmolality of 600 mOsm/L. Can you attribute her condition to any of her drugs?

The usefulness of chlorpropamide in the treatment of diabetes insipidus has only recently been discovered. The antidiuretic effect of the drug is most likely due to its ability to potentiate the effects of very small amounts of antidiuretic hormone (ADH) on the tubular reabsorption of water by increasing tubular C-AMP. Centrally, it may enhance the release of ADH and override the inhibitory effects of waterloading on ADH release (79). Only recently have cases of inappropriate ADH occurring in patients receiving the drug for diabetes mellitus been reported (97,274). The authors feel this may be due to a defect in the feedback mechanism; that is, serum hypo-osmolality fails to turn ADH completely off. Even though these basal secretions may be minimal, potentiation by chlorpropamide could induce water intoxication. Certain patients may be predisposed to these effects: geriatrics, those with congestive heart failure, and those who are taking thiazides. Thiazides induce the secretion of ADH by causing a negative sodium balance and by contracting extracellular volume. Additionally, therapeutic waterloads given to patients with urinary tract infections or prior to urinary tract manipulation should be used with caution in patients receiving chlorpropamide.

The drug-induced inappropriate ADH activity is reversible. Improvement occurs within a week after the medication is discontinued. It is estimated that it can occur in approximately 4% of those patients receiving the drug.

Although tolbutamide also appears to have some

Table 6
SULFONYLUREA-INDUCED BLOOD DYSCRASIAS

Blood Dyscrasia	Drug	Comments	Reference
Thrombocytopenia	Tolbutamide CPA 250 mg q.d.	2 patients with petechiae and hepatosplenomegaly 15 days onset; 3 cases	(22) (100,191)
Leukopenia	Tolbutamide	1 patient	(22)
Neutropenia	CPA	—	(248)
Agranulocytosis	CPA	3 fatal cases; all taking less than 500 mg daily	(150,248, 282)
Pancytopenia	Tolbutamide	Fatal	(49)
Pure Red Cell Aplasia	CPA	1.125 gm daily x 3 mos. Reversible	(219)
Immune Hemolysis	CPA Tolbutamide/Phenacetin Tolbutamide	1 patient with "innocent bystander" reaction 0.5 gm tid x 3 mos. 1 gm daily x 1 year	(175) (177b)
Hemolysis in G 6PD deficiency	Tolbutamide	1 gm daily x 12 days. Presence of acidosis and urinary tract infection may also have been contributing factors.	(31)

antidiuretic activity (125), Moses et al (192) have demonstrated that tolazamide, acetohexamide and glyburide may actually have a diuretic effect (79, 97, 125, 274).

56. What is the current status of phenformin in the United States and what are the indications for its use?

As of October 23, 1977, the general use of phenformin was banned by the Food and Drug Administration (FDA) and it was no longer available in pharmacies for dispensing. This action was primarily based upon the association of lactic acidosis with phenformin (see Question 60). In view of the fact that there is still some question as to whether phenformin will be permanently withdrawn from the market, pertinent information regarding this drug will be retained in this edition (7a,7b,7c).

Prior to this action and the findings of increased cardiovascular mortality in diabetics treated with phenformin by the UGDP study, phenformin was considered by many clinicians to be the drug of choice for obese diabetics. This was based upon the rationale that insulin and drugs which depend upon insulin for their action (i.e. sulfonylureas) promote lipogenesis. The weight gain and increased obesity which would presumably occur would produce a state of insulin resistance and increase insulin requirements. Thus, a vicious cycle would be established.

Since phenformin promotes the peripheral utilization of glucose independent of insulin and decreases the gastrointestinal absorption of carbohydrates, it theoretically minimizes lipogenesis and the accumulation of fat. The drug may also decrease towards normal the delayed, but excessive insulin response to hyperglycemia found in such patients. It may thereby ameliorate the appetite-stimulating postprandial hypoglycemia.

The anorexic effect of the drug is also claimed to be useful in the treatment of obese diabetics. The actual weight loss which can be expected from this drug is unpredictable. Some show no effect on weight while others show a weight loss in these patients which is proportional to the degree of obesity. At any rate, no one claims that ingestion of the drug results in a profound loss of weight, although most agree that anorexia would be an added benefit in the treatment of obese patients. Finally, the malabsorption of glucose ascribed to the drug may be of benefit in these patients (9,136,201,222,225,275).

However, since the drug has been withdrawn from general use, its indications have narrowed considerably. According to the FDA (7b):

"There is a small group of maturity-onset nonketotic diabetics in whom use of insulin poses special hardships and for whom the benefits of phenformin clearly outweigh the risks. This group may be defined as patients:

1. who are symptomatic, *and*
2. whose symptoms are not controlled with diet and sulfonylureas alone or who cannot take sulfonylureas because of nontolerance or allergy; *and*
3. whose symptoms are controlled by the addition of phenformin to their regimen; *and*
4. who have none of the underlying risk factors which contraindicate the use of phenformin; *and*
5. (a) whose occupation is such that the risk of hypoglycemia from insulin would threaten their jobs or be a hazard to them or others; *or* (b) who cannot take insulin because of serious mental or physical disability and there is no practicable way for them to receive assistance from relatives or friends."

A mechanism for making phenformin available only to those patients meeting *all* of the criteria above was to be established by the FDA (7b). As of October 1977, no arrangement which was acceptable to the manufacturers, the FDA, and the American Medical Association could be agreed upon and discussions were discontinued. It is unclear whether the drug will be made available on a limited basis in the future (7c).

57. Compare phenformin with the sulfonylureas with respect to mechanism of action, efficacy, and potency.

Mechanism of Action: Although extensive studies on the biochemical effects of phenformin have been done, the exact mechanism of its action is still unknown. Unlike its sulfonylurea counterparts, phenformin does not stimulate the beta cells of the pancreas to produce insulin nor is its activity fully dependent upon the presence of insulin, for it still may produce hypoglycemia in pancreatectomized animals. It also differs from the sulfonylureas in that it does not lower blood sugar levels in normal, nondiabetic subjects.

Initially, it was hypothesized that phenformin increased the peripheral utilization of glucose by blocking its oxidative metabolism and indirectly augmenting its anaerobic metabolism (270). Although this theory is useful in explaining phenformin-induced lactic acidosis, it has fallen into some disfavor. Most of the studies supporting this theory were done *in vitro* using phenformin concentrations unattainable *in vivo*. Searle et al (236) note that changes in the rate of glucose oxidation to CO_2 are insignificant following administration of phenformin to normal and diabetic patients.

Recent studies have demonstrated that phenformin inhibits the oral absorption of glucose in therapeutic doses (55,135,285). This may account for its major mechanism of action. Although many other theories have been proposed, it must be emphasized that not one of these fully explains the observed pharmacologic effect of phenformin. A combination of several activities may be useful in explaining its mode of action in the future.

Efficacy: The efficacy of phenformin is comparable to but not better than that of the sulfonylureas. The percentage of patients controlled initially range from 70-90%. Clinical trials are not as abundant as for tolbutamide and the high incidence of gastrointestinal side effects have discouraged its widespread use. One study claims that 70% of patients were controlled initially, that 12% developed secondary failure and that 56% were finally controlled. This figure is substantially better than the overall success rate of 20% quoted for the sulfonylureas (92,136).

Potency: The absolute potency of phenformin as judged by its ability to control diabetes in patients who developed secondary failure to tolbutamide therapy is similar to that of chlorpropamide. Its duration of action is much shorter than that of CPA.

58. Discuss the absorption, metabolism, excretion and duration of action of phenformin.

There is a severe lack of information concerning the pharmacokinetics of phenformin in the literature. The most recent edition of a prominent pharmacology text states that phenformin is adequately absorbed from the gastrointestinal tract. The site of absorption is not specified (263a). Approximately 45-55% of an oral dose (50 mg) is recovered in the urine. One-third of this appears as the para-OH metabolite (activity unknown) and two-thirds as unchanged drug (28,29). Small amounts of the drug enter the enterohepatic circulation, but the fecal elimination in man has not been quantitated. Since virtually all of an intravenous dose is recovered in the urine, the contribution of biliary excretion and subsequent fecal elimination must be small. These data also indicate that the oral absorption of biguanides is incomplete. The liver is the main site of metabolism and the kidney the main organ of excretion. The overall elimination of phenformin follows first order kinetics; the composite half-life of drug and metabolite is 3.2 hours. Since a significant portion of phenformin is recovered from the urine as unchanged drug, it is reasonable to predict that it will accumulate in patients with renal dysfunction. In any case, the drug is absolutely contraindicated in such patients due to their predisposition to lactic acidosis (see Question 60).

Radding et al (217) administered a single 100 mg dose of phenformin in tablet and time-released capsule form to diabetics. He noted that the hypoglycemic effects had dissipated in 6-8 hours following administration of the tablets and in 14 hours following the capsules.

59. The gastrointestinal side effects of phenformin are common and predictable. How do they present clinically, and how can they be minimized?

The anorexia, metallic taste, nausea, vomiting and diarrhea associated with phenformin are dose-related and severe enough to limit the maximum useful dose of the drug to 200 mg. Earlier, incidences of 25-40% were reported. This figure has been markedly reduced (3-7%) since the introduction of the time-disintegrated capsule.

It was found that these dose-related gastrointestinal effects could not be ascribed to direct irritation but were of central origin. It was also found that more frequent administration of smaller doses decreased the incidence of these effects, presumably because the drug never reached sufficiently high levels in the brain to trigger the emetic zone. It is assumed that the continual release of small amounts from the time disintegrated capsules maintains a sufficient blood level to produce a hypoglycemic effect but prevents an excessively high level in the brain, thus decreasing the incidence of side effects. Gastrointestinal effects can be avoided by:

(a) administration of time disintegrated capsules,

(b) gradually increasing the dose using no more than 50 mg initially, and

(c) administration with meals, not to prevent irritation, but to slow absorption (115,276).

60. A 60-year-old obese male with a 4 year history of diabetes moderately well regulated on diet and 50 mg of phenformin three times daily was admitted with a 3 day history of nausea, vomiting, diarrhea, weakness and tachypnea. Other medical problems include emphysema and mild renal failure.

On physical examination, the patient was oriented but appeared acutely ill. Temperature, pulse and blood pressure were within normal limits. The respiratory rate was 32/minute.

Significant laboratory values included the following: Na 140 mEq/L; K 6.2 mEq/L; Cl 103 mEq/L; HCO_3 5 m Eq/L; Arterial pH 6.8; Creatinine 3.2 mg/100 ml; Blood Glucose 130 mg/100 ml; Serum Acetones negative; Serum Lactate 150 mg/100 ml (normal: 6-16 mg/100 ml); and Serum Pyruvate 5.0 mg/100 ml (normal 0.4-1.2 mg/100 ml).

A diagnosis of lactic acidosis was made. What is the relationship between phenformin and lactic acidosis? What are the predisposing factors for lactic acidosis? How can this patient be managed?

The most notorious side effect associated with phenformin is its assumed cause/effect relationship with lactic acidosis. *Lactic acidosis* is defined as a metabolic acidosis characterized by a significant reduction in the arterial pH and an accumulation of serum lactate (253), a product of anaerobic metabolism. It is a condition which is highly lethal (50% mortality) and resistant to therapy. Lactic acidosis occurs when there is an increased production or decreased utilization of lactate. Decreased utilization of lactate occurs when tissues are unable to oxidize lactate to pyruvate (these two substances are normally present in the serum in a ratio of 10:1). Phenformin may predispose a patient to lactic acidosis by augmenting anaerobic metabolism or by decreasing the kidney's ability to handle an acid load.

Signs and symptoms are generally acute in onset and commonly include nausea, vomiting, diarrhea and hyperventilation. Hypovolemia, hypotension, confusion and coma may also occur; death is usually secondary to cardiovascular collapse.

Typical *laboratory findings* include a low serum bicarbonate and pCO_2; a low arterial pH; an elevated potassium; a normal or low serum chloride; elevated lactate and pyruvate levels; an increased L/P ratio (normal — 1:10) and an anion gap of 30 mEq/L or greater.

Treatment is empirical and includes one or more of the following measures:

(a) Correction of any underlying cause of anoxia and elimination of factors predisposing to lactic acidosis.

(b) Administration of large doses of sodium bicarbonate in an attempt to correct acidosis. Doses vary due to individual rates of lactate production but have ranged from 66 mEq in 6 hours to 3000 mEq in 48 hours. The frequent determination of arterial pH is also essential.

(c) Hemodialysis may be effective in patients who are refractory to bicarbonate or in those who cannot tolerate large sodium and fluid loads (186). Hemodialysis is used in an attempt to dialyze lactic acid and phenformin, provide a large buffer reservoir and to remove sodium and fluid overloads. The value of a peritoneal dialysis is equivocal (253) even when the lactate contained in the dialysis fluids is replaced with acetate.

(d) Glucose (20% IV at 100 cc/hour) and insulin (10U regular SQ q 4 hours) have resulted in a dramatic fall in serum lactate and pyruvate after unsuccessful therapy with bicarbonate. Glucose and insulin are administered in an attempt to improve the metabolic utilization of lactate and pyruvate.

Since 1959 when phenformin was originally marketed in the United States, the FDA has received 240 case reports of lactic acidosis in patients taking this drug. Since then, its advisory committee on endocrinology and metabolism has reviewed the evidence on several occasions. As late as 1974, the committee concluded that the data did not establish phenformin as a cause of lactic acidosis in the absence of predisposing factors such as alcohol ingestion, renal failure or severe cardiovascular disease. In October 1976, the committee again reviewed the 190 case reports then received by the FDA and other data. At that time they concluded that there was a definite causative association between phenformin and lactic acidosis. Furthermore, patients at risk for lactic acidosis frequently were not identifiable in that they apparently had normal renal function; lactic acidosis also occurred following the ingestion of usual therapeutic doses of phenformin. On the basis of their findings, they concluded that the risk to benefit ratio was too great and recommended that the drug be removed from the general market. In January 1977, the FDA decreased the maximum recommended dose from 200 mg to 100 mg and narrowed the indications for use (7a).

In August 1977, after fact-finding hearings, the Secretary of the Department of Health, Education and Welfare ordered an end to the general marketing of phenformin within 90 days (October 23, 1977). This was primarily based upon the fact that the estimated incidence of phenformin-induced lactic acidosis is 0.25 to 4 cases per 1000 users per year. Since at that time there were approximately 336,000 users of phenformin in the U.S. and since the overall mortality from this condition is 50%, approximately 50-700 deaths per year could be attributed to phenformin. It is important to note that the incidence of death associated with this drug exceeds that associated with other drug-induced adverse effects (e.g. penicillin anaphylaxis, oral contraceptive thromboembolism, or chloramphenicol aplastic anemia) by 5 to 80 times (7b).

A recent review of 330 cases of lactic acidosis in diabetics taking biguanides (175b) and the author's review of that literature reveals the following characteristics of phenformin-related lactic acidosis:

a. Almost all of the cases reported in the world literature have been associated with phenformin ingestion. Although metformin is heavily prescribed in European countries, only 12/237 patients were taking metformin alone. Four others were taking metformin in combination with phenformin. Thirty of 327 patients were taking buformin. Furthermore, none of the patients taking metformin had a serum creatinine level less than 3.0 mg/100 ml. Thus, the incidence of metformin-induced lactic acidosis is apparently lower than that of phenformin or buformin which is prescribed much less frequently than the other two biguanides. Metformin-induced lactic acidosis is also consistently related to decreased renal function in contrast to that induced by phenformin (175b,193a).

b. A predictable dose relationship cannot be established. Almost all patients were taking normal, therapeutic doses of phenformin when lactic acidosis developed. The average dose was 125 mg (56, 68, 175b). Lactic acidosis has also been observed following the acute ingestion of 2.5 gm. Symptoms may occur from 2 to 14 hours after the ingestion of such large doses (213, 253).

c. The development of lactic acidosis cannot be correlated with the duration of therapy, although where it could be determined, a majority of cases occurred within the first two years of therapy (175b).

d. Almost all patients had concurrent illnesses or conditions which could predispose them to lactic acidosis. Clinical *renal dysfunction* was present in at least 35% of the cases. This may result in accumulation of lactate and active drug. It is important to point out that since blood urea nitrogen and serum creatinine levels are frequently insufficient to detect renal dysfunction, especially in elderly patients, these parameters could not be dependably used to detect patients at risk for developing lactic acidosis. *Liver dysfunction* was present in 15% of the cases and could have resulted in an impairment of drug and lactate metabolism. Any condition which produces tissue anoxia promotes anaerobic metabolism and can increase the production of lactate. These include cardiovascular disease (present in 44%), pulmonary disease (present in 19%), shock (present in 24%), hemorrhage, anemia and ischemia. Infectious processes (present in 19%) are also associated with lactic acidosis. Alcoholism or recent alcohol ingestion was documented in a few of the reported cases. Alcohol increases lactate production and decreases its utilization; it also appears to have a synergistic effect with phenformin in elevating blood lactate levels (140, 145, 175b). Also see the chapter on *Acid-Base Disorders.*

61. Several drugs may induce hypoglycemia because of their own pharmacologic or toxic effects. These may therefore potentiate both insulin and oral hypoglycemics. Name these drugs and discuss the clinical significance of this effect.

Seltzer (238) extensively reviewed the matter of drug-induced hypoglycemia and the reader is referred to his article for a more complete discussion of this topic. A list of drugs reported to cause hypoglycemia with references is provided below. More commonly implicated agents are given more thorough consideration.

Acetaminophen. Hypoglycemia is associated with the ingestion of large doses (7-35 gm) and hepatic necrosis.

Alcohol. See below.

Anabolic Steroids. See below.

Chlorpromazine + orphenadrine (238).

EDTA in combination with insulin (238).

Fenfluramine. See below.

Haloperidol. Single case in a nondiabetic (238).

Isoniazid. See MAO inhibitors.

Manganese in combination with insulin (contained in alfalfa extract) (238).

Monoamine Oxidase (MAO) inhibitors. See below.

Oxytetracycline in combination with insulin (238).

Pentamidine. See below.

Potassium para-aminobenzoate (12 gm) in fasting nondiabetics (238).

Propranolol. See below.

Salicylates. See below.

Theophylline. See below.

Alcohol levels just high enough to cause mild intoxication can induce hypoglycemia in susceptible individuals — that is, those who have no glycogen reserve. It is important to note that chronic alcoholics are notorious for neglecting their nutritional requirements. Generally a 2 to 3 day fast is required before hypoglycemia can be induced in non-diabetic individuals; however, symptoms of hypoglycemia have been observed in non-fasting, non-obese, non-diabetic subjects who were given enough alcohol to produce an average serum level of 1 mg/ml (194a). Obese individuals appear to be relatively resistant to the hypoglycemic effects of alcohol. At least part of alcohol's effect is related to its ability to impair gluconeogenesis (27,102,103,148). Alcohol also increases the amount of insulin secreted in response to glucose in nondiabetics (185,194a). The effect is clinically significant, and the combination of alcohol and insulin appears to be especially dangerous. Five insulin-dependent diabetics had severe hypoglycemic reactions following alcoholic orgies. Three suffered irreversible neurologic damage and two died in irreversible hypoglycemic coma (16). Reversible hypoglycemia precipitated by alcohol and sulfonylureas has also been reported (239).

Anabolic Steroids in therapeutic doses can reduce the blood glucose of both diabetic and nondiabetic patients. Although symptomatic hypoglycemia has never been reported, it is a potential hazard in patients who are taking insulin or oral hypoglycemic agents. More specific observations are noted below (169, 247, 257).

(a) Testosterone can decrease the fasting blood sugar, glycosuria and insulin requirements in some diabetic patients.

(b) Dianabol, a 17-alpha alkylated oral derivative of testosterone, decreased the blood sugar by 8.8-12.6% in a group of nondiabetic men. The effect lasted for the duration of therapy but blood sugars never fell below 55 mg% and no symptoms of hypoglycemia were reported.

A dose of 10-20 mg for 2 weeks may increase the insulin response to glucose by three times. This may be due to a decreased destruction of insulin secondary to the hepatic effect of the androgens. This effect is reversible and a normal insulin response has been observed 10 days after the drug has been discontinued.

(c) Durabolin is without effect in normals but can have a hypoglycemic effect in some diabetics.

(d) Methandrostenolone (30 mg x 5 days) has induced hypoglycemia and decreased insulin requirements in emaciated patients. It has been reported to decrease the fasting blood sugar by 50%.

Clofibrate. A 4 week course of clofibrate (1 gm bid) was given to 14 adult onset diabetics between a 2 week and 4 week control period. Both the fasting blood glucose and the glucose tolerance were improved by 20% after 14 and 28 days of therapy. This effect was independent of the mode of antidiabetic therapy used by the patients, the presence or absence of hypertriglyceridemia, or serum levels of clofibrate. With the exception of one one patient, the glucose tolerance test returned to control levels after clofibrate was discontinued. Barnett et al reviewed the findings of other investigators and concluded that the conflicting reports may have been related to the lack of consideration of other variables which may affect glucose tolerance (25a).

Fenfluramine (40 mg administered 30 minutes before meals) consistently lowered postabsorptive hyperglycemia by 32-35% in maturity onset diabetics for a period of two hours. This was also observed in juvenile diabetics to a lesser extent. Hypoglycemia has not been reported to date. The drug increases glucose uptake by skeletal muscle but does not elevate lactate levels as does phenformin or stimulate insulin secretion as does tolbutamide (265).

Monamine Oxidase (MAO) Inhibitors have been known to potentiate both insulin and sulfonylurea induced hypoglycemias — apparently by blocking the homeostatic response to hypoglycemia (12,60). It has been suggested that this effect may be confined to the hydrazine type MAO inhibitors (60). Although MAO inhibitors are seldom used, it is of interest that isoniazid (INH) has a hydrazine type structure and has been reported to potentiate the effect of tolbutamide. 500 mg of INH with 3.0 grams of tolbutamide produced a 17-53% drop in the blood sugar after 4 hours. Tolbutamide alone produced a maximum drop of 43% (237). Hypoglycemia with other MAO inhibitors has

been known to occur as early as 11 days after the start of therapy. Insulin doses have been decreased as much as 30 units.

Pentamidine, given in therapeutic doses (4 mg/kg/day) caused 15/164 patients to develop blood sugars of less than 60 mg/100 ml. No mechanism was postulated (280).

Propranolol (40-120 mg/day) has reportedly induced severe hypoglycemic episodes in juvenile diabetics and nondiabetic patients. Patients who were not diabetic were generally predisposed to hypoglycemia. One was an elderly man who had had mild postgastrectomy hypoglycemia (162); others had fasted or may have had poor dietary intake prior to the episode (176,290). Hypoglycemia in two children who accidentally ingested 150 mg of propranolol has also been reported (132). Propranolol inconsistently produces hypoglycemia in insulin-dependent diabetics (162, 183, 221), presumably by blocking the glycogenolytic effects of sympathomimetics released in response to hypoglycemia. It may be anticipated that some symptoms of hypoglycemia will be masked as well (8). Another theoretical mechanism is inhibition of gluconeogenesis (8,10). Hypoglycemia in patients taking sulfonylureas has not been reported. Perhaps this is due to the diminished secretion of insulin in response to sulfonylureas caused by propranolol (208). (See Question 4.)

Salicylates (5-6 grams) can decrease ketonuria and glycosuria in mild to moderate diabetics and induce hypoglycemia in nondiabetics (230). Serum levels of 10-40% may decrease the fasting blood sugar of a diabetic by 28% (112). Similar doses may potentiate the action of both insulin and sulfonylureas necessitating a reduction in their doses. The mechanism of this hypoglycemic effect is unclear but it is not through the release of insulin or any augmentation of its effects. Salicylates appear to increase the peripheral uptake of glucose, increase the rate of glycolysis and decrease gluconeogenesis. Hyperglycemia has occasionally been reported in salicylate toxicities involving levels greater than 40 mg%, but this is not a consistent finding (7,72,84,112,130,239,242).

REFERENCES

1. ____: Final labeling approved for oral hypoglycemics. FDA Drug Bull May 1972.
2. ____: Alcohol insensitivity to sulfonylureas. Brit Med J 2:586, 1964.
3. ____: Phenformin and lactic acidosis. Calif Med 110:348, 1969.
4. ____: Oral hypoglycemics — FDA warning. Clin Alert 292:Nov, 1970.
5. ____: Clinitest Package Insert, Ames Drug Co., Elkhart, Ind.
6. Nicotinic acid and diabetes mellitus. Nutr Rev 22:166, 1964.
7. ____: Salicylates and carbohydrate metabolism (editorial). Diabetes 9:416, 1960.
7a.____: Phenformin: New labeling and possible removal from the market. FDA Drug Bull 7:6, May-July, 1977.
7b.____: Phenformin: removal from the general market. FDA Drug Bull 7:14, Aug 1977.
7c.____: Status of withdrawal of phenformin. FDA Drug Bull 7:19, Sept-Oct 1977.
7d.____: Report of the committee for the assessment of biometric aspects of controlled trials of hypoglycemic agents. JAMA 231:583, 1975.
7e.____: Insulin regimen for diabetic ketoacidosis. Brit Med J 1:405, 1977.
7f. ____: Federal Register Vol 40 No 130, July 7, 1975.
8. Abramson EA et al: Effects of propranolol on hormonal and metabolic responses to insulin induced hypoglycemia. Lancet 2:1386, 1966.
9. Abramson EA et al: Treatment of the obese diabetic. A comparative study of placebo, sulfonylurea and phenformin. Metab 16:204, 1967.

10. Abramson EA et al: Role of beta-adrenergic receptors in counter-regulation in insulin induced hypoglycemia. Diabetes 17:141, 1968.

11. Adam PA et al: Diagnosis and treatment: should oral hypoglycemic agents be used in pediatric and pregnant patients? Pediat 42:819, 1968.

12. Admitt PI: Hypoglycemic action of monoamine oxidase inhibitors (MAOI's). Diabetes 17:628, 1968.

12a. Alberti KGMM et al: Diabetic coma: A reappraisal after five years. Clin Endocrinol Metab 6:421, 1977.

12b. Alberti KGMM: Low-dose insulin in the treatment of diabetic ketoacidosis. Arch Int Med 137:1367, 1977.

12c. Alberti KGMM et al: Small doses of intramuscular insulin in the treatment of diabetic "coma". Lancet 2:515, 1973.

13. Alexander RW: Prolonged hypoglycemia following acetohexamide administration: Report of two cases with impaired renal function. Diabetes 15:362, 1966.

14. Ames Co.: False positive and false negative reactions with various tests for glucosuria, available on request. Elkhart, Ind.

15. Anderson OO et al: Carbohydrate metabolism during treatment with chlorthalidone. Brit Med J 2:798, 1966.

16. Arky RA et al: Irreversible hypoglycemia (alcohol induced). JAMA 206:575, 1968.

17. Arky RA et al: Alcohol hypoglycemia VII. Further studies on the refractiveness of obese subjects. Metab 17:977, 1968.

17a. Altszuler N et al: On the mechanism of diazoxide-induced hyperglycemia. Diabetes 26:931, 1977.

18. Baird I et al: Tolazamide in the treatment of diabetes mellitus. Practitioner 198:264, 1967.

19. Baird WR et al: Cholestatic jaundice from tolbutamide. Ann Int Med 53:194, 1960.

20. Baker H: Drug reactions X: Adverse cutaneous reactions to oral hypoglycemic agents. Brit J Derm 82:634, 1970.

21. Baker L et al: Hyperglycemia and acetonuria simulating diabetes. Am J Dis Child 3:59, 1966.

22. Balodimos MC et al: Nine years' experience with tolbutamide in the treatment of diabetes. Metab 15:957, 1966.

23. Balodimos MC et al: Acetohexamide therapy of diabetes mellitus. Metab 17:669, 1968.

24. Balodimos MC et al: Tolazamide in the treatment of diabetes mellitus: clinical experience and review of the literature. Curr Ther Res 13:6, 1971.

25. Barjon P et al: Hyperglycemic coma without ketoacidosis in two hypertensive patients treated with intravenous diazoxide. Sem Hop Paris 49:581, 1973.

25a. Barnett D et al: Effect of clofibrate on glucose tolerance in maturity onset diabetes. Brit J Clin Pharmacol 4:455, 1977.

26. Barrett JC et al: Tolbutamide in the therapy of insulin resistance. Diabetes 2(Suppl):35, 1962.

27. Becker CE: Medical Staff Conference: The clinical pharmacology of alcohol. Calif Med 113:37, 1970.

28. Beckmann R: The fate of biguanides in man. Ann NY Acad Sci 148:820, 1968.

29. Beckmann R: Resorption and biological degradation of phenformin. Diabetologia 3:368, 1967.

30. Belmonte MM et al: Urine sugar determination by the two drop clinitest method. Diabetes 16:557, 1967.

30a. Binder C: Absorption of injected insulin. Acta Pharmacol Toxicol 27:6, 1969.

31. Bird GWG et al: Haemolytic anaemia associated with antibodies to tolbutamide and phenacetin. Brit Med J 1:728, 1972.

32. Block MB et al: Spontaneous hypoglycemia in diabetic patients with renal insufficiency. JAMA 213:1863, 1970.

33. Boshell BR et al: Insulin resistance. Response to insulin from various animal sources including human. Diabetes 13:144, 1964.

34. Breckenridge A et al: Glucose tolerance in hypertensive patients on long-term diuretic therapy. Lancet 1:61, 1967.

35. Bressler R et al: Insulin treatment of diabetes mellitus. Med Clin N Amer 55:861, 1971.

36. Bressler R et al: Evaluation of tolazamide in the treatment of diabetes mellitus. Curr Ther Res 7:219, 1965.

37. Brook R et al: Failure of probenecid to inhibit the rate of metabolism of tolbutamide in man. Clin Pharmacol Ther 9:314, 1968.

38. Brotherton PM et al: A study of the metabolic fate of chlorpropamide in man. Clin Pharmacol Ther 10:505, 1969.

39. Burda CD: Sulfonylurea hypothyroidism in diabetics. Lancet

2:1016, 1965.

40. Burke G et al: Effect of long term sulfonylurea therapy on thyroid treatment in man. Metab 16:651, 1967.

40a. Cahill GH et al: "Control" and diabetes. NEJM 294:1004, 1976.

41. Camerini-Davalos RA: Prevention of diabetes mellitus. Med Clin N Amer 49:865, 1965.

42. Camerini-Davelos R et al: Clinical experiences with tolbutamide. Five years' experience with tolbutamide. Diabetes 11(Suppl): 74, 1962.

43. Campbell GD: Chlorpropamide and foetal damage. Brit Med J 1:59, 1963.

44. Canessa I et al: Clinical evaluation of chlorpropamide in diabetes mellitus. Ann NY Acad Sci 74:752, 1959.

45. Carliner NH et al: Thiazide and phtalimidine induced hyperglycemia in hypertensive patients. JAMA 191:535, 1965.

46. Cawein MJ et al: Levodopa and tests for ketonuria. NEJM 283:649, 1970.

47. Cerasi E et al: The effect of an adenosine 3'5' monophosphate diesterase inhibitor (aminophylline) on the insulin response to glucose infusion in prediabetic and diabetic subjects. Horm Metab Res 1:162, 1969.

48. Cervantes-Amezeua A et al: Long term use of chlorpropamide in diabetes. JAMA 193:759, 1965.

49. Chapman I et al: Pancytopenia associated with tolbutamide therapy. JAMA 186:595, 1963.

50. Charles MA et al: Nonketotic hyperglycemia and coma during intravenous diazoxide therapy in uremia. Diabetes 20:501, 1971.

51. Chazen JA et al: Etiologic factors in thiazide induced or aggravated diabetes mellitus. Diabetes 14:132, 1965.

51a. Chiles R et al: Excessive serum insulin response to oral glucose in obesity and mild diabetes: Study of 501 patients. Diabetes 19:458, 1970.

52. Chirman S: Hyperglycemia during IV fluid therapy. Calif Med 107:149, 1967.

53. Christensen LK et al: Sulphaphenazole induced hypoglycemic attacks in tolbutamide treated subjects. Lancet 2:1298, 1963.

54. Christensen LK et al: Inhibition of drug metabolism by chloramphenicol. Lancet 2:1397, 1969.

54a. Clements RS: Medical grand rounds: Ketoacidosis. South Med J 69:218, 1976.

55. Cohen BD et al: Carbohydrate metabolism in uremia; blood glucose response to the sulfonylureas. Am J Med Sci 254:608, 1967.

56. Cohen RD et al: The relation between phenformin therapy and lactic acidosis. Diabetologia 9:43, 1973.

57. Coleman WB et al: Insulin allergy. Ann All 29:283, 1971.

58. Collens WS et al: Cholestatic jaundice following use of sulfonylurea drugs. NY State J Med 65:907, 1965.

59. Conn JW et al: Influence of adrenal cortical steroids on carbohydrate metabolism in man (review). Metab 5:114, 1956.

60. Cooper AJ et al: Modification of insulin and sulfonylurea hypoglycemia by monoamine oxidase inhibitor drugs (editorial). Diabetes 16:272, 1967.

61. Cranston WI et al: Effect of oral diuretics on raised arterial pressure. Lancet 2:966, 1963.

62. Culp HW et al: The $NADPH_2$ dependent reduction of acetohexamide and related carbony compounds by a rabbit kidney enzyme. Fed Proc 24(2):426, 1965.

63. Cummings NP et al: Plasma glucose and insulin responses to oral glucose with chronic DPH therapy. Pediat 51:1091, 1973.

64. Curtis J et al: Chlorthalidone-induced hyperosmolar hyperglycemic nonketotic coma. JAMA 220:1592, 1972.

65. Czyzyk A et al: Effect of biguanides on intestinal absorption of glucose. Diabetes 17:492, 1968.

66. Dahl JR: Diphenylhydantoin toxic psychosis with associated hyperglycemia. Calif Med 107:345, 1967.

67. D'Alena P et al: Adverse effects after glycerol orally and mannitol parenterally. Arch Ophth 75:201, 1966.

68. Davidson MG et al: Phenformin hypoglycemia and lactic acidosis. NEJM 275:886, 1966.

69. De Mowbray RR: Risk of changing from ox to pig insulin (letter). Lancet 2:1027, 1966.

70. Diamond MT: Hyperglycemic hyperosmolar coma associated with hydrochlorothiazide and pancreatitis. NY State J Med 72:1741, 1972.

71. Diamond S: Ethacrynic acid and diabetes. JAMA 206:1793, 1968.

72. Dixon AJ editor: *Salicylates, An International Symposium*, J & A Churchill, Ltd., London 1963.

73. Dolger H et al: The diagnostic and therapeutic value of tolbutamide in pregnant diabetes. Diabetes 11(Suppl):97, 1962.
74. Dollery CT: Ch 13, Diuretic drugs, in *Side Effects of Drugs,* edited by L Meyler and A Herxheimer, Williams & Wilkins Co., Baltimore, 1968, p 212.
75. Dolovich J et al: Insulin allergy and insulin resistance: case report with immunologic studies. J Aller 46:127, 1970.
76. Donaldson JB: Current concepts in the treatment of diabetes mellitus. Med Clin N Amer 49:1349, 1965.
77. Dowling HF et al: Toxic reactions accompanying second courses of sulfonamides in patients developing toxic reactions during a previous course. Ann Int Med 24:629, 1946.
77a. Drash A: The control of diabetes mellitus: Is it achievable? Is it desirable? J Pediat 88:1074, 1976.
77b. Duck SC et al: Cerebral edema complicating therapy for diabetic ketoacidosis. Diabetes 25:111, 1976.
78. Duncan TG et al: The comparative clinical effectiveness of tolbutamide and acetohexamide. Metab 17:218, 1968.
78a. Dunphy T: Guidelines for use of oral hypoglycemic agents. Bulletin of the Hospital Pharmacy and the Drug Information Analysis Service. Vol 24, May 1976, University of California, San Francisco, 94143.
79. Early LE: Chlorpropamide antidiuresis. NEJM 284:103, 1971.
80. Edwards CC: Oral hypoglycemic agents, Report of the Food and Drug Administration. Diabetes 19(Suppl 2,viii, 1970.
80a. Engerman R et al: Relationship of microvascular disease in diabetes to diabetic control. Diabetes 26:760, 1977.
81. Fabrykant M et al: Nature and prevention of local skin lesions from insulin administration. Metab 3:1, 1954.
82. Fajans SS: What is diabetes? Definition, diagnosis and course. Med Clin N Amer 55:793, 1971.
83. Fajans SS et al: Further studies on diazoxide suppression of insulin release from abnormal and normal islet tissue in man. Ann NY Acad Sci 150:261, 1968.
84. Fang V et al: Hypoglycemic activity and chemical structure of the salicylates. J Pharm Sci 57:2111, 1968.
85. Fariss BL et al: Diphenylhydantoin induced hyperglycemia and impaired insulin release. Diabetes 20:177, 1971.
86. Farquhar JW et al: Hypoglycemia in newborn infants of normal and diabetic mothers. S Afr Med J 42:236, 1968.
87. Feinstein AR: Clinical biostatistics. VIII. An analytic appraisal of the University Group Diabetes Program (UGDP) study. Clin Pharmacol Ther 12:167, 1971.
87a. Feinstein AR: The persistant clinical failures and fallacies of the UGDP study. Clin Pharmacol Ther 19:78, 1976.
88. Feldman JM et al: Inhibition of glucose oxidase paper tests by reducing metabolites. Diabetes 22:115, 1973.
90. Felig P: Pathophysiology of diabetes mellitus. Med Clin N Amer 55:821, 1971.
91. Felig P et al: The glycemic response to arginine in man. Diabetes 21:308, 1972.
91a. Felig P et al: Insulin, glucagon and somatostatin in normal physiology and diabetes mellitus. Diabetes 25:1091, 1976.
91b. Felig P: Diabetic ketoacidosis. NEJM 290:1360, 1974.
91c. Felig P: Insulin: rates and routes of delivery. NEJM 291:1031, 1974.
92. Ferguson DB: The oral hypoglycemic compounds. Med Clin N Amer 49:929, 1965.
93. Ferguson MJ: Saluretic drugs and diabetes mellitus. Am J Cardiol 7:568, 1961.
94. Field JB: Treatment of resistant diabetes mellitus. Mod Treat 4:16, 1967.
95. Field JB et al: Potentiation of acetohexamide hypoglycemia by phenylbutazone. NEJM 277:889, 1967.
96. Field JB: Chronic insulin resistance. Acta Diabetologica Latina 7:220, 1970.
97. Fine D et al: Hyponatremia due to chlorpropamide. Ann Intern Med 72:83, 1970.
98. Finnerty RA: Hyperglycemia after diazoxide. NEJM 285,1487, 1971.
99. Fitzgerald MG et al: Alcohol sensitivity in diabetics receiving CPA. Diabetes 11:40, 1962.
100. Fitzpatrick WJ: Thrombocytopenia occurring during chlorpropamide therapy. Diabetes 12:457, 1963.
101. Free AH: A test for blind diabetics to estimate urine glucose. Diabetes 22(Suppl 1):319, 1973.
102. Freinkel N et al: Alcohol hypoglycemia: current concepts on its

pathogenesis. Diabetes 14:350, 1965.
103. Freinkel N et al: Effects of alcohol on carbohydrate metacolism in man. Psychosom Med 28:551, 1966.
103a. Gabbay KH: The sorbitol pathway and the complications of diabetes. Seminars in medicine. NEJM 288:831, 1973.
103b. Gabbay KH: Glycosylated hemoglobin and diabetic control. NEJM 295:443, 1976.
104. Gailani S et al: Diabetes in patients treated with asparaginase. Clin Pharmacol Ther 12:487, 1971.
105. Galloway JA et al: Metabolism, blood levels and rate of excretion of acetohexamide in human subjects. Diabetes 16:118, 1967.
106. Galloway JA et al: A comparison of acid regular and neutral regular insulin. Diabetes 22:471, 1973.
107. Galloway JA et al: New forms of insulin. Diabetes 21:637, 1972.
107a. Gedik O et al: Effects of hypocalcemia and theophylline on glucose tolerance and insulin release in human beings. Diabetes 26:813, 1977.
107b. Gerard MJ et al: Serum glucose levels and alcohol consumption habits in a large population. Diabetes 26:780, 1977.
107c. Genuth SM et al: Constant intravenous insulin infusion in diabetic ketoacidosis. JAMA 223:1348, 1973.
108. Gerich JE et al: Clinical and metabolic characteristics of hyperosmolar nonketotic coma. Diabetes 20:228, 1971.
108a. Gerich JE et al: Effects of somatostatin on plasma glucose and glucagon levels in human diabetes mellitus. NEJM 291:544, 1974.
108b. Gerich JE et al: Prevention of human diabetic ketoacidosis by somatostatin. NEJM 292:985, 1975.
108c. Gerich JE: Somatostatin. Its possible role in carbohydrate homeostasis and the treatment of diabetes mellitus. Arch Int Med 137:659, 1977.
108d. Gerich JE et al: Clinical evaluation of somatostatin as a potential adjunct to insulin in the management of diabetes mellitus. Diabetologia 13:537, 1977.
109. Ghafghazi T et al: Chlorpromazine and epinephrine hyperglycemic mechanisms. J Pharm Sci 57:1690, 1968.
110. Gharib H: Steroid diabetes (review). Minn Med 52:669, 1969.
111. Gifford H et al: Falsely negative enzyme paper tests for urinary glucose. JAMA 178:423, 1961.
112. Gilgore S: The influence of salicylate on hyperglycemia. Diabetes 9:392, 1960.
113. Goldberg EM et al: Hyperglycemic nonketotic coma following administration of dilantin. Diabetes 18:101, 1969.
114. Goldner MG et al: Hyperglycemia and glycosuria due to thiazide derivatives administered in diabetes mellitus. NEJM 262:403, 1960.
115. Goldner MG et al: Phenformin in the management of diabetes. General clinical concepts. Diabetes 9:220, 1960.
116. Goldschmid A et al: Sulfated insulin in resistant juvenile diabetes. Lancet 2:405, 1968.
117. Goldstein MJ et al: Jaundice in a patient receiving acetohexamide. NEJM 275:97, 1966.
118. Goodman JI: Role of phenformin (DBI) as an adjuvant in oral antidiabetic therapy. Metab 14:153, 1965.
119. Gorden P: Glucose intolerance with hypokalemia. Diabetes 22:544, 1973.
120. Graber AL et al: Clinical use of diazoxide and mechanism for its hyperglycemic effects. Diabetes 15:143, 1966.
121. Grant AM et al: The hyperglycemic activity of triamterene. Pharm Res Commun 1:224, 1969.
122. Gregory DH et al: Chronic cholestasis following prolonged tolbutamide administration. Arch Path 84:194, 1967.
123. Guthrie RA et al: Insulin resistance in diabetes in juveniles. Pediat 40:642, 1967.
124. Hadley WB: Insulin treatment of diabetes mellitus. Med Clin N Amer 49:921, 1965.
125. Hagen GA et al: Hyponatremia due to sulfonylurea compounds. J Clin Endocrin Metab 31:570, 1970.
126. Hamff H et al: Effects of tolbutamide and chlorpropamide on patients exhibiting jaundice as a result of chlorpropamide therapy. Ann NY Acad Sci 74:820, 1959.
127. Hamwi GJ et al: The effects of chlorpropamide on endocrine function in patients with diabetes mellitus and its effects in other endocrine disorders. Ann NY Acad Sci 74:1003, 1959.
127a. Hansen JM et al: Drug interactions with oral sulphonylurea hypoglycaemic drugs. Drugs 13:24, 1977.
128. Hanno G et al: Study of antithyroid effect of tolbutamide. J En-

docrin 25:343, 1962.

129. Haunz EA et al: Liver function in chlorpropamide therapy. JAMA 188:237, 1964.

129a. Heber D et al: Low-dose continuous insulin therapy for diabetic ketoacidosis. Prospective comparison with conventional insulin therapy. Arch Int Med 137:377, 1977.

130. Hecht A et al: Reappraisal of the hypoglycemic action of ASA. Metab 8:418, 1959.

131. Hershman JM et al: Effect of sulfonylurea drugs on the binding of tri-iodothyronine and thyroxine to thyronine binding globulin. J Clin Endocrin Metab 28:1605, 1968.

132. Hesse B et al: Hypoglycemia after propranolol in children. Acta Med Scand 193:551, 1973.

133. Hiles B: Hyperglycemia and glucosuria following chlorpromazine therapy (letter). JAMA 162:1651, 1956.

133a. Hirsch JI et al: Clinical significance of insulin adsorption by polyvinylchloride infusion systems. Am J Hosp Pharm 34:583, 1977.

134. Hollis WC: Aggravation of diabetes mellitus during treatment with chlorothiazide therapy. JAMA 176:1651, 1956.

135. Hollobaugh SL et al: Studies on the site and mechanism of action of phenformin. Diabetes 19:45, 1970.

136. Hooper M: Diabetes mellitus treated with phenformin. Analysis of 94 cases with particular reference to weight changes. Brit J Clin Pract 21:389, 1967.

137. Hughes JE et al: Marijuana and the diabetic coma. JAMA 214:113, 1970.

138. Hunton RB et al: Hypothyroidism in diabetics treated with sulfonylureas. Lancet 2:449, 1965.

138a. Ingelfinger FJ: Debates on diabetes. NEJM 296:1228, 1977.

139. Inoue S: Effects of epinephrine on asthmatic children. J Alter 40:337, 1967.

140. Isaacs P: Alcohol and phenformin in diabetes (letter). Brit Med J 3:773, 1970.

141. Jackson RL et al: Neutral regular insulin. Diabetes 21:235, 1972.

142. Jackson WPU et al: Effect of furosemide on carbohydrate metabolism, blood pressure and other modalities; a comparison with chlorothiazide. Brit Med J 2:333, 1966.

143. James RC et al: Evaluation of some commonly used semiquantitative methods for urinary glucose and ketone determinations. Diabetes 23:474, 1974.

144. Janovsky RC: Diabetogenic effects of nicotine acid. Ohio State Med J 64:1137, 1968.

145. Johnson HK et al: Relationships of alcohol and hyperlactatemia in diabetic subjects treated with phenformin. Am J Med 45:98, 1968.

145a. Job D et al: Effect of multiple daily insulin injections on the course of diabetic retinopathy. Diabetes 25:463, 1976.

146. Johnson PC et al: Metabolic fate of chlorpropamide in man. Ann NY Acad Sci 74:459, 1959.

147. Jori A et al: Mechanism of hyperglycemic effect of chlorpromazine (letter). J Pharm Pharmacol 18:623, 1966.

148. Kalkoff RK et al: Insulin resistant diabetics with autoantibodies induced by exogenous insulin. Diabetes 18:445, 1969.

149. Karam JH et al: Insulin resistant diabetics with autoantibodies induced by exogenous insulin. Diabetes 18:445, 1969.

150. Karlin H: Fatal agranulocytosis following chlorpropamide treatment of diabetes. NEJM 262:1077, 1960.

150a. Kaufman IA et al: The management of diabetic acidosis. West J Med 127:104, 1977.

151. Kater RM et al: Increased rate of clearances of drugs from the circulation of alcoholics. Am J Med Sci 258:35, 1969.

152. Kaye R et al: Limitations to the use of oral hypoglycemic agents in juvenile patients with diabetes. J Pediat 66:844, 1965.

153. Keen H: Minimal diabetes and arterial disease: Prevalence and the effect of treatment. In Early Diabetes, edited by R. Camarin-Davalos and HS Cole. Acad Press NY 1970, p 437.

154. Kemball ML: Neonatal hypoglycemia in infants of diabetic mothers given sulfonylurea drugs in pregnancy. Arch Dis Child 45:696, 1970.

154a. Kitabchi AE et al: The efficacy of low dose versus conventional therapy of insulin for treatment of diabetic detoacidosis. Ann Int Med 84:633, 1976.

154b. Kidson, W et al: Treatment of severe diabetes mellitus by insulin infusion. Brit Med J 2:691, 1974.

154c. Kleeman CR et al: Chapt 24: Diabetic acidosis and coma in Clinical Disorders of Fluid and Electrolyte Metabolism edited by MH

Maxwell and CR Kleeman, McGraw Hill, NY, 1972.

155. Klein JP: Diphenylhydantoin intoxication associated with hyperglycemia. J Pediat 69:463, 1966.

155a. Klimes I et al: Effect of glucose on the glucagon response to L-dopa in normal and diabetic subjects. Diabetes 27:396, 1978.

156. Klink DD et al: Disulfiram-like reaction to CPA (Diabinese). Wisc Med J 68:134, 1969.

157. Klumpp TG: Nalidixic acid. False positive glycosuria and hyperglycemia. JAMA 193:122, 1965.

158. Knowpp RH et al: DPA and an insulin-secreting islet adenoma. Arch Int Med 130:904, 1972.

159. Knowles HC: Diabetes mellitus in childhood and adolescence. Med Clin N Amer 55:975, 1971.

159a. Kogut MD: Management of diabetic ketoacidosis in children. West J Med 127:138, 1977.

160. Kohner EM et al: Effect of diuretic therapy on glucose tolerance in hypertensive patients. Lancet 1:986, 1971.

160a. Koivisto VA et al: Effects of leg exercise on insulin absorption in diabetic patients. NEJM 298:79, 1978.

161. Kostis J et al: Unusual color reaction in glycosuria testing during cephalothin administration (letter). JAMA 196:805, 1966.

162. Kotler MN et al: Hypoglycemia precipitated by propranolol. Lancet 2:1389, 1966.

163. Krall LP et al: Combined sulfonylurea-biguanide therapy of diabetes mellitus. In Tolbutamide . . . After 10 Years International Congress Series no. 149, edited by WJH Butterfield and W Van Esterling, Excerpta Medica Foundation, NY 1967, p 303.

163a. Kraegen EW et al: Carrier solutions for low-level intravenous insulin infusion. Brit Med J 3:464, 1975.

164. Kristensen KAB: IV tetracycline and "dipstick" urine test. NEJM 283:660, 1970.

165. Kristensen M et al: Accumulation of chlorpropamide caused by Dicoumarol. Acta Med Scand 183:83, 1968.

166. Kristensen M et al: Potentiation of the tolbutamide effect by Dicoumarol. Diabetes 16:211, 1967.

166a. Kumar D et al: Use of dexamethasone in traeatment of insulin atrophy. Diabetes 26:296, 1977.

167. Kytomaki O et al: Effects of L-dopa on plasma growth hormones and insulin. Acta Neurol Scand (Suppl) 51:125, 1972.

168. Lampe WTH: Hypoglycemia due to acetohexamide. Treatment by peritoneal dialysis. Arch Int Med 120:239, 1967.

169. Landon J et al: The effect of anabolic steroids on blood sugar and plasma insulin levels in man. Metab 12:924, 1963.

170. Larsson Y et al: Possible teratogenic effect of tolbutamide in pregnant prediabetic patients. Lancet 2:1425, 1960.

171. Leonards JR: Evaluation of enzyme tests for urinary glucose. JAMA 163:260, 1957.

172. Lvein SR et al: Diphenylhydantoin, its use in detecting early insulin secretory defects in patients with mild glucose intolerance. Diabetes 22:194, 1973.

173. Levine R et al: Carbohydrate homeostasis II. NEJM 283:237, 1970.

174. Lieberman P et al: Allergic reactions of insulin (Systemic desensitization). JAMA 215:1106, 1971.

174a. Little JA: Insulin antibodies and clinical complications in diabetics treated for five years with lente or sulfated insulins. Diabetes 26:980, 1977.

174b. Lightner ES et al: Low dose intravenous insulin infusion in patients with ketoacidosis: Biochemical effects in children. Pediat 60:681, 1977.

175. Logue GL et al: Chlorpropamide-induced immune hemolytic anemia. NEJM 283:17, 1970.

175a. Lundquist GAR: Glucose tolerance in alcoholism. Brit J Addict 61:51, 1965.

175b. Luft D et al: Lactic acidosis in biguanide-treated patients. A review of 330 cases. Diabetologia 14:75, 1978.

176. Mackintosh TF: Propranolol hypoglycemia. Lancet 1:104, 1967.

177. Madison LL et al: Ethanol induced hypoglycemia (mechanism of suppression of hepatic gluconeogenesis). Diabetes 16:252, 1967.

177a. Madison LL: Low-dose insulin: A plea for caution. NEJM 294:393, 1976.

177b. Malacarne P et al: Tolbutamide-induced hemolytic anemia. Diabetes 26:156, 1977.

178. Malherbe C et al: Effect of diphenylhydantoin on insulin secretion. NEJM 286:339, 1972.

179. Malone DN: Insulin mixture and hypoglycemia. Brit Med J 3:106,

1970.

179a. Malone JI et al: Good diabetic control — a study in mass delusion. J Pediat 88:943, 1976.

180. Marble A: Ch 11, Insulin in the treatment of diabetes. In *Joslin's Diabetes Mellitus,* Ed 11, edited by A Marble, et al. Lea & Febiger, Phila, 1973.

180a. Mattson JR et al: Insulin therapy in patients with systemic insulin allergy. Arch Int Med 135:818, 1975.

181. McGavack TH et al: Some clinical experiences with the arylsulfonylureas in the management of diabetes mellitus. Metab 5:919, 1953.

182. McKiddie MT et al: Relationship between glucose tolerance, plasma insulin and corticosteroids in patients with rheumatoid arthritis. Metab 17:730, 1968.

182a. McMahon FG et al: The comparative pharmacology of hypoglycemic drugs. Curr Ther Res 4:330, 1962.

183. McMurtry RJ: Propranolol, hypoglycemia and hypertensive crisis. Ann Int Med 80:669, 1974.

184. Mehnert H: Clinical results after 10 year treatment with tolbutamide. In *Tolbutamide . . . After 10 Years,* International Congress Series no 149, edited by WJH Butterfield and W Van Westerling. Exceprta Medica Foundation, NY, 1967, p 281.

185. Metz R et al: Potentiation of the plasma insulin response to glucose by prior administration of alcohol. Diabetes 18:517, 1969.

185a. Metz SA et al: Induction of defective insulin secretion and impaired glucose tolerance by clonidine. Diabetes 27:554, 1978.

186. Milisci RE et al: Phenformin induced lactic acidosis recovery with massive bicarbonate therapy and hemodialysis. Am J Med Sci 265:447, 1973.

187. Miller DL et al: Transfer of tolbutamide across the human placenta. Diabetes 11(Suppl):93, 1962.

188. Millichap JG: Hyperglycemic effect of diphenylthydantoin. NEJM 281:447, 1969.

189. Molnar GD et al: The effect of nicotinic acid in Diabetes mellitus. Metab 13:181, 1964.

190. Moret VB: Zur diabetogenen wirkung der sakeretika. Deutsch Med Wschr 90:1136, 1965.

191. Morley A et al: A case of thrombocytopenia associated with chlorpropamide therapy. Med J Aust 2:988, 1964.

192. Moses AM et al: Diuretic action of three sulfonylurea drugs. Ann Intern Med 78:541, 1973.

193. Mroczek WJ et al: The value of aggressive therapy in the hypertensive patient with azotemia. Circ 40:893, 1969.

193a. Nattrass M et al: Biguanides. Diabetologia 14:71, 1978.

194. Nelson C: Glucose urine testing systems. Drug Intelligence and Clin Pharm 8:422, 1974.

194a. Nikkila EA et al: Ethanol-induced alterations of glucose tolerance, post-glucose hypoglycemia, and insulin secretion in normal, obese and diabetic subjects. Diabetes 24:933, 1975.

195. Nora JJ et al: The route of insulin administration in the management of diabetes mellitus. J Pediat 64:547, 1964.

196. Nunes WT: *A Manual of Diabetes for the House Officer,* Ed 1. C.C. Thomas, Springfield IL 1963, p 23.

197. O'Brien JP et al: Abnormal carbohydrate metabolism in renal failure. Metab 14:1294, 1965.

198. O'Donovan CJ: Analysis of long term experience with tolbutamide (Orinase) in the management of diabetes. Curr Ther Res 1:69, 1959.

199. Paasiviki J: Long-term tolbutamide treatment after myocardial infarction. Acta Med Scand 507(Suppl):1, 1970.

199a. Page M et al: Treatment of diabetic coma with continuous low-dose infusion of insulin. Brit Med J 2:687, 1974.

199b. Page M et al: Treatment of diabetic ketoacidosis. NEJM 294:1183, 1976.

200. Paley RG et al: Dermal reactions to insulin therapy. Diabetes 1:22, 1952.

201. Patel DP et al: Phenformin in weight reduction of obese diabetics. Lancet 2:282, 1964.

202. Peaston MJ et al: A case of combined poisoning with chlorpropamide, acetylsalicylic acid and paracetamol. Brit J Clin Pract 22:30, 1968.

202a. Penhos JC et al: Insulin resistant hyperglycemia produced by aminophylline. Endocrinol 90:131, 1972.

203. Peters BH et al: Hyperglycemia with relative insulinemia in diphenylhydantoin. NEJM 281:91, 1969.

203a. Peterson I et al: Insulin absorbance to polyvinylchloride surfaces

with implications for constant infusion therapy. Diabetes 25:72, 1976.

204. Petitpierre B et al: Chloramphenicol and chlorpropamide. Lancet 1:789, 1970.

205. Petitpierre B et al: Behavior of Chlorpropamide in renal insufficiency and under the effect of associated drug therapy. Int J Clin Pharmacol 6:120, 1972.

205a. Petty G et al: Insulin adsorption by glass infusion bottles, polyvinylchloride infusion containers and intravenous tubing. Anesth 40:400, 1974.

206. Phillips GB et al: Alcoholic diabetes. JAMA 217:1513, 1971.

207. Podgainy H et al: Biochemical basis of the sulfonylurea induced antabuse syndrome. Diabetes 17:679, 1968.

208. Podolsky S et al: Hyperosmolar nonketotic diabetic coma; a complication of propranolol therapy. Metab 22:685, 1973.

209. Podolsky S et al: Potassium depletion in hepatic cirrhosis. A reversible cause of impaired growth hormone and insulin response to stimulation. NEJM 288:644, 1973.

209a. Pond SM et al: Mechanisms of inhibition of tolbutamide metabolism: phenylbutazone, oxyphenbutazone, sulfaphenazole. Clin Pharmacol Ther 22:573, 1977.

210. Porte D Jr: Sympathetic regulation of insulin secretion. Its relation to diabetes mellitus. Arch Int Med 123:253, 1969.

211. Portioli I et al: Sulfonylureas and hypothyroidism (letter). Lancet 1:681, 1969.

211a. Posner JB et al: Spinal-fluid pH and neurologic symptoms in systemic acidosis. NEJM 277:605, 1967.

212. Powell T et al: Diabetes mellitus treated with chlorpropamide and tolbutamide. Diabetes 15:269, 1966.

213. Proctor DW et al: Fatal lactic acidosis after an overdose of phenformin. Brit Med J 4:216, 1967.

214. Prout TE et al: The UGDP controversy. Clinical trials versus clinical impressions. Diabetes 21:1035, 1972.

215. Pyke DA: Advances in the treatment of diabetes. Practitioner 119:498, 1967.

216. Rabkin R et al: Effect of renal disease on renal uptake and excretion of insulin in man. NEJM 282:182, 1970.

217. Radding RS et al: Phenethylbiguanide: clinical experiences with the time disintegrated capsules in stable diabetes mellitus. Metab 11:404, 1964.

218. Rapport ML et al: Thiazide induced glucose intolerance treated with potassium. Arch Int Med 113:405, 1964.

218a. Rayfield EJ et al: L-dopa stimulation of glucagon secretion in man. NEJM 293:589, 1975.

219. Recker RR et al: Pure red blood cell aplasia with chlorpropamide (review). Arch Int Med 123:445, 1969.

219a. Rehfeld JF et al: Carbohydrate metabolism in alcohol-induced fatty liver. Gastroet 64:445, 1973.

220. Reichel J et al: Intrahepatic stasis following administration of chlorpropamide. Am J Med 38:654, 1960.

221. Reveno WS et al: Propranolol and hypoglycemia. Lancet 1:920, 1968.

222. Ricketts HT: Weight change with orally administered "antidiabetic" drugs. JAMA 213:1676, 1970.

223. Ricketss HT (editor): Editorial statement on the University Group Diabetes Program. Diabetes 19 (Suppl 2):iii, 1970.

224. Roberts HJ: Diabetogenic hyperinsulinism: pathogenesis and implications of sulfonylurea induced hypothyroidism. J Am Geriat Soc 15:674, 1967.

225. Roginsky MS et al: Double blind study of phenethylbiguanide in weight control of obest nondiabetic subjects. Am J Clin Nutr 19:223, 1966.

225a. Rossini AA: Why control blood glucose level? Arch Surg 111:229, 1976.

226. Root MA et al: Immunogenicity of insulin. Diabetes 21:657, 1972.

227. Rubenstein AH et al: Role of kidney in insulin metabolism and excretion. Diabetes 17:161, 1968.

228. Rull JA et al: Prolonged and recurrent tolazamide induced hypoglycemia. Diabetes 16:352, 1967.

229. Runyan JW: Influence of thiazide diuretics on carbohydrate metabolism in patients with mild diabetes. NEJM 267:541, 1962.

230. Samaan N et al: Diabetogenic action of benzothiadizines. Serum insulin-like activity in diabetes worsened or precipitated by thiazide diuretics. Lancet 2:1244, 1963.

231. Scharf J et al: Tolbutamide and hypothyroidism. Lancet 1:250, 1968.

232. Scheller JC et al: Frequently asked questions about insulin.

Hosp Pharm 6:7, 1971.

233. Schiff D et al: Neonatal thrombocytopenia and congenital mal-formations associated with the administration of tolbutamide to the mother. J Pediat 77:451, 1970.

234. Schless GL et al: Oral hypoglycemic therapy associated with hypothyroidism. Ann NY Acad Sci 148:813, 1968.

235. Schor S: The University Group Diabetes Program: a statistician looks at the mortality results. JAMA 217:1671, 1971.

236. Searle et al: Body glucose kinetics in nondiabetic human sub-jects after phenethylbiguanide. Diabetes 22:50, 1966.

236a. Seedat YK: Effect of potassium on blood sugar and plasma insu-lin level in patients undergoing peritoneal dialysis and hemo-dialysis. Lancet 2:1167, 1968.

237. Segarra RO et al: Experiences with tolbutamide and chlor-propamide in tuberculous diabetic patients. Ann NY Acad Sci 74:656, 1959.

238. Seltzer H: Drug induced hypoglycemia. Diabetes 21:955, 1972.

239. Seltzer H: A summary of criticisms of the findings and conclu-sions of the University Group Diabetes Program (UGDP). Diab-etes 21:976, 1972.

239a. Semple PF et al: Continuous intravenous infusion of small doses of insulin in treatment of diabetic ketoacidosis. Brit Med J 2:694, 1974.

239b. Shen SW et al: Clinical pharmacology or oral antidiabetic agents (2 parts). NEJM 296:493 and 787, 1977.

239c. Sherwin RS: Low-dose insulin therapy in diabetic ketoacidosis. A valid physiologic approach, not a panacea. Arch Int Med 137:1361, 1977.

239d. Shaw KM et al: Small doses of intramuscular insulin in the treatment of diabetic "coma". Lancet 2:1115, 1974.

240. Shipp JC et al: Insulin resistance: clinical features, natural course and effects of adrenal steroid treatment. Medicine 44:165, 1965.

240a. Siperstein MD: Pitfalls in the diagnosis of diabetes mellitus. Adv Int Med 1975 (in publication).

240b. Siperstein MD et al: Control of blood glucose and diabetic vas-cular disease. NEJM 296:1060, 1977.

240c. Sirtore CR et al: Metabolic responses to acute and chronic L-dopa administration in patients with parkinsonism. NEJM 287:729, 1972.

240d. Skillman TG: A current concept of the pathophysiology of the hyperglycemia of diabetes mellitus. W Virg Med J 72:247, 1976.

240e. Skillman TG et al: Diabetes Mellitus, Upjohn Co, Kalamazoo Mich, 1977.

241. Skinner NS Jr et al: Studies on the use of chlorpropamide in patients with diabetes mellitus. Ann NY Acad Sci 74:830, 1959.

242. Smith MJH & Smith PK, editors: The Salicylates: A Critical Bib-liographic Review. Interscience Publishers, NY 1966.

243. Sodoyez JC et al: Reduction in the activity of the pancreatic islets induced in normal rodents by prolonged treatment with derivatives of sulfonylurea. Diabetes 19:603, 1970.

244. Soeldner JS et al: Hypoglycemia in tolbutamide treated dia-betes. Report of 2 cases with measurement of serum insulin. JAMA 193:398, 1965.

245. Solomon HM et al: Effect of phenyramidol and bishydroxycou-madin on the metabolism of human subjects. Metab 16:1029, 1967.

245a. Sonksen PH: The evolution of insulin treatment. Clin Endocrinol Metab 6:481, 1977.

246. Spenney JG et al: Hyperglycemia, hyperosmolar, nonketotic diabetes, complications of steroid and immunosuppressive therapy. Diabetes 18:107, 1969.

246a. Sperling MA: The contribution of hyperglycemic hormones to the pathogenesis of diabetes mellitus. Am J Dis Child 131:1145, 1977.

247. Srikantia SG et al: Effect of C-17 aklylated steroid methandro-stenolene on plasma lipids of normal subjects. Am J Med Sci 254:201, 1967.

248. Stein JH et al: Agranulocytosis caused by chlorpropamide. Arch Int Med 113:186, 1964.

249. Storvick W et al: Effect of storage temperature on stability of commercial insulin preparations. Diabetes 17:499, 1968.

250. Stowers JM et al: Studies on the mechanism of weight reduction by phenformin. Postgrad Med J 45(Suppl):13, 1969.

251. Stowers JM et al: Clinical and pharmacologic comparison of chlorpropamide and other sulfonylureas. Ann NY Acad Sci 74:689, 1959.

252. Stowers JM et al: Pharmacology and mode of action of the sul-fonylureas in man. Lancet 1:278, 1958.

253. Strauss FG et al: Phenformin intoxication resulting in lactic acidosis. Johns Hopkins Med J 128:278, 1971.

253a. Strauss MB: Diabetic regimens — procrustean beds? NEJM 281:1481, 1969.

254. Sugar SJN: Diabetic acidosis during chlorothiazide therapy. JAMA 175:618, 1961.

255. Sussman KE: The use and abuse of oral hypoglycemic agents. Rocky Mountain Med J 64:54, 1967.

256. Sussman KE et al: Failure of warning in insulin induced hypog-lycemic reactions. Diabetes 12:38, 1963.

257. Tainter ML et al: Anabolic steroids in management of the diabe-tic patient. NY State J Med 64:1001, 1964.

258. Tantillo JJ et al: Antigenicity of "single peak" insulin prepara-tions in diabetics (Abstr). Diabetes 22(Suppl 2(:293, 1973.

258a. Tattersall R: Brittle diabetes. Clin Endocrinol Metab 6:403, 1977.

259. Taylor JA Pharmacokinetics and biotransformation of chlor-propamide in man. Clin Pharmacol Ther 5:710, 1972.

259a. Teuscher A: Treatment of insulin lipoatrophy with monocompo-nent insulin. Diabetologia 10:211, 1974.

260. Thomas RC et al: The metabolic fate of tolbutamide in man and in the rat. J Med Chem 9:507, 1966.

261. Thonnard-Neumann E: Phenothiazines and diabetes in hos-pitalized women. Am J Psych 124:978, 1968.

262. Traisman HS et al: A comparative clinical evaluation on a new proprietary method for urine testing in juvenile diabetics. Clin Pediat 12:357, 1973.

263. Tranquada RE: Subcutaneous lipomas at sites of insulin injec-tion. Diabetes 15:807, 1966.

263a. Travis RH et al: Chap 71, Insulin and oral hypoglycemics, in The Pharmacological Basis of Therapeutics, 4th ed MacMillan Co., London, 1970.

264. Treasure T et al: Hyperglycemia due to phenytoin toxicity. Arch Dis Child 563:Aug 1971.

265. Turtle JR et al: Hypoglycemic action of fenfluramine in diabetes mellitus. Diabetes 22:858, 1973.

266. Tzagournis M et al: Mortality from coronary heart disease during phenformin therapy. Ann Int Med 76:587, 1972.

267. Ueda H et al: Disappearance rate of tolbutamide in normal sub-jects and in diabetes mellitus, liver cirrhosis and renal disease. Diabetes 12:414, 1963.

267a. Unger R: Diabetes and the alpha cell. Diabetes 25:136, 1975.

267b. Unger R et al: Role of glucagon in diabetes. Arch Int Med 137:482, 1977.

267c. University Group Diabetes Program: Effects hypoglycemic agents on vascular complications in patients with adult onset diabetes: IV. A preliminary report on phenformin results. JAMA 217:777, 1971.

267d. University Group Diabetes Program: Effects of hypoglycemic agents on vascular complications in patients with adult onset diabetes: III. Clinical implications of UGDP results. JAMA 218:1400, 1971.

267e. University Group Diabetes Program: A study of the effects of hypoglycemic agents on vascular complications in patients with adult onset diabetes: II. Mortality results. Diabetes 19(Suppl 2):789, 1970.

268. Waife SO, editor: Diabetes Mellitus, 7th ed. Eli Lilly & Co., In-dianapolis, Ind, 1973.

269. Waitzken L: Glucose tolerance in man during chlorpromazine therapy. Diabetes 19:186, 1970.

270. Walker RS et al: Phenethyldiguanide. Brit Med J 2:1049, 1960.

270a. Ward FR et al: The inhibitory effect of somatostatin on growth hormone, insulin and glucagon secretion in diabetes mellitus. J Clin Endocrin Metab 41:527, 1975.

271. Watkins JD et al: Observation of medication errors made by diabetic patients in the home. Diabetes 16:882, 1967.

272. Watson BM et al: A treatment for insulin induced fat atrophy. Diabetes 20:628, 1971.

272a. Weber ME et al: Continuous intravenous insulin therapy in se-vere diabetic ketoacidosis: Variations in dosage requirements. J Pediat 91:755, 1977.

273. Weisenfield S et al: Adsorption of insulin to infusion bottles and tubing. Diabetes 17:766, 1968.

274. Weismann PN: Chlorpropamide hyponatremia. NEJM 284:65, 1971.

275. Willer C: Phenformin in weight reduction of obese diabetics.

Lancet 1:53, 1965.

276. Weller C et al: The phenformin timed-disintegration capsule (DBI-TD[R]) in the management of previously treated diabetic patients. Metab 11:1134, 1962.

277. Weller JM et al: Effect of furosemide on glucose metabolism. Metab 16:532, 1967.

278. Welles JS et al: Metabolic reduction of 1 - (p-acetylbenzene sulfonyl) - 3 - cyclohexylurea (acetohexamide) in different species. Proc Soc Exp Biol Med 107:583, 1961.

279. Wentworth SM et al: The use of purified insulins in the treatment of patients with insulin lipoatrophy. Diabetes 22(Suppl 1):290, 1973.

280. Western KA et al: Pentamidine isothionate in the treatment of pneumocystis acrinii pneumonia. Ann Int Med 73:695, 1970.

281. Weyer EM et al: Diazoxide and the treatment of hypoglycemia. Ann NY Acad Sci 140(part 2):191, 1968.

282. White LLR: Fatal marrow aplasia during chlorpropamide therapy. Brit Med J 1:691, 1962.

283. Wilansky DL et al: Modification of latent diabetes by short term phenformin administration. Metab 16:199, 1967.

284. Williams RH: Recent advances relative to diabetes mellitus. Ann Int Med 63:512, 1965.

285. Wingate DL et al: Effect of phenformin on water and glucose transport across isolated human ileum. Diabetes 22:175, 1973.

286. Wishinsky H et al: Protein interactions of the sulfonylurea compounds. Diabetes 11(Suppl 1):18, 1962.

286a. Witters LA et al: Insulin antibodies in the pathogenesis of insulin allergy and resistance. Am J Med 63:703, 1977.

287. Wolcott GJ et al: Levodopa and tests for ketonuria (Letter). NEJM 283:1522, 1970.

288. Wolff FW et al: Diabetogenic activity of long-term administration of benzothiadizines. JAMA 185:586, 1963.

289. Wolff FW et al: Reversal of diazoxide effects by tolbutamide. Lancet 1:1137, 1967.

290. Wray R et al: Propranolol induced hypoglycemia and myocardial infarction. Brit Med J 2:592, 1972.

291. Yalow R et al: Reaction of fish insulins with human insulin antiserums. NEJM 270:1171, 1964.

292. Young BA et al: Risk of changing from ox to pig insulin (letter). Lancet 2:910, 1966.

293. Yu T et al: Hypoglycemic and uricosuric properties of acetohexamide and hydroxyhexamide. Metab 17:309, 1968.

293a. Yue D et al: New forms of insulin and their use in the treatment of diabetes. Diabetes 26:341, 1977.

294. Zinn WJ et al: The effects of dextrothyroxine in diabetes. Calif Med 101:240, 1964.

295. Zucker P et al: Prolonged symptomatic neonatal hypoglycemia associated with maternal chlorpropamide therapy. Pediat 42:824, 1968.

Chapter 25

Diseases of the Thyroid

Betty J. Dong

The emphasis of this chapter is on the rational use, clinical application, and risks and benefits of the various pharmacologic agents used in the treatment of hypo- and hyperthyroidism. The reader is referred to standard medical textbooks for more detailed diagnostic information.

1. Review the physiology of the thyroid gland with respect to hormone synthesis, metabolism and regulation.

Triidothyronine (T_3) and *thyroxine (T_4)* are the two biologically active thyroid hormones produced by the thyroid gland, and their production is under negative feedback control by the pituitary and hypothalamus. Thyroid stimulating hormone (TSH), which is released from the pituitary in response to low circulating levels of thyroid hormone, promotes hormone synthesis and release by increasing glandular activity. When sufficient synthesis has occurred, high circulating hormone levels block further production by inhibiting TSH release. As the levels of hormone drop, the hypothalamic-pituitary centers again become responsive by releasing TSH (186).

Of the two active thyroid hormones, T_3 is more potent then T_4, but its serum concentration is lower. Formerly, all T_3 was thought to have been produced intrathyroidally, but recent findings indicate that about 80% of the total daily T_3 production results from the peripheral conversion of T_4 to T_3 through monodeiodination of T_4 (32d,371b,300,332). T_4 also has intrinsic biological activity and does not function solely as a prohormone; approximately 35-40% of secreted T_4 is converted to T_3. Certain chronic and acute diseases can modify the rate of conversion of T_4 to T_3 and the serum level of T_3 (300).

T_3 and T_4 exist in the circulation in the free (active) and protein-bound (inactive) forms. Nearly 100% of T_4 is bound: 80% to thyroxine binding globulin (TBG), 15% to throxine binding pre-albumin (TBPA) and 4-5% to albumin, while only 0.02% is free (257b). This affinity for plasma proteins accounts for its slow metabolic degradation and long half-life of 7 days (271b). In contrast, T_3 is considerably less strongly bound and about 0.2% exists as free hormone. Its lesser protein-binding affinity accounts for its three-fold greater metabolic potency and its shorter half-life of 1.5 days (257b, 271b).

CASE A–EVALUATION OF THYROID FUNCTION TESTS:

RF is a 42-year-old obese woman who has been suffering from fatigue, sluggishness, and hair loss for the past six months. Her other medical problems include bronchitis and congestive heart failure (CHF). On physical examination her thyroid was palpable, but not enlarged, and her reflexes were normal. She takes digoxin 0.125 mg daily and SSKI 5 gtts tid. Her laboratory data were as follows:

PBI 13 mcg/100 ml	**TT_4 9 mcg/100 ml**
(nl 4-8)	*(nl 5.3-14.5)*
BMR + 15 (nl ± 15)	**RT_3U 28% (nl 25-35)**
Cholesterol 385 mg%	**TSH 4 μ IU/ml**
Photomotogram	*(nl less than 10)*
300 millisec (nl 250-350)	

2. Briefly explain and discuss the use of the above tests in the evaluation of this patient's thyroid status. Which of these tests are influenced by disease states and drug therapy?

This patient's complaints may be indicative of hypothyroidism, but further information is required. The PBI, BMR, and cholesterol are relatively non-specific measures of thyroid function. In addition, the presence of CHF and the ingestion of iodides (both organic and inorganic) can interfere with accurate interpretations of the BMR and PBI (315). However, the TSH, TT_4 and RT_3U, which more accurately reflect thyroid function indicate that RJ is euthyroid.

The **BMR (Basal Metabolic Rate)** is an indirect measurement of the ability of thyroid hormone to stimulate O_2 consumption (189). The normal range is -15 to $+15$. Since the BMR is a nonspecific evaluation of oxygen consumption, its use has declined with the advent of more specific and reliable determinants of thyroid function.

The **PBI (Protein Bound Iodine)** is a measure of the iodine content of precipitated plasma protein and provides an indirect estimate of the circulating levels of thyroxine (T_4) (67e,189,315). Both inorganic compounds, such as SSKI, and organic iodine, such as that in IVP dyes, will elevate the PBI (66,315). Although the PBI is still used as a measure of the iodoproteins in certain thyroid disorders, it has largely been replaced

by more specific tests. Likewise, the **BEI (Butanol Extractable Iodine)** and the **T_4 by column (Thyroxine by Column Chromatography)**, which also depend on iodometry (315), have been superseded by the iodine-independent TT_4 by Murphy Pattee.

The **TT_4 by Murphy Pattee** utilizes a displacement technique to measure the amount of thyroxine bound to a specific binding protein in the patient's serum. Since the size, shape, and charge of the T_4 molecule rather than iodine content determines the results of this test, the TT_4 is not affected by iodides or organic dyes (189,315,123). Since thyroxine is 65% iodine by weight, the following conversion can be used to express the results of the TT_4 in terms that correspond to PBI or iodine content:

$$T_4I \text{ (T_4 iodine)} = TT_4 \times 0.65$$

The **Resin T_3 Uptake (RT_3U)** approximates the binding capacity of TBG (Thyroxine Binding Globulin). Radioactive labeled triiodothyronine (T_3) is added to the patient's serum and given time to equilibrate (67e,189,199). Since T_3 has less affinity for TBG than T_4, it will not displace T_4 from the protein and will only bind to available sites. Following equilibration, a resin is added to absorb the unbound T_3. In hyperthyroidism most binding sites on the TBG are occupied and the RT_3U is high; the converse is true in hypothyroidism. Thus, the RT_3U has a direct relationship to the serum thyroxine and an inverse relationship to the levels of circulating TBG. It is not a very sensitive indicator of thyroid function and should be interpreted in conjunction with the TT_4.

Since all of these tests (PBI, BEI, T_4 by Column, TT_4 by Murphy Pattee, and RT_3U) are indirect measures of *protein-bound* thyroxine, alterations in the levels of TBG or in the degree of protein binding will influence their results (see Questions 3 and 4). **The Free Thyroxine Index (FTI)** should be calculated to compensate for any influence that drugs or disease states may have on protein levels or the protein binding of thyroxine:

$$FTI = RT_3U \times TT_4$$

Cholesterol levels may be used as an adjunct to confirm thyroid dysfunction but are not diagnostic in themselves. In hypothyroidism the cholesterol level is elevated since its rate of degradation is decreased in relation to its synthesis (67e,189). Conversely, cholesterol levels may be decreased in hyperthyroidism. However, many extrathyroidal factors influence the plasma cholesterol.

A **photomotogram** measures the speed of the ankle jerk. The time from the beginning of the hammer tap to half relaxation is measured by interruption of a light beam which is directed on a photocell. Normal values are 250 to 350 milliseconds; lower values are seen in hyperthyroidism and higher values in hypothyroidism.

This test is not diagnostic in itself but is useful in the confirmation of a diagnosis (189).

The *plasma TSH (Thyroid Stimulating Hormone)* level is determined by radiommune assay and is one of the most sensitive tests used in the diagnosis of hypothyroidism (211,263). The main application of the TSH level is early detection of mild or borderline hypothyroidism, since TSH levels may be clearly elevated while thyroxine levels are normal. It is also used to distinguish between primary hypothyroidism which is characterized by increased TSH levels and secondary hypothyroidism which is characterized by undetectable or minimal TSH levels even though other thyroid function tests are grossly abnormal (199). Since TSH has a chemical structure similar to HCG, LH, and FSH, false elevations may be reported in pregnant or the postmenopausal women (67e,253a).

3. RC is a 45-year-old black male whose chief complaints are fatigue, dry skin, and constipation. His other medical problems include alcoholism for 10 years, cirrhosis, grand mal seizures treated with phenytoin 300 mg daily and phenobarbital 30 mg tid, and rheumatoid arthritis for which he takes aspirin 5 gr, 20 tablets daily. The results of his thyroid function tests were: TT_4 4.2 mcg/100 ml; RT_3U 40%; and TSH 6 μIU/ml. How should these laboratory findings be interpreted?

He is not hypothyroid as evidenced by the normal TSH level. A number of factors could account for the decreased TT_4 and increased RT_3U. Phenytoin can displace T_4 from its binding sites, causing spuriously low values for TT_4 and high values for RT_3U (257a, 67e, 233). Anti-inflammatory doses of salicylates can displace thyroxine from both TBG and TBPA causing lowered values for TT_4 and no change in or increased RT_3U values (9,112,240,372a). Furthermore, this patient may have decreased TBG production because of his cirrhosis. Other factors which have been reported to lower TT_4 and increase RT_3U by decreasing TBG and TBPA are stress, severe infections, and a hereditary decrease in TBG.

Thus, RC is taking several drugs which can displace thyroxine from its plasma protein binding sites, and he may have decreased plasma proteins available for binding because of his liver disease. In order to correct for these alterations in protein binding, the FTI (Free Thyroxine Index) should be calculated as described in the previous question. FTI = 4.2 × .40 = 1.68. Therefore, RC is euthyroid.

4. BR is a 23-year-old sexually active female who comes to clinic for evaluation of extreme nervousness, diaphoresis, and scanty menstrual periods. Although she appears healthy, the idea of hyperthyroidism is entertained on basis of a TT_4 of 16

mcg/100 ml and an RT_3U of 20% Comment.

BR is not hyperthyroid as evidenced by calculation of a normal FTI (see Question 2). The elevated TT_4 and the depressed RT_3U are consistent with the increased TBG levels observed in pregnancy and oral contraceptive users (144). Since TBG and therefore bound T_4 levels are increased by estrogens, values for PBI, T_4 by column and BEI will be elevated. Conversely, since there is an absolute increase in the amount of protein, the RT_3U will be decreased. However, thyroid function is not changed, since free thyroxine levels are not affected. Thyroid function tests should return to normal 2-4 weeks after discontinuation of BCPs, although some investigators report that 2-4 months may be required (144). Progesterone-only BCPs do not appear to affect protein binding; consequently they do not alter thyroid function tests (also see chapter on *Oral Contraception*).

5. GM is a 45-year-old teacher who presents with symptoms suggestive of hypothyroidism. He also complains of a headache. A diagnosis of hypothyroidism is confirmed by low TT_4, RT_3U and FTI values. Skull x-rays reveal an enlarged sella turcica and the possibility of secondary hypothyroidism is entertained. What laboratory tests can be used to distinguish between primary and secondary hypothyroidism?

Primary hypothyroidism results from a disturbance within the thyroid gland, while secondary hypothyroidism is caused by pituitary or hypothalalmic disturbances. TSH levels are elevated in primary hypothyroidism, and minimal or undetectable TSH levels are present in secondary hypothyroidism. See Question 2.

With the availability of the TSH level, there is little justification for the *TSH stimulation test* which has also been used to differentiate primary from secondary hypothyroidism. In primary hypothyroidism exogenous TSH will cause a rise in thyroid activity. The response is measured by comparing the RAI uptake before and after the administration of 10 IU bovine TSH (thytropar). In primary hypothyroidism there is no rise in RAI uptake; in secondary hypothyroidism RAI increases by 10%.

The *TRH (Thyrotropin-Releasing Hormone Test)* is a very useful test to measure pituitary responsiveness (199). A test dose of 400 mcg TRH is given as an IV bolus and samples of serum are taken at 0, 15, 30, 60, 90, 120 minutes for determination of TSH. In euthyroid patients a prompt increase in TSH is observed, with peak levels in 20-30 minutes. In hypothalmic hypothyroidism the pituitary responds sluggishly to exogenous TRH and produces a slow but continuous rise in TSH. In patients with primary hypothyroidism, the basal levels are elevated and the pituitary is hyperresponsive; TSH levels often reach 100-200 μIU/ml 30 minutes after TRH administration. In hypothyroid patients with hypopituitarism, no response of TSH to TRH would be expected. Thus, the TRH test will not only differentiate primary from secondary hypothyroidism it also differentiates hypopituitary from hypothalamic hypothyroidism. Patients receiving adequate T4 replacement treatment or chronic cortisone or L-dopa treatment do not respond to the TRH test (263a,365,323).

Origin of Deficiency	FTI	TSH Level	TSH Levels After TRH Stimulation
Thyroid	Low	High	Exaggerated
Pituitary	Low	High	No response
Hypothalamic	Low	High	Sluggish Response

Table 1
COMMON THYROID FUNCTION TESTS

Test	Measure	Normals	Comments
PBI	Iodine of precipitated proteins—approximates thyroxine iodine.	4.0-8.0 mcg/100 ml	Organic and inorganic iodides cause false elevation. Influenced by alterations of protein or protein binding.
BEI	Iodine of precipitated proteins—butanol extraction.	3.5-7.5 mcg/100 ml	No interference with inorganic iodides. Organic iodides will cause false elevation. Influenced by alterations of protein or protein binding.
T4I (by column)	Thyroxine iodine of precipitated proteins, utilizing anion exchange resin and column chromotography.	3.0-7.5 mcg/100 ml	Inorganic and many organic iodides do not interfere. May see false elevation with some radiocontrast dyes. Influenced by alterations of protein binding.
TT4 by Murphy Pattee	Displacement of thyroxine by competitive protein binding. Measured as total thyroxine.	5.3-14.5 mcg/100 ml	Specific for thyroxine. No interference by iodides. Influenced by alterations of protein or protein binding.
RT3U	Labeled T3 remaining on resin after saturation of binding sites. Indirect measure of binding sites.	25-35%	Influenced by alterations of protein or protein binding sites.
FTI	The product of the TT4 x RT3U gives the free thyroxine serum level as if measured by dialysis.	1.3-5.3	Compensates for alterations in protein binding.
RAIU	Radioactivity of the thyroid after a trace dose of I[131].	1 hr. = 0–5% 5 hr. = 5–15% 24 hr. = 11–35%	Lowered by dietary or medicinal iodide intake. See Question 22.
TSH Level	TSH by radioimmune assay.	Less than 10 μ IU/ml	Most sensitive index of hypothyroidism. FSH,LH and HCG may cause false elevations.
T3 by RIA (radioimmunoassay)	T3 levels. Directly related to TBG concentrations.	100-200 ng/100ml	Also influenced by alterations in protein binding. See Question 32.
TGAB	Antibodies to thyroglobulin by radioimmune assay.	0–8%	Elevated in Graves' and Hashimoto's; may be undetectable with remission. See Question 22.
Antimicrosomal by TRC	Antibodies to microsomal antigen by tanned red cell technique.	Titers 1:00	More sensitive of the two antibody techniques. Titers will be detectable even after remission. See Question 22.
T3 Suppression Test	Measures hypothalmic-pituitary-thyroid negative feedback axis.	Suppression of RAI to 50% of baseline RAIU after T3 therapy	Lack of suppression is seen in Graves' disease and indicates autonomous functioning of the gland. See Question 42.

CASE B – HYPOTHYROIDISM: MW is a 23-year-old music student who thinks that her neck has become increasingly "fatter" over the past three to four months. She describes herself as gaining weight, feeling mentally sluggish, and tiring easily and finds that she is unable to hit the high notes like she used to. On physical examination a puffy facies, yellowish skin, delayed DTR's (deep tendon reflexes), and a firm enlarged thyroid are noted. Laboratory data included TT_4 4mcg%, RT_3U 25%, TSH 20 μIU, TGAB 55%, antimicrosomal by TRC 1:2500, Hct (Hematocrit) 33%, Hgb (Hemoglobin) 12 gm%, RBC 3,500,000/mm^3 MCV 104 and a RAIU at 24 hours was 7%.

6. What do MW's symptoms and laboratory data suggest? What are the common clinical features of this disorder?

MW presents with many of the clinical features of *hypothyroidism.* These include weight gain, mental sluggishness, easy fatigability, lowering of the voice pitch, a puffy facies, a yellowish tint of the skin, delayed DTR's, and an enlarged thyroid. The diagnosis of hypothyroidism is substantiated by her laboratory findings of a borderline low TT_4 and RT_3U, an elevated TSH value, positive antibodies, and a low radioactive iodide uptake. Other symptoms of hypothyroidism not displayed by this patient include cold intolerance; dryness of the skin, nails and scalp; constipation; memory impairment with delirium and psychosis; menorrhagia (amenorrhea with galactorrhea may also occur); impotence or sterility; and muscle cramps with stiffness (108).

The general appearance of hypothyroidism is very characteristic in its severe form. The face is puffy and expressionless and has been described as "mask-like." Swelling of the eyelids is prominent, and ophthalmopathy may be present due to orbital edema and mucous. Drooping of the eyelids results from decreased sympathetic tone to the eye muscle. The tongue may be large and thickened and may interfere with swallowing. Characteristically, these patients lose the lateral aspects of their eyebrows, and the skin becomes cool, dry, rough, and scaly due to increased deposits of mucopolysaccharides. A yellowish tint to the skin and hands results from the deposition of carotene because the hepatic conversion to vitamin A is impaired. Cutaneous vasoconstriction and myxedema may make the skin appear pale and waxy. Impaired water excretion can occur (68). Goiter results from constant TSH stimulation of the gland in response to the low circulating thyroxine levels. This goiter may also be compounded by lymphocytic infiltration of the tissue due to an autoimmune reaction as in Hashimoto's thyroiditis.

Thyroid deficiency affects every bodily system by slowing down all normal body processes and mental faculties. Because its onset is often insidious and not easily recognized, it may progress to myxedema coma.

7. What are the causes of hypothyroidism? Briefly discuss the etiology and pathogenesis of MW's hypothyroidism.

A variety of etiologies may be responsible for hypothyroidism; these are listed in Table 2.

Table 2
CLASSIFICATION OF HYPOTHYROIDISM

I. Nongoitrous (no gland enlargement)
  A. Primary hypothyroidism (dysfunction of the gland)
    1. Idiopathic atrophy
    2. Iatrogenic destruction of the thyroid
      a) Surgery
      b) Radioactive iodine therapy
      c) X-ray therapy
    3. Post-inflammatory thyroiditis
    4. Cretinism (congenital hypothyroidism)
  B. Secondary hypothyroidism: Deficiency of TSH due to pituitary dysfunction
  C. Tertiary hypothyroidism: Deficiency of TRH due to hypothalamic dysfunction

II. Goitrous hypothyroidism (enlargement of the thyroid gland)
  A. Dyshormonogenesis: Defect in hormone synthesis, transport or action
  B. Hashimoto's thyroiditis
  C. Drug-induced: Iodides, lithium, thiocyanates, phenylbutazone, sulfonylureas
  C. Congenital cretinism: Maternally-induced
  E. Iodide deficiency
  F. Natural goitrogens: Rutabagas, turnips, cabbage

The presence of a firm goiter and thyroid antibodies, as well as clinical symptoms of hypothyroidism, strongly suggest Hashimoto's thyroiditis which may have been exacerbated by the ingestion of her medications. She has no history of prior antithyroid drug usage, surgery, or radioactive iodine treatment, which are the most common forms of iatrogenic hypothyroidism.

Hashimoto's thyroiditis or chronic lymphocytic thyroiditis is the most common cause of hypothyroidism other than iatrogenic destruction of the gland (353a). Hashimoto's thyroiditis is associated with an underlying defect or block in extrathyroidal organo-binding of iodide so that inactive or insufficient amounts of active hormones are produced with resultant hypothyroidism. Characteristically, the goiter is painless, enlarged, firmer in consistency than normal, and infiltrated with lymphocytes and plasma cells. Often, Hashimoto's occurs in conjunction with other autoimmune disorders such as pernicious anemia (299) or rheumatoid arthritis (18,238). The rate of occurrence in women is four times that in men and a familial tendency has been noted (67b). Antibodies to thrroid have been identified in Hashimoto's thyroiditis (235), but low titers may be found in other thyroid disease, in relatives of patients with either Graves' or Hashimoto's thyroiditis, and in some apparently normal persons (135, 135a, 135b).

Hashimoto's thyroiditis may be related to Graves' disease, a frequent cause of hyperthyroidism (see Question 23). Both diseases share some common clinical features: antibody titers, lymphocytic infiltration of the thyroid gland, a familial tendency, and a predilection for women. In fact, both diseases may coexist in the same gland (86), and thyrotoxicosis can precede the onset of Hashimoto's thyroiditis (36), suggesting that Graves' disease and Hashimoto's thyroiditis may be the same disease manifesting in differing ways.

8. Could MW's hematological status be related to her thyroid disease? What kinds of anemia have been associated with hypothyroidism?

MW appears to have a macrocytic anemia. Levels of B_{12} and folate should be determined since both B_{12} and folate deficiency have been associated with hypothyroidism. Hines et al reported folate deficiency in 8 of 40 hypothyroid patients in whom the hematological picture was corrected by the administration of thyroid and folate (152); impaired absorption of folate may be responsible. Pernicious anemia occurs in about 8 to 10% of all hypothyroid patients and is correctable by return to a euthyroid state and B_{12} administration (340,340a). Antibodies to the mucosa of the gastric fundus and intrinsic factor are present in thyroiditis as they are in a true pernicious anemia.

Anemia would be expected in hypothyroidism since thyroid hormones stimulate erythropoiesis. Three major types of anemia have been observed in hypothyroidism: a) A mild *normochromic normocytic* anemia is found in 25% of hypothyroid patients. It is unresponsive to iron therapy but is easily reversed by thyroid administration (88). b) *Hypochromic microcytic* anemia appears in 4 to 15% of hypothyroid patients (340). Contributing factors may include achlorhydria (75) and menorrhagia (110). This anemia will respond to iron therapy without correction of the hypothyroidism. c) A *macrocytic* anemia, as observed in this patient, may also appear in hypothyroidism.

Reports of the incidence of anemia in hypothyroidism range from 23 to 60% (66a, 179, 194, 340). Clinical symptoms may not be present (340).

9. What thyroid preparation should be used to treat MW's hypothyroidism? Are there significant differences, advantages or disadvantages among the various thyroid preparations?

The principle objective of thyroid hormone therapy is attainment and maintenance of a euthyroid state. Any of the commercially available preparations can accomplish this. The preparations can be classified as either synthetic (levothyroxine, L-triiodothyronine, liotrix) or from animal extract (dessicated thyroid, thyroglobulin).

Desiccated thyroid (USP) is derived from pork thyroid glands, although beef and sheep thyroid are also used. It is generally standardized by its iodine content (0.17 to 0.23%) and usually has a $T_4:T_3$ ratio of 2:1. Potency may vary with changes in the relative proportion of the two active hormones or from changes in the amount of organic iodine present. Inactive preparations containing small amounts of T_3 and T_4 or even iodinated casein instead of hormone have been identified as have preparations of greater than expected activity (207,267). Armour brand thyroid is standardized biologically; however, improper or prolonged storage may result in loss of potency. In addition to its variable potency, allergic reactions to the animal protein in desiccated thyroid may occur. The only apparent advantage of this preparation is its low cost. Patients already well maintained on desiccated thyroid need not be switched to other preparations, but desiccated thyroid is not a good choice for the initiation of thyroid therapy.

Thyroglobulin (Proloid) is a purified extract of hog gland standardized biologically to give a $T_4:T_3$ ratio of 2.5:1. It has no advantages over desiccated thyroid and is more expensive.

The synthetic preparations differ from one another in their relative potency, onset of action, and biological half-life:

L-thyroxine (Synthroid, Letter) or T_4 is one of the most commonly used thyroid preparations. Its advantages include stability, uniform potency, relatively low cost, and lack of allergenic foreign protein. The long half-life of five to seven days makes once-a-day dosing possible and may even allow the creation of special convenience schedules such as omission of medication on weekends. Although most patients absorb 60 to 65%, absorption may vary considerably (143). Therapeutic effect is easily monitored by use of TT_4 and RT_3U.

L-triiodothyronine (Cytomel) or T_3 has a relatively short half-life of one day which necessitates multiple daily dosing to insure a uniform response. Other disadvantages include a higher incidence of cardiac effects, difficulty in monitoring therapeutic/toxic effects with conventional TT_4/RT_3U laboratory tests, and its high cost. For these reasons, L-triiodothyronine is not recommended for routine thyroid hormone replacement. It is widely used as a diagnostic agent in the T_3 suppression test.

Liotrix (Euthroid, Thyrolar) is a combination of synthetic T_4 and T_3 in a ratio of 4:1. It is stable and has a

Table 3
THYROID PREPARATIONS

Drug	Composition	Grain Equivalent	Comments
Thyroid USP	Desiccated hog, beef, or sheep thyroid gland. Standardized by iodine content.	1 grain	Unpredictable $T_4:T_3$ ratio; unstable, deteriorates upon prolonged storage. Produces normal laboratory function tests.
Thyroglobulin (Proloid)	Thyroglobulin extract. Standardized biologically to give a $T_4:T_3$ ratio of 2.5:1	1 grain	No advantage over thyroid extract but more expensive.
L-thyroxine (Letter, Synthroid)	Synthetic T_4	100 mcg	Stable, predictable potency but variable absorption. May be more potent than desiccated thyroid because of its stability. When changing from desiccated thyroid to synthetic T_4, may want to lower the T_4 dose by ½ grain to avoid toxicity.
L-triiodothyronine (Cytomel)	Synthetic T_3	25 mcg	Need to use TSH levels to monitor therapeutic response. Requires multiple daily dosing schedule. Complete absorption.
Liotrix (Euthroid) (Thyrolar)	$T_4:T_3$ in 4:1 ratio 60 mcg T_4: 15 mcg T_3 50 mcg T_4: 12.5 mcg T_3	Euthroid-1 Thyrolar-1	No real need for liotrix since T_4 is converted to T_3 peripherally. Expensive, stable, and predictable content. Euthroid is 20% more potent than Thyrolar. This should be considered when changing from one preparation to the other.

predictable potency but is relatively more expensive than the other thyroid preparations. It is important to note that Euthroid is 20% more potent than Thyrolar when corresponding grain equivalents are compared. This preparation was once recommended as the drug of choice for thyroid replacement since it approximates the normal secretion of the human thyroid gland. However, since a significant amount of T_4 (30%) is converted peripherally to T_3 there is no rationale or need for such an expensive preparation (280,332).

10. What would be an appropriate dose of thyroxine for MW? How should her therapy be monitored?

Many textbooks recommend that thyroxine be given in a replacement dose of 200 to 300 mcg per day because the thyroid gland normally secretes 100 to 300 mcg per day. Also, it has been suggested that TT_4 laboratory values be maintained in the high upper limits of normal to make up for lack of T_3 administration, but this is not necessary since T_4 is converted peripherally to T_3 (32d,271b,332). Re-evaluation of the replacement dose of thyroxine in 44 patients with hypothyroidism showed that the average required dose was 169 mcg per day (2.25 mcg/kg) and that 89% of the patients were euthyroid on 100-200 mcg daily (329). These replacement doses correlated well with body weight, and 96% of the patients who were corrected to a euthyroid state had thyroxine (TT_4) laboratory values within the normal range (329). Others have found normalization of TSH levels by a thyroxine replacement dose of 200 mcg or less (58a). Doses of 300 mcg daily of T_4 may be excessive and result in hyperthyroidism (32e,92a).

In the absence of risk factors necessitating small dose increments (old age, cardiac disease, and long duration of disease) MW can be started with the full replacement dose of thyroxine. Based on her weight of 70 kg and a daily dose of 2.25 mcg/kg MW can be initiated on 0.15 mg daily (70 kg × 2.25 mcg/kg = .157 mg) and monitored both for toxicity and therapeutic response. TT_4, RT_3U, and FTI should be evaluated at least one month after the initiation of therapy because T_4 has a half-life of seven days, and three or four half-lives are needed to reach steady state. These laboratory data, in combination with her subjective and objective symptoms provide appropriate monitoring parameters. TSH levels can also be used if desired and should be normal in 10 to 14 days (282a). A more conservative approach would be to initiate 0.1 mg daily for one or two weeks and then increase the dose based on absence of toxicity (hyperthyroidism), realizing that MW's replacement dose will most likely be 0.1 to 0.16 mg/day. Appropriate dose titration can be obtained by having the patient not take any drug on certain days. For example: a) Take 0.15 mg every day except Sunday. Total dose = 0.13 mg daily (0.15 mg × 5 days/7 days); b) Take 0.15 mg every day except weekends. Total dose = 0.11 mg daily; c) Take 0.2 mg every day except Sunday. Total dose = 0.16 mg daily.

With the correct dose, a diuresis should develop

within two to three days, particularly in severe cases of hypothyroidism, and reversal of symptoms should occur within one to two weeks. Some symptoms such as anemia and hair and skin changes will take several weeks to be corrected (67e).

11. RF, a 45-year-old school teacher, comes to clinic complaining of fatigue and vague muscular aches and pains which she attributes to insufficient thyroid medication. On physical examination the gland was palpable but not enlarged and deep tendon reflexes were 2+ and brisk. She has been taking triiodothyronine (Cytomel) 25 mcg three times per day. Because a recent TT4 was 1.4 ml%, the dose was increased to 100 mcg daily. She denies taking any other medications. Comment.

This low TT4 value does not provide adequate justification for increasing RF's thyroid replacement. Since she is receiving triiodothyronine or T3, the TT4, which is a measure of bound T4, will always be low and will never reach normal levels. In fact, her vague complaints may be related to hyperthyroidism since she is receiving the equivalent of 0.3 mg of thyroxine (T4) daily (see Question 10 and Table 2). A TSH level should be performed to rule out hypothyroidism. Regardless of the outcome, she should be switched to thyroxine to facilitate monitoring and simplify her dosing regimen.

12. PB is a 70-year-old male with long-standing hypothyroidism treated with L-thyroxine 0.2 mg daily. He is currently in the hospital with a stroke and paralysis which has left him unable to take anything by mouth. What considerations should be made with regard to the administration of thyroid hormone to this man?

Because of the long half-life of L-thyroxine (5 to 7 days) one might delay the administration of thyroxine until he is able to take oral medications again. A delay of up to two weeks would be permissible. However, if parenteral administration is required, L-thyroxine can be given IM or IV. The IM route is not recommended since absorption may be slow and unpredictable, particularly in the presence of compromised circulation. When administering L-thyroxine intravenously, one should be aware that oral absorption is incomplete (usually 60 to 65%) and can vary from 30 to 90% (143); therefore, parenteral doses should be adjusted accordingly.

13. PK is a 35-year-old pregnant woman who receives L-thyroxine 0.15 mg daily for Hashimoto's thyroiditis. What effect, if any, might PK's thyroid disease have on her pregnancy? How should this be monitored and treated?

Inadequately treated maternal hypothyroidism has been associated with abnormal fetal development and difficulty in maintaining pregnancy (42a). However, the importance of maternal thyroid function on fetal development needs further study since women who were myxedematous throughout pregnancy gave birth to normal children (154,187).

In 244 hypothyroid women the stillbirth rate was twice that observed in euthyroid women (249). Spontaneous abortions, congenital defects, and undifferentiated developmental retardation have also been reported (122.) Offspring of mothers who have low plasma thyroxine levels during pregnancy may be at increased risk of mental retardation (205,205a). Fetal abnormalities from maternal hypothyroidism may be associated with poor placental maturation rather than lack of transplacental passage of maternal hormones which is negligible (67e). Maternal antibodies from Hashimoto's thyroiditis can cross into the fetal circulation and persist for several months (28,262), and this has been reported to cause congenital hypothyroidism (110b,333).

In the absence of restrictive factors such as cardiac disease, maternal thyroid supplementation should be initiated with 0.2 mg L-thyroxine daily and increased as needed. Supplements in the range of 0.3 to 0.4 mg of L-thyroxine are not unusual for the pregnant hypothyroid patient because TBG levels are increased in pregnancy and more T4 is bound. Laboratory values of TT4 and FTI should be in the upper limits of normal if replacement is adequate. A better indication of correct replacement is a TSH level of less than 10 μU/ml. Adequate treatment during pregnancy usually produces a normal baby but abortion and congenital abnormalities may still occur due to poor placental development.

14. PK delivered an apparently healthy baby at term without difficulty. The baby's postpartum serum T4 level was 5 mcg%. At home he became lethargic, had a weak cry, sucked poorly, and failed to thrive. What is your assessment of the situation? (Include treatment plan and prognosis.)

The symptoms are suggestive of hypothyroidism. The early clinical findings of congenital hypothyroidism include dry skin, lethargy, poor feeding, hoarse voice, delayed development, constipation, large tongue, neonatal jaundice, and piglike facies. Respiratory difficulties, delayed skeletal maturation, and choking are common findings (21a,132,197,204).

The postpartum level of T4 is low and should be verified by further diagnostic procedures. Normal T4 levels postpartum are 6 to 14 mcg%, rising to 10 to 20 mcg% in the next few days and returning to the normal range of 4 to 10 mcg% by two months of age. Values for FTI are also elevated in normal infants and do not fall to adult levels before 12 months. On the other hand, T_3 levels are below adult levels at birth but rise to normal adult levels within a few days (254). TSH levels can be used to document hypothyroidism since a TSH surge should occur on the first day or two of life (90). X-ray examination of the knee, revealing a moth-eaten appearance termed epiphyseal dysgenesis is virtually pathognomonic of early hypothyroidism (197). An x-ray of the knee, several measurements of TT_4 and TSH levels will confirm the diagnosis of congenital hypothyroidism.

Insurance of normal development is determined by the age at which treatment is started, the adequacy with which it is maintained, and the degree of initial athyreosis. Either T_4 or T_3 can be used for replacement. The dose of T_4 or T_3 required for replacement of thyroid hormone depends on the age of the infant. The following approximations can be used: 0-12 months requires 50-75 mcg of T_4; 12-24 months requires 75-125 mcg of T_4; 2-4 years requires 100-150 mcg of T_4; and 4-12 years requires 100-300 mcg of T_4. Equivalent doses of T_3 can be used (see Table 3). Small doses of T_4 or its equivalent can be used initially if the baby is extremely sensitive to the effects of thyroid. The dose can be increased gradually by 12½ mcg of T_4 every one to two weeks as tolerated until the therapeutic dose is achieved. If vigorous treatment is needed, intravenous doses of T_4 100 mcg can be given and then followed by daily maintenance doses (141). One should take care to watch for symptoms of excessive doses of thyroid hormone such as hyperactivity and irritability. The TSH level provides the most reliable index of therapeutic efficacy.

Mental, as well as growth development does not seem to be affected if treatment is initiated prior to 3 months of age. When treatment was instituted before 3 months of age, 81% of 22 patients achieved "normal intellect" (204). In contrast, when treatment was detained until 6 months to one year of age, normal mental development was impaired despite subsequent treatment (319). Others have noted impaired mental development in spite of early diagnosis and treatment (277).

CASE C – UNRESPONSIVENESS TO THYROID HORMONE: RT is a 45-year-old female who complains of sluggishness and cold intolerance. Her present medical problems include Hashimoto's thyroiditis treated with desiccated thyroid 4 grains daily, hypercholesterolemia treated with cholestyramine 4 gm four times daily, and arteriosclerotic heart disease which has resulted in decreased mental acuity. Her laboratory data include a cholesterol level of 280 mg%, a TSH of 15 µU/ml, an FTI of 1.0, and positive antithyroglobulin and antimicrosomal antibodies. She admits that she has increased the dose of thyroid since she feels better on the higher dose.

15. Comment on her symptoms and her apparent resistance to thyroid.

Her complaints and laboratory values confirm hypothyroidism which has been inadequately treated despite thyroid therapy. Anemia due to her thyroid condition should be excluded as a contributory cause of her complaints (see Question 8). Factors which should be considered as possible causes of a therapeutic failure include noncompliance, error in diagnosis, poor absorption, inactive preparation, rapid metabolism, and tissue resistance (143,280). The last two factors are extremely rare. In this case, noncompliance and error in diagnosis do not appear to be reasonable explanations. The possibilities of poor absorption and an inactive product should be examined further. Since cholestyramine binds thyroxine and delays its absorption, the two drugs should be administered at least one hour apart (252). RT should be questioned as to the time of administration of her thyroid and cholestryramine. Evidence for incomplete or malabsorption of the hormone may be obtained by comparing the patient's response to the oral and parenteral thyroxine. Gastrointestinal disorders such as steatorrhea may also interfere with the enterohepatic circulation of orally administered thyroid and lead to excessive fecal loss (153). RT may also be receiving an inactive product (see Question 9). After instruction regarding the proper spacing of her thyroid medication and cholestyramine, the thyroid medication should be changed to an equivalent dose of L-thyroxine, and therapeutic response should be re-evaluated in one month. (See Question 10 and Table 3.)

16. Could RT's hypothyroidism be responsible for her other medical problems?

Hypercholesterolemia has been associated with hypothyroidism. Although the rate of cholesterol synthesis is normal in hypothyroidism, elevated levels of cholesterol can result from a delayed rate of removal. Similarly, slow removal of triglycerides may result in hyperlipidemia. Hypercholesterolemia is frequently observed before the appearance of clinical hypothyroidism. Treatment with thyroxine alone should lower the cholesterol levels provided there are no other contributing etiologies. In fact D-thyroxine (Choloxin) has been recommended as an agent for the treatment of hyperlipidemia.

The association between hypothyroidism, arteriosclerosis, and heart disease is difficult to interpret since most of the data have come from patients 60 years of age and older (325,346). Bastenie et al found severe coronary atherosclerosis in 84% of myxedema patients on autopsy as compared to 46% in controls (15,15a). Because of the rarity of coronary infarcts observed, they suggested that hypometabolism may actually protect against myocardial infarcts. However,

Nickerson found no evidence of atherosclerosis in the hearts of patients with myxedema (245). Others (15,94,91a) suggest that subclinical hypothyroidism may be a predisposing factor in coronary artery disease. Such patients with subclinical hypothyroidism may have a chronic thyroiditis with chronic hyperlipidemia. Bastenie et al reported that 70% of patients admitted for MI's had evidence of underlying thyroiditis on the basis of biopsy and the presence of thyroid antibodies (15), but Heinomen was unable to confirm these findings (146).

With such equivocal data it is difficult to accurately define the relationship between heart disease, arteriosclerosis, hypercholesteremia, and hypothyroidism. Further studies are needed to adequately elucidate this issue. In RT, treatment with L-thyroxine should decrease the cholesterol levels if secondary hypercholesterolemia is the cause of the problem.

CASE D – IMPENDING MYXEDEMA COMA: RB is a 65-year-old alcoholic who arrived at the emergency room in acute agitation and complaining of chest pain unrelieved by nitroglycerin. His medical problems include alcoholic cardiomyopathy, angina, and hypothyroidism. Although he has been repeatedly advised to take his thyroxine regularly, he continues to take it sporadically. An FTI drawn 4 months ago was 1.0. He was given chlorpromazine 25 mg IM along with morphine sulfate 10 mg IM. After the injection the nurse noticed increased mental depression, lethargy, and shallow breathing. His oral temperature was 34.5°C and he exhibited chills and shakes.

17. What is happening? Comment on the administration of chlorpromazine and morphine to RB.

Chlorpromazine and morphine may be responsible for what appears to be impending myxedema coma. In severely myxedematous patients, respiratory depressants (anesthetics, narcotic analgesics, phenothiazines, sedative-hypnotics) alone or in combination with the hypothermic effects of the phenothiazines (229) can aggravate the pre-existing hypothermia and carbon dioxide retention of hypothyroidism and precipitate myxedema coma (251,358). Tranquilizers such as chlorpromazine should not be given; small doses of less depressive sedative-hypnotics such as the benzodiazepines should be used only when absolutely necessary. Myxedematous patients are inherently sensitive to the respiratory depressant effects of narcotic analgesics, especially morphine. A dose as small as 10 mg may induce coma in a hypothyroid patient or cause death in a patient who is already comatose. If morphine is required, the dose should be decreased to ⅓ to ½ the usual analgetic dose and the respiratory rate should be closely monitored (67e).

18. Briefly comment on the clinical features and pathogenesis of myxedema coma.

Myxedema coma is the end stage of long-standing uncorrected hypothyroidism. The classic features are hypothermia, delayed deep tendon reflexes, and an altered sensorium which may range from stupor to coma. Other predominant features may include carbon dioxide retention, severe hypoglycemia, hyponatremia, and paranoid psychosis (29). Unless appropriate treatment is instituted, death is likely (245). Since myxedema coma frequently occurs in the elderly, it is frequently difficult to distinguish the signs and symptoms from senility.

Precipitating factors include cold weather or hypothermia; stressful situations such as surgery, infection, trauma; coexisting disease states such as myocardial infarction, diabetes, hypoglycemia, fluid and electrolyte abnormalities (especially hyponatremia); and medications such as respiratory depressants and diuretics (94).

19. How should RB be treated?

Emergency treatment of myxedema coma is directed toward thyroid replacement, maintenance of vital function and elimination of precipitating factors. Immediate and aggressive therapy with large replacement doses of thyroxine are necessary to prevent mortality which occurs at a rate of 60 to 70% (94, 157, 246). L-thyroxine 500 mcg IV should be given initially to saturate the TBG (29,157,282a,289a). The initial dose can be modified upward or downward depending on the patient's size and presence of restrictive factors. In RB the dose may be adjusted downward to 200 mcg because of his cardiac disease. If the proper therapy has been instituted, consciousness and decreased TSH levels are achieved within 24 hours along with restoration of normal vital signs. Maintenance doses should be regulated by the patient's response; however, minimal maintenance doses in the absence of untoward effects should be about 50 mcg of T_4 daily or about 5 mcg of T_3 every six hours (120).

Supportive measures include assisted ventilation, glucose for hypoglycemia, restriction of fluids for hyponatremia, and the use of blood or plasma expanders to prevent circulatory collapse and maintain blood pressure. The use of blankets to treat the hypothermia is not advised since vasodilation will occur and further compromise the cardiovascular components of shock. Although steroids have not been shown to be clearly beneficial in primary myxedema, they may be life saving in patients with hypopituitarism presenting as myxedema coma. Since it is difficult to distinguish between primary and secondary myxedema, the use of hydrocortisone 50 to 100 mg every six hours is recommended (29,120,289a).

CASE E – HYPOTHYROIDISM WITH CHF: EB is a 45-year-old male admitted with complaints of substernal chest pain with pressure, shortness of breath, dyspnea on exertion, and orthopnea. The intern's impression was congestive heart failure (CHF) complicated by myocardial infarction. Significant past medical history revealed Graves' Disease treated with radioactive iodine (RAI) ablation three years ago with recurrence of symptoms. On physical examination cardiomegaly, obesity, facial edema and puffiness, delayed DTR's, and pretibial edema were noted. Pertinent laboratory findings included a TT_4 of 1.8 mcg%; RT_3U of 15%; CPK of 150; SGOT of 80; and an LDH of 250. Chest x-ray revealed cardiomegaly and pleural effusions, and an ECG showed bradycardia and flattened T-waves with ST depression. Diuretics and digitalis were instituted without reversal of the cardiac abnormalities.

20. Comment on these clinical findings. What recommendations can be made with regard to EB's cardiac status?

EB's history of RAI therapy, low thyroid function tests, symptoms, and physical findings confirm the presence of severe hypothyroidism. Several cardiac abnormalities suggestive of CHF have been associated with hypothyroidism. "Myxedema heart" is often suggestive of CHF since the symptoms are similar: cardiomegaly, dyspnea, edema, pleural effusions, and abnormal cardiogram. Low output failure is a result of the decreased cardiac output, decreased stroke volume, and decreased myocardial contractility. The cardiac enlargement results from dilation of the chambers, loss of muscle tone, and deposition of mucopolysaccharides in the myocardium (67, 67a, 116). Characteristic ECG changes include slow rate and voltage, flattened or inverted T-waves, an occasional prolongation of the PR interval and a widened QRS complex (54).

Although EB's enzyme elevations (SGOT, CPK, and LDH) are suggestive of an MI, they may be due to the altered metabolism, and liver and cardiac status may be normal (59,93). The enzymes can be fractionated to determine their origin.

If EB's cardiac abnormalities are caused by hypothyroidism rather than organic disease, treatment with adequate thyroxine will restore the heart size, reverse the ECG findings, and normalize the serum enzyme elevations within 2 to 4 weeks. The angina may develop or worsen with thyroxine therapy (67e,177). In the absence of organic disease, digitalis is not effective and may even be harmful. Hypothyroid patients are noted to have an increased sensitivity to digitalis which may lead to digitalis toxicity unless the maintenance dose is decreased. (See Question 26 and 27).

21. How should thyroid hormone therapy be initiated in EB? Is triiodothyronine (Cytomel) the agent of choice in patients with cardiac disease?

Patients with long-standing hypothyroidism, cardiac disease, or advanced age tend to be extremely sensitive to the cardiac effects of thyroid hormone. Normal therapeutic doses in these individuals may result in severe angina, myocardial infarction, cardiac failure, or tachycardia (177).

Treatment should, therefore, be cautiously initiated with minute amounts (0.025 mg) of T_4 and increased by increments of 0.05 mg of T_4 or its equivalent every 2 to 4 weeks. The rapidity with which the increments can proceed is determined by how well each increased dose is tolerated. If cardiac toxicity occurs with increased dosage, a longer interval or smaller increments can be employed. In some patients with severe cardiac sensitivity, complete euthyroidism may never be achieved. The correct dose appears to be a compromise between prevention of myxedema and induction of cardiac toxicity.

Triiodothyronine (Cytomel) has been suggested by some to be the agent of choice in patients with cardiac abnormalities. The onset of action of T_3 is 1 to 3 days as compared to 3 to 5 days for T_4. After therapy is withdrawn, the effects of T_3 are diminished in 3 to 5 days while 7 to 10 days are needed for thyroxine. Thus, if toxicity occurs, T_3 will rapidly disappear upon cessation of therapy, an advantage in the cardiac patient. Nevertheless, T_3 is not recommended for therapy here since it is biologically more potent and requires finer, more difficult regulation of dosage to insure smooth and uniform blood levels. Furthermore, it appears to have a higher incidence of cardiac toxicity, especially the aggravation of angina (67e,180).

CASE F – GRAVES' DISEASE: SK is a 38-year-old female physician who is admitted for a possible myocardial infarction. Her complaints include chest pain unrelieved by NTG, nervousness, palpitations, muscle weakness, weight loss despite increased appetite, epistaxis, and easy bruisability. Her other medical problems include: deep vein thrombosis treated with warfarin (Coumadin) 5 mg daily – last prothrombin time (PT) was 26 seconds; angina treated with nitroglycerin 0.4 mg; and atrial fibrillation (AF) treated with digoxin 0.375 mg daily. On physical examination (PE) she is a thin, flushed, hyperkinetic, and nervous female. Blood pressure is 180/90; pulse is 102; respiration is 30; and temperature is 37.5°C. Other findings include lid lag with stare, minimal proptosis with tearing, decreased visual acuity, a diffusely enlarged thyroid gland without nodules, a bruit in the left lobe of the thyroid, warm, moist skin with multiple bruises, tachycardia, slight diarrhea, acropachy, 2+ pitting edema, a fine tremor, proximal *muscle weakness, and irregular menses. Her family history is significant in that her mother had a thyroidectomy for overactive thyroid. Laboratory data included: TT_4 = 30 mcg%, RT_3U = 45%, RAIU at 24 hours was 80%, PT = 40 seconds, TDI = 100%, antimicrosomal trc = 1:6400, TgAb = 65%, and a scan that showed a diffusely enlarged gland which was 3 to 4 times the normal size.*

22. Briefly discuss and interpret the significance of these laboratory tests as they relate to SK's thyroid status.

The TT_4 and RT_3U are abnormally elevated. The calculated FTI which compensates for any alterations in protein binding is also elevated (see Question 2).

The **RAIU (Radioactive Iodine Uptake)** is a measure of iodine utilization by the gland. A tracer dose of I^{131} is administered, and the radioactivity of the gland is measured at one, five, and twenty-four hours following ingestion. The normal values will depend on the dietary iodine sufficiency of each geographical area (271). Some hyperthyroid patients will have peak uptake values within the first few hours after the tracer is administered and the uptake will then fall progressively to lower, even subnormal levels. Therefore, an uptake at 1, 5, and 24 hours is needed. The RAIU indirectly reflects not only the need for iodine but also the thyroid function. As a measurement of thyroid activity the test is said to have a clinical accuracy of between 70 to 95% and gives much better results in the hyperthyroid than in the hypothyroid ranges. Any condition which affects the thyroid requirement for iodine will alter the RAI uptake (117,315). Therefore, iodine deficiency resulting from rigorous diuretic therapy or from iodine deficient diets will cause a falsely increased RAIU due to depletion of total iodide pools. Likewise, administration of exogenous iodine or iodide will expand the total body iodide pool resulting in a decreased RAIU. SK's RAIU is abnormally elevated without any evidence for false positive interference. All of these tests indicate that SK is hyperthyroid.

A **scan of the gland** is performed simultaneously with the I^{131} uptake or after ingestion of 99^mTc per technetate. The scan allows an estimate of gland size, outlines the radioactivity of the gland, and exposes hypermetabolic (hot) areas and hypometabolic (cold) areas. The possibility of carcinoma must be considered if cold areas are present, and since carcinomas may exist with thyrotoxicosis, a scan is of utmost importance in the assessment of thyroid disease (189, 199). (See Questions 64 and 65.)

The **antithyroglobulin (TgAb) and antimicrosomal antibodies** to the thyroid gland are detected by radioimmune assay and by the tanned red cell (trc) agglutination method respectively. (See Table 1.) The presence of these antibodies in SK indicates the presence of an autoimmune process, although it does not determine the nature of the clinical disease. About 95% of patients with Graves' disease and 80% of patients with Hashimoto's thyroiditis will have positive antibodies (28b). Also, 5 to 10% of asymptomatic individuals will have positive antibodies (70).

Long Acting Thyroid Stimulator (LATS) is an immunoglobulin of the IgG type which is often found in the blood of patients with active disease and is considered to be the causative agent of Graves' disease. It is postulated that LATS displaces TSH from its receptor site, binds to the TSH receptor site and stimulates the thyroid like TSH (322). However, this view is currently in disfavor since only 50 to 70% of patients with active disease contain measurable LATS via the McKenzie mouse assay (stimulated mouse thyroid) and some patients may have LATS without evidence of hyperthyroidism (184,220,221a,231). The presence of other thyroid stimulators which are specific for human thyroid have been identified in virtually 100% of patients with Graves' disease. These are also circulating IgG molecules which have been called *LATS protector, HTS (human thyroid stimulator), TSI (thyroid stimulating immunologlobulin),* and more recently **TDI (thyrotropin displacing immunolglobulin).** All of these are thought to be antibodies specifically directed against human thyroid antigen that exhibit cross reactivity with similar thyroid components in other species such as the mouse (2,180). Normal TDI values at the University of California are 100% ± 20. On the basis of the positive TDI and presence of antibodies SK has Graves' disease.

23. Identify and discuss the etiology, incidence, and pathogenesis of SK's thyroid disorder.

The causes of hyperthyroidism are listed in Table 4.

Table 4
CAUSES OF HYPERTHYROIDISM

Graves' disease (toxic diffuse goiter)

Toxic uninodular goiter (Plummer's disease)

Toxic multinodular goiter

Nodular goiter with hyperthyroidism due to exogenous iodine (Jod-Basedow)

Exogenous thyroid excess through self-administration (Factitious hyperthyroidism)

Tumors (thyroid adenoma, follicular carcinoma, thyrotropin secreting tumor of the pituitary, and hydatiform mole with secretion of a thyroid stimulating substance)

Thyrotoxicosis occurring in conjunction with ocular and skin changes, positive antibodies and TDI, a diffuse goiter, and a positive family history strongly suggest the presence of Graves' disease (221a). Graves' disease occurs predominantly in females (5:1 ratio) and has a peak onset between the ages of 30 and

40 (67e). A familial association with Graves' has been well documented, but the exact mode of genetic transmission has not been established (31). Graves' disease appears to have a close relationship to Hashimoto's thyroiditis since both disorders occur genetically in the same family and may coexist within the same thyroid gland (353) (also see Question 7). Although the exact etiology of Graves' is unknown, it is strongly suspected that both humoral and cell mediated immunological mechanisms are involved (221a,353). Precipitation of Graves' disease has been associated with severe emotional stress (23), with the administration of thyroid hormone for weight reduction (34), and with the administration of iodides, especially in endemic goiter areas (57,328,344a,350).

24. Discuss the symptoms of Graves' disease as presented by SK.

In addition to symptoms clearly related to hyperthyroxinemia, the manifestations of ophthalmopathy, dermopathy, acropachy (clubbing of the fingers and toes with characteristic bony changes), and diffuse toxic goiter are characteristic of Graves' disease, although all of these need not be present (136a, 253, 322). SK's proptosis appears to be the ophthalmopathy of Graves' disease (see Question 52), and diffuse toxic goiter and acropachy were noted as well. Her symptoms of excessive thyroid hormone include lid lag (lid falls behind movement of the eye and narrow white rim of sclera becomes visible between the upper lid and cornea), lid retraction, palpitations, tachycardia, diarrhea, decreased menses, nervousness, tremor, muscle weakness, heat intolerance, weight loss despite increased appetite, increased perspiration and flushing of the skin (253,322). Clinically, there is increased metabolism of all body systems and functions.

25. Could SK's hypoprothrombinemia be related to her thyrotoxic state? What effect could this have on subsequent management of her thyrotoxicosis?

Increased sensitivity to the hypoprothrombinemic effect of warfarin has been observed in thyrotoxic patients (219,259,307,344b). This may be related to a shortened warfarin plasma half-life (219) as well as an increased turnover and disappearance of the clotting factors (188,165). The opposite occurs in hypothyroid states.

Therefore, thyrotoxic patients will need less warfarin while myxedematous patients will require more warfarin to achieve the same hypoprothrombinemic response. The anticoagulant response to warfarin should be monitored carefully in patients with thyrotoxicosis and the dose adjusted as the thyroid status changes.

One of the thioamides may be considered for treatment of SK's Graves' disease, but the use of thioamides, especially propylthiouracil has resulted in hypoprothrombinemia and bleeding (107, 115, 125, 241). Depression of the bone marrow and thrombocytopenia as well as depression of clotting factors II, VII, III, IX, X, and XIII, and vitamin K are responsible. The effects on the clotting factors and vitamin K appear to be due to a subclinical hepatic alteration in the synthesis of the clotting factors (107), although toxic hepatitis has also been reported (16, 87, 210, 227, 261, 288, 311, 335) with both PTU and methimazole. The duration of therapy before the onset of symptoms has been 2 weeks to 18 months. The bleeding is responsive to vitamin K or blood transfusions. Prothrombin times may remain depressed for up to two months after discontinuation of therapy (115).

26. What are the effects of thyrotoxicosis on cardiac status and management of cardiac disease?

Thyrotoxicosis increases cardiac demands by elevating heart rate (HR), stroke volume (SV), and cardiac output (CO) (35). Exacerbation or precipitation of angina, atrial fibrillation (AF), or high output congestive heart failure (CHF) can occur (116,193,194a). Myocardial infarction (MI) has also been reported (43). On physical examination, tachycardia, cardiomegaly, an elevated systolic blood pressure, decreased diastolic pressure, and widening of the pulse pressure are common findings (67,67a,67e). Electrocardiogram manifestations include tachycardia, increased voltage, and a prolonged PR interval.

The presence of thyrotoxicosis does not alter the therapeutic management of heart disease but may make it more difficult to control. Congestive heart failure (CHF) requires larger than normal doses of digitalis to be effective (see Question 27). CHF may be the only presenting symptom of thyrotoxicosis in the elderly patient (330). Correction of atrial fibrillation in thyrotoxicosis is often unsuccessful until euthyroidism is achieved. Then the fibrillation may revert spontaneously or respond to antiarrhythmic therapy (296). If no organic disease is present, reversal of the thyrotoxicosis may eliminate the cardiac symptoms.

27. After treatment with radioactive iodine (RAI) SK's daily dose of digoxin was increased to 0.5 mg because of persistent atrial fibrillation. After 3 months she returns with complaints of nausea and vomiting; the gland was palpable and considerably decreased in size. The ECG showed ST depression, AV block and occasional bigeminy. Comment on her current symptoms. Why was such a large dose of digoxin required initially?

The gastrointestinal symptoms of nausea and vomiting, together with the ECG changes of block and bigeminy strongly suggest digitalis toxicity. Continuation of the high dose of digoxin required initially during her thyrotoxicosis after apparent resolution of her hyperthyroidism increases the likelihood of digitalis toxicity.

The atrial fibrillation (AF) of hyperthyroidism is often resistant to digitalis. A comparison of the response to digitalis in euthyroid patients with AF before and after exogenous T_3 administration demonstrated that the daily digoxin requirement of 0.2 mg for a ventricular rate of 70 was increased to 0.8 mg (99). Higher doses without side effects are better tolerated by the hyperthyroid individual (99,237). Fifty percent more ouabain was required to produce ventricular arrhythmias in thyrotoxic dogs than in euthyroid animals (237).

The observed altered resistance to digitalis in thyrotoxic patients has been attributed to changes in intrinsic myocardial function, to an increased volume of distribution (Vd) and to increased glomerular filtration (63,73). Conversely, hypothyroid patients are inordinately sensitive to the effects of digitalis and require smaller doses for a therapeutic response.

Regardless of the mechanism of the altered sensitivity to digitalis, one should be aware that higher than normal doses may be required in thyrotoxicosis, and that the initial dose will need reduction as euthyroidism or hypothyroidism results.

CASE G – HYPERTHYROIDISM UNSUCCESSFULLY TREATED WITH IODIDES: CR is a 27-year-old Chinese male law student with a two to three month history of intermittent heat intolerance, sweats, tremor, and severe muscle weakness which has limited his ability to climb stairs at school. His appetite has increased remarkably despite weight loss, and he is bothered by the pounding of his heart. His hyperthyroid state was first discovered after a bout of periodic paralysis which occurred after dinner. There is no family history of thyroid disease and he denies taking any thyroid medications or having had any radiation to his neck. He has previously received iodide drops with improvement in his symptomatology, but exacerbation of his disease occurred despite continued administration of iodides. His only other medical problem is rheumatoid arthritis for which he takes ASA 5.4 gm daily.

Pertinent physical findings include a blood pressure of 170/110 mm Hg, a pulse of 110 beats per minute, hyper-reflexia, lid lag, and a diffusely enlarged gland which is four times normal (about 100 grams). Available laboratory data included the following: TT_4 15 mcg%, RT_3U 40%, RAIU at 5 hr 85% and at 24 hr 85%, and antimicrosomal antibodies (trc) = 1: 1600.

28. What considerations do you have regarding the interpretation of his laboratory findings?

CR's laboratory findings verify the presence of a

hyperthyroid state. However, the serum TT_4 is only at the upper limits of normal and is out of proportion to the severity of his disease state and his other laboratory findings. The possibility of T_3 toxicosis should be considered since elevations of T_3 may not be accompanied by elevations of T_4. The decreased TT_4 could also be explained by displacement of T_4 from TBG by aspirin. (See Questions 3 and 33.)

29. Has periodic paralysis and muscle weakness such as that experienced by CR been associated with thyrotoxicosis? Is there any specific treatment for this disorder?

Several muscular dysfunctions have been associated with thyrotoxicosis. Although the exact mechanism is not clear, muscle weakness and myopathy have been reported to occur in 10 to 100% of patients with hyperthyroidism (82,82a,278). The muscle weakness may only be apparent when climbing stairs, getting out of a chair, or holding an object. In more extreme cases of muscle involvement, muscular atrophy may co-exist with the weakness. The onset of the myopathy can be rapid, occurring within weeks, or insidious.

Thyrotoxic periodic muscle paralysis is a very rare complication and seems to have a familial tendency for the Oriental race (217,255). The paralysis can be precipitated by muscular exertion, carbohydrate load, psychological stress, or exposure to cold. It has been associated with low potassium levels (312a). Correction of the thyrotoxicosis as well as avoidance of precipitating factors constitute the main therapy. Propranolol has also proved to be of surprising value in improving many of the neuromuscular manifestations of hyperthyroidism (173,269,292,360).

30. Discuss the use of iodides in the treatment of thyrotoxicosis. Why did the iodide drops eventually become ineffective in CR?

Pharmacologic doses of iodides were first noted by Plummer (1923) to ameliorate the symptoms of thyrotoxicosis by inhibiting the release of thyroid hormone and by blocking organification (273, 344, 372). The inhibitory effect of iodides on organification, known as the Wolff-Chaikoff effect, is similar to that of the thioamides. However, despite chronic administration of 5 to 10 mg of iodides daily, the normal gland is able to "escape" from this block after 7 to 14 days so that goiter and hypothyroidism do not occur (20, 32, 344, 372). The Wolff-Chaikoff effect depends on the establishment of high intrathyroidal concentrations of inorganic iodide and is not overcome by TSH stimulation. It is postulated that the normal gland "adapts or escapes" by decreasing iodide transport or through an iodide leak (357b); both of these mechanisms would decrease intrathyroidal iodide and thereby decrease the organification block. Patients who already have high intrathyroidal iodine (i.e. Graves' disease) or patients with underlying defects in organic binding mechanisms (i.e. Hashimoto's thyroiditis) may be unduly sensitive to this effect of iodides and show the Wolff-Chaikoff effect with smaller doses (31a,32a,32b).

Stable iodine can be administered orally as either Lugol's solution containing 8 mg of iodide per drop or as saturated solution of potassium iodide (SSKI) containing 50 mg of iodide per drop. The minimum effective dose is 6 mg although larger doses are usually given (98).

When Lugol's solution was given for long-term primary suppressive treatment in 20 patients, 35% (7 patients) had poor responses, 35% were maintained in remission for one year after withdrawal of treatment, and 30% (6 patients) were controlled on the iodide, suggesting that a small percentage of patients (those with small goiters and mild disease) are suitable for such therapy (136). Males, older persons, and those with nodular goiters may be less responsive to iodide therapy (194,250). Amelioration of symptoms is seen within two to seven days (67e). Nagataki et al described 12 hyperthyroid patients in whom control was maintained effectively for 6 weeks with iodides. However, half of the patients "escaped" between the 6th and 14th week despite continued therapy (242).

The advantages of iodide therapy are that it is simple, inexpensive, relatively nontoxic, and there is no glandular destruction. The disadvantages include "escape", relapse after discontinuation of treatment, allergic reactions, and subsequent interference with RAI or thioamide therapy. Thus, the primary use of iodides is in preparation for surgery, in thyroid storm, and as an ameliorative measure while awaiting the therapeutic effects of RAI and thioamides. However, patients with mild disease and small glands may deserve a therapeutic trial with iodides in hopes of remission.

31. How should CR's hyperthyroidism be treated?

The three major treatment modalities are the thioamides, radioactive iodine (RAI), and surgery (133, 162, 164, 338). Potassium perchlorate is no longer used because of the risks of aplastic anemia and nephrotic syndrome associated with its use. In most cases any of these three modalities may be employed, and it is controversial which is the optimal means of therapy. Often, the final decision is empiric depending on the physician's available resources. However, the final decision should rest upon the patient armed with the knowledge of the advantages and disadvantages of each modality.

The **thioamides** are the preferred treatment for children, pregnant women, and young adults. However, the large number of tablets required and the long duration of treatment requires a highly motivated patient. Usually a good prognosis of remission is associated with a small gland and mild disease (312). Keeping the above variables in mind, thioamides may be tried in CR; however, his relatively large gland and the severity of his disease makes the prognosis for remission somewhat less favorable. (Also see Questions 43 and 50.)

Surgery is considered the treatment of choice when there is suspicion of malignancy, esophageal obstruction, failure with thioamides, or a large multinodular gland which does not regress with oral suppressive therapy. This is a safe, effective, and widely used treatment modality for hyperthyroidism (26). The patient's fear of surgery, economical status, and the relatively small risk of post-operative complications may make this a less desirable alternative. (Also see Questions 48 and 51.)

Radioactive iodine (RAI) is the preferred treatment for debilitated or elderly patients who are not good surgical canddates as well as those with recurrent hyperthyroidism after surgery (327). Because of fears of inducing genetic damage or neoplasia, many clinics have restricted the use of RAI to adults over some arbitrary age, such as 20 to 35 years. However, after more than 25 years of clinical experience with RAI, it is generally accepted that this is a safe and efficient treatment modality. There is no evidence of genetic damage after ingestion of I^{131} (67e); the dose of radiation to the gonads is only about five times that of a barium swallow (357c); and the incidence of leukemia or malignancy is no higher in recipients of I^{131} than in those receiving medical or surgical treatment for hyperthyroidism (72a,274,293). The advantages of RAI are that it is painless, effective, and requires no hospitalization. The disadvantages are fears of radiation and a high incidence of hypothyroidism. (Also see Questions 45-47 and 51.)

All of the above treatment modalities are applicable in CR. However, his personal preference may aid in selecting one modality over another.

CASE H – T₃-TOXICOSIS: BJ is a 45-year-old white female who complains of insomnia, palpitations, and increasing chest pain. Other medical problems are angina and systemic lupus erythematosus (SLE). Her past medical history is significant in that she underwent a subtotal thyroidectomy for Graves' disease one year ago after an exacerbation of her SLE by propylthiouracil. (See Question 36.) Her family history is significant in that several relatives have Graves' disease. On physical examination a palpable, nontender, left thyroid lobe, a mild tremor, and marked proptosis were noted. Medications were NTG and prednisone 10 mg daily. Laboratory findings included the following: TT₄ 4.3 mcg%, RT₃U 36%, FTI 1.5, TgAb

*28%, antimicrosomal antibodies 1:1600, T₃ by RIA 550
ng%, and an elevated RAIU.*

32. Briefly explain and discuss the use of the T₃ by RIA (Radioimmune assay).

Serum T_3 levels by radioimmune assay are valuable in the recognition of T_3 toxicosis (see Question 33). Normal levels are 100 to 200 ng% although this may vary among laboratories. The concentration of circulating T_3 is quite low compared to T_4 because it has less affinity for the binding proteins and has a larger intracellular distribution. However, adjustments in T_3 levels do need to be made when there are alterations in the binding proteins. T_3 levels are only useful in the diagnosis of hyperthyroid states (189).

33. What is your assessment of BJ's thyroid status? Discuss the etiology, pathogenesis, and significance of her thyroid disease. How should she be managed?

BJ seems to have a variant type of hyperthyroidism known as T_3 toxicosis (106,168). The clinical features include signs and symptoms of thyrotoxicosis, normal levels of TT_4, FTI, and TBG, increased or normal RAIU, nonsuppressibility of RAIU following T_3 administration, and elevated T_3 levels through preferential secretion and peripheral conversion of T_4 to T_3.

T_3 toxicosis has been associated with Graves' disease, nodular goiters, and thyroid carcinomas (331) and it may occur in children (230). The prevalence may be higher in iodine deficient areas since incidences as high as 12.5% have been reported in endemic goiter areas (155b).

Elevations of T_3 levels may precede elevation of T_4 levels and the development of overt hyperthyroidism. It has been suggested that T_3 toxicosis represents a preliminary stage of classical T_4 toxicosis and may be useful for early diagnosis or as an indication of relapse following withdrawal of thioamide therapy (155c, 209, 310).

34. How should BJ be treated?

If she is not pregnant, the treatment of choice for this lady is radioactive iodine. Thioamides are not a good choice because of her previous history of adverse reaction. She has already undergone thyroid surgery, and the incidence of morbidity and mortality increases with a second operation which is more difficult because of adhesions from the prior surgery. Also, the presence of cardiac disease increases the risks of surgery. RAI therapy is safe, convenient, and inexpensive.

35. JE is a 23-year-old premedical student complaining of insomnia, nervousness, fatigue and profuse sweating which necessitates several changes

of clothing daily. The diagnosis of Graves' disease is made and PTU is started. Evaluate the use of thioamides in the management of Graves' disease. How should a patient on thioamides be monitored?

The thioamides act by blocking the organification of thyroid hormone synthesis (306). Theoretically, propylthiouracil (PTU) may be more efficacious than methimazole, since it also blocks the peripheral conversion of thyroxine (T_4) to triiodothyronine (T_3) and this may play a significant role in its therapeutic effectiveness (104,254). Abuid et al demonstrated a significantly greater fall in the T_3 concentration and the T_3/T_4 ratio in hyperthyroid patients treated acutely with PTU and iodide than with methimazole and iodide (1). Because of its short half-life PTU must be dosed every six hours, or every four hours in severe hyperthyroidism; methimazole can be given every eight hours. Methimazole is ten times more potent than PTU on a milligram per milligram basis (345).

Initially, high blocking doses of PTU (400 to 800 mg daily) or methimazole (40 to 80 mg daily) should be given in divided doses depending on the degree of toxicosis. On rare occasions doses of 1200 mg daily of PTU or its equivalent may be required in patients with large goiter (four times normal size) or with severe disease. After the initial period of high-dose therapy the daily dose can be gradually reduced to that which maintains the patient at a euthyroid state, generally 100 to 300 mg PTU daily or its equivalent. In most toxic patients the euthyroid state will occur four to six weeks after the initiation of thioamides. This delay is to be expected because alleviation of symptoms will depend on the elimination of thyroxine stores; the half-life of thyroxine is seven days and elimination of all thyroxine requires roughly five half-lives, or 35 days.

Prior to the administration of thioamides, a baseline TT_4, RT_3U, and white blood cell count (WBC) with differential should be obtained. The thyroid function tests are used to monitor the efficacy of therapy while the WBC with differential is used to ascertain the development of agranulocytosis. A baseline WBC with differential is helpful since hyperthyroidism per se is associated with a relative reduction in the neutrophil count. All patients should be told to report rash, fever, sore throat, or any type of flu-like symptoms which may be signs of agranulocytosis (see Question 39). A repeat TT_4 and RT_3U should be obtained after one month of therapy and one month after any change in the dosing regimen of thioamides since circulating thyroxine levels should decline within one month (67e). Clinically, the therapeutic effect of thioamides should be evident by amelioration of symptoms and by a decrease in gland size (4b).

Thioamide therapy should be continued for at least a year. Some recommend two years of treatment, claiming a higher rate of remission. On the other hand, a recent study suggests that low remission rates may be possible with relatively short-term therapy (126). There is a scarcity of good data regarding the optimal treatment period.

After the withdrawal of antithyroid drugs the patient should be checked at intervals of one to two months for recurrence of hyperthyroidism.

36. After one week JE notices monoarticular swelling, joint pain, and diffuse myalgias. Laboratory data show an ESR of 30 and a positive LE preparation. Could PTU be responsible for her arthritic complaints?

Both PTU and methimazole have rarely been associated with the development of *lupus and lupus-like syndromes.* The incidence is less than 0.1% (5,25,196). Lupus-like syndromes include skin ulcers (356), splenomegaly (295,356), migratory polyarthritis (163a), pleuritis and pericarditis (25,369), periarteritis (215), and renal abnormalities (5,369). Serological abnormalities may also occur and include hyperglobulinemia (5,369), positive LE preparations (5), and antinuclear antibodies (ANA) (5,49,163a). Recovery occurs after adequate steroid therapy and withdrawal of the thioamides. Since cross-reaction between methimazole and PTU is likely to occur, these patients should be treated with surgery or RAI. JE's treatment should be monitored with this side effect in mind, but the occurrence of this syndrome is infrequent enough that a trouble-free course of therapy can be anticipated.

37. After taking PTU 400 mg daily for three weeks, JE continues to complain of insomnia, sweating, and fatigue and her gland is still enlarged. What considerations and recommendations do you have regarding her complaints?

The onset of action of the thioamides is slow because they block the synthesis rather than the release of thyroid hormone. Therefore, hormone secretion will continue until the large stores are depleted, and this may take four to ten weeks. However, some improvement should have been noted after one week. One must ascertain whether the response is inadequate due to patient noncompliance, inadequate dose, or inappropriate dosing interval. After these factors have been considered, an increase in dose may be justified using the patient's symptoms, gland size, and laboratory values as a guide. The RAIU should be low if iodide trapping has been blocked by suffcient doses of thioamides.

While awaiting the onset of the thioamides, iodides and/or propranolol can be used to ameliorate some of her symptoms. (See Question 30 and 44.)

38. JH is an 18-year-old Chinese female with

Graves' disease who has been taking PTU 400 mg daily for three weeks. She returns to the clinic complaining of a pruritic area over the pretibial aspects of both legs. She denies further rash, but on closer inspection you notice mild maculopapular erythematous patches on her body. She denies any other medications. What are your considerations and recommendations at this time?

JH may be experiencing a drug rash from PTU; however, the possibility of pretibial myxedema or the dermopathy of Graves' disease must also be considered due to the location of the pruritic area. This abnormality occurs in about 4% of patients with Graves' disease and is associated with infiltrative exophthalmos. It appears as thickening of the skin due to mucopolysaccharide infiltration, accentuation of hair follicles, and erythema with pruritus and is responsive to topical corticosteroids (101,184a).

PTU and methimazole have both been associated with the production of a *maculopapular pruritic rash* (218). If the rash is mild, drug therapy can be continued while the symptoms are treated with an antihistamine and a topical steroid; such rashes generally subside spontaneously. Alternatively, another thioamide can be substituted since there is little cross-sensitivity with regard to this side effect.

39. JH continues taking PTU and returns in three weeks with a generalized maculopapular pruritic rash associated with fatigue, fever, and a sore throat. What might be happening? How would you confirm your suspicions? Characterize the clinical features associated with this disorder?

The PTU should be discontinued, because *agranulocytosis* or *granulocytopenia* (defined as less than 250/mm³ and 1500/mm³ respectively of neutrophils and granulocytes) may have occurred. This is one of the most severe adverse hematological reactions associated with the thioamides (290). A WBC with differential would confirm the diagnosis. The onset of fever, malaise, gingivitis, and sore throat is so abrupt that routine WBC tests are not of value in monitoring for this adverse reaction.

Reports of the incidence of agranulocytosis or granulocytopenia range from 0.5 to 6% (14,19,52,348). There is no predilection for age or sex, but the risk for this hypersensitivity reaction may be dose-related (218,363). McGavack et al (218) found no reactions in 900 patients receiving less than 25 mg of methimazole daily but a 5.4% incidence of granulocytopenia including one death occurred in patients receiving more than 30 mg daily. Likewise, in 931 patients taking PTU, a 2.8% incidence of decreased granulocytes was seen with doses less than 150 mg daily and a 4.5% incidence was noted in those taking more than 250 mg daily (218). Wibert et al reported two cases of agranulocytosis among 25 patients receiving 120 mg methimazole daily, an incidence of 8% (363).

Agranulocytosis usually occurs within the first few months of therapy, although it can occur later (14, 56, 172, 198, 218). Fatality may result from overwhelming infection. The drug should be discontinued and the patient monitored for signs of infection and antibiotics should be instituted if necessary. If the patient recovers, granulocytes will begin to reappear in the peripheral blood within a few days to three weeks; a normal granulocyte count occurs shortly thereafter (14, 61a, 80, 218).

Although it would be best to proceed with another form of treatment, rechallenge with the same drug may or may not produce a similar reaction. Some cases of granulocytopenia have resolved despite continuation of thioamides (5,348). Very little information is available regarding cross-sensitivity between agents; both instances of cross-sensitivity and the lack thereof have been reported (14).

40.WG is a 23-year-old male with Graves' disease who has been euthyroid for three months while taking methimazole 10 mg tid. He has trouble remembering to take it three times a day and has heard about single-day dosing. Is WG an appropriate patient for such a regimen?

The plasma half-life of the thioamides is short: 1 to 2 hours for PTU (175,302,316) and 2 to 6 hours for methimazole (271a) and the half-lives do not change with the thyroid status (223,349). However, several clinical studies have demonstrated that single daily doses of methimazole or PTU are therapeutically effective, particularly in patients who are initially made euthyroid with multiple dosing (13,126a). Some patients with mild disease may be effectively treated with a single dose regimen throughout therapy (126,174).

The success rate of this approach depends upon the size of the gland and severity of the disease and has been reported to be 39% (126), 68% (13), 83% (174), and 93% (126a). Methimazole has been suggested as the preferred agent for once daily dosing because of its longer duration of action (13,174,357c). In spite of its short plasma half-life, a single 30 mg dose of methimazole has a duration of action of 24 hours (357c). Apparently, the duration of action of the antithyroid agents is not correlated with the plasma half-life but rather with the size of the dose and the intrathyroidal concentration of the drug (280).

Since this patient is now euthyroid as a result of treatment with a divided daily dosage schedule, he could be tried on a single daily dosing regimen and observed for exacerbation of his Graves' disease.

CASE I – PROGNOSIS OF THIOAMIDE THERAPY:
BJD is a 35-year-old white female who has been clinically euthyroid and has been taking PTU 100 mg daily for over two years. Despite treatment her goiter never appeared to shrink in size. After the following laboratory values were obtained, thyroxine 0.1 mg daily was initiated. A TT_4 was 6 mcg% and a RT_3U was 23%. A T_3 suppression test showed the following results:

RAIU	Baseline RAIU	After T_3 100 mcg Daily for 7 Days
2 hr	6%	8%
5 hr	15%	14%
24 hr	33%	25%

After two months the thyroxine and the PTU were discontinued.

Table 5
TREATMENT OF HYPERTHYROIDISM

Modality	Drug	Dose	Mechanism Of Action	Toxicity	Indications
THIOAMIDES	Propythiouracil 50 mg tablets	400-800 mg/d initally, maintenance of 100-300 mg daily.	Blocks organification of hormone synthesis, Blocks peripheral conversion of T_4 to T_3 (PTU only).	Skin rashes, gastrointestinal symptoms, arthralgias, hepatitis, blood dyscrasias, hypoprothrombinemia.	Children, young adults, pregnancy. Contraindication to surgery or RAI therapy.
	Methimazole (Tapazole) 5 and 10 mg tablets	40-80 mg/d initially, maintenance of 10 to 30 mg daily.			

(continued on following page)

Table 5 (continued)
TREATMENT OF HYPERTHYROIDISM

Modality	Drug	Dose	Mechanism Of Action	Toxicity	Indications
IODIDES	Lugol's Solution 8 mg/drop (5% Iodine 10% Potassium iodide) Saturated Potassium Iodide (SSKI) 50 mg iodide per drop.	Only 6 mg/day is effective although 5-10 drops tid are usually given for 10 to 14 days prior to surgery orally.	Decreases the vascularity of the gland and increases firmness.	Hypersensitivity reactions: skin rashes, mucous membrane ulcers, anaphylaxis, metallic taste, rhinorrhea, parotid and submaxillary swelling.	Preoperative preparation prior to surgery; can be used long-term for patients with mild disease and small goiters.
	Sodium Iodide (NaI) USP 1 gm/10cc 2 gm/20cc	0.5-2 gm IV over 24 hr.	Blocks release of thyroid hormone.		Thyroid storm.
ADRENERGIC ANTAGONISTS	Propranolol (Inderal) 10, 40, 80 mg tablets, 1 gm/10 cc IV	10 to 40 mg orally every six hours. 0.5-1 mg IV slow.	Blocks the effects of thyroid hormone peripherally, no effect on the underlying disease.	Related to symptoms of beta blockade: bradycardia, CHF, blocks hyperglycemic response to hypoglycemia, CNS symptoms at high doses.	Symptomatic relief while awaiting onset of action of thioamides, RAI; preoperative preparation for surgery; thyroid storm.
	Reserpine	1-3 mg IV every 8 hrs.	Catecholamine depletion.	Effects of sympathetic blockade: nasal congestion, hypotension; CNS effects.	Thyroid Storm (Propranolol is drug of choice).
	Guanethidine (Ismelin)	20-50 mg orally every 8 hours.	Catecholamine depletion.	Severe postural hypotension, effects of sympathetic blockade.	
SURGERY	Preoperative preparation with iodides or propranolol 10 to 14 days prior to surgery.		Subtotal, total thyroidectomy.	Cosmetic scarring. Hypothyroidism, hypoparathyroidism. Risks of surgery: vocal cord damage, poor wound healing, infection, risks of anesthesia.	Obstruction, choking, malignancy, pregnancy in 1st or 2nd trimester. Contraindication to RAI or thioamides.
RADIOACTIVE iodine	I^{131} or I^{125} radioactive isotope	80 to 100 microcurie per gram of thyroid tissue.	Destruction of the gland.	Hypothyroidism; fear of radiation-induced leukemia, genetic damage, and malignancy; rarely, radiation sickness.	Adults, elderly patients who are poor surgical risks, cardiac disease, patients with a history of prior thyroid surgery, contraindications to thioamide usage.

(continued on following page)

Table 5 (continued)
TREATMENT OF HYPERTHYROIDISM

Modality	Drug	Dose	Mechanism Of Action	Toxicity	Indications
MISCELLANE-OUS AGENTS	Prednisone	50-140 mg daily in divided doses.	Decrease LATS, decrease T_4 levels, suppression of inflammatory processes.	Complications of steroid therapy.	Ophthalmopathy, Thyroid Storm.
	Lithium (Eskalith) 300 mg capsules	600-1200 mg daily in divided doses.	Similar to the effects of iodides in blocking hormone release.	Increased incidence of toxicity with serum levels above 1.5 mEq per liter; toxicity increased with hyponatremia, diuretics; gastrointestinal disturbances, tremor, confusion, slurred speech, seizures, coma.	Alternative to iodides and thioamides as a last resort when other modalities are contraindicated.

41. What is the rationale for the addition of thyroxine to the regimen? What laboratory value might be beneficial in clarifying the need for thyroxine therapy?

Thyroxine was added as an attempt to decrease the size of the goiter which was assumed to be a result of excess TSH production due to large doses of PTU. The reported TT_4 and RT_3U are normal and thus of no value in supporting this assumption. However, an elevated TSH level (Question 2) would help ascertain if this was the primary reason for the goiter. If so, the easiest solution to this problem would be to decrease the dose of PTU; in cases where titration of the proper dose of PTU is difficult, the combination of T_4 and PTU can be used.

42. Briefly discuss the use and significance of the T_3 suppression test in this patient.

The *T_3 suppression test* is used to determine whether the thyroid gland is functioning under normal TSH-dependent negative feedback mechanisms or whether the gland is functioning autonomously (independently of TSH). The administration of a 5 to 7 day course of triiodothyronine (T_3) (75-100 mcg daily) will suppress TSH secretion (decrease RAIU) of a gland operating under normal feedback control while an autonomously functioning gland will not be suppressed. Therefore, by comparing the RAIU before and after T_3 administration it is possible to determine whether the gland is TSH-dependent or autonomous. A fall from the baseline RAIU to 50% or to less than 20% are the two most commonly employed indices of suppression. In BJD's case the results of the suppression test indicate that the gland is not suppressed and is functioning independently of TSH. This lack of return of T_3 suppressibility after treatment with PTU may indicate a poor prognosis for permanent remission of the disease.

McKenzie et al found that suppressibility at the end of a course of antithyroid drug treatment was associated with a relapse rate of 50%, while the relapse rate was 78% among those with nonsuppressible thyroid function (221a). Although Alexander et al found a lower relapse rate (26%) among those with suppressible thyroid function (4a,4c), 10% of their patients with nonsuppressible results remained euthyroid upon discontinuation of drug therapy. Cassidy found that remission could be predicted with 96% accuracy when the RAIU was 30% of baseline or less, and the likelihood of relapse could be predicted with 89% accuracy when the uptake was 50% or more; uptakes of 30 to 59% did not allow a reliable prediction (47).

43. What factors have been identified with remission and relapse after completion of treatment with thioamides?

It is widely believed that permanent remission can be expected in 50 to 60% of the patients treated with antithyroid drugs (322a), but others have found permanent remission to occur much less frequently (167a, 336a, 357). Unfortunately, the number of patients who will remain in remission after drug treatment is probably less than 40%; relapse rates as high as 80% have been reported (336a).

A number of clinical features are associated with a

higher rate of permanent remission. These include small goiters, mild and short duration of symptoms and disease, reduction in goiter size during treatment, and thyroid suppressibility (149, 149a, 312, 321, 336a, 368) (see Question 42). Although further study is needed, the initial absence of HLA-B8 antigen may be an indication that drug treatment will be successful; the presence of HLA-B8 antigen in thyrotoxic patients is associated with a 1.8 times greater probability of relapse after thioamide therapy (167).

Excess dietary iodide has been reported to increase the likelihood of relapse (4,357), but others (312b,336) have been unable to confirm these findings. More study is needed to determine the relationship between iodide intake and the rate of relapse.

It is not clear why some patients remain in permanent remission while others relapse, since antithyroid drugs do not change the basic abnormality present in Graves' disease; even patients who remain euthyroid continue to have mild or subclinical disease (38).

44. A 25-year-old female is referred for evaluation of bulging eyes and swollen neck. She appears clinically euthyroid although she admits that she had palpitations, diarrhea, mild tremor, and menstrual irregularities prior to starting propranolol for high blood pressure. A TT_4 was 28 mcg% and a RT_3U was 40%. How can these findings be explained? How is propranolol used in the treatment of thyrotoxicosis?

Since many of the signs and symptoms of thyrotoxicosis are mediated by sympathetic overactivity (17,194a), propranolol may be masking some of the symptoms of thyrotoxicosis even though the underlying metabolic defect continues unabated (128,359). Propranolol is sometimes used for this purpose while awaiting the effects of thioamides which may require four to six weeks, or after RAI which may require three to six months. In the interim propranolol will decrease nervousness, palpitations, fatigue, weight loss, diaphoresis, heat intolerance, and tremor. Patients generally remain mildly symptomatic and fail to regain weight; thyroid function tests are not affected. Nevertheless, remission of the disease has occurred on propranolol alone and it has been used as the only treatment for thyrotoxicosis (212,222a,269). It is also used as a pre-operative preparation for thyroidectomy (192,200,226,264,268), in the management of thyroid storm (37,65), and in the treatment of thyrotoxicosis during pregnancy (39,42,42a,188a).

CASE J – RAI THERAPY: BJ is a 35-year-old female with newly diagnosed Graves' disease complicated by CHF and angina. Thioamide therapy was discontinued after one week of PTU because of severe granulocytopenia. After a few days treatment with Lugol's solution, 5 drops daily, she received RAI

therapy. Three months later, she is still symptomatic.

45. Was pretreatment prior to RAI therapy indicated? What can be used?

Pretreatment before RAI therapy is recommended in patients with cardiac disease and in severely toxic patients to deplete stored hormones and prevent leakage of hormones from the damaged gland (67e,327). However, iodides should not be used prior to RAI therapy because they decrease the amount of RAI taken up. This effect persists for a few days to a week. Iodides can be instituted one day after RAI therapy if needed to control symptoms of hyperthyroidism. The thioamides can be used prior to RAI therapy to achieve a euthyroid state, but they should be discontinued one week before and for one to seven days after treatment to facilitate optimum uptake and retention of I^{131} by the gland. Goolder et al found that pretreatment with thioamides may lower the cure rate and increase the need for subsequent doses of RAI (113). Propranolol can be used before, during, and after RAI therapy without interfering with its uptake. (See Question 44.) In BJ, the iodides should have been discontinued; propranolol might have been instituted cautiously in light of her CHF.

46. When do the effects of RAI therapy become evident? When should a second dose of RAI be administered?

Although earlier beneficial results may be observed, three to six months are required for attainment of the euthyroid state in approximately 60% of patients treated with a single nonablative dose of RAI; the remainder become euthyroid over one year after two or more doses. This slow onset is a disadvantage, but control can be obtained more quickly by administration of a thioamide, propranolol, or iodides 1 to 14 days after the I^{131} dose (110a). If a second dose is considered, it should not be given before six months, and it is often recommended to wait a full year before repeating I^{131} administration. It is inadvisable to give a second dose before the major effects of the first dose have become apparent. Although the use of iodides prior to RAI may have decreased the amount of I^{131} taken up by this patient's thyroid, it would still be advisable to wait at least six months before a second dose is given.

47. BR is a 54-year-old white female who returns to thyroid clinic after being lost for follow-up for one year. She was initially treated with RAI three years ago but required a repeat dose of RAI a year ago for recurrence of hyperthyroidism. She currently has no other medical problems and is on no medications. She is a mildly obese, puffy-faced female wrapped in several layers of clothing. She complains of fatigue

and lack of energy. Her reflexes are delayed and her skin is cool and dry. What is a likely explanation of her symptoms? Can this complication be prevented?

BR should be evaluated for hypothyroidism secondary to RAI therapy; TT_4, RT_3U, and a TSH level would aid in the diagnosis. The symptoms of hypothyroidism are sometimes attributed to aging, resulting in delay of the correct diagnosis.

Iatrogenic hypothyroidism is the major complication of I^{131} therapy. The incidence of myxedema after RAI is often reported as 7 to 8% but it increases at a constant rate of 2.5% per year and is therefore much higher (40,110a,279). Various reports have determined the incidence of iatrogenic hypothyroidism to be 26% after 7 years (22), 28.8% after 10 years (119), 70% after 10 years (250) and 45% after 14 years (78).

Prevention of iatrogenic hypothyroidism has been directed toward calculation of a dose that will produce neither recurrent hyperthyroidism nor hypothyroidism. Low dose I^{131} therapy (131) as well as different radioactive isotopes have been used in hopes of avoiding these problems (50,279). Although the incidence of hypothyroidism after one year was only 7% when a low dose of I^{131} was given, 54% of the patients remained hyperthyroid (279). Furthermore, hypothyroidism eventually occurred despite the minimal dose employed. The I^{125} isotope has been used to decrease the incidence of hypothyroidism (127, 127a, 216a), but the results have been disappointing. Thus, predictable destruction of the thyroid tissue is impossible. The appearance of iatrogenic hypothyroidism may be inevitable with time, but since it is so easily managed, it may be an acceptable therapeutic endpoint. Since hypothyroidism after RAI therapy is latent and often insidious, patients should be made aware of and closely monitored for subsequent hypothyroidism (40,110a).

CASE K – SURGERY: JL is a 45-year-old male referred for management of Graves' disease and mild proptosis. He has a large visible multinodular goiter which causes a choking sensation and difficulty in swallowing. His symptoms of palpitations, diarrhea, tremors, and heat intolerance have become increasingly bothersome.

48. How should this patient be managed?

The therapy of choice for JL's hyperthyroidism would be surgery, because large goiters usually respond poorly to RAI or antithyroid drug treatment. His difficulty swallowing and choking further support surgery as the treatment of choice (26,140,338a).

Both subtotal and total thyroidectomies have been advocated (48,265,265a,303,338a). Subtotal thyroidectomies have been performed successfully in 90% of patients treated. The difficulty in this approach is re-

moving enough tissue to prevent recurrence of hyperthyroidism while at the same time preventing hypothyroidism. Because any remnant tissue is a potential site for recurrent disease, total thyroidectomy is advocated to eliminate this possibility; however, the occurrence of hypothyroidism is thereby assured. Recurrence of hyperthyroidism after surgery should be treated with RAI because the incidence of surgical complications is increased ten-fold with a second surgery (338a).

The reported incidence of hypothyroidism after thyroidectomy ranges from 4 to 42%. Many patients develop hypothyroidism within one year of surgery, but there is an insidious rise in incidence over the following 10 years (13a,29,119,149). Post-operative adhesions, damage to the parathyroids and laryngeal nerves, infection, poor wound healing, and the risks of anesthesia and surgery itself may decrease the attractiveness of this form of therapy. However, surgery can be a safe and effective form of treatment with little morbidity or mortality when performed by expert hands (55). Patients should be monitored for hypoparathyroidism and hypothyroidism post-operatively.

49. Lugol's solution 5 drops tid was given to JL prior to surgery with rapid amelioration of his symptoms. One week later he returned clinically euthyroid, complaining of a purplish pruritic rash and neck pain. The Lugol's solution was discontinued and the rash regressed. Comment. What is Lugol's solution and what is the rationale for its use? What recommendations do you have for alternative treatment?

JL has experienced an allergic reaction to the Lugol's solution. Lugol's solution is an unpleasant tasting solution containing 5% iodine and 10% potassium iodide; it contains 8 mg of iodide per drop. SSKI (Saturated Solution of Potassium Iodide) is a more palatable and more often used preparation containing 50 mg iodide per drop. Iodide is used as preoperative preparation for surgery because the prepared thyroid gland is less vascular and friable, facilitating a smoother and less complicated surgery. Iodides also help achieve a euthyroid state which is beneficial in decreasing postoperative complications (see Question 30). It is important that the patient be brought to surgery in a euthyroid state to prevent rapid postoperative rises in T_4 levels and subsequent toxic thyroid storm.

The combination of a thioamide and thyroxine is a suitable alternative to iodide. Heiman et al reported low morbidity and mortality rates when a combination of antithyroid drug and thyroxine was used for preoperative preparation (145). They recommend this combination as the method of choice, because the patient is brought to a euthyroid state, the thyroid is free of thyroxine stores, and thyroxine administration prevents TSH stimulation.

Propranolol can be used alone or in combination with the above drugs prior to surgery. There are conflicting reports of its efficacy for this purpose (200, 264), but most are positive (192,226,268). The primary utility is production of a euthyroid state. Propranolol is less effective in decreasing friability and vascularity than are the iodides or thioamides, but it can be used when these other drugs are contraindicated.

50. A 32-year-old woman who is 3 months pregnant is referred for management of her Graves' disease. She is concerned about how the disease and its management may affect the baby. What information can you supply to this lady regarding the treatment of thyrotoxicosis in pregnancy?

Hyperthyroidism has been estimated to occur in 0.02 to 1.4% of the pregnant population (111,320). Pregnancy may ameliorate the symptoms of thyrotoxicosis, but typically the disease is moderate enough to warrant therapy. Untreated, symptomatic thyrotoxicosis may result in a fetal mortality rate of 10% (67e). Special precautions should be taken during therapy to avoid hypothyroidism which is detrimental to both the mother and the fetus. (Also see Question 13.)

The use of radioactive iodine and the chronic administration of iodides during pregnancy are contraindicated since these will cross the placenta to produce fetal goiter (46,102a) and athyreosis (120a); as little as 12 mg of iodide daily has produced neonatal goiters (102a) and neonatal death (42a,102a). Also, long-term use of propranolol should be avoided as it has been associated with fetal respiratory depression, intrauterine growth retardation, impaired response to anoxia, and postnatal bradycardia and hypoglycemia (42,208a,343a).

Either surgery or the thioamides can be used. Surgery should only be performed in the first or second trimester because surgery in the third trimester can precipitate labor (42a). Iodides and propranolol can be used preoperatively without adverse effects on the fetus. PTU may be the thioamide of choice, because maternal ingestion of methimazole has produced scalp defects (228a) and aplasia cutis (232). In order to avoid fetal thyroid suppression, PTU is used in daily doses of 300 mg or less. Neonatal goiter from PTU is unlikely if the doses remain below 100 mg daily (42d). There is no rationale for administering thyroid hormones to prevent fetal goiter since they do not cross the placenta and may make maternal management more difficult (148,306a).

It is advisable to maintain the mother in a mildly hyperthyroid state to avoid fetal hypothyroidism. Laboratory indices should also be in the upper ranges of normal. If the mother is not toxic throughout pregnancy, a normal child can be expected. Occasionally, fetal eye findings and thyrotoxicosis may occur in the newborn.

Both PTU and iodides are excreted in breast milk; hence women taking these agents should be warned against nursing.

51. Bernice is a 12-year-old Chinese female referred for evaluation of hyperkinesis. She has been doing poorly in school because of hyperactivity, nervousness, and difficulty concentrating. Significant physical findings included a wide pulse pressure, fullness of the neck, tachycardia and hyperactivity. The diagnosis of Graves' disease was confirmed by a positive TDI and elevated TT₄. What is the preferred method of treatment for Graves' disease in children? What are the potential risks associated with each modality?

Thyrotoxicosis occurs considerably less frequently in children than in adults. Selection of the optimal method of treatment in children still remains controversial; all three treatment modalities — surgery, thioamides, and RAI — have been advocated (61,163).

Surgery: Several investigators have recommended subtotal thyroidectomies as the treatment of choice (8,142,142a,298) despite the high rate of recurrent hyperthyroidism of 14 to 15% (142). Total thyroidectomies in children have been associated with an unacceptable incidence of parathyroid damage (8). As in the adult, myxedema after surgery is a frequent complication (142,142a,298), incidences as high as 50% have been reported (8). The rapid surgical correction of thyrotoxicosis must be weighed against the risks of a permanent scar, the morbidity of surgery, and mortality. (See Question 48).

Thioamides: In one series, sixteen children out of 34 remained in remission after antithyroid drug therapy (163). The rate of success may approach 70% although figures lower than 59% have been reported (142). Some investigators claim that relapse after drug therapy is less frequent in children (67e); others question the adequacy of medical therapy due to the uncertainty of remissions, problems in patient compliance, and the frequency and severity of adverse effects. The prescribed regimen is similar to that of the adult. A course of PTU 120-175 mg/m² daily or its equivalent is given for one to two years (67e).

Radioactive Iodine (RAI): Although the number of studies using RAI in children is limited, the proposed risks of an increased incidence of thyroid cancer, leukemia, or genetic damage have not yet been demonstrated (72a,274,293). Benign thyroid nodule formation has been observed in children exposed to radiation fallout (141a), but such nodules were not detected in a nine year follow-up of 30 children who received RAI for hyperthyroidism (51). Papillary carcinoma occurred in one of 25 children treated with RAI (182), but other preliminary reports have found no increase in the incidence of thyroid cancer in children treated with RAI. More study is needed. The incidence of hypothyroidism following RAI in children is quite high (46% to 81%) (294,324,324a).

CASE L – OPHTHALMOPATHY OF GRAVES' DISEASE: VS is a 50-year-old lady who first developed "large eyes with stare", weakness, diaphoresis, and thyroid enlargement in 1965. She was diagnosed as having Graves' disease and treated with RAI with some regression of eye symptoms. She is clinically euthyroid although physical examination revealed severe bilateral conjunctival edema and injection, proptosis of the right eye, incomplete lid closure, and decreased visual acuity. She complains of photophobia, tearing, and extreme irritation.

52. Describe the symptoms of the infiltrative ophthalmopathy of Graves' disease.

The eye signs of Graves' disease are the most striking abnormality of this disorder. Fortunately, no more than 1 to 2% of patients are affected (134). The eye involvement can occur at any time and is usually bilateral, although unilateral involvement may occur. Following I^{131} or surgery the ocular symptoms usually subside or remain stable; some cases will progress during the euthyroid period (134,138,362).

It is unknown why the eye and its muscles are attacked in Graves' disease. Histologic examination reveals lymphocytic infiltration, increased mucopolysaccharide content, fat, and water in all retrobulbar tissue. Ocular symptoms include edema, chemosis, excessive lacrimation, photophobia, corneal protrusion (proptosis), scarring, ulceration, extraocular muscle paralysis and loss of eye movements, and blindness from retinal and optic nerve damage (72,129).

53. What considerations and recommendations do you have regarding the management of her ocular symptoms?

Since the pathophysiology of the ocular symptoms is not well understood, treatment is limited to symptomatic and empiric measures once the euthyroid state is achieved (7). Periorbital edema and chemosis are worse in the morning after being in the horizontal position, elevation of the head while in bed and treatment with diuretics and salt restriction may be helpful. Protective glasses are useful in decreasing photophobia and external irritation. Topical corticosteroid drops are effective in decreasing local irritation, but they should be used cautiously since they increase the risk of infection. Ocular irritants such as smoke and dust should be avoided. Incomplete lid closure predisposes to corneal scarring and ulceration, so lubri-

cant eyedrops containing methylcellulose should be applied several times daily and at night to keep the bulbs moist. Taping the eyelids shut at night may prevent drying and scarring. Lateral surgical closure of the lids (tarsorrhaphy) may be required to improve lid closure.

When the ophthalmopathy is severe and progressive, a more aggressive approach should be taken. Systemic corticosteroids have been used with both dramatic effect and marginal results in the emergency treatment of progressive exophthalmos with decreasing visual acuity. Prednisone doses of 35 to 80 mg daily have been effective, but doses as large as 100 to 140 mg daily may be required (6,33). X-ray therapy to the pituitary (21,103,150) and to the orbit (74, 159a, 206, 337) have shown both beneficial and nonbeneficial results. Some have recommended x-ray therapy to the orbit in conjunction with systemic steroids as the initial treatment of choice.

When the above measures and thyroid ablation fail to arrest the progression of visual loss and exophthalmos, then surgical decompression should be considered.

CASE M – THYROID STORM: A 48-year-old white woman was admitted to the hospital with a three week history of fatigability, weakness, dyspnea on exertion, shortness of breath, and palpitations. One year prior to admission she began noticing a preference for cold weather and an increase in nervousness and emotional lability. After her husband died a few days ago, she experienced increased irritability, insomnia, tremor, and a 104°F fever which she attributed to an upper respiratory tract infection. She denies any current medication. On admission a TT₄ was found to be 30 mcg%.

54. What do these symptoms indicate? What is the pathogenesis?

It appears that the patient is experiencing thyroid storm, a life threatening medical emergency (244, 289, 355). The incidence is 2 to 8%, and immediate treatment should be initiated to decrease the high mortality rate. (See Question 55.)

The pathogenesis of storm is not well understood, but the condition has been described as an "exaggerated" or decompensated form of thyrotoxicosis. The term "decompensated" implies failure of body systems to adequately resist the effects of thyrotoxicosis. It cannot be completely attributed soley to the release of massive quantities of hormones which may occur after surgery or following RAI therapy. Catecholamines also have an important role; the increased quantities of thyroid hormone in conjunction with increased sympathetic and adrenal output contribute to many of the manifestations of storm. Although thyroid hormones seem to have an independent action, amelioration of many of the symptoms of hyperthyroidism may be accomplished by catecholamine blocking agents such as reserpine and guanethidine.

The clinical manifestations of thyroid storm (212a) are the acute onset of high fever (sine qua non), tachycardia, tachypnea, and the following organ systems involvement: cardiovascular—tachycardia, pulmonary edema, hypertension, and shock; central nervous system — tremor, emotional lability, confusion, psychosis, apathy, stupor, and coma; gastrointestinal — diarrhea, abdominal pain, nausea and vomiting; and liver — enlargement, jaundice, and nonspecific elevations of bilirubin and prothrombin time. Hyperglycemia was a clinical finding in 12 out of 18 episodes (212a).

55. How should thyroid storm be treated?

Accurate, continuous, and immediate treatment of storm may decrease the mortality tremendously. Mortality rates as low as 7% and survival rates as high as 50% have been reported (67e).

Treatment of thyroid storm should be directed against four major areas (166):

Decrease in the synthesis and release of hormones: Large doses of thioamides, either PTU 600 to 1200 mg daily or methimazole 30 to 60 mg daily, should be given in divided doses. Theoretically, PTU may act more rapidly since it can prevent the peripheral conversion of T_4 to T_3, a dominant source of the hormone. Iodides, which rapidly block further secretion of thyroxine, should be given at least one hour after thioamide administration so as to avoid blocking the latter's therapeutic effect. Iodides can be administered as an intravenous drip of sodium iodide (NaI) 1 to 3 gm over 24 hours or orally as Lugol's solution 30 drops daily. Such a combination may ameliorate symptoms within one day.

Reversal of the peripheral effects of the hormones and the catecholamines: Depleting agents such as reserpine and guanethidine are effective in decreasing tachycardia, agitation, and tremulousness. Reserpine in doses of 1 to 3 mg IM/IV every 8 hours (30,44,69) or guanethidine 20 to 50 mg orally every eight hours can be tried (102,212a). Intravenous administration is preferred over intramuscular injection since absorption from IM sites is poor if circulatory collapse is present. Propranolol has been used with success in decreasing the tachycardia and agitation (266,359. It may prove to be the agent of choice, since it has been reported to be effective in patients refractory to reserpine and guanethidine (37,65).

Supportive treatment of vital functions: This may include sedation, oxygen, intravenous glucose, vitamins, treatment of infections with antibiotics, digitalization to maintain the cardiac status, rehydration, and

treatment of hyperpyrexia with cooling blankets, sponge baths and the judicious use of antipyretics. If hypoadrenalism is suspected, hydrocortisone 100 to 200 mg every six hours intravenously should be given (287). Pharmacologic doses of steroids acutely depress serum T_3 levels and may be beneficial in storm (67c,77,362a,367).

Elimination of the precipitating causes of storm: Factors which have been associated with the induction of thyroid storm include infection (most common), trauma, inadequate preparation prior to thyroidectomies, surgical operations, stress, diabetic acidosis, pregnancy, emboli, abrupt discontinuation of antithyroid medications, drug therapy, and RAI therapy.

56. RN is a 30-year-old nurse who complains of nervousness, fatigue, heat intolerance, palpitations, and irregular menses. Physical examination revealed a nonpalpable thyroid, brisk deep tendon reflexes, and sweaty, flushed skin. She denies any ingestion of medications or pain upon swallowing. Laboratory data show a TT₄ of 15 mcg%, a RT₃U of 40%, a RAIU of 3% at 24 hours, negative thyroid antibodies, and a sedimentation rate of 10 mm/hr. What is your assessment of the situation?

The classic presentation of thyrotoxicosis without goiter and a minimal RAIU in a patient with access to thyroid hormone raises the possibility of thyrotoxicosis factitia (self-administration of thyroid hormone). The low sedimentation rate and lack of pain or swelling rules out the possibility of subacute thyroiditis (114, 137). (See Question 63.)

57. MB is a 56-year-old white male who complains of sluggishness, cold intolerance, fatigue, and a "run-down" feeling which doctors have attributed to the depressive phase of his illness. He had previously been well controlled on imipramine 300 mg daily but lithium carbonate 400 mg daily was added four months ago because of unreasonable mirthfullness and uncontrollable gift buying tendencies. On physical examination, a puffy face and a large goiter were prominent. What is happening?

Although the incidence of goiter and hypothyroidism in the manic depressive population is not known, the possibility of lithium- and possibly impramine-induced hypothyroidism should be considered. Thyroid function tests should be drawn to document these suspicions.

The antithyroid effects of lithium were first demonstrated in the management of manic depressive patients. Lithium acts like the iodides by inhibiting the release of hormonal and nonhormonal iodine from the gland (323a,334,334a). It may also affect the pituitary-thyroid axis (190). The exact mechanism of lithium's effect on the gland has not been clarified although it is known that lithium is highly concentrated by the gland. The effects of lithium on indices of thyroid function include a low PBI and TT_4 (426), elevated TSH levels (42b,191), and an increased RAIU (42b,58,304).

Lithium-induced goiter with (45, 89, 202, 285, 313, 313a) or without (301) hypothyroidism appears in a small percentage of the population after 5 months to 2 years of therapy. The goiters respond to discontinuation of lithium or to suppression with thyroid hormone despite continuation of lithium therapy. In two patients the goiter had to be surgically removed due to pressure symptoms (301).

In this case, imipramine may be having a synergistic effect with lithium, because antithyroid effects have also been attributed to imipramine (89, 92, 275, 275a, 275b).

In most cases of lithium-induced thyroid abnormality a prior history of compromised thyroid function, such as thyroiditis or strong family history of thyroid disease, was present (285,304,313a). Therefore, baseline TT_4, RT_3U, antibodies, RAIU, and scan should be obtained prior to the initiation of lithium therapy. Patients should also be questioned regarding a family history of thyroid disease, and the concurrent use of tricyclic antidepressants should be noted.

58. CD is a 64-year-old woman who was admitted to the hospital in a state of florid thyrotoxicosis. Her only other medical problem is manic depressive illness which has been well controlled on lithium for 10 years. Prior to the onset of hyperthyroidism she had stopped the lithium because of feelings of fatigue which she attributed to the drug. She slowly noticed development of nervousness and tremor and finally frank thyrotoxicosis. Could lithium be responsible for the induction of thyrotoxicosis in this lady?

Lithium is known to cause goiter and hypothyroidism (Question 57) but paradoxically it has also been associated with the development of thyrotoxicosis (11,64,291). Like iodides, lithium inhibits hormone release from the thyroid (334,334a). Therefore, it is likely that lithium could have been suppressing frank hyperthyroidism which became evident after lithium withdrawal.

59. Has lithium been used in the management of thyrotoxicosis?

Lithium's antithyroid action is comparable to that of the thioamides (185,191,334,334a). After one to two weeks of lithium therapy, T_4 levels have been reported to decline 20 to 35% (185,191,334,334a). Lithium's effect is enhanced by the concurrent administration of thioamides because they block accumulation of iodides which would diminish lithium's effect on the gland (334,334a). Although escape was not seen when lithium was used alone for 6 months (191), it is rec-

ommended that thioamides be used concomitantly to prevent iodide buildup and escape (334,334a).

Lithium has been recommended as an adjunct to RAI therapy since it does not interfere with RAI uptake and increases the retention of RAI by the thyrotoxic gland by inhibiting its rate of disappearance (42b, 105, 342). Burrow et al found that the thyroidal half-life of I^{131} is increased by lithium (42b). This would be beneficial in localizing the dose of radiation to the gland.

Because of the limited clinical experience with lithium in thyrotoxicosis, its use should be restricted to situations where rapid suppression of thyroid hormone secretion is needed and where iodides are contraindicated. It should not be considered as an alternative to thioamides but rather as an adjunct.

60. A 54-year-old Vietnamese male presents with a 5 to 6 month history of weakness, fatigue, tremor, heat intolerance, and palpitations. On physical examination a 40 gram multinodular gland was noted. He denies any family history of thyroid disease or ingestion of any thyroid medication. The only interesting finding was that the onset of his complaints occurred after an intravenous pyelogram (IVP). Could the iodine from the IVP be responsible for his symptoms? Have iodides produced hyperthyroidism?

Iodide-induced hyperthyroidism, known as Jod-Basedow phenomenon, was first described in the 1800's when patients residing in iodide deficient areas became toxic upon adequate iodide supplementation (83). Other reports have appeared since (57,328,350). Both T_3 toxicosis and classical T_4 toxicosis have occurred following iodide ingestion (3,248a) or injection of roentgenographic contrast media (29a,313b).

Although it has been presumed that both iodide deficiency and large multinodular goiter are essential for the production of Jod-Basedow phenomen, it has also been reported among patients residing in iodine sufficient areas (344) and in patients with normal glands (297) following the administration of iodide. Large doses of iodides should be avoided in patients with nontoxic multinodular goiter.

61. MW is a 37-year-old male who complains of polyuria, polydipsia, palpitations, heat intolerance, and muscle weakness. He has a family history of diabetes and thyroid disease. Laboratory indices show an FTI of 7, an FBS (fasting blood sugar) of 330, and 3+ glucosuria. Treatment was initiated with tolbutamide 500 mg four times a day and PTU 300 mg every six hours. What is the relationship between diabetes and thyrotoxicosis? How will this affect his management?

Thyrotoxicosis can activate or intensify diabetes by increasing metabolism and subsequent insulin demand. Despite the increased need, insulin's effect on carbohydrate metabolism is enhanced (81). Diabetes may disappear after return to a euthyroid state if thyrotoxicosis was the precipitating factor. Consequently, the diabetes should be reassessed as the euthyroid state is approached (67e).

62. MW returns to the clinic 8 weeks later concerned about the size of his goiter which seems larger to him. He also compalins of extreme fatigue, sweating, dizziness, and depression which he attributes to his personal problems. Laboratory values show an FTI of 0.8, a TSH of 22 microIU, and an FBS of 70 mg%. What is your assessment of his complaints and laboratory findings?

MW is hypothyroid as evidenced by his laboratory findings. Thyroid oversuppression has occurred because the large initial dose of PTU was not decreased after 4 to 6 weeks. Large doses of sulfonylureas inhibit thyroid hormone formation as evidenced by impairment of RAI uptake (33a). This effect has been observed with large doses of chlorpropramide (317) but not with tolbutamide in daily doses of 1 to 2 gm. Hypothyroidism appears to be more common among diabetics treated with sulfonylureas than those treated by other means (161). (Also see the *Diabetes* chapter.)

MW's complaints of dizziness, sweating and fatigue suggest a hypoglycemic reaction which is confirmed by his low blood sugar. Hypoglycemia may occur in hypothyroid patients treated with insulin or hypoglycemic agents because hypothyroidism delays the metabolism of insulin (81). The tolbutamide should be discontinued and his diabetes should be re-evaluated after correction of his hypothyroid state.

63. HS is a 34-year-old woman who has suffered for the past three weeks with nervousness, palpitations, weight loss, and tremor unassociated with eye symptoms. She had similar symptoms four years ago which cleared spontaneously after a few months. On physical examination her thyroid was diffusely enlarged, firm, without nodules, and the left lobe was slightly tender. There was no family history of thyroid disease or history of irradiation to the gland. Thyroid function tests included the following: PBI 17 mcg%, TT$_4$ 9 mcg%, RT$_3$U 25%, RAIU 2% at 24 hours, and negative thyroid antibodies. Comment.

The clinical findings of hyperthyroidism, a tender or painful gland, an elevated PBI out of proportion to the TT$_4$, a low RAI uptake, and a history of spontaneous remission strongly suggest the possibility of subacute thyroiditis (DeQuervain's thyroiditis), an inflammatory condition of the thyroid (121,353a).

The etiology may be viral since it frequently follows an upper respiratory infection or sore throat. Patients with subacute thyroiditis but without any evidence of a viral infection have significant titers of viral antibodies against Coxsackie, adenovirus, influenza, and mumps. Of these, the Coxsackie antibodies are the most often found and changes in their titers most closely approximate the course of the disease (84,353b).

The alterations seen in the thyroid function can be explained by the pathophysiology of the disease state. The inflammatory destruction of the gland results in the leakage and release of iodoproteins and other iodinated proteins from the colloids which cause an increase of T$_4$ and T$_3$ levels. The PBI is elevated out of proportion to the T$_4$ because most of the liberated material is iodoprotein other than thyroxine. The RAIU is low and can approach zero because of the inability of the damaged thyroid to pick up iodine. This explains the paradox of the increased TT$_4$, PBI, and decreased RAIU. Hypothyroidism with elevations of TSH can occur if the gland becomes hormone-depleted and is unable to synthesize more. The disease usually remits within 1 to 2 weeks although it may continue with fluctuating intensity for 3 to 6 weeks. Recurrence is common and thyroid function usually returns to normal although permanent hypothyroidism may occur (374).

Treatment is mainly symptomatic and consists of rest and analgesics for the pain. T$_3$ replacement can also be given to prevent hypothyroidism and to suppress further TSH stimulation of the inflamed gland. If symptoms do not subside and the gland remains inflamed; prednisone 20 mg daily for one to two weeks can be given and then tapered.

64. HK is a 20-year-old female who noted a lump in the right side of her neck. There is no history of radiation, no family history of thyroid disease, no local symptoms, and no symptoms suggestive of hypo- or hyperthyroidism. The right lobe of the thyroid is occupied by a 3 x 3 cm firm, immovable nodule while the left lobe is barely palpable. All thyroid function tests are within normal limits although the gland is not suppressible. A scan shows a large "hot" nodule occupying the right lobe and a nonexistent left lobe. What is a "hot" nodule? How should this patient be managed?

"Hot" nodule is a term used to describe an area of the thyroid which is concentrating iodine or "hyperfunctioning" as shown on scan. It appears as an area of greater density than the rest of the gland. The hyperfunctioning autonomous nodule typically suppresses activity in the remainder of the gland, but it need not produce clinical or chemical evidence of hyperthyroidism and may remain unchanged for years. Some nodules may develop into toxic goiters causing overt symptoms of toxicosis. Most "hot" nodules are benign although malignancies have been reported (67d,100,159,178,228).

Treatment of the "hot" nodule will depend upon the

existing clinical situation. If the "hot" nodule has suppressed the other lobe of the thyroid, is not causing toxic symptoms, and is the only source of thyroid production, the patient should be left alone and closely monitored for signs of toxicity (41). If the other parts of the gland have not been suppressed by the functioning "hot" nodule, thyroid suppression therapy may be tried to shrink the nodule. A toxic "hot" nodule is treated either by surgery or radioactive iodine ablation. Since the normal thyroid tissue is suppressed, the RAI will be concentrated only by the "hot" nodule, sparing the suppressed tissue. After treatment, the suppressed tissue should begin functioning again.

65. SA is a 29-year-old female with a left thyroid nodule discovered on routine physical examination. She has no history of neck radiation, a negative family history of thyroid disease and no symptoms suggestive of hypo- or hyperthyroidism. A hard, nontender 3 x 4 cm nodule occupies the left lobe of the gland. Thyroid function tests are within normal limits. The scan shows a cold nodule; the echo reveals a solid mass ruling out the possibility of a cyst. Antibodies are negative. What is a "cold" nodule? How should this patient be managed?

A *"cold" nodule* is a "hypofunctioning" area of the thyroid which fails to collect radioiodine. It is depicted on the scan as a lighter or less dense area as compared to the rest of the gland. The possible considerations include Hashimoto's thyroiditis, benign adenomas, cysts, and malignant tumors. The absence of antibodies and solidarity of the mass by echo rules out the possibility of cyst or Hashimoto's thyroiditis. Most "cold" nodules turn out to be benign adenomas rather than cancers. The incidence of malignancy in a cold nodule varies between 10 and 20% (224). A history of irradiation increases the likelihood of cancer in a nodule and favors surgery (281). The nature of the nodule is important. Fixation of the nodule to the strap muscles or trachea, a hard bulging characteristic, any pain or tenderness, or voice hoarseness may indicate malignancy (124).

The appropriate treatment depends on a number of judgmental factors made by the physician and the patient. Absolute guidelines are not available although the following indicators can be used (376). Recent growth of a solid nodule, presence of disturbing symptoms such as a choking sensation, a history of irradiation to the neck and upper head as a child, males, young age (under 30), a positive family history of thyroid disease, or failure of regression of the nodule on thyroxine are all signs which favor surgery (124). Nodules in women over 30 without disturbing local signs, with no known history of radiation exposure, with no recent growth, or of a long standing nature are more likely to be benign and can be followed or excised surgically. Suppression therapy with thyroxine to decrease TSH secretion may shrink the nodule. However, a decrease in size does not eliminate the possibilty of malignancy (109,151). A positive response, i.e. shrinkage of the nodule, should be seen after a trial of thyroxine 0.2 mg daily for 3 to 6 months; otherwise surgery should be strongly considered.

66. HT is a 25-year-old white female who had thymic radiation at age 7. She is asymptomatic, has no family history of thyroid disease, and has never taken thyroid. On physical examination the thyroid was palpable and no nodules were found. What is the significance of irradiation to the thyroid at a young age? How should this patient be managed?

It is now known that there is an association between external radiation administered to the head, neck, and upper thorax of infants, children, and adolescents and the subsequent development of abnormal and neoplastic changes in the thyroid gland. Any irradiation above 50 rads to the area of the thyroid during childhood should be of concern. Numerous articles report a 1 to 7% incidence of neoplastic changes occurring 10 to 30 years after the initial irradiation (53, 76, 147, 281). Other abnormalities found include Hashimoto's thyroiditis, benign adenomas, and Graves' disease. All patients with a history of thyroidal irradiation during childhood should be evaluated for thyroid abnormalities. Examination of the thyroid gland manually, as well as a thyroid scan, antibodies, TT_4, RT_3U, and RAIU should be performed. In the absence of any abnormality the patient should be re-evaluated yearly.

REFERENCES

1. Abuid J et al: Triiodothyronine and thyroxine in hyperthyroidism — comparison of the acute changes during therapy with antithyroid agents. J Clin Invest 54:201, 1974.
2. Adams DD et al: Evidence to suggest that LATS protector stimulates the human thyroid gland. J Clin Endocrinol Metab 33:47, 1971.
3. Ahmed M et al: Triiodothyroxine thyrotoxicosis following iodide ingestion. J Clin Endocrinol Metab 38:574, 1974.
4. Alexander WD et al: Influence of iodine intake after treatment with antithyroid drugs. Lancet 2:866, 1965.
4a. Alexander WD et al: Thyroidal suppressibility after stopping long term treatment of thyrotoxicosis with antithyroid drugs. Metab 18:58, 1968.
4b. Alexander WD et al: Sequential assessment during drug therapy of thyrotoxicosis. Clin Endoc 2:43, 1973.
4c. Alexander WD et al: Prediction of the long term results of antithyroid drug therapy for thyrotoxicosis. J Clin Endocrinol Metab 30:540, 1970.
5. Amrhein JA et al: Granulocytopenia lupus-like syndrome and other complications of propylthiouracil therapy. J Ped 76:54, 1970.
6. Apers RC et al: Prednisone treatment in Endocrine Ophthalmopathy. Mod Probl Ophthal 14:414, 1975.
7. Aranow H et al: Management of thyrotoxicosis in patients with

ophthalmopathy—antithyroid regimen determined primarily by ocular manifestations. J Clin Endocrinol Metab 25:1, 1965.

8. Arnold MB et al: Concerning the choice of therapy for childhood hyperthyroidism. Ped 21:47, 1958.

8a. Astwood EB: The use of antithyroid drugs during pregnancy. J Clin Endocrinol Metab 11:1045, 1951.

9. Austen FK et al: Salicylates and thyroid function — depression of thyroid function. J Clin Invest 37:1131, 1958.

10. Ayd FJ: Prolonged perphenazine therapy and thyroid function. Am J Psych 120:592, 1963.

11. Bafaqueen HH et al: Lithium and thyrotoxicosis. Lancet 1:409, 1976.

12. Bahley RH et al: Thyroid crisis. Surg Gynecol Obstet 59:41, 1934.

13. Barnes HV et al: A simple test for selecting the thioamide schedule in thyrotoxicosis. J Clin Endocrin Metab 35:250, 1972.

13a. Barnes HV et al: Choosing thyroidectomy in hyperthyroidism. Surg Clin N Am 54:289, 1974.

14. Bartels EC: Agranulocytosis during propylthiouracil therapy. Am J Med 5:48, 1948.

15. Bastenie PA et al: Clinical and pathological significance of asymptomatic atrophic thyroiditis — a condition of latent hypothyroidism. Lancet 1:915, 1967.

15a. Bastenie PA et al: Preclinical hypothyroidism — a risk factor for coronary heart disease. Lancet 1:203, 1971.

16. Becker CE et al: Hepatitis from methimazole during adrenal steroid treatment for malignant exophthalmos. JAMA 206:1787, 1968.

17. Becker FO et al: Sympathetic blockade in hyperthyroidism. Arch Int Med 129:967, 1974.

18. Becker KL et al: Connective tissue disease and symptoms associated with Hashimoto's thyroiditis. NEJM 268:277, 1963.

19. Beebee RT et al: Fatal agranulocytosis during treatment of toxic goiter with propylthiouracil. Ann Int Med 34:1035, 1951.

20. Begg TB et al: Iodide goiter and hypothyroidism. Quart J Med 32:251, 1963.

21. Beierwaltes WH: Irradiation of the pituitary in the treatment of malignant exophthalmos. J Clin Endocrinol Metab 11:512, 1951.

21a. Beierwaltes WH et al: Congenital hypothyroidism. J Mich State Soc 58:927, 1959.

22. Beling U et al: Incidence of hypothyroidism and recurrence following I^{131} treatment of hyperthyroidism. Acta Radiol 56:275, 1961.

23. Benson PF et al: Emotion and nonspecific infection as possible aetiological factors in Graves disease. Lancet 2:196, 1968.

24. Bernstein RS et al: Intermittent therapy with L-thyroxine. NEJM 281:1444, 1969.

25. Best MM et al: A lupus-like syndrome following propylthiouracil administration. J Ky Med Assoc 62:47, 1964.

26. Black BM: Surgery for Graves disease. Mayo Clin Proc 47:966, 1972.

27. Blizzard JJ et al: Prolongation of the PR-interval as a manifestation of thyrotoxicosis. JAMA 173:1845, 1960.

28. Blizzard RM et al: Maternal autoimmunization to thyroid as a probable cause of athyreotic cretinism. NEJM 263:327, 1960.

29. Blum BM: Myxedema coma. Am J Med Sci 264:433, 1972.

29a. Blum M et al: Hyperthyroidism after iodinated contrast medium. NEJM 291:24, 1974.

30. Blumenthal M et al: Carcinoid syndrome following reserpine therapy in thyrotoxicosis. Arch Int Med 116:819, 1965.

31. Boas NF et al: Hereditary exophthalmic goiter — report of eleven cases in one family. J Clin Endocrinol Metab 6:575, 1940.

31a. Boyle JA et al: Phenomenon of iodide inhibition in various states of thyroid function. J Clin Endocrinol Metab 25:125, 1965.

32. Braverman LE et al: Changes in thyroidal function during adaption to large doses of iodides. J Clin Invest 42:1216, 1963.

32a. Braverman LE et al: Enhanced susceptibility to iodide myxedema in Hashimoto's. J Clin Endocrinol Metab 32:515, 1971.

32b. Braverman LE et al: Induction of myxedema by iodide in patients euthyroid after radioactive or surgical treatment of diffuse toxic goiter. NEJM 281:816, 1969.

32c. Braverman LE et al: The metabolism of thyroid hormones as related to protein binding. J Chron Dis 14:484, 1961.

32d. Braverman LE et al: Conversion of thyroxine (I_4) to triiodothyronine (T_3) in athyreotic human subjects. J Clin Invest 49:855, 1970.

32e. Braverman LE et al: Effects of replacement doses of sodium L-thyroxine on the peripheral metabolism of thyroxial and

triiodothyronine in man. J Clin Invest 52:1010, 1973.

33. Brown J et al: Adrenal steroid therapy of severe infiltrative ophthalmopathy of Graves Disease. Am J Med 34:786, 1963.

33a. Brown J et al: Mechanism of antithyroid effect of sulfonylurea in the rat. Endocrin 63:473, 1958.

34. Brunn E: Exophthalmic goiter developing after treatment with thyroid preparations. Acta Med Scand 122:13, 1945.

35. Buccino RA et al: Influence of the thyroid state on the intrinsic contractile properties and energy stores of the myocardium. J Clin Invest 46:1669, 1967.

36. Buchanan WW et al: Association of thyrotoxicosis and autoimmune thyroiditis. Brit Med J 1:843, 1961.

37. Buckle RM: Treatment of thyroid crisis by beta adrenergic blockage. Acta Endocrin 57:168, 1968.

38. Buerklin EM et al: Pituitary — thyroid regulation in euthyroid patients with Graves disease previously treated with antithyroid drugs. J Clin Endocrinol Metab 43:419, 1976.

39. Bullock JL et al: Treatment of thyrotoxicosis during pregnancy with propranolol. Am J Ob Gyn 121:242, 1975.

40. Burke et al: Hypothyroidism after treatment with sodium iodide ^{131}I. JAMA 210:1051, 1969.

41. Burman KD et al: Clinical observations on the solitary autonomous thyroid nodule. Arch Int Med 134:915, 1974.

42. Burrow GN: Hyperthyroidism during pregnancy. NEJM 298:150, 1978.

42a. Burrow GN: The thyroid in pregnancy. Med Clin N Am 59:1089, 1975.

42b. Burrow GN et al: Effect of lithium on thyroid function. J Clin Endocrinol Metab 32:647, 1971.

42c. Burrow GN et al: Innunosuppressive therapy for the eye changes of Graves disease. J Clin Endocrinol Metab 31:307, 1970.

42d. Burrow GN: Neonatal goiter after maternal propylthiouracil therapy. J Clin Invest 25:403, 1965.

43. Burstein et al: Myocardial infarction in thyrotoxicosis. Acta Med Scand 166:379, 1960.

44. Canary JJ et al: Effects of oral and intramuscular administration of reserpine in thyrotoxicosis. NEJM 257:435, 1957.

45. Candy J: Severe hypothyroidism — an early complication of lithium therapy. Brit Med J 3:277, 1972.

46. Carswell F et al: Congenital goiter and hypothyroidism produced by maternal ingestion of iodides. Lancet 1:1241, 1970.

47. Cassidy CE: Use of a thyroid suppression test as a guide to prognosis of hyperthyroidism treated with antithyroid drugs. J Clin Endocrinol Metab 25:155, 1965.

48. Catz B et al: Total thyroidectomy in the management of thyrotoxic and euthyroid Graves disease. Am J Surg 118:434, 1969.

49. Cetina JA et al: Antinuclear antibodies and propylthiouracil therapy. JAMA 220:1012, 1972.

50. Cevallos JL et al: Low-dosage ^{131}I therapy of thyrotoxicosis (diffuse goiters). NEJM 290:141, 1974.

51. Chapman EM et al: Use of radiodine in the diagnosis and treatment of hyperthyroidism — 10 years experience. Med 34:261, 1955.

52. Chevalley J et al: A four year study of the treatment of hyperthyroidism with methimazole. J Clin Endocrinol Metab 14:948, 1954.

53. Clark DE: Association of irradiation with cancer of the thyroid in children and adolescents. JAMA 159:1007, 1955.

54. Cohen RD et al: Exercise electrocardiogram in myxedema. Brit Med J 2:327, 1966.

55. Colcock BP et al: The mortality and morbidity of thyroid surgery. Surg Gynec Obstet 114:131, 1962.

56. Colwell AR et al: Propythiouracil-induced agranulocytosis, toxic hepatitis and death. JAMA 148:639, 1952.

57. Connolly RJ et al: Increase in thyrotoxicosis in edemic goiter area after iodination of bread. Lancet 1:500, 1970.

58. Cooper TB et al: Preliminary report of longitudinal study on the effects of lithium on iodine metabolism. Curr Ther Res 11:603, 1969.

58a. Cotton GE et al: Suppression of thyrotropin (h-TSH) in serum of patients with myxedema of varying etiology treated with thyroid hormones. NEJM 285:529, 1971.

59. Craig FA et al: Serum creatinine phosphokinase activity in altered thyroid states. J Clin Endocrinol Metab 25:723, 1965.

60. Cranswick EH et al: Two year follow up study of protein binding iodine elevation in patients receiving perphenazine. Am J Psych 122:300, 1965.

60a. Cranswick EH et al: An abnormal thyroid finding produced by a phenothiazine. JAMA 181:554, 1962.

61. Crile G Jr et al: Radioactive iodine treatment of Graves disease. Results in 32 children under 16 years of age. Am J Dis Child 110:501, 1965.

61a. Croke AR et al: Agranulocytosis occurring during methimazole (Tapazole) therapy. JAMA 148:45, 1952.

62. Crowley WF Jr et al: Noninvasive evaluation of cardiac function in hypothyroidism. NEJM 296:1, 1977.

63. Croxson MS et al: Serum digoxin in patients with thyroid disease. Brit Med J 3:566, 1975.

64. Cubitt T: Lithium and thyrotoxicosis. Lancet 1:1247, 1976.

65. Das G et al: Treatment of thyrotoxic storm with intravenous administration of propranolol. Ann Int Med 70:985, 1969.

66. Davis PJ: Factors affecting the determination of the serum protein bound iodine. Am J Med 40:98, 1966.

66a. Dawson MA et al: Anemia in hypothyroidism. South Med J 63:966, 1970.

67. Degroot LJ: Thyroid and the heart. Mayo Clin Proc 47:864, 1972.

67a. Degroot LJ et al: The thyroid state and the cardiovascular system. Mod Concepts Cardiovas Dis 38:23, 1969.

67b. Degroot LJ et al: Hashimoto's thyroiditis a genetically conditioned disease. NEJM 267(267, 1962.

67c. Degroot LJ et al: Dexamethasone suppression of serum T_3 and T_4. J Clin Endocrinol Metab 42:976, 1976.

67d. Degroot LJ et al: Thyroid carcinoma and radiation — a Chicago epidemic. JAMA 225:487, 1973.

67e. Degroot LJ et al: The Thyroid and its Diseases. 4th ed., J Wiley & Sons, New York, 1975.

68. Derubertis F et al: Impaired water excretion in myxedema. Am J Med 51:41, 1971.

69. Dillon PT et al: Reserpine in thyrotoxic crisis. NEJM 283:1020, 1970.

70. Dingle PR et al: The incidence of thyroglobulin antibodies and thyroid enlargement in a general practice in north east England. Clin Exp Immunol 1:277, 1966.

71. Dische S: The radioisotope scan applied to the detection of carcinoma in thyroid swellings. Cancer 17:473, 1964.

72. Dobyns BM: Present concepts of the pathologic physiology of exophthalmos. J Clin Endocrinol Metab 10:1202, 1950.

72a. Dobnyyns BM et al: Malignant and benign neoplasms of the thyroid in patients treated for hyperthyroidism — a report of the cooperative thyrotoxicosis therapy follow up study. J Clin Endocrinol Metab 38:976, 1974.

73. Doherty JE et al: Digoxin metabolism in hypo- and hyperthyroidism. Ann Int Med 64:489, 1966.

74. Donaldson SS et al: Super voltage orbital radiotherapy for Graves ophthalmopathy. J Clin Endocrinol Metab 37:276, 1973.

75. Doniach D et al: Autoimmunity in pernicious anemia and thyroiditis — a family study. Ann N Y Acad Sci 124:605, 1965.

76. Duffy BJ Jr et al: Cancer of the thyroid in children — a report of 28 cases. J Clin Endocrinol Metab 10:1296, 1950.

77. Duick DS et al: Effect of single dose dexamethasone on the concentration of serum triiodothyroxine in man. J Clin Endocrinol Metab 39:1151, 1974.

78. Dunn JT et al: Rising incidence of hypothyroidism after radioactive iodine therapy to thyrotoxicosis. NEJM 271:1037, 1964.

79. Eggen PC et al: The histological appearance of hyperfunctioning thyroids following various pre-operative treatments. Acta Pathol Micro Scand 81:16, 1973.

80. Eisenmenger WJ et al: Leukopenia following the use of propylthiouracil. JAMA 135:510, 1947.

81. Engbring NA: Current treatment of hyperthyroidism. Wisc Med J 67:265, 1968.

82. Engel AG: Neuromuscular manifestations of Graves disease. Mayo Clin Proc 47:919, 1972.

82a. Engel AG: Thyroid function and periodic paralysis. Am J Med 30:327, 1961.

83. Erman AM et al: Modification of thyroid function induced by chronic administration of I_2 — in presence of autonomous thyroid tissue. Acta Endocrin 70:463, 1972.

84. Eylan E et al: Mumps virus and subacute thyroidism. Lancet 1:1062, 1957.

85. Fairhurst BJ et al: Hyperthyroidism after cholecytography. Brit Med J, 3:630, 1975.

86. Fatourechi V et al: Hyperthyroidism associated with histologic Hashimoto's thyroiditis. Mayo Clin Proc 46:682, 1971.

87. Fedotin MS: Liver disease caused by propylthiouracil. Arch Int Med 135:319, 1975.

88. Fein HG et al: Anemia in thyroid disease. Med Clin N Am 59:1133, 1975.

89. Fieve RR et al: Lithium and thyroid function in manic depressive psychosis. Am J Psych 125:527, 1968.

90. Fischer DA et al: Acute release of thyrotropin in newborn. J Clin Invest 48:1670, 1969.

91. Fischer MG: Methimazole induced jaundice. JAMA 223:1028, 1973.

92. Fischetti B: Pharmacological influences on thyroid activity. Arch Ital Sci Farmacol 12:33, 1962.

93. Fleisher GA et al: Serum creatine kinase lactic dehydrogenase and glutamic-oxalacetic transaminase in thyroid diseases and pregnancy. Mayo Clin Proc 40:300, 1965.

93a. Fleischer N et al: Preliminary observations on the effect of synthetic thyrotropin releasing factor on plasma thyrotropin levels in man. J Clin Endocrinol Metab 31:109, 1970.

94. Forester CF: Coma in Myxedema. Arch Int Med 111:734, 1963.

95. Fowler PBS et al: Premyxoedema and coronary artery disease. Lancet 1:1077, 1967.

95a. Fowler PBS et al: Hypercholesterolemia in borderline hypothyroidism. Lancet 2:488, 1970.

96. Franco J et al: Propranolol and I^{131} in treatment of diffuse thyroid hyperplasia with hyperthyroidism. J Nucl Med 11:219, 1970.

97. Franco PS et al: Response to thyrotropin releasing hormone compared with thyroid suppression tests in euthyroid Graves disease. Metab 22:1357, 1973.

97a. Fredrickson DS et al: The effect of massive cortisone therapy on measurement of thyroid function. J Clin Endocrinol Metab 12:541, 1952.

98. Friend DG: Iodide therapy and the importance of quantitating the dose. NEJM 263:1358, 1960.

99. Frye RL et al: Studies on digitalis — the influence of triiodothyronine on digitalis requirement. Circ 23:376, 1961.

100. Fijimoto Y et al: Occurrence of papillary carcinoma in hyperfunctioning thyroid nodule report of a case. Endocrin Jap 19:371, 1972.

101. Gabrilove JL et al: Generalized and localized (pretibial) myxedema — effect of thyroid analogues and adrenal glucocorticoids. J Clin Endocrinol Metab 30:825, 1960.

102. Gaffney TE et al: Effects of guanethidine on triiodothyronine induced hyperthyroidism in man. NEJM 265:16, 1961.

102a. Galina MP et al: Iodide during pregnancy — an apparent cause of neonatal death. NEJM 267:1124, 1962.

103. Gedda PO et al: The hyperophthalmopathic type of Graves disease. Acta Med Scand 148:385, 1954.

104. Geffner DL et al: Prophylthiouracil blocks extrathyroidal conversion of T_4 to triiodothyronine and augments thyrotropin secretion in man. J Clin Invest 55:224, 1975.

105. Gershengorn MC et al: Use of lithium as an adjunct to radioiodine therapy of thyroid carcinoma. J Clin Endocrinol Metab 42:105, 1976.

106. Gharib H: Triiodothyronine. JAMA 227:302, 1974.

106a. Gharib H et al: Serum levels of thyroid hormones in Hashimoto's thyroiditis. Mayo Clinic Proc 47:175, 1972.

107. Gilbert DK: Hypoprothrombinemia as a complication of propylthiouracil. JAMA 189:855, 1964.

108. Gilliland PF: Myxedema recognition and treatment. Postgrad Med 57:61, 1975.

108a. Gladstone GR et al: Propranolol administration during pregnancy — effects on the fetus. J Pediat 86:962, 1975.

109. Glassford GH et al: The treatment of nontoxic nodular goiter with desiccated thyroid — results and evaluation. Surg 58:621, 1965.

110. Goldsmith RE: Radiosotope therapy for Graves disease. Mayo Clin Proc 47:953, 1972.

110b. Goldsmith RE et al: Familial autoimmune thyroiditis maternal fetal relationship and the role of generalized autoimmunity. J Clin Endocrinol Metab 37:265, 1973.

111. Goluboff LG et al: Hyperthyroidism associated with pregnancy. Obstet Gyn 44:107, 1974.

112. Good BF et al: Studies on the effects of salicylates in hyperthyroidism. Aust Ann Med 33:143, 1967.

112a. Good BF et al: The effect of salicylate and related drugs on thyroxine binding in man. Aust J Exp Biol Med Sci 43:291, 1965.

113. Goolder AWG et al: Treatment of thyrotoxicosis with low doses of radioactive iodine. Brit Med J 3:442, 1969.

114. Gorman CA et al: Metabolic Malingerers. Am J Med 48:708, 1970.

115. Gotta AW et al: Prolonged intraoperative bleeding caused by propylthiouracil induced hypoprothrombinemia. Anesthes 37:562, 1972.

116. Graettinger JS et al: A correlation of clinical and hemodynamic studies in patients with hyperthyroidism with and without congestive heart failure. J Clin Invest 38:1316, 1959.

117. Grayson RR et al: Factors which influence the radioactive iodine thyroidal uptake test. Am J Med 28:397, 1960.

118. Green DE et al: Glucocorticoid induced disappearance of the long acting thyroid stimulation in Graves ophthalmopathy. J Clin Invest 42:939, 1963.

119. Green M et al: Thyrotoxicosis treated by surgery or iodine [131] with special reference to development of hypothyroidism. Brit Med J 1:1005, 1964.

120. Green WL: Guidelines for treatment of myxedema. Med Clin N Am 52:43, 1968.

120a. Green H et al: Cretinism associated with maternal sodium iodide I[131] therapy during pregnancy. Am J Dis Child 122:247, 1971.

121. Greene JN: Subacute Thyroiditis. Am J Med 51:97, 1971.

122. Greenman GW et al: Thyroid dysfunction in pregnancy, fetal loss and follow up evaluation of surviving infants. NEJM 267:426, 1962.

123. Greenspan F: Thyroid physiology in relation to tests of thyroid function — in Laboratory Tests, in Diagnosis and Investigation of Endocrine Function. 2nd ed., edited by R Escamilla. FA Davis Co, Philadelphia, 1971, p 63.

124. Greenspan FS: Thyroid nodules and thyroid cancer. West J Med 121:359, 1974.

125. Greenstein R: Hypoprothrombinemia due to propylthiouracil therapy. JAMA 173:1014, 1960.

126. Greer MA et al: Short term antithyroid drug therapy for the thyrotoxicosis of Graves disease. NEJM 297:173, 1977.

126a. Greer MA et al: Treatment of hyperthyroidism with single daily dose of PTU. NEJM 272:888, 1965.

127. Greig WR: Iodine-125 treatment for thyrotoxicosis. Lancet 1:755, 1969.

127a. Greig WR: Radioactive iodine therapy for thyrotoxicosis. Brit J Surg 60:758, 1973.

128. Grossman WM et al: Effects of β-blockade on peripheral manifestations of thyrotoxicosis. Ann Int Med 74:875, 1971.

129. Haddad HM: Endocrine Exophthalmus. JAMA 199:559, 1967.

130. Hadden DR et al: Propranolol and iodine [131] in the management of thyrotoxicosis. Lancet 2:852, 1968.

131. Hagan GA et al: Comparison of high and low dosage levels of ^{131}I in the treatment of thyrotoxicosis. NEJM 277:559, 1967.

132. Hahn HB Jr: Congenital Nongoitrous hypothyroidism. Postgrad Med 57:71, 1975.

133. Haibach H et al: Hyperthyroidism in Graves disease. Arch Int Med 136:725, 1976.

134. Hales IB et al: Ocular changes in Graves disease. Q J Med 29: 113, 1960.

135. Hall R: Immunological aspects of thyroid function. NEJM 266: 1204, 1962.

135a. Hall R et al: Evidence for genetic predisposition to formation of thyroid autoantibodies. Lancet 2:187, 1960.

135b. Hall R et al: A study of the parents of patients with Hashimoto's disease. Lancet 2:1291, 1962.

136. Hamburger JI: Clinical Thyroidology. 2nd printing, Northland Thyroid Lab, Southfield, Michigan 1974, p 206.

136a. Hamburger JI: Hyperthyroidism Concept and Controversy. Charles C. Thomas, publisher, Illinois, 1972, p 196.

136b. Hamburger JI: Solitary autonomously functioning thyroid lesions — diagnosis clinical features and pathogenetic considerations. Am J Med 58:740, 1975.

137. Hamilton CR et al: Unusual types of hyperthyroidism. Med 52:195, 1973.

138. Hamilton HE et al: The endocrine eye lesion in hyperthyroidism. Arch Int Med 105:676, 1960.

139. Hamilton RD: Ophthalmopathy of Graves disease — a comparison between patients treated surgically and patients treated with radioiodide. Mayo Clin Proc 42:812, 1967.

140. Hardin WJ et al: Indications for thyroid surgery. Postgrad Med 57:121, 1975.

141. Hayek A et al: Thyrotropin behavior in thyroid disorders of childhood. Pediat Res 7:28, 1973.

141a. Hayek A et al: Long term results of treatment of thyrotoxicosis in children and adolescents with radioactive iodine. NEJM 283:949, 1970.

142. Hayles AB et al: Exophthalmic goiter in children. J Clin Endocrinol Metab 19:138, 1959.

142a. Hayles AB: Problems of childhood Graves disease. Mayo Clin Proc 47:850, 1972.

143. Hays MT: Absorption or oral thyroxine in man. J Clin Endocrinol Metab 28:749, 1968.

143a. Hays MT: Absorption of triiodothyronine in man. J Clin Endocrin 30:675, 1970.

144. Heath H et al: Conjugated estrogen therapy and tests of thyroid function. Ann Int Med 81:351, 1974.

145. Heiman P et al: Surgical treatment of thyrotoxicosis — results of 272 operations with special reference to pre-operative treatment with antithyroid drugs and L-thyroxine. Brit J Surg 62:683, 1975.

146. Heinonen OP et al: Symptomless autoimmune thyroiditis in coronary heart disease. Lancet 1:785, 1972.

147. Hempelmann LH: Risk of thyroid neoplasms after irradiation in childhood. Science 160:159, 1968.

148. Herbst AL et al: Hyperthyroidism during pregnancy. NEJM 273:627, 1965.

149. Hershman JM: The treatment of hyperthyroidism. Ann Int Med 64:1306, 1966.

149a. Hershman JM et al: Long term outcome of hyperthyroidism treated with antithyroid drugs. J Clin Endocrinol Metab 26:803, 1966.

150. Hertz S et al: Graves disease with dissociation of thyrotoxicosis and ophthalmopathy. West J Surg Obstet Gyn 49:493, 1941.

151. Hill LD et al: Thyroid suppression. Arch Surg 108:403, 1974.

152. Hines JD et al: Megaloblastic anemia secondary to folate deficiency associated with hypothyroidism. Ann Int Med 68:792, 1968.

153. Hiss JM et al: Thyroxine metabolism in untreated and treated pancreatic steatorrhea. J Clin Invest 41:988, 1962.

154. Hodges RE et al: Pregnancy in myxedema. Arch Int Med 90:863, 1952.

155. Hollander CS et al: Triiodothyronine toxicosis developing during antithyroid drug therapy for hyperthyroidism. Johns Hopkins M J 131:184, 1972.

155a. Hollander CS et al: Clinical and laboratory observations in cases of triiodothyronine toxicosis confirmed by radioimmunoassay. Lancet 1:609, 1972.

155b. Hollander CS et al: T_3-toxicosis in an iodine deficient area. Lancet 2:1276, 1972.

155c. Hollander CS et al: Hypertriiodothyroninemia as a premonitory manifestation of thyrotoxicosis. Lancet 2:731, 1971.

156. Hollister LE et al: Thyroid function and psychotherapeutic drugs. JAMA 185:890, 1963.

157. Holvey D et al: Treatment of myxedema with intravenous thyroxine. Arch Int Med 113:89, 1964.

158. Hoover MJ et al: Thyroid function in patients in clinical remission after medical treatment thyrotoxicosis. J Clin Endocrinol Metab 40:807, 1975.

159. Horst W et al: 306 cases of toxic adenoma — clinical aspects findings in radiodine diagnostics radiochromatography and history — results of I[131] and surgical treatments. J Nucl Med 8:515, 1967.

159a. Horst W et al: Radiojoddiagnostik und strahlentherapie der endokrinen ophthalmopathie. Otsche Med Wschr 85:730, 1960.

160. Howitt G et al: Betasympathetic blockade in hyperthyroidism. Lancet 1:628, 1966.

161. Hunton RB et al: Hypothyroidism in diabetics treated with sulfonylurea. Lancet 2:449, 1965.

162. Howard JE: Treatment of thyrotoxicosis. JAMA 202:706, 1967.

163. Hung W et al: Medical therapy of thyrotoxicosis in children. Pediat 30:17, 1962.

163a. Hung W et al: A collagen like syndrome associated with antithyroid therapy. J Pediat 82:52, 1973.

164. Ibarra JD et al: Treatment of hyperthyroidism. Postgrad Med 57:84, 1975.

165. Ikkala E et al: Plasma coagulation factors in thyrotoxicosis. Acta Endocrin 40:307, 1962.

166. Ingbar SH: Management of emergencies — thyrotoxic storm. NEJM 274:1252, 1966.

167. Irvine WJ et al: Correlation of HLA and thyroid antibodies with

clinical course of thyrotoxicosis treated with antithyroid drugs. Lancet 2:898, 1977.

167a. Ito K et al: A comparative evaluation of the treatment of hyperthyroidism. Endocrin Jpn 21:131, 1974.

168. Ivy HK et al: Triiodothyronine (T3) toxicosis. Arch Int Med 128:529, 1971.

169. Jackson GL: Treatment of hyperthyroidism in pregnancy. Penn Med 76:56, 1973.

170. Jackson IMD: Management of thyrotoxicosis. Am J Hosp Pharm 32:933, 1975.

171. Jacobs HS et al: Total and free triiodothyronine and thyroxine levels in thyroid storm and recurrent hyperthyroidism. Lancet 2:236, 1973.

172. Juliar B et al: Fatal agranulocytosis occurring during propylthiouracil therapy. JAMA 139:646, 1949.

173. Kammer GM et al: Acute bulbar muscle dysfunction and hyperthyroidism — a study of 4 cases and review of the literature. Am J Med 56:464, 1974.

174. Kammer H et al: Use of antithyroid drugs in a single daily dose. JAMA 209:1325, 1969.

175. Kampmann J et al: Pharmacokinetics of propylthiouracil. Acta Pharmacol Toxicol 35:361, 1974.

176. Karlan MD et al: Carcinoma of the thyroid following treatment of hyperthyroidism with radioactive iodine. Calif Med 101:196, 1964.

177. Keating FR et al: Treatment of heart disease associated with myxedema. Prog Cardiovasc Dis 3:364, 1961.

178. Kendall LW et al: Prediction of malignancy in a solitary thyroid nodule. Lancet 1:1071, 1969.

179. Kiely JM et al: Erythrokinetics in myxedema. Ann Int Med 67:533, 1967.

180. Knox AJS et al: Circulating lymphocytes from patients with Graves disease to produce thyroid simulating immunoglobulin (TSI). J Clin Endocrinol Metab 43:330, 1976.

181. Kock H et al: Protein bound iodine and abortion. Am J Ob Gyn 95:897, 1966.

182. Kogut MD et al: Treatment of hyperthyroidism in children — analysis of forty five patients. NEJM 272:217, 1965.

183. Koutras DA et al: Effect of T4 on exophthalmos in thyrotoxicosis. Brit Med J 1:493, 1965.

184. Kriss J: The long acting thyroid stimulator. Calif Med 109:203, 1968.

184a. Kriss J et al: Therapy with occlusive dressings of pretibial myxedema with fluocinolone acetonide. J Clin Endocrinol Metab 27:595, 1967.

185. Kristensen O et al: Lithium carbonate in the treatment of thyrotoxicosis. Lancet 1:603, 1976.

186. Labhart A: Clinical Endocrinology Theory and Practice, Springer Verlag, 1974, p 135.

187. Lachelin GCL: Myxedema and pregnancy. J Ob Gyn Brit Common 77:77, 1970.

188. Lamberg BA et al: Liver function in thyrotoxicosis — studies on the cholesterol and prothrombin levels in the blood during the treatment of thyrotoxicosis. Acta Endocrin 15:82, 1954.

188a. Langer A et al: Adrenergic blockage — a new approach to hyperthyroidism during pregnancy. Obstet Gyn 44:181, 1974.

189. Larsen PR: Tests of thyroid function. Med Clinic N Am 59:1063, 1975.

190. Lauridsen UB et al: Lithium and the pituitary — thyroid axis in normal subjects. J Clin Endocrinol Metab 39:383, 1974.

190a. Lavietes PH et al: Thyroid therapy of myxedema — a comparison of various agents with a note on the composition of thyroid secretion in man. Ann Int Med 60:79, 1964.

191. Lazarus JH et al: Treatment of thyrotoxicosis with lithium carbonate. Lancet 2:1160, 1974.

192. Lee TC et al: Use of propranolol in surgical treatment of thyrotoxic patients. Ann Surg 177:643, 1973.

193. Leonard JJ: The thyroid state and the cardiovascular system. Mod Concepts Cardiovasc Dis 37:23, 1969.

194. Lerman J et al: Treatment of the anema of hypothyroidism. Endocrin 16:533, 1932.

194a. Levey GS: The heart and hyperthyroidism. Med Clin N Am 59:1193, 1975.

195. Ley GS et al: Myocardial adenylcyclase — activation by thyroid hormone and evidence for two adenylcyclase systems. J Clin Invest 48:1663, 1969.

196. Librick L et al: Thyrotoxicosis and collagen like disease in 3

197. sisters of American Indian extraction. J Pediat 76:64, 1970.

197. Lightner ES: Congenital hypothyroidism — clues to an early clinical diagnosis. J Fam Pract 5:527, 1977.

198. Livingston HJ et al: Agranulocytosis and hepatocellular jaundice — toxic reactions following propylthiouracil therapy. JAMA 135:422, 1947.

199. Lizarralde G: Function tests and the physiology of thyroid homeostatis. Cont Educat Fam Physician 7:70, 1977.

200. Ljunggren JG et al: Preop treatment of thyrotoxicosis with a β-adrenergic blocking agent. Acta Chir Scand 141:715, 1975.

201. Loeliger EA et al: The biological disappearance rate of prothrombin factors VII IX X from plasma in hypo- hyper- and during fever. Thromb Diath Haemorrh 10:267, 1974.

202. Luby ED et al: Lithium carbonate induced myxedema. JAMA 218:1298, 1971.

203. Mackin JF et al: Thyroid storm and its management. NEJM 291:1396, 1974.

204. Maerpaa J: Congenital hypothyroidism — aetiological and clinical aspects. Arch Dis Child 47:256, 1972.

205. Man EB et al: Thyroid function in human pregnancy — development and retardation of a 4 year old progeny of euthyroid and of hypothyroxinemic women. Am J Obsete Gyn 109:12, 1971.

205a. Man EB et al: Thyroid function in human pregnancy. Am J Obsete Gyn 125:949, 1976.

206. Mandeville FB: Roentgen therapy of orbital-pituitary portals for progressive exophthalmos following subtotal thyroidectomy. Radiol 41:268, 1943.

207. Mangieri CN et al: Potency of United States pharmacopeia desiccated thyroid tablets as determined by the antigoitrogenic assay in rats. J Clin Endocrinol Metab 30:102, 1970.

208. Marchant B et al: The accumulation of ^{35}S antithyroid drugs by the thyroid gland. J Clin Endocrinol Metab 34:847, 1972.

209. Marsden P et al: Hormonal pattern of relapse in hyperthyroidism. Lancet 1:944, 1975.

210. Martinez-Lopez JI et al: Drug induced hepatic injury during methimazole therapy. Gastroent 43:84, 1962.

211. Mayberry WE et al: Radioimmunoassay for human thyrotrophin. Ann Int Med 74:471, 1971.

212. Mazzaferri EL et al: Thyroid storm — a review of 22 episodes with special emphasis on the use of guanethidine. Arch Int Med 124:684, 1969.

213. McArthur JW et al: Thyrotoxic crisis. JAMA 134:868, 1947.

214. McConahey WM et al: On the increasing occurrence of Hashimoto's thyroiditis. J Clin Endocrinol Metab 22:542, 1962.

215. McCormick RV: Polyarteritis occurring during propylthiouracil therapy. JAMA 144:1453, 1950.

216. McDouglas IR et al: Radioactive iodine (I^{131}) therapy for thyrotoxicosis. NEJM 285:1099, 1971.

216a. McDougal IR: I^{125} therapy in Graves' disease — long term results in 325 patients. Ann Int Med 85:720, 1977.

217. McFadzean AJS et al: Periodic paralysis complicating thyrotoxicosis in Chinese. Brit Med J 1:451, 1967.

218. McGavack TH et al: Untoward hematologic responses to the antithyroid compounds. Am J Med 17:36, 1954.

219. McIntosh TJ et al: Increased sensitivity to warfarin in thyrotoxicosis abstracted. J Clin Invest 49:632, 1970.

220. McKenney JF: Methods postitis. Postgrad Med 57:103, 1975.

221. McKenzie JM et al: Reconsideration of thyroid stimulating immunoglobulin as cause of hyperthyroidism in Graves' disease. J Clin Endocrinol Metab 42:778, 1976.

221a. McKenzie JM: Graves' disease. Med Clin N Am 59:1177, 1975.

222. McLarty DG et al: Results of treatment of thyrotoxicosis following relapse after antithyroid drug therapy. Brit Med J 11:203, 1969.

222a. McLarty DG et al: Remission of thyrotoxicosis during treatment with propranolol. Brit Med J 2:332, 1973.

222b. McLarty DG et al: Effect of lithium on hypothalmic pituitary thyroid function in patients with affective disorders. Brit Med J 3:623, 1975.

223. McMurray JF Jr et al: Pharmacdynamics of propylthiouracil in normal and hyperthyroid subjects after a single oral dose. J Clin Endocrinol Metab 41:362, 1975.

224. Messaris G et al: Incidence of carcinoma in cold nodules of the thyroid gland. Surg 74:447, 1973.

225. Mestman JH et al: Hyperthyroidism and pregnancy. Arch Int Med 134:434, 1974.

226. Michie W et al: Beta blockage and partial thyroidectomy for

thyrotoxicosis. Lancet 1:1009, 1974.
227. Mikas AA et al: Fulminant hepatitis and lymphocyte sensitization due to propylthiouracil. Gastroent 70:770, 1976.
228. Miller JM et al: The thyroid scintigram — the hot nodule. Radiol 84:66, 1965.
228a. Milham S Jr et al: Maternal methimazole and congenital defects in children. Teratology 5:125, 1972.
229. Mitchell JRA et al: Hypothermia after chlorpromazine in myxedematous psychosis. Brit Med J 2:932, 1959.
230. Mitsuma T et al: T_3-thyrotoxicosis in children. J Pediat 81:982, 1972.
231. Miyai K et al: Concentration of long acting thyroid stimulator (LATS) by subfractionation of gamma globulin from Graves' disease serum. J Clin Endocrinol Metab 26:504, 1966.
232. Muytaba Q et al: Treatment hyperthyroidism in pregnancy with propylthiouracil and methimazole. Obstet Gyn 46:282, 1975.
233. Molholm HJ et al: The effect of diphenylhydantoin on thyroid function. J Clin Endocrinol Metab 39:785, 1974.
234. Morgan EH et al: Plasma iron binding capacity and iron stores in altered thyroid metabolism in the rat. J Exp Phys 48:176, 1963.
235. Mori T et al: Measurement by competitive binding radioassay of serum antimicrosomal and antithyroglobulin antibodies in Graves' disease and other thyroid disorders. J Clin Endocrinol Metab 33:688, 1971.
236. Morreale de Escobar G et al: Extrathyroid effect of some antithyroid drugs and their metabolic consequences. Recent Prog Horm Res 23:87, 1967.
237. Morrow DH et al: Studies on digitalis — influence of hyper- and hypothyroidism on the myocardial response to ouabain. J Pharm Exp Ther 140:324, 1963.
238. Mulhern LH et al: Hashimoto's disease. Lancet 2:508, 1966.
239. Murray IPC et al: Iodide goiter. Lancet 1:922, 1967.
240. Musa BU et al: Effects of salicylates on the distribution and early plasma disappearance of thyroxine in man. J Clin Endocrinol Metab 28:1461, 1968.
241. Naeye RL et al: Hemorrhagic state after propylthiouracil treatment. Am J Clin Path 34:254, 1960.
242. Nagataki S et al: Effects of iodides on thyroidal iodine turnover in hyperthyroid subjects. J Clin Endocrinol Metab 30:369, 1970.
243. Nelson JC et al: Serum TSH levels and the thyroidal response to TSH stimulation in patients with thyroid disease. Ann Int Med 76:47, 1972.
244. Nelson NC et al: Thyroid crisis — diagnosis and treatment. Ann Surg 170:263, 1969.
245. Nickerson JF et al: Fatal myxedema with and without coma. Ann Int Med 53:475, 1960.
246. Nicoloff JT: Treatment of hypothyroidism and myxedema coma. Mod Treat 6:465, 1969.
246a. Nicoloff JT et al: Simultaneous measurement of thyroxine and triiodothyronine peripheral turnover kinetics in man. J Clin Invest 51:473, 1972.
247. Nielsen TP et al: Serum digoxin and thyroid hormone. Ann Int Med 81:126, 1974.
248. Nikkila EA et al: Thyroid function in diabetic patients under long term sulfonylurea treatment. Acta Endocrin 33:623, 1960.
248a. Nilsson G: Self-limiting episodes of JodBasedow. Acta Endocrinologia 74:475, 1973.
249. Niswander KR et al: The Women and Their Pregnancies. Philadelphia: W.B. Saunders, 1972.
250. Nofal MM et al: Treatment of hyperthyroidism with sodium iodide ^{131}I. JAMA 197:605, 1966.
251. Nordqvist P et al: Myxoedema coma and CO_2 retention. Acta Med Scand 166:189, 1960.
252. Northcutt RC et al: The influence of cholestyramine on thyroxine absorption. JAMA 208:1857, 1969.
253. Odell W: Symptoms physical fundings and etiology of hyperthyroidism — in symposium on hyperthyroidism. Calif Med 113:40, 1970.
253a. Odell W et al: Radioimmunoassay of thyrotropin in human serum. J Clin Endocrinol Metab 25:1179, 1965.
254. Ohalloran MJ et al: Thyroid function assay in infants. J Pediat 81:916, 1972.
255. Okihiro MM et al: Thyrotoxic periodic paralysis in Hawaii — its predilection for the Japanese race. Nuerol 15:253, 1965.
256. Oltman JE et al: Further report on protein-bound iodine in patients receiving perphenazine. Am J Psych 121:176, 1964.
256a. Oltman JE et al: Protein bound iodine in patients receiving per-

phenazine. JAMA 185:726, 1963.
257. Oppenheimer JH et al: Propylthiouracil inhibits the conversion of L-thyroxine to L-triiodothyronine — an explanation of the antithyroxine effects of propylthiouracil and evidence supporting the concept that triiodothyronine is the active thyroid hormone. J Clin Invest 51:2493, 1972.
257a. Oppenheimer JH et al: Depression of PBI levels by diphenylhydantoin. J Clin Endocrinol Metab 21:252, 1961.
257b. Oppenheimer JH: Role of plasma proteins in the binding, distribution and metabolism of the thyroid hormone. NEJM 278:1153, 1968.
258. Ormston B et al: Thyrotropin response to thyrotropin releasing hormone in ophthalmic Graves' disease — correlation with other aspects of thyroid function thyroid suppressibility and activity of eye signs. Clin Endocrin 2:369, 1973.
259. Owens JC et al: Effect of dextrothyroxine in patients receiving anticoagulants. NEJM 266:76, 1962.
260. Paris J et al: Iodide goiter. J Clin Endocrinol Metab 20:57, 1960.
261. Parker LH: Hepatitis and propylthiouracil. Ann Int Med 82:228, 1975.
262. Parker RH et al: Thyroid antibodies during pregnancy and in the newborn. J Clin Endocrinol Metab 21:792, 1960.
263. Patel YC et al: Radioimmunossay of serum thyrotropin — sensitivity and specificity. J Clin Endocrinol Metab 33:768, 1971.
263a. Patel YC et al: Serum thyrotropin (TSH) in pituitary and hypothalmic hypothyroidism normal or elevated basal levels and paradoxical responses for thyrotropin releasing hormone. J Clin Endocrinol Metab 37:190, 1973.
264. Pegg CAS et al: The surgical management of thyrotoxicosis. Brit J Surg 60:765, 1973.
265. Perzik SL: Total thyroidectomy in the management of Graves' disease. Am J Surg 131:284, 1976.
265a. Perzik SL et al: The place of total thyroidectomy in the management of thyroid disease. Surg 62:436, 1967.
266. Pietras RJ et al: Cardiovascular response in hyperthyroidism — the influence of adrenergic blockade. Arch Int Med 129:426, 1972.
267. Pileggi VJ et al: Determination of thyroxine and triiodothyronine in commercial preparations of desiccated thyroid extract. J Clin Endocrinol Metab 25:949, 1965.
268. Pimstone B et al: Use and abuse of b-adrenergic blockade in surgery of hyperthyroidism. South African Med J 44:1059, 1970.
269. Pimstone N et al: Beta adrenergic blockade in thyrotoxic myopathy. Lancet 2:1219, 1968.
270. Pineda G et al: Influence of iodine deficiency upon PBI in hyperthyroidism. J Clin Endocrinol Metab 30:120, 1970.
271. Pittman JA et al: Changing normal values for thyroidal radioactive uptake. NEJM 280:1431, 1969.
271a. Pittman JA et al: Methimazole — its absorption and excretion in man and tissue distribution in rats. J Clin Endocrinol Metab 33:182, 1971.
271b. Pittman CS et al: The extra thyroidal conversion rate of thyroxine to triiodothyronine in normal man. J Clin Invest 50:1187, 1971.
272. Plimstone BL et al: Parallel assays of thyrotrophin long acting thyroid stimulator and exophthalmos producing substance in endocrine exophthalmos and pretibial myxedema. J Clin Endocrinol Metab 24:976, 1964.
273. Plummer HS et al: Results of administering iodine to patients having exophthalmic goiter. JAMA 80:1955, 1923.
274. Pochin EE: Leukemia following radioiodine treatment of thyrotoxicosis. Brit Med J 2:1545, 1960.
275. Prange AF Jr et al: Effects of imipramine and reserpine on body in euthyroid and hyperthyroid growing rats. J Pharmacol Exp Ther 151:409, 1962.
275a. Prange AJ Jr et al: Enhancement of imipramine by thyroid stimulating hormone — clinical and theoretical implications. Am J Psych 127:191, 1970.
275b. Prange AJ et al: Enhancement of imipramine antidepressant activity by thyroid hormone. Am J Psych 126:457, 1969.
276. Prout TE: Thyroid disease in pregnancy. Am J Ob Gynecol 122:669, 1975.
277. Raiti S et al: Cretinism — early diagnosis and its relation to mental prognosis. Arch Dis Child 46:692, 1971.
278. Ramsay ID: Muscle dysfunction in hyperthyroidism. Lancet 2:931, 1966.
279. Rapoport B et al: Low dose sodium iodide ^{131}I therapy in Graves'

disease. JAMA 224:1610, 1973.

280. Refetoff I: Thyroid hormone therapy. Med Clin N Am 59:1147, 1975.

281. Refetoff S et al: Continuing occurrence of thyroid carcinoma after irradiation to the neck in infancy and childhood. NEJM 292:171, 1975.

282. Reveno WS et al: Observations on the use of antithyroid drugs. Ann Int Med 60:982, 1964.

282a. Ridgway EC et al: Acute metabolic responses in myxedema to large doses of intravenous L-thyroxine. Ann Int Med 77:549, 1972.

283. Rifkin A et al: The effect of lithium on thyroid functioning — a controlled study. J Psych Res 10:115, 1974.

284. Robayo JR: Pharmacokinetics in drug therapy — propranolol hydrochloride as adjunct therapy in the treatment of thyrotoxicosis. Am J Hosp Pharm 33:169, 1976.

285. Rogers MP et al: Clinical hypothyroidism occurring during lithium treatment — two case histories and a review of thyroid function in 19 patients. Am J Psych 128:158, 1971.

286. Roitt IM et al: Thyroid autoimmunity. Brit Med Bull 16:152, 1960.

287. Roizen M et al: Thyroid storm. Calif Med 115:5, 1971.

288. Rosenbaum H et al: Agranulocytosis and toxic hepatitis from methimazole. JAMA 152:27, 1953.

289. Rosenberg I: Thyroid storm. NEJM 283:1052, 1970.

289a. Rosenberg I: Hypothyroidism and coma. Surg Clin N Am 48:353, 1968.

290. Rosove MH: Agranulocytosis and antithyroid drugs. West J Med 126:339, 1977.

291. Rosser R: Thyrotoxicosis and lithium. Brit J Psychiat 128:61, 1976.

292. Rothberg MP et al: Propranolol and hyperthyroidism — reversal of upper motor neuron signs. JAMA 230:1017, 1974.

293. Saenger EL et al: Incidence of leukemia following treatment of hyperthyroidism. JAMA 205:855, 1968.

294. Safa AM et al: Long term follow up results in children and adolescents treated with radioactive iodine (^{131}I) for hyperthyroidism. NEJM 292:167, 1975.

295. Sammon TJ et al: Disseminated intravascular coagulation complicating propylthiouracil therapy. Clin Pediat 10:739, 1972.

296. Sandler G et al: Thyrotoxic heart disease. Q J Med 28:347, 1959.

297. Savoie JC et al: Iodine induced thyrotoxicosis in apparently normal thyroid glands. J Clin Endocrinol Metab 41:685, 1975.

298. Saxena KM et al: Childhood thyrotoxicosis — a long term perspective. Brit Med J 2:1153, 1964.

299. Schiller KFT et al: Gastric pathological and immunological abnormalities in Hashimoto's thyroiditis. GNT 8:582, 1967.

300. Schimmel M et al: Thyroidal and peripheral production of thyroid hormones. Ann Int Med 87:760, 1977.

301. Schou M et al: Occurrence of goiter during lithium treatment. Brit Med J 3:710, 1968.

302. Schuppan D et al; Preliminary pharmacokinetics studies of propylthiouracil in humans. J Pharmacokin Biopharm 1:307, 1973.

303. Scott AC Jr et al: Total thyroidectomy in management of diffuse toxic goiter. J Clin Endocrinol Metab 9:1048, 1949.

304. Sedvall G et al: Effects of lithium salts on plasma protein bound iodine and uptake of ^{131}I in thyroid gland of man and rat. Life Sci 7:1257, 1968.

305. Segal RL et al: Myxedema following RAI of hyperthyroidism. Am J Med 31:354, 1961.

306. Selenkow HA et al: Clinical pharmacology of antithyroid compounds. Clin Pharmacol Ther 2:191, 1961.

306a. Selenkow HA: Antithyroid-thyroid therapy of thyrotoxicosis during pregnancy. Obstet Gynecol 40:117, 1972.

307. Welf T et al: Warfarin induced hypoprothrombinemia potentiation by hyperthyroidism. JAMA 231:1165, 1975.

308. Shafer RB et al: Acute changes in thyroid function in patients treated with radioactive iodine. Lancet 2:635, 1975.

309. Sheline GE et al: Thyroid nodules occurring late after treatment of thyrotoxicosis with radioiodine. J Clin Endocrinol Metab 22:8, 1962.

310. Shenkman L et al: Recurrent hyperthyroidism presenting as triiodothyronine toxicosis. Ann Int Med 77:410, 1972.

311. Shipp JC: Jaundice during methimazole (Tapazole) administration. Ann Int Med 41:701, 1955.

312. Shizume K et al: Long term results of antithyroid drug therapy for Graves' disease — follow up for more than 5 years. Endocrin

Jap 17:327, 1970.

312a. Shizume K et al: Studies on electrolyte metabolism in idiopathic and thyrotoxic periodic paralysis. Metab 15:138, 1966.

312b. Siersbaek-Nielson K et al: Low remission after long term antithyroid treatment of Graves' disease in relation to iodine intake. Acta Endocrinol (KBH) Suppl 199:170, 1975.

313. Shopsin B et al: Lithium induced thyroid disturbance — case report and review. Comprehensive Psych 10:215, 1969.

313a. Shopsin B: Effect of lithium on thyroid function. Dis Nerv Syst 31:237, 1970.

313b. Silas AM et al: Hyperthyroidism after use of contrast medium. Vrit Med J 4:162, 1975.

314. Simone JV et al: Blood coagulation in thyroid dysfunction. NEJM 273:1057, 1965.

315. Sisson J: Principles of and pitfalls in thyroid function tests. J Nucl Med 6:853, 1965.

316. Sitar DS et al: Pharmacokinetics of propylthiouracil in man after a single oral dose. J Clin Endocrinol Metab 40:26, 1975.

317. Skinner NS Jr et al: Studies on the use of chlorpropamide in patients with diabetes mellitus. Ann N Y Acad Sci 74:830, 1959.

318. Slingerland DW et al: Effect TRH in hyperthyroidism patients treated with antithyroid drugs — in programs of the seventh international thyroid conference. Excerpta Medica Internat Cong Series 361:78, 1975.

319. Smith DW et al: Mental attainments of hypothyroidism children — review of 128 cases. Pediat 19:1011, 1957.

320. Smith L: Medical staff conference — thyrotoxicosis and pregnancy. Calif Med 112:41, 1970.

321. Smith RW: Hyperthyroidism management. Brit Med J 1:745, 1970.

322. Solomon D et al: Hyperthyroidism. Ann Int Med 69:1015, 1968.

322a. Solomon DH et al: Prognosis of hyperthyroidism treated by antithyroid drugs. JAMA 152:201, 1953.

323. Spaulding SW et al: L-dopa suppression of thyrotropin releasing hormone response in man. J Clin Endocrinol Metab 35:182, 1972.

323a. Spaulding SW et al: The inhbiiting effect of lithium on thyroid hormone release in both euthyroid and thyrotoxic patients. J Clin Endocrinol Metab 35:905, 1972.

324. Starr P et al: Late results of I^{131} treatment of hyperthyroidism in seventy-three children and adolescents. J Nucl Med 5:81, 1964.

324a. Starr P et al: Later results of I^{131} treatment of hyperthyroidism in 73 children and adolescents — 1967 follow up. J Nucl Med 10:586, 1969.

325. Steinberg AD: Myxedema and coronary artery disease — a comparative autopsy study. Ann Int Med 68:338, 1968.

326. Steinberg FU: Subacute granulomatous thyroiditis — a review. Ann Int Med 52:1014, 1960.

327. Sterling K: Radioactive iodine therapy. Med Clin N Am 59:1217, 1975.

327a. Sterling K et al: T_3 thyrotoxicosis — thyrotoxicosis due to elevated serum triiodothyronine levels. JAMA 213:571, 1970.

328. Stewart JC et al: Thyrotoxicosis induced by iodine contamination of food — a common unrecognized condition. Brit Med J 1:372, 1976.

329. Stock JM et al: Replacement dosage of L-thyroxine in hypothyroidism. NEJM 290:529, 1974.

330. Summers VK et al: Thyrotoxicosis and heart disease. Acta Med Scand 169:661, 1961.

331. Sung LC et al: T_3 thyrotoxicosis due to metastastic carcinoma. J Clin Endocrinol Metab 36:215, 1973.

332. Surks MI et al: Determination of iodothyronine absorption and conversion of L-thyroxine (T_4) to L-triiodothyronine (T_3) using turnover rate techniques. J Clin Invest 52:805, 1973.

333. Sutherland JM et al: Familial non goitrous cretinism apparently due to maternal antithyroid antibody. NEJM 263:336, 1960.

334. Temple R et al: The use of lithium in Graves' disease. Mayo Clin Proc 47:872, 1972.

334a. Temple R et al: The use of lithium in the treatment of thyrotoxicosis. J Clin Invest 51:2746, 1972.

335. Tennenbaum JI et al: Toxic hepatitis during treatment with methimazole (Tapazole) report of a case with apparent recovery. Ohio St Med J 58:306, 1962.

336. Thalassinos NC et al: Effect of potassium iodide on relapse rate of thyrotoxicosis treated with antithyroid drugs. Lancet 2:183, 1971.

336a. Thalassinos NC et al: Five year follow up of thyrotoxicosis treated with antithyroid drugs. Endokrinologie 63:325, 1974.

337. Thomas HM et al: Progressive exophthalmos following thyroidectomy. Bull Johns Hopkins Hosp 59:99, 1936.

338. Thomas ID: Hyperthyroidism — diagnosis and treatment. Drugs 11:119, 1976.

338a. Thomas CG: Surgery of the thyroid. Med Clin N Am 59:1247, 1975.

339. Tomkins GM et al: Effect of thyroid hormone on adrenal steroid metabolism. Ann N Y Acad Sci 86:600, 1960.

340. Tudhope GR et al: Anemia in hypothyroidism. Q J Med 64:513, 1960.

340a. Tudhope GR et al: Deficiency of Vitamin B_{12} in hypothyroidism. Lancet 1:703, 1962.

341. Turner GM et al: No tetratogenicity with propranolol. Brit Med J 4:281, 1968.

342. Turner JG et al: Lithium as an adjunct to radioiodine therapy for thyrotoxicosis. Lancet 1:614, 1976.

343. Turner P et al: Effect of adrenergic receptor blockade on tachycardia of thyrotoxicosis and anxiety state. Lancet 2:1316, 1965.

343a. Turnstall ME: The effect of propranolol on the onset of breathing at birth. Brit J Anesth 41:792, 1969.

344. Vagenakis AG et al: Adverse effects of iodides on thyroid function. Med Clin N Am 59:1075, 1975.

344a. Vagenakis AG et al: Iodide induced thyrotoxicosis in Boston. NEJM 287:524, 1972.

344b. Vagenakis AG et al: Enhancement of warfarin induced hypoprothrombinemia by thyrotoxicosis. Johns Hopkins Med J 131:69, 1972.

345. Vanderlaan WP: Antithyroid drugs in practice. Mayo Clin Proc 47:962, 1972.

346. Van haelst L et al: Coronary artery disease in hypothyroidism. Lancet 2:800, 1967.

347. Van Pilsum JF et al: Evidence that the goitrogen methimazole interferes with the extrathyroidal utilization of exogenous thyroxine. Endocrin 92:135, 1973.

348. Van Winkle W Jr et al: Clinical toxicity of thiouracil. Survey of 5745 cases. JAMA 130:343, 1946.

349. Vesell ES et al: Altered plasma half lives of antipyrine propylthiouracil and methimazole in thyroid dysfunction. Clin Pharmacol Ther 17:48, 1975.

350. Vidor GI et al: Pathogenesis of iodine induced thyrotoxicosis — studies in northern Tasmania. J Clin Endocrinol Metal 37:901, 1973.

351. Vigheri R et al: Effect dexamethasone on thyroid hormone response to TSH. Metabolism 24:1209, 1975.

352. Vinik AI et al: Sympathetic nervous system blockade in hyperthyroidism. J Clin Endocrinol Metab 28:725, 1968.

353. Volpe R et al: The pathogenesis of Graves' disease and Hashimoto's thyroiditis. Clin Endocrin 3:239, 1974.

353a. Volpe R: Thyroiditis current views of pathogenesis. Med Clin N Am 59:1163, 1975.

353b. Volpe R et al: Circulating viral and thyroid antibodies in subacute thyroiditis. J Clin Endocrinol Metab 27:1275, 1967.

354. Wahner HW: T_3 hyperthyroidism. Mayo Clin Proc 47:938, 1972.

355. Waldstein SS et al: A clinical study of thyroid storm. Ann Int Med 52:626, 1960.

356. Walzer RA et al: Immunoleukopenia as an aspect of hypersensitivity to propylthiouracil. JAMA 184:743, 1963.

357. Wartofsky L: Low remission after therapy for Graves' disease — possible relation of dietary iodine with antithyroid therapy results. JAMA 226:1083, 1973.

357a. Wartofsky L et al: Inhibition of iodine of the release of thyroxine from the thyroid glands of patients with thyrotoxicosis. J Clin Invest 49:78, 1970.

357b. Wartofsky L et al: "A method for assessing the latency, potency, and duration of action of antithyroid agents in man", in Further Advances in Thyroid Research, vol 1, edited by K Fellinger et al, Vienna Verlag der Wiener Medizinischen Academia, 1971 p. 121.

357c. Webster EN et al: Radiation hazards — measurements of gonadal dose in radiographic examination. NEJM 257:811, 1957.

358. Weg JG et al: Hypothyroidism and alveolar hypoventilation. Arch Int Med 115:302, 1965.

359. Weiner L et al: Influence of beta-sympathetic blockage (propranolol) on the hemodynamic of hyperthyroidism. Am J Med 46:227, 1969.

360. Weinstein R et al: Propranolol reversal of bulbar dysfunction and proximal myopathy in hyperthyroidism. Ann Int Med 82:540, 1975.

361. Weintraub M et al: Effect of dextrothyroxine in kinetics of prothrombin activity — proposed mechanism of the potentiation of warfarin by d-thyroxine. J Lab Clin Med 81:273, 1973.

362. Werner SC: Eye changes of Graves' disease — medical aspects. Mod Prob Ophthal 14:409, 1975.

362a. Werner SC et al: Remission of hyperthyroidism (Graves' disease) and altered pattern of serum thyroxine binding induced by prednisone. Lancet 2:751, 1966.

363. Wiberg JJ: Methimazole toxicity from high doses. Ann Int Med 77:414, 1972.

364. Wielsen ES et al: Value of early triiodothyronine suppression test in the prognosis of thyrotoxicosis. Scand J Clin Lab Invest 31:395, 1973.

365. Wilber JF et al: The effect of glucocorticoids on thyrotropin secretion. J Clin Invest 48:2096, 1969.

366. Willcox PH: Twelve years experience of antithyroid treatment. Postgrad Med J 38:275, 1962.

367. Williams DE et al: Acute effects of corticosteroids on thyroid activity in Graves' disease. J Clin Endocrinol Metab 41:354, 1975.

368. Wils JA et al: Incidence of remission after antithyroid drug treatment in Graves' disease. Acta Endocrin (KBH) Supp 138: 173, 1969.

369. Wing ES et al: Observations on the use of propylthiouracil in hyperthyroidism. Bull Johns Hopkins Hosp 90:201, 1952.

370. Wise PH et al: Single dose block replace regimes in treatment hyperthyroidism. Am Hosp J 90:273, 1975.

370a. Wise PH et al: Single dose block replace drug treatment in hyperthyroidism. Brit Med J 4:143, 1973.

371. Woeber KA et al: Effects of salicylates and its noncalorigenic congeners on the thyroidal release of I^{131} in patients with thyrotoxicosis. J Clin Endocrinol Metab 24:1163, 1964.

372. Wolff J: Iodide goiter and the pharmacological effects of excess iodide. Am J Med 47:101, 1969.

372a. Wolff J et al: Salicylates and thyroid function — the effect on thyroid pituitary interrelation. J Clin Invest 37:1144, 1958.

373. Wong ET et al: Suppressibility of thyroid function desite high levels of long acting thyroid stimulator. Ann Int Med 76:77, 1972.

374. Woolner LB et al: Granulomatous thyroiditis (DeQuervain's thyroiditis). J Clin Metab 17:1202, 1957.

375. Worley RF et al: Hyperthyroidism during pregnancy. Am J Obstet Gyn 119:150, 1974.

376. Wright HK et al: Current therapy of thyroid nodules. Surg Clin N Am 54:277, 1974.

Chapter 26

Oral Contraception

Betty J. Dong
James C. Eoff

The ideal contraceptive, one which is safe and completely reliable, still remains to be developed. Diaphragms, intrauterine devices, and oral contraceptives constitute the major forms of antifertility devices available for women today. Although numerous risks have been associated with their usage, the oral contraceptives are the most effective method of fertility control with the exception of sterilization. Since their introduction in the 1960's, oral contraceptives have gained wide-spread usage and publicity. Since their development, oral contraceptives have been used by over 150 million women and are currently being used by at least 50 million women. It is estimated that about 10 million women in the United States currently use oral contraceptives. Hundreds of articles have been published discussing their pharmacology and adverse effects. Unfortunately, thromboembolic events associated with birth control pills have received considerable attention at the expense of more commonly encountered problems. This chapter emphasizes the practical aspects which are relevant to the clinical practitioner.

1. Review the hormonal physiology of the female reproductive cycle.

The 28 day menstrual cycle can be divided into three phases:
    a. the follicular or pre-ovulatory phase,
    b. the ovulatory phase and
    c. the lutenizing or post-ovulatory phase.

The follicular phase (first 14 days) of the cycle occurs immediately following the onset of menstruation. During this period immature primordial follicles within each ovary respond to follicle stimulating hormone (FSH) released from the anterior pituitary in response to low estrogen levels after menstruation. Each ovary is capable of developing several primordial follicles; but only one follicle is able to mature into an ovum while all the others regress. As the follicle matures, theca and granulosa cells form within the follicle and begin to produce increasing amounts of estrogen, a hormone responsible for endometrial growth, size and tortuosity of glands, and for increased thickness and hyperemia of the mucosa. This increase in estrogen levels depresses FSH through a negative feedback mechanism and blocks its release until the next cycle.

Just prior to ovulation the granulosa cells begin to secrete small amounts of progesterone, and a temporary drop in the production of estrogens occurs. Elevated levels of a second pituitary hormone, LH (lutenizing hormone), are believed to trigger the ovulatory process which takes place about the 14th or 15th day of the cycle. The ovum is expelled, and a corpus luteum is formed from the ruptured follicle under the influence of LH.

The corpus luteum is responsible for the production of estrogens and progesterones for the remainder of the cycle. During this period, progesterone causes a secretory endometrium, increased tortuosity of glands and increasing thickness of fluid in preparation for implantation of the egg. As progesterone levels rise, LH secretion is shut off by a feedback mechanism. On about the 25th day of the cycle, if implantation has not occurred, the corpus luteum begins to regress, and the levels of progesterone and estrogens decline. With regression of the corpus luteum the inhibitory action of estrogen and progesterone on the pituitary gonadotrophic hormones is released; and another group of follicles begins to mature as the next cycle begins. Endometrial sloughing and bleeding occur around the 28th day of the cycle. (277, 381, 209)

2. A 22-year-old woman has taken Ortho Novum SQ prior to pregnancy; since the sequential birth control pills have been removed from the market, the physician prescribed Ortho Novum 1/50 following the birth of her child. Would Micronor be an effective alternative? How do these three preparations differ with respect to hormonal composition, mechanism of action and efficacy?

Ortho Novum 1/50, a combination birth control pill (BCP), contains as estrogen and progesterone for the entire 21 days of the cycle. The pregnancy rate for combined BCP's is 0.1 per 100 woman years; if one pill is missed the risk of pregnancy is still negligible. The low failure rate is attributed to its mechanisms of action:

a. the estrogens suppress FSH secretion, blocking follicular development of ovulation;
b. the progesterone suppresses LH secretion so no ovulation can occur even if follicular development is attained;
c. presence of progesterone early in the cycle thickens cervical mucus which interferes with sperm migration;
d. the progesterone causes a disturbance in the endometrium, making it unsuitable for implantation of the egg;
e. there may be alteration in tubal transport of the ova through the fallopian tubes. (42,353)

Ortho Novum SQ, an example of the sequential BCPs which were recently removed from the market, contained estrogen the first 14 days and an estrogen-progesterone combination the last seven days of the cycle; it thus closely approximated the normal cycle.

One major difficulty with the sequentials was that a single missed pill increased the likelihood of pregnancy. Progesterone alteration of the endometrium and cervical mucus are protective features which were unavailable in the sequentials. The sequential agents prevented conception only by suppressing follicular development, thereby inhibiting ovulation. If used properly, the failure rate was 0.5 per 100 woman years; this increased to 4 per 100 woman years if only one pill was missed (65).

Micronor, Ovrette, or Nor QD, better known as the "mini-pill", is a contraceptive containing only 0.35 mg of norethindrone, a progestin. It is taken daily without interruption. Unlike the sequentials, it lacks the protective actions of the estrogen component. The following mechanisms of actions have been proposed:

a. alteration of cervical mucus increases difficulty of sperm penetration;
b. alterations in the endometrium prevent ova implantation;
c. subtle changes in the hypothalmic-pituitary ovarian system inhibit ovulation in 30-40% of women using the "mini-pill." (349, 350)

If poor compliance is a major factor, the "mini-pill" would not be a suitable alternative, as it requires daily dosing to be effective and has a failure rate of 2.54 per 100 woman years (60, 35, 166, 566).

3. Why were the sequential oral contraceptives removed from the market?

The manufacturers voluntarily stopped marketing sequential oral contraceptives in 1976 at the request of the FDA, primarily because of reports indicating the sequential BCPs posed an increased risk of endometrial cancer compared with the combination BCPs. Furthermore, the sequentials were considerably less effective than the combined BCPs, especially with missed doses, and were also associated with a higher risk of thromboembolic disorders due to their higher estrogen content (227, 228). These problems will be discussed in more detail in Questions 30 and 37.

4. The differences among the various BCPs are dictated by their progesterone content. What are the major pharmacological differences in the available progesterones?

Modifications in the structure of steroids alter their estrogenic or progestational activity as well as their anabolic and androgenic properties. Most of the progestin agents used in oral contraceptives exhibit some degree of both estrogenic and antiestrogenic activity in animal assays. In ratios of progestin to estrogen of 20:1 to 50:1, progestins will potentiate estrogen potency; however, higher ratios inhibit estrogen potency. (42,71,91)

The **19-norsteroids** have progesterone-like effects on the endometrium and also inhibit ovulation by gonadal suppression, an effect which is not shared by the substituted 17-hydroxprogesterone compounds. The 19-norsteroids are norgestrel, norethindrone and its acetate, norethynodrel, ethynodiol diacetate, and lynestrenol. Most combination type birth control pills contain one of the 19-norsteroids as the progesterone component.

Norethindrone (Brevicon, Modicon, Ovcon, Ortho Novum, Norinyl, Micronor, Nor QD) is a strong progestational agent (can delay onset of menses) with significant androgenic (acne, hair growth) and anabolic (weight gain) properties. It is also somewhat antiestrogenic.

Norethindrone acetate (Norlestrin, Loestrin, Zorane). The addition of an acetate group to norethindrone results in a compound with double the progestational potency. It is the most potent anabolic agent available with androgenic effects and minimal antiestrogenic properties. In fact, patients receiving Norlestrin may demonstrate excess estrogen effects.

Ethynodiol diacetate (Ovulen, Demulen) is a potent progestin similar to norethindrone, but it is less androgenic, has no anabolic properties, and may demonstrate estrogen activity of clinical importance.

Norethynodrel (Enovid, Enovid E) differs structurally by a double bond which results in an "estrogenic progestin," with about 0.3% being converted to estrogen. It is neither anabolic nor androgenic.

Norgestrel (Ovral, Lo Ovral) is the most potent progestational agent available, having ten times the potency of norethindrone. It has little or no androgenic and anabolic properties but is quite antiestrogenic.

All of these progestins are converted to estrogens to some extent, but only norethynodrel and ethynodiol diacetate possess estrogen activity of clinical importance.

17-hydroxyprogesterone is an intermediate product in the biosynthesis of the steroids. The addition of groups at C-6 hinder the catabolism of the compound and enhance its biological effects. The derivatives include *chlormadinone acetate, medroxyprogesterone acetate* (Provera) and *megestrel acetate.* All these potent progestin compounds are antiestrogenic with low virilization and low anabolic potentials. (119, 207, 276, 277, 278, 458, 527).

5. An intern would like to prescribe a BCP with low estrogen content. Some preparations contain 50 mcg of mestranol while others contain 50 mcg of ethinyl estradiol. Are there any differences between mestranol and ethinyl estradiol?

Estrogenic activity is measured by the ability of the drug to induce cornification of vaginal epithelium. In this regard ethinyl estradiol has been shown to be ten times more potent than mestranol (116). Animal studies have shown ethinyl estradiol to be two to three times more potent than mestranol in inhibiting ovulation and gonadotropin release from the pituitary (116).

However, recent human data indicate that in doses of 50 to 100 mcg per day, no difference could be detected between various doses or between drugs, indicating that a plateau in endometrial response is reached (91,189,191). Mestranol and ethinyl estradiol also have equipotent antiovulatory effect in doses of 50 to 100 mcg in humans (189). Furthermore, there appears to be a synergism between these estrogens and progestins in so far as their antiovulatory effect is concerned, thus explaining the high contraceptive effectiveness observed with very low-dose combination regimens. (91,115,118,190,293)

In comparing effects on plasma gonadotropins, no change occurred in median FSH levels at the end of the first cycle regardless of the estrogen dose. After the second cycle, a stable, dose-related fall is obtained with the 80 or 100 mcg per day doses. The addition of progestins causes a prompt, stable, further fall in FSH level. By contrast, median LH levels rise in the first cycle with all estrogen regimens and then fall progressively in dose-related fashion in cycles two through six. The addition of a progestational agent results in greater LH suppression by ethinyl estradiol when compared to mestranol at 50 mcg per day. All other indices and dosages show ethinyl estradiol and mestranol to be essentially equipotent under these experimental conditions. Long-term administration of oral contraceptives produces comparable gonadotropin suppression. There was a suggestion of slightly less FSH suppression with agents using 50 to 75 mcg per day of estrogen than from those with 100 mcg per day.

In neither of these estrogens is there a direct relationship between contraceptive potency and effects on blood coagulation.

6. Some contraceptives are estrogen dominant, while others are progesterone dominant. Rate the contraceptives with respect to their estrogenic or progestogenic dominance.

The estrogen component of oral contraceptives has been implicated as the responsible agent in thromboembolic disease, endometrial cancer, and other adverse effects. Some authors attempt to rate estrogen potency entirely on the basis of the type and amount of estrogen. Results obtained in this manner do not correlate well with clinical observations (119).

The effect of the progestin component in oral contraceptives must also be considered in rating estrogenic activity. Progestins may possess estrogenic activity, anti-estrogenic activity, or in many cases, both types of activity (42).

A ranking of relative estrogen and progesterone dominance of oral contraceptives is presented in *Table 1* (91,137,258,263).

Table 1
ESTROGEN AND PROGESTERONE
DOMINANCE OF ORAL CONTRACEPTIVES

	Estrogen Dominance		Progesterone Dominance	
very high	Oracon Ortho Novum SQ Norquen		Ortho Novum 10 mg Norlestrin 2.5 mg Ovral	
high	Norlestrin 2.5 mg Enovid E Enovid 5 mg		Ortho Novum 2 mg Norinyl 2 mg Brevicon Modicon	*high*
intermediate	Norlestrin 1 mg Ovulen		Lo/Ovral Norinyl 1/50 Ortho Novum 1/50 Demulen	*moderately high*
low	Norinyl 2 mg Ortho Novum 2 mg Demulen Ortho Novum 1/80 Norinyl 1/80		Ovulen Norlestrin 1 mg Ortho Novum 1/80 Norinyl 1/80	*intermediate*
very low	Brevicon Loestrin Modicon Ortho Novum 1/50 Norinyl 1/50 Ovral Ortho Novum 10 mg Lo/Ovral		Enovid 5 mg Enovid E	*low*
			Ortho Novum SQ Norquen Oracon	*very low*

7. A 27-year-old woman is placed on Ovulen for dysmenorrhea. After one week she complains of intolerable morning nausea, bloating, and ankle edema. Her breasts are swollen and tender to the touch. Lately she has noticed a whitish discharge from the vagina. How should this patient be treated?

These symptoms are due to estrogen excess. Nausea tends to occur during the first month of use but usually disappears by the third or fourth cycle. The patient should be instructed to take the pill at night with meals since this seems to decrease the incidence of nausea. The bloating, swollen breasts and ankle edema are explained by increased reabsorption of salt and water by the kidney. Salt restriction and intermittent use of diuretics can afford the patient further relief. The whitish discharge, or leukorrhea, is a normal physiological reaction of the glands that line the inner portion of cervix to the estrogen component of the pill. However, bacterial and fungal infections should be ruled out. Other excess estrogen side effects not exhibited by this patient are decribed in *Table 2* (79).

Symptoms of excess estrogen usually decrease with the passage of time. However, if they persist beyond three months, the patient should be switched to a less estrogenic pill. The progestins norethynodrel (Enovid) and ethynodiol diacetate (Ovulen, Demulen) should not be used because of their estrogenic properties. Norlestrin should also be avoided since estrogen side effects may occur. Drugs of choice in this patient would be low estrogen dose (50 mcg) combinations. Ovral, which is strongly anti-estrogenic, is a suitable alternative.

8. A 48-year-old postmenopausal woman has been taking Ovral for endometriosis for one month. She now complains of hot flashes at night, increased nervousness, and irritability. How should she be treated?

The symptoms in this patient are due to estrogen deficiency complicated by her postmenopausal state and the very potent anti-estrogen progestin in Ovral, norgestrel. Switching to a less progestational agent would be the initial therapy. If symptoms persist, Enovid or a similar product should be considered. Other symptoms of estrogen deficiency not evident in this patient are listed in *Table 2* (119,178,278,365).

9. A 22-year-old tall, slender, depressed woman is seen in the outpatient clinic with complaints of abnormal hair growth on the chin and breast which she has removed by electrolysis. Past drug history revealed the use of tetracycline 250 mg/day from 1971 to 1975 for acne and then again in 1976. Physical examination was normal except for slight hair growth as noted above. She also noticed increased perspiration, but no voice changes. She has been taking Norlestrin 2.5 mg for three years. Are these symptoms the result of the Norlestrin?

The symptoms (acne, perspiration, hirsutism, depression) in this patient could well be due to the androgenic effects of the progesterone, norethindrone acetate, in Norlestrin. Medical problems such as adrenocortical insufficiency should be ruled out. The selection of a more estrogenic pill without androgenic tendencies would be a better choice in this patient who possesses masculine features. Norethindrone and its acetates (Norlestrin, Ortho Novum) should not be used in this patient, nor should Ovral, since it is highly anti-estrogenic. Rather, an estrogen dominant progestin such as norethynodrel (Enovid) should be selected. Other symptoms of progestin excess not seen in this patient are listed in *Table 2*.

Table 2
SIDE EFFECTS ASSOCIATED WITH HORMONAL EXCESS AND DEFICIENCY

Estrogen Excess
nausea
fluid retention
breast tenderness
leukorrhea
hypermenorrhea
dysmenorrhea
fibroid growth
chloasma
suppression of lactation
latent diabetic syndrome
headaches
hypertension
visual changes
thrombophlebitis

Estrogen Deficiency
early cycle spotting
early cycle breakthrough bleeding
predisposition to moniliasis
oligomenorrhea
amenorrhea
decreased vaginal secretion
hypoplastic uterus
nervousness, irritability
hot flashes

Progestin Excess
tiredness and fatigue
depression
alopecia
acne
appetite increase
steady weight gain
early cycle spotting
early cycle breakthrough bleeding
predisposition to moniliasis
oligomenorrhea
amenorrhea

Progestin Deficiency
late cycle spotting
late cycle breakthrough bleeding
dysmenorrhea
amenorrhea

The side effects related to estrogen excess and progestin deficiency tend to decrease in severity with time.

10. A 21-year-old woman who has taken Enovid E for three months has complaints of late cycle spotting and heavy, prolonged flow accompanied by clots and cramping. Are these complaints caused by the estrogen or progestin component?

These are signs of progestin deficiency. Symptoms of progestin deficiency usually decrease with successive months of use, but since they have been persistent in this patient, she should be switched to an oral contraceptive with greater progestogenic potency. Ovral or Ortho Novum 2 mg would be acceptable choices.

11. Is there an oral contraceptive that contains only a progestin which is not taken every day like the "mini-pill"?

There are experimental studies using high dose progesterone (d-norgestrel 1.0 mg daily dose) administered on a "21 days on and 7 days off" schedule (71, 431, 432). Cyclic administration of progesterone in this manner has good contraceptive efficacy but does not disturb the cycle or produce prolonged amenorrhea as does the continuous administration of low-dose progesterone (431,432).

12. Has a long-acting hormonal contraceptive been developed for women?

Although the long acting injectable form of medroxy progesterone acetate (MPA, Depo Provera) was initially approved for contraceptive use, the FDA has since withdrawn its original recommendation (412, 454). The major advantage of the 150 mg implant dose was that it only had to be administered once every three months, making it extremely valuable for developing countries; there are an estimated 1 million women now using injectable progesterones for contraceptives in underdeveloped countries (17).

The major concerns over its use are: (a) Return of fertility after use of MPA is variable and unpredictable, and (b) chronic administration to dogs has produced mammary nodules (412).

13. An 18-year-old woman was raped by 3 youths earlier this evening. History reveals she is currently using no means of contraception, and this is the 13th day of her cycle. She requests protection from the possibility of pregnancy. Is there a "morning after" type of oral contraceptive?

The FDA has approved the use of high doses of the estrogen, diethylstibestrol (DES), as a "morning after" pill. The use of DES in this manner is to be reserved for an emergency measure (in situations such as rape, incest, or where in the physician's judgment, the patient's physical or mental well-being is in jeopardy); it should not be used routinely as a contraceptive. The drug is started preferably within 24 hours and not later than 72 hours after exposure. To insure efficacy, patients must be warned to take the full course of the drug in spite of the nausea which frequently occurs. The originally suggested dosage was 100 mg per day for 3 days, but poor compliance with this regimen because of nausea has resulted in recommendation of a dosage schedule adjusted to 50 mg daily for 5 days (25 mg bid x 5 days). High doses of estrogen given in the early post-ovulatory period prevent ovum implantation. (13, 20,

225, 288, 354).

While nausea is encountered in approximately half of the patients, no serious side effects have been noted except for one case of acute pulmonary edema. The incidence of ectopic pregnancy may be elevated and may be as high as one out of ten cases. (224)

Morris reported 29 pregnancies occurred from 9000 mid-cycle exposures treated with estrogens, a 0.3 per cent pregnancy rate. However, most of these might be attributed to errors in timing or insufficient doses of estrogens. (352)

There is at present no positive evidence that the restricted postcoital use of DES carries a significant carcinogenic risk. However, because existing data support the possibility of delayed appearance of carcinoma in women whose mothers had been given DES later in pregnancy, and because teratogenic and other adverse effects on the fetus in early pregnancy are poorly understood, voluntary termination of pregnancy should be seriously considered if such therapy fails. (21, 82, 563)

Haspels has suggested the use of conjugated estrogens (Premarin) 10 mg daily for 10 days, and claims equal success with less nausea (224).

14. Demulen is prescribed for a patient to be taken "as directed". What instructions should have been given?

In the 21 day cycle, the first day of menstruation is considered day one. The pill is started on day five and continued for 21 days. No pills are taken the next seven days. Menstruation usually begins two or three days after the last pill. The exception to the above dosing schedule is the 28 day cycle in which seven inert tablets are added at the end of the 21 active tablets; this eliminates the need for counting. (278, 314)

15. A patient has completed the first month (21 days) of her new prescription for Demulen. She has waited seven days, and menses has not started. Should she continue the pill, or wait for menses?

Until recently, the standard recommendation was to resume therapy on the eighth day after the last pill, regardless of whether or not menses had occurred or was currently taking place; if no menses occurred for two cycles, a pregnancy test was performed. However, with the advent of evidence linking congenital limb defects with *in utero* exposure to BCPs this has become an unresolved question. Some clinicians feel that it would be best to continue with the traditional recommendation of continung therapy past the first skipped cycle followed by a pregnancy test in the event of a second incomplete cycle. However, others feel that the risk to the fetus warrants discontinuation of the pill until pregnancy is ruled out.

In this particular case, the patient is just starting BCPs and skipped cycles are common. Therefore, we would recommend continuing therapy for one more cycle. If a patient has been on oral contraceptives for several months without such problems, we would use more caution and stop the pill until pregnancy is ruled out.

16. A 32-year-old woman has been taking Ovral for seven years. She skipped her last period and was instructed to continue taking the Ovral for one more cycle. At the end of the second missed period, she went to the physician and had a positive pregnancy test. Are there any dangers associated with fetal development if oral contraceptives are taken during pregnancy?

There have been several recent articles that clearly indicate an increased incidence of fetal malformation in women who became pregnant while using oral contraceptives (220, 268, 281, 375, 376, 377). Congenital malformations of the heart and skeleton, exophthalmus, spina bifida, and virilization of the female fetus have been observed (58, 316, 425, 564). Both the combination and progestin-only preparations have been implicated (378). The incidence of malformed children with limb defects is definitely increased in pregnancies with a history of exposure to an oral contraceptive in early pregnancy. In one series the affected children were all males (253).

Although BCP-induced chromosome defects have been shown in animals, they have not been observed in the human fetus (281, 316). However, the observed rate of congenital abnormalities in a recent study was noted to be 6.8 per 1000 in a group taking oral contraceptives compared with 4.1 per 1000 in a group who never used such preparations (281).

Some clinicians feel that congenital effects may be possible for several months after discontinuation of the oral contraceptives. Therefore, Reid has suggested that patients stop taking the pill two or three months before a pregnancy is planned (420).

Another related concern is the association of diethylstilbesterol (DES) and vaginal adenocarcinoma in females whose mothers used the drug in pregnancy, an effect which may be delayed as much as 20 years (230, 231). The frequent occurrence of vaginal adenosis and cervical-vaginal ridges in these young women obviously implies a teratogenic drug effect. The FDA now warns against the use of DES for suspected miscarriage during pregnancy but does allow for its use as a "morning after" contraceptive.

17. What advice can you offer a patient who has missed doses?

The patient should make up missed doses as soon as possible so that adequate suppression of follicular develoment can be maintained. If one or two doses are forgotten, the patient should double the dose for one or two days. Breakthrough bleeding is common when more than one pill is missed. If three pills are missed, some other means of contraception should be used and therapy should resume after menses. Jackson (224) found no evidence of escape ovulation when the missed pill was taken 10-12 hours later. If one to five pills are missed, the pregnancy rate rises to 7.2% while the rate increases to 31.2% if 6-19 pills are missed. The possibility of pregnancy also seems greater if the pills are missed early in the cycle and if the patient is a relatively new user. A secondary means of contraception (e.g., a diaphragm and foam) is recommended for the remainder of the cycle as an added protection. When switchng to a lower dose pill, additional contraceptive methods during the first cycle are indicated since the pituitary can escape from the influence of estrogen suppression and ovulation may occur (69, 249, 278).

18. A 22-year-old patient has a prescription refilled for Ovral that has been refilled monthly for 8 months. How often should the young uncomplicated patient return for a routine physical examination?

A routine pelvic examination, PAP smear, breast examination and blood pressure check should be performed annually for women under age 35. The blood pressure of patients with a family history of hypertension should be checked every three to six months. The blood sugar of patients predisposed to diabetes should be evaluated six months after the initiation of therapy and annually thereafter. After the age of 35, patients should be evaluated more frequently, perhaps at six-month intervals. (181)

19. A 24-year-old woman gave birth to her second baby one week ago. How soon after delivery should she reinstitute BCPs to assure adequate contraception?

In the absence of lactation the earliest time at which ovulation occurs post-partum is about six to eight weeks (93, 468, 511). Oral contraceptives should be started about three to four weeks post-partum. Some clinicians recommend that if a woman is more than four weeks post-partum it is advisable to give 10 tablets to induce menstruation, then start medication when withdrawal bleeding ensues (278).

Waiting a month to six weeks before resuming oral contraceptive therapy allows for normal recovery of the hypothalamic-pituitary-gonadal axis and for the establishment of successful lactation if this is desired. Patient compliance with the usual four to six weeks postpartum moratorium on coitus would obviate the necessity for contraceptive protection during this period.

For women who breast feed, the period of postpartum infecundity is often increased by three-fourths of the average period of lactation (93). Although lactation is associated with prolonged amenorrhea and ovulation suppression (108, 112), (sucking and prolactin release tend to inhibit production and secretion of FSH and LH), there is still a 7-10% risk of conception during post-partum amenorrhea. This risk increases rapidly after menstruation has returned (511). Das and Mitra (112) reported that 12 women out of 110 resumed menstruation after puerperium without an appreciable period of amenorrhea. Therefore, this period of lactation amenorrhea should not be considered infertile (252).

20. The patient in the previous question is planning to breast-feed her child. What effect do birth control pills have on lactation and which type should be used?

Some clinicians claim that combination estrogen-progestogen oral contraceptives may adversely affect lactation. Over 40 studies have examined the effects of combined oral agents on the quantity and/or quality of mother's milk. However, most are not authoritative, because population samples were small, the variables were inadequately controlled, and because lactation suppression was poorly defined or measured. Nevertheless, nearly all studies report that combination BCPs appeared to decrease the volume of milk produced or to shorten the duration of lactation in some women. There appears to be less effect on milk production if lactation is established when oral contraceptives are begun. (93, 365)

The estrogen component has been blamed for the adverse effects combination pills may have on lactation. Large doses of estrogens have been used for years, with varying degrees of success, to suppress lactation in women who do not want to breast-feed. The combination type BCPs however, contain much less estrogen than is used for intentional lactation suppression. Recent studies imply that anticipation of suppressed lactation and refusal to let the child suckle may be at least as important in suppressing lactation as the estrogen component of combination pills. Thus, if a woman takes high doses of estrogen and does not permit suckling, lactation is suppressed, but if a woman takes oral BCPs and permits frequent suckling, the initiation of lactation is usually unaffected.

Extensive, careful research is needed to clarify this adverse effect. In the meantime, many clinicians and researchers have suggested that breast-feeding women who wish to use oral contraceptives should receive low estrogen combination type BCPs or progestogen-only pills or injections.

Progestin-only contraceptives do not seem to affect adversely either the quantity or quality of maternal milk. In some women, progestins may even produce a greater volume of milk and extend the duration of lactation. The 19-nor progestins, however, resemble the combination type BCPs in their effect on lactation. These progestins are metabolized *in vivo* to estrogens and have been reported both to inhibit the volume of milk and to shorten the duration of lactation.

The effects of the pill on the breast fed baby need further study. At present there is no evidence that hormones transmitted through the milk to the baby are in sufficient dose to cause ill effects. Oral contraceptives only minimally alter the composition of milk and assays of maternal milk have detected steroid levels of not more than 1%. A single case of breast enlargement occurring in a male infant is the only report of estrogen transmission that may have affected a child. (45) However, we recommend that other forms of contraception (foams, diaphragms, etc.) be used in lactating women because a small quantity of hormones do appear in the milk and the effects, if any, on the nursing infant have not been determined. The absence of negative data at this time is not a compelling reason to risk possible future ill effects in the child, particularly since alternative modes of contraception are available.

21. A patient who has been taking oral contraceptives for three years prior to her present pregnancy asks if there is an increased chance of having a female offspring.

Crawford and associates observed an increased incidence of female offspring among a group of 30 infants (23 female and 7 male) born to mothers who had used oral contraceptives (106). However, when the sex distribution of 624 infants born to mothers who had used contraceptives were compared to 835 births occurring in the same hospital, they found no significant difference between the sex distribution of the two groups (106). Another study by Keseru concluded (273) that there was a significant shift toward female births, but Oechsli indicated no significant difference (385).

In the most valid study to date, Rothman studied 6109 live births and concluded that oral contraceptives have no bearing on the sex of subsequent offspring (435). Sex of offspring was not related to total duration of oral contraceptive use, duration of use since any previous pregnancy, or interval between termination of use and conception (435).

22. Should a patient undergoing elective surgery stop taking oral contraceptives prior to surgery?

Two studies indicate a positive correlation between preoperative use of oral contraceptives and postoperative venous thrombosis (206, 526). Therefore, some clinicians recommend the discontinuation of oral contraceptives at least two weeks before a planned surgery (447, 529).

23. A 21-year-old woman who has been taking Ovulen-21 for approximately one year complains of nausea, vomiting and vague pains in the abdomen and legs. The adverse effects vary monthly and seem to parallel any new information that reaches the lay press. Could her symptoms be purely psychological in nature?

There have been many recent reports with regard to adverse effects of oral contraceptives, and as these reports reach the lay press, clinicians must be prepared to objectively evaluate complaints from their patients. One study of 147 women, noted that over 60% experienced various side effects from oral contraceptive placebos (36). Only one-third of these users of placebos were totally asymptomatic (36).

One solution to the problem of adverse effects is that of appropriate selection. The answer may not be as simple as changing the estrogen-progestin balance of the medication, but in a more precise manipulation of the dosage. The patient may be getting the correct medication, but not enough or too much of it. Most of the minor side effects can be managed by manipulating the dose or the products used. (132)

Table 3
ABSOLUTE AND RELATIVE CONTRAINDICATIONS TO BCPs

ABSOLUTE CONTRAINDICATIONS:
Present or past thromboembolic disease
Present or past cerebrovascular accident
Breast mass — before histological diagnosis
Active liver disease
History of cholestatic jaundice during pregnancy
History of severe mental depression
Young patient — prior to cessation of growth
Poor motivation — inability to understand and follow directions
Vascular headaches
Renal disease

RELATIVE CONTRAINDICATIONS (CAUTIONS):
Hypertension
Diabetes Mellitus
Rheumatic Heart Disease
Puerperium
Family history of breast cancer
Severe varicose veins
Convulsive disorders
Oligo- or amenorrhea

24. Are there any factors which predispose women to the various adverse effects of oral contraceptives?

As illustrated in Question 18 and Table 3, several diseases and/or conditions seem to predispose certain patients to major adverse effects. Several important considerations are the age of the patient, the duration of oral contraceptive therapy, and the amount of estrogen contained in the various products. Certainly a 45-year-old woman who has used a potent estrogen for 10 years will be more predisposed for various adverse effects than a younger patient who has taken a low dose of estrogen for a shorter length of time.

A family history of diabetes, hypertension, and cardiovascular disease must be weighed against the risks of pregnancy. Patients with the aforementioned diseases would be at greater risk for adverse effects. If factors such as obesity, smoking, and lack of exercise are included, it becomes difficult to make specific statements as to the risk of adverse effects of oral contraceptives. Risks will always vary with the patient, the underlying diseases, the specific oral contraceptive agent, and the duration of usage.

25. A 26-year-old woman has complained of irregular bleeding (spotting and extra periods) for ten years. Menarche at age 12 was accompanied by occasional cramping, but by age 16 her menstrual periods had become irregular and increasingly uncomfortable. Significant past medical history included three instances of dilatation and curettage to regulate bleeding; these were without success. She was placed on Ovulen, as a last resort. Her history thereafter was as follows:

> **1st month: breakthrough bleeding (BTB) for most of the month after starting the pill.**
> **2nd month: no problems.**
> **3rd month: BTB after second week on the pill.**
> **4th month: skipped one pill during midcycle resulting in spotting.**
> **5th month: BTB again in second week.**

Past medications include thyroid 1/2-2 gr daily (1962-1971). Other present medications include Chlortrimeton for congestion and multivitamins. The plan is to do a T-3 and T-4 test and have the patient return in a week. Define breakthrough bleeding and spotting. Why do they occur? How can they be prevented?

Breakthrough bleeding (BTB) and spotting are bleeding episodes which occur at times other than during the normal menstrual cycle. BTB is more copious and similar to menstrual discharge. Spotting indicates minimal discharge or staining. BTB develops in 5-8% of patients taking the pill. It is caused by degeneration of the endometrial tissue resulting from inadequate nutrition. Normally, estrogens, which are responsible for maintenance of the endometrium, are gradually increased with progesterone after ovulation. Therefore, a gradual increase of both estrogen and progesterone are necessary for maintenance of an intact endometrium. Early cycle BTB or spotting is usually a result of estrogen insufficiency, since too little exogenous estrogen is present to maintain a proliferative endometrium. Many of the 19-nortestosterone progestins are anti-estrogenic at the tissue level; thus, BTB and spotting may also be caused by too large a dose of progestin. Fluctuations in estrogen levels due to missed pills can also cause BTB and spotting; therefore, these patients should be instructed either to double the dose until the end of the cycle at the first sign of spotting or staining or simply to make up the missed dose. Late cycle BTB and spotting are most often a result of progestin deficiency and require a stronger

progestogenic pill.

If BTB occurs, the pill should be discontinued and the flow considered a regular menstrual period. The pill should be resumed five days after the onset of the flow. If BTB recurs after more than three cycles, a different preparation should be selected. This patient's early and mid-cycle bleeding due to estrogen insufficiency indicates that a more estrogenic pill such as Enovid-E should be selected. If BTB occurred very late in the cycle, (denoting progestin deficiency), a more potent progestin such as norgestrel (Ovral) or norethindrone (Ortho Novum 2 mg; Norlestrin 2.5 mg) would be appropriate. Persistent or recurrent menstrual dysfunctions require a thorough search for underlying causes and the endometrium should be evaluated by biopsy or curettage. (119, 278, 365).

26. A 29-year-old woman who took BCPs for four years has not had a menstrual period since she discontinued usage two years ago. Her earlier history of irregular periods was improved when she took oral contraceptives. One year ago a 3 month trial of Clomid induced spotting but was otherwise unsuccessful. How prevalent is post-pill amenorrhea, and how should it be managed?

The true incidence of prolonged amenorrhea or the "oversuppression syndrome" which occurs after discontinuation of the pill is difficult to establish but varies between 2 and 7% (216, 245, 423, 463). Golditch (188) noted an incidence of 2.2 per 1000 woman/years among 20,000 women using different brands of contraceptives. This complication cannot be correlated wth the type of steroid (188, 216), the duration of therapy (153, 213, 439), or the physical status of the individual; but it does seem to be related to pre-existing menstrual dysfunction (171, 188, 213, 316). Women who had irregular periods before treatment are more at risk (197).

The mechanism is presumed to be suppression of the hypothalamic-pituitary axis with inhibition of hypothalamic gonadotropin releasing factor and decreased gonadrotropin release from the pituitary (30, 77, 188, 213, 327, 406, 407, 550).

Post-pill amenorrhea seems to be a self-limiting condition with 90-95% of patients spontaneously resuming menses 6 (majority) to 18 months after its onset (171, 213, 217, 423, 515). If menses does not occur within 6 months of the onset of amenorrhea, most clinicians recommend further patient evaluation because it may represent other associated conditions such as hyperthyroidism, granulomatous disease, or tumors (188, 216, 335).

When remission does not occur and other causes of amenorrhea cannot be established, the drug of choice is clomiphene 50 mg/day for 5 days starting on any day of the menstrual cycle (188, 216, 464). If there is no response, the dosage may be increased by 50 mg increments each cycle until a total of 200 mg/day has been reached; 50-60% of patients will resume menses after therapy (188). Ergokryptine, an ergot alkaloid, has been studied in post pill galactorrhea-amenorrhea. It apparently inhibits the secretion but not the synthesis of pituitary prolactin which may be related to the amenorrhea (216). Human chorionic gonadrotropin (HCG) and human menopausal gonadotropin have been recommended as an adjunct to clomiphene therapy. Others have found the use of corticosteroids effective. (188, 216, 239).

Pyridoxine (vitamin B-6) in doses up to 600 mg per day has been used successfully to treat post-pill galactorrhea-amenorrhea. It is postulated that pyridoxine increases dopaminergic activity which increases prolactin secretion and decreases galactorrhea. (335)

27. A 23-year-old patient became pregnant while taking Overett. What is the incidence of ectopic pregnancy secondary to the "mini-pill"? Have the combination type of oral contraceptives been implicated in causing ectopic pregnancy?

Ectopic pregnancy occurs with increased frequency in women using low dose progestin products and implants (64, 226, 244). Apparently, these contraceptives, like intrauterine devices (IUDs), are more effective in preventing uterine than extrauterine implantation.

A possible increased risk of ectopic pregnancy also exists after discontinuing either combined or sequential oral contraceptives (543). However, the data are still inconclusive and confirmatory long term studies will be needed.

28. A 26-year-old medical student with one child is currently using an IUD for contraception. After a normal pregnancy she was started on Ortho Novum 1/50. No problems occurred during the first 11 months, but she noticed vaginal itching and a whitish discharge after the 12th cycle. A diagnosis of moniliasis was made, and she was successfully treated with the Mycostatin suppositories and Mycolog cream. She continued taking the same birth control pill and soon thereafter developed a recurrence of her infection. This time she was switched to Ortho Novum SQ only to be plagued by recurrence three months later. As a last resort she switched herself to Enovid E and had no further complications. The patient stopped the pill herself when she detected a small pea-sized lump in her right breast which regressed in size after discontinuing the pill. Discuss the incidence and association of the pill with moniliasis. How should it be treated?

The reported frequency of BCP-induced moniliasis ranges from 8.5% (250) to 91.3%, as compared to less than 10% in women not currently taking BCPs (255, 355, 399, 430, 532, 534, 553). Although there are a few reports which have not demonstrated a greater inci-

dence of moniliasis in women taking the pill (113, 121), the majority of evidence to date indicates there is an increased incidence of moniliasis in women who take BCPs.

Several studies show that there is a higher incidence of monilial infection associated with the combination agents (61.3%) than with the sequentials (37.5%) (121, 250, 485, 533), but one report noted an increase of monilial infection only if the duration of usage was more than a year. Apparently, there is a latent period of nine months before moniliasis becomes a problem (88, 89).

The mechanism whereby BCPs influence yeast infections is not known. A more susceptible vagina as in pregnancy and an alteration of glucose tolerance have been offered as explanations. However, there is not an increased occurrence of yeast infections in diabetics. Spellacy and workers (485) could not document significant differences in blood glucose or plasma insulin in those with or without moniliasis. The increased glycogen content of the vagina mucous membrane and the formation of acid by the action of lactobacillus may both contribute to the growth of Candida (88). Moniliasis secondary to the pill may represent a side effect of excess progestogen or estrogen deficiency; thus, the patient's changeover to a more estrogen dominant pill alleviated her infection. (24, 119, 304, 553)

Fortunately, pill-induced vaginitis responds to conventional treatment as demonstrated by this patient. However, medical treatment may not be efficacious until the pill has been discontinued (88, 409, 562).

29. Was the birth control pill responsible for the breast lump in this patient?

That the breast is a hormone sensitive organ, is evidenced by the breast hypertrophy and enlargement which occurs during pregnancy in response to estrogens. Nevertheless, it is not possible to determine the actual relationship between the pill or prolonged estrogen therapy and benign or malignant breast disease. Human carcinogens rarely make themselves known until at least 10 years after first exposure, so the consequences of the pill will remain obscure for some time. However, the carcinogenic effects of certain contraceptives on the mammary tissues of animals has led to the withdrawal of chlormadinone (C-Quens) and medroxyprogesterone (Provest) from the market.

At the present time there does not appear to be a BCP associated increased risk of breast tumors. Recent British and American studies indicate there may be a reduced risk of benign breast lesions in patients taking oral contraceptives. These reports do not conclusively prove the ability of oral contraceptives to protect against breast tumors, but it at least strengthens the concept of a lack of such risk (131, 156, 311, 374, 391, 506, 523). Additionally, two retrospective studies noted that oral contraceptives are not causative factors for benign breast lesions (445, 524). A history of oral contraceptive or estrogen use was given no more frequently by patients with cystic disease and fibroadenomas than their respective controls. In fact, fewer patients with cystic disease had used the pill than did the controls (445).

Oral contraceptives may cause rapid cellular growth and increased secretory activity in pre-existing benign lesions. Goldenberg (186) and Brown (72) have reported unusual hyperplastic and secretory changes in the epithelium of mammary fibroadenomas of women on the pill; and Wiegenstein and associates (552) have described an unusual number of cases of multiple breast fibroadenomas involving women on the pill.

It is probable that in this patient, the pill made detectable a mass which was present before the onset of contraceptive therapy.

The frequency of carcinoma of the breast is about 4% in women under 35 years of age. This has not changed with the advent of the oral contraceptives. Fechner (158) could not establish an association between the hormones and the induction of carcinoma in five cases of infiltrating ductal carcinoma of the breast in women who were taking the pill. Despite a lack of evidence linking the pill to breast cancer, it would seem advisable to find other means of contraception in the following high risk individuals:

    a. women with a strong family history of cancer;
    b. women with a history of cancer in one breast;
    c. women with recurrent chronic cystic mastitis;
    d. women with abnormal mammograms.

30. Have oral contraceptives been associated with other types of cancer?

There have been several reports describing adenocarcinoma of the endometrium in patients using oral contraceptives (269, 319, 320, 321, 415, 469, 473, 487, 544, 567). Further information is needed to define clearly the relationship between chronic use of high estrogen dominant oral contraceptives (the sequentials) and endometrial cancer appearing in young women (under 40). In one review of 21 cases of endometrial adenocarcinoma, 5 patients had taken predominately combined BCP's, and 11 patients took sequential BCPs, a ratio directly opposite that of the past usage of combined and sequential agents in the American population (469).

From 1971 to 1975, 63 newly diagnosed cases of adenocarcinoma of the endometrium were linked to estrogen usage in a survey of an affluent retirement community. The estimated risk for use of any estrogen was 8.0 times greater than non-pill users; and for conjugated estrogen use it was 5.6 times greater than non-pill users. Higher risks were associated with higher doses of estrogen, thus leading to the conclusion that estrogens should be given only at the lowest effective dose for the shortest possible time (321). Since chronic estrogen use increases the risk of adenocarcinoma of the endometrium on a dose-related basis, the FDA recommended to manufacturers that the sequential oral contraceptives be voluntarily removed from the market.

Due to the interest generated in the carcinogenic potential of estrogens, several investigators studied the relationship of estrogens and carcinoma of the cervix (444). An increased risk of carcinoma of the cervix was not noted in oral contraceptive users as compared to non-users. However, cervical carcinoma is a slowly developing disease and probably requires about 10 years for identification (140). Since the pill has been used less than 20 years, there is actually no proof that oral contraceptives have any relationship to cervical carcinoma.

31. A patient is switched to Enovid-E for her breakthrough bleeding. Her thyroid function tests include the following: T-4 = 12.5 mcg/100 cc and T-3 uptake = 20%. Do BCPs affect thyroid function and testing?

Tests which measure protein bound thyroxine are affected by BCPs (22, 146, 200, 428, 554). Estrogens increase the thyroid binding globulin and thereby increase circulating thyroxine. As a result, values for protein bound iodine, T-4 by column, and T-4 by Murphy Pattee will be elevated; and the T-3 resin uptake will be decreased. However, the uptake of radioactive iodine in the thyroid is, as a rule, normal and thyroid *function* is not changed because active free thyroxine levels are not affected. The free thyroxine index (FTI) can be calculated by taking the product of T-3 uptake and either the T-4 by Murphy Pattee or protein bound iodine (PBI). Normal values for the FTI at the University of California are 1.3 to 5.3. Other thyroid tests such as the I-131 uptake and thyroid stimulating hormone suppression test are not affected and remain within normal limits. (However, Rodriguiz, et al (428) reported low values for I-131 in 40% of users.) Thyroid function tests should return to normal two to four weeks after discontinuing the BCP although some investigators report that two to four months (165, 210) may be required.

The "mini-pill," norethindrone, does not alter protein binding or thyroid function tests (411). However, in a single study (49), subjects who received continuous low dose norethindrone exhibited a significant decrease in serum free throxine levels as compared to pretreatment values. It is postulated that norethindrone and, presumably, progesterones are capable of suppressing throxine production and/or release. The same results were observed when norethindrone was combined with mestranol. Injectable progestin contraceptives do not appear to influence tests of thyroid function (48, 149). Further research is needed to clarify the direct effect of progesterones on thyroid production.

32. A resident wants to know if Cushing's syndrome

can be caused or exacerbated by birth control pills. He is seeing a 28-year-old woman referred from screening clinic to rule out Cushing's disease. He is puzzled because the laboratory values showed decreased urinary 17-ketosteroids and the chart entry reads "R/O Cushing's, may be due to BCP." Your comment.

The estrogen component of the oral contraceptives can alter adrenal function testing by increasing transcortin, cortisol binding globulin (48, 303, 344). Therefore, patients on the pill show increased plasma cortisol levels resembling those seen in Cushing's syndrome (125). Due to increased binding, smaller amounts of free cortisol are available for metabolism, causing urinary excretion of 17-hydroxy-corticoids and 17-ketosteroids to decrease (48, 74, 146, 531). The birth control pill should be stopped weeks before evaluation of adrenal function in order to obtain a true value. The metapyrone test also will be altered in users (26, 305, 343), but the dexamethasone suppression test, which seems to be unaffected, can be used to exclude Cushing's disease (460).

The "mini-pill," which contains only progesterone, has not been shown to increase transcortin or increase plasma cortisol levels (48, 303). It has generally been accepted that the oral contraceptives do not alter adrenal responsiveness but only affect adrenal testing (343). However, Beck and associates (48) suggest that both the estrogen containing contraceptives and the "mini-pill" may alter adrenocortical function. Twenty subjects receiving either norethindrone combined with mestranol (10 subjects) or norethindrone alone had statistically significant decreases in cortisol secretion rates after therapy as compared to before therapy. Progesterone was suggested as the responsible component. Although both long and short term progestational therapy can suppress ACTH production, this aspect requires more study before a definite conclusion concerning adrenocortical suppression can be made (26).

33. A 28-year-old mildly obese diabetic woman wishes to start BCPs. Her diabetes was first diagnosed when an abnormal fasting blood sugar noted during the third trimester of her second pregnancy failed to regress after delivery. Family history revealed a father and sister with diabetes. Presently, her diabetes is controlled by diet alone and her urine sugars have been negative. How significant is the diabetogenic effect of oral contraceptives? Has one component been implicated?

Oral contraceptives do not alter fasting blood sugar in the majority of healthy users, but they definitely impair the oral and the I.V. glucose tolerance test (GTT) in predisposed patients (73, 483, 509, 520, 560). Phillips and Duffy (402) found that the results of one hour glucose tolerance tests in 4,815 healthy women taking the pill were 11 mg% higher than those of non-users. Although 11% is not a clinically significant increase, the implication is that the one hour tolerance in BCP users is comparable to that of women seven or eight years older, and this might reflect accelerated arteriosclerosis or other degenerative processes.

A delay in the time required to reach peak insulin levels and higher peak insulin levels were observed in women who take BCPs (50, 185, 477, 480, 483). Although there appear to be no alterations in growth hormone (480, 565), increased blood pyruvate, lactate, and cortisol levels have been observed (124, 560). Thus, various changes in hormone levels may contribute to the diabetogenic effect of BCPs, but further studies are required for confirmation.

Mestranol seems to be more responsible for deterioration of the GTT than ethinyl estradiol or the natural estrogens (Premarin) (122, 123, 380). Impairment of carbohydrate metabolism also seems to be more frequent if combinations rather than sequentials are used. Spellacy (480) studied 62 users for six to eight years and noted that the sequential group had 74.2% normal, 22.6% borderline abnormal, and 3.2% abnormal GTT's while the combination group had 22.6% normal, 38.7% borderline abnormal and 38.7% abnormal GTT's.

Susceptible persons to BCP-induced abnormal GTT's include:

    a. persons with a family history of diabetes;

    b. mothers of infants with birth weights greater than 8-9 lbs.;

    c. women who have an abnormal GTT during pregnancy; and

    d. obese subjects.

Posner (410) found no spontaneous recovery of GTT as long as BCPs were administered. Szabo (505) observed irreversible deterioration of the GTT in four of five women who had an abnormal GTT during pregnancy and resumed the pill after delivery; therefore, the pill *may* cause permanent diabetes in susceptible persons. However, most studies indicate that GTT returns to normal after discontinuation of BCPs.

Although more studies are needed, the "mini-pill" may be the pill of choice in patients with diabetes or latent diabetes since carbohydrate metabolism (as determined by GTT) appears to be unaltered by these agents (60, 70, 302, 366, 479, 482). Plasma glucose curves are only slightly affected, but plasma insulin levels can be significantly raised after treatment with the "mini-pill". It appears that the progestin, megestrol acetate, increases peripheral insulin resistance, and therefore more insulin is released to maintain glucose homeostasis (35). A trial with the "mini-pill" may be instituted if the patient is aware of its inherent disadvantages (see Question 2).

The total ultimate effect of BCPs on carbohydrate metabolism is not completely understood at this time.

Although some of the evidence appears to be contradictory, the clinician may minimize the risks by identifying those patients more liable to permanent carbohydrate intolerance.

34. A 22-year-old woman whose juvenile diabetes is controlled on NPH insulin would like to use the pill. The resident is hesitant because of the diabetogenic effects of the oral contraceptives. Your comment.

Oral contraceptives can certainly impair glucose tolerance and aggravate control of diabetes. Some feel, however, that since the beta-cells of these patients have no endogenous insulin, no further damage can be done to the pancreas. Although diabetic control may be made more difficult and insulin dosage may need readjustment, oral contraceptives are not absolutely contraindicated.

35. A 35-year-old woman with a seven year history of arthritis in the wrist, hands, arms, and legs, is seen in the outpatient clinic. She has been sporadically taking 6-12 aspirin daily for her arthritis. She also has been on Norlestrin for one year to prevent further pregnancies. No complications except BTB have occurred while on the pill. A complete blood count reveals a marked anemia. What are the possible etiologies of the anemia?

This patient's anemia may be caused by a number of factors acting alone or in combination. Aspirin-induced blood loss could be significant; the patient should be advised to take aspirin with warm water and/or antacids. Rheumatoid arthritis is associated with an anemia of unknown etiology. BTB, if severe, may also be contributory. (395).

The BCP's have been reported to cause folic acid (313, 336, 342, 363, 416, 440, 499, 513, 557) and/or vitamin B-12 megaloblastic anemia in a small percentage of susceptible persons (467, 547, 561). BCPs may block the enzymatic conversion of dietary polyglutamic folate to its absorbable monoglutamate form. The absorption is decreased by 50% (499); Castren and Ross (87) found that even though folate levels were lower in 30 healthy women after birth control therapy, these levels were not low enough to induce anemia. In another study of 526 women, the mean serum folate level for women taking oral contraceptives was not significantly lower than that in the control group (394).

Generally, there is a lack of evidence that oral contraceptives produce folate deficiency anemias in otherwise healthy subjects.

The studies on the effects of BCPs on vitamin B-12 are sparse. Wertalik and co-workers (547) noted that 15% of their 20 patients clearly had deficient levels of B-12. However, Prasad (413) found no significant alterations of vitamin B-12 serum levels due to BCP. It is postulated that oral contraceptives in some way increase the tissue avidity for vitamin B-12 resulting in a redistribution of the vitamin (298). However, further studies are needed to show that oral contraceptives can by themselves induce B-12 deficiency without other additional factors such as malnutrition or intercurrent disease. (260, 238, 466, 494)

36. A 24-year-old woman was hospitalized with shortness of breath, slight fever, and a tender swollen right calf which is 18 cm in diameter. Prior to admission she had been taking BCPs, aspirin for fever, and Actifed for sinus congestion. Significant laboratory values on admission included a prothrombin time (PT) of 14 seconds, ABG's: $pO_2 = 40$; $pCO_2 = 50$; $pH = 7.32$. A heparin infusion of 10,000 units in 250ml D5W every six hours was started on admission, and warfarin (Coumadin) was begun on the following day. After ten days she was discharged on warfarin 5 mg daily, and at this time her PT was 23 seconds. Four weeks later, her PT was 10 seconds. The intern would like to increase her dose of warfarin to 7.5 mg/day. Your comments.

It is possible that the patient resumed taking her BCPs. BCPs can increase clotting factors and therefore decrease the PT (214, 259, 337, 367, 456). The estrogen component is responsible for these effects with the sequential causing more pronounced changes of clotting factors than the combination type agents (348). Usually the BCP affects the clotting time if used for more than one or two cycles. Factors VII and X increase slowly but are increased in all users by the end of the third cycle. About 75% of users show an increase in prothrombin and IX, while all show increases in XII (135). Factors I,II,V, and VIII also are increased in most cases (193).

Although oral contraceptives affect specific clotting factors, the major mechanism by which they induce or facilitate intravascular coagulation is obscure. Oral contraceptives have been reported to reduce the activity of antithrombin III (100,243,143,154,530,400,569), which is the major inhibitor of activated factor X and thrombin and therefore an important factor in the pathogenesis of thromboemboli. In a recent study (548), oral contraceptives did not decrease the quantity of plasma antithrombin III although Xa inhibitory activity was significantly reduced among patients taking oral contraceptives. Depression of Xa inhibitory activity in the presence of a normal amount of antithrombin III does not necessarily mean that blood is actively clotting (hypercoagulability state), but rather that there is an increased risk of thrombosis following surgery, trauma, or other events that can initiate the thrombotic process.

Women using hormonal contraception have a slightly higher platelet count, increased platelet aggregation after long term use, slightly shorter partial thromboplastin time, accelerated thromboplastin generation, and elevation of coagulation factors (135). The presence of fibrinogen-fibrin complexes (6), and the presence of cryofibrinogen (intermediate complex developing after action of thrombin on fibrinogen), in 21% of 256 BCP users (306, 405) implies the occurrence of intravascular clotting.

Natural estrogens may not affect coagulation factors, and suggestions have been made to utilize natural estrogens in oral contraceptives (379, 380).

This patient should be questioned about the use of the pill before her dose of warfarin is increased. She should not be reinstated on the pill, and an alternate means of contraception should be used.

37. A 24-year-old white woman was hospitalized with a diagnosis of deep vein thrombosis. No predisposing factors were found, but she had taken Norlestrin 1 mg for three years. Review the relationship of the pill to thromboembolic disease.

Although the association between the pill and thromboembolic phenomena requires further study, there is increasing evidence that the administration of BCPs increases the likelihood of these occurrences. Clinical and epidemiologic studies relating the use of oral contraceptives to thromboembolic disease present conflicting viewpoints depending on the methods of design and statistical analysis. Retrospective studies suggest that such an association exists; however, these findings are not confirmed by most prospective studies. A summary of these results is presented.

In a retrospective study, Inman and Vessey (246) noted that 16 of 26 deaths secondary to pulmonary embolism occurred in otherwise healthy women taking the pill and concluded that the risk of death from pulmonary or cerebral thrombosis was increased seven to eight fold in BCP users. Similarly, Vessey and Doll (521) found that 45% (26/58) of healthy women with a diagnosis of deep vein thrombosis were using the pill as compared to 9% (10/116) of the controls. The use of the pill in women with a previous history of thrombophlebitis did not appear to increase the chance of recurrence, but the risk of venous thrombophlebitis was nine times greater in users than in non-users. Extending their study another year, Vessey and Doll (522) reaffirmed their previous results. Of 84 patients with deep vein thrombosis or pulmonary emboli, 42 (50%) had used oral contraceptives during the month preceding their illness while only 23 of the 168 controls (14%) had done so. An increased incidence of cerebral thrombosis was noted, and no differences in risk could be attributed to either the type of preparation or duration of use.

The results of the Collaborative Group for Study of Stroke (98) indicate that the estimated risk of cerebral ischemia or thrombosis is nine times greater in users of BCPs than in non-users, and more prevalent among white than black women. The Boston Collaborative

Program (66) estimates the risk of thromboembolic disorders with BCP usage to be eleven times that of non-users; and Masi (331) estimates a six fold increase in risk with these agents. These retrospective studies suggest a very strong association between the oral contraceptives and deep vein thrombosis or pulmonary emboli.

On the other hand, Drill and Calhoun (127) prospectively found an incidence of thrombophlebitis of 0.55 cases per 1000 women, considerably less than expected for women in the same age group (2.2 cases/1000 women per year). Based on these findings, they concluded that the pill does not cause thromboemboli. Their later prospective studies reaffirmed these results (129,130,192). These studies have not been as well accepted as Vessey's studies because of their poor design, lack of adequate controls, and variable patient populations and follow-ups.

The Royal College of General Practitioners' (436) six year prospective survey of 46,000 oral contraceptive users confirmed an increased incidence of venous thrombosis and cardiovascular disease in patients who use BCPs. However, these results have been criticized and invalidated on close statistical analysis, making this large study inconclusive. The Royal Australian College of General Practitioners' (437) showed no increased risk of thrombosis among users of BCPs than among non-users in each age group studied.

In an attempt to clarify existing data, Fuertes-de la Haba (176) designed a prospective study eliminating all the previously criticized variables. From this study, as well as from his later study (193) involving 9,898 women over an eight year period increases in the incidence of thromboembolic disease were not evident. Two other brief reports by the Boston Collaborative Group (66,67) also failed to confirm an increased incidence of thrombophlebitis in women taking the pill.

In a most extensive review and close analysis of all the reports of BCP induced thrombophlebitis, Goldzieher and Doizer (193) argue that early retrospective studies do not measure the incidence of thromboembolic disease in oral contraceptive users or non-users but rather actually measure the incidence of oral contraceptive use in women with thromboembolic disease as contrasted to oral contraceptive use in women with some other condition. Since virtually all the evidence supporting the causal relationship between oral contraceptives and thromboembolism is retrospective, conclusions must be examined carefully.

Retrospective studies and changes in the clotting system provide evidence for the association between various thromboembolic diseases and the pill. However, most prospective studies, which are needed to document a direct causal relationship, have not confirmed that such a risk exists for women on the pill. It is our opinion that more studies are needed to document the suggested relationship between the pill and thromboembolic diseases to predict which women might be prone to such occurrences. (4,5,214,241,338)

38. What pharmacological effects of BCPs could be responsible for an increased risk of thromboembolic disease?

The estrogen component seems to be the factor responsible for the "hypercoagulable state". The progestogen component has not been implicated since studies on blood clotting and platelet function have not revealed the same abnormalities induced by the estrogens. Therefore, the progestogen minipill may prove to be a safer form of contraception.

Although coagulation parameters, platelet function, and vessel anatomy change with the use of the oral contraceptives, none specifically predispose for thromboembolic disease. Similar changes occur in the 3rd trimester of pregnancy, but *despite these changes,* the incidence of thromboemboli during this period of pregnancy actually decreases, and the incidence increases during the postpartum period when coagulation abnormalities are disappearing.

Oral contraceptives elevate several clotting factors (135,193,348), decrease Antithrombin III (174, 400, 530, 569), decrease Xa inhibitory activity (548), and increase platelet count and platelet aggregation (135).

Statistically, patients with blood type O appear to be protected against formation of thromboemboli (256) as compared to those with blood type A, B, and AB. Blood type A is most common in patients with thromboembolic disease (256,356), and patients with blood group A antigen exhibit a greater "hypercoagulability" of blood when receiving BCPs (154). Interestingly, individuals with this blood type have slightly lower levels of antithrombin III (154).

Decreased venous blood flow and venous distensibility like that occurring in pregnancy (198,199), and an increased viscosity of blood occurs with the use of oral contraceptives (29). Changes in vessel anatomy which might predispose to thrombosis are endometrial proliferation, intimal thickening, and focal nodular thickening of the wall (248).

39. How can the risk of thromboembolic disease be reduced in users of BCPs?

To minimize BCP-induced thromboembolic disease, many clinicians suggest using the lower dose estrogenic preparations, since the estrogen component of BCPs is responsible for the changes in coagulation parameters (247, 348). The sequentials were associated with a higher risk of thromboembolic disorders probably due to their high estrogen content (227, 228). However, others do not believe the amount of estrogen is significant in the incidence of thromboembolic disorders (127, 193). Although this remains controversial,

based on information to date, the lower dose estrogenic products should be used when indicated (see Question 5 and 7).

Other risk factors to consider are the duration of use of BCPs and the age of the user. Although it is difficult to separate these risk factors, the age of the user appears to be more important with regard to increased incidence of thromboembolic disorders (193). More clinicians are recommending that patients age 35 or 40 currently taking BCPs should probably consider another means of contraception. A history of hypertension, severe varicose veins, obesity, and smoking would also be considered risk factors.

40. Do oral contraceptives increase the risk of myocardial infarction?

There have been several reports that indicate there is an increased risk of myocardial infarction in women taking oral contraceptives (4, 287, 322, 324, 325, 361, 387, 414, 418, 562, 535), but this observation requires confirmation.

Hartveit (223) and Oliver (388) studied the effect of oral contraceptives on coronary thrombosis and concluded that BCPs themselves did not cause myocardial infarction but probably affected women predisposed to ischemic heart disease. A controlled study (324) of 153 women less than 50 years of age who died of myocardial infarction showed a significant age-related association between oral contraceptives and myocardial infarction. The relative risk for the group 30 to 39 years of age was 2.8 times that of non-pill users and for the group 40 to 44 years of age was 4.7 times that of non-pill users (324). Another study (323) compared the frequency of use of oral contraceptives in 63 women (25 to 44 years of age) discharged from the hospital with a diagnosis of myocardial infarction with controls who were discharged from the same hospitals and were matched for age, marital status, and year of admission. The results also showed a positive association; 29% of the myocardial infarction patients and 8% of the controls used oral contraceptives. The risk increased 2.7 times in the 30 to 39 age group and 5.7 times in the 40 to 44 age group. Based on an additional 54 cases who died from myocardial infarction (322) in the 40 to 44 year age group, these investigators later revised their earlier estimate of a five fold increase in risk in this age group to a three-fold increase in risk. However, the total mortality attributable to complications associated with the use of oral contraceptives remained considerably greater among women over the age of 40.

The Boston Collaborative Drug Surveillance Program also studied the association between estrogen use and myocardial infarction in pre-menopausal women (67). Among 34 pre-menopausal women with myocardial infarction, 11.8% were currently using oral contraceptives and 5.9% were on other estrogen-containing drugs. Among 1,213 control subjects, oral contraceptives were used by 6.5% and 2.1% were on other estrogen products. Thus the crude relative risk for oral contraceptive users was 1.9 and for other estrogen users was 2.8 compared to non-users. However, after standardization for age of subjects and consideration of other factors (cigarette smoking, hypertension, angina, and diabetes) the relative risk for oral contraceptive users was 1.3 and for other estrogen users, 2.1.

Smoking, diabetes, obesity, history of pre-eclampsia, and hyperlipidemia are all factors that increase the risk of myocardial infarction, and it may have been the synergism of these factors which produced the increasing reports of myocardial infarction in young women. (251)

Although further studies are needed to confirm or refute the association between oral contraceptive use and increased risk of myocardial infarction careful consideration should be given to the implications of this potential adverse effect. Women over 40 years of age using oral contraceptives should be followed more closely and regularly, and discontinuation of oral contraceptives should be considered if other risk factors for cardiovascular disease are present.

41. A 24-year-old nurse is seen in the medical clinic with complaints of headache and lower back pain. She presents with a two-year history of hypertension which has been sporadically treated with Aldomet 750 mg/day; she has had no therapy for two weeks. Presently her blood pressure is 160/115. Significant laboratory findings show moderate renal deterioration (creatinine - 1.6 mg/100 ml; BUN - 30 mg/100 ml; creatinine clearance - 53 ml/min.). Medications include Aldomet and Ovulen for the last two years. Last year her physician discontinued her BCP for two weeks. However, because there were no significant changes in her blood pressure, the pills were resumed. Comment on the use of BCPs in this patient.

There is no doubt that the pill can induce or exacerbate preexisting hypertension in susceptible individuals (80, 105, 136, 205, 279, 295, 296, 297, 301, 317, 332, 368, 439, 471, 478, 484, 516, 538, 540, 542). The trial period off the pill was too short to negate the effects on the blood pressure. Pill-induced hypertension usually declines gradually over one to six months (three months average) after the medication is withdrawn (105, 475, 538). Likewise, the blood pressure increases slowly and elevation may not become significant for several (3-36) months (471, 538, 541). The pill should be discontinued for at least three months and pill-induced hypertension ruled out before further evaluation of the blood pressure is undertaken.

42. What is the mechanism for pill-induced hypertension?

The most widely circulated theory of BCP-induced

hypertension involves the renin-angiotensin system (78, 297, 478, 507, 518). Normally, a decrease in blood pressure leads to a release of the enzyme, renin, from the juxtaglomerular apparatus into the plasma. The renin then works on plasma renin substrate (angiotensinogen) to release angiotensin I, which is converted into active angiotensin II by enzymes in the kidney. Angiotensin II increases blood pressure by its potent vasopressor effects, and by stimulating the release of aldosterone which increases sodium and water reabsorption. Estrogen increases angiotensinogen two to five fold resulting in an increased renin "activity" (11, 51, 53, 105, 297, 368, 508, 538). Normally, the increased angiotensin exerts a negative feedback effect on the juxtaglomerular apparatus to shut off renin release and reduce the amount of angiotensin to normal. Hypertension occurs in women who are unable to suppress renin release in the presence of increased renin substrate (450). Normotensive BCP users also have increased renin substrate but do not have increased renin activity.

Other mechanisms have been suggested. The renal sodium retaining effects of the estrogens result in increased blood volume and cardiac output. Increased sympathetic activity may also be responsible for oral contraceptive-induced hypertension. When plasma dopamine-B-hydroxylase is used as an index of sympathetic activity (426), the levels are noted to be increased in pill users and are even higher in those users who develop hypertension.

Although there is no concensus on the exact mechanisms by which oral contraceptives produce hypertension, the risk of hypertension due to oral contraceptives is well accepted, and predisposed patients should use these agents only with close monitoring, if at all. (365)

43. What is the incidence and significance of oral contraceptive hypertension? Has one component been implicated as the cause?

The incidence of hypertension due to the BCP is highly variable; it ranges from 1% (475) to 15-18% (450, 516). A value of 5-6% (105, 439, 478) is probably more realistic. The elevation in blood pressure is often mild (in the range of 2.3-5.0 mm Hg), but malignant hypertension has been reported (221, 512).

The estrogen component seems to be primarily responsible for the BCP-induced changes in the renin-angiotensin system (see Question 42). There is no difference between mestranol (6%) or ethinyl estradiol (7%) in bringing about these changes (478). Crane and associates (105) described five patients who developed hypertension three months to five years after the ingestion of conjugated estrogens; four of these five patients became normotensive one to seven months after the conjugated estrogens were discontinued.

Progesterone, though not clearly implicated, may also contribute to blood pressure changes. Medroxyprogesterone (150 mg every month) was shown to produce a rapid increase in the diastolic and systolic blood pressure in 24% of users; 15.7% of these remained in the normotensive range despite elevations in the systolic pressure of more than 20 mm Hg (309). Spellacy and Birk (478) studied the effects of medroxyprogesterone (MP), ethynodiol diacetate, and norgestrel on blood pressure and found that MP elevated diastolic, while norgestrel decreased the diastolic pressure. The effects of progesterone on blood pressure require further study.

44. A patient who has been taking Demulen for several years suddenly develops severe lower abdominal pain and bloody, watery diarrhea. Could these symptoms be related to the oral contraceptives?

Yes, ischemic colitis and thrombosis of the mesenteric and the celiac artery and of the hepatic veins are significant complications of BCPs (56, 139).

The possibility of mesenteric vascular disease, sometimes with necrosis and infarction of the bowel, should always be considered in women with acute gastrointestinal complaints. Since more than 20 such cases have been reported, the association may not be as fortuitous as has been suggested (42, 139, 148, 329, 528).

45. A 34-year-old woman was admitted to the emergency room at 9pm with an acute attack of severe epigastric pain in the right upper quadrant accompanied by nausea, vomiting and low grade fever. The patient has no history of peptic ulcer disease. She was hospitalized and an UGI series and cholecystography showed a large number of gallstones and the patient was scheduled for surgery. The patient had been taking Ovulen for the past eight years. Has chronic use of birth control pills increased the incidence of gallstones?

Oral contraceptives appear to be associated with an increased incidence of cholecystitis and cholelithiasis (66, 67, 218, 242, 408, 436, 446). According to the Boston Collaborative Drug Surveillance Program, the annual attack rate of surgically proven gallbladder disease is about 79 per 100,000 in otherwise healthy women who do not use oral contraceptives and about twice that (158 per 100,000) in those who do (67). The Royal College of General Practitioners (436) also noted a two-fold increase in the incidence of gallbladder disease among oral contraceptive users.

Supersaturation of gallbladder bile with cholesterol and changes in bile acid composition may be responsible (54). Cholesterol gallstones usually occur in bile that contains more cholesterol than can be solubilized by the available bile acids and phospholipids (16). Chemical gallstone disease predates the radiologic appearance of gallstones by months or years, and there

may be an additional lag of several years before the gallstones become symptomatic (472). Therefore, the risk may be greater than that estimated by the Boston Collaborative Drug Surveillance Program.

46. A 42-year-old woman presented with a three month history of epigastric pain, anorexia and weight loss. She had been taking Ortho Novum 1/50 for the past 8 years. On examination her liver was found to be grossly enlarged, and laparotomy revealed a large mass in the right lobe and nodules in the left lobe. Histological examination revealed hepatocellular carcinoma (malignant hepatoma). Comment on the association of BCP and liver tumors.

More than 100 cases of BCP-associated liver tumors (described as benign hepatoma, hepatic adenoma, or focal nodular hyperplasia) have been reported since Baum (46) first reported seven cases in 1973. The incidence of benign liver tumors is unknown, but hepatologists agree that these lesions are very uncommon (370). In the past three years, such lesions have occurred with increasing frequency in young women (3, 10, 27, 40, 44, 46, 55, 68, 94, 95, 114, 103, 138, 187, 219, 236, 240, 272, 282, 283, 334, 345, 393, 465, 491, 492). Although the majority have been benign, malignant forms have been documented (182, 392).

In a recent review by Nissen (370), oral contraceptive use for periods varying from 6 months to 10 years was common to 67 cases of hepatoma. Hepatitis and known hepatotoxins were excluded as etiologic factors in all documented cases. Thus, the appearance of these tumors probably represents a cause and effect phenomenon. Eighteen of these patients presented with intrahepatic or extrahepatic rupture and hemoperitoneum with hemorrhagic shock due to vascular changes within their liver tumors; five died as a result of preoperative or postoperative blood loss.

The mean duration of oral contraceptive use is approximately six years in patients with liver cell adenomas. This accounts for the latency period between the beginning of widespread use of oral contraceptives in the mid 1960's and recognition of BCP-associated liver cell tumors in the 1970's.

Experimental and clinical data link estrogens and progesterones to other forms of liver damage. An increased incidence of hepatocellular carcinoma in male rats and the development of variations in liver cell size, cellular swelling, and opening up of sinusoids in female rats occurred with norethynodrel (315). While BCP-induced hepatomas seem to occur only after several years of continued usage, the oral contraceptives do have immediate effects on the liver. Estrogens stimulate hepatic synthesis of plasma proteins affecting the rough endoplasmic reticulum (3, 142), and progesterones stimulate formation of hepatic drug metabolizing enzymes by affecting the smooth endoplasmic reticulum (3). Estrogens may also stimulate regeneration of liver tissue (142).

Since the synthetic estrogens and progesterones used in many of the oral contraceptive preparations are 17-alkyl substituted steroids, similar in structure to anabolic steroids, it is not surprising that deleterious effects on hepatic function were noted soon after oral contraceptives were introduced in 1960. Androgenic anabolic steroids, which may cause jaundice and cholestasis, have also been associated with the development of hepatocellular carcinomas (275) and peliosis hepatis (41) after long-term use. Further evidence that oral contraceptives may be implicated in the evolution of hepatic tumors in humans is based on reports that liver cell adenomas occasionally reoccurred in women who reinstituted oral contraceptive use after resection of an adenoma (333) and unpublished reports that unresectable tumors decreased in size when oral contraceptive agents were withdrawn.

47. Mrs. G. presents a prescription for Periactin for pruritus which has bothered her for the past week. She also requests refills for the following medications: BCPs, Bonine for nausea and Kaopectate for her light stools. Comment.

With symptoms of nausea, pruritis, and light stools, BCP-induced cholestatic jaundice should be considered. Mrs. G. should be questioned as to the onset of her symptoms and the duration of her birth control usage.

Hepatic dysfunctions induced by the BCP are usually benign, reversible, and cholestatic (146,310). Ockner and Davidson (382) reported 40 cases of jaundice caused by oral contraceptives. Characteristically malaise, anorexia, nausea, and pruritus occur two weeks to several months (usually less than four weeks) after beginning the pill; later, dark urine and jaundice appear. Cessation of birth control therapy usually results in complete clinical remission within a few weeks to a month.

No one component of the pill has been implicated. However, anabolic steroids, estriol, estradiol, and particularly steroids alkylated at C-17 can produce cholestatic jaundice (45, 109, 146, 264, 340, 382). BCP-induced jaundice of pregnancy appears to occur more frequently in Scandinavia and Chile where recurrent jaundice of pregnancy is common (146, 337). Haemmerli and Wyss (211) calculate that the risk of oral contraceptive jaundice is 2,000 to 8,000 times greater in women with a history of jaundice of pregnancy.

48. What laboratory tests can be done to document suspicions of cholestatic jaundice?

Bilirubin is usually elevated to 3-10 mg/100 ml and this is due to the direct, conjugated portion. Transaminase values (normal 5-40 U) are moderately elevated (100-300 U). Occasionally the SGOT and SGPT may go as high as 1100 U and 1500 U respectively, thereby mimicking viral hepatitis (222, 337, 382, 510). Unlike other types of drug induced cholestasis, alkaline phosphatase may or may not be elevated (222, 510). A liver biopsy reveals canalicular and hepatocellular degeneration and necrosis, and minimal or absent inflammatory reactions (267, 382, 510).

The pill can also cause asymptomatic alterations in liver function tests. Mild increases in BSP retention (16% or less) have been reported in 21% of women on oral contraceptives who had no other clinical findings (146, 346, 514). Elevations in transaminases are observed in 0% (422,503) to 6% (299) to 15-18% (141) of women taking BCPs. The SGOT has not exceeded 82 U and the SGPT 140 U in asymptomatic women (382). Alkaline phosphatase is elevated in fewer than 2% of subjects (141, 299, 346).

Asymptomatic disturbances in bromsulphthalein do not necessitate discontinuation of the BCP, but alterations in transaminases and alkaline phosphatase warrant closer observation (382, 452). In our opinion, women without a history of jaundice in pregnancy and with elevated transaminases can be kept on the pill, but liver function should be closely monitored. The patient should then be warned of the symptoms and told that they are reversible if the BCP is discontinued.

49. A 22-year-old woman complains of throbbing headaches, accompanied by an aura, which have occurred at the end of each month since she has been taking Ovulen (1 year). There is no family history of headaches and no other drugs except aspirin have been taken. Are these headaches related to the pill?

This might be pill-induced migraine due to hormone withdrawal (289, 517). The patient should be specifically questioned as to when the headaches occur, since hormone withdrawal headaches tend to occur on the first or second day off the pill each month. Although both progesterone and estrogen withdrawal have been implicated, the latter seems more important. In eight women with migraine, estradiol injections given three to six days before the onset of menses delayed the onset of headache three to nine days. Most women experienced the headache when the plasma estradiol levels dropped below 20 mcg/100 ml. No delay in onset of headaches was noted with progesterone injections. (18, 140, 203, 476)

50. A 26-year-old woman presents with a three year history of headaches. The headaches begin with a blurred vision. An aura of about an hour's duration, characterized by nausea and vomiting, precedes the actual throbbing headache. The headaches seem to start early in the morning and last about two to three days. They occur twice a month with no relation to periods. There is a family history of a sister and an

aunt with migraine. A physical exam showed marked dermatitis and moderate proptosis with lid lag. Analgesics do not relieve the attacks; however, lying in a dark room seems to help. The patient is currently taking aspirin and has been taking Ovral for two years. A diagnosis of migraine due to oral contraceptives was made, the pill was discontinued, and a diaphragm was fitted. What is the incidence and significance of migraine due to BCPs?

The occurrence of headaches as a complication of the pill is a well-recognized phenomenon. However, because there is poor literature documentation of a causal relationship and good clinical studies are lacking, the incidence is difficult to ascertain. Grant (202) reported an incidence of 11%, while Goldzieher and associates (194) noted an incidence of 3.2% in 166 patients. In the latter study more than half of these patients had headaches prior to oral contraceptive treatment.

The headaches encountered are often typical of classical migraine (31, 120, 401, 462), although nonspecific or tension headaches may also occur (117, 120). Of 41 patients in a neurologic clinic, 20 patients with a prior history of migraine noted an increased severity and number of attacks while on the pill and 21 patients without previous history of migraine developed headaches while under the contraceptive regimen (401). Shafey and Scheinberg (462) reported 50 patients who developed or had an exacerbation of classical migraine; auras were present in half of the patients. One-third of these patients developed migraine *de novo* on the pill. Similarly, Desrosiers (117) described 32 of 46 patients (69.5%) with a history of previous attacks who developed increased incidence and severity of migraine symptoms on the pill. He noted that the migraine attacks seemed to appear between the last pill and the first day of menses, while tension headaches occurred throughout the cycle with no definite pattern. Others agree with this temporal relationship (83, 120).

While many patients have headaches on the pill, others have noted an improvement while taking the medication (339). Whitty and co-workers (551) reported striking results — complete freedom of headache attacks in 51-83% of chronic headache patients using the pill. In this regard it is interesting to note that progesterones have been used successfully in the treatment of migraine (300).

A study of 886 non-pregnant migraine sufferers (110) (241 pill takers, 290 ex-takers and 355 non-takers) found that more than a third of the patients who were taking the pill noted worsening of their migraines, and more than a third of those who had used the pill previously noted improvement upon stopping the pill. A significant increase in migraine at mid-cycle was most marked among those with severe attacks. (110)

The etiology of these headaches is unknown, although various mechanisms have been postulated. It has been suggested that they may be due to withdrawal of both progesterones (300) and estrogens (476). Other factors such as sodium and water retention secondary to the estrogen component and ordinary tension may be contributory factors.

Dalton (110) suggests that several factors may cause worsening of migraine among pill takers: age, especially after 30 years; parity; length of menstrual cycle outside the conventional 27-30 days; menstrual pattern of migraine; relief of migraine during the last trimester of pregnancy; and onset of migraine after a pregnancy. He concludes that any woman on the pill who develops migraine at mid-cycle should adopt another method of contraception.

Desrosiers (117) tentatively concluded that a combination of weak progesterone and weak estrogen or a strong combination of both preparations resulted in the lowest incidence of headache attacks. However, Dalton (110) found that an increase in migraine on the pill is unrelated to either the dosage, type of estrogen or progestogen which confirms clinical experience that deterioration of migraine on the pill is not likely to be improved by changing to a different pill.

Diuretics and conventional headache regimens have been used in treatment (117); however, response to appropriate drug therapy has sometimes been ineffective until the pill has been discontinued (462). Discontinuation is appropriate as headaches may be a forewarning of impending stroke or cerebral thrombosis (461, 532).

51. A 28-year-old woman with a history of depression wishes to use BCPs. Her physician is reluctant, as he feels that her condition might be aggravated. She takes only Elavil, 150 mg at bedtime. What is the mechanism of pill-induced depression? How should it be managed?

The literature on the pill and depression is inconsistent. Pill-induced depression and loss of libido are common reasons for discontinuing the pill (326). While oral contraceptives often alleviate premenstrual depression (233, 291), some women will become seriously depressed with continued use (19, 234, 235, 290, 308, 312). The incidence of depression secondary to the pill is difficult to ascertain but seems to be in the range of 5-6%. Of 261 women (168 on BCPs and 93 using other means of contraception) in which depression was evaluated through a self rating scale, 6.6% of the women on the pill were found to be more severely depressed than those using other means of contraception (235). These results tend to agree with those of other investigators (183, 233, 312). Wearing (536) reported a 16% incidence of depression in 62 patients and noted that depression became more prominent the longer the patient remained on the pill. According to one study, some symptoms of depression are seen in as many as 45% of women taking the pill (167). Predominant symptoms include pessimism, dissatisfaction, crying and tension (235). These can occur throughout the cycle but are the most commonly seen one to five days prior to menstruation.

Other investigators have been unable to correlate the pill to depression (37, 307, 360). A highly critical double blind placebo controlled study involving 398 women over 1,523 cycles found no significant increase in the incidence of nervousness and depression in BCP users (195). Women with a history of depressive disorder, severe premenstrual or gestational depression are those most likely to develop depression when using the pill (312, 234, 291, 233).

The cause of contraceptive depression remains obscure. Psychological factors have been suggested as have pills with a high progestogen content (12, 312). In one report (204), the incidence of depression and loss of libido was 28% in women on strongly progestational preparations, 7% in women on strongly estrogenic preparations, and 5% in women on sequentials (12, 312). A recent hypothesis for depression is that brain amine metabolism is altered as a result of abnormal tryptophan metabolism which is caused by pyridoxine (B-6) deficiency (1,2,42,427,556). Theoretically, the administration of pyridoxine could correct altered trytophan metabolism and alleviate pill-induced depression; an uncontrolled study provides some support for this thesis (47, 308, 555). In a double blind crossover study involving 22 healthy women with no predisposing causes for depression, 11 had clinical evidence of B-6 deficiency while the remainder did not (1). As expected, only the half with evidence of B-6 deficiency responded to its administration. Although contraceptive depression is still controversial, a trial of 25-50 mg daily of pyridoxine might be beneficial.

The physician is certainly right to be cautious and reluctant to use BCPs in this patient who is currently requiring management of depression with tricyclic antidepressants. This patient should not use BCPs but rather some other means of contraception. However, if she refuses to discontinue her BCPs, 50 mg of pyridoxine daily should be added in an attempt to prevent the depression.

52. A 30-year-old woman wishes a refill of Ortho Novum 1/80 #63. She mentions that she was vacationing in sunny Florida last month and got a bad case of sunburn which won't go away. You notice a brownish-like macular pigmentation on the forehead and malar regions. She would like to know what you have in the way of a skin lightening agent. Your comments.

The patient should be informed that the pigmentation may be a side-effect of BCPs. This is known as chloasma or the "mask of pregnancy" and seems to be aggravated by sunlight (51, 351, 413, 421). She should

be assured there is no danger; however, she should be referred to her physician for further evaluation. No lightening agents available over-the-counter have demonstrated any efficacy, although a sunscreening agent prior to sunlight exposure may be helpful. Taking the BCP at night may theoretically be helpful since circulating hormone levels will be minimal during the day when the skin is exposed to sun. One study evaluating the use of 2-5% hydroquinone cream (Eldoquin) in this condition, noted temporary improvement in 18/20 patients after one month of therapy (28, 486).

53. Is chloasma or melasma a significant complication of the pill?

Chloasma is one of the most common cutaneous complications of oral contraceptives; however naturally occurring estrogens (Premarin) apparently do not produce this particular effect (254). The true incidence is difficult to assess since reports range from 0-40% (14, 421). Carruthers (85) noted an incidence of 4% following one year of use which increased to 37% by the fifth year of use. Resnik (421) reported an incidence of 29%.

Chloasma or melasma appears to be more prevalent in geographical areas with more sunlight and may be more marked in dark skinned races. There is a positive correlation between the duration of therapy as well as the estrogen and progesterone content. Estrogens stimulate the melanocytes while the progesterones cause their spread (84).

The areas of hyperpigmentation are symmetrically distributed, irregular-shaped brown macules that most commonly occur on the forehead, malar eminences, lower cheeks and upper lip. The pigmentation tends to develop slowly and can appear from 1-20 months after starting therapy (85). Melasma in pregnancy may be predictive of susceptible individuals (254, 421). One study showed that 87% (52/61) of persons who developed melasma from BCPs had this condition during pregnancy (421). BCP induced melasma fades more slowly than that of pregnancy and may be permanent (14). In seven patients no improvement in the pigmentation was noted 3½ years after discontinuing the pill (421).

54. A 30-year-old woman who stopped taking Ortho-Novum 1/50 two months ago asks the community pharmacist if her recent diffuse hair loss is due to the pill or some other cause such as her shampoo.

Two types of alopecia have been associated with the use of BCPs. Hair loss may occur while the patient is maintained on therapy (15, 104, 413) or may occur one to four months following the cessation of BCPs (208, 519). Hair loss is diffuse; alopecia areata (patchy baldness) has not been associated with these agents. The reason for contraceptive induced hair loss is not clear. During pregnancy normal hair loss is retarded and then increases 1-4 months following delivery. Hair studies show that 95% of the scalp hairs remain in the growing (anagen) phase during pregnancy; however, in the postpartum period 25-55% of the hairs go into the resting phase (telogen); invariably hair loss results. It is believed that estrogens tend to maintain the hair in the anagen phase and that lower postpartum levels cause the hair to go into the telogen phase.

It is tempting to ascribe a similar mechanism to hair loss following the cessation of oral contraceptive therapy. However, careful studies on the effects of oral contraceptives on hair cycles have shown that the changes do not resemble those seen in pregnancy (15, 208). Some have suggested that the progesterone may give rise to a male baldness pattern. Carefully controlled studies are required to provide concrete evidence of the association of BCPs with alopecia.

55. An 18-year-old woman is seen in Dermatology Clinic for a one month outbreak of papulopustules on the lower cheeks and chin. No history of any contact sensitivity can be documented. She is not taking any drugs, but she discontinued taking Ovulen about three months before the eruption. Is acne pill-related? Can BCPs be used in the treatment of acne? Which type would you recommend?

Although the pill improves acne by suppressing levels of androgens, post-contraceptive acne is a common complaint (280, 389, 537). It is usually seen in women who have been on the pill at least one year and occurs three to four months after the pill has been discontinued (280). These lesions are self-limiting and usually subside in 6-12 months without treatment. The cause is thought to be a compensatory hypersecretion of gonadotropins as there is increased oiliness after treatment. Fortunately, these eruptions respond to conventional acne therapy if the patient wishes treatment (280).

Acne can also occur during treatment with BCPs and is a sign of progestational excess. Therefore, reports of severe acne attributed to Ovral (179, 280, 559) are not surprising; these cases responded dramatically to cessation of the BCP. Patients who experience this sign of progesterone excess can be given a less dominant pill such as Demulen. (See also Question 6; Tables 1 and 2.)

Birth control pills are efficacious in the control of acne as well (396, 397, 498). Estrogens decrease the size of the sebaceous glands or depress production of ovarian and adrenal androgens by inhibiting the pituitary function (498). Estrogens further depress sebaceous activity by increasing the synthesis of proteins that bind androgens. The ideal pills for the treatment of acne were the sequentials which are no longer available; the current pill of choice for acne treatment contains an estrogenic progestin without androgenic potential such as norethynodrel (Enovid-E) or ethynodiol-diacetate (Demulen) (396). Improvement with the pill is slow and is not apparent for one to four

months following the onset of therapy (254). Despite its proven efficacy in acne, its use is not recommended since serious complications may result from long-term use of these agents.

56. A 24-year-old woman with a two year history of lupus erythematosus (LE) is admitted to the hospital with an acute flareup. She presents with fever, malaise, ten pound weight loss, anorexia, joint symptoms and characteristic malar rash. Electron microscopy of renal biopsy revealed wire loop changes and deposits of complement and immunoglobulins on the glomerular membrane. Urinalysis revealed 3+ proteinuria, 10-12 RBC/HPF and RBC casts. Lab findings consisted of a hematocrit (HCT) of 33%, positive antinuclear antibodies (ANA), a positive LE prep, and an erythrocyte sedimentation rate (ESR) of 60. Drugs on admission included 10-15 aspirin daily for joint pain, Maalox, and Ovulen for two weeks. Have birth control pills been implicated in the exacerbation or initiation of collagen vascular diseases?

In rare cases, oral contraceptives may exacerbate lupus erythematosus (90, 404). More commonly, positive LE and ANA preparations have developed in healthy pill users, although the significance of this is unclear (134, 180). Schleicher (453) reported the occurrence of positive LE preps with arthralgias in ten healthy young women who had taken the pill for six months to three years. These signs and symptoms remitted spontaneously four to eight weeks after the pill was discontinued. The LE prep again became positive six to nine weeks after the birth control pill was restarted in two users. Similar findings were reported by Bole and associates (62) in eight patients on the pill. In this study the ANA disappeared in 5/8 patients and the LE cell disappeared in 5/6 patients after the birth control pill was discontinued. In addition, five patients were found to have elevated IgM levels which remained high after the birth control pill was discontinued. Kay and associates (270) studies 82 patients who had taken the pill for one year, and found a positive ANA in four, a positive rheumatoid factor in nine, and C-reactive proteins in 30 women. No rheumatic symptoms were noted in these users (270). Splekin and Plotz (489) also reported the development of arthritis, arthralgia and myalgia in 22 women who had been on the pill for three months to one year. These symptoms disappeared two to six weeks after cessation of the pill.

57. Has erythema nodosum ever been reported as a complication of oral contraceptives?

Although several cases have been reported in the literature (57, 59, 61, 111, 180, 265, 274, 275, 488, 501), the actual incidence in the clinical setting is undetermined. BCP-induced erythema nodosum seems to be a hypersensitivity reaction to the progesterone component of the pill (39). Baden and Holcomb (39) found that by switching to a BCP with a different progestational agent and the same estrogen, the reaction could be avoided although others (274) could not confirm these findings. Agents which have been implicated include norethynodrel, norethindrone and norgestrel (147).

There has also been one report of a young woman simultaneously developing erythema nodosum (EN) and serological signs of lupus erythematosus while taking an oral contraceptive. Both the EN and LE disappeared following cessation of medication but recurred with reinstitution of therapy (147).

58. A 28-year-old patient has had rheumatoid arthritis for six years with minimal complaints or complications. She presents with uncontrolled arthritic type pains which occurred three months after starting Ortho Novum 1/80. Can oral contraceptives adversely affect rheumatoid arthritis?

Although several reports link oral contraceptives to other rheumatic diseases (eg, lupus, erythema nodosum), there is no direct relationship between oral contraceptive usage and rheumatoid arthritis (61, 488). However, rheumatoid arthritis is a chronic disease characterized by spontaneous exacerbations and remissions that is not completely understood. Since the psychological well being of the patient is important to control this disease, it may be that psychological changes, produced by the pill, could exacerbate rheumatoid arthritis.

Since the trial use of BCPs seems to have caused an exacerbation of her rheumatoid arthritis, the BCP should be discontinued and the patient observed for disappearance of symptomatology. If rheumatic complaints subsequently subside, one more trial of BCPs could be recommended, but the patient would probably be better advised to use some other means of contraception.

59. A 23-year-old female enters a pharmacy for some contact lens wetting solution and a refill for her BCPs. She also wants something for dryness and itchiness of her eyes. What ophthalmic disturbances have been associated with BCP use?

Increased discomfort from the wearing of contact lenses can be a complication of the pill (81, 92, 421, 438, 441). The literature is devoid of well-documented cause and effect studies, although many isolated cases have been observed. Pregnancy may result in loss of contact lens tolerance both for scleral and corneal lenses. The well-fitted contact wearer may have fewer complications than the poorly-fitted or newly-fitted wearer (421). The underlying cause has been attributed to a change in the lubricant quality of tears resulting in contact lens discomfort (421, 438). The actual effects on the contact lens wearer are hard to assess, but lid edema, corneal staining and edema (81, 451), photophobia, and changes in visual acuity have been associated with the

pill (284, 398). Some have felt that corneal edema may be caused by estrogen water retention leading to changes in keratometry values. Others have suggested that these effects may not be due to the pill but to environmental changes and pollution (92).

Oral contraceptives have also been associated with a number of neuro-ophthalmic sequelae (101, 102, 150, 157, 170, 386, 429, 443, 532), including optic neuritis, retinal edema (201), pseudotumor cerebri, and the flashing light syndrome (52). Patients occasionally complain of blurred or double vision. Papilledema has also been observed (532). Walsh (532) collected 69 cases of patients with visual and neurologic symptoms while on the pill. The earliest onset of symptoms relative to the initiation of contraceptive therapy was within 58 hours, the latest after a few years. Twenty patients had pure ocular involvement secondary to central vein occlusion. One group of investigators (443) noted that more than half of the 100 patients with serious ophthalmic sequelae had a predisposing medical history (e.g. hypertension, migraine preceding the onset of symptoms). This group recommended that, because of the possibility of stroke, the occurrence of transient neurologic symptoms associated with the pill were indications for its immediate discontinuation.

Another aspect of ocular disturbances associated with the pill occurs in patients with myopia and astigmatism (442). Marked changes in astigmatic error may occur in these patients, resulting in frank keratoconus (conical protrusion of the cornea). These changes may not be apparent until six months after the pill has been started.

Glaucoma has occurred in three patients on the pill, one with a positive family history. However this relationship appears to be coincidental at present.

60. A patient who has been controlled with Ovulen-21 for 14 months has a sudden attack of blindness in the right eye and is carried to the emergency room. Could oral contraceptives be a complicating factor? What is the treatment for this condition?

Five articles describe cases of arterial occlusion in the retina, and thrombosis of the central retinal vein has been mentioned in several other articles (170, 196). Ischemia of the retina, due to acute occlusion of the central retinal artery has been noted in the literature as a cause of partial and total loss of sight (196).

Immediate treatment with IV heparin, papaverine, oral warfarin and xanthiol nicotinate as well as local massage, resulted in recovery of eyesight in one patient but was unsuccessful in another (170). Steroids have also been used with limited success (170).

61. A 24-year-old female on birth control pills complains of a ten pound weight gain. Was the weight gain caused by her BCPs?

Weight gain can be caused by either the estrogen or

progesterone component depending on the duration of pill usage. Estrogens can cause a transient or cyclic weight gain early in the cycle due to salt and water retaining effects (42). The patient may be switched to a lower estrogenic preparation or treated temporarily with diuretics. Progesterone can also cause weight gain with prolonged use due to its anabolic and appetite-stimulating properties (42). Usually the weight increases slowly and the gain is minor (5-10 lbs, although 30 lb gains have been reported), so that it is usually unnecessary to change pills.

62. An 18-year-old woman with a history of chronic asthmatic bronchitis is placed on Ovral. After her first bedtime dose, she awakens in the night with symptoms of shortness of breath and dyspnea. Are some patients allergic to oral contraceptives?

Aggravation of bronchial asthma as well as eczema and vasomotor rhinitis have been observed (7,43,55,163). Oral contraceptives were implicated in eight of 75 patients with vasomotor rhinitis and six patients with hypertropic rhinitis (55).

One case of angioneurotic edema has been reported with Ovulen (558). Oral contraceptives may help relieve or aggravate the asthmatic symptoms (558). Their use is certainly not contraindicated in this disease but should be monitored closely when therapy is initiated.

63. A 28-year-old woman was admitted to the hospital with a chief complaint of cough. She had tuberculosis three years ago and was treated with isoniazid (INH) and aminosalicylate calcium for one year. She presents with a right upper lobe infiltrate and right hilar adenopathy. Sputum cultures were positive for mycobacterium tuberculosis. The patient was given INH, 300 mg daily; ethambutol hydrochloride, 800mg daily; and Rifampin, 600mg daily. Six months later she was discovered to be six weeks pregnant. She was receiving oral contraceptives at the time (Ovral) and denied missing any doses. Have any of the antitubercular drugs been implicated in reducing the effectiveness of oral contraceptives?

There are twelve studies to date concerning pregnancy or menstrual abnormalities associated with rifampin ingestion (470). In 1973, five cases of pregnancy occurred in women receiving both oral contraceptives and rifampin (372) were subsequently reported (177). However, as early as 1971, Reimers and Jezek reported menstrual disorders in 62 of 88 women (70%) receiving oral contraceptives and rifampin (422).

By comparison only four percent of women receiving oral contraceptives and other anti-tuberculous drugs experienced menstrual abnormalities (97). These problems have resulted in the following warning on rifampin package inserts:

"It has been reported that the reliability of oral contraceptives may be affected in some patients being treated for tuberculosis with rifampin in combination with at least one other antituberculous drug. In such cases, alternative contraceptive measures may need to be considered; menstrual disturbances have also been noted."

This drug interaction is not completely understood and the mechanism is still controversial. Of several theories, the most prominent are the enzyme induction theory and the competitive action theory. Rifampin may stimulate hepatic hydrolases, which in turn increase the biliary elimination of exogenous estrogens. There is evidence for the increased breakdown of exogenous estrogens in the presence of rifampin, with estrogen serum levels decreasing below the concentration necessary for contraception (63, 212, 330, 358, 372, 504).

The competitive action theory is actually the reverse of the enzyme induction theory. According to this theory, rifampin blocks the elimination of estrogens (372). Such a situation would favor conception (372). Of 11 patients who were taking rifampin and oral contraceptives and who had menstrual irregularities, urine estrone and estriol levels were increased in five, decreased in three, and unchanged in three (372,373).

64. Are there any other drugs that affect oral contraceptive activity or are affected by oral contraceptives?

Some antiepileptic drugs may decrease the effectiveness of oral contraceptives by inducing enzymatic metabolism of the hormone. Increased spotting and three pregnancies have been observed in recipients of BCPs and antiepileptic drugs (292). Loss of seizure control is believed due to the fluid retention which accompanies oral contraceptives.

Abundant animal data indicate that the barbiturates increase the metabolism of estrogens and decrease their half lives (424). Of 51 oral contraceptive users who received phenobarbitone, thirty experienced breakthrough bleeding (BTB) and one pregnancy was reported. It seems likely that BTB and spotting were the clinical correlates of the enzyme induction which occurred due to phenobarbitone. (65, 424).

ORAL CONTRACEPTIVES

BRAND
Combinations:

Loestrin 1/20 (21's;28's*)	Norethindrone acetate 1mg	Ethinyl estradiol (20mcg)
Zorane 1/20 (28's)	Norethindrone acetate 1mg	Ethinyl estradiol (20mcg)
Loestrin 1.5/30 (28's)	Norethindrone acetate 1.5mg	Ethinyl estradiol (30mcg)
Zorane 1.5/30 (28's)	Norethindrone acetate 1.5mg	Ethinyl estradiol (30mcg)
Lo-Ovral (21's)	Norgestrel 0.3mg	Ethinyl estradiol (30mcg)
Brevicon (21's;28's)	Norethindrone 0.5mg	Ethinyl estradiol (35mcg)
Modicon (21's;28's)	Norethindrone 0.5mg	Ethinyl estradiol (35mcg)
Ovcon-35 (28's)	Norethindrone 0.4	Ethinyl estradiol (35mcg)
Norlestrin 1/50 (21's;28's;28's*)	Norethindrone acetate 1mg	Ethinyl estradiol (50mcg)
Ovcon-50 (28's)	Norethindrone 1mg	Ethinyl estradiol (50mcg)
Zorane 1/50 (28's)	Norethindrone 1mg	Ethinyl estradiol (50mcg)
Norelstrin 2.5/50 (21's;28's)	Norethindrone acetate 2.5mg	Ethinyl estradiol (50mcg)
Ovral (21's;28's)	Norgestrel 0.5mg	Ethinyl estradiol (50mcg)
Demulen (21's;28's)	Ethynodiol diacetate 1mg	Ethinyl estradiol (50mcg)
Norinyl 1/50 (21's;28's)	Norethindrone 1mg	Mestranol (50mcg)
Ortho Novum 1/50 (21's;28's)	Norethindrone 1mg	Mestranol (50mcg)
Otho Novum 10mg (20's)	Norethindrone 10mg	Mestranol (60mcg)
Enovid 5mg (20's)	Norethynodrel 5mg	Mestranol (75mcg)
Norinyl 1/80 (21's;28's)	Norethindrone 1mg	Mestranol (80mcg)
Ortho Novum 1/80 (21's;28's)	Norethindrone 1mg	Mestranol (80mcg)
Norinyl 2mg (21's)	Norethindrone 2mg	Mestranol (100mcg)
Ortho Novum 2mg (21's)	Norethindrone 2mg	Mestranol (100mcg)
Enovid-E (20's;21's)	Norethynodrel 2.5mg	Mestranol (100mcg)
Ovulen (20's;21's;28's)	Ethynodiol diacetate 1mg	Mestranol (100mcg)

Progestin only:

Micronor	Norethindrone 0.35mg	None
Nor-Q-D	Norethindrone 0.35mg	None
Ovrette	Norgestrel 0.075mg	None

Sequentials (no longer available in the United States):

Norquen (20's)	Norethindrone 2mg	Mestranol (80mcg)
Ortho Novum SQ (20's)	Norethindrone 2mg	Mestranol (80mcg)
Oracon (21's;28's)	Dimethisterone 25mg	Ethinyl estradiol (100mcg)

Indicates 21 hormone pills and 7 iron pills. Usually ferrous fumarate 75mg. All other 28 day cycles contain 7 inert tablets.

REFERENCE

1. Adams PW et al: Effects of pyridoxine HCL (vitamin B6) upon depression associated with oral contraception. Lancet 1:897, 1973.
2. Adams PW et al: Vitamin B6, depression, and oral contraception. Lancet 2(879):516, 1974.
3. Achlercrentz H et al: Some aspects of the interaction between natural and synthetic female sex hormones and the liver. Am J Med 49:630, 1970.
4. Adstedt B et al: Thrombosis and oral contraceptives: possible predisposition. Brit Med J 4:631, 1973.
5. Alkjaersig N et al: Association between oral contraception use and thromboembolism: a new approach to its investigation based on plasma fibrinogen chromatography. Am J Obstet Gyn 122:199, 1975.
6. Alkjaersig N et al: Thromboembolism and oral contraceptive medication (Abstr.). J Clin Invest 49:3a, 1970.
7. Aitken DA et al: Allergic reaction to quinestrol. Brit Med J 2:177, 1970.
8. Altschuler SL et al: Amenorrhea following rifamprin administration during oral contraceptive use. Obstet Gynecol 44:771, 1974.
9. Ameriks JA et al: Hepatic cell adenomas, spontaneous liver rupture, and oral contraceptives. Arch Surg 110:548, 1975.
10. Ammentorp PA et al: Hepatocellular adenoma and oral contraceptives. Ohio State Med J 72:283, 1976.
11. Amorosa L: Contraceptives, hypertension and renin. NEJM 286:1163, 1972.
12. Anon: Depression with oral contraceptives. Brit Med J 1:344, 1966.
13. Anon: DES as a "morning after" contraceptive. Med Letter 15:2, 1973.
14. Anon: Drug reaction VII: adverse cutaneous effects to oral contraceptives. Brit J Derm 81:946, 1969.
15. Anon: Hair loss and contraceptives. Brit Med J 2:499, 1973.
16. Anon: Iatrogenic gallstones. Brit Med J 2:859, 1976.
17. Anon: Injectable progestogens-Official debate but use increases. Population Reports 4:1, 1975.
18. Anon: Medical news: Plasma estradiol levels linked to migraine during menstrual period. JAMA 221:845, 1972.
19. Anon: Notes and comments: Depression with oral contraceptives. Brit Med J 1:344, 1966.
20. Anon: Postcoital contraception: An appraisal. Population Reports 5:141, 1976.
21. Anon: Postcoital DES. FDA Drug Bulletin, May, 1973.
22. Anon: Oral contraceptives and tests of thyroid function. Brit Med J 2:1545, 1966.
23. Anon: Thromboembolism and oral contraceptives, (Editorial). Brit Med J 1:213, 1974.
24. Anon: Vaginitis and the pill. JAMA 196:731, 1966.
25. Ansari AH et al: Electroencephalographic recording during progestation treatment. Fertil Steril 21:873, 1970.
26. Ansari AH et al: Pituitary-adrenocortical effect of short and long-term progestational therapy. Am J Obst Gyn 103:514, 1969.
27. Antoniades K et al: Liver cell adenoma and oral contraceptives: Double tumor development. JAMA 234:62—, 1975.
28. Arndt KA et al: Topical use of hydroquinone as a depigmenting agent. JAMA 194:965, 1965.
29. Aronson HB et al: Effect of oral contraceptives on blood viscosity. Am J Obst Gyn 10:997, 1971.
30. Arrata WSM et al: The oversuppression syndrome. Am J Obst Gyn 112:1025, 1972.
31. Ask-Upmark E: Progestin, thrombophlebitis, and migraine. Acta Med Scand 181:737, 1967.
32. Ask-Upmark E et al: Vertebral artery occlusion and oral contraceptives. Am Heart J 90:1, 1975.
33. Astedt B: New aspects of the thrombogenic effect of oral contraceptives. Am Heart J 90:1, 1975.
34. Atkinson EA et al: Intracranial venous thrombosis as complication of oral contraception. Lancet 2:914, 1970.
35. Aznar R et al: Effect of oral contraceptives on glucose tolerance tests. Contraception 13:299, 1976.
36. Aznar R et al: Incidence of side effects with contraceptive placebo. Am J Obst Gyn 105:1144, 1969.
37. Baaker CB et al: Side effects of oral contraceptives. Obst Gyn 28:373, 1966.
38. Badaracco MA et al: Recurrence of venous thromboembolic disease and use of oral contraceptives. Br Med J 1:215, 1974.
39. Baden HP et al: Erythema nodosum from oral contraceptives. Arch Derm 98:634, 1968.
40. Baek S et al: Benign liver cell adenoma associated with use of oral contraceptive agents. Ann Surg 183:239, 1976.
41. Bagheri SA et al: Peliosis hepatitis associated with androgenicanabolic therapy. Ann Int Med 81:610, 1974.
42. Balin H et al: Pharmacophysiologic and clinical aspects of oral contraceptives. Seminars in Drug Treatment 3:121, 1973.
43. Barnes J: Allergy to oral contraceptives. Practitioner 198:873, 1967.
44. Bart, CK et al: Letter: Oral contraceptives and benign liver tumor. Lancet 1:479, 1976.
45. Bassivala VM et al: The effect of oral contraceptives on concentrations of various components of human milk. Contraception 7:307, 1973.
46. Baum JK et al: Possible association between benign hepatomas and oral contraceptives. Lancet 2:926, 1973.
47. Baumblatt MJ et al: Pyridoxine and the pill. Lancet 1:833, 1970.
48. Beck RP et al: Thyroid function studies in different phases of the menstrual cycle and in women receiving norethindrone with and without estrogen. Am J Obst Gyn 112:369, 1972.
49. Beck RP et al: Adrenocortical function studies during normal menstrual cycle and in women receiving norethindrone with and without mestranol. Am J Obst Gyn 112:364, 1972.
50. Beck RP et al: Comparison of the mechanisms underlying carbohydrate intolerance in subclinical diabetic women during pregnancy and during postpartum oral contraceptive steroid treatment. J Clin Endocrin 29:807, 1969.
51. Berckerhoff R et al: Effects of oral contraceptives on the renin-angiotensin system and on blood pressure of normal young women. Johns Hopk Med J 132:80, 1973.
52. Behrman S: Homonymous hemianopia after oral contraceptives. Brit Med J 4:684, 1967.
53. Bell C et al: Effects of chronic oral contraceptive treatment on the conversion of angiotension I to angiotension II in the rat. J Pharm Exp Ther 193:160, 1975.
54. Bennion LJ et al: Effects of oral contraceptives and the gall bladder bile of normal women. NEJM 294:189, 1976.
55. Berg JW et al: Hepatomas and oral contraceptives. Lancet 3:349, 1974.
56. Bernardino ME et al: Erythema nodosum secondary to oral contraceptive usage: A case report. J Am Podiatry Assoc 66:417, 1976.
57. Berstein MZ et al: Erythema nodosum secondary to oral contraceptive usage: A case report. J Am Podiatry Assoc 66:417, 1976.
58. Bishun N et al: A cytogenetic study in women who had used oral contraceptives and in their progeny. Mutat Res 33:299, 1975.
59. Blomgren SE: Erythema nodosum. Sem Arthr Rheum 4:1, 1974.
60. Board JA: Continuous norethindrone 0.35 mg as an oral contraceptive agent. Am J Obst Gyn 109:53, 1971.
61. Bole Jr GG et al: Rheumatic symptoms and serological abnormalities induced by oral contraceptives. Lancet 1:323, 1969.
62. Boles GG et al: Rheumatic symptoms and serological abnormalities induced by oral contraceptives. Lancet 1:323, 1969.
63. Bolt HM et al: Rifampicin and oral contraception. Lancet 1:1280, 1974.
64. Bonnar J: Progestagen only contraception and tubal pregnancies. Brit Med J 1:287, 1974.
65. Borrell U: Contraceptive methods, their safety, efficacy and acceptability. Acta Obst Gyn Scand (Suppl.1)G11, 1966.
66. Boston Collaborative Drug Surveillance Program: Oral contraception and venous thromboembolic disease, surgically confirmed gallbladder disease, and breast tumors. Lancet 1:1399, 1973.
67. Boston Collaborative Drug Surveillance Program: Surgically confirmed gallbladder disease, venous thromboembolism and breast tumors in relation to postmenopausal estrogen therapy. NEJM 290:15, 1974.
68. Brander WL et al: Multiple hepatocellular tumors in a patient treated with oral contraceptives. Virchows Arch Pathol Anat 370:69, 1976.
69. Briggs M et al: Changing from a high to low dose and contraceptives. Brit Med J 1:575, 1975.

70. Briggs MH et al: Preliminary studies on the metabolic effects of a continuous dose prostagen only oral contraceptive. African J Med Sci 3:105, 1972.

71. Brogden RN et al: Progestagen only oral contraceptives: A preliminary report of the action and clinical use of norgestrel and norethisterone. Drugs 6:169, 1973.

72. Brown JM: Histological modification of fibroadenomas of the breast associated with oral hormonal contraceptives. Med J Aust 1:276, 1970.

73. Buchler D et al: Effect of estrogens on glucose tolerance. Am J Obst Gyn 95:479, 1966.

74. Bulbrook RD et al: Excretion of urinary 17-hydroxy corticosteroids and 11-deoxy-17 oxosteroids by women using steroidal contraceptives. Lancet 2:1033, 1969.

75. Burch H: Changing approaches to anorexia nervosa. Internat Psych Clin 7:3, 1975.

76. Burke M: Pregnancy, pancreatitis and the pill. Brit Med J 4:551, 1972.

77. Buttram VC et al: Post pill amenorrhoea. Int J Fertil 19:37, 1974.

78. Cain MD et al: Effects of oral contraceptive therapy on the renin-angiotensin system. J Clin Endocr 33:671, 1971.

79. Carey HM: Principles of oral contraceptives. Part II: side effects of oral contraceptives. Med J Aust 2:1242, 1971.

80. Carmichael SM et al: Oral contraceptives, hypertension, and toxemia. Obst Gyn 35:371, 1970.

81. Caron GA: Contact lens and oral contraceptives. Brit Med J 1:980, 1966.

82. Carrington ER: Relationship of stilbestrol exposure in utero to vaginal lesions in adolescence. J Pediat 85:295, 1974.

83. Carroll JD: Migraine-general management. Brit Med J 2:756, 1971.

84. Carruthers R: Chloasma and the pill. Brit Med J 3:307, 1967.

85. Carruthers R: Chloasma and the pill. Med J Aust 2:17, 1966.

86. Carter DE: Effect of oral contraceptives on plasma clearance. Clin Pharm Ther 18:700, 1975.

87. Castren OM et al: Effect of oral contraceptives on serum folic acid content. J Obst Gyn Brit Commonwealth 77:548, 1970.

88. Catterall RD: Candida albicans and the contraceptive pill. Lancet 2:830, 1966.

89. Catterall RD: Influence of gestogenic contraceptive pills on vaginal candidosis. Brit J Vener Dis 47:45, 1971.

90. Chapel T et al: Oral contraceptives and exacerbation of lupus erythematous. Am J Obst Gyn 110:366, 1971.

91. Chihal HJ et al: Estrogen potency of oral contraceptive pills. Am J Obstet Gyn 121:75, 1975.

92. Chizek DJ et al: Oral contraceptives; their side effects and ophthalmological manifestations. Survey Ophth 14:90, 1969.

93. Chopra JG: Effect of steroid contraceptives on lactation. Am J Clin Nutr 25:1202, 1972.

94. Christopherson WM et al: Liver tumors and oral contraceptives. Lancet 1:1076, 1976.

95. Christopherson WM et al: Liver tumors in women on contraceptive steroids. Obst Gyn 46:221, 1975.

96. Chumnijarakij T: Incidence of postpartum deep vein thrombosis in the tropics. Brit Med J 1:245, 1974.

97. Cohn HD: Rifanipin and the pill. JAMA 228,828, 1974.

98. Collaborative Group for the Study of Stroke in Young Women: Oral contraceptives and increased risk of cerebral ischemias or thrombosis. NEJM 288:871, 1973.

99. Collaborative Group for the Study of Stroke in Young Women: Oral contraceptives and stroke in young women, associated risk factors. JAMA 231:718, 1975.

100. Conard J et al: Anti-thrombin III in women using oral contraceptives. Path et Biol 22:77, 1974.

101. Connell EB et al: Ophthalmologic findings with the oral contraceptives. Obst Gyn 31:456, 1968.

102. Connell EB et al: Eye examinations in patients taking oral contraceptives. Fert Steril 20:67, 1969.

103. Contostaulos DL: Benign hepatomas and oral contraceptives. Lancet 2:1209, 1973.

104. Cormia FE: Alopecia from oral contraceptives. JAMA 201,635, 1967.

105. Crane MG et al: Hypertension, oral contraceptive agents, and conjugated estrogens. Ann Int Med 74:13, 1971.

106. Crawford JS et al: Pre-pregnancy oral contraception and sex ratio among subsequent potency. Lancet 2:453, 1973.

107. Crawford JS et al: Pre-pregnancy oral contraceptives and

108. Cronin TJ: Influence of lactation on ovulation. Lancet 2:422, 1968.

109. Dalen E et al: Occurrence of hepatic impairment in women jaundiced by oral contraceptives and in their mothers and sisters. Acta Med Scand 195:459, 1974.

110. Dalton K: Migraine and oral contraceptives. Headache 15:247, 1976.

111. Darlington LG: Erythema nodosum and oral contraceptives. Brit J Derm 90:209, 1974.

112. Das SK et al: A clinico-pathological study of lactational amenorrhea. J Obst Gyn (India) 16:156, 1966.

113. Davis B: Vaginal moniliasis in private practice. Obst Gyn 34:40, 1969.

114. Davis M et al: Histological evidence of carcinoma in a hepatic tumour associated with oral contraceptives. Brit Med J 4:496, 1975.

115. Delforge JP' ET AL: A histometric study of two estrogens, ethinyl estradial and its 3-methyl ether derivative (mestranol) their comparative effect upon the growth endometrium. Contraception 1:57, 1970.

116. Desaulles PA et al: A comparison of the antifertility and sex hormonal activities of sex hormones and their derivatives. Acta Endocrin (Kbh) 47:444, 1964.

117. Desrosiers HH: Headaches related to contraceptive therapy and their control. Headache 13:117, 1973.

118. Dickey RP: Established potency of three new low dose oral contraceptives. Am J Ob Gyn 125:976, 1976.

119. Dickey RP et al: Oral contraceptives: selection of the proper pill. Obst Gyn 33:273, 1969.

120. Diddle AW et al: Oral contraceptives, medication and headaches. Am J Obst Gyn 105:507, 1969.

121. Diddle AW et al: Oral contraceptive medication and vulvovaginal candidiasis. Obst Gyn 34:373, 1969.

122. DiPaola G et al: Oral contraceptives and carbohydrate intolerance. Am J Obst Gyn 101:206, 1968.

123. DiPaola G et al: Estrogen therapy and glucose tolerance. Am J Obst Gyn 107:124, 1970.

124. Doar JWH et al: Effects of obesity, glucocorticoids, and oral contraceptive therapy on plasma glucose and blood-pyruvate levels. Brit Med J 1:149, 1970.

125. Dodek OL et al: Effects of enovoid on cortisol metabolism. Am J Obst Gyn 93:173, 1965.

126. Drill VA: Benign cholestatic jaundice of pregnancy and benign cholestatic jaundice from oral contraceptives. Am J Obst Gyn 119:165, 1974.

127. Drill VA et al: Oral contraceptives and thromboembolic disease. JAMA 206:77, 1968.

128. Drill VA et al: Oral contraceptives and thromboembolic disease II: estrogen content of oral contraceptives. JAMA 219:593, 1972.

129. Drill VA et al: Thromboembolic disorders and oral contraceptives. JAMA 207:1151, 1969.

130. Drill VA: Oral contraceptives and thromboembolic disease I. Prospective and retrospective studies. JAMA 219:583, 1972.

131. Drill VA: Oral contraceptive relation to mammary cancer, benign breast lesions and cervical cancer. Ann Rev Pharmacol 15:367, 1975.

132. Drill VA: Save metabolic actions and possible toxic effects of hormonal contraceptives. Acta Endocrin 75:169, 1974.

133. Driskell JA et al: Vitamin B6 status of young men, women, and women using oral contraceptives. J Lab Clin Med 87:813, 1976.

134. Dubois EL et al: LE cells after oral contraceptives. Lancet 2:679, 1968.

135. Dugdale M et al: Hormonal contraception and thromboembolic disease, effects of the oral contraceptives on hemostatic mechanisms. J Chron Dis 23:775, 1971.

136. Dunn FG et al: Malignant hypertension associated with use of oral contraceptives. Brit Heart J 37:336, 1975.

137. Edgren RA: Potencies of oral contraceptives. Am J Obst Gyn 125:1029, 1976.

138. Edmondson HA et al: Liver-cell adenomas associated with use of oral contraceptives. NEJM 294:470, 1976.

139. Egger G et al: Ischaemic colitis and oral contraceptives, case report and brief review of the literature. Acta Hepatogastroenterol (STUTTG) 21:221, 1974.

140. Eicher E: Estrogen deprivation headaches. Obst Gyn 32:294, 1968.

141. Eisalo A et al: Liver-function tests during intake of contraceptive

respiratory-distress syndrome. Lancet 1:858, 1973.

tablets in premenopausal women. Brit Med J 1:1416, 1965.

142. Eisenfeld AJ et al: Estrogen receptors in the mammalian liver. Science 191:862, 1976.

143. Ekberg O: Inherited antithrombin deficiency causing thrombophilia. Thromb Diath Haemorr 13:516, 1965.

144. El Ashiry GM et al: Effects of oral contraceptives on the gingiva. J Periodont 42:273, 1971.

145. Elgart ML et al: Photosensitization. Med Ann D.C. 40:501, 1971.

146. Elgee NJ: Medical aspects of oral contraceptives. Ann Int Med 74:409, 1970.

147. Elias PM: Erythema nodosum and serological lupus erythematosus. Simultaneous occurrence in a patient using oral contraceptives. Arch Dermatol 108:718, 1973.

148. Ellis DL et al: Mesenteric venous thrombosis in two women taking oral contraceptives. MM J Surg 125:641, 1973.

149. El Mahgoub S et al: The effects of injectable contraceptives on the direct thyroid function tests. J Egypt Med Asso 55:192, 1972.

150. Ellis PP: Ocular pharmacology and toxicology. Arch Ophthal (Chicago) 78:534, 1967.

151. Elwan O et al: Steroid contraceptives: neuro-psychiatric and electroencephalographic complications. J Int Med Res 1:534, 1973.

152. Enzell K et al: Cryptogenic cerebral embolism in women taking oral contraceptives. Brit Med J 4:507, 1973.

153. Evrad JR et al: Amenorrhea following oral contraception. Am J Obst Gyn 124:88, 1976.

154. Fagerhol MK et al: Antithrombin III concentration and ABO blood groups. Lancet 2:664, 1971.

155. Falliers CJ: Oral contraceptives and allergy. Lancet 2:515, 1974.

156. Fasal E et al: Oral contraceptives as related to cancer and benign lesions of the breast. J Natl Cancer Inst 55:767, 1975.

157. Faust JM et al: Ophthalmologic findings in patients using oral contraceptives. Fert Sterl 17:1, 1966.

158. Fechner RE: Breast cancer during oral contraceptive therapy. Cancer 26:1204, 1970.

159. Fechner RE: Fibroadenomas in patients receiving oral contraceptives. Am J Clin Patho 53:857, 1970.

160. Fechner FE: Fibrocystic disease in women receiving oral contraceptive hormones. Cancer 25:1332, 1970.

161. Fechner RE: Benign breast disease in women on estrogen therapy; a pathologic study. Cancer 29:273, 1972.

162. Fiser RH: Complications of oral contraceptive agents — a symposium. Contraceptives and lipid metabolism. West J Med 122:35, 1975.

163. Fisher AA: Allergic reactions to contraceptives and douches. Med Aspects Hum Sex 9:110, 1975.

164. Fisher DA: Complications of oral contraceptives — a symposium. Liver disease and abnormalities of laboratory tests. West J Med 122:40, 1975.

165. Florshein WH et al: Effects of oral ovulation inhibitors on serum protein bound iodine and thyroxine binding protein. Proc Soc Exp Biol Med 117:56, 1964.

166. Foley M et al: Clinical trial and laboratory investigation of a low-dose progestogen-only contraceptive; exluton. Int J Fertil 18:246, 1973.

167. Fortin JN et al: Side effects of oral contraceptive medication; a psychosomatic problem. Can Psychiat Assoc J 17:3, 1972.

168. Foster ME et al: Pancreatitis, multiple infarcts and oral contraception. Postgrad Med J 51:667, 1975.

169. Frederick WC et al: Spontaneous rupture of the liver in patient using contraceptive pills. Arch Surg 108:93, 1974.

170. Friedman S et al: Acute ophthalmologic complications during the use of oral contraceptives. Contraception 10:685, 1974.

171. Friedman S et al: Amenorrhea and galactorrhea following oral contraceptive therapy. JAMA 210:1888, 1969.

172. Fries H ET AL: Dieting, anorexia nervosa and amenorrhea after oral contraceptive treatment. Acta Psychiat Scand 49:669, 1973.

173. Fries H et al: Psychological factors, psychiatric illness and amenorrhoea after oral contraceptive treatment. Acta Psychiat Scand 49:653, 1973.

174. Frigoletto FD et al: Hypercoagulability in the dysmature syndrome. Am J Obst Gyn 111:867, 1971.

175. Fuertes-De La Haba A et al: Measured intelligence in offspring of oral and nonoral contraceptive users. Am J Obst Gyn 125:980, 1976.

176. Fuertes-De La Haba A et al: Thrombophlebitis among oral and nonoral contraceptive users. Obst Gyn 38:259, 1971.

177. Gallagher JD et al: Does Rifampin inhibit oral contraception? TB Today 1:6, 1974.

178. Garcia CR et al: Clinical considerations of oral hormonal control of human fertility. Can Obst Syn 7:844, 1963.

179. Gibbs WP: Letter: acne and ovral. Arch Derm 109:912, 1974.

180. Gill D: Rheumatic complaints of women using antiovulatory drugs. An evaluation. J Chron Dis 21:435, 1968.

181. Glass RH: Oral contraceptive agents. West J Med 122:66, 1975.

182. Glassberg AB et al: Letter: Oral contraceptives and malignant hepatoma. Lancet 1:479, 1976.

183. Glick ID: Mood and behavioral changes associated with the use of the oral contraceptive agents. Psychopharmacologica 10:363, 1967.

184. Glueck CJ et al: Estrogen-induced pancreatitis in patients with previously covert familial type V hyperlipoproteinemia. Metabolism 21:657, 1972.

185. Gold EM et al: Insulin production on overt (maturity onset) diabetes; absence of hyperinsulinaemia despite hyperglycemia induced by contraceptive steroids. Metabolic Effects of Gonadal Hormones and Contraceptive Steroids; HA Salhonick et al. Plenum Press, New York, p.144, 1969.

186. Goldenberg VE et al: Florid breast fibroadenomas in patients taking hormonal oral contraceptives. Am J Clin Path 49:52, 1970.

187. Goldfarb S: Sex hormones and hepatic neoplasis. Cancer Res 36:2584, 1976.

188. Golditch IM: Postcontraceptive amenorrhea. Obst Gyn 39:903, 1972.

189. Goldzieher JW: Comparative studies of the ethynyl estrogens used in oral contraceptives. II antiovulatory response. Am J Ob Gyn 122:619, 1975.

190. Goldzieher JW: Comparative studies of the ethynyl estrogens used in oral contraceptives. III effect on plasma gonadotropins. Am J Ob Gyn 122:625, 1975.

191. Goldzieher JW: Comparative studies of the ethynyl estrogens used in oral contraceptives. I endometrial response. Am J Ob Gyn 122:619, 1975.

192. Goldzieher JW: Oral contraceptives; a review of certain metabolic effects and an examination of the question of safety. Fed Proc 29:1220, 1970.

193. Goldzieher JW et al: Oral contraceptives and thromboembolism: a reassessment. Am J Obst Gyn 123:878, 1975.

194. Goldzieher JW et al: New oral contraceptives. Am J Obst Gyn 90:404, 1964.

195. Goldzieher JW et al: Nervousness and depression attributed to oral contraceptives: a double blind placebo controlled study. Am J Obst Gyn 111:1013, 1971.

196. Gombos GM et al: Retinal vascular occlusion induced by oral contraceptives. Ann Ophthalmol 7:215, 1975.

197. Good AE et al: Prolonged over-suppression syndrome. Med Clin North Amer 58:861, 1974.

198. Goodrich SM et al: Effect of estradiol 17B on peripheral venous distensibility and velocity of venous flow. Am J Obst Gyn 96:407, 1966.

199. Goodrich SM et al: Peripheral venous distensibility and velocity of venous blood flow during pregnancy or during oral contraceptive therapy. Am J Obst Gyn 90:740, 1964.

200. Goolden AWG et al:Thyroid status in pregnancy and in women taking oral contraceptives. Lancet 1:12, 1967.

201. Goren SB: Retinal edema secondary to oral contraceptives. Am J Ophth 64:447, 1967.

202. Grant E: Relationship of arterioles in the endometrium to headache from oral contraceptives. Lancet 1:1143, 1965.

203. Grant E: Relation between headaches from oral contraceptives and development of endometrial arterioles. Brit Med J 2:402, 1968.

204. Grant E et al: Effect of oral contraceptives on depressive mood changes and on endometrial monamine oxidase and phosphatases. Brit Med J 3:777, 1968.

205. Greenblatt DJ et al: Oral contraceptives and hypertension. A report from the Boston Coolaborative Drug Surveillance Program. Obst Gyn 44:412, 1974.

206. Greene GR et al: Oral contraceptive use in patients with thromboembolism following surgery trauma or infection. Am J Public Health 62:680, 1972.

207. Greenhill JP: Control of Conception: Oral Contraceptives in Office Gynecology, 9th edition, Year Book Publishers, Chicago, p. 201, 1971.

208. Griffins WAD: Diffuse hair loss and oral contraceptives. Brit J Derm 88:31, 1973.

209. Guyton AC: Textbook of Medical Physiology. 5th ED, W.B. Saunders Co., Philadelphia, 1976.

210. Haden HT: Thyroid function test. Physiological basis and clinical interpretation. Postgrad Med 40:129, 1966.

211. Haemmerli P et al: Recurrent intrahepatic cholestasis of pregnancy. Medicine 46:299, 1967.

212. Hakin J et al: Effect of rifampin, isoniazid, and streptomycin on the human liver: A problem of enzyme induction. Gut 12:761, 1971.

213. Halbert DR et al: Amenorrhea following oral contraceptives. Obst Gyn 34:161, 1969.

214. Handin RI: Thromboembolic complications of pregnancy and oral contraceptives. Prog Cardiovas Dis 16:395, 1974.

215. Hansen P: Drug Interactions. Lea and Febiger, Philadelphia, p. 158, 1971.

216. Hanson FW: "Post-pill" amenorrhea. Diagnosis and management. Postgrad Med 53:156, 1973.

217. Hanson FW: Safety of contraceptive methods: amenorrhea. J Reprod Med 53:156, 1973.

218. Harden K: Letter: Latrogenic gall stones. Brit Med J 1:1074, 1976.

219. Hargreaves T: Oral contraceptives and liver function. J Clin Path (Suppl. 3) 23:1, 1970.

220. Harlap S et al: Letter: Birth defects and oestrogens and progesterones in pregnancy. Lancet 1:682, 1975.

221. Harris PWR: Malignant hypertension associated with oral contraceptives. Lancet 2:466, 1969.

222. Hartley RA et al: Topics in clinical medicine: the liver and oral contraceptives. Johns Hopkins Med J 124:112, 1969.

223. Hartveit F: Complications of oral contraceptives. Brit Med J 1:160, 1965.

224. Haspels AA: Postcoital estrogen in large doses. IPPF Med Bul 6:3, 1972.

225. Haspels AA: The effect of large doses of estrogen post coitum in 2000 women. European J Obs Gyn Repr Bio 3:113, 1973.

226. Hawkins DF: Letter: Progestogen-only contraception and tubal pregnancies. Brit Med J 1:387, 1974.

227. Heber KR: Low dose estrogen oral contraceptives. Contraception 10:241, 1974.

228. Heber KR: Letter: Withdrawal of serial C. Med J Aust 1:412, 1976.

229. Hempel EB et al: Medicinal enzyme induction and hormonal contraception. Zbl. Bynak 95:1451, 1973.

230. Herbst AL et al: Adenocarcinoma of the vagina. NFJM 284:878, 1971.

231. Herbst AL et al: Clear-cell adenocarcinoma of the vagina and cervix in girls: analysis of 170 registry cases. Am J Obst Gyn 119:713, 1974.

232. Herson J et al: Physical complaints of patients with sickle cell trait. J Repro Med 14:129, 1975.

233. Herzberg BN et al: Changes in psychological symptoms accompanying oral contraceptive use. Brit J Psychiat 116:161, 1970.

234. Herzberg BN et al: Oral contraceptives, depression, and libido. Brit Med J 3:495, 1971.

235. Herzberg BN et al: Depressive symptoms and oral contraceptives. Brit Med J 4:142, 1970.

236. Hilliard JL et al: Hepatic adenoma: a possible complication of oral contraceptive therapy. Southern Med J 69:683, 1976.

237. Holcomb FD: Erythema nodosum associated with use of an oral contraceptive. Obst Gyn 25:156, 1965.

238. Holmes R: Megaloblastic anemia precipitated by use of oral contraceptives. NC Med J 31:17, 1970.

239. Horowitz BJ et al: The oversuppression syndrome. Obst Gyn 31:387, 1968.

240. Horvath E et al: Benign hepatoma in a young woman on contraceptive steroids. Lancet 1:357, 1974.

241. Hougie C: Thromboembolism and oral contraceptives. Am Heart J 85:538, 1973.

242. Howat JM et al: Gallstones and oral contraceptives. J Int Med Res 3:59, 1975.

243. Howie PW et al: Antithrombin III and oestrogen content of oral contraceptives. Lancet 1:1185, 1973.

244. Huntington KM: Progestagen-only contraception and tubal pregnancies. Lancet 1:360, 1974.

245. Ingerslev M et al: Secondary amenorrhoea and oral contraceptives. Acta Obst Gyn Scand 55:233, 1976.

246. Inman WHW et al: Investigation of deaths from pulmonary, coronary, and cerebral thrombosis and embolism in women of childbearing age. Brit Med J 2:193, 1968.

247. Inman WHW et al: Thromboembolic disease and the steroidal content of oral contraceptives; a report to the committee on safety of drugs. Brit Med J 2:203, 1970.

248. Irey NS et al: Vascular lesions in women taking oral contraceptives. Arch Path 89:1, 1970.

249. Jackson JL: The missed pill: preliminary report in Progress in Conception Control, ed: D.L. Moyer. Lippincott & Co., Philadelphia, 1968.

250. Jackson JL et al: Comparative study of combined and sequential antiovulatory therapy on vaginal moniliasis. Am J Obst Gyn 126:301, 1976.

251. Jain AK: Cigarette smoking, use of oral contraceptives, and myocardial infarction. Am J Obst Gyn 126:301, 1976.

252. Janerich DT et al: Fertility patterns after discontinuation of use of oral contraceptives. Lancet 1:1051, 1976.

253. Janerich DT et al: Oral contraceptives and congenital limb-reduction defects. NEJM 291:697, 1974.

254. Jelinek JE: Cutaneous side effects of oral contraceptives. Arch Derm 101:181, 1970.

255. Jensen HK et al: Incidence of candida albicans in women using oral contraceptives. Acta Obst Gyn Scand 49:293, 1970.

256. Jick H et al: Venous thromboembolic disease and 'A', 'B', 'O' blood type. Lancet 1:539, 1969.

257. Johnson LF et al: Association of androgenic anabolic androgenic steroid therapy with development of hepatocellular carcinoma. Lancet 2:123, 1972.

258. Jones DE et al: Oral contraceptives — Clinical problems and choices. Am Fam Phys 12:115, 1975.

259. Jones JR et al: Alteration of some human coagulation — components by hormonal contraceptives. Gyn Invest 5:60, 1974.

260. Kahn SB et al: Correlation of folate metabolism and socioeconomic status in pregnancy and in patients taking oral contraceptives. Am J Obst Gyn 108:931, 1970.

261. Kakkar VV et al: Proceedings: Surgery, the contraceptive pill and postoperative deep vein thrombosis. Brit Surg J 62:162, 1975.

262. Kane FJ: Psychotic reactions to oral contraceptives. Am J Obst Gyn 102:1053, 1968.

263. Kaplan NM: Clinical complications of oral contraceptives. Adv Int Med 20:197, 1975.

264. Kappas A: Estrogens and liver. Gastroent 52:113, 1967.

265. Kariner DH: Erythema nodosum and oral contraceptives. Obst Gyn 42:323, 1973.

266. Karrer M et al: Two thousand woman years experience with a sequential contraceptive. Am J Obst Gyn 102:1029, 1968.

267. Kate R et al: Jaundice during treatment with oral contraceptives. Gastroent 50:853, 1966.

268. Kaufman RL: Birth defects and oral contraceptives. Lancet 1:1396, 1973.

269. Kaufman RH: Severe atypical endometrial changes and sequential contraceptive use. JAMA 236:923, 1976.

270. Kay DR et al: Antinuclear antibodies, rheumatoid factor and C-reactive protein in serum of normal women using oral contraceptives. Arthr Rheum 14:239, 1971.

271. Kay C : Oral contraceptives and health: Thromboembolic Diseases. Lancet 2:1138, 1974.

272. Kelso DR: Benign hepatomas and oral contraceptives. Lancet 1:315, 1974.

273. Keseru TL et al: Oral contraception and sex ratio at birth. Lancet 1:369, 1974.

274. Kirsby JF et al: Oral contraceptives and erythema nodosum. Obst Gyn 40:409, 1972.

275. Kirsby JF et al: Oral contraceptives and erythema nodosum. Obst Gyn 40:407, 1972.

276. Kistner RW: Oral contraceptives. Safety factors in prolonged use of progestin-estrogen combinations. Part I. Postgrad Med 39:207, 1966.

277. Kistner RW: Gynecology. Principles and Practices. 2nd Ed. Year Book Medical Publishers, Chicago, p. 670, 1971.

278. Kistner RW: The Pill. Facts and Fallacies About Today's Oral Contraceptives. Delacorte Press, New York, 1969, p.339.

279. Kleiger RE et al: Pulmonary hypertension in patients using oral contraceptives. A report of six cases. Chest 69:143, 1976.

280. Kligman AM: Pimples following the pill. Arch Derm 105:298, 1972.

281. Klinger HP et al: Contraceptives and the conceptus. I. Chromosome abnormalities of the fetus and neonate related to maternal

contraceptive history. Obst Gyn 48:40, 1976.

282. Knapp WA et al: Letter: Hepatomas and oral contraceptives. Lancet 1:270, 1974.

283. Knowles DM et al: Letter: Systematic contraceptives and the liver. Ann Int Med 83:907, 1975.

284. Koetting RA: The influence of oral contraceptives on contact lens wearers. Am J Optom 43:268, 1966.

285. Koide SS et al: Unusual signs and symptoms associated with oral contraceptive medication. J Repro Med 15:214, 1975.

286. Kright GM et al: The effects of hormonal contraceptives on the human periodontium. J Periodont Res 1:18, 1974.

287. Kubik MM et al: Myocardial infarction and oral contraceptives. Br Heart J 35:127, 1973.

288. Kuchera LK: Postcoital contraception with diethylstilbestrol. JAMA 218:562, 1971.

289. Kudrow L: The relationship of headache frequency to hormone use in migraine. Headache 15:36, 1975.

290. Kutner SJ et al: Types of oral contraceptives, depression. and premenstrual symptoms. J Nerv Ment Dis 155, 1972.

291. Kutners JS et al: History of depression as a risk factor for depression with oral contraceptives and discontinuance. J Nerv Ment Dis 155:163, 1972.

292. Laenger H et al: Epileptic drugs and faulure of oral contraceptives. Lancet 2:600, 1974.

293. Langer A et al: Choice of an oral contraceptive. Am J Obst Gyn 126,153, 1976.

294. Langhorne WH: Arterial thrombosis, smoking, and oral contraceptives. South Med J 67:523, 1974.

295. Laragh JH: Oral contraceptives and hypertensive disease. A cybernetic overview. Circ 42:983, 1970.

296. Laragh JH: The pill, hypertension and toxemias of pregnancy. Am J Obst Gyn 109:210, 1971.

297. Laragh JH: Oral contraceptive hypertension. Postgrad Med 52:98, 1972.

298. Larson-Cohn U: Oral contraceptives and vitamins: A review. Am J Obstet Gynecol 121:84, 1975.

299. Larsson-Cohn U: Oral contraception and liver function tests. Brit Med J 1:1414, 1965.

300. Larsson-Cohn U et al: Headache and treatment with oral contraceptives. Acta Neurol Scand 46:267, 1970.

301. Lasing AM: Hypertension in young females receiving anovulatory steroids. Ann Surg 171:731, 1970.

302. Lauris RE: Fertility control with continuous microdose norgestrel. J Reprod Med 8:165, 1972.

303. Layne DS et al: The secretion of metabolism of cortisol and aldosterone in normal and in steroid treated women. J Clin Endocrin Metab 22:107, 1962.

304. Lazar A: Gynecological moniliasis, incidence with various contraceptive methods. J Med Soc New Jersey 68:37.

305. Leach RB et al: Inhibition of adrenocortical responsiveness during progestin therapy. Am J Obst Gyn 92:762, 1965.

306. Lee RS: Cryofibrinogen and oral contraception in women. J Amer Osteopath Assoc 72:1161, 1973.

307. Leeton J et al: The relationship of oral contraceptives to depression. Aust NZ J Obst. Gyn., 11:237, 1971.

308. Leeton J: Depression induced by oral contraception and the role of vitamin B6 in its management. Aust NZ J Psychiatry 8:85, 1974.

309. Leiman G: Depo-medroxyprogesterone acetate as a contraceptive agent: its effects on weight and blood pressure. Am J Obst Gyn 114:97, 1972.

310. Lesser PB: Drug induced intrahepatic cholestatic jaundice: case reports. Milit Med 139,43, 1974.

311. Lewinson E: The pill, estrogens and the breast. Cancer 28:1400, 1971.

312. Lewis A et al: An evaluation of depression as a side effect of oral contraceptives. Brit J Psychiat 115:697, 1969.

313. Lewis FB: Folate deficiency due to oral contraceptives. Minn Med 57:945, 1974.

314. Liggins GC: Hormonal steroid contraceptives II: clinical considerations. Drugs 2:461, 1971.

315. Lingeman DB: Liver cell-neoplasma and oral contraceptives. Lancet 1:64, 1974.

316. Littlefield LC, Chromosone breakage studies in lymphocytes from normal women, pregnant women and women taking oral contraceptives. Am J Obst Gyn 121:976, 1975.

317. Low J et al: Oral contraceptive pill hypertension. J Reprod Med 15:201, 1975.

318. Lyon FA: Letter: Sequential oral contraceptives. Fertil Steril 27:346, 1976.

319. Lyon FA: The development of adenocarcinoma of the endometrium in young women receiving long-term sequential oral contraception. Am J Obstet Gynecol 123:299, 1975.

320. Lyon FA et al: Endometrial abnormalities occurring in young women on long-term sequential oral contraception. Obstet Gynecol 47:639, 1976.

321. Mack TM et al: Estrogens and endometrial cancer in a retirement community. NEJM 294:1262, 1976.

322. Mann JI et al: Fatal myocardial infarction in older women. Brit Med J 2:445, 1976.

323. Mann KI et al: Myocardial infarction in young women with special reference to oral contraceptive practice. Brit Med J 2:241, 1975.

324. Mann JI et al: Oral contraceptives and death from myocardial infarction. Brit Med J 2:245, 1975.

325. Mann JI et al: Oral contraceptives and myocardial infarction in young women: a further report. Brit Med J 3:631, 1975.

326. Marcotte DB et al: Psychophysiologic changes accompanying oral contraceptive use. Brit J Psychiat 116:165, 1970.

327. Marshall JC et al: Luteinizing hormone secrition in patients presenting with post-oral contraceptive amenorrhoea: Evidence for a hypothalamic feedback abnormality. Clin Endocrinol (OXF) 5:131, 1976.

328. Marshall R: Postmenopausal vaginal bleeding during estrogen therapy. JAMA 227:76, 1974.

329. Martel AJ et al: Hemorrhage and stenosis of the jejunum following course of progestational agent. A case report. Amer J Gastroent 57:261, 1973.

330. Martin JV et al: Enzyme inducation as a possible cause of increased serum-triglycerides after oral contraceptives. Lancet 1:1107, 1976.

331. Masi AT et al: Cerebrovascular disease associated with the use of oral contraceptives. Ann Int Med 72:111, 1970.

332. Masi AT: Editorial: Pulmonary hypertension and oral contraceptive usage. Chest 69:45, 1976.

333. Mays ET et al: Hepatic changes in young women ingesting contraceptive steroids. Hepatic hemorrhage and primary hepatic tumors. JAMA 235:730, 1976.

334. McAvoy JM et al: Benign hepatic tumors and their association with oral contraceptives. Arch Surg 111:761, 1976.

335. McIntosh EN: Treatment of women with the galactorrhea-amenorrhea syndrome with Pyridoxine (Vitamin B-6). J Clin wendocrin Met 42:1192, 1976.

336. McLean FW et al: Relationship between oral contraceptives and folic acid metabolism. Am J Obst Gyn 104:745, 1969.

337. McQueen EG: Hormonal steroid contraceptives III: Adverse reactions. Drugs 2:20, 1971.

338. McQueen EG: Hormonal steroid contraceptives IV: Adverse reactions and management of the patient. Drugs 2:138, 1971.

339. Mears E et al: Anovlar as an oral contraceptive. Brit Med J 2:75, 1962.

340. Medline A et al: Pruritus of pregnancy and jaundice induced by oral contraceptives. Am J Gastroent 65:156, 1976.

341. Mehrotra TN et al: Hyperlipidaemia and pancreatitis associated with oral contraceptive therapy. J Assoc Physicians India 23:161, 1975.

342. Merritt G: Letter: Oral contraceptives, serum folate, and hematologic status. JAMA 234:591, 1975.

343. Mestman GH et al: Adrenal pituitary responsiveness during therapy with an oral contraceptive. Obst Gyn 31:378, 1968.

344. Metcalf MG et al: Plasma corticosteroid levels in women receiving oral contraceptive tablets. Lancet 2:1095, 1963.

345. Meyer P et al: Letter: Hepatoblastoma associated with an oral contraceptive. Lancet 2:1387, 1974.

346. Miale JB et al: The effects of oral contraceptives on the results of laboratory tests. Am J Obstet Gynecol 120:264, 1974.

347. Mills J et al: Chromosomes and oral contraceptives: Aberrations in relation to neoplasia. Clin Oncol 1:141, 1975.

348. Mink IB et al: Progestational agents and blood coagulation. V. Changes induced by sequential oral contraceptive therapy. Amer J Obstet Gynec 119 :401, 1974.

349. Moghissi KS et al: Effect of microdose norgestrol on endogenous gonadotrophic and steroid hormones, cervical mucus properties, vaginal cytology and endometrium. Fert Steril 22:424, 1971.

350. Moghissi KS et al: Contraceptive mechanism of microdose norethindrone. Obst Gyn 41:585, 1973.

351. Monash S: Intermediate pigmentation in sunlight and artificial light. Arch Derm 87:686, 1963.

352. Morris JM: Interception: The use of postovulatory estrogens to prevent implantation. Am J Ob Gyn 115:101, 1973.

353. Morris JM: Mechanisms involved in progesterone contraception and estrogen interception. Am J Ob Gyn 117:167, 1973.

354. Morris JM: Postcoital anitfertility agents and their teratogenic effect. Contraception 2:85, 1970.

355. Mourad M et al: Vaginal moniliasis and the pill. J Egypt Med Assoc 57:378, 1974.

356. Mourant AE et al: Blood groups and blood clotting. Lancet 1:223, 1971.

357. Mueller H et al: Letter: Thromboembolism, oral contraceptives, and oestrogen concentration gradient. Lancet 1:683, 1975.

358. Mumford JP: Drugs affecting oral contraceptives. Brit Med J 2:333, 1974.

359. Mungall IP et al: Pancreatitis and the pill. Postgrad Med J 51:855, 1975.

360. Murawski BJ et al: An investigation of mood states in women taking oral contraceptives. Fert Steril 19:50, 1968.

361. Naysmith JH: Oral contraceptives and coronary thrombosis. Brit Med J 1:250, 1965.

362. Ndeti CS et al: Salt to lower blood pressure. NEJM 286:782, 1972.

363. Necheles TF et al: Malabsorption of folate polyglutamate associated with oral contraceptive therapy. NEJM 282:858, 1970.

364. Neilan L: Estrogen therapy intrahepatic cholestasis: Characteristics of high-risk patients. J Am Med Wom Assoc 31:97, 1976.

365. Nelson J: Clinical evaluation of side effects of current oral contraceptives. J Reprod Med 6:50, 1971.

366. Nelson J: The use of the minipill in private practice. J Reprod Med 10:139, 1973.

367. Newman RL: A study of blood coagulation parameters. Am J Obstet Gynecol 125:108, 1976.

368. Newton MA et al: High blood pressure and oral contraceptives. Am J Obst Gyn 101:1037, 1968.

369. Nilsson L et al: Clinical studies on oral contraceptives. A randomized double blind, crossover study of different preparation. Acta Obst Gyn Scand 46:1, 1967.

370. Nissen ED et al: Association of liver tumors with oral contraceptives. Obstet Gynecol 48:49, 1976.

371. Nissen ED et al: Liver tumors and oral contraceptives. Obstet Gynecol 46:460, 1975.

372. Nocke-Finck L et al: Effects of antibiotics on estrogen excretion in women taking oral contraceptives. Acta Endocrinol 177(suppl):136, 1973.

373. Nocke-Finck L et al: Effects of rifampin on the menstrual cycle and on estrogen excretion in patients taking oral contraceptives. Dtsch Med Wochenschr 98:1521, 1973.

374. Nomura A et al: Benign breast tumor and estrogenic hormones: A population-based retrospective study. Am J Epidemiol 103:439, 1976.

375. Nora AH: A syndrome of multiple congenital anomalies associated with teratogenic exposure. Arch Environ Health 30: 17, 1975.

376. Nora JJ et al: Birth defects and oral contraceptives. Lancet 1:941, 1973.

377. Nora JJ et al: Can the pill cause birth defects? NEJM 291:731, 1974.

378. Nora JJ et al: Preliminary evidence for a possible association between oral contraceptives and birth defects. Teratology 7: 24, 1973.

379. Notelovitz M et al: Effect of natural oestrogens on coagulation. Brit Med J 3:171, 1974.

380. Notelovitz M et al: The effect of natural estrogens on coagulation. S A Med J 49:101, 1975.

381. Novak ER et al: Textbook of Gynecology, 9th edition, Williams and Wilkins, Baltimore, pp.644-653, 1975.

382. Ockner R et al: Hepatic effects or oral contraceptives. NEJM 276:331, 1967.

383. Odell WD: An analysis of the reported association of oral contraceptives to thromboembolic disease. West J Med 122:26, 1975.

384. Odell WD et al: The pharmacology of contraceptive agents. Ann Rev Pharmacol 14:413, 1974.

385. Oechsli FW: Oral contraception and sex ratio at birth. Lancet 1:1004, 1974.

386. Ovffret G et al: Contraceptive agents and cataract. Bull Soc Ophtalmol Fr 74:1119, 1974.

387. Oliver F: Ischaemic heart disease in young women. Brit Med J 4:253, 1974.

388. Oliver MF: Oral contraceptives and myocardial infarction. Brit Med J 2:210, 1970.

389. Olson RL et al: Postcontraceptive ance. Letter to editor. Arch Derm 105:928, 1972.

390. O'Reilly RA: Problems of haemorrhage and thrombosis in pregnancy. Clin Haemat 2:543, 1973.

391. Ory H et al: Oral contraceptives and reduced risk of benign breast disease. NEJM 294:419, 1976.

392. O'Sullivan JP et al: Letter: Oral contraceptives and malignant hepatic tumours. Lancet 1:1124, 1976.

393. O'Sullivan JP: Oral contraceptives and liver tumours. Proc R Soc Med 69:351, 1976.

394. Paine CJ et al: Oral contraceptives, serum folate, and hematologic status. JAMA 231:731, 1975.

395. Pal B: Oral contraceptives: Metabolic and nutritional effect. J Appl Nutr 26:33, 1974.

396. Palitz LL: Abstract of a preliminary report on norethynodrel (Enovid) in the control of acne in females. Arch Derm 86:237, 1962.

397. Palitz LL et al: Enovia for acme in the female skin. 3:243, 1964.

398. Parsons CP et al: Observation in some contact lens wearers using oral contraceptives. Contacts 22:3, 1967.

399. Perl G: Monilial vulvovagninitis following the pill. Mt Sinai J Med NY 37:699, 1970.

400. Peterson R et al: Changes in antithrombin III and plasminogen induced by oral contraceptives. Am J Clin Path 53:468, 1970.

401. Phillips BM: Oral contraceptives and migraine. Brit Med J 2:99, 1968.

402. Phillips N et al: One hour glucose tolerance in relation to the use of contraceptive drugs. Am J Obst Gyn 116:91, 1973.

403. Pilegram LO et al: Oral contraceptives and increased formation of soluble fibrin. Brit Med J 3:556, 1974.

404. Pimstone BL: Systematic LE exacerbated by oral contraceptives. S Afr J Obst Cyn 4:62, 1966.

405. Pindyek J et al: Cryofibrinogenaemia in women using oral contraceptives. Lancet 1:51, 1970.

406. Pinkerton GD et al: Post-pill anovulation. Med J Aust 1:220, 1976.

407. Pinkerton GD et al: Post-pill infertility. Med J Aust 1:223, 1976.

408. Popper H: Cholestasis. Ann Rev Med 19:39, 1968.

409. Porter PS et al: Yeast vulvovaginitis due to oral contraceptives. Arch Derm 93:402, 1966.

410. Posner et al: Changes in carbohydrate tolerance during long term oral contraception. Obstet Gyn 123:119, 1975.

411. Powell LW et al: Failure of a pure progestogen contraceptive to affect serum levels of iron, transferrin, protein bound iodine and transaminase. Brit Med J 3:194, 1970.

412. Powell LC et al: Effect of depo-medroxyprogesterone acetate as a contraceptive agent. Am J Obst Gyn 110:36, 1971.

413. Prasad AS et al: Effects of oral contraceptives on nutrients III, Vitamin B-6, B-12 and folic acid. Am J Obstet Gyn 125:1063, 1976.

414. Preston SN: Myocardial infarction and the pill. J Reprod Med 16:1, 1976.

415. Prins RP: Vaginal embryogenesis, estrogens and adenosis. Obs and Gyn 48:246, 1976.

416. Pritchard JA et al: Maternal folate deficiency and pregnancy wastage. Am J Obst Gyn 109:341, 1971.

417. Prust FW et al: Massive colonic bleeding and oral contraceptive "pills". Am J Obstet Gynecol 125:695, 1976.

418. Radford DJ et al: Oral contraceptives and myocardial infarction. Brit Med J 3:428, 1973.

419. Ravn J: Long-term contraception with the lynestrenol "mini-pill" Curr Med Res Opinion 1:605, 1973.

420. Reid IS: Abnormalities with oral contraceptives. Lancet 2:373, 1976.

421. Resnik S: Melasma induced by oral contraceptive drugs. JAMA 199:601, 1967.

422. Reimers D: Simultaneous use of rifampicin and other antituberculous agents with oral contraceptives. Prax Pneumol 25:255, 1971.

423. Rice-Wray E et al: Return of ovulation after discontinuance of oral contraceptives. Fert Steril 18:212, 1967.

424. Roberton YR et al: Interactions between oral contraceptives and other drugs: A review. Curr Med Res 3:647, 1976.

425. Robertson-Rintoul J: Oral contraception: Potential hazards of hormone therapy during pregnancy. Lancet 2:515, 1974.

426. Rockson SG: Plasma dopamine-beta-hydroxylase activity in oral contraceptive hypertension. Circulation. 51:916, 1975.

427. Rockwell DA: Letter: More on oral contraceptives. West J Med 122:255, 1975.

428. Rodriguez G et al: Thyroid status in long term high dose oral contraceptive users. Obst Gyn 39:779, 1972.

429. Roever S: Clinical observations of vision abnormalities of patients taking oral contraceptives. Amer J Optom 46:552, 1969.

430. Rohatiner JJ et al: Genital candidasis and oral contraceptives. J Obst Gyn Brit Commonwealth 77:1013, 1970.

431. Roland M et al: A regimen for fertility control with a cyclic progestogen. Obs Gyn 41:595, 1973.

432. Roland M et al: Further study of a d-Norgestrel for fertility control. Obs Gyn 46:308, 1975.

433. Rose MB: Superior mesenteric vein thrombosis and oral contraceptives. Postgrad Med J 48:430, 1972.

434. Rosenberg L et al: Letter: Myocardial infarction and estrogen therapy in premenopausal women. NEJM 294:1290, 1976.

435. Rothman KJ: Gender of offspring after oral contraceptive use. NEJM 295:859-861, 1976.

436. Royal College of Gen. Practitioners: Oral Contraceptives and Health. Pittman Pub. Co., N.Y., 1974.

437. Royal Australian College of Gen. Practitioners: Anovulants: Thrombosis and other associated changes. Med J Aust 2:440, 1974.

438. Ruben M: Contact lens and oral contraceptives. Brit Med J 1:1110, 1966.

439. Russell RP et al: Pill and hypertension. Johns Hopkins Med J 127:287, 1970.

440. Rysser JE et al: Megaloblastic anemia due to folic acid deficiency in a young woman on oral contraceptives. Acta Haematol (Basel) 45:319, 1971.

441. Sabell A: Oral contraceptives and the contact lens wearer. Brit J Physiol Opt 25:127, 1970.

442. Sabistron DW: Ocular complications of the pill. New Zealand Med J 75:388, 1972.

443. Salmon ML et al: Neuro-ophthalmic sequelae in users of oral contraceptives. JAMA 206:85, 1968.

444. Sandmire HF et al: Carcinoma of the cervix in oral contraceptive steroid and IUD users and nonusers. Am J Obstet Gynecol 125:33o, 1976.

445. Sartwell PE et al: Epidemiology of benign breast lesions: lack of associations with oral contraceptive use. NEJM 288:551, 1973.

446. Sartwell PE et al: Letter: Contraceptives and gallstones. NEJM 294:1186, 1976.

447. Sartwell PE: Letter: Preoperative discontinuation of contraceptives. NEJM 290:576, 1974.

448. Sartwell PE et al: Pulmonary embolism mortality in relation to oral contraceptive use. Prev Med 5:15, 1976.

449. Sartwell PE et al: Thromboembolism and oral contraceptives: an epidemiological case-control study. Am J Epidemiol 90:365, 1969.

450. Saruta T et al: A possible mechanism for hypertension induced by oral contraceptives. Arch Int Med 126:621, 1970.

451. Sarwar M: Contact lenses and oral contraceptives. Brit Med J 1:1235, 1966.

452. Schaffner F: The effect of oral contraceptives on the liver. JAMA 198:1019, 1966.

453. Schleicher E: LE cells after oral contraceptives. Lancet 1:821, 1968.

454. Schmidt AM: FDA approved injectable contraceptive. FDA Drug Bulletin, September 1974.

455. Schoolwerth AC et al: Nephrosclerosis postpartum and in women taking oral contraceptives. Arch Int Med 136:178, 1976.

456. Schrogie JJ et al: Effect of oral contraceptives on vitamin K-dependent clotting activity. Clin Pharmacol Ther 8:670, 1967.

457. Scott JW et al: Massive norethynodrel therapy in the treatment of endometriosis. Am J Obst Gyn 95:1166, 1966.

458. Seddon RJ: Hormonal steroid contraceptives I: physiological and pharmacological considerations. Drugs 2:399, 1971.

459. Seed M et al: The pill and its effects — metabolic research at St. Mary's. Times 72:509, 1976.

460. Seidenstricker JF et al: Screening test for Cushing's syndrome with 11-hydroxycorticosteroids. JAMA 202:87, 1967.

461. Shafey S et al: Neurologic syndromes occurring in patients receiving synthetic steroids (oral contraceptives). Neurol 16:205, 1966b.

462. Shafey S et al: Vascular headaches and oral contraceptives. Ann Int Med 65:863, 1966a.

463. Shearman RP: Prolonged secondary amenorrhea after oral contraceptive therapy. Lancet 2:64, 1971.

464. Shearman RP: Secondary amenorrhoea after oral contraceptives — treatment and follow-up. Contraception 11:123, 1975.

465. Sherlock S: Hepatic adenomas and oral contraceptives. GUT 16:753, 1975.

466. Shojania AM: Effect of oral contraceptives on vitamin B-12 metabolism. Lancet 2:932, 1971.

467. Shojania AM et al: Effect of oral contraceptives on folate metabolism. Am J Obst Gyn 111:782, 1971.

468. Shuman J: Contraceptive provision in the immediate post partum period. Obst Gyn 40:403, 1972.

469. Silverberg SG et al: Endometrial carcinoma in young women taking oral contraceptive agents. Obst Gyn 46:503, 1975.

470. Skolnick JL et al: Rifampin, oral contraceptives and pregnancy. JAMA 236:1381, 1976.

471. Slick GL et al: Hypertension, renal vein thrombosis and renal failure occurring in a patient on an oral contraceptive agent. Clin Nephrol 3:70, 1975.

472. Small DM: Hormone use to change normal physiology — is the risk worth it? NEJM 294:219, 1976.

473. Smith DC et al: Association of exogenous estrogen and endometrial carcinoma. NEJM 293:1164, 1975.

474. Smith M et al: Progestogen-only oral contraception and ectopic gestation. Br Med J 4:104, 1974.

475. Smith R: Hypertension and oral contraceptives. Am J Obst Gyn 113: 482, 1972.

476. Somerville BW: The role of estradiol withdrawal in the etiology of menstrual migraine. Neurol 22:355, 1972.

477. Spellacy WN et al: Carbohydrate metabolic studies after six cycles of combined type oral contraceptive tablets. Diabetes 16:590, 1967.

478. Spellacy WN et al: Effect of intrauterine devices, oral contraceptives, estrogens and progestogens on blood pressure. Am J Obst Gyn 112:912, 1972.

479. Spellacy WN et al: Effects of norethindrone on carbohydrate and lipid metabolism. Obst Gyn 46:560, 1975.

480. Spellacy WN et al: Glucose, insulin and growth hormone studies in long term users of oral contraceptives. Am J Obst Gyn 106:173, 1970a.

481. Spellacy WN et al: Human growth hormone levels in normal subjects receiving an oral contraceptive. JAMA 202:451, 1967.

482. Spellacy WN et al: Medroxyprogesterone acetate and carbohydrate metabolism. Fert Steril 21:457, 1970b.

483. Spellacy WN et al: Plasma insulin and blood glucose levels in patients taking oral contraceptives. Am J Obst Gyn 95:474, 1966.

484. Spellacy WN et al: The development of elevated blood pressure while using oral contraceptives: a preliminary report of a prospective study. Fert Steril 21:301, 1970.

485. Spellacy WN et al: Vaginal yeast growth and contraceptive practices. Obst Gyn 38:343, 1971.

486. Spencer MC: Topical use of hydroquinone for depigmentation. JAMA 194:962, 1965.

487. Sperling MA et al: Complications of systemic oral contraceptive therapy: neoplasm — breast, uterus, cervix and vagina. West J Med 122:42, 1975.

488. Spiera H et al: Rheumatic symptoms and oral contraceptives. Lancet 1:571, 1969.

489. Splerin H et al: Rheumatic symptoms and oral contraceptives. Lancet 1:571, 1969.

490. Srinivasan S et al: The alteration of surface charge characteristics of the vascular system by oral contraceptive steroids. Contraception 9:291, 1974.

491. Stauffer JQ et al: Editorial: Systemic contraceptives and liver tumors. Ann Int Med 85:122, 1976.

492. Stauffer JQ et al: Focal nodular hyperplasia of the liver and intrahepatic hemorrhage in young women on oral contraceptives. Ann Int Med 83:301, 1975.

493. Statement by the Committee on Safety of Drugs: Combined oral contraceptives. Brit Med J 2:231, 1970.

494. Stephens MEM et al: Oral contraceptives and folate metabolism. Clin Sci 42:405, 1972.

495. Stern MP et al: Cardiovascular risk and use of estrogens or estrogen-progestagen combinations. Stanford Three-Community Study. JAMA 235:811, 1976.

496. Stolley PD: Assessing rare and delayed side-effects of contraceptive steroids. J Steroid Biochem 6:937, 1975.
497. Stolley PD et al: Thrombosis with low-estrogen oral contraceptives. Am J Epidemiol 102,197, 1975.
498. Strauss JS et al: Effect of cyclic progestin-estrogen therapy on esbum and acne in women. JAMA' 190:815, 1964.
499. Streiff RR: Malabsorption of polyglutamic folic acid secondary to oral contraceptives. Clin Res 17:345, 1969.
500. Struve FA et al: Electroencephalographic correlates of oral contraceptive use in psychiatric patientsl. Arch Gen Psych 33:741, 1976.
501. Stumbo, WG: Erytheme nodosum secondary to the use of oral contraceptive — a case report. J Ky Med Ass 71:433, 1973.
502. Susens GP: Letter: Oral contraceptives and myocardial infarction. NEJM 293:938, 1975.
503. Swabb LI: Oral contraceptives and liver damage. Brit Med J 2:755, 1964.
504. Syvalahti EK et al: Rifampin and drug metabolism. Lancet 2:232, 1974.
505. Szabo AJ et al: Glucose tolerance in gestational diabetic women during and after treatment with a combination type oral contraceptive. NEJM 282:646, 1970.
506. Taber BZ: Breast cancer and oral contraception. J Reprod Med 15: 97, 1975.
507. Tapia HR et al: Effect of oral contraceptive therapy on the renin-angiotensin system in normotensive and hypertensive women. Obst Gyn 41:643, 1973.
508. Tapla HR et al: Effect of oral contraceptive therapy on the renin angiotensin system in normotensive and hypertensive women. Obst Gyn 41:643, 1973.
509. Taylor M et al: Effect of oral contraceptives on glucose metabolism. Am J Obst Gyn 102:1035, 1968.
510. Thulin KE et al: Seven cases of jaundice in women taking an oral contraceptive, Anovlar. Brit Med J 1:584, 1966.
511. Tietze D: Manual of Contraceptive Practice. Williams & Wilkins, Baltimore, MD, 1964.
512. Tobon H: Malignant hypertension, uremia and hemolytic anemia in a patient on oral contraceptives. Obst Gyn 40:681, 1972.
513. Toghill RJ et al: Folate deficiency and the pill. Brit Med J 1:608, 1971.
514. Tyler ET: Current status of Los Angeles oral contraception studies. Appl Thera 6:507, 1964.
515. Tyson JE: Neuroendocrine dysfunction in galactorrhea-amenorrhea after oral contraceptive use. Obst Gyn 46:1, 1975.
516. Tyson JE: Oral contraceptives and elevated blook pressure. Am J Obst Gyn 100:875, 1968.
517. Utian WH: Estrogen, headache and oral contraceptives. S Af Med J 48:2105, 1974.
518. Vagnucci H et al: Perspectives on the renin-angiotensin-aldosterone system in hypertension. Metabolism 23:273, 1974.
519. Vallings R:Oral contraceptives and alopecia arcata. Br Med J 2:1005, 1965.
520. Vermeulen A et al: Effect of oral contraceptives on carbohydrate metabolism. Diabetologia 6:519, 1970.
521. Vessey M et al: Investigation of relation between use of oral contraceptives and thromboembolic disease. Brit Med J 2:199, 1968.
522. Vessey MP et al: Investigation of relation between use of oral contraceptives and thromboembolic disease. A further report. Brit Med J 2:651, 1969.
523. Vessey MP et al: Oral contraceptives and breast cancer. Progress report of an epidemiological study. Lancet 1:941, 1975.
524. Vessey MP et al: Oral contraceptives and breast neoplasia: a retrospective study. Brit Med J 3:719, 1972.
525. Vessey MP et al: Oral contraceptives and thromboembolism. Brit Med J 1:37, 1974.
526. Vessey MP: Postoperative thromboembolism. Brit Med J 3:123, 1970.
527. Vessey MP et al: Randomised double-blind trial of four oral progestagen only contraceptives. Lancet 1:915, 1972.
528. Vessey MP: Thromboembolism, cancer and oral contraceptives. Clin Obs Gyn 17:65, 1974.
529. Von Kaulla KN: Bed rest, elective surgery and oral contraceptives. JAMA 218:888, 1971.
530. Von Kaulla E et al: Oral contraceptives and low antithrombin III activity. Lancet 1:36, 1970.
531. Wallace EE et al: Edrenal functions during long term Enovid administration. Am J Ob Gyn 87:991, 1963.
532. Walsh FB et al: Oral contraceptives and neuro-ophthalmolgic interest. Arch Ophth 74:628, 1965.
533. Walsh H et al: Oral progestational agents as a cause of candida vaginitis. Am J Ob Gyn 101:991, 1968.
534. Walsh H et al: Candida vaginitis associated with use of oral progestational agents. Am J Ob Gyn 93:904, 1965..
535. Waxler EB et al: Myocardial infarction and oral contraceptives. Am J Cardiol 28:96, 1971.
536. Wearing MP: The use of norethindrone (2mg) with mestranol (0.1mg) in fertility control. Canad Med Aso J 89:239, 1963.
537. Weigand D et al: Cutaneous Medicine Case Studies. Medical Examination Publishing Co., New York, 1971, p. 60.
538. Weinberger MH et al: Hypertension induced by oral contraceptives containing estrogen and gestagen. Ann Int Med 71:891, 1969.
539. Weindling H et al: Laboratory test results altered by the pill. JAMA 229:1762, 1974.
540. Weir RJ: Blood pressure and the pill. Am Heart J 92:119, 1976.
541. Weir RJ: Blood pressure in women after one year of oral contraceptives. Lancet 1:467, 1971.
542. Weir RJ et al: Blood pressure in women taking oral contraceptives. Brit Med J 1:533, 1974.
543. Weiss DB et al: Ectopic pregnancy and the pill. Lancet 2:196, 1976.
544. Weiss N: Risk and benefits of estrogen use. NEJM 293:1200, 1975.
545. Weissman FG: Case 1: Oral contraceptives. Drug Intell Clin Pharm 6:138, 1972.
546. Weissman MM et al: Oral contraceptives and psychiatric distrubance: evidence from research. Brit J Psychiat:122, 1973.....
547. Wertalik LF et al: Decreased serum B-12 levels with oral contraceptive use. JAMA 221:1371, 1972.
548. Wessler, S et al: Estrogen containing oral contraceptive agents — A basis for their thrombogenicity. JAMA 236:2179, 1976.
549. West J et al: The electroencephalograph and personality of women with headaches on oral contraceptives. Lancet 1:1180, 1966.
550. Whitelaw MJ et al: Irregular menses, amenorrhea and infertility following synthetic progestational agents. JAMA 195:780, 1966.
551. Whitty CWM et al: Effect of oral contraceptives on migraine. Lancet 1:856, 1966.
552. Wiegenstein L et al: Multiple breast fibroadenomas in women on hormonal contraceptives. NEJM 284:676, 1971.
553. Wilson JR et al: Obstetrics and Gynecology, 4th ed, CV Mosby Co., St. Louis, MO. 1971.
554. Winikoff D: Oral contraceptives and thyroid function tests. Med J Aust 1:1059, 1971.
555. Winston F: Letter: Supplementary pyridoxine given to women using oral contraceptives. Am J Ob Gyn 122:793, 1975.
556. Winston F: Oral contraceptives, pyridoxine, and depression. Am J Psych 130:1217, 1973.
557. Wiseman A: Clinical management of complaints associated with the use of oral contraceptives. Clin Ob Gyn 1968.
558. Wolf, RL: Angioneurotic edema. JAMA 201,892, 1968.
559. Woodward RK: Letter: Acme stimulation by ovral. Arch Dermatol 110:812, 1974.
560. Wynn V et al: Some effects of oral contraceptives on carbohydrate metabolism. Lancet 2:715, 1966.
561. Wynn V: Vitamins and oral contraceptive use. Lancet 1:561, 1975.
562. Yaffee H et al: Moniliasis due to norethynodrel with mestranol. NEJM 272:647, 1965.
563. Yaffe SJ et al: Stilboestrol and adenocarcinoma of the vagina. Pediatrics 51:297, 1973.
564. Yasuda M et al: Prenatal exposure to oral contraceptives and transposition of the great vessels in man. Teratology 12:239, 1975.
565. Yen SSC et al: Effect of contraceptive steroids on carbohydrate metabolism. J Clin Endocr 28:1564, 1968.
566. Zanartu J et al: Low dose oral progesterones to control fertility. I. clinical investigation. Ob Gyn 43:87, 1974.
567. Zeil HK et al: Increased risk of endometrial carcinoma among users of conjugated estrogens. NEJM 293:1167, 1975.
568. Ziegler J: Ovulation suppressor contraception and depression. Ann Int Med 74:791, 1971.
569. Zuck TF et al: Implications of depressed antithrombin III activity associated with oral contraceptives. Surg Gyn Obst 133:609, 1971.
570. Zuck TF et al: Thrombotic predisposition associated with oral contraceptives. Obs Gyn 41:417, 1973.

Chapter 27

Clinical Use & Toxicity of Glucocorticoids

Donald T. Kishi

1. Describe endogenous hydrocortisone secretion.

Hydrocortisone (HC, Cortisol) is the major glucocorticoid produced in the body. The biosynthesis and secretion of HC is regulated by the hypothalamic-anterior pituitary-adrenocortical (HPA) axis. The hypothalamus secretes corticotrophin releasing factor (CRF) which travels to the anterior pituitary via the hypophyseal portal system. The CRF then stimulates the anterior pituitary secretion of adrenocorticotrophic hormone (ACTH). ACTH enters the general circulation and stimulates the zonae reticularis and fasciculata of the adrenal cortices to synthesize and secrete HC. ACTH and HC levels follow a diurnal or circadian rhythm.

In the normal individual, HC levels begin to rise between 2 a.m. and 6 a.m.; peak levels occur between 6 a.m. and 8 a.m. The levels decrease throughout the day until approximately midnight when minimal levels occur. The rise and fall of HC levels do not occur in smooth transitions; rather, there are multiple minor peaks and valleys throughout the day (95). These minor peaks and valleys can be partially explained by the release of CRF in response to stressful stimuli. Another influencing factor in the diurnal and minor variations of plasma ACTH and HC levels is the negative feedback inhibition of the HPA axis; that is, as HC or synthetic glucocorticoid levels increase, ACTH secretion decreases. Whether this feedback inhibition is exerted at the level of the hypothalamus or the anterior pituitary is not known. Of note is the fact that stress can overcome the negative feedback inhibition; however, this ability of stress to override the negative feedback inhibition is dose dependent (51, 52). The diurnal rhythm of the HPA axis may not be found in patients who have impaired consciousness (50), temporal lobe or other forebrain disease (96), Cushing's syndrome, or anorexia nervosa (21). Since the diurnal rhythm is in part a function of the awake-sleep or activity-inactivity cycle, individuals who work at night would be expected to have an inverted diurnal rhythm. Induction of inversion of the diurnal cycle requires one or two weeks. The average amount of HC secreted daily varies with the age, sex, and size of the individual: adult males — 20.4 mg; adult females — 17.4 mg; and childen 12.5 mg/m². In stress situations, the adrenal cortices can secrete up to 300 mg/24 hours (91, 120).

2. Describe the metabolism and excretion of HC.

Total plasma HC levels range from 7-20 mcg/100 ml. In this range approximately 90% of the HC is bound to protein. HC is metabolized by the liver to the dihydro and tetrahydro metabolites which are conjugated to glucuronides and sulfates. This is the rate limiting step in HC clearance. Approximately 200 mcg of unaltered HC is excreted in the urine each day (4). This represents approximately 1% of the usual daily HC production. Following IV administration of radio tagged HC, less than 1% was excreted unchanged and 90% excreted in the metabolite or conjugated form (141). This low fraction of HC renal excretion in normal patients can be attributed to the high degree of protein binding and passive tubular reabsorption of HC (15). Renal clearance is increased in states of elevated plasma HC levels (15, 81). Phenytoin and phenobarbital can induce hepatic enzymes which increase the metabolic clearance of HC. Similarly, in hyperthyroid patients HC synthesis, metabolism, and excretion are increased; the converse is true in hypothyroid patients (116).

3. What is the significance of the fact that hydrocortisone is so highly protein bound?

HC is reversibly bound to corticosteroid binding globulin (CBG or transcortin), CBA (corticosteroid binding albumin) and, to a minimal extent, to erythrocytes and leukocytes. At normal levels, CBG binds the majority of circulating HC. As the concentration of HC is increased the CBG sites become saturated; consequently, the CBA bound and the unbound fractions increase. This is of significance since it is the unbound fraction of HC which is metabolically active (15).

In hypo- or dysproteinemic states, the total endogenous HC levels are decreased. This decrease has not been correlated with inadequate or decreased HC effect. Conversely, in conditions associated with increased CBG (pregnancy, estrogen therapy) the total plasma HC levels are elevated. This elevation has not been associated with excessive HC effect (130, 143). The effect of decreased or increased total endogenous HC levels due to changes in binding protein are insignificant since the HPA axis apparently regulates the free HC level (15). However, when exogenous glucocorticoids are given to patients with altered protein binding capacities, the effect on glucocorticoid action is significant (102).

4. What is the effect of hepatic dysfunction on glucocorticoid metabolism?

(a) *Prednisone and cortisone biotransformation:* Prednisone and cortisone are biologically inactive until biotransformed to prednisolone and hydrocortisone, respectively. This biotransformation is the result of the enzymatic action of hepatic 11-beta-hydroxydehydrogenase. The efficiency of this reaction for prednisone is 100% and for cortisone 50-70% (23, 87, 141). Powell et al (145) reported a significant difference in plasma prednisolone levels when 20 mg of prednisone and 20 mg of prednisolone were administered to patients with acute hepatitis or active chronic hepatocellular disease. Peak plasma prednisolone levels occurred one hour later following prednisone. The authors concluded that hepatic dysfunction decreased the efficiency of the biotransformation of prednisone to prednisolone. Since the same enzyme is involved, one might speculate that hepatic dysfunction could further decrease the conversion of cortisone to hydrocortisone; however, in the only patient studied, the biotransformation of cortisone to hydrocortisone was normal (87).

(b) *Plasma half-life:* Powell et al (145) compared the half-life of intravenous prednisolone in three control patients and three patients with liver disease (two inactive and one active). The half-lives in the control patients were 150, 180, and 195 minutes. The half-lives in the patients with liver disease were 195, 220, and 250 minutes. Similarly, Araki et al (6) compared the half-life of intravenous prednisolone in cirrhotics and normals; in cirrhotics, the average half-life was 157 minutes and in normals, 115 minutes. With dexamethasone, the t½ in cirrhotics was 125 minutes and in normals, 110 minutes. Since the correlation between plasma half-life of glucocorticoids and the duration of action is unclear, the significance of this increase in half-life is open to conjecture.

(c) *Protein binding:* Hypoalbuminemia and decreased levels of CBG are found in patients with liver disease. Consequently, there is an increase in unbound glucocorticoid. The following relationships between percent binding and serum albumin concentrations have been demonstrated for prednisolone.

Albumin (gm%)	% Bound
4.0	65
3.5	55
2.5	45

The significance of decreased binding of prednisolone relates primarily to the incidence of side effects; that is, at serum albumin concentrations of 2.5 gm%, the incidence of side effects (facial plethora, hemorrhage, psychoses, hyperglycemia, myopathy) was doubled (102).

5. Prednisone and cortisone are physiologically inactive substances. What are the implications of this lack of activity?

Prednisone and cortisone are inactive until biotransformed to prednisolone and hydrocortisone, respectively. This biotransformation occurs primarily in the liver and is mediated by the enzyme 11-beta-hydroxydehydrogenase. The activation of prednisone and cortisone occur at an efficiency rate of 100% and 50-70%, respectively (23, 88, 141).

The implications of this are the following:

(a) The intra-articular use of cortisone esters is valueless since the activating enzyme is not present in synovial tissue and fluid (148).

(b) There are no topical or parenteral preparations of prednisone, cortisone or their esters commercially available.

(c) Biotransformation may be affected in liver disease

as noted in the previous question.

6. Compare the various synthetic glucocorticoids and hydrocortisone.

See Tables 1 and 2.

Table I
COMPARISON OF VARIOUS GLUCOCORTICOIDS WITH HYDROCORTISONE

Glucocorticoid	Anti-inflammatory Potency	Equivalent Potency (mg)	Sodium Retaining Potency
Hydrocortisone	1.0	20	2
Cortisone	0.8	25	2
Prednisolone	4.0	5	1
Prednisone	3.5	5	1
Methylprednisolone	5.0	4	0
Triamcinolone	5.0	4	0
Paramethasone	10.0	2	0
Betamethasone	25.0	0.60	0
Dexamethasone	30.0	0.75	0

Table 2
HALF-LIVES AND DURATIONS OF ACTION OF VARIOUS SYSTEMIC GLUCOCORTICOIDS

Glucocorticoid	T½ (minutes)	Duration HPA suppression (hours)*
Hydrocortisone	80-118	24-36
Cortisone	30	24-36
Prednisolone	115-212	24-36
Prednisone	60	24-36
Methylprednisolone	78-188	24-36
Triamcinolone		48
Paramethasone		48
Dexamethasone**	110-210	more than 48
Bethamethasone		more than 48

* The duration of action is based on a single patient who received a single dose of the various glucocorticoids at different times. The dose of each glucocorticoid was equivalent to 5 mg of prednisone. The duration of effect was measured as the length of time urinary 17-ketosteroid levels remained depressed following the dose of the particular glucocorticoid. These values have been extrapolated to be equivalent to the duration of anti-inflammatory effect. The values cited are open to question since the study involved a single patient who received single doses of the various glucocorticoids. Another consideration before accepting these values is that the duration of suppression of ACTH secretion is related to the glucocorticoid dose (50).

** Meikel et al (124) reported on a patient who became Cushingoid while receiving dexamethasone 0.25 mg tid. If one accepts that the tissue effect of dexamethsone persists for longer than 48 hours after a single dose, development of glucocorticoid side effects is not surprising. However, the authors attributed the adverse effects in their patient to a decreased metabolic clearance of the drug as evidenced by a half-life of 450 minutes.

7. Compare ACTH with the glucocorticoids.

The subject of ACTH versus glucocorticoid therapy remains controversial. The **advantages** of ACTH include the following:

(a) The adrenal cortex is stimulated rather than suppressed. However, the remainder of the HPA axis can be suppressed by long term administration (147).

(b) Withdrawal symptoms are less frequent.

(c) Fewer catabolic effects are seen, since ACTH stimulates the secretion of androgens (170). This effect may be advantageous in conditions associated with myopathic changes.

(d) There is no growth suppression.

The **disadvantages** of ACTH as compared to the glucocorticoids include the following:

(a) It must be administered parenterally at least once daily.

(b) Severe allergic reactions can occur (e.g. anaphylaxis). The synthetic corticotrophin, cosyntropin, is reputedly less antigenic.

(c) The amount of circulating cortisol is dependent on and limited by the secretory capacity of the adrenal cortex.

(d) Refractory states can occur.

(e) Since ACTH stimulates both aldosterone and cortisol secretion (170) sodium retention may prove to be a significant disadvantage in cardiac or hypertensive patients.

8. What are fludrocortisone and desoxycorticosterone?

Fludrocortisone and desoxycorticosterone are commercially available mineralocorticoids. Fludrocortisone is the 9-alpha derivative of hydrocortisone and possesses 125 times the mineralocorticoid and 12-15 times the anti-inflammatory potency of the parent compound. Fludrocortisone is equipotent with aldosterone when both compounds are administered intravenously. It possesses greater mineralocorticoid effects when administered orally. Fludrocortisone is available only in the oral tablet dosage form. Desoxycorticosterone is a precursor of aldosterone and possesses 1/30 the mineralocorticoid potency. Like aldosterone, desoxycorticosterone is essentially devoid of anti-inflammatory effects. Unlike fludrocortisone, it is available in parenteral and sublingual tablet dosage forms (158, 188).

9. If it is suspected that a patient has adrenocortical insufficiency, what rapid screening test can be done on an outpatient basis to confirm the diagnosis?

Two rapid screening tests can be used for establishing adrenocortical insufficiency. The basis for both these tests is that ACTH stimulates the adrenal cortex to produce hydrocortisone.

Cosyntropin Test: Cosyntropin (Cortrosyn) is a synthetic peptide unit of natural ACTH which retains full ACTH activity. It differs from the natural product in that it is less allergenic. One-tenth (0.1) mg of cosyntropin is approximately equivalent to 10 units of natural ACTH. After a baseline plasma cortisol level is drawn, 0.25 mg of cosyntropin is administered intramuscularly. One-half to one hour after the injection a second plasma cortisol is drawn. If the patient has normal adrenocortical function, there will be a doubling of the baseline plasma cortisol level. If the patient has adrenocortical insufficiency, the plasma cortisol level will not be elevated to greater than twice the baseline value. This test does not distinguish between adrenocortical and pituitary etiologies of adrenocortical insufficiency (122).

ACTH Screening Test: After a baseline plasma cortisol level is drawn, 25 U of ACTH is administered intramuscularly. One hour after the injection a plasma cortisol level is drawn. If the patient has normal adrenocortical function, the plasma cortisol will increase by 25 mcg % (range: 11.3-47.8 mcg %). If the patient has adrenocortical insufficiency (Addison's disease), the plasma cortisol will only increase by about 0.5 mcg % (range 1.5-2.5 mcg %). This test does not distinguish between adrenocortical and pituitary etiologies of hypocortisolism (118).

10. Describe the ACTH infusion test for adrenal insufficiency. Why should this test be done over a five day period?

On days 1 and 2, baseline 24 hours urine samples for corticosteroids (17-OHCS) are collected. On days 3, 4 and 5, 40 U of ACTH are administered in saline over an 8 hour period (usually between 8 a.m. and 4 p.m.). Three consecutive 24 hour urine samples for 17-OHCS are collected.

In normals, urinary 17-OHCS levels/24 hours will be elevated above the baseline values by 2-4 times. In patients with primary adrenocortical insufficiency (defect in the adrenal glands), urinary 17-OHCS levels/24 hours will not increase significantly beyond the baseline values even after the third day of ACTH infusion. In patients with secondary adrenocortical insufficiency (defect in the pituitary gland), urinary 17-OHCS levels/24 hours will progressively increase during serial ACTH challenges. These serial challenges are necessary to stimulate atrophic adrenal cortices in patients with severely compromised pituitary ACTH production. It should be noted that patients with minimal pituitary ACTH production may not have atrophic adrenal cortices. These individuals may respond to exogenous ACTH normally, but may be unable to produce increased levels of endogenous ACTH during periods of stress. Thus, this test provides only indirect and inconclusive evidence of pituitary function. It is thus necessary to test pituitary function directly. This may be done by using the metyrapone test (192).

11. Describe the metyrapone (Metopirone) test for adrenal insufficiency. What precautions should be observed before utilizing this test?

Metyrapone (SU4885) inhibits the enzyme 11-hydroxylase, which converts 11-desoxycortisol to cortisol (hydrocortisone). After metyrapone is administered, plasma cortisol levels fall and stimulate pituitary ACTH production. If pituitary function is intact, it responds by increasing ACTH production. Due to the metyrapone block, the adrenal cortex produces 11-desoxycortisol. When very high desoxycortisol levels are produced, blocked cortisol production is overcome. Both 11-desoxycortisol and cortisol are measured as 17-hydroxycorticosteroids in the urine.

Initially, two consecutive 24 hour urine samples are collected for baseline 17-OHCS levels. Thereafter, 750 mg of metyrapone is administered every 4 hours for 6 doses. A 24 hour urine sample for 17-OHCS is collected simultaneously. On the day following the metyrapone administration, another 24 hour urine for 17-OHCS is collected.

If pituitary function is normal, the 24 hour urine samples for 17-OHCS will be doubled on the day metyrapone is administered or on the day following. If pituitary insufficiency exists, it will not be able to respond to the metyrapone induced hypocortisolism and no ACTH will be secreted. Thus, urinary 17-OHCS levels should not change significantly from baseline values.

The metyrapone test should not be used prior to the ACTH infusion test, since there is a potential danger of inducing acute adrenal insufficiency in the individual with primary adrenal insufficiency. Also, if the test resulted in little or no increase in urinary 17-OHCS levels, the interpretation would not be diagnostic. That is, it would be unclear whether the low level was secondary to pituitary malfunction or the inability of the adrenal cortex to respond to the endogenous ACTH produced (191).

12. What is the dexamethasone screening test for adrenocortical hyperactivity? Describe the procedure, rationale, and interpretation of this test.

The basis for the dexamethasone suppression test is that the administration of exogenous glucocorticoids suppresses the hypothalamic-anterior pituitary-adrenal axis. One mg of dexamethasone is administered between 11 p.m. and 12 a.m. and a plasma cortisol level is drawn at 8 a.m. the following morning.

In normals the plasma 17-OHCS level is suppressed to less than 5 mcg%. A plasma 17-OHCS of 5 mcg% or more may be indicative of Cushing's syndrome (138). However, failure to suppress can also occur in patients who are under physical or emotional stress. Patients on phenytoin or phenobarbital may also fail to show suppression (26, 27).

13. Describe the procedure, rationale, and interpretation of the dexamethasone suppression test for adrenocortical hyperactivity (104).

The basis of this test is that dexamethasone and other exogenous glucocorticoids suppress the hypothalamic-pituitary-adrenal axis and thereby decrease endogenous cortisol production.

Two consecutive 24 hour urine samples are collected for baseline 17-OHCS values. Thereafter, 0.5 mg dexamethasone is administered every 6 hours for 8 doses. After administering the last 0.5 mg dose, 2.0 mg of dexamethasone is administered every 6 hours for 8 doses. Consecutive 24 hour urine samples for 17-OHCS are collected simultaneously.

Table 3 may be used for interpretation of this test.

14. Why is dexamethasone used in these tests rather than hydrocortisone or prednisone?

Because it is so potent on a mg for mg basis, the amount of dexamethasone required to suppress the axis will not increase plasma and urinary 17-OHCS levels significantly.

Table 3
INTERPRETATION OF THE DEXAMETHASONE SUPPRESSION TEST FOR HYPERACTIVITY

DEXAMETHASONE DOSE	NORMAL	BILATERAL ADRENAL HYPERPLASIA	ADRENO-CORTICAL TUMOR	ECTOPIC ACTH PRODUCING TUMOR
0.5 mg every 6 hours	S	NS	NS	NS
2.0 mg every 6 hours	S	S	NS	NS

S — Suppression of urinary 17-OHCS excretion compared to baseline.
NS — No suppression of urinary 17-OHCS excretion compared to baseline.

15. What factors influence the suppression of the adrenal-pituitary-hypothalamic axis during glucocorticoid therapy?

During glucocorticoid therapy, suppression of the adrenal-pituitary-hypothalamic (HPA) axis occurs. Suppression of this axis is related to dose, duration and continuity of therapy (1, 86).

Treadwell and associates (190) studied the metyrapone responsiveness of 41 patients on chronic glucocorticoid therapy. These patients were treated with an average daily dose of 3 to 35 mg of prednisolone or its equivalent for a period of 1 to 125 months. The total dose ranged from 0.180 grams to 59.4 grams of prednisolone or its equivalent.

The minimum total dose required to abolish metyrapone responsiveness was 4.6 grams of prednisolone. Three of the 28 patients who received greater than 7.0 gm of prednisolone maintained responsiveness to metyrapone. None of the patients who received 14.0 grams or more of prednisolone maintained metyrapone responsiveness.

All patients who were treated for 15 months or less maintained metyrapone responsiveness. Two of 22 patients treated for 30 months maintained some degree of metyrapone responsiveness. However, all patients treated for 35 months or more were unresponsive to metyrapone.

El Shaboury (187) states that adrenal suppression secondary to continuous glucocorticoid therapy occurs after 5 years or following a total dose of 15 grams of prednisone. The above findings can be used as broad guidelines for estimating the degree of HPA axis suppression secondary to glucocorticoid therapy. It must be remembered, however, that individual variability is a significant factor in the degree of axis suppression.

16. A patient who is obviously Cushingoid secondary to exogenous glucocorticoids is tapered off her medication. Describe the recovery of her HPA axis.

Graber et al (73) described the plasma ACTH and 17-OHCS levels in 6 patients following their tapered withdrawal from supraphysiologic doses of glucocorticoids. The duration of glucocorticoid therapy in these Cushingoid patients ranged from 1-10 years.

Phase I: During the first month following the discontinuation of their glucocorticoids, the patients had low plasma ACTH and 17-OHCS levels. Plasma and urine 17-OHCS levels were low in response to 50 U ACTH infused over an 8-hour period. Subjectively, the patients complained of weakness, malaise, anorexia, nausea, arthralgias, myalgias and despondency.

Phase II: During the second through the fifth months, the patients' plasma ACTH concentrations were either normal or supranormal; however, plasma 17-OHCS and adrenal responsiveness to ACTH infu-

sion remained low. The diurnal rhythm of ACTH secretion also returned in Phase II.

Phase III: During the sixth through the ninth months, both plasma ACTH and 17-OHCS returned to normal levels; however, adrenal responsiveness to ACTH infusions remained subnormal.

Phase IV: Following the ninth month, the patients had normal plasma ACTH and 17-OHCS levels and normal responses to ACTH infusion and metyrapone testing.

Based on this data the following conclusions can be made:

1. Recovery of pituitary function precedes adrenocortical recovery following discontinuation of long term glucocorticoid therapy.

2. Patients who are stressed can be at risk to develop adrenal insufficiency for up to 9 months following discontinuation of long-term glucocorticoid therapy.

17. How should a patient who has been receiving prednisone 20 mg tid for SLE be tapered off his glucocorticoid?

Tapering of glucocorticoid therapy is usually indicated after attenuation of an acute self-limited condition by the glucocorticoid, e.g. poison oak; when the patient is experiencing a severe glucocorticoid adverse reaction, e.g. psychosis; or after control of a chronic condition, e.g. SLE, has been achieved with glucocorticoid therapy. In the latter instance, the objectives of tapering would be to achieve the minimal effective dose and to minimize or prevent glucocorticoid adverse reactions.

Tapering of glucocorticoid therapy is not without risk. The two major concerns are loss of control or reactivation of the condition being treated, and the precipitation of adrenal insufficiency due to the withdrawal of glucocorticoids in a patient with a suppressed HPA axis. Consequently, the decision to taper a patient off glucocorticoids must be based on the risk vs benefit of tapering the dose.

Once the decision to taper glucocorticoids is made, patient acceptance and education become important. If the patient is unwilling to accept the minor discomforts he may experience with weaning, any attempt to taper the glucocorticoid will probably be met with noncompliance. The patient must be made aware of the benefits and the risks associated with and without tapering. Once tapering is initiated he should be versed in the signs and symptoms of adrenal insufficiency, what to do about them, and when to contact his physician. The patient should receive an identification card or bracelet concerning the state of his HPA axis. Although no standard protocol will be universally applicable, Bvyny (28) suggests the following approach:

(a) Decrease the dose of prednisone by 2.5 to 5.0 mg every three to seven days. If the disease flares up, increase the dose, then taper more gradually, switch to alternate day therapy, or add adjunctive therapy.

(b) Once the patient is at the physiologic dose of glucocorticoid, he should be switched to hydrocortisone 20 mg every morning. At this point the patient should receive education and an identification card and/or bracelet. The patient can also be given a preloaded dexamethasone syringe with instructions on how and when to administer the drug.

(c) After two to four weeks of hydrocortisone 20 mg every morning, a morning dose is withheld and a plasma cortisol level is drawn. The patient is instructed to taper the morning dose by 2.5 mg weekly until he achieves a morning dose of 10 mg per day. At this point the patient's plasma cortisol level should be evaluated every four weeks as described above. Once his morning plasma level is greater than 10 mcg/100 ml, the morning dose may be discontinued; however, stress supplementation should be maintained.

For stress supplementation for dental work, minor surgical procedures or severe infections, such as influenza, enteritis, or strep throat, Byyny (28) recommends increasing the hydrocortisone dose to 50 mg bid. For major stress such as trauma or operative procedures, the dose of hydrocortisone should be increased to 100 mg every 6 to 8 hours during and for three to four days following the stress. The dose should then be tapered until the physiologic range is reached. He should be periodically evaluated as outlined in the above paragraph.

(d) The patient should be seen monthly until his cosyntropin screening test is normal. (See Question 9.)

18. A patient with severe poison ivy is treated with prednisone 40 mg qid for 2 days. The lesions have cleared. How should her prednisone be discontinued?

Christy (36) reported that patients who received 4 to 6 grams of hydrocortisone for 24 to 48 hours did not manifest any signs or symptoms of acute adrenal insufficiency following the abrupt discontinuance of the hormone. Others (72) however, noted a withdrawal syndrome following a single dose of 40 mg of prednisone. Although this patient may develop some symptoms (myalgias, malaise, restlessness) upon discontinuance of her prednisone, it is doubtful that tapering her dose will be necessary. However, with the rapid discontinuance of the prednisone, a rebound flare of her poison ivy may occur.

19. Can the use of ACTH hasten the recovery of the HPA axis following withdrawal of glucocorticoid therapy?

No. Fleisher et al (60) attempted to hasten HPA axis recovery by administering ACTH gel or zinc ACTH every 2 to 3 days to patients who had just been withdrawn from chronic glucocorticoid therapy. Plasma cortisol and ACTH levels were taken monthly during the first nine months following withdrawal. When compared with patients not receiving long-acting ACTH injections, no difference between the treated and untreated patients' HPA axis recovery process was noted. Possible explanations for this lack of effect of exogenous ACTH include ACTH-binding antibodies and/or the possible suppression of a pituitary factor other than ACTH which is involved in the recovery of atrophied adrenal cortices.

20. A patient has been treated with daily ACTH injections for 2 years. Would there be any danger in discontinuing the ACTH therapy abruptly?

If chronic ACTH therapy is discontinued abruptly, there is a potential for the development of adrenocortical insufficiency. This seems to be enhanced if the patient is under stress. In a study by Reed and coworkers (147), patients on chronic daily ACTH injections for a period of one month to ten years did not develop overt signs of adrenocortical insufficiency after withdrawal of ACTH therapy. However, metyrapone testing of these individuals revealed some degree of pituitary unresponsiveness as reflected by abnormally decreased urinary 17-OH corticosteroids.

21. A physician writes an order for ACTH 40 units to be given by IV over one hour. Why should this order be questioned?

ACTH has a very short half-life (15 minutes) (170). Since the effect of ACTH on the adrenal cortex is related to its plasma level, rapid infusion will not result in an extended pharmacologic action (181).

22. Describe and discuss alternate day dosing of glucocorticoids.

When glucocorticoids are administered on an alternate day schedule, the patient's 48 hour requirement for steroids is administered as a single dose every other morning.

The objective of this regimen is to minimize suppression of the HPA axis and other adverse effects associated with chronic glucocorticoid therapy while maintaining the desired therapeutic effect.

Administration of the glucocorticoid in the morning mimics the normal diurnal variation of plasma hydrocortisone (high levels in the morning and low levels at night). Administration of the glucocorticoid on alternate days provides a rest period from elevated plasma glucocorticoid levels. This rest period allows the HPA axis to recover from the suppressive effects and other tissues to recover from the metabolic effects of the exogenous glucocorticoids.

Alternate day therapy is indicated whenever chronic or long term glucocorticoid therapy is anticipated.

However, it should only be instituted after the condition being treated has been controlled with multiple dose therapy. This dosing regimen should not be used for replacement glucocorticoid therapy in patients with adrenal insufficiency or in patients who have undergone bilateral adrenalectomy.

The major limitation to the use of this dosing regimen is the loss in control of the condition being treated. If the disease process cannot be controlled on this dosage regimen, it should not be utilized.

23. Mr. A.J. has been on prednisone (5 mg tid) for his rheumatoid arthritis. Is there any advantage or rationale for selecting one glucocorticoid over another for an alternate day dosing regimen?

The use of paramethasone, dexamethasone, or betamethasone in alternate day dosing regimens is irrational. Since these glucocorticoids have tissue and suppressive effects on the HPA axis in excess of 48 hours following a single dose, the value of alternate day dosing would be negated. The tissue and HPA suppressive effects of prednisone, prednisolone, methylprednisolone, and triamcinolone last 12 to 36 hours following a single dose. Triamcinolone has the longest biological half life of the intermediate acting steroids. These agents are most commonly used for alternate day therapy.

Hydrocortisone and cortisone are short acting steroids. Because the tissue effects of these two agents last less than 12 hours, they are considered unsuitable for alternate day therapy (46, 79).

24. How should the transition from multiple doses per day to alternate day be made?

(a) If a patient is on a multiple dose per day regimen, the total dose per day should be gradually consolidated into a single morning dose. For example, if the daily dosage regimen is 5 mg tid, a dosing schedule might look like this:

	6 AM	12 N	6 PM
	5 mg	5 mg	5 mg
Day 1	10 mg	0	5 mg
Day 2	12.5 mg	0	2.5 mg
Day 3	15 mg	0	0

(b) On alternating days the dose should be incrementally decreased and increased until the total 48 hour dose is given on alternating mornings. On the "off" mornings, no glucocorticoid is given. For example, if the daily morning dose is 15 mg, then a typical dosing schedule would be represented by the following:

	15 mg
Day 1	20 mg
Day 2	10 mg
Day 3	25 mg
Day 4	5 mg
Day 5	30 mg
Day 6	0 mg
Day 7	30 mg
Day 8	0 mg

In this example the patient is changed to an alternate day dosing regimen by 5 mg/day increments. However, a slower rate of change may be required by some. If the patient becomes symptomatic on the "off" days, a minimal dose of glucocorticoid should be given and gradually reduced.

(c) Once the alternate day dosing pattern is established, the dose should be gradually tapered to the lowest tolerated level (46).

25. Mr. A.J. has just received an unsuccessful trial of alternate day glucocorticoid therapy for his rheumatoid arthritis. The goal of therapy is to maintain control of the patient's disease with minimal HPA axis suppression. Suggest an alternate method of dosing.

If the disease cannot be controlled by the alternate day regimen, the next most logical method of dosing is to administer a single daily dose each morning. This is most compatible with the maintenance of a normal diurnal pattern of cortisol secretion so that the degree of HPA suppression is minimized. The degree of HPA axis suppression is less than that produced by divided daily doses (136).

26. What is the effect of glucocorticoids on lymphocytes?

(a) *Lymphocytopenia:* Glucocorticoids cause a decrease in circulating lymphocytes. However, there is a marked species variation based on the relative ease with which lymphoid depletion occurs following a given regimen of glucocorticoids. Based on this criterion, species have been classified as either glucocorticoid sensitive — hamsters, mice, rats, rabbits — or glucocorticoid resistant — ferret, monkey, guinea pig, man. Since the majority of studies use glucocorticoid sensitive species, extrapolation of this data to man should be done with caution (37).

The glucocorticoids cause a redistribution of lymphocytes from the circulation into other body compartments, particularly to the bone marrow, in mice (39) and guinea pigs (55). Circulating T-lymphocytes are decreased to a greater extent than B-lymphocytes (56, 205). In man following a single dose of hydrocortisone 400 mg IV (56), prednisolone 1.0 gm IV (38), methylprednisolone 1.0 gm IV (201) or prednisone 50 mg orally (205), the lymphocyte counts fell to 25-50% of baseline values. The peak depression occurred 4-6 hours after the dose and reverted to baseline values within 24 hours after the dose, with one exception. Following methylprednisolone, the lymphocytopenia persisted for 48 hours. Patients receiving alternate day prednisone had no lymphocytopenia on the "off" day (57).

(b) *Lymphocyte function:* The glucocorticoids decrease the blastogenic response of T-lymphocytes to mitogens (31) and antigens (82). However, macrophage migrating factor and macrophage aggregation factor production and release in the guinea pig are not influenced by glucocorticoids (11, 201). Glucocorticoids inhibit on-going antibody synthesis but do not interfere with the induction of antibody response if the antigen is introduced just prior to or during glucocorticoid therapy. IgG and IgA are decreased by glucocorticoids. IgG levels begin to decrease 2-6 days after institution of glucocorticoids. Following a 5-day course of methylprednisolone 16 mg every 4 hours, IgG levels were depressed to 50% of baseline; the levels remained depressed for 3 months.

(c) *Leukemic lymphocytes:* Human leukemic lymphocytes are more sensitive to glucocorticoids than normal lymphocytes (37).

27. What is the effect of glucocorticoids on polymorphonucleocytes (PMN's)?

Glucocorticoids cause a neutrophilia due to an influx of new PMN's from the bone marrow (19); mobilization of marginated PMN's (194); a decrease in migration of PMN's out of the circulation in response to macrophage aggregation factor (201); and prolongation of PMN half-life (42).

Glucocorticoids do not impair the phagocytic process but can inhibit the intracellular killing of bacteria (19). This inability to destroy is secondary to lysosomal stabilization and failure of lysosomes to fuse with phagocytic vacuoles (126). The effect of glucocorticoids on the PMN half-life is dose related. For patients on daily prednisone, (average daily dose 60.7±16.3 mg/day) the mean PMN half life was 15.8±5.1 hours. In untreated patients the mean PMN half-life is 6.6±0.2 hours. Similarly, in patients receiving alternate day steroid therapy, a variation in PMN half-life on the "on" day was prolonged and on the "off" day was approximately the same as that found in normal patients. The larger the dose on the "on" day, the longer the PMN half-life (42).

The glucocorticoid preparation used may also be of importance. In mice succinate-linked hydrocortisone and methylprednisolone did not enhance local infection; however, the phosphate-linked hydrocortisone did. The glucocorticoids were used in equivalent doses (25). In a similar study, acetate- and phosphate-linked steroids potentiated infections; however, succinate-linked glucocorticoids did not (58).

28. A patient with rheumatoid arthritis has been treated with hydrotherapy, paraffin, aspirin, and physical therapy. In spite of these measures, the arthritis has worsened. A trial of glucocorticoids is being considered. Comment on the use of glucocorticoids in the management of this disease.

The glucocorticoids should not be used as first line drugs in the treatment of rheumatoid arthritis. They are adjuncts to other anti-inflammatory agents and are indicated when an adequate trial of the salicylates has been ineffective.

Glucocorticoids provide symptomatic relief but are not curative; that is, degeneration continues in spite of therapy. The lowest dose which makes symptoms tolerable should be used. The side effects which accompany the long term use of doses that provide complete alleviation of symptoms are not worth the risk in these patients. Once these patients experience total relief, it may be difficult to reduce the dose. As with all chronic inflammatory conditions where glucocorticoids are used, periodic attempts to decrease the dose or discontinue therapy should be made.

Initially, one might use a single morning dose of 5 mg prednisone. The trial period for glucocorticoid therapy should approximate 4 weeks. If no beneficial response has occurred, it should be discontinued (70).

29. Can arthritis be treated with intra-articular glucocorticoids?

The use of intra-articular glucocorticoids should be reserved for patients with one or two severely affected joints. If multiple joints are involved, systemic glucocorticoids are more appropriate.

If intra-articular glucocorticoid therapy is indicated, a tertiary butyl acetate ester, such as triamcinolone acetonide or another insoluble parenteral preparation, should be used. Insoluble preparations are preferred over soluble preparations, since they persist in the synovial space longer and consequently have a longer duration of action. However, cortisone esters should not be administered by the intra-articular route since cortisone is inactive until bio-transformed to hydrocortisone. This biotransformation does occur in the synovial space, but only to a very limited degree (207).

The intra-articular dose is variable and is a function of the size of the joint. Usually between 0.1 and 1.0 ml is administered using aseptic techniques (70).

30. A patient with rheumatoid arthritis involving his elbows is currently receiving intra-articular glucocorticoid therapy. What are the potential therapeutic complications of intra-articular glucocorticoid administration?

(a) Infection may result from the introduction of organisms into the normally sterile synovial fluid (60).

(b) Aseptic necrosis of femur or humerus heads and

Charcot's arthropathy have been associated with repeated injections of intra-articular glucocorticoids. However, these adverse effects have also been noted following the administration of systemic glucocorticoids. It is recommended that the patient's activity be limited for 10 days following intra-articular injection of glucocorticoids in weight bearing joints (34, 129).

(c) Adrenal-pituitary-hypothalamic axis suppression may result from such use (158).

31. What is the role of glucocorticoids in the management of septic shock?

The role of glucocorticoids in the treatment of septic shock remains open to debate. Many early studies which concluded that glucocorticoids were ineffective used inadequate doses: less than 300 mg of hydrocortisone. On the other hand, study design has made supportive evidence questionable (149).

The proposed mechanisms by which the glucocorticoids exert a beneficial action in shock include the following (149, 204):

(a) Positive inotropic effect on the myocardium.
(b) Decrease in peripheral vascular resistance.
(c) Stabilization of lysosomal membranes.
(d) Maintenance of capillary integrity.
(e) Chemical inactivation of endotoxin.

Glucocorticoids have been beneficial in the treatment of septic shock when doses were massive; therapy was initiated early; and specific and supportive therapy (antibiotics, fluids and electrolytes, plasma expanders, and pressor agents) were used. Christy (36) advocates the use of 1.0 gm of hydrocortisone or its equivalent intravenously as a bolus every 4 to 6 hours for 24 to 48 hours.

Dietzman and Lillihei (45) recommend a single intravenous bolus of any one of the following glucocorticoids:

(a) Hydrocortisone — 50 to 150 mg/kg.
(b) Dexamethasone — 6 mg/kg.
(c) Methylprednisolone — 30 mg/kg.

Medical Letter consultants recommend a dose of 30 to 50 mg/kg of hydrocortisone every 4 hours (121).

32. A patient enters the hospital and is subsequently diagnosed as having staphylococcal endocarditis. The drug of choice for this condition is a penicillinase-resistant penicillin. This case, however, is complicated by the patient's history of penicillin allergy (anaphylaxis). Would the concomitant use of glucocorticoids to prevent anaphylaxis be rational and efficacious?

If the patient is allergic to penicillin, an alternative agent must be used or prevention of the allergic reaction must be attempted. Green et al (75) reported a case in which pretreatment with antihistamines and 15 mg of prednisone did not inhibit the development of an anaphylactic reaction to penicillin. Bernstein and Lustberg (18) reported a case in which a patient who was receiving prednisone 15 mg daily died as a result of anaphylaxis secondary to penicillin. Whether or not larger doses of glucocorticoids would suppress anaphylaxis is unknown. For this reason the use of an alternative antimicrobal agent such as vancomycin should be pursued. (Also see chapter on *General Principles of Antibiotic Therapy.*)

33. Mr. J. is being treated with prednisone for idiopathic thrombocytopenia. Shortly after initiation of prednisone therapy, Mr. J's wife, Mrs. J., is diagnosed as having tuberculosis. Consequently an intermediate PPD skin test is placed on Mr. J.'s forearm. Will the prednisone affect the interpretation of this test?

Yes. Prednisone and presumably all glucocorticoids and ACTH can alter a patient's response to the tuberculin PPD skin test. Seventy tuberculin (intermediate PPD) positive individuals were given prednisone 40 mg daily in 4 divided doses. The patients were given repeated intradermal intermediate PPD tests at 72 hour intervals. Of the 70 patients tested, the test became negative in 68. The average time required to develop tuberculin anergy was 13.6 ± 10.1 days following the initiating of prednisone therapy. No correlation could be established between the time required for skin test inhibition and sex, age, activity of the tuberculosis, or severity of the initial skin test. Four patients were noted to have increased sensitivity to the skin test at various times during prednisone therapy. Once prednisone was discontinued reconversion to a positive intermediate PPD skin test occurred in 6.0 ± 3.3 days. In two cases 15 and 21 days were required to regain sensitivity to skin testing. No correlation between age, severity of initial reaction, or disease activity and time required for reconversion was noted. However, a sex correlation was made: females reconverted in 5 ± 2.6 days whereas males reconverted in 6.9 ± 3.6 days. All patients in the study received concomitant isoniazid and streptomycin therapy (24).

34. A patient with rheumatoid arthritis unresponsive to salicylates is being considered for glucocorticoid therapy. Is the fact that this patient also has a positive PPD skin test a contraindication to the use of glucocorticoids?

"The patient with previous tuberculosis, an abnormal chest roentgenogram suggestive of inactive tuberculosis or a positive tuberculin reaction should be given isoniazid along with the steroid therapy" (5). Isoniazid is given in a daily dose of 300 mg for adults (or 10 mg/kg body weight but not more than 300 mg/day in children). The isoniazid is given during the steroid therapy and for 6 weeks following discontinuance of the steroid. If the patient has not had previous antitubercular therapy or is a recent skin test convertor, prophylactic isoniazid should be continued for 12 months following discontinuance of the steroid. Additionally, for the prophylaxis against isoniazid induced peripheral neuropathy, the use of pyridoxine should be considered.

35. Is there any rationale for the use of glucocorticoids in a patient with active tuberculosis?

In the patients with fulminant tuberculosis, the use of glucocorticoids in combination with anti-tubercular therapy may prove to be life saving. Stead (185) recommends the following regimen in combination with antitubercular therapy:

(a) Prednisone 40 mg daily for 1 to 2 weeks.
(b) Prednisone 20 mg daily for 8 weeks.
(c) Gradual withdrawal of the prednisone.

The use of glucocorticoids in combination with antitubercular therapy in patients with tuberculous meningitis has been beneficial (88, 166).

Some have said that glucocorticoids will decrease pleural fibrosis in patients with persistent tuberculosis. Others, however, have noted no beneficial effect of glucocorticoids on pleural fibrosis. Although their effect on the reduction of pleural fibrosis remains unclear, that they increase the rate of clearing of tuberculous pleural effusions has been accepted (61, 63, 69, 83, 99, 137, 175).

The use of glucocorticoids in patients with tuberculous peritonitis has been advocated to prevent late fibrotic complications such as constrictive pericarditis and bowel adhesions. The suggested regimen is prednisone 30 mg daily for three months with subsequent tapering during the fourth month (171).

Glucocorticoids were once advocated for use in patients sensitive to antitubercular agents (113, 169). However, with the introduction of newer drugs, this use appears to be outmoded except in some rare hypersensitive patients in whom no alternative therapy exists.

In all of the above instances, glucocorticoids are used only in conjunction with specific antitubercular agents.

36. A patient with carcinoma of the lung with cerebral metastases develops cerebral edema. Discuss the use of glucocorticoids in the treatment of cerebral edema.

There are two forms of cerebral edema — cytotoxic and vasogenic (94). The cytotoxic type occurs in both gray and white matter and results from direct cellular injury which causes intracellular swelling; however, this form of edema is not associated with changes in vascular permeability. The vasogenic type occurs primarily in the white matter and is associated with an increased vascular permeability and an enlarged ex-

tracellular space. In addition to these structural changes in the edematous tissues, there is an increase in sodium and a decrease in potassium (151).

In animal and human studies, dexamethasone has been reported to have the following effects on the CNS:

(a) decreased vascular permeability (155).
(b) correction of the altered sodium and potassium concentrations (160).
(c) decrease in CSF production (157).
(d) improved peritumor circulation (199).
(e) decrease in tumor weight (76).

French (39) reviewed 249 patients with cerebral edema of various etiologies who were treated with dexamethasone 4 mg every 6 hours, parenterally. He noted the onset of response in 12 to 24 hours with maximal neurological improvement in 3 to 4 days after therapy was initiated. There was also a gradation in response dependent on the etiology of the edema. Cerebral edema secondary to:

(a) hematoma was unresponsive.
(b) cerebral metastases responded better than edema associated with primary tumors (gliomas and astrocytomas).
(c) closed head trauma, subarrachnoid hemorrhage, pseudotumor cerebri, or irradiation responded well in a majority of cases.

French also noted that dexamethasone could mask postoperative hematomas.

French chose dexamethasone on the basis of potency and low sodium retaining properties. The dosing regimen of 4 mg every 6 hours is empirical and has been unchallenged — until recently. Renaudin et al reported that some patients with malignant brain tumors required 96 mg of dexamethasone per day before maximum benefit was achieved; however, no kinetic studies were done on these patients (150). Perhaps French's results might be modified if higher doses are used. Since the benefits of 16 mg of dexamethasone per day require 12 to 24 hours to become evident and 3 to 4 days for maximum benefit, osmotic dehydration therapy, e.g. mannitol, remains the therapy of choice in emergency situations such as cerebral herniation.

37. A 30-year-old chronic asthmatic has been managed with bronchodilators with decreasing success. Can and should glucocorticoids be used in this patient?

Before chronic glucocorticoid therapy is initiated in patients with chronic asthma, it should be established that adequate bronchodilator therapy has been ineffective, and that the patient will benefit from the chronic use of glucocorticoids. Walsh and Grant (195) have suggested that if the FEV_1 (forced expiratory volume at one second) does not improve by 30/ over the baseline FEV_1 after one week of therapy that the patient will not benefit from chronic prednisolone treatment. The authors also elaborated a plan for determining suitable dosing intervals by following the onset of FEV_1 decrease after discontinuance of the glucocorticoid. Their findings suggest the following relationship:

Onset of decrease in FEV_1 after discontinuation of glucocorticoid	Suggested dosing frequency
a. <24 hours	Daily
b. 24-48 hours	Alternate day
c. 48-96 hours	Two days out of four
d. >96 hours	Three days out of seven

The objective of glucocorticoid therapy is to achieve therapeutic benefits while minimizing adverse reactions. Attempts to taper the glucocorticoids should be made periodically (195).

38. A five-year-old child with asthma is being treated with glucocorticoids. What primary consideration should be made in this pediatric patient?

Linear growth retardation has been noted in children with Cushing's syndrome and in those treated with glucocorticoids. Disease may contribute to this growth inhibition, but it has been clearly demonstrated that the glucocorticoid therapy is the primary factor. Several mechanisms by which glucocorticoids inhibit growth have been proposed:

(a) Inhibition of growth hormone release (64, 131).

(b) Inhibition of the growth hormone action on bone (178).

(c) Inhibition of mucopolysaccharide production with a resultant decrease in cartilagenous bone matrix and epiphyseal proliferation (43).

(d) In Cushing's syndrome due to adrenocortical tumor or hyperplasia, osteoporosis has been noted in association with a decreased number of osteoblasts on the bone surface (62, 172). This decrease in bone forming cells may account for growth inhibition.

Glucocorticoid-induced growth suppression appears to be a dose related effect. However, no absolute dose for a given agent can be specified, since there appears to be a high degree of individual variability. Tables 4 and 5 represent a composite of some reported cases in the literature.

Table 4
GLUCOCORTICOID-INDUCED
GROWTH SUPPRESSION

Agent	Minimum Dose Reported to Produce Complete Inhibition of Growth	Reference
Cortisone	45 mg/M^2/day	(22)
Hydrocortisone	36 mg/M^2/day	(193)
Prednisone	12.9 mg/M^2/day	(193)
Prednisone	7 mg/M^2/day	(53)
Betamethsaone	0.9 mg/M^2/day	(53)

Table 5
GLUCOCORTICOID-INDUCED
GROWTH SUPPRESSION

Agent	Minimal Dose (mg/M^2/day)	Linear Growth in % of Normal	Number of Patients	Reference
Cortisone	40 mg	0-80	19/34	(22)
Cortisone	40 mg	0-80	6/10	(53)
Prednisone	4 mg	0-80	28/33	(53)
Prednisone	6 mg	50/ or less	20/28	(53)
Betamethasone	0.3 mg	0-80	9/11	(53)

Discontinuance of the glucocorticoid or a decrease in the dose below a critical level is followed by a major upswing in the growth rate. Blodgett and associates (22) reported that this critical level was approximately 30 mg/M^2/day for cortisone; 2.15 mg/M^2/day for prednisone; and 0.37 mg/M^2/day for betamethasone.

39. How might growth suppression by chronic glucocorticoid therapy be circumvented?

(a) Discontinuation of glucocorticoids is followed by a normal growth pattern (22).

(b) Alternate day regimens minimize growth suppression (176, 177).

(c) The use of ACTH concurrently or in place of glucocorticoids has been associated with an increased rate of growth as compared to glucocorticoids alone (66).

40. A 25-year-old Caucasian female with asthma is being managed with prednisolone 15 mg daily. The patient subsequently becomes pregnant. The activity of her disease does not allow for discontinuance of the prednisolone. What potential therapeutic complications should be considered?

(a) *Teratogenesis:* In a review article concerning the effects of maternal medications on the fetus and the newborn, Adamson and Joelsson (2) cite a 10% incidence of cleft palate in association with the use of cortisone during the first ten weeks of gestation. The authors also noted that it is during the tenth week of gestation that the palate closes. Warrell and Tayloer (197) reported 8 still births and 9 infants at risk (placental insufficiency and acute fetal distress) in 34 pregnancies in which the mothers received prednisolone (2.5 to 30 mg daily) before and throughout their pregnancy. The patients were receiving prednisolone for eczema, ulcerative colitis, urticaria, asthma, rheumatoid arthritis, or lupus erythematosus. In a control group of women with similar diseases there were no still births, three premature births, and one death secondary to status asthmaticus during labor. Although no specific data were presented, the authors state that none of the infants had clinical evidence of adrenal insufficiency.

(b) **Neonatal Adrenocortical Insufficiency:** Although this complication of glucocorticoid therapy is a possibility, there are no reported cases. One case of fetal adrenocortical necrosis was noted on post-mortem examination (2).

(c) **Maternal Adrenocortical Insufficiency:** During the stress of parturition and in post-partum stage, the patient who has been receiving glucocorticoids during pregnancy should receive supplemental glucocorticoids to prevent acute adrenal insufficiency.

41. A patient receiving glucocorticoids for ulcerative colitis is admitted to the surgery unit for a colectomy and colostomy. He receives adequate glucocorticoid pre- and post-operatively. What potential surgical complications might occur?

The glucocorticoids impair wound healing as a result of their anti-inflammatory and catabolic properties. Inhibition of vasularization and collagen deposition, as well as the stabilization of lysosomal membranes may also contribute to delayed wound healing.

In wounds sutured together (closed wound) the tensile strength of the wound is decreased if steroids are administered within three days of surgery (183). In open wounds the rate of epithelialization is decreased and contraction delayed. This effect is seen even if steroids are not initiated until after the inflammatory process has been established and contraction initiated (183).

Vitamin A has an antagonistic effect on glucocorticoid lysosomal membrane stabilization. Numerous animal studies have been performed to delineate the effect of vitamin A on glucocorticoid-induced delayed wound healing. Vitamin A inhibits the effect of glucocorticoids on collagen deposition and epithelialization of open wounds. On the other hand, Vitamin A does not antagonize glucocorticoid effects on wound contraction (184).

Vitamin A was used topically and systemically in the animal studies. However, no definitive dosing or topical concentrations were reported. A single case report using Aquasol A ointment (20,000 IU/oz) was cited (84). Controlled studies in humans are lacking.

42. A 23-year-old Caucasian female with ulcerative colitis has been managed with sulfisoxazole and hydrocortisone enemas for one year. Since the patient has been symptomless for two months, the physician decides to discontinue her medications. Should the patient be tapered off the steroid enemas or can they be stopped abruptly?

Glucocorticoids are absorbed to a significant degree when administered by rectal enema or suppository (see Table 6).

Since absorption is significant, the possibility of adrenal-pituitary-hypothalamic axis suppression exists. The common practice of administering glucocorticoid enemas and/or suppositories at bedtime enhances the possibility of suppression. Consequently, the patient's glucocorticoid enema should not be discontinued abruptly. Before discontinuance of therapy, the status of the axis should be determined and the appropriate measures taken based on the results of this testing.

43. When should glucocorticoid therapy be discontinued?

(a) When therapy is ineffective.
(b) When severe side effects develop:
    (1) Severe osteoporosis.
    (2) Gastrointestinal hemorrhage.
    (3) Poorly controlled diabetes.
    (4) Persistent infection.
(c) When it is possible to control the pathologic process on a daily dose of 37.5 mg of cortisone or less (189).

44. A patient with arthritis has been receiving prednisone 5 mg tid for approximately one year. He now complains of nonspecific upper abdominal pain. What adverse effects of prednisone must one consider?

(a) **Ulcer:** In the early 1950's, the glucocorticoids were still considered the "silver bullet" of rheumatoid arthritis therapy. It was also during this time that the glucocorticoids acquired their reputation of being ulcerogenic. A number of mechanisms for glucocorticoid-induced ulceration have been proposed: thinning of gastric mucus, decreased regeneration of gastric mucosal cells secondary to a slowing down of the mitotic process, and an increase in acid production. The majority of these studies are based on animal data (49, 68, 125, 146, 173, 174).

The initial reports of glucocorticoid-induced gastric ulceration were in patients with rheumatoid arthritis.

TABLE 6
RECTAL ABSORPTION OF GLUCOCORTICOIDS

Drug-Dosage Form-Vehicle	% Absorption	Ref.
Hydrocortisone Alcohol (enema, ? vehicle)	30-50%	(54)
Hydrocortisone Acetate (enema, ? vehicle)	30-50%	(54)
Prednisolone-21-phosphate (aqueous enema)	30%	(117)
Betamethasone phosphate (aqueous enema)	Adrenal suppression	(117)
Hydrocortisone acetate (suppository, ? base)	26%	)133)
Methylprednisolone	18-64%	(179)

Incidence rates in this patient population range up to 31% (47, 89). However, in other conditions such as asthma (148, 167), ulcerative colitis (141, 206), allergic disorders (10A), and dermatologic disorders (156) in which glucocorticoids were used, the incidence of ulceration did not exceed the 5-10% range which is found in the general population (85). This difference in the incidence of glucocorticoid associated ulceration in arthritics vs. non-arthritics can be explained on the following basis. Patients with rheumatoid arthritis usually receive other anti-inflammatory agents — aspirin, phenylbutazone or indomethacin — in addition to their glucocorticoid therapy. These other anti-inflammatory agents are well known gastric irritants and are capable of inducing ulcers when used without glucocorticoids. This is supported by a study by Atwater et al (9) who noted no difference in the incidence of ulcer in arthritics receiving glucocorticoids and those who did not.

In a review of prospective studies in which the authors compared the incidence of ulcers found in control groups and patients receiving systemic glucocorticoids for conditions other than rheumatoid arthritis, the following information was obtained (30):

i. Incidence of ulcer: In the control group, 1.8%; in the glucocorticoid treated group, 2.1%.

ii. Duration of therapy: Patients receiving glucocorticoids for more than 30 days have a higher incidence of ulceration than patients receiving glucocorticoids for 30 days or less (1.7% vs. 0.4%). Of note is the fact that the incidence of ulcer in the control group was also higher after 30 days.

iii. Daily dose: Patients who received the equivalent of 20 mg or less of prednisone per day had a slightly lower incidence of ulceration than patients who received greater than 20 mg of prednisone per day (1.3% vs. 1.7%).

iv. Total dose: Patients who received a total course of greater than 1000 mg of prednisone had a higher incidence of ulceration than patients who received less (5.3% vs. 0.1%). Of note is the fact that there was also a higher incidence of ulceration in patients who received over 1000 mg of placebo than in control patients who received less placebo (2.5% vs. 0%).

v. Liver disease and nephrotic syndrome: The incidence of glucocorticoid associated ulceration in patients with nephrotic syndrome (10%) and liver disease (11%) is higher when compared with their respective control groups. Since both these conditions are associated with hypoalbuminemia, it was postulated that the increase in ulceration was due to an increased percentage of the glucocorticoid being in the unbound state.

In conclusion, the precise relationship between peptic ulceration and glucocorticoid therapy is unclear. Patients who appear to be at risk are those who are being treated for nephrotic syndrome, liver disease, or are comatose post-craniotomy. Other predisposing factors include a total prednisone intake exceeding 1000 mg, a history of ulcer disease, concomitant use of known gastric irritants, and stress. Prophylactic antacids should be used until the relationship of glucocorticoids and ulcers is clarified.

(b) *Pancreatitis:* In some medical circles pancreatitis is not recognized as a complication of glucocorticoid therapy. Early reports of this pathologic entity were a result of post-mortem examination. Riemenschneider and associates (152) reported a 40% incidence of glucocorticoid-induced pancreatitis in nephrotic children. Carone and Liebow (32) reported a 28.5% incidence of pancreatitis in patients receiving glucocorticoid therapy for rheumatoid arthritis. In both of the above reports glucocorticoid pancreatitis was cited as the cause of death.

The mechanism for glucocorticoid-induced pancreatitis is not clear. Nelp (134) suggested that glucocorticoids induce hyperlipidemia and fatty necrosis of the pancreas. Alternatively they may alter the electrolyte content of pancreatic juices, resulting in inspissation and consequent pancreatic duct obstruction. Perforation of an ulcer and leakage of gastric juices onto the pancreas has also been suggested as a mechanism.

The danger of glucocorticoid pancreatitis is that its clinical presentation is similar to that of peptic ulcer disease so that it may be mistreated. In patients taking glucocorticoids, complaints of epigastric upper abdominal pain should not be attributed solely to peptic ulcer disease.

45. A 10-year-old child has ulcerative colitis which has been successfully managed with prednisone 40 mg per day. The physician begins to taper the dose in increments of 5 mg per day. On the third day following the completion of the tapering procedure, the patient becomes irritable and complains of headache and visual disturbances. Papilledema is noted on ophthalmologic exam. What might be happening to this child?

The patient's symptoms are compatible with intracranial hypertension. This syndrome may occur if glucocorticoids or ACTH are tapered too rapidly.

Post-glucocorticoid benign, intracranial hypertension has been reported primarily in pediatric patients. The pathogenesis of the syndrome is unclear. Objective findings include an enlarged subarachnoid space and ventricular enlargement in long standing cases. Severe visual loss may also occur if the condition is allowed to persist.

The syndrome is treated by re-instituting glucocorticoid therapy at one-half to one-third the original dose. The dose is then slowly tapered over a two to three month period. If visual deterioration is marked, high dose hydrocortisone (up to 400 mg/day) or operative decompression is recommended.

The most logical approach to this problem is to prevent its occurrence. Thus, following prolonged therapy, doses should be tapered over a one month period and abrupt decreases of 50% or more should be avoided (135).

46. A 60-year-old post-menopausal female is seen by her private physician for low back pain. On x-ray, a compression fracture of one of her lumbar vertebrae is noted. Of note is that she has been taking prednisone 10 mg/day for a chronic asthmatic condition for "years." Can this compression fracture be related to her prednisone therapy? If so, describe the mechanism by which it occurs, its reversibility, and treatment.

Post-menopausal females, men in the sixth decade, rheumatoid arthritic patients, diabetic patients and immobilized patients appear to have a predisposition to osteoporosis (136). The initiation of chronic glucocorticoid therapy in these patients carries the risk of this potential complication.

The osteoporosis occurs primarily in the axial skeleton: vertebral column and pelvic girdle. Spontaneous compression fractures of the lumbar vertebrae are most common. Fractures of the ribs and other bones can occur following minor trauma (154).

The mechanism for glucocorticoid-induced osteoporosis remains to be defined. However, they possess the following actions which may explain this adverse effect:

(a) *Negative calcium balance.* The glucocorticoids exert an anti-vitamin D action on calcium absorption from the intestine. Additionally, the glucocorticoids increase the renal clearance of calcium by decreasing its renal tubular reabsorption (78, 98).

(b) *Depression of new bone formation.* The glucocorticoids may inhibit the production of osteoblasts (48). This has been noted in Cushing's syndrome (62, 172).

(c) *Decreased collagen formation or increased collagen catabolism in bone matrix.* The evidence for increased bone resorption is conflicting (43).

(d) *Increased parathyroid hormone levels.* Fucik et al (67) measured the parathyroid hormone (PTH) levels of 11 patients who were taking prednisone, 15-80 mg/day for 1-50 months, and 11 ambulatory hospitalized patients who were given a single dose of 200 mg of hydrocortisone by 4-hour intravenous infusion. When the PTH levels of the chronic glucocorticoid patients were compared to those of the control patients, the treated group's levels were approximately double that of the control group. When the PTH levels of the hydrocortisone treated group were compared to their baseline levels, the post-treatment levels were ele-

vated. Within 15 minutes after the infusion was initiated PTH levels were elevated; at 1 hour the average was 152% of the baseline; at 3 hours the levels peaked at 172% of baseline. Of note is that parathyroid hyperplasia has been described in rats treated with glucocorticoids and in patients with Cushing's syndrome.

It should be noted that osteoporotic changes must be considerable before they are noted on radiologic exam. They may be asymptomatic until a fracture occurs. At this point the patient may complain that his back aches, that his clothes are too long, or that he has "shrunk." Therapy is relatively nonspecific and includes any of the following (100, 187):

Vitamin D—1500 IU daily
Calcium Lactate—1.0 gm tid
Sodium Fluoride—3.0 mg daily

Androgen or estrogen therapy (e.g., for elderly females: diethylstilbesterol 1 to 3 mg daily for three to five weeks with intervals of 7 to 10 days; for elderly males: testosterone proprionate 50 mg daily or testosterone enanthate 300 to 700 mg monthly).

High protein diet.

47. A patient, DM, has been initiated on prednisone 60 mg daily for SLE. She complains of polydipsia and polyuria. An FBS is drawn and her blood sugar is 395 mg%. Explain this finding.

Glucocorticoids cause hyperglycemia by stimulating gluconeogenesis and by inhibiting the peripheral utilization of glucose.

(a) *Gluconeogenesis* — Glucocorticoids are catabolic and cause a dose related hyperaminoacidemia. This increase in amino acid levels results in pancreatic alpha-cell stimulation and hyperglucagonemia which stimulates glycogenolysis (114). Hyperaminoacidemia also results in an increased amount of hepatic enzymes—glucose-6-phosphatase, fructose-6-phosphatase and phosphoenolpyruvate carboxykinase — which are involved in gluconeogenesis.

(b) *Glucose utilization* — Glucocorticoids decrease glucose utilization by interfering with glucose entry into the cell and by inhibiting phosphorylation. This action is secondary to peripheral insulin resistance induced by glucocorticoids (140).

Maximal hyperglycemia occurs 8 hours after a dose of glucocorticoid. The degree of glucose elevation does not appear to be dose related; however, Walton et al demonstrated that the duration of prednisone-induced hyperglycemia is related to the dose. Following 15 mg, 45 mg and 90 mg, the duration of hyperglycemia persisted for 10-12 hours, 12-16 hours and 18-24 hours, respectively.

Glucocorticoid therapy can aggravate preexistent diabetes or precipitate it in patients with or without a history of the disease (69). The hyperglycemia is usually mild; however, there are reports of diabetic coma and acidosis associated with glucocorticoid therapy (15, 142). Discontinuation of the glucocorticoid usually results in the reversal of the hyperglycemia; however, this may require several months.

In patients with glucocorticoid-induced hyperglycemia, dietary restriction and/or oral hypoglycemic agents can be used to manage the condition. While the dose of glucocorticoid is not a factor in precipitating the diabetic state, decreasing the dose can decrease the degree of hyperglycemia (128). Exogenous insulin can be used; however, a relative resistance to its effects has been noted. Consequently, it should not be surprising if large doses of insulin are required (44, 139).

Alternate day glucocorticoid dosing has also decreased glucose intolerance (168). Since glucocorticoids can aggravate preexisting diabetes, diabetic therapy may have to be revised. Since reversal of glucocorticoid-induced hyperglycemia may require months following discontinuation of therapy, diabetic therapy should be evaluated periodically to avoid hypoglycemic episodes (128).

48. A patient who has developed grand mal seizures is treated with phenytoin and phenobarbital. This patient has also had a bilateral adrenalectomy and is receiving replacement hydrocortisone (15 mg in the a.m., 7.5 mg in the early afternoon, and 2.5 mg in the early evening) and fludrocortisone 0.1 mg q.d. What potential problems might occur?

Phenytoin is capable of inducing hepatic microsomal steroid hydroxylases. Thus, the half-life of cortisol is decreased. In normal patients, endogenous cortisol production is increased to compensate for the increased metabolic clearance. The patient who is unable to compensate with an increase in endogenous hydrocortisone production may develop adrenocortical insufficiency.

Phenytoin (DPH) can interfere with the dexamethasone suppression test. This interference was attributed to the enhanced hepatic metabolism of dexamethasone by DPH. The net result is a decrease in circulating dexamethasone so that its suppression of the HPA axis is diminished (26).

Phenobarbital can also increase cortisol metabolism as evidenced by an increase in metabolite excretion (27).

49. A patient with CHF is to be treated for lupus. Which glucocorticoid should be used in this patient?

Depending on the specific agent used, the dose, and the physiologic status of patient, glucocorticoids can cause sodium retention or diuresis. Glucocorticoids induce sodium retention by increasing tubular cation

exchange (an aldosterone-like effect). Thus potassium, hydrogen, and ammonium ion excretion is increased. The glucocorticoids can cause a sodium diuresis by antagonizing aldosterone; increasing the GFR; and by correcting the pathological stimulus to hypersecretion of aldosterone. The net effect of the glucocorticoid depends on which of the two actions (sodium diuresis or retention) predominates. For example, in a normal patient the aldosterone-like effect of hydrocortisone predominates over its effect on the GFR. However, in diseases with high aldosterone levels, the anti-inflammatory action of the glucocorticoid may alleviate the underlying stimulus for aldosterone production. The net effect in the latter instance may be sodium diuresis (103).

Dose is a factor in the effect of glucocorticoids on sodium metabolism. For example, prednisolone in small doses can induce an increase in GFR which predominates over its aldosterone-like effect. However, the aldosterone-like action predominates following large doses of prednisolone so that sodium retention occurs (103). The sodium retentive effects of large doses of hydrocortisone usually persist only for a few days, after which sodium retention decreases in spite of continued therapy. Small doses, however, are associated with persistent sodium retention and potassium loss. This can be reduced if potassium supplements are given concurrently (43).

Structural modifications of the basic steroid molecule can alter the mineralocorticoid properties of the glucocorticoid (103).

It should be noted that all the glucocorticoids induce potassium loss regardless of mineralocorticoid activity, secondary to their protein wasting effects.

Thus, patients who have conditions such as CHF in which sodium retention can be an aggravating factor, glucocorticoids associated with a lesser degree of mineralocorticoid effects should be used. Digitalis glycosides should be administered with the awareness that all glucocorticoids cause potassium wasting. (See *Congestive Heart Failure* chapter.)

50. A 35-year-old female has been using topical glucocorticoids for approximately one year. The patient is scheduled for a cholecystectomy. Can topical glucocorticoids cause systemic effects including HPA axis suppression?

Yes. Topically applied glucocorticoids can cause systemic effects. The percutaneous absorption of topically applied glucocorticoids is, however, subject to many variables. The potency of the glucocorticoid once it is absorbed must also be considered. Evidence that topically applied glucocorticoids have systemic effects includes the following:

(a) cutaneous lesions distant from the site of application heal;

(b) there is an increase in serum cortisol following topically applied hydrocortisone;

(c) the number of circulating eosinophils is decreased;

(d) there are changes in urinary electrolyte concentrations;

(e) withdrawal symptoms occur following discontinuation of application and symptoms reverse upon resumption of application;

(f) symptoms of arthritis have been alleviated following topical glucocorticoid application;

(g) suppression of the hypothalamic-pituitary-adrenal axis has been demonstrated by the ACTH infusion test and the metyrapone test (165).

51. What factors may influence the percutaneous absorption of a topically applied glucocorticoid?

(a) The characteristics of the vehicle in which the glucocorticoid is applied.

(b) The concentration of glucocorticoid in the vehicle.

(c) The surface area to which the glucocorticoid is applied.

(d) The condition of the epidermal barrier at the time of application.

(e) The duration of contact of the glucocorticoid with the skin.

(f) The presence or absence of an occlusive dressing over the area to which the glucocorticoid has been applied (165).

(g) Hydrocortisone, when applied to various regions of the body in a dose of 4 mcg/cm^2, is absorbed to varying degrees depending upon the region of the body to which it is applied (112).

Region	% of Dose
Forearm (ventral)	1%
Forearm (dorsal)	1.1%
Foot arch	0.14%
Ankle (lateral)	0.42%
Palm	0.83%
Back	0.17%
Scalp	3.5%
Axilla	3.6%
Forehead	6.0%
Jaw Angle	13.0%
Scrotum	42%

52. Can topical glucocorticoids cause local effects?

Local glucocorticoid therapy has been associated with miliaria-like eruptions, furunculosis, diffuse erythema, burning sensations, and atrophic striae (35, 132). Occlusion may have been a factor in the above adverse reactions. In a recent report, seven patients who applied corticosteroids and employed occlusive dressings acquired severe burns after exposure to sun-

light. The causative factor was felt to be occlusion and not the glucocorticoid since the untreated normal skin under the occlusive dressing was more severely affected (33).

53. What is the objective of using an occlusive dressing over an area to which a glucocorticoid has been applied topically?

The objective of using an occlusive dressing (e.g., Saran Wrap) over the area of glucocorticoid application is to deliver more medication to the target site by enhancing percutaneous absorption. The occlusive dressing increases the temperature and degree of hydration of the striatum corneum locally. These local changes enhance percutaneous absorption (165).

54. A patient claims that she is allergic to hydrocortisone cream. She states that the cream made her dermatitis better initially; however, with continued use it made her dermatitis worse. Is this possible?

Yes. While this may seem paradoxical, contact sensitivity to topical glucocorticoids does occur. In most cases the reactions have been attributed to impurities, preservatives, ointment and cream base ingredients. Alami et al (3), however, reported 23 patients with contact sensitivity to hydrocortisone or hydrocortisone acetate when used in patch testing. The concentrations of the drugs used in the patch testing were 10% or greater. Since the patch reactions were directly proportional to the concentration of the drug, and since these drugs are used clinically in concentrations of less than 2%, the significance of the positive patch reactions is questionable.

55. Discuss the ophthalmic use and dangers of glucocorticoids.

The glucocorticoids have multiple therapeutic indications in ophthalmology. They find their major use in conditions affecting the superficial and/or anterior segment of the eye. For example, they are used to reduce scarring following burns or trauma; to inhibit the immune response following corneal transplantation; and to treat uveitis and allergic, non-pyogenic ophthalmic diseases (188). Cortisone is ineffective in the treatment of superficial ocular lesions because it has an innate lack of activity. However, in the treatment of lesions of the anterior segment of the eye, cortisone is effective by virtue of its tissue metabolism to cortisol (77). Ocular complications, however, may result from the use of glucocorticoids in the treatment of pathologically related or unrelated ocular or systemic diseases.

Increased Intraocular Pressure: The elevation of intraocular pressure (IOP) secondary to glucocorticoids occurs almost exclusively following ophthalmic application. Becker and Hawn (14) noted a 30% incidence of elevated IOP during the use of ophthalmic glucocorticoids in patients without a previous history of glaucoma. In contrast, Bernstein and Schwartz (17) noted that during systemic glucocorticoid therapy there was only an insignificant effect on IOP. Patients with a history of angle-closure glaucoma have not demonstrated a higher risk of IOP elevation during ophthalmic glucocorticoid therapy (64). Armally (7, 8) however, found the converse to be true in patients with a history of open-angle glaucoma or a familial history of glaucoma.

Although the mechanism of glucocorticoid-induced IOP elevation has not been defined, it is known that it is not secondary to sodium retention or mydriasis. Miller and associates (128) noted an increase in IOP associated with an increased resistance to aqueous humor outflow in the anterior segment of the eye in patients receiving glucocorticoids.

The elevation of IOP secondary to glucocorticoids occurs within a few days after the initiation of local ophthalmic therapy and within one to two years following systemic therapy (7, 8). Once an increase in IOP is noted one must weigh the risk of permanent ocular damage against the need for the drug. The use of miotics may decrease IOP but may not completely alleviate it. Cessation of therapy, however, usually leads to an alleviation of the elevated IOP within 4 to 5 days following discontinuance of therapy. Spiers (185), however, reported a case of persistent IOP elevation following discontinuance of therapy.

Cataracts. The development of posterior subcapsular cataracts has been associated with longterm ophthalmic and systemic glucocorticoid therapy (14). The incidence of cataracts for systemic therapy is estimated to be between 11 and 38% (71). The mechanism for the development of glucocorticoid cataracts is not known, however there is a relationship with dose and duration of therapy. Unlike glucocorticoid induced IOP

elevation, glucocorticoid cataracts are not reversible. Consequently, the Medical Letter (120) recommends that ocular exams be performed every 2 to 3 months during glucocorticoid therapy.

Adrenal Suppression. Suppression of the hypothalamic-pituitary-adrenal axis can occur during the use of ophthalmic glucocorticoids. Lindner and coworkers (108) noted that urinary steroid levels were suppressed by use of dexamethasone ophthalmic drops in high doses.

Ocular Infections. Topical or systemic glucocorticoids may reactivate a dormant herpes simplex infection and cause a superficial corneal ulceration. If such a situation should arise, it is recommended that the glucocorticoids be discontinued as rapidly as is feasible. Paradoxically, herpes zoster infections of the eye respond favorably to systemic and ophthalmic glucocorticoids (159). The use of glucocorticoids following ocular trauma or surgery predisposes to fungal and bacterial ophthalmic infections.

56. A 55-year-old arthritic patient has had his symptoms controlled on maximal doses of aspirin and prednisone 10 mg daily. While on vacation he has his prednisone prescription refilled. During the remainder of his vacation the patient notes that his arthritic symptoms are increasing in severity. Explain this loss of control.

Assuming that his prescription was filled properly, the loss of control could be attributable to a decreased bioavailability of the prednisone he received while on vacation. Cases similar to the above have been reported in the literature and have been attributed to slow dissolution rate of the preparation (29, 101). Bioavailability can account for a decrease in control of a previously stabilized patient, and adrenal insufficiency due to a decrease in available glucocorticoid can result. Conversely, a preparation with increased bioavailability can cause an unexpected increase in toxicity.

REFERENCES

1. Adams DA et al: Adrenocortical function during intermittent corticosteroid therapy. Ann Int Med 64:542, 1966.
2. Adamsons K Jr et al: The effect of maternal medications on the fetus and the newborn infant. Am J Gyn 96:437, 1966.
3. Alani MD et al: Allergic contact dermatitis to corticosteroids. Ann Allergy 30:181, 1972.
4. Amatruda TT et al: A study of the mechanism of the steroid withdrawal syndrome, evidence of integrity of the hypothalamic pituitary-adrenal system. J Clin Endocrin 20:399, 1960.
5. Anon: Committee on therapy: adrenal corticosteroids in man, in *Steroid Dynamics*, Pincus G et al (Ed). Academic Press New York, 1966, p. 463.
6. Araki Y et al: Dynamics of corticosteroids in man, in *Steroid Dynamics,* Pincus G et al (Eds). Academic Press, New York, 1966, p. 463.
7. Armally MF: Effects of corticosteroids on intraocular pressure and fluid dynamics, II. The effects of dexamethasone in the glaucomatous eyes. Arch Opth 70:492, 1963.
8. Armally MF: Inheritance of dexamethasone hypertension and glaucoma. Arch Opth 77:747, 1967.
9. Atwater EC et al: Peptic ulcer in rheumatoid arthritis. Arch Int Med 115:184, 1965.
10. Axelrod L: Glucocorticoid therapy Medicine 55:39, 1976.
10a. Baldwin HS et al: Evaluation of steroid treatment in asthma. J Allergy 32:109, 1950.
11. Balow JE et al: Glucocorticoid suppression of macrophage migration inhibitory factor. J Exp Med 137:1031, 1973.
12. Bar-Hat J et all: Adrenal function allergy: Effect of dexamethasone aerosols in asthmatic children. Pediatrics 33:245, 1964.
13. Becker B: Cataracts and topical corticosteroids. Am J Ophth 58:872, 1964.
14. Becker B et al: Topical corticosteroids and heredity in primary open angle glaucoma. Am J Ophth 57:543, 1964.
15. Beisel WR et al: Cortisol transport and disappearance. Ann Int Med 60:641, 1964.
16. Bennington JL et al: *Laboratory Diagnosis.* Macmillan, London, 1970, p. 251.

17. Bernstein HN et al: Effects of long term systemic steroids on ocular pressure and tonographic values. Arch Ophth 56:543, 1964.

18. Bernstein IL et al: Penicillin anaphylaxix occuring in patients on steroid therapy. Ann Int Med 47:1276, 1957.

19. Biship CR et al: Leukokinetic study: A nonsteady state kinetic evaluation of the mechanism of cortisone induced granulocytosis. J Clin Invest 47:249, 1968.

20. Blereau RP et al: Diabetic acidosis secondary to steroid therapy. NEJM 271:836, 1964.

21. Bliss EL et al: Endocrinology of anorexia nervosa. J Clin Endocrin 17:766, 1957.

22. Blodgett FM et al: Effects of prolonged cortisone therapy on the statural growth, skeletal maturation and metabolic status of children. NEJM 254:636, 1956.

23. Boland EW: The antirheumatic effects of hydrocortisone, hydrocortisone acetate, cortisone, and cortisone acetate. Brit Med J 1:559, 1952.

24. Bovornkitti S et al: Reversion and reconversion rate of tuberculin skin reactions in correlation with the use of prednisone. Dis Chest 38:51, 1960.

25. Brothers JR et al: Enhancement of infection by corticosteroids: Experimental clarification. Surg Forum 24:30, 1973.

26. Buchanan RA et al: Diphenylhydantoin: Interactions with other drugs in man (continued). In *Antiepileptic Drugs*, edited by DM Woodbury et al, Raven Press Publ., New York, 1972, p. 181.

27. Burstein S et al: Phenobarbital induced increases in 6-beta--hydroxycortisol excretion: Clue to its significance in human urine. J Clin Endocrin Metab 25:293, 1965.

28. Byyny RL: Withdrawal from glucocorticoid therapy. NEJM 295:30, 1976.

29. Campagna FA et al: Inactive prednisone tablets USP XVI (Communications) J Pharm Sci 52:605, 1963.

30. Cantu RC et al: Evaluation of the increased risk of gastrointestinal bleeding following intracranial surgery in patients receiving high steroid dosages in the immediage post operative period. Int Surg 50:325, 1968.

31. Caron GA: Prednisolone inhibition of DNA synthesis by human lymphocytes induced in vitro by phytohaemagglutinin. Int Arch Allergy Appl Immunol 32:191, 1967.

32. Carone FA et al: Acute pancreatic lesions in patients treated with ACTH and adrenal corticoids. NEJM 257:690, 1957.

33. Cattano AN: Photosensitivity following treatment of occlusive dressings. Arch Derm 102:276, 1970.

34. Chandler GN et al: Charcot's arthropathy following intra-articular hydrocortisone. Brit Med J 1(952, 1959.

35. Chernosky ME et al: Atrophic striae after occlusive therapy. Arch Derm 90:15, 1964.

36. Christy JH: Treatment of gram negative shock. Am J Med 50:77, Claman HN: Corticosteroids and lymphoid cells. NEJM 287:388, 1972.

37. Claman HN: Corticosteroids and lymphoid cells. NEJM 287:388, 1972.

38. Coberg AJ et al: Disappearance rates and immunosuppression of intermittent intravenously administered prednisolone in rabbits and human beings. Surg Gynecol Obstet 131:933, 1970.

39. Cohen JJ: Thymus derived lymphocytes sequestered in the bone marrow of hydrocortisone treated mice. J Immunol 107:841, 1972.

40. Conn HO et al: The nonassociation of adrenocortical steroid therapy and peptic ulcer. NEJM 294:473, 1976.

41. Cope CL et al: The reliability of some adrenal function tests. Brit Med J 2:1117, 1959.

42. Dale DC et al: Alternate day prednisone: Leukocyte kinetics and suscpetibility to infections. NEJM 291:1154, 1974.

43. David DS et al: Adrenal glucocorticoids after twenty years. A review of their clinically relevant consequences. J Chron Dis 22:637, 1970.

44. Debosa RC et al: Insulin hypersensitivity and physiologic insulin antagonists. Physiol Rev 38:389, 1958.

45. Dietzman RH et al: The nature and treatment of septic shock. Brit J Hosp Med 1:300, 1968.

46. Dluhy RG et al: Pharmacology and chemistry of adrenal glucocorticoids. Med Clin N Amer 57:1155, 1973.

47. DuBois EL et al: The corticosteroid induced peptic ulcer: a serial roentgenological survey of patients receiving high doses. Amer J Gastroent 33:435, 1960.

48. Duncan H: Bone dynamics of rheumatoid arthritis patients treated with adrenal corticosteroids. Arthr Rheum 10:216, 1967.

49. Dyre JC et al: Studies on the mechanism of the activation of peptic ulcer after nonspecific trauma. Effect of cortisone on gastric secretion. Am Surg 147:738, 1958.

50. Eik-Nes KB et al: Diurinal variation of plasma 17-OHCS in subjects suffering from severe brain damage. J Clin Endocrin 18:764, 1958.

51. Estep HL: Neuroendocrine aspects of surgical stress. In Bajusz E (Ed) *An Introduction to clinical neuroendocrinology* S Karger,Basel, 1967 p. 106.

52. Estep HL et al: Pituitary-adrenal dynamics during surgical stress. J Clin Endocrin 23:419, 1963.

53. Falliers CJ et al: Childhood asthma and steroid therapy as influence on growth. Am J Dis Child 105:127, 1963.

54. Farmer RG et al: Treatment of ulcerative colitis with hydrocortisone enemas: relationship of hydrocortisone absorption, adrenal suppression, and clinical response. Dis Colon Rect 13:355, 1970.

55. Fauci AS et al: Effect of hydrocortisone on guinea pig peripheral blood lymphocyte subpopulations. Fed Proc 33:750, 1974.

56. Fauci AS et al: The effect of in vivo hydrocortisone on subpopulations of human lymphocytes. J Clin Invest 53:240, 1974.

57. Fauci AS et al: (Abstract) Effect of alternate day prednisone therapy on human lymphocyte subpopulations. Clin Res 22:417A, 1974.

58. Fauvre RM et al: Comparative effects on corticosteroids on host resistance to infection in relation to chemical structure. J Exp Med 125:807, 1967.

59. Fleisher DS: Pituitary-adrenal responsiveness after corticosteroid therapy in children with nephrosis. J Pediat 70:54, 1967.

60. Fleisher NK et al: ACTH antibodies in the patients receiving depot porcine ACTH to hasten recovery from pituitary-adrenal suppression. J Clin Invest 46:196, 1967.

61. Fleishman SJ et al: Antitubercular therapy combined with adrenal steroids in the treatment of pleural effusions. Lancet 1:199, 1960.

62. Follis RN, Jr: The pathology of the osseous changes in Cushing's syndrome in an infant and in adults. Bull Johns Hopkins Hosp 88:440, 1951.

63. Forgaes P: The treatment of tuberculous pleurisy. Thorax 12:344, 1957.

64. Franta AG et al: Human growth hormone: Clinical measurement, response to hypoglycemia and suppression by corticosteroids. NEJM 271:1375, 1964.

65. French LA: The use of steroids in he treatment of cerebral edema. NY Acad Med Bull 42:301, 1966.

66. Friedman M et al: Effect of long term corticosteroids and corticotrophin on the growth of children. Lancet 2:568, 1966.

67. Fucik RF et al: Effects of glucocorticoids on function of the parathyroids in man. J Clin Endocrinol Metab 40:152, 1975.

68. Garb AE et al: Steroid-induced gastric ulcer. Arch Int Med 116:899, 1965.

69. Gerbeaux J et al: Primary tuberculosis in childhood. Am J Dis Child 110:507, 1965.

70. Gifford RH: Corticosteroid therapy for rheumatoid arthritis. Med Clin N Amer 57:1179, 1973.

71. Giles CL et al: The association of cataract formation and systemic corticosteroid therapy. JAMA 182:719, 1962.

72. Good TA et al: Symptomatology resulting from withdrawal of steroid hormone therapy. Arthr Rheum 2:299, 1959.

73. Graber AL et al: Natural history of pituitary-adrenal recovery following long term suppression with corticosteroids. J Clin Endocrin 25:11, 1965.

74. Grant SD et al: Suppression of 17-hydroxycorticosteroids in plasma and urine by single and divided doses of triamcinolone. NEJM 273:1115, 1965.

75. Green GR et al: Treatment of bacterial endocarditis in patients with penicillin hypersensitivity. Ann Int Med 67:235, 1967.

76. Gurcay O et al: Corticosteroid effect on transplantable rat glioma. Arch Neurol 24:266, 1971.

77. Hamashige S et al: Penetration of cortisone and hydrocortisone into ocular structures. Am J Ophth 40:211, 1955.

78. Harrison HE et al: Transfer of 45-Ca across intestinal wall in vitro in relationship to action of Vitamin D and cortisol. Am H Physiol 199:265, 1960.

79. Harter JG: Corticosteroids, their physiologic use in allergic disease. NY J Med 66:827, 1966.

80. Harter JG et al: Studies on an intermitten corticosteroid dosage

regimen. NEJM 269:591, 1963.

81. Hellman L et al: Tracer studies of the absorption and fate of steriod hormones in man. J Clin Invest 35:1033, 1956.

82. Hellman DH et al: Effect of cortisol on the transformation of human blood lymphocytes by antigens and allogenic leucocytes, in Schwarz MR (ed): *Proceedings of Sixth Leucocyte Culture Conference*. New York, Academic Press 1972, p. 581.

83. Houghton LE: Combined corticotrophin therapy and chemotherapy in pulmonary tuberculosis. Lancet 1:595, 1954.

84. Hunt TK et al: Effect of Vitamin A on reversing the inhibitory effect of cortisone on healing of open wounds in animals and man. Ann Surg 170:633, 1969.

85. Ivy AC: The problem of peptic ulcer. JAMA 132:1053, 1946.

86. Jasani MK et al: Studies of the rise if plasma 11-hydroxy-corticosteroids in patients with rheumatoid arthritis during surgery. Quart J Med 37:407, 1968.

87. Jenkins JS et al: The conversion of cortisone to cortisol and prednisone to prednisolone in man. Brit Med J 2:205, 1967.

88. Johnson JR et al: Corticotropin and adrenal steroids as adjuncts to the treatment of tuberculous meningitis. Ann Int Med 46:316, 1957.

89. Kemmerer WH et al: Peptic ulcer in rheumatoid arthritis patients on corticosteroid therapy. Arthr Rheum 1:122, 1958.

90. Karten I: Septic arthritis complicating rheumatoid arthritis. Ann Int Med 70:1147, 1969.

91. Kenny FM et al: Cortisol production rates II. Normal infants, children, and adults. Pediatrics 37:34, 1966.

92. Kinser JB et al: The use of ACTH, cortisone, hydrocortisone, and related compounds in the management of ulcerative colitis. Am J Med 22:264, 1957.

93. Kitazawa Y: Primary angle closure glaucoma. Arch Ophth 84:724, 1970.

94. Kaltzo I: Neuropathological aspects of brain edema. J Neuropath Exp Therap 26:1, 1967.

95. Krieger DT et al: Circadian variation of the plasma 17 hydroxycorticosteroids in central nervous system disease. J Clin Endocrin 26:929, 1966.

96. Krieger DT et al: Characterization of the normal temporal pattern of plasma corticoid levels. J Clin Endocrin 32:266, 1971.

97. Krupp MA et al: *Physician's Handbook*. Lange Medical Publications, Los Altos, California, 1968, p. 239.

98. Laake H: The action of corticosteroids on the renal reabsorption of calcium. Acta Endocrin 34:60, 1960.

99. Large SE et al: Aspiration in the treatment of primary tuberculous pleural effusion. Brit Med J 1:1512, 1958.

100. Lauler DP et al: Diseases of the adrenal cortex. In *Harrison's Principles of Internal Medicine*. McGraw-Hill Book Co., New York, 1970, p. 477.

101. Levy G et al: Studies on inactive prednisone tablets USP XVI. Am J Hosp Pharm 21:402, 1964.

102. Lewis GP et al: Prednisone side effects and serum protein levels. Lancet 2:778, 1971.

103. Liddle GW: Effect of anti-inflammatory steriods on electrolute metabolism. Ann NY Acad Sci 82: 854, 1959.

104. Liddle GW: Tests of the pituitary adrenal suppressibility in the diagnosis of Cushing's syndrome. J Clin Endocrin Metab 20:1539, 1960.

105. Liddle GW: Clinical pharmacology of anti-inflammatory steroids. Clin Pharmacol Ther 2:615, 1961.

106. Liddle GW: Delta-I-alpha-flourohydrocortisone: A new investigative tool in adrenal physiology. J Clin Endocrin 16:557, 1956.

107. Lindner WR: Adrenal suppression by aerosol steroid inhalation. Arch Intern Med 113:665, 1964.

108. Lindner WR: Ardrenal suppression by aerosol steriods. Arch Ophth 79:174, 1968.

109. Livanou T et al: Recover of the hypothalamo-pituitary-adrenal function after corticosteroid therapy. Lancet 11:856, 1967.

110. Long JB et al: The ability of ACTH and cortisone to alter delayed type bacterial hypersensitivity. Bull Johns Hopkins Hosp 87:186, 1950.

111. MacGregor RR et al: Alternate prednisone therapy. NEJM 280:427, 1969.

112. Maibach HI et al: Topical steriods. Med Clin N Amer 57:1253, 1973.

113. March K: Streptomycin-PAS. Hypersensitivity treated with ACTH. Lancet 2:606, 1952.

114. Marco J et al: Hypevxrglucagonism induced by glucocorticoid

115. Martin MM et al: Intermittent steroid therapy. NEJM 279:273, 1968.

116. Martin MM et al: Effect of altered thyroid function upon adrenocortical ACTH and methopyrapone (Su 4885) responsiveness in man. J Clin Endocrin 25:20, 1965.

117. Matts SGF et al: Adrenocortical and pituitary function after intrarectal steroid therapy. Brit Med J 2:24, 1963.

118. Maynard DE et al: A rapid test for adrenocortical insufficiency. Ann Int Med 64:552, 1965.

119. McCawley Q: Cortisone habituation. NEJM 273:976, 1965.

120. —: Adverse ophthalmic effects of corticosteroids. Medical Letter 10:22, 1968.

121. —: Treatment of shock associated with bacterial sepsis. Medical Letter 11:93, 1969.

122. —: Cosyntropin. Medical Letter 13:33, 1971.

123. —: A note on adrenocortical steroids increased intracranial pressure. Medical Letter 12:83, 1970.

124. Meikel AW et al: Cushing syndrome from low doses of dexamethasone. JAMA 235:1592, 1976.

125. Menguy R et al: Effect of cortisone on mucoprotein secretions by the gestric antrum in dogs. Pathogenesis of steroid ulcers. Surg 54:19, 1963.

126. Merkow LP et al: The pathogenesis of experimental pulmonary aspergillosis. Am J Pathol 62:57, 1971.

127. Miller D et al: Corticosteroids and the functions of the anterior segment of the eye. Am J Ophth 59:31, 1965.

128. Miller SE et al: Clinical features of the diabetic syndrome appearing after steroid therapy. Postgrad Med J 40:660, 1964.

129. Miller WT et al: Steroid arthropathy. Radiology 86:652, 1966.

130. Mills IH et al: The effect of estrogen administration on the metabolism and protein binding of hydrocortisone. J Clin Endocrin 20:515, 1960.

131. Morris HG et al: Plasma growth hormone concentration in corticosteroid-treated children. J Clin Invest 47:427, 1968.

132. Muller SA et al: Complications of topical corticosteroid therapy. Arch Derm 86:478, 1962.

133. Nabarro JDN et al: Rectal hydrocortisone. Brit Med J 2:272, 1957.

134. Nelp NB: Acute pancreatitis associated with steroid therapy. Arch Int Med 108:702, 1961.

135. Neville BGR et al: Benign intracranial hypertension following corticosteroid withdrawal in childhood. Brit Med J 3:554, 1970.

136. Nichols T et al: Diurinal variation in suppression of adrenal functions by glucocorticoids. J Clin Endocrin 25:343, 1965.

137. Paley SS et al: Prednisone in the treatment of tuberculous pleural effusions. Am Rev Tuberc 79:307, 1959.

138. Pavlatos FC et al: A rapid screening test for Cushing's syndrome. JAMA 193:720, 1965.

139. Perley M et al: Plasma insulin responses to glucose and tolbutamide of normal weight and obese diabetics and non-diabetic subjects. Diabetes 15:867, 1966.

140. Perley M et al: Effect of glucocorticoids on plasma insulin. NEJM 274:1235, 1966.

141. Peterson RE et al: The physiological disposition and metabolic fate of cortisone in man. J Clin Invest 36:1301, 1957.

142. Pierce LE et al: Hyperglycemic coma associated with corticosteroid therapy. NY State J Med 69:1785, 1969.

143. Pincus G et al: *Steroid Dynamics*. Academic Press, New York, 1966, p. 13, 387, 463-80.

144. Popov SE: Complications of ACTH and corticosteroid therapy. Fed Proc 11:23:T984, 1964.

145. Powell LW et al: Corticosteroids in liver disease: Studies on the biological conversion of prednisone to prednisolone and plasma protein binding. Gut 13:690, 1972.

146. Rasanan T: Fluctuations in the mitotic frequency of the glandular stomach and intestine under the influence of ACTH, glucocorticoids, stress, and heparin. Acta Physiol Scand 58:201, 1963.

147. Reed PI et al: Adrenocortical and pituitary responsiveness following long-term high dosage corticotrophin administration. Ann Int Med 61:1, 1964.

148. Rees HA et al: Long term steroid therapy in chronic intractable asthma. Brit Med J 1:1575, 1962.

149. Reichgott MJ et al: Should corticosteroids be used in shock? Med Clin N Amer 57:1211, 1973.

150. Renaudin J et al: Dose dependency of Decadron in patients with partially excised brain tumors. J Neurosurg 39:302, 1973.

151. Reulen HJ et al: Electrolytes, fluids, and energy metabolism in

human cerebral edema. Arch Neurol 21:517, 1969.

152. Riemenschneider TA et al: Corticosteroid induced pancreatitis in children. Pediat 41:428, 1968.

153. Roberts W: Rapid progression of cupping in glaucoma. Am J Ophth 66:520, 1968.

154. Rosenberg EF: Rheumatoid arthritis. Osteoporosis and fractures related to steroid therapy. Acta Med Scand 162 (Suppl): 211, 1958.

155. Rovit RL et al: Steroids and cerebral edema: The effects of glucocorticoids on abnormal capillary permeability following cerebral injury in cats. J Neuropath Exp Neurol 27:277, 1968.

156. Sanders SL et al: Corticosteroid therapy of pemphigus. Arch Derm Syph 82:717, 1960.

157. Sato O: The effect of dexamethasone on cerebrospinal fluid production in the dog. Brain, Nerve, Tokyo 19:485, 1972.

158. Sayers G et al: Adrenocorticotrophic hormone; adrenocortical steroids and their synthetic analogs. In The Pharmacologic Basis of Therapeutics, Ed. 4, edited by LS Goodman and A Gilman. The Macmillan Co., New York, 1970, p. 1604.

159. Scheie HF et al: Treatment of herpes zoster ophthalmicus with corticotrophin and corticosteroids. Arch Ophth 62:579, 1959.

160. Scheinberg LO et al: Cerebral edema in brain tumors: Ultrastructureal and biochemical studies. Ann NY Acad Sci 159:509, 1969.

161. Schrier RW et al: Steroid induced pancreatitis. JAMA 194: 564, 1965.

162. Schuster S et al: Pituitary and adrenal function during administration of small doses of corticosteroids. Lancet 2:674, 1961.

163. Schuster S et al: Adrenal suppression due to intraarticular corticosteroid therapy. Lancet 2:171, 1961.

164. Schwartz E: Prolonged therapy with adrenocorticosteroids in allergic diseases. NY State J Med 60:3973, 1960.

165. Scoggins RB et al: Percutaneous absorption of corticosteroids. NEJM 273:831, 1965.

166. Shane SJ et al: Tuberculous meningitis. NEJM 249:829, 1953.

167. Siegel SC: Corticosteroids and ACTH in the management of the atopic child. Ped Clin N Amer 16:287, 1969.

168. Siegel RR et al: Reduction of toxicity of corticosteroid therapy after renal transplantation. Am J Med 53:159, 1972.

169. Simpson DG et al: Hypersensitivity to drugs in the treatment of tuberculosis. Am Rev Resp Dis 86:738, 1962.

170. Singer B: Adrenal corticosteroids — physiological considerations. Brit Med J 1:36, 1972.

171. Singh MS et al: Tuberculous peritonitis: pathogenesis, diagnosis and therapy. NEJM 281:1091, 1969.

172. Sissons HA: The osteoporosis of Cushing's syndrome. J Bone Joint Surg 38B:418, 1956.

173. Skoryna SG et al: A new method of producing experimental gastric ulcers: the effects of hormonal factors on healing. Gastroent 34:1, 1958.

174. Smith AT et al: The acute effects of prednisone on the gastric mucosa. Am J Dig Dis 13:79, 1968.

175. Smith MHD: Adrenocortical steroids in the treatment of tuberculosis in children. NY Acad Sci 82:1004, 1959.

176. Sokya LF: The treatment of nephrotic syndrome in childhood: use of alternate day prednisone regimen. Am J Dis Child 113:693, 1967.

177. Sokya LF et al: Alternate day steroid therapy for nephrotic children. JAMA 192:225, 1965.

178. Sokya LF et al: Treatment of short statute in children and adolescents with human pituitary growth hormone. NEJM 271:754, 1964.

179. Spencer JA et al: The rectal absorption of 6-alpha C-14 H-3 pre-

dnisolone. Proc Soc Exp Biol Med 103:74, 1960.

180. Spiers F: A case of irreversible steroid induced rise in intraocular pressure. ActaOphth 43:419, 1965.

181. Spiro KMet al: Clinical and physiological implications of the steroid induced peptic ulcer. NEJM 263:286, 1960.

182. Stead WW: Mycobacterial diseases, in Harrison's Principles of Internal Medicine. McGraw Hill Book Co., New York, 1970, p. 865.

183. Stephens FO et al: Effect of delayed administration of corticosteroids on wound contraction. Ann Surg 173:214, 1971.

184. Stephens FO et al: Effect of cortisone and Vitamin A on wound infection. Am J Surg 121:567, 1971.

185. Summerskill WH et al: Clinical and experimental studies on the effect of corticotrophin and steroid drugs on bilirubinemia. Am J Med Sci 241:555, 1961.

186. Thetbald TJ et al: Treatment of subacute bacterial endocarditis in patients allergic to penicillin: report of four cases. Am J Cardiol 10:575, 1962.

187. Thomas P: Withdrawal of corticosteroid therapy, in Guide to Steroid Therapy. J.B. Lippincott Co., Philadelphia, 1968, p. 66.

188. Ibid., p. 195.

189. Thorn GW: Clinical considerations in the use of corticosteroids. NEJM 274:775, 1966.

190. Treadwell BLJ et al: Pituitary-adrenal function during corticosteroid therapy. Lancet 1:355, 1963.

191. Truelove SC et al: Cortisone in ulcerative colitis. Brit Med J 2:1041, 1955.

192. Tyler FH et al: Laboratory evaluation of disorders of the adrenal cortex. Am. J Med 53:664, 1972

193. Van Metre TE et al: Growth suppression in asthmatic children receiving prolonged therapy with prednisone and methylprednisolone. J Aller 30:103, 1959.

194. Vincent PC et al: The intravascular survival of neutrophils labeled in vivo. Blood 43:371, 1974.

195. Walsh SD et al: Corticosteroids in treatment of chronic asthma. Brit Med J 2:796, 1966.

196. Walton J et al: Alternate-day vs. shorter interval steroid administration. Arch Intern Med 126:601, 1970.

197. Warrell DW et al: Outcome for the fetus of mothers receiving prednisolone during pregnancy. Lancet 1:117, 1968.

198. Webel MS et al: Cellular immunity after intravenous administration of methylprednisolone. J Lab Clin 83:383, 1974.

199. Weinstein JD et al: The effect of dexamethasone on brain edema in patients with metastatic brain tumors. Neurology 23:121, 1973.

200. Weitzman ED etal: Acute reversl of sleepwaking cycle in man. Arch Neurol 22:483, 1970.

201. Western WL et al: Communications: Site of action of cortisol in cellular immunity. J Immunol 110:880, 1973.

202. Williams TW et al: Lymphocyte in vitro cytotoxicity: Correlation of derepression with release of lymphotoxin from human lymphocytes. J. Immunol 103:170, 1969.

203. Williams TW Jr et al: Management of bacterial endocarditis — 1970. Am J Cardiol 26: 186, 1970.

204. Wilson RF et al: The hemodynamic effects of massive steroids in Clinical shock. Surg Gyn Obst 127:769, 1968.

205. Yu DTY et al: Human lymphocyte subpopulations. Effect of corticosteroids. J. Clin Invest 53:565, 1974.

206. Zetzel L et al: ACTH and adrenalocorticosteroids in the treatment of ulcerative colitis. Am J Dig Dis (New Series) 3,916, 1958

207. Ziff M et al: The effects in rheumatoid arthritis of hydrocortisone and cortisone injected intra-articularly. Arch Int Med 90:774, 1952.

Chapter 28

Epilepsy

Patrick D. Ginn

Although seizures have many causes, the majority of the one and a half million epileptics in the United States have idiopathic epilepsy or convulsions of unknown etiology. Idiopathic epilepsy occurs most frequently in children between the ages of two and five and at puberty.

The prognosis of seizure patients depends upon variables such as age of onset and the promptness of seizure control. Fortunately, in about 75% of patients with convulsive disorders, attacks can be controlled or reduced in frequency by the use of anticonvulsant medications.

The treatment of patients with seizure disorders is based on a thorough study of the patient to determine the presence of underlying lesions or metabolic defects which can be corrected. When these have been ruled out or treated, attention is directed to the prevention of seizures with drugs. While there are no ideal anticonvulsants, several can prevent grand mal, petit mal and febrile seizures and, to a lesser extent, psychomotor seizures.

Generally, medications are prescribed empirically. If one drug does not prove successful, another is tried. However, changing drugs too frequently is not advisable and each drug should be given an adequate trial to arrive at an optimum dosage. In some patients, a combination of two or more anticonvulsants will produce better results than one alone. A therapeutic response for any patient must be determined to some extent by trial and error. Medications do not cure convulsive disorders but are important in symptomatic treatment.

1. R.I. is a 14-year-old female who presents to her physician with a seizure disorder. With the exception of the normal childhood diseases, past history only reveals that the patient may have suffered a slight concussion with no apparent sequelae eight years ago.

Several weeks ago, the patient experienced a "strange feeling" lasting several minutes. This feeling which she describes as a *deja vu* phenomenon occurred again the next day and on several occasions during the ensuing two weeks. On the morning of the patient's visit to her physician, she again experienced this peculiar sensation. Immediately following this experience, she suddenly lost consciousness, her body became rigid, and her arms and legs began to jerk wildly. Her companion reports that this activity continued for several minutes after which the patient slept for two hours.

What symptoms does this patient present with that are typical of a seizure disorder? What are the different types of epileptic seizures?

The patient's feeling of *deja vu* may be symptoms of psychomotor epilepsy. The major motor symptoms (rigidity, jerking of extremities) and loss of consciousness may indicate grand mal involvement.

It is difficult to classify seizures in a simplified manner because clinical manifestations are so variable. Complete breakdowns of types of epileptic seizures and of types of epilepsies are listed in Table 1 and Table 2, respectively.

For simplicity, seizures are divided into: (a) generalized convulsions (grand mal, major epilepsy); (b) petit mal; (c) psychomotor epilepsy; and (d) "other" types (2).

Grand mal or major convulsions are characterized by a loss of consciousness and by tonic spasms of the trunk and extremities. This is followed in a few seconds or minutes by repetitive generalized clonic jerking.

Petit mal attacks are brief impairments of consciousness often associated with a flickering of the eyelids and a mild twitching of the mouth. This type of seizure is most common in children.

Psychomotor or temporal lobe epilepsy is characterized clinically by attacks of impairment of consciousness and amnesia. These attacks are often associated with semi-purposeful movements of the arms or legs, and sometimes with psychic disturbances such as hallucinations and *deja vu* phenomena (2).

Medications commonly used to treat these seizure disorders are listed in Table 3.

TABLE 1
INTERNATIONAL CLASSIFICATION OF EPILEPTIC SEIZURES

I. PARTIAL SEIZURES (seizures beginning locally)
  A. Partial seizures with elementary symptomatology (generally without impairment of consciousness)
      1. Motor symptoms (includes Jacksonian seizures)
      2. Special sensory or somatosensory symptoms
      3. Autonomic symptoms
      4. Compound forms
  B. Partial seizures with complex symptomatology (generally with impairment of consciousness). Also known as temporal lobe or psychomotor seizures.
      1. Impairment of consciousness only
      2. Cognitive symptomatology
      3. Affective symptomatology
      4. "Psychosensory" symptomatology
      5. "Psychomotor" symptomatology (automatisms)
      6. Compound forms
  C. Partial seizures which secondarily become generalized

II. GENERALIZED SEIZURES (bilaterally symmetrical and without local onset)
      1. Absences (petit mal)
      2. Bilateral massive epileptic myoclonus
      3. Infantile spasms
      4. Clonic seizures
      5. Tonic seizures
      6. Tonic-clonic seizures (grand mal)
      7. Atonic seizures
      8. Akinetic seizures

III. UNILATERAL SEIZURES (or predominantly unilateral)

IV. UNCLASSIFIED EPILEPTIC SEIZURES (due to incomplete data)

ABSTRACTED FROM: Gastaut, H: Clinical and Electroencephalographical Classification of Epileptic Seizures, Epilepsia 11: 102-113, 1970.

TABLE 2
INTERNATIONAL CLASSIFICATION OF EPILEPSIES

1. GENERALIZED EPILEPSIES
    1. Primary generalized epilepsies (includes petit mal and grand mal seizures)
    2. Secondary generalized epilepsies
    3. Undetermined generalized epilepsies

II. PARTIAL (FOCAL, LOCAL) EPILEPSIES (includes Jacksonian, temporal lobe and psychomotor seizures)

III. UNCLASSIFIABLE EPILEPSIES

ABSTRACTED FROM: Gastaut, H: Clinical and Electroencephalographical Classification of Epileptic Seizures, Epilepsia 11: 102-113, 1970.

2. What are the incidences of the various types of epileptic seizure disorders?

In a statistical survey of nearly 2,000 patients, 51% of all epileptic patients had generalized convulsions, 8% had minor seizures referred to as petit mal, and 1% had psychic or psychomotor seizures. The remaining 40% had two or all three types, the most prominent being psychomotor.

3. What may have been the cause(s) of the seizure activity in the patient described in Question 1? What are the general causes of seizures?

As is the case with many patients with seizure disorders, this patient's history does not provide a definitive etiology for her seizures. Obviously, one possibility in this particular case is cerebral trauma that may have occurred during the automobile accident eight years prior to the first major motor seizure.

Seizures have been defined as "intermittent disorders of the nervous system presumably due to a sudden, excessive, disorderly discharge of cerebral neurons." (2). This discharge results in an almost instantaneous disturbance of sensation, a loss of consciousness, convulsive movements, or some combination thereof. Generally, any type of cerebral lesion may cause seizures. These lesions may be in the form of cerebral tumors, cerebrovascular disease, cerebral infections or degenerative disease. Congenital maldevelopment of the brain may cause seizures in the first weeks or months of life.

Seizures may be caused by metabolic disorders such as metabolic alkalosis, hypokalemia, water intoxication, hypoxia, pyridoxine deficiency, phenylketonuria, argininosuccinic aciduria, uremia, hypocalcemia, and hypoglycemia (2,95). Seizures of this type require therapy specific to the disorder.

Some drugs may induce seizures. Examples include: camphor, pentylenetetrazol, picrotoxin, penicillin in doses greater than 10 million units, and withdrawal from sedative hypnotics, alcohol, or anticonvulsants (53). (See chapter on *Drug Abuse*.) Acetylcholine may cause seizures at high concentrations since it is found in increased amounts in the cerebral spinal fluid (CSF) after a seizure.

Fevers can also cause seizures. Although a seizure may be a symptom of a brain or metabolic disease, it is more frequently a solitary expression of abnormal cerebral function in an individual who is otherwise in perfect health (2).

4. The parents of the patient in Question 1 are understandably concerned about the prognosis of their child's disorder. Exactly what is the prognosis of childhood epilepsy? How long should anticonvulsant therapy be continued after a seizure-free period?

To determine the frequency of relapse and to identify any prognostic criteria, 148 seizure-free epileptic children who had been treated for four years with anticonvulsant medications were followed for 5 to 12 years after drug withdrawal (61). Seizures recurred in 36 children (24%). There was no relationship between relapse and sex, race, heredity, puberty or previous seizure frequency. If the onset of epilepsy was at an early age (before eight years) and there was prompt seizure control, the recurrence rate was 13%. It was at least twice as high in cases with late onset, prolonged duration, or in those who had neurologic, psychologic and/or electroencephalographic abnormalities. Relapse rates were lowest in patients with grand mal attacks (8%), febrile seizures (12%) and petit mal epilepsy (12%). The relapse rate was 25% in patients with psychomotor attacks. The highest relapse rate occurred in children with Jacksonian seizures (53%) and multiple-seizure types (40%) (61).

The recurrence of seizures upon withdrawal of medication is always a possibility. Livingston notes that epileptics with generalized motor seizures receiving barbiturates and hydantoins are those most adversely affected by a sudden withdrawal of medication (83a,83b). He also states that the longer anticonvulsant medication is continued in epileptic patients, the less likely recurrence of seizures will take place after withdrawal of the drug. It is his policy that all patients be maintained on effective and well-tolerated dosages for at least four years after the last seizure plus one or two years during which the medication is gradually withdrawn.

5. The above patient is diagnosed as having epilepsy and a treatment program utilizing anticonvulsant medications is begun. Many factors influence the success or failure of treatment of any disorder. What are the most common causes of treatment failures in the therapy of convulsive disorders?

The primary causes of treatment failure are: (a) inadequate dosage; (b) changing drugs too frequently without allowing an adequate time trial (see Question 8); and (c) failure of the patient to take the prescribed dosage. Non-compliance is probably the most common reason for treatment failure.

6. The specific diagnosis in the above case is major motor (grand mal) and psychomotor epilepsy. What drugs would you recommend for treatment of grand mal epilepsy?

Most consider phenytoin (diphenylhydantoin, DPH, Dilantin) the drug of choice for treatment of tonic-clonic seizures in adults and older children. Phenobarbital (PB) is the drug of choice for infants and preschool children because of the frequency of adverse effects with phenytoin in this age group.

7. While explaining to the above patient how to take the phenytoin that has just been prescribed for her, she appears to lose consciousness, and has a grand mal seizure. What should be done?

Grand mal seizures are the most common epileptic emergency. Maintaining the patient's airway and protecting her from injury should be the primary concern. The head should be cushioned. At the onset of a seizure, a tongue depressor wrapped with gauze may be placed between the patient's teeth to keep her from biting her tongue. A hard object should never be used.

During the tonic phase, the teeth are clenched, and the muscles are in a state of continuous tension or contraction. At this stage, no attempt to insert anything into the mouth should be made since this would damage the teeth and surrounding tissues. The clonic phase is described as spasm, in which rigidity and relaxation alternate in rapid succession (55).

As a general rule, this is all that needs to be done during the course of a grand mal seizure. When the seizure is over, the patient will become comatose. At this time, she should be placed in a semi-prone position or on her side to keep the airway open and prevent aspiration or oral or pharyngeal contents.

8. The above patient was given 300 mg of phenytoin (DPH) daily; however, she had another seizure three weeks later. What should be done? If two drugs are given, can the dosage of DPH be reduced?

One must first consider whether or not the drug used has been given an adequate trial. That is, have the maximal effects of the present dose been observed? This can be estimated by recalling a simple rule of pharmacokinetics for drugs which are eliminated according to first order kinetics: if a constant dose of a drug is given at constant time intervals, the amount that accumulates in the body will be maximal or will plateau in approximately five half-lives. This patient was started on 300 mg daily three weeks ago. If we assume that the half-life of DPH is one day, then a steady state will have been reached in approximately five days (five x 1 day).

There are two alternatives in this patient's therapy. The dosage of DPH can be raised or a second drug can be added. First, serum DPH levels should be drawn. If the levels are below the therapeutic range, the dose of DPH should be increased. It will then take another five half-lives to observe the maximal effect of this increase in dose. If therapeutic blood levels are present but clinical control still has not been achieved, a second drug should be added.

A combination of DPH and PB is often more effective than either of the drugs used alone. When used in combination, these drugs must be given in full therapeutic doses. Also see Question 9 for a discussion of phenytoin and phenobarbital interaction.

Primidone (Mysoline) and carbamazepine are other major drugs used for grand mal attacks. Occasionally, mephenytoin (or a combination of this drug and DPH) will succeed where DPH alone has failed. This indicates that different phenytoins may be additive, but further clinical substantiation is needed (2). Complete control is never achieved in some patients.

9. The above patient is placed on phenobarbital (PB) in addition to phenytoin (DPH). Discuss the interaction between these two agents.

Phenobarbital induces hepatic microsomal enzymes, thereby increasing DPH metabolism. However, PB also competes with DPH for the same metabolic

TABLE 3
DRUGS COMMONLY USED IN SEIZURE DISORDERS

SEIZURE DISORDER	Drug	DAILY DOSE (mg) Adults	Children	USUAL THERAPEUTIC SERUM CONCENTRATION (mcg/ml)	t 1/2	TIME TO PLATEAU*
Tonic-Clonic	phenytoin (DPH)	300-400	4-7/kg	10-20	7-42 hrs	5-10 days
(grand mal)	phenobarbital (PB)	150-250	3-8/kg	10-35	2-4 days	14-21 days
	primidone	500-1500	10-25/kg	6-12	3-12 hrs	4-7 days
	carbamazepine	600-1200	15-30/kg	6-8	7-30 hrs	2-4 days
Absences	ethosuximide	750-2000	20-30/kg	40-80	2-3 days	5-8 days
(petit mal)	clonazepam	1-20	0.01-0.2/kg	0.013-0.072	20-35 hrs	5-10 days
	trimethadione	900-2100	10-25/kg	6-41	12-24 hrs	2-5 days
Complex Partial	phenytoin	300-400	4-7/kg	10-20	7-42 hrs	5-10 days
(psychomotor)	primidone	500-1500	10-25/kg	6-12	3-12 hrs	4-7 days
	phenobarbital	150-250	3-8/kg	10-35	2-4 days	14-21 days
	methsuximide	750-2000	20-30/kg	——	2-4 hrs	——

*Steady state level achieved if patient started on maintenance therapy (without loading dose), or if maintenance dose is increased secondary to poor clinical control.

pathway. In normal doses, enzyme induction occurs and competitive inhibition is negligible. Large doses of PB, and perhaps normal doses in patients with impaired liver function, may elevate serum DPH levels (58). Therefore, DPH levels can be increased, decreased, or unchanged by concomitant PB administration. The clinical consequence of concurrent administration of these two drugs depends upon which of the above described mechanisms has the most influence. Patients whose DPH-metabolizing enzymes are relatively "saturated" are most likely to manifest increased serum DPH levels following PB administration. Also, other drugs the patient may be taking (e.g. carbamazepine) may have already maximally induced the microsomal enzymes. DPH may also increase PB plasma levels, but this is probably not of sufficient magnitude to cause adverse effects (58).

To determine the significance of this interaction in the above patient, DPH blood levels before and after the institution of the PB should be measured. If the patient has a high DPH blood level, large doses of PB should probably be avoided.

10. The same patient develops petit mal seizures. Which drug(s) should be used for the treatment of these seizures?

As a general rule, drugs effective in the treatment of grand mal and psychomotor epilepsy are relatively ineffective in the treatment of patients with petit mal attacks. Most authors recommend ethosuximide as a drug of first choice. This drug in doses of 750-1,500 mg/day is effective and has fewer side effects than trimethadione, paramethadione and phensuximide. After the initial administration of 250 mg/day, the dose should be increased every week until a therapeutic effect is achieved. Trimethadione (Tridione) in a dose of 300-1,800 mg daily is effective in some patients. Methylphenylsuccinimide (300 mg tid-qid) and acetazolamide have also been used in the treatment of petit mal (2,45).

This patient should probably receive ethosuximide in addition to her DPH and PB.

Statements in the literature concerning the exacerbation of petit mal seizures by PB and DPH, as well as the exacerbation of grand mal by ethosuximide and trimethadione, require more substantiation.

11. Which drugs might be effective in the treatment of this patient's psychomotor seizure attacks?

Drugs that are effective against grand mal seizures are also useful for psychomotor seizures. DPH (300-500 mg/day) and primidone (750-1,000 mg/day) produce the best results. On the whole, however, they are not as effective for the treatment of psychomotor seizures as for grand mal seizures (2).

12. E.C. is a 35-year-old male who was first diagnosed as having epilepsy at age 18. His seizures have never been well controlled on medication and he now presents to the emergency department suffering from an apparent generalized major motor seizure. His wife states that unlike previous seizures which have lasted approximately 5 minutes, this episode began 20 minutes ago and has not stopped. Define status epilepticus. Can drugs induce status epilepticus?

Status epilepticus refers to recurrent convulsions that occur so rapidly that consciousness is not regained between seizures. This is a medical emergency. Most epileptic-related deaths are due to uncontrolled, recurrent seizures or an injury sustained during a seizure. Fever, circulatory collapse, brain damage, and nephrosis may be encountered in fatal cases. Sudden withdrawal of high dose sedative-hypnotics or anticonvulsants may induce status epilepticus. Drug withdrawal seizures may be single as well as multiple. They generally occur 12-36 hours after discontinuation of the drugs (2,55).

13. How should the patient in Question 12 be managed?

No drug exists that safely controls recurrent convulsions of all etiologies. A major hazard in the treatment of status epilepticus is that consciousness and vital functions may be suppressed to a point that threatens life. Nevertheless, anticonvulsant drugs should be given parenterally in full therapeutic doses since repeated administration of small, subtherapeutic doses is less effective. Modern means of resuscitation are usually adequate to cope with the complications of overtreatment.

Diazepam (Valium) is the current drug of choice for the initial treatment of status epilepticus. A 10 mg dose is given intravenously (IV) at a rate not exceeding 1 ml/min (5 mg/min). Like DPH, parenteral diazepam contains 40% propylene glycol, a cardiotoxic agent when given too rapidly intravenously. Following IV diazepam, there is a rapid fall in serum concentration that correlates well with the transitory therapeutic effect. It may be necessary to repeat the dose of diazepam in 15 to 30 minutes (66) should seizures recur. It may be necessary to give two or three 10 mg doses of diazepam over a period of 30 to 60 minutes before good control is achieved.

Diazepam is not appropriate for chronic seizure control because it requires frequent administration. DPH is useful for this purpose. For a rapid effect, a loading dose of 500 to 1,000 mg of DPH is given IV at a rate that does not exceed 50 mg/min. Thereafter, daily maintenance doses of 300 to 500 mg are administered to maintain therapeutic levels. (See Question 21.)

Some doses of medication commonly used in the

treatment of status epilepticus follow (2,55):

(a) *Diazepam:* 10-20 mg IV every 10 to 20 minutes; no more than 100 mg in 12 hours.

(b) *DPH:* 500-1000 mg IV at a rate which does not exceed 50 mg/min.

(c) *PB:* 300-400 mg IM stat; then 100-200 mg every 2 hours, maximum 1000 mg/24 hours. After IM injection of a single large dose (10 mg/kg) of PB to infants, therapeutic serum concentrations are achieved in 30 to 90 minutes (12).

(d) *Amytal or other short-acting barbituates:* 500 mg IV over 5 to 10 minutes.

(e) *Thiopental:* 300-600 mg IV or IM.

14. Are recurrent seizures in children treated with the same drugs that are given to adults?

Yes. Diazepam is given in a dose of 0.04-0.2 mg/kg. Phenobarbital in a dose of 3-7 mg/kg daily should also be given parenterally to achieve prolonged control (55). (See Question 16.)

15. What is the incidence and cause of febrile seizures?

Febrile seizures are the most common pediatric neurologic disorder. They affect about 500,000 children in the U.S. each year and occur most frequently in children between six months and three years of age. In the majority of these patients, the initiating cause is a respiratory or gastrointestinal infection.

In Millichap's series (94), the mean temperature at the onset of a seizure was 40.0°C (104.0°F); the range was 38.5° to 41.4°C (101.3° to 106.5°F). Whether genetic factors influence febrile seizures is not yet clear (89,92,94,101).

16. An 8-year-old patient with a persistent fever of 101°F secondary to infection suffers a convulsion. This situation poses several problems: How and when does one treat fevers? If a seizure occurs, does one treat the fever and/or the seizure? Finally, should anticonvulsant drugs be given chronically to a patient who has had a febrile convulsion?

Temperature elevations of one or two degrees ordinarily do not require antipyretic therapy. In fact, such treatment may obscure the beneficial effects of other concurrent therapy aimed at correcting the underlying cause (e.g., antibiotics).

When febrile convulsions occur, lowering the body temperature is vital. Antipyretic drugs such as aspirin and acetaminophen reduce temperatures and may therefore prevent seizures. Generally, 1 grain/yr of age is administered every four hours to pediatric patients. This may cause unpleasant diaphoresis which may be accompanied by an alarming fall in blood pressure; subsequently, fever and chills may recur. These latter effects can be mitigated by giving large amounts of fluids, and by administering the antipyretics regularly

and frequently (2 to 3 hour intervals). Other cooling measures may have to be employed at higher temperatures (22,36,54,89,94). Sponging the body with alcohol compresses and cooling blankets are more effective than immersion. However, Millichap claims that cold water induces constriction of superficial skin vessels and is deleterious. Since alcohol sponging is also considered dangerous, sponging with tepid water is advocated (see chapter on *General Care – Fever*).

Anticonvulsants, specifically phenobarbital, are also used to treat febrile seizures; however, there is significant controversy concerning their use. Some authors feel that the use of PB as needed for fevers is effective; however, others have shown that even with high oral doses (10 mg/kg), a period of 12 hours is required for the drug to reach therapeutic blood levels (100). Even after intramuscular administration of PB (10 mg/kg), therapeutic levels are not achieved for 30-90 minutes (12). Therefore, if one desires acute control of a seizure disorder, a parenterally administered loading dose of PB should be given. Phenobarbital blood levels should be obtained periodically to assure that a therapeutic range has been reached. Blood level data are the only accurate means of evaluating whether the dose is sufficient to achieve the desired clinical response.

Treatment of febrile convulsions with DPH has been relatively unsuccessful.

It is important to treat the underlying infection causing the elevated temperature. Moreover, if the seizures are not abolished with the cooling measures or anticonvulsants, one must rule out other etiologies. (See Question 3.)

The use of continuous anticonvulsant, after febrile seizures have been controlled is controversial. Some consider withholding treatment until a second episode occurs an unnecessary risk and treat these children with PB for up to 3 years. Others advocate anticonvulsant therapy only if convulsions develop and oppose chronic therapy. However, they recommend that patients with a history of febrile convulsions be treated with antipyretics at the first sign of temperature elevation.

17. A 16-year-old female with a history of febrile seizures is hospitalized for evaluation of a fever 101°F, anorexia, nausea, vomiting, and a cramping, localized right lower quadrant abdominal pain of seven days duration. Diarrhea with blood and mucous has been present for six days. She has not ingested food or medications for two days and is now NPO pending work-up of possible regional enteritis. Medications being administered parenterally include DPH 100 mg IM tid. Is this an adequate dose? Discuss the wisdom of intramuscular DPH for this young lady.

Due to the high alkalinity of parenteral phenytoin (pH 12), intramuscular administration of this drug is not only painful, but also hazardous as tissue necrosis can occur (140). Furthermore, the IM absorption of phenytoin is erratic, and therapeutic levels are not attainable for several days (19,21,116), resulting in reports of seizures occuring during IM phenytoin in patients previously controlled on the oral preparation. One parenteral dosing regimen designed to immediately attain and maintain therapeutic plasma levels of DPH in patients unable to tolerate oral medication has been developed (100a). In accordance with this regimen the above patient should receive an IV dose of 10.7 mg/kg immediately followed by an IM dose of 12.7 mg/kg. This should be followed by daily IM maintenance doses of 8.6 mg/kg until oral medication can be tolerated. Due to the delayed absorption of phenytoin from IM depots, lower than normal doses may be required for a period when switching back from IM to oral administration of DPH. Two studies recommend doses equal to one-half the normal oral dose for a period of time equal to the IM period (139a, 139b).

Although absorption by the oral route is complete (100), it is slow. O'Malley and co-workers, using 500 mg orally in adults, found that peak levels were attained at five hours on the average (99). Suzuki and co-workers noted that it took about 18 hours for the elimination rate after oral administration to equal that following intravenous administration indicating that absorption continued for this period of time (128).

Another study examined DPH blood levels in patients given a one gram oral loading dose, followed by daily maintenance doses. Therapeutic DPH plasma levels were reached in eight hours, and steady state levels were reached in 48 to 72 hours (129). If daily maintenance doses of 300-500 mg/day are administered without a loading dose, six to ten days will be required to achieve therapeutic blood levels (36,100,138).

The manufacturer recommends that DPH not be added to standard parenteral solutions due to the risk of precipitation. It is generally recommended that the drug be injected directly into the vein at a rate not exceeding 50 mg/min. Nevertheless, this author has witnessed uncomplicated phenytoin infusions (100 mg DPH in 100 cc normal saline over one hour), which suggest that this incompatibility may be related to factors such as diluent, concentration, and infusion time. Definitive data are needed.

18. Can the signs and symptoms of DPH toxicity be correlated with blood levels?

Both the therapeutic and toxic effects of phenytoin (DPH) correlate well with serum concentration. The "therapeutic range" of total plasma DPH concentra-

tion is generally thought to be 1-2 mg% (10 to 20 mcg/ml) for both the anticonvulsant and antiarrhythmic actions. For some children, the range may be somewhat broader at 0.5-2 mg% (72). Signs of toxicity increase with increasing serum levels; 50% of patients have side effects at levels of 3 mg% or more. The earliest sign of DPH intoxication is nystagmus which usually appears with levels over 2 mg%. Above a blood level of 3 mg%, ataxia is commonly observed. Above 4 mg%, toxicity is manifested by mental changes such as sedation, irritability, inability to concentrate and slurred speech. Coma may occur when the levels exceed 5 mg%.

Because some patients have levels between 3 and 5 mg% without showing signs of toxicity, the absence of nystagmus and ataxia does not assure levels in the accepted therapeutic range (2,45,71,78,129,133, 100).

Avoidance of high levels may be more important than has been recognized since an excess of the drug may increase seizure frequency. Lascelles et al (74) reduced the dose in 26 patients when DPH concentration in the blood was above 2.5 mg% and in 18, there was a reduction of seizure frequency. Since serum concentrations of 1-2 mg% appear to be safe and effective, higher concentrations should be avoided even when neurologic signs are absent (74).

19. A 13-year-old boy with idiopathic grand mal seizures is not controlled on 400 mg DPH which he has taken daily for two months. A blood sample indicates that he has a subtherapeutic DPH level of only 5 mcg/ml. The dose is increased to 800 mg daily over the next month, but a second blood sample indicates that the DPH level has remained essentially unchanged (6 mcg/ml). Because the seizures continue to occur, the patient's medication is changed from the capsule to a liquid suspension. After receiving 900 mg DPH suspension daily for four days, he became ataxic, developed slurred speech and complained of diplopia. A blood level at this time was 35 mcg/ml. What has occurred?

This patient exemplifies one of a group of patients that this author has observed who seem to absorb the capsular form of DPH very poorly. When switched to the oral suspension, these patients generally obtain much higher blood levels. The exact reason for this poor absorption is not known, but it may well be related to the physical characteristics of the capsule DPH preparation. It is possible, for example, that as the capsule dissolves and the DPH makes contact with stomach acid, it begins to precipitate as the free acid and forms a relatively insoluble layer around the remaining drug. This may then limit the dispersion and absorption of the drug. Literature concerning this point is scarce; therefore, this theory remains conjectural.

20. A 12-year-old patient with idiopathic epilepsy was given an adequate loading dose of DPH during his hospitalization and was discharged free of seizures. A DPH blood sample was within the therapeutic range and the patient was given a prescription for DPH suspension. One week later the patient had a seizure, but it was decided not to change the drug regimen at this time. Although he had no recurrence, by the end of the next week, he was exhibiting signs and symptoms of DPH toxicity. The patient had finished the last dose of his first prescription on the morning of his return visit. Could this patient's peculiar response have been explained by the dosage form of DPH?

Suspensions must be shaken well before each use. When inadequately mixed, underdosage can occur when patients utilize the initial portion of a bottle, and overdosage can occur as the more concentrated suspension in the lower portion of the bottle is consumed. These apparently diverse responses to the drug were due to the patient's failure to shake the suspension thoroughly before each use. Dilantin suspension is difficult to disperse, so it is necessary to instruct the patient to shake the bottle vigorously and to check the bottom for undispersed drug before measuring the dose. Clinicians should also be aware that Dilantin oral suspension is available as 125 mg/5 ml and as a pediatric suspension of 30 mg/5 ml. Cases have been reported wherein patients mistakenly received the wrong strength preparation. Therefore, usage of these suspensions now tends to be avoided.

21. What are the methods of "loading" with oral, IM, and IV phenytoin (DPH)? Should the loading dose be given all at once or in divided doses?

A loading dose of DPH should be administered only by the oral or IV routes, because absorption by the IM route is delayed and unpredictable.

The intravenous preparation of DPH contains 40% propylene glycol and 10% ethyl alcohol in water and is adjusted to pH 12 with sodium hydroxide. Massive doses of DPH (1000 mg over 10 minutes IV followed by 500 mg IM) have caused sudden deaths, because the parenteral DPH preparation has potent effects on cardiac conduction. These consist of marked hypotension; alteration of S-T segments and T waves; and prolongation of the P-R intervals and QRS complexes. Cardiovascular effects occur when the parenteral DPH preparation is injected faster than 50 mg or 1 ml per minute. Hypotension is caused by both DPH and the propylene glycol solvent. The latter is responsible for the ECG alterations, which may actually be prevented by DPH.

Oral administration of a single 1 gm dose of DPH has little advantage over giving this amount in divided doses over 8 to 12 hours. The rate at which therapeutic

blood levels are achieved in both cases is limited by the rate of absorption from the gastrointestinal tract. In one study, patients were loaded orally with 1 gm of DPH by giving 400, 300, and 300 mg amounts within an 8 to 11 hour period. Therapeutic plasma levels of DPH were reached 6 to 12 hours following the loading dose (129).

22. A patient states that he has difficulty taking his phenytoin (DPH) regularly throughout the day. Is it possible for him to take his DPH as a single daily dose?

Once-a-day dosing is adequate for most patients (15), because DPH's plasma half-life is about 22 hours. However, the half-life varies considerably among individuals (7 to 42 hours); thus, it is important to tailor the dose of the drug to each patient and to monitor each patient by the use of DPH blood levels. These individual variations may be due to: (a) differences in liver metabolism; (b) variation in the degree of dose-dependent kinetics among individuals; (c) differences in the plasma concentration of DPH at which enzyme induction occurs; or (d) differences in the level at which rate-limiting drug metabolizing enzyme reactions become saturated (15). Also see the chapter on *Clinical Pharmacokinetics* wherein the kinetics of DPH are discussed extensively.

Occasionally, larger doses of DPH may cause gastrointestinal irritation. Drinking a glass of water generally reduces the irritation considerably.

23. If a once-daily dosage regimen is adopted, at what time of the day should DPH be taken?

Peak levels will be reached 8 to 12 hours after the drug has been taken. Since toxic effects occur most often at this time, the drug should be taken in the evening so that peak levels and toxicities will occur while the patient is asleep (15).

24. What are some advantages and disadvantages of once-daily phenytoin (DPH) dosing?

Socially and psychologically, once-a-day dosing is advantageous for school-age children and for working adults. A second advantage is increased compliance. On the other hand, missing one dose on a once-daily regimen would be much more serious than missing one dose on a multi-dose regimen. Also, gastrointestinal irritation may be more pronounced with the larger dose.

25. A uremic patient has just had a convulsive episode. Should the dose of phenytoin (DPH) be altered in uremic patients? How is DPH normally metabolized and eliminated? Can the elimination of DPH be enhanced by altering urine pH?

Although DPH is handled quite differently in the

uremic patient, the clinical importance of this difference is not clear. Uremic patients have a shorter plasma half-life, lower blood levels, and accumulate the principle metabolite, 5-phenyl-5-parahydroxyphenylhydantoin (HPPH) (77). The unbound fraction of DPH is two to four times greater in uremic patients (9), and it is the free or unbound plasma concentration that is responsible for the pharmacologic activity. Although elevated free levels would require a reduction in the dose of DPH, the half-life is also decreased; therefore, the overall change in dose requirements for these patients is not known. It appears that lower serum levels in uremic patients may provide adequate levels of free drug to produce therapeutic effects. Currently, dose reductions are not recommended. Also see chapter on *Clinical Pharmacokinetics.*

Although 62% of the total DPH dose appears in the urine, only 5% is excreted unchanged. Some of the metabolites are lost in the feces after being excreted in the bile. Unchanged DPH and its metabolites are eliminated into the urine by glomerular filtration and tubular secretion (the latter process is the most important of the two). The rate of DPH filtration is limited by its high level of plasma binding (80 to 90%).

Theoretically, alkalinization of the urine should enhance the excretion of unchanged DPH. The higher pH allows more of the drug to exist in the ionized form; consequently, less is reabsorbed by the renal tubules. However, since the fraction of DPH that is eliminated in the urine unchanged is small (5%), alkalinization will have a negligible effect on the total rate of elimination. Complete excretion of a single oral or IV dose of DPH normally takes 72 to 100 hours.

26. A patient taking 500 mg of DPH daily enters the hospital with serum hepatitis. Does the dose need to be altered?

Since DPH is metabolized primarily in the liver, diseases of the liver may theoretically delay its elimination. However, since it is currently impossible to predict to what extent liver disease will affect the metabolic rate, this patient's current dose should be maintained and he should be monitored closely for signs of DPH toxicity (45).

Recent data suggest that the percentage of unbound DPH is increased with liver disease (as in uremia), and that the amount of bound DPH is directly proportional to the serum albumin concentration (8,105).

It should also be noted that DPH can rarely induce hepatitis (35,59,88,103).

27. A 20-year-old woman was seen by her physician because of fever, skin rash, malaise, and tender bilateral neck swelling of a week's duration. Four weeks prior to this presentation, the patient suffered a grand mal seizure. A full neurologic evaluation failed to disclose any localized disorder, and the patient was advised to take phenytoin (DPH) 200 mg twice daily. Suspecting an allergic reaction to the phenytoin, the physician withdrew the medication. The patient's symptoms subsided within the next several days. Discuss the above and other phenytoin-induced allergic reactions.

The above case is typical of DPH-induced lymphadenopathy (which may mimic malignant lymphoma). This *pseudolymphoma* syndrome usually occurs within seven to ten days after administration of the medication and is accompanied by fever, rash, lymphocytosis, and eosinophilia (50a,2a,111a,43a,98a, 25a,64a,115a). Additionally, leukopenia may occur (26a). Cervical lymph nodes are involved most commonly, and hepatosplenomegaly may be present (2a).

There is question as to whether phenytoin may actually induce true lymphoma. In laboratory animals DPH is thought to act as a hapten to interfere with T-cell (post-thymic lymphocyte) mediated immunity, thus stripping the organism of its biologic defense mechanisms against certain tumors (69a).

Other phenytoin-induced hypersensitivity reactions include various dermatoses such as erythema multiforme and Stevens-Johnson syndrome (31,106). Acute systemic lupus erythematosus (SLE) has also been associated with the administration of DPH. This is characterized by positive LE cells and characteristic vascular lesions throughout the body (75,123).

All of these side effects tend to occur within the first year of therapy, although they occasionally appear after several years. Fortunately, these adverse effects are rare and are usually quickly reversible if DPH is discontinued.

28. A young patient taking phenytoin (DPH), phenobarbital (PB), and primidone develops gingival hyperplasia. Which of the drugs caused the condition? Are there any measures the patient can take to minimize this effect?

Gingival hyperplasia occurs in approximately 20% of the patients (particularly children and adolescents) receiving DPH (44,110,144). It is not a dose-related effect and generally occurs within the first year of therapy. Hyperplasia may be related to significant DPH alterations in the connective tissue repair process (117,118). This side effect has not been reported with other hydantoins. Once gum hyperplasia occurs, it can be irreversible even if phenytoin is discontinued. The gums must be surgically resected. Moreover, if the patient continues to take phenytoin after the resection, hyperplasia may recur.

A number of different measures have been advocated for prevention and/or treatment of gum hyperplasia. A positive pressure appliance used after gingival resection appeared to prevent the recurrence of DPH-induced hyperplasia for an extended period (120). Both positive and negative results have been obtained with the use of systemic antihistamine therapy (42,13) and topical steroid application (112,127). Whether good oral hygiene (e.g. brushing gums, water pic, floss) minimizes gum hypertrophy is controversial. Nevertheless, until more conclusive data are available regarding its possible benefits, this method of protection should be routinely advocated for all patients receiving phenytoin. If gingival hyperplasia occurs despite rigorous dental hygiene, then alternative anticonvulsants (e.g. phenobarbital) should be considered.

29. After three years of uncomplicated DPH therapy, a patient developed an increased frequency of seizures, ataxia, nystagmus, slurred speech and EEG changes. After six months of uncomplicated DPH therapy, a second patient developed left hemiparesis, hemianesthesia and increased seizure frequency. These symptoms worsened when the dose of DPH was increased and cleared when DPH was discontinued. Comment on these two cases and discuss the neurological side effects associated with phenytoin.

These two cases exemplify an unusual type of toxicity, *DPH encephalopathy*, characterized by increasing seizures, EEG changes, alteration in mental function and certain motor and sensory disturbances. It is usually associated with toxic doses (but may appear in patients on usual doses) and is generally reversible upon discontinuation of DPH (100,122,68,5).

A number of other neurological problems may be associated with DPH therapy. *Purkinje cell damage* has been observed in rats given supratherapeutic doses (100-200 mg/kg per day) for two weeks. However, subsequent animal studies did not verify these initial findings. Purkinje cell damage has been observed only in patients who have had severe grand mal epilepsy. Hence, present data suggest that DPH does not produce any significant changes in the density and substructure of Purkinje cells unless the doses are so high that coma with prolonged hypoxia develops.

There are a small amount of data which suggest that *peripheral neuropathy* may be induced by DPH when it is given in toxic doses for prolonged periods (several years). One study suggests that this may respond to Vitamin B-12 (37).

DPH-induced permanent *neurological deterioration* (ataxia, impaired speech, bizarre behavior, increased seizure frequency, EEG changes), indistinguishable from a degenerative central nervous system disease was observed in four out of ten patients receiving large doses of DPH for at least ten years (135). All ten patients were previously mentally retarded. This complication does not appear to be a complication of long term ingestion of therapeutic doses.

30. A 48-year-old patient has been treated with diet and tolbutamide for five years for adult-onset diabetes. One year ago, the patient was started on DPH 300 mg each day for a convulsive disorder. The patient has followed her diet and has taken her medications regularly, but now she consistently demonstrates glucosuria. Comment.

It is possible that DPH is responsible for the *hyperglycemia*. It is proposed that DPH has a "membrane-stabilizing" effect on the pancreas that inhibits insulin release and leads to clinical diabetes (38). Clinically, hyperglycemia is probably not a significant problem in patients who are taking chronic, non-toxic doses of DPH. Nevertheless, close monitoring is warranted in those patients who are: (a) receiving high doses of DPH; (b) taking other diabetogenic medications; or (c) diabetic risks. Also, see *Diabetes* chapter.

31. M.B. is a 20-year-old female who has suffered from progressive fatigue, weakness, hirsutism, edema, glucosuria, amenorrhea, and osteoporosis over the past two years. Hypocalcemia and bone biopsy findings characteristic of osteomalacia are also present. The patient has been treated with phenytoin (DPH) for the past six months. What was the rationale for the use of DPH? What additional risks might it present to this patient?

The fatigue, weakness, hirsutism, edema, glucosuria, amenorrhea, and osteoporosis are symptoms compatible with a medical diagnosis of Cushing's syndrome. DPH has been effective in treating adrenal hyperfunction in a small group of patients; however, it only provided temporary improvement. The failure of DPH to maintain a depressed steroid level was attributed to activation of a negative feedback mechanism (i.e. accelerated cortisol clearance, increased ACTH output, and subsequent increased cortisol output by the adrenal cortex).

Additional risks to this patient include *hypocalcemia* and *osteomalacia* which have been associated with the long-term use of anticonvulsant drugs. A greater than 20% reduction in serum calcium has been observed in some patients and is associated with an elevated alkaline phosphatase (41,26,27,100). *Hypomagnesemia* and radiological findings of rickets in children have also been reported (25b).

It is currently postulated that DPH produces hypocalcemia by interfering with vitamin-D metabolism. Normally, vitamin D_3 is hydroxylated in the liver to 25-OH D_3, which is further hydroxylated in the kidneys to 1,25-dihydroxycholecalciferol. Though much less is known about the metabolism of vit-D$_2$, it is assumed that it follows a similar pattern (25b). One proposed mechanism of DPH interference involves induction of liver enzymes operative in the primary hydroxylation of vitamin-D. However, more study is needed to clarify the exact mechanism of phenytoin's interference.

Finally, the *hirsutism* noted in this patient may have been aggravated by DPH. Hirsutism is growth of body hair which occurs in a generalized distribution; it infrequently occurs after 2-3 months of therapy and regresses after discontinuance of the drug. Most reports involve young female patients (81).

32. P.B., a 20-year-old male epileptic who has taken phenytoin (DPH) 300 mg daily for several months, now presents with symptoms of weakness, sore tongue, anorexia, diarrhea, pallor, and a rapid pulse. Laboratory findings include a low hemoglobin and hematocrit, and a blood smear reveals macrocytosis. Could these symptoms be related to the DPH?

The diagnosis in this case was folic acid deficient megaloblastic anemia. DPH causes *folic acid deficiency* in 58% of patients by preventing the conversion of dietary folate (polyglutamate) to the absorbable monoglutamate form. However, few patients ever develop clinical megaloblastic anemia; those who do, respond to treatment with folic acid in the monoglutamate form. As little as 25 mcg each day has produced a satisfactory response (100).

A further complicating factor relates to potential interactions between DPH and folic acid. Replacement of folic acid in folate-deficient patients receiving DPH increases the metabolism of DPH, resulting in decreased DPH serum levels and potential increases in seizure frequency. Apparently by the same mechanism, folate therapy appears to ameliorate symptoms of DPH toxicity. Doses of 10-15 mg abolished typical signs of DPH toxicity such as nystagmus, ataxia and confusion. This group of patients had been difficult to manage in that they had a tendency to alternate between frequent seizures on lower doses of DPH and toxicity when placed on slightly higher doses (100). Additionally, there is evidence to suggest that at least some of the anticonvulsant effect of DPH is due to depletion of folate, the replacement of which may directly reverse some of the anticonvulsant activity of DPH. This effect appears significant only with long term (several months) folic acid therapy (108b).

Prophylactic folic acid therapy given concurrently with DPH is controversial and is not recommended since the actual incidence of anemia secondary to DPH therapy is less than 1% (59a). Also, large doses of folic acid may obscure the diagnosis of pernicious anemia. (See *Anemias* chapter.)

33. M.B. is a 24-year-old epileptic female who has taken phenytoin 300 mg daily since age 14. She has been seizure free for four years and is planning to have a child. Will pregnancy affect her seizure disorder? Are anticonvulsants teratogenic? Should anticonvulsants be discontinued during pregnancy?

The effect of pregnancy on epilepsy is unpredictable. The results of one study indicated that 50% of women with idiopathic epilepsy had no change in the number of seizures during pregnancy; 45.2% had an increase in frequency of seizures; and 4.8% had fewer seizures (66b). A recent study explored the possibility that the effect of previously adequate anticonvulsant drug therapy was reduced (73a). Plasma anticonvulsant levels were monitored during pregnancy in 11 epileptic women taking phenytoin and/ or PB or primidone. On the basis of the plasma level, the phenytoin requirement increased in all ten women taking this drug during pregnancy. The requirement fell again during puerperium. Plasma PB levels decreased during pregnancy in all five women taking a constant daily dose of phenobarbital or primidone. These findings should be considered if epileptics are to be protected against seizures during pregnancy and against anticonvulsant overdosage during the puerperium.

Most data have suggested a small but significant increase in the rate of fetal malformations and complications to gravid epileptics. Also, since the incidence of malformations with epileptics taking medication (mean 6.4%) is greater than the incidence with epileptics not taking medication (mean 3.2%) anticonvulsant medications may be the major teratogenic factor (9a). DPH therapy during the first trimester results in a significant incidence of congenital malformations which is two to three times greater than normal (115). A recent prospective study of 35 infants exposed prenatally to hydantoins showed that 11% had features of the *"fetal hydantoin syndrome"* with serious sequelae, while an additional 31% were affected to a lesser extent (56a). Features of this syndrome include craniofacial abnormalities, limb defects, and deficiencies in growth and development including intelligence (56a). In addition, hypoprothrombinemia and hemorrhage have occurred in the newborns of mothers who received DPH during pregnancy. Vitamin K effectively treats and prevents this disorder (49).

To determine whether phenytoin should be discontinued during pregnancy, one must evaluate the risks versus the benefits of continuing therapy. The patient in question, M.B., has been seizure-free for four years and may therefore do well temporarily without DPH. Furthermore, if one believes the above findings documenting teratogenic problems in up to 42% of the offspring, then the risk to the fetus appears high. Obviously, more data are needed since earlier studies found an overall low risk of anticonvulsant teratogenicities.

Another alternative is to switch to another anticonvulsant such as PB. It is presently unclear whether PB is a teratogen. However, based upon available information one would certainly have to conclude that it is much less hazardous in pregnancy than DPH.

34. DPH (phenytoin) is not an ideal anticonvulsant drug due to its troublesome side effects in certain patients. How do analogs of DPH compare with regard to their relative toxicity and spectrum of anticonvulsant activity?

The answer to this question is limited by the lack of controlled trials. The evaluation of uncontrolled trials is compromised by several factors: (a) combinations of anticonvulsants were administered; (b) drugs were administered for varying periods of time; (c) many different seizure patterns were treated; and (d) the age of patients varied within the trial groups.

Based upon existing studies, *mephenytoin* may be superior to DPH in controlling clonic and tonic seizure patterns, but its use is severely limited by its toxicity. Leukopenia is reported in 23% of the patients taking the drug (1). The incidence of skin rash is 9%, and drowsiness occurs in 16% of the patients (84).

Ethotoin appears to be less toxic than DPH, but also less effective (51). Controlled trials are necessary to establish its purported value in patients who have infrequent grand mal seizures and a hypersensitivity to DPH.

Initial trials indicate that *albutoin* may have a low degree of toxicity and a lower anti-epileptic potency than DPH (100), but gastric distress occurs erratically with its use.

35. Can phenobarbital's (PB) anticonvulsant and toxic effects be correlated with blood levels?

The therapeutic anticonvulsant level of PB in the serum is about 10-25 mcg/ml. In the normal adult without renal or hepatic disease, these levels can be achieved with a daily dose of 1-2.5 mg/kg. Children require doses that are two to three times higher (130) because they eliminate the drug faster than adults. Because it has a long half-life (2-4 days), PB can be given once daily to most patients (100).

Toxic levels of PB are not well defined. Drowsiness occurs in the first weeks of therapy, but wanes even while blood levels rise. Blood levels of 4-6 mg% may be associated with somnolence, nystagmus and unsteadiness, but there are individual variations (2,16,86,104,114,72).

36. An epileptic has developed reduced renal function. Should his dose of phenobarbital be changed?

This question is difficult to answer since the litera-ture concerning this problem is scarce (109). Most researchers feel that the half-life of PB may be increased in a patient with impaired renal function since as much as 30% of this drug may be recovered in the urine unchanged. The rate of accumulation with varying degrees of renal impairment is not known, so one must rely upon repeated blood level determinations and clinical response to accurately assess therapy in these patients.

37. An epileptic is admitted to the emergency room suffering from what appears to be an overdose of phenobarbital (PB). Alkaline osmotic diuresis is suggested as treatment to enhance renal excretion. Is this valid therapy?

This therapy is effective for acute intoxication only. PB is filtered by the glomerulus, and is reabsorbed in the renal tubules. In the unionized form, the molecule can diffuse back across the renal tubular wall. The pKa of PB (a weak acid) is 7.23. When urinary pH is above the pKa, the drug is predominantly in the ionized form and will not be reabsorbed; therefore, alkalinization of the urine is useful for the treatment of acute PB poisoning. This maneuver is not effective for shorter-acting barbiturates.

Reabsorption of PB by the renal tubule is also influenced by the rate of urine flow. Since less is reabsorbed at higher rates of flow, the use of osmotic diuretics is effective. Infusion of 3-4 liters per day of isotonic or hypotonic sodium bicarbonate solution, or a solution containing both urea and sodium lactate, has reduced the duration of coma by as much as one-half to two-thirds when poisoning was due to long and intermediate acting barbituates. The usual dose of sodium bicarbonate necessary to render the urine alkaline is 6-12 gm daily (45,80,136,119). These agents must be used in epileptics with caution since both alkalinization and hydration increase the tendency toward seizure (2,93). (Also see *Poisonings* chapter.)

38. A patient who has been taking warfarin 5 mg each day for six months is now started on phenobarbital (PB) and phenytoin (DPH) for a convulsive disorder. Discuss the potential drug interactions. (Also see Question 9.)

PB and other barbiturates induce hepatic microsomal enzymes and enhance the metabolism of coumarin anticoagulants. Heptobarbital has been reported to interfere with the oral absorption of bishydroxycoumarin; however, alteration of warfarin absorption by barbiturates has not been demonstrated (58).

It has been estimated that the chronic administration of barbiturates will decrease the plasma half-life and the average plasma concentration of coumarins by approximately 50%; however, this is not a reliable clinical figure (67). Frequent measurement of the prothrombin time and appropriate adjustment of the anticoagulant dose are essential when barbiturates are given to patients receiving coumarins. When barbiturates are discontinued, their effects on coumarin metabolism subside slowly. The time course of disappearance has not yet been accurately determined (67).

Whether warfarin and phenytoin interact is unclear. However, a bishydroxycoumarin-phenytoin interaction is documented. Administration of bishydroxycoumarin for one week quadrupled the serum half-life of DPH and markedly raised its serum level. This effect on DPH half-life occurs in a few hours, and in some subjects DPH serum levels remained abnormally elevated one week after the withdrawal of bishydroxycoumarin. Bishydroxycoumarin probably inhibits the enzyme that is responsible for the parahydroxylation of DPH in the liver.

39. When is primidone indicated?

Primidone is effective as an anticonvulsant for the treatment of generalized (grand mal) and psychomotor seizures. Generally, when control is not achieved with the combination of DPH and a long-acting barbiturate such as PB, primidone may be added. It is almost always used in combination with other drugs for the treatment of major motor seizures and is considered one of the drugs of first choice for psychomotor type seizures.

40. What is a therapeutic and toxic blood level of primidone?

The therapeutic blood level of primidone appears to be over 0.5 mg% (5 mg/L). Side effects are thought to be dose-related, and may occur with levels over 1.5 mg%. (See Question 42.) However, more blood level data on primidone are needed to confirm these figures.

Due to primidone's relatively short plasma half-life (see Table 3), blood levels tend to fluctuate and are influenced by the time interval between the last dose and the time when the blood sample is drawn. Therefore, to insure that the sample is drawn at a time when the blood level is at its lowest, it should be taken just prior to the next scheduled dose after steady state has been reached.

41. Discuss primidone's side effects.

Dose-dependent side effects include sedation, dizziness, nausea, vomiting, ataxia and diplopia. These effects are seen quite frequently and can be minimized by starting therapy with small (250 mg/day) and divided doses, and then gradually building to therapeutic levels. Other reported side effects include personality changes and folic acid deficiency (3,100).

42. A patient taking relatively high doses of phenytoin (DPH) and phenobarbital (PB) continues to have occasional seizures. Primidone is suggested as a third drug to be added to the regimen, but objection is raised because "primidone is metabolized to PB and therefore will be of no added benefit to this patient." Is this a valid objection? Discuss the potential interactions which may occur.

Primidone is converted to two major metabolites: PEMA (phenyl-ethyl malonamide) and PB. PB usually appears in the serum of patients taking only primidone 24 to 96 hours after initiation of therapy. The prevailing opinion (which is based upon incomplete clinical evidence) is that unmetabolized primidone and its major metabolites are all active anticonvulsants. On an anecdotal basis, many neurologists are familiar with subjects who had been uncontrolled with standard anticonvulsant regimens (including PB) and who responded well to the addition of primidone (100). A patient who is allergic to PB will also be allergic to primidone.

The ratio of phenobarbital to primidone in most patients taking primidone alone is one, but this may vary. A recent report suggests that this ratio may be as high as four in patients who are also taking DPH. Apparently, DPH induces enzymes responsible for the oxidation of primidone. In this same report, patients who were taking all three drugs (PB, primidone, and DPH) exhibited average PB levels in excess of 5 mg% even though the phenobarbital doses were, in some instances, less than 1 mg/kg (40).

43. S.R. is a 16-year-old epileptic who experienced his first major motor seizure at age ten. Phenytoin (DPH), phenobarbital (PB), and primidone have been administered in various combinations since that time. Although DPH has reduced the frequency of seizures, both PB and primidone were ineffective and the seizure disorder remains poorly controlled. Is carbamazepine a reasonable alternative for this patient? What are the potential hazards of this medication?

Carbamazepine is as effective in reducing seizures as is phenytoin or PB (24,132,134). In one double-blind crossover study of hospitalized patients with severe seizures, carbamazepine and phenytoin were equally effective in controlling frequency of seizures (24). In another trial of 37 patients resistant to standard agents, carbamazepine reduced the frequency of grand mal seizures by 55% and psychomotor seizures by 83% (111). The drug appears ineffective for petit mal epilepsy. Therefore, it is a reasonable alternative for this patient.

Up to 70% of patients experience symptomatic side effects such as vertigo, ataxia, drowsiness, stomatitis, nausea, and dry mouth which generally subside in two to seven days (108a,24,111,132,134). Paresthesias in the area of the trigeminal nerve are also not uncommon (108a). These effects are dose related. For example, in one study a dose of 600 mg daily produced vertigo in 43% of patients while 400 mg daily produced this effect in only 18% of patients (65a).

Adverse effects are minimized by starting with small divided doses, and gradually increasing to maintenance levels over a week or more. To minimize side effects, it has been recommended that an initial dose of 200 mg daily be followed by daily increments of no more than 100 mg (65a). A maintenance dose of 17 mg/kg/day in two daily doses is usually adequate. Doses above 1200 mg daily are generally not recommended.

There exists some uncertainty regarding the extent of carbamazepine's potential for agranulocytosis. However, ten reports of fatal aplastic anemia have been associated with the use of this agent, as well as several cases of thrombocytopenia (111). The onset of these complications has occurred from three weeks to two years after initiation of therapy.

Other possible effects for which there is little documentation include: cholestatic jaundice (83), reversible renal failure (83), aggravation of coronary artery disease (6), lenticular opacities (83), hypersensitivity pulmonary reactions (28a), lupus (83), exfoliative dermatitis (83), Stevens-Johnson syndrome (83) and an anti-diuretic action (137).

There are no reports of death secondary to carbamazepine overdose (82). Severe CNS depression requiring only supportive treatment has been observed. Several days may pass before the patient regains consciousness, but no residual effects have been reported. On the basis of its structural similarity to the tricyclic antidepressants, one might consider monitoring the ECG to detect possible cardiac effects.

44. An 8-year-old child presents to his physician with a history of "black-out spells". During the past several weeks the patient has been observed to temporarily "lose consciousness." Although he does not fall during the episodes, the patient is motionless and does not speak or respond to commands from others. The patient recalls these episodes only as "blank places" in his normal stream of consciousness.

A diagnosis of petit mal epilepsy is made and ethosuximide is prescribed. What dose of ethosuximide (Zarontin) will produce a therapeutic blood level? How should the drug be dosed?

The half-life of *ethosuximide* ranges from 24-60 hours, so once-a-day dosing is usually sufficient (14b). Maximum clinical control is achieved when the plasma level ranges from 40-100 mcg/ml, although there is considerable individual variation (14b). The initial dose of 20 mg/kg daily will produce a plasma level of 60 mcg/ml (100).

45. What are the toxicities and side effects of ethosuximide?

Ethosuximide, considered the drug of choice for petit mal seizures, is a relatively safe anticonvulsant. Gastric disturbances including nausea, vomiting, and anorexia are the most frequent complications and occur in approximately 30% of patients (14a). Central nervous system (CNS) symptoms, including fatigue, lethargy, headache, dizziness, hiccups, and euphoria, occur in 15-20% of patients. The gastrointestinal and CNS symptoms are dose related and are usually transient (14a). Goldensohn described patients who developed parkinsonian symptoms and photophobia in association with ethosuximide therapy (48). An acute dystonic reaction responsive to diphenhydramine has also been reported (66a).

Allergic reactions are rare and usually occur within the first year or two after therapy is started. These include non-specific skin rashes, urticaria and a single case of Stevens-Johnson syndrome (97). A few cases of systemic lupus erythematosus associated with ethosuximide have been reported (28). Hematopoietic reactions, including leukopenia and pancytopenia, are also observed rarely (14a,42). About 10% of the patients develop eosinophilia (111).

46. The patient in Question 44 has been given an adequate therapeutic trial of ethosuximide without clinical response. This drug is discontinued and clonazepam is now prescribed. In general, how effective is clonazepam as an anticonvulsant?

Initial data indicate that IV *clonazepam* is extremely effective in treating status epilepticus in doses of 1-8 mg (7,46,65). It has been effective even in rare cases that were resistant to IV diazepam (up to 30 mg) and/or phenobarbital (46). When and if the IV preparation is commercially available, it may replace IV diazepam as the drug of choice for status epilepticus.

Studies of clonazepam effectiveness have involved patients with a variety of long standing seizure disorders poorly controlled by available anticonvulsants. In a United States (US) Collaborative Study involving 300 patients in 14 different US centers, clonazepam was effective in all types of seizures (65). The best results have been noted in petit mal and petit mal variant type seizures and in minor motor seizures (myoclonic and akinetic). Less dramatic but encouraging results have been noted in patients with partial complex (psychomotor) epilepsy. Several studies, including the US Collaborative Study, have shown clonazepam to be effective in a significant percentage of patients with infantile spasms, a disorder for which present treatment is generally considered unsatisfactory (32,65).

However, several other investigators report poor results (57,87b).

Although clonazepam may benefit some patients with generalized tonic-clonic seizures (grand mal), the drug increases seizure frequency in others (6a,87a,97a). Therefore, it is not generally indicated in the treatment of grand mal.

Tolerance develops to the anticonvulsant effects of clonazepam in about 33% of patients (14,39,57,87b) after one to six months of administration (14).

47. Two days later the patient's mother calls the physician complaining that her child has been extremely drowsy since taking the clonazepam. Is this a transient effect and can it be minimized? What are other side effects of clonazepam?,

The adverse effects associated with clonazepam are primarily related to the central nervous system. *Drowsiness* and *ataxia* are by far the most commonly occurring adverse effects. Drowsiness is reported to occur in 50% of the patients and ataxia in 30%. These effects are most prominent during initiation of therapy and are often transient, dissipating over a period of several weeks. To minimize these effects, it is important to start with low doses and increase at three-day intervals to maintenance dosage levels over a period of three to four weeks. Divided daily doses (three times daily) also minimize these initial effects (14a).

Behavioral changes such as euphoria, confusion, hyperkinesis and aggressive behavior have been reported in as many as 25% of clonazepam treated patients, and appear to most commonly affect patients with a history of psychiatric disturbances (7,62,52). Increased frequency of grand mal seizures is reported in 7% of the seizure population (6a,87a,97a). Many of these patients can be controlled by adding or adjusting the dose of other anticonvulsants. Increased saliva production has been reported in 5% of the patients, and may cause respiratory distress symptoms in some infants (65).

48. If this patient later becomes tolerant to the sedative effects of clonazepam, can the drug then be given in one daily dose?

Like other benzodiazepines, the drug has a relatively long serum half-life (20 to 35 hours) (65a,34,97b). However, one study reports an effective duration of action of only six to eight hours requiring administration three times daily (39). It is unclear whether this study was performed at steady state. Nevertheless, present data suggest that optimum therapy requires divided daily therapy.

	Initial Dose	Maintenance Dose
INFANTS & CHILDREN	0.01 - 0.05 mg/kg/day	0.1 - 0.2 mg/kg/day
ADULTS	1 - 1.5 mg/day	5 - 10 mg/day (Maximum recommended dose is 20 mg/day.)

CASE HISTORY FOR STUDY

1. At age 3, Mary develops an upper respiratory infection. Following a seizure, she is taken by her mother to the local emergency department where her temperature is found to be 104°F. During the examination Mary had a second, generalized tonic-clonic seizure. Discuss the treatment of status epilepticus in this 3-year-old, 40 pound child.

2. Six months later, Mary again spikes a temperature and has a seizure. Should Mary be given prophylactic anticonvulsants? If so, which drug is indicated and how long should treatment be continued?

3. At age 15 Mary begins to experience intermittent "dizzy spells" with feelings of deja vu; however, she fails to bring this to the attention of her physician. At age 16 Mary has a major motor seizure while sitting in the school library. What immediate action, if any, should be taken?

4. Mary visits her physician and a complete workup results in a diagnosis of epilepsy with both psychomotor and major motor involvement. The decision is made to administer anticonvulsants. Which drug(s) is indicated? What dose would you recommend?

5. Mary is given phenytoin suspension 100 mg qid with no loading dose. If she is well controlled and has no more seizures over the next several years, should anticonvulsant therapy be discontinued? If so, how should one taper the dose? If Mary continues to take phenytoin, should chronic folic acid, calcium, and vitamin D be administered? What are the long-term neurological complications of phenytoin therapy?

6. Two days after starting phenytoin suspension, Mary has a second seizure and revisits her physician. Should the drug or the dosage be changed? Would blood levels be useful at this point?

7. Mary is taken off of phenytoin. Primidone plus phenobarbital are substituted. How should these drugs be initiated?

8. The patient appears to respond and after two months has had no major motor seizures and only occasional psychomotor seizures. Both primidone and phenobarbital blood level determinations are taken at this time. A month later Mary has another grand mal seizure followed in two days by another. The physician now adds phenytoin capsules to the regimen of primidone and phenobarbital. A loading dose of 800 mg phenytoin orally over 6 hours fol-

lowed by 200 mg bid is prescribed. Would further blood level determinations be useful at this time? Would primidone and phenobarbital levels now be the same as they were a month earlier?

9. Mary returns to the physician in three months with several complaints. She has developed hypertrichosis, a very bad case of acne, arthralgias in numerous areas of the body, fever, and lymphadenopathy. The patient is very depressed. Assess these complaints. Could they be related to her medication?

10. Phenytoin is discontinued and carbamazepine 1200 mg daily is added to the regimen. Mary experiences marked sedation and confusion after initial doses of carbamazepine. Later that evening she is found comatose in her bedroom. Empty medication bottles are scattered about. How should this apparent overdose involving PB, primidone, phenytoin, and carbamazepine be treated?

11. The patient recovers and is now given carbamazepine alone in gradually increasing doses with good results. Years later, Mary is married and is now considering having children. She has had no seizures for five years. Discuss the teratogenicity of anticonvulsants.

REFERENCES

1. Abbott JA et al: Mesantoin in the treatment of epilepsy; a study of its effects on the leukocyte count in seventy-nine cases. NEJM 250:197, 1954.
2. Adams DR: The convulsive state and idiopathic epilepsy. In *Harrison's Principles of Internal Medicine*. Bennett IL Jr et al editors. 8th edition. McGraw Hill, New York, 1977; p 127-135.
2a. Bajoghli M: Generalized lymphadenopathy and hepatosplenomegaly induced by diphenylhydantoin. Pediat 28:943, 1961.
3. Baker H et al: Lesions in folic acid metabolism induced by primidone. Experientia 18:224, 1962.
4. Barnett HL et al: Nephrotic syndrome occurring during Tridione therapy. Am J Med 4:760, 1948.
4a. Baylis EM et al: Influence of folic acid on blood-phenytoin levels. Lancet 1:62, 1971.
5. Bazemore RP et al: On the problem of diphenylhydantoin-induced seizures. Arch Neurol 31:243, 1974.
6. Beermann B et al: Advanced heart block aggravated by carbamazepine. Brit. Heart J 37:668, 1975.
6a. Birket-Smith E et al: Preliminary observation on the effect of a new benzodiazepine (R05-4023) in epilepsy. Acta Neurol Scand 48:385, 1972.
7. Bladin PF: The use of clonazepam as anticonvulsant — clincial evaluation. Med J Aust 1:685, 1973.
8. Blaschke TF et al: Influence of acute viral hepatitis on phenytoin kinetics and protein binding. Clin Pharmacol Ther 17:685, 1975.
9. Blum MR et al: Altered protein binding of diphenylhydantoin in uremic plasma (letter). NEJM 286:109, 1972.
9a. Bodendorfer T: Fetal effects of anticonvulsants drugs and seizure disorders. PRN 10:5, 1976, Memorial Hos Med Cntr Long Beach, Calif.
10. Booker HE et al: Myasthenia gravis syndrome associated with trimethadione. JAMA 212:2262, 1970.
11. Borofsky LG: Diphenylhydantoin in children. Neurol 23:967, 1973.
12. Brachet-Liermoin et al: Absorption of phenobarbital after the intramuscular administration of single doses in infants. J of Pediat 87:624, 1975.
13. Breg WR et al: Ineffectiveness of antihistamine therapy for gingival hyperplasia due to diphenylhydantoin sodium. NEJM 257:1128, 1957.
14. Browne TR: Clonazepam: a review of a new anticonvulsant drug. Arch Neurol 33:326, 1976.
14a. Browne TR et al: Ethosuximide in the treatment of abscence (petit mal) seizures. Neurol 25:515, 1975.
14b. Buchanan RA et al: Ethosuximide dosing regimens, Clin Pharmacol Therap 19:143, 1976.
15. Buchanan R et al: The metabolism of diphenylhydantoin (Dilantin) following once daily administration. Neurol 22:126, 1972.
16. Buchthal F et al: Aspects of the pharmacology of phenytoin (Dilantin) and phenobarbital to their dosage in the treatment of epilepsy. Epilepsia 1:373, 1959.
17. Buchthal F et al: Accumulation of phenobarbital in man. Epilepsia 4:199, 1963.
18. Burrill K et al: Effect of diphenylhydantoin on insulin secretion in man. NEJM 286:339, 1972.
19. Butler TC et al: Phenobarbital: studies of elimination, accumulation, tolerance and dosage schedules. J Pharmacol Exp Ther 111:425, 1954.
20. Butler TC et al: Metabolic conversion of primidone (Mysoline) to phenobarbital. Proc Soc Exp Biol Med 93:544, 1956.
21. Cantu RC et al: Comparison of blood levels with oral and intramuscular diphenylhydantoin. Neurol 18:782, 1968.
22. Carter S: Diagnosis and treatment; management of the child who has had one convulsion. Pediat 33:431, 1964.
23. Cereghino JJ et al: The efficacy of carbamazepine combinations in epilepsy. Clin Pharmacol Ther 18:733, 1975.
24. Cereghino JJ et al: Carbamazepine for epilepsy. Neurol 24:401, 1974.
25. Chao DHC et al: Diamox in epilepsy. J Pediat 58:211, 1961.
25a. Choovivathanavanich P et al: Psudolymphoma induced by diphenylhydantoin. J Pediat 76:621, 1970.
26b. Christiansen C et al: Actions of Vitamins D_2 and D_3 and 25- OHD_3 in Anticonvulsant Osteomalacia. Brit Med J 2:363, 1975.
26. Christy NO et al: Effects of diphenylhydantoin upon adrenal cortical function in man. Neurol 9:245, 1959.
26a. Cohen BL et al: Leukopenia and an unusual component of diphenylhydantoin hypersensitivity. Clin Ped 12:622, 1973.
27. Costa PJ et al: Effects of diphenylhydantoin (Dilantin) on adrenal cortical function. Arch Neurol Psych 74:88, 1955.
28. Cucinell SA et al: Drug interactions in man. 1. Lowering effect of phenobarbital on plasma levels of bishydroxycoumarin (Dicumarol) and diphenylhydantoin (Dilantin). Clin Pharmacol Ther 6:420, 1965.
28a. Cullinan SA et al: Acute pulmonary hypersensitivity to carbamazepine. Chest 68:580, 1975.
29. Dabbous IA et al: Occurrence of systemic lupus erythematosus in association with ethosuximide therapy. J Pediat 76:617, 1970.
29a. Davis JP et al: Effect of Trimethyloxazolidinedione and dimethyloxazolidinedione on seizures and on blood. Res Publ Assoc Res Nerv Ment Dis 26:423, 1947.
30. Dawson KP et al: Value of blood phenytoin estimation in management of childhood epilepsy. Arch Dis Child 46:386, 1971.
31. deHass AML et al: Experiences with x-ethyl-x-methylsuccinimide in the treatment of epilepsy. Epilepsia 1:501, 1959/60.
32. Demermuth G et al: The effect of clonazepam (R05-4023) in the syndrome of infantile spasms with hypsarhythmia and in petit mal variant or Lennox syndrome — preliminary report. Acta Neurol Scand (Suppl) 26, 1973.
33. Denhoff E et al: Clinical studies of the effects of 3,5,5-trimethyloxazolidine-2-4-dione (tridione) on the hematopoietic system, liver and kidney. Pediat 5:695, 1950.
33a. Dent CE: Osteomalacia with Long-term Anticonvulsant Therapy in Epilepsy, Brit Med J 4:69, 1970.
34. Dreifuss F et al: Serum clonazepam concentrations in children with absence seizures. Neurol 25:255, 1975.
35. Duma RJ et al: Hypersensitivity to diphenylhydantoin (Dilantin): a case report with toxic hepatitis. South Med J 59:168, 1966.
36. Eden AN et al: Clinical comparison of three antipyretic agents. Am J Dis Child 114:284, 1967.
37. Eisen AA et al: Peripheral nerve function in long-term therapy with diphenylhydantoin. Neurol 24:411, 1974.
38. Fariss BL et al: Diphenylhydantoin-induced hyperglycemia and impaired insulin release. Diabetes 20:177, 1971.
39. Fazio C et al: Treatment of epileptic seizures with clonazepam: a reappraisal. Arch Neurol 32:304, 1975.
40. Finchman RW: The influence of diphenylhydantoin on primi-

done metabolism. Arch Neurol 30:259, 1974.

41.   Frame B: Hypocalcemia and osteomalacia associated with anticonvulsant therapy. Ann Int Med 74:294, 1971.

42.   Gaillard RA: Antihistaminic therapy for gingival hyperplasia due to Dilantin. NEJM 256:76, 1957.

43.   Gallagher BB et al: The relationship of the anticonvulsant properties of primidone to phenobarbital. Epilepsia 11:293, 1970.

43a.   Gams RA et al: Hydantoin induced pseudolymphoma. Ann Int Med 69:557, 1968.

44.   Gardner A et al: An investigation of gingival hyperplasia resulting from Dilantin therapy in 77 mentally retarded patients. Exp Med Surg 20:133, 1962.

45.   Garrettson LK: Pharmacology of anticonvulsants. Ped Clin N Amer 19:179, 1972.

46.   Gastant H et al: Treatment of status epilepticus with a new benzodiazepine more active than diazepam. Epilepsia 12:197, 1971.

47.   Gastant H et al: Clinical and electroencephalographical classification of epileptic seizures. Epilepsia 11:102, 1970.

47a.   German J et al: Trimethadione and human teratogenesis. Teratology, 3:349, 1970.

48.   Goldensohn ES et al: Ethosuximide in the treatment of epilepsy. JAMA 180:840, 1962.

49.   Woodbury DM et al: Drugs effective in the therapy of epilepsies. In The Pharmacological Basis of Therapeutics, 5th Ed., edited by LS Goodman and A Gilman. Macmillan Co., New York, 1975, p 204-209.

50.   Greenberg LM et al: Erythema multiforme exudativum (Stevens-Johnson syndrome) following sodium diphenylhydantoin therapy. Ann Ophthal 3:137, 1971.

50a.   Greene DA: Localized cervical lymphadenopathy induced by diphenylhydantoin sodium. Arch Otolaryngol 101:446, 1975.

51.   Gruber CM Jr et al: Comparison of the effectiveness of phenobarbital, primidone, diphenylhydantoin, ethotoin, methabital and methyl phenylethylhydantoin in motor seizures. J Clin Pharmacol Exp Ther 3:23, 1962.

52.   Guldenpfennig W: Clinical experience with a new benzodiazepine in the treatment of epilepsy. S Afr Med J 47:998, 1973.

53.   Gutnick MJ et al: Penicillinase and the convulsant action of penicillin. Neurol 21:759, 1971.

54.   Hammill JF et al: Febrile convulsions. NEJM 274:563, 1966.

55.   Hahnemann F: Epileptic under attack; how to defend a helpless patient. Emer Med 2:17, 1970.

56.   Hansen JM: Carbamazepine-induced acceleration of diphenylhydantoin and warfarin metabolism. Clin Pharmacol Ther 12:539, 1971.

56a.   Hanson JW, et al: Risks to the offspring of women treated with hydantoin anticonvulsants, with emphasis on the fetal hydantoin syndrome, J Pediat: 88:662, 1976.

57.   Hanson RA et al: A new anticonvulsant in the management of minor motor seizures. Dev Med Child Neurol 14:3, 1972.

58.   Hansten PD: Drug Interactions, 3rd edition. Lea and Febiger, Philadelphia, 1976, pp 36-37, 202. pp 28-29, 139.

59.   Harinasuta U et al: Diphenylhydantoin sodium hepatitis. JAMA 203:1015, 1968.

59a.   Hawkins CF et al: Macrocytosis and megaloblastic anaemia caused by anticonvulsant drugs. Q J Med 27:45, 1958.

60.   Heathfield KWG et al: Treatment of petit mal with ethosuximide. Br Med J 2:565, 1961.

61.   Holowach J et al: Prognosis in childhood epilepsy. NEJM 286:169, 1972.

62.   Hooshmand H: Toxic effects of anticonvulsants: general principles. Pediat 53:551, 1974.

63.   Huisman JW: The estimation of some important anticonvulsant drugs in serum. Clin Cham Acta 13:323, 1966.

64.   Hutt SJ et al: Perceptual-motor behavior in relation to blood phenobarbitone level — a preliminary report. Develop Med Child Neurol 10:626, 1968.

64a.   Hyman GA et al: The development of Hodgkin's disease and lymphoma during anticonvulsant therapy. Blood 28:416, 1966.

64b.   Jensen ON et al: Subnormal serum folate due to anticonvulsive therapy. A double-blind study of the effect of folic acid treatment in patients with drug-induced subnormal serum folates. Arch Neurol 22:181, 1970.

65.   Joseph C et al: An evaluation of the efficacy and safety of clonazepam in the treatment of infractable seizures. Results of a collaborative study, Department of Medical Research, Hoffman-La Roche, Inc. Data on file.

65a.   Kaplan SA et al: Pharmacokinetic profiles of clonazepam in dog and humans and of flunitrazepam in dog. J Pharm Sci 63:527, 1974.

65b.   Killian JM et al: Carbamazepine in the treatment of Neuralgia: Uses and side effects. Arch Neurol 19:129, 1968.

66.   Kiorboe E et al: Zarontin (ethosuximide) in the treatment of petit mal and related disorders. Epilepsia 5:83, 1964.

66a.   Kirschberg GJ: Dyskinesia — an unusual reaction to ethosuximide. Arch Neurol 32:137, 1975.

66b.   Knight AH et al: Epilepsy and pregnancy: A study of 153 pregnancies in 59 patients, Epilepsia 16:99-110, 1975.

67.   Koch-Weser J et al: Drug interactions with coumarin anticoagulants. NEJM 285:547, 1971.

68.   Koolker JC, Sumi SM: Movement disorder as a manifestation of diphenylhydantoin intoxication. Neurol 24:68, 1974.

69.   Koutsoulieris E: Granulopenia and thrombocytopenia after ethosuximide. Lancet 3:310, 1967.

69a.   Kruger GR et al: Is phenytoin carcinogenic? (Letter) Lancet 1:372, 1972.

70.   Kutt H et al: Diphenylhydantoin metabolism, blood levels and toxicity. Arch Neurol 11:642, 1964.

71.   Kutt H et al: Diphenylhydantoin and phenobarbital toxicity — the role of liver disease. Arch Neurol 11:649, 1964.

72.   Kutt H et al: Usefulness of blood levels of antiepileptic drugs. Arch Neurol 31:283, 1974.

73a.   Lander CM et al: Plasma anticonvulsant concentrations during pregnancy. Neurol 27:128, 1977.

74.   Lascelles PT et al: The distribution of plasma phenytoin levels in epileptic patients. J Neurol Neurosurg Psychiat 33:501, 1970.

75.   Lee SL et al: Activation of systemic lupus erythematosus by drugs. Arch Int Med 117:620, 1964.

76.   Lennox W et al: Epilepsy and Related Disorders. Little Brown and Co., Boston, 1960.

77.   Letteri JM et al: Diphenylhydantoin metabolism in uremia. NEJM 285:648, 1971.

78.   Levy LL et al: Diphenylhydantoin activated seizures. Neurol 15:716, 1965.

79.   Levy RH et al: Pharmacokinetics of carbamazepine in normal man. Clin Pharmacol Ther 17:657, 1975.

80.   Linton L et al: Methods of forced diuresis and its application in barbiturate poisoning. Lancet 2:377, 1967.

81.   Livington S et al: Hypertrichosis occurring in association with dilantin therapy. J Pediat 47:351, 1955.

82.   Livington S: Carbamazepine overdosage. JAMA 233:1259, 1975.

83.   Livingston et al: Carbamazepine (Tegretol) in epilepsy. Nine-year, follow-up study, with special emphasis on untoward reactions. Dis Nerv Syst 35:103, 1974.

83a.   Livingston S: Comprehensive Management of Eiplepsy in Infants, Childhood, and Adolescence, Charles C Thomas, Springfield, Ill, 1972, p 167.

83b.   Livingston S: Drug treatment of convulsive disorders, NEJM 286:464, 1972.

84.   Loscalzo AE: Mesantoin in the control of epilepsy. Neurol 2:403, 1952.

85.   Louis S et al: The cardiocirculatory changes caused by intravenous Dilantin and its solvent. Am Heart J 74:523, 1967.

86.   Lous P: Blood serum and cerebrospinal fluid levels and renal clearance of Phenemol treated epileptics. Acta Pharmacol 10:166, 1954.

87.   Lous P: Plasma levels and urinary excretion of three barbituric acids after oral administration to man. Acta Pharmacol Toxicol 10:147, 1954.

87a.   Lund M et al: Clonazepam in the treatment of epilepsy. Acta Neurol Scand (Suppl) 82, 1973.

87b.   Martin D et al: Clinical experience with clonazepam (Rivotril) in the treatment of epileptics in infancy and childhood. Neuropediatriae 4:245, 1973.

88.   McGee FE et al: Diphenylhydantoin (Dilantin) hypersensitivity. South Med J 63:885, 1970.

89.   Meloff K: Seizures and fever. Pediat Neurol 50:107, 1971.

90.   Merlis JK: Proposal for an international classification of the epilepsies. Epilepsia 11:114, 1970.

91.   Mikkelsen B et al: Clonazepam in the treatment of epilepsy. Arch Neurol 33:322, 1976.

92. Miller LJ et al: Febrile convulsions in families, findings in an epidemiologic survey. Clin Pediat 5:604, 1966.

93. Millichap JG: Anticonvulsant action of Diamox in children. Neurol 6:552, 1956.

94. Millichap JG: *Febrile Convulsions.* Macmillan, New York 1968, p 86,135.

95. Millichap JG: Drug treatment of convulsive disorders. NEJM 286:464, 1972.

96. Monnet P et al: Systemic erythematosus lupus caused by ethosuximide in a 6-year-old girl. Lyon Med 220:467, 1968.

97. Muller K: Erythema exsudativum multiforme majus (Stevens-Johnson Syndrome) in folge Suxinutin-Uberempfindlichkeit. Z. Kinderheilkd 88:548, 1963.

97a. Muthe-Kaas AW et al: Clonazepam in the treatment of epileptic seizures. Acta Neurol Scand (Supp) 97, 1973.

97b. Naestoft J et al: Assay and pharmacokinetics of clonazepam in humans. Acta Neurol Scand, Suppl 53, 49:103, 1973.

97c. Nichols MM: Fetal anomalies following maternal trimethadione ingestion. J Pediat 82:885, 1973.

98. Niedermeyer E et al: Classical hysteria seizures facilitated by anticonvulsant toxicity. Psychiat Clin 3:71, 1970.

98a. Oates RK et al: Phenytoin and the pseudolymphoma syndrome. Med J Aust, 2:371, 1971.

99. O'Malley WE et al: Oral absorption of diphenylhydantoin as measured by GLC. Trans Am Neurol Assoc 94:318, 1969.

100. Penry JK et al: *Antiepileptic Drugs.* Raven Press, New York, 1972, pp 116-122, 219-224.

100a. Perrier D, et al: Maintenance of therapeutic phenytoin plasma levels via intramuscular administration. Ann Int Med 85:318, 1976.

101. Peterman MG: Febrile convulsions. J Pediat 41:536, 1952.

102. Peterson H: Association of trimethadione therapy and myasthenia gravis. NEJM 274:506, 1966.

103. Pezzimenti J et al: Anicteric hepatitis induced by diphenylhydantoin. Arch Int Med 125:118, 1970.

104. Plaa GL et al: Hydantoin and barbiturate blood levels observed in epileptics. Arch Int Pharmacodyn 128:375, 1960.

105. Porter RJ et al: Plasma albumin concentration and diphenylhydantoin binding in man. Arch Neurol 32:298, 1975.

106. Rallison ML et al: Lupus erythematosus and Stevens-Johnson syndrome; occurrence as a reaction to anticonvulsant medication. Am J Dis Child 101:725, 1961.

107. Ramsey ID: Carbamazepine-induced jaundice. Brit Med J 4:155, 1967.

108. Raun-Jonsen A et al: Excretion of phenobarbitone in urine after intake of large doses. Acta Pharmacol 27:193, 1969.

108a. Redpath TH et al: The side effects of carbamazepine therapy. Oral Surg 26:299, 1968.

108b. Reynolds EH: Anticonvulsants, folic acid, and epilepsy. Lancet 1:1376, 1973.

109. Ricket G et al: Drug intoxication and neurological episodes in chronic renal failure. Brit Med J 1:394, 1970.

110. Robinson L: The gingival changes produced by Dilantin sodium. Dis Nerv Syst 3:88, 1942.

111. Rodin EA et al: The effects of carbamazepine on patients with psychomotor epilepsy: results of a double-blind study. Epilepsia 15:547, 1974.

111a. Rosenfeld S et al: Syndrome simulating lymphosarcoma induced by diphenylhydantoin sodium, JAMA, 176:491, 1961.

112. Sackler AM et al: Hydrocortisone acetate in the treatment of Dilantin gingival enlargement. NYS Dent J 20:125, 1954.

113. Salcman M et al: Acute carbamazepine encephalopathy. JAMA 231:915, 1975.

114. Sataniemi E et al: The clinical significance of microsomal enzyme induction in the therapy of epileptic patients. Ann Clin Res 2:22.

115. Schneider S: Side effects of diphenylhydantoin in childhood. West J Med 120:403, 1974.

115a. Schreiber MM et al: Pseudolymphoma Syndrome. Arch Derm 97:297, 1968.

116. Serrano EE et al: Plasma diphenylhydantoin values after oral and intramuscular administration of diphenylhydantoin. Neurol 23:311, 1973.

117. Shafter W et al: Effects of Dilantin sodium on the tensile strength of healing wounds. Proc Soc Exp Biol Med 98:348, 1958.

118. Shapiro M: Acceleration of gingival wound healing in non-epileptic patients receiving diphenylhydantoin sodium. Exp Med Surg 16:41, 1958.

119. Sharpless SK: Hypnotics and sedatives in *The Pharmacological Basis of Therapeutics,* 4th ed., edited by LS Goodman and A Gilman, MacMillan Co., New York, 1970, p 110.

120. Sheridan PJ et al: Effective treatment of Dilantin gingival hyperplasia. Oral Surg 35:42, 1973.

121. Sherwin AL: Improved control of epilepsy by monitoring plasma ethosuximide. Arch Neurol 28:178, 1973.

122. Shuttleworth E et al: Choreo-athetosis and diphenylhydantoin intoxication. JAMA 230:1170, 1974.

123. Siegal S et al: Diphenylhydantoin (Dilantin) hypersensitivity with infectious mononucleosis-like syndrome and jaundice. J Aller 32:447, 1961.

124. Simpson JR: Collagen disease due to carbamazepine (Tegretol). Brit Med J 2:1434, 1966.

125. Sloan LL et al: Visual effects of Tridione. Am J Ophthal 30:1387, 1947.

126. Sparberg M: Diagnostically confusing complications of diphenylhydantoin therapy. Ann Int Med 59:914, 1963.

127. Spira A: Some tissue reactions associated with 5, 5-diphenylhydantoin (Dilantin) sodium therapy. Brit Dent J 95:289, 1953.

127a. Stamp TCB: Plasma levels and therapeutic effect of 25-hydroxycholecalciferol in epileptic patients taking anticonvulsant drugs, Brit Med J 4:9, 1972.

128. Suzuki T et al: Kinetics of diphenylhydantoin disposition in man. Chem Pharm Bull 18:405, 1970.

129. Svensmark D et al: 5, 5-diphenylhydantoin (Dilantin) blood levels after oral and intravenous dosage in man. Acta Pharmacol 16:331, 1960.

130. Svensmark D et al: Diphenylhydantoin and phenobarbital. Serum levels in children. Am J Dis Child 108:82, 1964.

131. Anon: Drugs for epilepsy, The Medical Letter 18:25, 1976.

132. Anon: Carbamazepine in the management of seizure disorders, The Medical Letter 17:76, 1975.

133. Triedman HM et al: Determination of plasma and cerebrospinal fluid levels of Dilantin in the human. Trans Am Neurol Assoc 85:160, 1960.

134. Troupin AS et al: Carbamazepine as an anticonvulsant: a pilot study. Neurol 24:863, 1974.

135. Vallarta JM et al: Progressive encephalopathy due to chronic hydantoin toxicity. Am J Dis Child 128:27, 1974.

136. Waddell WJ et al: The distribution and excretion of phenobarbital. J Clin Invest 36:1217, 1957.

137. Wales JK: Treatment of diabetes insipidus with carbamazepine. Lancet 948, 1975.

138. Wallis W et al: Intravenous diphenylhydantoin in treatment of actue repetitive seizures. Neurol 18:513, 1968.

139. Werk EE et al: Effect of diphenylhydantoin on adrenal cortisol metabolism in man. J Clin Invest 43:1824, 1964.

139a. Wilder BJ et al: Oral and intramuscular phenytoin, Clin Pharmacol Therap, 19:360, 1976. 16:507, 1974.

139b. Wilder BJ et al: Oral and Intramuscular phenytoin, Clin Pharmacol Therap, 19:360, 1976.

140. Wilensky AJ et al: Inadequate serum levels after intramuscular administration of diphenylhydantoin. Neurol 23:318, 1973.

141. Yahr M: The treatment of convulsive disorders. Med Clin N Amer 56:1225, 1972.

142. Zackai EH et al: The fetal trimethadione syndrome. J Pediat 87:280, 1975.

143. Zidar BL et al: Diphenylhydantoin-induced serum sickness with fibrin-platelet thrombi in lymph node microvasculature. Amer J Med 58:704, 1975.

144. Ziskin D et al: Dilantin hyperplastic gingivitis; its cause and treatment; differential appraisal. Am J Orthod 27:350, 1941.

Chapter 29

Parkinsonism

Sam K. Shimomura

Parkinsonism is a neurological disease characterized by tremor, akinesia, rigidity, and disorders of posture and equilibrium. The onset is slow and progressive, with symptoms manifesting themselves over several months to several years. The tremor of parkinsonism, which is probably the most obvious outward sign, is regular and rhythmic; it is most conspicuous when the patient is at rest, but it is absent during sleep. The rigidity, caused by the hypertonicity of the muscles acting against each other, may assume a characteristic "cogwheel" quality. Bradykinesia is the most incapacitating. An early sign of Parkinson's disease is a loss of facial movement resulting in a mask-like face. Changes in handwriting are also one of the initial signs of parkinsonism; the script becomes small and illegible as the tremor worsens. Postural instability is one of the later findings in the disease and may progress to the characteristic festinating gait of parkinsonism. Other signs and symptoms are sialorrhea, seborrhea, constipation, and changes in speech and mentation (13,40,64).

An estimated 200,000 to 400,000 persons in the United States are afflicted with this neurological disorder, and an estimated 40,000 new cases become apparent each year (51,64,67). Parkinson's disease is slightly more common in men than in women (13).

A detailed analysis of 672 cases of idiopathic parkinsonism by Hoehn et al (28) showed that the mean age of onset of the disease was 55.3 years, and two-thirds of these patients developed the disease between the ages of 50 and 69. The age of onset was the same for men as for women. The mortality rate was found to be nearly three times that of the general population of the same age, sex, and race. The mean duration of illness from diagnosis to death was 9.4 years for primary parkinsonism. The most common cause of death is not the disease itself, but arteriosclerotic heart disease, bronchopneumonia, and malignant neoplasms. The study by Hoehn was performed before the introduction of levodopa in 1967, and although it is too soon to make firm conclusions as to the impact of levodopa on the natural evolution of the disease, preliminary data indicate that mortality has been cut in half and the life span extended by at least two years (39,68). Further studies are needed to determine whether levodopa is responsible for this improvement or whether the patients benefited from generally improved and more attentive medical care.

Although the biochemical basis of Parkinson's disease is complex, the primary defect appears to be a neurotransmitter imbalance, i.e. an excess of acetylcholine and a deficiency of dopamine in the basal ganglia. Other neurotransmitters such as norepinephrine, gamma aminobutyric acid, histamine and serotonin may have some modifying influence on the primary transmitters (45,12). Excess acetylcholine has an excitatory effect on the central nervous system and appears to be responsible for the tremor associated with parkinsonism. This is supported by studies which demonstrate that centrally-acting cholinesterase inhibitors, such as physostigmine, aggravate parkinsonism, while centrally-acting anticholinergics such as benztropine alleviate the symptoms of this disease (20). Anticholinergics have been employed in the treatment of parkinsonism for over 100 years and were the mainstay of therapy until the introduction of levodopa.

The finding that reserpine produced a Parkinson-like syndrome by depleting the brain of dopamine provided insight into the biochemical basis of Parkinson's disease. Coupled with autopsy findings that showed an absence or deficiency of dopamine in the basal ganglia, the evidence is quite strong that dopamine deficiency is a central feature of the biochemical basis of parkinsonism. A number of drugs which act through the dopaminergic system have been shown to be effective to varying degrees in parkinsonism. Dopamine, which is given as its precursor, levodopa, directly increases the dopamine content in the brain and is currently the most effective treatment for parkinsonism. Several investigational drugs, e.g. bromocriptine, piribedil, as well as apomorphine and its congener n-propylnoraporphine are reported to directly stimulate dopamine receptors. Other drugs (e.g. amphetamines and amantadine) may increase dopamine at the receptor either by releasing intact striatal dopamine stores or by blocking dopamine reuptake (45,17,31).

Although this chapter emphasizes the drug therapy of idiopathic parkinsonism, drugs are only a part of an overall therapeutic regimen that also includes physiotherapy, exercise, psychological support, and occasional surgical intervention. Currently, there is no cure for this disease, and the goal of therapy is to provide maximum relief of symptoms and to maintain the independence and mobility of the patient.

The patient with Parkinson's disease is an excellent candidate for drug therapy monitoring by a pharmacist, especially in an outpatient setting. Because the disease is chronic, the clinician can come to know the patient and his or her problems from frequent contact over many years. The drugs used for this disease require careful dose adjustment and have a high potential for adverse reactions and drug interactions. Therefore, a sympathetic and knowledgeable pharmacist can contribute to the education of the patient regarding his or her drug therapy, thus insuring greater compliance, fewer complications and a better prognosis.

1. When is levodopa indicated? What is the proper way to initiate levodopa treatment in a parkinsonian patient?

Levodopa in combination with a decarboxylase inhibitor is clearly the drug of choice for parkinsonism. Since levodopa has many annoying, although rarely serious side-effects, it should be reserved for those patients whose signs and symptoms interfere with their work or other demands of daily living. Those patients with milder forms of the disease can often be adequately controlled with anticholinergic agents or amantadine.

In the past, therapy with levodopa was started with very small doses such as 250 mg three or four times a day and gradually increased by 250 mg every 2 to 3 days. As tolerance to the nausea and vomiting and other side-effects developed, the dose was gradually increased over a period of several months to 5 to 6 gms per day. Some patients responded adequately to as little as 2 gms per day, while others required the maximum recommended dose of 8 gms. Once an optimum dose of levodopa was reached, a maintenance phase followed during which the full benefits of the drug most often occurred.

The addition of carbidopa to levodopa therapy has reduced the induction phase to as little as one or two weeks and the maintenance dose to a quarter of the dose of levodopa alone.

Tablets containing 100 mg of levodopa and 10 mg of carbidopa (Sinemet 10/100) or 250 mg levodopa and 25 mg of carbidopa (Sinemet 25/250) are available. Levodopa is available alone in 250 or 500 mg tablets or capsules. Because peripheral dopa decarboxylase is saturated by approximately 100 mg of carbidopa per day, larger doses are unnecessary.

The induction phase of combined levodopa/carbidopa therapy is started with approximately 100 mg of levodopa three times a day and increased by 100 mg every day or every other day until a dose of 600 mg per day is reached. Then the patient may be switched to 250 mg three times a day. If needed, the patient may be titrated to a maximum dose of 2.0 gms of levodopa and 100 mg of carbidopa.

2. What are the advantages and disadvantages of using a decarboxylase inhibitor such as carbidopa in conjunction with levodopa?

Levodopa is metabolized to dopamine by the enzyme L-aromatic amino acid (dopa) decarboxylase. Since dopamine does not cross the blood-brain barrier, most of the levodopa administered orally is wasted by conversion to dopamine in the periphery. By combining levodopa with a decarboxylase inhibitor, which does not cross the blood-brain barrier, a larger proportion of levodopa is available to enter the brain.

The advantages of combining a decarboxylase inhibitor with levodopa are: (a) the dose of levodopa can be reduced by about 75 percent; (b) a number of the peripheral side-effects such as nausea, vomiting and cardiac arrhythmias are reduced since less levodopa metabolites such a dopamine, norepinephrine and epinephrine are being formed; (c) the patient can be titrated to an optimal dose of levodopa in a matter of weeks rather than months because the necessity for developing a tolerance to the peripheral side-effects is diminished; (d) pyridoxine will not antagonize the therapeutic efficacy of levodopa when used with this combination; (e) fluctuations in control of the patient's symptoms are somewhat improved by the longer duration of action of the combination and (f) the number of patients who improve and the degree of improvement are slighly greater because relatively larger doses can be tolerated due to the fact that the peripheral side effects are minimized (23,38).

On the other hand, the prevalence of orthostatic hypotension remains unchanged since it appears to be mediated by a central action of dopamine. Central nervous system side effects, such as abnormal involuntary movements and mental changes, tend to occur earlier and be more severe since more of the active drug crosses the blood-brain barrier (10,29).

3. LOL is a 66-year-old woman who was started on levodopa three years ago for her parkinsonism. She did well for the first two years of levodopa therapy, but has markedly deteriorated over the past year. She is now bed-bound, and unable to sit, turn, speak or swallow. What is the long-term efficacy of levodopa?

Initially, about 75% of parkinson patients respond favorably to levodopa therapy, but after a period of two to three years, the response diminishes, becomes more uneven and is accompanied by more side-effects. Marsden, et al. report that one-third of 400 patients followed over five years continue to benefit from the drug; another third have lost some of their initial response but are still better than before treatment; and the remaining third lost all initial benefits and are worse off than before therapy (39a).

Delaney and Fermaglich report similar findings in their 70 parkinson patients treated with levodopa. They found that 63 patients (90%) were improved during the first year. After five years only thirty-seven patients (52.9%) remained improved and thirty-three (47.1%) experienced a worsening of their condition (18a).

The causes of this fall-off in efficacy of levodopa are

unknown. Hypotheses include: (a) inadequate or diminished cerebral dopa decarboxylase leading to decreased conversion of levodopa to dopamine; (b) loss of striatal dopamine receptors and (c) loss of output pathways from the striatum or loss of other motor pathways.

While levodopa does not reverse or even stop the progression of parkinsonism, it does allow many parkinsonian patients the opportunity to live a more self-sufficient existence for a longer period of time. Several studies indicate that there may be a reduction in mortality and an extension of the life span (39,61a,68).

4. An 82-year-old male patient in a nursing home is being treated with papaverine for cerebral arteriosclerosis. During the past three months, there has been a gradual onset of tremors without noticeable rigidity or bradykinesia. The patient was started on levodopa. After a month, the patient was receiving two grams per day without any effect on his tremors. Why is this 82-year-old gentleman an apparent treatment failure?

There are a number of possible causes for this patient's apparent failure to respond to levodopa. First, not every elderly patient with tremors is afflicted with parkinsonism. Silversides (59) studied 2,915 residents of eight Toronto Metropolitan Homes for the Aged and found that 133, or 4.5%, had been diagnosed as suffering from parkinsonism. However, reexamination revealed that only 81 of 133 or 61% of these patients actually had Parkinson's disease. This patient should be examined by a neurologist to rule out other possible causes of tremor. Then, if the patient does have Parkinson's disease, his drug therapy should be reexamined. In general, anticholinergic agents are more effective in alleviating the tremor, while levodopa is more effective in reducing the akinesia and rigidity. It is also important to remember that levodopa has a very slow therapeutic onset when it is given without a decarboxylase inhibitor. Although some benefit would be expected within a month, some patients may require several months and a dose of 8 grams per day to achieve maximum effect. Also, at least a quarter of parkinsonism patients may not respond at all to levodopa (68).

Another important consideration in any instance of treatment failure is poor adherence to the dosage regimen by either the patient or the staff taking care of him.

Drug interactions are another cause of treatment failure. (See Table 2.) Most clinicians are aware that pyridoxine, reserpine, and phenothiazines are notorious for negating the beneficial effects of levodopa, but only recently has the deleterious effect of papaverine on levodopa therapy been appreciated.

Duvoisin (19) and Posner (52) report that papaverine in doses of 100 mg per day can reverse the beneficial effects of levodopa over a period of several weeks. Once the papaverine is discontinued, the expected response to levodopa reappears in five to seven days. The exact mechanism is unknown, but there is some evidence to suggest that papaverine may block the dopamine receptor in the striatum. Not only should papaverine be avoided in parkinsonism patients, but it should probably be avoided in all patients since there is no evidence to indicate that it is effective for cerebral arteriosclerosis.

In conclusion, in this patient the best course of action would be to discontinue the papaverine and levodopa and to reassess the patient's diagnosis. If he does indeed have parkinsonism, he would probably do better on a trial of anticholinergic agents since they appear to be more effective than levodopa against tremor. If this therapy is not sufficient, or his condition progresses, amantadine or levodopa with carbidopa can be added.

5. M.G. is a 65-year-old woman who has just been diagnosed as having parkinsonism. She has been started on levodopa, but she has difficulty swallowing the tablets or capsules. What can be done to help her?

Although only 15 to 20% of patients with Parkinson's disease complain of swallowing problems, a study using cinefluoroscopy showed that approximately 95% of the parkinsonism patients studied had swallowing disturbances (37). This difficulty in swallowing is responsible for the sialorrhea seen in advanced parkinsonism. The inability to cope with oral secretions may predispose the patient to pulmonary aspiration and pneumonia. Unfortunately, levodopa and levodopa/carbidopa (Sinemet) are not available as oral suspensions or in an injectable form.

If a patient is unable to swallow the large levodopa capsules, the white, odorless, tasteless powder can be emptied and mixed with soft food or a liquid.

If a patient requires a liquid formulation for administration through a nasogastric tube, a suspension in cherry syrup or other vehicle can be prepared. The concentration of levodopa should not exceed one gram in 5 to 10 ml. The suspension should be buffered with citric acid and sodium citrate to a pH between four and five because an alkaline pH will enhance deterioration.

The suspension is generally stable for 24 hours if it is stored in a dark, tightly-closed, refrigerated container. If the color of the suspension changes to a darker shade, it should be discarded because this indicates decomposition of the levodopa (9,65).

6. What are the common side effects of levodopa?

Levodopa causes numerous side effects, most of which are more annoying than serious. They primarily affect the gastrointestinal, cardiovascular and central nervous systems (81,17,68).

Cardiac arrhythmias such as sinus tachycardia and premature ventricular contractions appear to be caused by dopamine, norepinephrine and other metabolites of levodopa. Carbidopa decreases the peripheral metabolism of levodopa and seems to decrease the prevalence of its cardiac effects. However, orthostatic hypotension is not reduced by carbidopa (23). Parkinson patients tend to have low blood pressure and the addition of levodopa may aggravate the hypotension, especially early in therapy.

Levodopa causes mental changes manifested as depression, paranoia, agitiation, delusions, hallucinations, insomnia, dementia and loss of memory. Drug-induced mental changes are often difficult to distinguish from those caused by old age or the disease itself. These side effects can usually be controlled by a reduction of dose.

Abnormal involuntary movements occur in over half the patients taking levodopa for over six months and present as grimacing, chewing movements, bobbing of the head and neck, rocking movements of the trunk and active tongue movements.

Other side effects such as the gastrointestinal side effects and "on-off" effect are covered in Questions 7 and 8.

7. A 66-year-old patient with severe parkinsonism is being treated with levodopa, 2.0 gm/day. His disease is still poorly controlled and attempts to increase his dose cause severe nausea and vomiting. What can be done to decrease his nausea and vomiting?

Prior to the introduction of the dopa decarboxylase inhibitor, carbidopa, nausea and vomiting were frequently encountered when levodopa therapy was initiated. These effects were minimized by slowly increasing the dose of levodopa, dividing the total daily dose into four to six doses, and administering the drug with antacids (6,14,67).

The addition of carbidopa to levodopa (Sinemet) has greatly reduced the incidence and severity of this nausea and vomiting. Carbidopa inhibits the conversion of levodopa to dopamine in the periphery thereby enabling a reduction in the dose of levodopa by 75% and decreasing dopamine levels peripherally (38).

Thus, this patient should be switched to one-fourth the dose of levodopa in combination with carbidopa (Sinemet). If necessary, the dose may be increased to achieve optimal therapeutic effects.

8. What is the "on-off" effect seen in patients on long-term levodopa therapy?

The "on-off" effect has been described as "the sudden and abrupt onset of a marked inability to move (akinesia, "off" effect) that may last minutes to hours, followed by an equally abrupt return of the ability to move that is often accompanied by abnormal involuntary movements" (36a). A common form of the "on-off" effect is deterioration which occurs at the end of the dosing interval. In these patients, the duration of levodopa's therapeutic effects decreases from about four hours initially to two to three hours or less. Over a period of time, relief after each dose becomes shorter and shorter, and swings from good to bad become more violent. After five years, end-of-dose deterioration occurs in up to 40% of levodopa-treated patients (39a). The cause of the "on-off" effect may partly be due to fluctuating blood levels since continuous intravenous adminstration of levodopa tends to smooth out the abrupt changes in response. However, the disappearance of the "on-off" effect was sustained only when the patients remained in a supine position. Movement to a semivertical position or cold pressor stimulation exacerbated the hypokinesis. This suggests that other factors besides the pharmacokinetics of levodopa are responsible for the "on-off" effect (56a).

9. A 50-year-old male with no symptoms or family history of gout was placed on levodopa for parkinsonism. A few months later, his uric acid was found to be 9.5 mg%. Does levodopa cause gout or interfere with the laboratory determination of uric acid?

Levodopa can cause a false elevation of serum and urinary uric acid when the colorimetric method (Sigma Analytical Kit SMA 12/30 and No. 680) is used. In a study of 20 patients receiving three to seven grams of levodopa per day, 18 were noted to have elevated levels of uric acid averaging 20% above pretreatment levels. When the uricase method was used, all the patients showed normal values for serum and urinary uric acid (15).

In another study (40), blood uric acid sample testing was repeated 625 times and was found to be abnormal in 31% of the cases. When the researchers compared uric acid levels obtained by the uricase method and the colorimetric method, the former gave significantly lower levels. However, even by the uricase method, a few of the uric acid levels were slightly above normal. A number of other researchers have reported similar findings (51,33,48).

Thus far, only two cases of gout have been attributed to levodopa. One patient complained of a greatly swollen right ankle four days after initiation of levodopa therapy, and another case of clinical gout was seen after only two days of therapy. The same article described a third patient who developed elevated levels of uric acid but no symptoms. The validity of this report is open to question, because pretreatment evaluation of uric acid was not obtained and subsequent uric acid determinations were performed by the colorimetric method (30).

In conclusion, the uric acid determination should be repeated with the more specific uricase method. Further studies are needed to determine whether levodopa can actually produce significant elevation of uric acid and clinical symptoms of gout.

10. Is levodopa a true aphrodisiac?

It is probably inaccurate to describe levodopa as a true aphrodisiac, because it only causes a transient, nonspecific stimulation of sexual drive in a limited number of patients. It is not a predictable effect that occurs in every patient who receives the drug.

When the effects of levodopa on sexual function were studied in eight sexually impotent parkinsonism males, the most obvious effects noted were an increase in frequency of spontaneous erection during the night and a slight transient increase in degree of penile erection. An increase in libido was noted in only two of these patients (7).

The hypersexuality which may occur in levodopa-treated parkinsonian patients may sometimes be a dramatic complication of therapy. After administration of levodopa, some patients have been known to make little effort to avoid exposing themselves, while other have made amorous advances towards the hospital staff and other patients (56). On the other hand, an increased libido may be a welcome side effect, allowing a formerly impotent patient to resume satisfactory sexual intercourse.

In a study by O'Brien (47), six of nine male patients on a dose of 4 to 6 grams of levodopa daily reported spontaneous penile erections generally not related to a sexual object and not accompanied by sexual fantasies. The reactions were a source of embarrassment to the patients and were generally not revealed unless these patients were questioned. Three of the men reported increased libido.

Bowers et al (10) interviewed 19 patients with Parkinson's disease to assess the effects of levodopa on sexual behavior. Seven patients (six males and one female) reported an activation of sexual behavior. The authors feel that this activation of sexual behavior can be grouped into three general patterns. First, patients experience an overall improvement in function with attendant psychosocial consequences; the second pattern seemed to be a specific stimulation of sexual drive that is relatively independent of overall functional improvement, and the third pattern of sexual activation involved loss of sexual inhibitions secondary to an acute brain syndrome.

The aphrodisiac effect of levodopa has been greatly exaggerated in the lay press. This effect is most commonly associated with functional improvement of the patient which allows him or her to once again think actively about and engage in sexual activity. However, some patients may exhibit symptoms that result from a psychiatric side effect of levodopa therapy.

11. A 62-year-old male recently developed classic signs of Parkinson's disease, e.g. tremors, rigidity, and bradykinesia. In reviewing his past medical history, it was noted that he had a malignant melanoma removed three years ago. What effect, if any, will levodopa have on a patient with a history of cancer?

Levodopa may have a beneficial effect in certain types of cancers and may be contraindicated in others. Levodopa provided relief from bone pain caused by metastatic breast cancer in 10 of 30 women. These 10 patients also showed resolution of bone scan activity and roentgenographic evidence of bone recalcification (44).

The beneficial effects of levodopa in breast cancer may be related to its ability to suppress prolactin. However, the role of prolactin in mammary carcinogenesis is unclear (11); other mechanisms may be involved since the bone pain from prostatic cancer and metastatic hypernephroma has also responded to levodopa (46).

On the other hand, a temporal relationship has been demonstrated between the administration of levodopa and the recurrence of melanoma in four cases reported in the literature (36,53,61).

Levodopa is a common intermediate in the biosynthesis of melanin as well as catecholamines. Melanin synthesis begins with the hydroxylation of tyrosine to levodopa and levodopa to dopaquinone, followed by stepwise conversion to melanin. Elevation of levodopa levels may enhance melanin production and result in stimulation of tumor growth. Levodopa may also influence melanomas indirectly by stimulating growth hormone, which may stimulate melanoma growth.

Although this effect of levodopa must still be proven, it should be avoided in this patient because of the highly malignant nature of melanoma (36,53,61). Furthermore, it would seem prudent to use levodopa cautiously or avoid it completely in patients with pigmented lesions or a history of malignant melanoma.

12. How soon would you expect to see improvement in a parkinson patient after starting treatment with amantadine? What is its long-term efficacy?

Amantadine is an antiviral agent that produces moderate improvement in parkinsonism within 24 hours after therapy is initiated.

The usual dose is 100 mg with breakfast for about one week and then 100 mg with breakfast and lunch. If significant improvement is not observed within two or three weeks, the drug should be discontinued. After an almost immediate onset of action, there is a relative fall-off in therapeutic effect over a period of two to three months in about one-half of the patients. Brief courses of therapy may allow prolonged benefit (39b).

13. D. B. has been taking amantadine for five months. She now has developed a reddish-blue discoloration on her arms and legs. Has amantadine been associated with this type of dermatological condition?

Amantadine has been reported to cause livido reticularis, a condition characterized by a diffuse, rose-colored mottling of the skin; it is usually confined primarily to the lower extremities, but in some patients it also appears on the arms. A mild ankle edema commonly occurs in conjunction with the livido reticularis and the skin discoloration is most noticeable when the patient stands or is exposed to cold. The condition is reversible in two to six weeks upon discontinuation of the amantadine and is relatively benign clinically, even when the amantadine is continued.

The reported prevalence of amantadine-induced livido reticularis has been quite high in several studies. In 1970, Shealy et al (57) first reported this adverse reaction in 10 of 18 female patients receiving 100 to 200 mg of amantadine for a period of a month or more. Shortly after this, Vollum et al (62) reported livido reticularis in 21 of 21 women and 15 of 19 men who were receiving amantadine. However, Vollum also observed some degree of livido reticularis in 32 of 51 untreated control patients who did not have Parkinson's disease. Silver and Sach (58) noted this adverse effect in 10 or 34 patients. Although livido reticularis occurred in a high percentage of patients in these three studies, other studies of large groups of patients being treated with amantadine for parkinsonism did not mention this reaction. Also, although amantadine has been used for a number of years in a large number of patients for prophylaxis of influenza, there have been no reports of livido reticularis (2). The only large study looking for this side effect reported a prevalence of only eight cases out of 430 patients studied (54).

Amantadine may produce this adverse effect by causing a release of norepinephrine from peripheral nerve terminals which, in turn, causes vasoconstriction. The impaired peripheral blood flow could result in the appearance of livido reticularis and pedal edema (49).

In conclusion, the skin discoloration seen in D. B. appears to be a benign, reversible side effect that does not generally require discontinuation of the amantadine.

14. What other side effects have been attributed to amantadine?

In general, amantadine is a safe drug with few significant side effects in the dosage range of 200 to 300 mg usually employed. Most are mild, transient, and readily reversible upon discontinuation of the drug. In a study of 430 patients, Schwab et al (54) noted confusion, disorientation, depression, nervousness, and insomnia in 49 patients; dizziness and lightheadedness in 26 patients; and gastrointestinal complaints in 21 patients. Other side effects reported less frequently were dryness of the mouth, rash, livido reticularis, lethargy, drowsiness, ataxia, visual difficulties, headache, and edema. In only 22 patients (5.1%) was it necessary to discontinue therapy.

Hallucinations and convulsions have been reported following large doses of amantadine (22a,54a).

15. A patient has heard that there is a special diet for people receiving levodopa for the treatment of parkinsonism. What are the details of such a diet?

Parkinsonism patients should follow normal good eating habits. However, a number of years ago, a low-pyridoxine diet plan was developed, since excessive amounts of pyridoxine were reported to reverse the therapeutic effects of levodopa (63,69,12). Pyridoxal phosphate is a cofactor of the enzyme dopa-decarboxylase which converts levodopa to dopamine and thereby enhances the peripheral metabolism of L-dopa. Since dopamine cannot cross the blood-brain barrier, peripheral metabolism of levodopa results in mininished amounts of levodopa that are available to enter the brain (35). The amount of pyridoxine found in the average diet is estimated to be less than 1 mg per day, which is much less than the 5 to 10 mg per day needed to nullify levodopa effects (63,69). With the addition of carbidopa, a decarboxylase inhibitor, to levodopa (Sinemet), even large doses of pyridoxine will not adversely interact with levodopa (23). Therefore, restriction of pyridoxine is unnecessary when this combination is used.

High protein intake has been reported to neutralize the therapeutic effect of levodopa and sometimes precipitates an "on-off" phenomenon, i.e. the episodic loss of symptomatic control. Since levodopa is absorbed and transported like other amino acids, it has been postulated that high protein diets interfere with the absorption of levodopa. Although in experimental studies protein has been restricted to 0.5 gm/kg/day, it is probably sufficient to recommend diets that do not exceed the recommended dietary allowance of 0.8 gm/kg/day of protein (26,43,55).

Since constipation is often a problem in the elderly Parkinson patient, bran or other high fiber food may be included in the diet. Meat and other foods may have to be cut up for those patients who are severely incapacitated by the disease. In addition, a semi-soft diet may be necessary if dysphagia is a problem (55).

16. A 68-year-old woman with open-angle glaucoma, well-controlled on topical therapy, now complains of tremors and rigidity. Will anticholinergic agents and levodopa aggravate her glaucoma?

One of the great myths concerning drugs is that systemic anticholinergics and sympathomimetic agents aggravate or even cause open angle glaucoma. This misconception has arisen because of a lack of distinction between narrow angle and open angle glaucoma and topical versus systemic therapy. Patients with an abnormally narrow angle between the iris and cornea may experience a dangerous rise in intraocular pressure with topical and, more rarely, with systemic, anticholinergic or sympathomimetic agents.

However, patients with open angle glacoma can safely use systemic, anticholinergic drugs and levodopa in conjunction with their normal topical therapy, i.e. cholinergic drops that cause miosis. Before starting anticholinergic or sympathomimetic therapy, however, all patients should be screened for a narrow-angle anterior chamber to prevent precipitating a first attack of acute, angle-closure glaucoma (3,32,23).

17. D. B. is a 56-year-female with a 10 year history of adult onset diabetes and a five year history of Parkinson's disease. Her diabetes has been well controlled on diet and tolbutamide 500 mg tid, and her parkinsonism was controlled with amantadine and trihexyphenidyl. However, she now requires the addition of levodopa/carbidopa. Do levodopa or amantadine alter glucose levels?

Oral administration of amantadine causes no significant changes in plasma insulin or blood sugar concentrations. Levodopa increases growth hormone and serum cholesterol (approximately 10%), and it has been shown to decrease glucose tolerance with a delayed and exaggerated insulin response in experimental studies (34,60). However, levodopa has never induced diabetes nor has it significantly altered the insulin requirement of a previously diagnosed diabetic (68).

18. Will levodopa interfere with testing for urinary glucose in this patient?

Levodopa may cause a false negative reading in the presence of glycosuria when the glucose oxidase method (Clinistix) is used and a false positive "trace" reading with the copper reduction method (Clinitest). In one study, six of 25 urine specimens taken from patients receiving 0.75 to 3 grams of levodopa daily and fortified with glucose to 1% produced a negative glucose oxidase test. In addition, the glucose oxidase reaction was inhibited in 13 of 17 specimens from patients receiving 3.5 to 5.0 grams of levodopa. Further-

more, 19 of 43 specimens obtained from patients receiving levodopa produced a trace reaction with the Clinitest copper reduction test in the absence of glycosuria (24).

The chemical responsible for the false negative glucose oxidase test and the false positive "trace" copper reduction test is 3,4,dihydroxyphenylacetic acid (DOPAC), a metabolite of levodopa. It is a potent reducing agent which keeps the indicator dye, orthotoluidine, used in Clinistix in its reduced form, thus producing a false negative reaction for glucose.

In spite of this interference, Testape or Clinistix can still be used in testing for glucose in patients on levodopa. The Testape appears to act as a mini-ascending chromatography system which separates the glucose from the DOPAC. Since glucose migrates faster than DOPAC, it is present above the area where the tape is dipped and a positive reaction can be read. Similarly, if only part of the test area of the Clinistix is dipped in the urine sample, a positive reaction can be observed above the immersed portion (24).

19. Will levodopa interfere with her testing for urinary ketones?

False positive readings for urinary ketones have been reported with Ketostix and Labstix in patients receiving 0.5 to 7.0 grams of levodopa daily. Most investigators report Acetest to be unaffected by levodopa (50,16,66). However, Dawson (18) reported one patient on 2.5 grams of levodopa who was noted to have a false positive reading to Acetest as well as to Ketostix and Labstix.

Levodopa and its metabolites, dopamine and 3,4 dihydroxyphenylacetic acid (DOPAC), have all produced a color reaction with Ketostix and Labstix, but not generally with Acetest tablets (16).

20. D. B., the patient discussed in Question 17, now complains of peripheral neuropathy secondary to her diabetes. Will the addition of phenytoin be helpful?

Ellenberg (22) treated 60 patients with diabetic peripheral neuropathy with phenytoin. Based on symptomatic relief of paresthesias and pain, he claimed "excellent" results in 41 of these patients and "fair response" in 10. Although this was an uncontrolled trial with no objective therapeutic endpoints, no other effective treatment is available. Therefore, it is often worth trying phenytoin. If no improvement is noted within 24 to 96 hours, the phenytoin should be discontinued. Phenytoin has been reported to cause glucosuria, hyperglycemia, and diminished glucose tolerance but not to a degree that is generally clinically significant. (Also see chapter on Diabetes.)

Another important consideration in this patient is the recently reported interaction between phenytoin and levodopa (42). Five parkinsonism patients on levodopa or levodopa/carbidopa were given 100 mg of phenytoin, which was gradually increased to 300 to 500 mg per day over a period of several days. After a few days, hypokinesia, rigidity, and the postural instability of parkinsonism re-emerged. Tremor was the only major sign of parkinsonism that did not return. When phenytoin was discontinued, all patients returned to their previous state of control within two weeks. The mechanism for this interaction is unknown, although there are experimental data which suggest that phenytoin can interfere with either the binding of dopamine or the reactivity of the brain to the dopamine.

It is, therefore, apparent from the available information that the potential beneficial effects of phenytoin must be weighed against the possible interaction with levodopa, and if it is decided that phenytoin is to be tried, the patient should be informed of this possible interaction.

21. Since a number of Parkinson patients are becoming refractory to the therapeutic effects of levodopa or are unable to tolerate its side-effects, are there any alternative modes of therapy on the horizon?

The most promising group of new drugs for the treatment of parkinsonism is the direct dopamine receptor agonists. While levodopa requires conversion in the brain to its active form, dopamine, this group of drugs acts directly to stimulate intact post-synaptic receptors, thereby by-passing the degenerated nigra. Five dopamine agonists have been investigated in parkinson patients thus far; apormorphine, N-propylnoraporphine, piribedil, and the ergot alkaloids, lergotrile and bromocriptine. Apormorphine has limited clinical usefulness because of its nephrotoxicity and short duration of action. A derivative of apormorphine, N-propylnoraporphine has less nephrotoxicity, but tolerance quickly develops to its therapeutic effects (17a). Piribedil is only slightly effective in man and causes frequent central nervous system side-effects such as drowsiness and confusion (61b). Preliminary studies of lergotrile indicate that it has moderate antiparkinson effects and is particularly effective against tremor. Further studies are needed to determine its maximal therapeutic efficacy and long-term effects (36b). Bromocriptine is the most promising of the dopamine agonists. It appears to be as effective as levodopa and is often useful in parkinsonian patients no longer responding to levodopa. Other advantages of bromocriptine over levodopa are its longer half life (six to eight hours versus two to four hours), greater efficacy against tremors, and reduction of the "on-off" phenomena and abnormal involuntary effects. On the other hand, orthostatic

hypotension and mental changes were increased with bromocriptine (33a,36a,48a).

22. What drugs may produce a Parksinson-like syndrome?

Methyldopa. A few isolated case reports have appeared in the literature describing a Parkinson-like syndrome following the administration of methyldopa. The patients were generally over 50 years old and received from one to three grams of methyldopa a day for one to four months. The tremor, rigidity and other signs and symptoms of parkinsonism disappeared rapidly when the drug was discontinued (26a, 49a, 52a).

Reserpine may cause cogwheel rigidity, mask-like facies, tremor, rigidity, shuffling gait and other signs and symptoms of parkinsonism when given in large doses (usually greater than 5 mg per day). In a study of 19 patients given reserpine for psychiatric problems, 12 developed Parkinson-like symptoms three to 23 days after receiving between 3 to 13 mg intramuscularly and from 0.5 mg to 5 mg orally daily. Parkinson-like side effects are not a problem when reserpine is used in low doses, as in the treatment of hypertension (52b).

Phenothiazines and related drugs. A survey of 3,775 patients on phenothiazines found that 15.4% had Parkinson-like symptoms, 21.2% had akathisia and 2.3% had dyskinesias for a total of 38.9% with extrapyramidal symptoms. Twice as many females (19.6%) as males (11.0%) developed Parkinson-like symptoms. Ninety percent of the cases of parkinsonism developed within the first 72 days. Phenothiazine-induced extrapyramidal side effects can be treated with anticholinergic agents such as benztropine and diphenhydramine (6a).

23. A 64-year-old man is admitted to the hospital for abdominal surgery. He has had progressive left-sided Parkinson's disease since age 35 which progressed to his right side two years before admission. His symptoms have been well controlled on levodopa, 2.0 gm/day. Are there any special problems in drug therapy for a parkinsonism patient undergoing surgery?

Levodopa can be given preoperatively until the patient is not allowed to receive anything by mouth, usually the night before surgery (4). Levodopa has a short half-life of one to three hours; therefore, very little will be present on the day of surgery (8). The patient may be restarted after surgery at a lower dose of levodopa and titrated slowly up to his previous dose as soon as he is able to tolerate oral medication.

Although no interactions have been reported between levodopa and general anesthetics, some of the halogenated anesthetics are known to sensitize the heart to exogenous catecholamines (27). The metabolites of levodopa, such as dopamine, norepinephrine, and epinephrine, theoretically may predispose the patient to cardiac arrhythmias.

Phenothiazines should probably be avoided as preoperative medications and as post-operative anti-nauseants because they nullify the effects of levodopa and exacerbate the signs and symptoms of parkinsonism by blocking dopaminergic receptors (8). If an anti-emetic is needed, an antihistamine-type such as diphenhydramine (Benadryl) would be preferable.

Aminoglycoside antibiotics such as gentamicin may cause neuromuscular blockade in a Parkinson patient if they are given for an infection during the postoperative period. A patient similar to the one described here was reported to have had marked deterioration of his neurological status after receiving gentamicin in relatively modest doses in the post-operative period. He became flaccid and unable to exhibit any voluntary muscular movements other than very weakly squeezing his right hand and blinking his eyes. Within four hours after discontinuation of the gentamicin, he was fully oriented, able to speak and raise his arms and follow other commands. He was rechallenged with gentamicin and experienced a similar episode of neuromuscular blockade. Fortunately, despite the profound neurological blockade, the respiratory muscles were spared, and he did not require mechanical ventilation. The mechanism for this adverse reaction is unknown, but it could be related to the curariform effects of gentamicin being potentiated by the patient's disease or antiparkinson medication, i.e. amantadine and trihexyphenidyl (29).

CASE HISTORY FOR STUDY

A. M. is a 63-year-old female with complaints of anxiety, nervousness, weakness of the right hand, agitation, and tremors. She also has a five-year history of angina that has been treated with sublingual nitroglycerin and a two-year history of hypertension that has been untreated. Her blood pressure on physical examination was 200/112 reclining and 202/105 sitting. At the time of her initial visits she was given diazepam, 2 mg tid. This drug helped her nervousness, but did not alleviate her tremors.

Two weeks later, she returned to the clinic with the same complaints, which she feels are exacerbated by stressful situations in that many of the symptoms were initially noted at the time of her husband's death six months ago. She also says that the symptoms are worsened by pressure at work and that she "feels all tied up." Her friends have told her that her voice is changing. On physical examination, the patient is a well-developed, well-nourished, white female in no acute distress. She has noticeable tremors in both hands and cogwheel rigidity of both arms. There is a slight masklike facies. The rest of her history and physical are non-contributory. Her laboratory tests are normal, except for a glucose tolerance test which indicates that she is a borderline diabetic.

a) What signs and symptoms does A.M. have that are consistent with a diagnosis of parkinsonism?

b) What symptoms might she develop as her parkinsonism progresses?

c) What medications should the pharmacist inquire about in the drug history to rule out drug-induced parkinsonism?

d) What drugs should be used to treat her parkinsonism?

e) Will starting levodopa early prevent the progression of her disease?

f) Will any of the drugs used for parkinsonism aggravate her borderline diabetes or interfere with the testing of her urine for glucose or ketones?

g) What drugs should be used to treat her hypertension? Which antihypertensive agents will interfere with her Parkinson's disease and diabetes?

h) Will any of the drugs used to treat parkinsonism interfere with her therapy or diagnosis of hypertension?

i) Will sedatives and tranquilizers which may be prescribed for her psychological problems interfere with her Parkinson's disease? Does stress exacerbate parkinsonism?

j) Which antiparkinson or antihypertensive agent will aggravate her angina?

TABLE 1
ANTIPARKINSON DRUGS

Drug	Dose	Side Effects
Anticholinergics:		
Trihexyphenidyl (Artane) 2 and 5 mg tablets 5 mg time-released capsules 2 mg/5 ml elixir	1 to 5 mg tid, start with low doses. Doses over 20 mg a day are rarely tolerated.	Blurred vision, dry mouth, vertigo, drowsiness, muscle weakness, mild confusion. In toxic doses tachycardia, hallucinations, agitation, elevation of body temperature. Contraindicated in narrow angle glaucoma.
Biperiden (Akineton) 2 mg tablets	2 mg 3 to 4 times/day	See above.
Cycrimine (Pagitane) 1.25 and 2.5 mg tablets	Initially 1.25 mg 2 to 3 times/day. Usual range 3.75 to 15 mg daily in divided doses.	See above.
Procyclidine (Kemadrin) 2 and 5 mg tablets	Initially 2.5 mg 2 or 3 times/day. Usual dosage range 10 to 20 mg daily in 3 or 4 doses.	See above.
Benztropine (Cogentin) 0.5, 1.0 and 2.0 mg tablets	Initially 0.5 to 1 mg daily with slow increase to 1 to 2 mg per day. Maximum dose 6 mg in divided doses.	See above.
Diphenhydramine (Benadryl) 25 and 50 mg capsules	Initially 25 mg at bedtime and 75 mg daily in divided doses. Usual range 75 to 150 mg daily with 300 mg per day maximum.	Drowsiness, confusion, dizziness, atropine-like effects.
Chlorphenoxamine (Phenoxene) 50 mg tablets	Initially 50 mg TID. May increase to 100 mg QID.	See above.
Dopaminergic Drugs:		
Levodopa (Larodopa, Dopar, Levopa, Bendopa) 100 mg, 250 mg, 500 mg	Initially 300 to 500 mg a day with slow increase to 2 to 8 grams per day.	Nausea, vomiting, anorexia, hypotension, abnormal movements, behavioral changes, cardiac arrhythmias.
Levodopa/Carbidopa (fixed ratio 10:1) (Sinemet) 100 mg/10 mg or 250/25mg tablets.	300/30 to 1500/150 mg per day. Maximum dose 2000/200 mg per day.	Same as above, except less nausea, vomiting, and cardiac arrhythmias.
Amantadine (Symmetrel) 100 mg capsules syrup containing 50 mg/5 ml	100 mg with breakfast for 5 to 7 days and then 100 mg with breakfast and lunch.	Hyperexcitability, tremor, slurred speech, ataxia, depression, hallucinations, insomnia, livido reticularis.

TABLE 2
DRUG INTERACTIONS WITH LEVODOPA

Drug	Adverse Effect	Probable Mechanism	Reference
Benzodiazepines e.g. chlordiazepoxide and diazepam	decreased antiparkinson effect in an occasional patient	unknown	31a 54a
Methyldopa	may increase or decrease antiparkinson effect	may increase effect because it is a decarboxylase inhibitor. The mechanism for inhibiting effect unknown, but may act as a false transmitter for dopamine in the brain	61c
Monoamine oxidase inhibitors e.g. isocarboxazid, pargyline, phenelzine, tranylcypromine	hypertensive crisis	increase in storage and release of dopamine, norepinephrine or both	31b
Phenothiazines e.g. chlorpromazine and prochlorperazine	decreased antiparkinson	Inhibition of dopamine reuptake and blockade of dopamine receptors	4a, 68
Pyridoxine	decreased antiparkinson effect. Does not occur in patient receiving the combination of levodopa/carbidopa	increased decarboxylation of levodopa in the periphery	21
Phenytoin	decreased antiparkinson effect	unknown	42
Papaverine	decreased antiparkinson effect	unknown	19, 52

REFERENCES

1. Al-Hujaj M et al: Hyperuricemia and levodopa. NEJM 285:589, 1971.
2. AMA Department of Drugs: *AMA Drug Evaluations,* 2nd ed. Action Mass.: Publishing Sciences Group Inc., 1973 p 747.
3. Anon: Effects of systemic drugs with anticholinergic properties for glaucoma. Med Letter 16:28, 1974.
4. Anon: Manufacturer's official package circular for Larodopa (Roche).
4a. Ayd, F.J.: A survey of drug-induced extrapyramidial reactions. JAMA 175:1054, 1961.
5. Barbeau A: L-dopa therapy in Parkinson's disease: a critical review of nine years' experience. Can Med Assoc J 101:59, 1969.
6. Barbeau A et al.: Side effects of levodopa therapy, Ch 8 in *Recent Advances in Parkinson's Disease* edited by F H McDowell and C H Markham, Philadelphia, F A Davis Co, 1971 p 205.
6a. B.C.D.S.P.: Drug-induced extrapyramidal symptoms. JAMA 224:889, 1973.
7. Benkert O et al: Effects of L-dopa on sexually impotent patients. Psychopharmacologica 23:91, 1972.

8. Bianchine JR: Drug therapy of parkinsonism. NEJM 295:814-18, 1976.
9. Blacow NW: *Martindale The Extra Pharmacopoeia,* London, The Pharmaceutical Press, 1972 p 74.
10. Bowers MB et al: Sexual behavior during L-dopa treatment for Parkinsonism. Amer J Psych 127:1691, 1971.
11. Buckman MT et al: Prolactin in clinical practice. JAMA 236:871-74, 1976.
12. Cabot EE: Physician's advice needed in diet for parkinsonism. Modern Hospital 116:142-43, 1971.
13. Calne DB: *Parkinsonism: Physiology, Pharmacology and Treatment* Edward Arnold Ltd, London, 1970.
14. Calne DB et al: Antiparkinson drugs pharmacological and therapeutic aspects. Drugs 4:49, 1972.
15. Cawein MJ et al: False rise in serum uric acid after L-dopa. NEJM 281:1489, 1969.
16. Cawein MJ et al: Levodopa and tests for ketonuria. NEJM 283:659, 1970.

17. Cohen MM et al: Pharmacotherapy of Parkinson's disease. Am J Hosp. Pharm 34:531, 1977.

17a. Cotzias GC et al: Treatment of Parkinson's disease with aporphines. NEJM 294:567, 1976.

18. Dawson WL: Levodopa and tests for ketonuria. NEJM 283:264, 1970.

18a. Delaney, P et al: Parkinsonism and levodopa: A five-year experience. J Clin Pharmacol 16:652, 1976.

19. Duvoisin RC: Antagonism of levodopa by papaverine. JAMA 231:845, 1975.

20. Duvoisin RC: Cholinergic-anticholinergic antagonism in parkinsonism. Arch Neurol 17:124, 1967.

21. Dovoisin RC et al: Pyridoxine reversal of L-dopa effects in parkinsonism. Trans Am Neurol Assoc 94-81, 1969.

22. Ellenberg M: Treatment of diabetic neuropathy with diphenylhydantoin. NYJ Med 68:2653, 1968.

22a. Fahn S et al: Acute toxic psychosis from suicidal overdose of amantadine. Arch Neurol 25:45, 1971.

23. Falck RL: Carbidopa and levodopa evaluation. Drug Intell Clin Pharm 10:84, 1976.

24. Feldman JM et al: Levodopa and tests for urinary glucose. NEJM 283:1053, 1970.

25. Friedman JM et al: Inhibition of glucose oxidase paper tests by reducing metabolites. Diabetes 19:337 (May), 1970.

26. Gillespie et al: Diets affecting treatment of parkinsonism with levodopa. J Am Diet Assoc 64:525, 1973.

26a. Groden BM: Parkinsonism Occurring With Methyldopa Treatment. Brit Med J 1:1001, 1963.

27. Franz, DN: Drugs for Parkinson's disease: Centrally acting muscle relaxants. In the *Pharmacological Basis of Therapeutics* Ed 5, edited by Goodman LS and Gilman A. Ch. 14 The Macmillan Co., New York, 1975.

28. Hoehn MM et al: Parkinsonism: Onset, progression and mortality. Neurology 17:427, 1967.

29. Holtzman JL: Gentamicin and neuromuscular blockade. Ann Intern Med 84:55, 1976.

30. Honda H et al: Gout while receiving levodopa for parkinsonism JAMA 219:55, 1972.

31. Hornykiewicz D: Parkinson's disease and its chemotherapy. Biochem Pharmacol 24:1061, 1975.

31a. Hunter KR et al: Use of levodopa with other drugs. Lancet 2:1283, 1970.

31b. Hunter KR et al: Monoamine oxidase inhibitors and L-dopa. Br Med J 3:388, 1970.

32. Ignoffo R et al: Glaucoma. J Am Pharm Assoc NS12:520-34, 1972.

33. Jonas S: Hyperuricemia and levodopa. NEJM 285:1488, 1971.

33a. Kartzinal R et al: Studies with bromocriptine. Neurol 26:508-513, 1976.

34. Kitomaki O et al: Effects of L-dopa on plasma growth hormone and insulin. Acta Neurol Scand (Supp) 51:125, 1972.

35. Kott E et al: Excretion of dopa metabolites. NEJM 284:395, 1971.

36. Lieberman AN et al: Levodopa and melanoma. Neurol 24:340, 1974.

36a. Lieberman et al: Treatment of Parkinson's disease with bromocriptine, NEJM 295:1400, 1976.

36b. Lieberman A et al: Studies on the antiparkinsonian efficacy of lergotrile. Neurol 25:459, 1975.

37. Logemann JA et al: Dysphagia in parkinsonism. JAMA 231:69, 1975.

38. Markham CH et al: Carbidopa in Parkinson's disease and in nausea and vomiting of levodopa. Arch Neurol 31:128-33, 1974.

39. Markham CH et al: Parkinson's disease and levodopa. West J Med 121:188, 1974.

39a. Marsden CD et al: Success and problems of long-term levodopa therapy in Parkinson's disease. Lancet 1:345, 1977.

39b. Mawsdsley C et al: Treatment of parkinsonism by amandatine and levodopa. Clin. Pharmacol. Ther. 13:575, 1972.

40. McDowell F: Clinical laboratory abnormalities. Clin Pharm Ther 12 (part 2): 335, 1971.

41. McDowell FH: The diagnosis of parkinsonism syndrome. Ch 6 *Recent Advances in Parkinson's Disease* FH McDowell, CH Markham, eds, FA Davis Co., Philadelphia, 1971.

42. Mendez JS et al: Diphenylhydantoin blocking of levodopa effects. Arch Neurol 32:44, 1975.

43. Mens I et al: Protein intake and treatment of Parkinson's disease with levodopa. NEJM 292:181, 1975.

44. Minton JP: The response of breast cancer with bone pain to L-dopa. Cancer 33:358, 1974.

45. Moskowtiz MA et al: Catecholamines and neurologic diseases. NEJM 293:274, 332, 1975.

46. Nixon DW: Use of L-dopa to relieve pain from bone metastases. NEJM 292:647, 1975.

47. O'Brien CP et al: Mental effects of high-dosage levodopa. Arch Gen Psych 24:61, 1971.

48. Paladine WJ: Gout and levodopa. NEJM 286:376, 1972.

48a. Parkes SD et al: Bromocriptine treatment in Parkinson's disease. J Neurol Neurosurg and Psych 39:184, 1976.

49. Pearce LA et al: Amantadine hydrochloride: Alteration in peripheral circulation. Neurol 24:46, 1974.

49a. Peaston MJT: Parkinsonism associated with alpha/methyldopa therapy. Brit Med J 2:168, 1964.

50. Pocelinko R et al: Doped dipsticks. NEJM 281:1075, 1969.

51. Pollock M et al: The prevalence, natural history, and dementia of Parkinson's disease. Brain 89:429, 1966.

52. Posner DM: Antagonism of levodopa by papaverine. JAMA 233:768, 1975.

52a. Prescott LF: Methyldopa and parkinsonism. Brit Med J 2:687, 1964.

52b. Richman A et al: An extrapyramidal syndrome with reserpine. Canad Med Assoc J 72:457, 1955.

53. Robinson E et al: Levodopa and malignant melanoma. Arch Path 93:556, 1972.

54. Schwab RS et al: Amantadine in Parkinson's disease. Review of more than two years' experience. JAMA 222:792, 1972.

54a. Schwab RS et al: Amantadine in the treatment of Parkinson's disease. JAMA. 203:1168, 1969.

54b. Schwarz GA et al: Newer medical treatments in parkinsonism. Med Clin N Amer 54:773, 1970.

55. Selvey NP: Diet for patients receiving levodopa therapy for parkinsonism. JAMA 236:1169, 1976.

56. Shapiro SK: Hypersexual behavior complicating levodopa therapy. Minn Med 56:58, 1973.

56a. Shaulson I et al: On-off response. Neurol 25:1144, 1975.

57. Shealy CN et al: Livido reticularis in patients with parkinsonism receiving amantadine. JAMA 212:1522, 1970.

58. Silver DE et al: Livido reticularis in Parkinson's disease patients treated with amantadine hydrochloride. Neurol 22:665, 1972.

59. Silversides JL: Parkinsonism may be diagnosed too freely in elderly patients. JAMA 235:1091, 1976.

60. Sirtori CR et al: Metabolic responses to acute and chronic L-dopa administration in patients with parkinsonism. NEJM 287:729, 1972.

61. Skibba JL et al: Multiple primary melanoma following administration of levodopa. Arch Path 93:556, 1972.

61a. Sweet, RD et al: Five year's treatment of Parkinson's disease with levodopa: Therapeutic results and survival of 100 patients. Ann Intern Med 83:456, 1975.

61b. Sweet RD et al: Piribedil, a dopamine agonist in Parkinson's disease. Clin Pharmacol Ther 16:1077, 1974.

61c. Sweet RD et al: Methyldopa as an adjunct to levodopa treatment of Parkinson's disease. Clin Pharmacol Ther 13:23, 1972.

62. Vollum DI et al: Livido reticularis during amantadine treatment. Brit Med J 2:627, 1971.

63. Von Woert MH: Low pyridoxine diet in parkinsonism. JAMA 219:1211, 1972.

64. Wagner SL: The management of Parkinson's syndrome. Med Clin Amer 56:693, 1972.

65. Williams FF: DISS-Drug Information Sharing Service. Hosp Pharm 8:361, 1973.

66. Wolcott GT et al: Levodopa and tests for ketonuria. NEJM 283:1522, 1970.

67. Yahr MD: The treatment of parkinsonism. Med Clin N Amer 56:1377, 1972.

68. Yahr MD: Levodopa. Ann Intern Med 83:677, 1975.

69. Yahr MD et al: Pyridoxine and levodopa in treatment of parkinsonism. JAMA 220:861, 1972.

Chapter 30

Psychoses

Glen L. Stimmel

Psychotic disorders comprise a major component of psychiatric practice in which drug therapy plays a major role in treatment. This chapter will include functional psychoses, and exclude drug-induced and toxic psychoses and psychoses of organic origin. Schizophrenia is presented as the primary representative of functional psychoses since it is the most common, and since neuroleptic drugs are primarily used in its treatment. Neuroleptic drugs are sometimes used to treat psychotic depression and psychosis associated with organic brain syndrome. Comments regarding the efficacy, limitations, adverse effects, and precautions of neuroleptic use in the treatment of schizophrenia apply to these other indications as well.

The following cases are descriptions of patients whom the author has managed or is presently managing in his clinical practice. The overall approach to clinical practice is conservative. This approach is the natural result of the clinical pharmacist having direct decision-making responsibility rather than merely consulting on a therapeutic problem without responsibility for consequences. The effective clinical practitioner should have a solid literature information base, coupled with clinical experience to fill the gaps that presently exist in the literature.

The following case history is typical of many schizophrenic patients and will serve as a basis for the questions that follow.

Case History (K.K.)

K.K., a 40-year-old divorced, unemployed, male presently living with his mother, was hospitalized on the acute psychiatric ward after he made a bomb threat and acted in a bizarre manner toward two neighbors. (Admission date September 1975).

History of Present Illness: Patient is unclear regarding the events leading to this hospitalization. He states that he was brought to the hospital unjustly because his mother called the police. He feels that a car in the neighborhood had been tampered with, painters in his room had used a mixture of gasoline and paint, and too many people had been using his toilet, causing it to back up. His mother states that he has shown flagrant bizarre behavior during the past year, causing neighbors to fear him. During the past several months he has become progressively more withdrawn, having no social contacts. During the past two weeks he has slept on the floor and refused to eat, thinking that his food is poisoned.

Previous illnesses: In 1964 the patient lost his job due to nervousness. He apparently has been disturbed since his divorce in 1962. He was hospitalized in state institutions in 1967, 1970, and 1974, but he refuses to give any details. He has been treated with Stelazine and Thorazine in the past, but the dates, dosage, and duration of therapy are unknown. The patient denies alcohol and drug abuse.

Family History: There is no family history of mental illness.

Personal History: Normal adjustment was present during his high school years. He married at age 21, fathered three sons, and separated from his wife four years later. According to his mother, he has never been the same since his first episode of nervousness in 1964.

Physical Exam on Admission: The examination is unremarkable.

Mental Status Exam on Admission: A disheveled 40-year-old male with long uncombed hair and long thin fingernails. The patient is suspicious and restless. He displays much movement during the interview. The patient requests photographs not to be made during the interview because he does not want "them people to get the wrong idea." He is very guarded and refuses to provide any details he considers personal. However, he makes many bizarre references to plumbing, paint, a car, San Diego, and unfit food. His associations are markedly loose; thinking is very concrete. Much paranoid ideation is present. He denies hallucinations. His insight and judgment are poor. He is oriented x 3.

Provisional Diagnosis: Schizophrenia, chronic undifferentiated.

1. What is schizophrenia? Is it synonymous with psychosis?

Schizophrenia is a cluster of related difficulties in behavior, thoughts, and feelings. It has a chronic fluctuating course. Clinical manifestations in a patient may be similar to or very different from other schizophrenics. Schizophrenic patients may be floridly psychotic, yet at other times they may be in total control of behavior, thoughts, and feelings. Mendel, in seeking to establish precision in the diagnosis of schizophrenia, has identified the following three basic disabilities of function which are the trademark of schizophrenia (71). Whether in psychotic exacerbation or remission, schizophrenics show difficulties: 1) in **anxiety management,** 2) in **interpersonal relationships,** and 3) in regard to personally lived history **(historicity).** The symptoms of psychosis are secondary to these three disabilities and essentially represent attempts at restitution, or are the physiological or psychological consequences of these disabilities. Thus, schizophrenia is a chronic disorder with either an acute or insidious onset. It is characterized by periods of exacerbation and remission and life-long disabilities in anxiety management, interpersonal relationships, and in the failure of historicity.

Schizophrenia is best described as being one type of psychosis. The term psychosis refers to impaired mental functioning which interferes grossly with the capacity to meet ordinary demands of life. Schizophrenia is the most common of functional psychoses, and it occurs more frequently than the major affective disorders, paranoid states, and reactive psychoses. In addition to functional psychoses, there are a wide variety of organic psychoses such as the dementias, alcoholic psychoses, psychoses associated with cerebral, intracranial, or cerebrovascular disturbances, endocrine and metabolic disorders, systemic infection, drug or poison intoxication, and childbirth (3).

A common misconception involves the relationship of schizophrenia to the Dr. Jekyll — Mr. Hyde concept. Schizophrenic patients do not have split or multiple personalities. The "split personality" derived from the literal translation of schizophrenia actually refers to the difficulty of a schizophrenic patient in handling the coexistence of opposing thoughts or feelings, which typically results in indecision and ambivalence. Multiple personality best fits in the diagnostic category of a type of hysterical neurosis (3).

2. Identify those factors in K.K.'s premorbid personality and past psychiatric history consistent with a schizophrenic diagnosis. How do these factors influence K.K.'s prognosis?

Both the age of onset and the course of K.K.'s disorder, combined with the presenting symptoms of this admission, are consistent with a diagnosis of schizophrenia. At age 29, K.K.'s first overt symptomatology is within the typical age of onset, which ranges from late adolescence to the early thirties (65). The chronic course of his disorder, with exacerbations represented by at least three previous psychiatric hospitalizations over seven years, further supports a schizophrenic diagnosis (71).

K.K.'s premorbid personality is more positive than many schizophrenic patients because he had a normal adjustment through high school and had married. The majority of schizophrenic patients perform poorly in school, rarely date, have few friends, are socially isolated, and are rarely married (65, 88).

K.K.'s prognosis is probably in the middle of the spectrum. He will probably not recover sufficient functional abilities to live independently and be gainfully employed, but he may do well in a structured living and work setting such as a board and care home and workshop. Prognosis depends not upon the illness or subtype of schizophrenia, but rather on the patient's other assets such as premorbid personality, intelligence, genetic background, social and family supports, and physical factors such as beauty. The difference between good and poor prognosis is the difference in the patient's premorbid condition and how he is prepared to handle life with schizophrenia, which is related to how he might handle life without schizophrenia (71).

3. Describe the subtypes of schizophrenia.

Many classification systems have been proposed for schizophrenia, based upon symptomatology, presumed etiology, and premorbid condition. The most recently proposed classification incorporates only the useful parts of previous attempts, eliminating much past confusion. In the class of schizophrenia, which includes all those chronic illnesses of psychotic proportions, the following three categories have been identified (71):

A. Chronic intermittent Schizophrenia — This illness is characterized by at least a six month history of intermittent episodes of acute exacerbation and prolonged remission, but at all times the patient shows difficulty in his anxiety management, interpersonal relationships, and failure in historicity. The category includes both the chronic differentiated schizophrenias, which show a similar symptom pattern during acute exacerbations, and the chronic undifferentiated schizophrenias, which show varied symptom complexes during acute exacerbations.

B. Chronic Latent Schizophrenia — This illness is characterized by patients who do not show major psychotic symptoms during exacerbation, but exhibit the three disabilities of function previously mentioned. The natural history of their problems is life-long and there are periods of exacerbation and remission.

C. Chronic Paranoid Schizophrenia — This illness is characterized by a primarily paranoid approach to the world and to thinking, without evidence of other overt psychotic symptoms. The three chronic disabilities of function are again present, accompanied by the primary symptom of paranoid thought processes.

4. List the target symptoms of schizophrenia present in this patient. Which ones respond well to drug treatment? How long will it take for the patient to respond to therapy?

K.K. on this admission shows the following schizophrenic target symptoms: agitation, delusions, loose associations, paranoid ideation manifested by suspiciousness and guarding, concrete thinking, and poor judgment and insight.

Except for the delusional systems and paranoid ideation of long duration which have been well encapsulated within the personality, the majority of identified target symptoms should respond to neuroleptic drugs. Table I lists common schizophrenic target symptoms which are useful for the regular assessment of drug response.

Evidence of neuroleptic response may take several weeks. In a study of 44 schizophrenic patients, chlorpromazine in daily doses averaging 475 mg had no more antipsychotic effect than placebo during the first five days of treatment (45). Although sedation is an immediate effect to which tolerance develops, the onset of antipsychotic effect becomes noticeable during the second week of therapy and significant at three weeks (1, 73). Response can be hastened by aggressive high dose therapy and/or parenteral administration of the potent neuroleptic drugs (see Question 11).

5. What is the role of drug therapy in the total treatment plan for schizophrenia? What is the therapeutic endpoint for the treatment of K.K.'s acute exacerbation? What are the goals of maintenance therapy?

Neuroleptic drugs do not alter the natural course of schizophrenia, but at best they will ameliorate psychotic symptoms during acute exacerbation and suppress acute symptoms during maintenance therapy. The neuroleptic drugs have specific antipsychotic effects in reducing and often eliminating psychotic symptoms (94). In reviewing the basic disabilities of function in schizophrenia (see Question 1), it can be seen that amelioration of psychotic symptoms corrects only one aspect of the disorder. Neuroleptic drugs cannot correct difficulties in the interpersonal relationships and the inability to use personal experiences in making judgments and directing behavior. Management of these disabilities requires a supportive reality-based therapist and social services to aid in coping with day-to-day living, work, and financial matters. Thus, drug therapy is a vital part of a treatment program for a schizophrenic patient, but it is only one part of a total treatment plan.

Table I
COMMON TARGET SYMPTOMS OF SCHIZOPHRENIA

loose associations	lack of insight
bizarre behavior	poor judgment
delusions	concrete thinking
hallucinations	distractibility
inappropriate affect	insomnia
bizarre or disheveled	suspiciousness
appearance	

The therapeutic endpoint for K.K.'s neuroleptic drug therapy during this acute exacerbation is amelioration of the target symptoms (see Question 4). With these symptoms under control, other treatment modalities can be mobilized to provide a more stable work and living situation following discharge.

The therapeutic goal for maintenance neuroleptic therapy after discharge is to maintain K.K. free of psychotic symptoms and prolong the remission period. Supportive care and a more stable work* and living situation, along with neuroleptic drug therapy, should break the present pattern of frequent psychotic exacerbations as evidenced by past psychiatric hospitalizations.

6. Identify the common chemical classes of neuroleptic drugs available in the U.S. and comment on the major differences between them.

Several new chemical classes of neuroleptic drugs have been introduced to the U.S. market. Table II lists the more commonly used neuroleptic drugs and their chemical classification. Some general comments can be made regarding differences among the classes of drugs. These will help to place the newer drugs in proper perspective relative to the phenothiazines.

A. *Phenothiazines:* The oldest, most diverse and best understood neuroleptic drugs are the phenothiazines. Chlorpromazine has been traditionally used as the standard neuroleptic drug to which newer agents are compared. Three major subclasses of phenothiazines have been identified (aliphatic, piperidine, and piperazine) whose differences in adverse effects are described in Question 8.

B. *Thioxanthenes:* The thioxanthenes, best represented today by thiothixene, have no clinically significant differences from the phenothiazines (97). Because the chemical difference is so slight between the two classes, adverse effects including pigmentation are similar to phenothiazines (8, 96). Thioxanthenes are another effective neuroleptic drug class which offers no advantages over previously available agents.

C. *Butyrophenones:* The butyrophenones, represented at present by haloperidol, are chemically very distinct from the phenothiazines and differ significantly in their adverse effects. The butyrophenones offer the best treatment alternative for patients who are phenothiazine resistant, allergic, or suffer from long-term phenothiazine or thioxanthene pigmentary effects (10). Haloperidol's lack of sedation, anticholinergic and cardiovascular effects make it a useful first choice for patients in whom these effects are contraindicated (see Question 8).

D. *Dibenzoxazepines:* Loxapine, a relatively new neuroleptic in the United States, is the first neuroleptic introduced from this class. Although structurally different from phenothiazines, the piperazine side chain is a prominent feature. Not surprisingly, loxapine in most aspects is very similar to the piperazine phenothiazines and as yet offers no clinically useful advantage over previously available neuroleptic drugs (95, 101).

E. *Dihydroindolones:* Molindone is the first neuroleptic from this class brought to market in the United States. Interest in this new class of neuroleptic drugs is high, because there is no clear chemical similarity to the phenothiazines. In fact, molindone is structurally closer to reserpine. At present there is no evidence to show a clinically useful difference in molindone, since it most closely resembles piperazine phenothiazines (11). But because of chemical uniqueness, the dihydroindolones hold the greatest promise for clinically significant unique properties in the future.

7. Describe the antipsychotic mechanism of action of neuroleptic drugs.

Although the exact mechanism of antipsychotic activity of neuroleptic drugs has not been identified, much data are accumulating to suggest central post-synaptic dopaminergic blockade as the mechanism of action (94). It has been shown that the antipsychotic, extrapyramidal and antiemetic effects of neuroleptic

Table II
CLASSIFICATION OF NEUROLEPTIC DRUGS

Phenothiazines	
Aliphatic	
chlorpromazine	(Thorazine)
Piperidine	
thioridazine	(Mellaril)
Piperazine	
trifluoperazine	(Stelazine)
fluphenazine	(Prolixin)
Thioxanthenes	
thiothixene	(Navane)
Butyrophenones	
haloperidol	(Haldol)
Dibenzoxazepines	
loxapine	(Loxitane)
Dihydroindolones	
molindone	(Moban)

drugs are related to their interaction with central dopaminergic receptors. It is proposed, although not yet well established, that two different dopaminergic systems are affected by neuroleptic drugs: a nigro-neostriatal system, which might be the physiological substrate for the extrapyramidal effects, and a mesolimbic system, which might be responsible for the antipsychotic effect (104). Other evidence suggests that the corpus striatum, in addition to a motor regulatory function, has a function in the integration of more complicated forms of behavior, and thus may be the site of neuroleptic antipsychotic activity (104). An understanding of the neuroleptic drugs' effects on neurotransmitters is useful in explaining and predicting many clinical effects of neuroleptic drugs (98).

8. Based upon K.K.'s past history and presenting symptoms, what would be the neuroleptic of choice?

A drug such as trifluoperazine (Stelazine) would be the most appropriate choice. The reasons for this choice can be found in the following discussion.

For any class of drugs, the following three factors must be taken into consideration when choosing the most appropriate drug for a given patient: efficacy differences, relative differences in adverse effects, and past history of response.

A. *Efficacy:* Among all the commonly used neuroleptic drugs listed in Table II, there is no significant difference in their antipsychotic effect when given in equivalent doses. Chlorpromazine, thioridazine, fluphenazine, and haloperidol are all equally effective in ameliorating psychotic symptoms. Thus, differences in efficacy do not play any part in choosing a drug for a given patient (21, 41, 48, 60).

B. *Adverse Effects:* The major determinant initially in choosing a neuroleptic drug is the differences in their adverse effects. Although most neuroleptic drugs have the same adverse effects, the incidence varies greatly among individual drugs. Thus, to some degree it is possible to tailor the drug to the patient. Table III lists the differences in incidence of common adverse effects of neuroleptic drugs. As can be seen, some adverse effects can be used clinically, while others can be avoided. If sedation is desirable because a patient is very agitated or is not sleeping, then either chlorpromazine or thioridazine would be a logical choice. In a patient with a past history of severe extrapyramidal effects, thioridazine might be most appropriate. For the patient with chronic constipation, prostatic hypertrophy, or glaucoma, thioridazine is best avoided because of its significant anticholinergic effects. Patients who will require high dose long-term therapy should be given a piperazine phenothiazine or haloperidol because of their low incidence of pigmentary effects.

However, all drugs posses some disadvantages with respect to their adverse effects. This explains why several neuroleptic drugs are widely used. The drug, with its adverse effects, must be tailored to the patient based upon presenting symptomatology and significant preexisting medical conditions.

C. *Past History of Response:* Determining a patient's past history of neuroleptic response is an important variable in choosing a drug to restart therapy. The patient who complains about chlorpromazine slowing him down and making him groggy would not be a good candidate for chlorpromazine again. There may often be no pharmacological basis for patients' attitudes toward neuroleptic drugs, but a positive or negative attitude will significantly affect patient compliance.

The choice of neuroleptic for K.K. requires matching the drug and its side effects to the clinical symptomatology present, as well as considering his past neuroleptic drug history. Drugs with a moderate or high degree of sedation are not necessary since K.K. is not agitated or having difficulty sleeping, and thus sedation would be an undesirable effect. Of the less sedating neuroleptic drugs, an appropriate choice would be trifluoperazine since he has taken it in the past, has no memory of adverse effects, and apparently responded to it.

K.K. was started on trifluoperazine 10 mg bid, which was eventually titrated to 40 mg bid over two weeks with good clinical response apparent at the end of the five weeks.

Table III
RELATIVE INCIDENCE OF NEUROLEPTIC ADVERSE EFFECTS

	Sedation	Extra-pyramidal	Anti-cholinergic	Cardio-vascular	Pigmentation
chlorpromazine	high	mod	mod	high	high
thioridazine	high	low	high	high	high
trifluoperazine	low	high	low	low	low
fluphenazine	low	high	low	low	low
thiothixene	low	high	low	low	low
haloperidol	very low	very high	very low	very low	none

CASE HISTORY B.H.

B.H., a 25-year-old single unemployed, male, presently living with his parents, was involuntarily hospitalized on the acute psychiatric ward because his parents could no longer handle his worsening agitation, violent outbursts, and bizarre behavior at home. (Admission date September 1974).

History of Present Illness: In 1970 he left home and went to San Francisco to live for one year. Upon returning home, his parents noted unusual behavior and thoughts. The patient resented people and school, complained of auditory hallucinations, severe insomnia, and was hostile without reason. After six months at home, he improved somewhat but became socially withdrawn. Over the next 2-3 years, he lost all contact with friends, his bizarre behavior continued and ultimately he dropped out of college. Over the last few weeks prior to admission the patient began hearing frightening voices coming from outside his head. "They are mad at me, oppressing me, laughing at me, and making plans against me." The patient felt his own thoughts had been pushed out by voices which had assumed control of him. He is depressed because the voices have taken over, and he has lost all his energy. The patient denies suicidal ideation and recent use of drugs.

Previous Illnesses: He was hospitalized at a private psychiatric facility in 1971 and again in 1972 and was diagnosed schizophrenic. He eloped both times and had no follow-up care.

Family History: There is no family history of mental illness.

Personal History: He is the younger of two children and has a 30-year-old sister. His childhood was apparently normal, although his parents state that he had few friends and dated infrequently during adolescence. He used LSD and marijuana during high school. He was an above average student and attended a prominent Southern California college for two years. He has never been employed.

Physical Exam on Admission: The physical examination is unremarkable.

Mental Status Exam on Admission: This well-groomed 25-year-old male sat slumped in his chair during the interview. He shows depressed affect which is appropriate to thought content. His associations are tight. He denies delusions and suicidal ideation. His thought content centers on auditory hallucinations. His insight and judgment are fair. Oriented x 3.

Provisional Diagnosis: Schizophrenia, acute exacerbation.

9. How would a differential diagnosis be made between amphetamine psychosis and an acute schizophrenic exacerbation?

Although B.H. denies recent drug use before admission, there is a past history of this and the presenting clinical picture is consistent with one type of amphetamine psychosis. An acute, toxic amphetamine psychosis following one or two extremely large doses is not generally confused with schizophrenia because of the organic component which is present — delirium, disorientation, confusion and visual hallucinations. It is the non-toxic amphetamine psychosis, occurring with prolonged amphetamine usage, that can resemble schizophrenia. The subtle differences between non-toxic amphetamine psychosis and paranoid schizophrenia are that the former often lacks the thought disorders and affective components typically found in schizophrenia (4, 93, 94).

To differentiate between amphetamine psychosis and schizophrenic exacerbation in this case is difficult, although B.H.'s premorbid personality and past psychiatric hospitalizations seem to suggest schizophrenia. For amphetamine use to cause all the past and present difficulties., B.H. would have had to use large doses over a very long period of time. His hospital course and subsequent outpatient aftercare will verify the correct diagnosis.

10. What would be the neuroleptic of choice for B.H.?

B.H.'s two major target symptoms, auditory hallucinations and withdrawn behavior, should respond well to neuroleptic drug therapy. The depressed affect is directly related to the presence of the voices, because he feels they have gained control over him. The outbursts and bizarre behavior at home can also be viewed as an attempt to handle the voices. Since there is no evidence of outbursts or agitation on admission, a sedating neuroleptic is not indicated. Two hospitalizations over a three year period without follow-up care suggest B.H. is functional while living at home between acute exacerbations. For these reasons, the very limited target symptoms should respond to rapid high-dose neuroleptic therapy. Thus, a drug like haloperidol would be an appropriate choice.

11. Should B.H.'s neuroleptic be administered intramuscularly or orally?

Rapid parenteral neuroleptic drug therapy is certainly indicated for B.H. He is young, has no medical contraindications and has target symptoms which should respond to aggressive drug treatment. Although he could do quite well with less aggressive oral neuroleptic therapy, he would need to remain hospitalized for an extended period of time. A NIMH Collaborative Study utilizing seven public mental hospitals studied high dose chlorpromazine therapy (79). The results indicated that high dose (2000 mg daily) was significantly more effective than low dose (300 mg daily) in chronic schizophrenic patients under 40 years old with less than ten years of hospitalization. More recently, the use of high doses of the more potent neuroleptics has been reported to promote rapid improvement in decompensated schizophrenic patients (35). Using fluphenazine hydrochloride as an example, the patient is started on 10-20 mg orally the first day and the fluphenazine is increased by 10-20 mg increments daily or every other day. Typical effective doses are 50-100 mg daily. Another method of rapid tranquilization calls for administering neuroleptic drugs on a one to two hourly basis in an attempt to obtain an initial stage of control of psychotic behavior within the first six hours of treatment (78). For rapid control of symptoms of acute schizophrenia parenteral haloperidol 2 or 5 mg intramuscularly (IM) every thirty minutes for four doses followed by oral haloperidol resulted in maximal efficacy as compared to lower doses or to chlorpromazine 25 mg IM at the same intervals (82). Injectable haloperidol 5 mg every 6-8 hours is equivalent to injectable chlorpromazine 50 mg every 6-8 hours in highly agitated, acute psychotic patients, indicating the sedative effects are not essential for treating agitated patients (87).

B.H. should respond rapidly to high dose therapy with the potent neuroleptics. High dose neuroleptic therapy for B.H. is more important than the route of therapy chosen. An appropriate initial dose for B.H. would be haloperidol 5 mg IM every two hours to a maximum daily dosage of 40-50 mg or significant adverse effects, then conversion to oral haloperidol.

12. After one day of haloperidol 5 mg IM every two hours for seven doses followed by two weeks of haloperidol 30 mg po bid, B.H. continued to be isolated, affect was blunted, and now was grandiose. He denied the presence of voices, claiming they had never been present. The patient stated he was in the hospital because he had been working hard of a vital research project and insisted there was nothing wrong with him at all. His only complaints were continued initial insomnia and nervousness during the day.

What is the maximum daily dose for haloperidol? Should the dosage continue to be increased? If so, by how much? When should haloperidol be abandoned and another neuroleptic drug begun?

Although the FDA has set the maximum daily dose of haloperidol at 100 mg (70), there are no absolute daily maximum dosages for any neuroleptic drug. B.H.'s remaining target symptoms are ones which are generally slow to show response or are not responsive at all. While the haloperidol dosage could be further increased toward 80-100 mg daily, only little additional response should be expected. Denial of past symptoms

following remission is not uncommon in insightful patients and is not a sign of worsening. If acute symptoms were still present following several weeks of 80-100 mg daily of haloperidol, it would be appropriate to consider substituting another neuroleptic. B.H. does not exhibit acute symptomatology now, and he should remain on his present dosage of haloperidol. Table IV lists common dosage ranges for acute and maintenance doses of neuroleptic drugs. When the maximum dosage (as listed in Table IV) for acute psychotic episodes has been used with little or no response after several weeks, another neuroleptic drug should be substituted.

13. List the advantages and disadvantages of once-daily bedtime dosing of neuroleptic drugs.

Once-daily bedtime dosing of neuroleptic drugs is becoming more common and should be encouraged (9, 34, 97). Advantages of this dosing pattern as compared to divided dosage include:

a. Enhanced compliance.
b. Reduced adverse effects.
c. Reduced cost.
d. Elimination of need for a hypnotic.
e. Reduced drug administration time and costs.

There are some disadvantages of once-daily bedtime dosing as compared to a divided dosage schedule:

a. Some patients require the daytime sedative properties of neuroleptics.
b. Some patients on high doses refuse to ingest many tablets at once.
c. Some patients remain convinced they need their "tranquilizer" during the daytime also.
d. Haloperidol, specifically, may interfere with the onset of sleep and should thus be given in the morning (10).
e. Geriatric patients, with compromised metabolism, may not be able to tolerate once-daily dosing.

In reality, when those patients described under disadvantages are excluded, there remain the vast majority of patients taking neuroleptic drugs who could significantly benefit from once-daily bedtime therapy.

Table IV
COMMON NEUROLEPTIC DOSES

	Acute Dose mg/day	Maintenance Dose mg/day
chlorpromazine	400 - 1000	200 - 800
thioridazine	400 - 800	200 - 800
trifluoperazine	20 - 100	10 - 40
fluphenazine	20 - 80	10 - 40
thiothixene	20 - 100	10 - 40
haloperidol	20 - 100	10 - 40
loxapine	50 - 200	20 - 80
molindone	50 - 200	20 - 80

14. Eleven weeks after admission, B.H. was discharged from the hospital. He continued to deny the symptoms which required his hospitalization, claiming he only had some family misunderstandings. His affect was only slightly blunted. Isolation and withdrawal from other patients and strangers continued but was not present with staff members. The discharge plan included board and care home placement, a slow push into activities to avoid a fail situation, and haloperidol 40 mg bid.

How long will B.H. need to remain on neuroleptic drug therapy?

The need for long-term maintenance neuroleptic therapy for chronic schizophrenic patients is well established (16, 37, 61, 80). Significantly higher incidences of psychotic exacerbations appear in patients whose neuroleptic therapy is terminated than in patients on maintenance therapy. However this evidence is primarily based on studies of 4-8 month duration and provides few guidelines for long-term maintenance therapy of several years or even decades. One study of 8 years duration did show a significant difference with chlorpromazine after four years, but noted that the effect of maintenance therapy seems to decrease with the passage of time (37). Although maintenance neuroleptic therapy consistently shows significant prolongation of symptom remission, there remains up to one-half of the patients studied who showed no exacerbation of psychotic symptoms after four to eight months off drugs. Unfortunately, no reliable predictors of relapse can distinguish between patients who will maintain remission and those who will relapse (61, 84).

The value of maintenance neuroleptic therapy can also be assessed in terms of schizophrenic subtypes and prognosis groups (Questions 2, 3). The chronic latent schizophrenic will probably not benefit greatly from neuroleptic maintenance therapy. Also, extremely poor prognosis and extremely good prognosis schizophrenic patients will not benefit greatly. Long-term maintenance therapy is of greatest benefit to the chronic intermittent schizophrenic patient with a fair to good prognosis (68, 71).

B.H. probably fits best into the category of chronic intermittent schizophrenia with a good prognosis and should significantly benefit from maintenance haloperidol therapy. The dosage should be gradually reduced over several months to a maintenance level of about 20 mg daily. Drug holidays should be instituted yearly (Question 43), and an extended drug holiday might be tried if no signs of relapse are evident after two or three years of maintenance therapy.

15. M.T., a 42-year-old female, is referred to the pharmacist in the community mental health center for evaluation of her drug therapy. The patient was recently discharged from a state mental hospital after twelve years on a back ward for chronic schizophrenic patients. She was discharged with the following medications, which she has been maintained on for the past three years: trifluoperazine 5 mg qid; thiothixene 10 mg bid; thioridazine 50 mg tid; chloral hydrate 1000 mg hs; D.O.S.S. 100 mg hs.

Comment on the appropriateness of M.T.'s drug regimen.

M.T.'s drug therapy is clearly not optimal. Multiple neuroleptic drugs are often used to favorably influence efficacy and adverse effects. In long-term institutional facilities such as state mental hospitals or correctional facilities, such polypharmacy is often the result of adding another drug for each new problem encountered without reviewing those already in use and eliminating unnecessary ones. M.T.'s multiple neuroleptic drug therapy and impossible dosing schedules deserve correction. First, there is no evidence available to suggest that several neuroleptic drugs are better than one if equivalent doses are used (18, 40, 72). Nevertheless, a frequent justification for combinations is that adverse effects will be minimized. A close look at neuroleptic pharmacology will not verify such an assumption. Using M.T. as an example, the common assumption is that there is less potential for extrapyramidal effects to occur with her present therapy compared to an equivalent dose of trifluoperazine alone. Although potentially true, it is only true because of thioridazine's high inherent anticholinergic effect. It would be pharmacologically more correct, however, to use an anticholinergic agent to reduce potential extrapyramidal effects rather than to use a drug with many effects only for its anticholinergic activity (98). The use of one neuroleptic also allows the best flexibility for future dosage adjustments and simplifies the management of severe adverse effects or toxic manifestations should they occur.

Second, the dosing schedules of qd, bid, tid and qid will virtually assure noncompliance. Simplification of M.T.'s drug therapy should consist of substituting one neuroleptic in equivalent dosage for the previous three neuroleptic drugs. The choice of neuroleptic depends upon the degree of sedation desired. If the neuroleptic is given once daily at bedtime, the chloral hydrate can be withdrawn. The anticholinergic activity of the neuroleptic chosen should be assessed to determine if the D.O.S.S. will continue to be needed. Thus, M.T. can be switched from the present inappropriate drug therapy to one neuroleptic dosed at bedtime and possibly some D.O.S.S. then as well.

Case History (N.O.)

N.O., a 27-year-old female, was admitted to a psychiatric ward with an acute schizophrenic episode. Past history reveals three previous hospitalizations over the last four years. Her outpatient medication compliance is poor, and insight into her illness is poor. The patient attends outpatient follow-up only if individual therapy sessions are continued. During this hospitalization, she was placed on haloperidol, and she responded well to 20 mg bid after three weeks. The treatment team now decides this patient should be tried on the long-acting fluphenazine for outpatient follow-up.

16. What factors make this patient a good candidate for depot fluphenazine therapy?

Several factors make N.O. a potentially good candidate for a long-acting fluphenazine preparation. Her high frequency of psychotic episodes clearly suggests the need for maintenance neuroleptic therapy, and her past history of noncompliance to medication on an outpatient basis makes oral medication a poor choice. Her positive response to continued individual contacts can be coordinated with scheduled injection appointments which will favorably influence compliance. Lastly, her poor insight into her illness contributes to her noncompliance of oral medication. Patients who cannot understand the need for their medication and are aware only of adverse effects often comply poorly.

The only other indication for long-acting fluphenazine, not present in N.O., is for patients who may not absorb or metabolize neuroleptic drugs which are administered orally. Up to 40% of chronic drug-refractory schizophrenics treated with oral chlorpromazine have low serum levels, and many respond when given parenteral neuroleptics (2, 30, 69). Although still inconclusive, some evidence for the above has been suggested as being due to either induction of hepatic enzymes (22) or significant metabolism within the gastrointestinal tract (29). Because on a practical basis these patients cannot be given parenteral hydrochloride preparations of neuroleptics for long-term therapy, the long-acting fluphenazine is clearly indicated.

17. Of the two preparations available, fluphenazine enanthate and fluphenazine decanoate, which is the better choice for N.O.?

The decanoate ester of fluphenazine offers several advantages over the enanthate, and thus should be the only preparation used. The two preparations are identical in terms of efficacy, just as are all the other neuroleptics. The differences of clinical significance are duration of effect and incidence of extrapyramidal effects. By comparing the peak in fluphenazine-induced EEG changes, it has been shown that the enanthate peaks at one week while the decanoate ester peaks at two weeks (51). A later study demonstrated the duration of clinical effect of decanoate to be about two weeks longer than that of the enanthate ester (102). Enough evidence has accumulated to also state that the decanoate ester has a significantly lower incidence of extrapyramidal effects when compared to the enanthate (44).

Because of these two advantages, the decanoate ester of fluphenazine should be used whenever a long-acting injectable neuroleptic is desired.

18. How should the conversion be made from oral to parenteral depot fluphenazine in this patient? Is there a conversion ratio?

There is no exact conversion factor between oral fluphenazine and the long-acting injections. The dosage of a long-acting fluphenazine preparation is best estimated as if it were a separate drug (44).

Formulae for conversion exist in the literature, but all suffer from many questionable assumptions. One such formula for fluphenazine enanthate is (49):

1) Multiply the daily dose of fluphenazine or its equivalent by the dosing interval intended.
2) Divide by 4 (assume that parenteral fluphenazine is four times more potent than oral).
3) Reduce by one-third (assume that in 1-2 days a slight excess of fluphenazine will be released before a steady lower plateau occurs and to avoid possible exacerbations of extrapyramidal effects).

For example: For oral fluphenazine 10 mg daily,

fluphenazine enanthate =

$$\frac{10 \times 14}{4} - \frac{1}{3}\frac{10 \times 14}{4} = 25 \text{ mg approximately.}$$

A practical, useful conversion this author developed from extensive clinical use of the long-acting fluphenazine is to take the daily dose of oral fluphenazine or its equivalent, increase it to the next 0.5 cc amount of fluphenazine decanoate, and give that amount weekly or every other week. This approach is based on the facts that 20 mg - 80 mg of fluphenazine orally is needed for treatment of an acute psychotic episode, and that the typical dosage range for fluphenazine decanoate is 25 mg - 100 mg. N.O. is taking 40 mg daily of haloperidol, which is essentially equal to 40 mg daily of fluphenazine (Table V). Fluphenazine decanoate is available as 25 mg per cc, so N.O. should receive 50 mg of fluphenazine decanoate weekly.

Table V
APPROXIMATE EQUIVALENT NEUROLEPTIC DOSES

chlorpromazine	100
thioridazine	100
trifluoperazine	5
fluphenazine	2
thiothixene	5
haloperidol	2
loxapine	10
molindone	10

The conversion of N.O. from haloperidol to fluphenazine decanoate is not simply a matter of stopping one drug and starting the other. The pharmacologic activity of fluphenazine decanoate is slow in onset (51), and thus the oral neuroleptic should be slowly tapered and discontinued after the injection is given. Patients just resolving after an acute psychotic episode may decompensate if the oral neuroleptic is discontinued the day the injection is given. The literature offers little help in defining an appropriate transition period. In this author's experience, an appropriate transition for N.O. would be to give 50 mg of fluphenazine decanoate on day one, reduce the haloperidol in half on day three, and discontinue the haloperidol and give the second injection of fluphenazine decanoate 50 mg on day seven. The dosing interval can then be lengthened depending upon the patient's continued response. Acute schizophrenic patients need more frequent injections than do chronic schizophrenic patients (43). In other words, the weekly dosing interval for N.O. can be slowly lengthened to every two weeks and then possibly to every three weeks as N.O. moves toward chronic maintenance therapy.

19. Could fluphenazine decanoate have been used for treatment of N.O.'s acute psychotic episode?

While the efficacy of long-acting fluphenazines for chronic maintenance therapy of psychosis is widely accepted, their usefulness in the treatment of acute psychotic episodes is not as well established. Fluphenazine enanthate was included in a list of neuroleptics to be used in high dosage for rapid "loading" of decompensated schizophrenic patients. One case of clinical efficacy is described where fluphenazine enanthate 50 mg IM every other day was added to 100 mg daily of oral fluphenazine (35). Another study suggests fluphenazine enanthate, alone or combined with another oral neuroleptic during the acute psychotic episode, is more effective than chlorpromazine alone (19). Although difference in efficacy can be attributed to inequivalent doses, the study does suggest that fluphenazine enanthate is effective in the treatment of acute psychoses.

Despite these reports, the use of long-acting fluphenazine for treatment of acute psychotic episodes cannot be recommended. Philosophically, it makes little sense to use a long-acting preparation when initial neuroleptic therapy requires dosage titration. Dosage flexibility is sacrificed and, if toxicity occurs, the effects remain for days and often weeks.

One case of delayed severe extrapyramidal disturbance following frequent depot fluphenazine administration has been reported (105). A 28-year-old male was given 25 mg IM of fluphenazine enanthate three times per week for eight doses in addition to chlorpromazine 200 mg orally bid and benztropine 4 mg IM three times

per week. The patient was then discharged and took no more medication. Five days after discharge he became very weak and was hospitalized two days later, mute and immobile. Cogwheel rigidity and dystonias were treated vigorously with benztropine, but 24 days were required for full resolution of extrapyramidal effects. Similar cases have been experienced by this author and other clinicians.

Although the depot fluphenazines may be efficacious for acute psychotic episodes, it does not seem appropriate to chose them over oral or intramuscular hydrochloride preparations of neuroleptic drugs. The latter are equally effective, allow greater flexibility in dosage titration, and do not risk delayed severe extrapyramidal effects.

Case History (C.B.)

C.B., a 26-year-old male, came to the psychiatric outpatient clinic complaining of insomnia and auditory hallucinations of one week's duration. He had been maintained as an outpatient for nine months after his last psychotic episode, but he has been off neuroleptic medication for the past two months at his own insistence. The decision is made to restart trifluoperazine therapy. Trifluoperazine HCl 5 mg IM is given, with a prescription for 10 mg po tid. Two hours later, the patient returns to the clinic complaining of his neck being bent to the right side and so stiff that he cannot straighten it. He states he had not yet taken a tablet.

20. Identify this neuroleptic adverse effect.

This adverse effect should be identified as torticollis, a dystonic reaction involving the muscles of the neck unilaterally. Acute dystonic reactions are of sudden onset and usually take place within 24 to 48 hours from the start of medication. The incidence is greater in younger people and in males (23, 39). In a study of drug-induced extrapyramidal reactions in which 3,775 patients who had received phenothiazines a minimum of three months were surveyed (7), dystonias occurred in 2.3%. The trifluoromethyl halogen present in some piperazine phenothiazines caused the greatest incidence of dystonia. The male-female ratio was 2:1 and 90%developed within the first 4.5 days of therapy.

A later study of 1,152 psychiatric inpatients who received a phenothiazine, thioxanthene, or a butyrophenone reported a 10.1% incidence of dystonia (100). Torticollis was the most frequent, followed in order by swollen tongue, trismus, oculogyric crisis and opisthotonus. Haloperidol was most frequently associated with dystonia followed by the piperazine phenothiazines, chlorpromazine and thioridazine. The higher incidence of dystonia (10.1%) in the most recent survey was attributed to the introduction of haloperidol and fluphenazine enanthate.

21. What is the best treatment for neuroleptic-induced dystonia?

Parenteral anticholinergic agents are the most efficacious and rational treatment for neuroleptic-induced dystonias. Of all the extrapyramidal effects, dystonias are most responsive to treatment. Improvement is observed within ten minutes, and peak effects occur in 30 minutes (5, 7, 92).

The choice of intravenous (IV) versus intramuscular (IM) anticholinergic therapy is difficult due to the lack of good clinical data. Response to the treatment of post encephalitis oculogyric crisis with benztropine methanesulfonate occurred within 15 minutes following IV therapy and 30 minutes following IM therapy (76). Diphenhydramine is equally effective in the treatment of acute dystonic reactions.

Methylphenidate has also been suggested as an effective treatment for dystonia. One case of phenothiazine-induced torticollis and truncal torsion responded to methylphenidate 20 mg IV and another case of severe torticollis responded to methylphenidate 50 mg IV within 3-4 minutes (38).

For C.B., optimal treatment of his dystonia would be either benztropine 2 mg IM or diphenhydramine 50 mg IM, which can be repeated once after 30 minutes if full response is not achieved. His dystonic reaction does not contraindicate the continued use of trifluoperazine, but an oral anticholinergic agent should be added.

Case History (E.B.)

E.B., a 21-year-old male, walked into the outpatient psychiatric clinic asking for medication. He claims to have just moved to California from Texas, has not been taking neuroleptic drugs for eight months, but wishes to start therapy again. He states he formerly took three thiothixene capsules daily for several months, but stopped because "they slowed me down." In the past he was on thioridazine ("can't get it on with girls"), chlorpromazine ("makes me too fuzzy-headed"), and haloperidol ("makes me jittery"). The patient was last hospitalized one year ago for an acute psychotic episode, and had been hospitalized three prior times during a two year period. The decision was made to start the patient on trifluoperazine 5 mg bid for several days, then titrate the dosage upward depending on adverse effects.

22. What factors make E.B. a good candidate for prophylactic antiparkinsonian agents?

The issue of prophylactic anticholinergic agents has received much attention in the literature, yet clinicians still vary greatly in their clinical use of these agents. It has been clearly established that after three months of neuroleptic therapy, the vast majority of patients do not need anticholinergic agents. One study of 403 patients

withdrawn from antiparkinson agents showed 82% did well without them (64), and similar studies show that the majority of patients do not need antiparkinson drugs (32, 75). The remaining area of controversy is the initial three months of therapy (33, 85, 97).

For E.B., there are several factors which justify initial antiparkinson prophylaxis with trifluoperazine therapy. First, E.B. has experienced extrapyramidal effects in the past and discontinued the thiothixene because of adverse effects. A study of why schizophrenics are reluctant, and thus noncompliant, with medication revealed that 89% of the noncompliant patients experienced extrapyramidal effects as compared to only 20% of the compliant patients. The overall conclusion was that reluctance to take neuroleptic medication was significantly associated with extrapyramidal effects, most notably akathisia (103). Second, E.B. has experienced a variety of significant neuroleptic adverse effects, and he would thus be more likely to discontinue therapy if he experiences a significant adverse effect from trifluoperazine. Third, E.B. is being started on trifluoperazine, which has a high incidence of extrapyramidal effects (Table III), particularly dystonias and akathisia. Prophylactic antiparkinson coverage would not be indicated if he were being started on chlorpromazine or thioridazine. Because of the three factors identified above, E.B. should be given prophylactic anticholinergic coverage to maximize the possibility of compliance. Benztropine 2 mg daily is sufficient. It will not significantly add to peripheral anticholinergic effects and should be discontinued after three months if no extrapyramidal effects occur.

23. Explain the rationale for using anticholinergic agents to treat neuroleptic-induced extrapyramidal disorders.

Extrapyramidal effects are a result of postsynaptic dopaminergic blockade by neuroleptics in the corpus striatum (94). A simplified model of the corpus striatum has been described which focuses on the relative influences of striatal cholinergic and dopaminergic systems and how neuroleptic drugs alter these systems (98). Normal motor activity depends upon a balance between the striatal cholinergic and dopaminergic systems. Neuroleptic drugs upset the balance by diminishing dopaminergic activity in the striatum, causing a net cholinergic excess which is clinically manifest as extrapyramidal effects. Theoretically, the balance could be restored by levodopa, just as it is given in Parkinson's disease to restore balance by replacing deficient dopamine (55). Clinical studies, however, have shown levodopa to be ineffective in reversing neuroleptic-induced extrapyramidal effects (15, 109) only because peripheral adverse effects prevent the administration of the large doses needed to overcome neuroleptic blockade of striatal dopaminergic receptors.

Because the diminished dopaminergic activity in the striatum cannot be restored in neuroleptic-induced parkinsonism, the only treatment alternative is to restore the balance by diminishing the cholinergic influence. This alternative is the pharmacological basis for treating neuroleptic-induced extrapyramidal effects with centrally active anticholinergic drugs such as trihexyphenidyl and benztropine. Although both the dopaminergic and cholinergic striatal systems are diminished, normal striatal function can be restored if the two systems are balanced (98).

24. Why do neuroleptic drugs differ in their ability to cause extrapyramidal effects, and why is the incidence of extrapyramidal effects not directly dose related?

As shown in Table III, the individual neuroleptic drugs differ in their propensity for causing extrapyramidal side effects. An explanation for this variation was readily available once the inherent anticholinergic activity of neuroleptic drugs was quantified. It has been suggested that all neuroleptic drugs have about the same tendency to elicit extrapyramidal effects by virtue of their striatal dopaminergic receptor blockade, but they differ in incidence of extrapyramidal effects only because they differ in inherent anticholinergic activity (94). When the anticholinergic and extrapyramidal effects in Table III are compared, an inverse relationship is noted. Haloperidol causes a high incidence of extrapyramidal effects because it has low inherent anticholinergic activity. Thioridazine is associated with a low incidence of extrapyramidal effects because it is also a potent anticholinergic agent.

As high dose therapy became acceptable treatment for some patients, practitioners noted that the incidence of extrapyramidal effects was not strictly dose related. When ten patients who were previously refractory to treatment were given high doses of fluphenazine (300-1200 mg daily) the incidence and severity of extrapyramidal effects was no worse than in patients receiving 15-20 mg of fluphenazine daily (83). The same paper reviewed several other studies, particularly French studies, which also reported that the incidence of extrapyramidal effects was virtually the same with 20 mg as with greater than 100 mg daily. A review of haloperidol indicates that the incidence of extrapyramidal effects may in fact be less with high dose therapy than with low or moderate dose therapy (10). An explanation of this seemingly surprising fact is simplified when the striatal dopaminergic-cholinergic systems are considered. Taking trifluoperazine as an example, significant dopaminergic blockade is present with low doses. As the dosage is increased to high levels, dopaminergic blockade remains, but anticholinergic activity increases significantly, since it is purely dose related. With increasing anticholinergic activity, extrapyramidal effects are stabilized or even decreased (98).

25. E.B. tolerated the trifluoperazine well and within two weeks was receiving 20 mg hs. Six weeks after the trifluoperazine had been started, the patient complained of persistent anxiety, nervousness, and difficulty in falling asleep. During the interview the patient was visibly agitated and unable to sit still for more than five or ten minutes. He asked for more medication.

How would a differential diagnosis be made between re-emerging psychosis and akathisia?

The differential diagnosis between re-emerging psychosis and akathisia is extremely difficult in some patients. Akathisia is the most common extrapyramidal effect (incidence of 21.2%) induced by phenothiazines (7). The incidence today is probably much higher since the introducton of fluphenazine enanthate and haloperidol. Akathisia is described as a subjective desire to be in constate motion, typically manifest in the patient's constant pacing or inability to sit still. Mild akathisia may be virtually impossible to distinguish from anxiety, while the patient with severe akathisia may be restless to the point of agitation and panic (39, 103).

Akathisia may occur early in treatment and can often be mistaken for psychotic agitation. In E.B.'s case, it is difficult to distinguish, since we have no knowledge of his past clinical manifestations of psychosis or of the target symptoms which were present when neuroleptic therapy was reinstituted. An educated guess, based on available information, would be that E.B. is experiencing akathisia. The time course of six weeks is consistent with akathisia as is the presenting symptomatology. Trifluoperazine is more likely to cause akathisia as compared to other extrapyramidal manifestations, and no other symptoms present are suggestive of psychosis. For these reasons, akathisia should be the provisional diagnosis, and anticholinergic therapy should be instituted.

26. Assuming E.B. is experiencing akathisia, how can it best be treated?

The use of parenteral antiparkinson agents, such as benztropine 2 mg or diphenhydramine 50 mg, may produce an immediate response. It is not unusual, however, for akathisia to show little response to this treatment, because it is the most difficult extrapyramidal effect to treat successfully (23). If anticholinergic agents have been pushed to maximal dosage levels without adequate response, oral diphenhydramine or diazepam can be added as an adjunct. As a last resort, the dosage of the neuroleptic must be lowered or the neuroleptic drug changed (39, 97).

27. Are there clinically significant differences among the available antiparkinson anticholinergic drugs?

Table VI lists the more commonly used antiparkinson agents and their relative potencies. It is important to note that benztropine is twice as potent as trihexyphenidyl, a fact frequently overlooked because both agents are available as a 2 mg tablet. Among these four drugs, differences in efficacy or adverse effects have not been established. The only documented clinically significant difference is in duration of effect, with benztropine having the longest duration. It can be dosed once daily in the majority of patients (74), while the other three agents must be dosed three or four times daily. Benztropine, diphenhydramine, and biperiden are available for parenteral administration.

Case History (M.H.):

M.H., a 58-year-old female diagnosed as a chronic schizophrenic, was hospitalized for recurrence of hearing threatening voices, agitation and feelings that the board and care manager was poisoning her food. Past psychiatric history includes numerous hospitalizations dating back to 1949. Although she had been taking chlorpromazine 400 mg daily for the past four years and had taken trifluoperazine 20-30 mg daily for several years before the chlorpromazine, numerous other neuroleptic drugs had been added or substituted at various times. She discontinued her chlorpromazine 400 mg at bedtime two months prior to this admission. An OTC drug history reveals that she has been taking milk of magnesia about two times weekly for several years, and Sleep-Eze 3-4 capsules at bedtime for the past month.

The patient was started on fluphenazine 10 mg bid and benztropine 2 mg bid. On day 5, the patient complained of muscle stiffness, dry mouth and constipation. She still heard voices, although the intensity was less. She was still agitated and suspicious.

28. How can the complaints of muscle stiffness, dry mouth and constipation be minimized?

At the present time, M.H. is experiencing both peripheral anticholinergic effects and an extrapyramidal effect. Because she is still psychotic, the dosage of her neuroleptic cannot be reduced and, in fact, will probably need to be increased because of only partial response. Increasing the dose of benztropine will probably alleviate the muscle stiffness but will worsen the anticholinergic effects. Lowering the dose of benztropine will decrease anticholinergic effects but will worsen the muscle stiffness. Resolution of this double-bind situation depends almost entirely upon the patient. M.H. should be asked which of the adverse effects are most bothersome; the benztropine can then be adjusted accordingly. In most cases, and when pa-

tients cannot aid in the decision-making, the extrapyramidal effect should be treated. Anticholinergic effects, even if worsened, can be easily treated symptomatically (97), and extrapyramidal effects have been shown to be primarily responsible for neuroleptic noncompliance (103). Occasionally, however, a patient who reads a great deal or whose hobby requires near vision may choose to be a bit stiff rather than suffer cycloplegia. Dry mouth can be minimized by chewing sugarless gum, and if severe, pilocarpine 5 mg tid orally might be tried. Constipation is best treated with a stool softener such as D.O.S.S., because the most common complaint is hard dry stools (97).

29. On day six, M.H. had still shown little response. Thioridazine 100 mg bid and 400 mg hs was added to the fluphenazine 10 mg bid and benztropine 2 mg bid. Two hours after the bedtime dose of thioridazine, the patient got up from bed, confused, disoriented, and agitated. She picked at her bedclothes and complained that bugs were crawling under her skin.

Comment on the use of thioridazine as an adjunct to the fluphenazine.

The use of a second neuroleptic in this situation is probably the only indication for multiple neuroleptic therapy. A patient such as M.H., whose primary neuroleptic drug is nonsedating, can appropriately be given a sedating neuroleptic at bedtime for temporary treatment of insomnia. Sedating neuroleptics should not be considered as common hypnotics. Only when temporary use of sedation and additive antipsychotic activity is desirable should sedating neuroleptics be added. When the insomnia is relieved, the thioridazine should be discontinued and the fluphenazine dosage adjusted accordingly. Although no published studies have specifically addressed this issue, basic pharmacology supports the idea that sedating neuroleptic drugs will be as efficacious as hypnotics for acute short-term use. Patients do not develop psychological habituation to neuroleptic drugs as readily as to hypnotics.

30. Explain the cause of the symptoms observed in M.H. two hours after the bedtime dose of thioridazine.

Table VI
ESTIMATED EQUIVALENT DOSES
OF ANTIPARKINSON AGENTS (mg)

benztropine	(Cogentin)	2
trihexyphenidyl	(Artane, Tremin)	5
biperiden	(Akineton)	4
procyclidine	(Kemadrin)	5
diphenhydramine	(Benadryl)	50

M.H. has experienced acute central anticholinergic toxicity. The dose of thioridazine, a highly anticholinergic neuroleptic, was excessive and additive to the anticholinergic activity of the benztropine and fluphenazine. The acuteness of the syndrome coupled with the organic picture of disorientation, confusion, and tactile hallucinations differentiates it from worsening of the schizophrenia. A review (71) of anticholinergic intoxications in adults from a variety of sources reveals the classic physiologic manifestations of mydriasis, dry mucous membranes and tachycardia; mental status changes include a high incidence of disorientation, confusion, agitation, and picking or plucking movements (91, 106). Complete neuropsychiatric recovery within 24 hours of ingestion was reported in more than one-third of the cases. Drug treatment is rarely indicated, but if agitation must be controlled, benzodiazepines are indicated. Neuroleptic drugs are contraindicated because of their inherent anticholinergic activity. Treatment for M.H. consisted of discontinuing all medication for 24 hours. The syndrome cleared and neuroleptic therapy was reinstituted in an equivalent dosage but with less anticholinergic activity.

Case History (H.H.)

H.H., a 36-year-old female, was being followed in a psychiatric day treatment facility for schizophrenia. She had been discharged from the hospital three months earlier after treatment of an acute psychotic episode, and her haloperidol had been reduced from 100 mg daily to a present level of 25 mg bid. She is also being treated for mild hypertension; hydrochlorthiazide 50 mg bid and KCl 10% 30 cc daily has kept her in control.

After having been absent from the clinic for three days, the patient comes in this morning markedly agitated and delusional regarding her neighbors. After an assessment of her symptomatology, she is given chlorpromazine 200 mg orally stat. Thirty minutes later the patient complains of feeling faint after getting up to walk to the day room and falls to the floor. Blood pressure sitting is 85/55.

31. Explain the mechanism of neuroleptic-induced hypotension.

The most frequent neuroleptic-induced cardiovascular effect is orthostatic hypotension. It occurs more frequently and is more severe following the ingestion of aliphatic and piperidine phenothiazines. It is infrequently associated with piperazine phenothiazines and is rarely associated with haloperidol (10, 36, 52). The mechanism by which neuroleptic drugs cause hypotension is not clearly understood. Neuroleptic drugs have alpha adrenergic blocking effects, which may contribute to orthostatic hypotension by creating exaggerated venous pooling and loss of reflex vasoconstriction on assuming an upright position. Some evidence suggests a central effect and direct arterial effect of neuroleptics which also contributes to vasodilatation. Patients who have a decreased vascular volume from acute hemorrhage, dehydration, or treatment with diuretic agents are more prone to the hypotensive effects of neuroleptic drugs (36).

The exact incidence and severity of neuroleptic-induced hypotension is difficult to determine, because most studies report only daily pressures without description of technique or patient position. In a study of 56 patients receiving neuroleptic drugs, 21 (37.5%) had a postural decrease in systolic blood pressure between 20-40 mmHg sometime during the first 72 hours of treatment and 5 (8.9%) had greater than a 40 mmHg decrease (51).

32. How should H.H.'s hypotension be treated?

Patients who develop hypotension from neuroleptic drugs generally do not develop a shock-like syndrome. The hypotension, as experienced by H.H., can be treated by placing her in a Trendelenburg position. Drug treatment is only indicated when the patient develops shock. Epinephrine should never be used, because the neuroleptic alpha-adrenergic blockade permits unopposed beta (vasodilation) activity of epinephrine. When drug therapy is indicated, a pure alpha agonist, such as norepinephrine, should be used to overcome the alpha blockade (36, 107).

33. How could have this episode have been prevented?

Prevention of neuroleptic-induced hypotension is not difficult. First, H.H. should have been recognized as a patient at greater risk because of her diuretic therapy. A piperazine phenothiazine or haloperidol could have been used rather than chlorpromazine which has a high incidence of hypotensive effects. If chlorpromazine was felt to be the only indicated drug, H.H. should have remained in a sitting or recumbent position for at least one hour if possible and should have been instructed to arise very slowly. All patients, especially those being started on aliphatic and piperidine phenothiazines, should be warned about the possibility of orthostatic hypotension and instructed to sit or stand slowly to allow time for maximum circulatory compensation to occur (52). Fortunately, tolerance does develop, most often after the first week of therapy at a constant dosage level.

34. K.L., a 26-year-old Caucasian male, had been maintained on trifluoperazine 20 mg bid since his last hospitalization ten months earlier. Because of recent insomnia and loose associations, chlorpromazine 200 mg hs was added. Three weeks later, the patient

played basketball for about one hour on a sunny afternoon and came to the clinic the next morning complaining of severe sunburn. His face and arms were noted to be severely erythematous with slight edema.

What is the mechanism of chlorpromazine photosensitivity? How can it be prevented?

Phenothiazine photosensitivity is thought to occur because the tricyclic structure absorbs light energy from direct sunlight. Free radicals are released, which can result in altered biologic activity in tissues. Clinically, areas of the body exposed to sunlight become erythematous and sunburned. Chlorpromazine has been implicated most frequently (3%) based upon reported cases. Thiothixene has also been implicated (6). Thioridazine, however, while definitely causing skin pigmentation, has not been found to cause photosensitivity (13).

Prevention of neuroleptic photosensitivity is simple. Patients should be warned of this potential effect and, especially during summer months, should wear protective clothing or use a sunscreening preparation such as benzophenone (66).

Case History (N.H.)

N.H., a 19-year-old Caucasian female, was discharged to an outpatient psychiatric clinic following six weeks of hospitalization for her first psychotic episode. During hospitalization the patient required large doses of neuroleptics and received 1800 mg daily of chlorpromazine by the second week. She responded well and was discharged on chlorpromazine 1000 mg hs. After two months as an outpatient, the dosage was decreased to 800 mg hs. Further dosage reduction was slowed because of questionable bizarre behavior and thought disorder on two occasions. Four months after discharge the dosage was reduced to 600 mg daily. During the fifth month, the patient was seen three times because her mother was concerned about recent peculiar behavior. The patient's makeup was noted to be excessive and she had begun wearing long-sleeved, high-necked blouses. She had become more withdrawn from family and friends. At the end of the fifth month, the patient arrived late for her appointment because she had overslept and had not had time to put on any makeup. It was noted that her face, neck, and arms had a slate-gray color.

35. What is the incidence of skin pigmentation with neuroleptic drugs? Are there differences among individual drugs?

The incidence of neuroleptic-induced skin pigmentation is reported to be about 1%, although the incidence is highly dependent upon the neuroleptic used, its dosage, and the patient's exposure to the sun (12, 42). Development of pigmentation is directly related to the total dose of neuroleptic ingested. Thus, the less potent neuroleptic drugs (chlorpromazine and thioridazine) will have a higher incidence than the potent phenothiazines (fluphenazine, trifluoperazine), only because larger amounts of the former are given. Haloperidol is the only neuroleptic drug which reportedly does not cause skin pigmentation. Pigmentation was found in 30% of patients on chlorpromazine who had received either a total dose of 600 grams, a daily dose of 600 mg or greater for one year, or a total of 200 grams within one year (108). Thus, patients receiving high dose therapy which approaches these amounts should be evaluated periodically for the presence of eye pigmentation, and baseline slit lamp examinations should be performed.

36. Is there an association between pigmentation of the skin and pigmentation elsewhere?

Chlorpromazine-induced skin pigmentation has been well documented, as has corneal and lens pigmentation. A review of the literature reveals a significant association between skin and eye pigmentary changes. Pigmentary changes also were found in the liver and other internal organs of skin-pigmented patients (63). A common mechanism for skin and eye pigmentation is difficult to establish, however, because the former seems dependent upon an interaction of phenothiazine metabolites, melanin, and sunlight, and the cornea and lens contain no melanin. Nevertheless, the association between skin and eye pigmentation is of great clinical importance. Consensus of many studies suggests that if skin pigmentation is present, there is about 60% chance that there is significant corneal and lens pigmentation as well (63). Consequences of corneal and lens pigmentation are relatively insignificant clinically, because unlike thioridazine retinopathy, visual acuity is not compromised unless the pigmentation is severe (63). Thus N.H., because of her skin pigmentation, should be given a slit lamp examination to detect possible eye pigmentation.

37. How should N.H.'s pigmentation be treated?

Treatment of N.H.'s pigmentation, fortunately, is simple. She should be switched to a more potent phenothiazine such as fluphenazine, or optimally, to haloperidol which is devoid of pigmentary effects (see Question 35). Skin and eye pigmentation are reversible, although a significant reduction of ocular deposits may take as long as twelve months (63).

N.H. was switched from chlorpromazine to haloperidol, and the slate-gray pigmentation disappeared within four months.

38. G.Q., a 21-year-old single nulliparous female was seen in an outpatient psychiatric clinic for her regular monthly appointment. She has been receiving

fluphenazine decanoate 100 mg IM every week for nine weeks, along with benztropine 2 mg hs. All psychotic symptomatology has been ameliorated for the past six weeks except for mild suspiciousness and social isolation. Today she relates for the first time that she believes a man climbed through her window two months ago and raped her. Although she does not remember the incident, she believes that to be the only explanation for her being pregnant. She denies having ever dated, much less having sexual intercourse at anytime. Her evidence for believing herself pregnant is that she has missed two menstrual periods and for the past two weeks has had diffusely tender enlarged breasts with lactation. A pregnancy test was ordered, which came back positive.

Explain the etiology of this questionable pregnancy.

Although G.Q.'s belief that she was raped may sound delusional, it may be a genuine attempt by the patient to explain the occurrence of her symptoms of pregnancy. Few patients will ever consider neuroleptic drugs as the cause for their amenorrhea, lactation, and positive pregnancy test.

The incidence of neuroleptic-induced amenorrhea is extremely difficult to determine. A study of menstrual irregularities in 144 premenopausal women diagnosed as schizophrenic, but not treated with neuroleptic drugs, showed an 18% incidence of amenorrhea and a 31% incidence of delayed or prolonged cycles (86). In spite of this difficulty, the evidence for neuroleptic-induced amenorrhea is fairly clear. One review reports the incidence of menstrual changes as 16% with chlorpromazine, 3% with thioridazine and 4% with fluphenazine (62).

Galactorrhea has also been established as a neuroleptic effect. It is more common with high dose therapy and in premenopausal women, and may appear as early as eight days after the neuroleptic drug is begun. The incidence is highly variable (0 to 80%) due to different drugs, dosages, durations, and how the lactation is elicited (spontaneous versus squeezing of the nipple). Galactorrhea has been reported with chlorpromazine, thioridazine, trifluoperazine, fluphenazine, and thiothixene. It is often accompanied by amenorrhea (31, 50, 92). The mechanism of neuroleptic-induced galactorrhea is suppression of prolactin inhibitory factor in the hypothalamus (92).

Phenothiazines have been implicated in causing false positive results in frog pregnancy tests as well as in the newer immunologic pregnancy tests. A study of 76 patients receiving single neuroleptic drugs was done to determine the incidence of false positive immunologic pregnancy tests. Of four commercial tests employed on each urine specimen — Gravidex, HCG, Natatel, and UCG — the HCG test consistently gave false positive results. Incidence of HCG false positive tests for several specific drugs were as follows: chlorpromazine 10 of 20, thioridazine 8 of 21, trifluoperazine 1 of 3, fluphenazine 1 of 3, and thiothixene 1 of 7. There was only one false positive test of the 76 patients tested by the Natatel method. There were no false positive tests by the Gravidex and UCG methods (81).

39. D.R., a 41-year-old single male, came into the community mental health center asking for a refill of his medication. He had recently moved to San Francisco from Los Angeles where he had been treated as an outpatient at a Veterans Administration Clinic. For eight years he had been taking thioridazine 200 mg hs and claimed to be doing well. Upon further questioning, his only complaint was a medical one. For about the last eight years, he could maintain an erection and sometimes experience orgasm while masturbating but did not ejaculate. He described a very active sex life during his 20's and early 30's but now no longer feels virile or adequate. The patient last dated a woman six years ago. He blames the problem on his age but hopes he can be helped.

Explain thioridazine's possible role in this patient's complaint.

Disorders of male sexual function, including impotence, decreased libido, and ejaculation disorders, have been reported with many of the neuroleptic drugs (14, 93). Thioridazine has been particularly implicated in inhibition of ejaculation while not altering erection or orgasm. The proposed mechanism of ejaculation inhibition is hypothalamic sympathetic depression and peripheral alpha-adrenergic blockade. The central effect is common to all phenothiazines and thioxanthenes, but the significantly greater peripheral effects of thioridazine explain its high association with this disorder (93).

The potential causes for D.R.'s difficulty could be several, but all evidence is consistent with a classic case of thioridazine-induced ejaculation disorder. An appropriate first step in a differential diagnosis would be to switch the patient to another neuroleptic drug, preferably a piperazine phenothiazine or haloperidol.

Case History, (H.S.)

H.S., a 57-year-old female, was admitted to a psychiatric ward for barbiturate withdrawal. Past drug history revealed a 20-year history of sedative-hypnotic abuse and addiction, primarily involving meprobamate and pentobarbital. Trifluoperazine, in doses of 5-20 mg daily had also been prescribed continuously for "nerves" for the past eight years. There were two past hospitalizations for barbiturate withdrawal but no history of psychosis or psychiatric hospitalizations. Prior to this admission the patient was taking trifluoperazine 5 mg tid, pentobarbital 200 mg tid, and ethchlorvynol 2 grams hs. During withdrawal in the hospital, the trifluoperazine was discontinued. Approximately three weeks later, the patient was noted to have a fly-catching tongue movement of about 40-50 per minute and severe athetoid movements of the extremities. The patient adopted the habit of sitting on her legs and folding her arms across her chest to minimize the movement.

40. Explain the neurochemical basis for tardive dyskinesia.

The most widely accepted explanation for the etiology of tardive dyskinesia is that prolonged striatal dopaminergic receptor blockade by neuroleptic drugs produces a denervation hypersensitivity of those receptors (56). The tardive dyskinesia may not be clinically apparent during neuroleptic drug therapy, because the hypersensitive receptors are blocked. When the dose is significantly lowered or the neuroleptic drug is discontinued, the hypersensitive receptors are exposed to endogenous dopamine and the clinical manifestations of tardive dyskinesia appear (26, 39, 56).

Tardive dyskinesia must be differentiated from other neuroleptic-induced extrapyramidal disorders, because the biochemical basis is exactly opposite, and thus treatment is very different (see Question 23). Extrapyramidal effects result from diminished dopaminergic influence relative to cholinergic influence, while tardive dyskinesia results from increased dopaminergic influence relative to cholinergic influence. There is no excess of dopamine in tardive dyskinesia, but rather exaggerated response of the hyperactive dopaminergic receptors within the striatum (58, 98).

41. How can H.S.'s dyskinesia be treated?

Fortunately, H.S. does not require neuroleptic therapy at this time, and she should remain off neuroleptic drugs for as long as possible. Specific treatment approaches to tardive dyskinesia are easily predicted from an understanding of its mechanism. Successful tardive dyskinesia treatment would be to balance the striatal dopaminergic-cholinergic systems. Since the dopaminergic influence predominates, balance can be achieved by either decreasing the dopaminergic activity or increasing the cholinergic activity. Both treatment approaches have been tried in clinical studies of tardive dyskinesia management.

Drugs capable of decreasing dopaminergic activity include dopamine-depletors such as reserpine and dopamine blockers such as neuroleptics (54). Of the dopamine-depleting drugs, the most useful seems to be tetrabenazine. It is similar to reserpine but has a more rapid onset and shorter duration of action. It also apparently lacks some of reserpine's peripheral effects. Its beneficial effect, however, is often only tem-

porary. Of the dopamine-blocking agents, all neuroleptic drugs should be useful. Neuroleptic drugs are of benefit for short-term therapy but, as the offending agent, will only contribute to the dyskinesia in the long run. Cases treated with neuroleptic drugs have been reported in which the dyskinesia breaks through, requiring further increases in neuroleptic dose (57). Thus neuroleptic drugs should not be considered as a treatment alternative for tardive dyskinesia, but only as a method of temporarily masking the dyskinesis.

Deanol is a drug which can increase the cholinergic system in the striatum. Deanol has been used in several studies. As with dopamine depleting or blocking drugs, however, the efficacy of deanol is only temporary (17, 28, 59).

42. H.S. was discharged from the hospital three weeks after the dyskinesias began. She received no neuroleptic drugs, and was discharged on diazepam 5 mg tid and flurazepam 30 mg hs. The dyskinesias were still severe four weeks after discharge, significantly interfering with eating, talking and socializing. At the same time, the patient expressed great concern that her boyfriend of 15 years was threatening to leave her because of the dyskinesias. Neuroleptic therapy was then reinstituted, since stability of this long-standing support system for the patient was in jeopardy. Trifluoperazine 5 mg tid was begun, chlorpromazine 200 mg hs was added one week later, and the diazepam and flurazepam were discontinued. Within three weeks the tongue movement had decreased to about 10-20 per minute and the athetoid movement of the extremities decreased significantly. After four months of neuroleptic therapy, the dyskinesias decreased to the point where the patient had an infrequent tongue movement and no movement of the extremities.

Is H.S.'s tardive dyskinesia irreversible?

Reversibility of tardive dyskinesia seems to be primarily related to the duration of continuous neuroleptic drug therapy. Case reports and studies that mention duration and reversibility suggest that tardive dyskinesia remains reversible if the duration of neuroleptic drug therapy is no longer than two years. Tardive dyskinesia which develops or is discovered after more than two years, and certainly after five to ten years, is more likely to be irreversible. Neuroleptic dosage seems to be a less important factor, because cases of tardive dyskinesia have been reported at low and moderate doses (2a, 99).

Because H.S. had been on trifluoperazine continuously for eight years, her dyskinesia could be irreversible. The neuroleptics should be tapered in dosage and, if possible, discontinued to determine if the dyskinesia is reversible. If neuroleptics need to be continued, the dosage should be as low as possible to minimize further potential worsening of the dyskinesia.

43. How can tardive dyskinesia be prevented?

Because tardive dyskinesia is not easily treated once it becomes manifest, prevention becomes most important. Identification of patients at risk is a first step, but the only well-documented factor is long-term continuous neuroleptic therapy. The original group identified at greatest risk were older women on high dose long-term neuroleptic therapy with organic impairment (26, 39). A well-done study showed that tardive dyskinesia is also more likely to develop in patients with pseudoparkinsonian symptoms than in patients not exhibiting such manifestations (24). The majority of these factors have been questioned however (27). High dose therapy is not an important variable (Question 42). A more recent epidemiological study of tardive dyskinesia noted that factors such as sex, organic syndromes, and neuroleptic-induced extrapyramidal effects did not play a role in the prevalence of tardive dyskinesia. The only significant factor was age, with the incidence significantly higher in the older population (53).

Recommendations of the original paper on tardive dyskinesia prevention still hold true in light of the above findings (25). Patients on long-term neuroleptic therapy should be examined at least once every three months for dyskinesia or other types of neurological syndromes. Neuroleptic drugs should be completely withdrawn at least temporarily to unmask latent symptoms particularly in patients with incipient manifestations. There should be a gradual withdrawal of drugs followed by a four week drug-free period (24).

44. K.M., a 45-year-old female was admitted involuntarily to a psychiatric ward on 8-5-76. She had an eleven year psychiatric history with about twenty hospitalizations and had been consistently diagnosed with chronic undifferentiated schizophrenia. She had electroshock therapy on six different occasions and had been treated with a variety of neuroleptic agents, all with little effect on her illness. Since 1972, she had received fluphenazine enanthate 50 mg IM every two weeks and trihexyphenidyl 2 mg tid. Her last dose of fluphenazine enanthate was 8-2-76, three days prior to admission. One day prior to admission she had an exacerbation of psychotic symptoms characterized by agitation, hyperactivity, violence, loose associations, and delusions. Physical exam was unremarkable, pulse and blood pressure on admission were 85 and 140/90, respectively. Her complete blood count was within normal limits.

She was begun on chlorpromazine 100 mg qid and chloral hydrate 500 mg hs. The chlorpromazine was titrated upward to 400 mg qid by 8-10-76. On 8-11-76, she received chlorpromazine 75 mg IM at noon, because she refused the oral dose. Her last oral dose

was chlorpromazine 400 mg at 2200. From 0200 to 0330 on 8-12-76, the patient was reported to be noisy and agitated and was placed in restraints. At 0345, she was noted to be pulseless and in respiratory arrest. Cardiopulmonary resusitation was begun. During intubation she aspirated and was suctioned. EKG could not be interpreted and cardioversion was without result.

Is there a syndrome of "phenothiazine sudden death?"

Controversy continues regarding the validity of the syndrome termed "phenothiazine sudden death." Two major review papers address the issue, each reaching different conclusions. Medical literature from September 1963 to October 1966 on sudden or unexplained death involving phenothiazine drugs was reviewed (67). Sudden death was described as death in less than one hour; cases not involving phenothiazines and cases which did not have an autopsy were not included.

Of the 58 cases identified, mean age was 41 with 40 males and 18 females. Anatomical cause of death was listed as: none - 46, aspiration - 9, cardiac - 2, other - 1. Circumstances of death were: collapse and death - 24, found dead or dying - 21, unexpected death - 9, other - 4. Neuroleptic at time of death was: chlorpromazine - 23, thioridazine - 16, chlorpromazine and thioridazine - 6, trifluoperazine - 5, other or unknown - 11. Experimental studies were cited which indicate that thioridazine and, to a lesser extent, chlorpromazine, have potent and unpredictable cardiovascular effects, and many of the 58 deaths were apparently cardiovascular deaths. The authors concluded that sudden death caused by phenothiazines is a real entity comprised of two types. The first is aspiration and rapid asphyxia; the second is sudden cessation of cardiovascular competence on either an arrhythmogenic or a hypotensive basis.

A second, more recent, review of all cases called phenothiazine deaths and cases of lethal catatonia unrelated to phenothiazines in the English, German, French and Italian literature (77) reported 65 cases of phenothiazine deaths and 94 cases of lethal catatonia, and the two groups were compared according to several variables. These authors question whether phenothiazine sudden death exists, because such a group may include two previously known types of sudden autopsy-negative deaths: cardiac deaths among the general population and lethal catatonia among psychiatric patients. The survey raises doubts about the existence of phenothiazine death, but its existence could not be completely disproved.

Although there is still controversy and the syndrome is rare, unpredictable, and often unpreventable, the reported cases and that of K.M. suggest that three situations seem to deserve more careful attention. First, patients on high doses of chlorpromazine and thioridazine should be more carefully monitored, because the vast majority of cases involve these two drugs. Second, patients who complain of difficulty breathing after eating deserve more careful attention, because some cases involved asphyxia following meals. Third, agitated, hyperactive patients, especially those placed in restraints and medicated with one of the above two neuroleptic drugs, deserve more careful monitoring.

45. L.B., a 23-year-old male, is being discharged on thioridazine 400 mg hs following a good response to treatment of an acute psychotic episode. During the discharge interview, the patient asks if he can drink a few beers while taking thioridazine.

How should you respond to E.B.'s question?

It is well-known that alcohol and neuroleptic drugs, particularly sedating ones, will have an additive central nervous system depressant effect (46). The urge to impart the knowledge of this interaction should be resisted however. Telling L.B. he should not drink alcohol with his thioridazine will most probably cause him to not take the thioridazine rather than stop drinking beer. The best approach to this commonly asked question is to explain that he may become drowsy or drunk quicker while taking thioridazine so he should avoid driving, but drinking a few beers while on thioridazine is not prohibited. This approach will not adversely affect medication compliance and places an appropriate amount of responsibility on the patient for his drinking. The patient should also be warned about the possibility of becoming dizzy or faint due to the additive vasodilation effect of alcohol and the alpha adrenergic blocking effect of thioridazine.

CASE FOR STUDY I

J.C., a 35-year-old single male was brought to the psychiatric hospital by the police after he was found wandering on the Golden Gate Bridge. (March 1974).

History of Present Illness: Two months prior to admission the patient discontinued his trifluoperazine and benztropine because he believed he no longer needed it. Seven days prior to admission he began taking dextroamphetamine 20 mg daily because he began hearing voices and his thinking became confused. The voices increased in intensity, became more threatening, and told him to kill himself by jumping off the bridge.

Previous Illnesses: The patient had five previous psychiatric hospitalizations, the first one in 1965 and the others in 1966, 1968, 1972, and 1973. Diagnosis had consistently been chronic schizophrenia undifferentiated. Symptoms in past hospitalizations had been loose associations, bizarre behavior and threatening voices. No previous suicide attempts were reported but suicidal ideation was present during each past episode. Past hospitalizations have been brief, with the psychosis usually resolving within 1-2 months. The patient has been followed in group therapy and given medication maintenance in a community mental health center since

1968.

Drug History: Neuroleptic medications have been used almost continuously for the past nine years with intermittent antiparkinson medication. He uses ASA 10 gr about twice a week for headache. The patient denies the use of alcohol but admits to using dextroamphetamine 20-30 mg daily for several days in succession about once a month to "feel good." No drug or food allergies are reported. One episode of oculogyric crisis occurred in 1973 while on trifluoperazine, and the patient has had akathisia and muscle rigidity in the past. The patient states he cannot take chlorpromazine because it makes him too "groggy and zonked feeling." Past medication compliance is rated as fair.

Physical exam on admission is unremarkable except for involuntary lateral movements of the tongue.

Mental status exam on admission shows a 35-year-old white male, neat in appearance and grooming. Speech is somewhat pressured and associations are very loose. Mood is somewhat depressed but appropriate. He shows no evidence of delusions but admits to hearing threatening voices. He is oriented x 3 with normal intelligence.

CASE I Questions

1. List the target symptoms you would identify and regularly assess with time in this patient to determine drug therapy response.

2. Which neuroleptic drug would you choose for this patient and why?

3. Would an antidepressant be indicated in this patient? Explain.

4. If the tongue movement is tardive dyskinesia, what can be done about it at this time?

5. How would dextroamphetamine contribute to this patient's symptomatology? Explain the mechanism.

CASE FOR STUDY — II

N.Q., a 27-year-old unemployed female living at a board and care home, was brought to the hospital by the operator of the facility after she had been banging her head on the wall. (Nov 8, 1974).

History of Present Illness: Patient has an eight-year history of psychiatric hospitalizations with a diagnosis of schizophrenia and has apparently been doing well with follow-up and medication for the past two years. Because of apparent remission, the patient's social worker reopened the case concerning her two children, believing she could now assume responsibility for their care. On the stress of this situation, the patient again showed psychotic behavior. The children were then placed with the father, which apparently caused more stress to the patient. In July 1974 the patient was admitted to a state hospital; she was discharged within a month and was sent to live in a board and care facility. One week prior to admission, the father was given legal custody of the children, which apparently led to the behavior causing this admission.

Previous History: Medical - none. Psychiatric - She was hospitalized at the County Hospital in March 1968, May 1968, and October 1971, and admitted to state hospitals in 1969, February 1972, and July 1974.

Family History: There is no family history of mental illness.

Social History: The patient was raised by a grandmother in

Oklahoma until age 17 when she came to California to live with an aunt. She married at age 18 and separated after five years.

Drug History: The patient has been on various antipsychotic agents sporadically since 1967 and there is no history of drug abuse. Past drug reactions or allergies are denied, but validity is poor at this time. Past history reveals noncompliance as an outpatient after several hospitalizations.

On Exam: On admission the patient was dressed and groomed neatly, although she behaved in a silly and inappropriate manner, screaming and laughing intermittently. She appeared alert and oriented. Her affect was labile, appropriate to mood but inappropriate to circumstance. Her thought content was very disorganized. She experienced questionable delusions and hallucinations but nodded when asked if she was hearing voices.

Provisional Dx: Schizophrenia acute, questionable hebephrenic.

Treatment: Haloperidol.

Hospital Course

Tx and Progress: The patient was admitted in a withdrawn hebephrenic state refusing to answer questions.

11-10-74 Haldol 4 mg tid and Artane 2 mg bid. Agitated, hostile, sexually inappropriate, delusional, responding to voices.

11-13-74 Haldol 15 mg bid. Artane 2 mg bid Patient shows no response, still overtly psychotic.

11-15-74 Haldol 30 mg bid. Artane 2 mg bid, plus Haldol 5 mg IM twice. Patient still showing no response, in restraints.

11-21-74 Haldol 40 mg bid. Artane 2 mg bid. Patient much more in control, expressed concern that people could hear and see the bad thoughts going on in her head. Described auditory and visual hallucinations, felt she was being controlled by people.

12-9-74 Haldol 50 mg bid. Artane 2 mg bid. Patient showing fluctuating clinical course, voices continued and sometimes dictated her actions.

12-17-74 Haldol and Artane discontinued, start Prolixin 20 mg bid and Prolixin 5 mg IM bid for next three days.

12-18-74 Oculogyric crisis, successfully treated with Cogentin 2 mg IM stat. Cogentin 2 mg bid added to Prolixin. Patient c/o nervousness, pacing more.

12-20-74 Prolixin 20 mg bid, Prolixin decanoate 75 mg IM, Cogentin 2 mg bid. Patient now only occasionally c/o voices, socially appropriate, no complaints of adverse effects.

Diagnosis: Schizophrenia, chronic undifferentiated, presenting hebephrenic on this exacerbation.

Prognosis: Average in terms of being able to manage in a board and care home, work in a sheltered employment setting, perhaps competitive if closely followed and structure provided.

Condition on Discharge: Improved.

Disposition: Patient to live at board and care home, discharged on Prolixin decanoate 75 mg IM every three weeks and Cogentin 2 mg bid. Due for next injection 1-10-75.

Outpatient Follow-up

1-24-75 Prolixin decanoate 75 mg IM given, last injection was 12-20-74. Thought content shows some loose associations, voices again controlling her actions. Muscle stiffness noted. Cogentin 2 mg bid renewed.

1-31-75 Prolixin decanoate 75 mg IM given due to worsening mental status. Patient now c/o muscle stiffness, dry mouth, constipation.

2-27-75 Patient receiving Prolixin decanoate 75 mg IM weekly and Cogentin 2 mg bid. Thought content and mood appropriate, c/o voices only occasionally and able to handle them.

3-21-75 Patient missed injection on 3-7 and 3-14. Patient relates voices have become louder over past several days, and initial insomnia noted for same time period. Asked for hypnotic for sleep.
Given Prolixin decanoate 75 mg IM, Cogentin 2 mg bid, and Thorazine 200 mg hs.

CASE II Questions

1. From the mental status exam on admission, what target symptoms should be monitored?

2. On November 15, the patient showed no response although on a large dose of haloperidol. What is the most appropriate method to now treat the non-responding patient?

3. Are the patient's comments about people controlling her, etc. on November 21 signs of a worsening psychosis? Explain.

4. What is the most likely reason for the switch from haloperidol to fluphenazine on December 17?

5. Why is the patient nervous and pacing on December 18? How can it best be treated?

6. Is fluphenazine decanoate every three weeks an appropriate interval at discharge for this patient? Explain.

7. How can the adverse effects noted on January 31 best be managed?

8. Comment on the use of chlorpromazine for the initial insomnia noted on March 21.

REFERENCES

1. Abse D W et al: Evaluation of tranquilizing drugs in the management of acute mental disturbance. Am J Psychiat 116.973, 1960.
2. Adamson L et al: Fluphenazine decanoate trial in chronic inpatient schizophrenics failing to absorb oral chlorpromazine. Dis Nerv Syst 34:181, 1973.
2a. Allen R E, Stimmel G L: Neuroleptic dosage, duration, and tardive dyskinesia. Dis Nerv Syst in press.
3. American Psychiatric Association: Diagnostic and Statistical Manual of Mental Disorders, 2nd ed., Washington DC 1968.
4. Angrist B M et al: Psychiatric sequelae of amphetamine use in
Psychiatric Complications of Medical Drugs, Shader R I (Ed), Raven Press, New York 1972, p. 188.
5. Anon; Medical Letter 7:21, 1965
6. Appleton W S et al: Dermatological effects in Psychotropic Drug Side Effects, Shader R I and DiMascio A (Eds), Williams and Wilkins Co., Baltimore 1970, p. 77.
7. Ayd F J: A survey of drug-induced extrapyramidal reactions. JAMA 175:1054, 1961.
8. Ayd F J: Current status of thiothixene. Int Drug Therapy Newsl 2:1, 1967.
9. Ayd F J: Once a day dosing Int Drug Ther Newsl 7:33, 1972.
10. Ayd F J: Haloperidol: Fifteen years of clinical experience. Dis Nerv Syst 33:459, 1972.
11. Ayd F J: A critical evaluation of molindone (Moban): A new indole

derivative neuroleptic. Dis Nerv Syst 35:447, 1974.

12. Ban, T A et al: Skin pigmentation, rare side effect of chlorpromazine. Canad Psychiat Assoc J 10:112, 1965.

13. Berger H: Pigmentation after thioridazine. Arch Derm 100:487, 1969.

14. Blair J H et al: Effect of antipsychotic drugs on reproductive functions. Dis Nerv Syst 27:645, 1966.

15. Bruno A et al: Effects of L-dopa on pharmacological parkinsonism. Acta Psychiat Scand 42:264, 1966.

16. Caffey E M et al: Discontinuation or reduction of chemotherapy in chronic schizophrenics. J Chronic Dis 17:347, 1964.

17. Casey D E et al: Diethylaminoethanol in tardive dyskinesia. New Engl J Med 291:797, 1974.

18. Casey J F et al: Combined drug therapy of chronic schizophrenics. AM J Psychiat 117:997, 1961.

19. Chien C P et al: Depot phenothiazine treatment in acute psychosis: A sequential comparative clinical study. Am J Psychiat 130:13, 1973.

20. Clark M L et al: Drug treatment in newly admitted schizophrenic patients. Arch Gen Psychiat 25:404, 1971.

21. Cole J O: Phenothiazine treatment in acute schizophrenia. Arch Gen Psychiat 10:246, 1964.

22. Cole J O: Introduction to symposium on long-acting phenothiazines in psychiatry. Dis Nerv Syst 31 (suppl. 9): 5, 1970.

23. Coleman J H et al: Drug induced extrapyramidal effects — A review. Dis Nerv Syst 36:591, 1975.

24. Crane G E: Pseudoparkinsonism and tardive dyskinesia. Arch Neurol 27:426, 1972.

25. Crane G E: Prevention and management of tardive dyskinesia. Am J Psychiat 129:466, 1972.

26. Crane G E: Tardive dyskinesia in patients treated with major neuroleptics: A review of the literature. Arch Gen Psychiat 27:491, 1972.

27. Crane G E et al: Tardive dyskinesia and drug therapy in geriatric patients. Arch Gen Psychiat 30:341, 1974.

28. Curran D et al: Treatment of phenothiazine induced bulbar persistent dyskinesia with Deanol acetamidobenzoate. Dis Nerv Syst 36:71, 1975.

29. Curry S H: Chlorpromazine: concentration in plasma, excretion in urine, and duration of effect. Proc R Soc Med 64:285, 1971.

30. Curry S H et al: Double blind trial of fluphenazine decanoate. Lancet 2:543, 1972.

31. de Wied D: Chlorpromazine and endocrine function. Pharmacol Rev 19:251, 1967.

32. DiMascio A et al: Antiparkinson drug overuse. Psychosomatics 11:596, 1970.

33. DiMascio A: Towards a more rational use of antiparkinson drugs in psychiatry. Drug Therapy 1:23, 1971.

34. DiMascio A: Once or twice a day: Psychotropic drug regimen. Practical Psychiat 1:1, 1973.

35. Donlon P T et al: Rapid "digitalization" of decompensated schizophrenic patients with antipsychotic agents. Am J Psychiat 131:310, 1974.

36. Ebert M H et al: Cardiovascular effects in Psychotropic Drug Side Effects, Shader R I and DiMascio A (Eds), Williams and Wilkins Co., Baltimore 1970, p. 149.

37. Engelhardt D M et al: Phenothiazines in prevention of psychiatric hospitalization, IV. Delay or prevention — A reevaluation. Arch Gen Psychiat 16:98, 1967.

38. Fann W E: Use of Ritalin to counteract acute dystonic effects of phenothiazines. Am J Psychiat 122:1293, 1966.

39. FDA Task Force Report: Neurological syndromes associated with antipsychotic drug use. Arch Gen Psychiat 28:463, 1973.

40. Freeman H: The therapeutic value of combinations of psychotropic drugs, a review. Psychopharmacol Bull 4:1, 1967.

41. Goldberg S C et al: Prediction of response to phenothiazines in schizophrenia. Arch Gen Psychiat 26:367, 1972.

42. Gombos G M et al: Ocular and cutaneous side effects after prolonged chlorpromazine treatment. Am J Psychiat 123:872, 1967.

43. Grosser H H: Experience of psychiatric management of schizophrenia with fluphenazine decanoate. Dis Nerv Syst 31 (suppl. 9): 32, 1970.

44. Groves J E et al: The long-acting phenothiazines. Arch Gen Psychiat 32:893, 1975.

45. Hamill W T et al: The immediate effects of chlorpromazine in newly admitted schizophrenic patients. Amer J Psychiat 132:1023, 1975.

46. Hansten P D: Drug Interactions, 3rd ed, Lea and Febiger, Philadelphia 1976, p 159.

47. Hollister L E: Clinical Use of Psychotherapeutic Drugs, Charles C. Thomas, Springfield 1973, p 38.

48. Hollister L E et al: Specific indications for different classes of phenothiazines. Arch Gen Psychiat 30:94, 1974.

49. Hollister L E: Psychiatric disorders in Drug Treatment, Avery, G.S. (Ed), Adis Press, Sydney 1976, p 811.

50. Hooper J H et al: Abnormal lactation associated with tranquilizing drug therapy. JAMA 178:506, 1961.

51. Itil T M et al: EEG changes after fluphenazine enanthate and decanoate based on analog power spectra and digital computer period analysis. Psychopharmacologia 20:230, 1971.

52. Jefferson J W: Hypotension from drugs: Incidence, peril, prevention. Dis Nerv Syst 35:66, 1974.

53. Jus A et al: Epidemiology of tardive dyskinesia, Part I. Dis Nerv Syst 37:210, 1976.

54. Kazamatsuri H et al: Therapeutic approaches to tardive dyskinesia: A review of the literature. Arch Gen Psychiat 27:491, 1972.

55. Klawans H L: The Pharmacology of parkinsonism. Dis Nerv Syst 29:805, 1968.

56. Klawans H L: The pharmacology of tardive dyskinesias. Am J Psychiat 130:82, 1973.

57. Klawans H L et al: Neuroleptic-induced tardive dyskinesias in non-psychotic patients. Arch Neurol. 30:338, 1974.

58. Klawans H L et al: Effect of cholinergic and anticholinergic agents on tardive dyskinesia. J Neurol Neurosurg Psychiat 27:941, 1974.

59. Klawans H L: Deanol in L-dopa dyskinesia. Neurology 25:290, 1975.

60. Klein D F et al: Diagnosis and Drug Treatment of Psychiatric Disorders, Williams and Wilkins Co, Baltimore 1969, p 55.

61. Ibid, p. 68.

62. Ibid, p 97.

63. Ibid, p. 104.

64. Kleet CJ et al: Evaluating the long-term need for antiparkinson drugs by chronic schizophrenics. Arch Gen Psychiat 26:374, 1972.

65. Kolb L C: Modern Clinical Psychiatry, WB Saunders Co., Philadelphia 1973, p 308.

66. Korenyi C: The effect of benzophenone sunscreen lotion on chlorpromazine treated patients. Am J Psychiat 125:143, 1969.

67. Leestma J E et al: Sudden death and phenothiazines. Arch Gen Psychiat 18:137, 1968.

68. Leff J P et al: Trial of maintenance therapy in schizophrenia. Br Med J 3:599, 1971.

69. Lewis D M et al: Long-acting phenothiazines in schizophrenia. Br Med J 1:671, 1971.

70. Mc Neil Laboratories: Haldol package insert, 1975.

71. Mendel W.M: Precision in the diagnosis of schizophrenia. Psychiatria Fennica 1:107, 1975.

72. Merlis S et al: Polypharmacy in psychiatry: Patterns of differential treatment. Amer J Psychiat 126: 1647, 1970.

73. NIMH Psychopharmacology Service Center Collaborative Study Group: Phenothiazine treatment in acute schizophrenia: effectiveness. Arch Gen Psychiat 10:246, 1964

74. Neu C et al: Antiparkinson medication in the treatment of extrapyramidal side effects. Curr Ther Res 14:246, 1972.

75. Orlov P et al: Withdrawal of antiparkinson drugs. Arch Gen Psychiat 25:410, 1971.

76. Paulson G et al: Some remarks on the treatment of postencephalitic oculogyric crises with benztropine methanesulfonate. Int J Neuropsychiat 1:214, 1965.

77. Peele R et al: Phenothiazine deaths: A critical review. Am J Psychiat 130:306, 1973.

78. Polak P et al: Rapid tranquilization Am J Psychiat 128:132, 1971.

79. Prien R F et al: High dose chlorpromazine therapy in chronic schizophrenia. Arch Gen Psychiat 18:482, 1968.

80. Prien R F et al: Relapse in chronic schizophrenics following abrupt withdrawal of tranquilizing medication. Br J Psychiat 115:679, 1969.

81. Ravel R et al: Effects of certain psychotropic drugs on immunologic pregnancy tests. Am J Obst Gynec 105: 1222, 1969.

82. Reschke R W: Parenteral haloperidol for rapid control of severe disruptive symptoms of acute schizophrenia. Dis Nerv Syst 35:112, 1974.

83. Rifkin A et al: Very high dose fluphenazine for non-chronic treatment refractory patients. Arch Gen Psychiat 25:398, 1971.

84. Rifkin A et al: Long-term use of antipsychotic drugs in *Progress in Psychiatric Drug Treatment,* Klein D F Helman-Klein R (Eds), Brunner-Mazel, New York 1975, p. 387.

85. Rifkin A et al: Akinesia. Arch Gen Psychiat 32:672, 1975.

86. Ripley H S et al: The menstrual cycle with vaginal smear studies in schizophrenia, depression and elation. Am J Psychiat 98:567, 1942.

87. Ritter R M et al: Comparison of injectable haloperidol and chlorpromazine. Am J Psychiat 129: 110, 1972.

88. Rosebaum C P: *The Meaning of Madness,* Science House, New York 1970, p. 16.

89. Shader R I et al: Belladonna alkaloids and synthetic anticholinergics: Uses and toxicity in *Psychiatric Complications of Medical Drugs,* Shader R I (Ed), Raven Press New York 1972, p 103.

90. Shader R I et al: Galactorrhea and gynecomastia in *Psychotropic Drug Side Effects,* Shader R I and DiMascio (Eds), Williams and Wilkins, Baltimore, 1970, p. 4.

91. Shader R I : Ejaculation disorders in *Psychotropic Drug Side Effects,* Shader R I and DiMascia A (Eds), Williams and Wilkins, Baltimore, 1970, p. 72.

92. Sheppard C et al: Drug-induced extrapyramidal symptom: Incidence and treatment. Am J Psychiat 123:886, 1967.

93. Snyder S H : Amphetamine psychosis: A model schizophrenia mediated by catecholamines. Am J Psychiat 130:61, 1973.

94. Snyder S H et al: Drugs, neurotransmitters and schizophrenia. Science 184:1243, 1974.

95. Steinbrook R M et al: Lozapine: A double-blind comparison with chlorpromazine in acute schizophrenic patients. Curr Ther Res 15:1, 1973.

96. Sterlin C et al: The place of thiothizene in the treatment of schizophrenic patients. Canad Psychiat Assoc J 15:3, 1970.

97. Stimmel G L: Schizophrenia. J Am Pharm Assoc NS 14:257, 1974.

98. Stimmel G L: Neuroleptics and the corpus striatum: Clinical implications. Dis Nerv Syst 37:219, 1976.

99. Stimmel G L: Tardive dyskinesia with low dose short-term neuropleptic therapy. Amer J Hosp Pharm 33:961, 1976.

100. Sweet C: Drug-induced dystonia Am J Psychiat 132:532, 1975.

101. van der Velde C D et al: Effectiveness of loxapine succinate in acute schizophrenia: A comparative study with thiothixene. Curr Ther Res 17:1, 1975.

102. Van Praag HMM et al : Flupenazine enanthate and fluphenazine decanoate: A comparison of their duration of action and motor side effects Am J Psychiat 130:801, 1973.

103. Van Putten T: Why do schizophrenic patients refuse to take their drugs? Arch Gen Psychiat 31:67, 1974.

104. van Rossum J M et al: Pharmacology in *The Neuroleptics, Modern Problems in Pharmacopsychiatry,* Bobon D P et al (Eds), Volume 5, Karger, New York, 1970, p. 23

105. Warner A M et al: Delayed severe extrapyramidal disturbance following frequent depot phenothiazine administration. Am J Psychiat 132:743, 1975.

106. Warnes H: Toxic psychosis due to antiparkinson drugs. Canad Psychiat Assoc J 12:323, 1967.

107. Warnes H et al: Complications of psychotropic medications in high dosage. Psychiat Quarterly 45:87, 1971.

108. Wheeler R H et al: Ocular pigmentation, extrapyramidal symptoms and phenothiazine dosage. Br J Psychiat 115:687, 1969.

109. Yaryura-Tobias J A et al: Action of L-dopa in drug-induced extrapyramidalism Dis Nerv Syst 31:60, 1970.

Chapter 31

Affective Disorders

James H. Coleman

Hippocrates is generally credited with the first descriptions of an affective disorder, though the Old Testament describes the dysphoric mood of Job. Hippocrates is thought to have coined the term "melancholia", literally translated as "black bile". He thought that the influence of black bile and phlegm on the brain produced the depressive state which he labeled as melancholia (69).

In the second century A.D. Aretaeus made reference to melancholia and mania, noting that the conditions are often episodic but also occurred in a chronic, unremitting form. He, like Hippocrates, attributed the cause to humoral imbalance.

In 1896, Kraepelin separated the functional psychoses into two groups, the manic-depressive psychoses and dementia praecox. Undoubtedly his work was influenced by earlier endeavors of Falret and Baillarger who both gave very accurate clinical descriptions of recurrent attacks of depression and mania. Kraepelin felt that manic-depressive psychosis was independent of social and psychological forces and that the cause of the illness was "innate" (65).

Part of the controversy obscuring a clear understanding of the affective disorders is a result of semantics. Most efforts to classify the disorders revolve around dichotomies such as endogenous versus reactive, psychotic versus neurotic, or agitated versus retarded.

Most of the literature of the last few years equates reactive with neurotic depression and endogenous with psychotic. Generally, the former is milder and is a direct result of some precipitating event or the individual's response to some social or psychological stress and is less responsive to somatic therapy. This classification suffers from many shortcomings. The more recent classification of primary versus secondary avoids the inference about cause. Yet this classification has its faults as well. Many questions are still unanswered. No clear picture exists against which one can evaluate the actual importance of precipitating events.

1. What are the affective disorders?

The affective disorders are usually classed as primary and secondary affective disorders and can loosely be defined as **disturbances of mood.** The two obvious disturbances are depression and mania. However, not all depressive states are classified as affective disorders. There are depressive states that are symptoms of other disease states (pancreatitis) or that are normal reactions to external events or stress (death of a loved-one). The depressive phenomena with which we are concerned and which we are classifying as affective disorders include secondary depression and primary depression.

Secondary depression may be considered to be depression which can be traced to a pre-existing medical or psychiatric condition. It is not necessarily a reaction to the pre-existing condition but rather a depressive episode superimposed upon the pre-existing condition. For example, secondary depression is commonly diagnosed as secondary to an anxiety neurosis, alcoholism, hysteria, or even schizophrenia.

Primary depression includes recurrent unipolar depression and the depressive phase of bipolar, manic-depressive illness of which there may be many or few attacks over a lifetime. By convention, bipolar depression refers to depression which alternates with manic episodes. It is clinically indistinguishable from unipolar depression which refers to depressive episodes with no history of mania or hypomania.

Clinically, the opposite of depression is **mania.** Bipolar illness is often further broken down into bipolar type-I and type-II. Bipolar type-I refers to patients who experience depression alternating with mania, while bipolar type-II refers to depressions which alternate with hypomania or periods which might appear normal to the casual or untrained observer (36, 40, 59, 137).

With adherence to the above categorizations, further dissection of each of the affective disorders, with a presentation of the clinical signs and symptoms of each, and an attempt to present a rational approach to their treatment, will be undertaken in this chapter. To accomplish these goals, case histories and an analysis of each will be presented.

CASE A – PRIMARY DEPRESSION: H.T., a 36-year-old white male, presented to the outpatient clinic with the following constellation of symptoms: His mood was dysphoric. During the interview, he expressed ideas of hopelessness, self-reproach and suicidal thoughts. He stated that for the past three or four weeks he has felt increasingly worthless; he thought that people were talking about him and that his family was going to have him committed. He has refused to engage in social functions, preferring to remain alone in his room. He complained of sleep disturbances which included early morning awakening and tiredness on arising. His appetite has been poor, which has caused him to lose 7 to 10 pounds within the last three weeks. His job performance has been poor and he often misses work. He related these problems to his loss of energy and diminished ability to think, concentrate, or remember even simple tasks. He complained of some mild constipation and headaches almost every day. He became tearful several times during the interview, which seemed to add to his anxiety rather than provide any relief. There was no history of manic or hypomanic behavior. There was no history of recent family or object loss. His physical appearance was unkempt. There was mild psychomotor retardation and the affect was dull. All laboratory tests were essentially within normal limits.

2. Discuss the clinical signs and symptoms of depressive illness as they apply to this patient.

Though this case is unipolar depression, several important clinical manifestations of depression which apply to both unipolar and bipolar primary depression are evident. The symptom constellation can be divided into four primary categories: (a) emotional disturbances, (b) physiological disturbances, (c) intellectual disturbances, and (d) somatic complaints.

The *emotional problems* presented in this case include dysphoric mood, self-reproach, hopelessness, worthlessness, suicidal thoughts, social withdrawal and delusions. Other emotional disturbances might include self-pity, loss of interest in usual activities, anhedonia (absence of pleasure from acts that would ordinarily be pleasurable), excessive guilt and fearfulness.

The *physiological disturbances* observed included sleep disturbances, appetite disturbances, loss of energy, psychomotor retardation and gastrointestinal problems. Other physiological disturbances often observed include decreased libido, menstrual irregularities, tachycardia and shortness of breath.

The *intellectual disturbances* observed were diminished ability to think or concentrate and impoverished memory.

Somatic complaints included headaches, but backaches or other vague bodily complaints are commonly noted.

CASE B – SECONDARY DEPRESSION: M.J., a 23-year-old white male, had recently been treated and released from a psychiatric facility with the diagnosis of paranoid schizophrenia. This was the second hospitalization, the first occurring at the age of 18 while he was serving in the Marine Corps. At the time of the first episode he was diagnosed as suffering from a stress reaction and was treated with chlorpromazine for several days for what appeared, in retrospect, to be an attempt to provide sleep and rest. Treatment did not continue on an outpatient basis, and the patient completed his tour of duty with the Marine Corps. After release from his second hospitalization, he was maintained on trifluoperazine 30 mg daily. He presented to the outpatient department for his regular outpatient clinic visit where he related that he had become increasingly unable to cope with his job, and had lost interest in his family and friends. He stated that he was unable to concentrate on his work, that he was not resting well, often awaking several times throughout the night, and that he had become despondent and often cried when he considered the

fact that he had suffered a schizophrenic episode. Relating that he had read much about schizophrenia and how cure was so unlikely, he had developed a hopeless, helpless attitude and had lately been considering suicide. There was no sign of formal thought disorder or other symptoms of exacerbation of the schizophrenic process. Intensive questioning revealed that the patient had been compliant with his antipsychotic medication regimen. He had experienced no troublesome side effects. Because of his dysphoric mood, anhedonia, and other depressive symptoms, he was given the diagnosis of secondary depression (to schizophrenia). A tricyclic antidepressant, amitriptyline, was added to the antipsychotic regimen and improvement in his sleep pattern and energy were noted within 4-5 days. Ultimate resolution of the depressive episode was noted after approximately four weeks of treatment.

3. How does secondary depression differ from primary depression?

Secondary depression literally means a depression secondary to a pre-existing medical or psychiatric illness other than an affective illness. The cause can be an internal, metabolic or psychological reaction to the pre-existing medical or psychiatric illness or it may be psychodynamic in origin. While the onset of primary depression is usually abrupt, secondary depression is usually gradual in onset. Paranoid symptoms are more common in primary depressions and are usually observed as ideas of reference. There are very few consistently distinguishing characteristics between these two forms of depressive illness.

4. What is the catecholamine theory of affective disorders?

A multiplicity of psychological and sociological variables interface with the biological organism. However, for the purpose of this discussion the focus shall be on the biological variable.

At the present time the biogenic amines are the focus of attention as the major contributors to the pathogenesis of affective disorders. The biogenic amines are basically of two chemical types: Catecholamines, which include dopamine, norepinephrine and epinephrine, and the indolamines, which include tryptamine and serotonin. It is felt that in the affective disorders, norepinephrine and serotonin play the major roles. Schildkraut in 1965 formulated what is now known as the **Catecholamine Hypothesis** when he stated that, "Some, if not all depressions are associated with an absolute or relative deficiency of catecholamines, particularly norepinephrine, at functionally important adrenergic receptor sites in the brain. Elation conversely may be associated with an excess of such amines" (102). Similar evidence has accumulated for the role of serotonin (31,44,66). However, this may be a somewhat simplistic view. It has never been proven that there is a causal relationship between brain chemistry and behavior. There are many theories involving the biogenic amines, most of which focus on the premise that alterations in the levels or metabolic fates of the biogenic amines provoke some behavior. However, there is evidence to suggest that the converse may be true; that is, alterations in social and/or psychological events (stress, etc.) can induce major changes in brain amine levels (14,22,74). Rather than involve the reader of this text in the various hypotheses which are championed by an impressive array of researchers and clinicians, several references are listed for perusal (1, 2, 3, 15, 17, 18, 20, 25, 26, 39, 42, 56, 67, 70, 97, 108, 118, 132).

5. What is the permissive hypothesis of affective disorders?

The *Permissive Hypothesis* developed by Prange and others (87) offers an explanation of affective disorders based more on the role of serotonin than on the catecholamines. This hypothesis places depression and mania on a continuum rather than at polar opposites. Depressive illness is noted to be a less severe deviation from the normal than mania. Indeed, there are clinical and biological dysfunctions shared by both manic and depressed patients. For example, depressed patients suffer from CNS arousal such as insomnia, anorexia, agitation, increased residual sodium concentrations. These same conditions exist in the manic state but are more pronounced. Additionally, manic episodes are usually preceded and followed by mild depressive episodes; and occasionally manic and depressive symptoms occur simultaneously, which can only be explained by a continuum model. By placing the permissive influence on the CNS levels of serotonin, the role of the catecholamines becomes secondary and thus determines the type of affective disorder which will be observed. These data are presented in Table 1.

As noted above, it may be demonstrated that depression and mania are a continuum representing a state of CNS hyperarousal, mania representing a more severe arousal than depression. Whybrow and Mendels (132) reported that this CNS hyperarousal was commonly manifested by a lowered arousal threshold, disruption of rapid eye movement (REM) sleep patterns, and disappearance of delta or deep sleep. They subsequently postulated that this state of CNS hyperarousal could result from an intraneuronal hypernatremic condition. There are studies (4, 16, 28, 64, 73, 81, 111, 112) to indicate that intracellular sodium levels are increased during alcoholic inebriation, thus possibly producing some of the depressive symptomatology commonly associated with those individuals who consume large amounts of alcohol during drinking binges. Increases in intraneuronal sodium cause the resting membrane potential to be lowered, thus producing a state of hyperarousal. This phenomenon may in part explain the seizure diathesis commonly associated with chronic alcohol abuse. It becomes easy, utilizing this model, to understand why depressed individuals seeking to "drown their sorrows" find themselves in a worsened state after using alcohol. A disordered electrolyte state may precipitate a disorder in biogenic amine function, since several of the enzyme systems involved in normal biogenic amine function are sodium dependent. Aberrant biogenic amine function may in turn produce a disturbance of the diencephalic reinforcement mechanisms with subsequent impairment in mood, psychomotor activity, appetite, sleep and libido. So much of the research in this area is new, emerging, contradictory, and controversial that the reader is referred to the references cited to choose or reject as he deems appropriate (8, 13, 23, 27, 33, 41, 48, 51, 52, 53, 57, 60, 72, 75, 79, 82, 86, 88, 89, 100, 109, 110, 113, 117, 119, 120, 121, 127, 128, 131, 133, 135).

Table 1
PERMISSIVE HYPOTHESIS FOR AFFECTIVE DISORDERS

(IA = Indoleaminergic Transmission
CA = Catecholaminergic Transmission)

Normal IA	+	Normal CA	=	Normal
Reduced IA	+	Normal CA	=	Predisposition to Affective Disorder
Reduced IA	+	Reduced CA	=	Depression
Reduced IA	+	Increased CA	=	Mania

6. How are the antidepressants used to treat depressions such as those presented in cases A and B?

The antidepressants are a group of drugs which derive their name from the fact that clinically they serve to lift depression, restore a normal balance of mood, or improve ego functioning. They generally fall into three pharmacologic categories: (a) Tricyclic antidepressants, (b) Monoamine oxidase inhibitors, and (c) Stimulants. By far the greatest use is made of the tricyclic compounds.

The *tricyclic agents*, of which imipramine is the prototype, encompass six agents. These agents are the tertiary amines imipramine, amitriptyline, and doxepin and the secondary amines desipramine, nortriptyline and protriptyline (90).

The tricyclics appear to block the mechanism for norepinephrine reuptake into the presynaptic nerve ending following its release as a response to nerve stimulation (47). This produces an increased amount of norepinephrine in the synaptic cleft to produce an impulse within the postsynaptic neuron. Of the several mechanisms for the destruction of the released norepinephrine, the reuptake inactivation process is probably the most important physiologic means of terminating the amine's action. This is also true for serotonin. As can readily be seen, this theory of tricyclic action supports the catecholamine hypothesis. There is a latency period with any of the tricyclic drugs which varies from 10-20 days before beneficial effects on the mood are observed.

The tertiary amines appear to block the reuptake inactivation of serotonin while the secondary amines principally block norepinephrine (71). When the tertiary amines become demethylated they become secondary amines and block the reuptake inactivation of norepinephrine.

It was once thought that the tertiary amines had to become demethylated in order to exert their effect and this process of *in vivo* demethylation was responsible for the clinically observable latency period. Therefore, the demethylated derivatives, desipramine, and nortriptyline, were introduced to avoid this problem. However, these secondary amines act no faster than the tertiary amines; in fact, the tertiary amines are now considered pharmacologically active substances themselves.

When studying the individual characteristics of the various tricyclic agents, several striking differences are noted. For example, amitriptyline, doxepin and nortriptyline are more sedating than the others and perhaps exhibit slightly more antianxiety effect. On the other hand, protriptyline is stimulating. Table 2 (90) shows some of the other differences between these agents.

It is often tempting to pit the various attendant effects of the tricyclic agents against the presenting symptoms. For example, a retarded depression might be expected to respond better to an activating tricyclic than a sedating one, while a depressed individual who is experiencing marked insomnia would definitely benefit from an evening dose of a sedating tricyclic. However, this approach can be problematic and necessitates an accurate diagnosis. A few generalities concerning the use of the tricyclic agents which can be applied to clinical practice include the fact that men often respond better than women to imipramine (91), while the aged apparently respond better to amitriptyline than younger individuals (55). It is interesting to note that the sedation produced by the sedating tricyclics is immediate and may last for weeks. This can provide welcome relief for insomnia. Tricyclics, by abolishing REM sleep and prolonging stage IV, delta wave sleep, produce a more restful sleep.

CASE C – TRICYCLIC SIDE EFFECTS:

B.T., a 60-year-old black man, was diagnosed as suffering from primary unipolar depression. This was the first episode in several years. Past history is rather vague, but there appear to have been two or three other un-

Table 2
PHARMACOLOGICAL DIFFERENCES BETWEEN THE TRICYCLIC ANTIDEPRESSANTS

	Inherent toxicity	Guanethidine blocking	Anticholinergic effects	Sedation	Potency	Speed of action	Antianxiety effect	Antidepressant effect (under 60)	Antidepressant effect (over 60)
imipramine (Tofranil)	2	1	2	2	3	2	2	1	2
desipramine (Pertofrane, Norpramin)	2	1	2	2	3	2	2	1	2
amitriptyline (Elavil)	2	1	2	1	3	2	1	2	1
nortriptyline (Aventyl)	2	1	2	1	2	2	1	1	2
protriptyline (Vivactil)	1	1	2	3	1	2	2	1	2
doxepin (Sinequan)	3	2	3	1	3	2	1	2	1

Toxicity   Therapy
1. most
2. intermediate
3. least

treated episodes over the last thirty years. The patient was placed on a bedtime dose of amitriptyline 150 mg. After a week of therapy he complained of a dry mouth and blurred vision. He was reassured that these were only troublesome side effects and continued on the same therapy. After another week, the patient complained of constipation and difficulty urinating. He was given milk of magnesia which reduced the constipation. After three weeks of therapy he reported that he felt better, was sleeping well and had a good appetite. The urinary problem persisted, but was no worse than previously noted.

7. What are some of the more common side effects of tricyclic therapy and what can be done about them?

All of the side effects experienced by this patient were due to the significant **anticholinergic effects** caused by the tricyclic antidepressants. *Dry mouth* usually diminishes in intensity with continued treatment, but it may never totally disappear. Should it be bothersome, sugarless candy or gum may be recommended. *Constipation* usually responds to milk of magnesia, as in this case, or to dioctyl sodium sulfosuccinate 250 to 500 mg daily. Constipation is a common problem that can progress to paralytic ileus if not treated appropriately at the outset (47). (Also see the chapter on *General Care: Constipation and Diarrhea.) Benign prostatic hypertrophy* can be aggravated by tricyclic agents and must be carefully monitored. Should signs of prostatic hypertrophy appear, reduction in dosage is usually all that is necessary to provide relief. Many times, a mild discomfort from incomplete bladder emptying is all that develops and this never progresses to the point where disruption of therapy is indicated. This condition, though usually harmless, can be annoying, and requires reassurance to prevent the patient's discontinuation of treatment.

Generally, older subjects are more prone to experience the side effects of the tricyclic antidepressants and should be monitored more carefully. Other frequent side effects not noted in this patient include orthostatic hypotension, tachycardia, dizziness, and muscle tremors.

Tricyclic agents are capable of producing the **Parkinsonian syndrome** (90), which is often confusing when a patient is placed on lithium and a tricyclic concurrently. The tremor observed could result from either or both agents. It is well to remember that lithium tremors are much more common and short-lived than tricyclic induced tremors and that tricyclic tremors are usually attended by other Parkinsonian manifestations. Neither lithium-induced nor tricyclic-induced tremors are responsive to antiparkinsonian medication (125). They are generally not treatable by anything short of dosage reduction or discontinuation of therapy. The patient should be reassured that, though troublesome, they are not serious (90).

The average lethal dose is about 3.0 grams. Because suicide is not an uncommon occurrence in depressed individuals, the clinician should be aware of the treatment procedure for tricyclic overdosage (136). This is discussed in the chapter on *Poisonings.*

8. How should tricyclics be used in the treatment of depression?

In treating depression with tricyclic agents the usual starting dosage is 100-150 mg daily and can be increased up to 300-400 mg per day over the next 4-8 weeks as a maintenance dose if side effects do not become troublesome. Side effects may be minimized by giving the total daily dose at bedtime. Should sedation be desirable throughout the day, a sedating tricyclic may be given in divided daily doses, since the sedative side effect is separate from the antidepressant effect. Since most clinicians choose to give the total daily dose at bedtime, the pharmaceutical industry has developed larger dosage forms. These are convenient for the patient. The pamoate salt of imipramine offers no advantage over the hydrochloride salt forms. Prot-

riptyline and nortriptyline are exceptions to the the dosage recommendations listed above: Protriptyline is about five times as potent as the other agents in the class and nortriptyline is about twice as potent on a milligram for milligram basis. Therefore, the dosage of these agents are less, the upper limits of protriptyline being about 60-80 mg per day, while nortriptyline's upper limits approach 150-200 mg per day. Many clinicians do not administer these agents in appropriate dosage for adequate duration. The minimum effective dosage of imipramine or amitriptyline is 75-100 mg daily, though more commonly 150 mg daily is needed. Blood levels of tricyclic anti-depressants are being increasingly utilized to monitor therapeutic effects. Several weeks of continued therapy may be necessary before therapeutic effects become apparent (58, 63, 76, 77, 84, 107).

The majority of the depressions encountered clinically are unipolar and generally respond well to antidepressant treatment. However, some depressions are bipolar and present the clinician with another dilemma. The bipolar depressions respond to tricyclic therapy much like the unipolars, but tricyclics have been shown to precipitate manic episodes. This phenomenon has been referred to as the "switch" phenomenon by some investigators and can occur with short term (7-10 days) tricyclic therapy or with maintenance therapy (37). The fact that maintenance therapy involves a longer temporal exposure to the tricyclic means that the likelihood of this switch occurring becomes greater. Tricyclics have no prophylactic effect against the recurrence of manic episodes. Therefore, lithium is clearly indicated for prophylaxis of manic episodes when tricyclics are to be used for bipolar depression (93,94).

9. How long should maintenance therapy with tricyclics continue?

There are little hard data to support any stand on this issue. Prange (90) suggests a trial of dose reduction one month after remission seems complete, reinstating full dosage if symptoms reappear. Others (61) suggest reducing the dose by one-half for six months after remission before discontinuance, while others believe that maintenance therapy should continue after remission for as long as the depression symptoms initially existed. Regardless of which therapy one uses, it seems reasonable to assume that at some arbitrary point in time after remission has occurred, a trial of reduction of dosage is warranted if for no other reason than to reduce the risk of long term exposure to these chemical agents.

10. What is the mechanism of action of the monoamine oxidase inhibitors? How are they employed in the treatment of depression? Discuss the

dangers inherent in their use.

The *monoamine oxidase inhibitors* may be used to alleviate the depressions associated with both the primary and secondary affective disorders. Like the tricyclics, these agents act to increase the amount of biogenic amine available within the synaptic cleft. The mechanism of action differs from the tricyclics in that the monoamine oxidase inhibitors block the destruction of the biogenic amines by the enzyme monoamine oxidase in the presynaptic neuron. These agents are chemically classed as either hydrazines (phenelzine) or nonhydrazines (tranylcypromine and pargyline). They not only inhibit MAO in the brain, but elsewhere in the body as well. Consequently, the MAO-inhibited patient is in toxic jeopardy if he consumes certain dietary amines or amine-active drugs (47). Fatal results have been reported as a consequence of these interactions (122).

In acute MAO inhibitor toxicity it is tempting to control hypotension with sympathomimetic amines and CNS hyperexcitability with barbiturates. This action can lead to disasterous consequences. Because MAO inhibitors prevent the destruction of sympathomimetic amines, severe hypertensive crisis may ensue. Similarly, these agents may also prolong the CNS depressant effects of barbiturates, as well as narcotics, alcohol and anticholinergic agents. Conservative supportive treatment aimed at maintaining normal temperature, respiration, blood pressure and proper fluid and electrolyte balance has proven most successful (47).

In man, MAO activity in the brain increases with age, thus decreasing the central stores in biogenic amines and this may explain the occurrence of involutional depressive reactions in geriatric patients (98). While treating the elderly depressed patient with MAO inhibitors is indeed an appealing thought, the fact remains that they are potentially very toxic agents and the elderly are even more susceptible to untoward reactions than younger individuals.

Because of the inherent toxicity of these agents, *the tricyclics are preferred.* If there is good genetic inference (i.e., response of blood relatives) that the patient will respond to MAO inhibitors better than the tricyclics, or if a patient is found to be refractory to tricyclic action, the agents may be judiciously tried. There is some indication that when hysteria, obsessive-compulsive behavior, and anxiety neuroses accompany depression, the MAO inhibitors may be more effective than the tricyclics. Generally, indications for use of the MAO-inhibitors are the same as for the tricyclic agents.

11. How are the stimulants employed in the treatment of depression?

The stimulant class of antidepressants are infrequently used in psychiatry. They are attended by several serious complications such as addiction liability, short therapeutic effect, rapid development of tolerance, and a perception of unpleasantness by the depressed patient. Additionally, with the development of physical dependence, a withdrawal syndrome results upon discontinuation. This withdrawal itself is usually manifested by severe depression. Some clinicians use stimulants during the first 2-3 weeks of tricyclic therapy to elevate the CNS levels of the neurotransmitters as well as to provide a direct euphoriogenic effect until the antidepressant effect of the tricyclic develops (129).

Amphetamine is thought to cause the presynaptic neuron to leak neurotransmitters as well as to increase the amount of transmitter released with each impulse and even prevent the reuptake inactivation of neurotransmitters much like the tricyclics. This triphasic action can enhance the antidepressant effect, since it develops earlier than the tricyclic's effects (123).

Methylphenidate appears to interfere with the enzymatic destruction of imipramine, thus producing increased plasma and tissue levels (85,129). This probably has no advantage over an increased dosage of imipramine alone. Needless to say, stimulants should not be used in combination with MAO inhibitors because of the potentially fatal hypertensive crisis which could be produced by such a combination.

12. What other pharmacological agents have been used in the treatment of depression?

Other agents are mentioned, since they are the subject of investigations either singly or in combination with the other antidepressants. *L-Dopa,* an amino acid precursor of the catecholamines, has been tried as an antidepressant with poor results. This poor effect of L-Dopa strikes a blow at the catecholamine theory of depression. Because it raises the level of biogenic amines centrally, primarily dopamine, the lack of activity of L-Dopa is consistent with the permissive hypothesis. By increasing catecholamine activity without increasing indolamine activity, the affective disorder permission remains, but the type changes. Indeed, reports of depressions changing to mania have appeared (27).

L-tryptophan is a precursor of serotonin requiring the action of tryptophan hydroxylase to convert it to serotonin. This agent shows promise in the treatment of mania, but further studies are needed (90).

Triiodothyronine (T_3) has been tried as an adjunct to tricyclic therapy. Studies have shown that a two-week course of T_3 in a dosage of 25 mcg per day will enhance the therapeutic efficacy of tricyclics. It will occasionally shorten the lag time associated with tricyclic response and has converted non-responders to responders (92,130).

Prange (90) has reviewed the basis for the use of other more controversial experimental agents which are being investigated in affective states.

13. Can plasma levels of tricyclic antidepressants be utilized to insure proper dosing?

A frequent cause of failure with these agents in properly diagnosed cases is the failure to achieve proper levels of the drug within the patient. In other cases, the patient may be judged to be too sensitive to the adverse effects of the drugs when, in fact, the dosage was much too high. Plasma levels demonstrate marked inter-individual differences. For example, the same dose in two patients may produce a plasma level 200 times as high in one as in the other (43). Since each tricyclic has an optimal effective blood level, it is critical that this level be reached and maintained for the duration of treatment. Once plasma levels of the agents are known, a more rational decision can be reached concerning the proper dosage, less sedating.

Plasma levels reflect the central nervous system levels of these agents. The tricyclics are highly lipid soluble and tend to accumulate in fatty tissue, especially the brain. Therefore, blood tricyclic concentration tends to be low by comparison and would be even lower if these agents were not approximately 90% bound to plasma protein (5,24).

The tricyclics are metabolized to active and inactive metabolites with less than 10% excreted in the feces unchanged. The hepatic metabolism chiefly consists of N-demethylation, hydroxylation and subsequent conjugation with glucuronic acid (50). Tertiary compounds are metabolized to active secondary compounds. Other metabolites may be inactive as antidepressants, but may be responsible for some of the side effects. The use of gas-liquid chromatography and mass spectrometry makes it possible to measure levels of tricyclics and their metabolites in blood and urine with great accuracy, specificity and sensitivity.

At present, this approach is still experimental, but it holds great promise for the future (43).

14. M.A., a 30-year-old black female, was seen in the emergency room of city hospital in a very depressed, dysphoric state. She was withdrawn, displayed psychomotor retardation, bland affect, and episodic crying. Questioning revealed that her thought content was coherent and appropriate. She related that she felt worthless, hopeless and totally devoid of any pleasurable feelings or emotional responsiveness. She expressed ideas of reference, and indicated that she had heard her name being called on several occasions only to find no one was calling to her. She admitted suicidal intent. History revealed that this was the third episode of this

nature for the patient and that she was presently taking 250 mg of amitriptyline daily. There was a negative history for alcohol or other drugs. All routine laboratory tests were within normal limits (WNL). The patient was started on thiothixene 2 mg qid along with the tricyclic and began to respond after four days of therapy. Discuss how the major tranquilizers are applied to the treatment of depressive affective disorders.

Depressions, per se, do not constitute an indication for major tranquilizer therapy. Usually, depressions can be adequately managed with tricyclic antidepressant therapy. However, when a depressive reaction becomes so severe as to produce poor reality testing in the afflicted individual (manifested by delusions, hallucinations, feelings of unreality, depersonalization, paranoid ideation) a major tranquilizer has a definite place in the therapeutic regimen. Major tranquilizers apparently produce an ego boosting effect, improving self concept and alleviating to some degree the faulty ego functioning which causes one to become paranoid, hallucinate, etc. It is not intended that these agents be administred solely to produce rest, relaxation or sedation. Their effects, though helpful, can be achieved with the proper selection of a tricyclic antidepressant. Some reports have indicated that certain of the antipsychotic agents possess significant antidepressant properties (83). Those agents that have proven most efficacious in this respect are the more potent, less sedating agents. Small doses should be used to bolster ego functioning, because larger doses can produce a depersonalization syndrome in some patients, complicating the management of the case. Generally, because of the attendant adverse effects associated with major tranquilizers, they should only be used if antidepressants alone fail to achieve the desired clinical response.

CASE D – MANIA: Mr. W. is a 56-year-old caucasian male who has a long psychiatric history. Following the accidental death of his young daughter, Mr. W. experienced profound grief much beyond normal proportions. After over a year of depressive behavior, he was hospitalized and given electroconvulsive treatments (ECT). He responded briefly, but then began to relapse. Suddenly, after a period of mild depression lasting one or two days, Mr. W. became agitated, began drinking, and staying awake days at a time. This hyperactive state was described by his spouse as "going until he collapsed." At that time he was diagnosed as suffering from anxiety neurosis and alcohol abuse. He was treated with some unknown chemotherapeutic agents which kept him "knocked out all the time." Since this first episode 22 years ago, Mr. W. has had repeated episodes of profound depression for which he has received ECT and antidepressants. These episodes are usually diag-nosed as depressive neurosis or depressive neurosis complicated by alcohol abuse. During this same period of time, there have been three or four rather short-lived episodes of 2 to 3 weeks duration which the patient and his family described as "getting on the religious bandwagon." Mr. W. became very reli-gious, preaching to everyone, staying awake all night reading, feeling that he must save the world. Toward the end of these episodes he again began to con-sume alcohol and usually found himself in jail and ultimately in the hospital. The diagnoses assigned to these outbreaks ranged from alcohol abuse to paranoid schizophrenia. Prior to the last admission Mr. W. describes a day or two of feeling "a little blue" then, when working in the yard, he states that he felt as if his head "had exploded inside." He became an-gry, grandiose, loud, belligerent, suspicious, began drinking large quantities of alcohol, and abusing his family. He refused to go to bed and was later commit-ted to jail and ultimately to the hospital where he was given the diagnosis of manic-depressive illness, cir-cular. All admitting laboratory tests were WNL. Signif-icant family history revealed that the patient's father was an alcoholic and that his mother and maternal uncle had nondescript mental conditions which sounded much like depressive episodes. Treatment was begun with lithium carbonate and chlor-promazine. His behavior came under control in about five days. He was discharged two weeks after admis-sion to be followed as an outpatient on lithium and chlorpromazine.

15. What are the clinical manifestations of mania?

Mania is manifest clinically as euphoria, hyperactiv-ity and flight of ideas. Some manic patients are irrita-ble instead of euphoric. Flight of ideas is a rapid di-gression from one idea to another and, unlike the in-coherence and tangentiality of the schizophrenic's speech, is usually understandable, even though per-haps the associations are a little loose. Often this rapid speech is referred to as "pressure or push of speech." Psychotic symptoms (such as delusions of grandeur, hallucinations, ideas of passivity, ideas of reference, derealization and depersonalization), can occur dur-ing mania.

Occasionally depression and mania may occur si-multaneously, presenting as an odd mixture of both depressive and manic symptomatology.

Several additional points need to be considered in the presented case which may apply to other cases of manic-depressive illness:

(a) The patient began experiencing difficulty after a significant loss in his life which is inconsistent with the diagnosis of schizophrenia.

(b) He experienced mood swings and outbursts as-

sociated with alcohol. Careful history would have re-vealed that the mood swings preceded the patient's use of alcohol by several days. Yet, as is common with this type patient, his behavior was diagnosed as sec-ondary to alcohol abuse.

(c) Again, careful history would have revealed that the manic episodes were preceded by periods of nor-mal behavior and immediately preceded by mild de-pressions with agitation. The post-manic depressions which always followed were felt to be periods of re-morse which the patient was suffering because of his wild drinking sprees. These pre- and post-depressive episodes are almost always associated with manic episodes and provide valuable diagnostic information.

(d) The patient's alcohol use was episodic. These "binges" are more commonly associated with bipolar illness than with unipolar illness and certainly not characteristic of a chronic alcoholic or a schizophre-nic.

(e) There existed a positive family history for mental illness, though in this particular case it is not clear what type illnesses the relatives suffered.

(f) Oftentimes, behavior which looks paranoid can be manic. In this patient's case, other diagnostic signs indicated more of a manic-type behavior than para-noid schizophrenia. There was no formal thought dis-order. The patient was suspicious, but related that this was because he knew he would eventually find himself in jail because his family rejected his religiosity.

(g) Finally, the episodic nature of his condition would indicate that a primary affective disorder should have been considered. There were definite episodes of manic behavior interspersed with depressive behav-ior. Oftentimes agitated depressive behavior is dif-ficult to distinguish from manic behavior. As pointed out earlier (Question 5), the continuum model pro-poses that depression and mania share many signs of CNS hyperarousal, mania being a more severe state of hyperarousal than depression.

16. Discuss how the major tranquilizers are used in the treatment of manic episodes. (Refer to Case D).

Mania is best managed with lithium salts. However, since lithium generally takes 5-10 days to exert its an-timanic effect, it is often desirable to begin concomi-tant therapy with a major tranquilizer to calm the pa-tient. Chlorpromazine and haloperidol are often used for this purpose (21). It is not uncommon to begin patient on 400-600 mg of chlorpromazine or 20-40 mg of haloperidol along with 1200-1800 mg of lithium for rapid control. The dose of the major tranquilizer may then be tapered off as clinical response is achieved and adequate serum lithium levels are obtained.

The disadvantage of using a major tranquilizer over lithium for long-term control is that the major tran-quilizers must be used in large doses. They sedate the patient, causing dullness and sluggishness (54). Prien and his associates demonstrated that chlorpromazine and lithium were about equally effective therapeutically, but lithium did enjoy advantages over chlorpromazine mostly because of its lower incidence of side effects (95).

Haloperidol is frequently combined with lithium for rapid initial control of manic behavior. Since it is more potent than chlorpromazine and has fewer cardiovascular effects, it is superior to chlorpromazine. A recent report (30) indicating brain damage from the combination of lithium and haloperidol seems to be without basis. Ayd (9) and others have discounted the report, feeling that other causes accounted for the observations. The major tranquilizers are discussed extensively in the chapter on *Psychoses*.

17. How is lithium used to manage the affective illnesses?

It has been known for centuries that certain mineral waters produced a calming effect in some individuals. We now know that these waters contained lithium. Lithium replaces intracellular and intraneuronal sodium and thus stabilizes the neuronal membrane. It also prevents the release of norepinephrine and increases the active neuronal uptake of L-tryptophane, the precursor amino acid of serotonin (103,104). For a more detailed explanation of the mechanism of action, the reader is referred to a standard pharmacology text (47).

The use of lithium in the treatment of affective illnesses can best be described by one word, "prophylactic." Lithium prevents the recurrence of both manic and depressive episodes in bipolar patients, as well as the recurrence of depressive episodes in unipolar patients (10,11,105). Furthermore, a better response to lithium was obtained after patients had been on lithium for an extended time than was obtained during the first month of treatment. When exerting its prophylactic effect, lithium does so without significant sedation, hypnosis or intellectual impairment. It produces no tolerance or addiction. However, lithium has little effect in terminating an affective illness already underway (see Question 16).

Several studies (7,49,106) indicate that lithium is approximately equally effective in unipolar and bipolar patients. Statistical analysis of these studies bears out this conclusion (35).

Some investigators (34,93,94) found that in bipolar patients lithium had a larger quantitative effect in preventing the manic phase of the illness than it did in preventing the depressive phase of the illness. However, other studies (12,32) found essentially similar prophylactic effects against the manic and depressive phases in bipolar patients. Though these results do not agree, this author feels that lithium is equally ef-fective in both phases of the illnesses.

18. Is lithium effective in atypical affective states?

With respect to atypical affective states, such as cyclothymic personality and the so-called schizoaffective schizophrenia, the use of lithium has proven beneficial; however, it is much less effective in these states than in manic-depressive disorders. True schizophrenics develop central nervous sytem toxicity on lithium (114).

When manic-depressive disease co-exists with mental deficiency, lithium may have a moderately beneficial effect, but therapy must be closely monitored (80). Dunner and Fieve (38) described a subtype of manic-depressive patient who undergoes a very rapid cycle of four or more episodes per year. These patients respond very poorly to lithium therapy.

19. How should lithium be dosed and monitored initially and during maintenance therapy?

Though lithium alone will not bring a manic attack under control quickly, it is nonetheless important to achieve a rapid therapeutic blood level; 1200 to 1800 mg of lithium given in a divided (tid or qid) daily dose will usually achieve a blood level of 1.5 mEq/L quite rapidly (2 to 3 days). The level should be closely monitored and not allowed to exceed 2.0 mEq/L, since toxic effects rapidly become evident when this level is exceeded. After manic symptoms subside, lithium can be reduced to maintenance levels of 0.8 to 1.2 mEq/L. This may require 600 to 1800 mg per day, the average being about 1200 mg. It must be emphasized that there is wide individual variation in blood levels related to dosage. Application of lithium to depressive states does not require loading doses as described above for mania; however, the same blood levels are necessary for depressive maintenance therapy.

Initially, serum lithium levels should be monitored biweekly until the desired therapeutic level is reached. It is advisable to draw all serum samples before the morning dose to obtain consistent data. Once stabilized at a therapeutic level, serum lithium determinations can be made once per month or with patients who have demonstrated stable levels for several months, determinations may be made once per quarter.

20. What pharmacologic and pharmacokinetic principles are applicable to the use of lithium?

Serum lithium levels roughly correlate with therapeutic and toxic effects of the drug. Lithium **absorption** from the gastrointestinal tract is virtually complete (104). Apparently, food and other medications do not significantly impair absorption. This is good to remember, since lithium often causes gastric distress and concurrent administration with food or milk can be quite helpful. Absorption is complete in 6 to 8 hours, though peak serum levels are obtained in 2 to 4 hours. *Distribution* of lithium ion is roughly equal to total body water, but it later shifts intracellularly against a concentration gradient. It is not bound to plasma protein; therefore, it is freely filtered through the glomerular membrane, about 80% being reabsorbed, while the remaining 20% is excreted (124). *Excretion* of lithium is not appreciably affected by water loading, urinary acidification or diuresis, but it may be enhanced (up to 30% excreted) by *alkalinization* of the urine with sodium bicarbonate and even greater excretion may be achieved (100 to 200%) by infusing urea and sodium lactate. The half-life in the serum for an adult is about 24 hours, while in the elderly it may approach 36 hours.

Low *sodium intake* will cause serum lithium levels to rise and the converse, increased sodium intake, can cause serum levels to fall. Both sodium and lithium are reabsorbed by similar mechanisms in the renal tubule; therefore, restriction of sodium intake will allow more lithium to be reabsorbed and retained. *Fluid intake* can similarly effect serum lithium levels, marked increases in fluid intake lowers the level while reduced intake can raise the level. These changes in sodium and fluid intake must be quite pronounced for serious changes to occur in the serum lithium level (124). Some old reports dealing with the treatment of lithium toxicity recommend treatment with hypertonic saline. This does little in comparison to the use of urea and sodium lactate as mentioned above. Though rather large changes in sodium and fluid intake are necessary to produce significant serum lithium alterations, patients suffering from severe diarrhea, vomiting and dehydration should be carefully monitored for toxic signs.

21. Characterize the adverse side effects of lithium therapy. How can they be treated?

Lithium toxicity can be classified into three categories: Benign, serious and chronic. *Benign toxicity* includes a fine tremor that may persist and is unresponsive to anticholinergic therapy (125). Nausea, anorexia, stomach irritation and diarrhea are common complaints of lithium therapy which may be controlled by administering the drug with meals. Polyuria and excessive thirst are prominent within the first week of therapy due to sodium diuresis. Ataxia may appear, but is uncommon and usually transient.

Serious toxicity calls for discontinuation or reduced dosage. These toxicities include persistent vomiting and uncontrollable diarrhea, hypertonic muscles with hyperactive deep tendon reflexes and prominent muscular weakness. Chorea and choreoathetoid movements (writhing movements of the limbs) are serious toxic signs. Lethargy, drowsiness and impaired con-

sciousness that could progress to coma are signs that must be closely monitored and corrected at the onset. Opisthotonus (spastic hyperflexion of the neck), seizures and cardiac arrhythmias portend potentially fatal problems (124). The benign effects are often seen with therapeutic levels, while the serious toxicities generally appear with a serum level exceeding 2.0 mEq/L.

Chronic toxicities are extremely rare and include such conditions as non-toxic goiter, kidney tubular damage and a pitressin-resistant diabetes insipidus-like syndrome.

Toxicity can usually be averted by performing weekly serum determinations in the first 2-3 weeks and once per month thereafter until the patient is stabilized. After therapeutic response is achieved, quarterly determinations are usually sufficient. Again it should be noted that lithium toxicity is especially likely when a hyponatremic condition exists or when there is a decrease in creatinine clearance.

22. Discuss lithium's deleterious effect upon thyroid function.

Lithium possesses a goitrogenic effect, apparently producing *hypothyroidism*. Though the goiter is usually a diffuse, nontender thyroid enlargement that disappears when lithium therapy is discontinued, some cases of total abolition of thyroid function have been reported (99,115,116).

Although no clearcut data exists, it appears that the deleterious effect which lithium exerts on thyroid function is dose-related. Duration of therapy also appears to have a definite relationship to lithium's antithyroid effect. The literature is scant on this subject; however, it does not appear that lithium therapy for less than six months has been associated with the genesis of hypothyroidism. It is postulated that lithium contributes to or triggers some pre-existing thyroid defect (99,115,116). The effects of lithium on thyroid function are further discussed in the chapter on *Diseases of the Thyroid*.

23. A 28-year-old black male was admitted to the hospital for manic-depressive illness. He was in a manic state and quite agitated and hostile because of his confinement. He was placed on lithium 1800 mg daily and chlorpromazine 600 mg daily. Within four days the serum lithium level was 1.8 mEq/L and manic symptoms had subsided. Lithium dosage was reduced on the sixth day to 1200 mg daily and a maintenance serum level of 1.1 mEq/L was obtained. On the twelfth day of lithium therapy polyuria was noted. At that time, urinalysis revealed a clear urine which was negative for casts, cells, protein, glucose and bacteria. The specific gravity was 1.003. Urine volume was 3820 ml during the 24 hour collection

period. All other tests were essentially normal. What should be suspected?

Lithium can cause a *diabetes insipidus-like* syndrome manifested by high urine output of low specific gravity. Infusion of hypertonic saline paradoxically increases diuresis and water deprivation does nothing to improve urine concentration. This is not consistent with central impairment of ADH function. One proposed mechanism for this syndrome is a temporary hypokalemic nephropathy. There is no correlation between the polyuria and serum lithium levels. The syndrome may develop at any time during treatment with lithium, even after months of trouble-free lithium maintenance. Temporarily reducing the lithium dose or suspending therapy for a few days will correct the problem. Reinstitution of lithium at a lower level rarely reactivates the syndrome (6,68,96). Also see chapter on *Diseases of the Kidney.*

24. Following a clinic visit, a 24-year-old white female returned to her apartment and ingested sixty 300 mg lithium capsules. Within forty minutes she was seen in the emergency room and was noted to be comatose and exhibited hyper-reflexia, myoclonic movements, tremulousness and diarrhea. ECG recorded T-wave flattening. EEG recorded marked, diffuse delta (slow) waves punctuated with sharp spikes. Serum lithium level was 3.82 mEq/L and spinal fluid level was 1.8 mEq/L. The diagnosis was acute lithium toxicity. How should the case be managed?

Presenting signs and symptoms are obviously important in the assessment and subsequent monitoring of patients suspected of acute lithium toxicity. Those pharmacokinetic principles mentioned in Question 20 must be considered. Since this drug crosses the blood-brain barrier rather slowly, a high serum concentration does not necessarily mean a disasterous outcome. Indeed, it may be possible to promote a lithium diuresis before fatal amounts can enter the central nervous system.

Specific treatment of lithium intoxication includes the following:

(a) If the patient is conscious, gastric lavage or induction of vomiting should be performed.

(b) Urinary lithium excretion should be promoted utilizing osmotic diuretics such as 75 grams of 31% urea or alkalinization of the urine with agents such as sodium bicarbonate 245 mEq or acetazolamide 750 mg.

(c) In severe acute intoxication, hemodialysis may be life saving (124).

(d) Restoration of fluid and electrolyte balance is important. Because intoxication can persist for several days, supportive treatment is of practical value. Several reported deaths have been related to pulmo-

nary complications after acute lithium intoxication. Acute intoxication carries a much more favorable prognosis than chronic intoxication.

25. Can lithium be used in pregnant patients?

The use of lithium during pregnancy has been debated. In studies of pregnant women who took lithium, several congenital malformations have occurred, but a cause-effect relationship has not been established (46,134). In animal studies teratogenic effects have been observed at high dosage. For this reason the possible benefits derived from lithium therapy should be weighed against the possible hazards. If at all possible, lithium therapy should be suspended during the first trimester. Lithium is found in the milk of lactating women and can obviously be consumed by nursing infants. In one case, lithium was found in the serum of a nursing infant at a low level without apparent ill effects.

26. Can lithium be used in elderly patients?

The use of lithium in the geriatric population has been associated with a high incidence of toxic effects. The half-life of lithium in geriatric patients may be as long as 36 hours, probably secondary to decreased renal function in this age group. This may result in high serum levels. Furthermore, older persons appear to be somewhat more sensitive to the effects of lithium. Consequently, more frequent monitoring of serum levels is advisable for the geriatric patient (126).

27. Are there any important drug interactions with lithium?

Apparently, the tricyclics and monoamine oxidase inhibitors can be used concomitantly with lithium without adverse effect and with good therapeutic results.

The use of lithium with any agent which produces a sodium loss (e.g., a diuretic) may provoke a toxic response. Since both lithium and sodium compete for reabsorption in the renal tubule, a decreased sodium level will allow more lithium to be reabsorbed (47). This fact should be considered before placing the patient on a diuretic or low sodium diet. Individuals who perspire a great deal may experience similar problems.

An interesting reaction was reported when lithium and aldomet were used concurrently. Apparently, the combination of these drugs interferes with the serum lithium determinations. Patients presenting with clinical signs of toxicity may have a serum level which appears to be within the therapeutic range. Whether this combination interferes with accurate serum estimations of lithium or whether it causes higher intraneuronal levels, upsetting the intracellular-serum ratio, is not known (29). Until this problem is more clearly defined, the clinician should be aware of the potential problem and monitor clinical signs and symptoms very closely.

28. Are the so-called minor tranquilizers or sedative-hypnotics useful in the management of affective disorders?

Minor tranquilizers have no use in the treatment of manic episodes, nor in the management of any psychotic symptomatology. Generally, the same can be said for depressions. The biochemistry of depression is not compatible with the chemistry of this class of drugs. However, occasionally depression co-exists with severe, almost incapacitating, anxiety. In these few cases, small doses of an effective anxiolytic, such as diazepam, for a short duration are helpful.

Because these agents can produce habituation, physical dependency, tolerance, psychomotor impairment and other adverse effects, their use must be appropriately restricted, and they should only be used in low doses for brief intervals.

REFERENCES

1. Abraham K: Notes on the psychoanalytic investigation and treatment of manic depressive insanity and allied conditions (1911), in *Selected Papers on Psychoanalysis.*
2. Akiskal H et al: Overview of recent research in depression. Arch Gen Psych 32:285, 1975.
3. Akiskal H et al: Depressive disorders: Toward a unified hypothesis. Science 182:20, 1973.
4. Akiskal H et al: Diuretic-antidepressant combination in alcoholic depressives: Preliminary findings. Dis Nerv Syst 35:207, 1974.
5. Alexanderson B et al: Individual differences in plasma protein binding of nortriptyline in man: A twin study. Eur J Clin Pharmacol 4:196, 1972.
6. Angrist BM et al: Lithium induced diabetes insipidus-like syndrome. Comp Psych 11:141, 1970.
7. Angst J et al: Lithium prophylaxis in recurrent affective disorders. Brit J Psych 116:604, 1970.
8. Ashcroft G et al: 5-Hydroxytryptamine metabolism in affective illness: The effect of tryptophan administration. Psychol Med 3:326, 1973.
9. Ayd F: Lithium-haloperidol for mania: Is it safe or hazardous? Internat Drug Ther Newsletter 10:Nos. 8 and 9, 1975.
10. Baastrup P et al: Lithium as a prophylactic agent against recurrent depressions and manic-depressive psychosis. Arch Gen Psych 16:162, 1967.
11. Baastrup P et al: Prophylactic lithium. Lancet 1:1419, 1968.
12. Baastrup P et al: Prophylactic lithium: Double-blind discontinuation in manic-depressive and recurrent-depressive disorders. Lancet 2:326, 1970.
13. Baer L et al: The role of electrolytes in affective disorders. Arch Gen Psych 22:108, 1970.
14. Barchas J et al: Brain amines: Response to psychological stress. Biochem Pharmacol 12:1232, 1963.
15. Bart P: Depression: A sociological theory, in *Explorations in Psychiatric Sociology* edited by P Roman and H Trice. F. A. Davis Co., Philadelphia, 1974.
16. Beard J et al: Fluid and electrolyte balance during acute withdrawal in chronic alcoholic patients. JAMA 204:135, 1968.
17. Beck A: *Depression: Clinical, Experimental and Theoretical Aspects.* Harper and Row Publishers, Inc., New York, 1967.
18. Becker E: *The Revolution in Psychiatry.* Free Press of Glencoe, Collier-MacMilliam Ltd., London, 1964, pp. 108-135.
19. Belfer ML et al: Autonomic Effects, in *Psychotropic Drug Side Effects* edited by RI Shader and A DiMascio. Williams and Wilkins Company, Baltimore, Md., 1970, pp. 117-120.
20. Bibring E: The mechanism of depression, in *Affective Disorders* edited by P Greenacre. International Universities Press, New York, 1965, pp. 13-48.
21. Blinder M: Some observations on the use of lithium carbonate. Int J Neuropsych 4:26, 1968.
22. Bliss E et al: Brain amines and emotional stress. J Psych Res 4:189, 1966.
23. Bogdanski D et al: The effects of inorganic ions on uptake, storage and metabolism of biogenic amines in nerve endings, in Efron D (ed): *Psychopharmacology: A Review of Progress 1957-1967,* U. S. Government Printing Office, Washington, D.C., 1968, pp. 17-26.
24. Borga O et al: Plasma protein binding of tricyclic antidepressants in man. Biochem Pharmacol 18:2135, 1969.
25. Bowlby J: Grief and mourning in infancy and early childhood. Psychoanal Study Child 15:9, 1960.
26. Bunney W et al: Norepinephrine in depressive reactions. Arch Gen Psych 13:483, 1965.
27. Bunney W et al: The "switch process" in manic depressive illness: III. Theoretical implications. Arch Gen Psych 27:312, 1972.
28. Butterworth A: Depression associated with alcohol withdrawal. Q J Stud Alcohol 32:343, 1971.
29. Byrd GJ: Methyldopa and lithium carbonate: Suspected interaction. JAMA 233:320, 1975.
30. Cohen W et al: Lithium carbonate, haloperidol, and irreversible brain damage. JAMA 230:1283, 1974.
31. Coppen A: The biochemistry of affective disorders. Brit J Psych 113:1237, 1967.
32. Coppen A et al: Double-blind and open prospective studies of lithium prophylaxis in affective disorders. Psych Neurol Neurochir 76:500, 1963.
33. Crow T: Catecholamine-containing neurones and electrical self-stimulation: II. A theoretical interpretation and some psychiatric implications. Psychol Med 3:66, 1973.
34. Cundall R et al: A controlled evaulation of lithium prophylaxis in affective disorders. Psychol Med 2:308, 1972.
35. Davis J: Overview: Maintenance therapy in psychiatry: II. Affective disorders. Am J Psych 133:1, 1976.
36. *Diagnostic and Statistical Manual of Mental Disorders (DSM-II).* The Committee on Nomenclature and Statistics of The American Psychiatric Association, Washington, 1968.
37. Dorus E et al: Genetic determination of lithium ion distribution: 1. An in vitro monozygotic-dizygotic twin study. Arch Gen Psych 31:463, 1974.
38. Dunner D et al: Clinical factors in lithium carbonate prophylaxis failure. Arch Gen Psych 30:229, 1974.
39. Ferster C: Classification of behavior pathology, in *Research in Behavior Modification* edited by Krasner and L Ullman. Holt, Rinehart and Winston, Inc., New York, 1965, pp. 6-26.
40. Fieve R: *Physician's Guide to Depression.* PW Communications, Inc., New York, 1975.
41. Frazer A et al: Metabolism of tryptophan in depressive disease. Arch Gen Psych 29:528, 1973.
42. Freud S: Mourning and melancholia (1917), in *Collected Papers.* Hogarth Press, London, 1950, vol. 4, pp. 152-172.
43. Garattini S et al: Monitoring plasma levels of tricyclic antidepressant agents: An individualized approach to depression therapy, in *Physician's Guide to Depression* edited by R Fieve. PW Communications, Inc., New York, 1975.
44. Glassman A: Indolamines and affective disorders. Psychosom Med 31:107, 1969.
45. Glassman AH et al: The clinical pharmacology of imipramine: Implications for therapeutics. Arch Gen Psych 28:649, 1973.
46. Goldfield M et al: Lithium in pregnancy: A review with recommendations. Amer J Psych 127:888, 1971.
47. Goodman A and Gilman LS (eds): *The Pharmacological Basis of Therapeutics,* 5th Edition, MacMillan Publishing Company, Inc., New York, 1975.
48. Goodwin F et al: Depression following reserpine: A re-evaluation. Semin Psychiatry 3:435, 1971.
49. Grof P et al: Methodological problems of prophylactic trials in recurrent affective disorders. Brit J Psych 116:599, 1970.
50. Hammer W et al: Plasma levels of monomethylated tricyclic an-

tidepressants during treatment with imipramine-like compounds. Life Sci 6:1895, 1967.

51. Hauri P: Sleep in depression. Psych Ann 4:45, 1974.
52. Heath R (ed): *The Role of Pleasure in Behavior.* Paul B. Hoeber, Inc., New York, 1964.
53. Hokin-Nyverson M et al: Deficiency of erythrocyte sodium pump activity in bipolar manic depressive psychosis. Life Sci, to be published.
54. Hollister L: Drug therapy—mental disorders—antipsychotics and antimanic drugs. NEJM 286:984, 1972.
55. Hordern A et al: Amitriptyline in depressive states: Phenomenology and prognostic considerations. Brit J Psych 109:815, 1963.
56. Janowsky D et al: A cholinergic-adrenergic hypothesis of mania and depression. Lancet 2:632, 1972.
57. Jouvet M: Biogenic amines and the states of sleep. Science 163:32, 1969.
58. Kay D et al: A seven-month double-blind trial of amitriptyline and diazepam in ECT-treated depressed patients. Brit J Psych 117:667, 1970.
59. Klein D: A new classification of depressive disorders. Depression Notes No. 16, Sept 1975.
60. Klein D: Endogenomorphic depression: A conceptual and terminological revision. Arch Gen Psych 31:447, 1974.
61. Klein D and Davis J: *Diagnosis and Drug Treatment of Psychiatric Disorders.* Williams and Wilkins, Baltimore, 1969.
62. Klerman GL et al: Clinical pharmacology of imipramine and related antidepressant compounds. Pharmacol Rev 17:101, 1965.
63. Klerman G et al: Treatment of depression by drugs and psychotherapy. Amer J Psych 131:186, 1974.
64. Knott D et al: Diagnosis and therapy of acute withdrawal from alcohol. Curr Psych Ther 10:145, 1970.
65. Kraepelin E: *Manic Depressive Insanity and Paranoia.* E. S. Livingstone, Edinburgh, 1921.
66. Lapin et al: Intensification of the central serotoninergic processes as a possible determinant of the thymoleptic effect. Lancet 1:132, 1969.
67. Lazarus A: Learning theory and the treatment of depression. Behav Res Ther 6:83, 1968.
68. Lee RV et al: Nephrogenic diabetes insipidus and lithium intoxication—complications of lithium carbonate therapy. NEJM 284:93, 1971.
69. Lewis A: Melancholia: a historical review. In *The State of Psychiatry: Essays and Addresses.* Science House, New York, 1967.
70. Lewinsohn P: A behavioral approach to depression, in *The Psychology of Depression: Contemporary Theory and Research* edited by R Friedman and M Katz. US Government Printing House, Washington, DC, to be published.
71. Lidbrink P et al: The effect of imipramine-like drugs and antihistamine drugs on the uptake mechanisms in the central noradrenaline and 5-hydroxytryptamine neurons. Neuropharmacol 10:521, 1971.
72. Maas J: Adrenocortical steroid hormones, electrolytes and the disposition of catecholamines with particular reference to depressive states. J. Psych Res 9:227, 1972.
73. Mayfield D et al: Alcoholism, alcohol intoxication and suicide attempts. Arch Gen Psych 27:349, 1972.
74. Maynert E et al: Stress-induced release of brain norepinephrine and its inhibition by drugs. J Pharm Exp Ther 143:90, 1964.
75. Mendels J et al: Intracellular lithium concentration and clinical response: Toward a membrane theory of depression. J Psych Res 10:9, 1973.
76. Mindham R et al: An evaluation of continuation therapy with tricyclic antidepressants in depressive illness. Psychol Med 3:5, 1973.
77. Mindham R et al: Continuous therapy with tricyclic antidepressants in depressive illness. Lancet 2:854, 1972.
78. Mitchell JR et al: Antagonism of the antihypertensive action of guanethidine sulfate by desipramine hydrochloride. JAMA 202:973, 1967.
79. Naylor G et al: Erythrocyte membrane cation carrier in depressive illness. Psychol Med 3:502, 1973.
80. Naylor G et al: A double-blind trial of long term lithium therapy in mental defectives. Brit J Psych 124:52, 1974.
81. Ogata M et al: Electrolytes and osmolality in alcoholics during experimentally induced intoxication. Psychosom Med 30:463, 1968.
82. Olds J et al: Positive reinforcement produced by electrical stimu-

lation of septal area and other regions of rat brain. J Comp Physiol Psychol 47:419, 1954.
83. Overall J et al: Broad spectrum screening of psychotherapeutic drugs: Thiothixene as an antipsychotic and antidepressant. Clin Pharmacol Therap 10:36, 1969.
84. Paykel E et al: Effects of maintenance amitriptyline and psychotherapy on symptoms of depression. Psychol Med 5:67, 1975.
85. Perel J et al: In vitro metabolism studies with methylphenidate. Fed Proc 29:345, 1970.
86. Poschell B: Do biological reinforcers act via the self-stimulation areas of the brain? Physiol Behav 3:53, 1968.
87. Prange A et al: L-Tryptophan in mania: Contribution to a permissive hypothesis of affective disorders. Arch Gen Psych 30:56, 1974.
88. Prange A et al: Enhancement of imipramine antidepressant activity by thyroid hormone. Amer J Psych 126:457, 1969.
89. Prange A et al: Thyroid-imipramine clinical and chemical interaction: Evidence for a receptor deficit in depression. J Psych Res 9:187, 1972.
90. Prange A: The use of drugs in depression: Its theoretical and practical basis. Psych Ann 3:56, 1973.
91. Prange A: Published discussion of a paper by Freighner et al in Am J Psych 128:1230, 1972.
92. Prange AJ et al: Enhancement of imipramine by thyroid stimulating hormone: clinical and theoretical implications. Am J Psych 127:191, 1970.
93. Prien R et al: Lithium carbonate and imipramine in prevention of affective episodes. Arch Gen Psych 29:420, 1973.
94. Prien R et al: Lithium carbonate. Dis Nerv Syst 32:521, 1971.
95. Prien R et al: Comparison of lithium carbonate and chlorpromazine in the treatment of mania. Arch Gen Psych 26:146, 1972.
96. Ramsey TA et al: Lithium carbonate and kidney function. JAMA 219:1446, 1972.
97. Robertson J et al: Responses of young children to separation from their mothers. Courier Centre Inter Enfance 2:131, 1952.
98. Robison D et al: Aging, monoamines, and monoamine oxidase levels. Lancet 1:290, 1972.
99. Rogers M et al: Clinical hypothyroidism occurring during lithium treatment. Am J Psych 128:158, 1971.
100. Sachar E et al: Psychoendocrinology of ego disintegration. Am J Psych 126:1067, 1970.
101. Sacks MH et al: Cardiovascular complications of imipramine intoxication. JAMA 205:588, 1968.
102. Schildkraut, J: The catecholamine hypothesis of affective disorders: A review of supporting evidence. Am J Psych 122:509, 1965.
103. Schildkraut J et al: Effects of lithium ion on H3-norepinephrine. Life Sci 5:1479, 1966.
104. Schou M: Biology and pharmacology of the lithium ion. Pharmacol Rev 9:17, 1911.
105. Schou M et al: Lithium and manic depressive psychosis. Sandorama (special issue) 48, 1966.
106. Schou M et al: Pharmacological and clinical problems of lithium prophylaxis. Brit J Psych 116:615, 1970.
107. Seager C et al: Imipramine with electrical treatment in depression: a controlled trial. J Ment Sci 108:704, 1962.
108. Seligman M: Learned heplessness and depression, in *The Psychology of Depression: Contemporary Theory and Research* edited by R Freidman and M Katz. US Government Printing House, Washington, DC, to be published.
109. Seligman M: Fall into helplessness. Psychol Today 7:43, 1973.
110. Senay E: General systems theory and depression, in *Separation and Depression: Clinical and Research Aspects* edited by J Scott and E Senay. American Association for the Advancement of Science, Washington, DC, 1973, pp. 237-246.
111. Shaw D et al: Brain electrolytes in depressive and alcoholic suicides. Brit J Psych 115:69, 1969.
112. Shaw D et al: Electrolyte content of the brain in alcoholism. Brit J Psych 116:185, 1970.
113. Shaw D: Mineral metabolism, mania, and melancholia. Brit Med J 2:262, 1966.
114. Shopsin B et al: Pharmacology-toxicology of the lithium ion, in *Lithium: Its role in Psychiatric Research and Treatment* edited by S Gershon and B Shopsin. Plenum Press, New York, 1973, pp. 107-146.

115. Shopsin B et al: Lithium induced thyroid disturbance: Case report and review. Comp Psych 10:215, 1969.
116. Shopsin B: Effects of lithium on thyroid function — a review. Dis Nerv Syst 31:237, 1970.
117. Singh M: A unifying hypothesis on the biochemical basis of affective disorders. Psych Q 44:706, 1970.
118. Spitz R: Anaclitic depression: An inquiry into the genesis of psychiatric conditions in early childhood. Psychoanal Study Child 2:313, 1942.
119. Stein L: Neurochemistry of reward and punishment: Some implications for the etiology of schizophrenia. J Psych Res 8:345, 1971.
120. Stein L et al: Possible etiology of schizophrenia: Progressive damage to the noradrenergic reward system by 6-hydroxydopamine. Science 171:1032, 1971.
121. Stein L: Chemistry of reward and punishment, in *Psychopharmacology: A Review of Progress 1957-1967* edited by D Efron. US Government Printing Office, Washington, DC, 1968, 105-123.
122. Stockley I: Interactions of monamine oxidase inhibitors with foods and drugs. Pharm J 203:174, 1969.
123. Sulzer F et al: Biochemical and metabolic considerations concerning the mechanism of action of amphetamine and related compounds in *Psychotomimetic Drugs* edited by DH Efron. Raven Press, New York, 1970, pp. 83-94.
124. Thomsen K: Renal lithium elimination in man and active treatment of lithium poisoning. Acta Scand Psych Suppl 207:83, 1969.
125. Vacaflor L et al: Side effects and teratogenicity of lithium carbonate therapy. J Clin Pharmacol 10:387, 1970.
126. Van der Velde C: Toxicity of lithium carbonate in elderly patients. Am J Psych 127:1075, 1971.
127. Vogel G et al: The effect of REM deprivation on depression. Psychosomatics 14:104-107, 1973.
128. Von Bertalanffy L: *General Systems Theory.* George Braziller, New York, 1968.
129. Wharton R et al: A potential clinical use for methylphenidate with tricyclic antidepressants. Am J Psych 127:1619, 1971.
130. Wheatley D: Potentiation of amitriptyline by thyroid hormone. Arch Gen Psych 26:229, 1972.
131. White T et al: Effect of external N^+ and K^+ on the initial rates of noradrenaline uptake by synaptosomes prepared from rat brain. Biochem Biophys Acta 266:116, 1972.
132. Whybrow P et al: Toward a biology of depression: Some suggestions from neurophysiology. Am J Psych 125:45-54, 1969.
133. Whybrow P et al: Melancholia, a model in madness: A discussion of recent psychobiologic research into depressive illness. Psych Med 4:351, 1973.
134. Wilbanks G et al: Toxic effects of lithium carbonate in a mother and newborn infant. JAMA 213:865, 1970.
135. Wise C et al: Evidence of alpha-noradrenergic reward receptors and serotonergic punishment receptors in the rat brain. Biol Psych 6:3, 1973.
136. Wood C et al: Management of tricyclic antidepressant toxicities. Dis Nerv Syst 37:459, 1976.
137. Woodruff R et al: *Psychiatric Diagnosis.* Oxford University Press, New York, 1974.

Chapter 32

Drug Abuse

Darryl S. Inaba
Brian S. Katcher

Our society has only recently acknowledged a "drug problem" resulting from the use of psychoactive drugs. In reality, drugs have been used to produce altered states of consciousness in almost every society since the beginning of recorded history (47, 98,112).

"Drug abuse" and "drug addiction" are more socio-political terms than medical-pharmacological ones. As a result, the public ambiguously classifies drugs as "licit-illicit," "addicting-nonaddicting," "narcotic-nonnarcotic," or in short, "good" and "bad" (73). What is considered "drug abuse" varies greatly from culture to culture, from time to time, and from one situation to another within the same culture. For example, if barbiturates are taken to induce sleep under medical supervision, it is considered "drug use," whereas the same amount of barbiturate administered to produce euphoria is considered "drug abuse."

To avoid further confusion, we will adhere to the definition of drug addiction proposed by Jaffe (98): "a behavioral pattern of compulsive drug use, characterized by an overwhelming involvement with the use of a drug, the securing of its supply, and a high tendency to relapse after withdrawal."

Physical dependence will be separately defined from addiction, for within some individuals, addiction as defined here, has developed without physical dependence and conversely, physical dependence has developed without the development of addiction (98,193). Physical dependence then will be defined as "an altered physiological state produced by the repeated administration of a drug to prevent the appearance of a stereotype withdrawal or abstinence syndrome characteristic of a particular drug" (98).

Little is known about the mechanism of compulsive drug abuse, and although many theories have been offered, none are conclusive (32,76,97,118, 148,185,186). Moreover, the epidemiology of any drug abuse pattern is really a complex interaction between chemical, physical, psychological, and social variables. An appreciation of all these interactions is required by any health professional involved with the management of a "drug abuser."

Recent research has produced evidence of an endogenous opioid peptide in both man and animals. Referred to in literature as POP (Pituitary Opioid Polypeptide), endorphin, enkephalin, and beta-endorphin, the confirmation of endogenous peptides in man with opioid like activity will constitute a major breakthrough in the medical overview of opioid dependence and drug addiction (78,79,89,130,159). This would probably not, however, immediately change the current social interaction and medical treatment of the drug dependent individual.

The pharmacist's participation in this field has been on two basic levels: as an active participant in drug abuse treatment, prevention-education, research and screening, and as the community's or hospital's resident pharmacologist providing information about the toxicology of drugs.

The drug abuse scene has changed dramatically over the last three decades; it is the intent of this chapter to acquaint practitioners with the clinical picture, treatment modalities, and medical complications of the most common forms of drug abuse. An attempt will also be made to form a practical classification of these commonly abused drugs.

The drugs of abuse can be classed into four basic groups based upon their intrinsic pharmacological actions:

   (a) Depressants:
      (1) Opioid analgesics
      (2) Sedative-hypnotics and alcohol
   (b) Stimulants (primarily derivatives and analogues of the amphetamines and cocaine)
   (c) Psychotogens and marijuana
   (d) A miscellaneous group of inhalants, glue, and solvents.

Cases and questions will be presented to give a clinical picture of the pattern of addiction and physiologic dependence seen with each class and agents.

1. Frank Fixwell, a 25-year-old male, has been on a heroin "run" (daily use) for the past two years. His "Jones" (heroin habit) is now up to the $100 a day which he supports through various illegal activities. Although he had "kicked" (withdrawn off heroin) many times before, the longest that he managed to stay "clean" (abstinence from opiates) was only six weeks.

Eight to twelve hours after his last "fix" (injection of heroin) Frank became restless and started yawning. This was soon accompanied with a cluster of symptoms which Frank described as a "Super Flu." Frank had gone "cold turkey" (withdrawn off heroin without treatment) in jail and on his own before, and he knew that these symptoms would peak by the third day of abstinence and then subside to only minimal anxiety and restlessness by the seventh day.

Aware that his physical dependence is only one factor involved with his addiction to heroin, he seeks help in his attempt to abstain from this drug. What are the characteristics of the physiological withdrawal symptoms of heroin addiction?

The severity of opiate withdrawal symptoms that appear when the drug is discontinued is dependent upon many factors including the particular opiate, total daily dose, interval between doses, duration of use, and the health and personality of the addict.

Most opiate withdrawal symptoms will follow the general pattern described below and unlike withdrawal from barbiturate addiction, opiate withdrawal is seldom life threatening.

Six to twelve hours after the last dose of morphine or heroin (diacetylmorphine) the addict will develop symptoms of anxiety with yawning, sialorrhea, rhinorrhea, and lacrimation. There may also be profuse diaphoresis with concurrent "shaking" chills and pilomotor activity resulting in waves of "gooseflesh" of the skin (thus the term "cold turkey"). The gastrointestinal symptoms are those of anorexia, nausea, vomiting, and diarrhea with abdominal cramps.

These symptoms peak in severity 48 to 72 hours after the last dose. The most prominent symptoms are CNS hyperactivity, restlessness, and insomnia. Muscle spasms with kicking movements and pains in the bones, muscles of the back, and extremities are also characteristic.

During withdrawal the heart rate and blood pressure may be elevated; there is an increase in the levels of urinary 17-ketosteroids (50); leukocytosis is common; and the failure to take in food and fluids, combined with vomiting, sweating, and diarrhea, can result in marked weight loss, dehydration, ketosis, and acid-base imbalance. Occasionally, cardiovascular collapse during the peak phase of opiate withdrawal may occur.

The more dramatic symptoms subside in 5-10 days of abstinence even without treatment. However, there is some evidence (118) that the recovery process to restore complete physiological equilibrium may be complex and protracted. More data are needed to explain the especially high recidivism after acute detoxification from the opiates (68,69,98,189,190).

2. Are the withdrawal symptoms the same for all the opioid drugs?

Physiological withdrawal symptoms of all opioid drugs are qualitatively similar. However, there seem to be quantitative differences in the onset, duration, and overall severity of the abstinence syndromes produced by various opiate drugs.

Abstinence symptoms of meperidine appear within three hours after the last dose, peak within 8 to 12 hours and persist for 3 to 5 days. Although there seem to be fewer gastrointestinal symptoms than those produced by morphine and heroin withdrawal, there is reportedly a greater degree of restlessness, nervousness, and muscular twitching when the abstinence syndrome from meperidine is at its peak intensity (95).

Codeine, semisynthetic, and synthetic opioids also produce qualitatively similar abstinence syndromes to that of heroin and morphine. Opiates with a shorter duration of action tend to produce brief, more intense abstinence syndromes, while drugs eliminated from the body at a much slower rate produce withdrawal syndromes that are prolonged but mild (98). The abs-

tinence syndrome from methadone is consistent with the fact that it is a long-acting synthetic opiate. The symptoms are not apparent for 48-72 hours after the last dose. They are qualitatively similar to those of morphine and heroin but are less severe. Symptoms are most intense around the sixth day of abstinence. All observable symptoms except for persistent anorexia and lethargy subside and are minimal by the tenth to fourteenth day of abstinence (94).

3. J.B., a 21-year-old male who underwent bowel surgery, required morphine 10 mg sc q4h prn for two weeks. Is J.B. physiologically addicted to morphine?

Only mild symptoms of withdrawal, that may not even be recognized as such, will occur in patients who have received therapeutic doses of morphine several times daily for 1-2 weeks (98). However, withdrawal symptoms have been demonstrated in man receiving therapeutic doses of morphine, methadone or heroin four times daily after only 2-3 days if the narcotic antagonist nalorphine is administered (192). The role of physical dependence in the development of compulsive heroin or morphine abuse is apparently minor when one considers the number of patients who are made clinically dependent on the opiates during hospitalizations.

4. A 30-year-old female was admitted into the emergency room with violent shaking and chills. She admitted that she was a heroin addict and was forced into "doing some old cottons" because of an acute financial crisis. She now fears that she has contracted "cotton fever." What is "cotton fever" and what are other medical complications of heroin addiction?

When heroin is prepared for self administration, cotton is used as a filter to trap adulterants; thus, some of the drug also remains trapped within the cotton as well. These crude filters are saved, and when money or drug availability is poor, water is added to the "old cottons" to extract any remaining drug for intravenous use. "Cotton fever" is caused by an acute septicemia or an allergic reaction. The latter, caused by broken down cotton fibers or unknown foreign material may rarely result in anaphylactoid shock and death. The reaction is usually transient and will subside within 24 hours without treatment, although systemic shock requiring acute medical intervention may also occur.

Bacterial endocarditis, embolism, septic and aseptic abscesses, thrombophlebitis and cellulitis have also resulted from improper sterilization of injection apparatus and poor needle techniques.

The common practice of sharing "outfits" (needle and syringe) between friends has resulted in the transmission of viral hepatitis, syphilis, tetanus, and even malaria. Other complications of heroin addiction include the following: pulmonary emboli (caused by materials used to "cut" or dilute heroin); pulmonary edema; frequent upper respiratory tract infections (especially pneumonia); malnutrition and degenerative nerve changes (seen rarely and probably allergic in origin) (6,12,15,39,71,116,125,138).

5. What are the goals of the various treatment modalities available for the management of the opiate addict?

In a book published in 1868, H. B. Day (35) wrote that there was no agreement in the medical profession as to the proper treatment of opium disease. This statement is applicable today, as the treatment of heroin addiction is still one of legal, political, and medical controversy.

The ultimate goal of most detoxification programs is to transform the narcotic addict into a responsible, drug-free, emotionally stable, and productive member of society. Although many claims have been made, no program to date fulfills all of these goals. Furthermore, all programs either have a high recidivism rate or do not produce a drug-free state within the patient. Heroin addiction, or any chronic compulsive form of drug abuse, is a symptom of a wide variety of problems within different individuals. Therefore, no single treatment modality is universally effective.

The current available modalities are outlined below in a very general way. The two factors dealt with for each modality are those of opiate withdrawal and social rehabilitation.

6. Describe the methadone approach to the treatment of opiate addiction.

This modality, pioneered by Dole and Nyswander in 1965, has been useful primarily in the rehabilitation of chronic heroin addicts (42,43,44,45). By 1970, methadone substitution was considered the treatment of choice for opiate addiction by many researchers (98,152). Although skepticism ran high, the clamor of "drug experts" and politicians for increased methadone maintenance treatment programs (MMTP) resulted in the hasty fabrication of many such projects throughout the country. As might be expected, the effectiveness of these programs was not as good as the original ones. Also, methadone emerged as a drug of abuse and many deaths resulted from its excessive use (8,27,29,40,128,134). Thus the methadone approach is now more conservatively viewed as an important therapeutic modality rather than as a panacea of opiate abuse (49,151).

The basic pharmacology and addiction liability of methadone should be reviewed before considerations are made to incorporate this modality in the treatment of an opiate addict. Methadone is a synthetic, fully addictive, orally acting opiate with a prolonged duration of action (12-24 hours). Pharmacologically, it is qualitatively identical with morphine and other opioid analgesics (98).

Methadone plays a dual therapeutic role in the treatment of opiate addiction: that of acute detoxification and that of maintenance or long-term replacement therapy.

7. Dr. Jones, a local physician, has just seen a heroin addict who came to him for methadone treatment. Can Dr. Jones legally prescribe methadone to treat this patient's addiction? Can the pharmacist legally dispense it?

Methadone cannot be used without a special NDA (New Drug Application) permit. The drug is also under the more restrictive IND (Investigational New Drug) status if it is to be used in pregnant women or adolescents (144).

The Food Drug and Cosmetic Law (24CFR 130.40) allows for methadone detoxification treatment for no more than 21 days and methadone maintenance treatment in excess of 21 days if the ultimate goal is to produce a drug free patient (section 130.44). This law defines treatment programs and makes specifications for the inclusion of comprehensive patient services in addition to methadone therapy. It also allows private practitioners to develop detoxification and maintenance programs upon approval of the Federal Food and Drug Administration and the State Authority. A special permit is granted upon approval and after Federal forms FD 2632-2634 are filed.

The limitation on the dispensing of methadone only in specially licensed pharmacies was a matter of much controversy (144). A recent test case (Aug. 1976) before the Federal Courts has now acknowledged the legality of methadone dispensing by community pharmacies when a valid prescription is written for the treatment of pain (61). The use of methadone in the treatment of opioid addiction, however, is still limited to specific approved treatment facilities.

8. Dr. Dope has established a Methadone Treatment Medication Unit with Cure All Pharmacy. He is treating a heroin addict who claims to have a $75-100 per day "habit" of Haight-Ashbury "junk." The patient is to be started on methadone detoxification. What is the recommended methadone dose for treatment of this patient?

The quality of illicit heroin is highly variable and depends upon the geographical area from which it was obtained, its availability, and finally, the scruples of the local "connection" or "pusher." In the Haight-Ashbury of the time of this writing, a $10 to $25 "bag" or balloon filled with heroin contained 350 mg-400 mg of powder which contained 2-15% pure heroin. Thus, with generous reckoning, a $75 a day habit would equal about 120 mg of pure heroin (70). Since the quality of heroin varies greatly, it would probably be best to start methadone therapy empirically and regulate the dose on the basis of the patient's symptomatology.

Usually 1 mg of methadone can substitute for 4 mg of morphine, 2 mg of heroin, or 20 mg of meperidine (98). Reduction of the dose can be started immediately. A 20% daily reduction in dose is well tolerated and causes little discomfort. The majority of patients can be completely withdrawn from opioids in less than 10 days. Applying this formula to the above case, one would start with a dose of 60 mg methadone on the first day and progressively decrease it (48 mg, 38 mg, 30 mg, 24 mg, 19 mg, 15 mg, 12 mg, 10 mg) to 8 mg by the tenth day. At this time the methadone can be discontinued. The patient should be observed for a period of two or three days without medication, since the abstinence syndrome from methadone is not apparent for 48 to 72 hours after the last dose. This approach is highly controversial. Some recent research in methadone maintenance has shown that the dose of methadone is largely irrelevant to the size of the opioid habit, since 40 to 50 mg is sufficient to prevent the development of abstinence symptoms in the majority of addicts. The use of higher doses only affords the patient a **high** or euphoria from his daily dose of methadone (77,144). Therefore, large initial doses of methadone for allegedly large opiate "habits" are not only superfluous but also present the danger of methadone overdosage.

For habits which allegedly exceed 80 mg of pure heroin a day, a divided daily dose of 40 mg of methadone (10 mg qid) can be used initially to minimize its euphoriant properties. After two days of stabilization, the dose of methadone can be gradually reduced by 5 mg/day until the patient is on no drug by day 10.

For habits below 40 mg of heroin a day, 1 mg of methadone is administered for each 2 mg of heroin initially. Thereafter, the usual stepwise dose reduction can be instituted over the next few days of therapy. For such habits the initial dose of methadone rarely needs to exceed 15 to 20 mg (189).

Some methadone detoxification programs use adjuvant medication along with methadone therapy. Sedative-hypnotics, gastrointestinal medications, and even analgesics are used regularly in conjunction with methadone. These are usually unnecessary and an attempt should be made to differentiate between what Jaffe (98) terms "purposive" and "nonpurposive" symptoms of opioid abstinence syndromes. Purposive symptoms are subjective symptomatology that an addict will express in order to manipulate for some specific goal (i.e. narcotic prescriptions). Nonpurposive symptoms are more objective symptoms or pure physiologic signs of an abstinence syndrome (i.e. tremors). Other depressant drugs potentiate the euphoric properties of methadone.

9. What is methadone maintenance?

The clinician should acquaint himself with the role of methadone in maintenance or long-term replacement therapy. Foregoing the treatment of physiological addiction, heroin researchers have concentrated more directly upon the rehabilitation of heroin addicts with the deliberate substitution of one addicting drug for another. Although early results from methadone maintenance were somewhat variable, they were generally favorable and have constituted one of the most exciting developments in the treatment of heroin addiction in the past decade.

The ultimate goal of methadone maintenance is to produce a drug free individual. It was felt that methadone would enable an addict to escape from the illicit drug scene, thereby affording him the time to review his present life style, reorient his goals, and rehabilitate himself into a more responsible, drug free individual.

Early enthusiasm for methadone maintenance has now been tarnished by its recent use as a drug of abuse.

During methadone maintenance, the addict is stabilized on a dose that will be sufficient to suppress heroin withdrawal symptoms for 12 to 24 hours but will not produce the euphoria or the nodding high of opiate drugs. This dose will generally not exceed 50 mg (77). The drug is administered in single daily oral doses so that there is daily contact with the addicted patient. With the aid of daily counseling and rehabilitation it is hoped that the patient will eventually detoxify from methadone as well.

Recently, longer-acting methadone homologs such as d-acetylmethadol or 1-methadyl acetate have been developed. It is hoped that these homologs which have a duration of action from 72 to 96 hours will help to minimize the extensive medical and paramedical resources needed to carry out present treatment programs (99,100,152).

10. T.A., a 44-year-old male maintained on 120 mg of methadone per day, is in severe pain from an accident involving multiple fractures in his right leg. The attending emergency room physician would like to know what type and how much analgesic can be used with safety in this patient.

Although tolerance does develop to the analgesic effects of methadone in chronically maintained patients (98), clinical experience shows that conventional doses of meperidine or morphine are effective analgesics for such cases.

However, one must be wary of certain potent analgesics that are also narcotic antagonists, such as pentazocine (Talwin), which may produce opioid withdrawal symptoms when used in the methadone maintained patient (4,98).

Cushman (34) outlines two methods of handling methadone maintained patients who must undergo surgery.

(a) If the procedure is minor and pain is not expected to be severe or prolonged, full methadone maintenance dosages can be administered throughout the hospital stay including the day of surgery.

(b) If the procedure is major or if protracted pain is anticipated, methadone can be tapered preoperatively if possible and discontinued during the first few postoperative days. During this interval, analgesia and maintenance of the dependent state can be accomplished with frequent conventional doses of opioid analgesics. Methadone therapy can later be resumed by *gradually* increasing the dose to full maintenance levels.

Tolerance to the anesthetic effects of other CNS depressants is a different situation. Cross tolerance can occur in the methadone maintained individual so that higher doses of anesthetics may be indicated; however, these should be instituted with caution (6).

11. M.S., a 25-year-old female maintained on 100 mg of methadone a day, has had amenorrhea for a month and a recent positive test for pregnancy. She has not had intercourse for the last three months. Can these symptoms be due to her methadone therapy?

Although the hazards of pregnancy as well as amenorrhea, anovulation, and infertility among heroin and methadone addicted women have been somewhat over-emphasized in the past, these problems may occur and the gynecologist should be aware of them (17,19,21,169).

Horwitz and associates (88) studied the effect of differing doses of methadone on different pregnancy tests. A significant number of false positive and inconclusive tests were related to daily methadone doses when the Gravindex Slide test or the Pregnosticon Slide test were employed. High methadone doses (i.e. 200-240 mg/day) resulted in the highest percentages of false positive and inconclusive tests. However, there was minimal interference with the combination UCG-Pregnosticon tube test for pregnancy at all daily dosages of methadone studied.

In this case, the type of pregnancy test used should be established. Recommendations for a second test using the combined UCG-Pregnosticon tube test should be made. If the patient is not pregnant, methadone induced amenorrhea should be offered as a possible cause of her irregular menses. Other etiologies must also be ruled out.

12. J.R., a 28-year-old female, has been maintained on 100 mg daily doses of methadone for the past year. She is now 8 months pregnant and her obstetrician has made the following inquiries:
(a) Is methadone teratogenic?
(b) Will methadone cross the placental barrier and addict the child?
(c) Should J.R. be withdrawn from methadone?
(d) Will methadone be excreted into J.R.'s breast milk?
(e) What is the treatment of an opiate addicted newborn?

(a) Although the evidence is inconclusive, it appears that methadone is not teratogenic and that women on methadone maintenance frequently have regular menstrual periods, ovulate, conceive, and have normal pregnancies. Thirty-three per cent of babies delivered to methadone maintained mothers have been premature by weight, but no congenital anomalies have been reported. Also, four year follow-ups have demonstrated that these infants have normal physical and intellectual development (16,19).

However, there have been several reports concerning the hazards of pregnancy in the heroin addicted mother. The most commonly encountered problems included pre-eclampsia (10-15%); low birth weight (34-50%); and addiction (50-75%) of the newborn. These problems were potentiated by inadequate medical management of the addicted mother and her newborn (57).

(b) Methadone crosses the placental barrier and can cause CNS and respiratory depression as well as an opiate abstinence syndrome in the neonate. In one study, 50% of the infants born to methadone maintained mothers exhibited withdrawal signs of twitching and irritability. Half of these required treatment with phenobarbital or tincture of opium. Withdrawal signs in the newborn of a heroin addicted mother will become apparent a few hours after birth; however, in the infant of a methadone maintained mother, symptoms may be delayed for up to 3 days (16,19,182).

(c) At 8 months into pregnancy, J.R. should probably not be withdrawn from methadone because of the possibility of inducing methadone withdrawal symptoms. It is probably best to maintain her on methadone and take proper precautions to treat the neonate upon delivery for either narcotic depression or methadone addiction.

(d) Methadone is excreted into the breast milk of methadone maintained mothers. The quantities, though small, may be sufficient to cause some physical dependency in infants. Therefore, breast feeding is not advised for mothers on methadone maintenance (19).

(e) Opioid withdrawal in the neonate manifests itself in a wide variety of nonspecific signs which can readily be confused with meningitis, gastroenteritis, hypocalcemia, hypoglycemia, and intracranial hemorrhage. An accurate differential diagnosis is essential for all of these life-threatening disorders in the newborn.

In general, the most common withdrawal symptoms include restlessness, tremors, a high pitched cry, hypertonicity, increased reflexes, regurgitation and sneezing.

Management of the neonate's narcotic withdrawal syndrome entails careful attention to hydration with demand feeding, in addition to the management of the more obvious symptoms. Mild withdrawal symptoms need no treatment; however, moderate to severe symptoms may require 14 or more days of therapy.

Symptoms of physiological addition are usually apparent within 48 hours after birth. At this time treatment can be initiated with tincture of opium (10% opium) which is preferred over paregoric since the latter contains camphor. The initial dose is 1 to 2 drops per pound of body weight; this is increased until symptoms disappear. The tincture of opium is then gradually and totally withdrawn over a 1 to 2 week period (18,98,190). Methadone has also been used in a dose of 0.5 mg every 4 to 12 hours for 3 days. Doses of these drugs should be individualized so that neither withdrawal symptoms nor narcosis occur. Phenobarbital can be used to control major motor convulsions if they occur (190).

Prophylactic drug therapy should not be given to infants of addicts. Rather, therapy should begin when observable central nervous symptoms occur or when the infant is unable to sleep between feedings (57).

13. What is the "antagonist" or "heroin blockade" approach to the treatment of opioid addiction?

It has been proposed that methadone (80-150 mg or more) blocks the euphoriant effects of other opioids without producing euphoria itself. This dose produces a high degree of cross-tolerance to other opiates so that it is extremely difficult to achieve euphoric effects with intravenous injection of opioids (43).

However, this role of methadone has been questioned, since addicts have been able to obtain euphoric properties from doses of 60-100 mg of methadone. Furthermore, at lower maintenance doses of methadone which do not produce euphoria, addicts have been able to reach euphoric states through the intravenous administration of other opiates. Indeed, methadone in high blocking dosages has become a secondary drug of abuse (29,128).

The development of the true narcotic antagonists, cyclazocine and naloxone, has offered a more rational approach to heroin blockade therapy.

If opiate addiction results from a process of classical and instrumental conditioning and is positively reinforced by self administration and drug seeking behavior, then narcotic antagonists may break this addiction cycle. The advantages of the narcotic antagonist are that they (a) block the effects of heroin and other opiates; (b) prevent the development of physiologic dependence and (c) afford protection from opioid overdose deaths.

Of the two antagonists available for such therapy, cyclazocine has been the most extensively studied. The disadvantages of cyclazocine are that (a) some individuals experience unpleasant subjective effects ("like LSD"), (b) it is effective only on a short term basis because patients usually refuse to stay on the drug, (c) physiological dependence to cyclazocine may itself develop with daily doses of 4-8 mg, and (d) it is necessary to withdraw patients from all opiates before building up the dose of cyclazocine, since it can produce very severe withdrawal symptoms if it is given to an addict who is still physiologically addicted to opioids.

Naloxone (Narcan) has the advantage of being free from unpleasant subjective effects. Unfortunately, it has a short duration of action and a variable potency when taken orally. No physiologic dependence is induced by naloxone, but it is expensive; the need for close supervision in addition to the need for frequent administration of this drug, makes it somewhat impractical to use.

The use of narcotic antagonists in the treatment of opiate addiction is analagous to the use of disulfiram (Antabuse) in the alcoholic. It, therefore, seems reasonable that the narcotic antagonist will have limited value in the treatment of opiate addiction. As mentioned previously, it is important to treat the opiate addict and not just his use of opioid drugs. Cyclorphan and n-allyl opiate derivatives are other narcotic antagonists currently being studied (98,119,152,163), as are naltrexone (EN-1639A-Endo Lab.) and BC-2605 (Bristol Lab.) (3,22,120).

14. What is the "heroin maintenance" approach to narcotic addiction?

The British sought to humanize addict treatment and decrease crime by allowing private physicians to prescribe heroin to legally registered addicts. Unfortunately, addicts were not provided with adequate follow-up treatment and rehabilitative programs. Furthermore, they were not eligible for welfare, and daily intravenous doses of up to 250 mg of heroin were allowed.

It has been said that to support themselves, many of these licensed British addicts simply sold part of their heroin to novices, who soon became heroin-dependent. The latter eventually registered as addicts, perpetuated the cycle and thereby increased the population of heroin addicts. Although the number of reported British addicts did in fact increase, the number of narcotic-related crimes did not. It has been suggested that this approach did not actually increase the number of new addicts, but merely exposed those who had not entered into any available treatment program (46,116).

15. What is the "therapeutic community" approach to the treatment of narcotic addiction?

A modality that has been successful in the total rehabilitation of a heroin addict is the therapeutic community or what Smith and Gay (163) have termed the "third community" (the first community being the straight world in which an addict feels both different and alienated, and the second being the "hip drug scene" which advocates the use of psychoactive drugs as a means of problem solving and escape).

The first such program, Synanon, was founded in the early 1960's by Charles Dederick in Santa Monica, California. Dederick advanced the theory that the addict can change his deviant behavior patterns only by voluntarily joining a strongly disciplined but loving pseudo-family which helps him to re-experience the process of growing up (also termed as a total commitment to a new life style). The self-help regime utilizes all members of the "family" and includes physical labor. Synanon accomplishes its goals through techniques of group encounter and confrontation which they call "The Game." Synanon is an economically self sustaining organization with many branches throughout northern California. It offers its alternative life style to all members of society and not just drug addicts.

There have been many offshoots and variations on the Synanon theme. These include Daytop Village in Staten Island, New York; the Phoenix Complex in New York City; the Gateway House in Chicago, and the Family Awareness Houses in Arizona and California.

This is a long-term program, and although it can be successful, it appeals to relatively few addicts because of the live-in and total commitment aspects. Charles Dederick felt that Synanon would be effective for only one out of every 10 addicts and that Synanon members would never be able to return to the straight or hip worlds without going back to drugs. The biggest disadvantage of this approach is that it is suitable for only a few addicts. Of those addicts who are accepted and remain in such programs for more than a few weeks, 80 to 90% remain heroin-free and crime-free for at least one year. However, this number represents only a small per cent of the total number of addicts who need help. The programs lose their effectiveness if addicts do not join voluntarily (152,163,195).

Other short term therapeutic communities have

been organized like Synanon, but have placed more emphasis upon returning the addict to society. Odyssey House in New York, Walden House, Reality House, and Delancy Street in California and various other half-way houses throughout the country are oriented in this manner. Unfortunately, the same limitations and high recidivism rates that apply to Synanon also apply to these short-term therapeutic communities (157).

16. What is "pharmacologic" or "drug treatment" approach to the management of narcotic addiction?

Programs like the Haight-Ashbury Drug Detoxification, Rehabilitation and Aftercare Project in San Francisco provide outpatient, non-narcotic drug treatment of heroin withdrawal symptoms and place primary emphasis upon psycho-social counseling and social-vocational rehabilitation.

Outpatient treatment of heroin addicts was first instituted in the early 1900's and 44 centers were in operation between 1919 and 1923 (176). Though some clinics were reasonably successful, the New York Clinics were a disaster with respect to organization and supervision. These created such adverse publicity that all clinics were forced to close by 1923. Some authors now believe that these outpatient clinics did not receive a fair or adequate trial (46,70,124).

A small but significant re-emergence of the outpatient treatment clinics began in the late 1960's as the heroin problem reached epidemic proportions in certain communities. Now, with better organization and increased integration of "street professionals" (ex-addicts) with "paper professionals" (physicians, psychologists, pharmacists) these outpatient clinics are reasonably successful. They service a large number of the addict population in spite of the accessibility of numerous outpatient methadone maintenance programs.

The Haight-Ashbury Drug Detoxification Project, currently under the direction of Dr. John Newmeyer, is representative of these outpatient drug treatment programs. The medical regimen is set up to treat the symptomatology of each individual heroin addict. The symptomatology is broken down into four basic categories: (a) insomnia; (b) anxiety; (c) gastrointestinal complaints; and (d) musculoskeletal aches and pains.

A formulary of medications to treat these symptoms was established by first determining which of the non-narcotic drugs were acceptable to the patient population. Of these, only those drugs which afforded the highest therapeutic index and lowest addiction liability were included. Medications are dispensed on a daily basis; the single ingestion of a whole day's and night's dose of medication is not an uncommon experience. Thus, the medications used vary with the particular group of patients who are serviced by the program. Those in current use by the Haight-Ashbury Drug Detoxification Project include the following:

(a) chloral hydrate 1-1.5 gm or flurazepam (Dalmane) 30-90 mg for insomnia.

(b) diazepam (Valium) 15-40 mg or chlordiazepoxide (Librium) 20-60 mg for anxiety. Occasionally, doxepin (Sinequan) 75-300 mg is employed.

(c) belladonna alkaloids with ¼ gr phenobarbital, 4-8 tablets per day or prochlorperazine (Compazine) 30 mg for gastrointestinal complaints. Also, the balladonna alkaloids are effective for treatment of the rhinorrhea, sialorrhea and lacrimation of heroin withdrawal. Occasionally dicyclomine (Bentyl) 40-80 mg is employed.

(d) propoxyphene napsylate (Darvon N) 400-600 mg or chlorzoxazone with acetoaminophen (Parafon Forte) 4-8 tablets are used for pain.

These doses represent the daily dosages dispensed for acute heroin detoxification. The time spent in this phase should not exceed one to two weeks. The doses are then slowly reduced so that the addict is on no drug by one to two months. At this time he is encouraged to participate in social-vocational programs while his psycho-social counseling is actively continued.

This approach has been effective for the population of heroin addicts seen at the Haight Ashbury Clinic. Modification and adaptations of this type of program are necessary if one is to extend this therapy to differing populations of heroin addicts. The effectiveness of these programs may be attributed to their accessibility to the "street population." They further serve as a primary treatment "screen" for the heroin population (70).

New developments in this field have centered around the use of Darvon-N (propoxyphene napsylate) in doses of 0.6 to 2 gm per day as the sole drug treatment of opiate withdrawal symptoms (90,91,174,175).

17. Dr. Smith is treating a heroin addict in his inpatient detoxification ward at County General. The addict claims he has a $75 per day heroin habit and states that he has been taking 15 "reds" (secobarbital 100 mg) a day for the last 5 months. How should Dr. Smith manage this patient?

The problem of the multiple drug abuser is becoming fairly common. In an attempt to supplement their heroin or treat their withdrawal symptoms, heroin addicts may knowingly or unknowingly addict themselves to barbiturates, alcohol, or other sedative-hypnotics. Ultimately, simultaneous physical dependence to both types of depressant drugs may occur. Since withdrawal symptoms from heroin and barbiturates are clinically similar, the treatment of such cases is difficult to assess and may be fraught with danger if both drugs are withdrawn at the same time.

On an inpatient ward, Gay and associates (69) first withdrew the patient from the barbiturate using the phenobarbital method (see Question 21 and Table 1) while preventing the development of opiate withdrawal symptoms by maintaining the patient on 30-40 mg of methadone. Upon completion of the barbiturate withdrawal, they then withdrew the methadone in a stepwise reduction of 5 mg per day (189).

Patients who refuse to go to hospitals for fear of police intervention are treated on a different basis. They are withdrawn off heroin first using the non-narcotic drug treatment approach (70). Meanwhile, barbiturate addiction is maintained with subintoxicating amounts of phenobarbital (30 mg for each oral hypnotic dose of the short acting barbiturate allegedly ingested daily). After heroin withdrawal is complete, the phenobarbital is withdrawn in decrements of 30 mg/day (190).

18. T.F., a 21-year-old male, was brought to the emergency room in a comatose condition by friends. It was alleged that T.F. had "OD'd" (overdosed) on "junk" (heroin). A quick physical examination revealed a depressed respiratory rate of 6 per minute, cyanosis, and low body temperature. He had an increased heart rate (110 per minute), miotic symmetrical pupils, and a decreased blood pressure. Several "tracks" (needle scars) and some abcesses were noted on both arms. History, physical exam, the presence of Jaffe's (98) triad (coma, pinpoint pupils, and depressed respiration) were all consistent with an acute opiate overdose. What is the immediate treatment of choice in this situation?

Unlike the acute toxicity of other depressant drugs (i.e. barbiturates), there is a fairly safe and specific antidote for the opiate drug overdose. However, the use of these specific narcotic antagonists should not be viewed as the sole and primary management of this situation. The general principles of cardiopulmonary resuscitation should be considered the first step in the management of these cases (68,69,153).

The more traditionally used narcotic antagonists are nalorphine (Nalline) and levallorphan (Lorfan). These effectively antagonize the opioid's depressant effect, but frequent undesirable side effects and the intrinsic depressant properties of large doses limit their clinical usefulness. Their most common side effect is central nervous system excitation that can progress to acute psychosis. Other phenomena include increased narcosis, writhing, diaphoresis, and loss of urinary sphincter control. Because overdose from a mixture of depressant drugs is not an uncommon occurrence, the agonist properties of these two drugs may potentiate the CNS depressant actions of non-narcotic agents (e.g. barbiturates).

Unlike nalorphine and levallorphan, naloxone (Narcan) has little or no agonist properties of its own and is said to lack the hallucinogenic, miotic, and subjective effects as well. It does not produce tolerance or signs of physical dependence (85,102).

Naloxone also has a very high therapeutic index. A single 3000 mg oral dose has been tolerated with no reported side effects. The normal therapeutic dosage range for naloxone is from 5 to 25 mcg/kg. It is also stated to be 10 to 15 times as potent a morphine antagonist as nalorphine and 5 to 10 times as potent as levallorphan (60,85).

Other analgesics that have been abused and have caused respiratory depression upon acute overdose are pentazocine and propoxyphene. Reportedly, naloxone is capable of antagonizing the depressant effects of pentazocine and propoxyphene as well (59). The respiratory depressant effect of cyclazocine has also been effectively antagonized by naloxone (103). The limitations of naloxone include the following:

(a) Its duration of action (3-5 hours) is short relative to the narcotics so that there is a possibility of relapse, especially in the case of methadone overdosage (56,85,103).

(b) Naloxone is 5 to 8 times as potent as nalorphine in its ability to precipitate an abstinence syndrome in morphine-dependent subjects. Thus, large doses of naloxone may potentially precipitate severe withdrawal symptoms in an overdosed opiate addict. These precipitated symptoms are much more severe and difficult to manage than those induced by abstinence alone (102).

Both of these limitations apply to nalorphine and levallorphan as well. Thus, naloxone is the drug of choice in the treatment of the acute opioid toxicity. (Also see chapter on **Poisonings**.)

19. T.F. was brought to the emergency room by a friend who says he administered intravenous salt and milk solutions to T.F. in an attempt to revive him. What is the rationale of this maneuver and other types of "street therapy" in the treatment of the opiate overdose?

Of the many various "street" methods of resuscitation, two of the most commonly used and misunderstood are external stimulation and the intravenous administration of salt, milk, or vinegar solutions.

External stimulation techniques such as sharp slapping of the body, squeezing of sensitive areas (i.e. testicles or nipples), walking the victim around, placing him in a cold shower and applying ice to the testicles may all have some possible benefit in borderline cases. Since opiates only depress the automatic regulation of respiration but not its voluntary control, external stimulation of the conscious or semiconscious opioid overdosed patient may prevent apnea (98).

However, such procedures may result in an airway occluded with blood, mucous, or broken teeth, as well as broken bones and lacerations from over-vigorous application. Further, methods which produce hypothermia may exacerbate the pre-existing hypotension and complicate the management of the opioid overdosed patient (10,71).

Intravenous salt and vinegar solutions are thought to bind heroin and nullify its depressant effects. A volume of salt equal to the amount of heroin used is diluted with tap water and injected intravenously. These powerful sclerosing agents are painful and are frequently deposited outside the vein causing extreme pain. Thus, painful stimulation may again be of some benefit in arousing the borderline overdosed patient. Formation of painful abscesses, sclerosing of the veins, infections and the potentiation of pulmonary edema from a strongly hypertonic salt solution limit the usefulness of these methods (71).

Intravenous milk is also thought to reverse a heroin overdose. However, such therapy may result in microscopic embolisms, which may account in part for the lipoid pneumonia and foreign body granulomas found in the lungs of addicts (71,158).

Emetics and intravenous amphetamines are also commonly used street procedures in the management of narcotic overdose.

The force-feeding of milk and vinegar to induce vomiting is thought to stimulate the overdosed heroin addict and hasten his recovery time. Emesis may stimulate the autonomic nervous system and reverse to some extent the hypotension induced by a depressed vasomotor center. Such therapy in unconscious and semiconscious patients probably accounts for autopsy findings of milk aspirations in the lungs of opiate overdosed patients (10,158).

The "speed reversal" or the use of intravenous amphetamines and cocaine in the treatment of heroin overdose is thought to pharmacologically antagonize the depressant drug. The use of such drugs may precipitate life threatening convulsions which must be treated with depressant drugs, which may once again induce severe depression in the patient. Furthermore, cocaine has a narrow margin between stimulant and depressant effects, making it a very precarious antidote for the "street" treatment of opioid toxicity (71).

Each of these "street methods" for treating the acute opioid toxicity were described to point out the medical complications induced by such therapy. Medical professionals involved with the management of an acute heroin overdose must be cognizant of the fact that any one or a combination of "street methods" may have already been employed to complicate the overall medical status of the patient.

20. How long does it take to produce physiological

dependence to barbiturates and related sedative-hypnotics?

As pointed out in the discussion of hypnotics in the chapter on *General Care: Anxiety and Insomnia,* minor nocturnal EEG changes in the form of REM-rebound may occur after the cessation of only a few nights treatment with normal hypnotic doses of pentobarbital. However, dependence which gives rise to more obvious and more harmful signs of withdrawal requires larger doses for longer periods. After ingesting 600 mg of pentobarbital per day for one or two months, about 10% of subjects will have a single seizure on withdrawal. When subjects have ingested 900 mg to 2.2 gm per day for several months, seizures, orthostatic hypotension, and delirium occur with high frequency on withdrawal. All of the sedative-hypnotic drugs are capable of producing this abstinence syndrome (98,191). Meprobamate will induce dependence after 3.2 to 6.4 gm have been ingested for 40 days (98). Withdrawal symptoms have been seen after 80 to 120 mg of oral diazepam for 42 days (164). Table 1 lists the average dosage and time interval required for dependence on the most commonly abused hypnotic-sedatives.

During the mid 1970's there was a marked increase in methaqualone abuse in this country. Methaqualone (Sopor, Quaalude) was originally thought to be a non-addictive, non-barbiturate, and mildly toxic hypnotic drug. This is reminiscent of the early history of many sedative-hypnotics (i.e. meprobamate and glutethimide). Methaqualone is now known to cause full physical addiction and toxicity as seen in barbiturate abuse (92,165). It is estimated that 2 gm ingested daily for one month will produce withdrawal seizures (165).

Withdrawal from sedative-hypnotics is characterized by hyperexcitability of those physiological systems which have been depressed by the drug, and these effects may be present subclinically. It has been suggested that rebound tension and anxiety following only a few doses of short acting sedatives may be a motivating factor for the continued use of these agents. A single large dose of alcohol in mice first raises the seizure threshold above normal then lowers it to the subnormal levels after the effect wears off (98). Since any given drug abuser will often use a variety of CNS depressants in varying use patterns, these patients must always be treated with full awareness of possible sedative-hypnotic dependence (see also Question 17).

21. An 18-year-old woman comes to a free medical clinic in a state of extreme anxiety. She has a 12-month-history of intravenous "speed" (methamphetamine) use which has markedly decreased during the past three months when she began shooting "reds" (secobarbital) to treat the panic and paranoid reactions from the speed. Although they produced no "rush," they did provide some relief from her symptoms. After she developed several painful abcesses from missing the vein and heard stories of deaths from overdose, she began ingesting about 20 capsules per day. She has been taking these for the past two months. She would like help in kicking her "reds" habit. (a) What sequelae might occur if she discontinues her drugs abruptly at this point? (b) What treatment would you recommend for her dependence?

(a) Abstinence symptoms may be classified as minor and major. The minor symptoms, which appear within 24 hours and last three to 14 days for a drug like secobarbital or pentobarbital, include insomnia, anxiety, tremors of the upper extremities, twitching movements, muscular weakness, anorexia, nausea, and postural hypotension. Postural hypotension may be of value in differentiating the abstinence syndrome from ordinary anxiety states.

Major symptoms appear on the second or third day and last three to 14 days. Clonic-tonic seizures of the grand mal type may occur as isolated seizures or as status epilepticus. The psychoses that develop usually resemble the delirium tremens produced by alcohol withdrawal, with disorientation, agitation, delusions, and hallucinations. During the delirium, hyperthermia and agitation may lead to exhaustion and cardiovascular collapse. A number of deaths have been reported. With shorter acting barbiturates and meprobamate, symptoms reach their peak within 2 or 3 days. With long acting barbiturates and benzodiazepines, symptoms take about a week to appear and are milder (62,98,191).

(b) Treatment is substitution therapy which is directed at preventing major symptoms and minimizing minor symptoms. The patient is stabilized on any sedative-hypnotic and tapered slowly. Wikler (191) recommends first stabilizing the patient on pentobarbital, 200 to 400 mg (orally if possible) every 4-6 hours. The doses are adjusted to prevent abstinence phenomena and to minimize barbiturate intoxication. After two or three days of such stabilization the dose is tapered *slowly* at a rate not exceeding 100 mg per day.

Smith and Wesson (164) recommend phenobarbital rather than shorter acting barbiturates for substitution withdrawal, because there is a wider safety margin between easily observable toxic signs and serious overdose. Also, phenobarbital has the advantage of greater urinary excretion, a factor which may be a value in a population likely to have extensive liver damage. Furthermore, it is less likely to produce euphoria than the shorter acting barbiturates. Phenobarbital 30 mg is substituted for each 100 mg of secobarbital or pentobarbital, 10 mg of diazepam, 25 mg of chlordiazepoxide, 400 mg of meprobamate, 75 mg of methaqualone, 250 mg of chloral hydrate, 200 mg of ethchlorvynol, 100 mg of methyprylon, or 125 mg of glutethimide (165). A two day stabilization period is used for the short acting drugs, while more time is given for stabilization after switching from diazepam or chlordiazepoxide, since withdrawal symptoms from these drugs are delayed three to five days; seizures may appear as late as the eighth day. The daily dose of phenobarbital is given in four divided doses and the patient is monitored for slurred speech, nystagmus, or ataxia before each dose. The dose is omitted should any of these signs appear. Minor symptoms of withdrawal are treated with 200 mg of phenobarbital intramusculary and the daily dose is increased.

Once the patient is stabilized, the dose is tapered at a rate of 30 mg per day as long as withdrawal proceeds smoothly. Phenytoin is not incorporated into this withdrawal scheme since it will not prevent barbiturate induced seizures in animals.

Gay and co-workers (68,69) have modified this phenobarbital substitution regimen for outpatient use, since much of the population at the Haight-Ashbury Clinic refuses to be hospitalized. This approach extensively utilizes volunteer outreach personnel who are part of the community. The volunteers have had extensive personal use with drugs but have proven themselves to be current non-users. These outreach personnel provide a day to day patient monitoring that would be otherwise impossible without hospitalization.

Substitution dosing of phenobarbital must be done on a symptomatic basis rather than relying on history alone, because drug abusers give notoriously inaccurate histories; some may exaggerate their histories, while others may withhold information. Also, illicitly manufactured "reds" and "yellows" vary greatly in both purity and strength. General guidelines for phenobarbital substitution are given in Table 1.

22. Laura Lush enters the hospital at term and within one hour after the onset of regular labor pains. She is Para II and Gravida II both by C-section. By history she is a chronic alcoholic with several unsuccessful detox attempts and several documented seizures upon abstinence. What are some clinical considerations to be made in this case?

Although socially accepted and legal, alcohol by all pharmacologic, physiologic, sociologic and psychologic considerations constitutes the largest and most damaging drug abuse problem in the world. Statistics gathered by the National Institute on Alcohol abuse and Alcoholism (NIAA) in the United States are staggering (7,14). Alcohol ranks third behind heart disease and cancer as this country's biggest health problem. With 13,000 deaths due to alcohol each year (mostly from liver cirrhosis), alcohol accounted for almost 7% of all male deaths in 1971. This does not take into account the fact that alcohol is involved in at least 50% of each year's 55,500 automobile deaths. Also, alcohol usage was present in half of all murders and a fourth of all suicides in the U.S. The economic cost attributable to or associated with alcohol abuse in this country for 1971 was estimated to be $31.4 billion.

Despite these rather ominous statistics and its severe physiologic toxicology, ethanol abuse continues to be viewed more as a social problem than true drug abuse by our current society.

A complete presentation on alcoholism would probably consist of several volumes which is far beyond the scope of this one general chapter on drug abuse. However, the brief situation presented above should illustrate most of the current clinical considerations in dealing with the alcoholic patient.

Ms. Lush has gotten herself into an extremely precarious situation. It should first be recognized that true physiologic addiction does occur to alcohol and is similar in clinical characteristics to sedative-hypnotic dependence. The untreated mortality rate from Delirium Tremens (DT's) secondary to alcoholic withdrawal can be as high as 10 to 15% (13). DT's occur in up to 5% of hospitalized patients in withdrawal (150). Thus, some provisions should be made to prevent Ms. Lush from entering acute withdrawal while she is in the hospital (see Question 23).

Since the patient is secundipara via Caesarian sections, she will require another C-section here. Chronic alcoholics show cross-tolerance to general anesthetics and sedative-hypnotics but *not* to opioid drugs (98,105). Thus, an increased dosage of anesthetics or sedative-hypnotics may be required if Ms. Lush came in sober. If, on the other hand, she came in tipsy, it is important to note that a combination of ethanol with other depressant drugs results in synergistic effects increasing the potential for acute toxicity (84,141,149). The LD_{50} of alcohol alone without other drugs is 3 gm/kg or 0.5% in the blood. In most states the legal level of intoxication is set at 0.1% (150).

Alcohol is teratogenic; heavy drinking during the first trimester may affect normal fetal development, while heavy consumption near term may affect fetal nutrition and size (129a). The Food and Drug Administration has recently advised that pregnant women consume no more than two drinks on any given day, even if this is done only on an infrequent basis (61a). Neonates born to alcoholic mothers may also experience physical dependence and withdrawal (104).

Ms. Lush may also be suffering from a variety of medical problems related to her alcohol abuse. These include: cirrhosis; gastrointestinal ulcers and

TABLE 1
SEDATIVE-HYPNOTIC DEPENDENCE

GENERIC NAME	COMMON TRADE NAMES	COMMON STREET NAMES	ORAL SEDATING DOSE	PHYSICAL DEPENDENCE PRODUCING DOSE AND TIME NEEDED TO PRODUCE DEPENDENCE	TIME BEFORE ONSET OF PHYSICAL WITHDRAWAL	PEAK WITHDRAWAL SYMPTOMS (CONVULSIONS)	PHENOBARBITAL SUBSTITUTION PER EACH SEDATING DOSE
A. BARBITURATES							
SECOBARBITAL	Seconal, Seco-8	Reds, Red Devils, Seccies, F-40's, Mexican Reds	100 mg.	800-2200 mg X 35-37 days	6-12 hrs.	2-3 days	30 mg.
PENTOBARBITAL	Nembutal	Yellows, Yellow Jackets, Yellow Bullets, Nebbies	100 mg.	SAME	SAME	SAME	SAME
EQUAL PARTS OF SECO- & PENTOBARBITAL	Tuinal	Rainbows, Tuies, Double Trouble	100 mg. (Lilly F65)	SAME	SAME	SAME	SAME[1]
AMOBARBITAL	Amytal	Blue Heavens, Blue Dolls, Blues	65-100 mg.	SAME	8-12 hrs.	2-5 days	SAME[2]
B. NON-BARBITURATE SEDATIVE-HYPNOTICS							
GLUTETHIMIDE	Doriden	Goofballs, Goofers	125 mg.	1.5-3gm X 30 days	6-12 hrs.	2-3 days	30 mg.
METHAQUALONE	Quaalude, Sopor, Parest, Optimil, Somnafac	Ludes, Sopes, Soapers	75 mg.	2 gm X 30 days	6-12 hrs.	2-3 days	30 mg.
ETHCHLORVYNOL	Placidyl	—	200 mg.	1-1.5 gm X 30 days	6-12 hrs.	2-3 days	30 mg.
CHLORAL HYDRATE	Noctec, Somnos, Kessodrate	Jelly Beans, Miki's, Knockout Drops	250 mg.	Exact dose unknown 12 gm/day chronically has led to delirium upon sudden withdrawal	—	—	30 mg.
METHYPRYLON	Noludar	Noodlelars	100 mg.	3 gm x 30 days (est.)	6-12 hrs.	2-3 days	30 mg.
MEPROBAMATE	Equanil, Miltown, Meprotabs	—	400 mg.	1.6-3.2 g X 270 days	8-12 hrs.	3-8 days	30 mg.
DIAZEPAM	Valium	Vals	5-10 mg.	80-120 mg. X 42 days	12-24 hrs.	5-8 days	30 mg.[3]
CHLORDIAZE-POXIDE	Librium, Libritabs	Libs	10-25 mg.	300-600 mg. X 60-80 days	12-24 hrs.	5-8 days	SAME[3]
FLURAZEPAM	Dalmane	—	15-30 mg.	100-150 mg. X 30 days (Estimated)	8-24 hrs.	3-8 days	SAME[3]
CLORAZEPATE	Tranxene	—	7.5-15 mg.	150-180 mg. X 30 days (Estimated)	12-24 hrs.	5-8 days	SAME[3]
OXAZEPAM	Serax	—	15-30 mg.	Unknown	Unknown	Unknown	SAME[3]

[1]Note for 3 gr. Tuinal (Lilly F66) — 60 mg. of Phenobarbital would be equivalent to one (1) capsule.

[2]For 3 gr. Amytal (Lilly F33) — 60 mg. of Phenobarbital would be equivalent to one (1) capsule.

[3]Though 30 mg. will substitute for the benzodiazepines, this offers no pharmacological advantage over slow withdrawal of the addicting agent.

esophageal varices; cardiac and skeletal muscle damage; pellagra, peripheral polyneuropathies, Wernicke's encephalopathy, and Korsakoff's psychosis; hypoglycemia; fluid and electrolyte imbalances; infections; and traumatic injuries (13,98,108,129).

23. Acknowledging her ethanol dependence, Ms. Lush requests detoxification shortly after she is out of the recovery room. What are the clinical characteristics of alcohol withdrawal and how can it be managed?

When the body's metabolic capacity for ethanol (1 oz. whiskey, 4 oz. of wine, or 1½ beers per hour) is exceeded, physiologic addiction can occur in a matter of only a few days. Thus, withdrawal can occur after a few days of ingestion of 4 oz. whiskey every 3 hours (7,98).

Withdrawal symptoms are usually observable within 8 to 72 hours of total abstinence (13,98,150). Withdrawal symptoms have also been precipitated with only a slight decrease of the ethanol blood levels (i.e. 300 to 100 mg%) of an alcoholic (98).

There are acute, subacute and chronic phases of withdrawal (105). Though unpredictably progressive and overlapping, there are four stages of the acute treatment phase:

Stage I: Psychomotor agitation, autonomic hyperactivity (tachycardia, hypertension, hyperhidrosis), anorexia, insomnia.

Stage II: Hallucinations — auditory, visual, tactile or a combination of these; rarely olfactory. The hallucinatory experience is usually a frightening one and usually there is partial or total amnesia of the details.

Stage III: Delusions, disorientation, delirium, may be intermittent in nature — usually followed by amnesia.

Stage IV: Seizure activity.

Though Stages III and IV combined have been referred to as "Delirium Tremens" in the past, a more accurate description of the progressive signs and symptoms is much more appropriate to therapy.

The onset of major seizure activity is usually within 24 to 48 hours of withdrawal (13). Though generally self-limiting, seizures may occasionally progress to status epilepticus requiring definitive therapy such as intravenous diazepam (Valium).

The treatment of the acute withdrawal phase is best described as sedation while avoiding excessive sedation (108). Though chlorpromazine, hydroxyzine, chloral hydrate, barbiturates and paraldehyde have all been used clinically, most recent clinical studies have demonstrated the benzodiazepine sedative-hypnotics to be the most effective and accepted drugs during acute alcohol withdrawal (13,150). The most commonly used benzodiazepines are diazepam and chlordiazepoxide. Although both of these benzodiazepines have been extensively used both intravenously and in-

tramuscularly they are incompletely and slowly absorbed from IM injection sites (8a,66a,81a,169a). For the treatment of acute alcohol withdrawal some clinicians recommend diazepam 10 mg IV followed by 5 mg every five minutes until the patient is calm (not comatose) followed by maintenance doses of 5-10 mg po or slow IV at intervals of one to four hours (6a). Higher dosages may be necessary in patients who are excessive smokers (150). (Also see chapter on *General Care: Anxiety and Insomnia.*)

Though the phenothiazines and major tranquilizers may be of some benefit in alcoholic hallucinosis and alcohol paranoia, these drugs lower seizure threshold and can precipitate seizures in the alcoholic abstinence syndrome.

Special attention should be given to fluid and electrolyte status. Both overhydration and dehydration have been observed in the withdrawing alcoholic, the former being more typical in mild withdrawal. Plasma sodium, potassium, and magnesium should be evaluated; hypokalemia and hypomagnesemia occur frequently (13,108,150).

Multivitamin preparations are given on an empirical basis. However, even a few milligrams of thiamine will rapidly reverse sixth cranial nerve paresis. Doses of 50 to 100 mg of thiamine are usually given IM or by slow IV infusion. At least one dose of thiamine should be administered, but there is no evidence to justify daily routine administration (150).

Phenytoin will not prevent withdrawal seizures (13,150), but it should be used in conjunction with benzodiazepines in patients with pre-existing seizure disorders. Fructose therapy to increase the rate of ethanol removal has little clinical application (150).

Total abstinence from alcohol is extremely difficult due to its social acceptance, availability and ubiquity in our society. Thus, the most important and also the most difficult aspect of treatment is the chronic phase. Currently three basic approaches are employed:

(a) *Pharmaco-therapeutic approach:* Chronically administered medications are used to offset the underlying anxiety and/or depressed psyche of the chronic alcoholic. Though merely replacing one drug for another, some alcoholics stabilize into socially acceptable behavior when maintained on medications like diazepam 5-40 mg per day or doxepin 75-300 mg per day (13,108,150).

(b) *Pharmaco-aversion therapy:* Disulfiram (Antabuse) is used in daily maintenance doses of 250 to 500 mg to block the full metabolism of ethanol and produce unpleasant side effects or toxicity if ethanol is concurrently imbibed. Unfortunately, alcohol present in cough syrups, sauces and even after-shave lotions has been reported to cause serious Antabuse reactions in some patients. This approach is fully dependent upon total compliance of the patient and patients should therefore be fully informed that the long half-life of disulfiram will induce ethanol sensitivity for six to 12 days after ingestion (13). Metronidazole (Flagyl) is also capable of inducing a similar reaction with alcohol (13), although to a much lesser degree.

(c) **Didactic, Group Therapy and Support:** A prime example of a non-drug effective therapeutic modality is Alcoholic's Anonymous (AA). This approach concentrates on the toxic sequelae of alcohol abuse and reinforces its principles through the experiences and group support of its members (108). This program, which is extremely effective, requires its members to abstain completely from the use of alcohol. A brilliant analysis of the psychodynamic basis for this approach has been provided by Bateson (11a).

24. A 28-year-old undernourished male is admitted with a diagnosis of paranoid psychosis secondary to drug abuse. He has been using cocaine and methamphetamine intravenously for the past six months. He uses heroin, alcohol, and barbiturates occasionally. He was hospitalized because of a superficial knife wound received as the result of his acting upon a very complex paranoid delusional system which appears to have developed during the past few weeks and seems related to his "speed" use.

(a) Describe the pattern of use of intravenous methamphetamine and the development of paranoid psychosis. (b) How should this patient be treated initially?

(a) In the 1960's intravenous abuse of methamphetamine became an established and extensive form of drug abuse. The user begins with a 10-20 mg dose that is repeated at one to two hour intervals. Tolerance develops rapidly, and the continuous use necessitates the injection of 100-200 mg to perpetuate the effects. The initial "flash" is likened to an intense sexual orgasm, and there is a sensation of extreme mental and physical power. During long "runs" the subject may become disorganized, paranoid, and experience unpleasant hallucinations. He may become "hung-up" carrying out some nonsensical task for hours. Amphetamine-induced compulsive behavior is not focused on a single act such as repeated handwashing but reflects the enhanced concentration and high distractability brought about by the drug. Thus, a given subject may string beads for hours or days, doodle for hours, memorize the plots of all Italian operas, and so on depending on what stimulates his interest.

At later stages abusers may be using as much as 1 gm of the dissolved crystals at one or two hour intervals. "Speed runs" may last for several days with little or no sleep. The development of tremors, pain in the muscles and joints, and utter exhaustion necessitate termination of the injections. On discontinuance the subject falls into a prolonged semicomatose state.

Paranoid psychosis may result after a single large dose of amphetamines and inevitably follows the chronic use of high doses. Often, visual hallucinations originate in the peripheral visual field; these may be accompanied by auditory hallucinations. Initially the user may be able to attribute his paranoia to the amphetamines. He may even self-medicate his psychosis with heroin or barbiturates. It is quite common for drug abusers to treat unpleasant drug effects with other drugs. Later, as amphetamine abuse becomes more intense, he loses his "intellectual awareness" of his paranoia.

These paranoid thoughts, coupled with the physical hyperactivity brought about by the drug may predispose the subject to violence. Ellinwood (54) has reviewed the role of amphetamine induced paranoid psychosis in 13 homicide cases. Violence related to amphetamine abuse was well documented in the Haight-Ashbury district in San Francisco in 1968 and 1969.

These reactions can be produced by amphetamine, amphetamine-type drugs, and cocaine (1,26,52, 54,109,132).

(b) Treatment should begin with "talk down" therapy. Such counseling, along with benzodiazepines, has been effective in the vast majority of cases treated at the Haight-Ashbury Free Medical Clinic. Acute psychotic manifestations have also been treated with chlorpromazine (Thorazine). In cases of actual toxicity, phenothiazines raise the LD-50 and reverse many of the physical symptoms (55). If untreated, this psychosis would probably resolve over a period of several days to several weeks.

25. What sort of withdrawal course can be anticipated for this patient, and how may it be treated?

Within a week the most acute symptoms will be gone. There may be some residual confusion, memory loss and delusional ideas, but virtually all these effects will gradually resolve over a period of six to 12 months (109).

After withdrawal, abusers tend to become irritable and often experience depression. In spite of these symptoms it was long thought that there was no true withdrawal stage. However, Watson and co-workers (184) have demonstrated changes in brain chemistry and alterations in REM (rapid eye movement) sleep that correlate with the clinical depression seen on withdrawal. They found a significant decrease in urinary 3-methoxy-4-hydroxyphenylglycol (MHPG) which correlated with amphetamine withdrawal and the onset of depression. Interestingly, similar decreases in MHPG are seen in some nondrug-induced depressions, and urinary MHPG is increased in mania. Although the most intense phase of the depression ends in four to five days, residual effects may last for months. Patients are better able to cope with their depression if they are told it is related to transient chemical and electrophysiological changes. Some patients respond to tricyclic antidepressants (184).

The problem of effecting a true "cure" or change in the patient's drug taking behavior is far more difficult. There has been some work in developing an antagonist to the euphoric effects of amphetamine. Although alphamethyl-tyrosine seems to be effective in this regard, Renault and Schuster (136) point out that it is unlikely that anyone would willingly substitute this drug for amphetamine. It would seem that an enforced antagonist administration program would be prohibitively cumbersome, and the great cost and effort might be better applied to more direct approaches to changing drug taking behavior (136). Counseling directed at dependency producing behavior may be of benefit (58,65,194).

The approach to chronic amphetamine abuse detoxification used at the Haight Ashbury Free Medical Clinic is three phasic (28):

1) Initial detoxification — utilizing the traditional talk-down techniques along with sedative-hypnotic medication.
2) Initial abstinence — psychosocial counseling and rehabilitation, often with the employment of tricyclic antidepressants.
3) Long-term aftercare — prolonged follow-up with positive support therapy.

Chronic cocaine abuse is less frequent, but a similar approach may be used.

26. A 21-year-old male is admitted to the Emergency Room after having what seems to have been a grand mal seizure. He has no previous history of convulsions. On the morning of admission he had taken 50 mg of dextroamphetamine orally. Within an hour he developed an increasingly severe and incapacitating bilateral frontal headache. He has been taking 20 to 30 mg of oral amphetamine daily and has occasionally used intravenous methamphetamine for the past six months. Examination revealed moderate neck stiffness. Lumbar puncture revealed an opening pressure of 460 mm H$_2$O (normal 100-200) and grossly bloody fluid. Has amphetamine abuse been associated with intracranical hemorrhage? What is the mechanism of this phenomenon?

A number of cases of intracranial hemorrhage similar to the one described have been reported in the literature. The typical picture is severe headache immediately following a dose of amphetamine; this may later be followed by seizures or other neurologic symptoms. Examination reveals evidence of an intracranial hemorrhage (80,106).

The proposed mechanism is that a pre-existing vas-cular lesion such as an intracranial aneurysm or an arteriovenous malformation gives way under the acute hypertensive effects of the amphetamine. A more difficult question is whether this pre-existing vascular lesion is caused by amphetamine abuse. Rumbaugh and his colleagues (143) injected five Rhesus monkeys with methamphetamine in a dose of 1.5 mg/kg body weight intravenously every other day for a period of two weeks. This dose would be the equivalent of a human drug abuser injecting 50 to 100 mg intravenously, the lower dose range for human abuse. Angiograms after the injections showed decreased vessel caliber; and in two of the five animals this involved a decrease in both the small branch vessels and major arteries. The animals were sacrificed after two weeks, and gross pathologic findings were extensive. The cerebral cortex and basal ganglia of all five brains were quite soft and many small petechial hemorrhages were scattered throughout the brains. Large amounts of fresh blood were observed in the subarachnoid space of three of the five animals. Microaneurysms of small arteries were found on histological section, and it was presumed that these vessels ruptured causing the petechial hemorrhages and bloody cerebrospinal fluid. Other damaged arteries became occluded, resulting in areas of ischemia, infarction, and hemorrhage. The precise mechanism of the vessel wall changes is unknown (143).

These vascular changes were similar to the "necrotizing angiitis" described by Citron and co-workers (30) in fourteen drug abuse patients. These patients presented with a variety of symptoms ranging from no symptoms at all to renal failure, pulmonary edema, hypertension, and pancreatitis. Vascular changes were noted by selective angiography in the kidney, liver, pancreas, and small bowel. Although all these patients had abused a variety of drugs, methamphetamine was a common denominator in all these cases.

Rumbaugh and co-workers (142) reviewed cerebral angiographic changes in 19 drug abuse patients. Although many of these patients had abused amphetamines, some apparently had not, and they caution that since most abusers take a variety of drugs and use a variety of administration techniques, it is difficult to rule out changes due to other drugs and impurities. Also, anoxia, hypoglycemia, foreign protein sensitivity, and sepsis are other factors which may play a role (142). This criticism has been leveled against the conclusion of Citron and co-workers (30) that methamphetamine was the cause of all the vascular changes reported in their patients. Regardless of the role of other factors and drugs, it is clear that amphetamines are capable of causing vascular damage.

27. During a rock music concert, medical help was

sought for a pèrformer who had been up all night "snorting" cocaine, the last dose just prior to examination.

He exhibited the symptoms of chronic adrenergic overstimulation. He spoke in rapid staccato bursts and was initially quite suspicious and difficult to examine. He was pale, nervous and his extremities were visibly shaking. His pupils were dilated (5 to 6 mm) but reactive to light. His mucous membranes were pale and dry. He was intermittently retching and had previously vomited some bile-stained mucoid material. His apical pulse was 140, his peripheral pulse was also 140 but thready, weak and difficult to palpate. No rhythm irregularities were noted. His hands were pale, cold and dry. His blood pressure, also hard to determine, was 220/160 bilaterally by auscultation. Respirations were 40/minute and somewhat shallow.

How should cocaine toxicity be treated?

Response to cocaine in the CNS is biphasic, beginning with stimulation in the cortex, moving downward to stimulate lower portions of the cerebrospinal axis, eventually causing cortical depresssion, and finally medullary depression and respiratory failure. The stimulant effects may actually be the result of depression of inhibitory neurons (139). In addition, cocaine causes peripheral sympathetic stimulation by preventing the re-uptake of catecholamines (139,166). Thus, depending on the degree of toxicity, patients may present with a mixture of stimulation and depression (74). A rapid, shallow breathing pattern may ensue, Cheyne-Stokes respirations may appear, and death may occur due to central respiratory collapse. Further, intense vasoconstriction combined with hypermetabolism may lead to hyperpyrexia. Hyperreflexia, CNS anoxia, and tonic-clonic convulsions may supervene. A CNS hemorrhage may occur.

Treatment should be symptomatic with constant monitoring (75). This patient was first observed for 15 minutes while at rest, during which time his vital signs remained unchanged. He was given propranolol (Inderal) 1 mg intravenously. Within 60 seconds his pulse was 120, blood pressure was 200/120, and respirations were 32/minute. He was given five more 1 mg doses of propranolol at one minute intervals. Within ten minutes after the initial dose his pulse rate was 88, blood pressure was 140/86, and respirations were 18/minute. His peripheral tremors abated, and his color improved, although his extremities remained somewhat cold and dry. His pupils remained dilated (4 mm). He was given prochlorperazine (Compazine) 10 mg IM, whereupon his retching was immediately relieved and his anxiety markedly decreased. All signs remained normal thereafter. After another 15 minutes, speaking rationally and at a normal rate, he said he felt he could "go on now." He was given a prescription for a week's supply

of diazepam, and within another 15 minutes he was onstage and playing with his group.

Gay and his co-workers have used propranolol in 1 mg increments IV at one minute intervals up to a total of 8 mg with good results in a series of more than fifty cases of cocaine induced sympathetic overstimulation (75,135). In most cases the total dose should be limited to 5 mg. This treatment protocol is still experimental and somewhat controversial. Although it has been successful, risks such as bronchospasm and A-V block must be fully appreciated.

Stimulation is the most commonly seen manifestation of toxicity, but in every case the possibility of subsequent cocaine induced depressive effects must be considered. Other symptomatic treatments include: IV diazepam for convulsions, used with full awareness that CNS anoxia may already exist; establishing an airway and administering oxygen with assisted respiration; positioning the patient to insure cerebral blood return; and external cooling for hyperpyrexia. In short, treatment is symptomatic and should remain flexible and dynamic.

28. The patient described above was an experienced cocaine user. What factors might account for his successful dosing prior to the concert and his subsequent excess?

The lethal oral dose of cocaine for a 70 kg subject is considered to be 1.2 gm. The oral LD_{50} is about 500 mg. It has been estimated that the liver can detoxify one lethal dose in an hour (75,139).

Cocaine is rapidly hydrolyzed and inactivated in the stomach; much smaller doses are rapidly effective when the drug is absorbed through mucous membranes, accounting for the popularity of "snorting" or inhaling a "line" of up to 200 mg of street cocaine. Street cocaine is usually "stepped on" or cut, often with a local anesthetic such as procaine (23,75). A recent report of analysis of 939 alleged cocaine containing samples found cocaine in various amounts as the only detected drug in 67.5% of the samples (23).

Vasoconstriction limits the rate of absorption after "snorting" onto the nasal mucosa. Cocaine blood levels were recently studied after 1.5 mg/kg was applied as a 10% solution to the nasal mucosa of surgical patients receiving the drug prior to nasal intubation (181). Plasma levels increased rapidly for 15 to 20 minutes, peaked at 15 to 60 minutes, and gradually declined over the next 3 to 5 hours. Cocaine was obtained from the nasal mucosa as long as three hours after the initial dose. The plasma half-life of cocaine in this combined elimination and absorption situation was 2.5 hours.

In spite of limited absorption due to vasoconstriction, it is possible for the rate of absorption to surpass the rate of elimination (139), and this situation might be expected with repeated doses. Fortunately, excessive use is rare, because cocaine is extremely expensive. Sometimes referred to as "the champagne of drugs" or "the rich man's drug," cocaine sells on the street for $50 to $100 a gram and is doled out like rare old brandy. However, this case illustrates the recent popularity of cocaine among subjects wealthy enough to afford frequently repeated substantial doses. When possible, doses are repeated every forty minutes to maintain the most desired effect, probably related to increasing blood levels. Thus, doses may have accumulated to some extent and added to the stimulation experienced after being up all night. Moreover, sensitization to catecholamines by preventing their re-uptake (139,166) in the charged atmosphere of a rock concert and in a performer about to go on stage, no doubt resulted in the acute toxic effects described.

29. What are the psychotogenic drugs?

Many drugs from widely varying pharmacological classes are capable of inducing the "psychedelic experience" if administered in adequate dosages in the proper setting. Thus, the many differing drugs included in this classification will be based upon the intended use of such drugs by the drug abuse population.

Some of the drugs and natural products used to induce this "psychedelic experience" are listed in Table 2.

The feature distinguishing the psychotogens from other drugs of abuse is their capacity to reliably induce states of altered perceptions, thought, and feelings that can be further described as hallucinations, delusions, illusions, perceptual distortions, or in short, the "psychedelic experience" (63,64,98).

Of the different psychotogenic compounds, the most commonly abused and comprehensively studied continues to be LSD (lysergic acid diethylamide).

30. Describe the physiological effects and systemic toxicity of LSD.

The physiological reaction to LSD and many of the other psychotogens parallels that of anticholinergic drug reactions and is characterized by reflex hyperactivity; anxiety; mydriasis; increased blood pressure, pulse rate, and body temperature. Pilo-erection, muscular weakness, tremor, sweating, nausea, stimulation of uterine smooth muscle and hyperglycemia have also been reported in man. Deaths due to respiratory depression, convulsions, and marked hyperthermia have been reported in various species of laboratory animals who received massive doses of LSD (87,98).

31. Does tolerance, physical dependence and addiction develop with the psychotogens?

Although tolerance and some degree of cross toler-

ance between LSD, mescaline and psilocybin occurs (2,98), physical dependence does not occur and addiction, as defined by this chapter, is of rare occurrence.

In a 10 year follow-up on the medical use of LSD, McGlothlin and co-workers (122) further concluded that, "compulsive patterns of LSD use rarely develops . . . the nature of the drug effect is such that it becomes less attractive with continued use and in the long term, is almost always self-limiting."

32. What sort of clinical picture is seen in patients seeking medical care after ingesting LSD?

Patients taking LSD almost always seek medical help for drug-induced psychiatric reactions. The acute panic reaction more commonly known as the "bad trip," occurs soon after taking the drug. Neuropsychiatric sequelae to such reactions have been divided into four basic categories (107): (a) the prolonged "bad trip," acute anxiety or panic reaction; (b) post-LSD depression; (c) long-term schizophrenic or psychotic reactions; and (d) the "flashback" phenomenon.

33. A 24-year-old white female was seen at Emergency Hospital in an acutely agitated state. Approximately 4 hours ago she ingested a pill described as a "pink wedge" with her boyfriend.

Approximately one hour after ingestion she began having illusions with objects changing shape and color. She interpreted this perceptual alteration to be very pleasurable and decided to take five other "pink wedges" to friends. While walking across the city park, she noticed moving shadows and became quite frightened, feeling that the police were after her. To avoid detection, she "dropped her stash" (ingested the five "pink wedges") and then ran back to her Haight Street apartment. She gradually became more agitated and confused as her perceptual alterations intensified, but her boyfriend was able to maintain some control by talking to her and insisting that it was "all in her head" and would pass as the drug effect wore off. This technique worked for a few hours, but the patient finally insisted on going to the emergency hospital for a "downer" as she thought she might "go crazy."

Upon registration at the Emergency Hospital, the attending physician ordered her boyfriend to leave. At this, she became more agitated and had to be restrained by a uniformed ambulance attendant. Chlorpromazine 100 mg IM was given, and when the patient became delirious, an ambulance was called and the patient was taken under restraint to General Hospital where she was admitted to the Psychiatric Ward. Her week long hospital course was complicated by recurrent episodes of agitation and paranoia. In addition she was found to have two frac-

TABLE 2: ABUSED PSYCHOTOGENS OF SYNTHETIC AND NATURAL ORIGIN

COMMON NAME	SLANG NAMES	CHEMICAL CONSTITUENT OR COMPOSITION
LSD	acid, big D, sugar, trips, cubes, brown dot, sunshine, and a multitude of names depending on the dealer	lysergic acid diethylamide
MESCALINE (active constituent in Peyote cactus buttons)	mesc, big chief, cactus, peyote	3,4,5-trimethoxyphenethylamine
PSILOCYBIN (active constituent in Psilocybe mushrooms)	silly putty, the mushrooms, magic mexican mushroom	3 (2-dimethylamine) ethylindol-4-ol-dihydrogen phosphate
THC (one of the active cannabinoids in marihuana, hashish and kif from the Cannabis plant)	THC, grass, pot, weed, tea, mary jane, bhang, boo, bush, dope, hay, joint, dubie, J., reefer, roach, panama red, acapulco gold, hash, kif, hash oil, red oil.	tetrahydrocannabinol
PCP (Sernylan, Sernyl)	angel's dust, hog, peace pill, elephant, crystal, crystal joint, KJ's	phencyclidine or phenylcyclohexylpiperidine
STP, DOM	serenity-tranquility-peace pill	2,5-dimethoxy-4-methyl-phenethylamine
MDA	love drug	methylene dioxy amphetamine
DMA		3,4-dimethoxyphenyl-isopropylamine
TMA		trimethoxyamphetamine
MMDA		methoxymethylene + dioxyamphetamine
STP-LSD combination	wedge series: orange, purple, etc., wedges: harvey wallbanger	a single dose form combination of these two psychotogens
DMT	businessman's special	N,N-dimethyltryptamine
DET		diethyltryptamine
DOET		2,5-dimethoxy-4-ethylamphetamine
Morning Glory Seeds (Rivea corymbosa)		ololiugui and lysergic acid amide
Hawaiian Woodrose Seeds		lysergic acid amide
Nutmeg (Myristica fragrans)		myristicin
Kat (Catha edulis)		cathine
Ibogaine (Tabernantha iboga)		ibogine (an indole alkaloid)
Belladonna		various Belladonna alkaloids

tured ribs, which were treated by a consulting orthopedist without complications.

After her discharge from General Hospital, the patient had periodic recurrences of her bad LSD experience. She sought help at the Haight-Ashbury Clinic Psychiatric Annex because she thought she was "brain-damaged." Neurological examination was negative, and the patient was seen on a weekly basis and treated with supportive psychotherapy with emphasis placed upon reassurance and abstinence from drugs. The "flashbacks" gradually faded in frequency and intensity over the next year. What is the proper management and recommended drug therapy of this "bad trip" experience?

The above case history is typical of an acute toxic reaction to a psychotogenic substance also referred to as the "bad trip," "bum trip," "bummer," or "freak out." The term "toxic reaction" may be somewhat of a misnomer since many factors contribute to the reaction described above. These include the setting, mental status, and personality of the drug user. The "toxic" reaction is not, therefore, directly related to the dosage of the drug ingested but to a multitude of environmental and subjective factors. Furthermore, the "bad trip" cannot be reliably predicted or prevented in any given user as they have been experienced by users who have had previous "good trips." Thus, this acute anxiety reaction can be more accurately described as an adverse reaction to a psychotogenic drug rather than as a true toxic reaction (98).

A "bad trip" due to a psychotogenic drug is characterized by an acute anxiety reaction that may progress to a full scale toxic psychosis. A full description of this phenomenon has been presented in many references (81,110,160,172). Smith (161) has further classified the "bad trip" into three distinctive types:

(a) *Body trips:* These involve distorted perceptions of the subject's body dealing with his physical appearance. A feeling of ugliness or dirtiness may be the precipitant factors in this type of experience.

(b) *Environmental trips:* These include distortions of the visual field surrounding the individual. Often, frightening illusions and hallucinations develop to the point that subjects lose touch of reality and believe themselves to be going insane.

(c) *Mind trips:* These involve subconscious material which surface forth into the consciousness of the individual. Identity crisis and guilt feelings cause the subject to enter into feelings of depression, failure, disgust and suicidal states.

Under this system of classification, the experience of the above case can best be described as a bad environmental trip. The employment of many contraindicated methods of management in this particular case warrants discussion.

The initial management of the "bad trip" should consist of "talk down" therapy. The therapist attempts to convince the patient that his perceptual distortions and feelings of panic are temporary effects of the drug which should dissipate after it is metabolized. The subjective effects of LSD, which has a half life of 175 minutes, normally begin to clear 12 hours after ingestion (98). Unlike the case treated above, verbal contact should be made with the patient in a calm, reassuring, confident manner before any medication is given. This should be done in a more peaceful setting with less noise, fewer people, and less confusion than that which normally occurs in the emergency room of a hospital. It is more important to be supportive and friendly than it is to be a clinician in the management of a "bad trip." Time should be spent asking gentle questions in an attempt to redirect the patient's thoughts towards pleasant experiences. Reassurance and reality defining is often times all that is needed in the management of the "bad trip" (67,117,172).

Drug therapy of this initial anxiety reaction should only be considered after the patient is found to be refractory to the above procedures or if the patient insists that he needs something to bring him back to reality. Although chlorpromazine 50 mg IM initially, followed by 100 mg p.o. has been the recommended therapy of choice in the past, exacerbation of the anxiety state, orthostatic hypotensive episodes, precipitation of post-psychotic depression, an increased incidence of the "flashback" phenomenon, and potentiation of anticholinergic psychotogenic drugs now limit the usefulness of phenothiazine drugs in the initial management of the psychotogenic "bad trip" experience.

Furthermore, some clinical experience has suggested that the therapeutic effectiveness of the phenothiazines in the management of the "bad trip" may be more dependent upon the sedative qualities of these drugs rather than their antipsychotic properties (117,147,154,172,173).

This conclusion suggests that the minor tranquilizers or the sedative-hypnotic drugs such as the benzodiazepines, chloral hydrate, or barbiturates, may be effectively used in the initial management of the "bad trip" (11,111,154,172).

34. Can the above case be treated for a psychotogenic drug reaction purely from the history that the patient had ingested a drug known as a "pink wedge"?

Trade names, dosage forms, dosages, purity and strength of illicit drugs vary greatly from time to time, community to community and from dealer to dealer. Also drugs with low marketing potential are frequently misrepresented for drugs with higher marketing potential. It has been found by chemical analysis that many samples of LSD and phencyclidine have been sold as THC or tetrahydrocannabinol (the active constituent of marihuana). It would be best to initiate therapy in the overdosed drug abuser by the symptomatology of the patient, matching these with the history of the suspected drug ingested. The "pink wedge" in this case history was analyzed to be a combination of the two psychotogenic drugs LSD and STS (2, 5-dimethoxy-4-methylamphetamine, also known as DOM) (117).

35. What is the incidence rate for the bad trip phenomenon and how often does it progress to the more prolonged and severe type of toxic psychosis?

As mentioned previously, "bum trips" do not seem to be totally dose dependent either in occurrence, intensity or duration. Thus the overall incidence rate for this experience is somewhat of a controversy. An extensive study reported psychotic reactions lasting longer than 48 hours at an incidence of 0.08% in normal subjects and 0.18% in subjects undergoing psychotherapy. The total study population consisted of 5,000 patients who had taken LSD or mescaline an aggregate of almost 25,000 times (31). This low incidence rate was subsequently challenged (122, 160,179). In addition, the frequent adulteration of illicit drugs with a combination of other powerful psychotogens may be a significant factor in the precipitation of a "bad trip" accounting for observed higher incidence rates (161).

These "bad trip" panic reactions are the most common acute adverse reaction to LSD and other psychotogenic drugs. These reactions are generally temporary and last for approximately 24 hours with LSD. However, they can also become more prolonged, lasting for more than 48 hours, and sometimes progressing even further into a long lasting toxic psychosis (160).

Smart and Bateman (160) have estimated that approximately 50% of prolonged "bad trip" reactions resolve within 48 hours, while roughly 25% last from two to seven days and the remaining 25% for longer periods of time, occasionally for more than one year.

These estimates are also a matter of much controversy, since some researchers believe that the prolonged psychotic reactions to psychotogenic drugs are not due to direct toxic effects but are secondary to the unmasking of pre-existing psychotic behavioral traits (87,178).

36. The patient in the above case experienced "flashbacks" which gradually faded out in a year. What is the flashback phenomenon?

The "flashback" or "free trip" is a poorly understood phenomenon described as a transient, spontaneous recurrence of certain aspects of the psychotogenic drug experience following an earlier

intoxication after a period of relative normalcy (154). Flashbacks occur most frequently in the individual who has had a multitude of LSD experiences, has taken other psychoactive drugs (often major tranquilizers such as chlorpromazine), or is in the period of psychological stress (146,147,154). This phenomenon can occur sporadically or several times a day and can last from minutes to hours, or persist for as long as a year (114).

Theories attributing "flashbacks" to cumulative LSD toxicity in the CNS, persistence of a psychoactive LSD metabolite, and long-lasting retinal or optic pathway changes in the eye have been postulated. However, the more widely held view is that "flashbacks" are a mechanism learned while in the LSD state, whereby an individual reacts to stress in a novel way. It might be compared to "war neuroses" experienced by soldiers (81,154). "Flashbacks" are transient and gradually fade in frequency and intensity over time, provided the patient refrains from psychotogenic drugs.

Treatment should follow the same guidelines as the "talk down" therapy with major emphasis placed upon reassuring the patient that he is not "brain-damaged" or that he is not "going crazy." In view of the fact that different psychoactive medications may precipitate or exacerbate the "flashback" phenomenon, medication should be conservative and offered only when the patient exhibits extreme anxiety. Shick and Smith (154) recommend the use of the minor tranquilizers or sedative-hypnotic drugs rather than major antipsychotic tranquilizers.

37. A 19-year-old female admits to the use of LSD sometime during her second trimester of pregnancy. Her obstetrician has heard that LSD is teratogenic causing congenital deformities of extremities to infants born to mothers who have ingested LSD. What is the role of LSD in teratogenicity and chromosomal damage?

In an extensive review of the literature, Greenblatt and Shader (81) conclude that, "at the present time the volume and quality of evidence is not adequate to either confirm or rule out the possible adverse cytogenetic effects of LSD." Like almost all drugs, the question of LSD and pregnancy unfortunately remains unresolved.

Numerous studies on pregnant laboratory animals have been reviewed. In all of these studies huge dosages of LSD were administered, results were inconsistent, and the teratogenicity of LSD seemed to be related more to the particular strain of animal and the time of administration rather than upon the dose of the drug (81). Two studies involving a total of 273 pregnancies in mothers who ingested LSD during their pregnancy demonstrated a low, yet significant, increased incidence of severe congenital anomalies and spontaneous abortions. However, both studies involved "high risk" populations for these anomalies and also involved mothers who probably ingested other illicit drugs as well. These studies did indicate that LSD had no effect on the incidence of fetal anomalies when it was taken by the male partner or by the female partner prior to conception (81,123).

Five case histories have reported deformities resulting from maternal ingestion of LSD during the first trimester of pregnancy. These were in mothers who ingested drugs other than LSD during this time (9,25,51,86,196). Conflicting with these case studies are reports by Sato and Pergament (145) documenting a normal healthy infant born to a mother who ingested LSD on the 43rd and 57th day of pregnancy — and by Warren and co-workers (183), involving a normal child whose mother ingested large doses of LSD numerous times during pregnancy.

Most authors do not recommend the use of LSD during pregnancy especially during the first trimester period, though they feel that the literature and research do not substantiate LSD as being teratogenic (81,177).

Volumes of research have been published on the effects of LSD on the chromosomes of different laboratory animals and man. Most of the research was poorly controlled and conflicting (81). However, in one controlled study on the chromosomes of 40 patients who ingested LSD during the course of the experiments, the authors concluded that "there is no definite evidence that pure LSD damages chromosomes of human lymphocytes *in vivo*" (177).

38. Is LSD carcinogenic?

Two case histories have been published associating LSD usage with acute leukemia. One case involved a 19-year-old who developed acute leukemia and a "Philadelphia" chromosome (characteristic of chronic myelogenous leukemia) four months after the last of 15 LSD doses (83). The second case involved a 23-year-old who developed acute lymphocytic leukemia seven months after the last of numerous LSD doses (67).

Both patients had abused other drugs as well as LSD, and both had strong family histories for hematologic and malignant diseases. Thus, it would be fair to conclude that in the cases presented, the occurrence of acute leukemia after ingestion of LSD is probably more a matter of coincidence than of cause.

39. A 16-year-old was admitted to the Emergency Room in an agitated state. Admitting to having smoked "joints" (marihuana cigarettes) laced with PCP, she described her condition as similar to being on an "acid bummer" (LSD panic reaction). What is PCP?

Phencyclidine or PCP (also called Hog, Peace Pill, Crystal, Monkey Tranquilizer, and Angel's Dust) was originally intended to be used as a general anesthetic in man. However, the frequency and severity of CNS side effects soon limited its use to veterinary medicine (sold under the trade name of Sernyl). Its psychotogenic effect has been described as "sensory deprivation," and it appears to alter the response of the CNS to various sensory inputs. This may result in perceptual distortions and a toxic psychosis similar to the acute anxiety reaction seen with LSD. The biological half-life of PCP is only 30 to 60 minutes but subjective effects can last up to 48 hours and longer. Effects generally last longer than those produced by LSD (41,112a,177a).

Treatment of an acute reaction involves supportive care and reduction of sensory stimulation and should be along the same guidelines as the treatment of an LSD reaction. Chlorpromazine, diazepam, and intravenous sodium succinate (6 gm in 500 cc water infused over a 5 minute period) have been successfully used to treat the subjective effects of PCP (41). However, subsequent work noted that succinate was no more effective than saline alone (127a).

Large doses have produced seizures, spasticity, opisthotonus, deep coma, respiratory depression, cardiovascular instability and one fatality (112a). For the most part, PCP is not a preferred drug of abuse by the street population because of the frequency of "bad trips" associated with its use. Thus it is often sold as other more preferred drugs such as THC and mescaline to unsuspecting drug abusers (5).

40. What are other commonly abused psychotogens?

Mescaline (3,4,5-trimethoxyphenylethylamine) is the active component of the Peyote Cactus *(Laphophora williamsii)* which was ingested for religious practices by the Southwestern Plains Indians (37,66). The drug is generally taken orally as dried cactus buttons, tea, or gelatin capsules. Subjective effects are very similar to LSD and treatment of an acute anxiety reaction resulting from mescaline should be treated similarly. Oral doses of 5 mg/kg (generally 6-12 buttons) cause effects lasting for about 12 hours. Nausea, diaphoresis and static tremors are frequently seen with therapeutic doses (98). Available "street" or illicit mescaline is very rare although it is a highly preferred agent. Of 41 samples of "street" mescaline analyzed in the San Francisco area only two contained mescaline; the remaining samples contained LSD, PCP or no drug at all (5).

THC or delta 9-tetrahydrocannabinol is the major of a number of cannibinoids contained in the marihuana plant, *Cannabis sativa.* Although its effects are more of a sedative-hypnotic nature when smoked or ingested in moderate amounts, higher doses are capable of inducing adverse reactions similar to other psychotogens. Panic reactions, simple depressive reactions, toxic psychoses, prolonged psychotic reactions, and even "flashbacks" have been documented with its use (36,131,171,187). These adverse reactions are quite rare when placed in perspective of the many users of marihuana who do not develop adverse reactions.

Marihuana or hashish (dried pressed resin of cannabis) has been demonstrated to be fairly nontoxic with no long lasting mental or physical damage when smoked moderately for even long periods of time (82). However, this is still a matter of much controversy, since no controlled long term study has of yet been done on marihuana.

When smoked, a dose of 0.5-2.0 gm of crude marihuana gives effects that generally dissipate in three to four hours (188).

Synthetic THC was developed in 1965, however, it is very difficult and expensive to manufacture. Every sample of synthetic "street" THC in the Haight-Ashbury district of San Francisco was analyzed to be PCP. However, an extraction product of hashish (sold as "hash" oil or "red oil") has been analyzed to have a high concentration of THC.

Unlike other psychotogens, cannabis has sedative effects, does not produce sympathomimetic effects, and does not exhibit cross tolerance with other psychotogens. Thus, some authors have suggested a separate classification for cannabis other than that of a psychotogenic agent.

A critical literature review of marijuana abuse would constitute volumes of pages in itself. The basic conclusion of the *Commission on Marihuana and Drug Abuse* (33) is that the present penalties regarding the possession and use of cannabis far outweigh the extent of the crime and they therefore recommend an appropriate reduction in penalties.

Psilocybin, the "magic Mexican mushroom" was first reported in the medical literature by Heim in 1957. Later in 1958 Heim, with Hoffman and co-workers, isolated O-phosphoryl-4-hydroxy-N-dimethyltryptamine from Mexican mushrooms. This compound, which they named psilocybin, has been isolated in *Psilocybe cubensis, P. mexicana, Stropharia cubensis,* and one species of the *Conocybe* genera. Other hallucinogenic fungi have been studied, some of which contain another psychotogenic compound, bufotenine (24,155).

The subjective effects of psilocybin are similar to those of LSD and mescaline with a dose of 20 to 60 mg lasting from 5-6 hours (113). Like mescaline and THC, psilocybin is a sought after psychotogen, but very little of it is available to the illicit drug market. Of 22 psilocybin samples analyzed by Pharm Chem Laboratories in 1973, only one contained appreciable amounts of this drug (5).

MDA (3,4-methylenedioxyamphetamine) is a psychotogenic drug structurally similar to mescaline and STP which was first synthesized in the 1930's. Doses up to 150 mg are said to intensify feelings, facilitate insight, increase empathy, and heighten aesthetic enjoyment. However, it does not induce hallucinations, perceptual alterations, or cause depersonalization at this dosage (126,155).

Effects begin about 40 to 60 minutes after ingestion and generally persist for 6 to 10 hours. Marked physical exhaustion with free floating anxiety has been reported to last up to two days in some cases (96). Toxicity from MDA is somewhat more of an acute problem than it is for other psychotogens. One near fatal and two severe cases of adverse physical reactions consisting of dilated pupils, tachycardia, diaphoresis, rapid labored breathing, fever, generalized piloerection and muscular spasms have been reported in six persons who each ingested 500 mg of MDA (12).

MDA seems to be a "fad" drug with its abuse on the street related more to its unpredictable popularity than to its availability. Recently, N-methyl MDA derivatives have also appeared on the illicit drug market.

STP derives its initials from serenity, tranquility and peace which is inappropriate to the expected pharmacologic properties of DOM or 2,5-dimethoxy-4-methyl amphetamine. Its effects are similar to LSD and include dilated pupils, increased systolic blood pressure, and a slight increase in body temperature. Five mg of STP will produce hallucinogenic effects for five to six hours. Ten mg of the drug may last for 16 to 24 hours. More prolonged reactions (up to 72 hours), a higher incidence of acute panic reactions, and an increase in the occurrence of the flashback phenomenon has been reported with STP; thus, the drug has low preference in the drug abuse population (161,162,167). However, the recent appearance of a new 4-bromo STP derivative has been noted on the illicit drug market (156).

DMT (dimethyltryptamine) and DET (diethyltryptamine) are psychotogenic drugs with much shorter durations of action than those of other agents. Ineffective when taken orally, DMT must be smoked or inhaled into the lungs for psychotogenic effects. DMT has a 30 to 60 minute duration of action, and it also has a rapid onset; one minute when smoked and two to five minutes when snorted. The subjective effects of DMT approximate that of an LSD experience but are much shorter in duration. The popularity and availability of DMT as well as other tryptamine derivatives continues to remain below that of other psychotogenic drugs (155,170).

CASE FOR STUDY

A 20-year-old female is admitted into the Emergency Room comatose from a substance called "Gow" by her friends. She had also allegedly ingested an unknown number of pills from an unlabeled vial filled with a mixture of multi-colored tablets and capsules.

Vital signs upon admission were: blood pressure 80/60 mm Hg; pulse 110 faint, regular; Resp 10/min. Temp 99.8° F. On physical examination she was obtunded, icteric, and non-responsive to painful stimuli. The odor of alcohol was noted and there was evidence of recent emesis in her mouth and on her clothes. A few bruises with ecchymosis were noted on her head and neck. Otological examination however, was unremarkable. Her pupils were symmetri-

cally miotic. Pulmonary auscultation revealed a gargling stridor with a depressed respiratory rate. Cardiac auscultation showed the patient to be in sinus tachycardia with a regular thythm.

Examination of her arms found heavy bilateral antecubital venous puncture scars and multiple inflamed, indurated abscesses along her left flexor carpi radius muscle. A rigid muscle tonus with stiffness of her neck was also noticed.

————

A. What immediate clinical considerations and suggestions can be offered for the acute management of this patient?

B. What after-care and therapeutic plans should be developed for the chronic treatment of this patient?

REFERENCES

1. AMA Committee on Alcoholism and Addiction: Dependence on amphetamines and other stimulant drugs. JAMA 197:1024, 1966.
2. AMA Committee on Alcoholism Addiction: Dependence on LSD and other hallucinogenic drugs. JAMA 202:47, 1967.
3. Anon: Answers to the most frequently asked question about naltrexone (EN-1639A). Connection (Institute for Social Concern — Oakland, CA) 1:1, 1973.
4. Anon: Methadone in the management of heroin addiction. Medical Letter 14:13, 1972.
5. Anon: Pharmacy Chemistry Newsletter, published by Pharmacy Chemistry Laboratories, Palo Alto, CA 2:2, 1973.
6. Anon: Surgical complications in the drug addict. Mod Med 39:23, 1971.
6a. Anon: Treatment of alcohol withdrawal syndromes. Medical Letter 13:19, 1971.
7. Anon: Alcoholism: New victims, new treatment. Time, 75-81, April 22, 1974.
8. Aronow R et al: Childhood poisoning — an unfortunate consequence of methadone availability. JAMA 219:321, 1971.
8a. Assaf RAE et al: The influence of the route of administration on the clinical action of diazepam. Anesthesia 30:152, 1975.
9. Assemany SR et al: Deformities in a child whose mother took LSD. Lancet 1:1290, 1970.
10. Baden M: Narcotic abuse: A medical examiner's view. NY State J Med 72:834, 1972.
11. Barnett BE: Diazepam treatment for LSD intoxication. Lancet 2:270, 1971.
11a. Bateson G: The cybernetics of "self": A theory of alcoholism, in Steps to an Ecology of Mind, Ballantine Books, New York 1972, p 309.
12. Becker CE: Medical complications of heroin addiction. Calif Med 115:42, 1971.
13. Becker CE: The treatment of alcoholism. Rational Drug Therapy 6:1-8, 1972.
14. Berry RE: Estimating the economic costs of alcohol abuse. NEJM 295:620, 1976.
15. Bick RL et al: Malaria transmission among narcotic addicts. Calif Med 115:56, 1971.
16. Blatman S et al: Obstetrical aspects through the delivery room. Presented at the Third National Conference on Methadone Treatment, Nov. 1970.
17. Blinick G: Menstrual function and pregnancy in narcotic addicts treated with methadone. Nature 219:180, 1968.
18. Blinick G et al: Methadone maintenance, pregnancy and progeny. JAMA 115:477, 1973.
19. Blinick G et al: Methadone and pregnancy. In Fourth National Conference on Methadone Therapy, San Francisco, 1972. National Assoc for Prevention of Addiction to Narcotics. New York, 1972, p 129.
20. Blinick G et al: Methadone assays in pregnant women and progeny, Am J Obstet Gynecol 121:617, 1975.
21. Blinick G et al: Pregnancy in narcotic addicts treated by medical withdrawal: The methadone detoxification program. Am J Obst Gyn 105:997, 1969.
22. Blumberg H et al: Analgesic and narcotic antagonist properties of noroxymorphone derivatives. Toxicol Appl Pharm 10:406, 1967.
23. Brown JK et al: Status of drug quality in the street-drug market — an update. Clin Toxicol 9:145, 1976.
24. Buck RW: Mushroom toxins: A brief review of the literature. NEJM 265:681, 1961.
25. Carakushanski G et al: Lysergide and cannabis as possible teratogens in man. Lancet 1:150, 1969.
26. Carey JT et al: A San Francisco bay area 'speed' scene. J Health & Social Behavior 9:164, 1968.
27. Carroll T: Diversion, urinalysis and program abuse: Introductory comments. Fourth National Conference on Methadone Treatment. San Francisco, 1972. National Assoc. for Prevention of Addiction to Narcotics, New York, 1972, p 147.
28. Chambers, CD: Some considerations for the treatment of non-narcotic drug abusers, in Major Modalities in the Treatment of Drug Abuse, Brill and Lieberman editors, Little, Brown & Co, Boston 1970.
29. Chambers C et al: An empirical assessment of the availability of illicit methadone. Fourth National Conference on Methadone Treatment, San Francisco, 1972. National Assoc. for Prevention of Addiction to Narcotics, New York, 1972, p 149.
30. Citron BP et al: Nectroitizing angiitis associated with drug abuse. NEJM 283:1003, 1970.
31. Cohen S: A classification of LSD complications. Psychosom 7:182, 1966.
32. Collier HOJ: Tolerance, physical dependence and receptors: A theory of the genesis of tolerance and physical dependence through drug changes in the number of receptors. Adv Drug Res 3:171, 1966.
33. Commission on Marihuana and Drug Abuse: Marihuana: A Signal of Misunderstanding, U.S. Government Printing Office, Washington, D.C., 1972.
34. Cushman P: Methadone maintenance therapy for heroin addiction — Some surgical considerations. Am J Surg 123:267, 1972.
35. Day HB: The Opium Habit, With Suggestions As to Remedy. Harper & Brothers, New York, 1868.
36. Department of HEW: Marihuana and Health. Government Publications, Washington, D.C., January 31, 1971.
37. Der Marderosin A: Current status of hallucinogens. Am J Pharm 138:204, 1966.
38. Dimijan CG et al: Evaluation and treatment of the suspected drug user in the emergency room. Arch Intern Med 125:162, 1970.
39. Dismukes W et al: Viral hepatitis associated with illicit parenteral use of drugs. JAMA 206:1048, 1968.
40. Dobbs WH et al: Problems of controlling methadone diversion in an outpatient clinic: The case of Mary Jane. Fourth National Conference on Methadone Treatment, San Francisco, 1972. National Assoc. for Prevention of Addiction to Narcotics, New York, 1972, p 153.
41. Dodini LK: Clinical pharmacology of the "peace pill." Bulletin of hospital pharmacy and drug information analysis service, University of California, San Francisco 18:1, 1971.
42. Dole VP et al: A medical treatment for diacetylmorphine addic-

tion. JAMA 193:646, 1965.

43. Dole VP et al: Narcotic blockade. Arch Int Med 118:304, 1966.

44. Dole VP et al: Successful treatment of 750 criminal addicts. JAMA 206:2708, 1968.

45. Dole VP et al: Methadone treatment of randomly selected criminal addicts. NEJM 280:1372, 1969.

46. Edwards G: The British approach to the treatment of heroin addiction. Lancet 1:768, 1969.

47. Efron DH et al: *Ethno-Pharmacologic Search for Psychoactive Drugs.* Public Health Service Publications. No. 1645, U.S. Government Printing Office, Washington, D.C., 1967.

48. Einstein S: *The Use and Misuse of Drugs.* Wadsworth Publishers, Inc., Belmont, Calif., 1970.

49. Einstein S: Critical issues concerning methadone: Treatment, therapy, or what? *Fourth National Conference on Methadone Therapy,* San Francisco, 1972. National Association for Prevention of Addiction to Narcotics, New York, 1972, p 515.

50. Eisenman AJ et al: Urinary 17-Ketosteroid excretion during a cycle of addiction to morphine. J Pharmacol Exp Ther 124:305, 1958.

51. Eller JL et al: Bizarre deformities in offspring of user of lysergic acid diethylamide. NEJM 283:395, 1970.

52. Ellinwood EH: Amphetamine psychosis: I. Description of the individuals and process. J Psychedelic Drugs 2:42, 1969.

53. Ellinwood EH: Amphetamine psychosis: II. Theoretical implications. J Psychedelic Drugs 2:52, 1969.

54. Ellinwood EH: Assault and homicide associated with amphetamine abuse. Am J Psych 127:1170, 1971.

55. Espelin DE et al: Amphetamine poisoning. Effectiveness of chlorpromazine. NEJM 278:1361, 1968.

56. Fink M et al: Naloxone in heroin dependence. Clin Pharmacol Ther 9:568, 1968.

57. Finnegan LP et al: Comprehensive care of the pregnant addict and its effect on maternal and infant outcome. Contemporary Drug Problems 1:795, 1972.

58. Fischman VS: Stimulant users in the California rehabilitation center. J Psychedelic Drugs 2:92, 1969.

59. Fiut RE et al: Antagonism of convulsive and lethal effects induced by propoxyphene. J Pharm Sci 55:1085, 1966.

60. Foldes FF et al: Studies on the specificity of narcotic antagonists. Anesth 26:320, 1965.

61. Food and Drug Administration: Personal inquiry, 11/15/76.

61a. Food and Drug Administration: Fetal alcohol syndrome. FDA Drug Bulletin 7:18, 1977.

62. Fraser HF et al: Death due to withdrawal of barbiturates. Ann Int. Med 38:1319, 1953.

63. Freedman DX: On the use and abuse of LSD. Arch Gen Psych 18:330, 1968.

64. Freedman DX: The psychopharmacology of hallucinogenic agents. Ann Rev Med 20:409, 1969.

65. Frykman JH: Observations concerning treatment and care of drug abusers. J Psychedelic Drugs 2:105, 1969.

66. Frykman JH: *A New Connection.* Scrimshaw Press, San Francisco, 1971.

66a. Gamble JAS et al: Plasma diazepam levels after single dose oral and intramuscular administration. Anesthesia 30:164, 1975.

67. Garson OM et al: Studies in a patient with acute leukemia after lysergide treatment. Brit Med J 2:800, 1969.

68. Gay GR et al: Treating acute heroin toxicity. Hosp Physician 7:50, 1971.

69. Gay GR et al: A new method of outpatient treatment of barbiturate withdrawal. J Psychedelic Drugs 3:81, 1971.

70. Gay GR et al: Short-term heroin detoxification on an outpatient basis. Internat J Addictions 6:241, 1971.

71. Gay GR et al: Recognizing the battered flower child. Hosp Physician 8:43, 1972.

72. Gay GR et al: Outpatient barbiturate withdrawal using phenobarbital. Internat J Addictions 7:17, 1972.

73. Gay GR et al: *A Free Clinic Approach to Drug Abuse.* Proceedings of 2nd National Free Clinic Council, U.S. Government Printing Office, 1973.

74. Gay GR et al: Cocaine: history, epidemiology, human pharmacology, and treatment. A perspective on a new debut for an old girl. Clin Toxicol 8:149, 1975.

75. Gay GR et al: "An' ho, ho, baby, take a whiff on me:" La dama blanca. Cocaine in current perspective. Anesth Analg 55:582, 1976.

76. Goldstein A et al: Enzyme expansion theory of drug tolerance and physical dependence. Proc of Assoc Resp Nerv Mental Disorders 46:265, 1968.

77. Goldstein A: The pharmacologic basis of methadone treatment. *Fourth National Conference on Methadone Treatment,* San Francisco, 1972. National Assoc. for Prevention of Addiction to Narcotics, New York, 1972, p 153.

78. Goldstein A et al: A synthetic peptide with morphine-like pharmacologic action. Life Sciences 17:1643, 1975.

79. Goldstein A et al: On the role of endogenous opioid peptides: failure of naloxone to influence shock escape threshold in the rat. Life Sciences, 18:599, 1976.

80. Goodman S et al: Intracranial hemorrhage associated with amphetamine abuse. JAMA 212:480, 1970.

81. Greenblatt DJ et al: Adverse effects of LSD: A current perspective. Conn Med 34:895, 1970.

81a. Greenblatt DJ et al: Slow absorption of intramuscular chlordiazepoxide. NEJM 291:1116, 1974.

82. Grinspoon L: Marihuana. Scientific American 221:17, 1969.

83. Grossbard L et al: Acute leukemia with "Ph"-like chromosome in a LSD user. JAMA 205:791, 1968.

84. Hansten PD: Drug Interactions — 2nd Ed.: Lea and Febiger: Philadelphia, 1973.

85. Hasbrouch JD: The antagonism of morphine anesthesia by naloxone. Anesth Anal, Curr Res 50:954, 1971.

86. Hecht F et al: Lysergic-acid-diethylamide and cannabis as possible teratogens in man. Lancet 2:1087, 1968.

87. Hoffer A: LSD: A review of its present status. Clin Pharmacol Ther 6:183, 1964.

88. Horwitz CA et al: The effect of methadone on pregnancy tests. *Fourth National Conference on Methadone Treatment,* San Francisco, 1972. National Association for Prevention of Addiction to Narcotics, New York, 1972, p 111.

89. Hughes J et al: Identification of two related pentapeptides from the brain with potent opiate agonist activity. Nature 258:577, 1975.

90. Inaba DS et al: The yen for N: the use of propoxyphene napsylate in the treatment of heroin addiction. West J Med 121:106, 1974.

91. Inaba DS et al: I got a yen for that Darvon-N: a pilot study on the use of propoxyphene napsylate in the treatment of heroin addiction. Amer J Drug and Alcohol Abuse 1:67, 1974.

92. Inaba DS et al: Methaqualone abuse — "Luding out." JAMA 224:1505, 1973.

93. Ingall D et al: Diagnosis and treatment of the passively addicted newborn. Hosp Pract 5:101, 1970.

94. Isbell H et al: Liability of addiction to 6-Dimethylamino 4-4-diphenyl-3-heptanone (methadone, 'amidone' or 10820) in man. Arch Int Med 82:362, 1948.

95. Isbell H et al: Clinical characteristics of addiction. Am J Med 14:558, 1953.

96. Jackson B et al: Another abusable amphetamine. JAMA 211:830 (letter), 1970.

97. Jaffe JH et al: Pharmacological denervation supersensitivity in the central nervous system: A theory of physical dependence. Proc of Assoc Resp, Nerv and Mental Dis 46:226, 1968.

98. Jaffe JH: Ch 16, Drug addiction and drug abuse. In *The Pharmacological Basis of Therapeutics,* ed 5. Edited by L Goodman and A Gilman, Macmillan, New York, 1975, p 284.

99. Jaffe JH et al: Methadone and L-methadryl acetate. Use in management of narcotics addicts. JAMA 216:1303, 1971.

100. Jaffe JH et al: Methadryl acetate vs methadone. A double-blind study in heroin users. JAMA 222:437, 1972.

101. Jarvik ME: Ch 12, Drugs used in the treatment of psychiatric disorders. In *The Pharmacological Basis of Therapeutics,* Ed 4, Edited by L Goodman and A. Gilman, Macmillan, New York, 1970.

102. Jasinski DR et al: The human pharmacology and abuse potential of N-allylnoroxymorphone (Naloxone). J Pharmacol Exp Ther 157:420, 1967.

103. Jasinski DR et al: Antagonism of the subjective, behavioral pupillary, and respiratory depressant effects of cyclazocine by naloxone. Clin Pharmacol Ther 9:215, 1968.

104. Jones KL: Outcome in offsprings of chronic alcoholic women. Lancet 1:1076, 1974.

105. Kalant H et al: Tolerance to and dependence on some non-opiate psychotropic drugs. Pharmacol Rev 23:135, 1971.

106. Kane FJ et al: Neurological crisis following methamphetamine.

JAMA 210:556, 1969.

107. Kleber H: Prolonged adverse reactions from unsupervised use of hallucinogenic drugs. J Nerv Ment Disorders 144:308, 1967.

108. Knott DH et al: Alcoholism. Presented at 23rd Annual Scien. Assembly, American Academy of Family Practice, Miami, Fla., Oct. 1971.

109. Kramer JC: Introduction to amphetamine abuse. J Psychedelic Drugs 2:8, 1969.

110. Langs RJ et al: Lysergic acid diethylamide (LSD-25) and schizophrenic reactions. J Nerv Ment Disorders 147:163, 1968.

111. Levy RM: Diazepam for LSD intoxication. Lancet 1:1297, 1971.

112. Lewin L: Phantastica, Narcotic and Stimulating Drugs, Their Use and Abuse. E. P. Dutton and Co., New York, 1964.

112a. Liden CB et al: Phencyclidine — nine cases of poisoning. JAMA 234:513, 1975.

113. Lingeman R: Drugs From A to Z: A Dictionary. McGraw-Hill, New York, 1969.

114. Louria D: Lysergic acid diethylamide. NEJM 278: 435, 1968.

115. Louria D: The Drug Scene. Bantam Books, New York, 1968.

116. Louria D et al: Major medical complications of heroin addiction. Ann Int Med 67:1, 1967.

117. Martin CM: Caring for the "bad trip" — A review of current status of LSD. Hawaii Med J 29:555, 1970.

118. Martin WR: A homeostatic and redundancy theory of tolerance to a dependence on narcotic analgesic. Proc of Assoc Resp, Nerv, Ment Dis 46:206, 1968.

119. Martin WR: Opioid antagonist. Pharmacol Rev 19:463, 1967.

120. Martin WR et al: Naltexone, An antagonist for the treatment of heroin dependence. Arch Gen Psych 28:784, 1973.

121. Martin WR et al: The respiratory effects of morphine during a cycle of dependence. J Pharmacol Exp Ther 162:182, 1968.

122. McGlothlin WH et al: LSD revisited. 10 year follow-up of medical LSD users. Arch Gen Psych 24:35, 1971.

123. McGlothlin WH et al: Effect of LSD on human pregnancy. JAMA 212:1483, 1970.

124. Merry J: USA and British attitudes to heroin addiction and treatment centers. Brit J Addiction 63:247, 1968.

125. Morrison W et al: The acute pulmonary edema of heroin intoxication. Radiol 97:347, 1970.

126. Narango C et al: Evaluations of 3,4-methylenedioxy-amphetamine (MDA) as an adjunct to psychotherapy.

127. Medicina et Pharmacologia Experimentalis 17:359, 1967.

127a. Neubauer H et al: Sernyl, Ditran, and their antagonists, succinate and THA. Int J Neuropsych 2:216, 1966.

128. Newmeyer JA et al: Methadone for kicking and for kicks. Fourth National Conference on Methadone Treatment, San Francisco, 1972. National Assoc for Prevention of Addiction to Narcotics, New York, 1972, p 461.

129. O'Tolle VQ: Alcoholic liver disease — Part I and II. Drug Intell Clin Phar 6:314, 349, 1972.

129a. Oullette EM et al: Adverse effects on offspring of maternal alcohol abuse during pregnancy. NEJM 297:528, 1977.

130. Pasternak GW et al: An endogenous morphine-like factor in mammalian brain. Life Sci 16:1765, 1965.

131. Pillard R: Medical progress, marihuana. NEJM 283:294, 1970.

132. Post RM: Cocaine psychoses: a continum model. Am J Psych 132:225, 1975.

133. Post RM et al: Cocaine, kindling, and psychosis. Am J Psych 133:627, 1976.

134. Ramer BS: Have We Oversold Methadone: Fourth National Conference on Methadone Treatment, San Francisco, 1972. National Assoc. for Prevention of Addiction to Narcotics, New York, 1972, p 97.

135. Rappolt GT et al: Propranolol in the treatment of cardiopressor effects of cocaine. NEJM 295:448, 1976.

136. Renault PF et al: On the treatment of stimulant abuse. Persp Biol Med 15-561, 1972.

137. Richards KC et al: Near fatal reaction to ingestion of the hallucinogenic drug MDA. JAMA 218:1826, 1971.

138. Richter R et al: Transverse myelitis associated with heroin addiction. JAMA 206:1255, 1968.

139. Ritchie JM et al: Cocaine; procaine and other synthetic local anesthetics in The Pharmacological Basis of Therapeutics, ed 5. Edited by L Goodman and A Gilman. Macmillan, New York, 1975, p 386.

140. Robbins T: Characteristics of amphetamine addicts. Internat J Addiction 5:183, 1970.

141. Ruben E et al: Inhibition of drug metabolism by acute ethanol intoxication: a hepatic microsomal mechanism. Amer J Med 49:801, 1970.

142. Rumbaugh CL et al: Cerebral angiographic changes in the drug abuse patient. Radiol 101:335, 1971.

143. Rumbaugh CL et al: Cerebral vascular changes secondary to amphetamine in the experimental animal. Radiol 101:345, 1971.

144. Sampson P: Methadone — yes or no? JAMA 219:1275, 1972.

145. Sato H et al: lysergide a teratogen? Lancet 1:639, 1968.

146. Schwarz CJ: Paradoxical responses to chlorpromazine after LSD. Psychosom 8:210, 1967.

147. Schwarz CJ: Phenothiazine induced psychosis after LSD. Canad Med Assoc J 105:241, 1971.

148. Seevers MH et al: Physiological aspects of tolerance and physical dependence. In Physiological Pharmacology. Vol 1, The Nervous System, Part A: Central Nervous System Drugs, edited by WS Root and FG Hogmann. Academic Press, Inc., New York, 1963, p 565.

149. Seixas FA: Alcohol and its drug interactions. Ann Int Med 83:86, July 1975.

150. Sellers EM et al: Alcohol intoxication and withdrawal. NEJM 294:757, 1976.

151. Senay EC: Ch 9, Methadone: Some myths and hypotheses. In It's So Good Don't Even Try It Once – Heroin in Perspective, edited by DE Smith and GR Gay, Prentice-Hall, Inc., Englewood Cliffs, NJ, 1972, p 180.

152. Senay EC et al: Treatment methods for heroin addicts: A review. J Psychedelic Drugs 3:47, 1971.

153. Sheppard CW et al: Emergency treatment of acute depressant drug overdose. Missouri Med 109; 1972.

154. Shick J et al: Analysis of the LSD flashback. J Psychedelic Drugs 3:13, 1970.

155. Shulgin AT: Psychotomimetic agents related to the catecholamines. J Psychedlic Drugs 2:17, 1969.

156. Shulgin AT et al: 4-bromo-2, 5-dimethoxyphenylisopropylamine, a new centrally active amphetamine Analog. Pharmacol 5:103, 1971.

157. Shure E: Crimes Without Victims: Deviant Behavior and Public Policy. Prentice-Hall, Englewood Cliffs, NJ, 1965.

158. Siegel H et al: Continuing studies in the diagnosis and pathology of death from intravenous narcotism. J Forensic Sci 15:179, 1970.

159. Simantov R et al: A morphine-like factor 'Enkephalin' in rat brain: subcellular localization. Brain Research, 107:650, 1976.

160. Smart R et al: Unfavorable reactions to LSD: A review and analysis of available case reports. Canad Med Assoc J 97:1214, 1967.

161. Smith DE: Editor's Note. J Psychedelic Drugs 3:5, 1970.

162. Smith DE: Psychotomimetic amphetamines with special reference to STP (DOM) toxicity. J Psychedelic Drugs 2:73, 1969.

163. Smith DE & Gay GR, Ed: It's So Good Don't Even Try It Once, Heroin in Perspective. Prentice-Hall, Englewood Cliffs, NJ, 1972.

164. Smith DE et al: A new method for treatment of barbiturate dependence. JAMA 213:294, 1970.

165. Smith DE et al: Diagnosis and Treatment of Adverse Reactions to Sedative-Hypnotics. US Government Printing Office: 731-930, 1974.

166. Smith RB: Cocaine and catecholamine interaction. Arch Otolaryngol 98:139, 1973.

167. Snyder SH et al: DOM (STP), a new hallucinogenic drug, and DOET: Effects in normal subjects. Am J Psych 125:357, 1968.

168. Snyder SH et al: Drugs, neurotransmitters, and schizophrenia. Science 184:1243, 1974.

169. Stone ML et al: Narcotic addiction in pregnancy. Am J Obst Gyn 109:716, 1970.

169a. Sturdee DW: Diazepam, routes of administration and rate of absorption. Br J Anaesth 48:1091, 1976.

170. Szara S: Hallucinogenic effects and metabolism of tryptamine derivatives in man. Fed Proc 20:885, 1961.

171. Talbott J et al: Marihuana psychosis. JAMA 210:299, 1969.

172. Taylor RL et al: Management of "bad trips" in an evolving drug scene. JAMA 213:422, 1970.

173. Tec L: Phenothiazine and biperiden in LSD reactions. JAMA 215:980, 1971.

174. Tennant FS et al: Heroin detoxification — a comparison of propoxyphene and methadone. JAMA 232:1019, 1975.

175. Tennant FS et al: Treatment of Heroin Addicts with Pro-

poxyphene Napsylate. Presented Before Committee on Drug Dependence — National Academy of Sciences, Chappel Hill, North Carolina, May 23, 1973.

176. Terry CE et al: *The Opium Problem.* Bureau of Social Hygiene, Inc., New York, 1928.

177. Tjio JH et al: LSD and chromosomes: A controlled experiment. JAMA 210:849, 1969.

177a. Tong TG et al: Phencyclidine poisoning. JAMA 234:512, 1975.

178. Ungerleider JT et al: The "bad trip" — The etiology of the adverse LSD reaction. Am J Psych 124:1483, 1968.

179. Ungerleider JT et al: The dangers of LSD. An analysis of seven months' experience in a university hospital's psychiatric service. JAMA 197:389, 1966.

180. Ungerleider JT et al: A statistical survey of adverse reactions to LSD in Los Angeles County. Am J Psych 125:352, 1968.

181. Van Dyke C et al: Cocaine: plasma concentrations after intranasal application in man. Science 191:859, 1976.

182. Wallach RC et al: Pregnancy and menstrual function in narcotics addicts treated with methadone. The methadone maintenance treatment program. Am J Obst Gyn 105:1226, 1969.

183. Warren RJ et al: LSD exposure in utero. Pediat 45:466, 1970.

184. Watson R et al: Amphetamine withdrawal: Affective state, sleep patterns, and MHPG excretion. Am J Psych 129:263, 1972.

185. Way EL et al: Morphine tolerance, physical dependence, and synthesis of brain 5-hydroxytryptamine. Science 162:1290, 1968.

186. Way EL et al: Simultaneous quantitative assessment of morphine tolerance and physical dependence. J Pharmacol Exp Ther 167:1, 1969.

187. Weil A: Adverse reactions to marihuana, classification and suggested treatment. NEJM 282:997, 1970.

188. Weil, A: Clinical and psychological effects of marihuana in man. Science 162:1234, 1968.

189. Wesson DR et al: Managing narcotic and sedative withdrawal. Hosp Physician 8:52, 1972.

190. Wesson DR et al: Treatment techniques for narcotic withdrawal with special reference to mixed narcotic-sedative addiction. J Psychedelic Drugs 4:118, 1971.

191. Wikler A: Diagnosis and treatment of drug dependence of the barbiturate type. Am J Psych 125:758, 1968.

192. Wikler A et al: N-allylnormorphine: effects if single doses and precipitation of abstinence syndromes during addiction to morphine, methadone or heroin in man (post-addicts). J Pharmacol Exp Ther 109:8, 1953.

193. Wikler A et al: Effects of frontal lobotomy on the morphine-abstinence syndrome in man: An experimental study. Arch Neurol Psych 67:510, 1952.

194. Wilson WM et al: The Mendocino drug abuse program. J Psychedelic Drugs 2:102, 1969.

195. Yablonsky L: *Synanon: The Tunnel Back.* Penguin Books, New York, 1970.

196. Zellweger H et al: Is lysergic acid diethylamide a teratogen? Lancet 2:1066, 1967.

Chapter 33

Anemias

Robert J. Ignoffo
Nancy E. Korman

Anemia is defined as a reduction in red cell mass; however, it is difficult to measure the red cell mass accurately. Therefore, a more practical definition of anemia is that of a decrease in the red blood cell concentration per unit volume of blood, which is represented by a decrease in hemoglobin concentration.

Anemia is not a disease in the strict sense of the word, but rather a symptom due to many causes. Its occurrence is associated with several nutritional deficiencies, acute and chronic diseases, and exogenous factors such as drugs. As a result, anemia is one of the most common problems encountered in clinical medicine.

Since anemia can be caused by many pathologic conditions, it can be classified by pathophysiological mechanisms as seen in Table 1. This table categorizes anemia into the following groups: (a) anemia due to decreased red cell production, (b) anemia due to increased red cell destruction, and (c) anemia due to acute blood loss. Anemia due to decreased red cell production can be further subdivided into (i) anemias due to disturbances in *stem-cell* proliferation or differentiation, and (ii) anemia due to disturbances in *mature* or *differentiated* cells.

Anemias can also be classified according to morphological appearance. This latter approach is practical as well as simple and subdivides anemias into: (a) microcytic, hypochromic, (b) normocytic, and (c) macrocytic. By this type of classification, a simple microscopic evaluation of the peripheral blood smear can provide valuable information leading to the diagnosis of macrocytic anemias due to B_{12} or folic acid deficiencies, or to a microcytic anemia such as that of iron deficiency.

PATHOPHYSIOLOGY

Due to the reduction in red cell mass, anemic patients suffer from tissue hypoxia because of a low oxygen-carrying capacity. Tissue hypoxia occurs

Table 1
PHYSIOLOGIC CLASSIFICATION OF ANEMIA
(Modified from Wintrobe)

I. Deficient red cell production
  A. Deficiency of essential substances
    1. Iron, copper*, cobalt*
    2. Vitamin B_{12}; folic acid; pyridoxine*, riboflavin*; Vitamin E*; pantothenic acid*; protein deficiencies*
    3. Inadequate supply of plasma iron
      a. Block in discharge of iron from red cell (unknown cause) as in anemia of chronic disorders
      b. Absence of circulating transferrin
  B. Bone marrow failure—aplastic anemia; irradiation; tumor; cancer chemotherapeutic agents; sideroblastic anemias
  C. Endocrine deficiency—pituitary; thyroid; adrenal; testicular
II. Excessive red cell destruction
  A. Hemolytic anemias
    1. Intrinsic—hereditary spherocytosis; glucose 6 phosphate dehydrogenase (G6PD) deficiency; paroxysmal nocturnal hemoglobinuria (PNH); complement dependent abnormalities
    2. Extrinsic—Coombs positive; autoimmune reactions
III. Anemias with both increased destruction and decreased production
  A. Anemias of chronic disease (renal, liver, connective tissue disorders; infection; malignancy)
  B. Hemoglobinopathies (e.g. sickle cell)
  C. Thalassemias

* experimentally induced

when the oxygen tension in capillaries becomes too low to supply sufficient oxygen to distant cells. When oxygen-carrying capacity is decreased, oxygen extraction is enhanced which causes the capillary blood to become more desaturated on the arterial side and the oxygen tension on the venous side to be lower. It would appear then that an increased extraction of oxygen would be detrimental to the patient by increasing the area of hypoxic tissue.

Fortunately, the body compensates to offset the effects of the decreased oxygen-carrying capacity. It increases tissue perfusion to vital organs such as the brain, heart, and kidneys by shunting blood from non-vital organs such as cutaneous tissues. If the anemia is severe (i.e. hemoglobin less than 7 gm%), the body increases cardiac output. In addition, the kidney secretes increased erythropoietin which in turn stimulates red cell production. Even the respiratory rate is increased in an attempt to compensate for the decreased oxygen-carrying capacity of anemias. Of the compensatory mechanisms, increased vital organ tissue perfusion and increased erythropoietin secretion are the most efficient. The increased respiratory rate is relatively ineffective.

The body can also overcompensate for the decrease in oxygen-carrying capacity and produce complications. For example, excessive cardiac hyperactivity in severely anemic patients can result in systolic murmurs, angina pectoris, high-output congestive heart failure, pulmonary congestion, ascites, edema, and tachycardia. Thus, anemia is generally not well-tolerated in patients with cardiac disease. In addition, orthopnea and dyspnea are characteristic complications of anemia because of the increased respiratory compensatory mechanism.

Uncorrected tissue hypoxia per se can lead to a number of complications related to the cardiovascular system, central nervous system, and gastrointestinal system. These specific problems include: angina, intermittent claudication, muscular cramps; cerebral signs of headache, tinnitus, and faintness; and gastrointestinal signs of diffuse abdominal pain.

LABORATORY DIAGNOSIS

The usual diagnostic workup of anemia includes: hematocrit, hemoglobin, total iron binding capacity, as well as serum iron, folate, and B_{12} levels. Urinalysis is useful to determine the presence of hemoglobinuria or red blood cells. Stool guaiac tests should be performed to determine if gastrointestinal bleeding may be the cause of anemia. In most cases, these test results will provide enough information to manage the common "treatable" anemias, which are associated with iron, folate, and B_{12} deficiency. Normal values for common hematologic tests are given in Table 2.

Table 2
NORMAL HEMATOLOGIC VALUES

Hematocrit	
males	45% ±3%
females	41% ±3%
Hemoglobin	14.8 ±2 gm%
MCV	87 ± 5 microns^3
MCHC %	34 ±2%
Reticulocyte count	0.5 − 1.5%
Iron (Fe)	60 − 190 mcg%
Iron binding capacity (TIBC)	250 - 400 mcg%
Serum Vitamin B_{12}	>200 pcg%
Serum folate	7 − 18 mcg/ml
FIGLU (forminoglutamic acid excretion test)	<3 mg/24 hr
Haptoglobin	40 − 180 mg%
Serum hemoglobin	<5 mg%

If all of the above tests do not reveal an obvious cause for anemia, diseases such as collagen vascular disease, malignancy, chronic infection, endocrine disorders, drug-induced red cell destruction, and several other etiologies must be considered. The laboratory diagnosis of the treatable anemias is discussed in further detail below. Table 3 provides a relatively complex flow diagram for the workup of anemia.

Due to the several types of anemias encountered in clinical medicine, this chapter will limit discussion to the most common anemias, treatable anemias, and drug-induced anemias. Anemias secondary to congenital disorders will not be discussed. Before proceeding, the reader should review the basic hematologic laboratory tests in the chapter entitled *Interpretation of Clinical Laboratory Tests.*

1. B.R., a 52-year-old white male with a chief complaint of severe epigastric pain which is relieved by the ingestion of antacids or food, has been diagnosed as having active peptic ulcer disease. His laboratory data are as follows: hemoglobin 8 gm%, hematocrit 31.2%, MCHC 26%, MCV 76 cubic microns, serum iron 40 mcg%, iron binding capacity (TIBC) 450 mgc%, and 4+ stool guaiacs. Is this patient's blood picture compatible with iron deficiency anemia?

Before iron deficiency is manifested as anemia, a large amount of total body iron must be lost. Total body iron ranges from 3000 to 4000 mg, the majority of which is present in hemoglobin (67%). Ferritin and hemosiderin contain about 27% of the total body iron. The four other "iron compartments" of myoglobin iron, transport iron (transferrin), labile iron pool, and other tissue iron account for the remaining 6% of total body iron.

Table 3
LABORATORY DIAGNOSIS OF ANEMIA

Screening Procedures	Lab Classification	Consistent Lab Tests	Diagnosis

Screening Procedures: Hematocrit, Hemoglobin, Red Blood Cell Count, Peripheral Blood Smear → Indices, Red Cell Morphology

Macrocytic Anemia:

Hct↓ RBC↓
Hgb↓
MCV↑
Reticulocyte Count↓
Fe Normal
TIBC Normal
Fe/TIBC ratio 25-30%
→ Defective nuclear maturation with decreased production

Serum B$_{12}$↓ Schilling Test → Pernicious Anemia

or

Serum folate↓ FIGLU → Folate Deficiency Anemia

Normocytic Normochromic Anemia:

Hct↓ M/E ratio↓
Hgb↓ Retic. ct.↑
→ Acute Blood Loss

Haptoglobin↓
Bilirubin (indirect)↑
SERUM HGB↑
Hct↓ M/E ratio↓
Hgb↓ Retic. ct.↑
→ Hemolytic anemia

Coombs + → Autoimmune

Hct↓ Retic. ct.↓
Hgb↓ M/E ratio N1
→ Anemia of renal failure or chronic disease

Microcytic Hypochromic Anemia:

Hct↓ MCV↓
Hgb↓ MCHC↓
Fe↓ M/E ratio N1↓
TIBC↑ Retic N1 or
Fe/TIBC ratio <15%
→ Iron Deficiency Anemia

One ml of packed red cells contains approximately 1 mg of iron, and 1 ml of whole blood contains about 0.5 mg of iron. Thus, it is obvious that blood loss can lead to iron deficiency. This patient's 4 + stool guaiacs and diagnosis of peptic ulcer disease implicate gastrointestinal bleeding as the cause of the anemia.

Iron deficiency *without* anemia is usually diagnosed by laboratory tests, while iron deficiency *with* anemia may manifest either clinically or chemically. The first evidence of iron deficiency is the depletion of storage iron, which is distributed primarily in the reticuloendothelial system (the liver, spleen, gastrointestinal tract, and bone marrow). Thus, the serum iron and total iron-binding capacity are usually abnormal before clinical manifestations are apparent. Similarly, the bone marrow is depleted of hemosiderin granules which contain approximately 25 to 30% iron.

After the depletion of iron in the storage compartment, iron is not as readily available for heme and hemoglobin synthesis, and thus the effect on erythrocyte production is manifested in the peripheral blood smear. In severe deficiency, the red blood cells become hypochromic (low mean corpuscular hemoglobin concentration — MCHC) and microcytic (low mean corpuscular volume-MCV). These indices usually do not become abnormal until the hemoglobin concentration falls below 12 gm% in males or 10 gm% in females. In children, hypochromia may be evident earlier in the course of iron deficiency.

Other changes in the peripheral blood include neutropenia (10%), thrombocytopenia or thrombocytosis. The latter has been reported in 50 to 75% of patients with hypochromic anemia secondary to chronic blood loss. The reticulocyte count is usually normal or low in iron deficiency.

The bone marrow may be either hypo- or hyperplastic and is not characteristic by morphologic evaluation. However, a bone marrow aspirate may be diagnostic with regard to the *presence* or *absence* of hemosiderin granules.

Normal values for the common hematologic tests are given in Table 2. The ratio of the serum iron concentration to the total iron-binding capacity (TIBC) is termed transferrin saturation. With iron deficiency, this ratio falls to 15% or below. Most clinicians begin iron therapy when the Fe/TIBC ratio (transferrin saturation) falls below 10%, even if the peripheral indices (MCHC, MCV) are not abnormal.

This patient's corpuscular indices indicate that his anemia is hypochromic and microcytic. His serum iron is low and the transferrin saturation percentage $[(\text{serum iron/TIBC}) \times (100)]$ of 9% is also low. The low serum iron in the presence of an elevated TIBC, a low MCV and MCHC, the low Hgb, and the 4+ stool guaiac all support the diagnosis of an iron deficiency anemia.

Iron deficiency anemia is most commonly associated with a low serum iron and an elevated TIBC. If both the serum iron and TIBC are low, the picture is more consistent with the abnormalities found in various infections, inflammatory disorders, and neoplastic states. Except when due to blood loss, a low serum iron in the absence of an elevated TIBC should be supplemented with a bone marrow aspiration and specific iron stain before an anemia is attributed solely to iron deficiency (121,142,143).

2. How should this patient's iron deficiency anemia be treated based upon the limited data presented? What factors alter the absorption of iron?

The primary treatment of this patient should be directed towards control of the cause of anemia which in this case is probably due to gastrointestinal blood loss. The objective of iron therapy is to provide sufficient iron to correct the hemoglobin content of red blood cells and replenish iron stores (97). The iron therapy should be administered orally, because it is safer and considerably less expensive than parenteral forms of administration.

The oral absorption of iron is influenced by four main factors. First of all, the form of iron is important because the ferrous form is absorbed three times more readily than the ferric form. The presence of adjuvants (e.g. ascorbic acid) and the dose of iron also may affect absorption (7,27). Finally, the solubility of the iron salt would seem to be of significance.

The following is the solubility of various iron salts in water: ferrous sulfate 1 gm/1.5 ml; ferrous gluconate 1 gm/10 ml; and ferrous fumarate 1 gm/700 ml. Thus, it would appear, if all other factors were constant, that ferrous sulfate should be absorbed more readily than the gluconate or fumarate form. However, Brise and Hallberg (32) determined that mg for mg, all three of these preparations are absorbed almost equally. Therefore, even though factors such as solubility which influence iron absorption may differ significantly, the clinical response and side effects are relatively equivalent. Therefore, the choice of therapy should be based upon cost and availability.

The usual dose of ferrous sulfate is one tablet (325 mg) three times daily between meals. Actually, one can calculate the approximate daily dose of elemental iron which is required if no iron is being lost by bleeding (30). The calculations are based upon the fact that the maximal rate of hemoglobin regeneration is about 0.256 gm/100 ml per day.

Elemental Iron (mg/day)

$$= \frac{0.25 \text{ gm Hgb}}{100 \text{ ml blood/day}} \times \frac{5000 \text{ ml}}{\text{blood}} \times \frac{3.4 \text{ mg Fe}}{1 \text{ gm Hgb}}$$

$$= \frac{40 \text{ mg Fe/day}}{20\% \text{ absorption}}$$

$$= 200 \text{ mg Fe/day}$$

$$= 1000 \text{ mg FeSO}_4/\text{day since FeSO}_4 \text{ contains}$$

$$20\% \text{ elemental iron}$$

$$= 325 \text{ mg FeSO}_4 \text{ tid}$$

The number of tablets of ferrous sulfate, gluconate, and fumarate which must be administered daily to provide 180 to 200 mg of elemental iron differs as can be seen in Table 4.

This patient should receive iron therapy for approximately six months to insure adequate repletion of iron stores. During the first month of therapy, as much as 35 mg of elemental iron is absorbed daily; however, with time, a smaller percentage of iron is absorbed. By the third month, only about 5 to 10 mg of elemental iron is absorbed daily.

The iron tablets should be taken on an empty stomach because meals can decrease absorption by 40 to 50% (33). Since a smaller percentage of iron is absorbed with increasing doses (17,27,175) iron should be given in divided doses rather than one large daily dose. The doses should be spaced at least four hours apart because the absorption of oral iron returns to normal four hours after the last dose (35).

B.R. is taking antacids which may decrease iron absorption; therefore, he should be advised to take his iron one hour before the antacid dose. The mechanism of this interaction is unknown, but it may be that the antacid forms an insoluble complex with iron. This interaction has been reported with antacids containing calcium, magnesium, and aluminum cations (76). Antacids theoretically will also prevent conversion of ferric iron to the reduced absorbable ferrous state.

Table 4
IRON CONTENT OF VARIOUS IRON SALTS

Drug	Dose (mg)	Iron Content (mg)	% Fe	Daily Dose (tablets)
Ferrous Gluconate	325 mg	37	11	6
Ferrous Fumarate	200 mg	66	33	3
Ferrous Sulfate	325 mg	65	20	3
Fero-Gradumet (slow release FeSO₄)	525 mg	105	20	2

3. B.R. returns to his physician's office ten days after the institution of iron therapy and the following laboratory values are obtained: a stool guaiac is now negative, hemoglobin 9 gm%, hematocrit 35%, and the reticulocytes 8%. Do these laboratory values reflect the desired improvement in his anemia?

If doses of elemental iron are adequate, the reticulocyte response may begin within four days and peak between the 7th and 10th day of therapy. Thereafter, the reticulocyte count falls off rapidly to normal after 15 days of therapy (70). Therefore, the most convenient index to monitor in outpatients is the hemoglobin response. The hemoglobin should be increased by 2 gm% and the hematocrit by 6% in 3 weeks.

The improvement in hemoglobin, hematocrit, and reticulocyte count indicates that this patient's anemia is responding to iron therapy.

4. A patient requests Feosol Spansules, because a neighbor told her that they would not upset her stomach. Compare the side effects, effectiveness, and cost of sustained release iron preparations with sugar coated iron tablets.

Sustained-release preparations fall into three groups: (a) those claimed to increase gastrointestinal tolerance or decrease side effects, (b) those formulated to increase bioavailability, and (c) those with adjuvants claimed to enhance absorption. These preparations supposedly need only be given once daily and thus have the theoretical advantage of improving compliance.

Gastrointestinal side effects such as nausea and epigastric pain occur more commonly as the quantity of soluble elemental iron in contact with the stomach and duodenum increases. Many studies comparing the incidence of gastrointestinal effects caused by various iron salts have not been well controlled. However,

a double-blind controlled study (146) compared an equal quantity of 222 mg of elemental iron per day administered as one of three salts, gluconate, fumarate, or sulfate, to placebo. The incidence of gastrointestinal side effects with placebo was 13%. Each of the three iron salts caused a 25% incidence of gastrointestinal side effects. Therefore, no difference in gastrointestinal side effects between these three salts was seen when equivalent elemental doses of iron were administered. In another study (14), about 15% of patients taking 200 mg daily of elemental iron reported gastrointestinal intolerance; none of these patients experienced this problem with daily doses of 100 mg of elemental iron.

Anecdotal claims that sustained release iron preparations cause fewer gastrointestinal side effects have not been substantiated by controlled studies (144). Furthermore, sustained release iron products tend to transport iron past the duodenum and proximal jejunum and thereby reduce the absorption of iron (137). Thus, it is not surprising that clinical trials demonstrate poor absorption and poor hematological responses to ferrous sulfate sustained release capsules (19,28). Likewise, Ferro-Sequel, Vitron-C, Feosol Spansule, and enteric-coated ferrous sulfate release iron into gastric and duodenal fluids poorly (15,18). Fero-Gradumet is the only long-acting iron preparation which has been documented to induce an adequate hematologic response.

Cost should also be a factor in determining the oral iron preparation of choice. Table 5 compares the relative monthly cost of the various oral iron preparations. The sustained release preparations are exceedingly more expensive than ferrous sulfate, ferrous gluconate, and ferrous fumarate tablets. Thus, it is clear that the most efficacious, least expensive agents are ferrous sulfate, gluconate, or fumarate.

Table 5
COMPARATIVE COST OF VARIOUS IRON PREPARATIONS

Drug	Amt. (mg)	Iron Content (mg)	Monthly Cost ($)
Ferrous Sulfate	325	65	2.90
Ferrous Gluconate	325	37	4.00
Ferrous Fumarate	200	66	3.50
Ferrous Sulfate (enteric coat)	325	65	3.50
Feosol tablets	200	65	4.00
Feosol Spansules	150	50	7.50
Ferronord DLA	400	75	7.00
Fero-Gradumet	525	105	5.00
Mol-Iron Chronosule	390	78	5.75

Determined on the basis of 180-200 mg daily of elemental iron plus a prescription fee of $2.00. The fee will vary among pharmacies. The cost for each drug was based on American Druggist Redbook, 1976.

5. A 23-year-old white female with iron deficiency is treated with ferrous sulfate, 325 mg four times a day. After one month of therapy her hemoglobin remains stable at 10 gm%. Her physician adds ascorbic acid 100 mg twice daily. The only other medication this patient has been taking for this last month is tetracycline for acne. Comment on the lack of a hematologic response and the rationale and necessity for ascorbic acid.

The following factors play a large role in the treatment failures of iron deficiency anemia: (a) patient noncompliance; (b) chronic anemia secondary to infections, metabolic diseases, and inflammatory diseases; (c) malabsorption of oral iron; (d)continuing blood loss; (e) folic acid or vitamin B_{12} deficiency; (f) other anemias such as sickle cell or thalassemia; (g) inadequate dosage. Compliance can be determined by the presence of black stool and/or constipation. If these changes are not evident, then the patient is probably not taking her medication (3). The absorption of both iron and tetracycline is decreased when they are administered concomitantly. When the two drugs must be taken together, the iron should be taken three hours before or two hours after the tetracycline dose.

Ascorbic acid, when given orally, enhances the absorption of iron salts by maintaining iron in the reduced ferrous state. In addition, ascorbic acid complexes with trivalent iron in acidic media to form a soluble ascorbate chelate which enhances ferric ion absorption (41,151). Ascorbic acid in doses of 500 to 1000 mg increases iron absorption by 10%. This relatively small increase in iron absorption is not worth the addition of ascorbic acid to the regimen; in addition, the cost of therapy will be greatly increased. Small doses (100 mg) do not significantly increase absorption of iron. Table 6 lists a number of iron-vitamin C combinations. A comparison of costs reveals that these combinations are exceedingly expensive and thus unwarranted.

6. Why are women, especially pregnant women, more susceptible to iron deficiency anemia? When should pregnant women be treated with iron?

Most women of childbearing age have a borderline iron deficiency which becomes more evident during pregnancy when 85 to 90% develop clinically significant iron deficiency (18). The fetus diverts iron from the mother so that the pregnant female requires about twice the daily amount of iron (4 mg) as does the normal female (6,34). The greatest utilization of iron occurs around the beginning of the second trimester. A prophylactic dose of 325 mg (60 mg elemental iron) ferrous sulfate daily is sufficient. This does will not produce gastric irritation or worsen "morning sickness."

7. What is the incidence of iron deficiency in infants and children? How much iron should they receive?

Infants born at fullterm do not commonly have signs and symptoms of iron deficiency because sufficient iron is supplied to the infant by the mother during gestation. However, iron deficiency is the most common nutritional deficit in infants 6 months to 3 years of age (123). Infants develop this deficiency because of an increased requirement for iron arising from rapid growth, a three fold increase in blood volume, and low iron dietary content. Human and cow's milk contain only small quantities of iron. Table 7 lists the relative amounts of iron in infant foods. Generally, full term infants need about 1 mg of iron per day (128); however, premature infants require greater amounts of iron during their first year of life. If a true deficiency of iron develops, 10 to 20 mg of elemental iron should be administered in divided daily doses (64). A more precise method of determining the appropriate dose of iron for the treatment of anemia is found in the discussion to Question 2. Table 8 lists doses and the iron content of common oral pediatric iron liquid preparations and Table 4 lists the iron content of various tablet dosage forms.

Table 6
HEMATINICS CONTAINING VITAMIN C

Drug	Amt. Vit. C (mg)	Amount of Elemental Iron (mg)	Monthly Cost* ($)
Fero-Grad 500	500	105	6.80
Fergon W/C	200	50	6.00
Vitron C	125	66	5.25
Mol-Iron W/C	150	78	7.00
Theragran Hematinic	100	67	8.50
Iberet 500	500	105	8.50
Stuartinic	250	100	5.00
Ferrous Sulfate (plain)	—	65	2.90

*Based on 180-200 mg daily iron. Cost based on 1976 Redbook, including a prescription fee of $2.00.

Table 7
IRON CONTENT OF VARIOUS TYPES OF INFANT FOODS

Type of Food	Fe Content (mg/oz)
Breast milk	0.03
Whole milk	0.02
Pablum	9.0
Gerber	14.0
Vegetable purees	0.2
Meat	0.8

modified from Fairbanks (64)

Table 8
DOSE AND IRON CONTENT OF PEDIATRIC IRON PREPARATIONS

	Trade Name	Ferrous Sulfate (mg/ml)	Elemental Iron (mg/ml)	Prophylactic Dose (~20 mg)	Therapeutic Dose
Ferrous Sulfate					
elixir	Feosol	44	8.8	2.5 ml qd	5 ml bid-tid
drops	Fer-In-Sol	125	25	1 ml qd	1 ml tid-qid
syrup	Fer-In-Sol	18	3.6	3 ml qd	5 ml tid
Ferrous Gluconate					
elixir	Fergon	60	6.6	3 ml qd	5 ml bid-tid

There are other iron preparations which may be equally efficacious. The above preparations are not being endorsed.
*Modified from Levin (123).

8. A 55-year-old lady with hyperuricemia who has been treated with allopurinol 300 mg a day for about three months has developed iron deficiency of questionable etiology. Her physician wishes to start therapy with FeSO₄. Comment on the treatment of this patient's iron deficiency.

The manufacturer states that iron and allopurinol should not be used together because the latter has been shown to increase hepatic storage of iron in *animals.* Short-term and long-term allopurinol therapy has not produced an increase in iron absorption, serum iron levels, liver storage, or an alteration of ferro-kinetics. Therefore, the clinical significance of this drug-drug interaction is minimal and should not deter the clinician from properly dosing iron deficiency with ferrous sulfate (31,50,56,153).

9. G.W., a 39-year-old white male with a ten-year history of regional enteritis, develops an iron deficiency anemia. After two weeks of oral iron therapy the patient returns to clinic complaining of severe epigastric pain which he attributes to the iron. Laboratory studies reveal a reticulocyte count of 1% and a hemoglobin of 8.0 gm% unchanged from two weeks ago. Is parenteral iron indicated for this patient? In what circumstances is the use of parenteral iron therapy justified.

Although oral iron therapy is generally preferred, parenteral iron is indicated in some specific situations such as in this case. Patients with malabsorption syndromes (e.g. sprue), duodenal or upper small intestinal resection, ulcerative colitis, regional enteritis, patients with continued blood loss with inadequate maintenance of hemoglobin values by oral iron, and non-compliant patients are candidates for parenteral therapy.

10. Discuss the two available parenteral iron preparations. Is there a preferred parenteral product and/or route?

Available intramuscular preparations include iron-dextran (Imferon) and iron sorbitex (Jectofer). Iron sorbitex is only given intramuscularly, because iron from this complex is readily mobilized and may be toxic if given intravenously. To prevent iron overload no more than 100 mg of iron sorbitex should be given at one time.

Iron-dextran (Imferon) is a much more tightly bound complex and is more slowly released; it is the preferred product (162).

Intramuscular iron-dextran must be given by deep injection into the gluteal mass using a Z-track technique. Staining and pain at the site of injection are commonly encountered. Other problems of IM injection of iron include slow absorption of the drug from the muscle, sterile abscesses, and hematomas. Additionally, intramuscular iron-dextran may cause localized sarcomas (157a). The maximum volume of iron-dextran which can be administered into one intramuscular site is 2 ml (100 mg Fe). Thus, many injections are needed to complete a single course of therapy.

In contrast, intravenous administration of iron-dextran avoids many of the above problems of intramuscular injection. Slow absorption and sterile abscesses are not problems with IV dosing. Systemic reactions are not more common but do include fever, chills, backache, myalgia, dizziness, syncope, rash, urticaria, and anaphylaxis. Despite published opinions to the contrary, intravenous iron-dextran is not clinically more allergenic than the intramuscular preparation. In fact, if a patient is allergic to iron-dextran, the intravenous infusion can be stopped immediately, whereas the absorption of iron-dextran from IM sites continues over a prolonged period. Reactions resulting from IM injections will therefore be more difficult to control (36,186,197).

11. What is the total dose of parenteral iron-dextran needed to restore hemoglobin to normal and replenish iron stores in a 60 kg iron deficient patient with a hemoglobin of 8 gm% and a hematocrit of 31.2%?

Several formulae can be used to calculate iron deficits (145,162,183).

Eq. 1

$$\text{Iron deficit (mg)} = \text{B.W. (kg)} \times 70 \text{ ml/kg} \times (0.45 - \frac{\text{Hct}}{100})$$

where B.W. is the body weight and Hct is the observed hematocrit. Equation 1 calculates the packed RBC deficit in milliliters and is based upon the assumption that for each ml of blood which is lost, 1 mg of iron must be replaced. This is derived from the following information:

a. Blood volume is equal to 70 ml/kg.

b. Each gram of hemoglobin contains 0.35% iron. If the mean corpuscular hemoglobin concentration $(\frac{\text{Hgb}}{\text{Hct}} \times 100)$ is assumed to be 33 gm/100 ml of packed RBC's, then each milliliter or gram of packed RBC's contains approximately 1 mg of iron.

An additional amount of iron equalling 10 mg/kg (minimum 600 mg) must be added to this calculated amount to replete iron stores.

$$\text{Total iron (mg)} = 0.3 \times \text{B.W. (lb)} \times (100 - \frac{100 \text{ Hgb}}{14.8}) \quad \textbf{Eq. 2}$$

where B.W. is body weight and Hgb is the patient's observed hemoglobin value in gm%. Equation 2 provides in one calculation the total dose of iron necessary to replete stores and correct the hemoglobin and is the more commonly utilized formula.

$$\text{Total iron (gm)} = 0.255 (14.8 - \text{observed Hgb}) \quad \textbf{Eq. 3}$$

Equation 3 is based on an average 70 kg individual and assumes that 0.255 gm iron must be replaced for each gram of hemoglobin deficit. It does not take into account variations in weight and attendant alterations in blood volume.

The following chart compares total dose calculations for iron obtained at various body weights.

Weight (kg)	Equation 1* (mg)	Equation 2 (mg)	Equation 3 (mg)
50	1083	1516	1734
60	1180	1819	1734
80	1573	2425	1734

*Calculations include stores.

12. Describe the predicted hematological response with intravenous iron-dextran. Does it produce a response which differs from oral or intramuscular iron replacement?

The rate of hemoglobin regeneration is essentially equivalent whether iron is given orally, intramuscularly, or intravenously. The anticipated response to oral or intramuscular iron replenishment is a two to three fold increase in marrow production (96). At steady state, intravenous iron also increases marrow production 2 to 3 times normal; however, a transient increase in marrow production of as much as 4 to 8 times normal may occur during the first 7 to 10 days after an intravenous infusion. Thus, the response rate following intravenous administration may be slightly faster (96,186).

The reticulocyte count increases by about the fourth day, usually peaks at 5 to 15% in about a week, and returns to normal about one week later. The rate of rise in hemoglobin is approximately 1 gm% per week; and usually peaks about eight weeks after either parenteral or oral iron therapy. (Also see Question 3).

13. What parenteral form of Imferon should be employed to prepare an intravenous total dose infusion? What precautions should be taken?

Two dosage forms of Imferon are available and both contain 50 mg of elemental iron per milliliter. One is supplied in multiple dose vials and contains phenol 0.5% as a preservative. The package insert warns that this multidose vial should only be used for intramuscular injection. If a total dose of iron dextran (2.0 gm or 40 ml) is given to a patient, the amount of phenol given would be 200 mg. Phenol is well-absorbed from any route of administration, and systemic reactions consist of respiratory insufficiency, central nervous system depression, and circulatory failure (71). The toxic dose of phenol for adults is estimated to be 8 to 15 gm (63). Thus, a 200 mg dose of phenol is unlikely to produce systemic toxicity, although it would be prudent to avoid the phenol. Imferon is also available in ampules without preservatives like phenol and should be used for all IV Imferon dosing.

Intravenous infusions of Imferon (iron dextran) should be given in a manner such that systemic reactions such as thrombophlebitis, flushing, headache, nausea, vomiting, bronchospasm, urticaria and arthralgia are minimized or avoided. Moderate to severe local phlebitis occurs in 5% of patients (25). This incidence can be reduced to 2% if normal saline is used as the diluent. Mild phlebitis occurs in 15 to 25% of patients. The incidence of phlebitis is also minimized if the infusion time is confined to 4 to 5 hours (143,186). Phlebitis has not occurred after direct IV injection of undiluted iron dextran. The concomitant administration of heparin and hydrocortisone do not decrease the incidence of generalized reactions (143,186). Anaphylactoid reactions have been reported but are extremely rare. These reactions include bronchospasm, urticaria, and severe dyspnea. These symptoms respond readily to the intravenous administration of 0.3 to 0.4 ml of 1:1000 epinephrine plus 1000 mg hydrocortisone phosphate to combat shock, if present.

Intravenous infusion of iron-dextran has recently become very popular, but it appears that direct intravenous injection of undiluted iron dextran is equally efficacious and safe. Direct IV injection should not be given any faster than 50 mg/minute. The following protocol applies to both infusion and direct intravenous injection and will minimize systemic reactions (36,143).

(a) Exclude allergic patients (i.e., asthmatics).

(b) Precede infusion or injection by an antihistamine ½ hour before administration.

(c) For infusion, dilute iron-dextran in normal saline (if possible) or 5% dextrose to make a concentration not exceeding 5 gm% (50 mg/ml). Use an infusion set which delivers 60 drops per milliliter.

(d) Give a test dose: Infusion — 10 drops/minute for 20 minutes under supervision. Injection — 0.5 ml (25 mg).

(e) Increase the infusion rate to 45 drops/minute provided no reaction occurs.

(f) The direct injection should be given slowly, and should not exceed 50 mg/minute.

14. A 60-year-old woman with active rheumatoid arthritis has iron deficiency, and the physician feels that iron-dextran is indicated. Comment on the use of iron-dextran in this patient.

The administration of iron dextran to patients with rheumatoid arthritis may exacerbate rheumatic symptoms, such as joint pain, stiffness, swelling, and decreased joint movement (125). The explanation for this adverse effect is unclear, but it appears to be related to a delayed hypersensitivity reaction to the dextran in Imferon. During exacerbations of symptoms the erythrocyte sedimentation rate increases. Although Imferon seems to induce exacerbations of rheumatic symptoms, well-controlled studies are lacking. It remains to be seen if this association is clinically significant, but caution should be exercised when using iron dextran in this group of patients. Clock (22) claims that 80 to 90% of patients with active inflammatory disease will develop severe reactions.

The mild anemia that is commonly associated with rheumatoid arthritis does not usually respond to iron therapy unless the anemia is clearly one of iron deficiency. (Also see *Rheumatoid Arthritis* chapter.)

CASE A: D.L. underwent a subtotal gastrectomy seven years ago and is now hospitalized with symptoms of weakness, sore tongue, and emotional instability. Laboratory tests indicate the following: Schilling test less than 4% excretion, Hct 22%, Hgb 7 gm%, poikilocytosis, anisocytosis, MCV 105 cubic microns, MCHC 32%, WBC 4200/mm³, and platelets 105,000/mm³.

15. What is the Schilling's test?

A radioactive tracer dose of vitamin B_{12} is given orally, and the measurement of urinary excretion of radioactivity reveals the degree of absorption. In patients with pernicious anemia, 0 to 7% of the administered dose is excreted. The normal range is 15 to 40%. The patient should be fasted overnight and urine collected for 24 hours. Since very little radioactivity will be excreted, 100 mcg of unlabelled vitamin B_{12} is given parenterally two hours after the oral dose to serve as a "flushing dose." This allows the excretion of radioactive B_{12}. This test cannot be performed in patients with severe renal dysfunction since the excretion of labeled vitamin B_{12} depends on an adequate urinary output and an accurate urine collection (81,155,165). The Schilling test is an excellent test for measuring the absorption of vitamin B_{12}.

16. What forms of anemia are compatible with this patient's hematological picture?

Approximately 5% of patients with a history of gastrectomy develop megaloblastic anemia due to vitamin B_{12} deficiency, and 30% have malabsorption problems with this vitamin (127). In addition, 12% of these patients have impaired absorption of the vitamin B_{12}-instrinsic factor complex from the ileum because of abnormal gut flora (39).

Following gastrectomy, patients may also develop a quantitative deficiency of iron and a functional deficiency of folate. Iron deficiency in gastrectomy patients occurs due to a lack of gastric acid which normally would enhance iron absorption by increasing iron conversion to the ferrous state. In addition, the absorption of dietary iron is inefficient because the increased response to need, which occurs normally, does not take place in these patients. Folate deficiency occurs in association with vitamin B_{12} deficiency because vitamin B_{12}-dependent synthesis of methionine is blocked. Folate, which is normally converted to active tetrahydrofolate during methionine synthesis, becomes "trapped" as inactive N-5-methyl tetrahydrofolate. Thus, a modest, functional deficiency of folate coenzymes develops. Serum folate levels may be depressed by as much as one-half in 60% of patients who develop megaloblastic anemia after subtotal gastrectomy. However, there is inadequate evidence presented in this case to determine if this patient is iron or folate deficient. Thus a serum iron, TIBC, and folate should be obtained from this particular patient.

The laboratory findings in this patient are classical for pernicious anemia, but in reality such striking findings are only found in severe cases. The MCV is significantly increased and indicates a macrocytic anemia. Serum folate and B_{12} levels should always be obtained when the MCV is elevated. The red blood cell count would be expected to be reduced in greater proportion to the hemoglobin or hematocrit, and a bone marrow examination would reveal a hyperplastic marrow with a 30 to 50% red-cell component. The term "megaloblastic" refers to the fact that many of the red cells will be large and nucleated. A serum B_{12} level has not yet been obtained in this case but is usually less than 200 pcg/ml in pernicious anemia.

Anemia does not develop until the total body content is less than 200 mcg. Since the normal body store of vitamin B_{12} is approximately 500 mcg and since the body only loses about 5 mcg daily, years elapse before pernicious anemia develops secondary to a vitamin B_{12} deficiency (200). In situations where the absorption of this vitamin is affected by surgery or other malabsorptive states, hematopoietic and other systemic complications will not arise for 760 to 900 days. On the other hand, it may take as long as 10 to 15 years for megaloblastic anemia to develop in a patient with adequate intrinsic factor production who simply stops oral intake. In these latter patients, the vitamin B_{12} of the bile and pancreatic juices is effectively absorbed so that the amount excreted daily is less than those whose intrinsic factor is no longer functioning.

17. What are the symptoms of pernicious anemia, and are they compatible with the weakness, sore tongue, and emotional instability experienced by D.L.?

The onset of pernicious anemia which is due to a deficiency of vitamin B_{12} is insidious and in most instances, two of the following diagnostic triad of symptoms are encountered: weakness, sore tongue, and numbness or tingling in the extremities. Anorexia, pallor or pale yellow complexion, and shortness of breath on exertion, are also bothersome and may overshadow the diagnostic triad. In addition, the patient usually has not felt well for the past six months to a year.

A classical picture of the disease would be as follows. A formerly pleasant individual is now cantankerous with prematurely gray hair. He has a light, lemon yellow complexion, blue eyes, large ears, moderate scleral icterus, and vertigo. The main complaints are alternating constipation and diarrhea. Recurrent episodes of a sore, painful, red tongue, "pins-and-needles" sensations in the extremities, awkardness in lacing shoes or sewing, and ataxia may also be observed.

The central nervous system manifestations result from a diffuse but uneven degeneration of the white matter of the spinal cord and brain. The earliest change is swelling of the myelin sheaths of the large diameter nerve fibers. When the dorsal and lateral columns of the spinal cord are involved, the classic symptoms of ataxia, spasticity, and weakness are present. Mental signs are frequent and include irritability, apathy, somnolence, suspiciousness, and emotional instability (87).

18. What factors affect the oral absorption of vitamin B_{12} and what oral dose should this patient receive?

Intrinsic factor and passive diffusion are both essential elements in the absorption of vitamin B_{12}. Of the two, intrinsic factor is by far the most important. It binds and protects the dietary sources of this vitamin from degradation by gastrointestinal microorganisms, thereby allowing for absorption of this complex by the epithelial cells in the ileum. Passive diffusion, as the term implies, operates independently of intrinsic factor, and is important to absorption only when vitamin B_{12} is present in greater than normal concentrations.

The maximal amount of vitamin B_{12} which can be absorbed from a single oral dose or meal is 2 to 3 mcg, although between 5 to 15 mcg of this vitamin is absorbed daily from the average American diet. The percent of vitamin B_{12} absorbed decreases with increasing doses, and the chart below supports the concept that ideal receptor sites are saturated by increasing doses (38).

DOSE	% VITAMIN B_{12} ABSORBED
< 0.5 mcg	70
1-2 mcg	50
10 mcg	15
20 mcg	5
1000 mcg	1

Doses of 100 mcg or more must be ingested to absorb 5 mcg of vitamin B_{12}. Refractoriness to oral vitamin B_{12} occurs and is due to antibody production against vitamin B_{12}-intrinsic factor substances derived from hog mucosa (129). Therefore, preparations containing hog mucosal intrinsic factor are ineffective. Table 9 lists the commonly available vitamin B_{12} preparations and those preparations whose intrinsic factor is derived from hog mucosa.

Although some of the preparations which are listed in Table 9 do not contain intrinsic factors derived from hog mucosa, oral vitamin B_{12}-intrinsic factor preparations (e.g. Trinsicon) still cannot be recommended. These products are expensive, patient compliance is generally poor, and many patients often become refractory to therapy (129). The only conceivable indication for oral vitamin B_{12} is in a patient with a bleeding disorder who cannot receive intramuscular injections.

Table 9
VITAMIN B_{12} PREPARATIONS

Preparation	Amount B_{12} (mcg)	Intrinsic Factor (hog mucosa)
Vitamin B_{12} (various)	5-500	no
Redisol	25-250	no
Rubramin	25	no
Trophite	25	no
Rubrafolin	25	no
Rediface Forte	50	yes
Trinsicon	7.5	yes
Vitron C	10	yes
Mol-Iron Panhemic	7.5	yes

19. If D.L. is not to receive oral vitamin B_{12}, how should her pernicious anemia be treated?

This patient should receive parenteral vitamin B_{12} in sufficient doses to provide not only the daily requirement of approximately 5 mcg, but also about 2000 to 5000 mcg (average 400 mcg) to replenish liver stores. Since 30% of vitamin B_{12} is bound to plasma transcobalamin I and cellular binding sites, single intravenous doses in excess of 100 mcg exceed the binding capacity resulting in rapid renal excretion of the unbound fraction (11). Intramuscular administration of vitamin B_{12} leads to much slower systemic absorption and greater retention of this vitamin such that 11% of cyanocobalamin and 33% of hydroxycolalamin remain 28 days after administration of a 100 mcg dose (23).

To replenish this patient's deficiency, a loading dose of 1000 mcg of either cyanocobalamin or hydroxycobalamin should be given daily for four days (total 4000 mcg) followed by either:

(a) cyanocobalamin 100 mcg IM daily until remission or for 14 days (11).

(b) cyanocobalamin or hydroxycobalamin 100 mcg IM monthly (23); or

(c) cyanocobalamin or hydroxycobalamin 100 mcg twice weekly until the hematocrit is normalized (11).

Even though hydroxycobalamin provides higher and more sustained blood levels than cyanocobalamin, there is no clinical evidence that it is any more effective in normalizing the hematocrit (37). Regimen "b" appears to be the easiest to use since the patient may be treated as an outpatient after the loading dose has been administered.

20. When would D.L. begin to recognize subjective and objective improvement after therapy has been initiated?

If therapy is administered in optimal doses as described above and no complicating disease is present, the patient will become more alert within 48 hours. The soreness of tongue usually improves within 48 hours and the tongue returns to normal after two to three weeks (163). Reticulocytosis is related to the degree of anemia, but usually values peak after five to eight days of therapy. At this time the hematocrit begins to increase and returns to normal values after four to eight weeks of treatment (104).

21. Can vitamin B_{12} deficiencies be drug-induced?

A number of drugs can decrease the absorption of vitamin B_{12} and are listed in Table 10 below.

Table 10
DRUGS WHICH DECREASE ABSORPTION OF VITAMIN B_{12}

Drug	% of Patients with Decreased B_{12} Absorption	Ref.
Colchicine	92	(190)
KCl tablets (slow release)	36	(160)
Anticonvulsants	—	(121)
Phenformin	46	(182)
Neomycin	—	(108)
p-aminosalicylic acid	—	(95)

22. A 75-year-old female with hypothyroidism is admitted to General Hospital. For the past two months she has been feeling very weak. Lab data on admission include: Hct 20%, Hgb 7 gm%, MCV 119 cubic microns, negative stool guaiac. A bone marrow aspiration reveals megaloblastoid changes. Her peripheral smear shows ovalocytes and segmented PMN's. Four months prior to admission her hematologic values were normal. What is the etiology of this lady's megaloblastic anemia? Does hypothyroidism play a role in the development of megaloblastic anemia?

Macrocytic anemia in association with hypothyroidism may be due to either folate or vitamin B_{12} deficiency (81,98). The morphologic changes in the peripheral smear are typical: macrocytosis, ovalocytosis, segmentation of granulocytes, and decreased reticulocytes. Pernicious anemia occurs in 7.8% of hypothyroid patients and may be related to the occurrence of auto-antibodies directed against parietal cells or thyroid rather than dietary deficiencies. In many of these cases, the anemia is produced by folate deficiencies. Adequate hematologic response occurs when either vitamin B_{12} or folate is given along with thyroid. Other types of anemia are also associated with hypothyroidism. A normochromic normocytic anemia which is mild and which rarely produces a hemoglobin of less than 9 gm% also may occur. This anemia responds slowly to thyroid replacement, but will not respond to iron, folate or vitamin B_{12}. Iron deficiency anemia has also been demonstrated in hypothyroid patients and may result from decreased iron absorption as well as decreased plasma erythropoietin levels. The peripheral smear is characteristically microcytic and hypochromic in such cases.

In the above case, the megaloblastic anemia developed rather acutely over 2 to 3 months. It is difficult to implicate either folate or vitamin B_{12} deficiency until serum levels of each are determined. But without these values, it is more likely that the anemia is due to folate, since vitamin B_{12} deficiency anemia takes some 2 to 5 years to develop. If the hospital laboratory does not perform B_{12} or folate assays, there is a way to give both drugs in order to aid in the diagnosis of a deficiency of either (94). Very low doses of either vitamin B_{12} (1 mcg per day) or folate (100 mcg per day) are given for 10 days. If the anemia improves on low doses of vitamin B_{12} then the anemia is due to vitamin B_{12} deficiency. The typical hematological response to 100 mcg daily of cyanocobalamin includes reticulocytosis in 2 to 5 days, decreased plasma iron concentration, return to normal of white blood cells and platelets, and increased red blood cell count.

If the megaloblastic anemia is due to folate deficiency, the proper initial dose in therapeutic trials of folic acid is 0.1 mg daily since it will produce hematologic responses only in patients with folate deficiency. Doses greater than 0.2 mg daily may produce hematological responses in patients with vitamin B_{12} deficiency as well.

23. A 38-year-old alcoholic male with a history of variceal bleeding is hospitalized. His stool guaiacs are 4+, hematocrit 28%, hemoglobin 7 gm%, MCV 90 cubic microns, MCHC 33%, reticulocytes 0.5%, serum folate 0.8 ng/ml, B_{12} 800 pcg/ml, iron 20 mcg%, TIBC 350. A peripheral smear demonstrates macrocytosis, hypersegmented granulocytes, hypochromia, and microcytosis. Can the red cell indices be correlated with the peripheral smear? Once the bleeding has been stopped and the patient's status stabilized, how should his anemia be treated?

This patient's macrocytic RBCs and microcytic RBCs offset each other and the resultant MCV is read as being normal. The red cell indices only reflect average values and should be considered as one of several diagnostic tools. Accordingly, a peripheral blood smear should be examined to ascertain morphology and pathology. In this case, the patient appears to have a combined iron and folate deficiency anemia.

The estimated total body folate stores of 5 to 10 mg are capable of sustaining hematopoiesis for about two to four months (93). Therefore, 1 mg daily of folic acid daily for two to three weeks should be more than adequate to replace this patient's storage pool of folate. The patient should be reassessed after this course of therapy to determine response to therapy and to determine if the cause of the folate deficiency has been corrected. Actually, oral folate doses as small as 0.05 to 0.1 mg of folic acid can induce a hematological remission.

24. A patient with a three year history of grand mal seizures is being treated with phenytoin 100 mg four times daily and phenobarbital 30 mg four times daily. He has been feeling weak for the past month. One month prior to his clinic visit, he developed a urinary tract infection for which he has been treated with Bactrim (sulfamethoxazole and trimethoprim). His liver and renal function tests are normal, but the hemogram reveals a slight anemia (Hct 37%). Is there any association between the patient's clinical/laboratory findings and his drug therapy?

Dietary sources of folic acid (FA) are in the polyglutamate form and must be enzymatically deconjugated in the gastrointestinal tract to the monoglutamate form before they are absorbed. Once absorbed, the inactive dihydrofolate (FH_2) must be converted to active tetrahydrafolate (FH_4, folinic acid) by dihydrofolate reductase (DHFR):

The patient's weakness and slight anemia may be related to his phenytoin, phenobarbital, and trimethoprim. Phenytoin and phenobarbital impair folate absorption and trimethoprim inhibits the cellular utilization of folate.

Phenytoin, and other type "A" drugs (see Table 11), lower serum folate by inhibiting deconjugase enzymes in the gastrointestinal tract (100,158,178). Usually, drugs which lead to malabsorption of folate do not produce megaloblastic changes in red blood cells except when high doses are given for prolonged periods of time or when pretreatment folate stores are already decreased (188). Decreased serum folate occurs in 75% of patients taking anticonvulsants (118,156). Folate deficiency induced by type "A" drugs may be treated or prevented with the administration of 1 mg folic acid daily since all pharmaceutical products are in the readily absorbable monoglutamate form.

Trimethoprim, a constituent of Bactrim of Septra, may produce altered folate metabolism by binding to intracellular dihydrofolate reductase (DHFR), thus blocking the formation of active, tetrahydrofolate. In mammalian cells, this effect is significant only with high doses (195) or when the cells of patients already are deficient in folate (e.g. alcoholic patients or patients treated with methotrexate).

Several other type "B" drugs produce folate deficiency by dihydrofolate reductase inhibition (Table 11). Methotrexate, an antineoplastic agent, is the most potent inhibitor of DHFR in mammalian cells as compared to trimethoprim which is the least potent. Since the therapeutic effect of methotrexate is dependent upon DHFR inhibition, megaloblastic changes in red cells along with leukopenia and thrombocytopenia are common adverse effects. In contrast, other type "B" drugs given in usual doses are not toxic to hematologic elements (109,189).

Megaloblastic anemia and other toxic effects secondary to type "B" drugs are best treated with folinic acid (calcium leucovorin), which provides the active, reduced folate necessary to synthesize nucleic acids. Folic acid is ineffective in reversing toxicity because there is no DHFR to convert it to the active, reduced form of folinic acid (91,92). Active folinic acid 3 to 6 mg, orally or parenterally (91,92) three times daily for 2 to 3 days will rapidly reverse megaloblastic anemia from type "B" drugs (109,11). However, rescue from methotrexate must occur within 40 hours with folinic acid 9 to 12 mg per square meter every 6 hours for 12 doses (67a) (see chapter on *Cancer Chemotherapy*).

Table 11
DRUGS WHICH ALTER SERUM FOLATE LEVELS

Group A Drugs	Ref.	Group B Drugs	Ref.
Malabsorption		*Folate Antagonism*	
Phenytoin	100	Methotrexate	13
Primidone	118	Pyrimethamine	187
Barbiturates	118	Pentamidine	189
Oral contraceptives	178	Trimethoprim	174,195
(with mestranol)		Triamterene	42
Ethanol	189		
Isoniazid	117		
Cycloserine	117		
Glutethimide	147		

25. A 32-year-old white male presents with profound anemia and a history of diabetes mellitus. Hepatosplenomegaly is noted on physical examination, and liver biopsy shows fibrosis and increased iron stores. The clinical laboratory reports: Hgb 4 gm%, MCV 95 cubic microns, MCHC 25%, and a serum iron of 224 mcg%. A smear of peripheral blood demonstrates hypochromia, microcytosis, and abundant ringed sideroblasts. The patient has received multiple transfusions in an effort to correct the anemia. The nutrition of the patient is judged "adequate" and the patient denies excessive ingestion of ethanol. A workup of the anemia leads to the diagnosis of acquired sideroblastic anemia. Describe the appropriate pharmacologic therapy and anticipated hematologic response.

Sideroblastic anemia refers to a group of anemias which have in common a basic defect in hemoglobin synthesis. The anemia is usually hypochromic, microcytic, and ringed sideroblasts can be found in the bone marrow. Ringed sideroblasts are nucleated erythrocyte precursors containing large quantities of nonhemoglobin iron. Apparently, the defective hemoglobin synthesis is due to a failure of iron to be incorporated into protoporphyrin to form heme, and evidence of iron overload is frequently present on liver biopsy.

The sideroblastic anemias can be classified in many ways, but one common approach is to group them into two major categories of hereditary and acquired. Hereditary siderblastic anemia is rare, but appears to be transmitted as an X-linked recessive trait because of its predominant occurrence in males (101). Acquired sideroblastic anemias can be further classified into three sub-groups: drug-induced (see Table 12), secondary to diseases (for example leukemia, myelofibrosis, rheumatoid arthritis, uremia, infection), and idiopathic.

This patient's laboratory data are classically compatible with the usual abnormalities seen with sideroblastic anemia. His hemoglobin of 4 gm% represents severe anemia and is compatible with the finding that such sideroblastic anemias are commonly associated with hemoglobins of less than 6.5 gm%. It is not unusual for acquired sideroblastic anemias to be confused with iron deficiency anemia because of the hypochromasia and the microcytosis; however, this patient's high serum iron, or the presence of iron in bone marrow should preclude iron deficiency. Iron therapy for this patient would be absolutely contraindicated.

Patients with acquired (31a) or hereditary sideroblastic anemia (101,102) may respond to large pharmacologic doses of pyridoxine ranging from 50 to 200 mg daily. The response to therapy has been correlated with the degree of hypochromasia. If marked hypochromasia exists, hemoglobin values tend to only partially correct and stabilize at approximately 9 gm%. Reticulocytosis peaks in 4 to 10 days, and the serum iron, if initially elevated, decreases in most cases. If pyridoxine therapy is discontinued, a relapse of the anemia generally occurs within 10 days to 5 months (101). Some patients do not respond to pyridoxine therapy at all, and others may respond only after the addition of androgens (102).

Blood transfusions are usually required for patients

with hemoglobin values of less than 8 gm%, and it would be prudent to transfuse this patient whose hemoglobin value is 4 gm%. If acquired sideroblastic anemia is drug-induced, the offending agent must be discontinued.

Table 12
DRUGS ASSOCIATED WITH
SIDEROBLASTIC ANEMIA

Agent	Reference
chloramphenicol	8,148
cycloserine	75
ethanol	51,99
isoniazid and aminosalicylic acid	75,135
lead	47
pyrazinamide	130,136

26. L.D., a 58-year-old male with chronic renal failure secondary to hypertension, has been on a chronic hemodialysis program for the past year. His laboratory data six months ago were: Hgb 6.7 gm%, Hct 20%, MCV 89 cubic microns, MCHC 32.5%, serum ferritin 80 ng/ml. Normochromic and normocytic cells were noted on peripheral smear. His medications at that time included multivitamins one capsule daily, folic acid 1.0 mg daily, ferrous sulfate 325 mg tid, and nandrolone decanoate (Deca Durabolin) 100 mg IM weekly. Currently, this patient's hemoglobin is 8.9 gm% and his hematocrit is 28%. Is this blood picture compatible with the anemia commonly associated with chronic renal failure?

Uremia or chronic renal insufficiency are commonly associated with anemia (58), and the degree of anemia is inversely proportional to the severity of the uremia. As the BUN rises, the hematocrit decreases. The anemia is not due to aplasia, but is due to both a shortened erythrocyte survival time as well as to a lack of appropriate erythropoiesis. The shortened life span of the red cells results from the accumulation of waste products which inhibit the metabolism not only of red cells, but of normoblasts, platelets, leukocytes, and rapidly proliferating intestinal cells (60). The decrease in erythropoiesis is due to decreased renal production of erythropoietin which is responsible for stimulating red cell production in the bone marrow. With severe end stage renal disease, the production of renal erythropoietin ceases completely; however, a basal level of red blood cell production continues. The production of red blood cells independent of renal erythropoietin suggests either that an erythropoietin substance can be produced extra-renally, or that the bone marrow has a baseline production of red blood cells (59).

During long-term dialysis the possible induction of megaloblastic anemia may occur on the basis of folate deficiency. The dialysis procedure removes loosely bound circulating folate. Oral folic acid prevents the development of this folate deficiency (80). Long-term dialysis has also been associated with iron deficiency due to blood loss and multiple tests. Thus, these patients may benefit from iron therapy. On the other hand, dialysis has been reported to improve the rate of iron utilization possibly be reducing the toxic metabolites which impair the viability of mature red blood cells (60). Long-term dialysis of one to two years also improves the hematocrit and decreases transfusion requirements because of the lower level of available uremic toxins. Red cell survival, however, remains unchanged. (Also see *Diseases of the Kidney* chapter).

27. The above patient, L.D., was treated with Deca Durabolin. What is the benefit of androgens in the anemia of chronic renal disease?

Androgens possess an erythropoietic action. The mechanism of action is not well defined, but it appears that androgens stimulate the production of extrarenal sources of an erythropoietin-like substance (170). Although an erythropoietic response has been achieved in an anephric patient (52), a more significant response to androgens occurs when at least one kidney is present (168). Androgens must be converted to a biologically active metabolite to exert their erythropoietic action.

Males tend to require larger doses of androgens than females or children. This variation in responsiveness is due to a sex difference in metabolism of androgens (167).

Androgen therapy in the anemia of chronic renal failure is indicated for those patients undergoing chronic hemodialysis who develop symptoms secondary to a severe anemia. Androgen therapy will then obviate the need for multiple transfusions which increase the risk of hepatitis and suppress erythropoiesis.

A variety of androgenic-anabolic agents have been evaluated in the treatment of the anemia of chronic renal failure. Many studies purport to show the superiority, efficacy, or lack of efficacy of androgens in stimulating erythropoiesis, but these studies lacked blinding techniques, adequate controls, or were of inadequate duration (48,52,53,61,89,168,185,198). In several of the androgen trials, folate and iron stores were not considered and lack of androgen stimulated erythropoiesis might well have been due to lack of these essential substances.

The 17-alpha-alkylated androgens, testosterone esters, and non-17-alpha-alkylated androgens have been used for the treatment of the anemia of chronic renal failure. Table 13 lists some of these preparations, routes of administration and doses.

The androgenic effects of these agents do not seem to be responsible for their erythropoietic activity. Consequently, agents such as nandrolone which have more anabolic than androgenic activity have been

Table 13
ANDROGENS COMMONLY USED FOR ANEMIAS OF CHRONIC RENAL FAILURE

Type of Androgen	Generic Name	Route of Administration	Dose	Reference
17-alpha-alkylated androgens	Fluoxymesterone	Oral	10 mg/day for females, 30 mg/day for males	61
	Oxymetholone	Oral	100 mg/day	48
Testosterone esters	Testosterone enanthate	Intramuscular	400-600 mg weekly	157
	Testosterone enanthate	Intramuscular	200 mg twice weekly	52
	Testosterone-mixture of esters (Sustanon)	Intramuscular	250 mg weekly (except bilatilateral nephrectomy: 250 mg biweekly)	168
Non-17-alpha-alkylated androgens	Nandrolone decanoate	Intramuscular	100 mg weekly	89
	Nandrolone decanoate	Intramuscular	200 mg weekly	53,198

used with considerable success. Surprisingly, the only well-done studies of androgens in the treatment of anemia secondary to chronic renal failure used 100 mg (89) and 200 mg of IM nandrolone weekly (198). Both studies demonstrated a significant erythropoietic response to androgen therapy with only minimal side effects. However, three to six months may elapse before erythropoiesis can be adequately demonstrated (61).

The majority of side effects of androgen therapy are dose-related and include priapism, acne, cholestatic jaundice, increase in body weight, sodium retention, hematoma at the intramuscular injection site, and masculinization of females and children as evidenced by voice changes and hair growth (48,53,61,157,185). Cholestatic jaundice is a side effect associated with the C-17-alpha-alkyl substituted derivatives of testosterone, and as a result, all oral androgenic preparations share this problem. The testosterone esters and non-C-17-alpha-alkylated derivatives of testosterone are administered parenterally and are rarely associated with the development of cholestatic jaundice. The jaundice is usually mild, dose-related, and rapidly reversible upon discontinuance of the offending agent (164). The C-17-alpha-alkylated androgens are also rarely associated with the development of tumors which resemble adenocarcinomas. Although these resolved after the discontinuation of the androgen (54,167), and have occurred only in patients with aplastic anemia, all patients receiving long-term androgen therapy should be monitored for this potentially dangerous complication of therapy.

28. A 48-year-old white male with a history of alcoholism is admitted to the hospital. He has evidence of portal hypertension and ascites. His admission lab data include: Na 135 mEq/L, K 3.5 mEq/L, Cl 96 mEq/L, HCO$_3$ 26 mEq/L, Hct 28%, Hgb 8.5 gm%, MCV 110 cubic microns. What factors should be considered in the etiology and treatment of this alcoholic patient's anemia?

Patients with alcoholic cirrhosis present with multiple problems which may produce an anemia of chronic liver disease. Blood loss from esophageal and/or gastrointestinal varices may lead to iron deficiency anemia. Nutritional folic acid deficiency is also common among alcoholics and may lead to megaloblastic anemia. In this patient, folate deficiency needs to be documented because his MCV of 110 cubic microns suggests a macrocytic anemia. Although macrocytic anemia is typical in liver disease, variations in size and shape of red blood cells are not extremely changed; leukopenia is not observed. Red cell precursors are large, but these changes are not the same as those seen with megaloblastic maturation of vitamin B$_{12}$ or folic acid deficiencies since all stages of maturation are seen.

Folate deficiency in association with chronic alcoholism and liver disease is due to decreased absorption induced by the chronic ingestion of alcohol, and suppression of erythropoiesis by alcohol (79). If the anemia is due to folic acid deficiency alone, then hematologic response will follow administration of low doses of folic acid (82). However, it is not uncommon for folic acid deficiency to be superimposed on a true anemia of liver disease, in which a relatively severe bone marrow failure occurs. In patients with advanced liver disease, the rate of marrow production is increased in response to their anemia, but not to the same extent as would occur under normal conditions. This anemia is refractory to therapy, is enhanced by hypervolemia, and is characterized by increased red cell turnover and an inadequate bone marrow response.

The evaluation of anemia in patients with liver disease is difficult because a multitude of complications occur in these patients: folic acid deficiency, acute and chronic blood loss, iron overload, chronic alcoholism and renal failure. Folic acid deficiency may be diagnosed by administering physiologic amounts of folic acid (50 to 100 mcg) which should give a prompt hematologic response. Serum and red cell folate levels are also very helpful in making this diagnosis (82).

29. A 28-year-old veteran has returned from Vietnam to the United States. He has the diagnosis of malaria falciparum and is begun on primaquine and chloroquine therapy. One week later he feels extremely weak, his urine is dark brown, and the sclera of his eyes appear yellow. What may be the cause of these signs and symptoms?

The primary consideration in this case is the probable occurrence of drug-induced hemolysis with concurrent hyperbilirubinemia and jaundice. Primaquine is the classic drug which elicits hemolysis in hereditary G6PD deficiency. Hemolysis and anemia may be caused by a variety of oxidant drugs in patients with glucose-6-phosphate dehydrogenase (G6PD) deficiency (16,20,146), but the severity and incidence of the reaction varies substantially depending upon (a) the genotype of G6PD and (b) the racial characteristics of the subject exposed to the drug.

There are two types of G6PD enzymes, types A and B. The "normal" G6PD is type B and makes up the most common enzyme in all population groups. However, there are substantial differences in the occurrence of variant enzymes in various population groups. Approximately one-third of Black Americans have the type A G6PD variant and only have 5 to 15% of the needed enzyme activity within their red blood cells. Other groups, such as Mediterranean Jews or Chinese also have a high prevalence of G6PD deficient activity, and their cells often contain less than 1% of normal G6PD activity. The lower the enzyme activity, the more severe the hemolytic reaction.

Hemolysis occurs in G6PD deficiency, because G6PD is necessary to reduce nicotinamide adenine diphosphate (NADP) to NADPH at a normal rate. NADPH protects red blood cells from oxidation by keeping gluthathione (GSH) in a reduced state and thus prevents GSH from complexing with hemoglobin and denaturing it. Denatured hemoglobin precipitates within the red cell as Heinz bodies, and the red cells are lysed. Exposure to certain drugs (Table 14) with oxidant properties increases significantly the amount of GSH free radicals that can bind to sulfhydryl groups on the hemoglobin molecule. Therefore, the severity of the hemolysis after drug exposure is greater in those subjects who have very low levels of G6PD enzyme activity, and thus NADPH, than in those who have moderate to normal enzyme activity.

The bone marrow responds to hemolysis by producing young red cells. In type A G6PD deficiency, these young red cells have normal enzyme activity and are resistant to hemolysis. This response does not occur in Mediterranean, type B subjects. As a result, hemolysis is self-limiting in Black people, despite continued therapy with the offending agent, while chronic, severe hemolysis occurs in Caucasians with the variant type of G6PD deficiency (16,146) and drug therapy must be discontinued.

Table 14 lists the drugs and average doses that reportedly elicit hemolysis due to G6PD deficiency. Several oxidant drugs have not been reported to produce significant hemolysis in G6PD deficiency and these include: aspirin, ascorbic acid, chloroquine, dimercaprol, diphenhydramine, menadione, methylene blue, para-aminobenzoic acid, procainamide, probenecid, sulfadiazine, sulfamerazine, sulfisoxazole, sulfathiazole, sodium sulfoxone, tripelennamine, pyrimethamine, quinine, and quinacrine.

If primaquine were continued at the same dose, the clinical course of hemolysis would typically occur in three phases: the acute, recovery, and equilibrium

Table 14
DRUGS PRODUCING CLINICALLY
SIGNIFICANT HEMOLYSIS

Drug	Trade Name	Dose
Acetanilid		3.6 gm
Diaminodiphenylsulfone	Dapsone	25-200 mg
Furazolidone	Tricofuron	400 mg
Furmethonol	Altafur	1.0 gm
Nalidixic acid	NegGram	
Neoarsphenamine	Neosalvarsan	600 mg
Nitrofurantion	Furadantin, Macrodantin	400 mg
Nitrofurazone	Furacin	1.5 gm
Pamaquine		
Aminoquine,	Plasmoquine	30 mg
Pentaquine		30 mg
Primaquine		30 mg
Sulfacetamide	Sulamyd	
Sulfamethoxypyrimidine		
Sulfanilamide		3.6-5.0 gm
Sulfapyridine		4.0 gm
Sulfasalazine	Azulfidine	6.9 gm

phases. The acute phase generally begins 1 to 3 days after the start of drug administration. Heinz bodies are present at this time and the urine may be positive for hemoglobin. During the acute phase, systemic symptoms include weakness, mild abdominal or back pain, and slight jaundice. At 4 to 6 days after the initiation of drug administration, the reticulocyte count is increased, indicating bone marrow compensation. The recovery phase begins 7 to 10 days after drug administration with rising hemoglobin and hematocrit (after a nadir of 25 to 35% decrease of pre-drug levels). The patient should begin to feel better clinically. The equilibrium phase begins about 40 days after primaquine therapy and consists of full hematologic and clinical recovery. However, if the dose of primaquine is increased, a new episode of hemolysis will occur.

30. What are some of the general mechanisms by which red cells are destroyed?

The main mechanisms of hemolytic destruction probably are the result of an altered red cell membrane. This red cell abnormality may be caused intra- or extracellularly (191).

Altered red cells may be destroyed by (a) colloid osmotic lysis, (b) primary perforation of the red cell membrane, (c) fragmentation, and (d) red cell phagocytosis (81).

If destruction occurs in the plasma, the process is termed intravascular hemolysis. If the red cells are sequestered or trapped in certain regions of the circulation (spleen, liver, bone marrow), the process is termed extravascular hemolysis (81).

31. Describe the biochemical changes resulting from increased red cell destruction.

Red cell breakdown products (hemoglobin) are normally handled through the bilirubin-urobilinogen pathway. This process is called extravascular destruction and is diagrammed below:

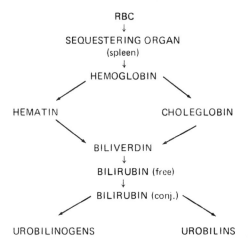

Increased hemoglobin catabolism is responsible for elevated levels of conjugated bilirubin and acholuric jaundice observed in hemolytic anemia. If intravascular hemolysis is the major site of destruction, hemoglobin is delivered directly to the plasma and hemoglobin elimination follows a different metabolic pathway. Haptoglobin is a collective term for alpha-globulins which bind hemoglobin in the plasma. The molecular relationship of haptoglobin to hemoglobin is 1:1 but depends on the concentration of each component. When haptoglobin is absent or completely saturated, hemoglobin circulates briefly then is either dissociated into heme and globin, removed in the liver, or excreted in the kidney. Unbound hemoglobin is filtered by the glomerulus and may exceed the reabsorption maximum in the proximal renal tubles resulting in hemoglobinuria (81,129).

As a result of the compensatory efforts of the bone marrow, increased numbers of young red cells or reticulocytes appear in the peripheral circulation. Reticulocytes which normally comprise 0.5 to 1.5% of the red cells increase to 10 or 20% in hemolysis. However, the reticulocyte count must always be related to the hematocrit. Thus, a reticulocyte count of 24% at a hematocrit of 15 gm% is equivalent to a reticulocyte count of 8% at a hematocrit of 45 gm% (81,97).

32. E.O., a 47-year-old man, was hospitalized with abdominal pain, vomiting, and diarrhea of one week duration. The patient had recently become depressed after a laryngectomy for squamous cell carcinoma of larynx. Since that surgery, he had not eaten routinely, but did ingest a fifth of whiskey per day. On admission, physical examination was significant for profound muscle weakness and tremulousness. Laboratory studies confirmed the diagnosis of acute pancreatitis. Approximately twenty-four hours after admission, serum phosphorous was noted to be less than 0.1 mg/dl. The initial hematocrit was 44%, and over the next five days it dropped to 25%. Serum bilirubin rose to 8.0 mg/dl and the reticulocyte count rose to 9%. Workup of the hemolytic anemia was negative, and included: direct and indirect Coombs, serum B$_{12}$, serum folate, cold agglutinins, G6PD and pyruvic kinase. What was the cause of the hemolytic anemia?

Severe hypophosphatemia, secondary to starvation and alcoholism, was initially manifested in this patient as muscular weakness. The hypophosphatemia was not treated for several days and a significant hemolysis ensued.

Hemolytic anemia secondary to hypophosphatemia is believed to be due to decreased levels of erythrocyte adenosine triphosphate (ATP) which maintains red cell membrane integrity and plasticity. ADP (adenosine diphosphate) is phosphorylated to ATP by inorganic phosphorous. The reservoir of phosphorous for phosphorylation is extracellular and is transmitted intracellularly by passive diffusion.

In vitro studies indicate that when ATP levels fall below 15% of normal, the erythrocyte membrane becomes rigid (105); however, it is unusual for ATP levels to fall below 40% of normal even in the presence of significant hypophosphatemia. Serum phosphorous levels must be extremely depressed (below 0.2 mg/dl) before ATP production is affected enough to induce hemolysis. An ATP level of 11% of normal was detected in a patient with a serum phosphorous of 0.1 mg/dl, and hemolytic anemia developed secondary to the hypophosphatemia (105).

Hypophasphatemia not only depresses ATP concentrations, but also levels of 2,3 diphosphoglycerate (2,3 DPG). Low levels of 2,3 DPG shift the oxy-hemoglobin saturation curve to the left, resulting in tissue anoxia (105).

33. How should the above patient's hypophosphatemic hemolytic anemia be treated?

The severe hemolytic anemia secondary to hypophosphatemia is readily reversible with the parenteral or oral administration of phosphates. Parenteral therapy may be preferred, especially if other signs of severe hypophosphatemia such as coma or convulsions are present. If oral therapy is utilized, 15 to 30 ml of Fleet's Phospho-Soda (80 to 160 mEq of phosphate) is given three times a day. If parenteral medication is necessary, 60 mEq of monobasic potassium phosphate is administered by continuous infusion over eight hours for a total of twenty four hours or longer (120) with careful monitoring of potassium values as well as clinical response. Oral or parenteral phosphate replenishment should not be overzealous, as hyperphosphatemia and the resultant hypocalcemia and metastic calcification must be avoided (72). Red cell survival improves within two to three days after correction of the serum phosphorous level (105).

34. What drugs can induce hypophosphatemic hemolytic anemia?

Drug-induced causes of hypophosphatemia include aluminum containing antacids, phosphate-poor total parenteral nutrition solutions, thiazide diuretics, estrogens, and androgens (67). As little as 90 ml of an aluminum-containing antacid, four times daily for thirty to ninety days, can produce symptomatic hypophosphatemia (126) by binding phosphate in the gastrointestinal tract. When phosphate-poor total parenteral nutrition solutions are administered, severe hypophosphatemia can develop within five to fourteen days (173). Phosphate is required for anabolism, and serum phosphorous will remain within normal limits when 20 mEq of phosphate is administered for each 1000 kilocalories (159,169).

35. Describe the direct and indirect Coombs' tests. When are these two tests employed? List the drugs associated with a positive direct Coombs' test.

The Coombs', or antiglobulin, test is an in vitro test used to detect coating antibodies against human erythrocytes. The two major types of erythrocyte coatings detected by this test are IgG, and C3b and C3d of the complement system. When these antibodies are present on the red blood cell surface, the antiglobulin reagents react to these proteins and the erythrocytes agglutinate (199).

Coombs' serum is prepared by the injection of human globulins into rabbits or goats. The test animals then produce antibodies to these human globulins. Subsequently, serum from these animals is collected. The direct Coombs' test is a one step procedure. A sample of the patient's red blood cells is collected and washed to remove any non-immunologically bound antibody. The washed erythrocytes are then combined with Coombs' serum. If agglutination occurs, the direct Coombs' test is positive. The direct Coombs' test is used in the diagnosis of hemolytic disorders of newborns such as erythroblastosis fetalis, hemolytic disorders of adults including acquired autoimmune hemolytic anemia, and hemolytic transfusion reactions (199).

The indirect Coombs' test is a two-stage procedure. The first step can be performed by two different methods. If one wishes to detect autoantibodies in the serum of a patient, red blood cells of known antigenic composition are exposed to the patient's serum containing unknown antibodies. After a sufficient contact time has passed, the exposed erythrocytes are washed and combined with Coombs' serum. If agglutination occurs, the indirect Coombs' test is positive and confirms that a now identified circulating antibody was present in the patient's serum. On the other hand, if one wishes to detect certain red blood cell antigens, serum containing specific known antibodies is combined with erythrocytes of unknown antigenic composition. After exposure these red cells are added to Coombs' serum. If agglutination occurs, the indirect Coombs' is positive and antigens coating the patient's

---

Table 15
POSITIVE DIRECT COOMBS' TEST
HEMOLYTIC ANEMIA SECONDARY TO DRUGS

Cephalosporins	Phenacetin
Isoniazid	Quinidine
Levodopa	Quinine
Mefenamic Acid	Rifampin
Methyldopa	Stibophen
Para-aminosalicylic Acid	Sulfonamides
Penicillins	Sulfonylureas

erythrocytes will have been identified. The indirect Coombs' test is used in the detection of autoantibodies in serum or certain weak antigens on red blood cells, such as D^u, or incomplete antigens, such as Duffy, Kidd, or Kell (199). Table 15 provides a list of the major drug-related causes of a positive direct Coombs' test.

36. A 42-year-old male was hospitalized with a ten day history of weakness, malaise, dark colored urine, and jaundice. Laboratory data included: hemoglobin 7.2 gm%, hematocrit 19%, WBC 9,600 per mm³, reticulocyte count 1.1%; the indirect bilirubin was 2.5 mg/dl; the direct Coombs' test was 2+ and the indirect Coombs' test was negative. A Cr⁵¹ red cell survival test resulted in a half life of 15 to 16 days (nl: 27 to 33 days). The diagnosis was idiopathic autoimmune hemolytic anemia. What are the causes of autoimmune hemolytic anemia and how is it treated?

Autoimmune hemolytic anemia is due to immunological factors in the red cell's environment and frequently is secondary to lymphomas, chronic lymphocytic leukemia, infections, rheumatoid arthritis, or other disorders. It also may be induced by drugs, or if no cause is readily discernible, it simply is categorized as idiopathic (40).

Prednisone in doses of 60 to 80 mg per day for 10 days is commonly used to treat autoimmune hemolytic anemia. Larger corticosteroid doses do not produce additional therapeutic benefits. Once a remission with steroids has been attained, the steroid should be tapered slowly over several months to a dose which will produce minimal side effects (10 mg prednisone daily) and prevent a recurrence of the anemia. As many as 84% of patients achieved partial or complete remission with a single course of corticosteroid therapy in one study. However, when the dose of prednisone was tapered to 10 to 15 mg per day, only 16% remained in remission. If the patient fails to respond to a ten day course of corticosteroid therapy, splenectomy is then a viable therapeutic alternative. Splenectomy can induce a remission in 44% of patients and is therefore sometimes utilized as an adjunct to steroid therapy in patients with relapsing autoimmune hemolytic anemia (40). Although splenectomized patients have twice the mortality of steroid-treated patients, the higher mortality associated with splenectomy may simply reflect the fact that patients who failed to respond to the corticosteroids tend to more severely affected (2). When splenectomy is contraindicated and when steroids result in therapeutic failure, cyclophosphamide 50 mg bid on alternate days is effective (40).

37. A 40-year-old white female was hospitalized with a systolic murmur, low grade fever, fatigue, night sweats, and joint pain. The diagnosis was sub-acute bacterial endocarditis and penicillin G five million units IV every 4 hours was instituted. After five days of therapy the hematocrit dropped from 39% to 27% and the hemoglobin dropped from 13 gm% to 9 gm%. The serum bilirubin rose from 0.8 mg% to 1.8 mg% (1.5 mg% indirect), the reticulocyte count rose from 2% to 9%, and the serum haptoglobin was 5 mg%. Additionally, the direct Coombs' test was positive and the indirect test was negative. What is the problem and what should be done?

This patient is experiencing the *haptene type* of hemolytic anemia which occurs in patients receiving more than 20 million units per day of intravenous penicillin. Not all patients receiving this dose develop IgG antibody (positive direct Coombs' test), nor do those who develop antibody necessarily have evidence of hemolysis (149,194,204).

A number of drugs which act as haptenes become antigenic when they combine with the red cell membrane. IgG antibody reacts with drug-red cell complex producing hemolysis (115,149). The direct Coombs' test is usually positive while the indirect is negative (44). The penicillins and cephalosporins bind to red cells strongly and are good examples of this type of immune-induced hemolytic anemia (176). The patient produces antibodies against the drug-red cell complex and thus coats them with immunoglobulins, with or without complement. The complement system may also be stimulated (114).

The symptoms of this patient are of mild to moderate severity; in many cases of haptene type hemolytic anemia, symptoms are not evident. In cases of severe hemolytic anemia, shaking chill, high fever, shock, jaundice, palpitations, dyspnea, cyanosis, cardiomegaly, anuria, as well as pain in the abdomen, back, or extremities may develop. Clinical signs of hemolytic anemia include hemoglobinuria, red urine, dark stools, hyperbilirubinemia (indirect), reticulocytosis, and splenomegaly (200).

The treatment of a haptene-type hemolytic anemia is discontinuation of the drug. Transfusion may be required depending on the degree of anemia. In this case, the patient does not need transfusions because he is asymptomatic from the hemolytic process. Corticosteroids are not effective in immune-induced hemolytic anemias (81).

38. A 61-year-old white female is started on quinine sulfate 300 mg three times daily for leg cramps due to arteriosclerotic vascular disease. Four days after the initiation of therapy she returns to her community pharmacy for some aspirin and kaolin-pectin suspension for what she believes to be the flu (chills, abdominal pain and diarrhea). She also asks if her new medicine (Quinine) can affect menstrual flow or cause break-through bleeding. Could any of her

complaints be associated with her quinine therapy?

Quinine has been reported to produce hemolytic anemia in many instances (138). The clinical findings of this drug-induced hemolysis may occur from 1 to 5 days after initiation of therapy and include fever, chills, and hemoglobinuria. The above patient may be having hemoglobinuria rather than "break-through" bleeding. The patient should stop her quinine therapy and be referred to her physician.

39. Describe the mechanism by which quinine produces red cell hemolysis.

Unlike haptene-induced hemolytic anemia from penicillin, quinine produces the *innocent bystander* type of hemolysis where the drug binds to an antibody (Ab), usually of the IgM type, to form an immune complex which then attaches to the erythrocyte membrane. Neither the drug nor the antibody alone have high affinity for the red cell. After attachment of the immune complex to the red cell membrane, complement (C') interacts with the drug-Ab-membrane and stimulates anti-C' antibodies which lyse the red blood cell with dissociation of the drug-Ab complex. The dissociated drug-Ab complex which was released into the plasma then goes on to initiate the reaction on other red cells. The small number of drug-Ab complexes accounts for a negative Coombs' test (anti-gamma globulin). However, the immune reaction becomes positive with anti-C' serum (69).

The dose of quinine need not be large to produce acute hemolysis, hemoglobinuria, and hemoglobinemia. However, prior drug exposure is required to elicit the reaction.

Several drugs produce hemolysis by the innocent bystander mechanism and are listed in Table 16. Most of these drug reactions are mediated by IgM (44), although some are of the IgG type (55). Most of these drugs also produce immune-induced thrombocytopenia. It has been proposed that IgM antibodies are responsible for hemolysis, while IgG antibodies are responsible for thrombocytopenic reactions (171).

As in haptene-induced hemolysis, discontinuing the drug results in rapid reversal of clinical symptoms. If the anemia is severe (hematocrit less than 20%), transfusions should be given.

Table 16
DRUGS WHICH INDUCE AN "INNOCENT BYSTANDER" TYPE OF HEMOLYTIC ANEMIA

Chlorpromazine	Phenacetin
Dipyrone	Quinidine
Insecticides	Quinine
Insulin	Rifampicin
Isoniazid	Stibophen
Melphalan	Sulfonamides
Para-aminosalicylic Acid	Sulfonylurea

40. A 67-year-old white male with Parkinson's disease was started on two grams of levodopa daily in March because of poor control with anticholinergics. By November, his hematocrit had dropped from 45% to 37%. By February of the following year, he noticed jaundice, weakness, and anorexia. His hematocrit was 19%, a reticulocyte count was 36%, total bilirubin was 5.6 mg% (4.1 mg% indirect), and Coombs' tests (direct and indirect) were 4+ positive. What type of anemia has developed? Explain the mechanism involved.

The autoimmune type of hemolytic anemia is evident in this case. It differs from the "haptene" and "innocent bystander" type in that the direct and indirect Coombs' with antiglobin G is positive (69). In addition, the IgG antibody can be obtained by eluting the Coombs' positive red cells which will then react with normal red blood cells without the addition of drug. These antibodies have an Rh-type specificity (81).

In a large study, the positive direct Coombs' test developed in 9% of patients receiving an average dose of five grams of levodopa (110). Most of these patients became positive between 90 and 360 days after therapy was initiated. Hemolytic anemia to both levodopa and alphamethyldopa is rare, but the clinical presentation and duration of antiglobulin response make it an interesting problem. (Also see the *Hypertension* chapter for a discussion of alphamethyldopa-induced hemolytic anemia). The symptoms and hematologic values (hematocrit and reticulocytes) usually return to normal within two months after discontinuing therapy; however, the Coombs' test can remain positive for many years (181,204).

41. A 26-year-old white female entered the hospital for an elective cholecystectomy. The patient claimed that she had never received penicillin and had no drug allergies. After the operation she was treated with 500 mg of cephalothin intravenously every six hours. After five days of therapy her hematocrit dropped from 37% to 27%, her hemoglobin dropped from 12 gm% to 9.8 gm%, and her reticulocyte count had increased to 23%. A Coombs' test was strongly positive. The patient was jaundiced with a bilirubin of 9.3 mg%, 6.2 mg% of which was direct. How does cephalothin hemolytic anemia differ from penicillin-induced hemolytic anemia?

The clinical presentation of cephalothin hemolytic anemia differs from penicillin-induced hemolytic anemia in several respects (74). It takes longer for symptoms and lab tests to return to normal after discontinuation of cephalothins in contrast to penicillin, and high doses are not needed to induce hemolysis. The specific antibody is IgG even though IgM antibodies can be elicited in most patients on cephalothin. Only two cases of cephalothin-induced hemolytic anemia have been reported, but in both patients the antibodies were IgG; thus the hemolytic reaction appears to have been due to these antibodies.

Although the direct Coombs' test is positive in 65% of patients taking cephalothin, the reaction is usually not associated with any laboratory evidence of hemolysis. In addition, the alteration of the red cell surface by cephalothin *in vitro* from earlier studies appears to have made a large percentage of the direct Coombs' test positive by a nonimmunological mecha-

nism. It was suggested that the positive reactions were due to the presence of antialbumin in antiglobulin sera. A more recent study by Spath (177) using sera without antialbumin demonstrated that only 4% of patients on cephalothin gave positive direct Coombs' tests if weak reactions were excluded.

In two cases reported by Gralnick (74) the hematocrit and reticulocyte count did not revert to normal when cephalothin was discontinued and one patient rapidly progressed to death.

REFERENCES

1. Allen DM: Oxymethalone therapy in aplastic anemia. Blood 32:83, 1968.
2. Allgood JW et al: Idiopathic acquired autoimmune hemolytic anemia: A review of 47 cases treated from 1955 through 1965. Am J Med 43:254, 1967.
3. Am Med Assoc: Council on foods and nutrition. JAMA 203:61, 1968.
4. Anon: Androgens in the anaemia of chronic renal failure. Brit Med J 3:417, 1977.
5. Bainton DF et al: The diagnosis of iron deficiency anemia. Am J Med 37:62, 1974.
6. Beal R: Hematinics: pathophysiological and clinical aspects. Drugs 2:190, 1971.
7. Beal R: Hematinics: clinical pharmacological and therapeutic agents. Drugs 2:207, 1971.
8. Beck EA et al: Reversible sideroblastic anemia caused by chloramphenicol. Acta Haematol 38:1, 1967.
9. Beck W: Folic acid deficiency. In *Hematology,* edited by W. Williams, McGraw-Hill, New York, 1972, p 279-283.
10. Beck W: General considerations in megaloblastic anemias. In *Hematology,* edited by W. Williams, McGraw-Hill, New York, 1972, p 256-278.
11. Beck W: Vitamin B$_{12}$ deficiency. In *Hematology,* edited by W. Williams, McGraw-Hill, New York, 1972, p 256-278.
12. Bennington J: *Laboratory Diagnosis,* Macmillan Co., New York, 1970, p 431.
13. Bertino J et al: Studies on the inhibition of dihydrofolate reductase by the folate antagonists. J Biol Chem 239:497, 1964.
14. Beutler E: *Clinical Disorders of Iron Metabolism* (Monograph). Grune & Stratton, New York, 1963.
15. Beutler E: Iron deficiency. In *Hematology,* edited by W. Williams, McGraw-Hill, New York, 1972, p 308.
16. Beutler E: Glucose 6-phosphate deficiency. In *Hematology,* edited by W. Williams, McGraw-Hill, New York, 1972, p 395.
17. Beutler E: Iron metabolism. In *Hematology,* edited by W. Williams, McGraw-Hill, 1972, p 129.
18. Beutler E: Iron Deficiency. In *Hematology,* edited by W. Williams, McGraw-Hill, 1972, p 316-19.
19. Beutler E & Meekreebs G: Doses and dosing. NEJM 274:1152, 1966.
20. Beutler E: Drug-induced hemolytic anemia. Pharmacol Rev 21:73, 1969.
21. Block M: In *Iron,* edited by W. Crosby, Medcom Series, New York, 1972, p 56.
22. Block M: Using IV iron, in *Iron: A Total Clinical Learning Experience,* edited by W. Crosby, Medcom series, New York, 1972.
23. Boddy K et al: Retention of cyanocobalamin, hydroxycobalamin after parenteral administration. Lancet 2:710, 1968.
24. Boddy K et al: Iron absorption in Addisionian pernicious anemia. Am J Clin Nutr 22:1555, 1969.
25. Bonnar J: Anemia in Obstetrics: an evaluation of treatment by iron dextran infusion. Brit Med J 3:1030, 1965.
26. Booth C et al: Site of absorption of vitamin B$_{12}$ in man. Lancet 1:18, 1959.
27. Bothwell T et al: The intestine in iron absorption. Am J Digest Dis 1:145, 1957.
28. Bothwell T et al: Factors affecting iron absorption. J Lab Clin Med 51:24, 1958.
29. Bothwell T & Finch C: *Iron Metabolism.* Little, Brown and Co., Boston, 1962.
30. Bothwell T: Iron deficiency. Med J Aust 2:433, 1972.
31. Boyett J et al: Allopurinol and iron metabolism in man. Blood 32:460, 1968.
31a. Brain MC: Sideroblastic anemia. *Textbook of Medicine* edited by PB Beeson and W McDermott. 14th Edition. WB Saunders, Philadelphia, 1975.
32. Brise H et al: Absorbability of different iron compounds. Acta Medica Scand 171(Suppl 376):23, 1962.
33. Brise H et al: Iron absorption studies. Acta Med Scand 171 (suppl 376): 1, 1962.
34. Brown E: Clinical pharmacology of drugs used in the treatment of iron deficiency anemia. Pharmacol Physicians 2:11, 1968.
35. Brown EB Jr et al: Studies in iron transportation and metabolism. XI. Critical analysis of mucosal block by large doses of inorganic iron in human subjects. J Lab Clin Med 52:335, 1958.
36. Cade J et al: The use of iron dextran by total dose infusion. Med J Aust 1:716, 1968.
37. Chalmers J et al: Comparison of hydroxycobalamin and cyanocobalamin in pernicious anemia. Lancet 2:1305, 1965.
38. Chanarin I: Absorption of cobalamins. J Clin Path 5 (Suppl 24):60, 1971.
39. Chanarin I: *The Megaloblastic Anemias.* Blackwell Scientific Publ., Oxford, England, 1969, pp 282-305.
40. Chaplin H et al: Autoimmune hemolytic anemia. Arch Intern Med 137:346, 1977.
41. Conrad M et al: Ascorbic acid chelates in iron absorption, a role for hydrochloric acid and bile. Gastroent 55:35, 1968.
42. Corcino J et al: Mechanism of triamterene induced megaloblastosis. Ann Intern Med 73:419, 1970.
43. Crichton R: Ferriten: Structure, synthesis and function. NEJM 284:1413, 1971.
44. Croft J et al: Coombs' test positivity induced by drugs. Ann Intern Med 68:176, 1968.
45. Crosby W: Mucosal block: an evaluation of concepts relating to control of iron absorption. Semin Hemat 3:299, 1966.
46. Cummings et al: Effects of two oral iron preparations on results of the benzidine test for occult blood in stools. J Clin Path 21:41, 1968.
47. Dacie JV et al: Siderocytes, sideroblasts and sideroblastic anemia. Acta Med Scand 179 (suppl 445):237, 1966.
48. Davies M et al: Oxymetholone in the treatment of anaemia in chronic renal failure. Brit J Urol 44:387, 1972.
49. Davis P: Trimethoprim — sulfamethoxazole and folate metabolism. Path 5:23, 1973.
50. Davis P et al: Effect of allopurinol on radioiron absorption in man. Lancet 2:470, 1966.
51. Davis RE et al: Pyridoxal and folate deficiency in alcoholics. Med J Aust 2:537, 1974.
52. DeGowin RL et al: Erythropoiesis and erythropoietin in patients with chronic renal failure treated with hemodialysis and testosterone. Ann Intern Med 72:913, 1970.
53. Doane BD et al: Response of uremic patients to nandrolone decanoate. Arch Intern Med 135:972, 1975.
54. Editorial: Liver tumours and steroid hormones. Lancet 1:481, 1973.
55. Eisner E et al: Quinine-induced thrombocytopenic purpura due to an IgM and IgG antibody. Transfusion 12:317, 1972.
56. Emmerson B: Effects of allopurinol on iron metabolism in man. Ann Rheum Dis 25:700, 1966.

57. Ersley A: Anemia of chronic disorders. In *Hematology,* edited by W. Williams, McGraw-Hill, New York, 1972, pp 371-379.
58. Erslev A: Anemia of chronic renal disease. Arch Intern Med 126:774, 1970.
59. Eschback J: Disorders of red blood cell production in uremia. Arch Intern Med 126:812, 1970.
60. Eschback J: Erythropoiesis in patients with renal failure undergoing chronic dialysis. NEJM 276:653, 1967.
61. Eschbach JW et al: Improvement in the anemia of chronic renal failure with fluoxymesterone. Ann Intern Med 78:527, 1973.
62. Eschbach JW et al: Iron balance in hemodialysis patients. Ann Intern Med 87:710, 1977.
63. Esplin D: Antiseptics and disinfectants; fungicides; ectoparasiticides, in *Pharmacologic Basis of Therapeutics,* edited by L Goodman and A Gilman, MacMillan Co., New York, 1970, pp 1035-37.
64. Fairbank V: Iron deficiency, in *Hematology,* edited by W. Williams, McGraw-Hill, New York, 1972, pp 311:312, 318.
65. Fairbanks VF: Iron deficiency: still a diagnostic challenge. Med Clin N Amer 54:903, 1970.
66. Fischer D: Acute iron poisoning in children. JAMA 218:1179, 1971.
67. Fitzgerald F: Hypophosphatemia. West J Med 122:482, 1975.
67a. Frei E et al: A new approach to cancer chemotherapy with methotrexate. NEJM 292:846, 1975.
68. Fried W et al: The erythropoietic effect of androgens. Ann NY Acad Sci 149:356, 1968.
69. Garratty G: Drug-related problems, in *A Seminar on Problems Encountered in Pretransfusion Tests.* American Assoc. of Blood Banks, Washington, D.C., 1972, pp 33-58.
70. Giorgio A: Current concepts of iron metabolism and iron deficiency anemia. Med Clin N Amer 54:1399, 1970.
71. Gleason M et al: Section 3, therapeutics index: phenol, in *Clinical Toxicology of Commercial Products.* Edited by M Gleason et al. Williams and Wilkins Co., 1969, p 189-191.
72. Goldsmith R et al: Inorganic phosphate treatment of hypercalcemia of diverse etiologies. NEJM 274:1, 1966.
73. Goldstein A: Drug idiosyncrasy and pharmacogenetics, in *The Principles of Drug Action,* edited by A Goldstein, Harper and Row, New York, 1968, pp 444-452.
74. Grainick H: Hemolytic anemia associated with cephalothin. JAMA 217:1193, 1971.
75. Haden HT: Pyridoxine-responsive sideroblastic anemia due to antituberculous drugs. Arch Intern Med 120:602, 1967.
76. Hall G et al: Inhibition of iron absorption by magnesium trisilicate. Med J Aust 2:95, 1969.
77. Hallberg L et al: Iron absorption studies. Acta Med Scand (Suppl 358) 168:1, 1960.
78. Hallberg L et al: Studies on oral iron therapy. Acta Med Scand (suppl) 459, 1966.
79. Halsted CA: The effect of alcoholism on the absorption of folic acid. J Lab Clin Med 69:116, 1967.
80. Hampers C: Megaloblastic hematopiesis in uremia and in patients on long-term dialysis. NEJM 176:551, 1967.
81. Harris J: *The Red Cell.* Harvard Press, Cambridge, Mass., 1972, pp 559-573.
82. Ibid: pp 727-733.
83. Ibid: p 526.
84. Ibid: pp 259-71.
85. Ibid: pp 517-519.
86. Ibid: pp 350-51.
87. Ibid: pp 335-37.
88. Ibid: pp 746-48.
89. Hendler ED et al: Controlled study of androgen therapy in anemia of patients on maintenance hemodialysis. NEJM 291:1046, 1974.
90. Herbert V: Current concepts in therapy: megaloblastic anemia. NEJM 268:368, 1963.
91. Herbert V: Drugs effective in megaloblastic anemia. In *Pharmacological Basis of Therapeutics,* edited by L Goodman and A Gilman, MacMillan Co., New York, 1970, pp 1414-1444.
92. Herbert V: Drugs effective in megaloblastic anemia, in *Pharmacological Basis of Therapeutics,* edited by L Goodman and A Gilman, MacMillan Co., New York, 1970, pp 1397, 1440.
93. Herbert V: Experimental nutritional folate deficiency in man. Trans Act Am Phys 75:307, 1962.
94. Herbert V et al: Correlation of folate deficiency with alcoholism and associated macrocytosis, anemia and liver disease. Ann Intern Med 58:977, 1963.
95. Hess D et al: Para-aminosalicylic acid induced intestinal malabsorption. Clin Res 18:77, 1970.
96. Hillman R et al: Control of marrow production by the level of iron supply. J Clin Invest 48:454, 1969.
97. Hillman R et al: Erythropoiesis: normal and abnormal. Semin Hematol 4:327, 1967.
98. Hines J et al: Megaloblastic anemia secondary to folate deficiency associated with hypothyroidism. Ann Intern Med 68:792, 1968.
99. Hines JD: Reversible megaloblastic and sideroblastic marrow abnormalities in alcoholic patients. Brit J Haematol 16:87, 1969.
100. Hoffbrand A et al: Mechanism of folate deficiency in patients receiving phenytoin. Lancet 2:528, 1968.
101. Horrigan DL et al: Pyridoxine-responsive anemia: analysis of 62 cases. Adv Intern Med 12:103, 1964.
102. Horrigan DL et al: Pyridoxine-responsive anemias in man. Vitams Horm 26:549, 1968.
103. Illingworth P: Influence of iron preparations on occult blood tests. J Clin Path 18:103, 1965.
104. Issacs R et al: Standards for red blood cell increases after liver and stomach therapy in pernicious anemia. JAMA 111:2291, 1938.
105. Jacob HS et al: Acute hemolytic anemia with rigid cells in hypophosphatemia. NEJM 285:1446, 1971.
106. Jacobs A et al: Ferritin in serum: Clinical and biochemical implications. NEJM 292:951, 1975.
107. Jacobs A et al: Gastric acidity and iron absorption. Brit J Haematol 12:728, 1966.
108. Jacobson E et al: An experimental malabsorption syndrome induced by neomycin. Am J Med 28:524, 1960.
109. Jenkins GC et al: A hematological study of patients receiving long-term treatment with trimethoprim and sulphonamide. J Clin Path 23:392, 1970.
110. Joseph C: Occurrence of positive Coombs' test in patients with levodopa. NEJM 286:1401, 1972.
111. Kahn SB et al: Effects of trimethoprim on folate metabolism in man. Clin Pharmacol Ther 9:550, 1968.
112. Kasower N: Does 3,4-dihydroxyphenylalanine play a part in favism? Nature 215:285, 1967.
113. Kerr D et al: Gastrointestinal tolerance to oral iron preparations. Lancet 2:489, 1958.
114. Kerr R et al: Erythrocyte-bound C_5 and C_6 in autoimmune hemolytic anemia. J Immunol 107:1209, 1971.
115. Kerr R et al: Two mechanisms of erythrocyte destruction in penicillin-induced hemolytic anemia. NEJM 287:1322, 1972.
116. Kimber C et al: The mechanism of anemia in chronic liver disease. Quart J Med 34:33, 1965.
117. Klipstein F et al: Folate deficiency associated with drug therapy for tuberculosis. Blood 29:697, 1967.
118. Klipstein F: Subnormal serum folate and macrocytosis associated with anticonvulsant drug therapy. Blood 23:68, 1964.
119. Klipstein F: Folate deficiency secondary to disease of the intestinal tract. Bull NY Acad Med 42:638, 1966.
120. Klock JC et al: Hemolytic anemia and somatic cell dysfunction in severe hypophosphatemia. Arch Intern Med 134:360, 1974.
121. Lees F: Radioactive vitamin B_{12} absorption in the megaloblastic anemia caused by anticonvulsant drugs. Quart J Med 30:231, 1961.
122. Leonards J: Reduction of aspirin-induced occult blood loss in man. Clin Pharm Ther 10:571, 1969.
123. Levin R: Iron deficiency anemia in the pediatric patient. Am Pharm Assoc J NS 11:670, 1971.
124. Lipschitz DA et al: A clinical evaluation of serum ferritin as an index of iron stores. NEJM 290:1213, 1974.
125. Lloyd K: Reactions to total dose infusion of iron dextran in rheumatoid arthritis. Brit Med J 2:323, 1970.
126. Lotz M et al: Evidence for a phosphorous-depletion syndrome in man. NEJM 278:409, 1968.
127. Lous P et al: The absorption of vitamin B_{12} following partial gastrectomy. Acta Med Scand 164:407, 1959.
128. Lowe C et al: Iron balance and requirements in infancy. Pediat 43:134, 1969.
129. Lowenstein L et al: An immunologic basis for acquired resistance to oral administration of hog intrinsic factor and vitamin B_{12} in pernicious anemia. J Clin Invest 40:1656, 1961.

130. MacCurcy RK et al: Thrombocytopenia and sideroblastic anemia with pyrazinoic acid amide (Pyrazinamide) therapy. Chest 57:378, 1970.

131. Marchasin S et al: The treatment of iron deficiency anemia with iron dextran. Blood 23:354, 1964.

132. Mattila MJ et al: Interference of iron preparations and milk with the absorption of tetracyclines. In: Excerpta Medica International Congress Series number 254. Excerpta Medica, Amsterdam, 1972, p 128-133.

133. Mazur A et al: Haemochromatosis and hepatic xanthine oxidase. Lancet 1:254, 1967.

134. McCredie KB et al: Oxymetholone in refractory anemia. Brit J Haematol 17:265-73, 1969.

135. McCurdy PR et al: Pyridoxine-responsive anemia conditioned by isonicotinic acid hydrazide. Blood 27:352, 1966.

136. McCurdy PR et al: Reversible sideroblastic anemia caused by pyrazinoic acid (Pyrazinamide) therapy. Ann Intern Med 64:1280, 1966.

137. Middleton E et al: Studies on the absorption of orally administered iron from sustained-release preparations. NEJM 274:136, 1966.

138. Muirhead E et al: Drug dependent Coombs' (antiglobulin) test and anemia. Observation on quinine and phenacetin. Arch Intern Med 101:82, 1958.

139. Murray M et al: Gastric factor promoting iron absorption. Lancet 1:614, 1968.

140. Murray M et al: Does the pancreas influence iron absorption? Gastroent 51:694, 1966.

141. Nalts J et al: Erythropoiesis in anephric man. Lancet 1:941, 1968.

142. Neuvonen P et al: Interference of iron with the absorption of tetracyclines in man. Brit Med J 4:532, 1970.

143. Newcombe R: Precautions in the intravenous use of iron dextran. Postgrad Med J 43:372, 1967.

144. O'Sullivan D et al: Oral iron compounds, a therapeutic comparison. Lancet 2:482, 1955.

145. Package Insert — Imferon (Lakeside Co.)

146. Pannacciulli I et al: The course of experimentally induced hemolytic anemia in a primaquine-sensitive caucasian. A case study. Blood 25:92, 1965.

147. Pearson D: Megaloblastic anemia due to glutethimide. Lancet 1:110, 1965.

148. Petitpierre-Gabathuler MPI et al: Effects of chloramphenicol on heme synthesis. Acta Haematol 47:257, 1972.

149. Petz L et al: Coombs' positive hemolytic anemia caused by penicillin administration. NEJM 274:171, 1966.

150. Petz LD et al: Drug-induced hemolytic anemia. Clin Hematol 4:181, 1975.

151. Pollack S et al: Iron absorption: effects of sugars and reducing agents. Blood 24:577, 1964.

152. Pollar L: Heparin-retarded plasma clotting test. Angiol 5:21, 1954.

153. Powell L: Effects of allopurinol on iron storage in the rat. Ann Rheum Dis 25:697, 1966.

154. Presant C et al: Oxymetholone in myelofibrosis and CLL. Arch Int Med 132:175, 1973.

155. Rath C et al: Effect of renal disease on the Schilling test. NEJM 256:111, 1957.

156. Reynolds E et al: Anticonvulsant therapy, megaloblastic hemopoiesis and folic acid metabolism. Quart J Med 35:521, 1966.

157. Richardson JR et al: Erythropoietic response of dialyzed patients to testosterone administration. Ann Int Med 73:403, 1970.

157a. Robertson AG et al: Intramuscular iron and local oncogenisis. Brit Med J 1:946, 1977.

158. Rosenberg I et al: Impairment of intestinal deconjugation of dietary folate: a possible explanation of megaloblastic anemia associated with phenytoin therapy. Lancet 2:530, 1968.

159. Rudman D et al: Elemental balances during intravenous hyperalimentation of underweight adult subjects. J Clin Invest 55:94, 1975.

160. Salokannel S et al: Malabsorption of vitamin B_{12} during treatment with slow-release KCl. Acta Med Scand 187:431, 1970.

161. Sanchez-Medal L et al: Anabolic androgenic steroids in the treatment of acquired aplastic anemia. Blood 34:283, 1969.

162. Savin M: A practical approach to the treatment of iron deficiency. Rational Drug Therapy 11:1, 1977.

163. Schieve JR et al: Response of lingual manifestations of pernici-

164. Schiff L: Diseases of the Liver, 3rd ed, Lippincott, Philadelphia, 1969, p 551-2.

165. Schilling R et al: Intrinsic factor studies, III: further observations utilizing the urinary radioactivity test in subjects with achlorhydria, pernicious anemia, or a total gastrectomy. J Lab Clin Med 45:926, 1955.

166. Shahidi N: Testosterone-induced remission in aplastic anemia of both acquired and congenital types. NEJM 264:953, 1961.

167. Shahidi NT: Androgens and erythropoiesis. NEJM 289:72, 1973.

168. Shaldon S et al: Testosterone therapy for anaemia in maintenance dialysis. Brit Med J 3:212, 1971.

169. Sheldon GF et al: Phosphate depletion and repletion: Relation to parenteral nutrition and oxygen transport. Ann Surg 182:683, 1975.

170. Sheldon S: The use of testosterone in bilateral nephrectomized dialysis patients. Trans Amer Soc Artif Intern Organs 17:104, 1971.

171. Shulman N: Mechanism of blood destruction in individuals sensitized to foreign antigens. Trans Assoc Am Physicians 76:72, 1963.

172. Siliuk SJ et al: An analysis of hypoplastic anemia with special reference to oxymethalone in its therapy. Aust Ann Med 17:224, 1968.

173. Silvis SE et al: Paresthesias, weakness, seizures and hypophosphatemia in patients receiving hyperalimentation. Gastroent 62:513, 1972.

174. Sive J et al: Effect of trimethoprim on folate-dependent DNA synthesis in human bone marrow. J Clin Path 25:194, 1972.

175. Smith M et al: Absorption of inorganic iron from graded doses. Brit J Hemat 4:428, 1958.

176. Spath P: Studies on the immune response to penicillin and cephalothin in humans. Part I and II. J Immunol 107:854,860, 1971.

177. Spath P et al: Studies on the immune response to penicillin and cephalothin in humans. J Immunol 107:854, 860, 1971.

178. Streiff R: Malabsorption of polyglutamic folic acid secondary to oral contraceptives. Clin Res 17:71, 345, 1969.

179. Stojceski T et al: Studies on the serum iron-binding capacity. J Clin Path 18:446, 1965.

180. Sullivan L et al: Suppression of hematopoiesis by ethanol. J Clin Invest 43:2048, 1964.

181. Territo M et al: Autoimmune hemolytic anemia due to levodopa therapy. JAMA 226:1347, 1973.

182. Tomkin G et al: Malabsorption of vitamin B_{12} in diabetic patients treated with phenformin. Brit Med J 3:673, 1973.

183. Turner JW: Ch 12, Anemia and bleeding disorders, in Manual of Medicical Therapeutics, 20th ed., Little, Brown Co., Boston, 1973.

184. Vincent PC: Complications and treatment of acquired aplastic anemia. Brit J Hematol 13:977, 1967.

185. Von Hartitzsch B et al: Androgens in the anemia of chronic renal failure. Nephron 18:13, 1977.

186. Wallerstein R: Intravenous iron dextran complex. Blood 32:690, 1968.

187. Waxman S et al: Mechanism of pyrimethamine-induced megaloblastosis in human bone marrow. NEJM 280:1316, 1969.

188. Waxman S: Metabolic approach to the diagnosis of megaloblastic anemias. Med Clin N Amer 57:315, 1973.

189. Waxman S et al: Drugs, toxins, and dietary amino acids affecting vitamin B_{12} or folic acid absorption and utilization. Am J Med 48:599, 1970.

190. Webb D et al: Mechanism of vitamin B_{12} malabsorption in patients receiving colchicine. NEJM 279:845, 1968.

191. Weed R et al: Membrane alterations leading to red cell destruction. Am J Med 41:681, 1966.

192. Westlin W: Desferoxamine in the treatment of acute iron poisoning. Clin Pediat 5:531, 1955.

193. Whelby M et al: The role of bile in the control of iron absorption. Gastroent 42:319, 1962.

194. White J et al: Penicillin-induced hemolytic anemia. Brit J Hematol 3:26, 1968.

195. Whitman A: Effect of prolonged administration of trimethoprim-sulfamethoxazole. Postgrad Med J 45:46(Suppl), 1969.

196. Whitten C: Studies in acute iron poisoning: II. Further observations of desferoxamine in the treatment of acute experimental

ous anemia to pteroylglutamic acid and vitamin B_{12}. J Lab Clin Med 34:439, 1949.

iron poisoning. Pediat 38:102, 1966.
197. Will G et al: The treatment of iron deficiency anemia by iron-dextran infusion: a radio-isotope study. Brit J Haematol 14:61, 1968.
198. Williams JS et al: Nandrolone decanoate therapy for patients receiving hemodialysis: controlled study. Arch Intern Med 134:289, 1974.
199. Winetrobe M: Clinical Hematology, 7th ed., Lea and Febiger, Philadelphia, 1974, p 450, 89304.
200. Wintrobe M: *Principles of Internal Medicine,* 6th ed. McGraw-Hill, New York, 1970, p 1614, 1617.
201. Ibid: p 1632.
202. Ibid: p 1595.
203. Ibid: p 1615.
204. Worlledge S: Immunologic drug-induced hemolytic anemias. Semin Hematol 10:327, 1973.

Chapter 34

Cancer Chemotherapy

Robert J. Ignoffo

Since the discovery of aminopterin by Farber and co-workers (58) in 1948, the management of neoplastic disorders and their complications has significantly improved. Major cancer research developments have occurred in cell biology, investigative technology, and screening for new antineoplastic agents. Initial clinical studies of antitumor agents were primarily empirical, but due to rigorous basic research, concepts of chemotherapy have emerged that are currently based on the rational application of combination chemotherapeutic agents that are synergistic as well as minimally toxic to the host.

In the past, chemotherapy was often palliative, but today it is prolonging patient survival and producing cures in several malignant disorders. (See Table 1.) Most of the antineoplastic drugs discussed in this chapter are commercially available; however, some investigational agents will be included, because they represent new developments and may eventually be released for general use.

The Role of Pharmacists in the Management of Cancer Patients:

Pharmacists should be more knowledgeable about

Table 1
DISEASES WHERE CHEMOTHERAPY HAS SIGNIFICANTLY PROLONGED SURVIVAL

Disease	Therapy
Burkitt's lymphoma	Cyclophosphamide
Choriocarcinoma	Methotrexate; actinomycin D
Acute lymphocytic leukemia	Vincristine and prednisone for induction; methotrexate, 6-MP for maintenance; VAMP*; POMP
Hodgkin's disease	MOPP
Lymphosarcoma	CVP
Mycosis fungoides	Nitrogen mustard
Embryonal testicular carcinoma	Actinomycin D; mithramycin; vincristine; methotrexate
Wilm's tumor	Surgery, radiotherapy and actinomycin D, vincristine
Ewing's sarcoma	Radiotherapy and vincristine, cyclophosphamide
Rhabdomyosarcoma	Surgery, radiotherapy and cyclophosphamide, vincristine, actinomycin D
Retinoblastoma	Radiotherapy and triethylenemelamine

*VAMP and POMP: vincristine, prednisone, 6MP, methotrexate. MOPP: nitrogen mustard, vincristine, procarbazine, prednisone. CVP: cyclophosphamide, vincristine, prednisone.

the clinical use of cancer drugs. We have neglected becoming "experts" in this field because it changes so rapidly. However, if pharmacists are to be recognized as *total* health care practitioners, they must take the initiative to learn more about neoplastic disorders and more importantly, the drugs used in their treatment.

A number of pharmaceutical services may be readily applied to an oncology ward. The preparation and administration of cancer drugs involves knowledge of drug stability, acute systemic effects, and methods by which these may be minimized. Because some special therapeutic modalities, such as intrapleural and intrathecal drug administration are not standardized, unpredictable results may occur. Therefore, the pharmacist, experienced in the management of these specific problems, can provide a valuable service which can positively influence health care delivery.

Other types of services include in-service education, patient education, and drug information, all of which can be provided with minor changes in existing pharmaceutical services. For example, patient education can involve the distribution of patient primers to patients who are receiving a particular drug or drugs for their cancer.

Clinically-oriented pharmacy services to oncology units have been implemented in several cancer centers throughout the country (94,143,147). These services include distribution of cancer drugs, individual patient monitoring to ensure proper dosing of chemotherapy, and evaluation of patient responses to chemotherapy. The case histories in Section VI were developed to give the reader an idea of the types of problems frequently encountered on the oncology ward or in the outpatient clinic.

Applied therapeutics of the antineoplastic medications means maximizing tumor cell kill while minimizing toxic effects to normal tissue. Therefore, this chapter will emphasize methods used to prevent severe cytotoxic effects to the host rather than to the tumor. In some cases, detailed knowledge of the pharmacology of a particular drug can provide insight into its most effective and least toxic dosing regimen. This will be discussed as it applies to the specific problems posed in the case histories.

TUMOR CELL GROWTH

To understand current concepts of chemotherapy, cell biology with regard to cancer growth must be discussed. The factors which induce a normal cell to become neoplastic have been discussed in several reviews, and it appears that genetic, environmental, or infectious factors, or a combination thereof, may be associated with neoplastic formation. Regardless of the cause, the neoplastic cell continues to grow due to the lack of feedback control.

Tumor cells, contrary to popular belief, grow **more slowly** than many normal tissues. In fact, the most rapidly growing tumor cells, leukemia cells, grow more slowly than endogenous, rapidly proliferating body tissues (e.g. bone marrow and gastrointestinal tract). Therefore, the rate of growth as well as feedback control mechanisms are important aspects of an enlarging tumor burden.

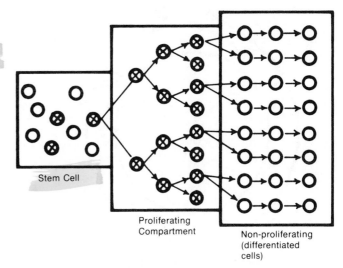

Stem Cell

Proliferating Compartment

Non-proliferating (differentiated cells)

Fig. 1. Proliferating cells in circled x's, which are sensitive to cell-cycle agents. Also note growth of tumor size from the stem cell and proliferating compartment.

Since all cells develop from a particular stem cell population, it is important to understand normal cell proliferation before abnormal cell growth can be discussed. In the adult, as well as the child, some body tissues continually renew their cell populations. The bone marrow, gastrointestinal tract, skin epithelial cells, and germinal cells are examples of cell renewal populations. This is illustrated in Fig. 1. This three-compartment model is important because cells in the non-proliferating compartment are relatively insensitive to chemotherapeutic agents compared to those that are dividing.

The classical model for cell growth is the cell cycle. A constantly dividing cell population repeats a cycle of growth (biochemical synthesis) that results in cell division as shown in Fig. 2. The **generation time (TG)** or **cell cycle time (Tc)** is that time it takes for one cell to traverse the cycle from one mitosis to a subsequent mitosis. If cells grow in a synchronous manner (all cells traversing the cycle at the same time), the population will increase in an exponential fashion. Fortunately, most cell populations do not expand in this manner because not all cells are proliferating at the same time. Thus, the term **growth fraction** becomes an important consideration in both normal and malignant growth.

The **doubling time (TD)** for a population of cells is defined as that time it takes to double the number of cells or mass of tissue and is related to the fraction of cells which are proliferating.

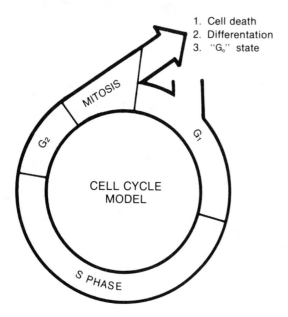

1. Cell death
2. Differentation
3. "G₀" state

CELL CYCLE MODEL

MITOSIS

G₂

G₁

S PHASE

Fig. 2. Phases of the cell cycle.

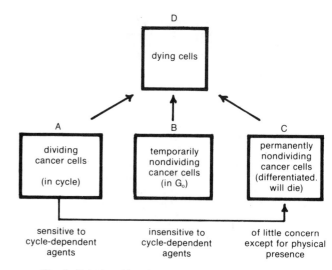

D
dying cells

A
dividing cancer cells
(in cycle)

B
temporarily nondividing cancer cells
(in G₀)

C
permanently nondividing cancer cells (differentiated, will die)

sensitive to cycle-dependent agents

insensitive to cycle-dependent agents

of little concern except for physical presence

Fig. 3. Relationship of cell compartments and cell loss.

Several other cell compartments influence cell growth because they decrease the fraction of cells which are present in the proliferating compartment. These compartments include differentiated cells, nutritionally deficient cells, hypoxic cells, dying or dead cells, and resting cells (G₀ phase). The relationship between these different types of cell compartments is shown in Fig. 3. The **G₀ or resting cells** are a very important group of cells which are temporarily non-dividing and generally refractory to several chemotherapeutic agents. These cells are in equilibrium with the **G₁ post-mitotic** phase and, under unknown circumstances, have the capability of returning to the cell cycle.

In contrast to normal cell growth, cancerous growth should not be regarded as abnormal growth (they divide by the same mechanisms as normal cells), but as an abnormality of the **regulation** of growth. Differentiated or mature cancer cells often function abnormally. For example, they are able to migrate to other sites or utilize greater amounts of nutrients.

Tumor cell growth, like many normal cells, follows a pattern of **exponentially decreasing (Gompertzian) growth.** Early growth is logarithmic up to a critical mass and is associated with a large growth fraction; these cells are very sensitive to chemotherapy. As the tumor becomes larger (above a certain size), the growth rate progressively diminishes and may eventually plateau. The plateau phase is characterized by a low growth fraction, a long doubling time, and an insensitivity to chemotherapy (114). It results from a decrease in cell nutrients, a decrease in vascular supply, and an increased cell loss. Cell loss can influence cell growth dramatically and is significant in most large tumors. Cell loss can occur through exfoliation from skin or pleura, migration via lymphatic and vascular

Number of Cancer Cells (logarithmic scale)	Clinical Event
10^{13} = 10 kg.	Death
10^{12} = 1 kg.	Severe Metastatic Disease
10^{11} = 100 gm.	Advanced Metastases
10^{10} = 10 gm.	Regional Spread of Cancer
10^{9} = 1 gm.	Clinical Detection (Symptoms)
10^{8} = 100 mg.	Subclinical Disease
10^{6} = 1 mg.	Subclinical Disease
10^{3} = 1 mcg.	Carcinoma in situ
10^{0} = 1 ng.	Neoplastic Transformation

Fig. 4 Clinical disease and tumor mass.

channels, or cell death. The tumor mass may grow, remain stable, or regress, depending on whether cell loss is less than, equal to, or more than cell input from the proliferating compartment. In addition, the growth fraction in different locations of the tumor mass may be variable, depending on local vascularization and nutrient supply.

All of the above concepts and definitions can be applied to the clinical setting. Relative tumor volume and clinical manifestations of disease are related in the following manner: the earliest clinical stage of disease is carcinoma in situ; the earliest lesion which can produce symptoms is 1 gram of tumor; 1 to 10 kg of tumor is lethal to the host. This is shown diagramatically in Fig. 4. The relative number of cells, tumor volume, mass, and growth fraction are depicted in Table 2.

In general, the earlier the stage (smaller tumor size), the better chance of cure and response. At 10^{9} tumor cells (1 gram) the chance of cure is very good in contrast to patients with tumor volumes of greater than 10 grams (10^{10} tumor cells).

What impact does cancer chemotherapy have on large tumor masses? A patient who presents with breast carcinoma which has spread to the lungs and liver probably has between a 10^{11} to 10^{12} tumor-cell burden (Fig. 4). With very effective chemotherapy (cell kill of 99.9%), 10^{9} tumor cells will remain. This patient would attain complete remission, but still would have 1 billion (10^{9}) cells remaining and would, therefore, require maintenance therapy. Relapse would probably

Table 2
THE RELATIONSHIP OF THE AMOUNT, SIZE, MASS, AND GROWTH FRACTION OF SOLID TUMORS

Number of Tumor Cells	Tumor Volume	Tumor Mass	Growth Fraction
1 x 10^{12}	1000 cm³	1 kg	<.10
1 x 10^{11}	100 cm³	100 mg	<.15
1 x 10^{10}	10 cm³	10 mg	<.20
1 x 10^{9}	1 cm³	1 mg	<.25

soon occur since the tumor may grow faster at a lower mass if the disease is considered to be rapidly growing.

CLASSIFICATION OF CHEMOTHERAPEUTIC AGENTS

The chemotherapeutic agents can be classified in a variety of ways: by biochemical mechanisms of action; by cell-cycle kinetic action(s); and by in vivo cell-culture, animal-model systems. The broadest classification is based on mechanisms of action and source of the drug. In this classification, drugs are distinguished that:

A. Interfere with the biosynthesis of DNA, RNA, and proteins:
   (1) Folic acid antagonists (methotrexate, Aminopterin)
   (2) Purine Antagonists (6 Mercaptopurine, 6-Thioguanine)
   (3) Pyrimidine Antagonists (5-Fluorouracil, FUdR, Ftorafur, Cytarabine, 5-Azacytidine, 6-Azauridine, Hydroxyurea, Guanazole)
   (4) Miscellaneous (Nitrosoureas [BCNU, CCNU, Methyl CCNU, Streptozotocin], Procarbazine)
B. Inhibit protein synthesis (L-asparaginase)
C. Interfere with replication, transcription, and translation of DNA
   (1) Alkylators (Nitrogen mustard, Cyclophosphamide)
   (2) Other alkylators (Pipobroman, Dibromodulcitol, Galaclitol, Diamminodichloroplatinum, Mitomycin C, Nitrosoureas, Imidazole carboxamide, ICRF-159)
   (3) Interfere with transcription (Actinomycin D, Daunomycin, Adriamycin, Carminomycin)
   (4) Translation inhibitors (Puromycin)
D. Enchance radiomimetic effects (Bleomycin, Streptonigran, Neocarzinostatin)
E. Interfere with the Mitotic Spindle (Vincristine, Vinblastine, VM-26).

Drugs can also be classified (30) on the basis of their effects on malignant and normal cells (Table 3 and Fig. 5). This classification is somewhat confusing because the terms "cell-cycle non-specific" and "cycle-specific" have different meanings to different investigators. In this chapter the term **cell-cycle specific (CCS)** will be used to refer to those agents that kill cells in a particular phase of the cell cycle and are schedule dependent. The term **cell-cycle non-specific (CCNS)** will be used for drugs that kill or inhibit cells in any phase of the cell cycle. This classification suggests that once an initial threshold concentration is surpassed, CCS agents are more toxic to tumor cells and this effect is schedule dependent, not dose-

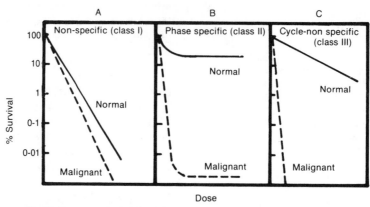

Fig. 5. Dose-survival curves for normal and malignant cells. (See text.)

dependent (Fig. 5B). In contrast, the effect of CCNS agents on tumor cells is dose-dependent (Fig. 5C).

Therapeutic response may be dependent on the **schedule** of drug administration (63). CCS agents are usually schedule-dependent, that is, maintaining a cytotoxic blood level for a period of time sufficient to kill tumor cells as they enter the S-phase produces more effective results. CCNS agents are most effective when given in large intermittent doses, because of the greater sensitivity ratio of tumor cells to normal cells. Note that an absolute fraction and not an absolute amount of cells are killed with each course of therapy (Fig. 5).

In order for tumor cells to be killed by a CCS agent, they must be in the appropriate phase of the cell cycle and exposed to a cytotoxic concentration of drug (schedule-dependency). In order for tumor cells to be killed or inhibited by a CCNS agent, they need only be exposed to an effective concentration, regardless of the duration of exposure (non-schedule dependent). This suggests that CCNS agents bind to nucleic acids or enzymes intracellularly and traverse the cell-cycle for the generation time of that cell.

Combination chemotherapy is most effective when the selected drugs act at different phases of the cell cycle. The effectiveness of sequential combinations may be influenced by using an agent which arrests cells at one phase of the cycle followed by one which kills cells maximally at the point of the block itself or in the phase immediately succeeding the blockade (Fig. 6).

PRINCIPLES OF CANCER CHEMOTHERAPY

In addition to cell kinetics of normal and malignant cells, other factors can influence the effectiveness of

Table 3
CELL-CYCLE SPECIFIC (CCS) AND
CELL-CYCLE NON-SPECIFIC AGENTS (CCNS)

Cell-cycle Specific (CCS)	Cell-cycle Non-specific (CCNS)
Azaserine	Actinomycin D
Azathioprine	Aminochlorambucil
Cytosine arabinoside	BCNU
Emetine	CCNU
Hydroxyurea	Chlorambucil
6-Mercaptopurine	Cyclophosphamide
Methotrexate	Daunomycin
Procarbazine	Dianhydromannitol
Vinblastine	Dimethylmyleran
Vincristine	DTIC
VM 26	5-Fluorouracil
	Iphosphamide
	Melphalan
	Methyl-CCNU
	Myleran
	Nitrogen mustard
	Nor-HN2
	Sarcolysin
	Thiotepa
	Triethylenemelamine

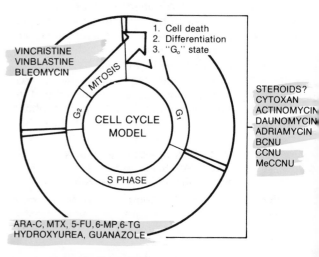

Fig. 6. The cell cycle and chemotherapy.

chemotherapy (Table 4). To design rational chemotherapy protocols, these factors must be considered:

A. Even when complete remissions are achieved with single agents, the duration of remission has been generally short compared to that achieved with combination therapy.

B. Treatment with chemotherapy should be started early when tumors have a high growth fraction.

C. Since chemotherapy is most effective when the tumor burden is small, tumor "debulking" with surgery or radiation should be performed when possible.

D. Once combinations of drugs have been shown to be effective in patients with advanced disease, their use as adjuvant therapy should be considered if they are relatively safe.

E. Drug scheduling is very important. For the same dose of drug, intermittent dosing with rest periods for bone marrow recovery are less toxic to host tissue than continuous daily dosing. An intermittent schedule can often be repeated for months once the maximum tolerable dose has been determined.

F. Alkylating agents tend to "eat" away at the bone marrow such that doses have to be decreased with each succeeding course.

G. Patients should be dosed to either response or toxicity, whichever comes first, before a change in therapy is considered.

H. Large bulky tumors (low growth fraction) are best treated initially with cell cycle nonspecific agents.

I. Drug resistance is often due to drug-induced mutation and selection of new cell genotypes. Several biophysical and biochemical mechanisms have been identified:

(1) *Decreased cell membrane permeability* — methotrexate (97), vincristine (46), and alkylating agents (164);

(2) *Increased intracellular degradation of active drug* — methotrexate (137) and alkylating agents (78);

(3) *Tumor-cell enzyme deficiency* — 5FU (99), 6MP (26), and cytarabine (36,83);

(4) *Altered enzymes* — increased dihydrofolate reductase in MTX-resistant cells (15,36);

(5) *Accelerated DNA repair mechanisms* — alkylating agents (41).

Future efforts in augmenting tumor cell kill should be aimed at allaying the onset of resistance.

Table 4
FACTORS INFLUENCING RESPONSE TO CHEMOTHERAPEUTIC AGENTS

1. Activity and sensitivity	5. Metabolism
2. Tumor kinetics	6. Resistance
3. Pharmacokinetics	7. Immunity
4. Drug scheduling	

INVESTIGATIONAL AGENTS AND CLINICAL TRIALS

Several drugs are currently undergoing clinical Phase I and II trials. Table 5 is provided to guide the reader to clinical information on these drugs.

Since Phase I through IV studies are commonplace for this ever-changing therapeutic class of drugs, a brief description of the various phases is given below;

Phase I — establishment of dosage schedule, maximum tolerated doses, toxicity parameters, and treatable or reversible toxicities;

Phase II — determines activity, new methods of administration, or new combinations;

Phase III — comparative effects of different therapies; and

Phase IV — observations by practicing physicians after the drug is commercially available.

Table 5
PROMISING INVESTIGATIONAL AGENTS

Alkylating Agents
Dianhydrogalactitol
Hexamethylmelanamine
Iphosphamide
Yoshi-864

Antimetabolic Agents
Baker's Antifol (triazinate)
Cyclocytidine
Ftorafur

Mitotic Inhibitors
VP-16
VM-26

Antitumor Antibiotics
Carminomycin
Chromomycin A₃
Daunomycin

Miscellaneous Agents
5-Azacytidine
Cis-Platinum
Cytembena
ICRF-159
Streptozotocin

CASE HISTORIES

Because of the voluminous amount of published information on neoplastic disorders, it is not within the scope of this text to describe the therapeutic details in the management of all known cancers. The reader is directed to the texts of Holland (85) and Clarysse (39) for detailed descriptions of such disorders. Two diseases, however, in which pharmacists should have a good knowledge of the pathophysiology and medical management are breast cancer and acute leukemia. Cases J, K, O and M, N illustrate many therapeutic considerations which arise in these two disorders. This section is divided into two parts. Questions 1

Table 6
LEUKOPENIC EFFECTS FROM CHEMOTHERAPY

Drug	Dose	Onset (days)	Nadir (days)	Recovery (days)	Comment
Busulfan	4-6 mg/d	7	14-21	28	
Chlorambucil	0.2 mg/kg/d	7	10-14	21	Delayed recovery
Cyclophosphamide	1-1.5 gm/m² every 3 weeks	7	10-14	21	
N-Mustard	6 mg/m² every 4-5 weeks	4-7	10	21-28	
Melphalan	12-18 mg/d every 6-7 weeks	7	10-18	42-50	Delayed recovery
Thiotepa	15-20 mg/wk	10	14	28	Weekly maintenance dose
Ara-C	100-150 mg/m²/d	4-7	14-18	21	
5 FU	15-20 mg/kg/wk	7-10	14	16-24	Weekly dosing has little BM toxicity
Methotrexate	15-25 mg twice weekly	4-7	14	21	Intermittent weekly dose has little BM toxicity
Mercaptopurine	2 mg/kg/d	7-10	14	21	
Actinomycin D	0.1 mg/kg/d x 5d	7	14	21-28	Significant thrombocytopenia
Adriamycin	60 mg/m² every 3 wks	10	14	21-24	
Bleomycin	10 mg/m² twice weekly	4-7	10	18	Essentially not marrow toxic
Mithramycin	25 mcg/kg/d x 10d	7	14	21-28	Significant thrombocytopenia & hypocalcemia. Leukopenia uncommon
Mitomycin-C	1.5-2.5 mg every 6-8 weeks	21	36	42-56	Delayed onset and duration of leukopenia and thrombocytopenia
Streptozotocin	1.0 gm/m² every 6-7 weeks	7	14	21	Leukopenia uncommon. Pulse dose every 6-7 wks.
BCNU or CCNU	100-150 mg/m²	14	21	42-50	
Vincristine	1-2 mg/wk	NA	NA	NA	Only bone marrow activity in patients with previous chemotherapy.
Vinblastine	5 mg/m²wk	7	10	17	
DTIC	200-400 mg/m² x 5d every 4 wks	7	10-14	24	
Procarbazine	100-150 mg/m² x 14 days every month	14	21	28	

WBC Nadir (3000-4000)

through 25 will illustrate chemotherapy-induced adverse effects, and Questions 26 through 49 will illustrate cancer-induced complications.

CASE A: BONE MARROW SUPPRESSION. A 55-year-old male with colon carcinoma and lung metastases is treated with mitomycin-C. His complete blood count (CBC) is shown below. His platelets have fallen to their lowest value (nadir) on day 21.

	Day 1	Day 21	Day 28	Day 42
WBC	4300	3500	4100	3100
Hematocrit	38.6	38.7		
Platelets	154,000	44,000	60,000	227,000
Mitomycin-C	25 mg	0	0	20 mg

1. Characterize the selective bone marrow toxicity of mitomycin-C. Do other chemotherapeutic agents have similar effects on the hematopoietic elements?

Mitomycin-C usually has a greater cytotoxic effect on platelets than leukocytes (47). No adequate explanation has been given for this differential effect, but it may be related to greater distribution of the drug into platelets.

Several drugs have similar differential effects on bone marrow elements. For example, busulfan predominantly produces leukopenia and cyclophosphamide spares the platelets. Table 6 delineates the differential effects on leukocytes of the most common cancer drugs.

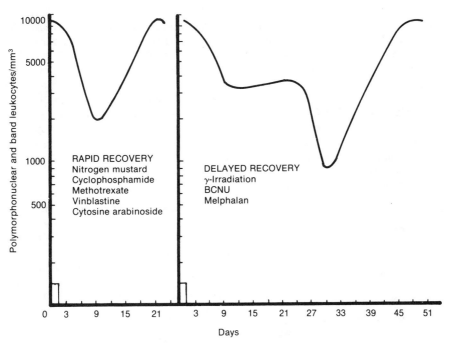

Fig. 7. Leucopenia from chemotherapy: patterns of toxicity and recovery. (Modified from Bergsagel, ref 14.)

2. Describe the time course for Mitomycin-C bone marrow suppression and recovery. Do other agents have different patterns of toxicity?

The bone marrow toxicity to Mitomycin C, like most cell-cycle non-specific agents, is directly related to the total dose of drug administered. After a single dose of 20 mg/m^2, the mean time to nadir is 25 and 30 days for leukopenia and thrombocytopenia, respectively (7,47). Recovery from leukopenia occurs in 1 to 2 weeks; thrombocytopenia in 2 to 3 weeks.

Other drugs have different patterns of toxicity and recovery. Fig. 7 and Table 6 provide the usual patterns seen for bone marrow suppression and recovery. Two patterns are observed (14). Following the administration of cyclophosphamide, cytarabine, methotrexate, nitrogen mustard, vinblastine, and adriamycin, the leukocyte count falls to its nadir in 8 to 10 days and recovers by day 17 to 21. Following administration of the nitrosoureas, melphalan, and thiotepa, the leukocyte counts decrease in two waves on day 8 to 10 and day 28.

3. Why is it important to be aware of the different patterns of bone marrow suppression?

The clinical importance of these facts is that the pattern of hematopoietic depression and recovery must be taken into consideration in determining the dosing interval for successive treatments. Similarly, predisposing factors to bone marrow suppression such as prior chemotherapy, prior irradiation (especially to large bones), and nutritional or physiologic status must be considered.

4. How should the dose of the cancer chemotherapeutic agent be adjusted in patients whose bone marrow is suppressed?

The following guidelines may be used to dose patients whose white count or platelets have been depressed by therapy:

Leukocytes	Platelets	% dose
>4,000	>120,000	100
3000 — 3999	100,000 — 119,999	75
2500 — 2999	75,000 — 99,999	25 — 50
<2,499	< 75,000	0

The patient in Case A received 75% dose of mitomycin-C on day 42 because the WBC count was 3,100. Some clinicians may have preferred to wait another week so that 100% of the dose could be given. Evidence indicates that it may be more effective to dose more frequently than to wait for a complete marrow recovery (136). The potential for toxicity, however, may be greater following frequent dosing, because a regenerating bone marrow has a greater fraction of proliferating stem cells which are more susceptible to the cytotoxic effects of the antineoplastic agents (27,136,160).

5. Are there any cancer drugs which "spare" the

bone marrow?

There are a number of drugs which, relatively speaking, spare the bone marrow (Table 7). These agents may be given to patients with moderate leukopenia in full or nearly full doses when other myelosuppressive agents are contraindicated.

CASE B. ADRIAMYCIN-DAUNOMYCIN CARDIOTOXIC-ITY. RA is a 61-year-old female with carcinoma of the cervix with metastases to the inguinal and peri-aortic lymph nodes. She has a significant past history of paroxysmal atrial tachycardia and myocardial infarction three years prior to admission. She is given adriamycin and cyclophosphamide. Two days after the first course of therapy she develops a tachycardia of 130 beats per minute, prolongation of the Q-T interval, ST-T wave changes, and atrial flutter with 2:1 atrio-ventricular block. Her arrhythmias continue for 72 hours after which they revert to normal sinus rhythm.

6. What is the clinical significance of adriamycin-induced arrhythmias and what should be done to manage this complication?

Several types of cardiac effects are attributed to adriamycin: electrocardiogram (ECG) abnormalities, arrhythmias, congestive heart failure (CHF), and cardiomyopathy (106). The subject of cardiomyopathy and congestive heart failure has been discussed in the chapter on Pediatric Hematology-Oncology. The incidence of arrhythmias and ECG changes from adriamycin is reported to be 15% and does not appear to be dose related (120). In patients with abnormal ECG's *prior to* the administration of adriamycin, the incidence of new ECG abnormalities increases to 43% (120). These ECG effects usually have not been considered predictive of CHF or cardiomyopathy. Some investigators, however, feel that persistent flattening or inversion of T-waves in the precordial leads or low QRS voltage may be correlated with the onset of cardiomyopathy (67,120). Therefore, a patient whose initial ECG is abnormal requires close cardiac monitoring during adriamycin therapy. The following recommendations should help to decrease the frequency of severe cardiac toxicity from adriamycin therapy:

A. Limit the total dose to 550 mg/m²;

B. Restrict the total dose to 450 mg/m² in patients who have had prior cardiac irradiation or those taking cyclophosphamide concurrently (120);

C. Patients with a history of heart disease should receive no more than 450 mg/m²; and

D. If the QRS voltage decreases by 40% in conjunction with *any* symptom of CHF, discontinue the adriamycin.

7. Compare and contrast daunomycin cardiotoxicity with adriamycin cardiotoxicity.

Some mention should be made of **daunomycin cardiac toxicity.** Van Hoff (159) reported that the total cumulative cardiotoxic dose is higher for daunomycin (800-1000 mg/m²) than for adriamycin (550 mg/m²). The incidence of daunomycin-induced cardiomyopathy is 0.69% (19 of 2,752) in adults compared to 1.6% (46 of 2,861) in children. The greater incidence in children may be related to the larger number antineoplastic agents used to treat acute lymphocytic leukemia or to their poorer clinical state compared to adults. The table below compares the incidence of CHF from daunomycin in children and adults with adriamycin-induced CHF:

Drug	Dose (mg/m²)	Incidence of CHF in Children	Incidence of CHF in Adults
Daunomycin	600	2%	1%
	800	5%	2%
	1050	17%	6%
Adriamycin	500-550	N.S.	9%
	551-600	N.S.	20%

N.S. — not studied

Data taken from references 120 and 159.

The data above show that daunomycin is significantly less cardiotoxic than adriamycin in adults. An acceptable cardiotoxicity risk for the use of daunomycin would be 5%, which corresponds to doses of 800 mg/m² for children and 1000 mg/m² for adults.

CASE C: BLEOMYCIN PULMONARY TOXICITY. A 72-year-old white male with metastatic thyroid carcinoma has a history of hypertension, chronic obstructive pulmonary disease, and allergies to penicillin and isoniazid. He is to receive bleomycin twice weekly and adriamycin every three weeks.

8. What potential bleomycin toxicity may be a significant problem in this patient?

The major complication limiting the dose of bleomycin is its pulmonary toxicity (167). Clinically, the onset is usually insidious and is characterized by a

Table 7
CHEMOTHERAPEUTIC AGENTS OR DOSAGE REGIMENS WHICH ARE RELATIVELY BONE-MARROW SPARING WHEN USED ALONE

Bleomycin
Corticosteroids
Cyclophosphamide (platelet-sparing only)
Ftorafur
Hexamethylmelamine
ICRF-159
Methotrexate with citrovorum factor rescue
Streptozotocin
Vincristine
VM-26

non-productive cough, dyspnea, and tachypnea. The earliest sign of pulmonary toxicity is fine bibasilar rales (51), while arterial blood gases and pulmonary function tests may show concurrent decreased oxygen consistent with restrictive pulmonary disease. The chest x-ray usually shows diffuse interstitial fibrosis. Unfortunately, pulmonary function tests are not predictive of impending pulmonary toxicity (167).

The incidence of mortality appears to be dose-related, occurring in 10% of patients who receive cumulative doses exceeding 550 mg. The incidence of clinical toxicity is approximately 5—10% in doses less than 450 mg (12). Patients over 70 years of age or those having received prior lung irradiation have an increased risk of pulmonary toxicity (12,16,167).

Therefore, the following guidelines should be used to minimize the risk of bleomycin pulmonary toxicity (48):

a. Do not exceed a total dose of 400 mg;

b. In patients over 70 years of age, restrict bleomycin to 150 mg/m²;

c. In patients who have received lung irradiation, limit the bleomycin dose to 150 mg/m²; and

d. Careful chest auscultation for bibasilar rales should be performed prior to each dose of bleomycin. Other antineoplastic drugs which should be used cautiously in patients with concurrent pulmonary disease are listed in Table 8.

CASE D: DRUG INDUCED FEBRILE REACTIONS. A 32-year-old white male with testicular carcinoma of the mixed cell type (embryonal and teratocarcinoma) presents to the hospital with fever, malaise, weight loss, and shortness of breath. Blood and urine cultures are negative. Chest x-ray (CXR) reveals three lesions in the left lung and two in the right lung. An abdominal mass is felt on physical examination and an exploratory laparotomy reveals 2 of 30 abdominal lymph nodes positive for testicular carcinoma. The patient is to receive a chemotherapy regimen consisting of the following:

Adriamycin 40 mg IV push
Bleomycin 30 mg/d x 5d by continuous infusion
Cyclophosphamide 800 mg IV push
Vinblastine 8 mg IV push
About four hours after injection of these drugs, the patient develops a fever of 39°C.

9. What association, if any, does chemotherapy have with this febrile episode?

Every chemotherapeutic agent this patient has received has been reported to produce febrile reactions. The drug most likely involved in this case is bleomycin. It produces fevers, chills, and malaise in one-third of patients (48). These episodes usually last two to three hours. In our experience acetaminophen and diphenhydramine diminish the severity but do not eliminate the febrile syndrome.

Table 9 lists other agents associated with fevers (131). The onset of fever occurs two to six hours after drug administration (16,167). Since many of these agents are used in combination, implicating one over another is impossible. The important point to consider, however, is that the febrile episode is most likely due to chemotherapy and not infection. If fever persists for longer than eight hours, infection must be ruled out by blood culture.

CASE E: HIGH-DOSE METHOTREXATE WITH CITROVORUM FACTOR RESCUE. RA is a 43-year-old male who presents with a diagnosis of osteogenic sarcoma of the right femur. Lymphangiogram reveals positive retroperitoneal lymph nodes. Chest x-ray is normal but whole-lung tomograms reveal two small lung nodules in the left lower lobe. All serum chemical values, renal function, and liver function tests are within normal limits. The hemogram is normal. The tumor board suggests the patient receive high-dose methotrexate (HDMTX).

10. What is the rationale for HDMTX with citrovorum factor (CF) rescue?

Table 8
PULMONARY TOXICITY FROM CHEMOTHERAPY

Drug	Presenting Symptom(s)	Pathology	Onset	Reversibility	Comment
Cyclophosphamide and Busulfan	Fever, Cough Dyspnea	Pulmonary Infiltrate	(8 mo-10 yrs.) 4 yrs.	—	Leads to restrict. lung disease
Methotrexate	Cough DOE	Interstitial infiltrate, Eosinophilia	2 wks-3 mo. after daily or intermittent schedule	+ in 2-3 days Cortico-steroids	Not dose related. Probably allergic pneumonitis
Bleomycin	Bibasilar rales, Cough DOE Tachypnea	Basilar infiltrates, Interstitial fibrosis	1 month after withdrawal	—	Dose related >200 mg/m² 10% <200 mg/m² 5%

This investigational regimen is used in the treatment of breast cancer, acute leukemia, lymphoma, and osteogenic sarcoma (53,109). The administration of high doses of methotrexate, greater than 150 mg, together with CF is more effective than treatment with conventional doses of the drug. This is because a very high blood concentration of methotrexate (MTX) destroys cells by a mechanism different from lower concentrations (less than 1 x 10^{-6} molar) and is more toxic to tumor cells than normal cells. Also, CF selectively "rescues" normal cells in low concentrations by enhancing MTX efflux from within these cells.

11. Describe the biochemical basis for the use of CF with MTX.

MTX inhibits dihydrofolate reductase (DHFR), an enzyme necessary for the synthesis of DNA, RNA, and proteins. When given in large doses 1-4 gm/M^2), serum MTX concentrations of 45-450 ug/ml (10^{-3} to 10^{-5} Molar) are achieved such that the drug will *passively* diffuse into cells. In low doses, MTX, like the active metabolites of citrovorum factor, is actively transported into cells. Some tumor cells which do not respond to low, conventional doses of MTX because they lack active transport mechanisms may respond to high doses of MTX.

Once methotrexate enters the cell, it binds DHFR until full saturation occurs (serum concentration of 10^{-4} Molar). After full saturation of intracellular DHFR, excess "free" methotrexate inhibits purine and

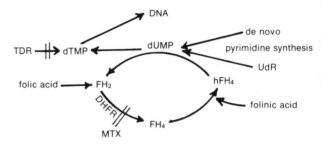

Fig. 8. Mechanism of action of methotrexate (MTX)
FH$_2$ = dihydrofolate; DHFR = dihydrofolate reductase
FH$_4$ = tetrahydrofolate; hFH$_4$ = methylene tetrahydrofolate
dUMP = deoxyuridylate; dTMP = thymidylate
UdR = deoxyuridine; TdR = thymidine

pyrimidine metabolism. Fig. 8 depicts the initial DHFR inhibition followed by thymidylate and guanylate inhibition, an effect which decreases DNA synthesis. In addition, "free" intracellular methotrexate prevents the influx of other folate compounds into tumor cells. This prevents low doses of citrovorum factor from "rescuing" tumor cells.

In "rescue" protocols, citrovorum is given at the end of a 4 to 30 hour methotrexate infusion in doses that achieve concentrations of 1 x 10^{-6} Molar. At this concentration, CF is transported actively into normal cells, especially bone marrow and gastrointestinal cells, but will not be transported across the membranes of tumor cells (70).

Citrovorum factor reverses the cytotoxic effects of MTX in equimolar concentrations by bypassing the metabolic block produced by MTX and by inducing efflux of free intracellular MTX, thereby dissociating MTX from DHFR and restoring DNA, RNA, and protein tetrahydrofolate (THF) synthesis (69). Citrovorum factor blood levels are not high enough to rescue tumor cells, but will rescue normal cells depending on the rate of folate (THF) influx. The rate of THF influx is dependent on the MTX blood level at the end of the infusion. At a MTX concentration of 1 x 10^{-4} M, 65% THF-inhibition will occur in the presence of a CF concentration of 1 x 10^{-6} M. As the MTX serum level falls, more CF will enter normal cells to reverse lethal toxicity. After 42 hours, CF will no longer reverse cell damage. Thus, the degree of cytotoxicity is determined to a large extent by the duration of time intracellular contents are exposed to "free" MTX, and any condition which inhibits the efflux of "free" MTX will enhance its toxicity. These conditions will be discussed in the following sections.

12. How should this combination (CF and MTX) be administered?

The maximum tolerated single dose of MTX without CF rescue is 2 mg/kg. The use of citrovorum factor increases the maximum tolerated dose of MTX to 250

Table 9
CHEMOTHERAPEUTIC AGENTS WHICH PRODUCE FEVER

AGENT	ROUTE OF ADMINISTRATION
Adriamycin	Intravenous
L-Asparaginase	Intravenous
Azathioprine	Oral
Bleomycin	Intramuscular; Intravenous
Chlorambucil	Oral
Cyclophosphamide	Intravenous
Cytosine Arabinoside	Intravenous
Dacarbazine	Intravenous
Dactinomycin	Intravenous
Daunomycin	Intravenous
6-Mercaptopurine	Intravenous; Oral
Methotrexate	Intramuscular; Intrathecal; Intravenous
Mithramycin	Intravenous
Procarbazine	Intravenous; Oral
Quinacrine	Intracavitary
Vinblastine	Intra-arterial; Intravenous
Vincristine	Intravenous

mg/kg. Since MTX concentrations greater than 1×10^{-7} M for more than 48 hours (attained following infusions of 1-4 gm/m² MTX) are associated with bone marrow and gastrointestinal toxicity, citrovorum factor rescue should be continued until MTX serum levels fall below this level (64,157). This method results in few episodes of bone marrow toxicity (6%).

13. Describe the clinical toxicity associated with HDMTX and CF. Discuss those factors which will alter the toxicity of this therapy.

High-dose methotrexate is associated with myelosuppression, nephrotoxicity, hepatotoxicity, and gastrointestinal toxicity. The plasma concentration and half-life of methotrexate are the principal determinants of toxicity (64,150). The plasma half-life in non-toxic patients ranges from 2.0-3.5 hours and 10-25 hours in toxic patients (150,156). The factors which primarily increase the plasma half-life of methotrexate or decrease its clearance are renal failure, a urine pH of less than 5.5, the presence of pleural effusions, or drugs which decrease renal clearance (see Case H).

The kidneys excrete 90% of methotrexate over 48 hours (50% in the first 8 hours). Therefore, patients with **severe renal dysfunction** are at increased risk for general systemic toxicity, unless very high doses of CF are given to neutralize the cytotoxic effects. Methotrexate, which is secreted by the kidney tubules, may precipitate out in the kidneys of patients with low creatinine clearances. Since methotrexate is a weak organic acid with a pKa 5.4, urinary alkalinization increases the solubility of the drug significantly (64,150) and decreases the risk of precipitation. In addition, low urine flow rates increase the risk of precipitation of MTX in the renal tubule.

In the presence of **pleural effusions,** the plasma half-life of MTX is prolonged due to a slow efflux of drug out of this "third" space (156,157). Table 10 shows that MTX concentrations in the pleural space are 10-50 times higher than corresponding plasma levels (157). Unless citrovorum factor is extended beyond the usual dosing period in this situation, toxicity will ensue.

Table 10
METHOTREXATE CONCENTRATIONS IN BLOOD AND PLEURAL FLUID (ref 156, 157)

Days following treatment	Methotrexate conc. (M)	
	Pleural fluid	Blood
1	5×10^{-6}	5×10^{-7}
3	3×10^{-6}	6×10^{-8}
7	6×10^{-8}	$<1 \times 10^{-9}$

14. How are MTX plasma levels used in the HDMTX regimens?

The above data suggest that when 50-200 mg/kg doses of MTX are given over a 6-20 hour infusion period, a single plasma level taken between 24-48 hours after the drug is administered may be predictive of imminent toxicity and might be used as a guide to increase the dose and prolong the administration of CF. Plasma MTX concentrations that are below 1×10^{-7} M at 48 hours have not been associated with toxicity (150,156).

15. What procedures should be followed to minimize toxicity from HDMTX?

The following guidelines have been developed by several institutions in an attempt to minimize toxicity from high-dose methotrexate regimens (64):

a. Obtain a baseline creatinine clearance, blood urea nitrogen (BUN), serum creatinine, and urinary pH. Avoid therapy in patients with severe renal dysfunction or pleural effusions.

b. If the urine pH is less than 7.0, increase it to a pH of 7.0 by using parenteral $NaHCO_3$ (44-88 mEq per liter of 5% dextrose). If sodium is contraindicated, use acetazolamide orally (250 mg qid).

c. Give vincristine 2 mg IV 30 minutes prior to MTX loading. Vincristine significantly increases the influx of MTX into tumor cells (70).

d. Give a loading dose of methotrexate (see Question 16 for calculation). Follow this with a 6-20 hour infusion of methotrexate to maintain a plasma methotrexate level of at least 1×10^{-5}M.

e. Begin calcium leucovorin (CF, folinic acid) with an initial dose of 10-12.5 mg/m² parenterally (IM or IV); subsequent doses can be given parenterally or orally at 10 mg/m². This dose attains serum concentrations of 1×10^{-6}M. Ninety percent of leucovorin is absorbed (127). Rescue is continued for 72 hours unless a 48 hour methotrexate level is less than 1×10^{-7}M.

f. Obtain a 48 hour serum methotrexate level. If the level is greater than 1×10^{-7}M, continue CF rescue for another 24 hours and obtain a 72 hour serum level. If MTX levels are still elevated continue CF rescue.

g. Avoid drugs which may decrease the renal clearance of MTX such as salicylates, probenecid and sulfonamides (see Case H).

h. Avoid drugs which may alter the cellular transport of MTX such as corticosteroids, cephalothin, phenytoin, tetracycline, and chloramphenicol (70).

16. Calculate a MTX loading dose and infusion rate for a 70 kg patient which will produce an approximate steady state plasma concentration (C_{pss}) of 1×10^{-5} M (45 mg/L). The apparent volume of distribution (Vd) of MTX is 1 L/kg, and its half-life is three hours.

Several pharmacokinetic parameters have been reported for methotrexate (86). From the data given in the question, the following regimen can be developed (also see Pharmacokinetics chapter):

Loading dose = $V_d \times C_{pss} \times$ patient's weight (kg)

$$\text{Maintenance dose} = \text{loading dose} \times \frac{0.693}{T\frac{1}{2}}$$

OR

$$\text{Loading dose} = 1 \text{ L/kg} \times 1 \times 10^{-5} \frac{\text{Mole}}{\text{L}} \times \frac{454 \text{ mg}}{\text{millimole}} \times$$

$$\frac{10^3 \text{ millimole}}{\text{mole}} \times 70 \text{ kg}$$

$$= 318 \text{ mg}$$

$$\text{Maintenance dose} = 318 \text{ mg} \times \frac{0.693}{3 \text{ hr}} \times 73 \text{ mg per hour}$$

A loading dose *must* be given to attain a 1 x 10^{-5}M concentration during the six hour infusion period. Without a loading dose, the predicted concentration after a six hour infusion would be 5 x 10^{-6} M, which is subtherapeutic.

CASE F: CHEMOTHERAPY IN RENAL FAILURE. A 48-year-old female with adenocarcinoma of the ovary has peritoneal spread of tumor with ureteral deviation indicating a possible urinary outlet obstruction. Her BUN and serum creatinine are abnormally high, 65 mg% and 5 mg% respectively. The following drugs are being considered for chemotherapy: adriamycin, cyclophosphamide, methotrexate, and vincristine.

17. Will any of the above agents have to be given in lower doses because of her renal failure?

Several chemotherapeutic agents are excreted by the kidney. However, since the effect of renal failure on the elimination of cancer drugs has not been well studied, there are no documented guidelines for their use in this situation. The data which are available on the renal excretion of these drugs are given in Table 11. Drugs for which some reasonable recommendations can be made include methotrexate, bleomycin, cis-platinum, cyclophosphamide, 6-mercaptopurine, 6-thioguanine, imidazolcarboximide, hydroxyurea, mithramycin, mitomycin-C, and streptozotocin.

When given in high doses (>2 mg/kg), 90% of **methotrexate** is cleared by the renal tubule. In patients with moderate to severe renal dysfunction (C_{cr} < 70 ml/min) MTX may produce excessive bone marrow toxicity. Investigators have suggested that the C_{cr} may be used to adjust the dose of drugs which are primarily excreted in the urine. However, this method may not be valid for MTX, because its plasma half-life is triphasic (distribution $T\frac{1}{2}$ of 0.8 hrs; plasma elimination $T\frac{1}{2}$ of 3.5 hrs; intracellular secretory $T\frac{1}{2}$ of 27

hours) (5,86) and it is this third half-life that accounts for MTX accumulation and best correlates with its intracellular toxicity. That is, toxicity is based not only on the concentration achieved, but on the duration that the level is maintained. Therefore, utilization of a dose-adjustment equation based on creatinine clearance and renal clearance of methotrexate may be risky until specific studies have been performed.

It has been recommended by some investigators that the dose of **cyclophosphamide** be decreased in patients with moderate to severe renal failure. Most of the administered cyclophosphamide (88%) is metabolized in the liver to active metabolites which are excreted in the urine within 30 hours (6,40). Only 15% of the parent compound is excreted in the urine during the first 24 hours; this is consistent with a low renal clearance of cyclophosphamide of 11 ml/min (40). It may be that the active metabolites (phosphoramide mustard, aldophosphamide, or acrobin) are responsible for the toxicity of this drug. Until studies define the impact which renal disease has on cyclophosphamide clearance, it is recommended that this agent not be used in patients with severe renal failure (< 20 ml/min). in patients with moderate renal failure and no oliguria in which therapy is absolutely necessary, assume that 100% of cyclophosphamide will be metabolized and excreted in the urine and lower the dose according to the following equation:

$$\text{adjusted dose} = \text{normal dose} \frac{\text{observed CL}_{cr}}{\text{normal CL}_{cr}}$$

Adriamycin is not excreted to any great extent by the kidney (6%); it is primarily (50%) excreted by the liver into the biliary system (13). Therefore, full doses of this agent may be used in this patient.

Vincristine is not excreted in the urine and may be given in usual doses in patients with renal dysfunction.

CASE G: CHEMOTHERAPY IN HEPATIC FAILURE. A 61-year-old white male with hepatocellular carcinoma presents with advancing jaundice and hyperbilirubinemia (6.5 mg/100 ml). The oncology staff wishes to administer adriamycin intravenously.

18. Does hepatic dysfunction affect the body clearance of adriamycin? What other antineoplastic agents are influenced by liver dysfunction?

Up to 85% of the administered dose of adriamycin is cleared by the liver. Normal doses in patients with liver dysfunction have led to severe bone marrow hypoplasia (12). The current recommendation for dosing adriamycin in patients with liver disease is given below:

Total Bilirubin >3.0 mg% — give 25% of the usual dose

Total Bilirubin 1.5 —2.9 mg% — give 50% of the usual dose

Total Bilirubin <1.5 mg% — 100% of usual dose

When dosed according to these recommendations, adriamycin plasma levels were comparable to those observed following usual dosage regimens, and the therapeutic effect was not significantly different from that observed in patients with normal liver function (12,13,17). Other cancer drugs which should be used cautiously in patients with increased serum bilirubin levels include 6-mercaptopurine, 6-thioguanine, 5-azacytidine, BCNU, streptozotocin, mithramycin, and methotrexate (38). Table 11 lists these agents along with suggested recommendations for their use in hepatic disease.

CASE H: DRUG INTERACTIONS. A 63-year-old female with squamous cell carcinoma of the nasopharynx also has a history of rheumatoid arthritis, gout, and chronic urinary tract infections. Her drug history reveals that she takes Anacin, 2 tablets qid, probenecid 250 mg tid, magnesium-aluminum hydroxide gel with each dose of Anacin, and cotrimoxazole (400:80 mg) 2 tablets bid. She is to begin chemotherapy with methotrexate, 40 mg IV once weekly, and bleomycin, 10 mg twice weekly.

19. Will any of the drugs prescribed for this patient interact with each other?

This case illustrates several drug interactions. Methotrexate is a weak organic acid and, like other organic acids, such as salicylates, thiazides, and sul-

fonamides, is secreted by renal tubular cells. Since 90% of administered methotrexate is excreted in the urine, any condition which retards its renal elimination may be expected to enhance its toxicity. Three drugs which this patient is receiving can decrease the renal clearance of methotrexate. Salicylates and sulfisoxazole decrease the renal clearance of methotrexate by 67% and 39%, respectively (112). Although probenecid decreases methotrexate clearance by 260% in the mouse model (24), no clinical reports have recognized this interaction. Patients taking methotrexate should avoid aspirin-containing compounds.

Two other effects of aspirin which may enhance potential side effects of MTX are gastrointestinal irritation and inhibition of platelet aggregation. Gastrointestinal irritation is common with aspirin and predisposes patients to the mucosal toxicity of MTX. Inhibition of platelet aggregation by aspirin may predispose patients to bleeding complications.

Another potential drug interaction exists between trimethoprim and methotrexate which are both dihydrofolate reductase inhibitors. Trimethoprim, however, has antifolate effects only on bacteria and not mammalian cells (93,126) and, therefore, should not be contraindicated in this patient. Salicylates can also completely antagonize the uricosuric effects of probenecid.

CASE I: "MOPP" THERAPY. A 38-year-old male with Hodgkin's disease, stage IVB is to receive "MOPP" chemotherapy. Other medications include prochlorperazine for nausea and vomiting; acetaminophen

Table 11
HALF-LIFE, ELIMINATION, AND DOSE ADJUSTMENT DATA FOR CANCER CHEMOTHERAPEUTIC AGENTS

Drug	Plasma T½ or Clearance	Metabolism	Excretion	Conditions Requiring Dose Reduction
Actinomycin D	85% clearance in 2 minutes	Unknown	Urinary: 12-20% in 24 hr. Biliary: 50-90% in 24 hr.	—
Adriamycin	Biphasic t ½ α = 1.1 hr. t ½ β = 16.7 hr.	Hepatic to adriamycinol and conjugation	Urinary: 5% of dose in 24 hr. Biliary: 85% of dose in 24 hr.	Hepatic dysfunction
L-Asparaginase	t ½ β = 8-30 hr.	Intracellular proteins	Unknown	—
Bleomycin	t ½ β = 1.5 hr.	Tissue metabolism in kidney, liver, blood	Urinary: 25-50% of dose (active and metabolites) — 20-40% of active drug	Pulmonary toxicity
Busulfan	90% blood clearance in 2-3 minutes	Unknown site metabolites inactive	Renal: 25-35% of methane sulfonic acid metabolites (inactive)	No effect of renal dysfunction
Carmustine (BCNU)	t ½ = 5 min; prolonged half-life	Active metabolites — unknown site of metabolism	Degradation products excreted in urine 80% in 24 hours	Renal dysfunction may increase the plasma half-life of active metabolites
Chlorambucil	Unknown	Unknown	Unknown	Unknown
Cyclophosphamide	t ½ = 4-6.5 hrs.	Hepatic metabolism (88%) to active metabolites	Renal excretion: 50-70% in 2 days (86% metabolites, 14% unchanged drug)	Renal dysfunction: probable increase in systemic toxicity from increased t ½ of alkylating metabolites

Cytarabine	$t \frac{1}{2} \alpha = $ 10 min. plasma $t \frac{1}{2} \beta = $ 130 min.	Hepatic deamination; blood deamination to inactive products uracil arabinoside	Renal excretion: 90% uracil arabinoside (inactive) 4-10% unchanged drug	Impaired liver function
Dacarbazine (DTIC)	$t \frac{1}{2} = $ 30-45 min.	Demethylation to amino imidazole carboxamide (active) (AIC)	Renal excretion: 50% of dose as metabolites and DTIC in 6 hrs. (50% DTIC, 50% AIC)	Renal dysfunction; phenytoin, phenobarbital enhance metabolism
Daunorubicin (DRB, daunomycin)	$t \frac{1}{2} = $ 30-50 hrs.	Hepatic metabolism to daunorubicinol	Renal excretion: DRB = 25% over 5 days Biliary excretion: 75%	Impaired hepatic function
Fluorouracil	$t \frac{1}{2} = $ 10-20 min.	Hepatic metabolism to urea and inactive uracils	Renal excretion: 10% of 5FU in 24 hrs.	Impaired hepatic function
Hydroxyurea	$t \frac{1}{2} = $ 2-5 hrs.	Hepatic and kidney metabolism to urea	Renal excretion: 80% of drug in 12 hrs.	Renal dysfunction

Lomustine (CCNU)	$t \frac{1}{2} = $ 5 min.
	Degradation products:
	$t \frac{1}{2}$ chloroethyl
	  group = 36 hrs
	$t \frac{1}{2}$ cyclohexyl
	  group = 24 hrs
	  (early) 72 hrs
	  (2nd phase)
		Metabolism = unknown
		site 100%
			Renal excretion:
			50% degradation
			products in 24 hrs.;
			75% degradation
			products in 4 days
				Unknown effect of
				hepatic or renal
				dysfunction

Mechlorethamine	$t \frac{1}{2} = $ minutes	Complete hydrolysis, chemical transformation to inactive drug	Renal excretion = <0.01% of drug	No effect of renal or hepatic dysfunction
Melphalan	$t \frac{1}{2}$ unknown; active compound in blood for 1-6 hrs.	Metabolism — unknown site	Renal clearance — none	No effect of renal dysfunction
Mercaptopurine (6-MP)	$t \frac{1}{2} = $ 1.5 hr.	Metabolism by xanthine oxidase and oxidation	Renal excretion: 50-70% of total dose 20-40% unchanged drug 20-80% metabolites	Decrease dose when CL_{cr} <20 ml/min. Concurrent allopurinol — decrease 6MP by 75%.
Methotrexate (MTX)	Triphasic half-life $t \frac{1}{2} \alpha = $ 0.75 hrs. $t \frac{1}{2} \beta = $ 2-4 hrs. (major half-life) $t \frac{1}{2} = $ 27 hrs.	Metabolism — minor; hepatic = 10%	Renal excretion = 90% of intact drug; Tubular secretion = CL_{MTX} = 120-180 ml/min.; 80% excreted in 8 hrs.	Renal dysfunction CL_{cr} <70 ml/min—avoid MTX Drug interactions: Probenecid, sulfonamides, salicylates decrease the renal clearance of MTX by 250%, 39%, and 63%, respectively
Mithramycin	Rapid plasma clearance	Metabolism	Renal excretion 25-40% of unknown products	Unknown effect of renal and hepatic dysfunction
Mitomycin C	$t \frac{1}{2} = $ 10-20 min.	Metabolism: major, unknown site	Renal excretion: 6%	Unknown effect of renal or hepatic dysfunction
Platinum (cis-Platinum)	Biphasic half-life $t \frac{1}{2} \alpha = $ 45 min. $t \frac{1}{2} \beta = $ 60-72 hrs.	Metabolism: unknown	Renal excretion: 20-33% in 24 hrs.; 25-44% in 48 hrs.	CL_{cr} <50 ml/min.: avoid
Procarbazine	$t \frac{1}{2} = $ minutes	Metabolism to inactive products	Renal excretion of inactive metabolites 20-70%	Gastrointestinal tolerance
Semustine (MeCCNU)	Undetectable in plasma	Active metabolites	Renal excretion 60% of metabolites in 48 hrs. (inactive)	No effect of renal dysfunction
Streptozotocin	$t \frac{1}{2} = $ 15 min.	Metabolism: major	Renal excretion: 10-20%	Drug is nephrotoxic; avoid with renal dysfunction
Thioguanine (6TG)	$t \frac{1}{2}$: unknown; peak plasma conc. in 6-8 hrs.	Metabolism to S-methy- lated product (inactive); not metabolized by xanthine oxidase	Renal excretion: 40% of a dose as S-methyl metabolite (inactive)	Hepatic dysfunction; renal dysfunction — — CL_{cr} <20 ml/min.
Thiotepa	Rapid plasma clearance	Metabolism	Inactive metabolites excreted in urine	—
Vinblastine	$t \frac{1}{2} = $ 30 sec.	Metabolism in liver	No renal excretion Biliary excretion	Biliary obstruction
Vincristine	$t \frac{1}{2} = $ 30 sec.	Metabolism in liver	Biliary excretion	Biliary obstruction

325 mg and codeine 30 mg for arthralgias; and diphenhydramine for pruritus.

20. What is MOPP therapy?

MOPP chemotherapy is the traditional regimen used in management of advanced Hodgkin's Disease. It consists of the following drugs and doses and the regimen is repeated every month.

Nitrogen Mustard	(M)	6 mg/m² IV push	Day 1 and 8
Oncovin	(O)	1.4 mg/m² IV push	Day 1 and 8
Procarbazine	(P)	100 mg/m² po	Day 1 — 14
Prednisone	(P)	60 mg/m² po	Day 1 — 14
(cycle 1 and 4)			

21. Are there any significant drug interactions with MOPP therapy? What are your recommendations if this patient asks about alcohol intake?

Procarbazine is a weak monoamine oxidase inhibitor (MAOI) and may, therefore, enhance the CNS depressant effects of sedative-hypnotics and analgesics. Actual reactions in our clinic and in others, however, have been uncommon. The ingestion of alcohol may produce a flushing syndrome, similar to disulfiram-alcohol reactions (72). We recommend that patients be cautious about alcohol intake during MOPP therapy. Only very small amounts of wine, beer, or mixed drinks should be taken during therapy, and only if no reaction has occurred after an initial "test" period.

Procarbazine may rarely produce hypertensive reactions when given with antidepressants, sympathomimetics, and tyramine-containing foods (72). We recommend avoiding these agents entirely, even though procarbazine is a relatively weak MAO inhibitor. Phenothiazine antiemetics can occasionally produce excessive sedation when used in these patients. This does not occur frequently enough to warrant the entire avoidance of their use in patients with severe nausea or vomiting.

22. The patient in Case H responded to adriamycin, vincristine, and reduced doses of cyclophosphamide (CTX). After two months of chemotherapy the patient underwent pelvic irradiation with 3,500 rads given over 20 days. She was then reinstituted on chemotherapy with the same agents. What potential problems may occur when chemotherapy is combined with radiation therapy?

Radiation enhances the effects of chemotherapy and vice-versa (128). Several cases of acute gastritis have been reported in patients who have received abdominal irradiation and adriamycin. Many of the chemotherapeutic agents (e.g. alkylators and antibiotics) are radiomimetic (128). Since pelvic irradiation may encompass the ureters in the radiated field, the chances of bladder toxicity from CTX may be enhanced. In a recent report, 34% of patients treated simultaneously with irradiation and CTX developed transient or severe urinary bladder toxicity compared to 8% who received the drug plus extrapelvic irradiation (88). It is suggested that another alkylating agent be substituted for CTX in such cases (88). If these patients at risk must receive CTX, maximal hydration to maintain a high urine flow (>100 ml/min) for 24-48 hours after administration should be used. It is well documented that hydration prevents chemical and hemorrhagic cystitis secondary to cyclophosphamide (36).

CASE J: BREAST CARCINOMA. LOCAL VESICANT REACTIONS. A 64-year-old female with breast carcinoma has been receiving adriamycin and cyclophosphamide every three weeks for advanced disease. One week after the administration of 60 mg of adriamycin by IV push in the left dorsum of the wrist, she comes to clinic complaining of redness and slight pain at the injection site.

23. Characterize the local reaction caused by adriamycin.

Severe local tissue necrosis following intravenous injections of chemotherapeutic agents has been reported for several drugs (75) (See Table 12), including adriamycin. Since adriamycin is efficacious in the treatment of several cancers, its increased use may result in more reports of this uncommon complication.

The incidence of drug extravasation ranges from 2 to 6% (154,162). The clinical course and histopathology of adriamycin-induced skin lesions has recently been described by Rudolph and co-workers (139). Characteristically, the onset of erythema, inflammation and vesicular ulceration at the site of injection is slow and may not be noted by the patient or physician for several days after drug administration. Progressive necrosis of the skin may continue for three months, resulting in severe local pain, staphylococcal infection, and occasionally, in local destruction of nerves or tendons.

Table 12
CHEMOTHERAPEUTIC AGENTS WHICH PRODUCE LOCAL TISSUE NECROSIS

Actinomycin-D (Cosmegen)
Chromomycin A₃
Daunomycin
Doxorubicin (Adriamycin)
Mechlorethamine (Mustargen)
Mitomycin C (Mutamycin)
Streptozotocin
Thiotepa
Vinblastine (Velban)
Vincristine (Oncovin)

24. How should local extravasations of vesicant agents be managed?

The following procedures should be used to treat these local reactions:

a. Apply topical soaks of 0.25% Dakin's Solution three times daily and cover the lesion *lightly* with gauze and tape.

b. Debridement of any necrotic tissue.

c. Those patients with progressive necrosis or in whom tissue necrosis is likely should be considered for wide surgical excision and subsequent skin grafting.

d. Patients with lesions filled with pus and large numbers of staphylococci on gram-stain should be given a one week course of dicloxacillin (1 gram per day) or an equivalent anti-staphylococcal antibiotic.

25. How may local reactions secondary to the extravasation of vesicant drugs be prevented?

It is important to prevent local reactions from vesicant chemotherapeutic agents by avoiding administration into the antecubital vein. Veins near joints should also be avoided, because it is difficult to observe extravasations at these sites, the range of motion may be compromised, and severe joint destruction or obstructive phlebitis of the elbow may lead to loss of nerve, vascular, and tendon function (162).

Factors which enhance the risk of local reactions include prior irradiation at the injection site, poor venous circulation, and the site of injection itself. "Recall phenomena," in which the local effects of prior irradiation are reactivated by systemic adriamycin have been reported (55,57).

Other drugs listed in Table 12 may produce similar problems if given in the antecubital vein. Though the antecubital vein is recommended by some investigators (139), our experience at the University of California Oncology Clinic, San Francisco, indicates that this injection site has few advantages and significant disadvantages. Our method for administering vesicant drugs is as follows:

a. Select a large vein on the dorsum of the hand or forearm which is easily palpable.

b. Avoid injecting drugs using straight needles.

c. Insert a 21-23 gauge scalp-vein needle ("Butterfly").

d. Inject 2-3 milliliters of normal saline or 5% dextrose observing for extravasation, then obtain a good blood return.

e. Inject the drug slowly, one milliliter at a time, drawing back on the syringe to observe for good blood return. If burning or stinging occurs, the injection should be discontinued and a different vein should be used.

f. Flush the "butterfly" line with 5 ml. of saline after drug administration.

g. If extravasation occurs, stop the injection; aspirate the drug solution with a new syringe and needle at the injection site (also aspirate the extravasated solution in the subcutaneous space); inject 25 mg of hydrocortisone hemisuccinate into the extravasated site; and apply hot compresses to enhance vascular absorption of the drug.

h. If nitrogen mustard is extravasated, it can be inactivated locally by injecting 1-2 milliliters of 4% sodium thiosulfate injection (4 ml of 10% U.S.P. solution diluted with 6 ml of sterile water) (118).

26. What is the incidence of breast cancer? What factors influence the prognosis and management of patients with breast cancer?

Breast cancer is the most common malignancy in the female population, accounting for 25% of recorded malignancies. Two-thirds of patients develop advanced metastatic disease and require systemic therapy. The staging of the disease is critical because of its relevance to prognosis. There are several features which influence survival and eventual management (39):

(a) Size of the primary tumor; (b) Presence of positive lymph nodes; (c) Cell-type and grade of malignancy; (d) Disease-free interval between primary diagnosis and subsequent dissemination; (e) Location of metastases (soft-tissue, osseous, and visceral); and (f) Menstrual status (pre-menopause, menopause, and post-menopause).

27. Discuss the role of surgery and radiation in the management of localized breast carcinoma.

Surgery. Early disease is primarily treated with radical mastectomy or modified radical procedures (135). The axillary lymph nodes, which drain outer quadrant lesions, are removed and examined for metastases. Extended radical mastectomy (excision of the internal mammary lymph nodes) is often performed for central or medial lesions, which tend to metastasize to internal mammary nodes (105).

Radiotherapy is occasionally used to treat localized axillary metastases to reduce tumor bulk and prevent distant metastases (11). However, complete sterilization of the local tumor by radiation does not appear to affect overall survival (59). The role of post-operative radiotherapy is controversial and in several studies increased mortality has been reported (148). Local radiotherapy is palliative in the treatment of focal osseous metastases (11).

28. Disseminated breast cancer is managed by altering the hormonal milieu and with cancer chemotherapeutic agents. What methods are used to modify the hormonal environment in these patients?

The growth of breast cancer may be altered by hormones such as estrogen or progestins of either ovarian or adrenal origin. Two types of hormone therapy are commonly used in the treatment of breast cancer: *additive therapy* consisting of estrogens, antiestrogen androgens, or progestins and *ablative therapy* consisting of oophorectomy, hypophysectomy, surgical adrenalectomy, and medical adrenalectomy (11,95). The effectiveness of hormone therapy can be correlated with the uptake of estrogen and progestins by disseminated breast cancer (52,117).

29. Which patients respond to estrogen therapy? What is the response rate?

Post-menopausal patients are candidates for *estrogen* therapy. Before one could establish the presence of hormone receptor proteins in malignant tissue, the over-all response rate to diethylstilbestrol or ethinyl estradiol was 30% (149). When ER (estrogen receptor) positive tumors are considered separately, the response rate is significantly increased to 60%; the response rate falls to 10% for ER negative tumors (89,117). Skin and soft-tissue metastases respond more frequently than visceral and bone metastases (95). The mean duration of estrogen-induced remission is 16 months (117), and the onset of response usually occurs within eight weeks (124).

30. What dose of estrogen should be used to treat breast cancer? What are the side effects of estrogen therapy?

The most commonly used estrogen, diethylstilbestrol, is initiated in doses of 5 mg daily. This dose is given up to three times daily if side effects are tolerated well. At the onset of therapy dose-related (nausea or anorexia) occurs in 50% of patients. Sodium retention, which may result in peripheral edema or complicate pre-existing cardiovascular disease also occurs (95). Since estrogens have been implicated in the development of a "hypercoagulable" state, it may increase the risk of thromboembolic complications (73). Therefore, patients with a significant history of cardiovascular stasis should be observed closely for such exacerbations.

31. Which breast cancer patients respond most favorably to androgen therapy?

Androgens are used in patients with bone metastases who have previously responded to other hormonal therapy since 50% of such patients respond to therapy (95). Patients with soft tissue and visceral metastases respond to a lesser degree (36% and 10% respectively). ER positive tumors are also more responsive to androgen therapy than those that are ER negative (117). The anti-tumor effect is dose-related (153), and there is no difference in response to par-

enterally or orally administered preparations (42,68). An adequate therapeutic trial of androgen is a minimum of six weeks.

32. Which androgens are most commonly used in the treatment of breast cancer? Describe the side effects most frequently encountered with this therapy.

The androgens most commonly used in the management of advanced breast cancer include: testosterone proprionate; fluoxymesterone (Halotestin®); and testolactone (Teslac®).

It is claimed that testolactone is less virilizing than testosterone or fluoxymesterone, but it may also be less effective (19% versus 30%). Other androgen side effects include nausea, vomiting, water retention, and, most significantly, hypercalcemia associated with acute activation of disease (46). Some clinicians feel that androgens should be discontinued during flares if hypercalcemia is present, but others interpret an acute flare of bone and skin lesions as a therapeutic response to androgen therapy and recommend that it be continued (95). In any case, if the serum calcium rises above 14 mg%, androgens must be discontinued until this imbalance has been corrected. Subsequent reinstitution of androgens will depend on the clinical situation.

33. Discuss the role and efficacy of tamoxifen, an antiestrogen, in the treatment of breast cancer. What are the side effects associated with this therapy?

Tamoxifen (triphenylethylene derivative), an investigational drug with *antiestrogen* activity has been effective in the therapy of advanced breast cancer (107,121,163). In doses of 10-20 mg twice daily, tamoxifen has produced an overall response rate of 40-55% (107,121). The drug appears to be particularly effective in patients with positive estrogen receptors (70%), and the median duration of response is 8 to 11 months. Most patients treated are postmenopausal although the drug appears to be equally effective in premenopausal patients (115).* Combining tamoxifen with chemotherapy in patients with positive estrogen receptors has resulted in a complete and partial response rate of 73% (82). The complete remission response was 24% which is significantly higher than that reported for adriamycin-vincristine therapy (8%) or a combination of cyclophosphamide, methotrexate, and fluorouracil (10%) (50).

---

*Theoretically, it would appear that an anti-estrogen, such as tamoxifen, should be most effective in estrogen-rich patients (premenopausal). Preliminary reports do indicate it is effective in such patients (115).

The side effects from tamoxifen are well-tolerated and consist of hot flashes (18%), nausea (15%), menstrual irregularities, mild leukopenia (20%), thrombocytopenia, and vaginal discharge or bleeding (5%). Hot flashes can be controlled with non-phenothiazine tranquilizers. Leukopenia and thrombocytopenia are mild. Only a few infectious or bleeding complications have been reported and the blood counts have often reverted to normal during continued tamoxifen therapy (121).

34. Discuss the efficacy and side effects of progestogens in the treatment of disseminated breast cancer. Describe the dose and routes of administration of the most commonly used agents.

The use of **progestational agents** in the treatment of breast cancer is not as well-defined as estrogen and androgen therapy. Progestins are active in patients with advanced disease, even where responses have not been produced by other hormonal manipulations (3,122). Very large doses of these agents produce regressions in 20-40% of patients (56,122). Soft-tissue metastases respond more frequently than do bone or visceral metastases (56). The preparations used most commonly are:

	Route	Usual Dose
Medroxyprogesterone acetate (Depo-Provera®)	IM	800-1000 mg per week
Noresthisterone (Delalutin®)	IM	
Megestrol acetate (Megace®)	p.o.	40 mg QID

Side effects from these agents occur infrequently and include occasional nausea, sodium retention, mild masculinization and sterile abscesses from intramuscular injections.

35. How effective is combination chemotherapy in the treatment of disseminated breast cancer?

Even though annual mortality from breast cancer has not changed in the last three decades, survival is prolonged and substantial palliation is available for the patient with advanced disease (31,32). This increased benefit is the result of the increased response rates to combination chemotherapy (80%) as compared to single agents (30-40%) (31,33). In addition to higher response rates, combination chemotherapy has resulted in complete clinical remissions not obtainable with single-agent chemotherapy (34,92).

The current "standard" combinations are listed in Table 13. The CMF regimen is equally effective as the adriamycin-cyclophosphamide (Adr-CTX) combination. CMF, however, does not produce as high a response rate as Adr-CTX in patients with liver, bone, or bone-marrow metastases (31,92). Due to the rapid in-

flux of new information, the CMF and Adr-CTX regimens, like all regimens, will be quickly replaced by new regimens with equal or better effectiveness.

Adjuvant chemotherapy is a new form of treatment for asymptomatic patients who are at high risk for rapid recurrence of tumor. In an effort to reduce the relapse rate in high risk patients, chemotherapy is added to ablative therapy (surgery or radiation) to eliminate the small numbers of residual tumor cells (micrometastases) in the body. Since the relapse rate for breast cancer patients with a small amount of regional spread (one to four lymph nodes positive) is high, adjuvant chemotherapy may be effective in delaying the onset of relapse and thus prolong survival. Two accepted programs of adjuvant chemotherapy are CMF and melphalan (L-PAM) (26,60). Decreased relapse rate in pre- and postmenopausal patients has been observed if they are given either CMF of L-PAM; however, survival is prolonged in the premenopausal group only. The combination of CMF is significantly more toxic to the bone marrow and gastrointestinal tract than melphalan.

CASE K: BREAST CANCER WITH MALIGNANT EFFUSIONS. *A 64-year-old female with breast carcinoma presents to the emergency room with shortness of breath (SOB) and weakness. A chest x-ray reveals a left pleural effusion which layers out on a decubitus (supine) view. Thoracentesis and drainage are productive of 700 ml of hazy pink fluid. The analysis of this fluid shows: protein 4.2 gm/100 ml, LDH 370 mg %, RBC's 115,000/mm³, WBC 2,500/mm³, with 65% lymphocytes, and specific gravity 2.025. Blood tests indicate that electrolytes, liver function tests, and renal function tests are within normal limits. The complete blood count (CBC) shows: WBC 3,200/mm³, platelets 165,000/mm³ and hematocrit 35.8%.*

Over the next two days the fluid reaccumulates, and a chest tube with suction apparatus is placed in the left chest. The patient is to receive intrapleural instillation of a schlerosing agent.

36. What is the pathogenesis of the patient's pleural effusion? What factors determine whether

Table 13
CHEMOTHERAPY OF ADVANCED BREAST CANCER (ref 22, 92)

"CMF" —	Cyclophosphamide	100 mg/m² Day 1-14
	Methotrexate	40 mg/m² Day 1, 8
	Fluorouracil	600 mg/m² Day 1, 8

Cycle repeated on Day 30

Adriamycin-Cyclophosphamide
	Adriamycin	40 mg/m² Day 1
	Cyclophosphamide	200 mg/m² Day 2-5

Cycle repeated on Day 21 to 28

local or systemic chemotherapy should be used?

It is important to determine the probable cause of pleural effusions as it influences whether or not local or systemic therapy is to be used. This patient's pleural fluid is considered to be an *exudate* rather than a *transudate* on the basis of the following criteria (111).

	Exudate	Transudate
Appearance	Cloudy or Blood-tinged	Clear
WBC/mm³	>1,000	<1,000
RBC/mm³	>100,000	<100,000
Sp. gr.	>1.016	<1.016
Total Protein	>3 gm/100ml	<3 gm/100ml

Not all of the above criteria need be satisfied. Exudative effusions are consistent with tuberculosis, bacterial and viral infections, pancreatitis, collagen vascular diseases, and malignancies, especially lung and breast carcinoma (111). Three out of four malignant effusions are positive for malignant cells on fluid cytology (111).

Once it is determined that the effusion is consistent with a malignant process, therapy depends on whether the fluid accumulation is due to serosal involvement by tumor in the pleura or venous or lymphatic obstruction by tumor which is common in patients with lymphomas (54). Local chemotherapy is most effective when the pleural fluid contains large numbers of cancer cells and accumulates on the basis of serosal involvement. Systemic chemotherapy or radiation should be used for patients with effusions caused by obstructive lesions.

37. Which agents can be used locally to treat pleural effusions? What is their mechanism of action?

The agents primarily used in the local management of effusions include nitrogen mustard, tetracycline, and thiotepa. Quinacrine (Atabrine) is no longer commercially available due to the high frequency of severe side effects (local pain, fever, and hypotension) that were associated with its use (23). Other agents such as talc, radioactive phosphate and gold are rarely used. All sclerosing agents work by producing an intense adhesive pleuritis and fibrosis which stops the leakage of pleural fluid.

These agents produce objective remissions in 50-80% of patients treated concurrently with closed thoracostomy tube drainage (62,161).

38. Discuss the dose and method of administration for the most commonly used sclerosing agents.

Nitrogen mustard is given via a thoracostomy tube in a dose of 0.4 mg/kg (max. 20 mg) diluted in 50 ml of normal saline. Since the drug is very sclerosing to mucosal surfaces, the patient should be rotated in various positions every 10 minutes for 60 minutes with the suction unclamped. The fluid and drug is suctioned off at the end of this period. Local pain can be severe, and thus, the patient should be premedicated with a potent analgesic and sedative. Approximately 30% of nitrogen mustard is absorbed systemically after intrapleural administration (54) so that it must be used with caution in leukopenic patients.

Thiotepa is given in doses of 30-45 mg using a similar protocol for patient rotation and drainage. Like nitrogen mustard, thiotepa produces a similar rate and duration of response (approximately nine months) (62). It is also systemically absorbed (author's personal observation).

Recently, *tetracycline* has supplanted quinacrine as an effective non-myelosuppressive sclerosing agent. It produces an 80% objective response rate for 6 to 10 months in effusions caused by breast cancer (138, 161). A dose of 500 mg diluted with 50 ml of saline is administered and is followed by another 20 ml of saline to clear the tubing of all medication. The same procedure for patient rotation described above is followed. Local pain and fever are common, so patients should be premedicated with analgesics and antipyretics.

39. Suggest a sclerosing agent for the patient described in Case K based upon her history and laboratory findings.

Because this patient has a modest leukopenia (WBC 3,200), she should not be treated with either nitrogen mustard or thiotepa because of systemic absorption and potential myelosuppression. Tetracycline is the drug of choice in this case since it has no significant effects on the bone marrow.

CASE L: MALIGNANT ASCITES. A 49-year-old female with ovarian carcinoma currently complains of shortness of breath, stomach pain, and anorexia. These symptoms are related to the presence of abdominal ascites which is currently being treated with weekly abdominal paracentesis. Her symptoms and abdominal fluid accumulation have worsened over the last three weeks despite the fact that she currently takes spironolactone 100 mg twice daily for ascites. Her abdominal fluid is positive on cytology for squamous carcinoma of the ovary.

40. How is malignant ascites managed? What is the current status of intracavitary administration of chemotherapeutic agents?

The management of ascites complicating malignant disease is often unsuccessful. The use of alkylating and sclerosing agents often results in severe abdominal pain, chemical peritonitis, and bone marrow suppression (10). Recently, it was shown that bleomycin benefited 36% of patients with malignant peritoneal effusions (127). Those with peritoneal effusions secondary to ovarian or breast carcinoma, however, had a 70% response rate. Bleomycin side effects were minimal and included fever (20%), but only 2% had pain, nausea, rash, or hypotension. Systemic absorption occurs to the extent of 25% of the administered dose. The duration of response after a mean dose of 120 mg ranges from 180 to 240 days (127).

CASE M: LEUKEMIA. A 51-year-old male with chronic myelocytic leukemia (diagnosed 33 months PTA) has a 2 week history of intermittent fever up to 103°F, chills, anorexia, and weight loss. He has been treated sequentially with busulfan, hydroxyurea, 6-mercaptopurine, and chlorambucil during the last two and one-half years. He had a splenectomy performed six months PTA for thrombocytopenia. Fifteen months PTA, a PPD and pleural biopsy for TB were positive for which he has received INH, rifampin, and ethambutol. He is admitted with the following laboratory data:

WBC 200,000, Blasts 50%, Polys 9%, Lymphs 32%, and Metamyelocytes 9%.

Plan: Daunomycin 45 mg/m² x 3d
      Cytarabine (ARA-C) 100 mg/m²/d x 7 by continuous IV infusion

His hospital course was as follows:

The patient's course was stormy after receiving chemotherapy and was complicated by mixed oral mucosal lesions caused by candida and severe stomatitis secondary to chemotherapy.

41. What is the significance of fever in a leukemic patient? How does neutropenia influence the interpretation of this symptom?

Fever represents a major diagnostic and therapeutic problem in patients with neutropenia secondary to chemotherapy or hematological malignancies. Approximately 75% of febrile episodes in leukemic patients with severe neutropenia are due to infection (18,20). Severe *neutropenia* is defined as neutrophil counts less than 100/mm³ and is commonly caused in these patients by bone marrow failure induced by acute blastic crisis or chemotherapy (134).

Fever in neutropenic patients should be regarded as an early sign of *infection* and justifies the initiation of antimicrobial therapy (134,142). Patients with acute leukemia are infected for over 50% of their hospital days when severe neutropenia is present (18). Approximately 70% of patients with acute leukemia die of untreated infectious complications (80), of which two-thirds are bacterial. The importance of the neutrophil count in infections is well documented (18) and the lower the neutrophil count, the higher the frequency of infection (See Fig. 9). A mortality of 80% has been reported in patients whose neutrophil count remained less than 100/mm³ during the first week of infection. The fatality rate was 60% if the neutrophil count was

	3/12	3/13	3/14	3/16	3/18	3/20	3/22	3/24	3/26	3/28	3/2
Daunomycin (mg)	75	75	75								
ARA-C (mg)	170	170	170		170	170	DC				
Allopurinol (mg)	600	600	600	300	300						
WBC(10³)	180	120	75	10	6.4	1.2	.9	.6	.7	.6	
PMNs	9%	12%	20%	36%	62%	10	–	–	–	–	
Blasts	50%	44%	40%	48%	21%			3%			
Platelets (10³)		87	74	46	14*	30	3*	185	23*	50	
Na	138	138	141	136	132		139	137	127	133	
K	3	4.5	3.8	4.1	3.2	2.5	3.0	2.9	3.3	3.6	
Stomatitis				++	++++	4+	4+	2+	1+		
Oral Mucosa Necrosis					++	+++	+++	++	–		
Temp (C°)		39.5	40°	39.5	39	39.5	38.5	37.1	37.1	37.0	
Blood Cultures		drawn	drawn	neg	neg	neg					
Oral Candida				present	present						
IV's with KCl (mEq)		90	90	90	120						
Nystatin oral susp.				given	given						
Amphotericin						1mg	15mg	15mg	15mg	DC	
Carbenicillin (gms)				24	24	24	24	24	24	24	DC
Gentamicin				240	240	240	240	240	240	240	DC

*Platelet transfusions

less than 1000/mm³ and did not increase in response to infection; it dropped to 27% if the neutrophil count increased (19).

42. What types of infections are encountered in leukemic patients? Why was carbenicillin and gentamicin used in this patient? Was it a rational combination?

The types of infections encountered in leukemic patients with neutropenia is shown in Table 14. Approximately 80% of these are due to gram-negative bacilli: *E. Coli, Pseudomonas aeruginosa,* or *Klebsiella-Enterobacter.* Prior to the use of effective antibiotics, the mortality from infections caused by gram-negative organisms was approximately 80% (18,134), and pneumonia and septicemia accounted for four out of five deaths in the severely neutropenic patient with leukemia.

The use of effective **antibiotics** has dramatically decreased the incidence of mortality in neutropenic patients with leukemia. Rodriguez (133) showed that although only 30% of febrile episodes were associated with positive blood cultures, 70% of the patients defervesced after the institution of antibiotics. No patients who received 7 to 10 days of antibiotic therapy died; however, 3 out of 30 patients whose antibiotics were stopped after 4 days because they did not defervesce, died (7% mortality rate).

It is imperative to institute empirical antibiotic therapy early to prevent the gram-negative organisms from producing fatal levels of endotoxin. Since both gram-positive and gram-negative infections occur in neutropenic patients, broad-spectrum coverage with empiric therapy is required. Table 15 shows that combinations of carbenicillin, a cephalosporin, and gentamicin are very active against most strains of gram-negative bacilli (102). Substituting tobramycin for gentamicin gives similar results (101). Amikacin is effective against *Pseudomonas, Enterobacter, E. Coli, Klebsiella,* and *Serratia* (18). In clinical studies amikacin was effective in 70% of neutropenic patients; however, the response rate was only 33% in patients with persistent neutropenia of less than 100/mm³ (19).

The use of synergistic antibiotic combination therapy is considerably more effective (80%) than non-synergistic combinations (50%) (142). Table 16 lists those drugs considered to be synergistic against common gram-negative organisms. For *Pseudomonas* infections, synergistic carbenicillin combinations are more effective than those without carbenicillin (18,142). This may be explained by the lack of bacteriocidal activity of gentamicin, tobramycin, and amikacin in patients with neutrophils of less than 1000/mm³ (Table 18).

Fifteen per cent of infections in these patients are due to gram-positive *Staphylococcus aureus* or strep-

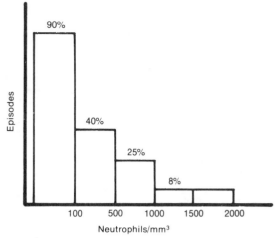

Fig. 9. Frequency of severe infections related to circulating neutrophils. (Modified from Bodey, ref. 19.)

tococci. Gentamicin has excellent *in vitro* activity against staphylococci as well as methicillin-resistant staphylococci (142). However, it remains to be seen if carbenicillin-gentamicin combinations are as active *in vivo* as they are *in vitro* against staphylococci.

Although the addition of cephalothin to carbenicillin and gentamicin does not improve the rate of response in *Pseudomonas* infections, it is a more effective combination for infections caused by *E. Coli* and *Klebsiella* (76).

In summary, several principles should be applied in management of a fever of unknown origin in severely neutropenic patients (134):

a. Carbenicillin should be part of the empiric regimen;

b. Synergistic combinations are most effective;

c. Antibiotic therapy should be continued for at least seven days whether a patient becomes afebrile or not;

d. In patients who fail to become afebrile after four days of double antibiotic therapy, a third antibiotic should be added (cephalosporin, clindamycin). If after one week of antibiotic therapy no response is observed, all antibiotics should be discontinued and the patient recultured; and

e. Since the incidence of fungal infection increases with prolonged granulocytopenia and antibiotic therapy (132), amphotericin should be considered in patients who remain febrile after 10 days of antibacterial therapy.

43. Discuss those adverse effects of antibiotics which are of particular importance in a leukemic patient.

The major drawback of multiple antibiotic therapy is the occurrence of **adverse reactions.** Nephrotoxicity, a qualitative platelet defect, urinary electrolyte loss,

Table 14
INCIDENCE OF BACTERIAL INFECTIONS
IN LEUKEMIC PATIENTS (ref 19)

	Acute Leukemia	Chronic Lymphocytic Leukemia
Staphylococcus aureus	10%	15%
Streptococci	5	15
Pneumococci	0	25
Hemophilus influenza	0	5
Escherichia coli	25	30
Pseudomonas aeruginosa	25	5
Klebsiella-Enterobacter	20	0
Other Gram-negative bacilli	15	5

Table 15
PERCENTAGE OF STRAINS INHIBITED BY GENTAMICIN,
CARBENICILLIN, CEPHALOTHIN,
AND THEIR COMBINATIONS (ref 102)

	GEN	CAR	CEP	CAR-GEN	CAR-CEP	CEP-GEN
Concentration (/ml)	0.7	25	6	25 + 0.7	25 + 6	6 + 0.7
E. coli	92	74	72	99	96	99
Klebsiella sp.	85	19	67	97	78	100
Proteus sp.	86	79	87	100	100	100
P. aeruginosa	24	70	5	95	81	78
Total	76	36	64	97	90	95

GEN = gentamicin; CAR = carbenicillin; CEP = cephalothin.

Table 16
PERCENTAGE OF STRAINS ON WHICH ANTIBIOTICS
ARE SYNERGISTIC (ref 102)

	Carbenicillin + gentamicin	Carbenicillin + cephalothin	Cephalothin + gentamicin	Ampicillin + gentamicin
E. coli	40	73	48	50
Klebsiella strains	52	58	73-	21
Proteus strains	42	76	81	54
P. aeruginosa	70	42	20	10
Total	50	60	55	45

Table 17
CLINICAL EFFECTIVENESS AND BACTERIOCIDAL ACTIVITY OF SERUM WITH SYNERGISTIC
AND NON-SYNERGISTIC COMBINATIONS OF ANTIBIOTICS (ref 102)

	Total number of patients	Number clinical successes	Percentage clinical successes*	Bactericidal activity of serum Trough concentration	Bactericidal activity of serum Peak concentration
Synergism	100	80	80.0	$\frac{1}{8}$ ($\frac{1}{2}-\frac{1}{16}$)	$\frac{1}{16}$ ($\frac{1}{2}-\frac{1}{64}$)
No synergism	105	52	49.5	$\frac{1}{2}$ ($\frac{1}{2}-\frac{1}{8}$)	$\frac{1}{4}$ ($\frac{1}{2}-\frac{1}{32}$)

*P<0.01

Table 18
EFFECT OF NEUTROPHIL COUNT ON RESPONSE TO ANTIBIOTIC THERAPY (ref 19)

Neutrophil count/mm³	Gentamicin Patients	Gentamicin % cured	Tobramycin Patients	Tobramycin % cured	Carbenicillin Patients	Carbenicillin % cured	Ticarcillin Patients	Ticarcillin % cured
Total	63	52	59	57	51	75	20	80
<100	22	23	21	24	16	75	12	92
101-1000	17	53	10	70	26	88	4	75
>1000	24	79	28	79	9	56	4	100
Decreased	32	31	23	39	29	72	—	—
Increased	31	74	36	70	22	82	—	—

ototoxicity, and allergic reactions are complications of carbenicillin and gentamicin therapy.

Carbenicillin should be included in empiric regimens for neutropenic patients even if there is a history of penicillin allergy. Anaphylaxis is uncommon if the drug is administered in small initial doses as in penicillin desensitization programs (19,76). It is recommended that diphenhydramine and hydrocortisone be administered parenterally prior to the first dose and be continued during carbenicillin therapy in this situation.

Similarly, carbenicillin should be used in leukemics with thrombocytopenia. Signs of bleeding are not a contraindication to carbenicillin therapy, because the drug inhibits aggregation of circulating and newly formed platelets only at very high concentrations (29).

Ticarcillin is similar to carbenicillin in structure, activity, and pharmacology. Studies in leukopenic patients indicate it has equal effectiveness to carbenicillin and thus can be used in combination with either gentamicin tobramycin, or amikacin. The usual intravenous dose of ticarcillin is 3.0 gm every 4 hours given as a 15-30 minute infusion.

The nephrotoxicity of gentamicin is discussed in the chapter on Antibiotic Therapy as well as in the chapter on Effects of Drugs on the Kidney. It should be stressed, however, that multiple courses of gentamicin can lead to a renal tubular defect which results in large urinary losses of magnesium, calcium and potassium. This syndrome of hypomagnesemia, hypocalcemia and hypokalemia has only been reported in patients receiving a total dose of more than 10,000 mg of gentamicin over several courses. The tubular defect has been associated with excessive parathyroid hormone and/or increased aldosterone serum levels. One patient at the University of California Moffitt Hospital exhibited urinary sodium and chloride losses of 250 mEq per day, along with 200 mEq of potassium. This patient's urinary electrolyte losses were reversed by 50% with the use of spironolactone 50 mg qid, as has been reported by other investigators (9).

44. What additional supportive care may be necessary in the management of this patient?

Granulocyte transfusions have been used at several institutions when patients have failed to respond to conventional broad-spectrum antibiotics (74). Initially, it was felt that HL-A matched granulocytes should be used (74), but recent evidence show that ABO matching is equally effective (1,8). Increased survival has been observed only in patients who live long enough to receive four or more daily transfusions.

It is difficult to decide when granulocytes should be transfused. Some institutions begin transfusions as soon as the white blood count falls below 1000/mm³.

Others wait until a febrile patient does not respond after 48-72 hours of antibiotic therapy. Eighty percent of the patients receiving early granulocyte transfusion (as soon as a leukemic patient becomes febrile) survived at least 21 days as compared to 20% of the controls in a recent study. Daily transfusions were given until the patients were afebrile for 72 hours.

Platelet transfusions can reduce severe visceral and CNS bleeding caused by thrombocytopenia (165,166). The risk of fatal CNS hemorrhage is minimal when the platelet count is above 20,000/mm³ (Fig. 10)(66). Ecchymoses and petechiae occur only occasionally when platelet counts are above 50,000/mm³. Therefore, patients should be prophylactically transfused when the platelet count falls below 20,000/mm³ or earlier if the patient has had a previous bleeding episode at platelet counts above this level. A rapid fall in platelets is more dangerous than chronic thrombocytopenia. Transfusion of pooled platelets should be used initially. If a one-hour, post-transfusion platelet count is not significantly increased, HL-A matched platelets should be considered. The life-span of transfused platelets is very short (4-6 days) and may be shortened further by excessive transfusions because of antibody formation.

Allopurinol is frequently used prophylactically in these patients to prevent the hyperuricemia that often results from the treatment of leukemia and lymphomas. It is extremely effective in preventing the formation of uric acid from nucleic-acids that are lib-

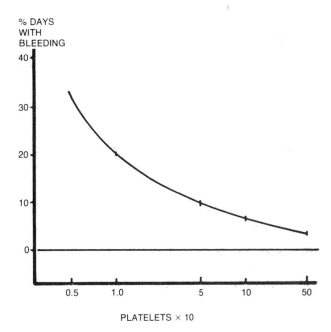

% DAYS WITH BLEEDING

PLATELETS × 10

Fig. 10. Relationship of the number of platelets and gross hemorrhage (defined as hematuria, melana, and hematemesis). (Modified from Gaydos, ref 66.)

erated by the rapid lysis of tumor cells (49,103).

Adequate hydration should be established by the oral or parenteral administration of fluids, and allopurinol 300 mg bid should be initiated two days prior to chemotherapy.

For patients with existing hyperuricemia and no renal failure the following treatment regimen is recommended:

a. Hydration with 3 liters of fluid per day

b. Allopurinol 300 mg bid

c. Alkalinize urine to pH greater than 7.0 with NaHCO₃ 2 grams qid p.o. and/or acetazolamide 250 mg qid p.o. plus 40-80 mEq KCl (79).

Patients with hyperuricemia in the presence of oliguria and urate stones should be treated as follows:

a. Diurese the patient with mannitol (12.5 to 25 gm IV over 5-10 min) and alkalinize the urine as above if diuresis is successful;

b. Remove the stones from ureters or renal pelvis surgically;

c. Hemodialyze the patient if necessary.

CASE N: MANAGEMENT OF LEUKEMIC MENINGITIS.

LC, a 40-year-old female with a 13 month history of acute myeloblastic leukemia, now in remission after ARA-C/6TG therapy, presents with a one week history of frontal headache and stiff neck. There is no evidence of fever, chills, photophobia, papilledema, anesthenia, paresthesias, seizures, diplopia, or syncope. Her physical exam is unremarkable except for neurological findings of decreased plantar reflexes, left arm weakness, stiff neck and headache. Pertinent laboratory data are as follows: Hct 36.7%, WBC 1,700 with 10% PMN's, and no blasts in peripheral blood. Electrolytes, renal and hepatic function tests, and urinalysis are normal.

The patient received a diagnostic lumbar puncture which revealed clear fluid and an opening pressure of 170 mm H₂O. The cell count was 90 WBC, 5 RBC and a cytocentrifuge revealed 94% blasts. Chemical analysis revealed 60 mg% protein and 50 mg% glucose and a negative India ink stain. Cultures were negative for acid fast bacilli and fungi. The impression was central nervous system leukemia.

45. What specific treatment should the patient receive?

Increased intracranial pressure is evidenced by papilledema, headache, and nuchal rigidity, and these symptoms are reversible with high dose **corticosteroids.** Although there is no evidence that fluorinated corticosteroids are more effective than non-fluorinated corticosteroids, dexamethasone in doses of 4 mg qid is most often used because of its minor sodium-retaining properties.

In addition to corticosteroids, **cranial irradiation**

along with the intrathecal administration of **methotrexate** or **cytosine arabinoside** are used to treat leukemic meningitis. Both agents appear to be equally effective in clearing the cerebral spinal fluid of leukemic cells. Doses of these agents are given below:

	Relative dose	Response Rate
Cytosine arabinoside	30-50 mg/m²	80% (8)
Methotrexate	10-12.5 mg/m²	80% (152)

46. Which of the chemotherapeutic agents administered intrathecally produces systemic toxicity? How may this be avoided?

Cytosine arabinoside (ARA-C) is metabolized by cytadine deaminase to inactive uracil arabinoside (ARA-U) or phosphorylated to arabinosyl cytidine triphosphate (ARA-CTP). ARA-CTP is the active metabolite which inhibits DNA synthesis. After intravenous administration of ARA-C, about 80% of the total drug is in the form of ARA-U, indicating that it is rapidly deaminated in the plasma (84). The alpha T½ of ARA-C is 15 minutes and the beta T½ is 2-3 hours after intravenous administration (see Pharmacokinetics Chapter) (84). In contrast, after intrathecal ARA-C administration, only 1-10% of the cerebral spinal fluid (CSF) drug concentration is present as ARA-U, indicating that there is very low ARA-C deaminase activity in the CSF. Since any ARA-C which is transported into the plasma is rapidly metabolized to the nontoxic metabolite, ARA-U, no systemic toxicity (bone marrow suppression) occurs after intrathecal administration of ARA-C.

Methotrexate exhibits three-compartment pharmacokinetics after intravenous administration with half-lives of 45 minutes, 2 hours, and 10-27 hours, respectively. After intrathecal administration, a triphasic curve is characterized by a distribution phase T½ of 30-45 minutes, and half-lives of 4.5 hours and 14 hours for the intervals of 4-36 and 48-96 hours, respectively (Fig. 11). Intrathecal doses of 12 mg/m² give CSF and plasma concentrations of 1×10^{-7} molar and 3×10^{-9} m at 48 hours, respectively (15a, 145). Plasma concentrations greater than 2×10^{-8} m, which may be exceeded for 20 hours by intrathecal MTX, are considered toxic to gastrointestinal and bone marrow stem cells (87). Clinically evident systemic myelosuppression has been observed in some of our patients after intrathecal MTX. Therefore, patients who are leukopenic at the time of intrathecal administration of methotrexate may be spared additional myelosuppression by the intravenous or intrathecal administration of 3-6 mg of calcium leukovorin 12-24 hours after intrathecal MTX (14a).

CASE 0: HYPERCALCEMIA SECONDARY TO BREAST CANCER. INTRACTABLE PAIN. A 62-year-old white

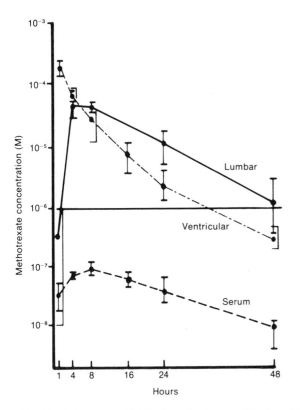

Fig. 11. Methotrexate distribution after intraventricular administration of 6.25 mg. per square meter. (Modified from Shapiro, ref 145.)

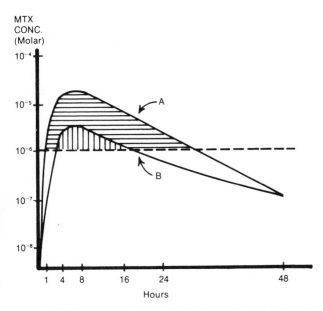

Fig. 12. MTX concentrations after lumbar administration of 12.5 mg/m²(A) and 6.25 mg/m²(B). (Modified from Shapiro, ref 145.)

female with metastatic breast carcinoma x 2 years to L4-6 region is experiencing severe back pain requiring potent narcotics (codeine, Percodan and most recently hydromorphone). She complains of severe nausea and vomiting about one-half hour after her pain medication. In addition, during the last week she has felt very apprehensive, tired and thirsty, and has noted an increased frequency of urination. Her daughter remarks that she has been somewhat confused in the last couple of days.

47. What can this woman be offered in the way of pain control with oral narcotics or other potent analgesic agents?

The particular patient above has not responded to several agents and has complaints of nausea and vomiting as well. Potent narcotics often produce nausea and/or vomiting via a central effect. The use of phenothiazine antiemetics used concurrently may be helpful in this case. In our experience, levallorphan, (Levodromoran) seems to produce a lesser degree of nausea and vomiting; however, it is not commonly used because of its expense.

A major problem in patient care is the management of chronic pain. Chronic pain is always present and, unlike acute pain, does not decrease with time unless the patient responds to his cancer therapy. In contrast to acute pain, chronic pain has an *aching* phase and an *agony* phase (112). The latter phase appears to be related to the psychological response the patient has to pain, either depression or anxiety. Therefore, the psychological component as well as the physical component must be considered in the management of pain in cancer patients.

Patients who fear the return of pain after an analgesic dose may exacerbate the physical component of the pain. These patients may benefit from antianxiety agents given with the analgesic.

The use of mild and potent analgesics is the mainstay of pain treatment. But one must consider adjunctive measures (antidepressants, antianxiety agents, psychosocial therapy) for successful pain control (158). In order to select the appropriate analgesic, the severity of pain must be determined. Table 19 lists narcotics and mild analgesics and their place in pain management. All efforts should be made to treat the patient with oral agents. It is better to treat the patient with an initial large dose to induce pain control, then maintain the analgesia with a lower dose if possible. Starting with a lower and usually ineffective dose may lead to greater patient anxiety (116,158).

Liquid formulations, such as Schlessinger's solution or Brompton's mixture, have been used successfully in pain management. These preparations (contents in Table 20) are very useful for the debilitated patient. Schlessinger's solution may be easily titrated by the patient since it is a concentrated preparation which is dosed in drops. It has the usual disadvantage of sedation. In contrast, Brompton's cocktail contains the CNS stimulant, cocaine, which is added to minimize the sedative effect of the morphine. Since cocaine absorption after oral administration is poor compared to its rapid absorption from mucous membranes (71), it should be more effective if the elixir is swished around the mouth for at least 15 seconds before it is swallowed. No prospective studies have been performed with either Schlessinger's or Brompton's cocktail, but they do appear to be helpful in the management of chronic terminal pain.

Recently, a study combining dextroamphetamine and morphine given intramuscularly to post-operative patients revealed significant analgesic response with minimal sedation and loss of alertness (61). A trial in cancer patients of similar therapy with oral narcotics and CNS stimulants is warranted.

48. What may be causing this patient's symptoms of thirst and polyuria? How should these be managed?

The symptoms of nausea, vomiting, polyuria, and polydipsia are consistent with hypercalcemia, a common complication of breast cancer. Many organ systems may be involved in hypercalcemia including the gastrointestinal, genitourinary, neurologic and central nervous systems. A serum calcium greater than 14 mg% constitutes a medical emergency because of the possibility of cardiovascular complications. Hypercalcemia is generally caused by the presence of osteo-

Table 19
ANALGESICS IN THE MANAGEMENT OF CHRONIC PAIN

Severity of Pain	Drug or Combination
Mild	Aspirin
	Acetaminophen
	Propoxyphene
Moderate	Aspirin with Codeine
	Acetaminophen with Codeine
Severe	Oral Morphine
	Schlessinger's Solution
	Brompton's Mixture
	Hydromorphone (Dilaudid)
	Oxycodone + APC (Percodan)
	Oxycodone + Acetaminophen (Percocet)
	Levorpharol (Levodromoran)
	Methadone (Dolophine)
Excruciating	Parenteral
	Morphine
	Meperidine (Demerol)
	Hydromorphone (Dilaudid)
Pain with Anxiety	Add Benzodiazepines
Pain with Depression	Add Antidepressants

lytic bone metastases and is most commonly seen in multiple myeloma, breast cancer, and leukemia (37,96,129). Occasionally, the underlying cause is due to the release of a parathyroid hormone-like substance in bronchogenic carcinomas. Other humoral substances such as prostaglandins which stimulate bone resorption may be released by particular tumors (129,144).

To prevent subsequent stupor, confusion, coma, renal failure, or cardiac arrythmias, immediate treatment is required as indicated in Table 21. General measures should include mobilization; adequate hydration with normal saline; low calcium intake (e.g. milk, cheese); and treatment of the underlying malignancy. ***Saline with furosemide*** diuresis is usually rapidly effective (123,151). In patients with hypercalcemia and osteolytic bone lesions, ***glucocorticoid*** therapy is the most effective long-term therapy (80% response) (90).

In resistant hypercalcemia which is presumably due to parathyroid-like hormone secreting tumors, ***mithramycin,*** which inhibits bone resorption is very effective (60%) (123,146). The effect of mithramycin occurs within two days after an intravenous dose of 25 mcg/kg is administered. If a favorable response is not seen in three days, the dose may be repeated. The usual toxic effects on the bone marrow, liver and kidney are seldom encountered after only one or two doses of the drug (146).

Hypercalcemia caused by increased prostaglandin release (renal cell carcinoma, squamous-cell lung cancer, and ovarian carcinoma) has been effectively treated with ***prostaglandin inhibitors*** such as aspirin and indomethacin (25,57,130,155). Indomethacin in a dose of 25 mg twice daily significantly reduces the serum calcium in three days in such cases.

When the patient's serum calcium has been decreased to near normal levels, the use of ***oral phosphates,*** such as Fleet's Phosphosoda or neutral phosphate (Neutro-Phos), in doses of 4 grams daily in divided doses is usually effective (37).

49. The patient above was initially treated with fluoxymesterone. She had a good response lasting

Table 20
NARCOTIC MIXTURES

Schlessinger's Solution

Morphine	3%
Ethyl Morphine	6%
Scopalamine	0.025%

Brompton's Cocktail

Morphine Sulfate	
Cocaine	
90% Alcohol	
qs to	1000 ml

10 months but relapsed when a new bone lesion developed in the eleventh thoracic vertebra. The patient was considered for adrenalectomy, but was not a good surgical candidate. An investigational drug, aminoglutethimide (Elipten) is to be started.

What is the rationale for aminoglutethimide? What complications may result from its use? What additional therapy should be included?

Adrenalectomy is an effective hormonal manipulation which affords palliation in 30% of patients with advanced breast cancer (77); however, because of the morbidity associated with this procedure, it is not recommended for many patients. Recently, medical adrenalectomy with 1-2 gm daily of aminoglutethimide produced objective remissions and pain relief from bone metastases in 55% of patients (140). Patients with bone or skin lesions responded best while those with liver metastases did not usually benefit.

Aminoglutethimide works by blocking the conversion of cholesterol to pregnenolone and thus inhibits the synthesis of all adrenal steroids. As a result, a decrease in cortisol secretion from this drug stimulates the pituitary to increase ACTH levels until the aminoglutethimide blockade is overcome. To prevent competitive antagonism by ACTH, dexamethasone is administered concurrently to prevent the compensatory rise in ACTH. Since aminoglutethimide decreases the half-life of dexamethasone from 260 minutes to 120 minutes, the usual daily dexamethasone replacement dose is 3 mg per day instead of 1 mg per day (140). This regimen is devoid of Cushing's side effects. Even with dexamethasone doses of 3 mg per day, our experience indicates that patients may eventually "escape"

Table 21
MANAGEMENT OF HYPERCALCEMIA IN MALIGNANT DISEASE

A. Mild cases:
1. Normal saline infusion for rehydration and increased urinary calcium (Na^+ competitively inhibits tubular reabsorption of Ca^{+2})
2. Loop Diuretics
   a. Furosemide, or
   b. Ethacrynic acid
3. Corticosteroids: if high Ca^{+2} due to osteolytic lesions
   a. Hydrocortisone 300-500 mg/liter every 8 hours, or
   b. Prednisone 40-100 mg in divided doses, taper after lowering of calcium
B. Severe cases (arrhythmias, CNS disorientation):
1. Normal saline, furosemide as in A.1 and A.2
2. Mithramycin 25 micrograms per kg I.V. Repeat in 48 hours if no response, or
3. Calcitonin (Calcimar) 2-8 units per kg by I.V. infusion over 24 hours (use plastic I.V. bag, avoid glass because of adsorption)
C. In cases of renal failure:
1. Hemodialysis
2. Peritoneal dialysis

the effects of aminoglutethimide. Therefore, the dose of dexamethasone should be increased by 50% to effectively inhibit the pituitary from overproducing ACTH.

This new modality appears to be a relatively well tolerated useful addition to the management of breast cancer. The agent may also be used to identify those patients who will benefit from surgical adrenalectomy since eight of nine patients who responded to this agent, versus none of nine patients who did not, responded to subsequent surgical adrenalectomy (125).

The major adverse effects of the aminoglutethimide/dexamethasone combination are lethargy, vertigo, ataxia, and total body rash. These side effects occurred in 25% of patients.

CASE P: HYPERALIMENTATION FOR CACHEXIC PATIENTS. MF is a 24-year-old man with mixed testicular carcinoma (embryonal and seminoma) with metastases to lung and abdomen. He currently complains of nausea, vomiting and a weight loss of 35 lbs over the last three months. On physical examination the patient is very cachectic and anxious. He weighs 32 kg (usual weight 60 kg) and has received several chemotherapeutic agents in the past 12 months. It is felt that the patient should again be treated with chemotherapy. His liver, renal, electrolytes, urinalysis are all WNL. A hemogram reveals: Hct 39%; Platelets 293,000; WBC 4,400. Prior to chemotherapy, the patient is placed on hyperalimentation.

50. What role does hyperalimentation play as an adjuvant to cancer chemotherapy?

Patients with malignant disease often have the severe problem of cachexia even in the presence of a normal dietary intake (45). Cancer cells appear to act as a nitrogen trap, extracting amino acid for protein metabolism from the host's nitrogen pool. Because cancer anabolism exceeds catabolism, amino acids are not recycled for use by the host. Since chemotherapy is often accompanied by emesis, this patient's nutritional status could be further compromised. In addition, adverse effects on the gastrointestinal tract are seen with methotrexate, 5FU, bleomycin, and cytarabine. Although not systematically studied, cancer chemotherapeutic agents could potentially cause malabsorption in man due to impaired assimilation of nutrients (141).

Cancer patients have been given hyperalimentaiton to enhance the effects of systemic chemotherapy on the tumor cell population (119). It appears that well-nourished patients receiving chemotherapy can tolerate much higher doses of chemotherapy with a much lower incidence of nausea, vomiting, diarrhea, weakness, and weight loss (45). Even though a well-controlled study of chemotherapy with and without

hyperalimentation has not been performed, the benefits from such therapy appear very promising (43,
44,45).

REFERENCES

1. Alavi JB: A randomized clinical trial of granulocyte transfusions for infection in acute leukemia. NEJM 296:706, 1977.
2. Anderson RJ et al: *Clinical Use of Drugs in Renal Failure.* Charles C. Thomas, Springfield, Ill., 1976.
3. Ansfield FJ: A clinical trial of megestrol acetate in advanced breast cancer. Cancer 33:907, 1974.
4. Ansfield FJ: Adjuvant radiotherapy for breast cancer. JAMA 235:67, 1976.
5. Azarnoff DL: Pharmacokinetics of methotrexate. Clin Pharmacol Therap 16:884, 1974.
6. Bagley CM: Clinical pharmacology of cyclophosphamide. Cancer Res 33:226, 1973.
7. Baker LH et al: Mitomycin C-phase I studies. Proc Amer Assoc Cancer Res 15:182, 1974.
8. Band PR et al: Treatment of central nervous leukemia with intrathecal cytosine arabinoside. Cancer 32:744, 1973.
9. Bar RS et al: Hypomagnesemia, hypocalcemia secondary to renal magnesium wasting — a possible consequence of high-dose gentamicin. Ann Int Med 82:646, 1975.
10. Baron JM: The management of malignant serous effusions, in *Chemotherapy of Malignant Neoplasms,* 2nd Ed., ed. by FJ Ansfield. Charles C. Thomas, Springfield, Ill., 1973, p 126.
11. Baum M: Surgery and radiotherapy in breast cancer. Semin Oncol 1:101, 1974.
12. Benjamin RS: Adriamycin chemotherapy — efficacy, safety and pharmacologic basis of an intermittent single high-dose schedule. Cancer 33:19, 1974.
13. Benjamin RS: Pharmacokinetics and metabolism of adriamycin in man. Clin Pharmacol Therap 14:592, 1973.
14. Bergsagel DE: An assessment of massive-dose chemotherapy of malignant disease. Canad Med Assoc J 104:31, 1971.
14a. Bertino JR "Rescue" techniques in cancer chemotherapy. Semin In Oncol 4:203, 1977.
15. Bertino JR et al: Increased levels of dihydrofolate reductase in leucocytes of patients treated with amethopterin. Nature 193:140, 1962.
15a. Bleyer WA et al: Clinical pharmacology of intrathecal methotrexate. Cancer Treat Rep 61:703, 1977.
16. Blum RH et al: A clinical review of bleomycin — a new antineoplastic agent. Cancer 31:903, 1973.
17. Blum RH et al: Adriamycin, a new anti-cancer drug with significant clinical activity. Ann Int Med 80:249, 1974.
18. Bodey GP et al: Quantitative relationships between circulating leucocytes and infection in patients with acute leukemia. Ann Int Med 64:328, 1966.
19. Bodey GP: Infections in cancer patients. Cancer Treatment Rev 2:89, 1975.
20. Boggs DR et al: Clinical studies of fever and infection in cancer. Cancer 13:1240, 1960.
21. Bonnadonna G et al: Update of clinical experience with adjuvant CMF in breast cancer. Presented at symposium on breast cancer. San Francisco, Calif., March, 1976.
22. Bonadonna G et al: Combination chemotherapy as an adjuvant treatment in operable breast cancer. NEJM 294:405, 1976.
23. Borja ER et al: Single-dose quinacrine (Atabrine) and thoracostomy in control of pleural effusion in patients with metastatic disease. Cancer 31:899, 1973.
24. Bourke RS: Inhibition of renal tubular transport of methotrexate by probecid. Cancer Res 35:110, 1975.
25. Brereton HD et al: Indomethacin — responsive hypercalcemia in a patient with renal-cell adenocarcinoma. NEJM 291:83, 1974.
26. Brockman RW et al: Resistance to purine analogs. Clinical pharmacology symposium. Biochem Pharmac 23:107, 1974, supplement 2.
27. Brown CH III: Effects of chemotherapeutic agents on normal mouse bone marrow grown *in vitro.* Cancer Res 31:185, 1971.
28. Brown RS et al: Hodgkins Disease: Immunologic, clinical and histologic features of 50 untreated patients. Ann Int Med 67:291, 1967.
29. Brown CH III et al: The hemostatic defect produced by carbenicillin. NEJM 291:265, 1974.
30. Bruce WR et al: Comparison of sensitivity of normal hematopoietic and transplant colony-forming cell to chemotherapeutic agents administered *in vivo.* J Nat Cancer Instit 37:233, 1966.
31. Canellos GP et al: Combination chemotherapy for advanced breast cancer: Response and effect on survival. Ann Int Med 84:389, 1976.
32. Canellos GP et al: Cyclical combination chemotherapy for advanced breast carcinoma. Br Med J 1:218, 1974.
33. Canellos GP: Combination chemotherapy for breast cancer. Cancer Chemother Rep 59:893, 1975.
34. Carter SK: Single and combination nonhormonal chemotherapy in breast cancer. Cancer 30:1543, 1972.
35. Chabner BA et al: Threshold methotrexate concentration for *in vivo* inhibition of DNA synthesis in normal and tumorous target tissues. J Clin Invest 52:1804, 1973.
36. Chabner BA: The clinical pharmacology of antineoplastic agents. NEJM 292:1107,1159, 1975.
37. Chopra D et al: Hypercalcemia and malignant disease. Med Clin N Amer 59:441, 1975.
38. Clarysse A: *Cancer Chemotherapy: Its Role in the Treatment Strategy of Hematologic Malignancies and Solid Tumors.* Springer-Verlag, New York, 1976, Chap 7, p 130.
39. Clarysse A: *Cancer Chemotherapy: Its Role in the Treatment Strategy of Hematologic Malignancies and Solid Tumors.* Springer-Verlag, New York, 1976, Chap 26, p 439.
40. Cohen JL: Pharmacokinetics of cyclophosphamide in man. Brit J Pharmacol 43:677, 1971.
41. Connors TA: Mechanisms of clinical drug resistance. Clinical pharmacology symposium, Biochem Pharmac 23:89, 1974.
42. Cooperative Breast Cancer Group: Results of studies — 1961-1963. Cancer Chemother Rep Suppl 1, 41:1, 1964.
43. Copeland EM et al: Intravenous hyperalimentation as an adjunct to cancer chemotherapy. Amer J Surg 129:167, 1975.
44. Copeland EM et al: Intravenous hyperalimentation in patients with head and neck cancer. Cancer 35:606, 1975.
45. Copeland EM et al: Cancer: Nutritional concepts. Semin in Oncology 2:329, 1975.
46. Creasey WA: Modifications in biochemical pathways produced by vinca alkaloids. Cancer Chemother Rep 52:501, 1968.
47. Crooke ST et al: Mitomycin-C: A review. Cancer Treatment Rev 3:121, 1976.
48. Crooke ST et al: Bleomycin, a review. J Med 7:333, 1976.
49. DeConti RC: Use of allopurinol for prevention and control of hyperuricemia in patients with neoplastic disease. NEJM 274:481, 1966.
50. DeLena M et al: Adriamycin plus vincristine compared to and combined with cyclophosphamide, methotrexate, and 5-fluorouracil for advanced breast cancer. Cancer 35:1108, 1975.
51. DeLena M et al: Clinical radiologic and histopathologic studies on pulmonary toxicity induced by treatment with bleomycin. Cancer Chemother Rep 56:343, 1972.
52. DeSombre ER: Prediction of breast cancer response to endocrine therapy. Cancer Chemother Rep 58:513, 1974.
53. Djerassi I et al: Management of childhood lymphosarcoma and reticulum cell sarcoma with high-dose methotrexate and citrovorum factor. Proc Amer Assoc Cancer Res 9:18, 1968.
54. Dollinger MR: Management of recurrent malignant effusions. Cancer 22:138, 1972.
55. Donaldson SS et al: Adriamycin activating a recall phenomenon after radiation therapy. Ann Int Med 81:407, 1974.
56. Edelstyn GA: Norethisterone acetate in advanced breast cancer. Cancer 32:1317, 1973.
57. Etcunabas E et al: Uncommon side effects of adriamycin. Cancer Chemother Rep 58:757, 1974.
58. Farber S: Temporary remissions in acute leukemia in children produced by folic acid antagonist, 4-aminopteroylglutamic acid. NEJM 238:787, 1948.
59. Fisher B et al: Postoperative radiotherapy in the treatment of breast cancer. Ann Surg 172:711, 1970.
60. Fisher B et al: L-phenylalanine mustard (L-PAM) in the management of primary breast cancer. NEJM 292:117, 1975.

61. Forrest WH et al: Dextroamphetamine with morphine for the treatment of postoperative pain. NEJM 296:712, 1977.
62. Fracchia AA et al: Intrapleural chemotherapy for effusion from metastatic breast carcinoma. Cancer 26:626, 1970.
63. Frei E III: Combination chemotherapy. Cancer Res 32:2593, 1972.
64. Frei E III et al: New approaches to cancer chemotherapy with methotrexate. NEJM 292:846, 1975.
65. Fujita H: Comparison studies in the blood level, tissue distribution, excretion and inactivation of anticancer drugs. Jap J Clin Oncol 12:151, 1971.
66. Gaydos LA et al: The quantitative relation between platelet count and hemorrhage in patients with acute leukemia. NEJM 266:905, 1962.
67. Gilladoga AC et al: Cardiac status of 40 children receiving adriamycin over 495 mg/m². Proc Amer Assoc Cancer Res and ASCO 15:107, 1974.
68. Goldenberg IS: Androgenic therapy for advanced breast cancer in women. JAMA 223:1267, 1973.
69. Goldman DI: Analysis of the cytotoxic determinants for methotrexate: A role for "free" intracellular drug. Cancer Chemother Rep Part 3, 6:51, 1975.
70. Goldman DI: Membrane transport of methotrexate and other folate compounds: Relevance to rescue protocols. Cancer Chemother Rep 6:63, 1975, part 3.
71. Goodman LS and Gilman A: *The Pharmocological Basis of Therapeutics.* 5th ed. MacMillan, New York, 1975, p 387.
72. Ibid pg 1295.
73. Ibid Pg 1446.
74. Graw RG et al: Normal granulocyte transfusion therapy: Treatment of septicemia due to gram-negative bacteria. NEJM 287:367, 1972.
75. Greenwald ES: *Cancer Chemotherapy.* 2nd ed. Medical Exam. Publ. Co., Flushing, N.Y., 1973.
76. Greene WH et al: Empiric carbenicillin, gentamicin, and cephalothin therapy for presumed infection. Ann Int Med 78:825, 1973.
77. Harris HS et al: Bilateral adrenalectomy in metastatic mammary cancer. Cancer 24:145, 1969.
78. Harrap KR et al: The selectivity of action of aklylating agents and drug resistance, III. Biochem Pharm 19:209, 1970.
79. Herrington RT et al: Uric acid nephropathy in leukemia. NEJM 266:934, 1962.
80. Hersh, E et al: Causes of death in acute leukemia: A ten-year study in 414 patients from 1954-1963, JAMA 193:105, 1965.
81. Herzig RH: Successful granulocyte transfusion therapy for gram-negative septicemia. NEJM 296:701, 1977.
82. Heuson JC: Current overview of EORTC clinical trials with tamoxifen. Cancer Treat Rep 60:1463, 1976.
83. Ho DH: Distribution of kinase and deaminase of 1-(Beta)-D-arabinofuranosylcytosine in tissues of man and mouse. Cancer Res 33:2816, 1973.
84. Ho DH et al: Clinical pharmacology of 1-Beta-D-arabinofuranosylcytosine. Clin Pharmacol Therap, 12:944, 1971.
85. Holland J: *Cancer Medicine.* Lea and Febiger, 1973.
86. Huffman DH: Pharmacokinetics of methotrexate. Clin Pharmacol Therap 14:572, 1973.
87. Hryniuk WM et al: Treatment of leukemia with large doses of methotrexate and folinic acid: Clinical-biochemical correlates. J Clin Invest 48:2140, 1969.
88. Jayalakshmamma B: Urinary bladder toxicity following pelvic irradiation and simultaneous cyclophosphamide therapy. Cancer 38:701, 1976.
89. Jensen EV: Estrogen receptors in hormone-dependent breast cancers. Cancer Res 35:3362, 1975.
90. Jessiman AG et al: Hypercalcemia in carcinoma of the breast. Ann Surg 157:377, 1963.
91. Johnson RK: The clinical impact of screening and other experimental tumor studies. Cancer Treat Rev 2:1, 1975.
92. Jones SE: Combination chemotherapy with adriamycin and cyclophosphamide for advanced breast cancer. Cancer 36:90, 1975.
93. Kahn SB et al: Effects of trimethoprim on folate metabolism in man. Clin Pharmacol Therap 9:550, 1968.
94. Kellick MG: Pharmaceutical services in a pediatric oncology day hospital. Am J Hosp. Pharm 33:1147, 1976.
95. Kennedy BJ: Hormonal therapies in breast cancer. Semin Oncol 1:119, 1974.
96. Kersinger A et al: Hypercalcemia of malignancy. Geriatrics 27:97, 1972.
97. Kessel D et al: Modes of uptake of methotrexate by normal and leukemic leukocytes and their relation to drug resistance. Cancer Res 28:75, 1968.
98. Kessel D et al: Uptake as a determinant of methotrexate response in mouse leukemia. Science 150:172, 1965.
99. Kessel D et al: Nucleotide formation as a determinant of 5-fluorouracil response in mouse leukemia. Science 156:1240, 1967.
100. Klastersky J et al: Clinical significance of *in vitro* synergism between antibiotics in gram-negative infections. Antimicrob Agents Chemother 2:470, 1972.
101. Klastersky J et al: Therapy with carbenicillin and gentamicin for severe infections caused by gram-negative rods. Cancer 31:331, 1973.
102. Klastersky J et al: The use of synergistic combinations of antibiotics in patients with hematological diseases. Clinics in Hematol 5:361, 1976.
103. Krakoff IH: The use of allopurinol in preventing hyperuricemia in leukemia and lymphoma. Cancer 19:1489, 1966.
104. Krick JA: Opportunistic invasive fungal infections in patients with leukemia and lymphoma. Clinics in Hematol 5:249, 1976.
105. Lacour J: Radical mastectomy versus radical mastectomy plus internal mammary dissection. Cancer 37:111, 1976.
106. Lenaz L: Cardiotoxicity of adriamycin and related anthracyclines. Cancer Treat Rev 3:111, 1976.
107. Lerner HJ: Phase II study of tamoxifen: Report of 74 patients with stage IV breast cancer. Cancer Treat Rep 60:1431, 1976.
108. Levine AS et al: Hematologic and marrow failure states: Progress in the management of complicating infections. Semin Hemat 11:141, 1974.
109. Levitt M et al: Improved therapeutic index of methotrexate with "leucovorin rescue." Cancer Res 33:1729, 1973.
110. Liegler DG et al: The effect of organic acids on renal clearance of methotrexate in man. Clin Pharmacol Therap 10:849, 1969.
111. Light RW et al: Cells in pleural fluid. Arch Intern Med 132:854, 1973.
112. Lipman AG: Drug therapy in terminally ill patients. Amer J Hosp Pharm 32:270, 1975.
113. Liu K et al: Renal toxicity in man treated with mitomycin-C. Ann Intern Med 77:239, 1972.
114. Lloyd HH: Estimation of tumor cell kill from Gompertz growth curves. Cancer Chemother Rep 59:267, 1975.
115. Manni A et al: Antiestrogen-induced remissions in stage IV breast cancer. Cancer Treat Rep 60:1445, 1976.
116. Marks R et al: Undertreatment of medical inpatients with narcotic analgesics. Ann Intern Med 78:173, 1973.
117. McGuire WL: Current status of estrogen receptors in human breast cancer. Cancer 36:638, 1975.
118. Merch, Sharp and Dome: Mustargen package brochure.
119. Meyer JA: Potentiation of solid tumor chemotherapy by metabolic alteration. Ann Surg 179:88, 1974.
120. Minow RA et al: Andriamycin cardiomyopathy: An overview with determination of risk factors. Cancer Chemother Rep 6:195, 1975.
121. Morgan LR et al: Therapeutic use of tamoxifen in advanced breast cancer: Correlation with biochemical parameters. Cancer Treat Rep 60:1437, 1976.
122. Muggia FM: Treatment of breast cancer with medroxy progesterone acetate. Ann Int Med 68:328, 1968.
123. Muggia FM et al: Hypercalcemia associated with neoplastic disease. Ann Int Med 73:281, 1970.
124. Nathanson I: Clinical investigative experience with steroid hormones in breast cancer. Cancer 7:754, 1952.
125. Newsome HH et al: Medical and surgical adrenalectomy in patients with advanced breast cancer. Cancer 39:542, 1977.
126. Niethammer D et al: The effect of trimethoprim on cellular transport of methotrexate. Brit J Haematol 32:273, 1976.
127. Nixon PF: Effective absorption and utilization of oral formyltetrahydrofolate in man. NEJM 286:175, 1972.
127a. Paladine W et al: Intracavitary bleomycin in the management of malignant effusions. Cancer 38:1903, 1976.
128. Phillips TL: Chemical modification of radiation effects. Cancer 39:987, 1977.

129. Powell D et al: Nonparathyroid humoral hypercalcemia in patients with neoplastic diseases. NEJM 289:176, 1973.

130. Powles TJ et al: The inhibition by aspirin and indomethacin of osteolytic tumor deposits and hypercalcemia in rats with Walker tumour, and its possible application to human breast cancer. Brit J Cancer 28:316, 1973.

131. Prince RA et al: Antineoplastic agents as a cause of fever. Drug Intell Clin Pharm 9:124, 1975.

132. Remington J: Opportunistic fungal infections in patients with lymphoma or leukemia. Clin Hematol 5:249, 1976.

133. Rodriguez V et al: Management of fever of unknown origin in patients with neoplasms and neutropenia. Cancer 32:1007, 1973.

134. Rodriguez V: Antibacterial therapy — special considerations in neutropenic patients. Clinics in Hematol: 5:347, 1976.

135. Rosemund GP: Role of mastectomy in breast cancer. Semin Oncol 1:97, 1974.

136. Rosenoff SH: Recovery of normal hematopoietic tissue and tumor following injury from cyclophosphamide. Blood 45:465, 1975.

137. Rothenberg SP: Alteration of methotrexate by leukemic cells loss of affinity for an anion exchange resin. Cancer Res 29:2047, 1969.

138. Rubinson R: Intrapleural tetracycline for control of malignant pleural effusion. South Med J 65:847, 1972.

139. Rudolph R et al: Skin ulcers due to adriamycin. Cancer 38:1087, 1976.

140. Santen RJ et al: Successful medical adrenalectomy with amino-glutethimide. JAMA 230:1661, 1974.

141. Schein PS et al: Nutritional complications of cancer and its treatment. Semin Oncol 2:337, 1975.

142. Schimpff SC et al: Empiric therapy with carbenicillin and gentamicin for febrile patients with cancer and granulocytopenia. NEJM 284:1061, 1971.

143. See K: Pharmacist as a provider of oncology ambulatory care services. Am J Hosp Pharm 33:1145, 1976.

144. Seyberth HW et al: Prostaglandins as mediators of hypercalcemia associated with cancer. NEJM 293:1278, 1975.

145. Shapiro WR et al: Methotrexate: Distribution in cerbrospinal fluid after intravenous, ventricular and lumbar injections. NEJM 293:161, 1975.

146. Slayton RE: New approach to the treatment of hypercalcemia: The effect of short-term treatment with mithramycin. Clin Pharmacol Therap 12:833, 1971.

147. Stephen SR: Pharmaceutical services for the cancer patient. Am J Hosp Pharm 33:1141, 1976.

148. Stjernsword J: Decreased survival related to irradiation postoperatively in early operable breast cancer. Lancet 2:1285, 1974.

149. Stoll BA: Hormonal Management in Breast Cancer. Pitman Med Co., London, 1969.

150. Stoller RG et al: Pharmacokinetics of high-dose methotrexate. Cancer Chemother Rep, part 3, 6:19, 1975.

151. Suki WN et al: Acute treatment of hypercalcemia with furosemide. NEJM 283:836, 1970.

152. Sullivan MP et al: Clinical investigations in the treatment of meningeal leukemia: Radiation therapy regimens vs. conventional intrathecal methotrexate. Blood 34:301, 1969.

153. Talley RW et al: A dose-response evaluation of androgens in the treatment of metastatic breast cancer. Cancer 32:315, 1973.

154. Tan C et al: Adriamycin, an antitumor antibiotic in the treatment of neoplastic disease. Cancer 32:9-17, 1973.

155. Tashjian AH: Tumor humors and the hypercalcemias of cancer. NEJM 290:905, 1974.

156. Tattersall MH et al: Clinical pharmacology of high-dose methotrexate. Cancer Chemother Rep, part 3, 6:25, 1975.

157. Tattersall MH et al: The pharmacology of methotrexate "rescue" studies, in Pharmacologic Basis of Cancer Chemotherapy, ed by MD Anderson Hosp. Williams and Wilkins, 1975, p 105.

158. Twycross R: Clinical experience with diamorphine in advanced malignant disease. Int J Pharmacol 9:184, 1974.

159. Van Hoff DD et al: Daunomycin-induced cardiac toxicity in children and adults. Ann Int Med 62:200, 1977.

160. Vogler WR: The effect of methotrexate on granulocyte stem cells and granulopoiesis. Cancer Res 33:1628, 1973.

161. Wallach HW: Intrapleural tetracycline for malignant pleural effusions. Chest 68:510, 1975.

162. Wang JJ et al: Therapeutic effect and toxicity of adriamycin with neoplastic disease. Cancer 28:837, 1971.

163. Ward HW: Anti-oestrogenic therapy for breast cancer: Trial of tamoxifen at two dose levels. Brit Med J 1:13, 1973.

164. Wheeler GP: Studies related to mechanisms of resistance to alkylating agents. Cancer Res 23:1334, 1963.

165. Whitecar JP et al: Replacement of platelets and granulocytes in patients with myelosuppression in Cancer Chemotherapy, II, ed. by Brodsky I. Grune and Stratton, New York, 1972, p 287.

166. Wintrobe ME: Clinical Hematology. 7th ed. Lea and Febiger, Philadelphia, 1974 p 1663.

167. Yagoda A et al: Bleomycin, an antitumor antibiotic: Clinical experience in 274 patients. Ann Int Med 77: 861, 1972.

Chapter 35

Pediatric Hematology — Oncology

William E. Evans

In the United States, cancer kills more children between 1 and 15 years of age than any other disease. For every million children under 15 years of age, approximately 71 die annually of cancer; 26 of acute lymphocytic leukemia (ALL), 7 of acute nonlymphocytic leukemia (ANLL) and one or less of chronic myelocytic leukemia (CML) (36). The most common childhood cancer is leukemia, usually occurring as the acute lymphoblastic form. Approximately 77% of childhood leukemia cases at St. Jude Children's Research Hospital are diagnosed as acute lymphocytic leukemia and 20% as acute non-lymphocytic. In American children less than 15 years of age, the incidence of Wilms' tumor, soft tissue sarcoma, carcoma of

bone, Hodgkin's disease, non-Hodgkin's lymphoma and neuroblastoma is reported to be similar to that of acute nonlymphocytic leukemia (244).

Prior to the introduction of aminopterin as treatment for acute leukemia in 1948, a child with acute leukemia had a median survival of about two to four months. The use of aminopterin to induce temporary remissions marked the beginning of the current era of therapy for acute leukemia, during which time numerous antineoplastic agents have been developed and become available for clinical use. Concurrent with the development of better treatment modalities for leukemia and other malignancies has been the improvement of therapy for the complications of treatment, such as infections. These developments coupled with an increased understanding of the biology of malignant diseases have led to improvement in the prognosis of many childhood malignancies. The most striking example of this is childhood acute lymphoblastic leukemia, where the therapeutic approach has changed from one of palliation of an almost universally fatal disease to current approaches aimed at long-term, disease-free survival and cure.

This chapter emphasizes the chemotherapy of childhood neoplastic diseases. Other components of treatment are also briefly described to provide a perspective of the total therapeutic approach to these diseases and the importance of chemotherapy in each. Results of clinical trials currently in progress will undoubtedly alter the current therapy of many childhood cancers and hopefully lead to further improvement in responses to treatment.

1. The immediate goal of remission induction therapy for children with acute lymphocytic leukemia is to rapidly reduce the number of leukemic cells and allow for normal marrow regeneration while producing the least drug-related toxicity. What are the drugs currently employed for remission-induction and their efficacy in single and multiple drug regimens?

Drugs that have been used for remission induction therapy in children with acute lymphocytic leukemia (ALL) include prednisone (corticosteroids), vincristine (VCR), L-asparaginase (L-ASP), daunomycin (DAUNO), cytosine arabinoside (ARA-C), methotrexate (MTX), cyclophosphamide (CYCLO) and 6-mercaptopurine (6 MP) (97,127,62,149). The ideal drug would be cytotoxic only to leukemic cells, have no effect on the proliferative activity of normal cells and be cell cycle nonspecific. Although no drugs presently possess all of these ideal characteristics, prednisone, vincristine and L-asparaginase most closely meet these criteria. As a single agent, prednisone will induce complete remission in approximately 50% of previously untreated children with ALL (241,141,227), while vincristine alone will induce remission in approximately 80% of patients. When administered in a multiple-drug induction regimen, these two agents induce remission in about 90% of children with previously untreated ALL (75). When prednisone is combined with either 6MP, MTX, CYCLO or DAUNO, remission induction rates range from 80-90%. Three- and four-drug regimens including prednisone and vincristine with either L-ASP, DAUNO or 6MP and MTX have resulted in induction rates of 90-98% (207, 6, 96, 98, 72, 71). Although a slight increase in the remission induction rate is achieved with these three and four drug regimens, the incidence of toxicity also increases. Since 6MP and MTX are useful in maintenance therapy regimens, three-drug induc-

tion regimens with PRED, VCR and L-ASP or PRED, VCR and DAUNO are preferable when more than two drugs are desired. A complete remission is usually achieved within four weeks when a combination of agents is used.

2. Allopurinol is routinely used as adjuvant therapy during remission induction. What is the rationale for its administration and what interaction may allopurinol have with antineoplastic drugs?

The accelerated degradation on nucleoprotein following leukemia cell lysis by chemotherapy often results in increased uric acid production. Uric acid nephropathy, which may occur in association with acute increases in uric acid production, is the most common cause of acute renal failure in leukemia (69). The administration of allopurinol will suppress uric acid formation by inhibiting xanthine oxidase, the enzyme that catalyzes the oxidative conversion of hypoxanthine to xanthine and xanthine to uric acid (245, 190). Sodium bicarbonate in doses of 4-6 gm/m^2-day or greater can be employed to alkalinize the urine, thereby increasing the solubility of uric acid and reducing the likelihood of uric acid precipitation in the renal tubules and collecting ducts (181). Adequate fluid intake sufficient to maintain good urine flow is also essential in preventing urate nephropathy.

The inhibition of xanthine oxidase by allopurinol suppresses the metabolic pathway responsible for the oxidative conversion of 6-Mercaptopurine (6MP) to 6-thiouric acid, a noncarcinostatic metabolite (53). The significance of this effect remains to be determined, since studies have been unable to show a change in the half-life or area under the plasma concentration-time curve of 6MP as a result of allopurinol administration (38). Current recommendations are that doses of 6MP be reduced by 50-75% when administered concomitantly with allopurinol, although the exact mechanism of the interaction remains to be clearly defined (38, 191, 144). Azathioprine, an immunosuppressive agent used primarily as an adjunct for prevention of rejection of kidney homografts, is converted *in vivo* to 6MP. Similar cautions and dosage adjustments should be observed when azathioprine is administered concomitantly with allopurinol.

Retrospective data from the Boston Collaborative Drug Surveillance Program indicate that cancer patients treated with allopurinol and cyclophosphamide have a greater incidence of bone marrow suppression than those treated with cyclophosphamide alone (28). Human studies by Bagley et al (10) demonstrated a significantly longer cyclophosphamide half-life in four patients who received allopurinol when compared to those receiving only cyclophosphamide. They were unable to demonstrate any difference in urinary excretion of intact cyclophosphamide, peak plasma levels of alkylating metabolites or the fraction of injected cyclophosphamide appearing as alkylating metabolites in the urine within 24 hours.

Alberts and Wetters (2), using the spleen colony assay system and survival duration studies in mice with P388 leukemia, showed a 1-log increase in the toxicity of cyclophosphamide to leukemia colony-forming units following pretreatment with allopurinol. Parallel survival studies demonstrated no difference in the antileukemic activity of cyclophosphamide resulting from allopurinol pretreatment. Their data also indicated that allopurinol had no effect on the toxicity of cyclophosphamide to normal bone marrow colony-forming units. There was no difference in the pharmacokinetics of cyclophosphamide following allopurinol pretreatment. Although the clinical significance and exact mechanism of the interaction between cyclophosphamide and allopurinol is presently unclear, caution should be used when these two drugs are administered concomitantly.

Allopurinol was originally synthesized as a potential antineoplastic agent, is reported to inhibit purine biosynthesis (191), and may be converted to a ribonucleotide that can inhibit enzymes regulated by purine or pyrimidine ribonucleotides (67, 125). However, there is currently no evidence that these effects are related to its apparent interaction with either 6-mercaptopurine or cyclophosphamide.

Allopurinol has also been reported to alter the effects of methotrexate (89,108). Grindey and Moran (89) demonstrated that the antitumor effects of methotrexate against early leukemic L1210 cells were partially reversed by the administration of allopurinol. They suggested that this interaction resulted from a decreased catabolism of preformed systemic purines. Hrynivk (108) using L5178Y murine lymphoblasts, reported that hypoxanthine partially protected these cells against the lethal effects of methotrexate. Further study is required before any clinical applications of these observations can be made.

3. W.J.T., a 4-year-old white boy with the diagnosis of acute lymphocytic leukemia, was placed on induction therapy consisting of prednisone 40 mg/m²/day X 28 days, vincristine 1.5 mg/m²/wk X 4 doses and daunomycin 25 mg/m²/wk IV X 4 doses. During the third week of therapy the patient's appetite and fluid intake decreased and his abdomen became distended. Approximately 12 hours after the onset of symptoms the patient became increasingly lethargic with a loss of deep tendon reflexes. Shortly thereafter he experienced a generalized seizure. Laboratory data revealed the patient to be hyponatremic (serum sodium 120 mEq/L), with a serum osmolality of 235 mOsm/L and excessive urinary loss of sodium (urine sodium 112mEq/L). Urine osmolality was 525 mOsm/L and the specific gravity was 1.030. Renal function tests were within normal limits (serum creatinine 0.5 mg/100 ml; BUN 9.1 mg/100ml). Other laboratory data included serum potassium 3.9 mEq/L, chloride 82 mEq/L, HCO₃ 25 mEq/L and glucose 110 mg/100ml. The patient was subsequently diagnosed as having inappropriate ADH syndrome and was successfully treated by fluid restriction. Discuss the component of this patient's induction chemotherapy which may be related to the inappropriate ADH syndrome.

The association between hyponatremia and vincristine therapy was first described by Fine et al (63); subsequently, cases of vincristine-induced inappropriate antidiuretic hormone secretion (IADHS) have been reported in both children (209, 214) and adults (185, 95). However, the syndrome of IADHS occurs infrequently with vincristine in acute childhood leukemia (94). Suskind et al (214) demonstrated increased levels of plasma antidiuretic hormone in a patient receiving vincristine who developed the syndrome of inappropriate ADH, and confirmed the diagnosis of IADHS by using both bioassay and radioimmunoassay. The precise mechanism by which vincristine produces an inappropriate secretion of ADH remains unclear. Others (209) speculate that the mechanism involves a direct toxic effect of vincristine on the supraoptic or paraventricular nuclei of the hypothalamus, the neurohypophyseal tract, or perhaps even on the posterior pituitary gland. There may be a close relationship between the dose-related neurotoxicity of vincristine and vincristine-induced inappropriate antidiuretic hormone secretion (34).

It is important to realize that many patients receiving vincristine therapy will develop symptoms of peripheral neuropathy as well as autonomic dysfunction (34, 104, 194). This is not always a sufficient indication for discontinuing therapy, although dose reduction may be necessary. The syndrome of inappropriate ADH does necessitate discontinuing vincristine therapy and subsequently modifying therapy once the IADHS is corrected. More extensive neurotoxicity of vincristine may be manifested by diplopia, 6th and 7th neuropalsy and seizures (104, 194). A complete review of the clinical spectrum of vincristine neurotoxicity may be found elsewhere (234).

For the patient presented above, the seizures were likely related to the severe hyponatremia (63, 209, 214), although seizures may occur secondary to the direct neurotoxicity of vincristine (120, 97).

In summary, inappropriate ADH secretion induced by vincristine is probably a dose-related, reversible toxicity which occurs infrequently. The mechanism may be a direct neurotoxic effect on the central nervous system at the sites of antidiuretic hormone storage and/or formation.

4. A.B., a 4-year-old white boy, was diagnosed as having acute lymphocytic leukemia. Remission induction therapy was begun with prednisone 40 mg/m²/day po in three divided doses for 28 days, VCR 1.5 mg/m²/wk IV for four doses and L-asparaginase (L-ASP) 10,000 U/m² for four doses. Immediately following the administration of the second dose of L-ASP, the patient rapidly became dyspneic and cyanotic. He shortly became unconscious and his blood pressure was unobtainable. The patient was treated with oxygen by mask, intravenous diphenhydramine and epinephrine. Following a second dose of epinephrine, the patient improved rapidly and the blood pressure returned to normal. Was this a drug-related reaction; how might it be prevented; and what is an alternative drug for future administration in this patient?

L-asparaginase is an enzyme with a molecular weight of approximately 130,000. The majority of L-asparaginase in clinical use today is obtained from *Escherischia coli*. Since this drug is a large molecular weight foreign protein, one of the most serious adverse effects is the occurrence of anaphylactic reactions (33, 168). The incidence of anaphylactic reactions to L-ASP ranges from 5-30% of treated patients (99, 164, 178). Peterson and associates (168 demonstrated passive hemagglutinating antibodies to L-ASP in all patients who had an allergic reaction at least one day before the reaction occurred; such antibodies were absent in all patients who did not manifest a reaction. Routine administration of a 50 unit intravenous test dose prior to each full dose of L-ASP may be useful in identifying patients at high risk for manifesting an anaphylactic reaction.

Asparaginase prepared from *Erwinia carotovora* also possesses antileukemic properties (33, 32), and it is presently the only asparaginase available for clinical use that is antigenically different from *E. coli* asparaginase (15, 230). *Erwinia carotovora* asparaginase may be administered to patients who are allergic to the *E. coli* asparaginase without a significant degree of immunologic cross reaction (165).

In general, the use of lower doses of L-asparaginase has resulted in a decreased incidence of hepatic, pancreatic, hematologic and anaphylactic toxicities without significantly compromising the drug's therapeutic effect (178). In patients who manifest an anaphylactic-type reaction to *E. coli* asparaginase, administration of *Erwinia carotovora* asparaginase should permit continued therapy with the enzyme.

5. What is the expected response to reinduction therapy for patients with acute lymphocytic leukemia who relapse while receiving maintenance chemotherapy or following termination of maintenance therapy ?

In general, the likelihood of response to reinduction therapy decreases with each relapse and with repeated attempts to induce remission (135). Aur et al (4) reported a median duration of complete and hematologic remission of 12 months following reinduction of remission. Six of the 16 children were surviving 46 to 50 months, with four of these patients receiving no chemotherapy. These patients were initially treated prior to 1969 and therefore had received less intensive therapy for initial remission induction and maintenance. The probability of response to reinduction therapy for hematologic relapse is probably greater in patients who receive less intensive initial therapy (110).

Results of reinduction therapy for patients who initially received preventive central nervous system (CNS) therapy and 31 months of combination chemotherapy indicate that of the 17 patients who developed recurrent acute lymphocytic leukemia *following cessation* of therapy, complete bone marrow remissions were achieved in 16 using vincristine, prednisone and adriamycin. The median duration of the second hematologic remissions was 216 days. The fact that the second hematologic remission was terminated by an equal number of CNS and hematologic relapses may indicate that a second course of preventive CNS therapy is needed. These responses were significantly better than those achieved in seven patients who relapsed *while receiving* maintenance chemotherapy. Reinduction of remission was achieved in only four of seven patients who relapsed while receiving maintenance chemotherapy, and the median duration of remission for these patients was only 50 days (184).

In conclusion, reinduction of remission can usually be achieved following relapse and is more easily achieved in patients who relapse following cessation of therapy. Likewise, the duration of the second remission is significantly longer in patients who relapse while they are off therapy versus those who relapse while receiving maintenance therapy. The fact that over 50% of these patients have a subsequent relapse indicates that they may require more therapy, including a second course of preventive CNS therapy. Randomized controlled studies evaluating the effectiveness of preventive CNS therapy during reinduction of a second remission should answer this question.

6. Intrathecal methotrexate and cranial irradiation are currently employed as prophylaxis for central nervous system leukemia. What are the complications and pharmacokinetics of intrathecally administered methotrexate?

Central nervous system prophylaxis with tumoricidal doses of cranial irradiation and intrathecal methotrexate produces a significant reduction in the frequency of CNS leukemia and a significant prolongation of complete remission (7, 8). Currently at the St. Jude Children's Research Hospital, all patients who attain remission after induction therapy are promptly entered on a program of CNS prophylaxis with cranial irradiation over two and a half weeks and intrathecal methotrexate 12 mg/m^2 twice weekly for five doses.

Neurological complications attributable to intrathecal MTX include encephalopathy, transverse myelitis, chemical arachnoiditis and transient paresis, (124,52). Fatal and permanent neurologic sequelae have been reported in patients receiving intrathecal MTX for the treatment of meningeal leukemia (124, 9, 13, 192, 202, 166, 157). Although there has been great concern about the toxicity of paraben preservatives in methotrexate preparations (192, 12), the toxicity caused by intrathecal MTX is probably not attributable to these agents (52). However, methotrexate is currently available without preservatives, and a freshly prepared preservative-free intrathecal preparation should be used. It has been suggested that the neurotoxicity of intrathecal MTX can be correlated with prolonged exposure of the CNS to excessive concentrations of MTX (21). Older children and children with active meningeal leukemia may be predisposed to MTX neurotoxicity because the ratio of the dose to cerebrospinal fluid volume is high and the elimination of the drug from the cerebrospinal fluid may be impaired. The half-life of intrathecal methotrexate in the cerebrospinal fluid is 12-18 hours in patients without neurotoxicity. Methotrexate levels in the cerebrospinal fluid of toxic patients range from 1.5 to 100 times higher than the corresponding mean value for non-toxic patients (21). It is conceivable that monitoring methotrexate levels in the cerebrospinal fluid (CSF) at the time of an intrathecal administration may assist in calculating subsequent doses and reducing toxicity. This author has used MTX CSF levels to monitor patients with active CNS leukemia who received maximum irradiation therapy and therefore required maximum, non-toxic doses of intrathecal MTX. This procedure enabled clinicians to dose such patients more precisely while avoiding toxicity.

The distribution of methotrexate in CSF is more reliable when the drug is administered intraventricularly via an indwelling intraventricular subcutaneous reservoir compared to intrathecal administration (201). However, the distribution of intrathecal MTX is sufficient to achieve therapeutic levels in the ventricular CSF and may be significantly better with larger volumes of intrathecal preparation. The volume of injected solution is an important factor in attaining widespread distribution following intrathecal administration. When the volume of injected solution is 10% of the estimated cerebrospinal-fluid volume, adequate distribution is obtained only at the level of the basal cisterns; whereas, when the volume is approximately 25% of the estimated CSF, distribution is obtained throughout the cerebral subarachnoid space and ventricular system (180).

Although subarachnoid and ventricular distribution of methotrexate may not be critical when cranial irradiation is given concomitantly for CNS prophylaxis, good cerebrospinal fluid distribution is essential if methotrexate alone is employed for the treatment or prophylaxis of CNS leukemia.

7. Regardless of the type or number of drugs used for remission induction therapy of acute lymphocytic leukemia, relapse occurs in the great majority of patients if therapy is stopped after remission induction. What drugs are best used as single agents to prolong remission, and what have been the results of combination chemotherapy regimens for maintaining remission?

The efficacy of individual drugs in maintaining remissions has been reviewed by Goldin (83). Methotrexate is the single most effective agent for prolonging the duration of remission of ALL. Intermittent, IV administration of high doses of methotrexate is superior to daily, oral administration of methotrexate (1, 167). Mercaptopurine is the next most effective single agent, followed by cyclophosphamide. Other less effective drugs include vincristine, cytosine arabinoside, daunomycin and L-asparaginase. In any given schedule, the efficacy of a single or multiple-drug regimen is related to dosage (83, 171, 105, 140). The development of resistance and subsequent relapse following remission maintenance therapy with single agents led to the evaluation of multiple-drug maintenance therapy. Combination chemotherapy for remission maintenance was designed to take advantage of the different mechanisms of action and toxicities of the effective maintenance-therapy drugs. The first controlled study of single versus combination maintenance chemotherapy reported that the median durations of remission in childhood ALL was the same whether methotrexate and mercaptopurine were given alone or in combination (71). Subsequently, prolongation of the remission period was reported in studies using multiple-drug maintenance therapy (206, 83). Another effort to improve remission maintenance therapy was the administration of "pulse doses" of drugs that had little apparent value in remission maintenance regimens (i.e. vincristine, prednisone). The rationale behind these "pulse doses" was that drugs with different mechanisms of action would further reduce the residual leukemia cell population. Both positive and negative results have been reported in studies evaluating the additive effects of pulse therapy (96, 95, 140, 155, 8).

The St. Jude Children's Research Hospital Total

Therapy Study VIII (207) was designed to answer the question: "does the advantage of multiple agent chemotherapy outweigh the disadvantage of dosage reduction of the more effective agents?" After attaining a complete remission and receiving preventive CNS therapy, patients were randomized to receive either (1) methotrexate (2) methotrexate + mercaptopurine, (3) methotrexate + mercaptopurine + cyclophosphamide or (4) methotrexate + mercaptopurine + cyclophosphamide + cytosine arabinoside. Dose adjustments were made to keep the leukocyte count between 2000 and 3500/mm^3. The group receiving only methotrexate was closed shortly after the initiation of the study because of an unusually high incidence of subacute leukoencephalopathy. Although this study is still in progress, preliminary results indicate that remission duration and the frequency of patients achieving two and a half to three years of continuous complete remission are similar for patients receiving two-, three- and four-drug maintenance therapy (207). As expected, patients receiving four-drug maintenance therapy had the greatest degree of immunosuppression, resulting in a higher incidence of infections, including *Pneumocystis carinii* pneumonia. Equal efficacy and reduced toxicity with the methotrexate and mercaptopurine combination suggest that this two-drug maintenance therapy is the best, although this protocol is still under active study.

8. L.C. is a 10-year-old white boy in whom acute lymphocytic leukemia was diagnosed in August, 1972. Remission was achieved after four weeks of induction therapy. He received preventive CNS therapy and was placed on a maintenance regimen of methotrexate 20 mg/m^2 IV weekly and mercaptopurine 50 mg/m^2 po daily. All therapy was discontinued after 2½ years of continuous, complete remission. What are the criteria and rationale for cessation of therapy?

It is clear that if therapy is stopped immediately after remission is induced, there is a high frequency of relapse regardless of the induction regimen used (241, 100, 101, 105). The proportion of patients in complete remission declines in an exponential fashion for the first 2-3 years of remission but levels off thereafter (206). There is also evidence that after a period of time, continued administration of maintenance chemotherapy may not eradicate, but only suppress, the remaining leukemia cells and a more resistant clone could eventually emerge and proliferate (128). Moreover, these drugs are immunosuppressive and place the patient at increased risk for fatal opportunistic infections despite leukemic control (204, 109). With approximately 50% of children with ALL achieving continued remissions for many years after cessation of therapy, potential delayed consequences of chemotherapy are

an additional concern. Delayed toxicities may include secondary malignancies; hepatic, pulmonary, skeletal and cardiovascular toxicities; prolonged immunosuppression; sterility; and adverse effects on the central nervous system (179). The actual significance of these potential delayed consequences of therapy cannot be determined until a larger number of patients with childhood ALL reach adulthood.

When single or multiple drug maintenance therapy is stopped after 6 weeks to 14 months of remission, 50% of patients relapse within 2 to 10 months (205). Patients who receive adequate prophylactic CNS therapy, multiple-agent chemotherapy, and who remain in remission for 2-3 years, have a 10% risk of relapse following cessation of therapy (203). A rebound lymphocytosis, which may be confused with relapse, occurs after remission maintenance chemotherapy for acute lymphocytic leukemia is discontinued (27). This rebound lymphocytosis varies in degree and duration and is accompanied by a recovery of immunocompetence (88).

In conclusion, current data indicate that patients should be continued on remission maintenance chemotherapy for 2 to 3 years, after which time the benefits of chemotherapy probably do not exceed the risks. It is important to note that some patients have had recurrence of disease as late as 11 years after diagnosis (61).

9. Prognostication of acute lymphocytic leukemia has been difficult, compared to solid tumors, because the disease is disseminated at the time of diagnosis. What factors have been identified as having a relationship to outcome of therapy?

Early attempts to identify prognostic criteria at the time of diagnosis suggest that a white blood cell count of more than 50,000/mm^3, massive hepatosplenomegaly, central nervous system involvement, and age less than one year or greater than ten years, were poor prognostic factors (73, 241). Also, the likelihood of inducing remission and the median duration of remission are less in Negro children as compared to Caucasian children. (237).

Simone (208) analyzed the relationship of a variety of initial features and the outcome of therapy in 363 children with acute lymphocytic leukemia. The criteria for evaluating the prognostic significance of a given feature was whether the patient attained or exceeded the median duration of complete remission, hematologic remission, or survival for all patients studied. In general, patients with more massive or extensive disease at diagnosis had a poorer response to therapy. Specific factors at the time of diagnosis associated with poor prognosis included: CNS involvement, spleen enlargement greater than 5 cm below the costal margin, initial leukocyte count above 100,000/mm^3, and mediastinal involvement. Children who were over ten years of age at the time of diagnosis and Negro children had a poorer prognosis. Also, children who were under two years of age at the time of diagnosis or who had hepatomegaly greater than 5 cm below the costal margin were less likely to attain at least three years of continuous, complete remission. It is important to realize, however, that with the exception of early CNS involvement, there were patients with each of the poor prognostic factors who had excellent responses to therapy.

Since the initial report of Sen and Borella (199) of the clinical importance of lymphoblasts with T-cell markers in childhood leukemia, several investigators have attempted to assess the prognostic value of cell surface markers. Specific surface markers on lymphoblasts have been related to the prognosis of acute lymphocytic leukemia in children (224). Patients were catagorized in one study as having T-marker lymphoblasts, B-marker lymphoblasts or null lymphoblasts. T-cells were identified by spontaneous rosette formation with sheep erythrocytes (E-Rosettes) and B-cells by the presence of surface immunoglobulin. Of 37 patients evaluated, eight had T-marker lymphoblasts, 28 had no markers, and one had B-marker lymphoblasts. Poor prognostic factors were found in 7 of 17 patients with null lymphoblasts and all of the patients with T-marker lymphoblasts. A mediastinal mass was not found in any patients with null lymphoblasts, but was found in the one child with B-marker lymphoblasts and in 5 of 7 patients with T-marker lymphoblasts. There was no statistically significant difference in the proliferative activity of the lymphoblasts among the three groups of patients as measured by the mitotic index and labeling index. In general, patients with T-marker lymphoblasts had a poorer prognosis than those with null lymphoblasts. The value of subtyping acute lymphocytic leukemia according to surface markers may become more clearly defined as additional studies are reported.

Generally, the prognosis of patients with cancer depends on the anatomical extent of the tumor, the sensitivity of the disease to therapy and the selectivity and toxicity of treatment. The ability to stratify patients according to prognosis is not only important to the patients and their family, but is also valuable in evaluating the efficacy of therapy.

10. What is the major complication of long-term administration of adriamycin, and what factors have been associated with an increased risk of developing this toxicity?

Adriamycin may produce several transient toxic effects including nausea, vomiting, stomatitis, alopecia, and myelosuppression. However, the use of adriamycin has been limited primarily by the severe dose-dependent cardiomyopathy that may occur with repeated administration (41, 139, 79, 40, 182).

The signs and symptoms of adriamycin cardiomyopathy are the same as those expected for congestive heart failure. The onset of symptoms may be insidious, followed shortly by rapidly progressive congestive heart failure.

The most clearly defined factor associated with the development of adriamycin cardiomyopathy is the cumulative dose of adriamycin which has been administered (41, 85, 138, 25, 17, 221). In a review of five series reporting 1758 patients who received adriamycin, cardiomyopathy developed in only 0.3% of all patients who received less than 500 mg/m^2 (156). The incidence was 11% when doses of 501-600 mg/m^2 were received. In a report of 50 children who received adriamycin in cumulative doses of 495-1695 mg/m^2, 16% had severe cardiomyopathy with congestive heart failure (80). None of 68 children who received cumulative doses of 200-495 mg/m^2 developed cardiomyopathy.

In a comparison of patients who developed fatal cardiomyopathy to those who developed nonfatal cardiomyopathy (156) it was noted that the median time from the first dose of adriamycin to the development of cardiomyopathy was shorter in the patients who died (244 days vs 330 days). When the median dose of adriamycin in mg/m^2 was calculated for these patients, it was found that the patients who died had received a median of 2.8 mg/m^2/day compared to 2.35 mg/m^2/day for those who developed nonfatal cardiomyopathy. The cumulative dose was similar for both groups. Although these doses are not statistically different, the data suggest that the administration of cumulative doses of adriamycin over 500 mg/m^2 in shorter time intervals may be associated with more severe cardiotoxicity.

The incidence of adriamycin cardiomyopathy is higher in patients who receive incidental cardiac irradiation (80, 141). This is most likely associated with the previous findings of cardiac fibrosis and myocardial necrosis observed after thoracic irradiation (18).

Another factor which may increase the risk of developing adriamycin cardiomyopathy is cyclophosphamide therapy. Cardiac necrosis has occurred (30) in patients receiving high-dose cyclophosphamide therapy (60-120 mg/kg). Appelbaum et al (3) reported an acute lethal myopericarditis in 4 of 15 patients receiving high-dose combination chemotherapy which included cyclophosphamide 45 mg/kg/day for four days. Pathological findings in those patients revealed nuclear changes resembling those in hearts of patients given anthracycline drugs. EKG changes compatible with cardiotoxicity have followed the administration of 120 mg/kg of cyclophosphamide over two days (158). Canine studies also demonstrated that 500 mg/kg of cyclophosphamide (equivalent on a surface area basis to 240 mg/kg in humans), when given as a single intravenous infusion, markedly decreases the voltage of the QRS complex after two to three hours; death from pulmonary edema and intractable cardiac failure occurs in another 30-90 minutes (163). In monkeys, 240 mg/kg of cyclophosphamide given over four days has resulted in a diffuse hemorrhagic diathesis most prominent in the myocardium (211). All of these data suggest that patients who have received high-dose cyclophosphamide therapy may be predisposed to adriamycin cardiomyopathy. This is supported by Minow's data (156): of 13 patients who had developed adriamycin cardiomyopathy at doses below 550 mg/m^2, 5 had received concurrent cyclophosphamide, 2 had prior radiation therapy and 2 had both prior radiotherapy and concurrent cyclophosphamide.

Other factors which possibly contribute to cardiac decompensation at lower doses of adriamycin include age, pre-existing heart disease, other cardiotoxic drugs (including high-dose methotrexate), severe pulmonary disease and dosage schedules (80). Hepatic dysfunction is known to prolong adriamycin's biological half-life and predispose to acute toxicity if proper dosage adjustments are not made (30).

Early recognition of adriamycin cardiotoxicity is essential so that adriamycin therapy can be discontinued. Chest roentgenograms should be taken frequently to detect cardiomegaly or pleural effusions. Monitoring of cardiac enzymes has not been effective in evaluating adriamycin cardiomyopathy (139). Increases in systolic time intervals (STI), (16, 183), and decreases in the ejection fraction measured by echocardiography, have been reported in patients with adriamycin cardiomyopathy (122). Minow (156) recommends discontinuance of adriamycin if there is a 40% decrease in QRS voltage in conjunction with the development of any cardiac abnormality. Despite these efforts to assess adriamycin cardiotoxicity, there is clearly a need for better methods to detect early myocardial damage produced by adriamycin.

The treatment of congestive heart failure secondary to adriamycin consists of prolonged digitalis and diuretic therapy and a salt restricted diet. Children with adriamycin cardiotoxicity are highly sensitive to digitalis therapy (80). These patients often require a total intravenous digitalizing dose of only 0.01-0.02 mg/kg of digoxin followed by a daily maintenance dose of 1/4 to 1/7 the total digitalizing dose.

11. Cyclophosphamide may be used for maintenance chemotherapy of acute lymphocytic leukemia in combination with other antineoplastic drugs. What toxicity may be encountered with cyclophosphamide that is rarely encountered with other antineoplastic drugs?

Cyclophosphamide has many side effects which are commonly encountered with other antineoplastic drugs including nausea, vomiting, anorexia, leukopenia and alopecia. Hemorrhagic cystitis is a complication that reportedly occurs in 2-40% of patients treated with the drug and is a toxicity peculiar to cyclophosphamide (210, 85, 145, 137, 121, 148).

In one study (137), 25 of 314 children with acute lymphocytic leukemia developed well documented hemorrhagic cystitis, which was usually mild and transient, although one death occurred secondary to bladder hemorrhage. There was no correlation between the total dose administered and the severity of the cystitis, nor was there a correlation between the frequency of cyclophosphamide-induced cystitis and age, sex or route of administration. Nineteen of the 25 cases occurred in the spring and summer months. It was suggested that this may have been related to a poorer state of hydration during these months resulting in a higher concentration of active metabolites in the urine. However, this could not be documented by urine specific gravity determinations. Also, cyclophosphamide-induced cystitis was found to be twice as frequent in black children as in white.

Johnson et al (121) reported a 25% incidence of transmural fibrosis and submucosal telangiectasia in the bladders of 40 children dying of neoplastic disease previously treated with long-term cyclophosphamide. The bladder changes were described as chronic and irreversible and were associated with total doses exceeding 6 gm/m^2. Interestingly, only 5 of the 10 children found to have bladder changes at autopsy had a documented history of cyclophosphamide-induced hemorrhagic cystitis. Another important finding was the lack of correlation between the frequency of other side effects of cyclophosphamide (i.e. leukopenia, gastrointestinal toxicity) and the occurrence of hemorrhagic cystitis.

Other investigators (118) reported a significantly increased frequency and severity of urinary-bladder toxicity in children receiving pelvic irradiation with simultaneous cyclophosphamide. The incidence of bladder toxicity was 34% in patients who received both pelvic irradiation and cyclophosphamide, compared to 8% in patients who received cyclophosphamide with radiotherapy outside the pelvic region. Since the reported frequency of urinary-bladder toxicity from pelvic irradiation ranges from 2.5-12% (189), cyclophosphamide and pelvic irradiation may act synergistically to produce bladder toxicity. The authors recommended that an alkylating agent other than cyclophosphamide be considered when patients are receiving or will receive radiotherapy to the pelvic region.

Patients receiving cyclophosphamide should be continuously evaluated for the development of hemorrhagic cystitis. The onset of hematuria should prompt immediate reconsideration of continued administration of cyclophosphamide. The following criteria were utilized by Lawrence et al (137) to establish a diagnosis of cyclophosphamide-induced hemorrhagic cystitis: (1) history of gross hematuria, (2) laboratory findings of gross or microscopic hematuria (at least 5 RBC/HPF on a centrifuged specimen) and/or a voiding cystogram consistent with cystitis (i.e. a contracted bladder with thickened mucosal folds), (3) platelet count greater than 50,000/mm³ and (4) no significant growth on urine cultures.

The initial therapy of cyclophosphamide-induced hemorrhagic cystitis is discontinuation of cyclophosphamide administration. Numerous methods have been employed to manage bladder hemorrhage including electrocautery (136), intravesicle hydrostatic pressure (106), colocystoplasty (148), cystectomy, epsilon aminocaproic acid locally or systemically (129), supravesical urinary diversion and irrigation with phenol (51), formalin (200), or silver nitrate (129, 173). A recent report (129) suggests that 0.5-1% silver nitrate irrigations after cystoscopic evacuation of clots produces fewer adverse effects yet appears to be as effective as more drastic measures such as cystectomy or colocystoplasty. It is important to realize that the control of bleeding is usually only temporary in that bleeding often recurs weeks to years later.

Current efforts to prevent the occurrence of cyclophosphamide-induced cystitis include the administration of intravenous fluids following weekly administration of intravenous cyclophosphamide and education of parents to have their children drink large amount of liquids the day of drug administration and void just before going to bed. These represent efforts to reduce the concentration of alkylating metabolites in the urine and reduce the duration of bladder exposure to these active metabolites.

12. The majority of drugs used to treat leukemia have their major therapeutic effect on cells within the mitotic cycle and have little effect on resting cells. In addition, most of these drugs have their principle effect on cells in a specific phase of the mitotic cycle.

Describe the principle laboratory studies performed to evaluate drug effects on cell kinetics and the effects of cytosine arabinoside, methotrexate, vincristine, cyclophosphamide, corticosteroids and L-asparaginase on acute lymphocytic leukemia cell kinetics.

The effects of chemotherapy on cell kinetics have been the subject of several excellent reviews (159, 151, 153, 131, 117). Chemotherapy-induced changes in the cell cycle can be measured by the *labeling index (LI)* and the *mitotic index (MI)* by obtaining serial marrow samples before and after the administration of drugs or drug combinations. The number of mitotic figures per 1000 nucleated cells (MI) is determined by microscopic examination of a bone marrow sample (117). The percentage of cells undergoing DNA synthesis (LI) is determined autographically using tritiated thymidine which is incorporated into DNA only during DNA synthesis (130). Other techniques are available for studying cell proliferation in acute leukemia, although the mitotic and labeling indices are the most widely used (152).

Two commonly used terms in dscribing the manipulation of cell kinetics by chemotherapy are "recruitment" and "synchronization". **Recruitment** refers to the process of recalling resting cells into the mitotic cycle at an accelerated rate. Since most drugs have little effect on resting cells, this process offers the theoretical advantage of providing more cells in a drug-sensitive state. **Synchronization** refers to the process of accumulating cells in a specific phase of the mitotic cycle (i.e. S phase). The administration of a cell cycle specific drug at a time when a maximum number of cells are in the susceptible phase should produce a greater therapeutic effect.

The mitotic cycle of dividing cells can be separated into four phases: (1) the interval between the completion of mitosis and the beginning of DNA synthesis (G_1); (2) the period of DNA synthesis (S); (3) the time between completion of DNA synthesis and the beginning of mitosis (G_2); and (4) mitosis (M). The utilization of cell kinetics in designing chemotherapy regimens requires an understanding of the subcomponents of the mitotic cycle and the effects of single and multiple drug regimens on the cell kinetics of the tumor being treated.

Cytosine arabinoside given in a dose of 5 mg/kg body weight by rapid intravenous injection markedly decreases the labeling index 1-4 hours after administration in patients with acute lymphocytic leukemia (132). The labeling and mitotic indices remain decreased for 24-72 hours, then gradually return to pretreatment levels. In the majority of patients, the labeling index rises to levels significantly greater than pretreatment values 24-96 hours after the drug has been given. These data indicate that partial synchronization of cells in the S phase of the mitotic cycle can be achieved with cytosine arabinoside.

Like cytosine arabinoside, methotrexate, administered in a dose of 1 mg/kg body weight by intravenous injection, produces synchronization of cells in the S phase (133, 56). The labeling index increases progressively until approximately 72 hours after the drug is administered. It is important to realize that methotrexate has a dose-dependent effect on the cell cycle (133, 55). In patients with acute myeloblastic leukemia, similar doses of methotrexate arrest cells in DNA synthesis for shorter periods of time.

Vincristine administered intravenously in a dose of 0.075 mg/kg produces a marked increase in the mitotic index at 24 hours in patients with acute lymphocytic leukemia (132). This marked increase in the number of mitotic figures indicates that vincristine arrests cells in mitosis. The labeling index does not change until 48 hours after the drug is given, at which time a significant decrease in the labeling index is found. One explanation for this phenomena is that cells in S phase and G_1 phase proceed through DNA synthesis and are subsequently arrested at mitosis while cells in G_0 are inhibited from entering the mitotic cycle. This would result in a marked depletion of cells in S phase at approximately 48 hours. Subsequent studies by McWilliams (154) support this theory by demonstrating that VCR impairs lymphocyte transformation when stimulated by phytohemaglutin *in vitro*.

Cyclophosphamide, a cell cycle non-specific drug, when given intravenously in a dose of 15 mg/kg to patients with acute lymphocytic leukemia, appears to inhibit DNA synthesis, arrest cells in mitosis and impair the entry of cells into S phase (133).

Corticosteroids have a lytic effect on acute lymphocytic leukemia cells; resting and proliferating cells seem to be equally affected (132, 56, 55). The result is a rapid reduction in the number of leukemic cells in most patients. The effects of corticosteroids on the mitotic cycle are manifested by a decreased flow of cells from the G_1 to the S phase. The duration of the effect on the mitotic cycle is approximately 24 hours after a single injection; recovery becomes evident in 48 hours.

L-asparaginase, administered intravenously in a dose of 1000-2000 units/kg body weight has an effect on acute lymphocytic leukemic cells similar to that of corticosteroids (133, 195). As seen with corticosteroids, cells in both resting and proliferating phases appear to be lysed. There is also an inhibition of cell passage from G_1 into the S phase.

13. Based on the effects of vincristine and cytosine arabinoside on acute lymphocytic leukemia cell kinetics, what would be the optimal schedule of administration of these two drugs in a combination regimen?

The administration of cytosine arabinoside to patients with acute lymphocytic leukemia will produce a significant increase in the labeling index 24-96 hours after the drug is given (132). The maximum increase in the number of cells in DNA synthesis may actually be too great to be accounted for simply by the entrance of cells from G_1 into the S phase. This indicates that in addition to synchronization of cells, recruitment of resting cells into the mitotic cycle also occurs.

A therapeutic advantage should be achieved if a second drug which has its effects on cells in S phase is given at a time following cytosine arabinoside administration when the labeling index is highest. Vin-

cristine produces a block as cells pass through mitosis (M) by causing a disruption of the microtubule and subsequent defective spindle formation (132). Cells are most sensitive to vincristine's effects on microtubules during the S phase even though the results do not become evident until they have completed S and G_2, and enter the M phase. It is for this reason that a greater cytotoxic effect of vincristine should be achieved if prior synchronization of cells in S phase has been accomplished with cytosine arabinoside.

Lampkin et al (133) demonstrated that the mitotic index remained significantly increased from two to four times longer when 0.05 mg/kg of vincristine was given after prior synchronization with cytosine arabinoside as compared to when 0.075 mg/kg of vincristine was administered alone.

It is equally important to realize that the administration of one drug may reduce the effectiveness of a second drug if an improper sequence of administration is employed. A theoretical example would be cytosine arabinoside administered 48 hours after vincristine in the treatment of acute lymphocytic leukemia. A profound decrease in the number of cells in S phase occurs approximately 48 hours after vincristine is administered (132). Although there is presently no consensus on the exact biochemical effects of cytosine arabinoside, it is regarded as an S-phase specific drug, since most of its proposed actions relate to DNA synthesis and function. Therefore, the administration of cytosine arabinoside at a time when a minimum number of cells are in the phase of DNA synthesis would decrease its effects.

The above are examples of how chemotherapeutic manipulation of cell kinetics can possibly alter the therapeutic response to drug combinations. The results of clinical studies where chemotherapeutic manipulation of cell kinetics have been used in designing drug therapy will provide greater evidence of the benefits of utilizing cell kinetic data in designing chemotherapy regimens.

14-18. What is the current role of chemotherapy in the treatment of acute nonlymphocytic leukemia, non-Hodgkin's lymphomas, neuroblastoma, osteosarcoma and rhabdomyosarcoma in children?

14. *Acute Nonlymphocytic Leukemia*

Despite the development and utilization of modern chemotherapy for acute leukemia, the prognosis for acute nonlymphocytic leukemia (ANLL) continues to be poor. The treatment of ANLL has not been nearly as successful as the 90% remission induction rate and 50% 5-year leukemia-free survival now obtainable with acute lymphocytic leukemia. In ANLL, remission is achieved in 30-70% of patients and the median duration of remissions is usually less than one year (231, 66, 23, 237, 14, 44, 108, 54).

There is currently no consensus among investigators and clinicians regarding the optimal therapy of ANLL. This recently became more apparent when daunomycin or cytosine arabinoside alone were reported to be as effective as multiple agents for inducing remission in adults (235, 211).

Choi and Simone reported a complete remission induction rate of 66% in 86 previously untreated children with ANLL who underwent treatment between 1968 and 1973 (36). Although these results are superior to the 34-38% induction rates in previous series spanning several years (102, 74), it is similar to the 50-60% induction rates of adult studies (23, 74, 14, 24, 37, 44, 188) and the 42-57% induction rate in children reported by the Argentine Study Group, (54, 19). Remission induction therapy included 6-azauridine, 6-mercaptopurine and vincristine for all patients. The details of therapy including the dose, sequence and duration of administration have previously been described (36, 231, 66). The median duration of remission was 6 months, which is similar to the 2-14 months median remission durations reported from series consisting primarily of adults (23, 102, 236, 14, 24, 92, 68, 93, 237).

Studies in acute myelocytic leukemia reporting predictive value of the initial tritiated thymidine labeling index (LI) for response to treatment suggests that cell kinetic data may be a valuable tool in designing and evaluating therapy of ANLL. Some studies have reported a positive correlation between complete response rate and a high initial labeling index (31, 237, 246, 70), while other studies have found no correlation between the initial thymidine labeling index and remission induction rate (197). Lampkin et al (134) obtained 90% complete remissions of acute myeloblastic leukemia by using cytosine arabinoside alone to synchronize and kill cells. Burke and Owens (31) obtained a better remission rate by utilizing cell kinetics in designing chemotherapy for ANLL, although their control group received only one drug, while the experimental group were administered three drugs. It is impossible to determine if the effect of combination chemotherapy alone could have explained their results. Other investigators have reported no increase in the remission rate with drug regimens designed to take advantage of cell recruitment and synchronization (143).

Attempts to prolong the duration of remission by administering maintenance chemotherapy have not been very successful, since a significant number of patients relapse within 4 months, an outcome that might occur with no maintenance therapy. Efforts have been made to prolong remission by a variety of non-chemotherapeutic measures, such as immunotherapy (93, 46, 14) irradiation of the liver and spleen (36), preventive craniospinal irradiation (36)

and splenectomy (66). Both positive and negative results have been reported in studies utilizing immunotherapy with allogeneic cells plus BCG or BCG alone to prolong remission duration (93, 46, 14). Irradiation of the liver and spleen has not only failed to prolong remission, but severely limits the subsequent dosage of chemotherapy (36). Equivocal results were obtained when splenectomy was performed in a small number of patients with ANLL (36). The value of splenectomy should be more clearly defined by studies currently in progress.

The poor response of childhood ANLL to current treatment regimens emphasizes the need for continued investigation of new approaches and modalities of therapy.

15. *Non-Hodgkin's Lymphoma*

Non-Hodgkin's lymphoma (NHL) is a neoplastic disease of lymphoreticular cells which exhibits a spectrum of clinical syndromes dependent upon the site of primary tumor involvement, extent of disease at diagnoses and to a lesser extent, histologic type. In recent years, the overall two-year survival in childhood NHL has been roughly 20-30% (82, 142, 160, 119). Patients with localized disease (Stages I and II) do significantly better than patients with generalized disease (Stages III and IV).

While these data suggest that the extent of the disease is an important determinant of outcome, there is no such consensus regarding the importance of histologic classification. Nodular lymphomas are rare in children, but have a good prognosis. However, greater than 95% of the cases of childhood NHL have a diffuse histologic pattern. It has been concluded by several investigators that either (1) the prognostic value of histology has not been established, (2) the histology exerts no independent prognostic influence, or (3) at least histology should not be used to determine management (242, 160, 142, 119). Most institutions presently use a modification of the Rapaport classification which is based on the histological classification by diffuse or nodular, and the cytological classification by lymphocytic or histocytic, although the functional classification of the non-Hodgkin's lymphomas is currently under revision.

The role of radiotherapy in the management of childhood NHL remains to be clearly defined. Radiotherapy is recognized as the only modality known to offer a significant chance for cure in malignant lymphoma (123, 162). However, its application for remission induction of childhood NHL is complicated by the usually aggressive clinical course of the disease characterized by apparent non-contiguous spread, a high frequency of bone marrow involvement and generalized rather than localized disease.

Since childhood NHL is often a generalized disease

at diagnosis, chemotherapy plays an important role in remission induction. Combination chemotherapy is superior to single-agent chemotherapy in malignant lymphomas, with the three most active agents against NHL being aklylating agents, vinca alkaloids, and corticosteroids. The combination of cyclophosphamide, vincristine, and prednisone has been shown to be superior to other single-agent or combination regimens for remission induction in adults, producing a 91% objective response rate (11). Other drugs currently being evaluated for induction therapy of childhood NHL include adriamycin, daunomycin, and methotrexate; in combination with cyclophosphamide, vincristine and prednisone.

Since 1971, treatment for children with NHL at Memorial Sloan-Kettering Cancer Center has consisted of the LSA-L$_2$ protocol (242). The initial results of the LSA-L$_2$ protocol have been excellent, with 80% of children with all stages of disease alive and free of disease at 40 months. This complex treatment protocol is divided into an induction phase, consolidation phase, and maintenance phase, and includes ten different drugs. The authors concluded that the main factor in the survival of children with NHL is therapy and that it must be early, aggressive, prolonged, and include surgery, irradiation and chemotherapy. However, comparison of the results of this series to others is difficult because of the large number of patients with Stage IV disease (40%) and the high percentage of patients with nodular lymphoma (14%). Many of the patients with Stage IV disease (on the basis of initial bone marrow involvement) would be considered leukemic by conventional criteria and would therefore be expected to have a very good response to therapy.

Convential therapy over the past two decades has cured roughly a third of all children with NHL (160, 82, 142, 172). Survival of children with localized disease is consistently better than children with generalized disease. Recent studies show that approximately 80-100% of children with Stage I disease are curable if an intensive multiple drug chemotherapy regimen is combined with radiation (242, 172, 5). This is in contrast to the less than 30% two-year survival of patients with Stage III and IV disease (172, 160, 82, 142). It has been recommended that treatment of children with NHL should be determined by the primary anatomic location and extent of disease (159, 161). Improvement in the response of children with generalized disease is unlikely to result from the application of therapeutic innovations introduced in the treatment of adults with NHL. Not only are there differences in histology and clinical behavior of the disease, there are examples of differences in chemotherapeutic sensitivity between adults and children (159, 161). Other components of therapy which are currently being evaluated in randomized studies are radiotherapy during induction for Stage III-IV patients and CNS prophylaxis (161).

16. Neuroblastoma

Neuroblastoma is the most common extracranial malignant solid tumor in infancy and childhood, comprising approximately 7-14% of childhood malignancies and 15-50% of neonatal malignancies (22, 47, 58, 224, 235). The age at diagnosis is a major determinant of prognosis, with cure being more frequently encountered in children under one year of age (126, 29, 48, 146, 216). Two-year survival is the most reliable indicator of prognosis, since most patients free of tumor for two years remain in remission indefinitely (216, 81, 91). It is also important to realize that neuroblastoma has the highest rate of spontaneous remissions of any human malignancy (60). Everson and Cole (60) compiled 29 cases of children with neuroblastoma that underwent spontaneous regression. Twenty-one of these children were less than six months of age at diagnosis and only four were older than one year.

Despite the progress that has been made during the past quarter century for other childhood cancers, the prognosis for neuroblastoma has remained uniformly poor. Treatment includes surgery, radiation therapy and chemotherapy. The roles of each of these components on therapy have been recently reviewed in detail (113). Another modality of therapy that is currently under investigation is immunotherapy with BCG plus irradiated tumor cells (86, 87).

Vincristine, nitrogen mustard, and cyclophosphamide have been used alone to treat patients with disseminated disease (198, 116). Comparison of the effectiveness of these drugs is difficult because of the differences in patient populations and definitions of response in published series (215, 169, 222, 223, 65). The response rate to combination chemotherapy with vincristine and cyclophosphamide is reported in three series to be 32, 28, and 38% (57, 170, 213). Sawitsky reported a 55% response rate with these two drugs and reported similar results whether the drugs were given sequentially, concurrently or in an alternate week schedule (196). Other drugs which have been reported to have antitumor activity for neuroblastoma include daunorubicin (193, 217, 220), adriamycin (26, 87) and dimethyl triazeno imidazole carboxamide (DTIC) (64).

Green et al (87) recently reported a 63% rate of complete remission in 33 children with unresectable neuroblastoma using sequential low-dose cyclophosphamide (150 mg/m^2/day X 7 days) followed by adriamycin (35 mg/m^2 on day 8). This remission induction rate is superior to previously reported series.

Additional investigations are required to determine the value of chemotherapy and/or immunotherapy in maintaining remissions and improving the survival of children with neuroblastoma.

17. *Rhabdomyosarcoma*

Rhabdomyosarcoma is the most frequently encountered soft tissue sarcoma in children. Rhabdomyosarcoma accounts for approximately 10% of all solid malignant tumors referred to childhood cancer centers.

The current treatment of rhabdomyosarcoma includes surgery, radiation therapy and chemotherapy. The roles of each of these modalities of therapy in the multidisciplinary treatment of rhabdomyosarcoma have been described elsewhere (177, 78).

At St. Jude Children's Research Hospital, chemotherapy is used in all patients in an attempt to prevent metastases or to erradicate microscopic residual disease following surgery or to erradicate gross residual disease which cannot be treated with radiation therapy. Dactinomycin, cyclophosphamide, vincristine and adriamycin, singly or in combination, have been found to produce regression of measurable lesions in childhood rhabdomyosarcoma. Each agent produces tumor regression in one-fourth to one-half of patients treated with a single agent alone. When administered to patients with resected rhabdomyosarcoma, these drugs have been reported to inhibit the formation of metastases (103). Current treatment protocols include the administration of all four of these drugs in a combination chemotherapy regimen. Treatment is continued for approximately 18 months, which represents the period of time in which recurrence of local disease or detection of metastases might be expected in 90% of the patients who would develop such recurrences or metastases.

The use of combined modality therapy including surgery, chemotherapy and radiotherapy has led to an increasing number of patients achieving complete remission, thus improving the chances of long-term disease-free survival of patients with resectable or partially resectable rhabdomyosarcoma (219). When three or four of these agents are combined, most patients demonstrate partial or complete regression (175, 176). Ghavimi (76) reported that 14 of 17 children with rhabdomyosarcoma (all stages) treated with vincristine, cyclophosphamide, dactinomycin, adriamycin and radiation therapy are surviving and free of disease from 4 to 27 or more months. Pratt et al (177) reported that 26 of 34 patients treated with surgery, supervoltage radiation and vincristine-cyclophosphamide-dactinomycin chemotherapy had complete responses. Six patients had partial or mixed responses and only two patients failed to respond. Seventeen of these 34 patients were surviving from 12 months to more than 5½ years. Fifteen of these 17 patients had no evidence of persistent or recurrent tumor. Comparable results have been obtained by other investigators using coordinated multidisciplinary therapy, indicating that this approach to treatment has greatly improved the survival rate of children with rhabdomyosarcoma (103, 90, 50, 107, 115, 240, 35, 77).

18. *Osteosarcoma*

Various approaches to the medical treatment of osteosarcoma have been attempted in the past 50 years. It has become clear that the *sine qua non* for survival following the diagnosis of osteosarcoma is amputation of the affected part. Previous results of the treatment of osteosarcoma, the most common malignant bone tumor in the pediatric age group, have been unsatisfactory. In the largest series of pediatric patients with this tumor, there was a 17% 5-year tumor-free survival rate, with a median post-amputation survival time of 8½ months for patients who died (147). Radiation therapy followed by delayed amputation did not extend the lives nor improve the results of treatment of patients with this tumor. Metastases were usually noted in the lungs during the first year following amputation of the extremity with the primary tumor. Development of pulmonary metastases and ultimate outcome were found to be unrelated to sex, race, preoperative duration of symptoms or preoperative radiation therapy.

In 1971, Jaffe adapted the use of high-dose methotrexate-leucovorin rescue to adjuvant chemotherapy for osteosarcoma after noting two complete and two partial responses in ten patients with pulmonary metastases (114). These investigators used high-dose methotrexate-oral leucovorin in a method first advocated by Djerassi for the treatment of acute lymphocytic leukemia and lung cancer (49). Jaffe et al have since advocated the addition of vincristine by injection 30 minutes to 2 hours prior to methotrexate infusions in an attempt to increase the intracellular concentrations of high-dose methotrexate. Current experience of these investigators is that 4 of 20 patients who have received adjuvant high-dose methotrexate with leucovorin rescue have developed pulmonary metastases (11).

Also in 1971, Wang (233), Cortes (43) and co-workers of Acute Leukemia Group B observed a response of pulmonary metastases following treatment with the antitumor antibiotic, adriamycin. They adapted the use of adjuvant adriamycin to their patients who were free of obvious pulmonary metastases at the time of the diagnosis, and currently report that 8 of 21 patients treated intensively over a 6-month period have developed pulmonary metastases (233).

Sutow and members of the Southwest Oncology Group (218) have treated 43 patients with combinations of agents including cyclophosphamide, vincristine, phenylalanine mustard, and adriamycin (CONPADRI I), of which 23 of 43 patients are surviving and free of tumor for more than two years. An additional group of 30 patients has received treatment with CONPADRI II, which is a modified CONPADRI I regimen and includes three pulses of methotrexate-leucovorin. Two patients had early deaths following the receipt of methotrexate and four patients developed pulmonary metastases, while 24 patients are free of metastatic osteosarcoma.

Wilbur and associates (239) at the Children's Hospital at Stanford have treated 13 patients with adjuvant chemotherapy programs consisting of methotrexate-leucovorin, vincristine, adriamycin and cyclophosphamide. Two of 13 patients developed pulmonary metastases.

At the Memorial Sloan-Kettering Cancer Center, Rosen and his associates (187) have treated nine patients with adjuvant high-dose methotrexate-leucovorin, vincristine, adriamycin and cyclophosphamide following amputation. Seven of these nine patients remain free of evidence of pulmonary metastases from 2 to 11 months after treatment. Additionally, Marcove, Rosen and associates (186) have treated 20 patients with a similar adjuvant chemotherapy program followed by *en bloc* resection of the affected bone and soft tissues with prosthetic bone replacement. One patient died prior to surgery, one required amputation and 17 of 19 patients with measurable primary tumors had partial or complete responses following chemotherapy prior to the replacement procedure. There has been no evidence of soft tissue recurrence 2 to 15 months postoperatively. Fifteen patients who had total femur-knee joint or proximal tibia-knee joint replacement remain well.

Adjuvant therapy for osteosarcoma at St. Jude Children's Research Hospital began in January 1973 and has continued to the present (174). Twenty consecutive patients with osteosarcoma of an extremity and with no evidence of pulmonary or bony metastases at the time of admission to the study have been treated. Chemotherapy was started after amputation, allowing time for satisfactory postoperative recovery. Patients received adriamycin on days 1 and 2, followed by cyclophosphamide on day 3 and methotrexate 100 mg/kg by 6-hour intravenous infusion on day 15, followed by intravenous and intramuscular leucovorin. The protocol is designed to administer ten monthly courses of these agents, representing the median time to the development of pulmonary metatases plus one standard deviation. Eleven patients have remained free of pulmonary or bony metastases for 12 to 40 months. These patients have received six to ten courses of chemotherapy as outlined. Five patients developed pulmonary metastases following completion of ten courses of chemotherapy. One patient died following her third infusion of methotrexate. Her death was associated with methotrexate toxicity; no evidence of tumor was found at autopsy. None of the patients developed local recurrence of tumor.

Clinical toxicity included nausea and vomiting, abdominal discomfort, mild acne, desquamative skin changes, alopecia, hyperpigmentation of dermal creases, chemical burns, and various infections. Laboratory evidences of toxicity included anemia, leukopenia, thrombocytopenia, megaloblastic changes of the bone marrow, abnormalities of liver function, transient increases of serum uric acid and blood urea nitrogen values, and minor electrocardiographic abnormalities.

A nationwide survey of centers with approved protocols for the administration of high-dose methotrexate reports 29 cases of drug-related deaths in 498 recipients (229). Attempts have been made to identify factors which predispose patients to serious life-threatening toxicity from high-dose methotrexate (112, 59). It has been reported that an increased risk of severe toxicity may be associated with dehydration, infection, fever, "third space reservoirs" (pleural effusion, ascites, edematous tissues), and persistently acidic urines (112, 59). Because of the potential of such chemotherapeutic regimens to cause severe toxic effects, it is suggested that treatment with high-dose methotrexate and leucovorin rescue be carried out in clinical centers with the resources needed to assess and manage these toxic effects, including the facilities for major supportive care and pharmacokinetic monitoring of methotrexate blood levels.

The pharmacologic rationale for the administration of high doses of methotrexate followed by leucovorin rescue is discussed in the chapter on **Cancer Chemotherapy.**

ACKNOWLEDGEMENTS — The author thanks Drs. R.J.A. Aur, A.A. Green, A.M. Mauer, S.B. Murphy, C.B. Pratt, G. Rivera, and J.V. Simone for the many helpful comments, personal communications of unpublished reports, and preprints received which materially assisted in the preparation of this manuscript.

REFERENCES

1. Acute Leukemia Group B: New treatment schedule with improved survival in childhood leukemia. JAMA 194:75, 1965.
2. Alberts DS and Wetters TD: The effect of allopurinol on cyclophosphamide antitumor activity. Cancer Res 36:2790, 1976.
3. Appelbaum FR et al: Acute lethal carditis caused by high-dose combination chemotherapy. Lancet 1:58, 1976.
4. Aur RJA et al: Response to combination therapy after relapse in childhood acute lymphocytic leukemia. Cancer 30:334, 1972.
5. Aur RJA: Therapy of localized and regional lymphosarcoma of childhood. Cancer 27:1328, 1971.
6. Aur RJA et al: A comparative study of central nervous system irradiation and early remission of childhood acute lymphocytic leukemia. Cancer 29:381, 1972.
7. Aur RJA et al: Central nervous system therapy and combination chemotherapy of childhood lymphocytic leukemia. Blood 37:272, 1971.
8. Aur RJA et al: Comparison of two methods of preventing central nervous system leukemia. Blood 42:349, 1973.
9. Back EH: Death after intrathecal methotrexate. Lancet 2:1005, 1969.
10. Bagley CM et al: Clinical pharmacology of cyclophosphamide. Cancer Res 33:226, 1973.
11. Bagley CM et al: Advanced lymphosarcoma: Intensive cyclical combination chemotherapy with cyclophosphamide, vincristine, and prednisone. Ann Intern Med 76:227, 1972.
12. Bagshawe KD et al: Intrathecal methotrexate. Lancet 2:1258, 1969.
13. Baum ES et al: Intrathecal methotrexate. Lancet 1:649, 1971.
14. Beard MEJ et al: Acute leukemia in adults. Semin Hematol 11:5, 1974.
15. Beard MEJ et al: L-asparaginase in treatment of acute leukemia and lymphosarcoma. Br Med J 1:191, 1970.
16. Benjamin RS: A practical approach to adriamycin (NSC-123127) toxicology. Cancer Chemother Rep 6:191, 1975.
17. Benjamin RS et al: Adriamycin chemotherapy, efficacy, safety, and pharmacologic basis of an intermittent single high-dosage schedule. Cancer 33:19, 1974.
18. Berdjis CC: The cardiovascular system. In: Pathology of Irradiation. Edited by CC Berdgis, Williams & Wilkins Co., 1971.
19. Bernard J et al: Acute promyelocytic leukemia: Results of treatment by daunorubicin. Blood 41:489, 1973.
20. Bland PR et al: Treatment of central nervous system leukemia with intrathecal cytosine arabinoside. Cancer 32:744, 1973.
21. Bleyer WA et al: Neurotoxicity and elevated cerebrospinal-fluid methotrexate concentration in meningeal leukemia. NEJM 289:770, 1973.
22. Bodian M: Neuroblastoma. Pediat Clin N Amer 6:449, 1959.
23. Bodney GP et al: Chemotherapy of acute leukemia. Arch Intern Med 133:260, 1974.
24. Boiron M et al: Daunorubicin in the treatment of acute myelocytic leukemia. Lancet 1:330, 1969.
25. Bonadonna G: Clinical trials with adriamycin, results of three years study. In International Symposium on Adriamycin. Edited by SK Carter, A Dimarco, M Ghione, New York, Springer-Verlag, pp. 139, 1972.
26. Bonadonna G et al: Therapeutic effects of adriamycin in the neoplastic disease of children and adults. Proc Amer Assoc Cancer Res 11:10, 1970.
27. Borella L et al: Immunologic rebound after cessation of long-term chemotherapy in acute leukemia. Blood 40:42, 1972.
28. Boston Collaborative Drug Surveillance Program: Allopurinol and cytotoxic drugs. Interaction and relation to bone marrow suppression. JAMA 227:1036, 1974.
29. Breslow N et al: Statistical estimation of prognosis for children with neuroblastoma. Cancer Res 31:2098, 1971.
30. Buckner CD et al: High-dose cyclophosphamide therapy for malignant disease-toxicity, tumor response and the effects of stored autologous marrow. Cancer 29:357, 1972.
31. Burke PJ et al: Attempted recruitment of leukemic myeloblasts to proliferative activity by sequential drug treatment. Cancer 28:830, 1971.
32. Campbell DH et al: Methods in Immunology. New York, WA Benjamin Inc p 143, 1964.
33. Capizzi RL et al: L-asparaginase. Ann Rev Med 21:433, 1970.
34. Casey EB et al: Vincristine neuropathy: Clinical and electrophysiological observations. Brain 96:69, 1973.
35. Cassady JR et al: Radiation therapy for rhabdomyosarcoma. Radiology 91:116, 1968.
36. Choi S and Simone JV: Acute non-lymphocytic leukemia in 171 children. Med Ped Onc 2:119, 1976.
37. Clarkson BD: Acute myelocytic leukemia in adults. Cancer 30:1572, 1972.
38. Coffey JJ et al: Effect of allopurinol on the pharmacokinetics of 6-mercaptopurine (NSC 755) in cancer patients. Cancer Res 32:1283, 1972.
39. Colebatch JH et al: Cyclic drug regimen for acute childhood leukemia. Lancet 1:313, 1968.
40. Cortes EP et al: Adriamycin in advanced bronchogenic carcinoma. Cancer 34:518, 1974.
41. Cortes EP et al: Adriamycin cardiotoxicity in adults with cancer. Clin Res 21:412, 1973.
42. Cortes EP et al: Amputation and adriamycin in primary osteosarcoma. NEJM 291:998, 1974.
43. Cortes EP et al: Doxorubicin in disseminated osteosarcoma. J Amer Med Assoc 221:1132, 1972.
44. Crowther D et al: Combination chemotherapy using L-asparaginase, daunorubicin and cytosine arabinoside in adults with acute myelogenous leukemia. Brit Med J 4:513, 1970.
45. Cutting, HO et al: Inappropriate secretion of antidiuretic hormone secondary to vincristine therapy. Amer J Med 51:269, 1971.
46. Cuttner J et al: Chemoimmunotherapy of acute myelocytic leukemia. Proc Amer Assoc Cancer Res 16:1175, 1975.
47. Dargeon HW: Neuroblastoma. J Pediat 61:456, 1962.
48. De Lorimer AA et al: Neuroblastoma in childhood. Amer J Dis Child 118:441, 1969.
49. Djerassi I: High-dose methotrexate (NSC 740) and citrovorum factor (NSC 3590) rescue: Background and rationale. Cancer Chemother Rep (3)6:3, 1975.
50. Donaldson SS et al: Rhabdomyosarcoma of head and neck in children: Combination treatment by surgery, irradiation and chemotherapy. Cancer 31:26, 1973.
51. Duckett JW et al: Severe cyclophosphamide hemorrhagic cystitis controlled with phenol. J Pediat Surg 8:55, 1973.
52. Duttera MJ et al: Irradiation, methotrexate toxicity, and the treatment of meningeal leukemia. Lancet 2:703, 1973.
53. Elion GB et al: Relationship between metabolic fates and antitumor activities of thiopurines. Cancer Res 23:1207, 1963.
54. Eppinger-Helft M et al: Sequential therapy for induction and maintenance of remission in acute myeloblastic leukemia. Cancer 35:347, 1975.
55. Ernest P et al: Perturbation of generation cycle of human leukemic blast cells by cytostatic therapy in vivo: Effect of corticosteroids. Blood 36:689, 1971.
56. Ernst P et al: Effect of anti-leukemic drugs on cell cycle of human leukemic blast cells in vivo. Acta Med Scand 186:239, 1969.
57. Evans AE et al: Vincristine sulfate and cyclophosphamide for children with metastatic neuroblastoma. JAMA 207:1325, 1969.
58. Evans AR: Congenital neuroblastoma. J Clin Path 18:54, 1965.
59. Evans WE et al: Prognostic factors contributing to and affecting recovery from toxicity associated with high-dose methotrexate. (Abstract) Amer Soc Hosp Pharm, Midyear Clinical Meeting, 1976.
60. Everson TC and Cole WH: Spontaneous Regression of Cancer. WB Saunders Co., Philadelphia, pp 11-87, 1966.
61. Feldman F et al: Acute leukemia relapse after prolonged remission. J Pediatr 76:926, 1970.
62. Fernbach DJ et al: Chemotherapy of acute leukemia in childhood: Comparison of cyclophosphamide and mercaptopurine. NEJM 275:451, 1966.
63. Fine RN et al: Hyponatremia and vincristine therapy. Amer J Dis Child 112:256, 1966.
64. Finklestein JZ et al: Combination chemotherapy for metastatic neuroblastoma. Proc Amer Assoc Cancer Res 15:175, 1974.
65. Finklestein JZ et al: Evaluation of high-dose cyclophosphamide regimen in childhood tumors. Cancer 23:1239, 1969.
66. Fleming I et al: Spleenectomy and chemotherapy in acute myelocytic leukemia of childhood. Cancer 33:427, 1974.
67. Fox RM et al: Orotinuria induced by allopurinol. Science

168:861, 1970.

68. Freeman CB et al: Active immunotherapy used alone for maintenance of patients with acute myeloid leukemia. Brit Med J 4:571,
1973.

69. Frei E et al: Renal complications of neoplastic disease. J Chron
Dis 16:757, 1963.

70. Frei E III et al: Cytokinetic evaluation of the effectiveness of
remission induction treatment in patients with acute leukemia.
Adv Biosci 14:15, 1975.

71. Frei E III et al: Studies of sequential and combination an-
timetabolite therapy in acute leukemia:6-mercaptopurine and
methotrexate, from the acute leukemia group B Blood 18:431,
1961.

72. Freireich EF et al: In The Proliferation and Spread of Neoplastic
Cells. Baltimore, MD, The Williams and Wilkins Company, p 441,
1967.

73. Freireich EJ: Factors influencing patient selection for
chemotherapy studies of acute leukemia. J Chron Dis 15:251,
1962.

74. Freireich EJ et al: The usefullness of multiple pretreatment patient characteristics for prediction of response and survival in
patients with adult acute leukemia. Adv Biosci 14:131, 1975.

75. George P et al: A study of "total therapy" of acute lymphocytic
leukemia in children. J Pediat 72:399, 1968.

76. Ghavimi F et al: Combination therapy in children with embryonal
rhabdomyosarcoma. Proc Amer Assoc Cancer Res 14:54, 1973.

77. Ghavimi F et al: Combination therapy of urogenital embryonal
rhabdomyosarcoma in children. Cancer 32:1178, 1973.

78. Ghavimi F et al: Multidisciplinary treatment of embryonal rhabdomyosarcoma in children. Cancer 35:677, 1975.

79. Gilladoga AC: Cardiac status of 40 children receiving adriamycin
over 495 mg/m^2 and animal studies. Proc Amer Assoc Cancer
Res 15:107, 1974.

80. Gilladoga AC et al: Cardiotoxicity of adriamycin (NSC-123127) in
children. Cancer Chemother Rep Part 3 6:209, 1975.

81. Gitlow SE et al: Biochemical and histologic determinants in the
prognosis of neuroblastoma. Cancer 32:898, 1973.

82. Glatstein E et al: Non-Hodgkin's lymphomas. VI. Results of
treatment in children. Cancer 34:204, 1974.

83. Goldin A et al: The chemotherapy of human and animal acute
leukemia. Cancer Chemother Rep 55:309, 1971.

84. Goldman RL et al: Hemorrhagic cystitis and cytomegalic inclu-
sions in the bladder associated with cyclophosphamide therapy.
Cancer 25:7, 1970.

85. Gottlieb JA et al: Fatal adriamycin cardiomyopathy: Prevention
by dose limitation. Proc Amer Assoc Cancer Res 14:88, 1973.

86. Green AA: Personal Communication, 1976.

87. Green AA et al: The response of neuroblastoma to sequential
low dose cyclophosphamide and adriamycin therapy. Proc Amer
Assoc Cancer Res 17:478, 1976.

88. Green AA et al: Immunological rebound after cessation of long-
term chemotherapy in acute leukemia II. In vitro response to
phytohemagglutin and antigens by peripheral blood and bone
marrow. Blood 42:99, 1973.

89. Grindey GB and Moran RG: Effects of allopurinol on the
therapeutic efficacy of methotrexate. Cancer Res 35:1702, 1975.

90. Grosfeld JL et al: Combined therapy in childhood rhabdomyosarcoma. An analysis of 42 cases. J Pediat Surg 4:637,
1969.

91. Gross RE et al: Neuroblastoma symatheticum; A study and report of 217 cases. Pediatrics 23:179, 1959.

92. Gunz V et al: The therapy of acute granulocytic leukemia in
patients more than fifty years old. Ann Intern Med 80:15, 1974.

93. Gutterman JV et al: Chemoimmunotherapy of adult leukemia.
Prolongation of remission in myeloblastic leukemia with B.C.G.
Lancet 2:7894, 1974.

94. Haggard ME et al: Vincristine in acute leukemia of childhood.
Cancer 22:438, 1968.

95. Haghbin M et al: Treatment of acute lymphoblastic leukemia in
children with "prophylactic" intrathecal methotrexate and intensive systemic chemotherapy. Cancer Res 35:807, 1975.

96. Haghbin M et al: Intensive chemotherapy in children with acute
lymphoblastic leukemia (L-2 Protocol). Cancer 33:1491, 1974.

97. Hardisty RM et al: Vincristine and prednisone for the induction
of remissions in acute childhood leukemia. Brit Med J 2:662,
1969.

98. Hart JS et al: The mechanism of induction of complete remission

in acute myeloblastic leukemia in man. Cancer Res 29:2300,
1969.

99. Haskell CM et al: L-asparaginase therapeutic and toxic effects in
patients with neoplastic disease. NEJM 28:1028, 1969.

100. Henderson ES: Combination chemotherapy of acute lymphocytic leukemia of childhood. Cancer Res 27:2570, 1967.

101. Henderson ES et al: Evidence that drugs in multiple combinations have materially advanced the treatment of human malignancies. Cancer Res 29:2272, 1969.

102. Henderson ES et al: Factors influencing prognosis in adult acute
myelocytic leukemia. Adv Biosciences 14:71, 1975.

103. Heyn RN et al: The role of combined chemotherapy in the treatment of rhabdomyosarcoma in children. Cancer 34:2128, 1974.

104. Holland JF et al: Vincristine treatment of advanced cancer: A
cooperative study of 392 cases. Cancer Res 33:1258, 1973.

105. Holland JF et al: Chemotherapy of acute lymphocytic leukemia
of childhood. Cancer 30:1480, 1972.

106. Holstein P et al: Intravesical hydrostatic pressure treatment:
New method for control of bleeding from the bladder mucosa. J
Urol 109:234, 1973.

107. Holton CP et al: Extended combination therapy of childhood
rhabdomyosarcoma. Cancer 32:1310, 1973.

108. Hryniuk WM: Purineless death as a link between growth rate and
cytotoxicity by methotrexate. Cancer Res 32:1506, 1972.

109. Hughes WT et al: Infectious disease in children with cancer.
Pediat Clin N Amer 21:3, 1974.

110. Jacquillat MW et al: Evaluation of 216 four-year survivors of
acute leukemia. Cancer 32:286, 1973.

111. Jaffe N et al: Adjuvant methotrexate and citrovorum-factor
treatment of osteogenic sarcoma. NEJM 291:994, 1974.

112. Jaffe N et al: Toxicity of high-dose methotrexate and citrovorum
factor in osteogenic sarcoma. Cancer Chemother Rep (3)6:13,
1975.

113. Jaffe N: Neuroblastoma: Review of the literature and an examination of factors contributing to its enigmatic character. Cancer
Treat Reviews 3:61, 1976.

114. Jaffe N et al: Recent advances in the chemotherapy of metastatic
osteogenic sarcoma. Cancer 30:1627, 1972.

115. Jaffe N et al: Rhabdomyosarcoma in children. Improved outlook
with a multidisciplinary approach. Amer J Surg 125:482, 1973.

116. James DH et al: Vincristine in children with malignant solid
tumors. J Pediat 65:534, 1964.

117. Japa J: A study of the mitotic activity of normal human bone
marrow. Brit J Exp Pathol 23:272, 1942.

118. Jayalakshmamma B and Pinkel D: Urinary-bladder toxicity following pelvic irradiation and simultaneous cyclophosphamide
therapy. Cancer 38:701, 1976.

119. Jenkin RDT: The management of malignant lymphoma in childhood. In Malignant Diseases in Children. Edited by TJ Deely,
Buttersworth, London, 1974.

120. Johnson FL et al: Seizures associated with vincristine sulfate
therapy. J Pediat 82:699, 1973.

121. Johnson WW et al: Urinary bladder fibrosis and telangiectasia
associated with long-term cyclophosphamide therapy. NEJM
284:290, 1971.

122. Jones SE et al: Echocardiographic detection of adriamycin heart
disease. Proc Amer Assoc Cancer Res 16:228, 1975.

123. Kaplan HS: Clinical evaluation and radiotherapeutic management of Hodgkin's disease and the malignant lymphomas. NEJM
278:892, 1968.

124. Kay HE et al: Encephalopathy in acute leukemia associated with
methotrexate therapy. Arch Dis Child 47:344, 1972.

125. Kelley WW et al: Allopurinol alteration in pyrimidine metabolism
in man. Science 169:388, 1970.

126. Kinnier, Wilson LM et al: Neuroblastoma, its natural history and
prognosis: A study of 487 cases. Brit Med J 3:301, 1974.

127. Krivit W et al: Induction of remission in acute leukemia of childhood by combination of prednisone and either 6-mercaptopu-
rine or methotrexate. J Pediat 68:965, 1966.

128. Krivit W et al: The need for chemotherapy after prolonged complete remission in acute leukemia of childhood. J Pediat 76:138,
1970.

129. Kumar APM et al: Silver nitrate irrigation to control bladder
hemorrhage in children receiving cancer therapy. J Urol 116:85,
1976.

130. Lala PK et al: A comparison of two markers of cell proliferation
in bone marrow. Acta Haematol (Basel) 31:1, 1964.

131. Lampkin BC et al: Cell kinetics and chemotherapy in acute leukemia. Seminar Hematology 9:211, 1972.

132. Lampkin BC et al: Drug effect in acute leukemia. J Clin Invest 48:1124, 1969.

133. Lampkin BC et al: Synchronization and recruitment in acute leukemia. J Clin Invest 50:2204, 1971.

134. Lampkin BC et al: Manipulation of the mitotic cycle in treatment of acute myeloblastic leukemia. Blood 44:930, 1974.

135. Lane DM et al: Remission induction in childhood leukemia with a second course vincristine and prednisone therapy. Cancer Chemother Rep 54:113, 1970.

136. Lapides J: Treatment of delayed intractable hemorrhagic cystitis following radiation of chemotherapy. J Urol 104:707, 1970.

137. Lawrence HJ et al: Cyclophosphamide-induced hemorrhagic cystitis in children with leukemia. Cancer 36:1572, 1975.

138. Lefrak EA et al: Adriamycin cardiomyopathy. Cancer Chemother Rep (Part 3) 6:203, 1975.

139. Lefrak EA et al: A clinopathologic analysis of adriamycin cardiotoxicity. Cancer 32:302, 1973.

140. Leikin SL et al: The use of combination therapy in leukemia remission. Cancer 24:427, 1969.

141. Leikin SL et al: Varying prednisone dosage in remission induction of previously untreated childhood leukemia. Cancer 21:346, 1968.

142. Lemerle M et al: Lymphosarcoma and reticulum cell sarcoma in children. Retrospective study of 172 cases. Cancer 32:1499, 1973.

143. Levi JA et al: Combination chemotherapy of adult nonlymphoblastic leukemia. Ann Intern Med 76:397, 1972.

144. Levine AS et al: Combination therapy with 6-mercaptopurine and allopurinol during induction and maintenance of remission of acute leukemia in children. Cancer Chemother Rep 53:53, 1969.

145. Liedberg C: Cyclophosphamide hemorrhagic cystitis. Scand J Urol Nephrol 4:183, 1970.

146. Makinen J: Microscopic patterns as a guide to prognosis of neuroblastoma in childhood. Cancer 29:1637, 1972.

147. Marcove RC et al: Osteogenic sarcoma under the age of twenty-one. J Bone Joint Surg 52:42, 1962.

148. Marsh FP et al: Cyclophosphamide necrosis of bladder causing calcification, contracture and reflux, treated by colocystoplasty. Brit J Urol 43:324, 1971.

149. Matthews RN et al: Daunorubicin results in childhood leukemia. Arch Dis Child 47:272, 1972.

150. Mauer AM: Cell kinetics and chemotherapy. Haematologica 60:393, 1975.

151. Mauer AM: Cell kinetics and practical consequences for therapy of acute leukemia. NEJM 293:389, 1975.

152. Mauer AM: Studies of leukemia cell proliferation. I. Reviews in leukemia and lymphomas. In *Advances in Acute Leukemia*. Edited by FJ Cleton, D Crowther, SS Malpas, Amsterdam, North Holland Publishing Company, pp. 69-94, 1974.

153. Mauer AM et al: Effects of chemotherapeutic agents on cell cycle and cellular proliferation: Basic and clinical considerations. Transplan Proc 5:1181, 1973.

154. McWilliams NB et al: Dose dependent vincristine effects. Clin Res 19:494, 1971.

155. Miller DR et al: Additive therapy in the maintenance of remission in acute lymphoblastic leukemia of childhood: The effect of initial leucocyte count. Cancer 34:508, 1974.

156. Minnow RA et al: Adriamycin cardiomyopathy — An overview with determination of risk factors. Cancer Chemother Rep (Part 3) 6:195, 1975.

157. Mott MG et al: Methotrexate meningitis. Lancet 2:656, 1972.

158. Mullins GM: High dose cyclophosphamide therapy in solid tumors. Cancer 36:1950, 1975.

159. Murphy SB: The management of childhood non-Hodgkin's lymphoma. Cancer Treat. Rep. (In press), 1976.

160. Murphy SB et al: A study of childhood non-Hodgkin's lymphoma. Cancer 36:2121, 1975.

161. Murphy SB: Personal Communication, 1976.

162. Nobler MP: Curative radiotherapy in the malignant lymphomas. Cancer 22:752, 1968.

163. O'Connell TX: Cardiac and pulmonary effects of high doses of cyclophosphamide and isophosphamide. Cancer Res 34:1586, 1974.

164. Oettgen HF et al: Toxicity of *E. coli* L-asparaginase in man.

Cancer 25:253, 1970.

165. Ohnuma T et al: *Ervinia carotovora* asparaginase in patients with prior anaphylaxis to asparaginase from *E. coli*. Cancer 30:376, 1972.

166. Pasquinucci G et al: Intrathecal methotrexate. Lancet 1:309, 1970.

167. Perrin JCS et al: Intravenous methotrexate (amethopterin) therapy in the treatment of acute leukemia. Pediatrics 31:833, 1963.

168. Peterson RG et al: Immunological responses to L-asparaginase. J Clin Invest 50:1080, 1971.

169. Pinkel D: Cyclophosphamide in children with cancer. Cancer 15:42, 1967

170. Pinkel D et al: Survival of children with neuroblastoma treated with combination chemotherapy. J Pediatr 73:928, 1968.

171. Pinkel D et al: Drug dosage and remission duration in childhood lymphocytic leukemia. Cancer 27:247, 1971.

172. Pinkel D et al: Non-Hodgkin's lymphoma in children. Br J Cancer 31:298, 1975.

173. Pool TL: Irradiation cystitis: Diagnosis and treatment. Surg Clin North Am 39:947, 1959.

174. Pratt CB et al: Adjuvant multiple drug chemotherapy for osteosarcoma of the extremity. Cancer (In press).

175. Pratt CB: Response of childhood rhabdomyosarcoma to combination chemotherapy. J Pediatr 74:791, 1969.

176. Pratt CB et al: Coordinated treatment of childhood rhabdomyosarcona with surgery, radiotherapy and combination chemotherapy. Cancer Res 32:606, 1972.

177. Pratt CB et al: Combination therapy including vincristine for malignant solid tumors in children. Cancer Chemother Rep 52:489, 1968.

178. Pratt CB et al: Low-dosage asparaginase treatment of childhood acute lymphocytic leukemia. Am J Dis Child 121:406, 1971.

179. Proceedings of the National Cancer Institute Conference on the delayed consequences of cancer therapy: Proven and Potential. Cancer 37:999, 1976.

180. Rieselbach RE et al: Subarachnoid distribution of drugs after lumbar injection. NEJM 267:1273, 1962.

181. Rieselbach RE et al: Uric acid excretion and renal function in the acute hyperuricemia of leukemia. Am J Med 37:872, 1964.

182. Rinehart JJ et al: Adriamycin in 87 patients with osteosarcoma. Cancer Chemother Rep Part 3 6:305, 1975.

183. Rinehart JJ et al: Adriamycin cardiotoxicity in man. Ann Intern Med 81:475, 1974.

184. Rivera G et al: Recurrent childhood lymphocytic leukemia following cessation of therapy. Cancer 37:1679, 1976.

185. Robertson GL et al: Vincristine neurotoxicity and abnormal secretaion of antidiuretic hormone. Arch Intern Med 132:717, 1973.

186. Rosen G et al: Chemotherapy en bloc resection and prosthetic bone replacement in the treatment of osteogenic sarcoma. Cancer 37:1, 1976.

187. Rosen G et al: Osteogenic sarcoma: Sequential chemotherapy in 45 consecutive patients. Proc Am Assoc Cancer Res 16:227, 1975.

188. Rosenthal DS et al: The treatment of acute grulocytic leukemia in adults. NEJM 286:1176, 1972.

189. Rubin P and Casarett GW: Urinary tract: The bladder and ureters. In *Clinical Radiation Pathology*. Philadelphia, WB Saunders Co. Vol 1, 1968.

190. Rundles RW et al: Allopurinol in the treatment of gout. Ann Intern Med 64:229, 1966.

191. Rundles RW et al: Effects of xanthine oxidase inhibitor on thiopurine metabolism, hyperuricemia, and gout. Trans Assoc Am Physicians 76:126, 1963.

192. Saiki JH et al:Paraplegia following intrathecal chemotherapy. Cancer 29:370, 1972.

193. Samuels LD et al: Daunorubicin therapy in advanced neuroblastoma. Cancer 27:831, 1971.

194. Sandler SG et al: Vincristine-induced neuropathy: A clinical study of fifty leukemia patients. Neurology 19:367, 1969.

195. Saunders EF: The effect of L-asparaginase on the nucleic acid metabolism and cell cycle of human leukemia cells. Blood 39:575, 1972.

196. Sawitsky A: Vincristine and cyclophosphamide therapy in generalized neuroblastoma. Am J Dis Child 119:308, 1970.

197. Scarffe JH et al:The relationship between the pretreatment proliferative activity of bone marrow blasts and prognosis in adult

acute myelogenous leukemia. Workshop on clinical usefulness of cell kinetic information for tumor chemotherapy. Oct. 14-15, 1974, Rijswijk, Neth. pp. 84-87.

198. Selawry OS et al: Vincristine treatment of cancer in children. JAMA Med Assoc 183:741, 1963.

199. Sen L and Borella L. Clinical importance of lymphoblasts with T-markers in childhood acute leukemia, NEJM, 293:828, 1975.

200. Shah BC et al: Intraversical instillation of formalin for the management of intractable hematuria. J Urol 110:519, 1973.

201. Shapiro WR et al: Methotrexate distribution in cerebrospinal fluid after intravenous, ventricular and lumbar injections. NEJM 293:161, 1975.

202. Shapiro WR et al: Necrotizing encephalopathy following intraventricular instillation. Arch Neurol 28:96, 1973.

203. Simone JV: Acute lymphocytic leukemia in childhood. Semin Hematol 11:25, 1974.

204. Simone JV: Fatalities during remission of childhood leukemia. Blood 39:759, 1972.

205. Simone JV: Treatment of children with acute lymphocytic leukemia. Adv Pediatr 19:13, 1972.

206. Simone JV et al: "Total Therapy" studies of acute lymphocytic leukemia in children current results and prospects for cure. Cancer 30:1488, 1972.

207. Simone JV et al: Combined modality therapy of acute lymphocytic leukemia. Cancer 35:25, 1975.

208. Simone JV et al: Initial features and prognosis in 363 children with acute lymphocytic leukemia. Cancer 36:2099, 1975.

209. Slater LM et al: Vincristine neurotoxicity with hyponatremia. Cancer 23:122, 1969.

210. Spechter JH et al: Folgen Am Hainbereitenden Und Harnableitenden System Wahrend Cyclophosphamide-therapy. Dtsh Med Wochenchi 90:1458, 1965.

211. Storb RC et al: Cyclophosphamide regimens in Rhesus monkeys with and without marrow infusion. Cancer Res 30:2195, 1970.

212. Stoutenborough KA et al: Cytosine arabinoside vs cyclophosphamide, vincristine, cytosine arabinoside, and prednisone in the treatment of acute non-lymphocytic leukemia in adults. Proc Am Assoc Cancer Res Abstract 16:1150, 1975.

213. Sullivan MP et al: Evaluation of vincristine sulfate and cyclophosphamide chemotherapy for metastatic neuroblastoma. Pediatrics 44:685, 1969.

214. Suskind RM et al: Syndrome of inappropriate secretion of antidiuretic hormone produced by vincristine toxicity (with bioassay of ADH level). J Pediatr 81:90, 1972.

215. Sutow WW and Valeriole F: In Clinical Pediatric Oncology. Sutow, Vietti and Fern bach (Eds) St. Louis: C.V. Mosby Co. 1973.

216. Sutow WW et al: Comparison of survival curves, 1956 versus 1962, in children with Wilms' tumor and neuroblastoma. Pediatrics 45:800, 1970.

217. Sutow WW et al: Daunomycin in the treatment of metastatic neuroblastoma. Cancer Chemother Rep 54:283, 1970.

218. Sutow WW et al: Further experience with multidrug chemotherapy in primary treatment of osteogenic sarcoma. Proc Am Assoc Cancer Res 16:232, 1975.

219. Sutow WW: Prognosis in childhood rhabdomyosarcoma. Cancer 25:1384, 1970.

220. Tan C et al: Daunomycin, an antitumor antibiotic, in the treatment of neoplastic disease. Clinical evaluation with special reference to childhood leukemia. Cancer 20:333, 1967.

221. Tan C et al: Adriamycin — an antitumor antibiotic in the treatment of neoplastic diseases. Cancer 32:9, 1973.

222. Thurman WG et al: Cyclophosphamide therapy for children with neuroblastoma. Cancer Chemother Rep 51:399, 1967.

223. Thurman WG et al: Cyclophosphamide therapy in childhood neuroblastoma. NEJM 270:1336, 1964.

224. Thurman WG and Donaldson MH: In Neoplasia in Childhood, Chicago, Yearbook Medical Publishers 1967.

225. Tsukimoto I et al: Surface markers and prognostic factors in acute lymphoblastic leukemia. NEJM 294:245, 1976.

226. Vietti TJ et al: Vincristine, prednisone and daunomycin in acute leukemia of childhood. Cancer 27:602, 1971.

227. Vietti TJ et al: The response of acute childhood leukemia to an initial and a second course of prednisone. J Pediatr 66:18, 1965.

228. Vogler WR et al: Correlation of cytosine arabinoside-induced increment in growth fraction of leukemic blast cells with clinical response. Cancer 33:603, 1974.

229. Von Hoff DD et al: The incidence of drug related deaths secondary to high dose methotrexate and citrovorum factor administration. Cancer Treat Rep (In press).

230. Wade HE et al: A new L-asparaginase with antitumor activity. Lancet 11:766, 1968.

231. Waiters TR et al: 6-azauridine in combination chemotherapy of childhood acute myelocytic leukemia. Cancer 29:1057, 1972.

232. Walters T et al: Poor prognosis in Negro children with acute lymphocytic leukemia. Cancer 29:210, 1972.

233. Wang J et al: Therapeutic effect and toxicity of adriamycin in patients with neoplastic disease. Cancer 28:837, 1971.

234. Weiss HD et al: Neurotoxicity of commonly used antineoplastic agents (second of two parts). NEJM 291:127, 1974.

235. Wells HG: Occurrence and significance of congenital malignant neoplasms. Arch Pathol 30:535, 1940.

236. Wiernik PH et al: Daunorubicin alone versus daunorubicin, pyrimethamine, cytosine arabinoside and thioquanine for the treatment of acute non lymphocytic leukemia. Cancer Treat. Rep. 60:41, 1976.

237. Wiernik PH et al: A randomized clinical trial of daunorubicin and a combination of prednisone, vincristine, 6-mercaptopurine, and methotrexate in adult acute non-lymphocytic leukemia. Cancer Res 32:2023, 1972.

238. Wiernik PH et al: Factors effecting remission and survival in adult acute non-lymphocytic leukemia (ANLL). Medicine 49:505, 1970.

239. Wilbur JR et al: Drug therapy and irradiation in primary and metastatic osteogenic sarcoma. Proc Am Assoc Cancer Res 15:188, 1974.

240. Wilbur JR: Combination chemotherapy for embryonal rhabdomyosarcoma. Cancer Chemother Rep 58:281, 1974.

241. Wolff JA et al: Prednisone therapy of acute childhood leukemia: Prognosis and duration of response in 330 treated patients. J Pediatr 70:626, 1967.

242. Wollner N et al: Non-Hodgkin's lymphoma in children: Results of treatment with LSA-L2 Protocol. Br J Cancer 31:337, 1975.

243. Wollner N et al: Non-Hodgkin's lymphoma in children.' A comparative study of two modalities of therapy. Cancer 37:123, 1976.

244. Young JL et al: Incidence of malignant tumors in U.S. children. J Pediatr 86:254, 1975.

245. Yu TF et al: Effect of allopurinol on serum and urinary uric acid in primary and secondary gout. Am J Med 37:885, 1964.

246. Zittoun R et al: Prediction of the response to chemotherapy in acute leukemia. Cancer 35:507, 1975.

Chapter 36

General Principles of Antibiotic Therapy

Robert M. Elenbaas
Joel O. Covinsky

with case discussions by
Unamarie Clibon and John K. Siepler

SUBJECT OUTLINE

INTRODUCTION

Since the introduction of the sulfonamides and penicillin into clinical medicine (1935 and 1941 respectively), an ever increasing number of antimicrobial agents have been added to our therapeutic armamentarium. Every day we are confronted (and too often confounded) by advertisements heralding the coming of the latest "wonder drug." Because dramatic cures have been effected by their administration and because they are considered by many practitioners to be essentially innocuous, probably no other single group of pharmacologic agents has been subjected to as much abuse and misuse as have the antibacterials. It is essential, therefore, that one possess a good working knowledge of the basic principles of antibiotic therapy, as well as specific factors affecting the use of these compounds. The literature is replete with discussions concerning the basic principles of antibiotic therapy (83, 84, 88, 129, 244, 245). Rather than unnecessarily duplicating these discussions, the reader is referred to these citations. (S)he should become thoroughly familiar with their contents before continuing with this chapter. The reader is also referred to other chapters for discussions of specific infections *(Endocarditis, Urinary Tract Infections, Tuberculosis, Venereal Diseases).* This chapter will only briefly review selected principles of antibiotic therapy and major discussions will be centered on specific problems in antibiotic therapy. Because the area of antibiotics is so broad, this chapter will depart from the question-answer format of the text to conserve space.

DIAGNOSIS OF BACTERIAL INFECTION

If through the clinical presentation of the patient, it appears that an infectious process exists, all attempts to *isolate and identify* the responsible microorganism should be made. Because many infections respond promptly to empiric administration of one or another of the commonly used antimicrobials, it may appear that sensitivity testing is unnecessary. However, when the diagnosis is uncertain, cases relapse, patients do not respond quickly to therapy, or the disease is severe and fulminating, laboratory assistance is essential and may be life saving. The selective factor involved in the choice of proper antibiotics is the relative sensitivity of the invading bacterium. As the tendency of many bacteria to become resistant to antimicrobials becomes a problem of ever-increasing importance, the selection of the correct antimicrobial agent with the aid of sensitivity testing becomes apparent.

The relationship between the results of *in vitro* sus-

ceptibility tests and response to treatment with an antibiotic is not always direct. The only absolute criterion by which one can judge the efficacy of a given antimicrobial is its effect in a specific patient. The basic limitation of all *in vitro* antimicrobial testing is that one is pitting a pure bacterial culture against an antimicrobial in a neutral environment. Despite this limitation, *in vitro* testing provides a rapid and relatively inexpensive means of determining which antimicrobial agents may be of clinical value and which are not likely to be useful. When tests are conducted carefully, with adequate standardization and control, clinical correlation is surprisingly good, especially with rapidly growing aerobic bacteria; in contrast, testing of acid-fast and anaerobic bacteria is less satisfactory.

The choice of method used to determine bacterial sensitivity largely depends on the facilities available and experience of the laboratory personnel. In any procedure the bacterial population of the inoculum must be standardized. The common *in vitro* methods of testing for bacterial sensitivity (Kirby-Bauer) utilize paper discs impregnated with predetermined quantities of specific antimicrobials (Table 1). The medium used in the petrie dishes can be either infusion or blood agar. For testing susceptibility to sulfonamide drugs, a medium free of para-aminobenzoic acid must be used, such as Mueller-Hinton agar. These discs are placed on the medium containing the organism to be tested and are incubated for 24-48 hours. The antibiotic will diffuse out of the disc into the surrounding medium and zones of bacterial growth inhibition will be formed around the disc containing drugs to which the organism is sensitive. The size of the zone surrounding the disc does not necessarily indicate relative susceptibility of the organisms to the different drugs, since zone size is also affected by factors such as drug con-

Table 1
COMMONLY UTILIZED ANTIMICROBIAL DISC SENSITIVITY CONCENTRATIONS
(mcg)

Ampicillin	10
Carbenicillin	50
Cephalothin	30
Chloramphenicol	30
Clindamycin	2
Colymycin	10
Dicloxacillin	1
Erythromycin	15
Nitrofurantoin	300
Gentamicin	10
Kanamycin	30
Methicillin	5
Nafcillin	1
Nalidixic Acid	30
Penicillin	10
Streptomycin	10
Tetracycline	30
Tobramycin	10

tent of the disc, ability of the agent to diffuse into the medium, and the rate of bacterial growth. Nevertheless, this method of bacterial-sensitivity testing is of practical importance to the clinician in deciding which therapeutic agent to employ (89). This is considered the method of choice for routine-semiquantitative testing. It is relatively inexpensive, rapid, reproducible, and when done properly very reliable. *These sensitivity reports must be interpreted in accordance with the concentration of antibiotic expected at the site of infection,* i.e., in the urinary tract vs. the plasma (216). The discs are generally designed to provide concentrations comparable to those achieved in the plasma. It should be stressed that the level of antimicrobial in the serum is of significance only insofar as it provides a measure of concentration of drug in the tissue (69).

It is sometimes necessary to precisely determine the smallest concentration of a given antimicrobial that will suppress the growth of a patient's organism. This requires serial tube dilutions of the antimicrobial in the culture media, following which all tubes are inoculated with standard suspensions of the test organism. A measure of the susceptibility of the organism to the antimicrobial is manifested by failure of the organism to grow in a given dilution. The least amount of antibiotic resulting in complete inhibition of growth is the end point and is recorded as the *minimum inhibitory concentration* (M.I.C.). (The concentration of antibiotic in the last clear tube is reported as the minimum inhibitory concentration.)

If an organism is sensitive to a concentration less than one half that achievable in blood, it should be considered a sensitive bacterium. If the minimum inhibitory concentration exceeds the achievable blood level, then the bacterium should be considered a resistant strain. While these general guidelines hold, it is important to realize that the dilutions of the antibiotic reflect a serum level at one point in time when in reality antibiotic serum levels are constantly changing. Thus, in using this type of data the laboratory results must be interpreted in light of the specific antibiotics under consideration.

Synergistic or antagonistic combinations of antimicrobials can be evaluated by mixing stock solutions of the agents before diluting. There is some question, however, whether this procedure correlates well with the *in vivo* activity of a combination of antibiotics. It is also possible to determine whether the antibiotic being tested has a bactericidal or bacteriostatic effect in a given concentration by subculturing the tube containing the minimum inhibitory concentration of antimicrobial. In those tubes showing additional growth in thioglycollate broth, a bacteriostatic action is surmised.

Since microorganisms differ quantitatively in their susceptibility to antimicrobials, and patients differ greatly in the rate of absorbing and eliminating drugs, it is sometimes necessary to determine the effectiveness of various dilutions of the patient's own serum against a stock strain of organism. A sample of the patient's serum is normally obtained one hour after the administration of the primary antibiotic being utilized. The goal is to determine the effectiveness of the various dilutions of the combination of the patient's own immune responses and the antibiotic in circulation. Recently, Klastersky (117) reported that peak titers of serum bacteriostatic activity equal to or greater than 1:8 correlated with clinical cure in 80% or more of cases. Since this method requires more time to perform than other sensitivity tests, it is more expensive. Thus, it is generally only utilized for those infectious processes which are more difficult to eliminate, such as bacterial endocarditis.

In life-threatening infections it may not be possible to await the results of bacterial culture and sensitivity (C&S) studies before initiating chemotherapy. In these instances the clinician must make an educated guess as to the responsible organism based on site of infection, specific patient characterisitics (i.e., — age, immunologic integrity, etc.), and microscopic examination of smears obtained from the blood, urine, cerebrospinal fluid (CSF), sputum, etc. Antiobiotic therapy must then be based on the usual sensitivity patterns of the suspected organism (159). Therefore, one must be aware not only of the usual sensitivity patterns of commonly encountered microorganisms (166), but also of specific sensitivity patterns which may exist in given geographical areas or hospitals. It is important to realize that the data gained by studying organisms in one institution may not be totally applicable to infections which originate outside that institution. In general, hospital acquired infections are more often caused by organisms which have been exposed to multiple antibiotics and thus have a higher propensity for resistance. In initiating therapy for any infection, then, it is important to consider where it was acquired. In all cases, samples of exudates or appropriate body fluids must be sent for culture and sensitivity determination prior to the initiation of drug therapy.

HOST FACTORS AFFECTING ANTIBIOTIC USE

It is not sufficient to have identified the infecting organism and its sensitivity pattern when planning the use of antibiotics. One must *always* consider certain patient-specific factors which may affect the selection and dosing of the therapeutic agent (245).

Allergy

In addition to reactions on previous administrations of a given antibacterial agent, one must consider the general "allergic history" of the patient. Individuals with a history of atopy are highly susceptible to the development of hypersensitivity reactions to antimicrobial agents, even if they have never been previously exposed to these compounds (214, 215). One must, therefore, administer antibiotics to these patients with due caution and watch them closely for the first signs of untoward reaction.

Age

The age of the patient being treated must obviously be considered, since it may influence the elimination, route of administration and untoward effects of some antimicrobial agents. The pediatric patient deserves special consideration, because renal function of premature and full-term infants is not fully mature. Although at 2 months of age the renal function of children approaches that of adults, complete maturity is probably not reached until the age of one year (7, 156). The kidney function of the geriatric patient is also frequently decreased, even though serum creatinine and blood urea nitrogen may be within normal limits. (Decreased production of these compounds accounts for the discrepancy.) Weinstein and Dalton (245) have discussed the effects of age and decreased renal function on the use of a number of common antimicrobials, and the reader is referred to that article.

Neonates possess immature levels of enzymes (glucuronyl transferase) responsible for hepatic metabolism of various drugs and endogenous compounds. The association between chloramphenicol or sulfonamide administration to neonates and the subsequent development of kernicterus is well-known (143, 181). (Also see chapter on *Pediatric Therapy.)*

Also well known is the relationship between tetracycline administration to young infants and tooth discoloration. Since the tetracyclines cross the placental barrier and attain significant concentrations in fetal tissues, developing teeth of the embryo may also be affected. This adverse effect may occur if tetracyclines are administered anytime during the last 4 months of pregnancy. Children are susceptible to tetracycline-induced dental injury until age 5-7, at which time formation of the tooth crowns have been completed (250). However, the effect of tetracycline administration on bone development would still have to be considered (85).

Neonates in the first 1-2 days of life and elderly patients (particularly over age 60) suffer from hypo- or achlorhydria (170, 194). Thus, acid labile antibiotics (e.g., penicillin) may be very well absorbed following oral administration in these patients. Although one might expect that the oral administration of penicillin may cure an infection in a very young infant or old adult when it would fail to do so in an older infant or young adult, clinical documentation of this is lacking.

Immunologic status of a patient may vary with age. While admittedly difficult to measure quantitatively, it is likely that the general humoral immune capacity undergoes a sharp rise in infancy, maintains a plateau throughout most of adult life, and gradually declines in later life. The fluctuations influence the need for the variable immunization requirement seen in the extreme age groups and their propensity for developing infection.

Pregnancy

Administration of antimicrobial compounds during pregnancy may hold potential dangers for both patient and fetus. A number of these agents pass the placental barrier, including ampicillin, cephalothin, chloramphenicol, methicillin, oxacillin, penicillin G, streptomycin, sulfonamides and tetracycline (245). Administration of streptomycin at any stage of pregnancy appears to be associated with 8th cranial nerve damage in the fetus (58). The effects of sulfonamide, chloramphenicol and tetracycline upon fetal development or the neonate already have been mentioned. Tetracyclines may have a particularly hazardous effect in pregnant women. Intravenous administration of greater than 2 gm per day to such patients (particularly those with some degree of concurrent renal insufficiency) appears to be associated with an unusually high incidence of fatal, fatty metamorphosis of the liver (146).

Diabetes Mellitus

The intramuscular absorption of penicillin G and, to a lesser extent, sulfisoxazole, is diminished in patients with diabetes mellitus. Peak blood levels of penicillin G in the diabetic population were noted to be only 65-70% those of the normal patients, following an IM dose of 10,000 u/kg (139). Additionally, this peak was delayed in the diabetic group (2 hrs. vs. 1 hr. in the control population). The half-life and degree of protein binding of penicillin G were the same in both groups, but urinary excretion during a given time was diminished in the diabetic patients. This suggested that a decrease in the rate, but not extent, of absorption from the intramuscular site was responsible for the lower blood levels observed. Therefore, when high blood levels of penicillin G (and possibly other antimicrobials) are needed to treat infections in diabetic patients, the drug should be given intravenously (139, 247).

An increasing amount of evidence, based on studies of insulin-deficient patients and experimental animal models, indicates that deficiencies of insulin may impair the ability of granulocytes to perform a number of vital defense functions. In the presence of ketoacidosis, energy dependent granulocytic processes such as chemotaxis (176) and phagocytosis (45) have been shown to be depressed (5). It is speculated that the intracellular killing of ingested microorganisms is dependent upon normal metabolic activity within the granulocyte (120). In the presence of insulin deficiency, several key glycolytic enzymes may be impaired resulting in an inability of leukocytes to generate sufficient high energy phosphate to maintain normal granulocyte function. This probably makes the diabetic patient more susceptible to infection and, when coupled with the increased incidence of neuropathies, provides a favorable setting for ascending infection in the urinary tract.

Host Immunity

One of the most important determinants of the effectiveness of antimicrobial agents is the functional state of the patient's immune response. The immune response against invading organisms depends on the body's recognition of a foreign antigen which stimulates specific lymphocytes. There are two distinct populations of immune responsive cells which are often referred to as the "B" and "T" cells. The immune response which depends on antibody production is mediated by B lymphocytes, which are presumably derived directly from the bone marrow. The B lymphocytes are the precursors of plasma cells, which are the antibody producing cells. The T lymphocyte depends on the thymus for development. They play a vital role in those immune responses in which antibody is *not* required, including delayed hypersensitivity reactions, graft rejections, and action against intracellular pathogens. In the laboratory, it is possible to distinguish B and T cells by their specific cell surface characteristics. On the surface of B cells are immunoglobulin molecules, which are released as antibodies after stimulation by specific antigens (bacteria).

Although T lymphocytes do not themselves produce antibodies, they initiate a critical function triggering the response of B lymphocytes to antigens. Macrophages also seem to participate in some acute reactions either by altering the antigen to make it available for recognition by the T or B cell or by directly affixing the antigen to the lymphocyte surface. Presumably in T and B cooperation, receptors on the surface of the T cell first recognize and then respond to a specific combining site on the surface of an antigen and then aid B cell receptors in reacting with another site on the same antigen (11, 41, 53, 62, 78, 110, 190).

The B lymphocytes of the humoral immune system eliminate foreign invaders by providing the antibody which interacts with the antigenic surface of the bacteria (cell wall). This antigen-antibody complex initiates the complement sequence; which consists of a group of nine proteins (C1 through C9). Antibodies of the IgG or IgM class characteristically are responsible for activation of the complement cascade. It appears that activation of complement fragments on the cell's surface leads to the formation of a functional "hole" in the bacterial cell membrane. The bacteria then loses its ability to maintain osmotic equilibrium and, as water follows solute into the cell, it undergoes osmotic lysis. Additionally, sequential interaction of the complement proteins leads to the production of a variety of biologically reactive materials, some of which possess potent chemotactic properties. These products mediate changes in vascular permeability, attract polymorphonuclear and mononuclear granulocytes into the area of immunologic reaction, and enhance phagocytosis in their function as opsonins; these effects are probably of greater importance than the "bacteriolytic" reaction *per se* (155a).

The complement pathway represents a sequence of reactions that, in general, is initiated by the union of an antigen with an antibody. It has been clear for many years, however, that the body is capable of destroying microorganisms and maintaining host integrity on first challenges with a microorganism. This response must take place before the elaboration of large amounts of specific antibody. In 1954, Pillemer published the results of a series of experiments which indicated that there is a mechanism capable of mediating the bactericidal and opsonic effect of complement but which does not require specific antibodies (191). This mechanism might be important in providing protection for the unimmunized host. Properdin is a serum protein which will react with and activate C3 in the presence of properdin factors A, B, and properdin convertase. While the exact molecular mechanism whereby the properdin system is activated is still under investigation, current evidence indicates the lipopolysaccharide (endotoxin) from gram negative organisms is capable of mediating fixation of the late components of the complement cascade. Thus, the complement cascade can be initiated even in the absence of humoral antibodies (155b).

Whereas complement activation plays a significant role in the humoral immune system in dealing with foreign invaders, the exact mechanism whereby the cellular immune system deals with the various pathogens is unclear. When a T cell is stimulated by a specific antigen, sensitized lymphocytes produce a number of soluble materials termed lymphokins which have areas of biological activities (i.e., macrophage inhibitory factor, macrophage aggravation factor, chemotactic factor, blastogenic factor, lymphotoxin factor, transfer factor, and interferon). Further clarification of the characteristics of these substances is necessary to determine how the many different molecules are produced and which of the various biologic events are induced by the same molecules. While many lymphokines have been described in terms of their activity *in vitro*, the biologic importance of each of these substances *in vivo* remains to be elucidated (61a).

In short, probably the most significant factor affecting the outcome of antimicrobial therapy is the state of the patient's immune system (host defense mechanisms). Patients suffering from immune system deficiencies or suppression secondary to disease or drugs may not respond favorably to appropriate antimicrobial therapy, even when extremely large doses are employed. Whereas pure agammaglobulinemic patients are especially susceptible to extracellular, pyogenic infections (pneumococcus and *Streptococcus*), they can usually cope normally with viral and fungal infections. In contrast, patients with a cellular immune deficiency are particularly prone to infections caused by organisms such as *Mycobacterium tuberculosis, pneumocystis carinni, pseudomonas aeruginosa,* and certain viral infections (i.e.; herpes, varicella, etc.) (61a). Treatment of infection in patients with immunosuppression deserves special consideration. As a rule bactericidal, rather than bacteriostatic, agents should be used. For this reason, agents such as tetracycline, erythromycin, chloramphenicol and the sulfonamides should be avoided if possible.

Hepatic Dysfunction

Available data describing the effect of liver disease on antimicrobial effectiveness or elimination are still quite limited. Several of these drugs are eliminated through the hepatobiliary system in varying degrees (ampicillin; cephalosporins; clindamycin, lincomycin, and tetracyclines). Even though the relationship between their administration and the development of toxicity in patients with liver disease is unclear, their use should be approached with caution.

Chronic chloramphenicol administration to patients with hepatic dysfunction has been observed to result in blood levels 3-16 times that found in normal patients (22). Additionally, the incidence of toxic effects (depression of erythropoiesis) is more frequent in patients with liver disease than in those without.

(Also see chapter on **Disease of the Liver.**)

Renal Dysfunction

A great number of commonly used antibiotic agents are eliminated totally or partially via the kidneys. Therefore renal function not only affects the choice of drug to be given, but may also affect the dose and risk of toxicity. Antibiotic induced nephrotoxicity is discussed later in this chapter.

Several nomograms designed to calculate the proper dosage of antimicrobials in the presence of renal dysfunction have been developed and the topic of antibiotic use in patients with renal insufficiency has been discussed in many papers (15, 60, 61, 101, 104, 106, 130, 146). Unfortunately, space within this chapter does not allow a complete discussion of antibiotic utilization in the presence of renal dysfunction. The reader is referred to the chapter on **Disease of the Kidney** and to the citations noted above. However, dosage consid-

erations of several antibiotics commonly utilized in individuals with renal insufficiency will be discussed here: carbenicillin, kanamycin, gentamicin, and tobramycin. Needless to say, an assessment of the adequacy of renal function must be determined and frequently monitored in patients receiving any of these antibiotic agents.

Carbenicillin: Like the other penicillin derivatives, carbenicillin is eliminated almost completely unchanged by the kidney. Although carbenicillin is not commonly associated with nephrotoxicity, neurological or hematological toxicities appear more likely if drug accumulation occurs in the presence of kidney insufficiency (106). It may, therefore, be necessary to modify the dosage regimen of carbenicillin in such patients. The elimination half-life (t½) of carbenicillin in patients with normal renal and hepatic function is about 1 hour; however, the t½ may prolong to approximately 23 hours in patients with concomitant oliguria and hepatic dysfunction. Hoffman and co-workers (101), following an investigation of carbenicillin pharmacokinetics in 40 patients, proposed the dosage guidelines described in Table 2. Following an initial loading dose of 4 gm, a maintainance dosage regimen may be determined from Table 2.

Kanamycin: The aminoglycoside antibiotics are characterized by a relatively narrow range between therapeutic and toxic serum concentrations. Therapeutic serum levels of kanamycin are between 10-30 mcg/ml; peak concentrations in excess of 30 mcg/ml should be avoided, since the nephro- and ototoxic effects of kanamycin are more likely when drug concentration exceeds this value (106). Careful attention must therefore be given to designing a dosage regimen appropriate for each individual patient; an evaluation of renal function must be the basis for determining this regimen. Several nomograms have been suggested as guides in selecting an appropriate kanamycin dosage regimen (61, 131, 157). All of these treatment schedules utilize serum creatinine as the

Table 2
RECOMMENDED DOSAGE REGIMEN FOR CARBENICILLIN*

Creatinine Clearance (ml/min)	Dosage
>30± hepatic dysfunction	4-5 gm every 4 hours
10-30	2-4 gm every 6-12 hours
<10	2 gm every 12 hours
<10 + hepatic dysfunction	2 gm every 24 hours
Intermittent hemodialysis	Additional 2 gm after each dialysis

*(for extraurinary-tract infections due to *Pseudomonas aeuriginosa*)

FIGURE 1: Estimation of Kanamycin Elimination Half-Life (t½) in Patients with Renal Insufficiency (146)

$$\text{Kanamycin } t\frac{1}{2} \text{ (min.)} = \frac{Vd \times 0.693}{0.6 \times \text{Creatinine clearance}}$$

Where: 0.6 x creatinine clearance = the relationship between kanamycin clearance & creatinine clearance, and

Vd = volume of distribution of kanamycin
= 0.2 x body weight (kg).

FIGURE 2: Nomogram for Determining Gentamicin Dosage in Patients with Renal Insufficiency (104)

1. Select a loading dose in mg/kg (*lean* body weight) to provide the peak serum level desired:

Loading Dose: (mg/kg)	Expected Peak Serum Level After 30 min. IV IV Infusion: (mcg/ml)
2.0	6-8
1.75	5-7
1.5	4-6
1.25	3-5
1.0	2-4

2. Select a maintenance dose (as a percentage of chosen loading dose) to continue peak serum levels indicated above according to patient's creatinine clearance & desired dosing interval:

Percentage of Loading Dose Required for Dosage Interval Selected*

Creatinine Clearance	8 hours	12 hours	24 hours
90	90%	-	-
80	88	-	-
70	84	-	-
60	79	91%	-
50	74	87	-
40	66	80	-
30	57	72	92%
25	51	66	88
20	45	59	83
15	37	50	75
10	29	40	64
7	24	33	55
5	20	28	48
2	14	20	35
0	9	13	25

*Shaded area indicates suggested dosage interval.

only measurement of renal function and estimate the elimination half-life of kanamycin by essentially multiplying the serum creatinine concentration by three. However, serum creatinine concentration is a poor predictor of creatinine clearance unless one also considers that creatinine excretion varies widely with sex, age, and body weight of the patient (113). It has been found that a much more accurate prediction of kanamycin half-life can be made by utilizing creatinine clearance (or an estimate thereof) as an assessment of renal function (146) (Figure 1). The most widely quoted formula (61) recommends administration of 7 mg/kg body weight at an interval equal to three times the elimination half-life. However, in patients with marked renal insufficiency the dosage interval may be so long that extended periods of subtherapeutic serum concentrations may result. Therapeutic, non-toxic serum levels, with less fluctuation in the maximum and minimum concentrations, may be achieved in patients with renal failure by administering an initial kanamycin loading dose of 7 mg/kg and a maintainence dose of 3.5 mg/kg at an interval approximately equal to the elimination t½ (106).

Gentamicin/Tobramycin: Gentamicin is a widely used and effective antibiotic in the management of gram-negative infections. Because it is eliminated almost entirely in unchanged form by the kidney, its administration to patients with renal insufficiency has resulted in drug accumulation and nephro- and ototoxicity (73, 107). These problems can be largely avoided if gentamicin dosage regimens are designed with a consideration of the drug's pharmacokinetics. The therapeutic serum level for gentamicin is generally considered to be between 4-8 mcg/ml; concentrations in excess of 12 mcg/ml should be avoided, since they appear to be associated with a higher incidence of toxicity (106). Several nomograms for determining gentamicin dosage in the presence of renal insufficiency have been described (52, 60, 104, 160). That of Hull and Sarubbi (104) appears to be most reliable in predicting gentamicin serum levels (Figure 2). Consideration of the patient's hematocrit is unnecessary when utilizing this nomogram to determine gentamicin dosage (as has been suggested by others (9, 201), because the minor error introduced by neglecting this parameter is not considered important.

Tobramycin, a newly released aminoglycoside antibiotic, has an antimicrobial spectrum almost identical to that of gentamicin. Additionally, the pharmacokinetic parameters describing tobramycin are quite similar to those of gentamicin; therapeutic and peak serum levels, elimination half-life and renal clearance are essentially identical (144). The elimination of both drugs is affected equally by changes in renal function (144). It appears, therefore, that those methods previously described for determining gentamicin dosage can be directly applied to the use of tobramycin.

Amikacin: Amikacin, a chemical derivative of kanamycin, is another new aminoglycoside agent similar in its antibacterial spectrum to kanamycin and gentamicin and very similar to kanamycin in its pharmacokinetic properties (47). Like the other aminoglycosides, its dosage must be modified in the presence of renal insufficiency; unfortunately, data describing the pharmacokinetics of amikacin in patients with decreased kidney function is sparse. Manufacturer recommendations for amikacin administration to such patients is based on the work of Sarubbi and Hull (not yet published at the time of this writing) (38) (Figure 3). Because the pharmacokinetics of kanamycin and amikacin appear so similar, one might expect that the nomogram pictured in Figure 3 could be utilized for kanamycin as well.

FIGURE 3: Amikacin Dosage in Patients with Renal Insufficiency. (38)

1. Select a loading dose in mg/kg (*lean* body weight) to provide the peak serum level desired:

Loading Dose:	Expected Peak Serum Level:
7.5 mg/Kg	20-30 mcg/ml
4 mg/Kg	10-20 mcg/ml

2. Select a maintenance dose (as a percentage of chosen loading dose) to continue peak serum levels indicated above according to patient's creatinine clearance & desired dosing interval:

Percentage of Loading Dose Required
For Dosage Interval Selected*

Creatinine Clearance (ml/min)	12 hours	24 hours
80	91%	-
70	88	-
60	84	-
50	79	-
40	72	92%
30	63	86
25	57	81
20	50	75
17	46	70
15	42	67
12	37	61
10	34	56
7	28	47
5	23	41
2	16	30
0	11	21

* Shaded area indicates suggested dosage interval

Neorological Disorders

The presence of neurologic disease, most notably epilepsy and myasthenia gravis, may increase the susceptibility of such patients to the development of neurological toxicities from some antibiotic agents. Very large doses of penicillin G have been associated with the occurence of twitching, somnolence, coma, myoclonic jerks, hyper-reflexia and seizures (183). Central nervous system (CNS) toxicities of penicillin G are typically observed with continuous intravenous administration of greater than 60,000,000 units per day. The presence of renal dysfunction and underlying brain disease are predisposing factors to the development of such toxicities.

Patients with myasthenia gravis may experience an exacerbation of their disease, with extreme generalized muscle weakness and even respiratory arrest, when given streptomycin, kanamycin, gentamicin, neomycin, polymyxin or colistin, which possess a curare-like activity. Other neurological toxicities of antimicrobial compounds are discussed elsewhere in this chapter.

ALLERGIC REACTIONS TO ANTIMICROBIAL THERAPY

Allergic reactions to antimicrobial agents are probably the primary factor limiting their effective use. Welch (248) reported 809 cases of adverse reactions to antibiotics. Of these, approximately 10% were fatal and 793 (98%) were caused by penicillin. However, this work was reported in 1957 before many of our currently used agents were available. Ten percent of all adverse drug reactions are caused by penicillin, and it is the most common cause of anaphylactoid reactions (249).

Penicillin Allergy

The subject of penicillin allergy will be reviewed principally because the mechanisms and terminology discussed also apply to other antibiotics and drug-induced allergic reactions. Allergic reactions to penicillin are estimated to occur in 2-5% of the general population; approximately 10% of patients who have **previously** been exposed to penicillin will experience an allergic reaction (193). Thus, the chance of a patient developing such a reaction to a given course of penicil-

Table 3
INCIDENCE OF PENCILLIN ALLERGY
VS ROUTE OF ADMINISTRATION

Drug/Route of Administration	Approximate Incidence of Allergic Reactions
Procaine Penicillin G: IM	5%
Aqueous Penicillin G: IM, IV	2.5%
Penicillin G: PO	0.3%

lin increases 2-5 times if(s)he has previously received the drug. Additionally, patients with a history of hives, asthma, hay fever, eczema and other drug sensitivities are more likely to experience severe, anaphylactoid reactions to penicillin. The importance of accurately determining a patient's history of previous allergic reactions or exposures to penicillin (including preparation and route of administration) becomes obvious. Penicilin preparations given by the parenteral route are associated with a higher incidence of sensitivity reactions than are oral or topical preparations (Table 3) (151).

Types of Allergic Reactions

Allergic (hypersensitivity) reactions may be divided into three groups, depending on their characteristics and mechanism of production (Table 4).

Immediate reactions generally occur within twenty minutes following administration of the drug. The onset of the reaction is often heralded by itching of the palms or axilla, apprehension, generalized weakness, coughing, sneezing, shortness of breath, or an unexplained rise in body temperature. The allergic reaction may be manifested only by flushing, generalized pruritis or urticaria. However, it may also be anaphylactoid in nature and include vascular collapse, shock, cardiac arrest, bronchospasm, laryngeal edema, respiratory depression or arrest. MacFarlane and McCarron (149) have attempted to clarify the definitions of "anaphylaxis," "anaphylactic shock," and "anaphylactoid reaction": *Anaphlactic shock* (synonym — anaphylaxis) is an immediate hypersensitivity-type adverse drug reaction which occurs within the first hour, usually within a few minutes, after the administration of a drug and is characterized by the sudden onset of *shock or cardiac arrest*, respiratory distress, and/or loss of consciousness. It is frequently accompanied by allergic manifestations in the skin. An *anaphylactoid reaction* is an immediate hypersensitivity-type adverse drug reaction which occurs within the first hour (usually within a few minutes) after the administration of a drug and is characterized by the sudden onset of respiratory distress and/or loss of consciousness. It is frequently accompanied by allergic manifestations in the skin. The World Health Organization has estimated that an anaphylactoid reaction or anaphlaxis occurs in approximately ten of every 10^6 penicillin injections and that 1/10 of these reactions are fatal. Between 90 and 115 deaths due to severe allergic reactions to penicillin occur yearly (243).

Accelerated reactions have their onset from 30 minutes to 48 hours after the administration of the causative agent. Many of the characteristics of an accelerated reaction are similar to those of an immediate reaction; however, the former are usually less severe and only occasionally include hypotension or laryngeal edema. Erythema, with or without fever, and urticaria are the most common manifestations.

Most allergic penicillin reactions are *delayed* in nature, and develop days, and occasionally even weeks, after the use of the drug. Reactions involving the skin and mucous membranes are the most common of all penicillin reactions and include erythema, urticaria, vesicular or bullous eruptions, and exfoliative dermatitis. Unfortunately, the exact incidence with which penicillin (or any other antimicrobial) produces these reactions is not known (24).

Mechanisms of Penicillin Allergy

The mechanisms of penicillin-induced allergic reactions have received considerable attention. It is generally agreed that compounds of low molecular weight are able to induce antibody formation only when attached to larger protein molecules. Most drugs (penicillin included) function as *haptens* and must irreversibly bind to protein macromolecules before they can be recognized by the immunologic system. The penicillin molecule itself is unable to form irreversible, covalent bonds and is thus not able to function as a hapten. However, many of the penicillin degradation products are able to form such bonds; these compounds are now considered to be the responsible haptenic determinants.

A variety of compounds have been implicated as the agents responsible for the development of penicillin allergy. The presence of a *macromolecular impurity* in commercial benzylpenicillin, ampicillin, cephalothin and cephaloridine has been demonstrated (11, 219). These substances are non-dialyzable, devoid of an-

Table 4
CLASSIFICATION OF ALLERGIC REACTIONS TO PENICILLIN

Modified from Ibister (105)

Immediate Reaction (developing within 2-20 minutes)
  Hypotension
  Diffuse urticaria
  Asthma
  Rhinitis
  Laryngeal edema

Accelerated Reaction (developing within 30 minutes 48 hours)
  Urticaria
  Laryngeal edema (occasionally)

Delayed Reaction (developing after 3 days)
  Skin rashes (erythema, urticaria, pruritis, angio-edema, bullous eruptions, exfoliative dermatitis, morbilliform, purpura, Stevens-Johnson syndrome, fixed drug eruption, contact dermatitis)

Hemolytic anemia	Allergic angiitis
Neutropenia	Fever
Thrombocytopenia	Lupoid hepatitis
Serum sickness	Nephropathy
Lupus-like syndrome	Loeffler's syndrome

tibacterial properties and are not polymers of penicillin or its degradation products. It is believed that these impurities result during the manufacturing process of penicillin G and are retained during fractionation and isolation processes. There is some evidence that purification of these products reduces the incidence of penicillin reactions (219), and it has been suggested that digestion of these compounds partially explains the lower incidence of allergic reactions associated with oral penicillin therapy (105). However these impurities are not totally responsible for the development of allergic reactions, and other compounds have been implicated.

Several *degradation products of benzylpenicillin* are capable of acting as haptens (Figure 4). The penicilloyl group has received considerable attention. It accounts for about 95% of the penicillin degradation products and thus has been named the "*major determinant.*" This name carries with it the unfortunate connotation that penicilloyl (also called benzylpenicilloyl; BPO) is the primary antigen involved in the production of allergic reactions. In actuality, penicilloyl does not appear to be responsible for immediate, life-threatening allergic reactions which are of primary concern to the clinician, although it is the mediator of accelerated urticarial reactions (Green, 1971). Penicillin G also combines with protein to form other antigenic determinants. Only because these determinants are formed to a lesser degree *in vitro,* they have been called the "minor determinants" (236). The **minor antigenic determinants** have not been well-identified. However, they are postulated to result from degradation products such as penicilloic acid, penicillenic acid, penicillenic disulfide, penamaldic acid, and penicillamine and are closely related to the production of anaphylaxis (116). All of these compounds have been observed in aqueous penicillin solutions upon storage and can be produced *in vivo* after parenteral administration of penicillin (105). Because penicillenic acid is both a minor determinant and may give rise to major determinant (penicilloyl), it has been proposed that the immunogenicity of various penicillin derivatives is related to their ability to form penicillenic acid (76). The role of major and minor determinants in skin testing for penicillin allergy is discussed below

Antibodies to Penicillin

Antibodies to penicillin antigenic determinants have been demonstrated in all five classes of immunoglobulins (IgG, IgA, IgD, IgM, IgE). Antipenicillin antibodies can be demonstrated in almost every patient who receives penicillin therapy. Penicilloyl-specific antibody production represents a natural immune response to penicillin but does not necessarily indicate a clinical allergy. These antibodies generally belong to the IgM or IgG classes. Formation of IgA and IgD antibodies have been demonstrated, but their role, if any, in the production of penicillin hypersensitivity has not been established. Antibodies belonging to the IgE class appear to be the most important mediators of penicillin hypersensitivity. Skin sensitization is caused by IgE antibodies which also mediate anaphylactic reactions. It is important to note that this group of antibodies may be detected by a wheal and flare reaction on direct skin testing (213).

Reaginic antibodies (IgE) to the minor antigenic determinants (and occasionally penicilloyl) have been demonstrated in immediate anaphylactic reactions. Delayed urticarial reactions seem to be related to IgE antibodies with penicilloyl specificity. Although the role of IgG and IgM antibodies in penicillin hypersensitivity is uncertain, IgG is able to perform as a "blocking antibody." That is, it may inhibit the formation of penicillin-IgE complexes depending on whether the IgG and IgE have identical specificities. If IgG combines with the penicillin antigenic determinant, it will not couple with IgE, and the allergic reaction will be blocked. However, because IgG tends to be penicilloyl-specific while IgE generally has an affinity for a wider range of antigens, penicillin allergy may persist in the presence of high titers of IgG (105, 220).

Despite the fact that IgG may function as a blocking antibody and inhibit IgE mediated reactions, it may also be responsible for the production of some allergic reactions. There is evidence that gamma-G antibodies may be responsible for the various penicillin-induced "cytopenias," including hemolytic anemia (18), in which circulating antibodies are directed against cell-fixed antigenic determinants. Additionally, penicilloyl-specific IgG may be responsible for the interstitial nephritis occasionally associated with methicillin and other penicillin administration (91). Furthermore, IgG, and possibly IgM, has been implicated in the production of some morbilliform skin eruptions (79). Most delayed maculopapular eruptions, however, appear to be mediated via cellular immunity (105). As one can easily ascertain from the above discussion, much remains to be elucidated regarding the

FIGURE 4:
THE DEGRADATION OF PENICILLIN (193)

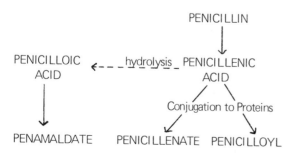

mechanisms of penicillin hypersensitivity and its various manifestations.

The Value of Skin Testing

Skin testing individuals with a past history of penicillin hypersensitivity to determine the relative risk of administering penicillin is currently receiving considerable attention. The simplest means of reducing the frequency of reactions to antibiotics (and to all medications for that matter) would, of course, be to prescribe them only when definitely indicated and to administer them only for the proper duration and by the proper route (58). Also, the importance of an accurate, thorough drug history cannot be overemphasized. The pharmacist's role in both of these areas is obvious.

Penicilloyl-polylysine (PPL) and minor determinant mixture (MDM) appear to offer the most promise as skin testing reagents in screening for patients likely to have immediate anaphylactic reactions to penicillin (1, 141). PPL is a conjugate of benzylpenicilloyl attached to a polylysine chain. The MDM generally contains benzylpenicillin and its derivatives sodium benzylpenicilloate and sodium benzylpenilloate. Patients with a history of penicillin allergy are scratch tested with MDM. The test is considered positive if erythema greater than 5 mm or a wheal greater than 3 mm develops within 5 minutes. If the scratch test is positive, no further testing is necessary. If, however, it is negative, intradermal injections of 0.02 ml of PPL and 0.02 ml of MDM should be placed on the forearm. The tests are read after 15 minutes; a wheal of 5 mm or greater in size is considered a positive reaction. Using this technique, Adkinson and associates (1) found that they could markedly decrease the incidence of penicillin reactions. They adminis-

Table 5
TEST FOR ALLERGY TO PENICILLIN AND RELATED ANTIBIOTICS

Adapted from Stewart (220)

TEST	ANTIBODY	SPECIFICITY
PPL; MDM	Cell fixed IgE	Penicilloyl; penicillenate; dimeric & polymeric conjugates; minor determinants; ampicillin dimers
Passive cutaneous anaphylaxis	Circultaing IgE	Same as PPL/MDM; Cephalosporoyl
Hemagglutination	IgG & IgM	Penicilloyl, cephalosporoyl
Direct Coomb's	Immunoglobulins	Nil
Indirect Coomb's	Immunoglobulins	Uncertain
Basophil degranulation	Cellular	?Penicilloyl
Lymphocyte transformation	Cellular	Penicilloyl, cephalosporoyl
Histamine-release from tissue	Cellular	Uncertain
Radio-isotope	IgG	Penicilloyl
Bacteriophage reduction	IgG, IgM, IgE	Penicilloyl

tered the skin testing materials to 218 patients, 66 of which gave positive histories of penicillin allergy, without any adverse incidents. Fifty of the "penicillin allergic" patients had negative skin tests to both PPL and MDM; of those challenged with penicillin therapy (46), none experienced adverse allergic reactions. Sixteen patients had positive responses to skin tests; only one subsequently received penicillin, and she experienced a mild accelerated urticarial reaction within 12 hours of therapy. Those patients with negative histories of penicillin allergy and non-reactive skin tests all tolerated penicillin administration without incident. The authors conclude that the routine use of PPL and MDM is a practical, safe, and useful method of predicting and preventing penicillin reactions.

Levine and Zolov (141) reported similar results in 218 patients with acceptable histories of penicillin allergy. They found that a negative reaction to both PPL and MDM almost completely excluded the possibility of an immediate anaphylactic reaction and markedly reduced the likelihood of an accelerated urticarial reaction. They subsequently treated 185 skin-test-negative patients without observing any notable hypersensitivity reactions.

Benzylpencilloyl-polylysine (BPL; PPL) is now commercially available as an aid in the detection of penicillin allergy (Pre-Pen); unfortunately, a minor determinant mixture is not yet available. Patients demonstrating a positive reaction to PPL alone are very likely to have an allergic reaction when administered therapeutic doses of penicillin. However, a negative reaction to PPL alone does not exclude the possibility of an immediate life-threatening anaphylactic reaction (165). Approximately 80% of positive reactors when tested with both PPL and MDM can be detected by administering only PPL (1,141). Although testing with PPL alone would thus identify the majority of individuals likely to suffer an immediate or accelerated allergic reaction, the number of "false negative" reactors is quite high. A solution of aqueous penicillin G can be used as a substitute for minor determinant mixture and, when combined with PPL, provides a more accurate skin-testing procedure than using PPL alone (186). When utilized in this way, skin-testing with aqueous penicillin G should first be performed by scratch using a concentration of 5 units per milliliter; if negative after 20 minutes, a second scratch test utilizing a solution of 10,000 units/ml should be performed. If this is also negative, a final test using a solution of 10,000 units/ml is carried out by intradermally injecting enough solution to raise a tiny blister (165).

It should be emphasized, however, that current skin testing procedures are not reliable in predicting late allergic reactions such as morbilliform rashes, serum sickness, etc. At present, those tests capable of determining cellular and delayed hypersensitivity are not readily applicable to the clinical situation (Table 5).

Treatment of Allergic Reactions

The treatment of an allergic reaction to an antibiotic, or any other drug, is obviously dependent on the type of reaction. Fortunately most hypersensitivity reactions to penicillins and other antibiotics consist only of urticarial, erythematous or morbilliform (maculopapular) eruptions. These reactions are rarely life-threatening (although occasionally erythema nodosum, erythema multiforme, or widespread vesiculobullous eruptions may occur) and may be treated by discontinuing the suspected causative agent; antihistamines may provide symptomatic relief, but corticosteroids are rarely indicated. Because patients are frequently receiving multiple drugs it may often be difficult to identify the responsible agent. Levine (140) has suggested the use of PPL and MDM skin testing procedures for the diagnosis of penicillin allergy. Almost all patients experiencing penicillin-induced urticarial reactions (whether immediate, accelerated or delayed) will have positive skin tests to these reagents when administered 4-6 days after penicillin therapy is discontinued. If both tests are negative, penicillin allergy cannot be completely ruled out, but a nonpenicillin etiology is strongly favored. One must, of course, examine the clinical setting for other causative factors. The primary reason for misdiagnosing "penicillin allergy" in children is viral exanthema (63). Many children treated with penicillin for malaise and upper respiratory symptoms in the prodromal phase of a viral exanthema are subsequently falsely labeled as having an allergic reaction to penicillin. This emphasizes the importance of administering antimicrobial agents only when clearly indicated. Additionally, a number of infectious diseases (meningococcus meningitis, disseminated gonorrhea) are frequently associated with cutaneous manifestations.

For more severe reactions (severe serum sickness or anaphylaxis), therapeutic intervention will be necessary. The following regimen has been suggested for the management of severe serum sickness reactions (116): (a) discontinue the causative agent; (b) salicylates, if needed, for joint symptoms; (c) diphenhydramine 25-50 mg four times daily for sedation and relief of itching; (d) local lotions (calamine) and soothing baths (Aveeno) to relieve pruritis; (e) prednisone 40 mg/day with gradual withdrawal only if symptoms are very severe; (f) epinephrine 0.2-0.4 mg subcutaneously if rapidly developing wheals and pruritis accompany the reaction.

Immediate anaphylactic reactions represent a life-threatening situation and must be dealt with correctly and promptly. Epinephrine, 0.3-1.0 mg administered subcutaneously, is the drug of choice and may be repeated every 5-15 minutes as indicated. If profound cardiovascular collapse exists, a 1:10,000 dilution may have to be given intravenously to assure accurate and prompt delivery. Corticosteroids and antihistamines do not appear to offer a great deal to the treatment of an immediate reaction but may be useful in accelerated or delayed reactions. If marked hypotension is present, vigorous resuscitation with intravenous normal saline is indicated. General supportive measures such as securing a patent airway and administering oxygen are not to be overlooked (116, 193). The treatment of allergic reactions such as hemolytic anemia or interstitial nephritis is primarily supportive (transfusion, dialysis, etc.).

In some patients experiencing allergic reactions to penicillins and other antibiotics, continued administration of the antimicrobial agent, though undesirable, may be indicated. With rare exception, one should select a suitable alternate agent to which the infecting organism is sensitive. However, care must be taken to select an agent from a different chemical group and preferably one to which cross-sensitivity with the original drug has not been demonstrated. The Medical Letter on Drugs and Therapeutics, *Handbook of Antimicrobial Therapy*, (166) is an excellent source to consult if one is unsure of the most appropriate alternate agent to select.

In cases of infective endocarditis where penicillin G is the drug of choice, the clinician may wish to either desensitize (which involves the production of blocking antibodies — IgG) or concomitantly administer steroids and antihistamines to the penicillin-allergic patient (See chapter on **Endocarditis**). However, Kasik and Thompson (116) have recommended that desensitization or the use of steroids be attempted only on the rarest occasions when an alternate drug is unfeasible or has been used without success.

Cephalosporins in the Penicillin-Allergic Patient

Based solely on microbiologic grounds, the cephalosporins often appear to be the alternate drugs of choice in penicillin allergic patients. However, one may not always be able to indiscriminately administer cephalosporins to such patients because of cross-sensitivity between penicillin and cephalothin or its derivatives. Although the evidence is confusing, the problem of cross-sensitivity does seem to be real.

Penicillin and the cephalosporins share a common beta-lactam structure. It has been proposed and substantiated that the cephalosporins are capable of forming a protein (cephalosporonyl) conjugate analogous to the penicilloyl haptenic determinants formed by penicillin (35, 75). It is unclear whether the cephalosporins form "minor determinants" in a manner similar to the penicillins; however, Levine (142) has presented indirect evidence that minor determinants of cephalothin may be involved in producing immediate reactions.

In 54 patients, 14 of which gave histories of penicillin

allergy, a total of 7 experienced allergic reactions to cephalothin; 5 of these patients were among those with penicillin-allergic histories. The investigators observed two anaphylactic reactions, both of which occurred in the penicillin-allergic patients. One occurred within 30 seconds and the other within one day of cephalothin therapy (228).

In another report, 9/22 patients with histories of penicillin allergy experienced hypersensitivity reactions to cephalothin, in contrast to 5/43 patients without histories of penicillin allergy. No immediate or accelerated reactions were observed. The difference in incidence of allergic reactions may be interpreted either as evidence of cross-sensitivity between penicillin and cephalothin, or as evidence that penicillin-allergic (atopic) individuals are more likely to develop sensitivity reactions to other drugs than are nonpenicillin-allergic (nonatopic) individuals.

Insufficient evidence exists to determine the incidence of allergic reactions to the other cephalosporins such as cephaloridine, cephalexin, cephazolin, or cephapirin, much less the frequency with which they cross-react with penicillin. Seven of 149 patients (4%) receiving cephaloridine in one study experienced hypersensitivity skin eruptions (37). Even though the evidence is inconclusive, one must use caution in administering cephalosporins to patients reporting histories of penicillin allergy. The decision to administer a cephalosporin to such a patient must be based, to a large extent, on the type of allergic reaction the patient experienced and the availability of other suitable alternatives. A patient who experienced an immediate or accelerated reaction to penicillin, or a penicillin-induced hemolytic anemia or nephritis, should not receive a cephalosporin antibiotic. Unfortunately, the decision is not as clear clear cut in the patient who suffered only a mild morbilliform eruption. If a cephalosporin is prescribed, appropriate measures to deal with an immediate reaction should be available.

Ampicillin Rash

Ampicillin rash deserves special consideration because of its frequent occurrence and somewhat atypical characteristics. Adverse cutaneous reactions to ampicillin have been succinctly summarized by Almeyda and Levantine (3) and have been the subject of several prospective studies involving a very large number of patients (10, 20, 56, 211). The overall incidence of rash in patients receiving ampicillin has been reported to be from 4-22% (20). However, the incidence is probably closer to 7% in patients without complicating factors (see below). Shapiro (211) found that the incidence of rash secondary to ampicillin administration in 422 patients was 7.7%, while only 2.7% of 622 patients receiving other penicillins developed rash. The route of administration does not seem to affect the incidence of rash in ampicillin-treated patients; oral administration of the other penicillins does, however, appear to be associated with a significantly lower frequency of rash than the parenteral route (20,211). There is also some indication that ampicillin induced rash may be directly related to dosage (4, 20).

Two main types of rash are commonly reported following ampicillin therapy. An **urticarial eruption,** which is similar to the rash associated with penicillin hypersensitivity, accounts for approximately 1/3 of ampicillin-induced eruptions and is thought to be a true hypersensitivity reaction. It may appear soon after the onset of treatment or may be delayed for as long as 3 weeks. Urticaria may occur independently or in conjunction with angioneurotic edema or a serum sickness syndrome. Although ampicillin-induced urticaria may be associated with positive PPL and MDM skin tests, anaphylaxis to ampicillin is relatively rare (3). Knudsen (125) has estimated that the incidences of ampicillin and penicillin-induced urticaria are not significantly different.

More commonly, ampicillin produces a characteristically erythematous, dull red, macular or maculopapular, mildly pruritic rash. It typically begins on the extensor aspects of the limbs, is accentuated over the knees and elbows, and eventually spreads in a symmetrical pattern to most parts of the body. This maculopapular rash accounts for approximately two-thirds of the ampicillin-induced eruptions. The rash develops after 5-14 days of treatment, although it may occasionally appear during the first day. It may develop after ampicillin administration has been discontinued. Mild eruptions generally subside 2-3 days after ampicillin is discontinued but may persist for a week or more in some cases (3). The mechanism of this **ampicillin rash** remains to be elucidated. There is growing evidence that it is not allergic in origin (20, 59) and that patients experiencing such an eruption should not be labeled as penicillin-allergic. Indeed, the typical "ampicillin rash," in itself, is not an absolute contraindication to subsequent treatment with ampicillin or any other penicillin (56). In an attempt to determine if the incidence of ampicillin rash was related to the commercial preparation administered, the Boston Collaborative Drug Surveillance Program (31) designed a prospective study involving 482 patients. They could discern no significant difference between the two preparations studied (Principen and Polycillin). However, Knudsen and associates (126) administered a commercially available ampicillin to 1077 patients and a "purified" preparation to another 1068. They found that macromolecular impurities (analogous to those described for penicillin) could be removed from the ampicillin preparation and that this resulted in a decrease in the incidence of rash by almost 50%. Unfortunately, such purified preparations are not commercially available in

Table 6
ANTIMOCROBIAL AGENTS ASSOCIATED WITH RENAL COMPLICATIONS (93)

Major Direct Nephrotoxicity

Amphotericin	Kanamycin
Bacitracin	Neomycin
Cephaloridine	Polymyxin B
Colistin	Vancomycin

Minor Direct Nephrotoxicity

Capreomycin *	Rifampin *
Cephalothin *	Streptomycin
Gentamicin	Sulfonamides

Hypersensitivity

Nitrofurantoin	PASA
Penicillin & derivatives	Sulfonamides

Anti-anabolic

Tetracyclines. **Doxycycline & Minocycline excepted.

* May cause rise in BUN without other evidence of nephrotoxicity

** May cause rise in BUN without other evidence of nephrotoxicity, Outdated tetracycline may produce Fanconi-like syndrome.

the United States.

A number of factors appear to influence the incidence of maculopapular ampicillin rash. Most notable among these is the association between *infectious mononucleosis* and the development of the typical ampicillin rash. A 100% incidence of ampicillin rash was first recorded by Patel (188) in 13 patients with infectious mononucleosis treated with the antibiotic for actual or suspected secondary infections. In contrast, only 9% of patients receiving no antibiotic, and 14% of patients receiving either penicillin G, cloxacillin, or tetracycline developed rash. Two other groups (164, 198) subsequently reported incidences of ampicillin rash of 95% and 69% respectively in patients with mononucleosis. Weary and associates (242) summarized the above three reports and concluded that skin eruptions developed in 14% of patients receiving no antibiotics, 28% of patients administered penicillin or tetracycline, and 84% of patients given ampicillin. They noted that, in contrast to the rash which spontaneously occurs in some patients with infectious mononucleosis, the ampicillin-induced eruption generally occurred later in the course of the illness, was usually more severe and somewhat more extensive, was of somewhat longer duration, and had a greater tendency to involve light-exposed areas, pressure points, and the palms and soles. The mechanism of this increased incidence of ampicillin rash is unclear. Mononucleosis (a disease characterized by the presence of atypical lymphocytes and antibodies) in some way renders patients hypersensitive to ampicillin. Cytomegalo-virus mononucleosis, a condition similar to EB-virus infectious mononucleosis but without tonsillitis or lymphadenitis and a negative heterophile agglutination test, has also been associated with a markedly increased incidence of ampicillin rash (123).

The Boston Collaborative Drug Surveillance Program (27) reported an apparently increased incidence of rash in patients receiving both ampicillin and *allopurinol.* They observed a 2.1% incidence of rash in patients receiving allopurinol alone, while 22.4% of patients administered both medications developed eruptions. However, data on serum uric acid levels was not available to these investigators, making it impossible to determine if the increased incidence of rash was due to an interaction of ampicillin with allopurinol, hyperuricemia, or both. An altered immunologic state of hyper-reactivity has been noted in *hyperuricemic* patients. Through retrospective questioning of hyper- and normouricemic individuals, 14.1% of patients with increased uric acid levels reported histories of penicillin allergy as compared to only 4.9% of normouricemic, control patients (80). Unfortunately, this report did not specifically distinguish between ampicillin and the other penicillins. Although inconclusive, this report lends some support to the belief that the increased frequency of rash is due to hyperuricemia rather than allopurinol alone. Pending further clarification, clinicians should be prudent in the administration of ampicillin to hyperuricemic patients, especially those receiving allopurinol.

Approximately 85% (10/12) of patients with *lymphatic leukemia* administered ampicillin also developed the typical ampicillin rash (49). It is interesting that all three disease states mentioned (infectious mononucleosis, hyperuricemia, leukemia) are accompanied by disturbances in immunologic reactivity and by increases in the incidence of ampicillin rash.

NEPHROTOXICITY

Several of the antibiotics most valuable in the treatment of infectious diseases have the unfortunate potential of producing *nephrotoxicity* (Table 6). However, if administration is discontinued as soon as the adverse effects are identified, the renal lesions are largely reversible. Therefore, renal function must be regularly monitored when patients receive any of the agents listed below. Pre-existing renal disease, dehydration, or the concomitant administration of other nephrotoxic drugs renders the individual more sensitive to the nephrotoxic effects of agents such as kanamycin, gentamicin, polymyxin B, etc. Since patients with severe renal disease should not be denied the potential life-saving effects of these drugs if indicated, their doses should be altered appropriately. The concomitant administration of two or more potentially nephrotoxic drugs should be avoided if possible; if they must be used concurrently, extreme caution should be exercised and the patient monitored closely (237). Since proteinuria frequently marks the onset of renal toxicity, patients receiving these drugs should be closely watched for its occurrence. (Also see chapter on *Adverse Effects of Drugs on the Kidney).*

Aminoglycosides

The commonly used aminoglycosides are well known for their potential nephrotoxic effects. Because **neomycin** is the most nephrotoxic of the aminoglycoside antibiotics (Table 7) (73), its parenteral use has been replaced by less toxic agents. Although it is now used only topically or orally, one should keep in mind that 1-2% of orally administered neomycin is absorbed and that accumulation may occur in patients with hepatic or renal disease. Oral doses of 4 gm daily in such patients may result in blood levels of sufficient magnitude to be ototoxic as well as nephrotoxic (132). As many as 25% of patients with hepatic and/or renal dysfunction may experience these toxic effects (93).

Nephrotoxicity following administration of **kanamycin** is generally manifested only by an abnormal urinary sediment and only occasionally by more severe abnormalities. Urinary sediment changes include proteinuria, microscopic hematuria and cylinduria (207). A mild rise in blood urea nitrogen and serum creatinine may also appear as early signs of nephrotoxicity (82). Should kanamycin administration continue, a decrease in renal blood flow, development of lesions in the proximal tubule characterized by a decrease in glomerular filtration rate and urinary osmolality, as well as acute renal failure, may occur (93, 237). Fortunately, reports of serious renal impairment secondary to kanamycin have been rare, and the lesions described have been, for the most part, entirely reversible. Most of the urinary abnormalities caused by kanamycin were reported during the early use of the drug when doses were frequently in excess of those now recommended for patients with normal or abnormal renal function. Finegold (82) demonstrated a direct relationship between a patient's age and the likelihood of developing kanamycin toxicity. Older patients (with normally decreased renal function) and patients with kidney disease who are likely to accumulate abnormally high serum levels of the drug are the most susceptible to its toxic effects. The need for careful monitoring of these patients and the application of biopharmacokinetic information to the use of agents like kanamycin is evident. It is important to remember that tubular secretion decreases with age, and this parameter is not evaluated by traditional measures of renal function (138).

Gentamicin is less nephrotoxic than kanamycin. Indeed, gentamicin has been implicated as a potentially nephrotoxic agent in only a small percentage of patients. Based on 1152 patients in published reports, the Schering Corporation has estimated the frequency of gentamicin-induced renal dysfunction to be 2% or less. Mild azotemia or slight elevations in BUN were the most common abnormalities reported (73). Wilfer and co-workers (252) reviewed 71 patients who received 77 courses of gentamicin therapy. Forty-two percent of gentamicin courses were associated with a fall in renal function as measured by a rise in BUN, creatinine, or both. In only 5 cases, however, could gentamicin be named as the most likdly causative agent; all other cases were complicated by other factors known to produce renal dysfunction, and it was impossible to determine the most likely etiology. Even though the association between gentamicin administration and renal abnormalities is not strong, renal function should be monitored regularly (including a baseline creatinine clearance), and extreme care must be taken when it is given to patients with pre-existing renal dysfunction (237).

Several recent reports suggest that the joint administration of gentamicin and cephalothin (23, 48, 121, 184) and tobramycin and cephalothin (118, 231) may potentiate the renal toxicity of these agents. Although not generally considered to be nephrotoxic, there is growing evidence that cephalothin may cause renal damage when given in high doses for prolonged periods (8-24 gm/day for 8-35 days) (99, 121). Prolonged treatment with high doses of gentamicin and cephalothin may result in their accumulation to high serum levels; indeed, most of the reported cases have been in patients with some degree of pre-existing renal failure given relatively large doses of both antimicrobials. Therefore, it would be prudent to administer cephalothin-gentamicin (or other aminoglycoside) combinations with caution, especially in patients with renal dysfunction. Another combination which has become popular in the last few years is clindamycin and gentamicin. While reports of possible increased renal toxicities with this combination have appeared, the data is insufficient to permit assessment at this time.

The comparative nephrotoxicity of tobramycin and amikacin with that of gentamicin and kanamycin is uncertain. Several reports have documented the nephrotoxicity of tobramycin (114, 162, 234) and amikacin (135). However, adequate studies to determine the relative incidence of nephrotoxicity between the newer aminoglycosides and gentamicin or kanamycin have yet to be performed.

Administration of **streptomycin** has been associated

Table 7
RELATIVE NEPHROTOXICITY OF AMINOGLYCOSIDE ANTIBIOTICS (73)

Neomycin	Most nephrotoxic
Polymyxin	
Colistin	
Kanamycin	
Gentamicin	
Streptomycin	Least nephrotoxic

with a very low incidence of renal abnormalities (207). Parenteral administration of more than 4 gm/day, in the early days of antituberculous therapy, was often associated with proteinuria, azotemia and a decreased glomerular filtration rate. This early nephrotoxicity may have been partially the result of impurities in the early streptomycin preparations (93).

Polymyxin-Colistin

Polymyxin B and colistin (colistimethate; polymyxin E) are closely related antibiotics occasionally useful in the treatment of gram-negative infections. With the advent and effectiveness of carbenicillin and gentamicin in the treatment of pseudomonas infections, and the effectiveness of the aminoglycosides against other gram-negative organisms, polymyxin and colistin are infrequently used. They are useful, however, in the treatment of infections caused by pathogens resistant to the above mentioned drugs. The nephrotoxic effects of polymyxin and colistin are identical, and include proteinuria, hematuria or cylinduria, impairment of renal concentrating ability, oliguric or non-oliguric renal failure with azotemia, and acute tubular necrosis (71, 128, 196). Renal dysfunction may occur in as many as 20% of patients and usually develops during the first 3-4 days of treatment (93). The lesions consist of proximal tubular necrosis (237). Early studies comparing the effectiveness of polymyxin B and colistin indicated that colistin was the less toxic agent (68); however, it is now largely felt that the nephrotoxic potential of the two drugs is essentially identical (180). In a small number of patients receiving recommended therapeutic dosages, Pedersen and associates (189) could demonstrate no difference in the nephrotoxic effects of polymyxin and colistin. They did observe, however, that polymyxin administration was associated with a 70% incidence of other side effects like paresthesia, skin rash, fever, and severe pain at the injection site; colistin produced only a 23% incidence of such reactions. Additionally, animal studies demonstrated a significantly higher incidence of renal toxicity with polymyxin than colistin. Because of these differences some recommend the use of colistin instead of polymyxin B.

Patients with pre-existing renal dysfunction appear more susceptible to the nephrotoxic effects of these compounds. Marked increases in blood urea nitrogen and serum creatinine may develop when such patients receive polymyxin or colistin, and may only slowly return to pre-treatment values after therapy is discontinued (77, 102). Although these agents are usually fairly well tolerated in patients with normal renal function (237), nephrotoxicity may occur in these patients as well (128). Adler and Segel (2) reported 4 cases of acute, non-oliguric, renal failure secondary to colistin. Three of these patients were concomitantly receiving

cephalothin, and the fourth had received cephalothin immediately prior to colistin. They point out that urine output alone should not be monitored as a sign of nephrotoxicity (since BUN and creatinine may increase without oliguria) and suggest that cephalothin may enhance the nephrotoxic potential of colistin, analogous to the discussion above concerning gentamicin and cephalothin. The general guidelines outlined above concerning the use of potentially nephrotoxic agents should be closely followed when the clinical situation necessitates administration of colistin or polymyxin B.

Methicillin (Penicillin)

It is now widely acknowledged that the administration of **methicillin** may be associated with a hypersensitivity-induced interstitial nephritis affecting the tubules but sparing the glomeruli (6, 36, 74, 91, 203, 208, 212, 254). Renal toxicity is characterized by spiking fevers, malaise, anorexia, eosinophilia, skin rash, hematuria, pyuria, albuminuria, and oliguria (237). Since skin rash, eosinophilia, and proteinuria generally herald the onset of renal toxicity, patients receiving methicillin should be monitored for these signs so that therapy can be discontinued should they develop. Interstitial nephritis is more common in patients receiving high doses (12-24 gm/day) for prolonged periods. It is postulated that the methicillin forms a haptenic complex with the renal epithelium and that this complex is recognized as a foreign body during an immune response. Immunofluorescent studies have demonstrated methicillin antigen (assumed to be dimethoxyphenyl-penicilloyl), IgG and the third component of complement deposited along the tubular basement membrane but not along the glomerular basement membrane (25). During this immunologic reaction the tubular cell is destroyed (6, 91). The lesion is usually reversible, and patients recover rapidly after therapy is discontinued. Occasionally, progressive renal damage occurs despite discontinuation of therapy (91). Although the role of corticosteroids in the management of this nephritis is uncertain, they may be useful in those patients not responding to a simple discontinuation of methicillin administration (255).

Penicillin G has also been associated with the development of interstitial nephritis, usually in daily doses of 20-60 MU (6,208). The administration of other penicillins to patients who have experienced methicillin or penicillin-induced nephritis should be strictly avoided. Since all of the penicillins have similar chemical structures, cross-sensitivity is not surprising. **Ampicillin** (91), **nafcillin** (187), and **cephalothin** (55, 66, 203) have all caused a recurrence of the nephropathy when given to such patients.

Amphotericin B

Until recently amphotericin B was the only agent

available for the treatment of severe systemic fungal infections. Even with the addition of 5-fluorocytosine, however, amphotericin continues to be the drug of choice. Nephrotoxicity is a regular and predictable complication of amphotericin administration; renal tubular acidosis results and is usually the factor limiting continued therapy. Nephrotoxicity is manifested by cast formation, decreased concentrating ability, defective acid excretion, diminished glomerular filtration rate, potassium loss and hypokalemia, azotemia, and an increase in BUN and serum creatinine (93). The GFR may often be diminished by as much as 80%. Amphotericin is generally administered in a dose of 0.5-1 mg/kg daily or every other day. A total dose of 2-4 gm will effectively treat most mycotic infections. Signs of renal toxicity will invariably develop during treatment; however at this dosage level nephrotoxicity is usually not permanent, and normal or near-normal renal function returns upon discontinuation of therapy (171). When the total dose is above 5 gm, permanent residual damage is more likely (44, 223).

Since profound systemic acidosis and hypokalemia may represent a component of the renal tubular acidosis caused by amphotericin, sodium bicarbonate by mouth and potassium supplementation are indicated. In general, amphotericin administration should be withheld when the serum creatinine rises above 3mg% and reinstituted (possibly at a lower daily dose or an every-other-day regimen) when the creatinine returns to a level below this amount. The recommendations outlined in Table 8 should be followed during amphotericin therapy.

Cephalosporins

The cephalosporins are a rapidly expanding class of antimicrobial agents. Cephalothin and cephaloridine are the oldest of these agents; however, newer compounds such as cephalexin, cephapirin, cephradine, and cephazolin are rapidly appearing on the market with various claims of superiority over their predecessors. **Cephalothin,** the most frequently used cephalosporin, is generally considered to have no nephrotoxic properties. However, evidence that renal damage may result from cephalothin administration is accumulating (43, 50, 99, 185). In the majority of cases described thus far there was evidence of pre-existing renal dysfunction, although concomitant heart failure was also common. Doses have generally been higher than recommended and have most commonly ranged from 8-25 gm/day. Additionally, there appears to be a relationship between the simultaneous use of cephalothin and gentamicin and an increased frequency of nephrotoxic reactions (23, 121, 184). The incidence of cephalothin nephrotoxicity can be minimized by (a) properly adjusting the dosage regimen in patients with renal failure; (b) not exceeding daily doses of 12 gms in patients with

normal renal function (particularly in the presence of dehydration or when potent diuretics are given); (c) avoiding sustained serum concentrations in excess of 100 mcg/ml (86); and (d) by close observation (especially in patients receiving an aminoglycoside concomitantly).

Mandell (152) has summarized much of the known data on the pharmacokinetics, indications, and adverse reactions of **cephaloridine.** Nephrotoxicity is a well-known effect of cephaloridine and appears to be dose related. The serious and occasionally fatal renal toxicity of this agent in patients with previously normal kidneys given doses exceeding 6 gm/day, or in whom plasma levels exceed 150-200 mcg/ml, has been repeatedly documented (100, 112, 115, 185, 218, 246). The lesion, characterized by proximal tubular necrosis, has also been observed in patients receiving 4 gm or less daily, who also have endocarditis, hypotension, or renal disease (122). Pre-existing renal dysfunction is a

Table 8
RECOMMENDATIONS FOR THE USE OF AMPHOTERICIN B

1. Reconstitute 50 mg vial with 10 cc sterile water (final concentration 5 mg/cc). Sterile water must contain no perservative or bacteriostatic agent: precipitation or pyrogenic reactions may result.

2. Use reconstituted solution as soon as possible. Should be stored no longer than one week under refrigeration.

3. Daily dose is diluted in 5% dextrose in water (D5W) and infusion begun immediately. Deterioration may occur if allowed to stand for prolonged period.

4. Dosage schedule:
   Day 1 - begin with 1 mg in 500 cc D5W over 4 hours
   Day 2 - 5 mg
   Day 3 - 10 mg   in 500 cc D5W over 4-6 hours
   Day 4 - 15 mg
   Day 5 and thereafter - 0.5-1.0 mg/Kg/day. Dose is governed by patient's tolerance to drug, renal function and clinical improvement. The *rate*-of administration may also be varied with tolerance. Manufacturer recommends that the solution be protected from light, but the dilution is probably stable for the duration of the infusion if used immediately.

5. Complications of therapy and their treatment:
   a. thrombophlebitis - use veins as distal as possible; use pediatric scalp vein needles; alternate veins; add 5 mg heparin to infusion solution.
   b. fever and chills - ASA or acetaminophen as needed
   c. nausea and vomiting - administer Compazine prior to infusion
   d. anorexia, myalgias, headache - ASA or acetaminophen as needed
   e. If b, c, and d persist may also vary dose and rate of administration or add 5-20 mg of hydrocortisone to the infusion
   f. hypokalemia - serial potassium determinations and supplementation as needed.
   g. azotemia - serial BUN determinations. Withold drug if BUN is greater than 50 mg% or creatinine is greater than 3 mg%.
   h. anemia - serial Hct determinations
   i. systemic acidosis - NaHCO$_3$ administration

6. Parameters to monitor while patient is on Amphotericin B:
   a. weight
   b. cumulative dose
   c. serum electrolytes: Na, K, Cl, HCO$_3$
   d. renal function: BUN, creatinine, creatinine clearance, urine volume
   e. urinalysis: pH, protein, RBC's, WBC's, casts
   f. blood cells: WBC, RBC, platelets, reticulocytes, hematocrit

major predisposing factor to the development of nephrotoxicity. Cephalothin is generally considered the cephalosporin of choice when parenteral administration is indicated because of its lower frequency of toxicity compared to cephaloridine. Because cephaloridine is less painful when given intramuscularly, it has traditionally been selected when this route is desired. If cephaloridine must be used, daily doses in excess of 4 gm should not be administered; in fact, doses greater than this are unnecessary. It should not be given to patients with shock, oliguria or azotemia. If possible, serum levels should be monitored to avoid untoward accumulation of the drug, and it should not be administered concomitantly with other nephrotoxic drugs (13, 152).

Two newer cephalosporins released for parenteral administration, **cephapirin** and **cephazolin,** should replace cephaloridine and possibly even cephalothin in clinical use. Cephazolin is associated with relatively little pain when injected intramuscularly (174). To date, they have not been associated with any renal toxicity (34, 200, 251); however, one should still monitor renal function in patients receiving either of these agents until additional clinical experience has accumulated.

HEPATOTOXICITY

A large number of antimicrobial drugs and chemicals are known to produce liver injury (Table 9). Most drugs causing hepatotoxicity appear to do so through a hypersensitivity-type reaction, although a few may function as true hepatotoxins (119). The types of liver abnormalities resulting from untoward reactions to drugs have been divided into three categories based on the pathologic lesion identified: hepatocellular, hepatocanalicular, and canalicular (8). Liver function tests performed in patients with the *hepatocellular* variety are identical to those seen in viral hepatitis: serum transaminase values are elevated (often to levels greater than 1000 IU/L) while alkaline phosphatase is only minimally elevated. Liver biopsy reveals diffuse

hepatocellular necrosis and inflammation. Hepatic toxicity of the hepatocellular variety carries the highest mortality rate, although it varies with the particular drug involved. Several antibiotics produce hepatocellular toxicity, including isoniazid, pyrazinamide, ethionamide, tetracycline, and some sulfonamides.

Hepatocanalicular toxicity mimics the biochemical abnormalities commonly observed in obstructive jaundice (cholelithiasis). Liver biopsy shows bile stasis and inflammation of the portal triads but only minimal hepatocellular necrosis. Erythromycin estolate (Ilosone) and some sulfonamides have produced this type of reaction.

The **canalicular-type,** apparently caused only by methyltestosterone and the anabolic steroids, consists largely of simple cholestasis. Liver function studies demonstrate only mild abnormalities of serum transaminases and alkaline phosphatase.

Isoniazid

Isoniazid (INH) is well-known for its ability to produce hepatocellular toxicity in patients receiving normal therapeutic doses. Most patients tolerate INH therapy without incident; however approximately 10% of individuals demonstrate mild and transient elevations in serum transaminase enzymes (SGOT, SGPT) during the first 2 months of treatment (46, 206). These elevations usually return to normal despite continued drug administration; however, liver biopsy performed during this time demonstrates a mild focal hepatitis. A severe hepatitis with jaundice has been estimated to occur in approximately 1% of the general population given isoniazid (87) but does not appear to be related to daily dose or duration of therapy. The incidence of severe hepatotoxicities is even higher (2.3%) in the INH-treated population over 50 years of age (173). The syndrome is characterized by a prodromal period (fatigue, weakness, anorexia, malaise and occasionally fever) which may occur after only 5 days of therapy. Prompt discontinuation of INH administration at the initial appearance of these prodromal symptoms mar-

Table 9
INCIDENCE OF HEPATIC INJURY, PRESUMED MECHANISM AND TYPES OF LESION PRODUCED BY ANTIBIOTIC AND ANTIMICROBIAL DRUGS
MODIFIED FROM WORK OF ZIMMERMAN (256)

AGENTS	INCIDENCE	MECHANISM	TYPE OF INJURY	HISTOLOGIC CHANGES
Antitubercular:				
INH	Low	Hypersensitivity & metabolic idiosyncrasy	Hepatocellular or hepatocanalicular	Necrosis or only bile casts with portal inflammation
Pyrazinamide	3-5%	Metabolic idiosyncrasy	Hepatocellular	Degeneration & necrosis
Ethionamide	3-5%	Metabolic idiosyncrasy	Hepatocellular	Degeneration & necrosis

Cycloserine	Low	Indirect toxicity	?Hepatocellular	?Degeneration & necrosis
PAS	1%	Hypersensitivity	Mixed hepatocellular	Necrosis, degeneration
Thiosemicarba-zone	High	Mild indirect toxicity	Cytotoxic-hepato-cellular	Fatty metamorphosis & necrosis
Rifamycin	Dysfunction dose-related jaundice	Mild indirect toxicity	Interference with bile secretion or bilirubin uptake from blood	No demonstrable lesion
Chloramphenicol	Very low	Hypersensitivity	Cytotoxic-Hepato-cellular jaundice or cholestatic	Diffuse degeneration & necrosis or only bile casts
Erythromycin estolate	low	Hypersensitivity	Cholestatic-Hepa-tocanalicular jaundice	Bile casts & portal inflammation, rich in eosinophils
Griseofulvin	Probably dose related	Mild indirect toxicity plus probable meta-bolic idiosyncrasy	Cytotoxic (also can provoke porphyria)	Fat & necrosis (experimental animals)
Nitrofurantoin	Low	Hypersensitivity	Predominantly hepatocellular	Bile casts & portal inflammation
Novobiocin	Very low	Mild indirect toxicity	Interferes with bilirubin con-jugation	No demonstrable lesion
Oxacillin	Low & dose related	Mild indirect toxicity plus(?) hypersensiti-vity	Cholestatic-hepa-tocanalicular jaundice	Bile casts
Penicillin	Very Low	Hypersensitivity	Cytotoxic-hepato-cellular	Necrosis
Sulfonamides	Low	Hypersensitivity	Mixed hepatocell-ular	Degeneration & necrosis
Sulfones	2-5%	Hypersensitivity plus indirect toxicity	Mixed hepatocell-ular	Degeneration & necrosis
Tetracyclines	Low with oral admin-istration. High with high dose parenteral administration	Indirect toxicity	Cytotoxic-hepato-cellular jaundice	Small-droplet (micro-vesicular) degenera-tion & fatty meta-morphosis & areas of necrosis
Triacetylolean-domycin	1%	Mild indirect toxicity plus metabolic idio-syncrasy or hyper-sensitivity	Mixed cholestatic & cytotoxic-mixed hepatocellular jaundice	Focal area necrosis & degeneration & bile casts
Xenazoic acid	Low	Hypersensitivity	Hepatocanalicular	?

kedly decreases the incidence of overt hepatitis. Conversely, continued isoniazid administration after symptoms of hepatitis develop results in more severe hepatic damage (150).

The mechanism of INH-induced hepatotoxicity is uncertain. Early reports speculated that a hypersensitivity reaction was responsible (94, 150, 217); however, more recent evidence discounts this mechanism and supports a direct hepatotoxic effect of the drug as being responsible. Individuals who are rapid acetylators have a higher incidence of INH-induced hepatitis; it has therefore been proposed that such individuals produce toxic hydrazine metabolites (acetylhydrazine) which covalently bind to tissue macromolecules in the liver and produce necrosis (172, 173). This is particularly important in evaluating the risk benefit ratio associated with utilizing INH prophylactically in patients with positive TB skin tests. Edwards (69a) found that in a population of 1.1 million military recruits with strongly positive skin tests, the incidence of actually developing tuberculosis was only 0.08%. The incidence of severe hepatotoxicity with INH is considerably higher than this, particularly in the rapid acetylator sub-group. With the development of a convenient method for the characterization of acetylation phenotype utilizing sulfamethazine (172), it may be possible to identify the population at greatest risk of developing hepatotoxicity. This subject needs further study before its clinical utility can be accurately determined.

The need for close monitoring of patients receiving INH and prompt discontinuation of treatment should hepatitis or its prodromal symptoms develop, is evident. However, it does not appear necessary to stop drug treatment in patients demonstrating only *mild* transaminase elevations. There does not appear to be any convincing evidence that pre-existing liver disease is a contraindication to isoniazid therapy, even though the package insert lists it as such (175). (Also see chapters on *Diseases of the Liver* and *Tuberculosis.)*

Erythromycin

Erythromycin estolate (Ilosone), the lauryl sulfate salt of erythromycin propionate, has been associated with the production of a hepatocanalicular-type hepatotoxicity (202). The lesions have typically been observed after 1-2 weeks of continuous therapy or following several repeated courses of the drug. The reaction is felt to be hypersensitivity induced (237). Jaundice, abnormal liver function tests (SGOT, SGPT), and eosinophilia are characteristic of the reaction and indicate obstructive cholestasis. The observed abnormalities rapidly reverse when drug administration is discontinued. Erythromycin estolate may cause serum transaminase elevations in as many as 25% of patients given the drug and up to 4% may develop obstructive jaundice (8). Only the estolate salt of erythromycin has

been associated with hepatotoxicity, and erythromycin base or other salts appear free of this untoward effect. Because of this difference, the routine use of erythromycin estolate should be avoided and the base or stearate salt administered instead. While it is true that the estolate yields higher blood levels of erythromycin than does the base or stearate salt, there is controversy as to the significance of this difference (129). (Also see chapter on *Diseases of the Liver.)*

Triacetyloleandomycin, similar in chemical structure and antimicrobial activity to erythromycin, also produces obstructive jaundice (202). Ticktin and Zimmerman (229) found that over half of their patients given this agent for 2 weeks or longer developed signs of hepatic dysfunction demonstrated by abnormal bromsulphalein (BSP) retention, cephalin flocculation, and transaminase elevations. Four percent of their patients developed jaundice. They speculated that the mechanism of triacetyloleandomycin-induced liver abnormalities was not mediated through a hypersensitivity reaction but because of its alarmingly high incidence, represented a direct hepatotoxic effect. Triacetyloleandomycin is now only rarely used in clinical medicine and does not appear to have any significant advantages over other agents.

Tetracycline

Tetracycline administration has been associated with the production of hepatic toxicity in over 70 reported cases during recent years; these have been summarized by MacFarlane and McCarron (148). In the early 1950's reports of tetracycline associated liver dysfunction (primarily fatty infiltration) appeared (136, 204). Most of these cases developed in patients receiving 2 gm or more of parenteral tetracycline daily. However, cases were also recorded of patients receiving large oral doses or a combination of oral and parenteral administration. It soon became apparent that the majority of cases occurred in pregnant women, often receiving tetracycline as treatment for acute pyelonephritis, following intravenous administration of greater than 2 gm/day (57, 209). Most cases occurred during the third trimester of pregnancy, although a few were reported during the second trimester or early postpartum period. The liver dysfunction closely resembles viral hepatitis, and initial symptoms consist of anorexia, nausea, vomiting, abdominal pain, weakness, and malaise followed by progressive jaundice. Premature labor, with a high fetal mortality, is common. Restlessness and central nervous system depression (occasionally with stupor or coma) may accompany the delivery period. Maternal mortality is also common; hematemesis, coma and shock are usually the terminal events. Although the majority of cases have occurred in pregnant women, tetracycline-induced liver dysfunction has also been reported in nonpregnant females,

males, and even children.

Laboratory studies demonstrate hepatic and renal insufficiency and pancreatitis. Hypoprothrombinemia, transaminase elevations, high BUN and serum creatinine, metabolic acidosis, elevation of serum amylase, and leukocytosis are common; hypoglycemia has been noted on occasion (57). It appears that hepatotoxicity from tetracycline is more likely when high blood and tissue concentrations of the drug are obtained, either because of administration of doses larger than recommended or accumulation secondary to pre-existing renal failure. Factors influencing the likelihood of tetracycline hepatotoxicity include daily dose, route of administration, duration of therapy, pregnancy, underlying hepatic or renal disease, and the concurrent use of other hepatotoxic drugs. Because there are no clear indications for parenteral tetracycline, it should not be given by this route except under unusual circumstances. Additionally, its antianabolic effect with subsequent elevation of BUN tends to contraindicate its use in patients with renal and hepatic dysfunction (28).

Nonspecific Elevations of SGOT

Nonspecific elevations of serum glutamic oxaloacetic transaminase (SGOT) have been reported following the administration of several antimicrobial agents. Ampicillin, oxacillin, cloxacillin, lincomycin, colistin, cephalothin and nalidixic acid all have this effect. SGOT elevations are transient and return to normal upon discontinuation of therapy; the significance of ths this effect is not clear (237).

OTOTOXICITY

A number of antibiotics are capable of producing ototoxic effects (Table 10). These may affect either the auditory (cochlear), or vestibular functions of the middle ear, or both.

Aminoglycosides

The aminoglycosides have notoriously been associated with severe deafness or vestibular dysfunction. Contrary to original speculations, the site of this toxicity does not appear to be the end-organ, cochlear nerve, or central nuclei. Instead, the aminoglycosides seem to exert their adverse effect at the level of the hair cell or vestibular apparatus. The mechanism is unexplained, although it has been speculated that they may interfere with oxygen supply to the hair cells. In contrast to the reversible ototoxicity of the salicylates and quinine, which appears to be caused by a constriction of blood vessels supplying the organ of Corti, the aminoglycosides cause nonreversible hearing loss (179).

Auditory toxicity may appear gradually with minor tinnitus and high tone hearing loss as the initial manifestations. If these symptoms are ignored, rapid, severe, and permanent deafness may result. Because the aminoglycosides are removed slowly from the middle ear, the hearing deficit may progress even though antibiotic administration has been discontinued (177). Vestibular dysfunction is not an infrequent complication. Vertigo is the primary manifestation during the acute state; this is followed by a chronic phase characterized by ataxia, to which the patient usually eventually adapts (237).

Dihydrostreptomycin was one of the first agents noted to produce ototoxicity and, as indicated in Table 10, affects primarily the auditory component resulting in deafness.

Since **Streptomycin** rarely produces deafness, and its ototoxicity is generally limited to vestibular function, it has replaced dihydrostreptomycin when there is clinical indication for their use (154). Streptomycin ototoxicity occurs when (a) excessive doses are given; (b) administration is continued for an extended period of time; or (c) drug therapy is allowed to continue after toxic signs develop. When administered in the usual dose (1 gm/day), streptomycin may be administered for over a month with little chance of toxicity; however, daily doses of 2-3 gm will almost certainly be associated with signs of vestibular dysfunction within 3-4 weeks (177). Concurrent renal disease may lead to drug accumulation and increase the likelihood of ototoxicity. It appears that the ototoxicity of streptomycin and dihydrostreptomycin is more closely related to daily dose (and serum level) than to total dose administered during a therapeutic course (137). Because early vestibular dysfunction may be very difficult to ascertain, the patient must be closely monitored. Baseline determinations of auditory and vestibular function should be done prior to therapy and repeated regularly during drug administration. Evaluation of auditory function is more reliable than evaluation of vestibular function, since one must rely on subjective reports of the patient for the latter. Nevertheless, simple balance and caloric tests are easily performed and documentation of vestibular dysfunction is possible (253).

Table 10
OTOTOXIC ANTIBIOTICS (168)

DRUG	VESTIBULAR TOXICITY	AUDITORY TOXICITY
Colistin	++	+
Dihydrostreptomycin	+	++++
Framycetin		++++
Gentamicin	++	+
Kanamycin	+	+++
Neomycin	+	++++
Streptomycin	+++	+
Vancomycin		+++
Viomycin	+++	++

Because of the serious renal and auditory toxicities, **neomycin** should no longer be given parenterally. Aminoglycosides which are less toxic should be used instead. However, ototoxicity caused by neomycin continues to occur and cases have been reported following its oral use and irrigation of the pleural cavity, mediastinum, and infected wounds (145). Of 495 retrospectively studied patients receiving neomycin, six developed significant hearing loss (31). All had received the drug orally for advanced hepatic cirrhosis, and at least three also had evidence of impaired renal function. Of four patients available for follow-up, none recovered auditory function. Generally, neomycin-induced deafness has an extremely poor prognosis (16). Even patients with normal renal function and low neomycin serum levels may develop ototoxicity with prolonged exposure, since even minimal oral absorption has been associated with auditory dysfunction in some patients (16). Daily doses of neomycin should not exceed 4 gm in individuals with renal insufficiency or ulcerative bowel disease, because serum levels may reach alarmingly high concentrations in such patients (237).

Kanamycin also produces irreversible hearing loss. Although it is definitely ototoxic, kanamycin is less toxic to the vestibular system than streptomycin and far less toxic to the auditory system than neomycin or dihydrostreptomycin (111). The ototoxicity of kanamycin generally involves the cochlear component of the middle ear. As with all the aminoglycosides, ototoxicity is more common in patients with some degree of renal insufficiency. Of 243 patients treated with kanamycin, the Boston Collaborative Drug Surveillance Program (BCDSP) reported that three of the four patients who developed deafness had some renal dysfunction (31). However, even patients with normal renal function may develop hearing loss when the daily dose, duration of therapy or total dose are excessive. Doses in excess of 7.5 mg/kg or 500 mg every 12 hours should be avoided and therapy should not be continued for more than 2 weeks unless absolutely indicated (237). Hearing loss is generally bilateral (164), and although it may be permanent, there is evidence that deafness may be reversible (155) if the drug is discontinued at the appropriate time. Hearing loss may progress after kanamycin has been discontinued, because the drug is only slowly removed from the endolymphatic system (177).

There is also some evidence to suggest that kanamycin ototoxicity may be potentiated by simultaneous or alternating administration of diuretics like ethacrynic acid or mannitol (31, 108, 195). Until more definitive data are available, it would be best to avoid concomitant use of these agents unless absolutely necessary. Jones (111) has reported a case of both maternal and fetal ototoxicity apparently resulting from the simultaneous administration of kanamycin and ethacrynic acid to a pregnant woman with chronic renal disease.

One must always be certain that the daily dose of kanamycin is appropriate for the patient's renal function, that therapy not be continued longer than indicated, and that drug administration be discontinued at the first sign of hearing loss. Baseline and repeat audiology tests are necessary if the clinician is to detect ototoxicity before significant permanent damage has occurred. Ideally, all elderly individuals and patients with decreased renal function should have these tests performed before and during kanamycin administration, but costs and equipment availability are often limiting factors.

As indicated in Table 10, ototoxicity from **gentamicin** primarily involves vestibular dysfunction, however, auditory damage may also occur (169, 230). The vestibular symptoms of severe vertigo and dysequilibrium are often preceded by slight postural vertigo with rapid head movements. If drug administration is discontinued early, additional loss may be prevented (177).

The estimated incidence of gentamicin ototoxicity is approximately 2%, and almost two-thirds of patients with ototoxicity have renal impairment (107). Sixty-six percent of gentamicin ototoxic patients demonstrated only vestibular dysfunction, 18% auditory plus vestibular, and 16% auditory dysfunction only. Symptoms of ototoxicity generally appear during the second week of treatment but can occur as early as the third day (107). In all reported cases, the onset of symptoms occurred within two weeks of gentamicin administration. In patients with normal renal function the daily dose was the only factor which could be correlated with the development of toxicity. However, in patients with renal insufficiency previous courses of ototoxic antibiotics, daily dose, and total dose all appeared to influence the production of ototoxicity. Gentamicin serum concentrations in excess of 12 mcg/ml appear to be associated with an increased incidence of ototoxicity (107). Interestingly, the duration of gentamicin therapy did not appear to affect the likelihood of toxicity.

As previously mentioned, vestibular dysfunction may be difficult to ascertain since bedridden patients may not be aware of vertigo. Therefore, routine tests of vestibular function should be performed before and during gentamicin therapy. Because symptoms may appear several weeks after treatment has been discontinued, follow-up examination performed for three to four weeks after drug therapy has been discontinued may be necessary. Additionally, audiology tests should be performed as described above in relation to kanamycin. Careful monitoring of patients for early signs of toxicity and proper attention to dosage based on pharmacokinetic parameters should allow one to markedly decrease the frequency of gentamicin-induced ototoxicity. Gentamicin is probably less ototoxic than kanamycin.

CENTRAL NERVOUS SYSTEM TOXICITY

Fortunately, central nervous system (CNS) toxicity is relatively uncommon following antimicrobial administration. Several antibiotics have been associated with the production of encephalopathy, including penicillin, cycloserine, amphotericin B, polymyxin B, colistin, and tetracycline (95, 177, 237). However, most of these adverse reactions have only been sporadically reported.

Penicillin G

Penicillin G is probably the most well known antibiotic for producing CNS disturbances. Since Johnson and Walker (109) first reported the epileptogenic properties of penicillin, numerous case reports describing seizure activity following penicillin administration have appeared (29, 133, 134, 138, 178). Although the vast majority of adverse reactions associated with penicillin are allergic in nature, encephalopathy is a direct toxic reaction. Penicillin encephalopathy is characterized by CNS stimulation and is manifest by delirium or coma with intense myoclonic and generalized seizures (177). Penicillin is very irritating when applied directly to the cerebral cortex and has, in fact, been used experimentally to induce seizure activity in animals. As expected, direct administration of penicillin into the cerebrospinal fluid, particularly by intraventricular or intracisternal injections, is more likely to cause neurotoxicity. Doses greater than 30,000 units should not be injected into the subarachnoid space in adults (95).

Penicillin normally crosses the blood-brain barrier poorly; however, in patients with meningeal irritation, or very high serum levels of penicillin, appreciable drug concentrations may be achieved within the CNS. Thus, most cases of penicillin encephalopathy following systemic administration of the drug have occurred in patients (a) receiving more than 60 million units per day, (b) with concomitant renal failure or (c) with pre-existing cerebral disease (21, 37). Daily doses of less than 20 million units have produced seizures in patients with renal dysfunction. Because penicillin crosses slowly into the cerebrospinal fluid (CSF), intermittent intravenous doses of penicillin are less neurotoxic than continuous infusions (177). Lerner, et al., (138) compared CSF levels of penicillin in patients with and without neurotoxicity. In the toxic group, CSF penicillin levels ranged from 12-61.4 U/ml; nine of ten patients had levels above 15 U/ml, and the majority had concentrations in excess of 25 U/ml. In the nontoxic group only one patient had a CSF penicillin level in excess of 7.8 U/ml (15.4 U/ml). Apparently, neurotoxicity from penicillin can be avoided if CSF levels are kept below 10 U/ml. It should also be noted that serum sodium concentrations in the toxic group were most often between 115 and 130 mEq/L, while most of the nontoxic patients had concentrations above 130 mEq/L.

Evidence of penicillin-induced CNS hyperexcitability generally appears within 24-72 hours after therapy is begun. Myoclonas of the face and extremities are often the initial symptoms and may be accompanied by delirium and generalized tonic-clonic grand mal seizures. Stupor and coma may be noted in severe cases. The seizure activity is usually continuous and does not respond well to anticonvulsant medicatons. Prompt improvement occurs 12-24 hrs after penicillin is discontinued (138).

The BCDSP (29) has reported a case of oxacillin induced seizures in a patient with normal renal function receiving 8 gm/day, and carbenicillin has also been associated with neurotoxicity (22, 133). All penicillins may share the epileptogenic potential of penicillin G.

Procaine Penicillin

A wide variety of unusual behavioral and neurologic reactons, sometimes designated as Hoigne's Syndrome, have been reported in patients shortly following an intramuscular injection of procaine penicillin G (167). The usual manifestations of this adverse reaction include visual and auditory disturbances, dizziness, tachycardia, palpitations, seizure activity, unusual tastes, combativeness, confusion, and fears of death (33). The reaction occurs immediately after injection and generally subsides within 5-10 minutes. A number of factors may contribute to these bizarre reactions, including inadvertent intravascular injection of the preparation with subsequent release of free procaine or (although less likely) micro-cerebral emboli of the procaine penicillin suspension. Green and associates (97) measured plasma procaine concentrations in 26 patients immediately after the IM injection of 4.8 million units of procaine penicillin G and observed levels of 3.6-11.0 mcg/ml. Although individual differences among patients exist, these concentrations are compatible with the production of neuropsychiatric symptoms and EEG abnormalities.

It has been estimated that adverse neurologic reactions occur once in every 120-400 injections (97, 233). Thus, the potential exists for a very large number of these reactions to occur. Because they are self-limiting, no specific treatment is necessary; however, the clinician must be able to accurately identify the reaction. Unfortunately, this adverse reaction is often misinterpreted as anaphylaxis. Since immunologic mechanisms are probably not involved, the patient should not be labeled as penicillin-allergic.

Cycloserine

Cycloserine is an antituberculosis agent which may still occasionally be used in cases of tuberculosis resistant to other drugs. The major factor limiting the effective use of cycloserine is the frequent occurrence of neurotoxicities. In doses exceeding 1 gm/day myoclonic jerking and epileptiform seizures are fairly common

(95). Convulsions occur in about 10% of all patients receiving effective antituberculous doses of cycloserine (54). Other adverse neurological reactions include dyskinesias, paresis, paresthesias, tremors, and psychotic manifestations. The urinary excretion of pyridoxine (vitamin B-6) is markedly increased in patients receiving cycloserine, and Cohen demonstrated that supplementation of this vitamin (50 mg tid) greatly decreases, and may even eliminate, the neurotoxicity of cycloserine (54). Although the incidence of convulsions, paresthesia, and tremors appears to be reduced by pyridoxine supplementation, the frequency of psychotic manifestations is not affected.

Tetracycline

Over the last fifteen years occasional reports of tetracycline-induced increased intracranial pressure have appeared in the literature (19, 81, 90, 92, 127, 153). Although only about 15 cases have been reported, this complication of tetracycline therapy is felt to be much more common (127). Benign intracranial hyptertension (also called pseudotumor cerebri, serous meningitis, meningeal hydrops and otic hydrocephalus) is characterized by headache, nausea, vomiting, papilledema, an increase in intracranial pressure, normal or small ventricles, and the absence of a space-occupying lesion (153). Intracranial infection, hypertensive encephalopathy, and hypercapnic respiratory failure are absent, and the cerebrospinal fluid is normal (19). In infants and young children, in which closure of the cranial sutures has not yet taken place, the syndrome is generally manifested by a bulging anterior fontanel; in fact, tetracycline-induced intracranial hypertension was first recognized in such patients. It was originally felt that intracranial hyptertension caused by tetracycline only occurred in infants; however a few cases have been reported in adolescent patients and adults (19, 92, 127). Benign intracranial hypertension has also been associated with hyper- and hypo-vitaminosis A, hypoparathyroidism, prolonged glucocorticoid therapy, chronic adrenal insufficiency, severe hypochromic microcytic anemia, pregnancy (127), and nalidixic acid therapy (26). The problem is one of differential diagnosis in which other causes of increased intracranial pressure must be ruled out, including intracranial mass.

The mechanism by which tetracycline induces an increase in intracranial pressure remains obscure; hypersensitivity has been suggested (19), though the evidence available is too scanty to draw any valid conclusions. It has been suggested that the immature blood-brain barrier of young infants may allow greater passage of tetracycline into the CSF accounting for the apparent predilection of children to develop this reaction (127). Although most cases develop within four days, Giles and Soble (92) described a 16-year-old

female who developed an increase in intracranial pressure after 5 months of drug administration for the control of acne. They did not state, however, if tetracycline therapy had been continuous during this period. Signs of intracranial hypertension abate within a few hours to three days after tetracycline administration is discontinued; however, papilledema may resolve somewhat more slowly, especially in adult patients (19). No permanent sequelae have been observed. In those patients re-exposed to tetracycline, symptoms promptly return (182).

NEUROMUSCULAR BLOCKADE

Skeletal muscle weakness, respiratory depression, and even respiratory paralysis following the use of the **aminoglycoside compounds** have been commonly reported. **Polymyxin**, **colistin**, and **bacitracin** have also produced a neuromuscular blockade, both clinically and experimentally (177, 237). McQuillen (163) summarized 123 patients with antibiotic-induced muscular weakness. The syndrome occurred immediately after a surgical procedure in all but 11 of the patients. Although the first reported case followed the intraperitoneal administration of neomycin (197), subsequent cases have followed the intravenous, intramuscular, oral, intrapleural, spray, intraluminal irrigation, and retroperitoneal administration of these antibiotics (163).

Several factors are known to potentiate the neuromuscular blocking properties of the above listed antibiotics. These include (a) the concurrent administration of other drugs with neuromuscular blocking activity (ether, d-tubocurarine, gallamine, triethiodide, decamethonium bromide, and succinylcholine), (b) administration of the antibiotic intravascularly or directly onto serosal surfaces; (c) accidental overdosage; (d) drug accumulation in patients with renal insufficiency; and (e) administration of the antibiotic to patients with neuromuscular disease (i.e., myasthenia gravis) (241). The mechanism by which the antibiotics produce neuromuscular blockade is unclear. Their action is often described as "curariform", although several noticeable differences exist between the blockade produced by curare and that produced by the aminoglycosides (14). In fact, differences even exist between the various antibiotics; the blockade of neomycin, streptomycin, and dihydrostreptomycin may be effectively antagonized by neostigmine, while that of polymyxin B and kanamycin appears to be made worse by the administration of neostigmine (192). It is generally thought that the antibiotics cause a deficient release of acetylcholine from motor nerve endings. Elmquist and Josefsson (70) found that neomycin produces both a decrease in the sensitivity of the postjunctional end-plate membrane to acetylcholine and a decrease in the amount of acetylcholine released. McQuillen, et al. (163) studied a patient with neuromuscular blockade secondary to kanamycin and colistin and concluded that the blockade was of pre-synaptic origin.

Although the neuromuscular blockade is rapidly re-versible, it must be recognized and dealt with quickly, since severe respiratory depression or arrest may oc-cur. Calcium chloride (1 gm IV) generally produces an immediate response demonstrated by an increase in muscle strength and respiratory rate. Calcium in-creases the release of acetylcholine from motor nerve endings and thus may be directly antagonistic to the action of the antibiotics. Neostigmine has also been used successfully; however, in cases of kanamycin-induced neuromuscular blockade neostigmine may ac-tually worsen the condition. Only two cases of gentamicin-induced neuromuscular blockade have been reported (98, 241); one patient was successfully treated with calcium chloride, the other was not treated. The effect of neostigmine on gentamicin-induced blockade remains to be determined. Because most cases of antibiotic-induced neuromuscular bloc-kade have occurred in the immediate post-operative period, the aminoglycoside or polymyxin antimicro-bials should be used cautiously in this situation. Pa-tients with neuromuscular disease should never be de-nied the potential life-saving properties of these agents when they are indicated. An awareness of the potential for adverse reaction, scrutinous monitoring of the pa-tient and, if necessary, respiratory assistance should allow the aminoglycosides to be used safely in such patients.

GASTROINTESTINAL COMPLICATIONS

All antimicrobial agents have been associated with the production of nausea, anorexia, and vomiting, but these symptoms are usually mild and do not significant-ly interfere with the planned course of therapy. Occa-sionally, vomiting or diarrhea may be sufficiently se-vere to necessitate discontinuance or alteration of an-tibiotic therapy. Stomatitis and glossitis occur rela-tively frequently with the use of broad spectrum agents like tetracycline. Superinfection with *Candida albicans* is often responsible. Termination of antimicrobial ad-ministration is usually all that is needed to treat a mild infection; however, specific therapy may be indicated if a severe infection is present (8). Orally-administered nystatin tablets will be ineffective against Candida stomatitis. Dissolving a nystatin vaginal tablet in the oral cavity twice daily is a very effective means of treat-ing oral candidiasis and appears to be more effective than the suspension.

Diarrhea is probably the most frequent complication of both oral and parenteral antimicrobial therapy. Al-though proliferation of Candida within the gastrointes-tinal tract may occasionally be responsible for the diarrhea (210), the majority of cases are thought to be due to changes in the bacterial flora. Lincomycin, and to a lesser extent, clindamycin, have been associated with a high incidence of diarrhea. As many as 50 % of patients treated with lincomycin (8) and up to 21% of patients given clindamycin (164) develop diarrhea. Re-cently, cases of antibiotic-induced **pseudomembra-nous colitis** have appeared. Ampicillin (205), penicillin (227), tetracycline (124, 199), chloramphenicol (199), lincomycin (14, 42, 64, 238) and clindamycin (42, 64, 122, 221, 226, 232, 238) have all been implicated. Diarrhea may begin during or up to several weeks after drug administration. The exact incidence with which any of these antimicrobials causes colitis is unknown; however, Tedesco (225), reported a 10% incidence of pseudomembranous colitis detected by proctoscopy following the use of oral or parenteral clindamycin. Pseudomembranous colitis should be considered a possibility in any patient developing a temperature, diarrhea or ileus during or shortly after antibiotic treatment. Any patient having more than 5 stools per day while receiving the above-named antibiotics should discontinue therapy. If drug administration must be continued, close monitoring including endos-copy is essential. Elderly, bedridden patients with un-derlying diseases of the bowel appear to be at a higher risk for developing serious colitis than do younger indi-viduals; however, cases have been reported in previ-ously healthy young patients. Additionally, attempts to control the diarrhea with agents like diphenoxylate-atropine (Lomotil) or other opiates may prolong and/or worsen the condition. Anticholinergics have been im-plicated in the development of toxic megacolon. Cor-ticosteroids, given systemically or as retention enemas, may help relieve the colitis. Preliminary evidence has indicated that cholestyramine may help to relieve the symptoms and shorten the course of the disorder; further study is planned (42). The condition may take as long as 4-6 weeks to resolve and attention must also be payed to the general management of patients with se-vere and protracted diarrhea, since many are elderly. Because of the apparently high incidence of pseudomembranous colitis associated with clindamy-cin use, The Medical Letter (164) has recommended that the drug be reserved for treatment of non-CNS, severe anaerobic infections or selected staphyloccal infections occurring in penicillin-allergic individuals. (Also see chapter on **General Care-Constipation and Diarrhea**.)

HEMATOLOGIC COMPLICATIONS

A large number of drugs and chemicals, including several antibiotics, are capable of producing blood dyscrasias. Table 11 lists those antibiotics known to produce hematological complications; Table 12 lists those antimicrobials specifically implicated in causing hemolytic anemia. Fortunately, significant hematologic complications of antimicrobial agents occur infrequently; however, they are largely unpredictable and, depending on the reaction, often associated with a high morbidity and mortality. Granulocytopenia (agranulocytosis) is the most common severe hematologic reaction to drugs. Should infection develop as the result of marked neutropenia the mortality rate is between 20-50%, even with prompt, appropriate antibiotic therapy (103). Aplastic anemia is the most frequently fatal of the blood dyscrasias, and next to agranulocytosis is the most commonly reported (224).

Chloramphenicol

Chloramphenicol is most infamous for its ability to produce aplastic anemia. Although the incidence of this complication is actually quite rare (approximately 1/40,000) (240), cloramphenicol is the drug most commonly implicated in cases of aplastic anemia (72). The mechanism of chloramphenicol induced **aplastic anemia** remains unclear; there is evidence, however, that it develops on the basis of a genetically determined biochemical predisposition. Because there is no way to predict those patients likely to develop this complication (224), it is important that the drug be administered properly only for relatively short periods of time and only when clearly indicated.

Table 11
HEMATOLOGIC COMPLICATIONS
OF ANTIMICROBIAL THERAPY (27, 224)

DISORDER	ANTIMICROBIAL
Anemia	
Aplastic anemia	chloramphenicol
	sulfonamides
"Iron deficiency"	chloramphenicol
Hemolytic	see Table 12
Granulocytopenia	chloramphenicol
	ampicillin
	sulfonamides
	ristocetin
Thrombocytopenia	sulfonamides
	ristocetin
Eosinophilia	Allergic response: may occur with all agents. Occurs frequently with streptomycin
Positive Coomb's test	penicillin
	cephalothin
Platelet inhibition	carbenicillin (39)
	other penicillins (?)

Table 12
ANTIMICROBIAL DRUGS AND
HEMOLYTIC ANEMIA (224)

MECHANISM	DRUG
Enzyme deficiency G6PD deficiency	Chloramphenicol (whites only), sulfisoxazole (large doses), sulfamethoxypyridazine, N-aceylsulfanilamide, nitrofurantoin, nalidixic acid, para-aminosalicylic acid
Glutathione peroxidase deficiency	sulfisoxazole nitrofurantoin
Hemoglobinopathy-Hemoglobin Zurich	sulfonamides
Immune mechanisms	penicillin and derivatives cephalothin (? other cephalosporins) isoniazid para-aminosalicylic acid
Unknown mechanism	streptomycin amphotericin B

Chloramphenicol may also produce an **"iron deficiency" anemia**. However, unlike the aplastic anemia described above, the reversible hematopoietic depression caused by chloramphenicol is a predictable, relatively benign condition. There appears to be no relationship between these two complications. The simple anemia of chloramphenicol is associated with an increase in serum iron, decrease in reticulocytes and vacuolization of the bone marrow cells. The mechanism of this reaction is unclear but appears to result from an inhibition of mitochondrial protein synthesis (237). Bone marrow depression may be more prevalent in patients with concomitant renal or hepatic dysfunction (222) and occurs regularly when serum concentrations of chloramphenicol exceed 25 mcg/ml (129). The aplastic anemia and anemia resulting from bone marrow depression of chloramphenicol are contrasted in Table 13.

Table 13
HEMATOLOGIC TOXICITY
OF CHLORAMPHENICOL (224)

BONE MARROW DEPRESSION	APLASTIC ANEMIA
Common	Rare (? genetic basis)
Dose related	Not dose related
Reversible	Usually fatal
Occurs concurrently with therapy	Late clinical onset
Cellular marrow	Aplastic or hypoplastic marrow
Vacuolization of early erythroid cells	
Reticulocytopenia	
Elevation of serum iron	

Hemolytic Anemia

Hemolytic anemia is an occasional complication of antimicrobial therapy and can be induced by various mechanisms. Glucose-6-phosphate dehydrogenase (G-6-PD) deficiency is associated with hemolytic anemia when patients with significant deficiences of the enzyme are exposed to certain oxidant antimicrobial agents. Glucose-6-phosphate dehydrogenase is the first enyzme of the pentose-phosphate pathway. This pathway is responsible for the reduction of nicotinamide adenine dinucleotide phosphate (NADP) to NADPH, which is an important source of reductive power to the red blood cell contributing protons and electrons for the reduction of glutathione. Reduced glutathione is needed to reduce hydrogen peroxide in red cells and protect hemoglobin and other cell proteins (including the cell membrane) from being oxidized. In normal erythrocytes under the stress of oxidant drugs, the rate of NADPH regeneration can be greatly accelerated by increasing the amount of glucose metabolized via the pentose phosphate pathway. Sufficient NADPH is therefore readily made available for reduction of oxidized glutathione and methemoglobin through the respective reductase reactions. Patients with G-6-PD deficiencies are incapable of sufficiently rapid regeneration of NADPH, thus, all reductive processes are impaired. Metabolic processes are diminished, normal vital functions can no longer be carried out, and hemolysis occurs as a consequence of the alterations in the lipoprotein membrane of the cell.

About 3% of the world population has glucose-6-phosphate dehydrogenase deficiency. This deficiency is genetically determined and is a sex-linked partially dominant characteristic with full expression in the homozygous female (3%) or in the hemizygous male (13%). About 20% of Black males appear to be heterozygous and experience a variable degree of hemolysis ranging from clinically undetectable to severe hemolysis when they are exposed to oxidant drugs. Among Caucasians, glucose-6-phosphate dehydrogenase deficiency is particularly prominent in those of mediterranean descent. Caucasians with this deficiency appear to be more prone to hemolytic anemia than Blacks. It is important to realize that the hemolytic process is related to the drug's blood level which may well depend on the metabolism, excretion, and interaction with other concurrent illnesses (infection and diabetic ketoacidosis both enhance hemolytic reactions) (18).

Immune complex injury also may be responsible for hemolytic anemias. Penicillin and its derivatives are most commonly associated with the immune complex variety. Penicillin-induced hemolytic anemia has only been reported following the administration of large doses, generally more than 20 million units per day. The hemolysis is accompanied by a reticulocytosis, de-crease in red-blood-cell life span, and a positive direct Coombs' test. Hyperbilirubinemia may or may not be present depending on the degree of hemolysis and hepatic function of the patient. A circulating IgG anti-penicillin antibody, capable of mediating hemolysis, can be demonstrated in the serum of these patients (65, 235). Evidence of hemolysis may persist for several weeks after the cessation of penicillin therapy. Treatment consists of discontinuing the offending agent, blood transfusion and supportive therapy as indicated. Corticosteroids may be helpful. (Also see chapter on **Anemias**.)

Carbenicillin

Shortly after its introduction into clinical medicine, reports of a carbenicillin-induced bleeding diathesis began to appear (147, 158, 239). Early studies on carbenicillin's effect on hemostasis suggested that it prevented the conversion of fibrinogen to fibrin. However, these reports utilized concentrations of carbenicillin greatly in excess of those commonly achieved during its clinical use. Brown and associates (39) administered therapeutic doses of carbenicillin to normal volunteers and infected patients and demonstrated that the hemostatic defect results from inhibition of platelet aggregation. This occurs 12-24 hours after carbenicillin therapy is initiated and may persist for the duration of the platelet's lifetime. It appears that carbenicillin or a metabolite not only has a permanent effect on circulating platelets but also affects megakaryocytes so that newly formed thrombocytes may also be defective, even though the drug is no longer present. The drug had little effect on fibrin formation or other phases of coagulation in usual doses. Patients receiving carbenicillin must be closely monitored for signs of bleeding. One measure of platelet function which seems to be affected in a dose-dependent manner is the template bleeding time. This test is said to be most useful for monitoring the hemostatic effectiveness of thrombocytes in patients receiving carbenicillin (39). Penicillin G in high concentrations also inhibits platelet aggregation *in vitro* (51); however, the defect has no clinical significance *in vivo* following the administration of therapeutic doses.

PENETRATION OF ANTIBIOTICS INTO CEREBROSPINAL FLUID*

Meningitis Case

A 49-year-old adult-onset diabetic was hospitalized with chills and fever. Four months prior to admission, he was treated for a **Klebsiella** *lung abscess; he has*

---

* This portion of the chapter was authored by Unamarie Clibon.

noted recurrent chills, fever, and hemoptysis over the past three months.

Physical examination revealed an oriented, alert male with a temperature of 38.9°C, a pulse of 110/min, a blood pressure of 140/82 mm Hg, and a respiratory rate of 30/min. Chest X-ray revealed left lower lobe consolidation; neurological examination was within normal limits. Blood and sputum cultures were obtained and IV cephalothin 1 gm every 4 hours was begun.

Twenty-four hours later stupor developed and a lumbar puncture was performed. The opening pressure was 250 mm H_2O (normal-125). Analysis of the cerebrospinal fluid (CSF) revealed a protein of 190 mg/100 ml (20-45), 80,000 WBC/mm_3 with 100% neutrophils (0.5 lymphs), and a glucose of 4 mg/100 ml (50-85). A gram stain showed gram negative rods, so antibiotic therapy was changed to gentamicin 5 mg/kg/day IV and 8 mg/day intrathecally (IT). Sputum and blood cultures taken on the day of admission and spinal fluid taken one day later subsequently grew Klebsiella sensitive to cephalothin, ampicillin and gentamicin.

The patient received six IT injections and a 14 day course of IV gentamicin. His lung consolidation cleared and his mental status slowly improved to normal. He was discharged three weeks after admission.

Which antibiotics produce effective CSF concentrations when administered systemically?

Although bacterial meningitis is primarily a childhood infection, this patient's stuporous condition and CSF findings confirm the diagnosis. Findings consistent with bacterial meningitis include an increased opening pressure as well as a low glucose, elevated protein, high WBC (neutrophils) count, and bacteria in the CSF. One must seriously consider the degree to which various antibiotics penetrate the meninges when selecting therapy for patients with meningitis.

Although many factors may enhance the passage of drug into the CSF (e.g. low serum protein binding and high lipid solubility), the presence of meningeal inflammation has the greatest influence (258, 277).

Of all antibiotics, *chloramphenicol* achieves the highest CSF concentration (30-50% of the serum concentration) (265). Even higher concentrations are achieved if the meninges are inflamed. Preliminary data indicate that *metronidazole* may also achieve high CSF levels (as % of serum concentrations) (262).

Sulfonamides also achieve CSF concentrations as high as 30-50% of serum concentrations in the presence of meningeal inflammation (280). As late as 1965 sulfonamides were recommended for the treatment of gram negative meningitis (278). They are no longer used because many organisms have developed resistance to them and there are now more effective antibio-

tics available (270).

Early data from healthy adult volunteers showed that **trimethoprim-sulfamethoxazole (TMP-SMZ)** achieved CSF concentrations a quarter to a third of those in the serum (257). Recent data from infants with meningitis confirm that CSF concentrations approximately 33% of those in the serum are achieved with parenteral administration (275).

In the absence of meningeal inflammation, **ampicillin** produces a CSF concentration that is 4% of its serum concentration. This increases to 11% when inflammation is present. Systemic ampicillin is effective in the treatment of bacterial meningitis if used in doses of 150-400 mg/kg/day (259).

Although **penicillin G** penetrates the inflamed meninges poorly (6% of its serum concentrations), high doses (12 to 20 MU/day) produce adequate CSF levels for sensitive microorganisms. Therefore intrathecal administration is not necessary (264). Mohr and associates (267) attribute poor responses in the treatment of neurosyphilis to inadequate CSF levels of penicillin obtained from the U.S. Public Health Service and World Health Organization recommended intramuscular dosages of benzathine penicillin G. They demonstrated more than spirocheticidal levels in the CSF after giving aqueous penicillin G 5 to 10 MU/day intravenously for ten days and strongly suggest that the recommended therapy be re-evaluated.

Methicillin is undetectable in the CSF unless the meninges are inflamed, in which case 2.9 - 10% of the serum concentration is achieved (269). Although a dose of 12 gm/day may be effective in the treatment of meningitis due to penicillinase-producing *Staphylococcus,* intrathecal administration may be necessary in fulminant cases (261). Salmon (276) suggests 25 to 50 mg daily depending on estimated CSF volume.

Carbenicillin passes relatively well into the CSF and attains levels of approximately 15% of its serum concentrations in the absence of inflammation, and 19% in meningitis (260). Because rather high concentrations are required to inhibit *Pseudomonas,* some suggest intrathecal administration in addition to systemic therapy (273).

The data for the **cephalosporins** are confusing because early reports used an assay which measured some inactive metabolites as well as active drug. Apparently, cephalothin produces CSF concentrations of 0-1.2% of its serum concentration and cephaloridine produces CSF levels of 1.1% of its serum concentrations when the meninges are not inflamed. In the presence of inflammation cephalothin and cephaloridine produce CSF concentrations which are 1.2-5.6% and 9.7% of their serum concentratins, respectively (266, 268, 269, 279). Cephalosporins are not recommended for the treatment of meningitis, because there have been numerous reports of patients who developed meningitis while taking cephalosporins (268). However, Fisher has reported success with a combination of cephalothin 12 gm/day intravenously and cephaloridine 12.5 to 50 mg/day intrathecally (263).

Of all the **aminoglycosides,** only gentamicin penetrates the meninges when they are inflamed (6% of serum concentrations). To acehive adequate CSF levels, gentamicin must be given intrathecally as well as systemically to patients with gram negative meningitis (271).

In summary, chloramphenicol, ampicillin, penicillin and methicillin achieve effective CSF levels when administered systemically; the cephalosporins and aminoglycosides do not. See Table 14.

How much gentamicin should be administered intrathecally (IT) and how often?

An IT dose of 4 mg of gentamicin provides therapeutic CSF concentrations for 18 hours (T½ 5.5 hours) (272). An 8 mg intrathecal dose of gentamicin maintains therapeutic concentrations in the CSF for 24 hours and does not accumulate when administered in this dosing interval. Therefore, 8 mg of gentamicin should be administered IT every 24 hours in addition to 5 mg/kg/day IV in adults as was done in the case presented. Some authors have noted better distribution of intrathecal lumbar injections to ventricular and cisternal areas if the volume of injection is at least 10-25% of CSF volume (274).

PENETRATION OF ANTIBIOTICS IN JOINT FLUID*

Septic Arthritis Case

A 28-year-old male stepped on a nail and developed an abscess on the plantar aspect of his right foot. The abscess was incised, drained and an embedded piece of sock was removed. Although he was treated as an outpatient with oral tetracycline, the infection progressed. X-rays of the right foot were consistent with osteomyelitis of the right distal first metatarsal. Culture of the drainage material and two of the six blood cultures yielded Pseudomonas aeruginosa. Therapy at this time included bed rest, immobilization of the right foot, gentamicin 120 mg every 8 hours and carbenicillin 30 gm/day intravenously. Antibacterial treatment was continued for 14 days, and the patient was discharged after three weeks of hospital care with full use of his right foot.

Four months later he was hospitalized complaining of a painful, swollen, hot, red right knee. Cultures of aspirated synovial fluid from the right knee grew out Pseudomonas aeruginosa.

* This portion of the chapter was authored by John Siepler.

Table 14
PENETRATION OF ANTIBIOTICS INTO THE CSF

Drug	% of Serum Concentration Uninflamed Mengines	% of Serum Concentration Inflamed Meninges
Chloramphenicol	30-50%	30-50% or more
Sulfonamides	up to 33%	33-50%
TMP-SMZ	25-33%	33%
Carbenicillin	15%	19%
Ampicillin	4%	11%
Penicillin G	0-trace%	6%
Methicillin	0%	2.4-10%
Cephalothin	0%(man),1.2%(dogs)	1.2-5.6%
Cephaloridine	1.1%	9.7%
Gentamicin	trace with serum concentrations of 4 mcg/ml	6% with serum concentrations of 8 mcg/ml
Kanamycin	0%	trace
Vanomycin	0%	trace

Which antibiotics best penetrate into a septic joint? Are bactericidal levels achieved in the synovial fluid?

Septic arthritis is an infectious disease with grave complications. If left unchecked or treated too late, serious joint damage may result, ending ultimately in amputation of the affected appendage.

Treatment of this disorder is controversial. Some instill antibiotics into the joint, whereas others treat with systemic antibiotics only.

A critical review of the literature produces some interesting findings. Following systemic administration, antibiotics diffuse into infected joint fluid slowly so that peak levels are reached two to four hours after a single dose. Diffusion out of the infected joint, however, is very slow. Concentrations of antibiotics which are higher than the corresponding serum concentrations may be demonstrated several days after the administration of a single dose. In contrast to serum levels, there is almost no fluctuation of antibiotic concentrations within the joint fluid. In other words, serum levels degrade as predicted by their half-lives, while joint fluid levels fall much more slowly.

Intra-articular administration of antibiotics carries the risk of introducing new organisms into the joint. If surgery or direct instillation are to be avoided, systemic antibiotics must penetrate into the joint to produce adequate levels. The penetration of specific antibiotics into the joint fluid is examined in more detail below.

Penetration of **penicillins** into infected joints has been extensively studied. Early studies which found penetration to be marginal are invalid because of the low doses used; additionally, serum joint fluid samples were drawn too soon after the administration of the penicillin (290, 293). It has been shown that ampicillin, methicillin, nafcillin, cloxacillin, and penicillin are concentrated in the joint fluid to at least 80-100% of the peak serum level (291, 294). If the penicillin being used achieves bactericidal serum levels, it will most likely achieve bactericidal concentrations in the joint as well. Questionable situations can be resolved by obtaining serum and joint fluid bactericidal levels.

Cephalosporins. Nelson (291) showed that an IM dose of cephalothin (20 mg/kg) produces a synovial fluid level of 2 to 5 mcg/ml. Parker et al (295) determined that after six to eight hours, cephaloridine joint fluid concentrations were 80-100% of serum concentrations. The newly released cephalosporins have not been studied in this regard. Cephalothin probably will not achieve bactericidal joint fluid levels for sensitive gram negative organisms, but doses of 8 to 12 gm/day will probably achieve adequate joint fluid levels for the treatment of *Staphylococcus aureus* infections.

Lincomycin and **Clindamycin** have been promoted for the treatment of osteomyelitis because they reportedly produce high concentrations in bone (288, 292). However, information concerning their penetration into synovial fluid is sparse. Cases of *Staphylococcus* septic arthritis cured with lincomycin have appeared in the literature; however, these did not contain specific data on its penetration into joint fluid (283, 296). Two studies indicate that lincomycin and clindamycin produce joint fluid levels that are 60-80% of serum concentration; therefore, MIC's for *Staphylococcus,* but perhaps not for *Bacteroides,* are obtainable in joint fluid (283, 296).

Penetration of systemically administered **Aminoglycosides** into the synovial fluid has not been well studied. Traditionally, septic arthritis due to gram negative bacteria is treated surgically with saucerization, insertion of irrigation and drainage tubes, and penicillin or aminoglycoside containing irrigations (287). Studies on the penetration of kanamycin are sparse, but Baciocco (281) found the kanamycin concentrations in the synovial fluid often approached those seen in the serum. Studies on the penetration of gentamicin give conflicting results. Dewart (284) found the concentrations in the synovial fluid to be less than 1.6 mcg/ml after administration of 240 mg/day of gentamicin. Marsh (289) indicated that inhibitory concentrations of gentamicin were achieved in a septic joint following an IM dose of 90 mg. No paired samples were obtained in either case, but Chow et al (282) report synovial fluid concentrations of gentamicin as high as 2.7 mcg/ml following 120 mg of gentamicin IV; they found that joint fluid concentrations never exceeded serum concentrations, and their patient required the addition of carbenicillin to sterilize the joint. Donovan (285) reports a case of *Serratia* arthritis successfully treated with amikacin, but no joint fluid concentrations were obtained.

In conclusion, the achievement of bacteridal levels in infected joints cannot be predicted for these antibiotics. Serum and joint fluid concentrations of the aminoglycoside used should be obtained in questionable situations.

REFERENCES

1. Adkinson NF et al: Routine use of penicillin skin testing on an inpatient service NEJM, 285:22, 1971.
2. Adler et al: Nonoliguric renal failure secondary to sodium colistimethate: a report of four cases. Amer J Med Sci, 261:109, 1971.
3. Almeyda et al: Drug reactions XIX. Adverse cutaneous reactions to the penicillins — ampicillin rashes, Brit J Dermatol, 87:293, 1972.
4. Annotations: Ampicillin rashes, Lancet, 2:993, 1969.
5. Bagdade JD: Impaired leukocyte function in patients with poorly controlled diabetes. Diabetes, 23:9, 1974.
6. Baldwin DS et al: Renal failure and interstitial nephritis due to penicillin and methicillin, NEJM, 279:1245, 1968.
7. Barnett HL et al: Physiologic and clinical significance of immaturity of kidney function in young infants, J Pediat, 42:99, 1953.
9. Barza M et al: Predictability of blood levels of gentamicin in man, J Infect Dis, 132:165, 1975.
10. Bass W et al: Adverse effects of orally administered ampicillin, J Pediatr, 83:106, 1973.
11. Batchelor FR et al: A penicilloylated protein impurity as a source of allergy to benzylpenicillin and 6-aminopenicillanic acid, Lancet, 1:1175, 1967.
12. Benacerraf B: Cellular hypersensitivity. Ann Rev Med, 20:141, 1969.
13. Benner EJ: Cephaloridine and the kidneys, J Infect Dis, 122:104, 1970.
14. Benner E et al: Pseudomembraneous colitis as a sequel to oral lincomycin therapy, Am J Gastroenterol, 54:55, 1970.
15. Bennett WM et al: A guide to drug therapy in renal failure, JAMA 230:1544, 1974.
16. Berk DP et al: Deafness complicating antibiotic therapy of hepatic encephalopathy, Ann Intern Med, 73:393, 1970.
17. Beutler E: Drug-induced blood dyscrasias. III. Hemolytic anemia, JAMA, 189:143, 1964.
18. Beutler E: Drug-induced hemolytic anemia, Pharmacol Rev, 21:73, 1969.
19. Bhowmich BK: Benign intracranial hypertension after antibiotic therapy, Brit Med J, 3:30, 1972.
20. Bierman CW et al: Reactions associated with ampicillin therapy, JAMA, 220:1098, 1972.
21. Bloomer HA et al: Penicillin-induced encephalopathy in uremic patients, JAMA, 200:121, 1967.
22. Blum P et al: Obvious seizures from carbenicillin, Minn Med, 54:697, 1971.
23. Bobrow N et al: Anuria and acute tubular necrosis associated with gentamicin and cephalothin, JAMA, 222:1546, 1972.
24. Bond CA: Drug-induced skin eruptions, University of Wisconsin, Personal Communication.
25. Border WA et al: Antitubular basement membrane antibodies in methicillin-associated interstitial nephritis, NEJM, 291:381, 1974.
26. Boreus LO et al: Intracranial hypertension in a child during treatment with nalidixic acid, Brit Med J, 2:744, 1967.
27. Boston Collaborative Drug Surveillance Program: Excess of ampicillin rashes associated with allopurinol or hyperuricemia, NEJM, 286:505, 1972.
28. Boston Collaborative Drug Surveillance Program: Tetracycline and drug-attributed rises in blood urea nitrogen, JAMA, 220:377, 1972.
29. Boston Collaborative Drug Surveillance Program: Drug-induced convulsions, Lancet, 2:677, 1972.
30. Boston Collaborative Drug Surveillance Program: Ampicillin rashes, Arch Dermatol, 107:74, 1973.
31. Boston Collaborative Drug Surveillance Program: Drug-induced deafness, JAMA, 224:515, 1973.
32. Box TRH: The hematological complications of commonly prescribed drugs, Appl Therap, 11:477, 1969.
33. Bradberry JC et al: Acute psychotic reaction to procaine penicillin, Amer J Hosp Pharm, 32:411, 1975.
34. Bran JL et al: Clinical and in vitro evaluation of cephapirin, a new cephalsoporin antibiotic, Antimicrob Agents Chemotherap, 1:35, 1972.
35. Brandiss MW et al: Common antigenic determinants of penicillin, cephalothin and 6-aminopenicillanic acid in rabbits, J Immunol, 94:696, 1965.
36. Brauninger GE et al: Nephropathy associated with methicillin therapy, JAMA, 203:125, 1968.
37. Brayton RG et al: Cephaloridine: Clinical trial in gram-positive and gram-negative infections, Antimicrob Agents Chemotherap, 1966.
38. Bristol Laboratories: "Product Brochure. Amikin. Amikacin Sulfate," Syracuse, New York, June, 1976.
39. Brown CH III et al: The hemostatic defect produced by carbenicillin, NEJM, 291:265, 1974.
40. Brown G at al: Drug rashes in glandular fever, Lancet, 2:1418, 1967.
41. Brtscher O: The control of humeral and associative antibody synthesis. Transplant Rev, 11:217, 1972.
42. Burbige EJ et al: Pseudomembranous colitis. Association with antibiotics and therapy with cholestyramine, JAMA, 231:1157, 1975.
43. Burton JR et al: Acute renal failure during cephalothin therapy, JAMA, 229:679, 1974.
44. Butler WT et al: Nephrotoxicity of amphotericin B. Early and late effects in 81 patients, Ann Intern Med, 61:175, 1964.
45. Bybee JD: the phagocytic activity of polymorphonuclear leukocytes obtained from patients with diabetes mellitus. J Lab Clin Med 64:1, 1964.
46. Byrd RB et al: Isoniazid toxicity. A prospective study in secondary chemoprophylaxis, JAMA, 220:1471, 1972.
47. Cabana BE et al: Comparative pharmacokinetics of BB-K8 and kanamycin in dogs and humans, Antimicrob Agents Chemotherap, 3:478, 1973.
48. Cabanillas F et al: Nephrotoxicity of combined cephalothin-gentamicin regimen, Arch Intern Med, 135:850, 1975.
49. Cameron SJ et al: Ampicillin hypersensitivity in lymphatic leukemia, Scot Med J, 16:425, 1972.
50. Carling PC et al: Nephrotoxicity associated with cephalothin administration, Arch Intern Med, 135:797, 1975.
51. Cazenave JP et al: Effects of penicillin G on platelet aggregation, release, and adherance to collagen, Proc Soc Exp Biol Med, 142:159, 1973.
52. Chan RA et al: Gentamicin therapy in renal failure: a nomogram for dosage, Ann Int Med, 76:773, 1972.
53. Clanman HN: Thymus-marrow cell combination. Synergism and antibody production. Proc Soc Exp Biol Med, 122:167, 1966.
54. Cohen AC: Pyridoxine in the prevention and treatment of convulsions and neurotoxicity due to cycloserine, Ann NY Acad Sci, 166:346, 1969.
55. Cohen SN et al: Drug-induced nephropathy, JAMA, 227:325, 1974.
56. Collaborative Study Group: Prospective study of ampicillin rash, Brit Med J, 1:7, 1973.
57. Combes B et al: Tetracycline and the liver, Progress in Liver Diseases, 4:589, 1972.
58. Conway N et al: Streptomycin in pregnancy: effect on fetal ear, Brit Med J, 2:260, 1965.
59. Corless JD et al: The rash associated with ampicillin therapy, South Med J, 63:1341, 1970.
60. Cutter RE et al: Correlation of serum creatinine concentration and Gentamicin half-life, JAMA, 219:1037, 1972.
61. Cutler RE et al: Correlation of serum creatinine concentration and kanamycin half-life, JAMA, 209:539, 1969.
61a.David JR: "Delayed hypersensitivity," in SCOPE monograph on Immunology, Medical Communications, Inc., New York, 1970, p. 22.
62. Davies AJ: The failure of thymus derived cells to produce antibodies. Transplant 5:222, 1967.
63. Davis LJ: The management of a patient with a history of penicillin hypersensitivity, J Okla State Med Assoc, 65:214, 1972.
64. Davis JS: Severe colitis following lincomycin and clindamycin therapy, Amer J Gastroenterol, 62:16, 1974.
65. Dawson RB Jr et al: Penicillin-induced immunohemolytic anemia, Arch Intern Med, 118:575, 1966.
66. Drago JR et al: Acute interstitial nephritis, J Urol, 115:105, 1976.
67. DuJovne CA et al: Experimental basis for the different hepatotoxicity of erythromycin preparations in man, J Lab Clin Med, 79:833, 1972.
68. Duncan DA: Colistin toxicity. Neuromuscular and renal manifestations. Two cases treated by hemodialysis, Minn Med, 56:31, 1973.
69. Eagle H: Speculation as to the therapeutic significance of penicillin blood levels, Ann Int Med 28:260, 1948.

70. Elmqvist D et al: The nature of the neuromusuclar block produced by neomycin, Acta Physiol Scand, 54:105, 1962.

71. Elwood CM et al: Acute renal failure associated with sodium colistimethate treatment, Arch Int Med, 118:326, 1966.

72. Erslev AJ: Drug-induced blood dyscrasias. I. Aplastic anemia, JAMA, 188:531, 1964.

73. Falco FG et al: Nephrotoxicity of aminoglycosides and gentamicin, J Infect Dis, 119:406, 1969.

74. Feigin RD et al: Hematuria and proteinuria associated with methicillin administration, NEJM, 272:903, 1965.

75. Feinberg JG: Allergy to antibiotics. I. Facts and conjecture on the sensitizing contaminants of penicillins and cephalosporins, Int Arch Allergy, 33:439, 1968.

76. Feinberg JG: "Experimental studies on penicillin allergy." Penicillin Allergy, Thomas Publishers, Springfield, Ill., 1970, p. 90.

77. Fekety FR et al: The treatment of gram-negative bacillary infections with colistin, Ann Intern Med, 57:214, 1962.

78. Feldmann M: Cell interactions in the immune response in vitro. V specific collaboration via complexes of antigen and thymus-derived cells immunoglobulins. J Exp Med 139:737, 1972.

79. Fellner MJ et al: Intercellular antibodies in blood and epidermis. A histochemical study of IgG immunoglobulins in patients with late reactions to penicillins and their comparison with similar antibodies in patients with pemphigus vulgaris, Brit J Dermatol, 89:115, 1973.

80. Fessel WJ: Immunologic reactivity in hyperuricemia, NEJM, 286:1218, 1972.

81. Fields JP: bulging fontanel: a complication of tetracycline therapy in infants, J Pediatr, 58:74, 1961.

82. Finegold SM: Kanamycin, Arch Int Med, 104:15, 1959.

83. Finegold SM et al: Drugs of choice for specific bacteria, Cal Med, 111:374, 1969.

84. Finegold SM et al: Chemotherapy guide, Cal Med, 111:362, 1969.

85. Finland M et al: Oral penicillin, JAMA, 129:315, 1945.

86. Foord RD: Cephaloridine and the kidney, Progress in Antimicrobiol and Anticancer Chemotherapy, 1:597, 1969.

87. Garibaldi RA et al: Isoniazid-associated hepatitis, Amer Rev Resp Dis, 106:357, 1972.

88. Garrod LP et al: Antibiotic and Chemotherapy, Williams and Wilkins, Co., Baltimore, ED. 3, 1972.

89. Gavan TL et al: Antimicrobial Susceptibility Testing, American Society of Clinical Pathologists Commission on Continuing Education, Chicago, Illinois, 1971.

90. Gellis S (ed.): Editorial comment, The Year Book of Pediatrics, 1956-1957, The Year Book Publishers, Chicago, 1956, p. 40.

91. Gilbert DN et al: Interstitial nephritis due to methicillin, penicillin and ampicillin, Annals of Allergy, 28:378, 1970.

92. Giles CL et al: Intracranial hypertension and tetracycline therapy, Am J Ophthamol, 72:981, 1971.

93. Glassock RJ: Complications of antibiotic therapy. Renal complications, Calif Med, 117:31, 1972.

94. Goldman AL et al: Isoniazid: a review with emphasis on adverse effects, Chest, 62:71, 1972.

95. Goldner JC: Neurotoxicity of antibiotics, Minn Med, 51:1629, 1968.

96. Green GR et al: Report of the penicillin study group — American Academy of Allergy, J Allergy Clin Immunol, 48:331, 1971.

97. Green RL et al: Elevated plasma procaine concentrations after administration of procaine penicillin G, NEJM, 291:223, 1974.

98. Hall DR et al: Gentamicin, tubocurarine, lignocaine and neuromuscular blockade, Brit J Anaesth, 44:1329, 1972.

99. Hansen PD: Cephalothin, gentamicin, colistin hazards, JAMA, 223:1158, 1973.

100. Hinman AR et al: Nephrotoxicity associated with the use of cephaloridine, JAMA, 200:148, 1967.

101. Hoffman TA et al: Pharmacodynamics of carbenicillin in hepatic and renal failure, Ann Int Med, 73:173, 1970.

102. Hopper J Jr. et al: Polymyxin B in chronic pyelonephritis: observation on the safety of the drug and its influence on renal function, Amer J Med Sci, 225:402, 1953.

103. Huguley CM Jr.: Drug-induced blood dyscrasias. II. Agranulocytosis, JAMA, 188:817, 1964.

104. Hull JH et al: Gentamicin serum concentrations: Pharmacokinetic predictions, Ann Int Med, 85:183, 1976.

105. Ibister JR: Penicillin allergy, Rev Allergy, 25:1201, 1971.

106. Jackson EA et al: Pharmacokinetics and dosing of antimicrobial agents in renal impairment, part I, Amer J Hosp Pharm, 31:36, 1974.

107. Jackson GG et al: Ototoxity of gentamicin in man: A survey and controlled analysis of clinical experience in the United States, J Infect Dis, 124:suppl:130, 1971.

108. Johnson AH et al: Kanamycin ototoxicity — possible potentiation by other drugs, South Med J, 63:511, 1970.

109. Johnson HC et al: Intraventricular penicillin. A note of warning, JAMA, 127:217, 1945.

110. Jondal M: Human lymphocytes subpopulations: Classification according to surface markers n/4 functional characteristics. Transplant Rev 16:163, 1973.

111. Jones HC: Intrauterine ototoxicity. A case report and review of literature, J Natl Med Assoc, 65:201, 1973.

112. Kabins SA et al: Cephaloridine therapy as related to renal function, Antimicrob Agents Chemotherap, 5:922, 1965.

113. Kampmann JP et al: Rapid evaluation of creatinine clearance, Acta Med Scand, 196:517, 1974.

114. Kaplan JM et al: Clinical pharmacology of tobramycin in newborns, Amer J Dis Child, 125:656, 1973.

115. Kaplan K et al: Cephaloridine. Studies of therapeutic activity and untoward effects, Arch Int Med, 121:17, 1968.

116. Kasik JE et al: Allergic reactions to antibiotics, Med Clin N Amer, 54:59, 1970.

117. Klastersky J: Antibacterial activity in serum and urine as a therapeutic guide in bacterial infections. J Infect Dis 129:187, 1974.

118. Klastersky J et al: Empiric therapy for cancer patients: Comparative study of ticarcillin-tobramycin, ticarcillin-cephalothin and cephalothin-tobramycin, Antimicrob Agents Chemotherap, 7:640, 1975.

119. Klatskin G: Toxic and drug-induced hepatitis. Ch 14. Diseases of the Liver, 3rd edition, edited by Leon Schiff, J. B. Lippincott and Co., 1969, p. 498.

120. Klebanoff SJ: Intraleukocytic microbicidal defects. Ann Rev Med, 22:39, 1971.

121. Kleinknecht J et al: Acute renal failure after high doses of gentamicin and cephalothin. Lancet, 1:1129, 1973.

122. Kleinknecht D et al: Nephrotoxicity of cephaloridine, Ann Intern Med, 80:421, 1974.

123. Klemola E: Hypersensitivity reactions to ampicillin in cytomegalovirus mononucleosis, Scand J Infect Dis, 2:29, 1970.

124. Klotz AP et al: Aureomycin proctitis and colitis: a report of five cases, Gastroenterology, 25:44, 1953.

125. Knudsen ET: Ampicillin and urticaria, Brit Med J, 1:846, 1969.

126. Knudsen ET et al: Reduction in incidence of ampicillin rash by purification of ampicillin, Brit Med J, 1:469, 1970.

127. Koch-Weser J et al: Benign intracranial hypertension in an adult after tetracycline therapy. JAMA, 200:345, 1967.

128. Koch-Weser J et al: Adverse effects of sodium colistimethate. Manifestations and specific reaction rates during 317 courses of therapy, Ann Intern Med, 72:857, 1970.

129. Kucers A: Erythromycin. The Use of Antibiotics. A Comprehensive Review with Clinical Emphasis, William Heinemann Medical Books Ltd, 1972, p. 212.

130. Kunin CM: A guide to use of antibiotics in patients with renal disease. A table of recommended doses and factors governing serum levels, Ann Int Med, 67:151, 1967.

131. Kunin CM: Antibiotic usage in patients with renal impairment, Hosp Prac, 7:141, 1972.

132. Kunin CM et al: Absorption of orally administered neomycin and kanamycin. With special reference to patients with severe hepatic and renal disease, NEJM, 262:380, 1960.

133. Kurtzman NA et al: Neurotoxic reaction to penicillin and carbenicillin, JAMA, 214:1320, 1970.

134. Lavy S et al: Convulsions in septicemia patients treated with penicillin, Arch Surg, 100:225, 1970.

135. Leonard JM et al: Gentamicin and carbenicillin-resistant Pseudomonas and Serratia infections: therapy with amikacin (BB-K8), Antimicrob Agents Chemotherap, Abst 328, 1974.

136. Lepper MH et al: Effect of large doses of aureomycin on human liver, Arch Int Med, 88:271, 1951.

137. Lerche S: Hearing impairment after prolonged dihydrostreptomycin treatment of surgical tuberculosis, Scand J Resp Dis, 53:27, 1972.

138. Lerner PI et al: Penicillin neurotoxicity, Ann NY Acad Sci, 145:310, 1967.

139. Lerner PI et al: Abnormalities of absorption of benzylpenicillin G

and sulfasoxazole in patients with diabetes mellitus, Am J Med Sc, 248:37, 1964.

140. Levine BB: Skin rashes with penicillin therapy: current management, NEJM, 286:42, 1972.

141. Levine BB et al: Prediction of penicillin allergy by immunological tests, J Allergy, 43:231, 1969.

142. Levine BB: Antigenicity and cross-reactivity of penicillins and cephalosporins, J Infect Dis, 128:suppl:364, 1973.

143. Lischner H et al: Outbreak of neonatal deaths among full term infants associated with administration of chloramphenicol, J Pediat, 59:21, 1961.

144. Lockwood WR et al: Tobramycin and gentamicin concentrations in the serum of normal and anephric patients, Antimicrob Agents Chemotherap, 3:125, 1973.

145. Lowry LD et al: Acute histopathologic inner ear changes in deafness due to neomycin: a case report, Ann Otol Rhin Laryngol, 82:876, 1973.

146. Lumholtz B et al: Dose regimen of kanamycin and gentamicin, Acta Med Scand, 196:521, 1974.

147. Lurie A et al: Carbenicillin-induced coagulopathy, Lancet, 1:1114, 1970.

148. MacFarlane MD et al: Fatty metamorphosis of the liver after I.V. tetracycline, Drug Intell Clin Pharm, 6:310, 1972.

149. MacFarlane MD et al: Anaphylactic shock and anaphylactoid reaction. Analysis of 62 cases, Drug Intell Clin Pharm, 7:394, 1973.

150. Maddrey WC et al: Isoniazid hepatitis, Ann Intern Med, 79:1, 1973.

151. Maheras MG: Penicillin hypersensitivity, Minn Med, 52:1811, 1969.

152. Mandell GL: Cephaloridine, Ann Intern Med, 79:561, 1973.

153. Maroon JC et al: Benign intracranial hypertension. Sequel to tetracycline therapy in a child, JAMA, 216:1479, 1971.

154. Martin WJ: Newer antimicrobial agents having current or potential clinical application, Med Clin N Amer, 48:255, 1964.

155. Matz GJ et al: the ototoxicity of kanamycin. A comparative histopathological study, Laryngoscope, 75:1690, 1965.

155a Mayer MM: The complement system, Scientific Amer, 229:54, 1973.

155b McCabe WR: Serum complement levels in bacteremia due to gram negative organisms, NEJM, 288:21, 1973.

156. McCance RA: Renal physiology in infancy, Am J Med, 9:229, 1950.

157. McCloskey RV et al: Evaluation of the Cutler-Orme method for administration of kanamycin during renal failure, Antimicrob Agents Chemother: 161-164, 1970.

158. McClure PD et al: Carbenicillin-induced bleeding disorder, Lancet, 2:1307, 1970.

159. McCracken GH et al: Antimicrobial therapy in theory and practice. II. Clinical approach to antimicrobial therapy, J Pediat, 75:923, 1969.

160. McHenry MC et al: Gentamicin dosages for renal insufficiency. Adjustments based on endogenous creatinine clearance and srum creatinine concentration, Ann Intern Med, 74:192, 1971.

162. McNitt T et al: A randomized comparative study of tobramycin and gentamicin in acute urinary tract infections, Antimicrob Agents Chemother, Abst 216, 1974.

163. McQuillen MP et al: Myasthenic syndrome associated with antibiotics, Arch Neurol, 18:402, 1968.

164. The Medical Letter on Drugs and Therapeutics, Colitis associated with clindamycin, 16:73, 1974.

165. The Medical Letter on Drugs and Therapeutics: Tests for penicillin allergy, 17:54, 1975.

166. The Medical Letter on Drugs and Therapeutics, Handbook of Antimicrobial Therapy, 1976.

167. Menke HE et al: Acute non-allergic reaction to aqueous procaine penicillin, Lancet, 2:723, 1974.

168. Meuwissen HJ et al: The ototoxic antibiotics: a survey of current knowledge. Clin Pediat, 6:262, 1967.

169. Meyers RM: Ototoxic effects of gentamicin, Arch Otolaryng, 92:160, 1970.

170. Miller RA: Observations on gastric acidity during first month of life, Arch Dis Childhood, 16:22, 1941.

171. Miller RP et al: Amphotericin B toxicity. A follow-up report of 53 patients, Ann Intern Med, 84:181, 1976.

172. Mitchell JR et al: Increased incidence of isoniazid hepatitis in rapid acetylators: possible relation to hydrazine metabolites, Clin Pharmacol Ther, 18:70, 1975.

173. Mitchell JR et al: Isoniazid liver injury: clinical spectrum, pathology and probable pathogenesis, Ann Intern Med, 84:181, 1976.

174. Moellering RC Jr. et al: The newer cephalosporins, NEJM, 294:24, 1976.

175. Mosley JW: Isoniazid toxicity, JAMA, 218:447, 1971.

176. Mowat A: Chemataxis of polmorphonuclear leukocytes from patients with diabetes mellitus. NEJM, 284:621, 1971.

177. Nelson JR: Complications of antibiotic therapy. Neurological complications, Calif Med, 117:37, 1972.

178. New PS et al: Cerebral toxicity associated with massive intravenous penicillin therapy, Neurology, 15:1053, 1965.

179. Nilges TC et al: Iatrogenic ototoxic hearing loss, Ann Surg 173:281, 1971.

180. Nord MN et al: Polymyxin B and colistin; a critical comparison, NEJM, 270:1030, 1964.

181. Odell GB: Dissociation of bilirubin from albumin and its clinical implications, J Pediat, 55:268, 1959.

182. O'Doherty NJ: Acute benign intracranial hypertension in an infant receiving tetracycline, Develop Med Child Neurol, 7:677, 1965.

183. Oldstone MBA et al: Central nervous system manifestations of penicillin toxicity in man, Neurology, 16:693, 1966.

184. Opitz A et al: Akute neireni 1suffizienz nach gentamycin-cephalosporin kombinationstherapie, Med Welt, 22:434, 1971.

185. Owens DR et al: The cephalosporin group of antibiotics, Adv Pharmacol Chemother, 13:83, 1975.

186. Parker CW: Drug allergy (Part III), NEJM, 292:957, 1975.

187. Parry MF et al: Nafcillin nephritis, JAMA, 225:178, 1973.

188. Patel BM: Skin rash with infectious mononucleosis and ampicillin, Pediatrics, 40:910, 1967.

189. Pedersen MF et al: A clinical and experimental comparative study of sodium colistimethate and polymyxin B sulfate, Invest Urol, 9:234, 1971.

190. Pernis B: Immunoglobulin spot on surface of rabbit lymphocytes. J Exp Med, 132:1001, 1970.

191. Pillemer L: The properdin system and immunity. I. Demonstration and isolation of a new serum protein, properdin and its role in immune phenomenon. Science 120:279, 1954.

192. Pittinger DB et al: Potential dangers associated with antibiotic administration during anesthesia and surgery, Arch Surg, 79:207, 1959.

193. Pitts JC III: Allergic penicillin reactions, J Kansas Med Society, 72:322, 1971.

194. Polland WS: Histamine test meals: analysis of 988 consecutive tests, Arch Int Med, 51:903, 1933.

195. Prazma J et al: Ethacrynic acid ototoxicity potentiation by kanamycin, Ann Otol Rhin Laryngol, 83:111, 1974.

196. Price DJE et al: Effects of large doses of colistin sulphomethate sodium on renal function, Brit Med J, 4:525, 1970.

197. Pridgen JE: Respiratory arrest thought to be due to intraperitoneal neomycin, Surgery, 40:571, 1956.

198. Pullen H et al: Hypersensitivity reactions to antibacterial drugs in infectious mononucleosis, Lancet, 2:1176, 1967.

199. Reiner L et al: Pseudomembraneous colitis following aureomycin and chloramphenicol, Arch Pathol, 54:39, 1952.

200. Ries K et al: Clinical and in vitro evaluation of cephazolin, a new cephalosporin antibiotic, Antimicrob Agents Chemotherp, 3:168, 1973.

201. Riff LJ et al: Pharmacology of gentamicin in man, J Infect Dis (suppl): 98, 1971.

202. Robinson MM: Hepatic dysfunction associated with triacetyloleandomycin and propionyl erythromycin ester lauryl sulfate, Amer J Med Sci, 243:502, 1962.

203. Sanjad SA et al: Nephropathy, an underestimated complication of methicillin therapy, J Pediatr, 84:873, 1974.

204. Sborov VM et al: Fatty liver following aureomycin and terramycin therapy in chronic hepatic disease, Gastroent, 18:598, 1951.

205. Schapiro RL et al: Acute enterocolitis. A complication of antibiotic therapy, Radiol, 108:263, 1973.

206. Scharer L et al: Serum transaminase elevations and other hepatic abnormalities in patients receiving isoniazid. Ann Intern Med, 71:1113, 1969.

207. Schreiner GE et al: Toxic nephropathy, Amer J Med, 38:490, 1965.

208. Schrier RW et al: Nephropathy associated with penicillin and homologues, Ann Intern Med, 64:116, 1966.

209. Schultz JC et al: Fatal liver disease after intravenous administration of tetracycline in high dosage, NEJM, 269:999, 1963.

210. Seelig MS: The role of antibiotics in the pathogenesis of candida infections, Am J Med, 40:887, 1966.

211. Shapiro S et al: Drug rash with ampicillin and other penicillins,

Lancet, 2:969, 1969.

212. Simenhoff ML et al: Acute diffuse interstitial nephritis. Review of the literature and case report, Amer J Med, 44:618, 1968.

213. Smith JW: The problem of penicillin allergy, Arizona Med, 28:395, 1971.

214. Smith JW et al: Studies on the epidemiology of adverse drug reactions. II. Evaluation of penicillin allergy, NEJM, 274:998, 1966.

215. Smith JW et al: Studies on the epidemiology of adverse drug reactions. V. Clinical factors influencing susceptibility, Ann Int Med, 65:629, 1966.

216. Stamey TA: Serum versus urinary levels of oxytetracycline in cure of urinary tract infections. *Proceeding of the twelfth interscience conference on antimicrobial agents and chemotherapy*. Atlantic City, NJ, September 1977, page 17.

217. Stead WW et al: Isoniazid hepatitis: backlash of progress, Ann Intern Med, 79:125, 1973.

218. Steigbigel NH et al: Clinical evaluation of cephaloridine, Arch Int Med, 121:24, 1968.

219. Stewart GT: Allergic residues in penicillin, Lancet, 1:1177, 1967.

220. Stewart GT: Allergy to penicillin and related antibiotics: antigenic immunological mechanisms, Ann Rev Pharmacol, 13:309, 1973.

221. Stroehlein JR et al: Clindamycin-associated colitis, Mayo Clin Proc, 49:240, 1974.

222. Suhrland LG et al: Chloramphenicol toxicity in liver and renal disease, Arch Intern Med, 112:747, 1963.

223. Takacs FJ et al: Amphotericin B nephrotoxicity with irreversible renal failure, Ann Intern Med, 59:716, 1963.

224. Tanaka KR: Complications of antibiotic therapy. Hematologic complications, Calif Med, 117:43, 1972.

225. Tedesco FJ et al: Clindamycin-associated colitis. A prospective study, Ann Intern Med, 81:421, 1974.

226. Tedesco, FJ et al: Diagnostic features of clindamycin-associated pseudomembraneous colitis, NEJM, 290:841, 1974.

227. Terplan K et al: Fulminating gastroenterocolitis caused by staphylococci. Its apparent connection with antibiotic medication, Gastroent, 24:476, 1953.

228. Thoburn R et al: Studies on the epidemiology of adverse drug reactions. IV. The relationship of cephalothin and penicillin allergy, JAMA, 198:345, 1966.

229. Ticktin HE et al: Hepatic dysfunction and jaundice in patients receiving triacetyloleandomycin, NEJM, 267:964, 1962.

230. Tjernstrom O et al: The ototoxicity of gentamicin, Acta Path Microbiol Scand, 81:suppl:73, 1973.

231. Tobias JS et al: Severe renal dysfunction after tobramycin/cephalothin therapy, Lancet, 1:425, 1976.

232. Unger JL et al: Clindamycin-associated colitis, Amer J Dig Dis, 20:214, 1975.

233. Utley PM et al: Acute psychotic reactions to aqueous procaine penicillin, South Med J, 59:1271, 1966.

234. Valdivicsco M et al: Therapeutic trials with tobramycin, Amer J Med Sci, 268:149, 1974.

235. Van Arsdel PP Jr. et al: Anemia secondary to penicillin treatment: studies on two patients with "non-allergic" serum hemagglutinins, J Lab Clin Med, 65:277, 1965.

236. Van Dellen RG et al: Penicillin skin tests as predictive and diagnostic aids in penicillin allergy, Med Clin N Am, 54:997, 1976.

237. Van Ommen A: Untoward effects of antimicrobial agents on major organ systems, Med Clin N Amer, 58:465, 1974.

238. Viteri AL et al: The spectrum of lincomycin-clindamycin colitis, Gastroenterology, 66:1137, 1974.

239. Waisbren BA et al: Carbenicillin and bleeding, JAMA, 217:1243, 1971.

240. Wallerstein RO et al: Statewide study of chloramphenicol therapy and fatal aplastic anemia, JAMA, 208:2045, 1969.

241. Warner WA et al: Neuromuscular blockade associated with gentamicin therapy, JAMA, 215:1153, 1971.

242. Weary PE et al: Eruptions from ampicillin in patients with infectious mononucleosis, Arch Dermatol, 101:86, 1970.

243. Webster B: Untoward reactions to antibiotic therapy, J Arkansas Med Soc, 66:206, 1969.

244. Weinstein L: "Chemotherapy of microbial diseases. General Considerations." Chapter 55. *The Pharmacological Basis of Therapeutics*. Edition 4. Edited by Goodman LS and Gilman A, The MacMillan Company, 1970, p. 1154-1176.

245. Weinstein L et al: Host determinants of response to antimicrobial agents, NEJM, 279:467, 1968.

246. Weinstein L et al: The cephalosporins. Microbiological, chemical,

and pharmacological properties and use in chemotherapy of infection, Ann Intern Med, 72:729, 1970.

247. Weinstein L et al: Absorption and excretion of penicillin injected into muscles of patients with diabetes mellitus, Nature (London), 192:987, 1961.

248. Welch HCN et al: Severe reactions to antibiotics, Antibio Med Clin Ther, 4:800, 1957.

249. Westerman GW et al: Adverse reactions to penicillin, JAMA, 198:173, 1966.

250. Weyman J: Tetracyclines and teeth, Practitioner, 195:661, 1965.

251. Wiesner P et al: Evaluation of a new cephalosporin antibiotic, cephapirin, Antimicrob Agents Chemotherap, 1:303, 1972.

252. Wilfert JN et al: Renal insufficiency associated with gentamicin therapy, J Infect Dis, 124:suppl:148, 1971.

253. Wilmot TJ: Vestibular analysis in streptomycin ototoxicity, J Laryngol Otol, 87:235, 1973.

254. Woodroffe AJ et al: Nephropathy associated with methicillin administration, Aust NZ J Med, 4:256, 1974.

255. Zacherle B: Methicillin induced interstitial nephritis — Medical Staff Conference, West J Med, 123:380, 1975.

256. Zimmerman JH: Drug-induced hepatic injury, Hypersensitivity to Drugs, 1:299, 1972.

Meningitis:

257. Avery GS(Ed): Dvaluations of new drugs. Orimetroprim-Sulphamethoxazole. Drugs 1:7, 1971

258. Barlow CF: Clinical aspects of the blood brain barrier. Ann Rev Med 15:187, 1964.

259. Barrett FF et al: Ampicillin in the treatment of acute suppurative meningitis. J Ped 69:343, 1966.

260. Bodey CP et al: Clinical pharmacological studies of carbenicillin. Am J Med Sci 257:185, 1969.

261. Callaghan RP et al: Septicemia due to colonization of spitz holter values. Brit Med J 1:860, 1961.

262. Feingold S: Unpublished data from grand rounds presentation at Audie Murphy VA Hospital, San Antonio, Texas, November 1976.

263. Fisher LS: Cephalothin and cephaloridine therapy for bacterial meningitis. Ann Int Med 82:689, 1975.

264. Hambleton G et al: Diagnosis and management of bacterial meningitis. Drugs 8:15, 1974.

265. Kelley RS et al: Studies on the absorption and distribution of chloramphenicol. Pediat 8:362, 1951.

266. Legner PI: Penetration of cephaloridine into cerebrospinal fluid. Am J Med Sci 262:321, 1971.

267. Mohr, JA et al: Neurosyphilis and penicillin levels in cerebrospinal fluid. JAMA 236:2208., 1976.

268. Mungi RJ et al: Development of meningitis during cephalothin therapy. Ann Int Med 78:347, 1973.

269. Oppenheimer S et al: Pathogenesis of meningitis. III. Cerebrospinal fluid and blood concentrations of methicillin, cephalothin and cephaloridine in experimental pneumococcal meningitis. Lab Clin Med 73:535, 1969.

270. Rahal JJ: Treatment of gram-negative bacillary meningitis in adults. Ann Int Med 77:295, 1972.

271. Rahal JJ et al: Intrathecal gentamicin. NEJM 291:533, 1974.

272. Rahal JJ et al: Intrathecal and intramuscular gentamicin in meningitis. NEJM 290:1394, 1974.

273. Richardson AE: Experiments with carbenicillin in the treatment of septicemia and meningitis. Postgrad Med J 44:844, 1968.

274. Rieselbach, RE et al: Subarachnoid distribution of drugs after lumbar injection. NEJM 267:1273, 1962.

275. Sabel KG et al: Treatment of meningitis and septicemia in infancy with a sulphamethoxazole/trimethoprim combination. Acta Paediatr Scand 64:25, 1975.

276. Salmon JH: Ventriculitis complicating meningitis. Am J Dis Child 124:35, 1972.

277. Schanker LS: Passage of drugs into and out of the central nervous system. Antimicrob Agents Chemother 5:1044, 1965.

278. Swartz MN et al: Bacterial meningitis — A review of selected aspects. NEJM 272:779, 1965.

279. Vianna NJ et al: Penetration of cephalothin into the spinal fluid. Am J Med Sci 254:216, 1967.

280. Weinstein L et al: The sulfonamides. NEJM 263:793, 1960.

Septic Arthritis:

281. Baciocco ES et al: Ampicillin and kanamycin concentrations in joint fluid. Clin Pharmacol Ther 12:858, 1972.
282. Chow A et al: Gentamicin and carbenicillin penetration into the septic joint. NEJM 285:178, 1971.
283. Deodhar SD et al: Penetration of lincomycin and clindamycin into the synovial cavity in rheumatoid arthritis. Curr Med Res Opin 1:108, 1972.
284. Dewart D et al: Serratia arthritis. JAMA 225:1642, 1973.
285. Donovan TL et al: Serratia arthritis. J Bone Joint Surg 58A:1009, 1976.
286. Evaskus DS et al: Penetration of lincomycin, penicillin, and tetracycline into serum and bone. Proc Sci Exp Biol Med 130:89, 1969.
287. Gyeco MN: Pseudomonal arthritis and osteomyelitis. J Bone Joint Surg 54A:1693, 1973.
288. Hnatko SI: Treatment of acute and chronic staphylococcal osteomyelitis and soft tissue infections with lincomycin. Can Med Assoc J 97:580, 1967.
289. Marsh DC: Transport of gentamicin into synovial fluid. JAMA 228:607, 1974.
290. Mirsh H et al: A study of diffusion of penicillin across the serious membranes of joint cavities. J Lab Clin Med 31:535, 1946.
291. Nelson JD: Antibiotic concentrations in septic joint effusions. NEJM 284:349, 1971.
292. Norden CW: Experimental osteomyelitis II: therapeutic trials and measurement of osteomyelitis in bone. J Infect Dis 124:565, 1971.
293. Ory EM et al: Penicillin levels in serum and some body fluids during systemic and local therapy. J Lab Clin Med 30:809, 1945.
294. Parker RM: Transport and choice of antibiotics in septic arthritis. Mod Treat 6:1071, 1969.
295. Parker RM et al: Antibacterial activity of synovial fluid during therapy of septic arthritis. Arthr Rheum 14:96, 1971.
296. Plott MA et al: Penetration of clindamycin into the synovial fluid. Clin Pharmacol Ther 11:577, 1970.

Chapter 37

Urinary Tract Infections

Julia K. Elenbaas

Urinary tract infections (UTI) are frequently encountered in both the community and hospital environment; they are the most common type of infection in females.

The treatment of a UTI is relatively straight forward, and usually successful if the proper antimicrobial agent is administered and the patient has no underlying complicating factors. The major therapeutic problem posed by UTI's is recurrence. Because recurrent infections tend to become asymptomatic, medical treatment may be overlooked by the practitioner or patient compliance may be poor. In addition, it is recognized that UTI is the most common cause of gram-negative sepsis.

This chapter will attempt to provide the reader with sufficient background information to understand the problems inherent in infections of the urinary tract. Antimicrobial agents which are used to treat urinary tract infections have been the subject of several excellent review articles and texts (15, 65, 102, 104, 119). Because the clinical pharmacology of most of these agents is discussed in other portions of this text, only those drugs used specifically in the treatment of urinary tract infections will be included in this chapter. The reader may consult the charts and tables at the end of this chapter for specific information regarding doses, urinary concentrations, and indications for those agents which have not been discussed in detail.

It is expected that the discussions which follow, in conjunction with the treatment protocol for UTI included in this chapter, will aid the clinician and student in understanding this infectious disease state, its treatment and potential complications.

1. Which population groups are predisposed to the development of urinary tract infections (UTI)?

Females: UTI is predominantly a problem in females. The incidence of bacteriuria in school age females is about 1%, 30 times greater than in males of the same age. This incidence increases at a rate of about 1-2% per decade once childbearing age is attained. 10-20% of females will experience a UTI in their lifetime. (65, 104).

Neonatal Males: The incidence of UTI in neonates is about 1%, and of these, most occur in males. Bacteremia at the time of bacteriuria is seen infrequently; however, slight to moderate vesicoureteral reflux is observed. These observations suggest that these infections are not of hematogenous origin (1).

Males: UTI becomes a problem to males after the age of 50, when prostatic obstruction and urethral instrumentation influence the infection rate. Infection at an earlier age in a male is very rare and requires careful evaluation (65, 104).

Pregnant Females: The incidence of bacteriuria in pregnancy (~5%) is not significantly different from that of the non-pregnant female (3-5%) (7,65). Bacteriuria may be diagnosed early in pregnancy but it rarely develops later (81). However, there is an increased incidence of acute symptomatic pyelonephritis in pregnancy if the bacteriuria is untreated. In an evaluation of 265 bacteriuric pregnant patients there was a 25% incidence of acute pyelonephritis in the untreated group and a 3% incidence in the treated group (73). Another study reported comparative rates of 19% and 0% (7). Early treatment has greatly reduced this complication of pregnancy. Factors which render the pregnant female more susceptible to symptomatic disease are not known, although hormones and anatomical changes have been suspected (4).

Diabetics: The prevalence of UTI in juvenile diabetics is 1-2%, which is similar to that in the general population of school-age children (31, 65, 89). Although it was once thought that UTI's were much more prevalent in the adult diabetics, results of recent studies are conflicting. Vejlsgaard found a prevalence of 9.3% bacteriuria in 269 diabetics, compared to 4.5% in 260 non-diabetics (121). Although bacteriuria was more frequent in the non-diabetic male than the diabetic male (2.1% versus 0.7%), it was significantly more frequent in diabetic females than non-diabetic females (18.8% versus 7.9%). The results were similar in diabetic and non-diabetic pregnant females (122). Ooi et al also found a higher incidence of bacteriuria in female diabetics (15.8%) compared to non-diabetic female controls (4.6%) (85). However, O'Sullivan did not find any significant difference in the incidence of bacteriuria between 150 diabetic and 150 non-diabetic outpatients (86). Autopsy histologic findings of chronic pyelonephritis are more common in diabetics, although its relation to bacterial infection is unknown (112). Regardless of whether or not UTI's occur more frequently in diabetics, these infections make insulin control more difficult and are a major complicating factor in the increased incidence of perinephritis and perinephric abscess observed in these individuals (88).

Hospitalized Patients: UTI is the most commonly acquired infection in the hospital and accounts for about 30% of all active nosocomial infections (95). Debilitating disease and decreased host resistance are the major factors contributing to this high incidence; however, 80% of UTI's can be related to urethral catheterization.

Paraplegic Patients: Catheterization leads to the high frequency of UTI in patients with spinal cord injuries. Although better catheter care and intermittent catheterization have decreased the incidence of this complication in these patients, many still suffer severe morbidity. *E. coli* is a relatively rare infecting organism, whereas organisms highly resistant to therapy, (e.g., *Klebsiella* and *Pseudomonas)* are common (29, 102).

2. Is there good correlation between pyuria, dysuria, urgency, frequency and flank pain and the presence of a UTI?

There is poor correlation between signs and symptoms and the actual presence or severity of UTI. Not all infected patients are aware they have bacteriuria; and all patients with dysuria or pyuria do not necessarily have a UTI.

Studies have been done on both symptomatic and asymptomatic persons. Several large scale surveys in healthy asymptomatic population groups document the presence of UTI (defined as the presence of 10^5 bacteria/ml of urine) (62). However, careful questioning reveals that many such patients are symptomatic. Also, patients with recurrent infections tend to become asymptomatic. Of those patients complaining of typical UTI symptoms, (dysuria, urgency, frequency and flank and lower abdominal pain), actual infection is confirmed in as few as 50% (9, 94).

The presence or absence of pyuria also correlates poorly with bacteriologically documented UTI. Pyuria is more frequently associated with infected urine, but many bacteriurics have no pyuria (2, 41, 69). Leukocytes will be present in any type of inflammatory reaction, not just that resulting from bacterial infection. Leukocytes from the vaginal flora of females are also frequent contaminants of collected urine specimens (33, 69). The presence of more than 5 WBC/HPF of centrifuged urine is suggestive of a renal abnormality other than infection. Although pyuria is not a valuable diagnostic tool for UTI, it may be associated with progressive renal parenchymal disease if an infection is confirmed (33).

3. What criteria are necessary to establish the diagnosis of a urinary tract infection?

The sole criterion used to confirm a UTI is the bacterial culture. A minimum of 10^5 colonies of bacteria/ml cultured from a midstream urine specimen is necessary to confirm the diagnosis. A single carefully collected specimen provides 80% reliability, and two repeat cul-

tures of the same organism is virtually diagnostic (65).

The presence of mixed flora (two or more organisms) is rare except in severely debilitated individuals. The presence of less than 10^5 colonies/ml of mixed flora frequently indicates contaminantion. Less than 10^5 colonies of a single organism may be indicative of contamination, dilution or a true infection, and a repeat specimen should be obtained (9, 65).

It is mandatory that the urine specimen be obtained prior to any antibiotic administration. In many cases the urine may become free of bacteria after one or two doses; it is virtually sterile after 24 to 48 hours (65).

4. What convenient methods of bacteriologic culture are available for office use?

New simplified culture methods are available which are as reliable as the traditional loop-and-pour plate method with regard to bacterial identification and quantification.

a. **Filter-paper method** (Testuria): A strip of paper of uniform porosity is dipped into the urine and spread onto a miniature agar plate. After incubation for 10-24 hours the plate is examined and the presence of more than 25 colonies is equivalent to 10^5 bacteria/ml of urine (66).

b. **Dip-slide method** (Clinicult); Each side of a glass slide is coated with culture media, one side supporting the growth of most aerobic organisms and the other side selective for gram-negative enteric bacteria. Uniform wetting of the slide is assumed and quantitative interpretation can be made after an 18-24 hour incubation period. Reliability is considered equal to the pour-plate technique (41, 66).

c. **Pad culture method** (Microstix); A plastic strip is dipped into urine and incubated overnight. The strip consists of two pads, one with a chemical reagent for the Griess nitrite test (discussed below) and the other containing dehydrated culture media designed with areas for gram-positive organism growth and gram-negative organism growth. The culture media contains colorless tetrazolium which becomes red when reduced by bacteria. Quantitative interpretation is based on the density of the red color. This is a major drawback of the method as there is difficulty in distinguishing counts of 10,000 to greater than 100,000 colonies/ml. However, the method is about 92% accurate (41, 66).

5. What role do chemical tests have in the detection of bacteriuria?

Chemical tests may be used to detect UTI's rapidly and early. Patients with recurrent UTI's may use them for self-screening or they may be used for mass screening. In one colorometric method (Griess Test, Bac-U-Dip) a reagent turns red when nitrite is present in the urine. Nitrite would be formed in the urine if at least 100,000 bacteria were present to reduce the normally occurring urinary nitrate to nitrite. Although the test is highly specific, there is a significant rate of false negative results (10-66%). Accuracy is improved if the first morning urine specimens are used and if positive results are formed on repeated testing. False positive results may also occur (41).

6. Evaluate the various methods available for obtaining urine specimens.

Voided Sample (midstream urine; clean catch): This is the most practical method and easiest to perform. The external urethral area must be thoroughly cleaned and rinsed before urine collection, because organisms are normally harbored here. Antibacterial cleansers should be avoided; if used, they should be thoroughly and completely rinsed off, because they may contaminate the specimen and inhibit bacterial growth during culture. The specimen is collected from the middle portion of the urine stream (hence "midstream"). This method is entirely satisfactory for specimen collection in males but is much less reliable in female patients because contamination is extremely difficult to avoid. Reliability is increased by testing more than one specimen.

Bladder Aspiration (supra-pubic aspiration): This method, although unpleasant from a patient's point of view, is generally not painful and is very reliable. A needle is inserted into the bladder transcutaneously and a urine sample is withdrawn. Since the needle goes directly into the bladder, sterility of the sample is insured. This procedure is not practical for routine office or clinic practice, but may be especially useful in cases where voided samples repeatedly yield questionable results (e.g., females with recurrent UTI, infants and paraplegics). Since contamination is negligible, any number of bacteria found by this method reflects infection.

Catheterization: This method is fairly reliable if performed carefully, however, so many factors influence the quality of the urine sample collection that results are frequently invalid. The preparation of the patient, type of catheter, method of flushing the catheter, and the individual performing the procedure can all influence the degree of contamination. An important limitation of this method is that a significant number of infections may result from the procedure itself, because organisms may be introduced into the bladder at the time of catheterization (87, 102).

7. A 20-year-old female (married, no children) with no previous history of UTI, complains of dysuria and urinary urgency. A urine sample shows gram-negative rods on gram stain. The physician prescribes sulfisoxazole 1 gm qid for 10 days and asks her to return to his clinic in two days. Culture and sensitivity (C & S) studies indicate: *Proteus mirabilis*

sensitive to ampicillin, cephalosporins, and kanamycin; intermediately sensitive to sulfa, penicillin G and nalidixic acid; resistant to tetracycline. The patient returns for her scheduled clinic appointment completely free of symptoms. Another urine specimen is obtained and shows no bacteria. The patient is instructed to continue the medication until all is gone. Is it wise to prescribe a drug to which the infecting organism is only "intermediately sensitive?"

Sensitivity studies are performed with paper discs impregnated with effective serum concentrations observed after administration of a standard dose of the antimicrobial agent in question. However, essentially all drugs useful in the treatment of urinary tract infections are primarily eliminated by the kidney. Because they are excreted unchanged, very high urine concentrations (20-100 times serum concentration) are achieved (see Table 1). Therefore, a particular organism which is only intermediately sensitive, or even "resistant" to the concentration of antibiotic found in the testing-disc, might be quite sensitive to the concentration of drug actually present in the urine (99). There is often a poor correlation between *in vitro* and *in vivo* sensitivity (32, 105).

When the renal parenchyma is infected (i.e., pyelonephritis as opposed to uncomplicated cystitis), the necessity of achieving adequate tissue concentrations of the antimicrobial agents is controversial. Although it is not clear whether renal parenchymal concentrations of antibiotics correlate best with blood or urine concentrations, vigorous treatment with a drug to which the organism is sensitive is usually advisable to reduce the risk of renal damage (15).

8. Drug treatment of urinary tract infections is often started before C&S results are known. What information must the clinician have to intelligently initiate such empiric therapy?

It is important to be able to predict the most likely infecting organism to select the most rational antibacterial agent. The majority of community acquired infections (approx. 90%) are caused by *E. coli* and a small fraction by *P. mirabilis* and *K. aerogenes*. Approximately 80% of community acquired *E. coli* remain sensitive to sulfonamides, and these agents (e.g., sulfisoxazole) are the drugs of choice. Those organisms resistant to sulfas are generally sensitive to ampicillin.

In the hospital environment, the incidence with which particular organisms cause infection and the sensitivity of these bacteria to antimicrobial agents is often markedly different from that seen in the community and frequently varies from one hospital to another. Therefore, the microbiology department of a particular hospital should be consulted to determine current trends in infections acquired in this setting. In general, however, *E. coli* is still the predominant infecting organism, but an increased incidence of infections caused by other gram-negative bacteria, especially *Proteus* and *Pseudomonas,* is also noted. Hospital acquired organisms tend to be more resistant to the commonly used antibiotic agents (especially sulfonamides) than those acquired in the community. If prompt treatment is required, a urinary bactericidal agent should be administered while awaiting C&S results. Ampicillin is considered the drug of choice for hospital acquired *E. coli* infections. Alternatively, an aminoglycoside could be used initially if a different gram-negative organism is suspected (11, 15).

When empirical antimicrobial therapy is used, the patient is in essence serving as her own "sensitivity study." In virtually all cases, if the infecting organism is sensitive, the urine will be sterile in 24 and certainly by 48 hours. If a urine specimen collected 48 hours after therapy was initiated is not sterile and the patient has been taking the medication properly, one can be quite certain that an inappropriate antibiotic is being used. An appropriate antimicrobial selected on the basis of C&S results, should be substituted. If, however, the urine specimen is sterile, one can be confident that the appropriate antimicrobial is being used (regardless of sensitivity studies) and the full course of therapy should be completed (65).

9. How long should therapy be continued in a patient who presents with a UTI for the first time? What should the duration of therapy be for a recurrent UTI?

Although the urine is sterile within 48 hours after appropriate therapy is initiated, a 7-14 day course is recommended for both hospital and community acquired infections (119). The effectiveness of a shorter treatment course is unknown and is complicated by the fact that a significant number of uncomplicated infections can clear spontaneously (15). Longer treatment does not add any significant benefit. A 14 day therapy is usually recommended for recurrent infections, since the optimal treatment regimen is still unknown (119). Turck et al observed that an additional six weeks of therapy benefitted 50% of patients with relapses; however, many of these patients had infected kidneys as well and thus required more vigorous treatment (116, 117). Generally 14 days of therapy is adequate for uncomplicated pyelonephritis.

10. See Question 7 for case presentation. The urine sample collected at the second visit was sterile and the patient became asymptomatic. However, three weeks later her symptoms reappeared. How should she be evaluated before her recurrent infection is treated?

One must determine if the recurrent infection represents a relapse or reinfection. A relapse generally occurs within six weeks and involves the same organism. A reinfection may occur any time after the resolution of the previous infection and generally involves a different organism. Over 80% of recurrent infections represent reinfections and these may occur within days after treatment of the previous infection (11).

One should first attempt to rule-out any cause for relapse. Poor compliance to prescribed treatment is a common cause of inadequate therapy because patients often become asymptomatic within one or two days of treatment. Inadequate therapy may also result if the original antibiotic selected was inappropriate or if the organism developed resistance to the prescribed agent. For these reasons repeat C&S's should be performed.

Structural abnormalities of the urinary tract should also be considered as a cause for relapse. Infected kidney stones and unilateral atrophic kidneys are the most common correctable abnormalities in females. Since *P. mirabilis* is the most common organism found in infected stones, repeated *Proteus* infections should make one suspicious of an infected stone which is "seeding" the bladder (11).

The three-week interval between infections in this patient makes both relapse and reinfection a possibility. Unless noncompliance has definitely been established, it is best to initiate empiric therapy with a different antibiotic. It is also important to note that tetracycline, ampicillin and sulfonamides alter the normal fecal flora within a few weeks so that resistant organisms from the altered flora may become responsible for new infections (71). (Also see Question 21). If the patient develops a history of recurrent infections, one must keep in mind that these frequently become highly refractory to therapy (119). It is therefore useful to keep records which accurately reflect the frequency, infecting organisms, and response to therapy of past infections.

11. What role do localization studies play in the diagnosis or treatment of urinary tract infections?

Localization studies help to differentiate whether bacteria gained access to the bladder from the kidney, from an external source via the urethra, or from the prostate or paraurethral glands. Several methods are used:

(a) Urethral catheterization differentiates renal from bladder infection. A sterile collection indicates the bacterial source is below the ureters.

(b) Expression of prostatic secretions rules out the presence of bacteria in the prostate.

(c) Raised hemagglutinating antibody titers indicate tissue inflammation; i.e., kidney or prostate involvement. Infections limited to the bladder do not cause significant antibody response.

(d) Bacterial serotyping is an indirect method of localization. Relapse caused by bacteria of the same serotype often indicates the presence of a focal seeding site somewhere in the urinary tract, whereas a different serotype suggests that a new organism is responsible.

(e) Radiology: Intravenous pyelograms are useful in revealing urinary tract abnormalities, such as polycystic kidneys, stones, papillary necrosis or chronic atrophic pyelonephritis. The micturating cystourethrogram might reveal reflux.

Localization methods are too involved to perform routinely and generally are not necessary for successful treatment. Many methods are primarily used as research tools to better understand UTI's. In persistent, recurrent, or difficult cases where physical defects have been ruled out by radiologic studies, some of these methods may be used to determine the cause of treatment failure and to decide which therapeutic alternative is indicated: surgery, more vigorous treatment or chronic antimicrobial prophylaxis. (15, 33, 69)

12. Is renal failure a significant consequence of chronic bacteriuria?

The relationship between chronic bacteriuria and progressive renal failure has not been definitely established. Although early studies presented data relating bacteriuria to renal abnormalities, scarring, and damage, many failed to consider concurrent vascular disease, primary urological and neurological abnormalities, and previous instrumentation, or failed to establish specific histologic criteria for progressive bacterial damage. Also, these studies looked at patients with symptomatic, chronic bacteriuria, rather than the more common asymptomatic population. (57)

Pyelonephritis with vesico-ureteral reflux in the female child is frequently associated with renal tissue damage at the time of kidney organ growth, and therefore, a clubbed calyx, kidney scarring, or, rarely, gross destruction may result (15). It is suggested that these consequences might be minimized by more intensive treatment than the usual 10-14 day regimen (45). On the whole, the risk of significant chronic renal disease in a child is small but definite (57).

Studies indicate that at any point in time, the asymptomatic patient has a 50% chance of having bacteria present in ureteral urine specimens (i.e., the kidney). Despite this significant frequency of pelvic bacteriuria, there is little evidence for concurrent chronic, progressive renal disease (104). Scarring, decreased concentrating ability, stones and some degree of pelvic atonicity are seen more frequently in the bacteriuric population and these lesions increase the risk of further deterioration.

Renal damage may occur with UTI and the damage might be associated with chronic renal disease, but a clear causal relationship has not been shown. It has been suggested that renal failure may be due to a primary defect, and the infections are secondary or incidental to the primary disease (57). Further studies are needed in this area.

13. Should all cases of asymptomatic bacteriuria be treated?

All cases of significant bacteriuria ($>10^5$ bacteria/ml urine) should be treated, whether or not the patient is symptomatic, because there is a higher incidence of renal scarring and stones in patients with bacteriuria than in normal patients. Treatment also prevents the development of symptomatic infection with generalized sepsis. Data collected by Kunin suggest that repeated treatment of recurrent urinary tract infections will eventually result in a decreased incidence of subsequent infections (65). Severe cases of pyelonephritis complicating pregnancy have been reduced by treating asymptomatic bacteriuria early in pregnancy (4).

Unfortunately, in some cases treatment of asymptomatic bacteriuria does not permanently eliminate bacteria within the urinary tract, and these patients must be continually retreated or placed on chronic suppressive therapy. Due to this apparent lack of success, some practitioners do not treat all cases of asymptomatic bacteriuria. Most agree that young patients should be treated aggressively; however, treatment might be withheld from the asymptomatic older patient when the expense, side effects, and potential complications of an additional drug might outweigh the benefit. (72, 119)

14. A 19-year-old recently married female presents with typical UTI symptoms. An examination of her urine sediment reveals many white blood cells and gram-negative rods. She has had three UTI's in the past few months, but had none prior to this time. Is there an association between sexual intercourse and UTI's?

The relationship between sexual intercourse and the occurrence of UTI's has been suggested by various studies. The frequency of infections is strikingly less in nuns than in a population of non-pregnant females. Also, some women are able to consistently relate the onset of infections to coitus.

Since UTI's are uncommon in males, transmission of an infection from the male to the female is unlikely. Occasionally, bacteria harbored under the foreskin of an uncircumcised male may be transmitted to his partner in intercourse (104).

Studies in adult females indicate that introital (vaginal vestibule and urethral mucosa) bacterial colonization by fecal bacteria plays a definite role in recurrent infection. The number of pathogenic enterobacteria increases immediately prior to infection and serotypic studies show them to be identical to the infecting bacteria. Sexual intercourse appears to facilitate innoculation of organisms from the introitus into the bladder via the urethra (103).

15. The patient described above would like to begin

taking oral contraceptives; would this further increase her risk for UTI's?

The urine cultures of 12,000 healthy women revealed a higher incidence of bacteriuria in those taking oral contraceptives; the incidence among these women was 2.4%, whereas the incidence among those who had never taken oral contraceptives was 1.6% (108). Although greater sexual activity among the oral contraceptive users would account at least in part for these findings, it was also noted that there was a positive correlation between the dose of estrogen and the frequency of bacteriuria. However, the overall incidence of bacteriuria noted in this study was low compared to that expected for the general population (2 to 10%). Furthermore, a smaller prospective study involving 82 women demonstrated no difference between oral contraceptive users and non-users with respect to bacteriuria, although the incidence was higher among those on progesterone alone (24).

Ureteral dilitation similar to that noted in pregnancy has been observed in women taking oral contraceptives (75), and the stasis of urine may facilitate the rise of bacteria from the lower tract and cause bacteriuria (83). However, ureteral dilitation is not consistently observed in UTI patients on oral contraceptives (23).

In conclusion, a causal relationship between the use of oral contraceptives and UTI has not been established, and more study is needed.

16. Postcoital urinary tract infections are often treated prophylactically by the administration of a single dose of antibiotic immediately after intercourse. Is this rational?

This form of antibiotic prophylaxis is often recommended when UTI is recognized to be sexual-intercourse-induced. The effectiveness of a single nightly dose of 50 mg nitrofurantoin in inhibiting bacterial growth was evaluated by Bailey et al in a double blind trial of 50 women with histories of recurrent infections. Of 37 women with normal intravenous pyelograms (IVP), only one became infected over a trial period of 10-183 weeks. Five of the 15 patients with abnormal IVP's became infected over 14-260 weeks of therapy (8).

Vosti evaluated five different drugs (nitrofurantoin, cephalexin, nalidixic acid, sulfonamide, penicillin) and found the frequency of bacteriuria to be decreased by all of them, but most significantly by nitrofurantoin and cephalexin. (123)

Theoretically, this single dose produces bactericidal activity in the urine before bacteria have a chance to multiply. The patient empties her bladder just after intercourse before taking the medication to minimize the number of bacteria present in the bladder and eliminate unnecessary dilution of the drug in the urine. Since most drugs effective in urinary tract infections are rapidly excreted by the kidney and reach high uri-

nary concentrations, this regimen appears reasonable and does lower the incidence of postcoital infections. However, it has the same drawbacks as any other type of antibiotic prophylaxis, and is not recommended in patients with abnormal urinary tract or renal function. It is also important to treat symptomatic infection with appropriate therapy before beginning prophylaxis.

17. A 24-year-old female presented to her local doctor complaining of dysuria, pyuria, urgency and frequency. Her temperature was 101°F, but she reported no flank pain. The patient's medical record indicated that she had a similar problem three years previously. At that time a urinary tract infection secondary to *E. coli* was documented and successfully treated with sulfisoxazole. She has had no signs or symptoms of a UTI in the three year interim.

A urine specimen was obtained for C&S. Gram negative rods thought to be *E. coli* were present on gram stain. The patient was given a prescription for penicillin G, 500 mg orally every six hours and instructed to return for a follow-up urinalysis in two days. Is penicillin G a reasonable drug to use for the treatment of this woman's urinary tract infection?

Penicillin G is almost completely excreted in an unchanged, active form by the kidney and thus achieves remarkably high concentrations in the urine. An oral dose of 500 mg produces a serum level of approximately 0.5-1.0 mcg/ml, a concentration too low to be effective against any gram-negative pathogen. However, the average urine concentration achieved by the same dose is about 150 mcg/ml, (99), and peak concentrations as high as 597 mcg/ml have been reported (52). These concentrations are bactericidal to many urinary pathogens. *E. coli* is generally sensitive to penicillin G in concentrations of about 50 mcg/ml (99, 53). It should be noted, however, that some strains may require higher urine concentrations.

Because *E. coli* is responsible for the majority of community-acquired urinary tract infections, penicillin G may often be an effective agent. Hulbert (53) compared the effectiveness of penicillin G, sulfamethoxazole, nalidixic acid, ampicillin, nitrofurantoin and tetracycline in 242 patients with UTI and found that penicillin G was equally effective as the other agents in treating an acute or recurrent infection. The follow-up procedures used by Hulbert do not allow accurate comparison of the frequency of recurrent infections among the various treatment groups. The data suggest, however, that the incidence of relapse or reinfection may be significantly higher in the penicillin-treated patients than in those who received sulfamethoxazole. Stamey and associates (99) also documented the effectiveness of penicillin G in the treatment of urinary tract infections secondary to *E. coli* . If penicillin G is administered for an *E. coli* infection, it is essential that its effectiveness be confirmed by collection of a sterile urine sample two days after initiation of therapy. It should be noted that some evidence exists to suggest that penicillin V is much less effective against gram-negative bacilli than is penicillin G (39). It should, therefore, not be given in this situation.

In spite of the evidence which has been presented here, no well-controlled studies exist comparing the effectiveness of penicillin G and sulfonamides in community-acquired UTI's. While penicillin G may be effective in such situations, sulfonamides should still be considered the drugs of choice until the necessary comparative data are available.

18. A 28-year-old female, with symptoms of dysuria and frequency, is diagnosed as having a UTI. A urine C&S revealed 10^5 E. coli sensitive to the entire antibacterial panel tested (including sulfonamides). She is given the following prescription: Sulfisoxazole 500 mg tabs. #82. Sig: 2 gm stat, then 1 gm qid for ten days. Is sulfisoxazole (Gantrisin) the sulfonamide of choice?

The specific sulfonamide administered to a patient with a UTI does not markedly affect clinical outcome but sulfisoxazole (Gantrisin) is often considered the agent of choice. Although one might predict that sulfisoxazole would be most efficacious because it is excreted into the urine more rapidly than sulfamethoxazole (Gantanol), sulfamethoxypyridazine (Kynex), or the other long-acting compounds, there is no concrete evidence to document its clinical "superiority." Cost is the major factor affecting one's choice of agent. (124)

19. What is the rationale and necessity for the "stat" 2 gm dose of sulfisoxazole? If sulfamethoxazole were used, would a loading dose be required?

The 2 gm loading dose is recommended in the manufacturer's product literature but is unnecessary and probably represents a "carry-over" from earlier days when long-acting sulfonamides were in use. A single oral dose of sulfisoxazole is well absorbed, and peak serum levels are reached in 30-120 minutes. The elimination half-life is 3-6 hours and 70% of the drug appears in the urine as the free, active form. Because it is rapidly absorbed and appears in high concentrations in the urine, a loading dose of sulfisoxazole is not particularly advantageous and need not be given.

Sulfamethoxazole is not as completely or rapidly absorbed as sulfisoxazole. Peak serum levels are achieved within 4-6 hours, the elimination half-life of sulfamethoxazole is approximately 9-12 hours, and about 50% of the drug appears in the urine as the free, active form. Because of its longer half-life, sulfamethoxazole is generally administered only twice daily. The long half-life and relatively slow excretion into the urine (as compared to sulfisoxazole) may

necessitate the administration of a loading dose (120, 124).

20. It is known that sulfonamides are more soluble in an alkaline than in an acidic medium and problems of sulfonamide-induced crystaluria have been reported. Should the urine be alkalinized in an attempt to prevent crystaluria secondary to sulfisoxazole administration?

The solubility of sulfisoxazole and its acetylated metabolite may vary as much as eight-fold with changes of one pH unit. At normal body temperature, sulfisoxazole has a solubility of 1200 mg% at pH 6.5 but a solubility of only 150 mg% at pH 5.5. Its acetyl derivative is less soluble at the same pH values, 450 mg% and 55 mg%, respectively. Thus a moderate fall in pH may markedly affect the urine solubility of sulfisoxazole.

Sulfisoxazole is one of the most soluble of the available sulfonamides. On the other hand, sulfamethoxazole (Gantanol) carries a somewhat greater risk of precipitating within the kidney, because it is less soluble than sulfisoxazole and also forms a larger fraction of a less soluble acetyl metabolite. The solubility of sulfamethoxazole is 509 mg% at pH 7 and 63 mg% at pH 5. The solubility of its metabolite is 256 mg% at pH 7 and 147 mg% at pH 5.

Nevertheless, crystaluria secondary to sulfisoxazole or sulfamethoxazole is not a major clinical problem and is not common enough to warrant routine alkalinization of the urine. Crystaluria, characterized by pain, hematuria, and even anuria if the renal pelvis or ureters become occluded, appears to be a greater problem with the less soluble sulfonamides such a sulfadiazine. Preventative measures such as a high fluid intake should be encouraged in patients taking sulfisoxazole and sulfamethoxazole. Also, the current vogue of ingesting large doses of vitamin C is to be discouraged since this vitamin acidifies urine (125).

21. A 35-year-old woman with a past history of several UTI's is noted to have bacteriuria on a routine urinalysis. Even though she is completely asymptomatic, a urine specimen is obtained for C&S, and an initial gram stain reveals gram-negative rods. All her previous infections were caused by serotypes of E. coli and were treated successfully with sulfisoxazole. Her last infection occurred one month ago. Would sulfisoxazole be a reasonable drug to select in this case if treatment were begun before C&S results were known?

Generally, therapy is withheld from a patient who is not in acute distress until culture and sensitivity results are obtained. Because sulfisoxazole was given to this patient only one month ago, it is probably not a good choice for empiric therapy.

There have been occasional reports of an increasing incidence of resistance of community-acquired infections to sulfisoxazole. Although this is not the general case, resistance can and does occur. Factors affecting the development of resistant organisms include the frequency of recurrent infections and the effect of sulfonamides on normal fecal bacterial flora. Despite the almost complete absorption of sulfisoxazole from the gastrointestinal tract, a significant change in bacterial flora occurs during its administration. The proportion of sulfonamide-resistant fecal bacteria can increase considerably (from 12% to 98%) during therapy. Because UTI's are most often caused by fecal bacterial contamination, the probability that a resistant organism will be responsible for the infection increases when the interval between infectious episodes is short. If there is a long interval between infections a normal gastrointestinal flora will be established; thus, there is a lower incidence of sulfonamide-resistant infections when several months elapse between each episode.

The alteration of fecal flora which occurs with sulfonamide, tetracycline and ampicillin administration makes these drugs poor choices for repeated use in cases of frequent reinfection, especially when C&S results are not known. The development of bacterial resistance may also limit the usefulness of these agents for chronic antimicrobial therapy (71).

22. A 65-year-old Black male with an eight year history of congestive heart failure (CHF) and an 11 year history of emphysema, was admitted to the hospital with increasing shortness of breath. During his stay he was given medication for his CHF, respiratory disease and chronic bronchial infection. His hematocrit was stable at 39-43% and his total serum bilirubin was reported to be 0.8 mg%. Sixteen days after admission a UTI due to *E. coli* was discovered and the patient was given sulfisoxazole 4 gm daily. Twenty days after admission, the hematocrit suddenly dropped to 25% and the hemoglobin to 8.4 gm%. There were no signs of bleeding, but his sclerae became icteric. Twenty-three days after admission, the hematocrit was still 25%, but the reticulocyte count had risen to 6.6%; the bilirubin was normal. Sulfisoxazole was discontinued and over a period of two and a half weeks the hematocrit steadily rose to 40%. Discuss the probable adverse drug reaction which occurred in this patient.

Several hematologic disorders may be associated with sulfonamide administration and are mediated by either a hypersensitivity reaction or by a genetic enzyme deficiency. In this case, hemolytic anemia due to glucose-6-phosphate dehydrogenase (G6PD) deficiency was confirmed by measuring red blood cell enzyme levels. G6PD deficiency is most prevalent in Black males and occurs in about 13% of those living in the United States. It occurs in approximately 1% of the White population. Although the enzyme deficiency is a

sex-linked, homozygous trait, anemia (usually of a mild degree with reticulocytosis) can occur in heterozygous females. Hemolysis may be benign and of short duration or may be prolonged, severe and fatal. Although not as prevalent in the White population, those males who are affected seem to develop a very severe, often fatal anemia on exposure to precipitating factors (16, 82, 124).

Acute hemolytic anemia induced by sulfonamides in G6PD deficient individuals does not appear to be dose-related. It is usually abrupt in onset and occurs within the first week of therapy. Typical symptoms include nausea, fever, vertigo, jaundice, hepatosplenomegaly and occasionally, hypotension. Hematocrit and hemoglobin values may fall precipitously and may be reduced to as low as 30-50% of normal; leukocytosis and reticulocytosis are common; and acute tubular necrosis may result from the hypotension and hemolysis. A mild hemolytic episode may be characterized only by reticulocytosis, without a significant fall in hemoglobin or hematocrit (16, 51).

Clinical illness as well as drug administration may also precipitate hemolysis in patients with G6PD deficiency. The combination of chronic illness (especially bacterial infections of the urinary or upper respiratory tract) and the chronic or repetitive use of certain drugs is especially important in the precipitation of hemolysis (16).

Other enzyme deficiencies, especially those associated with the pentose-phosphate shunt (as is G6PD) can be associated with hemolytic reactions. Anemia in a female with a deficiency of glutathione peroxidase who received sulfonamide and nitrofurantoin has been reported (107).

23. If the Black male described in the case above should, at a later date, acquire another UTI, which antibacterial agents should be avoided?

Of the antibacterial drugs known to cause hemolytic anemia in G6PD deficient individuals, sulfonamides account for the majority of cases. Other antibiotics used in the treatment of UTI and known to produce this untoward reaction include nitrofurantoin and nalidixic acid (16). Oxolinic acid (Utibid), although structurally similar to nalidixic acid, has not yet been associated with G6PD deficiency anemia.

24. What other hematological reactions may be caused by the sulfonamides?

Sulfonamides have also caused agranulocytosis, thrombocytopenia (occasionally with hemorrhage) and aplastic anemia (109, 124). The incidence with which sulfonamides produce these adverse reactions is not well known but is apparently very low. Agranulocytosis secondary to sulfisoxazole has been reported and is not related to the dose or blood level of the sulfonamide (50). It is thought to be a hypersensitivity reaction, may appear suddenly or after a period of progressive neutropenia, usually develops after ten days to six weeks of therapy, and is generally reversible.

25. List and discuss other adverse reactions which have been attributed to the sulfonamide. What is the incidence of these reactions?

Sulfonamide administration has been associated with a wide variety of adverse reactions. It appears that the type and incidence of reaction varies with the particular agent; however, it has been estimated that the risk that an untoward effect will develop is 18% with sulfathiozole, 6% with sulfadiazine, 9.5% with sulfamerazine, 6-10% with sulfamethoxypyridazine and 3-9% with sulfisoxazole (70).

Rash is one of the more common adverse effects noted after sulfonamide administration, and about 2% of patients treated with sulfisoxazole will develop a rash. A variety of hypersensitivity reactions involving the skin and mucous membranes have been reported, including morbilliform, scarlatinal, urticarial, erysipeloid, pemphigoid, purpuric and petechial rashes; erythema nodosum; exfoliative dermatitis; photosensitivity reactions; and the Stevens-Johnson syndrome (124).

Drug fever, which is usually acute in onset, may occur in as many as 3% of patients receiving sulfisoxazole and may be accompanied by headache, chills, malaise, pruritis and skin rash. It most often occurs between the seventh and tenth day of treatment and discontinuation of sulfonamide administration is generally followed by rapid defervescence (124).

Nausea, vomiting and anorexia occur in about 1-2% of patients given sulfonamides and may be so severe as to necessitate discontinuation of therapy. A multitude of other, less frequent, adverse reactions attributed to sulfonamide include allergic hepatitis (<0.1%), sleep disturbances, arthralgias, acute psychosis, peripheral neuritis with motor and/or sensory disturbances, goiter, and hypothyroidism (124).

26. The combination of sulfamethoxazole and trimethoprim is now available in the United States as Septra and Bactrim. Describe the synergism which occurs with this particular combination.

The effectiveness of the trimethoprim-sulfamethoxazole (tmp-smx) combination is based on its synergistic action against bacterial folic acid synthesis. The two agents affect folic acid metabolism at different sites: the sulfonamide inhibits bacterial conversion of PABA to dihydrofolic acid, and trimethoprim blocks the conversion of dihydrofolic acid to tetrahydrofolic acid by inhibiting the enzyme, dihydrofolate reductase (115).

Folic acid derivatives are essential for purine and DNA synthesis in both man and bacteria. Folic acid is absorbed from the gastrointestinal tract of man and incorporated into essential cellular components in this form. However, folic acid does not cross bacterial cell membranes and must be synthesized from para-amino-benzoic acid (PABA). Because of this difference in cellular metabolism between man and bacteria, the sulfonamides and agents like trimethoprim are able to "selectively" inhibit bacterial metabolism (14).

The synergy achieved by tmp-smx makes it effective against several systemic infections, including those caused by *Salmonella, Pneumocystis carinii,* and *Neisseria,* and chronic respiratory infections (61). Currently, it is only approved by the FDA for the treatment of chronic urinary tract infections. The degree of synergism and success of the combination against a given pathogen largely depends upon the sensitivity of the organism to the individual drugs. Individually, these drugs are basically bacteriostatic, but they are bactericidal in combination for many systemic infections (14). The high urinary concentrations achieved by these drugs makes the combination almost uniformly successful in the treatment of UTI, even against organisms which were originally highly resistant to either agent alone. In one study, 78% of patients with recurrent, persistent infections unresponsive to treatment with sulfamethoxazole and trimethoprim separately, responded to the combination (26). With the exception of *Pseudomonas,* most urinary pathogens seem susceptible to this drug combination.

27. The synergism achieved by Bactrim and Septra can occur with a combination of any sulfonamide and trimethoprim. Why was sulfamethoxazole selected for this particular combination?

Sulfamethoxazole was selected mainly because its elimination half-life is similar to that of trimethoprim. The kinetics of sulfamethoxazole were discussed in Question 19. Trimethoprim is well absorbed orally and its plasma half-life is about 10-13 hours (17). About 45% is bound to serum proteins (96). Approximately 70-80% of the absorbed drug is excreted unchanged by glomerular filtration (27).

Although the ratio of sulfamethoxazole to trimethoprim in the available products is 5:1 (400 mg sulfamethoxazole: 80 mg trimethoprim), potentiation of antibacterial activity occurs over a wide range of ratios. This ratio was selected because the *in vitro* activity of trimethoprim is 20-100 times that of sulfamethoxazole and administration of five times as much sulfamethoxazole will result in approximately equivalent activity *in vivo* (14, 17). Variable ratios have been highly effective for the treatment of UTI, probably because such high concentrations are achieved in the urine (14).

28. When is trimethoprim-sulfamethoxazole (tmp-smx) indicated in the treatment of urinary tract infec-

tions? Compare its efficacy with traditional antimicrobial therapy.

The FDA has approved tmp-smx for the treatment of chronic urinary tract infections; however, since this covers a large population, discrimination should be practiced until more studies are available.

The efficacy of a ten-day regimen of tmp-smx in the treatment of chronic urinary tract infections has been evaluated (25, 43, 44). In a multi-center, double-blind study of 163 patients with chronic infections, tmp-smx was somewhat better than ampicillin in eradicating and preventing recurrence of *E. coli* (44). Its effectiveness appeared equal to ampicillin against *P. mirabilis* and enterococci; however, the number of patients with these organisms was very limited. Cosgrove also observed a higher cure rate with tmp-smx than ampicillin after 12 weeks of observation following a ten-day regimen (25). In an earlier study comparing tmp-smx to its components individually, it was found that tmp-smx eradicates a larger number of sulfonamide sensitive organisms initially; however, the incidence of sterile urines 55 days after the ten-day treatment was not significantly different between the tmp-smx and sulfonamide group (43). This indicates that tmp-smx does not prevent recurrence. Harding and Ronald felt that tmp-smx was not superior to sulfonamide alone when treating sulfonamide-sensitive organisms (48). Therefore, tmp-smx should only be used when more traditional antimicrobials cannot be used.

In low doses, tmp-smx appears to be effective for chronic prophylaxis (49, 56). In a crossover study of 40 females comparing tmp-smx one-half tablet daily, to methenamine mandelate 500 mg qid, sulfamethoxazole 500 mg daily and placebo, Harding and Ronald found that the incidence of recurrence was significantly less in those patients treated with tmp-smx as compared to those treated with the other regimens over a one year period (49). Kalowski et al also observed that tmp-smx, one tablet daily, was superior to one gram of methenamine hippurate daily (56). The success rate is significantly decreased in patients with a renal abnormality or dysfunction (56, 84). It should also be emphasized that those infections which are not eradicated by a short-term therapeutic trial of tmp-smx are not likely to respond to a long-term regimen (84). An observation which would require further evaluation was the increased introital colonization with *S. faecalis* observed in patients on chronic tmp-smx (49).

In summary, tmp-smx should be limited to prophylactic use in patients with chronic urinary tract infections and to the intensive therapeutic treatment of UTI's when traditional antimicrobials cannot be used. It appears to be more effective than methenamine mandelate or sulfamethoxazole alone when used prophylactically. It is not as effective in the patients with urological abnormalities.

29. Discuss the toxic and adverse effects which may be caused by the trimethoprim-sulfamethoxazole combination.

Because relatively low doses of each drug are contained in this combination, toxicities occur infrequently. As expected, all adverse effects reported with the use of sulfamethoxazole alone can occur when it is combined with trimethoprim. Dyspepsia occurs in a few patients; a previous history of sulfonamide hypersensitivity is a contraindication to the use of tmp-smx, as is G6PD deficiency.

Hematologic complications such as leukopenia and thrombocytopenia have been reported following administration of this drug combination (36). Although these cases may be due to the sulfonamide, trimethoprim can also cause similar hematologic toxicities (14). As is the case with all drug combinations, it is not always possible to determine which drug is responsible for an observed complication.

The ability of the sulfonamides to inhibit folic acid synthesis occurs only in the bacterial cell and does not affect, to a significant degree, human cell processes. Although trimethoprim has a greater affinity for the bacterial and protozoal cell, when given in high doses, it may also affect folic acid utilization in man (61). Folate deficiency anemia has been reported when trimethoprim is administered in doses higher than recommended. It is not yet known whether this will be a complication in patients taking recommended doses for prolonged periods; in malnourished persons; or in people taking other agents affecting folate utilization (e.g., phenytoin).

Both trimethoprim and sulfamethoxazole are protein bound (trimethoprim 40%; sulfamethoxazole 70%). Cases of drug interactions with other protein-bound drugs have not been reported; however, caution should be taken when such agents are administered concurrently. Theoretically, tmp-smx could increase the toxicity of methotrexate by protein displacement or through its additive effects on folic acid metabolism (115).

Effects of administration have been studied in a limited number of pregnant women. Teratogenicity attributed to the drug combination has not been reported to date. Williams et al described its use in 43 pregnant patients, and Brumfitt and Pursell in 25 such patients (13,126). However, the total number of females taking the preparation during their first trimester (the period during which the fetus is most susceptible to teratogenic effects) was too small to make any conclusive statement about its safety. Fetal malformations have been associated with the use of other folic acid antagonists, so that it is probably best to avoid the use of tmp-smx in the pregnant patient.

Nephrotoxicity induced by tmp-smx has been suggested; however, all 16 patients in this report had prior underlying renal abnormalities and deterioration of function reflected by high serum creatinines (54). Rosenfield et al evaluated 18 patients with neurogenic bladders, but good creatinine clearances, who took tmp-smx for 60-80 days and observed no changes in renal function (92). It is recommended that tmp-smx be avoided or used cautiously in patients with renal failure. If tmp-smx must be given to a patient with renal dysfunction, the following dosage regimen is recommended:

Creatinine Clearance (ml/min)	Recommended Dosage Regimen
>30	2 tablets every 12 hours
15-30	1 tablet every 12 hours
<15	use not recommended

Tmp-smx has not had adequate clinical use to conclusively evaluate its potential for producing adverse effects. Although few cases have been reported thus far, the potential adverse reactions outlined above should always be kept in mind.

30. A 35-year-old female is placed on nitrofurantoin 100 mg qid for 14 days for a UTI caused by sensitive E. coli. She has had many UTI's since childhood including two severe cases of pyelonephritis. About half of her infections have occurred over the past year. E. coli has been the predominant pathogen, although P. mirabilis has been cultured on occasion. She has been successfully treated with sulfisoxazole, ampicillin, and nalidixic acid. Is nitrofurantoin an effective drug for the treatment of patients with frequent reinfections?

Nitrofurantoin does not significantly alter the fecal or introital flora, and the development of resistant organisms is uncommon. Eighty to ninety per cent of E. coli are sensitive to the drug. However, re-infection might involve organisms like P. mirabilis and Klebsiella which tend to be less sensitive to nitrofurantoin. Culture and sensitivity studies should never be neglected in patients with recurrent infections (61, 104).

Because the risk of developing resistant organisms is minimal with nitrofurantoin administration, it is generally a useful agent for the treatment of recurrent infections (providing the organism was originally sensitive).

31. If paper disc sensitivity studies indicate that an organism is only intermediately sensitive to nitrofurantoin, would it still be a reasonable agent to select for treatment?

Unlike most of the other agents discussed in this chapter, nitrofurantoin is strictly used in the treatment of urinary tract infections. Sensitivity studies are performed with discs containing 100 mcg of the drug, an amount which correlates with the average urinary concentrations achieved, NOT serum concentrations.

Sensitivity studies thus correlate bacterial susceptibility to the actual concentration of nitrofurantoin achievable in the urine. Nitrofurantoin should therefore not be used unless C & S results indicate that the infecting organism is sensitive to the drug (61, 104).

32. If the disc sensitivity studies confirm sensitivity of the infecting organism to nitrofurantoin, what other consideration must be made in this patient (see Question 30) before this drug is used?

In view of this patient's long history of severe urinary tract infections, renal function should be evaluated. Excretion of nitrofurantoin is linearly related to creatinine clearance (93). Adequate glomerular filtration is required to achieve adequate antibacterial concentrations in the urine. It has been reported that when the creatinine clearance is less than 80 ml/min, nitrofurantoin excretion becomes significantly decreased, and below 60 ml/min, excretion might be inadequate to inhibit growth of E. coli (34, 93).

Additionally, neurotoxicity characterized by a peripheral neuropathy is more common in uremic patients. Despite the decreased excretion of the drug found in renal failure, serum concentrations do not seem to increase proportionally. Although blood levels may rise from the average 1.8 mcg/ml to 6 mcg/ml, they seldom exceed this concentration, regardless of the severity of renal failure (93). It is postulated that nitrofurantoin is sequestered by and accumulated in peripheral neural tissue (34). Neuropathy may develop within days of drug initiation. Damage to sensorimotor fibers results in paresthesias and polyneuritis which begin distally and bilaterally (113). The prognosis for reversibility is related to severity of the symptoms and full recovery may require months. Permanent neuropathy occurred in 13 of 100 patients evaluated retrospectively (113).

33. The patient complains of nausea and gastrointestinal upset after the ingestion of each dose of nitrofurantoin. What alternatives in therapy might be considered?

Nausea is a fairly frequent complication of nitrofurantoin therapy and is probably the major factor limiting the use of this agent. The patient's compliance with the prescribed regimen is likely to be severely affected by this common side effect. Several alternatives are available to decrease or eliminate the drug-induced nausea.

(a) The daily dose of nitrofurantoin might be too large for this patient since nausea and vomiting appear to occur more frequently in small persons. The minimum effective dose of nitrofurantoin is generally stated to be 5 mg/kg/day; the average dose is usually 7 mg/kg/day. At daily doses above 7 mg/kg the incidence of nausea appears to increase markedly, so a dose in excess of this amount should not be prescribed (60).

(b) The macrocrystalline preparation of nitrofurantoin (Macrodantin) is better tolerated. Although the mechanism by which nitrofurantoin produces nausea has not been clearly defined, it appears to be a central effect, since it occurs after both parenteral and oral administration. The larger particle size of the macrocyrstalline preparation has a slower rate of dissolution and absorption, which results in a lower serum level and fewer gastrointestinal side-effects. Because this form is more slowly absorbed, there may be a delay of one hour before effective urine concentrations are reached. This minor delay does not affect the effectiveness of the treatment (22, 46).

Kalowski and co-workers compared the incidence of adverse reactions in patients treated with either crystalline or macrocrystalline nitrofurantoin (55). They observed that patients receiving the macrocrystalline preparation experienced significantly fewer side-effects than those receiving the crystalline form (17% vs 39%). Nausea and vomiting were the most common reactions noted; others included shaking chills, headache, "lightheadedness," skin rash and diarrhea. Although a cure rate of 86% was recorded for patients receiving the macrocrystalline form of the drug and 76% for those receiving the crystalline, this difference was not significant.

(c) Administration of nitrofurantoin with milk or meals will usually lessen the associated nausea. Administration with food undoubtedly slows the absorption of the drug (analogous to the macrocrystalline preparation) and thereby lowers the incidence of gastrointestinal upset.

(d) If nausea cannot be avoided, an alternate drug to which the organism is susceptible will have to be substituted (61).

34. The patient tolerated the macrocrystalline form taken with meals and continued her regimen. However, ten days later she began to complain of dyspnea, tachypnea, a distressing cough and wheezes. She has a past history of occasional milk asthma which responds to non-prescription ephedrine compounds but has never had symptoms of this severity. Examination revealed a temperature of 38.4°C, pulse 115/min, and soft inspiratory and expiratory rhonchi with a few bibasilar rales. Nitrofurantoin administration was stopped, and 250 mg aminophylline given IV without relief. Two days later she became afebrile, but the rhonchi and rales were more pronounced. Betamethasone 6 mg was then given IM, followed by oral doses through the next day; symptoms disappeared in two days.

Two weeks later when she took one 100 mg nitrofurantoin capsule, she developed severe tightening of the chest, respiratory distress and a temperature of 38.4°C. She took ephedrine-containing compounds

until she was seen by the physician the following day. By that time she appeared completely recovered. Discuss the apparent nitrofurantoin-induced respiratory reaction which occurred in this patient.

Over 200 cases of nitrofurantoin-induced hypersensitivity pulmonary reactions have been reported (47). Hailey et al reviewed the literature on nitrofurantoin pulmonary reactions and found that the condition is usually acute and develops several days after institution of therapy (47). The reaction occurs in patients of all ages but is more common in the elderly. Symptoms vary from a mild, flu-like syndrome to dyspnea, cough and fever and, infrequently, severe pulmonary edema and myocardial infarction. Eosinophilia usually appears a few days after the onset of symptoms. X-ray studies generally reveal pulmonary infiltration and pulmonary function tests indicate restrictive disease. Rash occurs in a few cases. Rapid recovery usually follows discontinuation of the drug; however, treatment with steroids may be beneficial and necessary in severe cases (47, 49). Oftentimes the reaction is misdiagnosed as pneumonia, and recovery is attributable to antibiotic therapy rather than discontinuation of the nitrofurantoin. However, rapid development of symptoms on subsequent exposure to the drug (sometimes within hours of the first dose) pinpoints nitrofurantoin as the etiologic agent (47). A few chronic cases have also been reported, with insidious development of pulmonary symptoms in patients on long-term nitrofurantoin therapy.

Failure to recover completely from either the acute or chronic pulmonary reaction is rare. The first case of death from the reaction was recently reported in an elderly patient who had taken nitrofurantoin intermittently for a few years and suffered two episodes of severe dyspnea prior to her death which was related to her resumption of nitrofurantoin therapy (67). Diffuse eosinophilic interstitial infiltration suggested a chronic immunologic process. When the wide use of nitrofurantoin is considered, this hypersensitivity reaction is relatively uncommon. However, awareness of its occurrence is important; because it is frequently misdiagnosed, patients are unnecessarily reexposed to nitrofurantoin.

35. A 40-year-old female with a ten year history of recurrent urinary tract infections is given nalidixic acid 1 gm qid for her present infection. The causative organism is E. coli, serotype 011, sensitive to the drug. Four days after initiating therapy, the patient's dysuria persists. A repeat urine culture is taken, nalidixic acid is stopped, and ampicillin 250 mg qid is started. Two days later C & S results indicate that the infection is due to E. coli, serotype 011, sensitive to nitrofurantoin, ampicillin, sulfisoxazole, and kanamycin, but resistant to tetracycline and nalidixic acid. A

third urine culture taken at this time is sterile, and the patient recovers following a 14 day course of ampicillin. What is the bacterial spectrum of nalidixic acid? What is the major limitation to its use in the treatment of UTI's?

Nalidixic acid is effective against a broad spectrum of gram-negative bacteria commonly infecting the urinary tract, including *E. coli, Proteus, Klebsiella* and *Enterobacter. Pseudomonas, Staphylococci* and *Strep. fecalis* are not sensitive to nalidixic acid at concentrations achievable in the urine. Nalidixic acid might be most useful for UTI's secondary to *Klebsiella* or indole-positive *Proteus,* and in penicillin allergic individuals who have *Proteus mirabilis* infections (100).

The major factor limiting the usefulness of nalidixic acid is the rapid development of resistant organisms. The frequency with which this occurs varies among reports. In an evaluation of 50 patients treated with nalidixic acid, 13 (26%) developed resistant strains of the same species and serotype which were sensitive to the drug prior to treatment (91). Others have reported a lower incidence (6-14%) (10, 90). The resistance generally appears within 2-3 days, is extremely stable and nontransferable, and is thought to result from a single step mutation (91). The resistant organisms proliferate in nalidixic acid concentrations exceeding 1000 mcg/ml. Brumfitt and Pursell demonstrated no increase in the incidence of nalidixic acid resistant strains within a community over several years; however, this fact does not negate the problem of resistance development, treatment failures within the individual, and the need for repeat urine cultures 2-3 days after initiation of the drug when it is used (12).

36. Oxolinic acid (Utibid) was recently marketed in the U.S. In view of its chemical similarity to nalidixic acid, what advantages does this product offer in the treatment of UTI?

Oxolinic acid covers the same bacterial spectrum as nalidixic acid. Lower MIC's are necessary to eradicate susceptible organisms and the drug needs to be given only twice daily, rather than four times daily as does nalidixic acid (6). The development of resistance is also a limitation in the use of oxolinic acid (21, 68). Since the problem of treatment failures far outweighs any advantage which maybe gained in the more convenient dosage regimen, the routine use of oxolinic acid as well as nalidixic acid is discouraged.

37. During a recent hospital stay a 40-year-old female contracted a UTI which was successfully treated with cephalothin (Keflin) 2 gm qid for 7 days. Because she had a past history of several UTI's, her physician decided chronic drug therapy was necessary and prescribed methenamine mandelate (Mandelamine) 1 gm qid. When is chronic drug therapy indicated to prevent recurrent urinary tract infections?

Chronic infections may be handled in one of two ways: by treating each recurrent infection with an appropriate antibacterial for 10-14 days; or, by administering chronic, low-dose prophylactic therapy.

The frequency of infections is probably the main determinant of whether or not chronic suppressive therapy should be used. There is no conclusive evidence that either method is superior, and there are no studies comparing the two treatment regimens. Data collected by Kunin suggest that repeated treatment of recurrent infections will eventually result in a decreased incidence of subsequent infections (65). The U.S. Public Health Cooperative Study demonstrated that the incidence of recurrent infections was significantly less (30%) in males taking chronic antimicrobials than males taking placebo (20%) over 1 year (35). A patient is placed on chronic prophylaxis if the frequency of infections is sufficient to warrant continued administration of an antimicrobial agent and to avoid the distress and discomfort of multiple infections. Before placing a patient on chronic suppressive therapy, however, any active infection which may exist must be completely eradicated by an appropriate course of antibiotic therapy. The low doses of antimicrobials used for chronic prophylaxis suppress bacterial growth but do not eliminate active infection. Also, certain bacteria (e.g., *Proteus)* may render the urine pH too alkaline for agents like methenamine to be effective.

The kidney should be ruled out as a source of recurrent infections, because low dose prophylactic therapy will not eliminate an infectious focus within the kidney. Anatomical deformities which predispose the patient to recurrent infections (i.e., obstruction, stones,) and are amenable to surgical corrections should also be ruled out. A poorer response was observed in patients with urologic abnormalities (35, 56).

Age should also be considered when contemplating chronic antimicrobial therapy. An asymptomatic, elderly patient taking many other medications is not a candidate for chronic prophylactic treatment (15, 72, 118). Since the relationship between recurrent bacterial infections and progressive renal disease is still unclear, most practitioners agree that suppressive therapy is indicated in the young patient (118).

Patient acceptance, compliance, and commitment to follow-up are important to the success of chronic suppressive therapy. Regular follow-up is necessary to determine the frequency of recurrence or the development of a resistant organism (104).

38. Which drugs are generally recommended for chronic antimicrobial therapy in patients with frequent recurrent infections?

The merits of chronic drug therapy have not been sufficiently evaluated, so the drugs and doses used vary among practitioners. When selecting a drug which will be administered chronically, one should consider the likelihood that resistant organisms will develop during treatment and the long-term toxicity of the agent. Methenamine salts and nitrofurantoin are recommended by Kunin because of their broad-spectrum of activity, minimal toxic potential, and the low incidence of bacterial resistance associated with their use (65). The U.S. Public Health Cooperative Study compared sulfamethizole, nitrofurantoin, methenamine mandelate and placebo in 249 males over a two year period. The side effects resulting from the long-term use of these agents were negligible and the emergence of resistant organisms was not significant (35). However, a surprisingly higher mortality rate unrelated to infection occurred in the sulfamethizole group. Methenamine was superior in delaying recurrence after one year of treatment, but the differences among all drugs and placebo became negligible on longer therapy. Another study found tmp-smx superior to both sulfonamide alone and methenamine in preventing recurrences in 40 females after one year (49).

Sulfonamides are generally not recommended for prophylaxis, because they alter fecal flora which increases the risk of a resistant infection (71). Methenamine and nitrofurantoin were considered equally effective in the U.S. Public Health Cooperative Study; however, the results on the population of males cannot be extrapolated to the more common female population. Both drugs must be used cautiously in patients with renal failure; nitrofurantoin is ineffective and more toxic in this situation (see Question 32) and methenamine provides an undesirable acid load to the azotemic patient (35). Further studies comparing and evaluating tmp-smx, nitrofurantoin and methenamine are needed.

39. Should an acidifying agent be administered with methenamine salts?

Upon exposure to an acid medium, methenamine is hydrolyzed to formaldehyde, the compound responsible for the antibacterial activity of the methenamine salts : methenamine mandelate (Mandelamine) and methenamine hippurate (Hiprex) (78).

If 4-5 gm of methenamine base are given daily and the fluid intake is limited there will be an adequate urinary formaldehyde concentration (97). Mandelic acid is said to be bacteriostatic in daily doses of 10 gm if fluid intake is restricted. Hippuric acid is a normal metabolic end product and is said to be bacteriostatic at pH5 (97).

Several reports indicate that the acid salts of methenamine are bacteriostatic up to a pH of 6.4 (37, 78). However, urine concentrations of formaldehyde measured intermittently after 1 gm methenamine twice a day were highest at pH~ 5.5 (58, 78). The amount of mandelic or hippuric acid in the available preparations

is not sufficient to provide any antiseptic effect but is said to aid the hydrolysis of methenamine to formaldehyde. It is also claimed that if fluid intake is limited, additional agents to acidify the urine are not needed. An increased urine volume (through increased fluid intake or administration of diuretics); low urinary specific gravity; or a pH greater than 6.5 will significantly decrease the formaldehyde concentration (58, 78). Concomitant administration of an acidifying agent will increase the formaldehyde concentration, but excessive formaldehyde can cause dysuria by direct irritation to the bladder and urethral mucosa.

Although it is unnecessary to acidify the urine if fluid intake is limited, fluid restrictions may be impractical or undesirable. Because urine pH may vary widely even while on this medication, addition of a urinary acidifying agent will yield a more constant and predictable urine pH and effective formaldehyde concentration. Urine pH should be monitored closely when therapy is administered whether or not an acidifying agent is used.

40. What agents will effectively acidify the urine?

Drugs which have been used for urinary acidification include ammonium chloride, methionine and ascorbic acid. Ammonium chloride will effectively lower urine pH when given in doses of 2 gm every 6 hours. Travis et al have indicated that for short term therapy, ammonium chloride is better than ascorbic acid in lowering urine pH (114). However, its effects are short-lived and may be reversed by the kidney; its use is not practical for chronic administration. Methionine is also an effective agent in doses of 12-15 gm per day; however, these doses are associated with gastrointestinal pain which limits its usefulness (114).

The most commonly used acidifying agent is ascorbic acid (vitamin C). The dosage regimen utilized can markedly influence the degree of acidification achieved. Two groups of patients received 2-8 gm/m²/day. The group receiving ascorbic acid every 4 hours around-the-clock most consistently had a urinary pH below 5.5. The other group, given the drug four times daily before meals, had wide fluctuations in urine pH. It was noted, however, that when ascorbic acid and methenamine mandelate were administered concurrently, a low urine pH was maintained even when the "four times daily" regimen was used (114).

Diet may influence the ability of vitamin C to lower urine pH. A high intake of fruits and fruit juices (except cranberry, plum and prune) may produce a more alkaline urine (80). Also, persons with chronic indigestion or peptic ulcer disease who take several ounces or tablets of absorbable antacids may inadvertently neutralize the effect of the ascorbic acid (40). Therefore, a patient taking ascorbic acid should be encouraged to check his urine pH with nitrazine paper several times during the day to insure consistent acidification.

41. A 41-year-old male experienced his first UTI at age 18, with symptoms of frequency, dysuria, nocturia, perineal pain, chills and fever, but no flank pain. Acute prostatitis was diagnosed, *E. coli* was cultured, and a sulfonamide was prescribed with successful results. After 12 asymptomatic years, an infection due to *E. coli* recurred and again responded to sulfonamide therapy. Two more *E. coli* infections occurred over the next eight years. The fourth infection responded initially to sulfonamides but recurred three weeks after the medication was discontinued. How is the diagnosis of bacterial prostatitis confirmed?

Chronic bacterial prostatitis is the major cause of recurrent UTI's in males. Except in males with spinal cord injuries, infectious stones, or obstructive abnormalities of the urinary tract, recurrent infection is almost assuredly due to persistence of bacteria in the prostate which seed the bladder. Normal males secrete a prostatic antibacterial factor; however, this substance is absent in men with chronic prostatitis (30). Even in the above exceptions, simple urinary tract infections will often eventually involve the prostate gland where bacteria are difficult to eradicate.

The most satisfactory method of confirming the diagnosis of bacterial prostatitis is by examination of expressed prostatic secretion. To assure accurate localization (i.e., to distinguish prostatic from urethral bacteria) segmented urine samples are taken. The first 5-10 ml of the voided sample represents urethral urine, the midstream sample represents bladder urine, and the last portion of the voided sample which is collected after prostatic massage, represents prostatic urine (99). The presence of bacteria in prostatic secretions and a higher bacterial count in the "prostatic urine sample" than the other two samples indicates that bacteria are originating from the prostate gland. The bacteria are similar to those of UTI in general (30).

42. Evaluate the treatment alternatives available to the patient described in Question 41.

Unfortunately, most antibiotics are acidic and do not cross the prostatic epithelium into the alkaline prostatic fluid. Until recently, erythromycin was the only agent which produced high prostatic concentrations, but it is ineffective against most prostatic pathogens (101).

Although not approved for this use in the United States, trimethoprim-sulfamethoxazole has been used extensively in Europe for the treatment of bacterial prostatitis and is currently being investigated in this country. Sulfamethoxazole does not distribute into prostatic fluid; however, high concentrations of trimethoprim which is effective against many of the common pathogens can be achieved in the prostate (101).

Drach suggests that any appropriate antibiotic can be used acutely, as penetration is probably enhanced in inflamed tissue (30).

Chronic low-dose therapy with agents such as nalidixic acid, nitrofurantoin or methenamine can be initiated to alleviate the symptoms of episodic bladder infection associated with chronic bacterial prostatitis. Infections eventually recur with greater frequency in most of these patients, although some become asymptomatic, even in the presence of chronic bacteriuria. Chronic, low-dose antibacterial therapy sterilizes the bladder; alleviates symptoms; confines bacteria to the prostate; and inhibits infection and damage to the rest of the urinary tract. Chronic bacterial prostatitis is one of the few indications for continuous antibiotic therapy.

43. What is the risk of urinary tract infection following urethral catheterization?

The most common type of hospital-acquired infection is the catheter-induced urinary tract infection. Catheterization and other forms of urologic instrumentation are involved in 75% of all hospital-acquired urinary tract infections, and catheter-associated urinary tract infection is said to account for 30% of all nosocomial infections. A more serious consideration is the fact that urinary tract infections are also the major cause of gram-negative bacteremia (38, 106).

The risk of infection is directly related to the type and care of the catheter, duration of catheterization, and the susceptibility of the patient. Diagnostic or single, short-term catheterization is associated with a much lower risk of infection than indwelling, long-term catheterization. Despite careful technique, there is always the risk of contaminating a sterile bladder with urethral bacteria. The incidence of infection following a single catheterization is 1% in healthy young women and 20% in hospitalized patients (102).

The risk of infection from an indwelling catheter is well-recognized. In the open drainage system the sterility of the unit is not maintained when the catheter and bag are disconnected for urine collection or bladder irrigation. Consequently, the most careful and aseptic insertion techniques will not prevent infection and 50% of patients are infected within 24 hours and nearly 100% of patients are infected after four days (3).

Infections can be dramatically reduced by the closed sterile drainage system, the most common type of catheter currently in use. The overall incidence of infection from the closed system with careful insertion and maintenance is about 20%; the risk increases to 50% after 14 days of catheterization (63). If the system is disconnected and sterility is broken, the infection rate is similar to that of an open system.

44. Does the prophylactic use of topical antimicro-

bial agents prior to and during catheter insertion decrease the risk of infection?

The urethral meatus and distal third of the urethra always contain bacteria. Bacterial contamination of the bladder from these sites which occurs when the catheter is inserted accounts for the infections following single diagnostic catheterizations and probably the early infections from indwelling catheters. For this reason, it is recommended that the periurethral area be carefully cleansed with soap and water followed by some type of antiseptic solution. An iodophor solution is often recommended, but benzalkonium chloride is not because it is ineffective against some gram-negative organisms (106). The instillation of antibacterial lubricants into the urethra is often advocated before catheterization; however, placebo-control studies fail to show that the incidence of infection is significantly reduced by their use (19, 64). The antibacterial effectiveness of the local lubricants lasts only 24-48 hours, and there is no evidence that they offer any added protection beyond that provided by the closed drainage system (3, 106). Also, the pericatheter space within the urethra appears to be less important than the catheter lumen as a route of bacterial access to the bladder (3, 65, 106). However, Kunin found that daily lubricant instillation, either with or without an anti-infective agent, appeared to have some protective effect (64).

45. Are constant bladder irrigations with antibacterial or antiseptic solutions effective in preventing infection? Discuss the hazards and limitations associated with their use.

Antibacterial instillation is quite effective in the open drainage system. Over a ten-day period, the incidence of infection was reduced from 100% to less than 20% (3). The antibacterial preparations frequently used are 0.25% acetic acid, nitrofurazone, and neomycin-polymixin (Neosporin GU irrigant). A limitation of *acetic acid* is that the urine pH must be maintained below 5.0 in order for it to have any antibacterial effect. Systemic acidosis might also be a hazard in older patients. Acetic acid is associated with about a 20% incidence of infection.

Nitrofurazone in a 1:6 solution is also associated with a 20% incidence of infection in patients on open drainage. Gross hematuria is a hazard associated with its use; one study found the incidence to be 19% (77). Although systemic absorption of nitrofurazone does not seem to occur, the solvent, polyethylene glycol, is detectable in the sera in levels of 10-716 mcg/ml (77). The significance of this absorption has not been elucidated.

Neosporin (40 mg)-polymixin (20 mg) seems to provide the greatest preventive effect, decreasing the incidence of bacteriuria to 6% in patients with open drain-

age catheterization. As with the other solutions, its effectiveness is greatest during the first ten days of catheterization, and it is not effective in eradicating a pre-existing infection. Resistant *Proteus* and enterococci are frequent pathogens in infections acquired after prolonged irrigation with neosporin-polymixin (77, 110). After ten days of irrigation, polymixin is not detectable in the sera; however, neomycin concentrations of 0.1 mcg/ml have been observed. Irrigations lasting as long as 78 days were not associated with any systemic effects (110).

Although it is speculated by many that the combination of bladder irrigation and closed drainage catheterization would be additive in preventing bladder inspection, the combined system has not been adequately evaluated. In two studies, the use of such combination in a total of 33 patients resulted in a 20% incidence of infection, which is similar to the incidence observed by Kunin following the use of closed catheterization alone (42, 59, 63).

46. What role does systemic anti-infective therapy have in the prevention of catheter-induced urinary infections?

The benefits of systemic antibiotics in preventing catheter-induced UTI's have not been clarified. A review of the literature indicates that studies prior to 1965 showed systemic therapy failed to reduce the incidence of bacteriuria; open-drainage systems, poor catheterization technique, and use of chloramphenicol as the agent of choice may account for the failures in these early studies (5, 76). More recent studies using closed drainage systems and diligent catheter care indicate that systemic antibiotics decrease the daily and overall incidence of infection in patients with sterile urines prior to catheterization (38, 59, 63, 98). The preventive effect of the antimicrobial agents is greatest for short-term catheterizations or during the first four to seven days of catheterization (38, 59, 63). Thereafter, the rate of infection increases; although the overall incidence is still decreased, the emergence of resistant organisms is significant (38, 59). Therefore, in deciding to use systemic antimicrobials one must consider the patient's underlying diseases or risk factors, duration of catheterization, and the potential complications of drug toxicity or resistant organisms which may result from the chronic use of antimicrobial agents. (See also Question 48).

47. What catheterization techniques minimize the complications of bacteriuria?

Recommendations for catheter care have recently been published by the Center for Disease Control (106). In summary, these recommendations emphasize the importance of asepsis and sterility at insertion, as well as proper maintenance. A closed drainage system should never be disconnected, because contamination is generally initiated from the collecting system (38, 111). Likewise, to avoid reflux the collection bag should be positioned to maintain a downward flow. Since cross-infection among catheterized patients can occur, catheterized patients should be separated. It is particularly important to separate bacteriuric catheterized patients from non-infected catheterized patients (74).

48. What is the appropriate treatment for a urinary tract infection contracted during catheterization?

There is no doubt that systemic antibiotic therapy selected specifically for the infecting organisms will result in a sterile urine. However, it is also recognized that reinfection, often by a resistant organism, occurs in a third to one-half of these cases if closed drainage catheterization is continued during therapy (20, 63). For this reason, it is generally recommended that systemic antimicrobial therapy be begun after the catheter is removed, or with catheter in place, if its removal is soon anticipated (28, 59, 65). Since bacteriuria is inevitable in long-term catheterization, Kunin suggests that the patient be left untreated if asymptomatic to avoid the complication of recolonization and potential bacteremia by highly resistant organisms (65). As mentioned earlier, prophylaxis in these patients probably provides minimal benefit and exposes the patient to possible risks; therefore, the strictest adherence to good catheter care is the primary concern in the chronically catheterized patient. Recatheterization with a new, sterile unit should be performed whenever contamination is suspected.

TABLE 1
AVERAGE URINE CONCENTRATIONS OF COMMONLY USED ANTIMICROBIALS IN PATIENTS WITH NORMAL RENAL FUNCTION

Drug	Dose (q 6°, unless otherwise stated)	Average Urine Concentration	Reference
Penicillin G	250 mg po	75 mcg/ml	a
	500 mg po	100 mcg/ml	a
Ampicillin	250 mg po	300 mcg/ml	a
Carbenicillin	1.0 Gm of ester po	640-2000 mcg/ml	b
Tetracycline	250 mg po	150 mcg/ml	a-1
Oxytetracycline	250 mg po	150 mcg/ml	a
Cephalexin	1.0 Gm po	2000-3000 mcg/ml	a
Chloramphenicol	500 mg po	100 mcg/ml	a
Kanamycin	500 mg/12 hr IM	100-600 mcg/ml	c
Streptomycin	500 mg/12 hr IM	400 mcg/ml	a
Gentamicin	0.8 mg/12 hr IM	100 mcg/ml	a
Colistin	75 mg/12 hr IM	50(?) mcg/ml	a
Sulfisoxazole	1 Gm q 4 hr po	2570 mcg/ml	d
Sulfamethoxazole	(see trimethoprim-sulfamethoxazole)		
Sulfamethizole	250 mg po	400-1100 mcg/ml	a-2
Nitrofurantoin	100 mg po	100 mcg/ml	a
Nalidixic Acid	1.0 Gm po	200 mcg/ml	a
Trimethoprim- sulfamethoxazole	160 mg 12 hr po +800 mg	78.4 mcg/ml 29.5 mcg/ml	e e

a. Stamey, T.A.: Urinary Infections, Williams & Wilkins, 1972, p. 32.24°collection; 1200-1500 ml urine out-put/24 hours.
a-1. Ibid., p. 278. Urine output unspecified.
a-2. p. 280. 24°collection; urine output unspecified.
b. Bran, J.L. et al: Human pharmacology and clinical evaluation of an oral carbenicillin preparation. Clin Pharmacol Ther 12:525, 1971. 6 hr. collection, urine output unspecified.
c. Kucers, A. Use of Antibiotics. William Heinemann Medical Books, Ltd., London, 1972, p. 131. Urine output unspecified.
d. Svec, F.A. et al: A new sulfonamide (Gantrisin). Studies on solubility, absorption and escretion. Arch Int Med 85:83, 1950. 1500 cc/urine output/24 hours assumed; includes metabolites
e. Bergan, T. et al: Human pharmacokinetics of a sulfamethoxazole-trimethoprim combination. Acta Med Scand 192:483, 1972. 4 to 5.5 hr. collection.

TABLE 2
DRUGS OF CHOICE FOR URINARY TRACT INFECTIONS

Infecting Organism	Community-Acquired DOC*	Community-Acquired Alternative	Hospital-Acquired DOC*	Hospital-Acquired Alternative
E. coli	Sulfonamide	Ampicillin Nitrofurantoin	Ampicillin	Nitrofurantoin Cephalosporin
P. mirabilis	Sulfonamide	Ampicillin Cephalosporin	Ampicillin	Cephalosporin Trimethoprim- Sulfamethoxazole Kanamycin
Proteus (other)	Sulfonamide	Carbenicillin Trimethoprim- Sulfamethoxazole Nalidixic Acid	Carbenicillin	Kanamycin Gentamicin Trimethoprim- Sulfamethoxazole
Klebsiella	Sulfonamide	Cephalosporin Trimethoprim- Sulfamethoxazole	Cephalosporin	Gentamicin Kanamycin Trimethoprim- Sulfamethoxazole
Aerobacter			Gentamicin	Carbenicillin Trimethoprim- Sulfamethoxazole
Pseudomonas			Carbenicillin	Gentamicin
Enterococcus	Ampicillin		Ampicillin	Nitrofurantoin

*DOC = Drug of Choice

TABLE 3

RECOMMENDED DOSAGE OF ANTIMICROBIALS IN URINARY TRACT INFECTIONS FOR PATIENTS WITH NORMAL RENAL FUNCTION

Drug	Dose	Dosing Interval
Sulfisoxazole	0.5-1.0 gm	q 4-6 hr
Sulfamethoxazole	1.0 gm	q 12 hr
Nalidixic Acid	1.0 gm	q 6 hr
Nitrofurantoin	100 mg	q 6-8 hr
Penicillin G	250-500 mg	q 6 hr
Ampicillin	250-500 mg	q 6 hr
Tetracycline	250-500 mg	q 6-8 hr
Cephalexin	250-500 mg	q 6-8 hr
Trimethoprim-sulfamethoxazole	2 tabs	q 12 hr
Kanamycin	7.5 mg/kg IM	q 12 hr
Gentamicin	1 mg/kg IM or IV	q 8 hr
Colistimethate	0.8-1.6 mg/kg IM	q 8 hr
Methenamine mandelate	1.0 gm	q 6 hr
Methenamine hippurate	1.0 gm	q 12 hr

APPENDIX
Treatment Protocol for Urinary Tract Infections
(see Figure 1)

The treatment of a urinary tract infection is generally straightforward and usually successful if a few basic rules are followed and the proper antimicrobial agent administered. Kunin (65) has expertly and succinctly outlined the basic rules for the treatment of a urinary tract infection:

(A) Sensitivity studies.

(1) uncomplicated infection — results are desirable but not essential prior to initiating therapy.

(2) recurrent infection — results are highly desirable to aid in selection of therapy. If unavailable; select another agent than that used previously.

(3) frequent recurrent infection — results are mandatory and likely to indicate bacterial resistance to multiple antibacterial agents.

(B) Useful agents

(1) uncomplicated infection — sulfonamides (avoid in presence of allergy or G6PD deficiency); ampicillin (avoid in patients with penicillin allergy); tetracycline (avoid in children less than 8 years and pregnant women).

(2) recurrent infection—ampicillin; cephalexin; tetracycline; nalidixic acid and nitrofurantoin. Nitrofurantoin has the particular advantage of minimal development of resistance with repeated usage.

(3) frequent recurrent infection — nitrofurantoin; methenamine mandelate (after active infection eradicated), occasionally nalidixic acid.

(C) Duration of treatment.

(1) uncomplicated infection — 10 to 14 days.

(2) recurrent infection — 10 to 14 days.

(3) frequent recurrent infection — 1-3 months. Discontinue treatment and observe for recurrences.

(D) Follow-up.

(1) uncomplicated infection —

a. Two days after initiation of therapy. Urine sediment should no longer reveal organisms (pyuria may persist).

b. One week after completion of therapy. Obtain urine culture to check that infection has been eradicated.

c. If reinfection does not occur. Check monthly for 3 months, then every 3 months for 9 months, then semiannually for one year.

(2) recurrent infection — same as above

(3) frequent recurrent infection — same as above.

A *treatment protocol,* which we have developed for the treatment of urinary tract infections in hospitalized patients; follows (see Figure 1). The protocol is designed to indicate the steps a clinician must follow in approaching a patient with a UTI. While the protocol was developed for us in hospitalized patients; the methods outlined are still valid in the ambulatory setting.

If the student will combine the "rules" outlined above, the information contained in this chapter, and the basic thought processes outlined in the protocol, he should have little trouble understanding the treatment of urinary tract infections and participating in the care of patients with this infectious disease state.

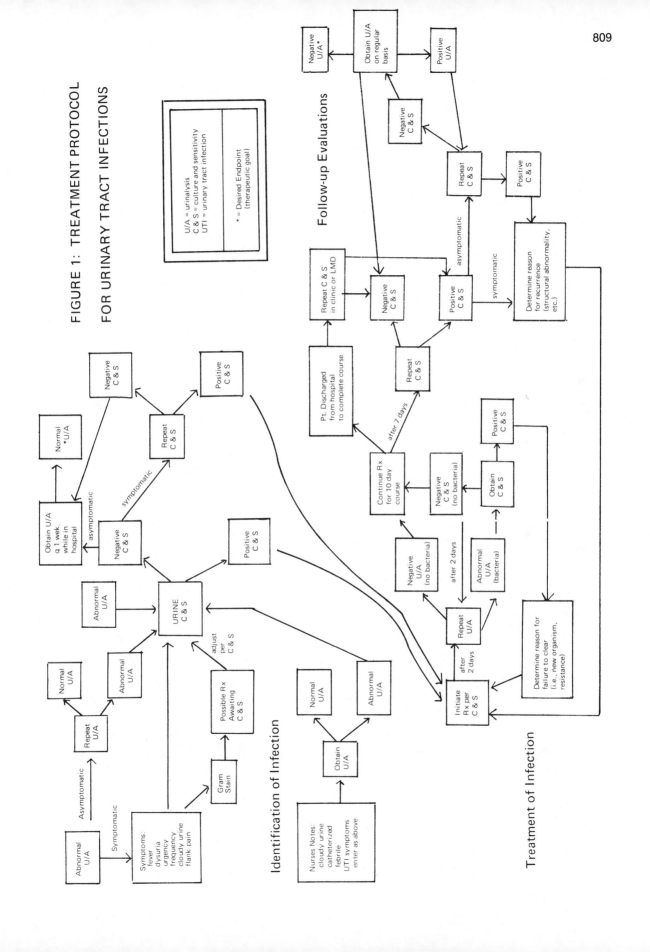

FIGURE 1: TREATMENT PROTOCOL FOR URINARY TRACT INFECTIONS

U/A = urinalysis
C & S = culture and sensitivity
UTI = urinary tract infection

* = Desired Endpoint (therapeutic goal)

Identification of Infection

Treatment of Infection

Follow-up Evaluations

809

REFERENCES

1. Abbot GD: Neonatal bacteriuria: A prospective study in 1,460 infants. Brit Med J 1:267, 1972.
2. Alwall N et al: A population study on renal and urinary tract disease III. Acta Med Scand 194:541, 1973.
3. Andriole VT: Hospital-acquired urinary infection and the indwelling catheter. Urol Clin N Amer 2:451, 1975.
4. Andriole VT: Urinary tract infections in pregnancy. Urol Clin N Amer 2:485, 1975.
5. Appleton DM et al: The prophylactic use of chloramphenicol in transurethral resections of the prostate. J Urol 75:304, 1956.
6. Atlas E et al: Nalidixic acid and oxolinic acid in the treatment of chronic bacteriuria. Ann Int Med 70:713, 1969.
7. Bailey RR: Urinary infections in pregnancy. N Zeal Med J 71:216, 1970.
8. Bailey RR et al: Prevention of urinary tract infection with low-dose nitrofurantoin. Lancet 2:1112, 1971.
9. Bailey RR et al: Problem of recurrent urinary tract infections. Drugs 8:54, 1974.
10. Barlow AM: Nalidixic acid in infection of the urinary tract. Brit Med J 2:1308, 1963.
11. Brumfitt W: Recent developments in the treatment of urinary tract infections. J Infect Dis 120:61, 1969.
12. Brumfitt W et al: Observations on bacterial sensitivities to nalidixic acid and critical comments on the 6 center survey. Postgrad Med J 47 (suppl):16, 1971.
13. Brumfitt W et al: Double-blind trial to compare ampicillin, cephalexin, co-trimoxazole and trimethoprim in treatment of urinary infection. Brit Med J 2:673, 1972.
14. Brumfitt W et al: Trimethoprim-sulfamethoxazole: The present position. J Infect Dis 128(suppl):S778, 1973.
15. Brumfitt W: Urinary infection. Med Soc Trans 90:105, 1974.
16. Burka ET et al: Clinical spectrum of hematolytic anemia associated with glucose-6-phosphate dehydrogenase deficiency. Ann Int Med 64:817, 1966.
17. Bushby SRM et al: Trimethoprim, A sulfonamide potentiator. Brit J Pharmacol Chemother 33:72, 1968.
18. Bushby SRM: Trimethoprim-sulfamethoxazole: In vitro microbiological aspects. J Infect Dis 128(suppl):S442, 1973.
19. Butler HK et al: Evaluation of polymixin catheter lubricant and impregnated catheters. J Urol 100:560-566, 1968.
20. Butler HK et al: Evaluation of specific systemic antimicrobial therapy in patients while on closed catheter drainage. J Urol 100:567, 1968.
21. Clark H et al: Emergence of resistant organisms as a function of dose in oxolinic acid therapy. Amer J Med Sci 261:145, 1971.
22. Conklin JD et al: Urinary drug excretion in man during oral dosage of different nitrofurantoin formulations. Clin Pharmacol Ther 10:534, 1969.
23. Corriere JN: Effect of anovulatory drugs on the human urinary tract and urinary tract infections. Obstet Gynec 35:211, 1970.
24. Corriere JN et al: Bacteriuria in young women. Urology J 2:539, 1973.
25. Cosgrove MD et al: Ampicillin vs. trimethoprim-sulfamethoxazole in chronic urinary tract infection. J Urol 111:670, 1974.
26. Cox Ce et al: Combined trimethoprim-sulfamethoxazole therapy of urinary tract infection. Postgrad Med J 45(suppl):65, 1969.
27. Craig WA et al: Trimethoprim-sulfamethoxazole: Pharmacodynamic effects of urinary pH and renal failure. Ann Int Med 78:491, 1973.
28. Dale GA: Iatrogenic urinary infections Urol Clin N Amer 2:471, 1975.
29. Dike AE: Bacteriology of urinary tract infections in paraplegics. J Clin Path 27:933, 1974.
30. Drach GW: Prostatitis: Man's hidden infection. Urol Clin N Amer 2:499, 1975.
31. Etzwiler DD: Incidence of urinary tract infections among juvenile diabetics. JAMA 191:81, 1965.
32. Eudy WE: Correlations between in vitro sensitivity testing and theraputic response in urinary tract infections. Urology 2:519, 1973.
33. Fairley KF: Diagnosis and treatment of pyleonephritis. Drugs 6:417, 1973.
34. Felts JH et al: Neural, hematologic and bacteriologic effects of nitrofuratoin in renal insufficiency. Am J Med 51:331, 1971.

35. Freeman RB et al: Long term therapy for chronic bacteriuria in men. Ann Int Med 83:133-147, 1975.
36. Frisch JM: Clinical experience with adverse reactions to trimethoprim-sulfamethoxazole. J Infect Dis 128(suppl):607, 1973.
37. Gandelman AL: Methenamine mandelate: Antimicrobial activity in urine and correlation with formaldehyde levels. J Urol 97:533, 1967.
38. Garibaldi RA et al: Factors predisposing to bacteriuria during indwelling urethral catheterization. NEJM 291:215-219 (Aug. 1), 1974.
39. Garrod LP: Relative antibacterial activity of three penicillins. Brit Med J 1:527, 1960.
40. Gibaldi M et al: Effect of antacids on pH of urine. Clin Pharmacol Ther 16:520, 1974.
41. Gillenwater JY: Diagnosis of urinary tract infection: Appraisal of diagnostic procedures. Kidney Int'l 8:S3, 1975.
42. Gladstone JL et al: Prevention of bacteriuria resulting from indwelling catheters. J Urol 99:458, 1968.
43. Gleckman RA: A cooperative controlled study of the use of trimethoprimsulfamethoxazole in chronic urinary tract infections. J Infect Dis 128 (suppl):S647, 1973.
44. Gleckman RA: Trimethoprim-sulfamethoxazole vs. ampicillin in chronic urinary tract infections. JAMA 233:427, 1975.
45. Govan DE et al: Management of children with urinary tract infections. Urinology 6:273, 1975.
46. Hailey FJ et al: Gastrointestinal tolerance to a new macrocrystalline form of nitrofurantoin: A collaborative study. Curr Ther Res 9:6000, 1967.
47. Hailey FJ et al: Pleuropneumonic reactions to nitrofurantoin. NEJM 281: 1087, 1969.
48. Harding GKM et al: Efficacy of trimethoprim-sulfamethoxazole in bacteriuria. J Infect Dis 128 (suppl):S641, 1973.
49. Harding GKM et al: A controlled study of antimicrobial prophylaxis of recurrent urinary infection in women. NEJM 291:597, 1974.
50. Haunz EA et al: Agranulocytosis due to Gantrisin. Report of a case with recovery. JAMA 144:1179, 1950.
51. Heinrich RA et al: A pharmacological study of a new sulfonamide in G6PD deficient subjects. J Clin Pharmacol 11:428, 1971.
52. Hulbert J: Urinary tract infections and oral penicillin G. J Clin Path 25:73, 1972.
53. Hulbert J: Gram-negative urinary tract infection treated with oral penicillin G. Lancet 2:1216, 1972.
54. Kalowski S et al: Deterioration in renal function in association with co-trimoxazole therapy. Lancet 1:394, 1973.
55. Kalowski S et al: Crystalline and macrocrystalline nitrofurantoin in the treatment of urinary tract infections. NEJM 290:385, 1974.
56. Kalowski S et al: Controlled trial comparing co-trimoxazole and methenamine hippurate in the prevention of recurrent urinary tract infections. Med J Aust 1:585, 1975.
57. Kass EH et al: Bacteriuria and renal disease. J Infect Dis 120:27, 1969.
58. Katul MG et al: Antibacterial activity of methenamine hippurate. J Urol 104:320, 1970.
59. Keresteci AG et al: Indwelling catheter infection. Can Med Assoc J 109:711, 1973
60. Koch-Weser J et al: Adverse reactions to sulfisoxazole, sulfamethoxazole and nitrofurantoin. Arch Int Med 128:399, 1971.
61. Kucers A et al: The Use of Antibiotics (ed 2), JB Lippincott Co., Philadelphia, 1975, pp. 490, 491, 462.
62. Kunin CM: Asymptomatic bacteriuria. Ann Rev Med 17:383, 1966.
63. Kunin CM et al: Prevention of catheter-induced urinary tract infections by sterile closed drainage. NEJM 274:1155, 1966.
64. Kunin CM et al: Evaluation of an intraurethral lubricating catheter in prevention of catheter-induced urinary tract infections. J Urol 106:928, 1971.
65. Kunin CM: Detection, Prevention, and Management of Urinary Tract Infections, Lea and Febiger, Philadelphia, 1972.
66. Kunin CM: New detection methods in urinary tract infections. Urol Clin N Amer 2:423, 1975.
67. Kursh ED et al: Nitrofurantoin pulmonary complications, J Urol 113:392, 1975.
68. Lampe WT: Oxolinic acid treatment of urinary tract infections, Pennsylvania Med 74:59, 1971.
69. Lang GG et al: Diagnosis and treatment of urinary tract infections. Med Clin N Amer 55:1439, 1971.

70. Lehr D: Clinical toxicity of sulfonamides. Ann NY Acad Sci 69:417, 1957.

71. Lincoln K et al: Resistant urinary tract infections resulting from changes in resistance pattern of fecal flora induced by sulfonamide and hospital environment. Brit Med J 3:305, 1970.

72. Lindemeyer RI et al: Factors determining the outcome of chemotherapy in infections of the urinary tract. Ann Int Med 58:201, 1963.

73. Little PJ: Incidence of urinary infection in 5000 pregnant women. Lancet 2:925, 1966.

74. Maki DG et al: Prevention of catheter-associated urinary tract infection. JAMA 211:1270, 1972.

75. Marshall S et al: Ureteral dilitation following use of oral contraceptives. JAMA 198:782, 1966.

76. Martin CM et al: Bacteriuria prevention after indwelling urinary catheterization. Arch Int Med 110:703, 1962.

77. Meyers MS et al: Controlled trial of nitrofurazone and neomycin-polymixin as constant bladder rinses for prevention of post-indwelling catherization bacteriuria. Antimicrob Agents Chemother 571, 1964.

78. Miller H et al: Antibacterial correlates of urine drug levels of hexamethylenetetramine and formaldehyde. Invest Urol 8:21, 1970.

79. Morgan LK: Nitrofurantoin pulmonary hypersensitivity. Med J Aust 2:136, 1970.

80. Mow TW: Effect of urine pH on the antibacterial activity of antibiotics and chemotherapeutic agents. J Urol 87:978, 1962.

81. Norden CW, Kass EH: Bacteriuria of pregnancy-A critical appraisal. Ann Rev Med 19:431, 1968.

82. Norden CW et al: Hemolytic effect of sulfonamides in patients with erythrocytes deficiency in glucose-6-phosphate dehydrogenase. NEJM 279:30, 1968.

83. O'Grady F Catell WR: Kinetics of urinary tract infections. Brit Med J 38:149, 1966.

84. O'Grady F et al: Long term treatment of persistent or recurrent urinary tract infection with trimethoprim-sulfamethoxazole. J Infect Dis 128 (suppl):S652, 1973.

85. Ooi BS et al: Prevalence and site of bacteriuria in diabetes mellitus. Postgrad Med J 50:497, 1974.

86. O'Sullivan DS et al: Urinary tract infections: A comparative study in diabetics and the general population. Brit Med J 1:786, 1961.

87. Pfau A et al: An evaluation of midstream urine cultures in the diagnosis of UTI in females. Urol Int'l. 25:326, 1970.

88. Plevin SN et al: Perinephrotic abscess in diabetic patients. J Urol 103:538, 1970.

89. Pometta D et al: Asymptomatic bacteriuria in diabetes mellitus. NEJM 276:1118, 1967.

90. Reese L: Nalidixic acid in the treatment of urinary infections. Canad Med Assoc J 92:394, 1965.

91. Ronald AR et al: A critical evaluation of nalidixic acid in urinary tract infections. NEJM 275:1081, 1966.

92. Rosenfield JB et al: Effect of long term co-trimazole on renal function. Med J Aust 2:546, 1975

93. Sachs J et al: Effect of renal function on urinary recovery of orally administered nitrofurantoin. NEJM 278:1032, 1968.

94. Sanford JP: Urinary tract symptoms and infections. Ann Rev Med 26:485 1975.

95. Scheckler WE et al: Prevalences of infections and antibiotic usage in eight community hospitals, in Proceedings of the International Conference on Nosocomial Infections, Center for Disease Control Aug 3-6, 1970, Chicago, AHA, 1971, p 299.

96. Schwartz DE et al: Assay and pharmacokinetics of trimethoprim in man and animals. Postgrad Med J 45:32, 1969.

97. Seneca H et al: Chemotherapy of chronic urinary tract infections with methenamine hippurate. J Urol 97:1094, 1967.

98. Shapiro SR et al: Catheter associated urinary tract infections: Incidence and a new approach to prevention. J Urol 112:659, 1974.

99. Stamey TA et al: Localization and treatment of urinary tract infections. Role of bactericidal urine levels in opposition to serum levels. Medicine 44:1, 1965.

100. Stamey TA et al: Clinical use of nalidixic acid: A review and some observations. Invest Urol 6:582, 1969.

101. Stamey TA: Chronic bacterial prostatitis and diffusion of drugs into prostatic fluid. J Urol 103:16, 1970.

102. Stamey TA et al: Urinary infections: A selective review and some observations. Calif Med 113:16, 1970.

103. Stamey TA et al: Recurrent urinary tract infections in adult women. Role of introital enterobacteria. Calif Med 115:1, 1971.

104. Stamey TA: Urinary Infection, Williams and Wilkins Co, Baltimore, 1972.

105. Stamey TA et al: Serum vs. urinary antimicrobial concentrations in cure of urinary tract infections. NEJM 291:1159 1974.

106. Stamm WE: Guidelines for prevention of catheter-associated urinary tract infections. Ann Int Med 82:386, 1975.

107. Steinberg M et al: Acute hemolytic anemia associated with erythrocyte glutathione-peroxidase deficiency. Arch Int Med 125:302, 1970.

108. Takahashi M et al: Bacteriuria and oral contraceptives. JAMA 227:762, 1974.

109. Thompson HT: Clinical evaluation of Gantrisin (NU-44S). J Urol 62:892, 1949.

110. Thornton GF et al: Bacteriuria during indwelling catheter drainage. JAMA 195:179, 1966.

111. Thornton GF et al: Bacteriuria during indwelling catheter drainage. JAMA 214:339, 1970.

112. Thornton GF: Infections and diabetes. Med Clin N Amer 55:931, 1971.

113. Toole JF et al: Nitrofurantoin polyneuropathy. Neurology 23:554, 1973.

114. Travis LB et al: Urinary acidification with ascorbic acid. J Pedi at 67:1176, 1965.

115. Trimethoprim-sulfamethoxazole. Drugs 1:7, 1971.

116. Turck M: Relapse and reinfection in chronic bacteriuria. NEJM 275:70, 1966.

117. Turck M: Relapse and reinfection in chronic bacteriuria. NEJM 278:422, 1968.

118. Turck M: Localizing site of recurrent urinary tract infections. Urol Clin N Amer 2:433, 1975.

119. Turck M: Therapeutic guidelines in the management of urinary tract infections and pyelonephritis. Urol Clin N Amer 2:943, 1975.

120. VanPetten GR et al: Studies on the physiologic availabilities and metabolism of sulfonamides. J Clin Pharmacol 11:27, 1971.

121. Vejlsgaard R: Studies on urinary infections in diabetics. Acta Med Scand 179:173, 1966.

122. Vejlsgaard R: Studies on urinary infections in diabetics. III. Acta Med Scand 193:337, 1973.

123. Vosti KL: Recurrent urinary tract infections. JAMA 231:934, 1975.

124. Weinstein L et al: The sulfonamides. NEJM 263:793, 1960.

125. Weinstein L: The sulfonamides, in Goodman LS, Gilman A (eds): The Pharmacological Basis of Therapeutics (ed 4), Macmillan Co, New York, 1970, pp1179,1189,1195.

126. Williams JD et al: Treatment of bacteriuria in pregnant women with sulfamethoxazole and trimethoprim. Postgrad Med J 45 (suppl):71, 1969.

Chapter 38

Infective Endocarditis

Steven L. Barriere

Infective endocarditis is a disease characterized by infected thrombi (vegetations) on the inner lining of the heart and the mucosa which underlies it. The primary sites of infection within the heart are the closing edges of valve leaflets and cusps.

The primary lesion in the pathogenesis of the infection is a thrombus formation which can rapidly become colonized in the presence of bacteremia (45, 59,65,121). The thrombus may form on the valve surface as a result of trauma to the endothelial cells because of congenital or acquired cardiac abnormalities that produce an abnormal flow of blood within the cardiac chambers and vessels (65,108,120,121). Direct trauma from cardiac catheterization has also led to endocarditis (45). Of all patients with endocarditis, it has been estimated that 50-75% have some underlying cardiac disease.

Endocarditis can occur where blood flow regurgitates through a narrow opening at a high velocity (such as an incompetent valve) and where blood flows from a relatively high pressure chamber to a relatively low pressure chamber (e.g. aorta back to ventricle or ventricle back to atrium). There is very little lateral pressure just distal to the valve and the poor perfusion of the distal surface may predispose it to endocarditis.

For example, a patient with rheumatic heart disease may have an incompetent mitral valve. This malfunction would allow backflow of blood into the left atrium from the left ventricle during systole (ventricular contraction). This abnormal flow of blood produces a low pressure, poorly perfused area on the atrial surface of the valve, and at the same time the high velocity regurgitant flow can be damaging to the atrial wall which faces the damaged valve. Thus two loci for infective endocarditis are generated (121).

Rheumatic heart disease (RHD) is one of the most common cardiac disorders leading to endocarditis. In most cases, acute rheumatic fever appears to be a complication of pharyngeal infection with group-A beta-hemolytic streptococci (S. pyogenes). Although the actual mechanism by which the streptococci damage the heart muscle is unclear, it has been shown that the organisms or their products reach the endocardium by way of the lymphatic system draining the pharynx (114). The presence of various antistreptococcal antibodies suggests that damage to the heart results because the body cannot immunologically differentiate between cross-reacting antigens of streptococcal protein and endocardium; thus, an inflammatory reaction is produced (99,104). Other forms of

Table 1
CLINICAL PRESENTATIONS OF
INFECTIVE ENDOCARDITIS

Features	Acute (Rapid)	Subacute (Indolent)
Duration/Onset	4-6 weeks or less	6-8 weeks or more
Pathogenesis	Usually normal valves or prosthetic valve	RHD, congenital, or prosthetic valve
Common Infective Agents	Staphylococcus aureus (> 50%) Pneumococcus (5%) Gram-negative bacilli Fungi (5-10%)	Streptococcus viridans (70-80%) Enterococcus (10%) Other Streptococci

cardiac disease predisposing to endocarditis include: ventricular septal defects, patent ductus arteriosus, and atherosclerotic disease.

Infective endocarditis has been classified into two forms based upon clinical presentation (Table 1). **Acute endocarditis** is a fulminant disease that rapidly destroys the endocardium. It has a mortality rate of 33 to 90% in treated cases, depending upon the infecting organism and the presence of other underlying diseases (11). **Subacute endocarditis** is a slowly progressive, benign form of the disease that is amenable to treatment; fatality rates for this form of the disease range from 5-10%. Endocarditis after prosthetic valve implantation carries a poor prognosis with a more than 40% mortality rate (see Question 20).

Certain microorganisms that in other settings are usually not pathogenic or invasive, such as *Streptococcus viridans* and certain group-D streptococci, may produce subacute disease on previously damaged endocardial sites. However, *Staphylococcus aureus* and pneumococcus *(Streptococcus pneumoniae)* are highly pathogenic and can produce disease in previously undamaged tissue or on prosthetic valves. It is important to note that any of these organisms can produce either type of clinical presentation. Factors which adversely affect the survival of patients with endocarditis are: virulent, drug-resistant organisms; old age; serious underlying disease; propensity of the organism to produce large vegetations which may embolize (such as fungi); presence of paravalvular infection; antimicrobial toxicity; cardiac surgery, and the presence of congestive heart failure (11, 59, 60, 64, 65, 112, 120, 128).

Bacteria must gain entrance to the circulation in sufficient numbers for a long enough period of time for endocarditis to occur. Entrance into the bloodstream may be by local infection spread through the lymphatics, direct invasion of the bloodstream from infected or colonized sites, or direct inoculation of contaminated material.

Spontaneous bacteremia occurs in normal individuals and is related to minor infected foci. This occurs commonly in patients with periodontitis, abscesses in the oral cavity, and tonsillitis. Traumatic procedures such as contamination from infected surgical sites, uterine dilatation and curettage, burns, insect bites and soft tissue infection can all produce significant bacteremia (59,64,65). Tooth brushing, chewing, and use of an oral irrigation device have also produced bacteremia. Any manipulation of the gastrointestinal or genitourinary tracts can produce invasion of the bloodstream with the flora residing in those areas (primarily gram-negative bacilli, anaerobes, and enterococci) (see Table 2). In most instances these bacteremias are cleared by the reticuloendothelial system and circulating macrophages. It is only with highly virulent organisms such as *S. aureus* that a single bacteremia may produce endocarditis in a patient without pre-existing cardiac disease (see Question 21). In general, multiple bacteremias are needed to initiate the infection, regardless of the state of the endocardium. The most common infecting organisms are the *Viri-*

Table 2
PATHOGENS COMMONLY PRODUCING ENDOCARDITIS:
SOURCE OF BACTEREMIA

Location	Organisms
Oropharynx	Strep. viridans Peptostreptococci Diphtheroids Bacteroides sp.
Skin	Staph. aureus Staph. epidermis
Gastrointestinal	Bacteroides sp. E. coli Pseudomonas sp.
Genitourinary	Enterococci Klebsiella Proteus sp. Pseudomonas Serratia

dans streptococci which produce more than one-third of all cases. These are followed, in approximate order of frequency, by staphylococci (primarily *S. aureus),* group D streptococci *(S. fecalis* and *S. bovis),* gram negative bacilli, and fungi (126). In areas with a significant population of intravenous drug abusers, the incidence of staphylococcal, fungal and gram-negative endocarditis is higher.

Endocarditis caused by Enterobacteriaceae is rare in the general population. The most commonly encountered organisms are *E. coli, Klebsiella, Enterobacter* and *Serratia* species. Fungal disease is caused by *Candida albicans* and *C. parapsilosis.*

Pseudomonas endocarditis is often found in individuals who abuse drugs intravenously, but it also occurs in patients following urinary tract infections and cardiac surgery (89). The intravenous abuse of medications has led to numerous reports of various types of endocarditis. The organisms most commonly reported are: *S. aureus* (7,67,86,108,109); gram-negative bacilli (5,69,78,89,91), especially *Serratia marcescens* and *Pseudomonas aeruginosa;* and fungi (52,82), predominantly the *Candida* species. The sources of the organisms in this form of endocarditis are the tapwater in which the illicit drug has been dissolved, the patients' skin, and the nasopharynx *(S. aureus)* (107, 109).

Anaerobic endocarditis is quite uncommon, but it has been seen after large bowel manipulation or surgery, and most often involves *Bacteroides fragilis* (75) and anaerobic streptococci. Even more rare are the 1 to 5% of cases of endocarditis caused by gram-negative organisms such as *Alcaligenes, Brucella, Herellea, Salmonella, Hemophilus, Pasteurella,* and meningococci (22,39,111). Spirochetes *(Spirillum minus),* rickettsia (including the agent of Q fever), and cell-wall-deficient organisms may be the cause of some cases of culture-negative endocarditis (47,76). Viral endocarditis has been described in animals (14).

Cardiac surgery has been plagued with the postoperative complication of endocarditis (17,41,100). The most common organism producing infection of prosthetic implants has been *Staphylococcus epidermidis.* Prophylactic antibiotics have met with limited success in the prevention of endocarditis in this setting (100) (See Question 21).

CASE A. ACUTE INFECTIVE ENDOCARDITIS. *A 44-year-old white male is admitted to the medical center by his private physician because of malaise, nausea, and fever for the last seven days. Admission was precipitated by the recent onset of chest pain and shortness of breath. He complained of a painful left knee, diffuse myalgias and a headache unrelieved by acetaminophen. Physical examination on admission revealed a well-developed, well-nourished man in*

some distress. There were non-tender hemorrhagic areas on his palms and soles and an erythematous, swollen area which was tender to palpation in his right axilla. No cardiac murmur was heard and he denied a history of heart disease or intravenous drug abuse. The rest of the physical examination was unremarkable. Upon further questioning, the patient admitted that he had had a "boil" in his axilla which he had lanced himself about one week prior to the onset of his symptoms. Laboratory data revealed a leukocyte count of 23,600/mm³, with a "shift to the left" in the differential; a normal hemoglobin, hematocrit, and platelet count; an erythrocyte sedimentation rate of 86 mm/hr; and microscopic hematuria on urinalysis.

1. What clinical manifestations of endocarditis are seen in this patient, and how might this patient's disease be classified? Describe the clinical manifestation of endocarditis in general.

The abrupt onset of signs and symptoms in this patient and the rapid clinical course are consistent with acute endocarditis. The constitutional symptoms of malaise, myalgias, and monoarticular arthralgia are common musculoskeletal manifestations of endocarditis (23). The headache, although probably a benign finding, should be investigated to rule out cerebral embolus. Embolism to the kidney and lung as suggested by his symptoms of hematuria, shortness of breath and chest pain also occurs commonly in the acute form. Pulmonary emboli, which may be septic, are caused by tricuspid valve infection. The lesions on the soles of his feet and palms are most likely Janeway lesions, which are also embolic in origin, and are a classic sign of endocarditis. The absence of cardiac murmurs is not unusual since they are only heard in about 30-35% of the cases of right sided endocarditis (59,65,101,105). Neurologic complications (59) are seen in 20 to 40% of patients and include major cerebral emboli, leading to hemiplegia, mental changes, aphasia, or ataxia. Acute brain syndrome is most common in older patients who may present with paranoia, hallucinations, and personality changes. Meningitis and brain abscess are rare sequelae of *S. aureus* endocarditis. Other neurologic symptoms which may occur, but which are not present in this patient include: seizures, neuropathy, visual disturbances, and involuntary movements. The increased ESR and elevated white blood cell count suggest acute infection. The absence of anemia is also consistent because an anemia of chronic disease is only seen in subacute form of endocarditis (see Case C). Other laboratory tests which might be useful in the diagnosis are complement levels, which would be depressed in patients with immune complex nephritis, and rheumatoid factor titers, which are elevated in about 50% of the cases of subacute disease.

2. Blood cultures taken on admission are positive the next day for penicillin-resistant *Staphylococcus aureus*. What is the role of the blood culture in the diagnosis and treatment of endocarditis?

The bacteremia produced by an infected heart valve is qualitatively constant (59,112,121,122). Therefore, the blood culture is probably the most important laboratory aid to the diagnosis of endocarditis. Classically, 4 to 6 blood cultures will give 90 to 95% certainty of isolating the infecting organism (12). Although cultures are nearly always positive in the presence of endocarditis, negative cultures do occur. These patients' sera should be tested for fungal and rickettsial antibodies if the history of the illness is compatible with those diagnoses. "Culture-negative" endocarditis may be due to inadequate culture technique, uremia, prior administration of antibiotics, or non-bacterial causes, as cited above (21,81). The site of infection can most often be determined from the history and physical examination, but newer techniques developed to aid in the diagnosis and monitoring of this disease include: cardiac catheterization, intracardiac phonography, angiography and echocardiography (80). These procedures might be most valuable in detecting right sided (tricuspid) endocarditis which only produces clinically detectable murmurs in 30 to 40% of patients (64). The mortality rate of treated culture-negative endocarditis is higher than that of patients with positive cultures (21), presumably due to a delay in diagnosis.

In addition to their importance for diagnosis, blood cultures are vital to evaluate the success of treatment. One of the end-points of therapy is to obtain negative blood cultures, and presumably, sterile heart valves.

3. The patient has no history of heart disease or drug abuse, and no detectable murmur. Aside from the signs and symptoms of endocarditis, why does the staphylococcal bacteremia suggest endocarditis in this patient?

Staphylococcal bacteremia in this patient makes the possibility of endocarditis likely, because the initial site of infection (lanced axillary abscess) was not obvious and because the source of the bacteremia is not readily removable. Several investigators (57,77,118) have recognized that the risk of developing endocarditis from *S. aureus* bacteremia is high, especially if the focus of the bacteremia is not easily identified or is not readily removable. Intravascular devices such as catheters have been implicated in producing endocarditis with a single inoculation of bacteria in experimental animals (118). Iannini et al (57) found no cases of endocarditis in 29 patients with *S. aureus* bacteremia when the focus of infection was identified and promptly removed. Watanakunakorn et al (118),

however, diagnosed eight cases of endocarditis out of 21 patients with bacteremia despite removal of the presumed focus. Finally, Nolan et al (77) found that the overwhelming majority of the cases of endocarditis in their series of 105 cases of *S. aureus* bacteremia occurred in those patients who developed secondary staphylococcal foci as a result of the bacteremia; these secondary foci were primarily in the lungs, joints or kidneys. Therefore, all patients with staphylococcal bacteremia should be followed closely. All possibly infected foci must be removed as soon as possible, and any secondary foci of infection must be identified and treated vigorously.

The staphylococcus in the aforementioned case was resistant to penicillin, and the organism could be inhibited in-vitro only by methicillin, vancomycin, gentamicin, and erythromycin. Methicillin was ordered in a dose of 2 gm every 4 hours intravenously. The patient became afebrile, and subsequent blood cultures were negative. However, after six days of therapy, signs and symptoms of methicillin-induced nephritis were evident. Vancomycin, 5 mg/kg every 8 hours intravenously was ordered.

4. Is vancomycin in this dose safe and adequate therapy for staphylococcal endocarditis in this patient? Why was it chosen instead of gentamicin or erythromycin? How should vancomycin be administered?

Assuming that the patient has normal renal function, this dosage of vancomycin will probably produce peak serum levels of 15-20 mcg/ml, which should be bactericidal for the staphylococcus. Gentamicin, and other aminoglycosides, although demonstrating adequate anti-staphylococcal activity *in vitro*, have not been demonstrated to be effective in the treatment of clinical infections caused by *S. aureus* and are therefore not effective in the treatment of endocarditis and other staphylococcal infections. The same is true for erythromycin. Erythromycin has been found to be effective *in-vitro* and *in-vivo* against *S. aureus*, but very high concentrations of the drug must be achieved to exert a bactericidal effect. In practice, with clinically achievable concentrations, the drug exerts only bacteriostatic activity which has been shown to be inadequate for the treatment of endocarditis. Bacteriostatic antibiotics can produce clinical improvement, but relapse of the infection can occur after treatment is discontinued. The organisms residing within the cardiac valve vegetations have a slowed rate of metabolism and reproduction. Therefore, antibiotics which only inhibit growth will have a minimal effect upon these organisms. Bacteriostatic antibiotics include the tetracyclines, erythromycins, sulfonamides, and often, lincomycin and clindamycin. However, these agents, particularly the tetracyclines, may be necessary for the treatment of those rare cases of endocarditis due to rickettsia or chlamydia (64).

The toxicity of vancomycin nearly always involves the eighth cranial nerve. Serum levels of 80 mcg/ml or greater have been associated with deafness. Nephrotoxicity seems to have been eliminated by a reformulation of the drug (see chapter on *Adverse Effects of Drugs on the Kidney).* Other significant adverse reactions attributed to vancomycin are thrombophlebitis, which may be obviated by slowly infusing a dilute solution of the drug intravenously, and vascular collapse, associated with too rapid infusion of the drug. The dose of vancomycin is widely advertised as 40 mg/kg/day intravenously; however, doses of 15-20 mg/kg daily will provide adequate and safe serum levels. The half-life of the drug is approximately 4-6 hours, and the drug is excreted entirely unchanged into the urine. The half-life of the drug in anuric patients may be as long as 7 days.

Doses of approximately 500 mg may be diluted in 100-200cc of intravenous solution and infused slowly over 30-60 minutes or longer, every 8-12 hours. Dosage regimens must be adjusted in direct proportion to creatinine clearance for patients with renal dysfunction.

5. Why is the bactericidal activity of serum important to assess in this patient with endocarditis?
The serum bactericidal test measures the ability of serial dilutions of a patient's serum to sterilize a standardized inoculum of the infecting organism (19). The test is potentially most useful in assessing the response of gram-negative endocarditis to aminoglycoside therapy, where the minimum bactericidal concentration of gentamicin or tobramycin may be only slightly lower than toxic levels of the antibiotic. Blood should be drawn at the expected peak serum level (1 hour after an intramuscular injection or as soon as possible after an IV infusion). This patient's blood should be drawn within 30 minutes after the infusion of vancomycin is complete. The outcome of therapy of many systemic infections including endocarditis positively correlates with elevated levels of

Table 3
RECOMMENDED ANTIBIOTIC TREATMENT SCHEDULES FOR INFECTIVE ENDOCARDITIS

Organism	Drug of Choice	Daily Dose	Duration	Alternate Drugs	Comments
S. viridans S. bovis	Penicillin G Penicillin V	6,000,000 u IV 2-4 gm po	4 weeks 4 weeks	a) Vancomycin, 15-20 mg/kg/day b) Cephalosporins	Oral therapy only under unusual circumstances.
Enterococcus (S. faecalis)	Penicillin G + Streptomycin or Gentamicin	10-20,000,000 u IV plus 1 gm IM or 3-5 mg/kg IM/IV	6 weeks	Ampicillin plus an Aminoglycoside; or Vancomycin plus/− Aminoglycoside	Important to distinguish from S. bovis. Consider gentamicin in a patient with renal failure; easier to monitor therapy.
Staphylococci	Nafcillin Penicillin G Dicloxacillin or Cloxacillin (optional)	6-9 gm IV 12,000,000 u IV 2 gm/day po	6 weeks 1-2 weeks at end of therapy	a) Vancomycin as above b) Cephalosporin in maximum doses c) Clindamycin 600-900 mg IV q 6-8 h	Additional oral therapy has not been shown to be of benefit. Bactericidal activity of serum must be demonstrated for Clindamycin, cephalosporins, or oral therapy.
Gram-negative*	Ampicillin Kanamycin Gentamicin Tobramycin Amikacin Carbenicillin	8-12 gm IV 15 mg/kg IV, IM 5-6 mg/kg IV, IM 5-6 mg/kg IV, IM 15 mg/kg IV, IM 30-40 gm IV (alone or in various combinations)	At least 6 weeks	Trimethoprim Sulfamethoxazole 10/50 mg/kg per day +/− Polymixin B 3 mg/kg/day	Surgery usually necessary. *Choice of antibiotic depends upon individual sensitivities
Fungi	Amphotericin B ± 5-fluorocytosine	Up to 1 mg/kg daily or every other day, as tolerated by the patient 150 mg/kg in four doses po	At least 6-8 weeks usually to total Ampho B dose of 2-4 gm	Surgery. None commercially available. Miconazole 25-30 mg/kg/day	Always requires surgery. Use of flucytosine depends upon demonstration of in-vitro sensitivity of patient's fungus, and clinical response to Amphotericin alone. **Investigational drug
Anaerobes B. fragilis Streptococci, Clostridia, Other Bacteroides	Carbenicillin Penicillin G	30-40 gm IV 10-20,000,000 u IV	At least 6 weeks	Clindamycin as above Chloramphenicol 30-50 mg/kg IV/PO Metronidazole 20-30 mg/kg PO/IV***	Static drugs are not as effective as penicillins. ***IV formulation is investigational. This drug is bactericidal, but may be carcinogenic.

antibacterial activity in the serum (19,62). A serum concentration retaining "cidal" activity to at least eight dilutions seems to provide the best prognosis. However, several reports of gram-negative endocarditis have shown poor correlation of *in-vitro* tests with clinical outcome (69).

The question of whether it is more important to achieve high, intermittent bactericidal levels through bolus injections or lower, but constant bactericidal serum levels through constant infusion is unanswered (50). Clinical cures have been achieved using both methods of treatment. Barza et al found by measuring antibiotic penetration into fibrin clots in-vivo that intermittent administration of the drugs yielded higher clot concentrations (8). However, Hamburger, et al found that constant infusion of a penicillin type of antibiotic yielded a higher percentage of cures in experimental endocarditis (50).

CASE B. DRUG ABUSE ENDOCARDITIS. A 19-year-old white male heroin and amphetamine abuser is admitted to the medical center with complaints of fever, chest pain, shortness of breath, and abdominal pain. He had been well until about 2 weeks prior to admission when he noted the onset of fever and right upper quadrant fullness and pain. He denied having dark urine and he was not jaundiced. Physical examination revealed a grade III/IV holosystolic murmur and coarse rales on chest auscultation. The neck veins were distended. An enlarged liver, which was nontender, and a spleen tip were palpated. Chest X-ray revealed small areas of fluffy infiltrate in the right middle lobe and a slightly enlarged heart. Endocarditis was suspected and blood cultures were taken. Laboratory tests were within normal limits except for a BUN of 56 mg% and a creatinine of 3.8 mg%.

6. What are the clinical manifestations of endocarditis in this patient and what are the most likely infecting organisms?

This patient manifests the classic signs of acute right sided endocarditis which may be due to a variety of organisms. Fever, chest pain, pulmonary infiltrates, and shortness of breath are all consistent with pulmonary embolism. An enlarged heart, liver enlargement, and a cardiac murmur may be heralding the onset of right sided cardiac failure due to tricuspid valve insufficiency. The enlarged spleen is also consistent with endocarditis. The tricuspid valve, in the right side of the heart is the valve most frequently involved in addicts who develop endocarditis.

Emboli to the kidney are a frequent cause of the renal dysfunction that is often seen in the course of bacterial endocarditis. This is manifested as an increase in the BUN and serum creatinine, hematuria, proteinuria, and a decrease in the creatinine clearance. The majority of autopsies that have been performed following fatal endocarditis have shown that these patients had some type of renal lesion (59). However, it is difficult to tell whether the renal dysfunction was due to the disease or to the therapy because many antibiotics are nephrotoxic themselves (e.g. penicillins, aminoglycosides). Another form of renal disease that has been seen is an acute glomerulonephritis. This may be due to the deposition of antigen-antibody complexes and the activation of the cellular immune system, which damages the glomerular basement membrane (GBM). Immunofluorescence demonstrates the presence of gamma-globulin and complement on the GBM (48,61,106). This is somewhat analogous to post-streptococcal glomerulonephritis. Arthritis and arthralgias have also been associated with the disease; these are rarely disabling (10,90).

Emboli to the retinal artery are also common. This embolic episode may be the presenting sign of endocarditis and is most often seen in fungal disease. Infarcts, or areas of necrosis secondary to ischemia, are also often due to embolic phenomena.

The parenteral injection of unsterilized material may cause transient bacteremia in a number of ways: bacterial cellulitis may occur at the site of injection which would allow the bacteria to reach the circulation by lymphatic drainage; direct inoculation occurs during passage of the needle through the skin; bacterial phlebitis produces a bacteremia; preparations of the drug may contain virulent microorganisms due to nonsterility. An abnormal endocardial surface would further predispose the addict to infection (59).

The most common micro-organisms isolated from drug users with endocarditis are: *S. aureus* (50 to 60%), gram-negative bacilli (15%), fungi (10%), and various aerobic and anaerobic streptococci (especially enterococci).

The most common site of infection in addicts with endocarditis is the tricuspid valve (70%), but mitral, aortic and multiple valvular infection are not uncommon. The most common features of endocarditis in these patients are: fever (100%), and pulmonary embolism (60 to 65%). Subcutaneous abscesses are frequently seen. Emphysema, septic arthritis and pericardial effusion are seen in 5% of cases or less (7,86).

7. Until the results of culture and sensitivity tests are available, what antibiotics should this patient receive?

The initial empirical regimen should include: a penicillinase resistant penicillin (nafcillin) (38) for *S. aureus* and an aminoglycoside such as gentamicin, tobramycin, or amikacin, which are active against most gram-negative bacilli. Some clinicians might also include penicillin G for streptococci, since nafcillin lacks significant bactericidal activity against enterococci by itself or in combination with aminoglycosides (Also see Question 12).

Empiric therapy would not ordinarily include antifungal therapy because of the toxicity of amphotericin B, and because *Candida* species are easily grown on routine culture media within 24-48 hours (52,82) so that specific antifungal therapy may be instituted without significant delay.

8. The patient has been doing well and has become afebrile on penicillin G, nafcillin and gentamicin. Blood cultures taken on admission now reveal *S. aureus* in all samples. The organism is sensitive to nafcillin, gentamicin, vancomycin, erythromycin, and clindamycin. How should this patient be managed? How long should he be treated?

If *S. aureus* is cultured, some authorities believe that the aminoglycoside, which has anti-staphylococcal activity, should be continued for the duration of therapy. Although enhanced bacterial killing can be demonstrated in vitro with this combination, there is no evidence to show that it is clinically superior to the penicillin alone (59,73,96). Collaborative studies have been undertaken to assess this combination therapy and have not demonstrated any advantage to the combination. In practice, if the bactericidal activity of the patient's serum were not adequate on nafcillin alone, the addition of the aminoglycoside may be considered to enhance bacterial killing.

The optimal duration of antimicrobial treatment of *S. aureus* endocarditis is unclear at present. It is the opinion of nearly all infectious diseases clinicians that therapy should be carried out for at least 4 to 6 weeks. The use of oral therapy after an initial period of parenteral treatment is a subject of debate. As long as adequate bactericidal activity ($\geq$ 1:8 dilutions) can be achieved in the serum on oral medication, clinical cure could be expected with perhaps 2 weeks of IV nafcillin, followed by 4 weeks or oral cloxacillin or dicloxacillin, provided patient compliance is assured. We have personally treated only a few patients in this fashion, and much more experience is needed before definitive recommendations can be made.

There are reports of successful use of cephalosporins in the treatment of endocarditis (84,85); however, there are a few papers purporting to demonstrate therapeutic failure with certain cephalosporins (cefazolin and cephaloridine) (20,84,92). These failures have been linked to the susceptibility of these drugs to staphylococcal beta-lactamase (32). There is no clinical evidence to support this contention, however, and it is this author's opinion that although the cephalosporins are not the drugs of first choice in the treatment of *S. aureus* endocarditis, they may be valuable for certain penicillin-allergic patients or for those who cannot tolerate a penicillin or vancomycin for other reasons. The cross-allergenicity of the penicillins and cephalosporins must be considered as well, and a patient with a history of an accelerated or immediate hypersensitivity reaction to a penicillin should never receive a cephalosporin. (See chapter on *General Principles of Antibiotic Therapy*.)

The alternative drug of first choice in the penicillin-allergic patient is vancomycin for *S. aureus* infection. The dose is 15 to 20 mg/kg/day in two or three divided dosages given intravenously. It is our experience that this dose is both safe and effective in the treatment of *S. aureus* endocarditis. Failures with this drug have been uncommon (42) (see Question 4 for a discussion of the use of vancomycin). Clindamycin is very active *in-vitro* against S. aureus, but several reports of treatment failure have appeared recently when the drug was used to treat endocarditis (110,117). This was primarily due to unreliable bactericidal activity.

Infective endocarditis in drug addicts is very difficult to treat, not only because of the virulence of the organisms, but because the addicts will often reinfect themselves. If the original valve has been replaced by a prosthetic device and the addict infects this valve, the prognosis is poor. (See Question 20 for a discussion of prosthetic valve endocarditis).

9. One week into the course of antibiotic therapy with nafcillin, the patient develops a morbilliform rash over his trunk and extremities. Since this is presumably an allergic reaction to the nafcillin, what are the alternative approaches to the further management of this patient?

Aside from alternative antibiotics as described above, there are three possible approaches to this patient's management.

a. *Desensitization with skin testing:* This is a dangerous practice, since anaphylaxis has occurred as a result of this process. Desensitization should only be used if the patient allergic to penicillin can *only* be treated with a penicillin. This procedure is, in fact, almost never necessary since there are other effective, bactericidal antibiotics available. Although presumably accurate methods of skin testing for immediate or accelerated reactions to penicillin have been described, their accuracy and utility is questionable (4).

b. *Prophylactic antihistamines and corticosteroids:* Antihistamines and steroids in moderately large doses have not been shown to be effective in preventing allergic reactions. Large doses of steroids can impair the allergic responses, but these large doses are hardly warranted when normal host defenses are crucial in the handling of infection or superinfection (46,87).

c. *Give the penicillin in the face of the allergic his-*

tory: This should only be attempted in patients whose prior allergic history is one of mild reactions, not anaphylaxis or exfoliative dermatitis. This should be done cautiously with epinephrine on hand for the administration of the first dose. Most mild allergic reaction are self-limiting and can be treated symptomatically while antibiotic therapy is continued. In this case, as in most, the use of an alternative bactericidal antibiotic such as vancomycin is the safest, most efficacious route to take.

CASE C. SUBACUTE INFECTIVE ENDOCARDITIS. A 68-year-old white male is admitted to the medical center three months after a transurethral prostatectomy. He has suffered from malaise and fever for the last month. He had been in good health until five years prior to admission when he suffered a myocardial infarction following several months of angina pectoris. He recovered, and the only residual damage appeared to be an apical pansystolic murmur, without evidence of regurgitation. During and after the prostate surgery, he was given cephalothin 1 gram every 6 hours, as prophylaxis. Physical examination now reveals a temperature of 101.5° F, petechiae in his conjunctivae, on his palate, and on his hands and feet. Examination of his fundi revealed no hemorrhages. He had firm, painful purplish lesions on his palms. There were no hemorrhages in his nailbeds, nor was there clubbing of the fingers. His liver and spleen were slightly enlarged, and the cardiac murmur which had been present for some time was noted to have increased in intensity. Laboratory data were unremarkable except for a hematocrit of 31%, hemoglobin of 10 gm%, leukocyte count of 10,400/mm³, and an erythrocyte sedimentation rate (ESR) of 62 mm/hr. Endocarditis is suspected and four blood cultures are taken.

10. What are the clinical manifestations of endocarditis in this patient, and how might the patient's disease be classified?

Although this patient presents with malaise and fever which are most commonly associated with acute disease, the overall clinical picture is more consistent with subacute bacterial endocarditis. Specific signs present in this patient which commonly occur in the subacute form include the conjunctival hemorrhages, as well as the petechiae in his mouth and extremities which are caused by microemboli to the capillary circulation. The lesions on the palms of his hands appear to be Osler's nodes. These are probably the result of a vasculitis at the site, from which the infecting organism can sometimes be cultured. Splenomegaly is also quite common in subacute disease, occurring in nearly half of all patients. Cardiac murmurs, especially new ones or those which have changed in intensity or

quality, in the presence of positive blood cultures are nearly pathognomonic for endocarditis. Laboratory data in this patient reveal an anemia which is probably the anemia of chronic disease. This anemia is characteristically normocytic and normochromic and is not responsive to any therapy except eradication of the infection. A slightly elevated leukocyte count, an elevated ESR and the time course of his symptoms and signs which have progressed over several months are also consistent with subacute disease.

11. What would the most common infecting organisms be in this patient's situation?

The most common organisms producing this type of disease are the streptococci: *S. viridans* and *S. fecalis* (Enterococcus). Other less common organisms are anaerobic and microaerophilic streptococci (15). A history of genitourinary manipulation in this patient leads one to think of the enterococcus and gram-negative bacilli as possible causes of the infection. However, the indolent clinical course of this patient and the rarity of endocarditis due to organisms such as E. coli and Proteus species, which would most commonly infect the urinary tract, make gram-negative bacillary endocarditis less likely. The disease produced by gram-negative bacilli is usually acute in its course and more fulminant. It is possible, however, for organisms such as Serratia or Pseudomonas to have caused this infection, and most empiric regimens would include coverage for these organisms. Since the enterococcus is a likely pathogen, the distinction should be made between *S. fecalis* and another Group D streptococcus, *S. bovis*.

Until recently *S. bovis* was not recognized to be an important cause of endocarditis, simply because it could not be distinguished from the enterococcus, both being members of Group D. In general *S. bovis* is very sensitive to penicillin G (MIC ≤0.1 mcg/,ml whereas *S. fecalis* is relatively insensitive (MIC ≥1.0 mcg/ml. *S. fecalis* is usually resistant to penicillinase resistant penicillins and clindamycin, while *S. bovis* is quite sensitive.

The clinical presentation of both organisms is similar. However, infection with *S. bovis* carries a more favorable prognosis due to its sensitivity to antibiotics (71,116).

12. Forty-eight hours after admission, all culture bottles are growing *S. fecalis*. How should this patient be managed?

In vitro studies demonstrate that enterococci generally are intermediately sensitive to penicillin G and ampicillin with MICs in the range of 1-2 mcg/ml (24,34,56,58,94). Clinical trials of penicillin G alone in the treatment of enterococcal endocarditis have met with poor results. These organisms are resistant to aminoglycoside antibiotics *in-vitro.* This resistance is divided into low and high level categories. Those organisms requiring less than 1000 mcg/ml of streptomycin for inhibition will be killed by the combination of penicillin or ampicillin plus streptomycin. Those organisms which have high level resistance (MIC > 1000 mcg/ml) will usually not respond to the combination *in-vitro* (94). This occurs in approximately 20% of all enterococci. Nearly all enterococci will be killed with the combination of penicillin G or ampicillin plus gentamicin (56). The time-honored combination of choice is penicillin-streptomycin (See Table 3 for dosage regimens); cure rates are 80 to 85% (24,34,58).

The combination is effective and synergistic due to the action by the penicillin component on the cell wall of the bacteria, which allows intracellular penetration of the aminoglycoside where it exerts its effect to inhibit protein synthesis. As mentioned in Question 7, penicillinase-resistant penicillins in combination with an aminoglycoside are not effective against the enterococcus in experimental infection (66).

In general, cephalosporins do not produce a synergistic effect against enterococci in combination with aminoglycosides, and may even produce antagonism (63). There is no evidence that ampicillin is superior to penicillin G in combination with an aminoglycoside in the treatment of enterococcal infection. The choice of the aminoglycoside in this patient might be gentamicin, because assay of serum levels are usually available, and therapy is more easily monitored for toxicity in this manner. This is especially important in patients with renal dysfunction as well as the elderly, such as our patient who will have decreased renal function due to age. Reduction of dose in proportion with estimated or measured creatinine clearance would be indicated. Routine audiometric or vestibular function testing is controversial. The doses of aminoglycoside required for this infection are not as high as for gram-negative bacillary infection, and the incidence of toxicity would be expected to be less. See Table 3.

The alternate drug of choice in the penicillin-allergic patient is vancomycin in the same dosage as for staphylococcal disease. Synergy is achieved by the addition of an aminoglycoside to vancomycin, but there is scant evidence that the combination is clinically superior (68,123).

CASE D. STREPTOCOCCAL ENDOCARDITIS. A 49-year-old female with a long history of rheumatic heart disease had a tooth extracted three months prior to her present admission. No prophylactic antibiotic therapy was given. Over the next two and one-half months she increasingly complained of night sweats, anorexia, and fatigue. Two weeks before admission she began developing shortness of breath, dyspnea on exertion, and a petechial rash. The physician sus-

pected endocarditis and instituted penicillin G in a dose of 5,000,000 units IV q6h. Subsequently blood cultures grew S. viridans.

13. What is the optimal antibiotic therapy for *Streptococcus viridans* endocarditis?

The optimal therapy for *S. viridans* endocarditis consists of intravenous penicillin G for four weeks. (See Table 3 for dosages.) The addition of streptomycin to this is controversial (59,60,64,112,120). Wolfe et al (127) state that no relapses have been noted with the addition of two weeks of streptomycin to four weeks of penicillin. However, it is our experience that penicillin alone for at least four weeks is equally effective. The phenomenon of "breakthrough" bacteremia is often seen clinically during the acute stages of treatment of intravascular infection and is associated with subinhibitory levels of antibiotic (3). For this reason, the interval between doses of antibiotics with short half-lives, such as the penicillins and cephalosporins, is usually no more than 4 hours. However, the exquisite sensitivity of the streptococci to penicillin, and a lag period of growth after antibiotic exposure may allow for prolonged antibacterial effect and allow for increased intervals between doses.

The penicillin may be infused rapidly over 10-15 minutes and is relatively non-toxic to patients with normal renal function. Rare side effects are severe allergic reactions, hemolytic anemia, interstitial nephritis, and neurotoxicity in the form of convulsions if the drug is allowed to accumulate in renal insufficiency (9). (See the chapter on *General Principles of Antibiotic Therapy).*

Alternate treatments of choice for the penicillin-allergic patient for *S. viridans* are vancomycin and the cephalosporins. (See Table 3).

14. The patient in Case D develops severe phlebitis and pain in her arm when the penicillin is given and desires to be treated with "pills." Is oral therapy of endocarditis feasible?

S. viridans endocarditis has been treated with oral penicillin V or ampicillin in doses of four to eight grams per day (49,83). This treatment may be given with or without the addition of an aminoglycoside administered intramuscularly for the first one to two weeks (54). Amoxicillin has also been used with or without gentamicin (43,98). Relapse rates for these shorter regimens with oral drug range from 6-17%. The higher relapse rates may have been due to poor patient compliance. As mentioned above, serum bactericidal activity must be adequate (≥ 1:8 dilutions) to assure the success of any therapy. Oral therapy should only be considered under unusual circumstances.

CASE E. FUNGAL ENDOCARDITIS. A 64-year-old man

was admitted to the medical center with a two-month history of fever and an eight month history of shortness of breath and weakness. Mitral insufficiency had been diagnosed 15 years earlier and this patient has already been treated twice for SBE. Physical examination reveals Roth's spots, Janeway lesions on the soles of the feet, splinter hemorrhages and absent pulses in the lower extremities. Chest X-rays and ECG suggested left ventricular failure. Blood cultures were taken and penicillin and gentamicin were begun for presumed SBE. The patient continues to deteriorate despite antibiotic therapy. Blood cultures taken on admission are reported to be growing yeast.

15. What fungi are most commonly associated with endocarditis and how may the diagnosis be confirmed if cultures are negative?

The fungi most commonly associated with endocarditis are: *Candida albicans, C. tropicalis,* and *C. parapsilosis* in heroin addicts. Aspergillus and other fungi are rare causes of this disease. Blood cultures are not as frequently positive as in bacterial infection (97) and therefore, clinicians must often rely on the titers of candida antibodies. Sustained and rising titers of these antibodies may indicate invasive disease, whereas low or transiently elevated titers occur in noninfected or superficially infected patients. Many clinicians avoid use of the precipitin test for Candida antibodies since many false positive results occur. The organism may be isolated from other sites in disseminated infection. If fungemia is present, however, the organisms will grow on routine blood culture.

16. The yeast are subsequently identified as C. albicans, and amphotericin B therapy has been instituted. How should the drug be administered and what toxicities might be expected from the drug?

The drug treatment of choice for fungal endocarditis is amphotericin B given intravenously. In addition, nearly all patients must undergo surgery to have vegetations scraped from the affected valve or to have the valve replaced. Amphotericin B is a toxic drug, especially when given over an extended period of time, as for endocarditis. Just a few toxicities are: hypokalemia, azotemia, renal tubular acidosis and anemia. See Table 3 in this chapter and Table 8 in *General Principles of Antibiotic Therapy* for information on dosage, duration of therapy, side effects and their amelioration. The presence of heart failure and the suggestion of emboli as indicated by the absence of pulses in the legs, are indications for valve replacement surgery. The patient should be treated with amphotericin B prior to, during, and after surgery for a prolonged period to avoid relapse (37).

Chemotherapy alone is insufficent for the treatment of fungal endocarditis. The vegetations formed on the

heart valve are quite large and friable, so that embolic episodes, as illustrated in this patient, occur often. In addition, it has been demonstrated that there is very little penetration of amphotericin B into avascular fibrin clots (93).

17. Are there any alternative antifungal agents for the treatment of endocarditis?

The addition of flucytosine to the regimen would depend upon whether there was adequate antifungal activity with amphotericin alone. In addition, *in vitro* sensitivity to flucytosine must be documented, as nearly 50% of all candida species are resistant (33).

Other antifungal agents not yet adequately tried in the treatment of endocarditis are clotrimazole and miconazole. Both of these are investigational at the present time. A new and promising drug which is currently in the developmental stages is the methyl ester of amphotericin B (55). The esterification renders amphotericin water soluble and apparently free from serious toxicity. However, the efficacy of this agent in the treatment of fungal infection, both in experimental animals (36) and in humans, have been disappointing. Miconazole, used intravenously, has shown promise in selected cases of fungal infection, but there is limited experience in the treatment of Candidal infection (103).

CASE F. GRAM-NEGATIVE BACILLARY ENDOCARDITIS WITH PERFORATED VALVE. The patient is a 39-year-old black male heroin abuser with a history of congenital heart disease. On admission to the hospital he complained of headache, hemiparesis, malaise, shortness of breath, and physical examination revealed a loud murmur, thought to be originating from a perforated mitral valve leaflet, as well as pulmonary edema, probably resulting from left sided heart failure. Temperature was 103°F and the white blood cell count was 21,400/mm³. The spleen was enlarged and fundoscopic examination revealed hemorrhages. Blood cultures were taken and the patient was given nafcillin and tobramycin intravenously. The following day, cultures were reported to be growing Serratia marcescens which was inhibited in vitro only by gentamicin, carbenicillin, tobramycin, and trimethoprim/sulfamethoxazole.

18. How should this patient be managed?

The most serious complication of bacterial endocarditis is perforation or rupture of the infected cardiac valve. This leads to progressive congestive heart failure, pulmonary edema, and ultimately death if untreated. In the preantibiotic era, this occurred in about 15% of all cases of endocarditis. The incidence of this complication has since *doubled* (18). This is probably related to infections caused by more virulent organisms which have become resistant to most of the less toxic, more commonly used antibiotics. These organisms produce severe necrotic infections of the heart valves. A perforated or ruptured heart valve is an emergency situation and the treatment of choice is surgery. Replacement of the infected valve, or even of a prosthesis which has become malfunctional, is lifesaving if congestive heart failure has not progressed too far. Recent advances in cardiac surgery and valve replacement have reduced mortality to 25 to 35% (13,30,79). One recent study reports mortality to be greatest in those patients with uncontrolled infection prior to surgery and urges early surgical intervention (16).

Suppressive antibiotic therapy is recommended prior to surgical replacement of the valve. This patient should receive intravenous doses of gentamicin or tobramycin of at least 5 to 6 mg/kg daily, with or without carbenicillin in doses of 400 to 500 mg/kg per day. Carbenicillin should be added if adequate serum bactericidal activity cannot be obtained with maximum aminoglycoside doses since synergy may be obtained with this combination (69). If this therapy is not adequate for any reason or if toxicity prevails, therapy with high dose trimethoprim/sulfamethoxazole may be tried.

Serratia marcescens endocarditis is becoming more prevalent. The organism is slowly becoming resistant to most antibiotics, and many strains isolated are sensitive only to amikacin and trimethoprim/sulfamethoxazole. Centers which are testing the efficacy of a new cephalosporin report that cefoxitin, a cephamycin cephalosporin, may be very effective in the treatment of resistant Serratia infections (70).

Gram-negative endocarditis is not always cured by chemotherapy alone (29,53,78,89,91,124). Surgery is often required as with fungal disease, especially if there is evidence of embolism or heart failure.

19. What other gram-negative organisms produce bacterial endocarditis, and how are these infections managed?

Other gram-negative organisms which produce endocarditis are: Klebsiella, Pseudomonas, and Hemophilus species (22,39). Hemophilus is relatively uncommon, and is quite sensitive to most antibiotics in vitro (29,39). Pseudomonas aeruginosa is very difficult to treat because relatively high concentrations of antimicrobials are required (89). Pseudomonas cepacia, an unusual organism which has been appearing more often in heroin addicts who develop endocarditis, is resistant to most of the usual antibiotics that are used to treat P. aeruginosa. Reports of cures using trimethoprim/sulfamethoxazole with and without polymyxin B have appeared (51,78). (See Table 3 for regimens). The anaerobic gram-negative organism

Bacteroides fragilis is very difficult to treat, since the drugs of choice for most infections would be clindamycin or chloramphenicol which are bacteriostatic. Large doses (30-40 grams per day) of carbenicillin have been effective in the treatment of B. fragilis endocarditis (1), as has metronidazole (40).

20. The patient discussed in Case F had valve replacement surgery and was treated for four weeks with gentamicin plus carbenicillin. When he was afebrile, blood cultures were negative, and the complications of his disease were resolved, he was discharged to be followed in the outpatient clinics. At his first clinic visit three weeks later, he presented with shortness of breath, fever, chills, a new cardiac murmur, and an elevated white blood count of 24,400/mm³. Blood cultures were taken and the patient was admitted to the hospital. Chest X-ray and fluoroscopy revealed that the mitral valve prosthesis was beginning to loosen, and left ventricular hypertrophy was present. How should this patient be managed for presumed prosthetic valve infection?

There are two major etiologies for the infection: inadequate therapy of the original infection and reinfection by continued illicit use of intravenous drugs. The incidence of postoperative infection following valve replacement not previously associated with endocarditis is only 1 to 4% (95,102,125). The mortality rate for infections involving the prosthetic valve is 50 to 60%. The most common infecting organisms in this situation are Staphylococcus epidermidis, diphtheroids, gram-negative bacilli, and fungi (59,102,125). To cover all possible etiologic organisms (Serratia and the organisms listed above), the patient should receive penicillin G, nafcillin and gentamicin until blood cultures and sensitivities are reported. All of the antibiotics should be given in the doses recommended in Table 3.

21. A patient who is about to undergo urogenital surgery had rheumatic fever as a child and was left with a cardiac murmur. Would it be reasonable to recommend prophylactic antibiotics in this situation? How should they be administered?

Several large, well-controlled, double-blind clinical trials have shown that the incidence of postoperative infection is more related to surgical technique and quality of nursing care than to the administration of prophylactic antibiotics (17,41). For example, a large study of infections occurring after open-heart surgery revealed a higher incidence of infection in patients who had received prophylactic antibiotics (100).

However, chemoprophylaxis is practiced and recommended in patients with pre-existing cardiac disease or prosthetic valves to prevent bacteremia and eradicate microorganisms after intravascular invasion (59). Prophylaxis is indicated in those patients who have congenital, rheumatic, or atherosclerotic heart lesions if they are to undergo a procedure which will produce a bacteremia and possibly implant bacteria on the damaged endocardium. Such procedures include dental work, abortion and delivery of a child, tonsillectomy and adenoidectomy, and urogenital and gastrointestinal surgery or manipulation (31). There is no proof that prophylaxis is effective in preventing endocarditis in these situations, but it appears to offer a reasonable approach to the problem. Experimental evidence suggests that bacteriostatic drugs do not prevent bacteria from implanting on heart valves (27); yet, a recent study demonstrated that chemoprophylaxis with a variety of antibiotics (static and cidal) prevented endocarditis from developing in 21 patients with prosthetic valves. Other studies have either met with mixed results (6) or have had questionable controls and methodology (74). The antibiotics used most commonly have been penicillinase-resistant penicillins and cephalosporins. It is, however, generally accepted that chemoprophylaxis should be employed when an invasive procedure is to be performed on a patient with a prosthetic valve, since the mortality rate from the resulting prosthetic valve infection is very high. If antibiotics are given, they should be started just prior to surgery and continued for no longer than 48 hours post-operatively. It is felt that this regimen prevents superinfection and provides antibacterial activity in the serum only during the time when bacteremia may occur.

Unless she is allergic to penicillin, this patient should receive penicillin G 2,000,000 units IV/IM or ampicillin 1 gram IM/IV plus gentamicin 1.5 mg/kg IV/IM, 30 minutes to an hour pre-operatively, and two more doses postoperatively at eight hour intervals.

The American Heart Association has recently presented endocarditis prophylaxis recommendations covering a variety of clinical situations (2).

CASE HISTORY FOR STUDY

J. G. is a 27-year-old 60 kg, white female who is admitted to the medical center with chief complaints of shortness of breath, cough, chest pain, fever, and night sweats. Other complaints include headache, weakness, dizziness, blurred vision, joint pain, and sore throat.

The patient admits to using intravenous drugs as recently as two days ago.

Physical examination reveals sinus tachycardia with a grade III/VI systolic ejection murmur. Echocardiography indicates vegetation on the trucuspid valve. Chest X-rays reveal bilateral pleural effusions and pulmonary infiltrates.

Cultures were taken of blood, sputum, pleural fluid, urine, and cerebro-spinal fluid (CSF).
Laboratory values on admission:

Temp: 39.5°C
WBC: 14,200/mm^3
Diff: 92P, 3L, 2M, 3 Bands
Hemoglobin: 10.7 mg%
Hematocrit: 31.6%
Platelets: 129,000/mm^3

Na$^+$/K$^+$: 131/3.5 mEq/liter
Cl$^-$/HCO$^-_3$: 97/27 mEq/liter
BUN: 25 mg%
Creatinine: 0.8 mg%
ESR: 70 mm/hr

a. What signs and symptoms of endocarditis are present in this patient? How might this patient's disease be classified?

b. What empirical therapy for suspected endocarditis should this patient receive until results of cultures and sensitivities are known?

The patient was given penicillin G 3.5 million units every 4 hours intravenously, methicillin 2 grams every 4 hours intravenously, and gentamicin 90 mg every 8 hours intramuscularly.

All cultures except for CSF grew *S. aureus* resistant to penicillin G.

c. What therapy should J. G. receive and for how long?

The penicillin and gentamicin were discontinued and methicillin was continued, to be given for four weeks intravenously, with two weeks or oral dicloxacillin for a total of six weeks of therapy.

Ten days later, after J. G. had been afebrile for 5 days, she spiked a temperature to 39°C that remained more or less constant. Eosinophilia to 19% was noted in the complete blood count, and pyuria, proteinuria, and hematuria were seen in the urinalysis.

d. What has happened, and should J.G.'s therapy be changed?

Methicillin was continued for 3 more days until the BUN and serum creatinine were noted to rise. At that time vancomycin, 20 mg/kg intravenously daily, was instituted to complete six weeks of therapy.

e. Should J.G.'s vancomycin therapy be modified in the face of renal insufficiency, and why?

REFERENCES

1. Al-Ibrahim MS et al: Treatment of bacteroides endocarditis with carbenicillin. Am J Med Sci 273:105, 1977.
2. American Heart Association: Prevention of bacterial endocarditis. Circulation 56:139A, 1977.
3. Anderson ET et al: Simultaneous antibiotic levels in breakthrough gram-negative rod bacteremia. Am J Med 61:493, 1976.
4. Anon: Penicillin allergy. Medical Letter 20:14, 1978.
5. Archer G et al: Pseudomonas endocarditis in drug addicts. Am Heart J 88:570, 1974.
6. Austin TW et al: Cephalothin prophylaxis and valve replacement. Ann Thor Surg 23:333, 1977.
7. Banks T et al: Infective endocarditis in heroin addicts. Am J Med 55:444, 1973.

8. Barza M et al: Penetration of antibiotics into fibrin loci in vivo: Intermittent vs constant infusion. J Infect Dis 129:73, 1974.

9. Barza M: Antimicrobial spectrum, pharmacology, and therapeutic use of antibiotics. Part II penicillins. Am J Hosp Pharm 34:57, 1977.

10. Bayer AS et al: Severe disabling polyarthritis associated with bacterial endocarditis. West J Med 123:404, 1975.

11. Bayer AS et al: Infectious disease emergencies: Part II — patients presenting with cardiac decompensation or circulatory insufficiency. West J Med 125:119, 1976.

12. Belli J et al: The number of blood cultures necessary to diagnose most cases of bacterial endocarditis. Am J Med Sci 232:284, 1956.

13. Black S et al: Role of surgery in the treatment of primary infective endocarditis. Am J Med 56:357, 1974.

14. Blailock ZR et al: Adenovirus endocarditis in mice. Science 157:69, 1967.

15. Block PJ et al: Actinobacillus actinomycetecomitans endocarditis: Report of a case and review of the literature. Am J Med Sci 266:387, 1973.

16. Boyd AD et al: Infective endocarditis, an analysis of 54 surgically treated patients. J Thor Cardiovasc Surg 73:23, 1977.

17. Brainbridge MV: Cardiac surgery and endocarditis. Lancet 1:1307, 1969.

18. Braniff BA et al: Valve replacement in active bacterial endocarditis. NEJM 276:1464, 1967.

19. Bryan CS et al: Gram-negative bacillary endocarditis: Interpretation of the serum bactericidal test. Am J Med 58:209, 1975.

20. Bryant RE et al: Unsuccessful treatment of staphylococcal endocarditis with cefazolin. JAMA 237:569, 1977.

21. Cannady PB et al: Negative blood cultures in infective endocarditis — a review. South Med J 69:1420, 1976.

22. Carruthers MM: Endocarditis due to enteric bacilli other than Salmonellae — case reports and literature review. Am J Med Sci 273:203, 1977.

23. Churchill MA et al: Musculoskeletal manifestations of bacterial endocarditis. Ann Intern Med 87:754, 1977.

24. Dowling HF: Present status of therapy with combinations of antimicrobials. Am J Med 39:796, 1965.

25. Doyle EF et al: Risk of bacterial endocarditis during antirheumatic prophylaxis. JAMA 201:129, 1967.

26. Dreyer NP et al: Heroin-associated infective endocarditis. Ann Intern Med 78:699, 1973.

27. Durack DT: Current practice in prevention of bacterial endocarditis. Brit Heart J 37:478, 1975.

28. Edit: Candida endocarditis. Brit Med J 3:264, 1975.

29. Elster SK et al: Hemophilus aprophilus endocarditis — review of 23 cases. Am J Cardiol 35:72, 1975.

30. English TAH et al: Surgical aspects of bacterial endocarditis. Brit Med J 4:598, 1972.

31. Everett ED et al: Transient bacteremia and endocarditis prophylaxis — a review. Medicine 56:61, 1977.

32. Farrar WE et al: Antistaphylococcal activity and betalactamase resistance of newer cephalosporins. J Infect Dis 133:691, 1976.

33. Fass RJ et al: Flucytosine in the treatment of cryptococcal and Candida mycoses. Ann Intern Med 74:535, 1971.

34. Fekety FR et al: Enhanced susceptibility of enterococci to the combination streptomycin plus penicillin of cephalosporin. Antimicrob Agents Chemother 6:156, 1966.

35. Friedberg CK: Vancomycin therapy for enterococcal and S. viridans endocarditis. Arch Intern Med 122:134, 1968.

36. Gadebusch HH et al: Amphotericin B and amphotericin B methyl ester ascorbate: I. Chemotherapeutic activity against Candida albicans, Cryptococcus neoformans, and Blastomyces dermatitidis in mice. J Infect Dis 134:423, 1976.

37. Galgiani JN et al: Fungal endocarditis: Need for guidelines in evaluating therapy. J Thor Cardiovasc Surg 73:293, 1977.

38. Geraci JE et al: Methicillin and other semi-synthetic penicillins in the therapy of staphylococcal endocarditis. Antimicrob Agents Chemother 5:627, 1965.

39. Geraci JE et al: Haemophilus endocarditis — report of 14 patients. Mayo Clin Proc 52:209, 1977.

40. Giamarellou H et al: Treatment of 48 patients with serious anaerobic infection with metronidazole. J Antimicrob Chemother 3:347, 1977.

41. Goodman JS et al: Infections after cardiovascular surgery. NEJM 278:117, 1968.

42. Gopay V: Failure of vancomycin treatment in staphylococcus aureus endocarditis. JAMA 236:1604, 1976.

43. Gray IR: The choice of antibiotic for treating infective endocarditis. Quart J Med 44:449, 1975.

44. Green GR et al: Treatment of bacterial endocarditis in patients with penicillin hypersensitivity. Ann Intern Med 67:235, 1967.

45. Greene JF et al: Septic endocarditis and indwelling pulmonary artery catheters. JAMA 233:891, 1975.

46. Grieco MH et al: Penicillin hypersensitivity in patients with bacterial endocarditis. Ann Intern Med 67:235, 1967.

47. Grist NR: Q-Fever endocarditis. Am Heart J 75:846, 1968.

48. Gutman RA et al: The immune complex glomerulonephritis of bacterial endocarditis. Medicine 51:1, 1972.

49. Hamburger M: Oral therapy for SBE caused by S. viridans. Heart Bull 15:111, 1966.

50. Hamburger M et al: Studies in experimental endocarditis in dogs v. treatment with oxacillin. J Lab Clin Med 70:786, 1967.

51. Hamilton J et al: Successful treatment of pseudomonas cepacia endocarditis with trimethoprim/sulfamethoxazole. Antimicrob Agents Chemother 4:551, 1973.

52. Harris PD et al: Fungal endocarditis secondary to drug addiction. J Thor Cardiovasc Surg 63:980, 1972.

53. Hausing CE et al: E coli endocarditis. Arch Intern Med 120:472, 1967.

54. Herrell WE: Two week treatment schedule for endocarditis. Clin Med 79:9, 1972.

55. Howarth WR et al: Comparative in vitro anti-fungal activity of amphotericin B and amphotericin B methylester. Antimicrob Agents Chemother 7:58, 1975.

56. Iannini PB: Effects of ampicillin-amikacin and ampicillin-rifampin on enterococci. Antimicrob Agents Chemother 9:448, 1976.

57. Iannini PB et al: Therapy of staphylococcus aureus bacteremia associated with a removable focus of infection. Ann Intern Med 84:558, 1976.

58. Jawetz E et al: Penicillin/streptomycin treatment of enterococcal endocarditis. NEJM 274:710, 1966.

59. Kaye D Edit Infective Endocarditis. Ed 1 University Park Press, Baltimore, 1976.

60. Kaye D: Changes in the spectrum, diagnosis, and management of bacterial and fungal endocarditis. Med Clin NA 57:941, 1973.

61. Keslin MH et al: Glomerulonephritis with SBE. Arch Intern Med 132:578, 1973.

62. Klastersky J et al: Effectiveness of carbenicillin-aminoglycoside and of cephalothin-aminoglycoside combinations against enterococci in vitro. Path Biol 23:345, 1975.

63. Klastersky J et al: Antibacterial activity in serum and urine as a therapeutic guide in bacterial infections. J Infect Dis 129:187, 1974.

64. Lerner PI et al: Infective endocarditis in the antibiotic era. NEJM 274:199, 259, 323, 388, 1966.

65. Lerner PI: Infective endocarditis. Med Clin N Amer 58:605, 1974.

66. Lincoln LJ et al: Penicillinase-resistant penicillins plus gentamicin in experimental enterococcal endocarditis. Antimicrob Agents Chemother 12:484, 1977.

67. Louria DB: Major medical complications of heroin addiction. Ann Intern Med 67:1, 1967.

68. Mandell GL: Enterococcal endocarditis. Arch Intern Med 125:258, 1970.

69. Mills J et al: Serratia marcescens endocarditis: a regional illness associated with intravenous drug abuse. Ann Intern Med 84:29, 1976.

70. Mills J: Personal Communication.

71. Moellering RC et al: Endocarditis due to Group D Streptococci. Am J Med 57:239, 1974.

72. Mulcahy JJ et al: Transurethral prostatic resection in patients with prosthetic cardiac valves. J Urol 113:642, 1975.

73. Murray HW et al: Combination antibiotic therapy in staphylococcal endocarditis. Arch Intern Med 136:480, 1976.

74. Myerowitz PD et al: Antibiotic prophylaxis for open heart surgery. J Thor Cardiovasc Surg 73:625, 1977.

75. Nastro LJ: Endocarditis due to anaerobic gram-negative bacilli. Am J Med 54:482, 1973.

76. Neu HC et al: Isolation of protoplasts in a case of enterococcal endocarditis. Am J Med 45:784, 1968.

77. Nolan CM et al: Staphylococcus aureus bacteremia. Am J Med 60:495, 1976.

78. Noriego ER et al: Subacute and acute endocarditis due to pseudomonas cepacia in heroin addicts. Am J Med 59:29, 1975.

79. Okies JE et al: Valve replacement in bacterial endocarditis. Chest 63:898, 1973.

80. Pazin GJ et al: Determination of site of infection in endocarditis. Ann Intern Med 82:746, 1975.

81. Pelletier LL et al: Infective endocarditis — a review of 125 cases from the University of Washington Hospitals 1963-72. Medicine 56:287, 1977.

82. Premsingh N et al: Candida endocarditis in two patients. Arch Intern Med 136:208, 1976.

83. Quinn EL et al: Clinical and laboratory observations in 27 patients treated with penicillin V orally for endocarditis. NEJM 264:835, 1961.

84. Quinn EL: Clinical experience with cefazolin and other cephalosporins in bacterial endocarditis. J Infect Dis 128Supp:386, 1973.

85. Rabinovich S et al: Treatment of bacterial endocarditis with cephalothin. NEJM 273:297, 1965.

86. Ramsey RG et al: Endocarditis in the drug addict. Am J Cardiol 25:608, 1970.

87. Raper AJ et al: Use of steroids in penicillin-sensitive patients with bacterial endocarditis. NEJM 273:297, 1965.

88. Reiner NE et al: Enterococcal endocarditis in heroin addicts. JAMA 235:1861, 1976.

89. Reyes MP et al: Pseudomonas endocarditis in the Detroit Medical Center 1969-72. Medicine 52:173, 1973.

90. Robinson MJ et al: Sequelae of bacterial endocarditis. Am J Med 32:922, 1962.

91. Rosenblatt JE et al: Gram-Negative bacterial endocarditis in heroin addicts. Calif Med 118:1, 1973.

92. Rountree PM et al: Cephaloridine and staphylococcal endocarditis. Brit Med J 1:373, 1967.

93. Rubinstein E et al: Tissue penetration of amphotericin B in candida endocarditis. Chest 66:376, 1974.

94. Ruben RW et al: Antibiotic synergism against Group D Streptococci in the treatment of endocarditis. Med J Aust 2:114, 1973.

95. Sande MA et al: Sustained bacteremia in patients with prosthetic cardiac valves. NEJM 286:1067, 1972.

96. Sande MA et al: Nafcillin-gentamicin synergism in experimental Staphylococcal endocarditis. J Lab Clin Med 88:118, 1976.

97. Seelig MS et al: Candida endocarditis after cardiac surgery. J Thor Cardiovasc Surg 65:583, 1973.

98. Seligman SJ: Treatment of enterococcal endocarditis with oral amoxicillin and intramuscular gentamicin. J Infect Dis 129Supp:213, 1974.

99. Sellers TF: An epidemiologic view of rheumatic fever. Prog Cardiovasc Dis 16:303, 1973.

100. Shafer RB et al: Bacterial endocarditis after open heart surgery. Am J Cardiol 25:602, 1970.

101. Silverman ME: Physical signs in infective endocarditis. Hosp Med 9:94, 1973.

102. Slaughter L et al: Prosthetic valvular endocarditis: A 12 year review. Circulation 47:1319, 1973.

103. Stevens DA: Miconazole in the treatment of systemic fungal infection. Am Rev Resp Dis 116:801, 1977.

104. Stollerman GH: Nephritogenic and rheumatogenic Group A Streptococci. Circulation 43:915, 1971.

105. Tompsett R et al: Reappraising clinical features of endocarditis. Postgrad Med 42:462, 1967.

106. Tu WH et al: Acute glomerulonephritis in bacterial endocarditis. Ann Intern Med 71:335, 1969.

107. Tuazon CU et al: Increased rate of carriage of Staphylococcus aureus among narcotic addicts. J Infect Dis 129:725, 1974.

108. Tuazon CU et al: Staphylococcal endocarditis in drug users. Arch Intern Med 135:1555, 1975.

109. Tuazon CU et al: Staphylococcal endocarditis in parenteral drug abusers — source of the organism. Ann Intern Med 82:788, 1975.

110. Tuazon CU et al: Relapse of Staphylococcal endocarditis after clindamycin therapy. Am J Med Sci 269:145, 1975.

111. Van Scoy RE et al: Coryneform bacterial endocarditis — difficulties in diagnosis and treatment, presentation of three cases, and review of the literature. Mayo Clin Proc 52:216, 1977.

112. Vogler WR et al: Bacterial endocarditis — A review of 148 cases. Am J Med 32:910, 1969.

113. Wang K et al: Bacterial endocarditis in IHSS. Am Heart J 89:359, 1975.

114. Wannamaker LW: The chain that links the heart to the throat. Circulation 48:9, 1973.

115. Watanakunakorn C et al: Some salient features of Staphylococcus aureus endocarditis. Am J Med 54:473, 1973.

116. Watanakunakorn C: Streptococcus bovis endocarditis. Am J Med 56:256, 1974.

117. Watanakunakorn C: Clindamycin therapy of Staphylococcus aureus endocarditis. Am J Med 60:419, 1976.

118. Watanakunakorn C et al: Staphylococcus aureus bacteremia and endocarditis associated with a removable infected intravenous device. Am J Med 63:253, 1977.

119. Watanakunakorn C et al: Prognostic factors in Staphylococcus aureus endocarditis and results of therapy with a penicillin and gentamicin. Am J Med Sci 273:133, 1977.

120. Weinstein L et al: Infective endocarditis — 1973. Prog Cardiovasc Dis 16:239, 1973.

121. Weinstein L et al: Pathoanatomic, pathophysiologic, and clinical correlations in infective endocarditis. NEJM 291:832, 1974.

122. Werner AS et al: Studies on the bacteremia of bacterial endocarditis. JAMA 202:127, 1967.

123. Westenfelder GO et al: Vancomycin-streptomycin synergism in enterococcal endocarditis. JAMA 223-37, 1973.

124. Williams JC et al: Serratia marcescens endocarditis. Arch Intern Med 125:1038, 1970.

125. Wilson WR et al: Prosthetic valve endocarditis. Ann Intern Med 82:751, 1975.

126. Wilson WR et al: Infective endocarditis — a changing spectrum? Mayo Clin Proc 52:254, 1977.

127. Wolfe JC et al: Penicillin-sensitive Streptococcal endocarditis. Ann Intern Med 81:178, 1974.

128. Youmans GP et al: Chapter 41 Bacterial endocarditis. In *The Biologic and Clinical Basis of Infectious Diseases,* WB Saunders, Philadelphia, 1975.

Chapter 39

Tuberculosis

Lloyd Y. Young
Steven L. Barriere

Mycobacterium tuberculosis is an aerobic acid-fast bacillus (AFB). It thrives in organs of relatively high oxygen tension such as the apices of the lungs, followed by the renal parenchyma, the growing ends of bones, and the cerebral cortex. The liver and spleen, which are low in oxygen tension, are generally not affected except in cases of massive overwhelming infection (95). The tubercle bacilli do not elaborate toxins and do not elicit a tissue reaction. Therefore, they mutliply unopposed by host defenses in previously uninfected individuals until a cell-mediated immune response develops. Three to ten weeks may elapse before the immune response is fully developed, and in that time, it is theoretically possible for one organism to father more than four trillion progeny (88). Generally, this immunity prevents further *M. Tuberculosis* multiplication. While many bacilli are destroyed by this host defense mechanism, considerable numbers of bacilli enter into a dormant stage and are resistant to further attack by the immune system. These dormant organisms are also unaffected by chemotherapy because the effectiveness of antitubercular drugs is based upon interruption of active metabolic processes. These dormant bacilli are capable at any given time of suddenly overcoming the general host defenses and producing symptomatic tuberculosis. In summary, *M. tuberculosis* is a relatively slow growing organism which is capable of remaining dormant for long periods of time and is relatively resistant to chemotherapy.

Tubercle bacilli are transmitted on airborne "droplet nuclei" produced by a person with pulmonary tuberculosis. These droplet particles must be small enough (less than 10 microns in diameter) to be kept airborne by normal air currents in a room. Larger particles usually fall to the floor, but are innocuous if inhaled because they are caught on the mucociliary defenses of the upper airways and cleared by the gastrointestinal tract (88,95). Crowded living conditions optimize spread of the disease because droplet nuclei become concentrated in room air where they can be inhaled by susceptible individuals. Transmission can be blocked by adequate ventilation and by chemotherapy of the source case (1,3,8,15,42,72). Tuberculosis (TB) is not transmitted by dishes, clothing, or bedding, and sterilization of these objects is of no practical value (9). Thus, tuberculosis is actually quite difficult to spread as infection requires almost constant *fresh* droplet nuclei exposure. Practically, only family household contacts and those sharing an enclosed environment with the source case are at major risk for infection (82a).

The risk of developing clinical tuberculosis has been estimated to be 3.3%; in other words, one newly infected person out of thirty will develop a symptomatic infection. Overall, between 5-15% of those infected will develop the disease within five years; and of those who do not develop clinical disease within five years, 3-5% will develop disease during their lifetime (53,88).

Unlike most infectious epidemics, tuberculosis has a normal cycle of approximately 300-400 years in any given geographic area. The present tuberculosis epidemic began in Europe in the 16th century and it is only now that the Western world is on the downward slope of the epidemic cycle. Although the new case rate for tuberculosis in the United States has declined from 53 per 100,000 population in 1953 (63), to 15 per 100,000 population in 1976, more than 32,000 new cases were reported in 1976 (9a). In 1976, Massachusetts spent 1.5 million dollars for approximately 47,000 clinic visits and for about 3,500 courses of chemotherapy in 45 clinics (53a). Therefore, the closing of TB sanatoriums and special hospitals does not mean that tuberculosis is uncommon. It only indicates that effective chemotherapy has made it possible to treat the disease in existing health care facilities (9a,53a).

1. A 29-year-old diabetic, alcoholic female was admitted to the Medical Center with a two-month history of bilateral pleuritic chest pain, night sweats, weakness, hemoptysis, fever, and a five pound weight loss. A PPD skin test is ordered by the admitting physician. What is the PPD test and how is it interpreted?

In the presence of either a clinical or a subclinical (dormant) mycobacterial infection, a delayed hypersensitivity reaction to the tubercle bacillus or to its cellular components develops in the host. Upon re-exposure to the tuberculin antigen, the host's cellular immunity responds with a characteristic inflammatory reaction at the site of exposure. Therefore, the tuberculin skin test is a valuable diagnostic tool for the detection of tuberculosis. The test is performed by injecting tuberculin or its purified protein derivative (PPD) intradermally. Most commonly, 0.1 ml of an "intermediate-strength" tuberculin test solution containing five tuberculin units (5TU) is injected into the skin of the forearm with a small gauge needle. A palpable induration of greater than 10 mm diameter 48-72 hours after administration is considered to be a positive reaction; a reading of 5-9 mm is interpreted as doubtful; and 0-4 mm is considered to be a negative reaction. This measurement is not based upon the erythematous zone of demarcation, but rather upon the palpable induration which represents a localized thickening of the skin due to edema and accumulation of sensitized lymphocytes (95).

A negative skin test may be the result of technical error but most frequently occurs in individuals who have had no prior infection with *M. tuberculosis* or who have been infected within 6-8 weeks, or who are anergic. Anergy may be due to severe debility, extreme old age, high fever, sarcoidosis, immunosuppressive drugs, lymphosarcoma, Hodgkin's disease, overwhelming disseminated (miliary) tuberculosis, recent virus infection, or vaccination (e.g., rubella, smallpox). Even the nutritional state of the patient is of concern as the number of positive skin tests in tuberculosis patients clearly increases with the correction of malnutrition (44,83). Therefore, a negative response to intermediate strength PPD (5TU) does not exclude active tuberculosis (89,95). If a "false-negative" skin test reaction is suspected, second strength PPD (250TU) is sometimes used. However, severe lymphangitis and local tissue necrosis have occurred following the use of second strength PPD. Furthermore, immunologic responsiveness to cross-reacting antigens (89) resulted in a 33.6% positive reaction in a non-tuberculous population who were given the second-strength PPD test. In view of this, the use of 250 TU PPD cannot be recommended.

A positive PPD (5 TU) does not imply active mycobacterial disease. It merely signifies that the person was probably previously infected with *M. tuberculosis* or rarely, an atypical mycobacterium. False positive reactions can also occur in patients sensitive to the diluent or other non-tuberculin constituents of the PPD test. Therefore, a positive skin test alone is not diagnostic of a tuberculosis infection. This must be confirmed by isolation of the bacilli and by radiological examination.

Until recently, the PPD (Mantoux) test was available as a soluble tablet which was dissolved with an accompanying diluent; this solution was supposedly stable for 30 days. However, it was discovered that most of the active agent was lost by adsorption to the sides of the glass vial or to the syringe, so the product was stabilized with Tween 80, a solutilizing agent. This stabilized solution should be administered within 30 minutes of its withdrawal from the vial (104).

2. What are some of the symptoms of tuberculosis in this patient? Does she have any risk factors for the contraction of TB?

Many patients with pulmonary tuberculosis have no acute symptoms, and cases are often found following routine chest X-rays ordered for another unassociated illness. The onset of clinical illness is frequently insidious with general complaints of malaise and weakness. Most patients have fever at some point in their illness but it may be low-grade or intermittent; it typically occurs in the late afternoon or evening. Chills or "night sweats" may accompany the fever. A history of cough, weight loss, hemoptysis, and chest pain should raise the index of suspicion for a diagnosis of tuberculosis.

Diabetes, gastrectomy, alcoholism, silicosis, a social history of crowded living conditions, travel or habitation in a country or area endemic with tuberculosis, household contact with a recent tuberculosis patient, reticuloendothelial disease, corticosteroid therapy and the ex-TB patient who has never received chemotherapy are all factors which increase the risk of tuberculosis.

In the previous case, both alcoholism and diabetes were specific clinical risk factors, and her history of chest pain, night sweats, weakness, hemoptysis, fever, and weight loss are all compatible with tuberculosis. This patient presented to the medical center with a sufficient number of "classic" symptoms of tuberculosis to cause the house officer to order a PPD test. However, the absence of "classic" symptoms of tuberculosis can lead to a misdiagnosis, as evidenced by a report from a private urban hospital where almost half of the cases of active tuberculosis were misdiagnosed over a one year span (63). More than one-third of their tuberculous patients had no sweats, chills, or malaise, and fewer than one-half had fever. Cough was evident in 80% of these patients, but only 25% had hemoptysis. Although dullness over the apices of the lungs and post-tussive rales are expected in tuberculosis, fewer than one-third of the above patients showed any abnormal pulmonary signs upon physical examination. As a result, tuberculosis was not suspected in 44% of the cases from one institution, nor was it diagnosed in up to 95% of cases in some other reports (63).

Since the focus of tuberculosis care has shifted from sanatoriums to general hospitals and ambulatory clinics, all clinicians must be made more aware of this disease which is still very much present in the United States (9a,53a).

3. A 65-year-old Chinese male came to the clinic for his yearly routine physical examination. On routine screening, he was found to have a strongly positive reaction to the intermediate strength PPD skin test;

he had negative reactions to PPD in previous years. A chest X-ray was negative. What are the current recommendations for using isoniazid in the prophylaxis of tuberculosis and should this patient be treated?

Preventive therapy of tuberculosis with isoniazid (INH) decreases the bacterial population in the person taking this drug. Therefore, INH preventive therapy is not really "prophylactic therapy," but in actuality reflects treatment of an infection. Such therapy clearly reduces future morbidity from tuberculosis in high risk groups. Benefits from preventive therapy usually outweigh the risks of iatrogenic drug reactions, because every positive PPD skin test reactor is at risk of developing clinical tuberculosis throughout a lifetime. New reactors are at a 4.2% per year risk of contracting active tuberculosis. Persons with abnormal chest X-rays but inactive disease are at a 1% per year risk (30,82).

The effectiveness of INH prophylaxis has also been demonstrated in children. In a large study of urban school children, 3,000 PPD skin test converters were treated with INH and compared prospectively with 1,200 untreated children (22). The incidence of tuberculosis in the untreated group was 60 times that of the treated children. This study provides further evidence for the necessity of closely following untreated converters.

Isoniazid 300 mg/day for adults and 10 mg/kg/day (not to exceed 300 mg/day) for children is the treatment of choice for preventive therapy of tuberculosis. This dose should be administered as a single daily dose for 12 months. Unfortunately, there are no data on the use of any drug other than INH for chemoprophylaxis.

The American Thoracic Society, the American Lung Association, and the Center for Disease Control have balanced the risks of developing active tuberculosis against the risk of INH toxicity and have jointly established the following guidelines and priorities for determining who should receive preventative therapy (7a):

a. *Household members or close associates of persons with newly diagnosed tuberculosis* are at high risk of developing active disease. During the first year, the risk is estimated to be 2.5%; however, this risk rises to 5% if upon initial evaluation the person is tuberculin positive.

b. *Positive tuberculin reactors with findings on chest X-ray consistent with nonprogressive disease, and persons without prior or adequate treatment for past tuberculosis disease* should be treated with INH. The risk of disease reactivation in these individuals is between 1.0-4.0%.

c. *Newly infected individuals* (those who have had skin test conversion within the last two years) are candidates for INH chemoprophylaxis because of a 5%

risk of developing active disease. A "booster" effect, lasting from one to two years, may increase the zone of induration on a repeat test and may be misread as a positive reaction. This booster effect occurs with increasing frequency in patients over the age of fifty and must be considered when determining whether a positive skin test conversion really represents a new infection. Borderline converters (i.e. change of less than 6 mm from the previous year), are probably not candidates for chemoprophylaxis due to the variability of testing techniques.

d. *Positive tuberculin reactors with the following special clinical situations* may require INH preventive therapy: (a) prolonged therapy with glucocorticoids, (b) immunosuppressive therapy, (c) leukemia, Hodgkin's disease, other hematologic or reticuloendothelial disease, (d) diabetes mellitus, (e) silicosis, (f) post-gastrectomy.

e. *Other positive tuberculin skin test reactors* should be considered on a case by case basis as to the advisability of chemoprophylaxis. Age is an important factor in the equation of benefits versus risk. Tuberculin reactors who are 35 years of age or greater are not to be routinely treated with prophylactic INH, because the risk of INH-induced hepatitis in this age group outweighs the potential benefits of therapy. These individuals, however, should receive chemoprophylaxis if other risk factors, as outlined above, are present. INH therapy is mandatory for children under six years of age and is highly recommended for tuberculin converters under 35 years of age, even in the absence of other risk factors because the probable benefits of INH outweigh the risk of hepatitis.

This 65-year-old Chinese patient fits into the third category of newly infected individuals because he has a negative chest X-ray and is a recent tuberculin converter. His positive reaction to the skin test must be interpreted in light of the possibility of a booster effect from previous skin tests because of his age. Furthermore, he is over 35 years of age and is at relatively high risk for developing liver disease from INH (68). Additionally, he has approximately an 80% chance of being a rapid acetylator of isoniazid because he is Asian (33). Rapid acetylators of INH hydrolyze more INH (45%) to hydrazine moieties than do slow acetylators (30% of a dose) and the primary hydrazine metabolite is thought to be hepatotoxic (67,68). For these reasons, this patient should not receive INH chemoprophylaxis; however, he should be followed by X-ray examinations for any change and observed for symptoms indicative of active tuberculosis (20).

4. A 29-year-old Asian male was skin tested with intermediate strength PPD because his sister, with whom he lives, developed active tuberculosis with isoniazid-resistant organisms. His skin test is mark-

edly positive but his chest X-ray, sputum smears, bacteriology, and clinical presentation do not indicate active disease. What is the incidence of primary infections with drug-resistant organisms? Should this patient receive INH chemoprophylaxis?

Data on primary resistance (to be distinguished from resistance that is acquired during treatment) show that 2.8% to 4.4% of patients studied had INH-resistant bacilli; 1.6% to 9.7% of isolated organisms demonstrated resistance to ethambutol; and only 0.8% to 1.6% were resistant to rifampin. Less than 1% of these bacilli were resistant to a combination of two drugs (45). In contrast, up to 50% of tuberculosis infections acquired from the Asian continent may be isoniazid-resistant (16b).

Primary drug-resistant bacilli (resistant bacilli in patients without a history of previous drug treatment) can be transmitted, and the National Communicable Disease Center has recently documented a multiple-case outbreak involving transmission of multiple drug-resistant tubercle bacilli (4b). Containment of such a tuberculosis outbreak involves not only aggressive treatment of active cases, but also prevention of future cases in tuberculin positive reactors. There is a major problem, however, with this principle of containment. No data are available concerning the efficacy or safety of antitubercular medications other than INH in the prevention of tuberculosis in positive tuberculin reactors. Therefore, transmission must be interrupted by treating active and potentially active cases with a combination of antitubercular drugs to which the organism is not resistant.

Since failures in the prevention of tuberculosis have occurred when INH-resistant organisms were cultured, Fairshter and associates have suggested chemoprophylaxis with either ethambutol and/or rifampin for INH-resistant cases (34). Byrd (16b) recommends the use of rifampin as the chemoprophylactic agent if isoniazid drug resistance is suspected. However, this 29-year-old male should receive INH 300 mg/day because other reports have documented successful treatment and prophylaxis of disease despite in vitro resistance (4b,47,62). Also, since 100% of organisms present in a drug-resistant patient are usually not resistant, it is possible that the transmitted organisms are susceptible to isoniazid (82b). Furthermore, should active tuberculosis develop in this patient, the bacilli would not have acquired resistance to effective alternative drugs (46). Since INH therapy may be ineffective, this patient should be monitored closely to ensure prompt detection of active disease and early institution of appropriate therapy.

Other close associates of his sister should be contacted and skin tested with 5TU PPD. Positive tuberculin reactors should be managed according to the principles described in Questions 3 and 4. Negative reactors should be retested in approximately three months (4d).

5. The 29-year-old male patient described in the previous question is to receive 300 mg/day of INH for 12 months; what are the principle INH side effects to which he will be exposed?

Since its introduction in 1952, isoniazid was considered to be almost perfect as an antitubercular agent because it was inexpensive, bactericidal, and well absorbed orally. Numerous studies documented its therapeutic efficacy and its remarkable record of safety when used in treatment of tuberculosis. After it was shown that INH, by itself, was effective and safe in preventing disease, the American Thoracic Society formally recommended in 1965 that INH be used for individuals with dormant infection who were at high risk of developing active disease. The premise that INH caused no serious side effects led to more widespread use of this drug, and at one point almost 500,000 people per year were receiving INH for preventive therapy (39a). Subsequently, a case report in 1970 (65a), conclusively confirmed previous suspicions that INH alone could cause abnormal liver function tests and hepatitis. Then in the same year, 19 of 2,321 Capitol Hill employees who were receiving INH chemoprophylaxis manifested clinical signs of liver disease (39a).

Hepatocellular toxicity induced by INH can occur at any time after initiation of therapy, but most commonly is noticed within the first three months of treatment. It usually begins with gastrointestinal symptoms (55% of patients) such as nausea, anorexia, vomiting, and abdominal discomfort. Some patients (35%) complain of a viral like illness, and others are asymptomatic until the onset of jaundice (10%). Hepatomegaly (33%), hyperbilirubinemia (25%), and prolonged prothrombin times (35%), are some of the manifestations of the INH-induced hepatitis which has been characterized as being clinically, biochemically, and histologically indistinguishable from viral hepatitis (68a). Unlike viral hepatitis which primarily affects young adults, INH hepatitis primarily affects older patients (20). Progressive liver damage is rare with INH in individuals less than 20 years of age. It occurs in up to 0.3% of individuals between the ages of 20-34 years; in up to 1.2% between 35-49 years of age; and in up to 2.3% of persons 50 years of age or older (4c).

Approximately 10 to 20% of INH recipients have biochemical evidence of liver injury (67,68) which is manifested as transaminase elevations (67,68). Most patients with mild subclinical hepatic damage do not progress to overt hepatitis and recover completely even while continuing INH therapy (68a). However, INH continuation in the presence of symptomatology can also result in severe hepatocellular toxicity (64) which is associated with a fatality rate as high as 12.3% (68a). It is difficult to predict which patients will have progressive liver disease and which will recover completely. Therefore, routine biochemical monitoring of serum glutamic oxaloacetic transaminase (SGOT), serum glutamic pyruvic transaminase (SGPT), serum bilirubin, and alkaline phosphatase is not considered to be useful by the Tuberculosis Advisory Committee (7a). However, if any of these tests are obtained for some reason and if the level exceeds three times normal, INH hepatitis is more likely and therapy with INH must be seriously reconsidered (7a,95). All patients should be monitored clinically and questioned monthly concerning the signs and symptoms of hepatitis.

One possible predictor for INH liver injury is the individual's acetylation phenotype. Asians may be more susceptible to isoniazid liver injury than Caucasians, because over 90% are genetically rapid acetylators of INH. When 25 non-Asians were phenotyped into rapid and slow acetylator groups (68) by the sulfamethazine method (80), 86% of the patients with "probable" isoniazid hepatitis were rapid acetylators. Patients with rapid acetylator phenotype apparently hydrolyze more INH to acetylhydrazine than slow acetylators, and the acetylhydrazine metabolite is converted to a potent acylating compound. This latter compound produces liver necrosis in animals (68a), and is postulated to be the hepatotoxic component of isoniazid in humans. (Also see chapters on *Diseases of the Liver* and *General Principles of Antibiotic Therapy*.)

Currently, the predominant evidence available seems to indicate that rapid acetylators are more prone to INH-hepatitis; however, a preliminary report (23a) disputes the postulate that rapid acetylation is a risk factor.

Isoniazid may also rarely cause a direct dose dependent *peripheral neuropathy* when usual recommended dosages of 5 mg/kg/day are used; however, as many as 20% of patients may experience this side effect with higher dosages (40). Alcoholics and others in poor nutrition are more susceptible to this adverse reaction of isoniazid (95). The peripheral neuropathy occurs as a result of INH competitive inhibition of pyridoxine in neural enzyme systems, and can be prevented by the concurrent administration of 10 mg of pyridoxine for every 100 mg of INH. *Convulsions*, responsive to large parenteral doses of pyridoxine, have also been reported in INH treated patients who had no history of a previous seizure disorder. The individuals had undetectable blood concentrations of pyridoxine (102).

INH has also been associated with *arthritic* symptoms (41a), *lupus erythematosus* (2), and an increased prevalence of antinuclear antibodies in as many as 50% of patients. Other less frequently reported reactions are dry mouth, epigastric distress, central nervous system stimulation and depression, psychoses, hemolytic anemia, agranulocytosis, acne, pellagra, spiking fevers and hypersensitivity reactions (40,51,102). Although not conclusive, isoniazid-induced lupus, pyridoxine-responsive neuropathies, acne, and pellagra may be more predominent in slow acetylators (18a) as compared to hepatitis which may be more prevalent in rapid acetylators (68a).

Phenytoin intoxication is a well documented and clinically significant adverse reaction which is due to an interaction between INH and phenytoin; it is also more common in slow acetylators. Apparently INH inhibits the hepatic metabolism of phenytoin and increases the blood levels of phenytoin. Patients should be observed for signs of such toxicity and the dosage of phenytoin decreased if necessary (43).

6. A 58-year-old Asian female enters the clinic with complaints of fatigue, weight loss, and a productive cough of three week's duration. Chest X-ray shows a right middle lobe infiltrate. A sputum smear reveals acid-fast bacilli (AFB) and appropriate laboratory studies are ordered to confirm the diagnosis. All three sputum cultures grow out *M. tuberculosis* six weeks later. Since AFB were noted on smear, isoniazid 600 mg (10 mg/kg/day) each morning is ordered because the physician believes that a larger dose of isoniazid is as efficacious as two drugs. Is he correct in his belief concerning the larger dose of isoniazid?

Effective treatment of tuberculosis is dependent upon a period of intensive drug therapy with at least two drugs, one of which is isoniazid (INH). Although nodular pulmonary tuberculosis can be treated with INH alone, single drug therapy is distinctly inferior to combination therapy of INH with another antitubercular drug (102). With cavitary tuberculosis, two or three drugs are definitely necessary (4a,102).

The concept of multiple drug therapy is based upon the principle that the number of drugs needed to control tubercle bacilli growth is related to the number of organisms involved in the disease process (88). A large mycobacterial population of 10^7 (88) to 10^8 (82a) organisms is present in cavitary tuberculosis. Since INH resistance occurs naturally in about 1 out of every 100,000 (10^5) organisms and streptomycin resistant mutations occur in 1 out of every 1,000,000 (10^6), it would be statistically predictable that treatment with only INH or streptomycin would permit the ultimate development of a drug-resistant strain (82a,88).

Although some clinicians prefer a three-drug regimen for all patients with tuberculosis (4a,102), there is ample evidence that even in advanced cavitary pulmonary tuberculosis, the combination of isoniazid and rifampin or isoniazid and ethambutol are as effective as any combination of three drugs (12,12a, 12b,25,53,71). INH 5-8 mg/kg/day in combination with either rifampin 10 mg/kg/day or ethambutol 15-25 mg/kg/day equals the therapeutic effectiveness of similar three-drug combinations that include para-aminosalicylic acid (PAS) and/or streptomycin (12a,12b,25). The treatment of miliary tuberculosis and tuberculous meningitis are, however, generally initiated with three drugs. Triple therapy is usually begun with isoniazid-ethambutol-rifampin or isoniazid-ethambutol-streptomycin. Streptomycin is often stopped when the sputum smear is negative or after eight weeks of therapy (4a,102).

High dosages of isoniazid will not significantly alter the statistical probability affecting the emergence of resistant organisms. Therefore, this patient should be treated with INH 300 mg/day, pyridoxine 50 mg/day, and ethambutol 25 mg/kg/day for the first 60 days followed by 15 mg/kg/day as *single daily doses* (see Table 2). Weinstein (102) recommends daily divided doses of INH to minimize the neurotoxic side effects. However, large single daily doses of INH are more likely to saturate acetyltransferase, and less isoniazid would be converted, theoretically, to hepatotoxic acetylated metabolites (68a). Most clinicians prefer single daily isoniazid doses to improve compliance.

7. Assuming the patient in Question 6 received INH, pyridoxine, and ethambutol as suggested, how often should the patient be monitored for effectiveness of therapy and does she need to be hospitalized for isolation?

The progress of a patient should be monitored clinically, bacteriologically, and radiologically. Patients on chemotherapy should be evaluated weekly until sputum smears are negative for acid-fast bacilli, and monthly thereafter until sputum cultures are negative. Thereafter, Stead recommends that patients be seen every four to six weeks for the next six months (95). Follow-up visits after the patient has finished the course of chemotherapy are not necessary (20,28,81). With appropriate therapy, sputum smears should be negative in about six to eight weeks; however, patients cease to be infectious in about two to four weeks when the numbers of organisms in their sputum are significantly reduced (1,8,15,42,72). The sputum culture takes longer than smears to become negative, but usually is negative within three to five months (82a). In general, healthy tuberculosis patients may continue their usual school or work activities when their sputum smears indicate that the numbers of bacilli are declining (53). Patients need not be hospitalized (3). In fact, some patients receiving effective chemotherapy can be immediately discharged to home or work (59).

8. When the patient in Question 6 is presented to the attending physician, a question is raised concerning the comparative efficacy and cost of the INH and ethambutol combination versus INH and PAS (para-aminosalicylic acid). How do these two different combinations compare to each other?

PAS is less expensive than ethambutol (EMB); however, the small economic savings hardly compensate for the high incidence of side effects associated with the use of PAS. Patients unwilling to tolerate troublesome side effects do not continue therapy, and higher health costs ensue because of the need for re-treatment. In one study, the patient drop-out rate from treatment with INH plus PAS was 33%, as compared to an 8% to 10% drop-out rate respectively for a low dose (6 mg/kg) and usual dose (15 mg/kg) of ethambutol plus INH (12a). Furthermore, the combination of INH and PAS was less effective than the INH and ethambutol treatment (12a). In other studies of two and three drug regimens, PAS was associated with the highest incidence of nausea, vomiting, diarrhea and epigastric distress (12b,25). It is for these reasons that PAS is no longer used as much because newer and better (i.e. rifampin, ethambutol) agents are available (see Table 1). However, according to an official statement of the American Thoracic Society, PAS may be preferable to ethambutol when used in combination with INH for the treatment of young children because the changes in visual acuity which can occur with ethambutol are difficult to monitor in this age group (6a).

Table 1
ORDER OF EFFECTIVENESS OF THE ANTI-TUBERCULAR AGENTS

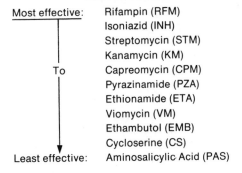

Most effective:	Rifampin (RFM)
	Isoniazid (INH)
	Streptomycin (STM)
	Kanamycin (KM)
	Capreomycin (CPM)
To	Pyrazinamide (PZA)
	Ethionamide (ETA)
	Viomycin (VM)
	Ethambutol (EMB)
	Cycloserine (CS)
Least effective:	Aminosalicylic Acid (PAS)

9. Although the combination of isoniazid and ethambutol is the most frequently used for the initial treatment of tuberculosis, many clinicians are beginning to switch over to a combination of INH and rifampin. Is this latter combination better?

Isoniazid and rifampin are the most potent tuberculocidal agents available and when used in combination are more effective than any regimen previously used for the treatment of pulmonary tuberculosis (36,71). The combination of INH and rifampin is even more effective than any three drug combination not containing rifampin (82a). However, many physicians prefer to limit the use of rifampin for far-advanced or difficult-to-treat cases of tuberculosis because of its expense and because of fear of the widespread development of resistant strains (85). It has been estimated that one month's treatment with rifampin costs about $50 (61a), and that rifampin resistant organisms have gradually increased to a level approaching 2% in some areas (95a).

Due to the problems of cost and resistance, investigators have been attempting to determine the smallest total amount of rifampin needed for successful tuberculosis treatment. One recent investigation suggests that initial therapy with INH, rifampin, and ethambutol for about three and one-half months, followed by continuation treatment with isoniazid plus ethambutol is as effective as other more standardized treatments (61a). The dose of rifampin appears to be important because less than 600 mg/day in combination with INH is associated with decreased effectiveness (62a).

There is also some concern that rifampin may increase the incidence of INH-hepatitis when used in combination with INH (4a,61,75a,82a), although this association needs more study. Additionally, the INH plus rifampin combination may result in more drug toxicity than INH plus ethambutol (80a).

10. How long should an active case of pulmonary TB, like the patient in Question 6, be treated?

Isoniazid, ethambutol, rifampin, and streptomycin are generally termed first-line or primary antitubercular agents. These agents affect metabolic processes of mycobacteria; INH primarily affects DNA synthesis; ethambutol and rifampin affect RNA synthesis; and streptomycin affects protein synthesis (88). Therefore, antitubercular drugs are only effective against replicating tubercle bacilli. Mycobacteria replicate very slowly and because they commonly become dormant, prolonged therapy is necessary for eradication. The official standard for duration of treatment is that 18-24 months of uninterrupted therapy with two or more drugs is necessary to completely eradicate all infectious mycobacteria (6a,95). Even though this may seem to be an inordinately long period of time, recurrences and relapses may still occur.

Patient non-compliance to therapy is a major problem. Patients commonly feel well in a very short period of time and do not feel obligated to continue therapy for the requisite 18-24 months (35). Such non-compliance may ultimately result in resistant organisms which require therapy with more toxic antitubercular drugs (e.g. capreomycin, cycloserine, ethionamide) to which the patient's mycobacteria have not been previously exposed. Therefore, alterna-

tives to standard chemotherapy regimens are constantly being evaluated.

Much interest has been generated by controlled studies carried out in Europe, East Africa and Asia in which daily and intermittent short-course regimens have been used (14,35,36,47-50,69,86,87). Short-course daily therapy with INH plus rifampin is also being studied under controlled investigational conditions in the United States (6a) as is short-course intermittent chemotherapy (25b). If these studies continue to confirm the data summarized below, future antituberculosis therapy may change dramatically.

Although various combinations of antitubercular medications have been used for varying lengths of time, nine and twelve-month regimens seem to be superior to those of six month's duration and equal in effectiveness to the standard 18-24 month's duration as assessed by culture negativity, relapse rates, and "cure" rates (14,36,49a). The British Thoracic and Tuberculosis Association demonstrated a 100% cure rate following a 12-month course of chemotherapy with daily isoniazid and rifampin plus daily streptomycin and ethambutol for the initial two months of treatment (14). Evaluations 9 to 12 months after treatment failed to uncover any incidences of relapse. In another study daily streptomycin, INH, and rifampin for six months demonstrated a 98% cure rate 30 months after treatment (89).

Intermittent short-course chemotherapy has also been evaluated with a variety of agents and schedules. Streptomycin plus high dosage INH once and twice weekly; streptomycin, INH and pyrazinamide daily for 4 weeks followed by once weekly streptomycin plus INH in high dosages (36); INH plus PAS twice weekly (98); and rifampin 600 mg plus INH 300 mg daily for one month followed by twice weekly rifampin 600 mg and INH 900 mg (25b) are all examples of new approaches to therapy in controlled investigative programs. The results of a controlled trial of 6-month and 9-month regimens of two times a week; three times a week; and daily streptomycin, isoniazid, and pyrazinamide for pulmonary tuberculosis demonstrate that all three 9-month regimens were equally effective in eliminating susceptible strains of bacilli from the sputum. The rate of relapse for the 9-month regimen by 30 months was 6% compared to 21% for the 6-month regimen. However, all the relapses were susceptible to drugs, and none involved drug-resistant strains (49a).

The implications of short-course chemotherapy are far-reaching and may well represent the new standard of therapy. These regimens will mean that health care services will be used more efficiently and chronic drug toxicity will be decreased. They are also safer because surviving organisms remain sensitive to drugs. The need for routine patient follow-ups after chemotherapy should also be decreased. Apparently, intensive chemotherapy for a short period eliminates the most active metabolizing bacilli and relies upon an effective immune host response to contain the less active mycobacteria.

The patient described in Question 6 should be treated for 18 months with the prescribed therapy. Although short-course chemotherapy is promising, its use is still investigational. This patient should then be monitored for relapse after her course of therapy, but aggressive follow-up is unnecessary (1,28,75,81,93). Some clinicians do not believe that any follow-up is needed as long as the patient is known to have been 75-80% compliant.

11. Six months after initiating therapy with INH 300 mg/day, pyridoxine 50 mg/day, and ethambutol 15 mg/kg/day, the patient in Question 6 complains of blurred vision during a routine clinic visit. Her laboratory evaluations include a serum uric acid of 9.7 mg%, a serum creatinine of 2.5 mg%, and an SMA SGOT of 82 units. Urinalysis revealed epithelial and red cell casts as well as urate crystals. She has been taking her ethambutol twice daily for the past six months due to a pharmacist's misinterpretation of her prescription. Can her medical problems be related to her medications?

The *elevated serum glutamic oxaloacetic transaminase* (SGOT) value of 82 units is of significance because this patient is receiving isoniazid. Statistically, this Asian lady would be more prone to develop INH-hepatitis because of her race and because her age places her in a high-risk group (7a). Her liver function should continue to be monitored; however, a biopsy or phenotypic studies are unnecessary at this point because about 10% to 20% of patients receiving INH alone will develop transient elevations in SGOT levels (7a,16c).

The patient's decrease in visual acuity is compatible with ethambutol-induced *optic neuritis* which can also be manifested as central scotomas, loss of green color vision, or less commonly as a peripheral vision defect. The intensity of these ocular defects is related to the duration of continued therapy after the first noted appearance of decreased visual acuity (102). This optic neuritis is dose related. It occurs in less than 2% of patients who receive 15 to 25 mg/kg/day of ethambutol; however, the incidence increases with higher doses or when usual doses are used in the presence of moderate to severe renal impairment (60,100). Recovery is complete when the drug is promptly discontinued.

When doses of ethambutol greater than 15 mg/kg/day are prescribed, some clinicians recommend monthly or bimonthly studies of visual acuity, visual fields, and tests for green color vision. Others prefer to have patients read the fine print of a newspaper and to immediately report changes in vision (100).

This patient's visual changes can probably be attributed to her ethambutol because she is receiving an inappropriately high dose due to an error, and she does have some moderate renal dysfunction. Her *hyperuricemia* (78) can also be attributed to her ethambutol (also see chapter on *Gout and Hyperuricemia*). Her elevated serum creatinine in conjunction with the red cell casts noted on urinalysis could possibly be due to a gouty nephropathy.

12. Will this patient (see Question 11) need to have her medications altered in light of her mild renal dysfunction?

Isoniazid dosing in renal failure has not been well studied, but current evidence suggests that modifications in dosage are not necessary (12c). In patients with normal renal function, from 1% to 36% of an administered dose is excreted into the urine as active, unchanged isoniazid. Therefore, the serum half-life of INH would be expected to be prolonged in renal impairment. However, variations in the serum half-life of isoniazid are significantly more dependent upon acetylation phenotype than upon renal function. Since this patient is Asian, and is therefore likely to be a rapid acetylator, alteration of her INH dosage with a creatinine of 2.5 mg% is probably unnecessary.

Ethambutol should be discontinued in this patient because it may well be the cause of her ocular and renal problems. Another first line antitubercular agent such as para-aminosalicylic acid (PAS), streptomycin (STM), or rifampin (RFM) should replace ethambutol as the companion drug to INH. PAS would not be a desirable alternative because it is the least active antitubercular drug (see Table 1); accumulates in renal insufficiency (102); and has a high incidence of troublesome side effects (see Question 7). Streptomycin would have been an effective agent, but it too accumulates in renal failure. This patient's renal impairment would further increase her risk to streptomycin induced ototoxicity. Furthermore, streptomycin must be administered intramuscularly and would be inconvenient for the patient as well as for the clinic staff. Therefore, in this situation, rifampin is the only reasonable alternative. Up to 15% of a dose of rifampin is excreted into the urine as active unchanged drug, but dosages need not be adjusted for renal impairment (102). Rifampin should not exacerbate this patient's present problems, although anecdotal data suggest that rifampin may potentiate INH induced hepatotoxicity (4a,75a,82a). All of the other antitubercular agents listed in Tables 1 and 2 are either reserved for retreatment of primary drug failures or are too toxic for general use.

Table 2
SUMMARY OF ANTITUBERCULAR DRUGS

Drug	Daily Dose	Peak Blood Levels	Primary Toxicities	Dosage Adjustment in Renal Impairment	Comments
Isoniazid (INH)	Adults: 5-8 mg/kg (300 mg) Children: 10-20 mg/kg	2-5 μg/ml	Peripheral neuropathy: hepatic dysfunction; skin rashes; fever; arthralgia, SLE syndrome.	No	Neuropathy preventable by pyridoxine 10 mg/INH 100 mg. Increases serum levels of phenytoin.
Ethambutol (EMB)	15-25 mg/kg	2-5 μg/ml	Retrobulbular neuritis; peripheral neuritis; headache; skin rashes.	Yes	Routine vision tests of questionable value. 80% excreted unchanged in urine.
Rifampin (RFM)	10-20 mg/kg (600 mg)	8 μg/ml	Hepatic dysfunction; thrombocytopenia.	No	Red discoloration of body secretions (perspiration, saliva, urine). Increased anticoagulant activity.
Streptomycin (STM)	Adults: 10-15 mg/kg Children: 20-40 mg/kg	20-40 μg/ml	Vestibular auditory dysfunction of 8th nerve; renal dysfunction; skin rashes; neuromuscular blockade.	Yes	Audiometric and neurological examinations recommended. 60-80% excreted unchanged in urine.
Kanamycin ((KM)	Adults: 10 mg/kg Children: 15 mg/kg	15-30 μg/ml	Auditory dysfunction primarily. (See also SM.)	Yes	(See STM)
Viomycin (VM)	10-15 mg/kg	20-40 μg/ml	(See SM)	Yes	(See STM)
Capreomycin (CPM)	10-15 mg/kg	30-35 μg/ml	(See SM)	Yes	(See STM)
Aminosalicylic Acid (PAS)	200-300 mg/kg	7-8 μg/ml	GI upset (10%); anemia in G6PD deficient patients; skin rashes; fever; hepatitis; hypothyroidism.	Yes	Must be taken with meals or antacids. 100% excreted into urine. False positive reaction with Clinitest. May increase levels of INH.
Cycloserine (CS)	15 mg/kg	10 μg/ml	CNS toxicity (psychosis and convulsions); headache; tremor; fever; skin rashes.	Yes	Contraindicated in epileptic patients. Some toxicity preventable by pyridoxine. 65% excreted unchanged in urine.
Pyrazinamide (PZA)	25-35 mg/kg	60 μg/ml	Hepatitis (3-6%); hyperuricemia; fever; skin rashes; arthralgias; hemolytic anemia.	Yes	SGOT monthly. Hyperuricemia. Nearly 100% excreted in urine.
Ethionamide (ETA)	15 mg/kg	20 μg/ml	Gi irritation (50%); hepatitis (esp. diabetics) gynecomastia; impotence; postural hypotension; difficulty in diabetic management.	No	Must be given with or antacids. SGOT monthly.

13. The patient described above is sent home from the clinic with a supply of rifampin and more isoniazid. She is advised to take two rifampin 300 mg capsules daily and to continue taking 300 mg/day of isoniazid. Three months later she returns to the clinic complaining of a flu-like syndrome of approximately four days duration. SMA-12 laboratory data reveal a serum uric acid of 6.4 mg%, a serum creatinine of 4.3 mg/100 ml SGOT of 140 U/ml, a lactic dehydrogenase (LDH) of 440 U/ml, and a total bilirubin of 2.5 mg/100 ml. The patient discontinued her rifampin a month prior to this clinic visit because her garments were being stained red from perspiration and her saliva looked bloody. Five days prior to this visit she restarted the rifampin and soon became ill with nausea, vomiting, malaise, arthralgia, and fever. Is her symptomatology drug-related?

Rifampin is an orange-red crystalline powder, readily absorbed by the gastrointestinal tract and excreted primarily by the liver and the kidney. It distributes throughout the body, is present in many body fluids in adequate concentrations, and is known to confer an orange-pink color to saliva, tears, urine and sweat (102). Therefore, this patient should have been alerted to this discoloration prior to the initiation of rifampin therapy. With marked rifampin overdosages, the skin discoloration is so intense that it is described as resembling a boiled lobster. If this distinct coloration is associated with severe liver damage as well, the rubric "red-man syndrome" is applied (85).

This patient's other reaction, the "flu-like syndrome," is frequently seen in patients who self-administer rifampin at irregular intervals. It may be associated with acute renal failure, hepatorenal syndrome, thrombocytopenia, or even on rare occasions with massive hemolysis (17,18,21,46,51,66,79). This syndrome does not appear to be as major a problem in patients who ingest rifampin two or three times weekly as part of a planned intermittent therapy regimen (25b,85). This reaction is thought to be associated with circulating rifampin antibodies, but it is not known if these antibodies mediate the tissue damage (85).

This patient's renal and liver impairment, flu-like syndrome, history of intermittent irregular rifampin ingestion, and orange-red perspiration are all consistent with rifampin adverse reactions. These reactions have resolved with supportive therapy and discontinuation of rifampin. Actually, milder reactions have resolved when regular administration of the drug was reinstituted (5). Since this patient's reaction seems rather severe, it may be wise to reinstitute ethambutol in place of rifampin and to treat the hyperuricemia with allopurinol in view of her past reaction to ethambutol. The INH should be continued; however, her physician should remember that INH is also hepatotoxic, and concurrent adverse drug reactions may be occurring in this patient. Another therapeutic alternative would be to discontinue all therapy in this patient, and to reinstitute therapy with INH and ethambutol in a controlled environment after her reactions have subsided.

In light of this patient's vague history of non-compliance to rifampin, it would be prudent to re-evaluate the status of her disease by smears, cultures, X-rays and drug sensitivity studies.

14. A 27-year-old American Indian male is seen in the outpatient tuberculosis clinic for a routine follow-up visit. Four months ago, he was placed on isoniazid, PAS, and streptomycin for severe cavitary tuberculosis of the right lung. However, he is still producing copious sputum, which on smear reveals many acid-fast bacilli. He has continued to lose weight because of his "lack of appetite" and "nausea." On questioning he admitted that he only took his medication intermittently. A review of his medical records revealed that he had visited the clinic weekly for his streptomycin injections, but he had never refilled his two-month supply of isoniazid and PAS, although he did take these medications sporadically. How should tuberculosis be treated in patients such as this?

Treatment failure should be considered whenever sputum cultures remain positive four to six months after initiation of therapy, or whenever chest X-rays indicate progression of the disease (82a). This patient can certainly be considered a treatment failure because many acid-fast bacilli were present on the sputum smear, which should have been negative about six to eight weeks after therapy was begun. Treatment failures can result from deficient host immune response, inappropriate therapy, or poor patient compliance. However, lack of patient compliance in completing an antitubercular course of therapy probably represents the most important factor contributing to the unsuccessful treatment of this disease (84,88). Factors such as education, cost of medication, age, sex, ethnic background, size of tablets, or even the number of tablets have no bearing on patient compliance (88). In most cases, it is the patient who suffers the consequences of non-compliance; however, with tuberculosis, society suffers as well. Therefore, it is essential to devise special treatment programs to render unreliable patients non-infectious.

Directly administered intermittent therapy provides one effective option for ensuring an adequate therapeutic regimen. In such programs, health personnel can even visit the patient at home or at work, if necessary, to administer the needed antitubercular medications two or three times weekly. Isoniazid, ethambutol, and streptomycin are effective when administered two or three times a week in doses two or three times larger than the usual daily doses (6a,23,50,84,86). In addition to these three medications, studies from East Africa and Asia have documented the efficacy and safety of pyrazinamide and ethionamide (47,49a,98).

The best clinical results have been obtained with a combination of daily chemotherapy for the first two to three months followed by fully supervised intermittent therapy (50,98). Although it is very clear that twice weekly intermittent therapy is adequate for success, some recommend a three-times-a-week regimen so that if one visit is missed, the patient would still be effectively treated (82a).

This patient has a history of non-compliance and would be an excellent candidate for intermittent therapy. Adequate sputum specimens should be collected prior to initiation of a retreatment chemotherapy program, and drug sensitivity tests should be performed. The results from susceptibility testing will be delayed for about three weeks, but therapy should begin immediately with at least two drugs which he has not previously received. *A single new potentially effective drug must never be added to a regimen that has already failed because the further development of resistance must be avoided* (6a, 82a, 95). Since this patient has been receiving isoniazid, PAS, and streptomycin, it would be logical to discontinue these medications. A combination of rifampin and ethambutol would be an excellent choice for this patient; it would also be reasonable to continue the isoniazid (INH) pending the results of sensitivity testing. The INH can later be discontinued should resistance be demonstrated by the test results. The INH can then be replaced with another agent to which the organism is sensitive.

15. A 64-year-old male is brought to the emergency room following a four-day period in which he progressively became disoriented, febrile to 105°F, and obtunded. Physical examination revealed a decorticate posture (opisthotonus) and a positive Brudzinski sign (neck resistant to flexion).

Glucose, thiamine, and naloxone were given intravenously without response. A lumbar puncture resulted in an opening pressure of 280 mm Hg, and 10cc of clear spinal fluid. Analysis of the CSF revealed an elevated protein concentration and a glucose concentration less than 20% of the serum level. Cell count revealed 760 white cells, 85% of which were lymphocytes. A smear of the spinal fluid revealed a few AFB. How is tubercular meningitis treated?

Treatment of tuberculous meningitis must be started *immediately* with at least two and probably three drugs because irreversible brain damage or death may occur as soon as two weeks after the onset of infection (not symptoms) (73). All of the four primary drugs useful in the treatment of pulmonary tuberculosis can be used in treatment with the possible exception of streptomycin (73). See Table 3 for a list of the most commonly used drugs, their cerebral spinal fluid (CSF) concentrations, and usual minimum inhibitory concentrations.

Table 3
CONCENTRATION LEVELS OF THE
COMMON ANTITUBERCULAR AGENTS

	Cerebrospinal Fluid Concentrations (μg/ml)	Minimum Inhibitory Concentrations
Isoniazid	2-5	0.05-0.2
Ethambutol	1-2	1-2
Rifampin	2-4	0.5
Pyrazinamide	60	20

Isoniazid is required in a dose of 5 to 10 mg/kg/day since it is the most active of these drugs and its use

has significantly reduced morbidity and mortality due to tuberculous meningitis (96). Doses of INH as high as 25 to 30 mg/kg/day have been given for meningitis with good results (102). Ethambutol (11,76,77) and rifampin (24,76,91,101) have both been used successfully as a second drug, in doses of 15 to 25 mg/kg/day and 10 mg/kg/day respectively. The route of administration in an unconscious patient must, by necessity, be through the nasogastric tube. Only isoniazid and streptomycin are available for parenteral administration at the present time. Only streptomycin must be administered intrathecally since inadequate CSF levels are obtained through systemic administration.

Corticosteroids may be indicated to reduce cerebral edema (73), but there are so few reports that the effect of dexamethasone on morbidity and mortality cannot be definitively assessed (16,74). However, morbidity has been decreased with the use of steroids in severe pulmonary disease (52). Patients with mild to moderate disease may become worse following steroid treatment.

16. What is the current status of BCG vaccination in the prevention of tuberculosis?

BCG (Bacillus of Calmette and Guerin) is a bovine mycobacterial vaccine. There are many different BCG vaccines available worldwide and all differ with respect to immunogenicity, efficacy, and reactogenicity. The vaccines now available in the United States have not been tested in controlled clinical trials in over 20 years, and their efficacy can only be inferred from earlier trials because of changes in production and multiple derivations from the original strain (4). Nevertheless, these vaccines are considered to be effective and are capable of conferring 80% protection against the development of clinical tuberculosis with 60% effectiveness remaining as long as 15 years after vaccination (27).

Adverse reactions to BCG vaccine vary according to the vaccine, dosage, age of the vaccine, and degree of patient monitoring; however, osteomyelitis, prolonged ulceration at the vaccination site, lupoid reactions, lymphadenitis, disseminated BCG infection, and death have all been reported (4). Therefore, in the United States, this vaccine is only used for a very few select groups of individuals who are repeatedly exposed to highly infectious, untreated patients. BCG vaccine is not to be used in routine prophylaxis because in most of the United States the risk of exposure to tuberculosis is relatively low and preventive chemotherapy, tuberculin testing, and X-ray screening of high risk groups are available at low cost.

Investigationally, BCG vaccine has been used as supplemental therapy for various carcinomas. Apparently the vaccine is capable of stimulating an active nonspecific immune response and thereby prolongs the duration of remission after chemotherapy, surgery or irradiation (38). The reader is also referred to the chapter on *Cancer Chemotherapy*.

CASE FOR STUDY:

The patient is a 63-year-old female immigrant from Hong Kong, who comes to the outpatient clinic with a three-week history of malaise, nocturnal diaphoresis, cough, hemoptysis, fever, and a ten-pound weight loss. Past medical history indicates that adult onset diabetes mellitus is being treated with tolbutamide, 1 gm/day, and a seizure disorder is being treated with phenytoin 300 mg/day.

The initial physical examination of this patient revealed an elderly Chinese woman with rales and rhonchi in her right middle lobe; the remainder of the examination is grossly within normal limits except for some mild bilateral nystagmus on lateral gaze. She is admitted to the hospital for evaluation and possible treatment, and a culture was taken of her sputum. A smear of sputum and Gram stain revealed acid-fast bacilli. Initial laboratory values revealed the following:

Hgb 10.9 mg%	BUN 45 mg/L	Albumin 2.5 gm%	SGOT 85 U
Hct 30.4%	Creatinine(s) 2.8 mg%	Total Protein 4.9 gm%	Glucose 285 mg%
WBC 8,200	Uric Acid 9.8 mg%	Alkaline phosphatase 154 U	LDH 340U
Retic 3.5%	Protime 12.4 sec		
	Control 12.2 sec		

a. What should be done to confirm the diagnosis of TB?

b. How should she be treated and what are some important considerations in the choice of a chemotherapeutic regimen for this patient?

c. What drug interactions might occur?

d. What adverse reactions to treatment might occur?

e. If this patient is noncompliant, what are the alternatives?

REFERENCES

1. Abeles H: The early discharge of tuberculous patients with sputum containing acid fast bacilli. Am Rev Resp Dis 108:975, 1973.
2. Alarcon-Segovia D: Drug-induced lupus syndromes. Mayo Clin Proc 44:664, 1969.
2a. Albert RK et al: Monitoring patients with tuberculosis for failure during and after treatment. Am Rev Resp Dis 114:105, 1976.
3. American Thoracic Society: Guidelines for work for patients with tuberculosis. Am Rev Resp Dis 108:160, 1973.
4. Anon: Recommendation of the Public Health Service Advisory Committee — BCG vaccinations. USPHS Morbidity and Mortality Weekly Report 24:69, 1975.
4a. Anon: Drugs for treatment of tuberculosis. Med Lett 19:97, 1977.
4b. Anon: Drug resistant tuberculosis in Mississippi. USPHS Morbidity and Mortality Weekly Report 26:417, 1977.
4c. Anon: Isoniazid-associated hepatitis: summary of the report of the tuberculosis advisory committee and special consultants of the director, Center for Disease Control. USPHS Morbidity and Mortality Weekly Report 23:97, 1974.
4d. Anon: Tuberculosis-Maryland. USPHS Morbidity and Mortality Weekly Report 25:93, 1976.
5. Aquinas SM et al: Adverse reactions to daily and intermittent rifampicin regimens for pulmonary tuberculosis in Hong Kong. Brit Med J 1:765, 1972.
6. Ashley MJ et al: The influence of immigration on tuberculosis in Ontario. Am Rev Resp Dis 110:137, 1974.
6a. Bailey WC et al: Treatment of mycobacterial disease (an official statement of the American Thoracic Society). Am Rev Resp Dis 115:185, 1977.
7. Barlow PB et al: Preventive therapy of tuberculous infection. Am Rev Resp Dis 110:371, 1974.
7a. Barlow PB et al: Preventive therapy of tuberculous infection. USPHS Morbidity and Mortality Weekly Report 24:71, 1975.
8. Bates JH: Ambulatory treatment of TB — an ideas whose time has come. Am Rev Resp Dis 109:317, 1974.
9. Bates JH et al: Effect of chemotherapy on infectiousness of tuberculosis. NEJM 290:459, 1974.

9a. Bates JH: The changing scene in tuberculosis. NEJM 297:610, 1977.
10. Bentz RR et al: The incidence of urine cultures positive for mycobacterium tuberculosis in a general tuberculosis patient population. Am Rev Resp Dis 111:647, 1975.
11. Bobrowitz ID: Ethambutol in tuberculous meningitis. Chest 61:629, 1972.
12. Bobrowitz ID: Ethambutol/isoniazid vs. streptomycin/isoniazid/ethambutol in the original treatment of cavitary TB. Am Rev Resp Dis 109:548, 1974.
12a. Bobrowitz ID et al: Ethambutol-isoniazid vs PAS-isoniazid in the original treatment of pulmonary tuberculosis. Am Rev Resp Dis 96:428, 1967.
12b. Bobrowitz ID et al: Ethambutol compared to streptomycin in the original treatment of advanced pulmonary tuberculosis. Chest 60:14, 1971.
12c. Bowersox DW et al: Isoniazid dosage in patients with renal failure. NEJM 289:84, 1973.
13. Brennan RW et al: Dilantin intoxication attendant to slow inactivators of INH, Neurol (Minneap.) 20:867, 1970.
14. British Thoracic and Tuberculosis Association: Short course chemotherapy in pulmonary TB. Lancet 1:119, 1975.
15. Brooks SM et al: A pilot study concerning the infection risk of sputum positive tuberculous patients on chemotherapy. Am Rev Resp Dis 108:799, 1973.
16. Busey JF et al: Adrenal corticosteroids and TB. Am Rev Resp Dis 97:484, 1968.
16a. Byrd RB et al: Treatment of tuberculosis by the nonpulmonary physician. Ann Intern Med 86:799, 1977.
16b. Byrd RB: Tuberculosis chemoprophylaxis (letter). Ann Intern Med 87:792, 1977.
16c. Byrd RB et al: Isoniazid chemoprophylaxis. Arch Intern Med 137:1130, 1977.
17. Campese VM et al: Acute renal failure during intermittent rifampicin therapy. Nephron 10:256, 1973.
18. Chan WC et al: Renal failure during intermittent rifampin therapy. Tubercle 56:191, 1975.
18a. Cohen LK et al: Isoniazid-induced acne and pellagra. Arch Dermatol 109:377, 1974.

19. Comstock GW: The modern epidemiology of tuberculosis. Am J Epidem 101:363, 1975.

20. Comstock GW et al: The competing risks of tuberculosis and hepatitis for adult tuberculin reactors. Am Rev Resp Dis 111:573, 1975.

21. Cordonnier D et al: Acute renal failure after rifampicin. Lancet 2:1364, 1972.

22. Curry FJ: Prophylactic effect of INH in young tuberculin reactors. NEJM 277:562, 1967.

23. Curry FJ: The effect of acceptable and adequate outpatient treatment on the length of hospitalization and on readmission for relapse or reactivation of pulmonary TB: Chest 63:536, 1973.

23a. Dickinson DS et al: The effect of acetylation status on isoniazid hepatitis. Am Rev Resp Dis 115 (April Suppl):395, 1977.

24. D'oliveira JJG: Cerebrospinal fluid concentration of rifampin in meningeal tuberculosis. Am Rev Resp Dis 106:432, 1972.

25. Doster B et al: Ethambutol in the initial treatment of pulmonary TB. Am Rev Resp Dis 107:177, 1973.

25a. Doster B et al: A continuing survey of primary drug resistance in tuberculosis, 1961-1968. Am Rev Resp Dis 113:419, 1976.

25b. Dutt AK et al: Treatment of pulmonary tuberculosis with short-course, intermittent chemotherapy using rifampin-isoniazid. Am Rev Resp Dis 115(April Suppl):396, 1977.

26. East African TB Investigation Centre: Short course treatment in pulmonary TB. E Afr Med J 52:472, 1975.

27. Editorial: BCG vaccination. Brit Med J 4:603, 1975.

28. Edsall J et al: Routine followup of inactive TB: a practice to be abandoned. Am Rev Resp Dis 107:851, 1973.

29. Edwards OM et al: Changes in cortisol metabolism following rifampin therapy. Lancet 2:549, 1974.

30. Edwards PQ: Screening for tuberculosis. Chest 68 Supp:451, 1975.

31. Eidus L et al: Pharmacokinetic studies with an isoniazid slow-releasing matrix preparation. Am Rev Resp Dis 110:34, 1974.

32. Ellard GA et al: Pharmacology of some slow release preparations of isoniazid of potential use in intermittent treatment of TB. Lancet 1:340, 1972.

33. Ellard GA: Variations between individuals and populations in the acetylation of isoniazid and it's significance for the treatment of pulmonary tuberculosis. Clin Pharmacol Ther 19:610, 1976.

34. Fairshter RD et al: Failure of INH prophylaxis after exposure to INH-resistant tuberculosis. Am Rev Resp Dis 112:37, 1975.

35. Fox W: General considerations in intermittent drug therapy of pulmonary TB. Postgrad Med J 47:729, 1971.

36. Fox W et al: Short course chemotherapy for pulmonary tuberculosis. Am Rev Resp Dis 111:325, 1975.

37. Freedman SO et al: Immunobiology of tuberculin hypersensitivity. Chest 68(Supp): 470, 1975.

38. Freireich EJ: Approaches to local immunotherapy. JAMA 234:1258, 1975.

39. Furey WW et al: Tuberculosis in a community hospital — a five year review. JAMA 235:168, 1976.

39a. Garibaldi RA et al: Isoniazid associated hepatitis: report of an outbreak. Am Rev Resp Dis 106:357, 1972.

40. Goldman IL et al: Isoniazid: a review with emphasis on adverse effects. Chest 62:71, 1972.

41. Goldstein RA et al: Rifampin in cell mediated immune responses in tuberculosis. Am Rev Resp Dis 113:197, 1976.

41a. Good AE et al: Rheumatic symptoms during tuberculosis therapy, a manifestation of isoniazid toxicity. Ann Intern Med 63:800, 1965.

42. Gunnels JJ et al: Infectivity of sputum positive TB patients on chemotherapy. Am Rev Resp Dis 109:323, 1974.

43. Hansten PD: Drug Interactions. Third edition. Philadelphia, Lea and Febiger, 1975, p. 140.

44. Harrison BDW et al: Tuberculin reaction in adult Nigerians with sputum positive pulmonary TB. Lancet 1:421, 1975.

45. Hobby GL et al: Primary drug resistance: a continuing study of drug resistance in tuberculosis in a veteran population in the U.S. Am Rev Resp Dis 110:95, 1974.

46. Hong Kong Tuberculosis Treatment Services/British Medical Research Council: The influence of age and sex on the incidence of the flu syndrome and rifampin dependent antibodies in patients on intermittent rifampin for tuberculosis. Tubercle 56:173, 1975.

47. Hong Kong TB Treatment Services/British Med. Research Council: Controlled trial of 6 and 9 month regimens of daily and intermittent streptomycin plus INH plus pyrazinamide for pulmonary TB in Hong Kong. Tubercle 56:81, 1975.

48. Hong Kong TB Treatment Services/Brompton Hospital/British Med. Research Council: A controlled trial of daily and intermittent rifampicin plus ethambutol in the retreatment of patients with pulmonary TB. Tubercle 56:179, 1975.

49. Hong Kong TB Treatment Services/East African and British Med. Research Councils: First line chemotherapy in the tretreatment of bacteriological relapses of pulmonary TB following short course regimens. Lancet 1:162, 1976.

49a. Hong Kong Chest Service/British Medical Research Council: Controlled trial of 6 month and 9 month regimens of daily and intermittent streptomycin plus isoniazid plus pyrazinamide for pulmonary tuberculosis in Hong Kong. Am Rev Resp Dis 115:727, 1977.

50. Hudson LD et al: Twice weekly tuberculosis chemotherapy. JAMA 223:139, 1973.

51. Jacobs NF et al: Spiking fever from isoniazid simulating a septic process. JAMA 238:1759, 1977.

52. Johnson JR et al: Corticosteroids in pulmonary TB. Am Rev Resp Dis 96:62, 1967.

53. Johnston RF et al: State of the art review; The impact of chemotherapy on the care of patients with tuberculosis. Am Rev Resp Dis 109:636, 1974.

53a. Kaplan AI: Tuberculosis treatment in Massachusetts in 1977. NEJM 297:616, 1977.

54. Kleinknecht D et al: Acute renal failure after rifampicin. Lancet 1:238, 1972.

55. Krakoff IH: Clinical pharmacology of drugs which influence uric acid production and excretion. Clin Pharmacol Ther 8:124, 1967.

56. Krebs A: Preliminary results of isoniazid prophylaxis for fibrotic lesions: efficacy of varying durations of treatment. Proc. of 22nd Conf. Int. Union Against TB. Tokyo, Japan, Sept., 1973.

57. Kutt H et al: Depression of para-hydroxylation of phenytoin by anti-tuberculous chemotherapy. Nuerol (Minneap.) 16:594, 1966.

58. Lal S et al: Effect of rifampicin & INH on liver function. Brit Med J 1:148, 1972.

59. Leff A et al: Outpatient treatment of advanced pulmonary tuberculosis without initial hospitalization. Am Rev Resp Dis 109:697, 1974.

60. Leibold JE: The ocular toxicity of ethambutol and its relation to dose. Ann NY Acad Sci 135:904, 1966.

61. Lees AW et al: Toxicity from rifampicin/INH and rifampicin/ethambutol. Tubercle 52:182, 1971.

61a. Lees AW et al: Ethambutol plus isoniazid compared with rifampicin plus isoniazid in antituberculous continuation treatment. Lancet 1:(8024)1232, 1977.

62. Lim BT et al: Ethambutol and capreomycin in the retreatment of advanced pulmonary TB. Am Rev Resp Dis 99:793, 1969.

62a. Long MW et al: Comparison of 12 versus 18 months of chemotherapy after sputum conversion among TB patients initially treated with three Rifampin-INH regimens: results of a USPHS trial. Am Rev Resp Dis 115(April Suppl):403, 1977.

63. MacGregor RR: A year's experience with tuberculosis in a private urban teaching hospital in the postsanatorium era. Am J Med 58:221, 1975.

64. Maddrey WC et al: Isoniazid hepatitis. Ann Intern Med 79:1, 1973.

65. Malaviya AN et al: Factors of delayed hypersensitivity in pulmonary TB. Am Rev Resp Dis 112:49, 1975.

65a. Martin CE et al: Hepatitis after isoniazid administration. NEJM 282:433, 1970.

66. Mattson K et al: Acute renal failure following rifampicin administration. Scand J Resp Dis 55:291, 1974.

67. Mitchell JR et al: Acetylation rates and monthly liver function tests during one year of isoniazid preventive therapy. Chest 68:181, 1975.

68. Mitchell JR et al: Increased incidence of isoniazid hepatitis in rapid acetylators. Possible relation to hydrazine metabolites. Clin Pharmacol Ther 18:70, 1975.

68a. Mitchell JR et al: Isoniazid liver injury-clinical spectrum, pathology, and probable pathogenesis. Ann Intern Med 84:181, 1976.

69. Mitchison DA et al: Laboratory aspects of intermittent drug therapy for tuberculosis. Postgrad Med J 47:737, 1971.

70. Murray FJ: Outbreak of unexpected reactions among epileptics taking INH. Am Rev Resp Dis 86:729, 1967.

71. Newman R et al: Rifampin in initial treatment of pulmonary

tuberculosis. Am Rev Resp Dis 103:461, 1971.

72. Oatway WH: Early discharge of patients with active TB. Am Rev Resp Dis 109:321, 1974.

73. Oill PA et al: Infectious disease emergencies: Part 1 — patients presenting with an altered state of consciousness. West J Med 125:36, 1976.

74. O'Toole RD et al: Dexamethasone in TB meningitis. Ann Intern Med 70:39, 1969.

75. Pamra SP et al: Relapse in pulmonary tuberculosis. Am Rev Resp Dis 113:67, 1976.

75a.Pessayre D et al: Isoniazid-rifampin fulminant hepatitis. Gastroent 72:284, 1977.

76. Pilheu JA et al: Ethambutol and rifampicin in tuberculous meningitis. Reports on rifampicin presented at the XXI International Tuberculosis Conference, Aug. 1974.

77. Place VA et al: Ethambutol in tuberculous meningitis. Am Rev Resp Dis 99:783, 1969.

78. Postlethwaite AE et al: Hyperuricemia due to ethambutol. NEJM 286:761, 1972.

79. Ramgopal V et al: Acute renal failure associated with rifampin. Lancet 1:1195, 1973.

80. Rao KVN et al: Sulphadimidine acetylation test for classification of patients as slow or rapid inactivators of isoniazid. Brit Med J 3:495, 1970.

80a.Ravikrishnan KP et al: Toxicity to isoniazid and rifampin in active tuberculosis patients. Am Rev Resp Dis 115 (April Suppl):405, 1977.

81. Reichman LB: Routine follow-up of inactive tuberculosis: a practice that has been abandoned. Am Rev Resp Dis 108:1442, 1973.

82. Reichman LB: Tuberculosis screening and chest x-ray films. Am Rev Resp Dis 112:448, 1975.

82a.Reichman LB et al: Practical management and control of tuberculosis. Med Clin N Am 61:1185, 1977.

82b.Reichman LB et al: Tuberculosis in the foreign born. Am Rev Resp Dis 116:561, 1977.

83. Rooney J Jr. et al: Further observation on tuberculin reactions in active tuberculosis. Am J Med 60:517, 1976.

84. Rothstein E: 31st VA-Armed Forces Pulmonary Disease Research Conference. Am Rev Resp Dis 106:125, 1972.

85. Sanders WE: Rifampin. Ann Intern Med 85:82, 1976.

86. Sbarbaro JA et al: High dose ethambutol: an oral alternate for intermittent chemotherapy. Am Rev Resp Dis 110:91, 1974.

87. Sbarbaro JA et al: Intermittent chemotherapy for adults with tuberculosis — statement by the American Thoracic Society. Am Rev Resp Dis 110:374, 1974.

88. Sbarbaro JA: Tuberculosis: the new challenge to the practicing clinician. Chest 68 Supp:436, 1975.

89. Second East African/British Medical Research Council: Controlled clinical trial of four 6-month regimens of chemotherapy for pulmonary tuberculosis. Am Rev Resp Dis 114:471, 1976.

90. Singapore Tuberculosis Service/British Med. Research Council: Controlled trial of intermittent regimens of rifampicin plus isoniazid for pulmonary tuberculosis in Singapore. Lancet 2:1105, 1975.

91. Sippel JE et al: Rifampin concentrations in CSF of patients with TB meningitis. Am Rev Resp Dis 109:579, 1974.

92. Smith J et al: Hepatotoxicity in INH/Rifampin treated patients, related to rates of INH inactivation. Chest 61:587, 1972.

93. Stead WW et al: Productivity of prolonged follow-up after chemotherapy for tuberculosis. Am Rev Resp Dis 108:314, 1973.

94. Stead WW: Goals and productivity of tuberculosis screening. Chest 68 Supp:446, 1975.

95. Stead WW et al: Tuberculosis, in *Harrison's Principles of Internal Medicine.* Edition 8, edited by MM Wintrobe et al. McGraw-Hill, New York, pp. 900-912, 1977.

95a.Stottmeier KD: Emergence of rifampin-resistant *Mycobacterium tuberculosis* in Massachusetts. J Infect Dis 133:88, 1976.

96. Sumaya CV et al: Tuberculosis meningitis in children during the isoniazid era. J Pediat 87:43, 1975.

97. Thomas PA et al: Chemoprophylaxis for the prevention of tuberculosis in the immunosuppressed patient receiving a renal allograft. Transplantation 20:76, 1975.

98. Tuberculosis Chemotherapy Centre, Madras: Controlled comparison or oral twice weekly daily isoniazid plus PAS in newly diagnosed pulmonary TB. Brit Med J 2:7, 1973.

99. U.S. Dept. of Health, Education and Welfare Public Health Service, Reported Tuberculosis Data 1973, Center for Disease Control, 1974.

100. VanScoy RE: Antituberculosis agents — isoniazid, rifampin, streptomycin, ethambutol. Mayo Clin Proc 52:694, 1977.

101. Visudhipan P et al: Evaluation of rifampicin in the treatment of tuberculosis meningitis in children. J Pediat 87:983, 1975.

102. Weinstein L: Chemotherapy of tuberculosis, Chapter 60. In *The Pharmacological Basis of Therapeutics,* 5th edition, edited by LS Goodman and A Gilman. Macmillan Co. New York, 1975, pp. 1201-1216.

103. Whitcomb ME: Transfer factor therapy in a patient with progressive primary tuberculosis. Ann Int Med 79:161, 1973.

104. Wijsmuller G et al: The tuberculin test effects of storage and methods of delivery on reaction size. Am Rev Resp Dis 107:267, 1973.

105. Youmans GP: Relation between delayed hypersensitivity and immunity in tuberculosis. Am Rev Resp Dis 111:109, 1975.

106. Youmans GP: Chapter 24, Tuberculosis in *The Biological and Clinical Basis of Infectious Diseases.* Edition 1, edited by Youmans GP et al. WB Saunders, Philadelphia, 1975.

Chapter 40

Venereal Diseases

Richard F. de Leon

The national venereal disease (VD) problem has reached epidemic proportions. In 1975, over one million cases of gonorrhea and 26,000 cases of primary and secondary syphilis were reported in the U. S. These figures represent increases of 10% for gonorrhea and 1% for syphilis when they are compared to the 1974 statistics. In addition, if the unreported cases are taken into account, it is estimated that as many as two million cases of gonorrhea and about 80,000 cases of syphilis actually occurred during 1975 (28). Also, the number of undetected carriers of gonorrhea and syphilis must also be included in considering the epidemiological implication of VD.

The VD Branch of the Center for Disease Control (CDC) estimates that there are 800,000 cases of asymptomatic, undetected gonorrhea in the U. S. female population and 500,000 cases of untreated or inadequately treated syphilis among both sexes.

There are many reasons for this upsurge in the incidence of syphilis and gonorrhea. Gonorrhea has a short incubation period that promotes its rapid spread, and poor reporting by physicians greatly hampers the location of contacts and carriers (55). In addition, asymptomatic carriers of gonorrhea escape detection because of inadequate screening procedures; there is no simple blood test that can be used for mass public screening. Another problem is that the resistance of gonococcus to antibiotic therapy has increased in a relatively short time. Fortunately, *Treponema pallidum* has not demonstrated resistance to antibiotic therapy. Although syphilis offers some degree of immunity to reinfection, gonorrhea infection confers no such resistance. There is no vaccine available to prevent infection from either *T. pallidum* or *Neisseria gonorrhoeae.*

Another reason for the increase in the incidence of gonorrhea and syphilis is the poor acceptance of condoms; and washing with soap and water and urinating after intercourse are not common practices. Perhaps the most significant reason for the increase in syphilis and gonorrhea is inadequate education.

Gonorrhea:

Gonorrhea is caused by *Neisseria gonorrhoeae,* a gram-negative diplococcus. In males, gonorrhea occurs four to ten days after contact with an infected source. A milky urethral discharge associated with meatal pain (especially when voiding) and urinary frequency are the first signs of infection. The discharge, which is caused by the irritating endotoxin released by the dying gonococcus, may become more profuse and blood-tinged as the infection progresses. Extension of the infection to the seminal vesicles, epididymis, and prostate may occur if the condition is untreated. Urethral stricture after repeated attacks, and sterility after epididymitis, are now rare complications of gonococcal infection, due to the effectiveness of antibiotics.

Patients with asymptomatic disease serve as reservoirs for the infection. At one time, only females were thought to have asymptomatic gonorrhea, but the significance of asymptomatic male carriers is becoming apparent (67,68,69). Fifty to 70% of infected women are asymptomatic (69); however, there is usually a purulent urethral discharge. Urgency, frequency, and dysuria may also occur.

Although lower genital tract symptoms in women may disappear within a month, the patient remains infected and becomes an asymptomatic carrier of gonorrhea if untreated. Eventually, salpingitis with fibrosis and scarring of fallopian tubes may result in sterility. Pelvic inflammatory disease (PID) is a further complication of untreated gonorrhea. Other complications include gonococcal arthritis and gonococcal ophthalmia neonatorum.

Syphilis:

Syphilis, like gonorrhea, is transmitted by direct contact. *T. pallidum,* the causative agent, invades the body by penetrating the epithelium. Then, after penetration, *T. pallidum* spreads via the lymphatic system, and regional lymph nodes may become tender. Dissemination occurs within a few days after its initial implantation.

Usually a primary chancre appears at the invasion site about three weeks after infection, but the incubation period can vary from 10 to 90 days. However, the chancre does not have a typical appearance or location and may be easily missed. The primary lesion usually heals two to six weeks after its appearance. Primary syphilis, the most infectious stage, begins with the initial infection and usually ends some six to eight weeks later (range six weeks to six months), when the patient enters the secondary stage of the disease process.

A widespread maculopapular skin rash, frequently involving the palms of the hands and the soles of the feet in addition to the trunk and extremities, marks the beginning of the secondary stage. Mucous membranes may also be involved; and the patient may complain of fatigue, malaise, headache, and fever during this time. If untreated, the lesions of secondary syphilis heal in 4 to 12 weeks. This is the beginning of the latent stage of the disease.

During the latent stage there are no clinical lesions, the darkfield examination is negative, and the cerebrospinal fluid examination is normal. Positive nontreponemal and treponemal serologic tests are the only manifestations of the disease during this stage. The latent stage is divided into the early latent (less than four years duration) and late latent (more than four years duration) phases. The early latent phase is infectious if there is relapse to the secondary stage, while the late latent stage is considered to be noninfectious.

The lesions of late syphilis involve virtually every organ system and tissue in man. The skeletal system is affected in about 5% of patients with late syphilis. Involvement of the cardiovascular and central nervous system (the most serious of complications) is responsible for 90% of deaths due to syphilis. The cardiovascular system may be affected as late as 20 to 30 years after acquisition of the infection. *T. pallidum* may invade the media of the ascending aorta, cause tissue destruction and loss of elasticity which ultimately may lead to aneurysm formation. Rupture of the aneurysm will cause death.

Neurosyphilis has a broad range of symptoms. Headache, vomiting, and malaise are symptoms of a meningitis that usually respond to appropriate therapy. Invasion of nervous system tissues by *T. pallidum* produces general paresis, tabes dorsalis, or optic atrophy. General paresis (dementia paralytica) usually occurs 10 to 25 years after the primary lesion. The disease begins with loss of memory, confusion, and impaired judgment, and progresses rapidly to the point where the patient is physically, socially and mentally disabled. General paresis is usually fatal within three years of its onset.

Tabes dorsalis (locomotor ataxia) may become evident 10 to 20 years after the primary lesion. Destruction of portions of the nervous system affect the patient's sense of joint position and results in a characteristic gait. "Lightning pains," sharp jabs of pain, are experienced by most patients with tabes dorsalis.

Syphilis may be transmitted from the infected mother to the fetus. Congenital syphilis may be manifested by severe dehydration and malnutrition. Roentgenographs of the long bones may demonstrate bone destruction and osteochondritis. Late congenital syphilis involving the CNS may appear as late as 20 years after birth. Eighth nerve deafness, optic atrophy, and juvenile paresis may also occur.

SYPHILIS

1. How is the diagnosis of syphilis made?

Darkfield microscopy provides the earliest means of diagnosing syphilis during the primary stage. The patient's immune response to the infection may not be sufficiently developed early in the disease process; consequently, serologic tests would be of no use.

Serous material obtained from the suspected syphilitic lesion is viewed through a microscope fitted with a darkfield condenser. Objects viewed through such equipment appear to be brightly illuminated when placed against a black background. A positive diagnosis is made if organisms of the characteristic morphology, and motility of *T. pallidum* are observed. Darkfield examination of oral lesions may be unreliable, since *T. microdentium,* a nonpathogen that is part of the normal flora of the mouth, is morphologically indistinguishable from *T. pallidum.*

Serologic tests provide the means for diagnosing syphilis in the absence of adequate histories or clinical manifestations. There are two types of tests used for the serodiagnosis of syphilis: nontreponemal tests and treponemal tests. The nontreponemal tests measure serum concentrations of reagin, a lipoidal antigen that is generated as part of a nonspecific immune response to an infectious or noninfectious disease (59).

Nontreponemal tests are not specific for *T. pallidum,* but they are inexpensive and useful for screening large numbers of people. The Venereal Disease Research Laboratory (VDRL) test is the most widely used nontreponemal test. The quantitative VDRL is much more useful than the qualitative test. Serum is geometrically diluted and the test is repeated on each dilution. The value reported is the most dilute serum concentration having a positive reaction.

Subsequent testing may be used to follow the progress of the disease or the effectiveness of therapy. If the titer of a patient receiving therapy increases by more than two dilutions, e.g., from a dilution of 1:4 to 1:16, the therapy is ineffective and another treatment regimen must be instituted. Usually, effective therapy will decrease the titer and eventually return the patient to a seronegative state. Quantitative VDRL tests are also required for those patients who remain serofast (i.e., have a consistent reactivity at the same titer for an indefinite period, perhaps for life); two dilution deviations in either direction from the "steady state" titer are indicative of disease relapse or return to seronegativity.

Reagin levels, usually negative or low in early primary syphilis, reach a peak during secondary syphilis. The reagin levels fall slowly during latent syphilis, so that the patient may eventually return to a seronegative state or may remain seropositive for life. The patient usually becomes seronegative 6 to 12 months after treatment for primary syphilis and 12 to 24 months after therapy for secondary syphilis.

The diagnosis of syphilis can be made on the basis of a positive medical history and physical examination, darkfield examinations, and a nontreponemal test. If all diagnostic components support the positive VDRL, then the more specific treponemal tests for syphilis should be employed. The VDRL must be repeated to rule out laboratory error.

Specific ***treponemal tests*** are used to help distinguish between a biologic false positive and a true positive test for syphilis, to assist in establishing a diagnosis of syphilis in those patients without clinical manifestations of syphilis, and to establish the diagnosis of syphilis in patients with evidence of the disease. The Fluorescent Treponemal Antibody Absorption (FTA-ABS) test is the test of choice for detecting syphilis in the early, primary, and latent stages of the infection. The Treponema Pallidum Immobilization (TPI) test is not used routinely because of its cost and complexity.

The FTA-ABS is based on an indirect fluorescent antibody reaction that occurs when a patient's serum is added to the antigen, *T. pallidum,* which is fixed to a glass slide. This preparation is stained with a fluorescein-labeled antihuman globulin. If any antitreponemal antibody is present in the patient's serum, the spirochetes will fluoresce. The FTA-ABS becomes positive earlier in primary syphilis and remains positive in more patients than does the VDRL.

2. What drugs should be used for the treatment of syphilis? What are the complications of therapy?

The drug of choice for the treatment of all stages of syphilis is penicillin (7,23). Every effort should be made to rule out penicillin allergy before choosing other antibiotics which have been studied much less extensively than penicillin in the treatment of syphilis.

If penicillin is contraindicated, the alternatives are tetracycline, erythromycin, clindamycin, cephaloridine, and cephalothin (Table 1). Since *T. pallidum* has not developed resistance to antibiotic treatment, drug regimens have not changed substantially over the years.

Primary, secondary, and latent syphilis (with a negative CSF) of less than one year's duration may be treated with a single intramuscular dose of 2.4 MU of benzathine penicillin G. Procaine penicillin G in oil with 2% aluminum monostearate is no longer available in the U. S., but in other countries a dose of 1.2 MU is injected into each buttock on the first visit and is followed by two additional doses of 1.2 MU in three-day intervals. Alternatively, aqueous procaine penicillin G can be administered intramuscularly 600,000 units daily for eight days (7). Late syphilis, neurosyphilis, and cardiovascular syphilis are treated with 2.4 MU of intramuscular benzathine penicillin G on the first visit. This dose is repeated twice at seven-day intervals. Aqueous procaine penicillin G 600,000 units intramuscularly daily for 15 days can be used as an alternative (7).

TABLE 1
ALTERNATIVE ANTIBIOTICS FOR
THE TREATMENT OF SYPHILIS

Antibiotic	Dose and Route	Frequency and Duration	Reference Source
Tetracycline	500 mg po	4 times daily for 15 days	(3,7)
Erythromycin	500 mg po	4 times daily for 15 days	(7)
Cephalothin	1.0 gm IM	Every 12 hrs for 20 days for primary syphilis	(62)
Cephalothin	1.0 gm IM	Every 12 hrs for 25 days for secondary syphilis	(62)
Cephaloridine	500 mg IM	Daily for 10 days for early syphilis	(36)

Once treatment is initiated, *T. pallidum* disappears from the infected lesions within 24 hours (34). Repeat physical examinations and quantitative VDRL tests should be performed at 1, 3, 6, 9, 12, 18, and 24 months (23). Return of lesions or a two-dilution increase in titer indicates the need for retreatment due to relapse or reinfection. In two years, all but a small percentage of patients with early syphilis become seronegative. If the disease is treated during the late stages, complete seroreversal may not occur; and while the disease process may have been halted, the damage that may have been done to the cardiovascular system or nervous system cannot be reversed.

The Jarisch-Herxheimer reaction is a benign, self-limiting complication of treponemal antibiotic therapy due to the sudden release of antigenic substances from rapidly killed treponemes. The resulting fever, malaise, and a worsening of the syphilitic lesions may be controlled with the use of antipyretics or corticosteroids. Penicillin allergy may also be a treatment complication. Incidence of penicillin allergy in venereal disease clinics is 6.61 cases per 1,000 patients (80), which is slightly below the 1% incidence in the general population (60).

3. A 27-year-old pregnant woman in the 19th week of gestation has a positive VDRL and a positive FTA-ABS. Is treatment indicated? How should she be treated?

Because transmission of syphilis to the fetus does not take place until the fifth month of gestation (36), treatment before the 18th week of gestation almost always prevents fetal infection. Therapy initiated after 18 weeks of gestation will cure the fetal spirochetemia, but may not prevent the development of congenital syphilis. If the mother is left untreated, the fetus may be aborted, stillborn, or may be born with congenital syphilis.

Pregnancy may cause false-positive reactions to both the nontreponemal (12,94) and the treponemal tests (82). A patient who is seropositive does not necessarily require therapy if, for example, she has been treated adequately, has no significant increase in titer (two dilutions or more), and has no signs of relapse. The patient who has recently become seropositive, has developed a two-dilution increase in titer, or shows signs of relapse or reinfection must be treated. During pregnancy, the patient should be followed with monthly quantitative VDRL titers to evaluate the effectiveness of therapy; thereafter, she should be followed as any other syphilitic patient.

The treatment of the pregnant patient with syphilis is the same as for other patients with the disease. Penicillin is the drug of choice (3). Primary, secondary, and latent syphilis of less than one year's duration may be treated with 2.4 million units of benzathine penicillin G given intramuscularly at a single session, or 4.8 million units total of aqueous procaine penicillin G given intramuscularly, 600,000 units daily for eight days (7). Latent syphilis of more than one year's duration, cardiovascular, late-benign, and neurosyphilis should be treated with three successive weekly intramuscular injections of 2.4 million units of benzathine penicillin G for a total of 7.2 million units. Aqueous procaine penicillin G may also be used if 600,000 units is given intramuscularly each day for 15 days (7).

Tetracycline should be avoided during pregnancy because of its effects on the fetus (tooth staining and damage to the long bones) (46,72) and its association with maternal liver and kidney damage (17,22). Erythromycin has been used with success in the treatment of pregnant patients with syphilis. Doses range from 250 to 500 mg orally 4 times daily for 15 days (3,36).

Erythromycin, however, achieves only 6 to 20% of the maternal blood levels in the fetus (88,95). This may explain why some patients treated with erythromycin aborted or gave birth to stillborn infants. Therefore, documentation of penicillin allergy is especially important before resorting to erythromycin. The estolate salt of erythromycin, like the tetracyclines, is not recommended because of potential adverse effects on mother and fetus (7). Clindamycin may be a more satisfactory alternative to penicillin than erythromycin, because it crosses the placental barrier more readily and predictably (73).

Cephaloridine may also be used for the pregnant syphilitic patient with penicillin allergy. Cephaloridine has been used in early syphilis in doses of 0.5 to 2 gms given intramuscularly daily for 3 to 32 days (27,31). A regimen of 0.5 gm given intramuscularly daily for 10 days was found to be effective in patients with early syphilis (30). For discussion of cross sensitivity with penicillin, see the chapter on **Principles of Antibiotic Therapy.**

If the VDRL performed on cord blood of the fetus is positive, both the FTA-ABS and FTA-ABS IgM should be performed. Because both the VDRL and FTA-ABS tests may become positive as a result of the passive transfer of antibodies in maternal blood to the fetus, the FTA-ABS IgM is the most reliable test for the detection of congenital syphilis (52). The test relies upon the detection of antitreponemal antibodies produced *in utero* by the fetus in response to *T. pallidum* infections. Since IgM does not cross the placenta, the presence of this antibody indicates that the fetus is infected by spirochetes. The newborn with congenital syphilis can be treated with intravenous aqueous penicillin G 100,000 units/kg divided into 10 daily doses; the maximum total dose is 3 million units (31). Infants with congenital syphilis should have a CSF examination before treatment and should return for repeat quantitative nontreponemal tests three, six, and 12 months after treatment. Additional guidelines for the treatment of congenital syphilis can be found with the Center for Disease Control (7).

GONORRHEA

4. What is the status of *N. gonorrhoeae* and *T. pallidum* resistance to antibiotics?

At present, evidence does not indicate that *T. pallidum* is developing resistance to the antibiotic agents used in its treatment. Although *T. pallidum* has occasionally persisted in the aqueous humor despite massive doses of penicillin (87,74a), it has not been possible to determine if this is due to antibiotic resistance.

The sulfa drugs were the mainstay treatment for gonorrheal infections until 1946, when resistance developed. When penicillin was introduced, the

minimum inhibitory concentration (MIC) for gonorrhea (0.003 to 0.030 U/ml) (77) was easily achieved with rather low doses of IM penicillin. In 1957 and 1958, reports of decreased gonococcal sensitivity to penicillin and treatment failures appeared (29, 93). At this time, the MIC of some strains of *N. gonorrhoeae* had increased to 0.20 U/ml (77).

Resistance to penicillin has since steadily increased throughout the world (1,8,37,53). In the Far East, the MICs for *N. gonorrhoeae* are among the highest in the world (0.25 to 0.50 U/ml) (45). This may be a result of the OTC availability of oral antibiotics in these countries.

Recent reports of penicillinase-producing strains of *N. gonorrhoeae* have caused concern. One hundred and fifty cases have been reported in the U. S., and additional cases have been identified in 16 different countries since May, 1977 (5,6,6a). Eleven of the U. S. isolates were linked to individuals who recently traveled through the Far East. This change in resistance mechanisms has initiated a worldwide search for penicillinase-producing strains of *N. gonorrhoeae*.

The CDC recommendation for the treatment of uncomplicated gonorrhea remains 4.8 million units of aqueous procaine penicillin G intramuscularly with 1 gm of probenecid orally (6). Spectinomycin should be administered to patients who remain positive on follow-up culture after initial treatment with recommended doses of penicillin, ampicillin, or tetracycline (6). All patients should be followed up with cultures in 3 to 7 days, rather than the usual 7 to 14 days after completion of therapy (6,6a).

The antibiotic resistance of *N. gonorrhoeae* is not limited to penicillin. Strains relatively insensitive to penicillin are usually highly resistant to streptomycin and moderately resistant to erythromycin, chloramphenicol, and tetracycline (74,78). Strains of *N. gonorrhoeae* resistant to spectinomycin have been reported in Denmark (79). In the U. S., three of the cases of penicillinase-producing *N. gonorrhoeae* (PPNG) were known to have been previously treated with 2-4 grams of spectinomycin and did not respond to therapy despite the fact that PPNG isolates from these failures were sensitive to spectinomycin *in vitro* (6a). Nonpenicillinase-producing gonococci with absolute resistance to spectinomycin have been detected in the U. S. (6b), and if spectinomycin is indiscriminately used resistance will increase.

The resistance to penicillin exhibited by most strains of *N. gonorrhoeae* is relative rather than absolute. Although the MIC has increased, antibiotic serum levels in excess of the MICs can still be achieved (19,47) by adding probenecid to the treatment regimen. This measure has reduced failure rates to less than 5%, even in areas where resistant strains are common (33,41,46,47). Probenecid blocks the renal tubular secretion of penicillin and ampicillin, resulting in a 50 to 100% increase in peak serum levels and a commensurate increase in the duration of effective serum levels (47). Eventually, it may be necessary to use alternate or additional antibacterial therapy and to prolong treatment to prevent the emergence of more resistant strains.

5. How is gonorrhea diagnosed?

In a male, a purulent urethral discharge occurring 4 to 10 days after sexual contact is sufficient evidence to make a presumptive diagnosis of gonorrhea (9). The subsequent demonstration of intracellular gram-negative diplococci in the gram stained exudate confirms the diagnosis. If the gram stain is negative, the exudate should be cultured on Thayer-Martin (TM) medium, an enriched chocolate agar to which vancomycin, colistimethate, and nystatin have been added (93). Cultures from both the oral and anal orifice should also be obtained if warranted by history.

The most useful test for the screening of women with asymptomatic gonorrhea is an endocervical culture, which is positive in 80% of cases (49). This test should be a part of every pelvic examination of sexually active women. After treatment, the anal canal should be cultured as a test of cure, since the organism persists here in approximately 25% of treatment failures. Nevertheless, diagnosing gonorrhea in women from cultures is a major problem because vaginal and rectal organisms commonly overgrow and obscure the gonococcus. Swarming overgrowths of Proteus and other organisms with colonial morphology resembling N. Gonorrhoeae that are not inhibited by the TM medium make diagnosis of gonorrhea sometimes difficult. Additionally, the vancomycin and colistin in the TM medium can inhibit as much as 8% of the cultures with a definite population of gonococci. Therefore, a completely satisfactory laboratory method for the diagnosis of gonococci is probably dependent upon the development of a specific diagnostic antiserum or a specific serological technique (7a).

6. How is uncomplicated gonorrhea (GC) treated?

Unless contraindicated, penicillin or ampicillin are the drugs of choice for the treatment of GC of the urethra, cervix, pharynx, or rectum. The treatment schedules recommended by the CDC should be adhered to in order to minimize the incidence of treatment failures.

Single-dose regimens administered at the time of examination are considered superior to multiple-dose regimens that depend upon patient compliance for the completion of the course of therapy. Long-acting penicillins such as benzathine penicillin should not be used for the treatment of gonorrhea, because they do not achieve adequate tissue levels, and low serum levels of penicillin serve only to select out resistant gonococci (100).

TABLE 2
CENTER FOR DISEASE CONTROL RECOMMENDATIONS FOR TREATMENT OF UNCOMPLICATED GONORRHEA

Drug	Regimen	Success Rate	Ref Source
Aqueous procaine penicillin G	4.8×10^6 units IM in two injections at one visit plus 1.0 gm probenecid 30 minutes before the injection.	96.8%	43
-OR- Ampicillin	3.5 gm po with 1.0 gm probenecid given simultaneously at one visit.	92.8%	43

If penicillin is contraindicated, the following drugs may be used as alternatives:

Spectinomycin	2 gm IM in one injection for men and women	94.8%	43
-OR- Tetracycline	1.5 gm po initially, followed by 0.5 gm po 4 times daily for 4 days for a total dosage of 9 gm.	96.2%	43

About 3% of patients with gonorrhea also have syphilis (26). Although the penicillin regimens recommended by the CDC effectively eradicate existing incubating syphilis (83), alternative antibiotics may not be effective in the recommended doses. For example, 15 grams of tetracycline must be taken to achieve the same effect (83), and spectinomycin is inactive against syphilis and may mask the incubating disease (81). Spectinomycin is recommended by the CDC for those patients who have failed to respond to penicillin or are allergic to penicillin, procaine, or probenecid. While the reports of gonorrhea strains resistant to spectinomycin are few, it is essential that the use of spectinomycin be limited, in order to delay the development of resistance and prolong its usefulness (79). Although a larger dose has been recommended for women, there is no evidence that a 4-gm dose is more effective than 2 gms (54). A 2-gm dose produces cure rates in excess of 95% in both sexes (70) and is a CDC recommendation (5).

Congeners of tetracycline (demeclocycline, doxycycline, and minocycline) have been used to treat uncomplicated gonorrhea. The primary advantage of the long-acting tetracyclines over the hydrochloride salt is that they may be given less frequently (twice daily), which may improve patient compliance. The long-acting tetracyclines are, however, no more effective than generic tetracycline hydrochloride in eradicating uncomplicated gonorrheal infections of the urethra and are frequently more expensive.

The following dosage regimens have been employed for the long-acting tetracyclines:

demeclocycline 600 mg po at once, then 300 mg po every 12 hours for 4 days for a total dose of 2 gm.

doxycycline 200 mg po at once, then 100 mg po every 12 hours for 3 days.

minocycline 200 mg po at once, then 100 mg every 12 hours for 3 days.

Although oral tetracyclines are widely used for the therapy of gonorrhea, the MICs of gonococci for tetracycline are higher than for penicillin, and clinical failures may be more common. Furthermore, tetracycline therapy permits viable gonococci to persist for longer periods after initiation of therapy, thereby allowing for transmissions to other contacts (7a). Therefore, penicillins are clearly the agents of choice if patients are not allergic to them.

7. How does one determine whether drug therapy of GC has been effective?

The absence of discharge and symptoms following therapy is inadequate proof of cure. For males, smears of genital and anal secretions should be made four to seven days after treatment. If the smear is positive, then retreatment is indicated. If it is negative, then a repeat culture on Thayer-Martin medium should be obtained; a positive culture is an indication for retreatment.

For women, repeat cultures should be taken from the endocervical canal, anus, and pharynx if warranted by history. Two successive negative cultures are required for proof of cure following antigonorrheal therapy.

TABLE 3
FAILURE RATES OF THE CEPHALOSPORINS WHEN USED IN A SINGLE DOSE FOR UNCOMPLICATED GONOCOCCAL URETHRITIS

		% Failure	Ref. Source
cefazolin	1 gm IM x 1	42%	(42)
	2 gm IM x 1	10-25%	(42,61)
	3 gm IM x 1	11%	(61)
cephapirin	4 gm IM x 1	80%	(96)
cephaloridine	2 gm IM x 1	5-17%	(51,56) (63,64,85)
cephalexin	2 gm po x 1	55%	(65)
	3 gm po with 1-2 gm probenecid	8-14%	(29,65,99)
cephalothin	2 gm IM x 1	50-80%	(59,86)

8. Are the cephalosporins effective alternatives to penicillin therapy in the treatment of uncomplicated gonococcal urethritis?

Although the cephalosporins have been used to treat penicillin-resistant GC, there is a high incidence of cross resistance (51,63,64). Also, the cephalosporins are not as effective as penicillin when given in single-dose regimens (see Table 3). Failure rates could be decreased by adding probenecid and/or by repeating doses of the cephalosporins. The use of cephalosporins in penicillin-allergic patients is controversial, since the question of cross-allergenicity between these two antibiotics has not been settled (71). (See chapter of **General Principles of Antibiotic Therapy.** For these reasons, cephalosporins are generally poor alternatives to penicillin in the treatment of GC urethritis.

9. How is pelvic inflammatory disease (PID) treated?

Pelvic inflammatory disease, which is a complication of GC, occurs in up to 10% of females with gonococcal infections (41,76). PID results when gonococci migrate from the cervix into the uterus and through the fallopian tubes into the peritoneal cavity (peritonitis). Abcess formation may occur in the pelvic or abdominal cavity and in one or both of the fallopian tubes.

Acute PID is manifested by severe cramp-like, nonradiating lower abdominal pain accompanied by chills, fever, and leukocytosis (11,40). Since cultures generally grow a variety of bacteria rather than a pure N. gonorrhoeae, broad spectrum penicillins or antibiotic combinations may be used. Treatment of these patients varies with the severity of the infection.

Mild infections may be treated on an outpatient basis with oral ampicillin 1.0 to 1.5 gm or tetracycline 500 mg four times daily for 7 to 10 days (57). Patients with moderate and severe infections should be hospitalized and treated with parenteral antibiotics. Patients with moderate infections should be given parenteral ampicillin 6.0 gm or cephalothin 8.0 gm each day for seven to ten days. Patients with severe infection should be given penicillin G 20 MU and an aminoglycoside parenterally each day. Treatment is continued for several days after the fever subsides.

10. How should the dermatitis and arthritis of gonococcemia be treated?

Gonorrheal bacteremia, another complication of GC, occurs in 1 to 3% of women and 1% of men. The most common manifestation of gonococcemia is the gonococcal arthritis-dermatitis syndrome. Symptoms include fever, chills (occasional), tenosynovitis, and skin lesions that are petechial, papular, pustular, and hemorrhagic in appearance. Blood cultures are positive for N. gonorrhoeae, but the skin lesions are not. Purulent synovial effusions may develop if treatment is delayed or inadequate (38).

The drug of choice for the treatment of gonococcal dermatitis is intravenous penicillin G 4.5 MU every two hours for two days, followed by 12 MU daily for 11 days

(10). Gonococcal arthritis, the most common cause of infectious arthritis (18), is five times more common in women than men (32). It tends to be polyarticular and most commonly involves the wrist or the knee. If untreated, erosion of the cartilage and adjacent bony structures may occur (48). Gonococcal arthritis should be treated with IV aqueous penicillin G 10 to 20 MU daily for seven to ten days or aqueous procaine penicillin G 6 MU every 12 hours for 14 days (44,75).

11. What are the characteristics and treatment for gonococcal carditis and meningitis (44,75)?

The incidence of gonococcal carditis has declined with the introduction of antibiotics. Involvement of the heart is a life-threatening complication of GC, because death may occur from septic emboli, valve damage, or congestive heart failure. Gonococcal carditis should be treated with massive doses of intravenous penicillin G until cultures are negative (48).

Gonococcal meningitis mimics meningococcal meningitis and may occur in adults with genitourinary gonorrhea or in infected newborns (13). Treatment may be accomplished with aqueous penicillin G 2 MU every two hours for two days, followed by 12 MU daily for 11 days (90).

12. A newborn has been diagnosed as having gonococcal ophthalmia neonatorum. Will topical antibiotics resolve the infection? How could it have been prevented?

Gonococcal ophthalmia, while primarily a neonatal disease (48), may occur in adults and older children as well (35). The infection is usually acquired as the fetus passes through the infected birth canal. An acute purulent conjunctivitis classically develops three to four days after birth, but the appearance of signs of conjunctivitis may be significantly delayed beyond this time. Corneal scarring, which leads to blindness, may occur at any age if due to a gonococcal eye infection (7a).

The incidence of gonococcal ophthalmia neonatorum has been reduced substantially since the routine administration of eyedrops of 1% silver nitrate to newborns has become widespread (2). Treatment failures have resulted when the drops have been applied incorrectly or the infection was well-established at the time of delivery. Topical antibiotics should not be used for the prophylaxis of gonococcal ophthalmia neonatorum, because they have not been shown to be efficacious and because their use may needlessly sensitize the infant to antibiotics (39).

Treatment of gonococcal ophthalmia neonatorum may include both topical and systemic antibiotics. Irrigation with penicillin G 200,000 U/ml saline has been used with IM procaine penicillin G 200,000 U/kg daily (39). Adults have been treated successfully with 2.4 to 4.8 MU of IM procaine penicillin G IM and topical broad spectrum antibiotics, such as Neosporin (36). The treatment of gonococcal ophthalmia with topical antibiotics alone is not recommended, because infections of the anus and respiratory tract may coexist.

13. What are the manifestations, significance, and treatment of oral gonorrheal infections?

Oral infections due to N. gonorrhoeae include pharyngitis (25,66,91), tongue ulceration (20), and a pharyngitis that leads to gonococcal septicemia with arthritis and dermatitis (14,49,58). Such infections occur in 5 to 11% of patients with urogenital GC (15,89,97).

The danger of oral GC is that the majority of cases are asymptomatic and may thus serve as reservoirs for the infection (15,89,97). The disease is transmitted from the genitals to the oropharyngeal tissues (97); the reverse may also occur (24). The symptoms of oropharyngeal gonococcal infection, range from a mild to moderate sore throat to an acute febrile tonsilitis (15).

These infections are particularly resistant to treatment, with the reported failure rates as high as 60% (15,97). The most successful regimen utilizes po tetracycline 2.0 gm daily for five days (97). In one study, failure occurred in 2 of 45 patients given the recommended doses of procaine penicillin (4.8 MU with and without probenecid) and in 7 of 13 patients given a single 4.0 gm dose of IM spectinomycin (97).

REFERENCES

1. Amies CR: Sensitivity of N. Gonorrhoeae to penicillin and other antibiotics. Brit J Vener Dis 45:216, 1969.
2. Anon: Prophylaxis of gonococcal ophthalmia. Medical Letter 12:38, 1970.
3. Anon: Treatment and prevention of syphilis and gonorrhea. Medical Letter 13:85, 1971.
4. Anon: Recommended treatment schedules for gonorrhea. USPHS Morbidity and Mortality Weekly Report 21:82, 1972.
5. Anon: Penicillinase-producing Neiserria gonorrhoeae. USPHS Morbidity and Mortality Weekly Report 25:261, 1976.
6. Anon: Follow-up on penicillinase-producing Neisseria gonorrhoeae. USPHS Morbidity and Mortality Weekly Report 25:101, 1976.
6a. Anon: Follow-up on penicillinase-producing Neisseria gonorrhoeae — worldwide. USPHS Morbidity and Mortality Weekly Report 26:153, 1977.
6.b Anon: Follow-up on antibiotic resistance to Neisseria gonorrhoeae. USPHS Morbitity and Mortality Weekly Report 26:29, 1977.
7. Anon: Syphilis — CDC recommended treatment schedules, 1976. USPHS Morbidity and Mortality Weekly Report 25:101, 1976.
7a. Anthony BF et al: Gonococcal infections — laboratory, clinical, and epidemiological aspects. West J Med 120:456, 1974.
8. Arya OP et al: Antibiotic sensitivity of gonococci and treatment of gonorrhea in Uganda. Brit J Vener Dis 46:149, 1970.
9. Ashamalla G et al: Recent clinicolaboratory observations in the treatment of acute gonococcal urethritis in men. JAMA

195:1115, 1966.

10. Barr J et al: Septic gonococcal dermatitis. Brit Med J 1:482, 1971.
11. Benson RC: Gynecology and obstetrics, in *Current Diagnosis and Treatment,* Ed by H Brainerd et al. Lange Medical Publications, Palo Alto, California, 1969, p 433.
12. Boak RA et al: Biologic false positive reactions for syphilis in pregnancy as determined by the treponema pallidum immobilization test. Surg Gyn Obstet 101:751, 1955.
13. Branham SE et al: Gonococcic meningitis. JAMA 110:1804, 1938.
14. Bro-Jørgensen A et al: Gonococcal tonsillar infections. Brit Med J 4:660, 1971.
15. Bro-Jørgensen A et al: Gonococcal pharyngeal infections — Report of 110 cases. Brit J Vener Dis 49:491, 1973.
16. Clark DO: Gonorrhea: Changing concepts in diagnosis and management. Clin Obstet Gyn 16:3, 1973.
17. Clendenning WE: Complications of tetracycline therapy. Arch Derm 91:628, 1965.
18. Cooke CL et al: Gonococcal arthritis. JAMA 217:204, 1971.
19. Cornelius CE III et al: Variations in serum concentrations of penicillin after injections of aqueous procaine penicillin G with and without oral probenecid. Brit J Vener Dis 47:359, 1971.
20. Cowan L: Gonococcal ulceration of the tongue in the gonococcal dermatitis syndrome. Brit J Vener Dis 45:228, 1969.
21. Curtis FR et al: A comparison of the in vitro sensitivity of gonococci to penicillin with the results of treatment. Brit J Vener Dis 34:70, 1958.
22. Dowling HF et al: Hepatic reactions to tetracycline. JAMA 188:307, 1964.
23. Drusin LM: The diagnosis and treatment of infections and latent syphilis. Med Clin N Amer 56:1161, 1972.
24. Evrard JR: Spread of gonococcal pharyngitis to the genitals. Am J Obstet Gyn 117:856, 1973.
25. Fiumara NJ et al: Gonorrheal pharyngitis. NEJM 276:1248, 1967.
26. Fiumara NJ: The diagnosis and treatment of gonorrhea. Med Clin N Amer 56:1105, 1972.
27. Flarer F: On the antitreponemic action of cephaloridine. Postgrad Med J 43 (suppl): 133, 1967.
28. Fleming WL et al: National survey of venereal disease treated by physicians in 1968. JAMA 211:1827, 1970.
29. Fowler W: Discussion. Postgrad Med J 46 (suppl): 106, 1970.
30. Glicksman JM et al: Parenteral cephaloridine treatment of patients with early syphilis. Arch Int Med 121:342, 1968.
31. Gonzaliez-Ochoa A et al: The treatment of early syphilis with cephaloridine. Postgrad Med J 43 (suppl): 134, 1967.
32. Goobar JE et al: Rheumatological manifestations of gonorrhea. AIR 7:1, 1964.
33. Gundersen T et al: Treatment of gonorrhea by one oral dose of ampicillin and probenecid combined. Brit J Vener Dis 45:235, 1969.
34. Guthe T: Treponemal disease, in Cecil-Loeb *Textbook of Medicine,* Ed. by PB Beeson and W McDermott, W.B. Saunders, Philadelphia, 1971, p 655.
35. Harbin T et al: Gonococcal conjunctivitis. Ann Ophth 6: 221, 1974.
36. Holder WR et al: Syphilis in pregnancy. Med Clin N Amer 56:1151, 1972.
37. Holmes KK et al: Studies of venereal disease: Probenecid-procaine penicillin G combination and tetracycline hydrochloride in the treatment of penicillin resistant gonorrhea in men. JAMA 202:461, 1967.
38. Holmes KK et al: The gonococcal arthritis-dermatitis syndrome. Ann Int Med 75:470, 1971.
39. Holmes KK: Gonococcal infection — clinical, epidemiologic, and laboratory perspectives. Adv Int Med 19:259, 1974.
40. Jacobsen L et al: Objectivized diagnosis of acute pelvic inflammatory disease. Am J Obstet Gyn 105:1088, 1969.
41. Johnson DW et al: Antibiotic treatment of asymptomatic gonorrhea in hospitalized women. NEJM 283:1, 1970.
42. Karney WW et al: Cefazolin in the treatment of gonorrhea. J Infec Dis 129 (suppl): 5399, 1973.
43. Kaufman RE et al: National gonorrhea therapy monitoring study: treatment results. NEJM 294:1, 1976.
44. Keiser H et al: Clinical forms of gonococcal arthritis. NEJM 297:234, 1968.

45. Keys TF et al: Single-dose treatment of gonorrhea with selected antibiotic agents. JAMA 210:857, 1969.
46. Kline AH et al: Transplacental effect of tetracycline on teeth. JAMA 188:178, 1964.
47. Krale PA et al: Single oral dose ampicillin-probenecid treatment of gonorrhea in the male. JAMA 215:1449, 1971.
48. Kraus SJ: Complications of gonococcal infection. Med Clin N Amer 56:115, 1972.
49. LaLuna F et al: Gonococcal pharyngitis and arthritis. Ann Int Med 75:649, 1971.
50. Lucas JB et al: Cephalothin therapy in male gonorrhea. Antimicrob Agents Chemother 5:686, 1965.
51. Lucas JB et al: Treatment of gonorrhea in males with cephaloridine. JAMA 195:919, 1966.
52. Mamunes P et al: Early diagnosis of neonatal syphilis. Am J Dis Child 120:17, 1970.
53. Martin JE Jr et al: Comparative study of gonococcal susceptibility to penicillin in the United States, 1955-1969. J Infect Dis 122:459, 1970.
54. McCormack W et al: Spectinomycin. Ann Int Med 84:712, 1976.
55. McKenzie-Pollock JS: Physician reporting of venereal disease in the United States. Brit J Vener Dis 46:114, 1970.
56. McLone DG et al: Cephaloridine treatment of gonorrhea in the female. Brit J Vener Dis 44:220, 1968.
57. Mead PB et al: Antibiotics in pelvic infections. Clin Obstet Gyn 12:219, 1969.
58. Metzger AL: Gonococcal arthritis complicating gonorrheal pharyngitis. Ann Int Med 73:267, 1970.
59. Miller SE: Ch 16, The laboratory diagnosis of venereal infections, in *A Textbook of Clinical Pathology,* 7th ed., Ed. by SE Miller. Williams and Wilkins Co., Baltimore, 1966, p. 757.
60. Minkin W et al: Incidence of immediate systemic penicillin reactions. Milit Med 133:557, 1968.
61. Nelson M: Cefazolin in the treatment of uncomplicated gonorrhea in men. J Infect Dis 128 (suppl): 5404, 1973.
62. Nicolis G et al: Cephalothin in the treatment of syphilis. Brit J Vener Dis 50:220, 1974.
63. Oller LZ: Cephaloridine in gonorrhea and syphilis. Brit J Vener Dis 43:39, 1967.
64. Oller LZ: Further experience with cephaloridine in gonorrhea. Postgrad Med J 43 (suppl): 124, 1967.
65. Oller LZ et al: Cephaloridine and cephalexin in venereologic practice. Postgrad Med J 46 (suppl): 99, 1970.
66. Owens RL et al: Rectal and pharyngeal gonorrhea in homosexual men. JAMA 220:1315, 1972.
67. Pariser H et al: Asymptomatic gonorrhea in the male. South Med J 56:688, 1964.
68. Pariser H et al: Gonorrhea — frequently unrecognized reservoirs. South Med J 63:198, 1970.
69. Pariser H: Asymptomatic gonorrhea. Med Clin N Am 56:1127, 1972.
70. Pedersen AHB et al: Spectinomycin and penicillin G in the treatment of gonorrhea: A comparative evaluation. JAMA 220:205, 1972.
71. Petz LD: Immunologic reactions of humans to cephalosporins. Postgrad Med J 47 (suppl): 64, 1971.
72. Pflug GR: Toxicities associated with tetracycline therapy. Am J Pharm 135:438, 1963.
73. Philipson A et al: Transplacental passage of erythromycin and clindamycin. NEJM 288:1219, 1973.
74. Phillips I et al: In vitro activity of twelve antibacterial agents against Neisseria gonorrhoeae. Lancet 1:263, 1970.
74a. Pirozzi DJ: Syphilis and penicillin. Ann Int Med 79:447, 1974.
75. Poske RM et al: Gonococcal arthritic, General Pract. 39:91, 1969.
76. Rees R et al: Gonococcal salpingitis. Brit J Vener Dis 45:205, 1969.
77. Reyn A et al: Effects of penicillin, streptomycin and tetracycline on N. gonorrhoeae isolated in 1944 and 1957. Brit J Vener Dis 34:227, 1958.
78. Reyn A et al: Relationships between the sensitivities in vitro of Neisseria gonorrhoeae to spiramycin, penicillin, streptomycin, tetracycline, and erythromycin. Brit J Vener Dis 45:223, 1969.
79. Reyn A et al: Spectinomycin hydrochloride in the treatment of gonorrhea. Observations of resistant strains of Neisseria gonorrhoeae. Brit J Vener Dis 49:54-59, 1973.
80. Rudolph AH et al: Penicillin reactions among patients in ve-

nereal disease clinics: a national surgery. JAMA 223:499, 1973.

81. Rudolph AH: Control of gonorrhea. Guidelines for antibiotic treatment. JAMA 220:1587, 1972.

82. Salo OP et al: False-positive serological tests for syphilis in pregnancy. Acta Derm Venerol 49:332, 1969.

83. Schroeter AL et al: Therapy for incubating syphilis — Effectiveness of gonorrhea treatment. JAMA 218:711, 1971.

84. Schroeter AL et al: The rectal culture as a test of cure of gonorrhea in the female. J Infect Dis 125:499, 1972.

85. Shapiro LG et al: Therapy of female gonorrhea with cephaloridine. Am J Obstet Gyn 108:471, 1970.

86. Smith EB: Cephalothin in gonococcal urethritis. Curr Ther Res 9:79, 1967.

87. Smith JJL: Treponemes in human aqueous humor and cerebrospinal fluid after penicillin therapy and transfer of syphilitic infection to the experimental animal, in *Spirochetes in Late Seronegative Syphilis, Penicillin Notwithstanding.* Charles C. Thomas, Springfield, Ill., 1969, p. 287.

88. South MA et al: Failure of erythromycin estolate therapy in utero syphilis. JAMA 190:70, 1964.

89. Stolz E et al: Gonococcal, oro- and nasopharyngeal infections. Brit J Vener Dis 50:104, 1974.

90. Taubin HL et al: Gonococcal meningitis. NEJM 285:504, 1971.

91. Thatcher RW et al: Asymptomatic gonorrhea. JAMA 210:315, 1969.

92. Thayer JD et al: The sensitivity of gonococci to penicillin and its relationship to "penicillin failures." Antibiot Chemother 7:306, 1957.

93. Thayer JD et al: Improved medium selective for cultivation of N. gonorrhoeae and N. meningitides. Pub Health Rep 81:559, 1966.

94. Tuffanelli DL et al: Fluorescent treponemal-antibody absorption tests: Studies of false positive reactions to tests for syphilis. NEJM 276:258, 1967.

95. Weinstein L: Ch. 60. Antibiotics: Miscellaneous antibiotic agents, in *The Pharmacological Basis of Therapeutics,* 4th ed., Ed. by LS Goodman and A Gilman, The Macmillan Co., New York, 1970.

96. Wiesner P et al: Evaluation of a new cephalosporin antibiotic, cephapirin. Antimicrob Agents Chemother 1:303, 1972.

97. Weisner PJ et al: Clinical spectrum of pharyngeal gonococcal infection. NEJM 288:181, 1973.

98. Wiesner PJ et al: Low antibiotic resistance of gonococci causing disseminated infection. NEJM 288:1221, 1973.

99. Willcox RR et al: Cephalexin in the oral treatment of gonorrhea by a double dose method. Postgrad Med J 46 (suppl): 103, 1970.

100. Willcox R: A survey of problems in the antibiotic treatment of gonorrhea with special reference to Southeast Asia. Brit J Vener Dis 46:217, 1970.

101. Willmott FE: Transfer of gonococcal pharyngitis by kissing? Brit J Vener Dis 50:317, 1974.

Chapter 41

Diseases of the Skin

C. A. Bond

There are many over-the-counter (OTC) products which cure or improve minor dermatological problems. In order to use these OTC products correctly and make appropriate suggestions for prescription medication, clinicians must have a thorough knowledge of the disease state and its response to treatment. They must also be familiar with the efficacy and potential toxicities of all dermatologicals, as well as the dermatological toxicities of drugs used for other conditions. Before proceeding, a few general approaches to dermatological problems should be summarized. These are some of the more commonly encountered types of dermatoses and their treatments:

Acute Lesions — Acute lesions are characterized by redness, swelling, heat, itching and oozing. Generally, the more severe the dermatitis, the milder the initial topical therapy should be. The initial treatment for acute lesions should be a wet dressing. A soft cloth soaked in either Burow's Solution (1:20 - 1:40), which has astringent and antiseptic effects, or normal saline applied to the lesion for 15 minutes will provide rapid relief. The dressings provide evaporative cooling which causes vasoconstriction and a slowing of the oozing process. Burow's Solution 1:40 can be prepared by dissolving one Domeboro packet or tablet in a pint of water. If large areas of the body are involved, the patient should take a cool bath several times a day. Other topical medications should generally be withheld until the acute inflammatory process subsides.

Subacute and Chronic Lesions — There are no absolute rules for treating subacute or chronic lesions. Generally, if the lesion is dry, an oleaginous or occlusive preparation should be used. If there are extensive, thick, or hyperkeratotic areas, a keratolytic may be incorporated into the vehicle or used separately. If there are extensive excoriations, cotton gloves should be used. In chronic conditions, the choice of preparation will often depend more on patient preference than on scientific selection.

Pruritus — Pruritus is the most common cutaneous symptom. It has many different causes and has been associated with numerous systemic diseases. Among these are obstructive biliary disease, anemia, hypertension, gout, various malignant diseases, thyroid disease (both hyper and hypo), diabetes mellitus, and pregnancy (usually the first trimester) (72). In the absence of a cutaneous dermatitis, a careful history and physical exam should be performed to rule out one of the systemic causes of pruritus.

Although often detrimental, scratching is the most commonly encountered method of relief for pruritus. By this means the receptor nerve endings are probably damaged or fatigued. Therefore, one would expect topically applied local anesthetics or antihistamines to be effective in dulling the sensation, but this approach is often disappointing, probably because of the poor absorption of the salt forms of the drugs through the intact epidermis and the low concentrations used in over-the-counter preparations. An additional drawback to the use of these agents is their ability to cause an allergic contact dermatitis.

Cold water is effective in the relief of pruritis as are products containing aluminum acetate (Burow's Solution), tannic acid, or calamine.

Moisturizing mixtures such as Keri Lotion, Lubriderm, or simply, mineral or baby oil can be advantageous in the treatment or pruritus caused by dry skin, which is often encountered in the elderly. Bathing should be restricted to avoid additional drying and the irritant effect of alkaline soaps, as well as the trauma of toweling.

Topical steroid applications can be very effective. They reduce inflammation and are often contained in a cream base which helps to soothe the affected area. However, atrophy of the skin may eventually result from prolonged use.

Systemic antihistamines evoke a favorable response for many patients suffering from pruritus, although their major beneficial effect may be due to sedation. There is disagreement concerning which antihistamines or anti-serotonin agents are most efficacious in the treatment of pruritus (47,60). There is some evidence that hydroxyzine may be more effective than diphenhydramine or cyproheptadine (11, 147), but additional study is needed to confirm these findings.

1. A 49-year-old psoriatic, who used betamethasone 0.1% cream twice daily and at bedtime under a "space suit" (plastic occlusive dressings) for many years, states that he is going to discontinue his corticosteroid cream because he feels it is not helpful. (55% of his body is involved with psoriasis). Besides a potential exacerbation of his psoriasis, what other problems might this patient encounter?

While absorption of topical corticosteroids is usually negligible, occlusive dressings can enhance the absorption and thus cause suppression of the adrenal cortex. If therapy is abruptly discontinued, adrenal insufficiency may occur. (157, 158)

2. Do any of the fluorinated corticosteroid creams differ significantly from one another or from hydrocortisone in their topical effectiveness or side effects? Are assay procedures available to determine the availability of a steroid from its base?

The various proprietary formulations of topical corticosteroids offer a range of potencies (table 2).

A human bioassay procedure based on the intensity of blanching of the skin is useful in predicting the bioavailability and clinical effectiveness of various corticosteroid topical preparations (167). Clinical response is also evaluated by applying the agents to areas of experimentally produced irritation (67, 83).

The side effects of topical corticosteroids are related to the potency of the steroid, its penetrability, and the duration of therapy. A slightly higher incidence of side effects is associated with the newer, more potent topical corticosteroids, but this is rarely a problem clinically, and if side effects do occur, they are usually reversible. Tables 1 and 2 list the side effects observed with topical corticosteroids and the relative potencies of various products (42, 62, 68, 141, 165, 167).

Hydrocortisone or a less potent fluorinated preparation should generally be used as the initial treatment of large areas of skin or when prolonged therapy is anticipated. More potent preparations should be used only after an inadequate response.

3. Is there any difference among ointment, cream, gel, and lotion bases with respect to the activity of corticosteroids contained within them?

If equal amounts of a corticosteroid are formulated in appropriate ointment, gel, cream, and lotion bases, the gel and ointment bases are generally more active (13, 14, 62). (See Table 2 as well as chapter on ***Glucocorticoids***.)

4. Combination antimicrobial topical ointments are often used for self-limiting, minor infections. What problems may arise from such use? Are these preparations effective?

There have been many reports of contact dermatitis caused by topical antimicrobials. Neomycin sensitivity has been reported in 50% of patients with allergic eczematous contact dermatitis (49), 6% of patients patch tested with common allergens (150), and 8% of randomly chosen subjects tested with both patch and intradermal methods (132). Also, a high incidence of sensitization was reported when preparations containing this agent were used in long-term treatment of leg ulcers (92). The steroid contained in many neomycin preparations does not prevent these allergic reactions, although it may decrease their severity.

If the patient has been sensitized to neomycin, the incidence of cross reactions to gentamicin is 40% (135), to streptomycin 10-90% (135, 51), and kanamycin 56% (136). (See also Question 33.)

Neomycin is generally considered effective against *Staphylococcus* and many gram-negative organisms; it is less effective against *Streptococcus*. Usually it is combined with bacitracin or polymyxin in topical preparations.

Hypersensitivity reactions, usually manifested by a rash, have followed the topical use of nitrofurazone

Table 1
TOPICAL CORTICOSTEROID SIDE EFFECTS

1) Systemic effects — see Question 1.
2) Delayed healing
3) Atrophy and fragility of the skin
4) Telangiectasia
5) Striae
6) Rebound pustulation
7) Increased incidence and spread of infections
8) Masking of infections such as *Tinea* or scabies

Table 2
POTENCIES OF TOPICAL CORTICOSTEROIDS

Most Potent:

Halcinonide (Halog) cream	0.1%
Fluocinolone acetonide acetate (Lidex) cream	0.05%
Fluocinolone acetonide acetate (Lidex) ointment	0.05%
Fluocinolone acetonide acetate (Topsyn) gel	0.05%

Very Potent:

Betamethasone diproprionate (Diprosone) cream	0.05%
Betamethasone-17-benzoate (Benisone, Fluorobate) gel	0.025%
Betamethasone 17-valerate (Valisone) lotion	0.1%
Betamethasone 17-valerate (Valisone) ointment	0.1%
Triamcinolone acetonide (Aristocort) cream	0.5%

Moderately Potent:

Fluocinolone acetonide (Synalar) cream	0.2%
Triamcinolone acetonide (Aristocort, Kenalog) ointment	0.1%
Fluocinolone acetonide (Synalar) ointment	0.025%
Flurandrenolide (Cordran) ointment	0.05%

Potent:

Fluocinolone acetonide (Synalar) cream	0.025%
Triamcinolone acetonide (Kenalog) lotion	0.025%
Triamcinolone acetonide (Kenalog) cream	0.1%
Flurandrenolide (Cordran) cream	0.05%
Betamethasone 17 valerate (Valisone) cream	0.1%

Less Potent:

Flumethasone pivalate (Locorten) cream	0.03%
Desonide (Tridesilone) cream	0.05%

Less potent than the above but clinically useful are preparations containing hydrocortisone, dexamethasone, or methylprednisolone.

(Furacin). Because the overall incidence of sensitization is relatively high, nitrofurazone is not recommended for the treatment of bacterial infections complicating serious burns.

Ethylenediamine, employed as a stabilizer in ointment preparations such as Mycolog (neomycin, nystatin, gramicidin and triamcinolone acetonide), has been associated with contact dermatitis (48). Tetracycline and oxyquinoline (e.g. Vioform) topical preparations can also cause sensitivity reactions.

If the skin infection is severe, deep, or is associated with fever and other systemic manifestations, systemic antimicrobials should be used. If a topical antibiotic preparation is indicated, it should be employed with full awareness of its sensitizing properties (37, 38, 134).

5. A patient with a history of chronic eczema will need routine vaccinations for travel. Should this patient be given any special instructions?

Smallpox vaccinations are contraindicated in patients with eczema and pemphigus, because they predispose the patient to severe disseminated vaccinia. Since the patient can also become infected through contact with a vaccinated person, none of the patient's family can be vaccinated unless they assume separate residence until the scab has fallen off. A letter of explanation should be obtained from the patient's physician so that difficulty getting back into the country can be minimized (41).

6. How effective is zinc sulfate in accelerating wound healing?

The evidence that oral zinc improves wound healing is unsatisfactory. Although oral zinc therapy may be useful in patients with dietary deficiency, zinc deficiency is probably only partially responsible for the delayed healing. A few studies indicate oral zinc benefits wound healing, but other factors (e.g. ascorbic acid deficiency) that could have been responsible for the delayed wound healing were not considered (36, 69, 159).

While dosages of zinc vary, it is generally thought that a 220 mg dose of zinc sulfate given orally tid for 7 to 8 weeks will improve wound healing in zinc deficient patients. If no improvement is noted by this time, the delay in wound healing should not be ascribed to a zinc deficiency. The only reported side effect with this regimen is nausea which can be minimized by taking the zinc with meals (10).

7. What is the effect of vitamin A on the healing of wounds in man and animals?

Vitamin A reverses the inhibitory effect of cortisone on the healing of open wounds in man and animals (79). Apparently, topical and systemic vitamin A stimulates the healing of cortisone-retarded wounds but does not enhance wound healing in subjects not receiving cortisone. Presumably, vitamin A restores the inflammatory process suppressed by corticosteroids.

The normal healing process in rats can be accelerated by topical administration of vitamin A acid and its derivatives (96, 97, 98). More extensive research is needed to evaluate the effects of vitamin A on wound healing in normal human subjects, since most of the research to date has been in animals. Recommendations on dosage for humans would be premature at this time.

8. What is sunburn? What wavelengths of light produce it?

Sunlight is composed of light in wavelengths from 2,900 angstroms (near ultraviolet) to about 25,000 angstroms (infrared). The visible region is between 3,900 and 7,000 angstroms. The ultraviolet radiation that is responsible for sunburn falls between 2,950 and 3,200 angstroms. At 2,950 angstroms about 10% of the ultraviolet light penetrates into the dermis; this increases as the wavelengths increase toward 3,200 angstroms. Other wavelengths of light are also absorbed and, if intense enough, can produce erythema and burning. This type of burning is different from sunburn in that it is due to generated heat rather than a photochemical reaction.

After initial exposure, erythema begins in two to eight hours and usually peaks in 24 hours (86). Tissue destruction is caused by a photochemical reaction in the epidermis and upper dermis. This denatures and coagulates protoplasm of the epidermal cells and produces a histamine-like reaction in the dermis (71, 181).

9. K.I., a 19-year-old female, requests information about which product she should purchase to prevent sunburn. Her current preparation, which is promoted for "tanning without burning," is not working well; she burned after being out in the sun for only two hours.

Currently, the best available sunscreening agents include opaque materials such as titanium dioxide or zinc oxide; para-aminobenzoic acid (PABA); esters of PABA; and the benzophenones. The opaque agents are very good for small areas (nose or lips) but are not practical for application to large areas of the body. Of the remaining agents, PABA is the most effective sunscreen; its major drawback is its tendency to stain fabrics. The esters of PABA (Blockout, Sea and Ski, etc.) are effective but offer less complete protection from sunburn than PABA. They do not stain fabrics but are more easily washed off by sweat and water. The benzophenones (eg, Uval and Solbar) are also effective in protecting the skin from sunburn. Because they absorb light at wavelengths greater than 3,200 angstroms, the benzophenones may also be useful in preventing photosensitivity reactions (43, 62).

10. Are different wavelengths of light responsible for sunburn and suntan? Can chemical blocking agents assure a suntan without a burn?

The same wavelengths of light which cause burning are responsible for melanocyte stimulation and increased skin pigmentation. The only satisfactory method of tanning without burning is short repetitive exposures to the sun. This stimulates melanocytes without exposing the skin to excess radiation. Sunscreening agents block penetration by ultraviolet light and should be used after limited exposure to the sun, before burning begins (62).

11. Warts are caused by a DNA virus of the *papova* group which can withstand extremes of temperature and live in liquid nitrogen for many months. Why is liquid nitrogen (-196°C) therapy effective for warts? How does this treatment differ from the over-the-counter (OTC) wart preparations?

The diseased tissue which is frozen by liquid nitrogen sloughs off with the virus intact within the nucleus of the epidermal cells. Surgery is slightly more effective with regard to recurrence but has the disadvantage of leaving a residual scar (149, 161).

12. Review the growth cycle of hair and the causes of hair loss.

Growth and replacement of hair is cyclic rather than continuous. Since hair growth is not synchronized, each hair follicle can be in a different phase of growth. There are three phases: (a) anagen is a 2 to 6 year period during which the hair is actively growing; (b) catagen is a short transition phase lasting from 2 to 3 weeks; (c) telogen is a resting phase of about 2 months during which the hair dies and is shed (93, 94).

There are many causes of hair loss, ranging from the most common basis for hair loss, heredity, to rather unusual causes such as the ingestion of certain drugs. The following is a list of common causes of hair loss (59):

(a) *Hereditary* — most common form; it primarily affects males.

(b) *Stress* or trauma.

(c) *Endocrine* — more common in women and may be seen 6 to 18 weeks postpartum in some women, or in women taking oral contraceptives. Other endocrine causes include hypoparathyroidism, hypothyroidism, hyperthyroidism, and hypopituitarism.

(d) *Drugs* — see Questions 13 and 14 below.

(e) *Infections* — most often seen with fungal infections of the scalp.

(f) *Nutritional disorders* — most commonly with protein deficiency states.

13. A 39-year-old female taking probenecid, colchicine, acetaminophen and multivitamins has noticed that her hair has become brittle. She also loses an excessive amount each time she brushes her hair. Could any of these drugs be responsible for her complaints? What is the mechanism? What other drugs have been associated with diffuse hair loss?

Colchicine, like any other drug which depresses cell turnover, can lead to hair loss. The hair becomes brittle and more susceptible to breakage as the hairshaft narrows from the effects of the drug (62). Other drugs that have been associated with hair loss include heparin, idoxuridine, most cytotoxic drugs, gentamicin, oral contraceptives, vitamin A (toxic amounts), amphetamines, dextran, trimethadione, gold salts, thiouracil, bismuth, and warfarin (26, 32).

14. Z.A. is a 46-year-old female who requests something for her weak hair. She has recently noticed more and more hair in her hair-brush. She is currently taking warfarin 5 mg po daily and was hospitalized 8 weeks earlier for thrombophleblitis in her left leg, for which she received a ten day course of continuous drip heparin. Could either of these drugs be related to Z.A.'s current problems?

Heparin and the oral anticoagulants produce alopecia by converting a large number of anagen follicles into the telogen phase of hair growth. The hair is usually lost two to three months after a patient starts taking these drugs and will regenerate if the agent is discontinued. Some patients lose large amounts of hair, while others lose imperceptible amounts (62, 156).

15. A 41-year-old male with an obvious case of dandruff and a prescription for Selsun wonders if there is a less expensive over-the-counter (OTC) product that may be effective? What type of general instructions should be given to a patient purchasing an OTC dandruff preparation?

While Selsun is regarded as a standard for the treatment of dandruff, other less expensive agents are equally effective. When selenium sulfide 2.5% (Selsun) was compared with zinc pyrithione 2% (Head and Shoulders), the latter was as effective in treating dandruff. Both were significantly better than a placebo (125).

While these results may reflect therapeutic equivalence, the physical washing of the scalp and the technique used are probably more important than the agent employed. Since most studies done to date are not double blind, it is difficult to draw conclusions regarding the efficacy of individual products in the treatment of dandruff.

The following is a list of general instructions for patients with dandruff (22):

(a) The scalp should be shampooed frequently: three times a week until the dandruff is under control, then twice a week thereafter.

(b) Agitation of the scalp while shampooing is desirable. A rubber scalp agitator may be employed for those with short or fragile fingernails.

(c) If a medicated shampoo is employed, contact time should be as long as possible — preferably about 5 minutes. Also, it may be desirable to shampoo at least

twice, the first shampooing to remove oil and dirt and to wet the scalp and the second to work the medicated shampoo down into the scalp. A third shampooing can also be employed if results are inadequate.

(d) If a selenium containing product is used:

(i) A second shampoo should be employed if the hair is still oily or greasy, as selenium is not a good degreasing agent.

(ii) Hair should be rinsed thoroughly and hands should be washed to lessen the chances of toxicity and staining.

(iii) Use should be stopped and a physician or pharmacist consulted if cutaneous irritation, conjunctivitis, or hair loss occur.

(iv) Selenium may discolor light colored hair brown to orange if not thoroughly rinsed.

16. O.T. is a 78-year-old female who has several dark facial lesions which have been diagnosed as actinic keratoses. How should these be treated?

Topical 5-fluorouracil (1% in propylene glycol) is the treatment of choice for actinic keratoses (precancerous lesions secondary to chronic exposure to the sun). It has a selective effect on keratoses and spares normal skin (186). Following application, tenderness, erythema, erosion, and scaling of the keratoses occur in three to four days. Treatment is continued for two to three weeks for face lesions, and six to eight weeks for hand lesions. The reaction subsides approximately two weeks after the medication is discontinued and leaves no scar or pigmentary changes. Patients should expect mild irritation and should avoid unnecessary exposure to sunlight, which can increase the inflammatory reaction to the drug. 5-fluorouracil is used less enthusiastically for skin carcinomas and warts (34, 76).

17. How does griseofulvin work? When is it indicated? How long must it be used? What precautions and advice should be given to a patient taking this drug?

Griseofulvin is incorporated into the stratum corneum where it acts as a barrier to further fungal invasion and reproduction. The drug is most useful in *Tinea* or ringworm infections. Prior to the introduction of this drug, scalp ringworm could only be treated with X-ray. Duration of treatment is approximately 4 to 6 weeks, or until the infected layers of skin are sloughed off. Griseofulvin is only moderately effective against body ringworm and is least effective in ringworm affecting the hands; feet or nails. In the latter case, 6 to 12 months may be required for full eradication, and treatment is not justified unless severe discomfort is caused by the disease (62, 180). The drug should be taken with milk or fatty foods, because absorption is increased. The patient should be aware that the effects of alcohol may be potentiated by griseofulvin.

18. A 21-year-old male requests a product for his athlete's foot. Both feet but not the toenails are infected, and he is currently using an undecylenic acid preparation. What would you recommend?

A tolnaftate containing product should be recommended, as it is one of the most effective topical preparations available for the treatment of fungal infections of the skin. Improvement occurs in one to ten weeks in 80-90% of patients infected with *T. cruris, T. corporis* or *T. vericolor.*

T. rubrum (puerpurum), which sometimes causes athlete's foot, is often resistant to other standard medications, but is sensitive to tolnaftate. The drug is also less irritating than the fatty acid/organic acid formulations. Treatment is unsuccessful in the presence of acute inflammation. In such cases, initial treatment should consist of 1:20 Burow's solution used 3 to 4 times daily. Highly resistant cases may have to be treated with griseofulvin, although the response is unpredictable. Tolnaftate solution or cream should be applied twice a day as the initial treatment. Some improvement should be noted within 5 days, and therapy should be continued for at least two to three weeks; up to six weeks of treatment may be required. A second or third course of therapy may also be required. The following is a list of recommendations which will improve the chances of therapeutic success in patients with athlete's foot:

(a) Avoid public showers or wear sandals while showering.

(b) Keep feet clean and dry. Dry carefully between toes, dust with powder.

(c) Change shoes and socks frequently.

(d) Wear shoes with good ventilation; sandals are probably best.

(e) If there are extensive callouses on the feet, a keratolylic cream should be used in conjunction with the antifungal agent (applied separately).

19. How do the newer anti-fungal agents such as haloprogin (Halotex), clotrimazole (Lotrimin), and miconazole (Micatin) compare with tolnaftate in the treatment of dermatophytes?

Haloprogin is a very effective topical agent in the treatment of dermatophytoses (athlete's foot). In double blind studies, haloprogin and tolnaftate were equally effective and significantly better than placebo (74, 88). Clotrimazole and miconazole are probably also as effective as tolnaftate (44). Clotrimazole, miconazole, or haloprogin should be used with mixed fungal infections or when the causative agent is unknown, because these agents are effective against both dermatophytes and *Candida,* whereas tolnaftate is only effective against dermatophytes. In addition, these agents are also effective in the treatment of *T. cruris,* which often causes jock itch (44, 109). In *T. versicolor* infections these agents are more effective and have

better patient acceptability than the selenium sulfide preparations which have been used in the past (109).

20. K.A., a 19-year-old female, presents you with a prescription for nystatin 100,000 units vaginal tablets p.v. bid for 14 days. She also asks for something to relieve the crusty, pruritic lesions on the corners of her mouth. K.A. is taking erythromycin 250 mg bid for acne. Comment on this situation.

Erythromycin, as well as other broad spectrum antibiotics, could have led to vaginal overgrowth by *C. albicans.* This could also account for the crusty, pruritic lesions on her mouth which are probably oral candidiasis. If infections recur, it may also be necessary to give oral nystatin to eliminate *Candida* from the GI tract and to stop the erythromycin.

While nystatin has been proven efficacious in vaginal candidiasis, two newer and somewhat more expensive preparations, clotrimazole (Gyne-Lotrimin) and miconazole (Monistat), have been shown to be as effective and possibly more effective than nystatin in vaginal candidiasis (33, 106, 140, 154). Nystatin is still recommended for treating candidia infections in pregnant women (45, 46).

The lesions on the lips could be treated by clotrimazole, miconazole, or nystatin creams. If the candida infection is within the oral cavity, it should be treated with nystatin suspension 400,000 - 600,000 units qid (4). The suspension should be held in the mouth for up to 5 minutes, because the drug is only effective when it is in contact with infected lesions. Many practitioners use a nystatin vaginal tablet dissolved in the mouth to treat oral candidiasis. To date there are no studies confirming the effectiveness of this dosage form, but this approach is sound because of the longer contact time in the mouth. The manufacturer has informed the author that there is nothing in nystatin vaginal tablets (Mycostatin) that would be considered deleterious if used orally.

21. T.T. is a 23-year-old male who contracted a case of scabies several days ago. How should this problem be treated?

The most efficacious product is gamma benzene hexachloride (Kwell, Lidane, Gamene) (4). Kwell lotion should be applied once and left on the skin for 24 hours before washing. A second treatment may be given 4 to 7 days later if needed. If the scalp is infected, Kwell shampoo should be applied for 5 minutes and then washed out. This may be repeated after 4 and 8 days if needed. Because Kwell is irritating to the skin, care should be taken when applying the drug around mucous membranes. If irritation occurs, the drug should be washed off at once. Because of the possibility of neurotoxicity from frequent topical application, the drug should not be applied more frequently than recommended (56).

Gamma benzene hexachloride is neurotoxic at sufficiently high systemic levels and penetrates skin to a significant degree. Several poorly documented cases of convulsions have already been reported to the FDA. Therefore, this drug should only be used for active disease and only in the recommended doses. Kwell Spray is an insecticide and must not be confused as being for human use (56).

22. Q.A. is a 22-year-old female who was recently diagnosed as having psoriasis. She currently has extensive silver-white dry scaling patches on most of her scalp, shins, elbows, and on parts of her stomach and back. About 30% of her body surface is involved. Outline the general approach to her therapy. What is the underlying pathological lesion of psoriasis?

If the lesions are not extensive, psoriasis should be treated conservatively with topical agents. Corticosteroid creams, the mainstays of topical therapy, are often used with occlusive dressings to increase their penetration into the skin. A variety of coal tar preparations are available and may be used by themselves or incorporated into corticosteroid creams. Ammoniated mercury is generally less effective than coal tar but can be substituted if necessary. Salicylic acid is sometimes incorporated into these preparations to help remove thick scales. Anthralin may be used, but it is usually reserved for more severe cases of psoriasis because of its harsh effects on uninvolved skin (53, 54, 55).

Systemic therapy is reserved for the most severe or resistant cases. Methotrexate is the most frequently used systemic agent.

The basic pathological lesion of psoriasis is due to a loss of control of the normal growth regulating mechanisms in the epidermis (43). The normal turnover time for a cell to proceed from the generative layer of the skin to the point where it sloughs off is 27 days. In the psoriatic, the turnover time is decreased to 3 to 4 days. Therefore, the cells do not mature and keratinization fails to reach completion. (53, 62, 163) The epidermis is thickened by the increase in mitotic activity of the generative layer. Along with the increased cell turnover, there is a corresponding increase in nucleoprotein synthesis as well as an increase in certain enzymes responsible for growth. Vascular changes are seen with the blood vessels becoming dilated and tortuous. The blood vessels extend further up into the skin than normal, which allows bleeding to occur when the lesions are subjected to trauma. Inflammation with leukocyte infiltrates is also seen to varying degrees and is secondary to the underlying psoriatic lesion.

23. How is methotrexate (MTX) used in the treatment of psoriasis? Is it effective? What criteria should be used in determining whether or not a patient should receive methotrexate?

Methotrexate is not curative, but it suppresses psoriatic lesions and induces prolonged remissions in up to 75% of patients (39). Because of its toxicity, MTX should be reserved for severe disabling cases of psoriasis refractory to more conservative forms of therapy. The following are relative contraindications to the use of MTX in psoriasis: history of significant renal function abnormalities; liver impairment or history of hepatic disease; pregnancy; anemia; leukopenia; thrombocytopenia; active peptic ulcer disease; active infection; and lastly, an unreliable patient.

Three dosage schedules are commonly used in the treatment of psoriasis:

(a) Large doses (10-25 mg; occasionally as much as 37.5 mg) may be administered weekly by the oral, intramuscular or intravenous route. As the dose is increased, more frequent blood counts are indicated.

(b) A large weekly dose may be administered over a 36 hour period. Usually, 2.5 to 5 mg is given orally every 12 hours for three doses or every 8 hours for four doses. The total dose should not exceed 37.5 mg/week.

(c) Low oral doses may be given daily with rest periods. Usually, 2.5 mg is given daily for 5 days followed by a minimum two day rest period; a second 5 day course is followed by a rest period of at least seven days.

The three schedules are about equally effective. However, a given amount of MTX is less toxic when given as a single dose. Thus, dosage regimen (c) produces more toxicity than does (a) or (b). If the cellular kinetics of psoriatics are considered, schedule (b) appears to be the most appropriate (179). This regimen is probably also the least toxic (3, 27).

All dosage regimens should be tailored to the individual patient. The goal of MTX therapy is not to cure psoriasis, but to achieve a tolerable level of disease activity with the lowest possible dose (152).

24. Doses of methotrexate used to treat psoriasis are lower than those used to treat cancer. What are the side effects of MTX in the doses used?

The side effects encountered with MTX as used in psoriatics are essentially the same as those found in patients treated for cancer, but less severe. The most commonly reported adverse reactions are dose related and include ulcerative stomatitis, leukopenia, abdominal distress, and nausea. Irreversible and sometimes fatal hepatotoxicity (cirrhosis and fibrosis) is not an uncommon complication in patients taking MTX chronically. Serum enzymes and other liver function tests do not correlate with the severity of liver damage and are generally not predictive. For this reason a liver biopsy is performed prior to the initiation of MTX and yearly thereafter in some institutions (70, 174). Alcohol may increase the prevalence and severity of this adverse reaction.

25. How does hydroxyurea compare to metho-

trexate in the treatment of psoriasis?

Currently, the most popular chemotherapeutic agent for the treatment of psoriasis is methotrexate (16). After MTX, hydroxyurea has received the most extensive evaluation. It is not as effective as MTX but has a wide margin of safety and is considerably less toxic (99, 120).

Other antineoplastic agents that have been used include triacetyl azauridine (20), and busulfan (110). More extensive studies must be completed before definitive statements can be made concerning the effectiveness of these agents.

26. A 36-year-old woman with ten year history of psoriasis is well controlled on MTX. She purchases aspirin for her stiff elbow. Comment.

Approximately 25% of psoriatics develop arthritis (55), which mimics but is not the same as rheumatoid arthritis (142, 183). Generally, therapy is the same for both rheumatoid arthritis and psoriatic arthritis.

The use of aspirin could cause a serious problem in this patient. Salicylates can decrease the renal clearance of MTX by as much as 35% (100) and can displace MTX from its plasma protein binding by 30% (31). Both actions increase levels of free MTX, making it more potent and toxic. Therefore, salicylates should be avoided in these patients. Alternatively, the dose of MTX can be empirically decreased by one-third to one-half.

27. What are the Goeckerman and Ingram regimens for the treatment of psoriasis?

These are the two most commonly employed treatment programs for inducing and prolonging remissions in patients with psoriasis. The Goeckerman regimen employs coal tar or its derivatives and ultraviolet light. A coal tar ointment (2-5% crude coal tar or its equivalent) is applied several times a day and removed 24 hours after the initial application; this is followed by exposure to ultraviolet light. In addition, a coal tar bath, using a water soluble preparation, is given at least once a day. With successive daily treatments, the exposure to ultraviolet light is gradually increased. This particular regimen produces a significant number of remissions lasting 6-18 months (32, 133.)

The Ingram regimen differs in that an anthralin paste is applied to each psoriatic plaque, and stockinet dressings are applied over the lesions. This regimen is very effective but requires close supervision because anthralin irritates normal skin (25).

Each of these regimens can be modified. Frequently, topical corticosteroids and occlusive dressings are used as adjuvants.

28. A 37-year-old male has been treated for severe psoriasis with topical and systemic steroids for several years. He is currently taking 20 mg of prednisone daily, but this is not controlling his disease. A decision is made to slowly withdraw the prednisone and begin MTX. What problems may be anticipated? Are systemic corticosteroids contraindicated in the treatment of psoriasis?

Even if the prednisone is tapered correctly, the patient may develop a severe rebound of his disease requiring large doses of steroids for control. This reaction can be quite severe and progress to widespread, life-threatening psoriatic erythroderma. The toxicities of chronic systemic corticosteroid therapy, as well as the threat of rebound, limit their use in psoriatics. In severe cases, short courses of systemic glucocorticoids may be used to supplement topical therapy. The increased level of control should be maintained with other therapy (e.g., MTX) (32, 54). It would probably be best to start the withdrawal of corticosteroids while gradually beginning MTX therapy. The patient should be monitored very closely for infections and toxicity while he is receiving both drugs.

29. Can antineoplastic agents be used topically to treat psoriatic lesions?

Topical nitrogen mustard has been shown to be very effective in the treatment of psoriasis (173). Unfortunately, up to 80% of the patients treated developed contact sensitivity, and therapy had to be discontinued (184).

30. Z.K. is a 33 year-old male who asks you to recommend a product for his poison ivy. He also wonders if family members could get poison ivy from him? Comment.

Poison ivy (Rhus) dermatitis is the major cause of allergic contact dermatitis in the United States, exceeding all other causes combined. It is estimated that 50 to 95% of the population is sensitive to the plant to some degree. The severity of the condition varies from mild discomfort to an extremely painful and debilitating condition. Rhus dermatitis is caused by sensitization to an allergic substance in the leaves, stems, and roots of poison ivy, poison oak, and poison sumac plants. All three plants contain the same sensitizing oleoresin, urushiol oil, which contains pentadecacatechol, the actual sensitizing agent. For this reason the dermatitis caused by the three different plants is identical. The ivy is a woody vine or shrub found in all parts of the U.S., except the Southwest and the Pacific coast. Poison oak grows on the Pacific coast as a low shrub, a large tree-like plant, or a vine. Both the ivy and the oak have leaves in groups of three. Poison sumac is a shrub or small tree native to most parts of the country; it does not have the three leaf pattern.

Direct contact with the plant is not necessary for the rash to occur. Highly susceptible persons may develop severe dermatitis merely from exposure to Rhus oleoresin carried by pollen or by smoke from burning leaves. The oleoresin may remain active for months on clothing, shoes, tools, and sporting equipment. Once the toxic substance comes in contact with the skin, it can be spread by the hands to other areas of the body (genitals, eyes, etc), or to people who may come into close contact with the exposed person. Although washing with soap and water will not prevent the dermatitis unless done within fifteen minutes of exposure, it will prevent spreading of the oleoresin (32, 62).

Poison ivy dermatitis can be contracted throughout the year, including the winter, when the dermatitis results from exposure to the roots. The virulence of the leaf sap varies little during the foliage period. The incidence of poison ivy is higher during the spring due to several factors: the leaves are tender and bruise easily, the call to the outdoors is stronger, and as summer progresses people become more aware of the condition and more cautious.

It is of primary importance to determine what parts of Z.K.'s body are affected. If the genital areas, eyes, or mouth are affected, the patient should be referred to a physician for evaluation and probably a brief course of systemic corticosteroid therapy. To help relieve the burning and itching sensation, cool wet compresses are very useful and can help reduce inflammation. Normal saline or Burow's solution (1:20-1:40), which is a good, inexpensive, astringent solution, can be used to saturate soft linens or old bed sheets. These wet dressings are applied to the affected part four times a day with applications lasting fifteen minutes to one hour. Topical application of bland drying agents like calamine lotion without phenol, starch baths, or oatmeal baths, will do no harm and may provide some relief. Agents that can sensitize the skin, such as topical antihistamines, antibiotics, and local anesthetics, should be avoided. Phenol, menthol and camphor should be used with caution due to their ability to irritate the skin. It is interesting to note that most of the commercial products promoted for the treatment of poison ivy contain one or more of the sensitizers or irritants mentioned above. Antihistamines may be used systemically for the pruritis if necessary (see the chapter introduction for a further discussion). Topical corticosteroids can also be of great benefit if the lesions are past the acute, weeping, inflammatory stage (61, 130, 138, 172).

31. Characterize drug eruptions. How often do they occur? Why is it so difficult to obtain accurate statistics with regard to the incidence and type of drug eruptions? Which drugs cause the highest incidence of cutaneous adverse reactions?

Clinically recognizable adverse drug reactions are manifested more often in the skin than any other organ or organ system (9). It has been estimated that between 1% (103) and 5% (12) of hospitalized patients will develop a drug eruption. Outpatient statistics are much

more difficult to obtain, as many drug eruptions are not reported, or when reported, they may only be described as a rash, not the type of eruption. In many cases the causative agent(s) may not be known.

Penicillin is the most frequently implicated drug (175). Other drugs which frequently induce eruptions are listed in Table 3.

The most common type of eruption encountered in clinical practice, and probably the one most often overlooked, is the *exanthematic eruption.* This type of reaction comprises both *morbilliform* (measles-like) and *scarlatiniform* (scarlet fever-like) eruptions (62). Since drug eruptions often mimic other types of dermatitis, it is necessary to have a good understanding of the mimicked disease state to make the proper diagnosis.

32. A 13-year-old girl, with a measles-like morbilliform rash on her arms and chest is taking phenytoin, tetracycline, and multivitamins. How can one distinguish whether the rash is drug related or if she actually has measles?

Both phenytoin and tetracycline have been reported to cause morbilliform rashes (62). If she has been taking these drugs for a long period of time, it is doubtful that they have caused the rash. If she has taken the drugs for a short period of time, she may be experiencing a drug eruption. Another clue to the origin of the eruption is the existence or lack of other clinical signs of measles (fever, cough). If a drug eruption seems likely after a thorough diagnostic work up, withdrawal of these agents should lead to improvement within several days (62).

33. *Eczematous eruptions* are often associated with contact sensisitivity. Is it possible for an eczematous eruption to occur when a drug is given systemically if the person has previously been sensitized to the drug by topical administration?

Eczematous eruptions from systemically administered drugs almost always reflect prior topical sensitization; this may result from topical contact with the same drug or one which is chemically similar. Prior sensitization may have occurred years before, and often is not remembered by the patient (61).

34. Characterize the *fixed drug eruption.* How long will it last after withdrawal of the offending agent?

Table 3
AGENTS WHICH FREQUENTLY
CAUSE DRUG ERUPTIONS (23, 175)

arsenicals	penicillins
barbiturates	quinine
bromides	salicylates
gold salts	streptomycin
hydantoins	sulfonamides
iodides	thiouracil
mercurials	

What drugs have been reported to cause this type of eruption?

Fixed drug eruptions are erythematous, sharply bordered, and have a tendency to be darker than the surrounding, unaffected skin. They may also be eczematous, urticarial, vesicular, bullous, or nodular. Because these lesions have a marked propensity to recur at the same location, the term "fixed" is used to describe them. Although the eruptions heal after withdrawal of the causative agent, there usually is a marked hyperpigmentation of the area which may take months to resolve. Apparently, one area of the skin has the ability to evoke an allergic response which other areas lack. Drugs associated with fixed eruptions are listed in Table 4.

35. A 27-year-old female presents to the emergency room with large, painful, fluid filled sacs (bullae) on her legs, which appeared about 12 hours earlier. She is currently taking Tylenol, Cafergot, multivitamins, birth control pills, and an occasional pentobarbital capsule. Can any of these drugs be responsible for her present condition? What drugs have been reported to cause *bullous eruptions*?

Bullous lesions may occur in combination with other drug eruptions, such as erythema multiforme or toxic epidermal necrolysis, or independently (23). In this patient the Tylenol, the ergot in the Cafergot, or the pentobarbital could have caused these eruptions.

36. A 47-year-old accountant complains of acne which he has not experienced since his teens. He is currently taking Afrodex, Tuss-Ornade, multivitamins, and Valium. Could any of these drugs have caused his present condition? What other drugs may produce *acneiform eruptions*?

Afrodex contains an androgen, Tuss-Ornade contains iodide, and the multivitamins contain vitamin B_{12}, all of which have been reported to cause acneiform eruptions.

37. A 19-year-old female presents with a fever, sore throat, and slight lymphadenopathy. Six days after ampicillin 250 mg qid was started, a diffuse maculopapular rash involving 40% of her body surface developed. There was no previous history of drug allergy. A diagnosis of infectious mononucleosis was made and subsequently confirmed by the Monospot Test. What is the relationship between the rash associated with mononucleosis and ampicillin? Would steroids improve the rash?

The incidence of rash when ampicillin is used in patients with mononucleosis is between 80-100% (177, 35). The ampicillin-related rash appears in 5-10 days,

Table 4
DRUGS IMPLICATED IN FIXED ERUPTIONS (23, 30, 153)

acetaminophen	hydralazine
acetanilid	licorice
aminopyrine	mandelic acid
amphetamine	meprobamate
antimonial compounds	mercury compounds
barbiturates	morphine
belladonna alkaloids	PAS
bromides	pentaerythritol tetranitrate
BSP	phenacetin
chloral hydrate	phenolphthalein
chlordiazepoxide	phenothiazines
chloramphenicol	phenylbutazone
codeine	phenytoin
diethylstilbestrol	quinacrine
digitalis	quinine
disulfiram	reserpine
ephedrine	saccharin
ergot	salicylates
ethchlorvynol	sulfonamides
gold salts	tetracyclines
	vermouth

Table 5
DRUGS IMPLICATED IN BULLOUS ERUPTIONS
(9, 32, 160)

acetaminophen	licorice
aminopyrine	mercury compounds
arsenicals	mesantoin
atropine	penicillin
barbiturates	phenolphthalein
bismuth	phenytoin
bromides	promethazine
chloral hydrate	quinine
digitalis	streptomycin
ergot	sulfonamides
gold salts	

Table 6
DRUGS IMPLICATED IN ACNEIFORM ERUPTIONS
(9, 75, 178)

ACTH	iodides
androgens	phenytoin
bromides	quinine
chloral hydrate	scopolamine
cod liver oil	thiouracil
disulfiram	thiourea
isoniazid	trimethadione
	vitamin B_{12}

starts on the trunk, and spreads to the face and extremities. Palms, exposed areas, and pressure points are most severely affected. The severity is proportional to the dose and duration of treatment. Steroids given before and during the appearance of the rash do not decrease the extent or influence the severity of the rash (131)

38. What is the *Jarisch-Herxheimer reaction*?
This drug eruption follows the administration of a

drug for an infectious disease and represents a toxic, or more likely an allergic response to products released from the dying microorganisms. The reaction is seen most often in patients with syphillis, nearly 50% of whom experience malaise, fever, and an exacerbation of existent skin lesions 8-24 hours following treatment with penicillin. This type of reaction can also be seen in patients who receive griseofulvin for *Tinea pedis* infections (62).

39. The Stevens-Johnson syndrome, toxic epidermal necrolysis and exfoliative dermatitis are *life-threatening eruptions* which can be produced by drugs. Briefly describe these eruptions and how they are treated. Can less severe drug eruptions progress to one of these life threatening forms?

The **Stevens-Johnson syndrome** is the most common type of severe drug reaction (148). It is classified as a serious variant of bullous erythema multiforme. This syndrome may involve mucous membranes, and constitutional symptoms such as fever and malaise are common. The skin can become hemorrhagic and pneumonia and joint pains may occur. Serious ocular involvement is common and can culminate in partial or complete blindness. In addition to drugs, this syndrome has been associated with infections, pregnancy, foods, deep X-ray therapy, and neoplasms.

Toxic epidermal necrolysis was first described by Lyell in 1956 and may be preceded by a prodrome characterized by malaise, lethargy, fever, and occasionally throat or mucous membrane soreness (23, 12). Epidermal changes follow and consist of erythema and massive bullae formation which easily rupture and peel. The skin appears scalded. Hairy parts of the body are usually not affected, but mucous membrane involvement is common. Approximately 30% of patients with toxic epidermal necrolysis succumb, often within 8 days after bullae appear (148). The usual cause of death is infection complicated by massive fluid and electrolyte loss. Even though the skin takes on a very grave appearance, healing occurs within 2 weeks in the remaining 70% of patients, usually with no scarring (62, 32). In addition to drugs, certain bacterial infections and foods are believed to cause this type of eruption. Most cases of toxic epidermal necrolysis in children are due to infection; *Staphylococcus aureus* has been implicated.

Exfoliative dermatitis is characterized by large areas of skin becoming scaly and erythematous and then sloughing off. Hair and nails sometimes are lost. In most patients, a generalized systemic toxicity also accompanies the eruption. Secondary bacterial infection may occur, and most fatalities are due to infection. Exfoliative dermatitis also may follow other drug eruptions; thus, a less severe eruption may culminate with an exfoliative dermatitis (9, 148). This type of eruption may take weeks or months to resolve, even after withdrawal of the offending agent (161, 32).

Treatment of life threatening drug eruptions is basically symptomatic (10). They can evolve from less severe eruptions, especially if the causative agent is not discontinued when the reaction first appears. After discontinuing the suspected agent(s), systemic corticosteroids should be quickly administered to stop or at least retard the inflammatory reaction. Parenteral replacement of fluids and electrolytes may be necessary; analgesics, antihistamines, and sedatives may also be of value (17, 62, 148).

Table 7
DRUGS IMPLICATED IN LIFE-THREATENING ERUPTIONS (9, 148, 161, 32, 62, 17)

Stevens-Johnson Syndrome:

allopurinol	phenobarbital
antipyrine	phensuximide
ASA	phenylbutazone
chloramphenicol	phenytoin
chlorpropamide	smallpox vaccine
hydralazine	sulfonamides
measles vaccine	tetracycline
penicillin	trimethadione

Toxic Epidermal Necrolysis:

acetazolamide	penicillin
aminopyrine	phenolphthalein
barbiturates	phenylbutazone
brompheniramine	phenytoin
dapsone	polio vaccine
diptheria innoculations	sulfonamides
gold salts	tetanus antitoxin
nitrofurantoin	tetracycline
	tolbutamide

Exfoliative Dermatitis:

actinomycin D	methantheline
allopurinol	methylphenidate
antimony compounds	PAS
arsenic	penicillin
barbiturates	phenacemide
boric acid (internally)	phenolphthalein
chlorpropamide	phenytoin
codeine	quinacrine
diethylstilbestrol	quinidine
gold salts	streptomycin
iodides	sulfonamides
mercury compounds	tetracycline
mesantoin	vitamin A

40. B.B. is a 17-year-old female who was recently started on SSKI for hyperthyroidism; she has noticed that her acne has become much worse. Do patients with pre-existing dermatological problems have a higher incidence of drug eruptions when treated with agents known to produce lesions similar to their underlying condition?

Some conditions predispose patients to cutaneous reactions to certain drugs. For example, those with acne are susceptible to acneiform eruptions due to iodides, bromides, androgens, and other steroid hormones. Patients with atopic dermatitis are more susceptible to eruptions produced by salicylates. Those with monilia infections are more susceptible to eruptions produced by iodides and bromides. Persons with purpuric or hemorrhagic conditions are more susceptible to reactions due to barbiturates, arsenicals, gold salts, sulfonamides, and salicylates, while those who have urticarial eruptions are more susceptible to reactions due to salicylates, bromides, and many other drugs (91).

41. Characterize photosensitivity reactions. Is there a difference between systemic or topical administration of photosensitizing medications? Which drugs can cause photosensitive reactions?

There are two types of *photosensitivity reactions,* both of which require the presence of drug and light. The first is a *photoallergic* reaction, in which light alters the drug so that it becomes antigenic or acts as a haptene. Photoallergic eruptions require previous exposure to the offending drug and are not dose related. They may be induced by chemically related compounds and appear in a variety of forms, including urticaria, bullous lesions and sunburn. These eruptions are usually caused by topical agents.

The second type of photosensitive eruption is known as a *phototoxic* reaction. In this reaction, light alters the drug to a toxic form which results in tissue damage that is independent of an allergic response. This eruption may occur on first exposure to a drug, is dose related, usually has no cross sensitivity, and almost always appears as an exaggerated sunburn. In some instances a drug may produce both photoallergic and phototoxic reactions (23, 50).

Table 8
DRUGS IMPLICATED IN PHOTOSENSITIVE ERUPTIONS (62, 71)

antimalarials	phenothiazines
barbiturates	psoralens
chlorpromazine	quinethazone
coal tar	quinine
gold salts	smallpox vaccine
griseofulvin	sulfonamides
mesantrol	sulfonylureas
nalidixic acid	tetracycline
norethynodrel	thiazides

42. Recent studies have clarified the sequence of events leading to clinically significant infections following burns. What are the primary sites of infection and major pathogens involved in burn wound sepsis?

For a very brief period of time after a severe burn the surface of the wound is sterile. Shortly thereafter, the area becomes colonized by a mixed flora in which Gram-positive organisms predominate. By the third post burn day, this bacterial population becomes dominated by Gram-negative organisms. By the fifth post burn day, these organisms have invaded tissue well beneath the surface of the burn. These organisms proliferate and eventually invade adjacent unburned tissue causing burn wound sepsis (113).

The organisms most commonly isolated from burn patients are *Staphylococcus aureus, Pseudomonas aeruginosa, Klebsiella-Enterobacter* species, *Proteus* and *Candida* (104).

43. A 9-year-old girl recently received third degree burns involving 20% of her body surface. An adverse reaction to one of her topical medications was suspected when all blood cultures were negative despite the fact that she appeared septic. Comment.

Approximately 50% of patients with fatal burn wound sepsis do not demonstrate any noteworthy spread of organisms beyond the immediate area of the wound itself (113). Thus, a positive blood culture is not necessary for the diagnosis of sepsis in these patients (111).

44. Would massive doses of systemic antibiotics be beneficial to this patient?

The avascular nature of the burn wound precludes delivery of effective concentrations of antimicrobial agents to the site of active bacterial proliferation (124). Therefore it is doubtful that treatment with systemic antibiotics would significantly affect the course of sepsis (112), but they should be given to decrease the chance of bacteria seeding out to various parts of the body. As expected, the fatality rate is high in these patients despite the administration of appropriate antibiotics.

45. D.K. is a 46-year-old painter who was recently burned in a paint fire. He currently has over 50% of his body covered with third degree burns. The resident caring for D.K. asks that since circulation is mandatory for delivery of antibiotics to infected burn areas, when should systemic antibiotics be started?

In both second and third degree burns, the affected area undergoes vascular occlusion at the time of thermal injury. In second degree burns (partial thickness burns), circulation to the burn area is restored within 24-48 hours if invasive infection does not occur. If infection occurs, progressive thrombosis of the reestablished circulation converts partial thickness skin destruction to one of full thickness skin loss. With third degree burns (full thickness burns), circulation is reestablished in about three weeks in the granulation tissue which is at the interface between the burned and unburned skin. Also, when the blood supply is occluded, both humoral and cellular defense mechanisms are effectively impeded, thus increasing the risk of infection in the necrotic tissue (111). While the question of whether or not to use systemic antibiotics has never been fully answered, it is advisable to use systemic antibiotics when the burn patient exhibits signs of bacteremic sepsis (1).

46. Silver nitrate is one of the most often used topical antiinfectants in the treatment of severe burns. What are its advantages and disadvantages?

The antibacterial action of silver nitrate is entirely due to the silver ion, which precipitates as silver chloride when it comes into contact with tissue, thus limiting its effectiveness and hindering its penetration beyond surface tissues. Vigorous debridement of the burn wound must accompany silver nitrate therapy to permit its continued access to the bacterial population. Silver nitrate is effective against pathogenic organisms, including *Pseudomonas aeruginosa,* and bacterial resistance has not been a problem. The main drawbacks of silver nitrate are the absorption of large volumes of distilled water from the dressings and the loss of electrolytes (calcium, chloride, potassium, and sodium) into the dressings. The dressings are also comparatively expensive and messy to use. Rare cases of methemoglobinemia have been reported (139).

47. Mafenide (Sulfamylon) is currently used extensively in the therapy of burn wounds. What local and systemic problems may be encountered with its use?

Pain of varying intensity and duration is experienced upon application of mafenide, and analgesic supplements may be required. The intensity of this pain is usually inversely proportional to the burn depth. Hypersensitivity, manifested by a maculopapular rash in the unburned areas, occurs in 3 to 5% of patients and can be controlled by antihistamines. A more serious side effect, metabolic acidosis, results from carbonic anhydrase inhibition. The immediate demand to clear this acid load is placed upon the lungs, resulting in hyperventilation, although this is less apparent in children. Mafenide penetrates the eschar to produce an effective concentration in adjacent, unburned tissue (112).

48. Is silver sulfadiazine a significant addition to the topical management of the burn patient? What is its mechanism of action? Is this agent more effective than silver nitrate or sulfadiazine alone?

Silver sulfadiazine combines the advantages of silver nitrate and sulfadiazine while eliminating several of the disadvantages of each product. The silver ion is firmly bound to the sulfadiazine which prevents rapid inactivation of the silver ion through precipitation with chloride. The silver ion is released slowly to produce its antibacterial effects, which in turn prevents too rapid absorption of sulfadiazine, thus protecting the patient from renal complications reported with systemic sulfadiazine (15, 111).

49. How effective are topical antimicrobials in the therapy of burn wounds?

Silver nitrate, mafenide, and silver sulfadiazine, when properly used, appear to be effective (114). The best results are obtained in patients who have burns on 30 to 50% or less of their body surface. These agents have improved the survival rates of patients with burns involving 50 to 70% of their body surface area. When more than 70% of body surface area is affected, no reduction in mortality is noted (111, 113, 114). Reduction in mortality is attributed to the control of bacterial flora and the elimination of burn wound sepsis.

50. M.M. is a 15-year-old female who recently noticed a worsening of her acne. She states that she has been eating a considerable amount of oily foods recently and wonders if there is an association. She also asks what causes acne. Comment.

The basic lesion of acne involves an inflammation of the pilosebaceous follicles of the skin. Only certain areas of the body are affected; the size of the sebaceous gland of most hair follicles is roughly proportional to the size of the hair (66), but in the areas of the body where acne occurs, there are large sebaceous glands present with small or rudimentary hairs. This combination is particularly favorable for the development of acne, which explains why acne occurs on the face, neck, or upper trunk, and not on the scalp or other hairy parts of the body.

At puberty under the influence of androgens, the sebaceous glands increase in size and activity. In response, the follicular walls hypertrophy. When this increase in keratinization occurs, the flow of sebum to the outside skin becomes mechanically blocked (66, 64). The pilosebaceous follicle starts to dilate and becomes filled with entrapped sebum and cellular debris. At this point the lesion is known as a *comedo* or blackhead. The follicular orifice of the blackhead usually remains partially open and allows varying amounts of sebum to reach the outside skin, but it can close off completely.

When the comedo forms, bacteria that are normally present on the skin and in the follicular canal are especially favored in this nutrient-rich environment of the plugged pilosebaceous gland. Organisms most often found in the pilosebaceous follicle are the acid-producing bacteria *Corynebacterium acnes, Staphylococcus albus* and the fungi *Pityrosporon ovale* (66, 155). Of these, *Corynebacterium acnes* and, to a lesser extent, the other bacteria produce lipolytic enzymes (144). These enzymes are capable of converting the sebum, which is normally composed of esterified long chain fatty acids, into short chain free fatty acids. It has been shown that free fatty acids, especially those of carbon chains between 8 and 14, have the ability to provoke a nonspecific type of inflammatory response. Thus, while these bacteria do not take an active role in producing acne, they act as mediators or catalysts in the inflammatory response.

As the free fatty acid content of the entrapped sebum builds up, an inflammatory reaction occurs with its characteristic leukocytic infiltrates. As this process continues, bacterial by-products and dead leukocytes cause the walls of the sebaceous gland and follicular canal to become thinner and more brittle. Trauma to this area can cause the pilosebaceous follicle to rupture, spilling its contents into the surrounding dermis. If this occurs, the follicular contents produce a foreign body reaction and a *cyst* generally will form. At this point, the hair follicle is usually destroyed and will not regenerate (66). Sometimes these cysts will rupture again and again, forming larger and larger cysts. When a large number of cysts occur in any given area, they can form interconnecting channels (62). This type of acne is known as *acne conglobata* and is a very severe form of the disease often leading to scarring. Systemic therapeutic agents should be used with this type of acne to lessen the chance of scarring.

The role of diet as a means of acne therapy has been exaggerated, and opinions on the usefulness of diet vary greatly from practitioner to practitioner. There is no evidence to support the value of eliminating various dietary items in helping the course of disease (7, 62, 64, 32). Some patients, though, insist they have flareups from certain foods. In such cases, those foods should be avoided.

51. M.M. asks you to recommend a product for the control of her acne. What are the goals of acne therapy and what are the agents available for the control of acne? She also asks if there would be any improvement in her acne if she started taking oral contraceptives.

The goal of acne therapy is to interrupt the degeneration of the pilosebaceous follicles so that cysts will not form and scarring will not occur. Treatment is directed toward keeping the skin clean and to the peeling of skin so that the follicular orifices are kept open and draining properly. Soaps or other cleansers have a major role.

It is important to maximize the keratolytic effects and minimize the keratoplastic properties of topical acne treatments. The most often used keratolytic is sulfur. It is used in concentrations of 3 to 12% and has keratoplastic properties at the 3% level but rapidly becomes keratolytic as the concentration is increased. Another popular agent is salicylic acid which is used in concentrations of 1/2 to 3%. Salicylic acid has keratoplastic properties below 2% and keratolytic effects above 2% concentration. Resorcinol is also used in many proprietary preparations and generally is used in concentrations of 2 to 20%. It is not uncommon to find several keratolytic agents used in combination in the same product. In such cases, adequate keratolytic effect is maintained in spite of low concentrations of each keratolytic agent (64).

The second class of compounds used in the topical treatment of acne are the potent keratolytic or peeling agents. These agents are designed to remove the skin from around the comedones and covering superficial acne pustules. This helps to keep sebaceous follicles patent and draining properly (64, 5). Benzoyl peroxide is one of the more popular nonprescription peeling agents. It is converted to hydrogen peroxide on the skin and acts as an oxidizing agent to promote peeling. Retinoic acid, one of the newer peeling agents, has proved to be very effective in promoting peeling despite its high irritant properties. Hot Vleminckx compresses and carbon dioxide slush are peeling agents which should be used only under close and expert supervision because of their low therapeutic indices (64, 62, 32).

Hot Vleminckx compresses are cloth compresses soaked in a hot, sulfurated lime solution applied to the skin for varying lengths of time. Carbon dioxide slush treatment uses pulverized carbon dioxide in a cloth bag that is soaked in acetone and applied to the skin. Both of these treatments can produce severe irritation if allowed to stay in contact with the skin too long.

Ultraviolet light treatments are sometimes used to produce mild peeling. The light treatments produce a mild burn which then causes peeling. There are also several types of mechanical peeling agents available. These agents contain an abrasive compound, usually a fine sand or small plastic balls and are used to produce peeling and also to help keep the skin clean.

When using any of the peeling agents, there should be a mild or tolerable level of irritation produced. There is considerable variation from patient to patient in the amount of peeling agent tolerated. In the case of retinoic acid, some patients can tolerate three or four applications per day while other patients may not be able to use the agent at all because of the severe irritation produced. Therefore, it is necessary to individualize treatment when using these agents.

Birth control pills are generally effective in the treatment of acne (128, 129, 169). The estrogen in the birth control pills counteracts the effects of endogenous androgens (see Question 50), causing a decrease in sebaceous gland size and sebum production (170, 169). Limitations to the use of birth control pills for acne are the age of the patient, complications, and the one to four month lag time seen when these agents are used (81). As one might expect, the birth control pills with higher estrogen components are more effective than those with low or no estrogenic component. Unless the acne is quite severe and other measures fail, the risk is generally not worth the benefit. See also chapter on *Oral Contraception*.

52. O.T.B. is a 16-year-old male taking 250 mg tetracycline p.o. daily for his acne. Because his 18-year-old sister was recently given 250 mg of tetracycline four times a day for a respiratory infection, he won-

ders if he too shouldn't be taking a higher dose of tetracycline. Comment.

Antibiotics used in treating acne do not pass the epithelial lining of the pilosebaceous follicle. Instead, they are sequestered in cells surrounding the sebaceous follicle and then shed into the sebum. Sequestration explains why low doses of antibiotics are effective and also accounts for the lag time observed between administration of various drugs and their therapeutic effects (65).

It appears that tetracycline, erythromycin, clindamycin, sulfadimethoxine, and trimethoprim-sulfamethoxazole are all equal in their effectiveness against acne (166, 2). Tetracycline is considered the drug of first choice and is relatively safe when used in doses under 1 gm/day (2). Erythromycin is probably the drug of second choice. The other agents, while effective, should be discouraged due to cost or toxicity (2).

53. B.B. is a 17-year-old female who has been taking 250 mg tetracycline daily for 2 years. She would like to know if tetracycline would work on her acne if she applied it topically to her face?

Topical preparations specially formulated to enhance the penetration of erythromycin, tetracycline, and clindamycin, have been shown to decrease C. acnes counts and bring about clinical improvement (146). When topical tetracycline was compared to orally administered tetracycline, they were judged to be equally effective and far superior to placebo (18). More study is needed to fully evaluate the effectiveness of topical antibiotics in acne, but these preparations may prove to be valuable alternatives to systemically administered antibiotics.

54. A 21-year-old female using retinoic acid for her acne notices the package label which states that retinoic acid is vitamin A acid. She wonders if vitamin A taken internally would also help her acne. Comment.

To date no controlled studies have demonstrated that systemic vitamin A is effective for acne (6). Vitamin A inhibits keratinization in vitro, but this process does not seem to be applicable in vivo. Thus, although systemic vitamin A might be useful on a theoretical basis, it appears to be ineffective (143).

55. What is the mechanism by which retinoic acid (vitamin A acid) produces its beneficial effects when applied topically? What side effects are commonly encountered? What instructions should be given to this patient regarding the use of vitamin A acid?

The exact mechanism of action of retinoic acid is unknown (101). It is a fairly potent irritant and causes redness and peeling of the skin. It is alleged to act deeper within the pilosebaceous unit than conventional agents to inhibit comedo formation and loosen keratinized cells (85).

The side effects encountered with this medication

are extensions of the therapeutic effects, namely severe irritation, redness, and inflammation (95). The goal of therapy is to produce a moderate (tolerable) degree of redness and irritation. Patients differ in their tolerance to retinoic acid, thus explaining why some are able to tolerate several applications daily while others are unable to use it at all.

The following instructions should be given to the patient (105, 126):

(a) It should be applied once a day as a light application. Areas around the eyes and mouth should be avoided, as they are particularly sensitive to the effects of vitamin A acid.

(b) Since washing appears to increase its potency, vitamin A acid should be applied at least 30 minutes, and preferably one hour after washing the face.

(c) No other acne preparations should be used, and the face should be washed no more than twice daily with a gentle soap.

(d) Increased effects from sunlight may be noted, and proper precautions should be taken.

(e) Some redness and peeling may begin within a week and persist for 3 to 4 weeks. If this becomes severe, the physician should be contacted.

(f) A flare in the acne may occur during the first month of therapy. This can be explained as the surfacing of the lesions beneath the skin, an expected part of the clearing process.

56. Discuss the pathogenesis of herpes simplex infections.

There are two types of infectious processes due to herpes simplex viruses. The first is a primary infection of a previously unexposed person. The patient usually experiences no clinical symptoms and, after this primary exposure, will have circulating antibodies against the virus. During this initial infection, the virus becomes fixed within the cells of the tissue it has invaded and goes into a dormant period.

The second type of infection involves a reactivation of the tissue-fixed virus. The recurrence usually surfaces at the site of the primary infection. The lesion is limited to the epidermis and produces an intradermal vesicle that does not extend below the basement membrane. Biopsy shows congestion of the dermis and ballooning degeneration of the epidermal cells. Multinucleated giant cells are often found and can usually be considered diagnostic of this type of infection. In the healing phase the corneum and vesicles are infiltrated with leukocytes (32, 84, 161, 182).

There are two naturally occurring variants of the herpes simplex virus. Type I primarily infects nongenital sites, and type II primarily infects genital sites. Both produce similar infections (116, 117, 118).

57. A patient complains that almost every time she has diarrhea she gets a cold sore. Could this be due to

herpes simplex virus? What other factors trigger herpes simplex infections? How often do herpes infections recur?

Diarrhea and other gastrointestinal disturbances can cause cold sores. Other factors that can activate herpes are fever, trauma, sunshine and menstruation. The type and amount of stimulus needed to produce an infection varies greatly from one patient to another. This explains why some people can suffer infections as often as once a month while others remain asymptomatic after initial exposure for the rest of their lives. Seventy-five percent of those who have had a primary infection will experience a recurrence of the infection during their lives (62).

58. C.T. is a 22-year-old female who has received six smallpox vaccinations over the last two months for recurrent cold sore infections. Comment on this situation.

The rationale for this type of treatment is induction of an immunologic response analogous to that produced by B.C.G. vaccine in certain malignant processes; theoretically this could decrease the number of cold sore infections. However, in a double blind study there was no difference between the number of herpes attacks in patients given repeated smallpox vaccinations and a control group. The dangers of using smallpox vaccine far outweigh any beneficial effect that could be gained from its use (89).

59. Is killed herpes virus vaccine effective in providing prophylaxis against herpes simplex infections? Why?

The results of a double blind study showed killed herpes vaccine to be no more effective than placebo (90). Herpes virus apparently grows intracellularly and spreads from cell to cell; thus it escapes the body's defense system (antibodies). Therefore, although antibody titers against herpes virus may be high, they have no access to the virus to destroy it (90).

60. Is idoxuridine (IDU) effective in the treatment of a cutaneous herpes simplex infection? How is it thought to work? How should it be applied if it is used?

Opinions vary greatly regarding the effectiveness of topical IDU for herpes simplex infections. IDU, when administered by dermajet or applied topically in a 5% suspension in dimethylsulfoxide (DMSO), a surface active agent, shortened the course of the illness (82, 102). Topical application of commercially available preparations (Stoxil or Herplex) has been ineffective. This may reflect the poor penetrability of IDU and its inability to reach the virus in adequate concentration.

IDU is a pyrimidine analog which inhibits the synthesis of DNA; theoretically it should inhibit the replication of the herpes virus as well. If used, IDU should be applied every 5 minutes during the first hour of the prodromal stage, then every hour for the next 12 hours

and finally every 2 hours for a total of 4 days of treatment. Additional application has no further benefit and may slow healing (24). It should also be noted that IDU has been given intravenously for herpes simplex encephalitis (121).

61. Is photodynamic inactivation effective in the treatment of cutaneous herpes simplex? How is it used?

Photodynamic inactivation of herpes infections is still being investigated. It has been reported that the use of heterocyclic dyes (0.1% neutral red, 0.1% proflavine, and 0.1% methylene blue) shortens the healing time of herpes infections but does not affect the number of recurrences (57, 58, 164). The procedure requires the sterile rupturing of early vesicles prior to application of the dye. The area is next exposed to fluorescent light at a distance of about 10 cm for 15 minutes. The area is re-exposed to this light source at 30 minutes, 8 hours, and again at 36 hours. It is theorized that the dye binds irreversibly to the viral nucleic acid which causes a disruption of the molecule when exposed to light.

This procedure is somewhat controversial, in that Rapp (145) has reported malignant transformation of cells in tissue cultures when exposed to light treated viruses. This has not been confirmed by other investigators (80). However, Meyers and co-workers (108) have reported a failure of neutral red in treating herpes simplex virus infections. This type of treatment will have to be studied further for both efficacy and toxicity before any conclusions can be made.

62. D.F. is a 26-year-old male who suffers from repeated herpes genitalis (type II) infections. He has had four infections within the last six months. Are there any effective treatments for recurrent herpes genitalis infections?

At present there are no proven treatments for recurrent herpes genitalis infections. All that can be done is to recommend symptomatic treatments consisting of systemic analgesics and sitz baths (63). There are reports of two experimental approaches that may be effective in the treatment of herpes genitalis; topical application of ethyl ether (123, 151) and phosphonoacetic acid (162). Both these compounds will need further study to confirm their usefulness.

63. Are over-the-counter (OTC) products for herpes simplex infections effective?

The OTC products available for cold sores usually contain one or more of the following: a drying agent, a local anesthetic, and/or an emollient. They are only palliative and do little to affect the course of the infection. For a more extensive review of these products, read the *APhA OTC Handbook*.

64. You receive a prescription for betamethasone

0.1% cream which is to be applied to cold sores qid.
Comment.

As a general rule, corticosteroids should be avoided in patients with viral infections, as they depress serum interferons and could thereby prolong the infection or make it worse. In cases with severe inflammation which may result in scarring, corticosteroids may be justified (32).

CASE FOR STUDY — ATOPIC DERMATITIS

P.K., a 23-year-old male, is currently being followed in the University Dermatology Clinic for his atopic dermatitis. The patient has 30% of his body covered by an eczematous rash with extensive involvement of the popliteal and antecubital fossas. His chief complaint is extreme pruritis over the involved areas, as well as cosmetic disfiguration in the antecubital fossas, around the neck, and on the forehead.

Family History: The patient's mother and aunt have bronchial asthma; one sister age 16 has hay fever; his father and younger brother, age 11, appear to have no atopic manifestations.

Past Medical History: An eczematous rash was first noted on P.K. one month after birth. The scalp, face and neck were the only areas affected, and the rash continued with varying degrees of severity until age 2½ years when it spontaneously resolved. P.K. developed hay fever at age 6 with occasional attacks of asthma (last attack, age 15). An eczematous rash reappeared at age 12 and has not disappeared since that time. His skin has followed a variable course, partially clearing in the summer and during periods of little stress, and worsening during the winter and periods of much stress.

Physical Exam: Well nourished, well developed white male with no physical abnormalities noted except for his skin. Skin: oozing, crusted, erythematous, hyperkeratotic, hyperpigmented, maculopapular, and finely vesicular eruptions on face, neck, dorsal aspects of both arms and legs, hands, and chest. There is some evidence of secondary bacterial infection in both antecubital fossas and on portions of the left leg.

Current medications:

1) Hydroxyzine 25 mg tid.

2) Hydrocortisone cream 1%, apply sparingly bid.
3) Cetaphil lotion, apply bid.
Allergies: **Penicillin, milk, fish, and chocolate.**

1. Discuss ways to alter the itch-scratch cycle in P.K. and thus improve his condition; include non-drug remedies.
2. Are there any additional drugs that P.K. should be given? Comment on the use of topical antibiotics for the areas that are infected.
3. What factors have been shown to aggravate atopic dermatitis?
4. What is the prognosis for P.K.? What are the chances of his children developing atopic disorders?

Atopic Dermatitis, Selected References

Baer RL: *Atopic Dermatitis,* L.B. Lippincott Co., Philadelphia, 1955.

Barker H: Disease of the skin — management of eczema. Brit Med J 4:605, 1973.

Ellis EF: Immunologic basis of atopic disease. Advances in Pediat 16:65, 1969.

Fitzpatrick TB: *Dermatology in General Medicine,* Ed. 1, McGraw Hill Book Co, New York, 1971, p. 680.

Kempe CH et al: Smallpox vaccination of eczema patients with a strain of attenuated live vaccinia. Pediatrics 42:980, 1968.

Prose PH: Pathologic changes in eczema. J Pediat 66:178, 1965.

Rostenberg A: Atopic dermatitis and infantile eczema, in *Immunological Diseases,* Samter M, editor, Little Brown and Co., Boston, 1965, p. 635.

Roth HL et al: A natural history of atopic dermatitis: A 20 year follow up study. Arch Derm 89:209, 1964.

Scholtz JR: Management of atopic dermatitis. Calif Med 100:103, 1964.

Solomon LM et al: Atopic dermatitis. Amer J Med Sci 252:478, 1966.

Wells J: Understanding atopic syndromes. Postgrad Med 58:67, 1975.

*Whyte HJ: Atopic dermatitis, in *Current Therapy,* ed Conn, R B, W B Saunders Co, Philadelphia, 25 ed, 1973.

* This year's edition is highly recommended.

REFERENCES

1. Abston S et al: Gentamicin for septicemia in patients with burns. J Infect Dis 124 (Suppl.):275, 1971.
2. Ad Hoc Committee on use of antibiotics in dermatology: Systemic antibiotics for treatment of acne vulgaris. Arch Derm 111:1630, 1975.
3. Almeyda J et al: Drug reations, XV Methotrexate, psoriasis, and the liver. Brit J Derm 85:302, 1971.
4. AMA Drug Evaluations, Science Group, Inc., Action, Mass., 1973. Vol. II.
5. American Society of Hospital Pharmacists: American Hospital Formulary. Washington DC, 1972.
6. Anderson JAD: Vitamin A in acne vulgaris: report by the S.E. Scotland Faculty of the Coll Gen Pract. Brit Med J 2:294, 1963.
7. Andrews CC: Acne vulgaris. Med Clin N Am 49:737, 1965.
8. Arndt KA: *Manual of Dermatologic Therapeutics,* Little, Brown and Co., Boston, 1974.
9. Baer RL et al: Types of cutaneous reactions to drugs. JAMA 202:710, 1967.
10. Bailey G et al: Toxic epidermal necrolysis. JAMA 191:979, 1965.
11. Baraf CS: Treatment of pruritis in allergic dermatoses: An evaluation of the relative efficacy of cyproheptadine and hydroxyzine. Curr Ther Res 19:32, 1976.
12. Barr DP: Hazards of modern diagnosis and therapy — the price we pay. JAMA 159:1452, 1955.
13. Barry BW et al: Comparative bioavailability of proprietary topical corticosteroid preparations: vasoconstrictor assays on thirty creams and gels. Br J Derm 91:323, 1974.
14. Barry BW et al: Comparative bioavailability and activity of proprietary topical corticosteroid preparations: vasoconstrictor assays on thirty-one ointments. Br J Derm 93:563, 1975.
15. Baxter DR: Topical use of 1.0% silver sulfadiazine, in *Contemporary Burn Management,* ed. by Polk HC Jr and Stone HH, Little, Brown and Co., Boston, 1971, p 227.
16. Bergstresser P et al: Systemic Chemotherapy for psoriasis. Arch

Derm 112:977, 1976.

17. Bianchine JR et al: Drugs as etiologic factors in the Stevens-Johnson syndrome. Am J Med 44:390, 1968.

18. Blaney DJ et al: Topical use of tetracycline in the treatment of acne. Arch Derm 112:971, 1976.

19. Burnett JW: The route of antibiotic administration in superficial impetigo, NEJM 268:72, 1963.

20. Calabresi P et al: Beneficial effects of triacetyl azauridine in psoriasis and mycosis fungoides. Ann Int Med 64:352, 1966.

21. Carruthers R: Oral zinc in cutaneous healing. Drugs 6:161, 1973.

22. Chesterman KW: An evaluation of O-T-C dandruff and seborrhea preparations. JAPhA 11:578, 1972.

23. Coleman WP: Unsual cutaneous manifestations of drug hypersensitivity. Med Clin N Am 51:1073, 1967.

24. Corbett MD et al: Idoxuridine in the treatment of cutaneous herpes simplex. JAMA 196:441, 1966.

25. Cormaish S: Ingram method of treating psoriasis. Arch Derm 92:56, 1965.

26. Crounse RG et al: Changes in scalp hair roots as a measure of toxicity from cancer chemotherapeutic drugs. J Invest Derm 35:83, 1960.

27. Dahl MD: Methotrexate hepatotoxicity in psoriasis, comparison of different dosage regimens. Br Med J 1:654, 1972.

28. Davis JE et al: Comparative evaluation of monistat and mycostatin in the treatment of vulvovaginal candidasis. Obstet Gyn 44:403, 1974.

29. Deneau DG et al: The treatment of psoriasis with azaribine. Dermatologica 151:158, 1975.

30. Derbes V: The fixed eruption. JAMA 190:765, 1964.

31. Dixon RL et al: Plasma protein binding of methotrexate and its displacement by various drugs. Fed Proc 24:545, 1965.

32. Domonkos AN: Andrews' Diseases of the Skin, 6th ed. WB Saunders Co., Philadelphia, 1971.

33. Dunster GD: Vaginal candidasis in pregnancy — trial of clotrimazole. Postgrad Med (Supp) 1:86, 1974.

34. Eaglstein WH et al: Flourouracil: mechanism of action in human skin and actinic keratoses. Arch Derm 101:132, 1970.

35. Editorial: Ampicillin rashes. Lancet 2:993, 1969.

36. Editorial: Zinc sulfate administered orally: wounds reported to heal faster. JAMA 196:33, 1966.

37. ————: Hypersensitivity skin reactions due to neomycin. Medical Letter 9:71, 1967.

38. ————: Nitrofurazone — atopical antimicrobial drug. Medical Letter 9:71, 1967.

39. ————: Methotrexate in the treatment of psoriasis. Medical Letter 14:41, 1972.

40. ————: Tinactin. Medical Letter 7:102, 1965.

41. ————: Pregnancy and other contraindications to smallpox vaccination. Medical Letter 7:37, 1965.

42. ————: Betamethasone valerate ointment (Valisone). Medical Letter 11:73, 1969.

43. ————: Topical sunscreening agents. Medical Letter 14:27, 1972.

44. ————: Newer antifungal preparations. Medical Letter 18:101, 1976.

45. ————: Miconazole — A new topical antifungal drug. Medical Letter 16:24, 1974.

46. ————: Gyne-Lotrimin for vaginal infections. Medical Letter 18:65, 1976.

47. ————: Cyproheptadine (Periactin) for allergic and pruritic dermatoses. Medical Letter 9:28, 1967.

48. Epstein E et al: Ethylenediamine-allergic contact dermatitis. Arch Derm 98:476, 1968.

49. Epstein E: Allergy to dermatologic agents. JAMA 198:517, 1966.

50. Epstein E: Photoallergy. Arch Derm 106:741, 1971.

51. Epstein S et al: Cross sensitivity to various "mycins." Arch Derm 86:101, 1962.

52. Esterby NB et al: The treatment of pyoderma in children. JAMA 212:1667, 1970.

53. Faber EM: Studies on the nature and management of psoriasis. Calif Med 114:1, 1971.

54. Faber EM et al: A current review of psoriasis. Calif Med 108:440, 1968.

55. Faber EM et al: Psoraisis — A questionnaire survey of 2,144 patients. Arch Derm 98:248, 1968.

56. FDA: Gamma benzene hexachloride alert. Bulletin on Drugs 28, June 1976.

57. Felber TD: Photodynamic inactivation of herpes simplex. JAMA 216:836, 1971.

58. Felber TD et al: Photodynamic inactivation of herpes simplex: Report of a clinical trial. JAMA 223:289, 1973.

59. Fenske NA et al: Major causes of alopecia. Postgrad Med 60:79, 1976.

60. Fischer RW: Comparison of antipruritic agents administered orally. A double-blind study. JAMA 203:418, 1968.

61. Fisher AA: Contact Dermatitis. Lea and Febiger, Philadelphia, 1967, pp. 82-90.

62. Fitzpatrick TB et al: Dermatology in General Medicine, McGraw Hill, New York, 1971.

63. Fleury F: Managing common vulvovaginal diseases. J Fam Practice 3:487, 1976.

64. Frank SB: Acne Vulgaris, Charles C Thomas, Springfield, 1971.

65. Freinkel RK et al: Effects of tetracyclines on the composition of sebum in acne vulgaris. NEJM 273:850, 1965.

66. Freinkel RK: Pathogenesis of acne vulgaris. NEJM 280:1161, 1969.

67. Gip L et al: The rapidity of effect of different types of topical corticosteroids: a double-blind comparison between diproderm ointment .05% and calmurilhydrocortisone 1%. Curr Therp Res 16:300, 1974.

68. Greaves MW: The pharmacological basis for the rational use of topically applied corticosteroids. Pharmacol for Physicians, 10:3, 1969.

69. Greaves MW et al: Effects of long-continued ingestion of zinc sulfate in patients with venous leg ulceration. Lancet 2:889, 1970.

70. Griesman FA et al: Methotrexate-associated liver disease in psoriatic patients. Northwest Med 71:609, 1972.

71. Hartman DL et al: Photodermatitis induced by drugs. Skin 3:198, 1964.

72. Hassar M et al: Treatment of pruritis. Rational Drug Therapy 9:1, Sept, 1975.

73. Hellgren L et al: On the effects of urea on human epidermis. Dermatologica 149:289, 1974.

74. Hermann HW: Clinical efficacy studies of haloprogin, a new topical antimicrobial agent. Arch Derm 106:839, 1972.

75. Hitch JM: Acneiform eruptions induced by drugs and chemicals. JAMA 200:879, 1967.

76. Honeycutt WM et al: Topical antimetabolites and cytostatic agents. Cutis 6:65, 1970.

77. Hoover JE (ed): Remington's Pharmaceutical Sciences, 14th ed., Mack Publishing Co., Easton, 1970.

78. Hughes W et al: Impetigo contagiosa: Etiology complications, and comparisons of therapeutic effectiveness of erythromycin and antibiotic ointments. Am J Dis Child 113:449, 1967.

79. Hunt TK et al: Effect of Vitamin A on reversing the inhibitory effect of cortisone on healing of open wounds in animals and man. Ann Surg 170:633, 1969.

80. Jarratt M et al: Photoinactivation therapy and herpes simplex: Reply to Dr. Pass. Arch Derm 110:642, 1974.

81. Jelinek JE: Cutaneous side effects of oral contraceptives. Arch Derm 101:181, 1970.

82. Juel-Jensen B E et al: Herpes simplex lesions of face treated with idoxuridine applied by spray gun: Results of a double-blind controlled trial. Brit Med J 1:901, 1965.

83. Kaidbey KH et al: Assay of topical corticosteroids. Arch Derm 112:808, 1976.

84. Kaplan AS: Herpes Simplex and Pseudorabies Viruses. Springer-Verlag, New York, 1969.

85. Kalivas J: Acne vulgaris — Fact, fancy and in between. Rational Drug Ther 7:1, 1973.

86. Kaminester L: Sunlight, skin cancer and sunscreens. JAMA 232:1373, 1975.

87. Kastrup EF (ed): Facts and Comparisons, Facts and Comparisons Inc., St. Louis, 1970.

88. Katz R et al: Haloprogin therapy for dermatophyte infections. Arch Derm 106:837, 1972.

89. Kern AB et al: Smallpox vaccinations in management of recurrent herpes simplex: Controlled evaluation. J Invest Derm 33:99, 1959.

90. Kern AB et al: Vaccine therapy in recurrent herpes simplex. Arch Derm 89:844, 1964.

91. Kirshbaum BA et al: Drug eruptions: A review of some of the recent literature. Am J Med Sci 240:512, 1960.

92. Kirton V et al: Contact dermatitis from neomycin and framycin. Lancet 1:138, 1965.

93. Kilgman AM: The human hair cycle. J Invest Derm 33:307, 1959.
94. Kilgman AM: Pathologic dynamics of human hair loss. Arch Derm 83:175, 1961.
95. Kilgman A M et al: Topical Vitamin A acid in acne vulgaris. Arch Derm 99:469, 1969.
96. Lee KH et al: Mechanism of action of salicylates VIII: Effect of topical application of retinoic acid on wound-healing retardation action of a few anti-inflammatory agents. J Pharm Sci 59:1036, 1970.
97. Lee KH et al: Mechanism of action of retinyl compounds on wound healing: Structural relationship of retinyl compounds and wound healing retardation action of salicylic acids. J Pharm Sci 58:773, 1969.
98. Lee KH et al: Studies on the mechanism of action of salicylates VI: Effect of topical application of retinoic acid on wound healing retardation action of salicylic acids. J Pharm Sci 58:773, 1969.
99. Leavell UW et al: Hydroxyurea — A new treatment for psoriasis. Arch Derm 102:144, 1970.
100. Leigler DG et al: The effect of organic acids on renal clearance of methotrexate in man. Clin Pharmacol Ther 10:849, 1969.
101. Logan WS: Vitamin A and keratinization. Arch Derm 105:748, 1972.
102. MacCallum FO et al: Herpes simplex virus skin infection in man treated with idoxuridine in dimethylsulphoxide: Results of double-bind controlled trial. Brit Med J 2:805, 1966.
103. MacDonald MG et al: Adverse drug reactions, Experience of Mary Fletcher Hospital during 1962. JAMA 190:1071, 1964.
104. Macmillan BC: Ecology of bacteria colonizing the burned patient given topical and systemic therapy: A five year study. J Infect Dis 124 (Suppl) 278, 1971.
105. Mandy SH: The art of tretinoin therapy in acne. Cutis 855, 1975.
106. Masterton G et al: Six day clotrimazole therapy in vaginal candidosis. Curr Med Res Opin 3:83, 1975.
107. McDonald C: Chemotherapy of Psoriasis. Int J Derm 14:563, 1975.
108. Meyers M et al: Failure of neutral-red photodynamic inactivation in recurrent herpes simplex infections. NEJM 293:945, 1975.
109. Millikan LE: Superficial and cutaneous fungal infections. Postgrad Med 60:52, 1976.
110. Moller H et al: Psoriasis treated with busulfan. Acta Derm Verner 50:445, 1970.
111. Moncrief JA: Burns. NEJM 288:444, 1973.
112. Moncrief JA: Topical therapy of the burn wound: Present status. Clin Pharmacol Ther 10:439.
113. Moncrief JA: Changing concepts in burn sepsis. J Trauma 4:233, 1964.
114. Moncrief JA et al: Topical antibacterial therapy in the treatment of burn wound. Arch Surg 92:558, 1966.
115. Moran JM et al: A clinical and bacteriologic study of infections associated with venous cut downs. NEJM 272:554, 1965.
116. Nahmias AJ et al: Infection with herpes simplex virus 1 and 2 (1st part). NEJM 289:667, 1973.
117. Nahmias AJ et al: Infection with herpes simplex virus 1 and 2 (2nd part). NEJM 289:719, 1973.
118. Nahmias AJ et al: Infection with herpes simplex virus 1 and 2 (3rd part). NEJM 289:781, 1973.
119. N.A.S. — N.R.C. Drug Efficacy Study Group, Federal Register 37:12857, 1972.
120. Newbold PC: Antimetabolites and psoriasis. Brit J Derm 86:87, 1972.
121. Noland DC et al: Idoxuridine in herpes simplex virus (type 1) encephalitis. Ann Int Med 78:243, 1973.
122. Norden CW: Application of ointment to the site of venous catheterization — a controlled trial. J Infect Dis 120:611, 1969.
123. Nugent GR et al: Treatment of labial herpes. JAMA 224:132, 1973.
124. Order SE et al: Vascular destructive effects of thermal injury and its relationship to burn wound sepsis. J Trauma 5:62, 1965.
125. Orentreich N et al: Comparative study of two antidandruff preparations. J Pharm Sci 58:1279, 1969.
126. Package insert: Retin-A. Johnson and Johnson, 1974.
127. Package insert: Neosporin Ointment. Burroughs Wellcome Co., 1974.
128. Palitz LL: Abstract of a preliminary report on norethynodrel (Enovid) in the control of acne in females. Arch Derm 86:237, 1962.
129. Palitz LL et al: Envoid for acne in the female skin. Skin 3:243, 1964.
130. Parker G et al: Poison ivy (Rhus) dermatitis. AFP 6:62, 1972.
131. Patel BM: Skin rash with infectious mononucleosis and ampicillin. Pediat 40:910, 1967.
132. Patrick J et al: Neomycin sensitivity in the normal (nonatopic) individual. Arch Derm 102:532, 1970.
133. Perry HO et al: The Goeckerman treatment of psoriasis. Arch Derm 98:178, 1968.
134. Pirila V et al: Twelve years of sensitization to neomycin in Finland. Report of 1760 cases of sensitivity to neomycin and/or bacteracin. Acta Derm Vener 47:419, 1967.
135. Pirila V et al: The pattern of cross sensitivity to neomycin. Dermatol 136:321, 1968.
136. Pirila V et al: On cross sensitization between neomycin, bacitracin, kanamycin and framycetin. Dermatol 121:335, 1960.
137. Place VA et al: Precise evaluation of topically applied corticosteroid potency. Arch Derm 101:531, 1970.
138. Poison ivy, poison oak, and poison sumac. Arch Environ Health 22:280, 1971.
139. Polk HC Jr: Aqueous silver nitrate (.5%) for topical wound care, in Contemporary Burn Management, ed. by Polk, HC and Stone, HH, Little, Brown and Co., Boston, 1971, p. 177-191.
140. Proost JM et al: Miconazole in the treatment of mycotic vulvovaginitis. Am J Ob Gyn 112:668, 1972.
141. Purdy MJ: Adverse effects of strong topical corticosteroids. Drugs 8:70, 1974.
142. Reed WB et al: Psoriasis and arthritis. Arch Derm 81:577, 1960.
143. Reisner RM: Systemic agents in the management of acne. Calif Med 106:28, 1967.
144. Reisner RM et al: Lipolytic activity of corynebacterium acne. J Int Derm 51:190, 1968.
145. Rapp F et al: Transformation of mammaliam cells by DNA-containing viruses following photodynamic inactivation. Virology 55:339, 1973.
146. Resh W et al: Topically applied antibiotics in acne vulgaris. Arch Derm 112:182, 1976.
147. Rhoades RB et al: Suppression of histamine induced pruritus by three antihistaminic drugs. J Clin Imm 55:180, 1975.
148. Rostenberg A et al: Life threatening drug eruptions. JAMA 194:660, 1965.
149. Rowson EEK et al: Human papova (wart) virus. Bact Rev 31:110, 1967.
150. Rudner ES et al: Epidemiology of contact dermatitis in North America 1972. Arch Derm 108:537, 1972.
151. Sabin A: Misery of recurrent herpes: What to do? NEJM 293:986, 1975.
152. Sams WM et al: Use of methotrexate in psoriasis. Arch Derm 105:383, 1972.
153. Savin J: Current causes of fixed drug eruptions. Brit J Derm 83:546, 1970.
154. Sawyer PR: Clotrimazole: A review of its antifungal activity and therapeutic efficacy. Drugs 9:424, 1975.
155. Scehadeh NH et al: The bacteriology of acne. Arch Derm 88:829, 1963.
156. Schiff BL et al: Cutaneous reactions of anticoagulants. Arch Derm 98:136, 1968.
157. Scoggins RB et al: Percutaneous absorption of corticosteroids. NEJM 273:831, 1965.
158. Scoggins RB et al: Relative potency of percutaneously absorbed corticosteroids in the suppression of pituitary-adrenal function. J Invest Derm 45:347, 1965.
159. Serjeant GR et al: Oral zinc sulfate in sickle cell ulcers. Lancet 2:891, 1970.
160. Shapiro S et al: Drug rash with ampicillin and other penicillins. Lancet 2:969, 1969.
161. Shelley WB: Consultations in Dermatology, WB Saunders, Philadelphia, 1972.
162. Shipkowitz NL et al: Suppression of herpes simplex virus infections by phosphonoacetic acid. Appl Microbiol 26:264, 1973.
163. Sidi E et al: Psoriasis, Charles C Thomas, Co., Springfield, Ill., 1968.
164. Smith EB: Management of herpes simplex infections of the skin. JAMA 235:1731, 1976.
165. Sneddon IB: Clinical use of topical corticosteroids. Drugs 11:193, 1976.
166. Stewart WD et al: Therapeutic agents in acne vulgaris: II D-alpha amino benzyl penicillin, erthromycin, and sulfadimetloxine. Can Med Assoc J 92:1339, 1965.
167. Stoughton RB: Bioassay system for formulations of topically

applied glucocorticosteroids. Arch Derm 106:825, 1972.

168. Stoughton RB: Perspectives in topical glucocorticosteroid therapy. Prog Derm 9:7, 1975.

169. Strauss JS et al: Systemic estrogen therapy of acne. Prog Derm 2:7, 1967.

170. Strauss JS et al: Effect of cyclic progestinestrogen therapy of sebum and acne in women. JAMA 190:815, 1964.

171. Subcommittee for the Task Force on Psoriasis: Guidelines for use of azaribine in the treatment of psoriasis. Arch Derm 112:338, 1976.

172. Taub S: Poison ivy dermatitis. Eye, Ear, Nose and Throat Monthly 51:76, 1972.

173. Taylor JR et al: Topical use of mechlorethamine in the treatment of psoriasis. Arch Derm 106:362, 1972.

174. Tobias H et al: Hepatoxicity of long-term methotrexate therapy for psoriasis. Arch Int Med 132:391, 1973.

175. Torok H: Dermatitis medicamentosa: A ten year study. Derm Int 6:57, 1969.

176. Volger WR et al: A double blind study of azaribine in treatment of psoriasis. Ann Int Med 73:951, 1970.

177. Weary PE et al: Eruptions from ampicillin in patients with infectious mononucleosis. Arch Derm 101:86, 1970.

178. Weary P et al: Acneiform eruptions resulting from antibiotic administration. Arch Derm 100:179, 1969.

179. Weinstein GD et al: Methotrexate for psoriasis. Arch Derm 103:33, 1971.

180. Whittle CH: Antifungal drugs. Pract 202:69, 1969.

181. Willis I: Sunlight and the skin. JAMA 217:1088, 1.

182. Wintrobe MM et al: *Harrison's Principles of Internal Medicine.* 7th ed., McGraw Hill, New York, 1974.

183. Wright V: Psoriatic arthritis. Arch Derm 80:27, 1959.

184. Zackheim HS et al: Topical therapy of psoriasis with mechlorethamine. Arch Derm 105:702, 1972.

185. Zaynoun ST et al: Topical antibiotics in pyodermas. Brit J Derm 90:331, 1974.

186. Selickson AS et al: Effects of topical fluorouracil on normal skin. Arch Derm 111:1301, 1975.

187. Zinner SH et al: Risk of infection with intravenous indwelling catheters: Effect of application of antibiotic ointment. J Infect Dis 120:616, 1969.

Suggested Readings in Dermatology

Braverman IM: *Skin Signs of Systemic Disease.* W.B. Saunders, Philadelphia, 1970.

Domonkos AN: *Andrews' Diseases of the Skin.* W.B. Saunders, Philadelphia, 1971.

Fitzpatrick TB et al: *Dermatology in General Medicine.* McGraw-Hill, New York, 1971.

Rode AJ et al: *Textbook of Dermatology,* 2nd ed. F.A. Davis, Philadelphia, 1973.

Arndt KA, *Manual of Dermatologic Therapeutics*, Little Brown and Co., Boston, 1974.

Journals:
Archives of Dermatology (Monthly)
British Journal of Dermatology (Monthly)

Chapter 42

Pediatric Therapy

Gary C. Cupit

Case History: Aminophylline in an Apneic Infant.

E.H. is a one-day-old 2,500-gram premature male infant born to a para 1 gravida 1 Caucasian mother. At birth the child showed appropriate development for a gestational age of 32 weeks. The infant was admitted to the newborn intensive care unit so that he could be observed closely. After approximately 24 hours, the child had episodes of apnea followed by bradycardia, occuring 12 to 15 times daily, and on one occasion, a generalized seizure was noted. At that time, phenobarbital, 5 mg/kg, was given as a single intramuscular (IM) injection, followed by 5 mg/kg/day given orally in two doses every 12 hours. Because of the severe apnea, intravenous theophylline was given in a dose of 5 mg/kg every six hours. After receiving four doses of this regimen, another seizure was observed. The possibility of increasing the phenobarbital to prevent recurring seizures is being considered.

1. What pharmacokinetic differences are observed in newborns compared with adults?

Newborn infants are no longer considered small adults. There are also qualitative differences between infants and children with regard to physiologic function. The immaturity of organs involved in drug metabolism and excretion may alter not only the pharmacokinetics, but also the toxicity of many drugs. Furthermore, tremendous variability exists in absorption, protein binding, distribution, metabolism, and excretion according to gestational age and birth weight. The complexity of variability is increased with the concomitant existence of congenital anomalies and pathological syndromes. However, it is important here to focus on the known consequences of the altered kinetic pattern.

The **absorption** of drugs from the gastrointestinal tract is regulated by pH-dependent diffusion and gastric emptying time. At birth, gastric pH is between six and eight, but falls to values of one to three in the first 24 hours. Afterwards, there is no acid secretion until the eighth or tenth day of life. During this one- to eight-day period, there exists a time of relative achlorhydria. Adult values for gastric acidity are not reached until three years of age (128). Also, gastric emptying time may be as long as six to eight hours in the newborn infant. Adult values are approached only after six to eight months.

Based on these findings, it is expected that the relatively higher bioavailability of penicillin G (45) and ampicillin (110) could be related to the relative achlorhydria that exists in the newborn period. However, it has been shown, for example, that the oral absorption of phenobarbital is both delayed and reduced in newborns up to 15 days old, and that it is more efficiently absorbed if given by intramuscular injection (122). Similarly, a delay in oral absorption has been reported for phenytoin (48) and acetaminophen (63).

In the newborn, several factors in combination lead to a decrease in **plasma protein binding**. This is related not only to the reduced plasma protein concentration, but to the presence of other factors (86): a qualitatively different albumin (fetal albumin demonstrates lower binding capacity for drugs); elevated concentrations of bilirubin and free fatty acids; a lower blood pH; and other endogenous competing substrates (121).

Another important factor which could have a significant effect on drug distribution in the newborn is the diminished concentration of a Y protein in the neonatal liver (66). This Y protein has been shown to be a major hepatic anion-binding protein, to which several antibiotics bind (57).

Although plasma albumin levels may be present at birth in the same concentrations as in adults, total plasma proteins and protein binding do not reach adult values until the child is 10 to 12 months of age (125).

The changes in the **volume of distribution** of drugs in the newborn are an important consideration. These changes have been linked to both the decrease in plasma protein binding of drugs (86) and the increase in extracellular fluid volume (27). Extracellular fluid volume decreases from 50% in prematures to 35% in 4- to 6-month-old infants, to 25% at one year, and 20% in adults. Total body water changes from 86% in prematures to 70% in full-term infants and to 55% in adults (27).

In terms of drug dosing, this means that the dose of a relatively water soluble drug would be decreased as the child's age and weight increased. As a result of an expanded apparent volume of distribution, a given plasma level in the newborn may reflect a plasma to

Table 1
ANTIBIOTIC DOSAGE SCHEDULES IN NEWBORN INFANTS

Drug	Infants Less Than One Week	Infants One to Four Weeks
Ampicillin Sodium	50-100 mg/kg (2)*	100-200 mg/kg (3)
Gentamicin Sulfate	5 mg/kg (2)	7.5 mg/kg (3)
Kanamycin Sulfate	15-20 mg/kg (2)	15-20 mg/kg (2)
Methicillin Sodium	100 mg/kg (2)	200-250 mg/kg (4)
Aqueous Penicillin G	50,000-100,000 u/kg (2)	50,000-100,000 u/kg (3)

*Number in parentheses reflects number of doses in which the daily dosage should be equally divided.

(Adapted from the data of: McCracken GH Jr: Pharmacologic basis for antimicrobial therapy in newborn infants. Clin Perinat 2:139, 1975)

tissue ratio higher than an adult's, resulting in a larger amount of drug in the body tissues than is reflected by the same concentration in adults.

The development of **drug metabolizing enzymes** and activity in humans is a poorly explored area. Several specific compounds have been studied to develop some understanding of this field.

In newborns, it has been reported that an increased half-life for *acetaminophen* exists, mainly because of decreased glucuronidation (120). This was studied further and it was found that the limited capacity for acetaminophen conjugation with glucuronic acid was partially compensated by a well developed capacity for sulfate conjugation.

Another drug with an increase in plasma half-life in newborns secondary to decreased metabolism is *diazepam*. Hydroxylation of the demethylated active metabolite is minimal in newborns and is related to the degree of maturation of the infant (77,87). In full-term newborns, the apparent plasma half-life of diazepam ranges from 20 to 45 hours, but premature newborns demethylate diazepam more slowly (87) so the half-life in these subjects is 40 to 100 hours.

This prolonged half-life of diazepam in newborns is altered by exposure of the infant in utero or in the first few days of life to compounds that increase the enzymatic activity of the liver. A prime example of such an induction is exposure of the fetus or the newborn to phenobarbital. After brief exposure to phenobarbital, the newborn infant, premature or full-term, has an apparent half-life for diazepam of 12 to 16 hours. This decrease in half-life is parallelled by an increase in the hydroxylating and conjugating activities of the liver as documented by urinary measurements of metabolites (106).

Other drugs for which a prolonged apparent half-life is observed secondary to decreased metabolism include: amobarbital (55), phenytoin (83), and salicylate (30, 64).

Another organ system that has a distinct effect on drug elimination is the kidneys. At birth, the **renal function** of premature and full-term infants is lower than that of children and adults. Renal function comparable to that of adults is not reached until the child is between six months and one year of age (86). And it should also be noted that glomerular filtration, tubular secretion, and tubular reabsorption do not mature at the same rate (67). Also, urinary pH is somewhat lower in newborns than in children and adults (73).

Compounds that are not extensively metabolized and are dependent on renal function for excretion are eliminated slowly in the newborn infant. For drugs eliminated in this manner, doses and dosage schedules should be adjusted and based on maturation of kidney function. Examples of these adjustments are shown in Table 1.

In contrast to the lower doses required for some compounds that are eliminated renally, other compounds require higher doses to achieve their action. A prime example of such compounds are the thiazide diuretics. The diuretic response may be limited by a lowered glomerular filtration rate (GFR) in the newborn and immature tubular function. Presently, saluretic compounds such as furosemide appear to be the diuretics of choice in the neonate; in infants with a depressed GFR, an osmotic diuresis after glucose administration may produce beneficial results (67).

2. How is theophylline used in newborn infants to treat apnea? What dosing considerations must be undertaken?

Apnea in the newborn period is a life-threatening condition. It is usually associated with periods of bradycardia following the apneic episode. Past treatment has been external stimulation, consisting of gently agitating or irritating the infant to resume spontaneous breathing.

Recently, consideration has been given to the use of pharmacologic agents in the treatment of apnea. Currently, the most promising agent is theophylline, which is thought to act centrally to stimulate spontaneous breathing (58). Since the recognition of this effect on respiration, theophylline has been given to apneic newborns in the form of suppositories (58), oral solutions (33, 118), and by intravenous infusion (3).

Theophylline disposition in newborns differs considerably from that in children and adolescents. The average half-life of 19.9 hours in newborns is greater when compared to a mean of 3.4 hours in children aged 1.3 to 4.4 years (69) and 3.7 hours in older children (33). The volume of distribution in newborns is also larger, averaging 0.91 L/kg compared to 0.48 L/kg in young children (69) and 0.42 L/kg in older children (33). This observed increase in the apparent volume of distribution may be accounted for either from increased total body water (50) or by diminished binding to plasma proteins (3).

The successful management of apnea with theophylline depends on the maintainence of appropriate therapeutic concentrations. In adults, the concentration that is thought to be desirable for the treatment of asthma is a plasma level of 5 to 20 mg/L (84), with toxicity more likely with levels above 20 mg/L. Presently, it is thought that the desired upper concentration limits in newborns are determined by toxiticity and not efficacy. The therapeutic concentration range of 10 to 20 mg/L in adults corresponds to 4.4 to 8.8 mg/L of unbound theophylline. These levels of unbound theophylline would correspond to total concentrations of 6.9 to 13.8 mg/L in newborn plasma (3). These levels appear to be desirable for the treatment of apnea in newborn infants (107).

Based on the pharmacokinetic data presented here, the initial loading dose of theophylline should be approximately 6 mg/kg with a constant infusion of 0.14 mg/kg/hour or 2 mg/kg every 12 hours (3, 33). (It must be recognized that this data is obtained from a small number of premature infants. Therefore, frequent serum determinations should be performed to assist in tailoring the dose to each patient.)

In the case previously presented, the dosage of theophylline which was given, which was 1 mg/kg/hr, was approximately seven times the recommended rate of infusion for newborns. One possible explanation for this infant's seizures, if infection, hypoxia, bleeding, and other causes are eliminated, is theophylline toxicity. (See the chapter on *Asthma* for further explanation.) Certainly, a serum level drawn at this time would be of value to eliminate this possibility. If this is the case, the discontinuation of anticonvulsants should be considered.

Case History: Hyperbilirubinemia

M.T. is a female infant, born after a 37-week gestation period to a para 0 gravida 2 mother. At birth the child's weight is 3,250 grams and the physical examination indicates nothing unusual. During the course of the infant and mother, nothing remarkable occurs until the infant's third hospital day. At this time serum bilirubin, which has been rising 12 hours after delivery, has been noted to have reached 16 mg/100ml. No evidence exists for sepsis or ABO (blood-type) incompatibility, and the infant is being bottle fed. Discussion is initiated at this time regarding the management of this situation.

3. What is the etiology of hyperbilirubinemia in newborn infants?

During the first week of life many newborn infants are hyperbilirubinemic by adult standards (serum conjugated bilirubin greater than 2 mg/100 ml). This transient hyperbilirubinemia is usually benign in full-term infants and has been termed physiologic jaundice. In the absence of hemolytic disease, "physiologic" jaundice may be defined as an elevation of the serum bilirubin not exceeding 12 mg/100 ml in full-term infants or 15 mg/100 ml in premature infants during the first week of life (74).

Full-term infants usually develop maximum serum bilirubin concentrations at three to four days of age; concentrations diminish thereafter. In the premature infant, physiologic jaundice peaks in five to seven days and bilirubin levels are higher than in term infants (49).

Any or all of the following factors may contribute to reduced bilirubin clearance in the neonatal period (116): overproduction of pigment, deficiency of hepatic uptake, maternal interference by factors transmitted placentally or through breast milk, or increased intestinal absorption of pigment excreted in bile.

4. Why is an elevated bilirubin more serious in an infant than in an adult?

Elevated plasma levels of unconjugated bilirubin occur almost exclusively in the newborn period and may result in neurologic damage. Although **kernicterus** is strictly a pathological diagnosis (i.e. the presence of bilirubin in the central nervous system), the term is now used to describe any neurological damage associated with hyperbilirubinemia.

Before considering the theories explaining the occurence of kernicterus in newborns, it is useful to review the metabolism of bilirubin in this age group and compare it to that of adults. The normal destruction of red cells by the reticuloendothelial system (RES) accounts for approximately 75% of daily bilirubin production in the newborn infant (31, 49). Once bilirubin leaves the RES it is tightly bound to albumin and transported to the parenchymal cells of the liver where it is conjugated by an enzyme system, bilirubin glucuronyl transferase (25). (Also see Figure 1 in the chapter on *Interpretation of Clinical Laboratory Tests*). After conjugation, bilirubin is rapidly excreted by the hepatic cell into the bile and excreted into the intestine. In the adult, conjugated bilirubin is reduced to urobilinogen, by normal gut flora and there is minimal enterohepatic circulation; however, the newborn infants lack this intestinal flora. Instead, their intestinal mucosa contains a large amount of betaglucuronidase, which hydrolyzes conjugated bilirubin to the unconjugated form which may be reabsorbed in the intestine and recirculated in the plasma (49).

As previously mentioned, unconjugated bilirubin in the plasma is firmly bound to albumin, and less than 1% is present in the free, diffusible form (91). Only the free (diffusible) bilirubin is able to enter intracellular fluid compartments and cross the blood-brain barrier where it may damage the central nervous system.

Several factors may predispose the newborn to elevated levels of free, unconjugated bilirubin. First, newborns, especially premature infants have low serum albumin levels. Second, acidosis is common in sick infants and the binding affinity of bilirubin for albumin decreases with a decreasing pH. (92). Finally, several exogenous or endogenous organic ions have been found to compete with bilirubin for albumin binding sites. Exogenous substances include drugs such as salicylates (114); sulfonamides (75); sodium benzoate (114) found in products such as caffeine with sodium benzoate and in the injectable form of diazepam; novobiocin, oxacillin, cephalothin (75); and possibly methylparaben (68, 100). However, many of these reports result from *in vitro* testing and their clinical importance is unknown at present. Recently, an *in vivo* test of methylparaben, a preservative for gentamicin injection, failed to corroborate the increased displacement of bilirubin that had been reported from previous *in vitro* studies. The explanation for the difference between *in vitro* and *in vivo* observations may be *in vivo* preservative catabolism or excretion (127). Endogenous anions that are competitive with bilirubin for albumin include fatty acids (40) and bile acids (29).

5. What is the current treatment for hyperbilirubinemia?

Essentially, three means exist for the treatment of hyperbilirubinemia: a) removal of bilirubin by mechanical means, such as exchange transfusion, b) acceleration of normal metabolic pathways for bilirubin by the use of phenobarbital, and c) utilization of alternative pathways such as phototherapy for bilirubin excretion.

a) The removal of bilirubin by **exchange transfusion** is done primarily when there is impending severe hyperbilirubinemia or hemolysis, complicating ABO incompatibility. Exchange transfusion removes red blood cells and bilirubin-laden plasma and provides fresh plasma with bilirubin-free albumin (74). Thus, during the exchange, bilirubin may be mobilized from the extravascular space. Even after a "two-volume" exchange, the serum bilirubin may remain at 45% of the pre-exchange level; this reflects the mobilization of extracellular bilirubin into the circulation (113).

It has also been shown that the administration of albumin in a dose of 1 gm/kg one to two hours before the exchange will enhance the removal of bilirubin (17,93).

b) **Phenobarbital**, a potent inducer of microsomal enzymes, increases bilirubin conjugation and excretion in the newborn (13). However, it is important to emphasize that in addition to enhancing the activity of hepatic bilirubin glucuronyl transferase (129), phenobarbital affects the entire hepatic transport system for organic anions, which may be viewed as a functional unit including uptake, biotransformation, and excretion (117,130).

The possible adverse effects of phenobarbital on the neonate have been reviewed extensively (124). Liver cells affected by phenobarbital may become more susceptible to hepatotoxic drugs; the increase in microsomal activity may accelerate the metabolism of some drugs, making them less effective (11); and sexual and behavioral development may be affected by a possible alteration in steroid metabolism (18). Another concern is that large doses of barbiturates in pregnant women have produced coagulation defects in newborns (88). Since the excretion of barbiturates in the newborn is extremely variable, levels may be present in some infants for days or weeks, while others excrete the drug within 48 hours (80). Parenteral barbiturates used as sedatives in labor can affect the infant and lead to a reduced oral intake after birth (56). Despite these reports of possible adverse reactions, no immediate or serious side effects have been reported from those clinical trials in which phenobarbital was given to mothers and infants (74).

The indications for the use of phenobarbital in the newborn are poorly defined. Phenobarbital in a daily dose of 5 mg/kg, requires 72 hours to achieve a lowering of serum bilirubin by 1 to 2 mg/100 ml whereas, the same effect is obtained after 8 to 12 hours of exposure to phototherapy. Phenobarbital is also less effective in low birthweight infants.

c) The evidence from several well controlled studies clearly indicates that **phototherapy** is an effective procedure in the treatment of hyperbilirubinemia of prematurity (34,41,70). In these patients, a 30 to 50% lower average serum bilirubin concentration may be attained in infants who are treated with light than in infants in the control group. This means that instead of a 20% incidence of serum bilirubin levels over 15 mg/100 ml, there may be an incidence of only 2% if phototherapy is used (71).

Photodegradation of bilirubin is thought to be the mechanism of action of phototherapy. The ability of bile pigments to absorb light is a function of their molecular structure. Free bilirubin, which is not bound to albumin, is especially susceptible to photo-oxidation (61). The lights which are most effective in photo-oxidizing bilirubin are those which have a high energy output near the absorption peak of bilirubin, which is 450 to 460 nm (109).

Adverse reactions to phototherapy have been a concern since its introduction. Reactions and dangers that have been reported include: effects on growth and development (74), loose stools and skin rashes (72), bronze discoloration (108), jaundice masked by the lights (113), retinal damage (74), and increased insensible water loss (94). Eute and Klein present a more extensive listing of complications (23). Despite this long list of possible complications, many of which are rare, the use of phototherapy has been amazingly hazard free.

In an effort to improve the effectiveness of phototherapy, several adjunctive measures have been tried. The use of twin banks of fluorescent lights above and below the infant has been advocated to increase the surface area of the infant exposed to radiation (47). The relative safety of this greater exposure remains to be evaluated. Riboflavin may enhance the photocatabolism of bilirubin *in vivo* (54,94) and it may soon be possible to administer pharmacologic doses (1.5 mg/kg of riboflavin phosphate) of this vitamin to reduce the intensity and duration of phototherapy. In two studies (119,126) it was shown that the concomitant use of phenobarbital and phototherapy was not more effective than phototherapy used alone.

Agar, a drug that interferes with the enterohepatic circulation of bilirubin has been used. However, in a recent trial with agar administered to low birth-weight infants (79), the results conflicted with earlier reports of success in lowering the serum bilirubin in term infants (97). At the present time, agar cannot be recommended for the treatment of hyperbilirubinemia.

6. A 27-year-old female complains of "burning urine" to her physician. Examination and diagnosis revealed signs and symptoms of an acute urinary tract infection. A prescription is given to the patient for sulfisoxazole, 500 mg. No. 80 with directions to take two tablets four times a day for ten days. When the patient is presented with the prescription by the physician, she informs him that she has a ten-day-old child who is being breast-fed.

What is the clinical significance of the excretion of pharmacologic compounds in breast milk?

To appreciate the complexity of determining whether drugs are excreted in breast milk, it is important to understand those factors related to their ability to cross from plasma into breast milk.

The composition of breast milk changes in three phases after the birth of the child. The milk differs in fat content, carbohydrate content, and pH during these phases, and the ability of a drug to cross from the plasma into breast milk is altered during each of these stages. In the first three to four post-partum days, colostrum is secreted. It is a yellow, alkaline fluid which has a greater specific gravity than breast milk. Colostrum has a lower carbohydrate and fat content than the breast milk that appears later. After a few days, colostrum is replaced by a transitional milk which assumes the characteristics of whole breast milk by the third week (90). The time of feeding also is important to the composition of breast milk. In the morning, the fat content is highest, a condition which favors the excretion of lipid soluble drugs.

Once a drug has achieved a therapeutic plasma concentration, it must cross the capillary endothelium into the alveolar cells of the breast where it can be excreted into the lumen with the milk. This process occurs by diffusion since a variation exists in the concentration gradient between plasma and milk. Drugs which are weak acids or bases cross membranes in the unionized form, so the pH difference between plasma (pH 7.4) and breast milk (pH 6.8) is important (62). Breast milk which is more acidic than plasma would "trap" drugs that are weak bases (12).

For example, erythromycin, a weak base with a pKa of 8.8, which has a ratio of ionized to unionized drug of 15 to 1 in the serum will readily pass into breast milk where the ratio of ionized to unionized molecules is 100:1 (62). From this data the concentration of erythromycin in breast milk should theoretically be six times its concentration in maternal plasma, and this has been confirmed in clinical studies (90).

Table 2 summarizes those drugs that are clinically significant when taken by breast feeding mothers.

When information is not available about a drug's excretion in breast milk, the risks should be weighed against the benefits. During the time of drug administration, the infant can be bottle fed and the mother can pump her breasts. Then, breast feeding can resume when the drug therapy has been completed.

7. Compare the nutrient needs of infants to adults.

During the first year of life, growth is greater than at any other time period. An infant doubles his birthweight at six months of age and triples it by one year of age.

The recommended daily dietary allowance (RDA) for total caloric intake is approximately 120 Cals/kg of body weight per day for infants in the first six months, and approximately 105 Cals/kg per day in infants six months to one year of age. As would be expected, the premature or low birthweight infant has a greater caloric need than the full-term infant, requiring as much as 130 Cals/kg per day (6). (Adults' caloric requirements are 40 Cals/kg/day.)

Of the total caloric intake, provision must be made for adequate intake of protein, carbohydrates, and fats. Protein intake should be approximately two to three

Table 2
DRUGS EXCRETED IN BREAST MILK

DRUG	AMOUNT EXCRETED	SIGNIFICANCE
Aspirin	Moderate amounts	May cause bleeding tendency by its platelet effects on the infant
Atropine Sulfate	Below 0.1 mg/100 ml	May cause atropine intoxication in infant
Bromides	0-6.6 mg/100 ml	Reactions include rashes and drowsiness
Chloramphenicol	Breast milk levels 50% of serum levels	Toxicity related to inability to glucuronidate and excrete chloramphenicol resulting in "gray baby" syndrome
Cyclophosphamide	Unknown	Nursing should be discontinued during all antineoplastic therapy
Diazepam	51 ng/ml after 96 hours therapy	May induce lethargy and weight loss
Erythromycin	3.6 - 6.2 ug/ml	Higher concentrations in milk than in plasma have been observed
Estrogens (Oral Contraceptives)	0.17 ug/100 ml	Possible gynecomastia in male infants; may inhibit lactation if given in early postnatal development
Isoniazid	0.6 - 1.2 mg/100 ml Milk levels equal serum levels	Monitor infants for signs of isoniazid toxicity
Lithium Carbonate	0.3 mEq/liter	Infant should be monitored for possible lithium toxicity
Meprobamate	Milk levels 2-4 times maternal levels	Monitor infant for intoxication if therapy must be continued
Nicotine	0.4 - 0.5 mg/liter; 11-20 cigarettes/day	Only if no more than 20 cigarettes per day are consumed
Penicillin G	6 units/100 ml	Parents should inform physician that infant has been exposed to penicillin
Potassium Iodide	3 mg/100 ml	Avoid, may affect infant thyroid
Sulfapyridine	3-13 mg/100 ml after 3 gm daily dose	Can cause skin rashes
Sulfisoxazole	Concentration equal to plasma level	May cause kernicterus during first month of life
Thiazides	Unknown	Avoid, based on manufacturers recommendations
Thiouracil	Higher in milk than in blood: 9-12 mg/100 ml	Avoid, may cause goiter or a-granulocytosis in nursing infants
Warfarin	Unknown	Infant must be monitored with mother

Data adapted from O'Brien, 1974 (90)

gm/kg/day, or 7 to 16% of the total intake per day. (Adult protein requirements are approximately 1 gm/kg/day.) Carbohydrates should range from 35 to 65% and fat, 30 to 50% of the total caloric intake. Of particular importance is the provision of the essential fatty acids, linoleic and arachidonic acids, in the fat intake (19).

8. What is the composition of the available infant formulas? How do they differ from breast milk?

All commercial formulas are patterned after the nutrient qualities of breast milk. Cow's milk is used as the base in many of the formulas because it is safe, inexpensive, and convenient. Any formula which is selected should have an adequate distribution of protein, carbohydrate, and fat; be readily digestible; and provide all the essential vitamins and minerals.

Metabolic studies have found that for the infant 7 to 16% of calories should be derived from protein, 30 to 50% from fat, and 35 to 65 per cent from carbohydrate (26). Human milk contains 7% protein, 55% fat, and 38% carbohydrate. Corresponding values for cow's milk are 20% protein, 50% fat, and 30% carbohydrate.

Human and cow's milk contain two different types of protein: casein (the protein in the curd) and whey. The predominant protein of cow's milk is casein, while in human milk it is whey. It should be noted that the high casein content of cows' milk can be responsible for the formation of a hard rubbery mass in the infant's stomach, and to prevent this, cow's milk formulas are usually heat- or acid-treated to prevent curd formation (2).

The fat in cow's milk differs from that found in human milk in two characteristics: the triglycerides of cow's milk consist of short- and long-chain fatty acids, while human milk contains primarily medium chain fatty acids. Also, human milk is composed of unsaturated fatty acids, while cow's milk primarily contains saturated fatty acids. Commercial formulas attempt to duplicate human milk by utilizing vegetable oils and medium-chain triglyceride (MCT) oils (6). Table 3 shows a breakdown of the composition of many infant formulas.

9. Discuss the common feeding disorders of infancy and the therapeutic use of formulas.

The classification of formulas under the heading of therapeutic formulas in Table 3 is useful in deciding how to respond to many disorders of infancy that affect feeding. Those disorders include milk allergy, fat restriction, congenital heart disease, and caloric and carbohydrate restrictions.

Milk allergy is a disorder that must be differentiated from milk intolerance. **Milk intolerance** generally presents as abdominal discomfort, "spitting up," and poor feeding habits. It can usually be relieved by diluting the formula or slowing the feeding rate. **Milk allergy,** how-

ever, is manifested by a rash, wheezing, and other allergic symptoms; in this condition, all forms of milk protein must be eliminated, and substitution of either soy or casein formulas are recommended. In "true" milk allergy, it has been reported that the soy protein formulas are frequently cross-allergenic with cow's milk protein (32). This may necessitate a change to a formula such as Nutramigen.

Infants who require **fat restriction** include those with cystic fibrosis of the pancreas and celiac disease. Often a formula such a Pregestimil has been useful in these disorders; however, it is possible to utilize pancreatic enzymes with a commercial milk formula.

Those infants with **congenital heart disease** (CHD) usually require a concentrated formula with a low sodium content. The formula must be concentrated, because many CHD infants tire before finishing feeding. Formulas such as SMA Improved, PM 60/40, or Lonalac may be concentrated to 100 Cals/100 ml without creating an excessive intake of solute.

Many infants may also develop a condition of **disaccharidase deficiency.** This may occur as a congenital defect, secondary to such conditions as cystic fibrosis or may result from severe diarrhea. During disaccharidase deficiency, the infant's ability to hydrolyze disaccharides is impaired. The increase in the quantity of undigested disaccharides in the colon creates an osmotic gradient, resulting in loose, watery stools. In these cases, a formula such as CHO-Free may be given to eliminate carbohydrates from the diet. Later, it may be possible to reintroduce carbohydrates slowly.

Infants with **galactosemia,** resulting from deficiency of the enzyme galactose-1-phosphate uridyl transferase, must have milk lactose eliminated from their diet. When this precursor is eliminated, the body may convert glucose only to the amount of galactose it requires (6). Formulas such as Nutramigen would be acceptable.

10. M.K., a two-month-old infant, returns to the clinic for his first scheduled well-baby visit. The mother inquires about immunizations for her baby.

What is the present status of immunizations in pediatrics and when should some of these immunizations be given?

Advancements in the field of immunizations have been remarkable over the past ten years. Recent developments have provided live viral vaccines against polio, measles, rubella, and mumps. In addition, bacterial vaccines against meningococcal disease, H. influenza infection, and pneumococcal infections are under evaluation.

Despite many of these advances, there was a decline in the number of immunized pre-school age children during the early 1970s. National surveys indicate that 40% of the 14 million one-to-four-year-old children are

Table 3
INFANT FORMULAS (ABBREVIATED CONTENTS)

	Cal/100 ml	Protein Gm/100 ml	Fat Gm/100 ml	CHO Gm/100 ml	Na mEq/100 ml	K mEq/100 ml	Type CHO	Source Protein	Type Fat
STANDARD FORMULAS									
Breast Milk	75	1.1	4.5	6.8	0.7	1.3	Lactose	Human Milk	Human Milk Fat
Whole Cow's Milk	69	3.5	3.5	4.9	2.5	3.6	Lactose	Cow's Milk	Butterfat
Enfamil	66	1.5	3.7	7.0	1.1	1.8	Lactose	Cow's Milk	Corn, Oleo, Coconut Oil
Similac	66	1.8	3.6	7.0	1.3	2.3	Lactose	Cow's Milk	Coconut, Corn Oil
SMA Improved	66	1.5	3.5	6.8	0.7	1.4	Lactose	Demineralized Whey	Safflower Oil
THERAPEUTIC FORMULAS									
Milk Allergy									
Isomil	66	2.0	3.6	6.8	1.4	1.8	Sucrose Malto-dextrins	Soy Isolate	Corn, Coconut Oil
Mull-Soy	66	3.1	3.6	5.2	1.6	4.0	Sucrose Invert Sugar	Soy	Soy Oil
Neo-Mull-Soy	66	1.8	3.5	6.4	1.7	2.5	Sucrose	Soy Isolate	Soy Oil
Nutramigen	66	2.2	2.6	8.6	1.3	2.6	Sucrose Arrowroot Starch	Hydrolyzed Casein	MCT Oil
Pro-Sobee	66	2.5	3.4	6.8	2.1	2.2	Corn syrup solids	Soy Isolate	Soy Oil
Medium-Chain Triglyceride (MCT) Formula									
Portagen	66	2.3	3.1	7.4	1.7	2.6	Sucrose Malto-dextrins	Casein	MCT Oil
Carbohydrate (CHO) or Fat Restriction									
CHO-Free Formula Base	40	1.8	3.5	0.02	1.6	2.2	None	Soy	Soy Oil
Pregestimil	66	2.2	2.8	8.8	1.9	2.3	Glucose	Hydrolyzed Casein	MCT Oil
Skim Milk	36	3.6	Trace	5.3	2.3	3.6	Lactose	Cow's Milk	None
Renal Solute Restriction									
PM 60/40	66	1.5	3.4	7.2	0.6	1.4	Lactose	Cow's Milk	Corn, Coconut Oil
Sodium Restriction									
Lonalac	66	3.4	3.5	4.8	0.1	2.6	Lactose	Casein	Coconut Oil

Adapted from Bender, 1975(6).

not immunized against polio, measles, rubella, pertussis, or diphtheria. Polio immunization dropped from a high of 88% of those eligible in 1964, to a low of 63% in 1974 (32).

An examination of the available immunizations and a discussion of their risks and benefits is appropriate in view of the present decline in immunization practices. An immunization schedule that is presently recommended is shown in Table 4.

Diphtheria-Pertussis-Tetanus (DPT): DPT is a combined product containing alum-precipitated diphtheria-tetanus toxoids and killed pertussis bacteria. The advantages of DPT over single antigens are: 1) greater antigenic stimulation with more pertussis response, and 2) decreased incidence of systemic reactions. tions.

Its disadvantages include local reactions and a slightly increased interval until antibodies are stimulated. Reactions may be decreased if the vaccine is injected intramuscularly rather than subcutaneously (53).

When immunization of DPT is completed, between 20 to 80% of infants will be protected from pertussis (115); protection against diphtheria and tetanus will approach 100 per cent. If a dose is missed, due to illness or other factors, the other doses may be given later without restarting immunizations. Intervals of six to nine months have been acceptable (53).

The incidence of serious systemic reactions to pertussis vaccine or DPT in this country is unknown. In Sweden, a study of severe reactions revealed that the incidence of neurological reactions was about one in 6,000 immunizations. Death or permanent damage occurred in one of 17,000 persons immunized (115). Other estimates have been placed at 1 in 50,000 to 1 in 100,000 (76).

If a convulsion, severe febrile reaction, or thrombocytopenia occur after innoculation, pertussis administration should be discontinued. Immunization should then be performed with DT. The "adult DT" should not be used for children under the age of six since "adult DT" is altered to contain 5 to 10% the amount of diphtheria toxoid in the regular preparation to reduce undesirable reactions. However, this vaccine may be safely used after children are six years of age. The recommended interval for DT boosters is ten years.

Poliovirus Vaccines: The number of children who are protected against all three types of polio in the United States has continued to drop. While epidemics of paralytic polio have been reported in the last few years, they have occurred mostly in unvaccinated individuals. In other parts of the world, polio cases have continued to rise over the last few years, particularly in the tropics and subtropics. This is a concern for Americans who travel abroad.

The live vaccine (attenuated, Sabin, oral) can be given as the monovalent form, containing one poliovirus type, or as the trivalent, containing all three types. In the trivalent form, dosages are adjusted so that Type 2 does not predominate over Types 1 and 3.

Recent controversy has arisen regarding the relative safety of oral polio virus vaccine (OPV) versus that of inactivated poliovirus vaccine (IPV). This controversy resulted from a 1974 court decision (Reyes versus Wyeth, No. 72-2251, U.S. Court of Appeals, 5th Circuit) that raised questions regarding the legal liability involved in the risk of paralysis secondary to OPV administration. Among the reported 111 cases of paralytic polio that were reported in the U.S. between 1969 and 1974, 15 occurred in OPV recipients and 27 in their contacts. Of the 15 OPV cases, 5 were immunodeficient. This incidence equates to a risk of one case of paralytic disease for every 9,000,000 doses of vaccine (28).

The arguments for continuance of OPV include (28) its efficacy in preventing polio and thus, efficacy in halting epidemics; its provision of intestinal immunity and lowering of wild virus growth; the practicality of oral administration; and the lack of need for "booster" doses to provide immunity through life.

Arguments for using IPV include (104) its demonstrated efficacy in the U.S. when it was the sole vaccine available; the Scandinavian experience (only IPV was used and, with 90% of the population immunized, neither paralytic polio nor wild virus were reported); the lack of side effects, especially paralytic polio; and the claimed long lasting immunity.

While the advantages of OPV are attractive, the recent litigation regarding its risks may make IPV an attractive alternative. Presently, with provision of good patient information and informed consent, OPV re-

Table 4
IMMUNIZATION AND TUBERCULIN TESTING SCHEDULE FOR INFANTS AND CHILDREN

Age	Vaccines
2 months	DPTa, TOPVb
4 months	DPT, TOPV
6 months	DPT, TOPV
1 year	Measlesc, Tuberculin Testd
1-12 years	Rubellac, Mumpsc
1.5 years	DPT, TOPV
4-6 years	DPT, TOPV
14-16 years	
Tde	

a — DPT: diphtheria-pertussis-tetanus.

b — TOPV: trivalent oral polio virus vaccine.

c — May be given at one year as Measles-Rubella or Measles-Mumps-Rubella combined vaccines.

d — Tuberculin testing frequency dependent on risk of exposure and prevalence of TB in the population group.

e — Td: combined tetanus and diphtheria (adult type).

mains a rational selection.

Measles-Mumps-Rubella: *Live measles vaccines* offer stimulation of antibodies in 95% of recipients, and immunity appears to continue undiminished for at least nine years as measured by antibody titers. Inactivated measles vaccines are no longer used since they afford protection of limited duration and have been associated with illness years later upon exposure to natural or "atypical" measles.

Mumps vaccine is a live attenuated viral strain grown in chicken fibroblasts. It is contraindicated in patients sensitive to eggs or neomycin. It has been shown that immunity persists undiminished for six to eight years. Administration of this vaccine to patients who have had mumps has resulted in no adverse effects (53).

Live attenuated rubella virus vaccines have now been developed. Although only 10 to 20% of women of childbearing age have not acquired natural immunity, infection in this group carries a high risk of fetal abnormalities. Presently, immunization programs are designed to protect women from exposure by immunizing children, and it is hoped that, in addition, women will maintain immunity from childhood into adulthood.

Recipients of the rubella vaccine may experience lymphadenopathy, transient arthralgias, or arthritis two to four weeks after immunization. Immunization is contraindicated in pregnancy or in women who may become pregnant during the next two months. Present data indicate that the risk to an unborn infant from immunizing the mother is not as great as previously thought (85).

Presently, it is recommended that measles, mumps, and rubella be given as a combined immunization. Data clearly show that there is no difference in antibody titers from giving separate immunizations or from combining them (123).

11. What is recommended for a four-year-old child who has not received any immunizations?

A basic schedule to "catch up" a child who is not current with his immunizations is as follows (96):

First visit:	DT (diphtheria-tetanus)
	TOPV (trivalent oral polio virus vaccine)
	Tuberculin-Tine Test
Two months later:	DT
	TOPV
	MMR (Measle-Mumps-Rubella)
One year later:	DT
	TOPV

Case History: Otitis Media

R.I. is a five-year-old male who comes to the outpatient clinic with a chief complaint of an earache. The history of his present illness includes two days of cough and sore throat, and his past medical history is unremarkable for any related conditions. A physical examination reveals a suppurative otitis media. Tympanocentesis is performed and appropriate cultures are taken. Antibiotic therapy is to be instituted.

12. Discuss the factors which predispose infants and children to otitis media.

Otitis media is a disease that is confined almost exclusively to the pediatric population. One study has shown that in 722 children followed from infancy through 7½ to 13½ years of age, 84% had at least one episode of otitis media and 40% had four or more episodes (10). This incidence is increased in premature infants (8) and in infants bottle fed in the supine position (5).

Children with chronic otitis media have evidence of eustacian tube dysfunction. Many of these children develop either eustachian tube obstruction and/or abnormal reflux of nasopharyngeal secretions into the middle ear (9). Eustachian tube obstruction results in high negative pressures within the middle ear when oxygen is absorbed from the middle ear cavity. Because of the pressure gradient between the nasopharynx and the middle ear, intermittent opening of the eustachian tube can result in nasopharyngeal secretions being aspirated into the middle ear.

The high incidence of otitis media in children is the result of factors which predispose to tubal obstruction and tubal reflux (42).

13. What organisms most commonly cause otitis media infections?

Specific therapy of otitis media is dependent on the bacterial etiology of the disease.

The most common agent that has been isolated from middle ear exudates is *Diplococcus pneumoniae* (pneumococcus). It has been isolated in 25 to 50% of the patients older than six weeks of age (44,89). *Hemophilus influenza* has been isolated from another 20% of patients less than five years of age (44,89). The importance of *Hemophilus influenza* in older children is becoming more evident since it has now been cultured from 12 to 14% of patients older than seven years of age (101). Streptococci have been implicated in fewer than 1% of the cases of otitis media. *Neisseria catarrhalis* has been reported to be a significant pathogen in 5 to 8% of the cases (52). The presence of *Staphylococcus aureas* and *S. epidermidis* are difficult to interpret in many middle ear infections, because cultures may have been contaminated with organisms from the external ear canal; however, the possibility that they are pathogens cannot be excluded. Recently, *S. epidermidis* was isolated in pure cultures in 10 of 130 patients seen for otitis media (24). In a study of neonatal otitis media, coliforms and *S. aureus* were the most common organisms obtained (8).

14. What antibiotics are most efficacious in the treatment of otitis media?

The use of antibiotics in the treatment of otitis media is not without controversy in that in spite of bacterial etiology, many of the infections are self-limiting (101). However, two studies have shown a significant, but less dramatic, difference between antibiotic and placebo treatment of otitis media (39,59). In view of the risk of severe complications that may result from untreated otitis media (e.g. mastoiditis, meningitis, brain abscess), appropriate treatment should be initiated as rapidly as possible.

In treating *Hemophilus influenza* infections, ampicillin or erythromycin and sulfonamides may be used (9, 43). The use of penicillin V or erythromycin singly has been shown to be no more effective than a placebo (9). Pneumococci, however, are extremely sensitive to oral penicillin V, parenteral penicillin G, or procaine penicillin (9). Recent data show that clinically, pneumococci respond to amoxicillin more effectively than to penicillin V (43). Streptococci appear to have the same sensitivity as pneumococci to penicillin, which would indicate that this should be the treatment of choice. Antibiotic concentrations that are achieved in middle ear fluid are shown in Table 5.

Dosage recommendations are:

Ampicillin:	50 mg/kg/day
Penicillin V:	50 mg/kg/day
Triple Sulfonamides:	100 mg/kg/day
Erythromycin:	25-50 mg/kg/day
Chloramphenicol:	50-100 mg/kg/day

For the penicillin-allergic patient, erythromycin and triple sulfonamides are recommended.

Antihistamines and decongestants also are given in the treatment of otitis media, because these agents are thought to diminish eustachian tube obstruction (81); however, their value remains unproven (101).

Case History: Minimal Brain Dysfunction (MBD)
B.D. is a seven-year-old male who is sent to a physician's office by his parents and teacher who say that his performance in school is deteriorating. He is described as being extremely active, yet poorly organized or controlled in a "socially acceptable" manner. His teacher has found that his attention span is extremely short and his memory pattern is erratic. Also, B.D. does not relate well to his classmates. There are periods of both impulsive and explosive behavior with little self-control. The consideration is made to evaluate this behavior disorder.

15. What is minimal brain dysfunction?

Minimal brain dysfunction (MBD) occurs in children of normal intelligence who have disturbances of func-

tions of the central nervous system which may be accompanied with learning and behavioral disabilities (38). It must be stressed that this disorder is not identifiable by a single disorder; it is composed of a number of variants. At least 100 clinical manifestations of MBD have been listed, including dyslexia, dysgraphia, dysarthria, hyperactivity, and temper tantrums (105).

16. What are the clinical characteristics of MBD?

The clinical manifestations of MBD result when a child fails to achieve a satisfactory level of developmental maturity and demonstrates this in several areas (65):
a. Disorders of activity
  (1) hyperactivity or hypoactivity
  (2) lack of motor coordination
  (3) sleep problems
b. Disorders of behavior and thought
  (1) attention span problems
  (2) memory disturbances
  (3) perceptual-concept difficulties
  (4) emotional instability
c. Disorders of classroom performance
  (1) reading
  (2) writing
  (3) mathematics

17. What is the medical management of children with MBD?

The treatment of MBD involves working on three levels, which include: counseling parents, teachers, and the child when necessary, individualized modification of the educational environment, and rational prescribing of stimulant medications

The use of stimulant medication as an adjunct to MBD therapy has been shown to be an asset (21,22). The medication acts by decreasing purposeless motor activity and enhancing attention span (21). The pharmacologic mechanism appears to be through the mediation of catecholamine metabolism, allowing increased amounts of norepinephrine available for neuro-transmission in the arousal center of the reticular matter of the brain stem (112). Presently known

Table 5
ANTIBIOTIC CONCENTRATIONS IN SERUM AND MIDDLE EAR FLUIDS

Drug	Dose	Mean Antibiotic Level (mcg/ml) Serum	Ear Fluid
Ampicillin (16)	34 mg/kg — IM	15.3	9.5
Penicillin V (51)	13 mg/kg — po	12.0	2.1
	26 mg/kg — po	14.0	6.3
Erythromycin Ethyl Succinate (4)	50 mg/kg/day	1.3	0.8
Sulfonamide (43) (Trisulfapyrimidines)	120 mg/kg/day	13.4	83.0
Amoxicillin (43)	30 mg/kg/day	4.8	2.2

medications that have proven useful include methylphenidate, imipramine and dextroamphetamine.

Methylphenidate is effective rapidly and has a great advantage of flexibility, safety, and efficacy. Dosages usually begin at 0.1 to 0.3 mg/kg/day in two divided doses and should be increased slowly to 0.7 mg/kg/day if needed (111). Treatment can be initiated by giving the child 5 mg in the morning and 5 mg on returning from school. If afternoon problems persist in school, another dose may be instituted at noon.

Imipramine was first noted to be beneficial in enuretic children, and the observation that it improved behavior was an incidental finding. Initial evaluation showed that imipramine improved alertness, handwriting, reading, and arithmetic in children with various behavior disorders (98). Subsequent studies have confirmed the usefulness of this medication (46,99). Initial doses are usually 12.5 to 25 mg given as a single dose in the evening after dinner. Doses may be increased to as high as 100 to 125 mg daily. The therapeutic effect is usually noted within twenty-four hours. Its efficacy is similar to methylphenidate and amphetamine. Specific advantages include the fact that it may be given as a single daily dose and that it may be used in patients with concurrent sleep problems or enuresis.

Dextroamphetamine is the most established medication and has been the treatment of choice. However, it is not used as frequently since its potential for drug abuse became apparent and because of reports of adverse effects on growth in children (102,103). In addition, it has been reported to be associated with significant personality deterioration in some patients (36). When other medications have failed, dextroamphetamine may be of some value.

Other medications have been used with varying success and are described comprehensively elsewhere (82). Anticonvulsants, e.g. phenytoin, are reported to reduce hyperactive and explosive behavior, but often produce drowsiness and diminished academic alertness. Many of the tranquilizers are also plagued with this side effect. Thioridazine may be an effective adjunct in an older child with anxiety and tension; Deanol has been found to be of little value; pemoline has just been released and for this reason it is difficult to assess its long-term utility.

As with all long-term medications, the patient must be monitored for appropriateness of therapy and adverse effects. Insomnia and anorexia are reported in over 25% of patients treated with stimulant medication, although these effects abate with time. Measures which may be used to diminish these effects include administering medications after breakfast or other meals and not administering a dose later than 4 p.m. in the afternoon.

A recent study has shown that there is no stunting of growth, as was previously reported, from the long-term use of methyphenidate, dextroamphetamine, or imipramine in children (37). Any slowing of growth when treatment is first started is compensated for later on, both while the patient is taking the medication, and after discontinuing it.

18. What factors influence compliance in the pediatric population?

Compliance in completing a prescribed medication regimen is the goal of medical treatment, but studies have shown that compliance varies from 89% in some private group practices to as low as 18% in institutional clinics (7,14,60).

There is an association of compliance with the degree of morbidity caused by an illness (35). If the child is asymptomatic, there is a 50% chance of his completing the course of medicine as prescribed (15).

A recent study attempted to identify additional factors that decrease patient compliance (78). In an analysis of 100 patients treated for otitis media, only 5% achieved full compliance. Factors limiting compliance included:

a. 15% — inadequate dispensing of medication at drug stores

b. 36% — incorrect therapy schedule

c. 37% — early termination of the medication by the parent

d. 7% — spilled medicine

e. 5% — medication shared with other children.

This compliance of 5% was raised to 51% by instituting the following measures:

1. Pharmacist's provision of verbal and written medication administration instructions
2. Dispensing a calibrated measuring device
3. Dispensing a calendar to record doses

This study showed the importance of detailed instructions, and the pharmacists' potential role was better defined.

REFERENCES

1. Ackerman BD: What should kernicterus mean as a clinical diagnosis? Pediatrics 46:15, 1970.
2. Ament ME: Therapeutic use of infant formulas. Drug Ther 14:15, 1972.
3. Aranda JV: Pharmacokinetic aspects of theophylline in premature newborns. NEJM 295:413, 1976.
4. Bass JW et al: Erythromycin concentrations in middle ear exudates. Pediatrics 48:417, 1971.
5. Beauregard WG: Positional otitis media. J Pediatr 79:740, 1971.
6. Bender KJ et al: Infant formulas. J Am Pharm Assoc 15:230, 1975.
7. Bergman AB et al: Failure of children to receive penicillin by mouth. NEJM 268:1334, 1963.
8. Bland, RD: Otitis media in the first six weeks of life: diagnosis, bacteriology, and management. Pediatrics 49:187, 1972.
9. Bluestone CD et al: Middle ear disease in children: pathogenesis, diagnosis, and management. Pediatr Clin Am 21:379, 1974.
10. Brownlee RC et al: Otitis media in children: incidence, treatment, and prognosis in pediatric practice. J Pediatr 75:636, 1969.

11. Burns JJ: Implications of enzyme induction for drug therapy. Am J Med 37:327, 1964.

12. Catz CS et al: Drugs and breast milk. Symposium Pediatr Pharmacol 19:151, 1972.

13. Catz C et al: Pharmacologic modification of bilirubin conjugation in the newborn. Am J Dis Child 104:516, 1962.

14. Charney E: How well do patients take oral penicillin? A collaborative study in private practice. Pediatrics 40:188, 1967.

15. Charney E: Patient-doctor communication. Implications for the clinician. Pediatr Clin N Am 19:263, 1972.

16. Coffey JD: Concentration of ampicillin in exudate from acute otitis media. J Pediatr 72:343, 1972.

17. Comley A et al: Albumin administration in exchange transfusion for hyperbilirubinemia. Arch Dis Child 43:151, 1968.

18. Conney AH et al: Increased activity of androgen hydroxylases in liver microsomes of rats pretreated with phenobarbital and other drugs. J Biol Chem 238:1611, 1963.

19. Davidson M: Formula feeding of normal term and low birth weight infants. Pediatr Clin N Am 17:913, 1970.

20. Diamond I: Bilirubin binding and kernicterus. in Advances in Pediatrics edited by Schulman. Chicago: Yearbook Medical Publishers, 1969.

21. Eisenberg L: Principles of drug therapy in child psychiatry with special reference to stimulant drugs. Am J Orthopsychiatry 41:371,1971.

22. Eisenberg L: The clinical use of stimulant drugs in children. Pediatrics 49:709, 1972.

23. Eute G et al: Hazards of phototherapy. NEJM 283:544, 1970.

24. Feigen RD et al: Assessment of the role of staphylococcus epidermidis as a cause of otitis media. Pediatrics 52:569, 1973.

25. Fleischner G et al: Recent advances in bilirubin formation, transport, metabolism and excretion. Am J Med 49:576, 1970.

26. Fomon S: Nutrition in infancy. In Infant Nutrition, Medcom, Inc. New York, 1972.

27. Friis-Hausen B: Body water compartments in children: changes during growth and related changes in body composition. Pediatrics 28:169, 1961.

28. Fulginiti VA: Controversies in current immunization policy and practices: One physician's viewpoint. Curr Probl Pediatr 6:3 (April) 1976.

29. Fulop M et al: The effect of bile salts on the binding of bilirubin by plasma proteins. Clin Sci 33:459, 1967.

30. Garrettson LK etal: Fetal acquisition and neonatal elimination of a large amount of salicylate. Study of a neonate whose mother regularly took therapeutic doses of aspirin during pregnancy. Clin Pharmacol Ther 17:98, 1975.

31. G artner LM et al: Formation, transport, metabolism and excretion of bilirubin. NEJM 280:1339, 1969.

32. Gerrard JW et al: Milk allergy: clinical picture and familial incidence. Can Med Assoc J 97:780, 1967.

33. Giacoia G et al: Theophylline pharmacokinetics in premature infants with apnea. J Pediatr. 89:829, 1976.

34. Giunta F: A one year experience with phototherapy for jaundice of prematurity. Pediatrics 47:123, 1971.

35. Gordis L et al: Why patients don't follow medical advice: A study of children on long-term antistreptococcal prophylaxis. J Pediatr 75:957, 1969.

36. Greenberg L et al: Side effects of dextroamphetamine therapy of hyperactive children. West J Med 120:105, 1969.

37. Gross MD: Growth of hyperkinetic children taking methylphenidate, dextroamphetamine, or imipramine/desimipramine. Pediatrics 58:423, 1976.

38. Haller JS et al: Minimal brain dysfunction: another point of view. Am J Dis Child 129:1319, 1975.

39. Halsted C et al: Otitis media: clinical observations, microbiology and evaluation of therapy. Am J Dis Child 115:542, 1968.

40. Hargreaves T: Effect of fatty acids on bilirubin conjugation. Arch Dis Child 48:446, 1973.

41. Hodgeman JE et al: Phototherapy and hyperbilirubinemia of the premature infant. Am J Dis Child 119:473, 1970.

42. Holborow C: Eustachian tubal function: changes in anatomy and function with age and the relationship of these changes to aural pathology. Arch Otolaryn 92:624, 1970.

43. Howard JE et al: Otitis media of infancy and early childhood: A double-blind study of four treatment regimens. Am J Dis Child 130:965, 1976.

44. Howie VM et al: Otitis media: a clinical and bacteriological correlation. Pediatrics 45:29, 1970.

45. Huang NN et al: Comparison of serum levels following the administration of oral and parenteral preparations of penicillin to infants and children of various age groups. J Pediatr 42:657, 1953.

46. Huessey HR et al: The use of imipiramine in children's behavior disorders. Acta Paedopsychiat 37:194, 1970.

47. Isenberg JN et al: Double-light phototherapy for neontal hyperbilirubinemia. Pediatrics 83:116, 1973.

48. Jalling B et al: Plasma concentrations of diphenylhydantoin in young infants. Pharmacologica Clinica 2:200, 1970.

49. Johnson JD: Neonatal hemolytic jaundice. NEJM 292:194, 1975.

50. Jusko WJ: Pharmacokinetic principles in pediatric pharmacology. Pediatr Clin N Am 19:81, 1972.

51. Kamme C et al: The concentration of penicillin V in serum and middle ear exudate in acute otitis media in children. Scand J Infect Dis 1:77, 1969.

52. Kamme C: Evaluation of the in vitro sensitivity of neisseria catarrhalis to antibiotics with respect to acute otitis media. Scand J infect Dis 2:117, 1970.

53. Kempe CH: Immunization update: with a word of caution. Drug Therapy 4:71 1974.

54. Kostenbauder HB et al: Riboflavin enhancement of bilirubin photocatabolism in vivo. Experientia 29:282, 1973.

55. Krauer B et al: Elimination kinetics of amobarbital in mothers and their newborn infants. Clin Pharmacol Ther 14:442, 1973.

56. Kron RE et al: Newborn sucking behavior affected by obstetric sedation. Pediatrics 37:1012, 1966.

57. Kunin CM: Clinical significance of protein binding of the penicillins. Ann NY Acad Sci 145:282, 1967.

58. Kuzemko JA et al: Apneic Attacks in the Newborn Treated with aminophylline. Arch Dis Child 48:404, 1973.

59. Laxdal OE et al: Treatment of acute otitis media: a controlled study of 142 children. Can Med Assoc J 102:263, 1970.

60. Leistyna JA et al: Therapy of streptococcal infections. Do pediatric patients receive prescribed oral medication? Am J Dis Chil 3:22, 1966.

61. Lester R et al: New light on neonatal jaundice. NEJM 280:779, 1969.

62. Levin R: Drugs excreted in breast milk. Bull Hosp Pharm — Univ Calif SF 19:1 (June) 1972.

63. Levy G et al: Pharmacokinetics of acetaminophen in the human neonate: formation of acetaminophen glucuronide and sulfate in relation to plasma bilirubin concentration and D-glucaric acid excretion. Pediatrics 55:818, 1975.

64. Levy G et al: Kinetics of salicylate elimination by newborn infants of mothers who ingested aspirin before delivery. Pediatrics 53:201, 1974.

65. Levy HB: Minimal brain dysfunction /specific learning disability: a clinical approach for the primary physician. South Med J 69:642, 1976.

66. Litwack G: Ligandin: A hepatic protein which binds steroids, bilirubin, carcinogens, and a number of orgnic anions. Nature 234:446, 1971.

67. Loggie JM et al: Renal function and diuretic therapy in infants and children: Pt. I, II, III. J Pediatr 86:485, 657, 825, 1975.

68. Loria CJ et al: Effect of antibiotic formulations in serum protein: bilirubin interaction of newborn infants. J Pediatr 89:479, 1976.

69. Loughnan PM et al: Pharmacokinetic analysis of the disposition of intravenous theophylline in young children. J Pediatr 88:874, 1976.

70. Lucey JF et al: Prevention of hyperbilirubinemia of prematurity by phototherapy. Pediatrics 41:1047, 1968.

71. Lucey JF: Phototherapy of jaundice 1969. Bilirubin metabolism, in birth defects, original articie series 6:63, 1970.

72. Lucey J: Neonatal phototherapy: uses, problems, and questions. Sem Hematol 9:127, 1972.

73. Mackinnon J et al: The assessment of organ function in the newborn. Brit J Hosp Med 14:395, 1975.

74. Maisels JM: Bilirubin: on understanding and influencing its metabolism in the newborn infant. Pediatr Clin N Am 19:447, 1972.

75. Malaka-zafiria K et al: The effect of anti-microbial agents on the binding of bilirubin by albumin. Acta Paediat Scand 58:281, 1969.

76. Malmgren B et al: Complications of immunization. Br Med J 2:1800, 1960.

77. Mandelli M et al: Placental transfer of diazepam and its disposi-

tion in the newborn. Clin Pharmacol Ther 17:564, 1975.

78. Mattar ME et al: Pharmaceutic factors affecting patient compliance. Pediatrics 54:100, 1974.

79. Maurer HM et al: Controlled trial comparing agar, intermittment phototherapy and continuous phototherapy for reducing neonatal hyperbilirubinemia. J Pediatr 82:73, 1973.

80. Melchier JC et al: Placental transfer of phenobarbitone in epileptic women and elimination in newborns. Lancet 2:860, 1967.

81. Miller GF: Influence of an oral decongestant on eustachian tube function in children. J Allergy 45:187, 1970.

82. Millichap JG: Drugs in the management of minimal brain dysfunction. Ann NY Acad Sci 205:321, 1973.

83. Mirkin BL: Diphenylhydantoin: placental transport, fetal localisation, neonatal metabolism, and possible teratogenic effects. J Pediatr 78:329, 1971.

84. Mitenko PA et al: Rational intravenous doses of theophylline. NEJM 289:600, 1973.

85. Modlin JF et al: Risk of congential abnormality after inadvertent rubella vaccination of pregnant women. NEJM 294:972, 1976.

86. Morselli PL: Clinical pharmacokinetics in neonates. Clinical Pharmacokinetics 1:81, 1976.

87. Morselli PL et al: Diazepam elimination in premature and full term infants and children. J Perinatal Med 1:133, 1973.

88. Mountain KR et al: Neonatal coagulation defects due to anticonvulsant drug treatment in pregnancy. Lancet 1:265, 1970.

89. Nilson BW et al: Acute otitis media: treatment results in relation to bacterial etiology. Pediatrics 45:351, 1969.

90. O'Brien TE: Excretion of drugs in human milk. Am J Hosp Pharm 31:844, 1974.

91. Odell GB et al: Studies in kernicterus II. The determination of the saturation of serum albumin with bilirubin. J Pediatr 74:214, 1969.

92. Odell GB: The distribution and toxicity of bilirubin. Pediatrics 46:16, 1970.

93. Odell GB et al: Administration of albumin in the management of hyperbilirubinemia by exchange transfusion. Pediatrics 30:613, 1962.

94. Oh W et al: Phototherapy and insensible water loss in the newborn infant. Am J Dis Child 124:230, 1970.

95. Pascale JE et al: Riboflavin and bilirubin response during phototherapy. Pediat Res 10:854, 1976.

96. Phillips CE: Advice on 'first shots' for unimmunized child. JAMA 225:14, 1973.

97. Poland RL et al: Physiologic jaundice: the enterohepatic circulation of bilirubin. NEJM 284:1, 1971.

98. Rappaport J: Childhood behavior and learning problems treated with imipramine. Int J Neuropsychiat 1:635, 1965.

99. Rappaport JL et al: Imipramine and methylphenidate treatments of hyperactive boys. Arch Gen Psychiatry 30:789, 1974.

100. Rasmussen LF Ahlfors, CE, and Wennberg, RP: The effect of paraben preservatives on albumin binding of bilirubin. J Pediatr 89:475, 1976.

101. Rowe DS: Acute suppurative otitis media. Pediatrics. 56:285, 1975.

102. Safer D et al: Depression of growth in hyperactive children on stimulant drugs. NEJM 287:217, 1972.

103. Safer DJ et al: Factors influencing the suppressant effects of two stimulant drugs on the growth of hyperactive children. Pediatrics 51:660, 1973.

104. Salk JE: Viral diseases: their control by immunologic means. Postgrad Med 30:99, 1961.

105. Schmitt BD: The minimal brain dysfunction myth. Am J Dis Child

129:1313, 1975.

106. Sereni F et al: Induction of drug metabolizing enzyme activities in the human fetus and newborn infant. Enzyme 15:318, 1973.

107. Shannon DC et al: Prevention of apnea and bradycardia in low-birth weight infants. Pediatrics 55:589, 1975.

108. Sharma R: A complication of phototherapy in the newborn: the "bronze baby." Clin Pediatr 12:231, 1973.

109. Sisson T et al: Factors influencing the effectiveness of phototherapy in neontal hyperbilirubinemia. In *Bilirubin Metabolism in the Newborn*, Edited by Bergsman. Birth Defects Original Article Series, 6:63, 1970.

110. Silverio J et al: Serum concentrations of ampicillin in newborn infants after oral administration. Pediatrics 51:578, 1976.

111. Sleator EK et al: Methylphenidate in the treatment of hyperkinetic children. Clin Pediatr 13:19, 1974.

112. Snyder SH et al: How amphetamine acts in minimal brain dysfunction. Ann NY Acad Sci 205:310, 1973.

113. Sproul A et al: Bilirubin equilibration during exchange transfusion in hemolytic disease of the newborn. J Pediatr 65:12, 1964.

114. Stern L: Drug interactions. Part II: Drugs, the newborn infant and the binding of bilirubin to albumin. Pediatrics 49:916, 1972.

115. Strom J: Further experience of reactions, especially of a cerebral nature in conjunction with triple vaccination. A study based on vaccinations in Sweden 1959-65. Brit Med J 4:320, 1967.

116. Thaler M: Neonatal hyperbilirubinemia. Semin Hematol 9:107, 1972.

117. Thaler M et al: Drugs and bilirubin. Pediatrics 47:807, 1971.

118. Uauy R et al: Treatment of severe apnea in prematures with orally administered theophylline. Pediatrics 55:595, 1975.

119. Valdes O: Controlled trial of phenobarbital and/or light in reducing neonatal hyperbilirubinemia in a predominently Negro population. J Pediatr 79:1015, 1971.

120. Vest MF et al: Detoxification in the newborn: the ability of the newborn infant to form conjugates with glucuronic acid, glycine acetate, and glutathione. Ann NY Acad Sci 111:183, 1963.

121. Wallace S: Factors affecting drug-protein binding in the plasma of newborn infants. Brit J Clin Pharm 3:510, 1976.

122. Wallin A et al: Plasma concentrations of phenobarbital in the neonate during prophylaxis for neonatal hyperbilirubinemia. J Pediatr 85:392, 1974.

123. Weibel RE et al: Long-term follow-up for immunity after monovalent and combined live measles, mumps and rubella virus vaccines. Pediatrics 56:380, 1975.

124. Wilson JT: Phenobarbitone in the neonatal period. Pediatrics 43:324, 1969.

125. Windorfer A et al: The influence of age on the activity of acetylsalicylic acid esterase and protein salicylate binding. Eur J Clin Pharmacol 7:227, 1974.

126. Wong YK et al: Relative roles of phototherapy and phenobarbital in treatment of nonhaemolytic jaundice. Arch Dis Child 48:704, 1973.

127. Woods JT et al: Gentamicin and albumin bilirubin binding: an in-vivo study. J Pediatr 89:483, 1976.

128. Yaffe SJ et al: Perinatal pharmacology. Annual Rev Pharmacol 14:219, 1974.

129. Yaffe SJ et al: Enhancement of glucuronide conjugating capacity in a hyperbilirubinemic infant due to apparent enzyme induction by phenobarbital. NEJM 275:1461, 1966.

130. Yeung CY et al: Phenobarbitone enhancement of bromsulfphalein clearance in neonatal hyperbilirubinemia. Pediatrics 48:556, 1971.

Chapter 43

Poisonings

Gary M. Oderda
Anthony S. Manoguerra

The purposeful taking of one's life or the accidental ingestion of a drug or chemical are all constituents of the poisoning problem. Statistics from the National Clearinghouse of Poison Control Centers (NCPCC) show that accidental ingestion by young children constitutes the majority of poisoning cases. Of 163,500 case reports submitted by Poison Control Centers in 1973, 71.5% were accidental. Most (62.2%) of the reported ingestions were in children four years of age and younger. (4) Internal medications and household products were ingested most commonly. These cases surely represent only a small fraction of the ingestions that actually do occur.

In an attempt to decrease the poisoning problem, the first Poison Control Center was opened in Chicago in 1952 by the American Academy of Pediatrics. Since then, over 500 other centers have been established across the country. Most centers are staffed by physicians, pharmacists, and nurses, and accept calls from the general public as well as medical personnel. Lay callers are told how the ingestion can be treated at home or are referred to a treatment facility if necessary.

Pharmacists can play an active role in the treatment of poisonings. Frequently, it is the community pharmacist who is contacted initially in the case of an ingestion. Thus, it is his/her responsibility to determine the potential severity of the ingestion and recommend treatment or make a referral to the proper agency. The objective of this chapter is to provide students and practitioners with useful information about the treatment of poisoning.

1. What is a poison?

A poison is any substance that produces injury or death when introduced into a living being. The amount of substance ingested frequently determines whether or not it is considered a poison. For example, although table salt is not usually considered a poison, death has occurred as a result of salt intoxication (7, 14,21,27,43,71,91). Most agents commonly considered poisons are toxic in small doses.

2. One of your patients has found his daughter with an empty medicine vial. What information is needed to assess this situation?

Identification of the agent is of primary importance. If the agent is innocuous, other considerations will be irrelevant. Identification of all ingredients is necessary to assess the situation. In situations of ingestion of household products which are not adequately labeled, one can call the manufacturer whose name and address should be on the label.

The *amount ingested* should be determined if possible. If the original number of tablets in the vial is known, then the amount ingested can be determined by a simple count. In most cases, only an estimate is possible. It is best to overestimate the ingested amount if one cannot be certain of the amount ingested.

The patient's *age and weight* are useful in evaluating the potential severity of the ingestion and in determining the proper dose of therapeutic agents which might be used.

The patient's *symptoms* must be ascertained to determined whether or not they correlate with the toxic effects of the ingested agent. If the signs and symptoms are not appropriate, one must consider that the patient may have ingested other agents. Symptomatology is the major determinant of treatment, as it is important to "treat the patient — not his poison." (56) Symptomatic and supportive care is the mainstay of therapy.

The *time since ingestion,* together with knowledge of the agent's bioavailability, onset of action and peak effect, is invaluable in assessing the situation. For example, if a patient is seen shortly after the ingestion, minimal symptoms may not mean that the amounts ingested were sub-toxic. This information is also useful in determining whether or not the patient's gastric contents should be emptied by emesis or lavage.

Once the above information is obtained, the patient's parent should be given instruction for home treatment or referred to an emergency facility. It may also be necessary to support or calm the parent, arrange for transportation, and relay the available information to the treatment center.

Poison Centers are available in most metropolitan areas to help with the interpretation of this information and to assist in evaluating whether there is need for treatment.

3. Clinical Toxicology of Commercial Products by Gosselin, et al (32) is the best reference textbook in the field of clinical toxicology. Before answering the following questions, examine the page entitled, "How to Use This Manual" in the fourth edition. The following questions test the reader's ability to use this valuable reference source.

3a. Describe the toxicity of doxylamine succinate.

Doxylamine succinate is an antihistamine closely related to diphenhydramine with an oral LD_{50} in mice of 470 mg/kg. It produces a high incidence of sedation. This answer was found in the blue *Ingredient Index,* location 1225.

3b. A two-year-old child has ingested a small amount of metadelphene. What are the ingredients? Where would one find toxicity and treatment information?

Metadelphene contains N, N,-diethyl m-toluamide, 95% and related isomers 5%. (pg. 436, yellow *Trade Name Index*) For further information on toxicity and treatment one would consult the index in front of the blue ingredients section under N,N,-diethyl m-toluamide (pg. 21) where he would be referred to location 1088 (pg. 212) in the *Ingredients Index.*

3c. C-4 Soluble Cresylic Disinfectant is a product manufactured by Coopers Creek Chemical. What is the major ingredient? Describe the toxicity and expected symptoms seen following a topical exposure.

This product contains 75% of a combination of cresylic acids and soap (pg. 179, yellow *Trade Name Index*). Cresylic acid is a combination of o-,m- and p-hydroxytoluene. It is similar in toxicity to phenol, although perhaps slightly more corrosive. (See Cresols location 470, pg. 129, blue *Ingredients Index*). Pain and numbness occur following contact with the skin. After initial blanching, an opaque eschar forms over the burn. This eventually sloughs off, leaving a brown stain (pg. 273, white *Therapeutics Index* under Phenol).

3d. A 3-year-old child ingests 15cc of a nail polish remover that had been transferred to another container. The original container is unavailable and thus the trade name and ingredients are unknown. What are the likely ingredients?

Nail polish removers generally contain over 50% of a solvent (usually acetone or ethyl acetate), 0.1-1.0% essential oils, and 10-20% water. The oily products also contain 2-10% of lanolin, oils, or cetyl alcohol. These products may also contain other solvents, benzene, castor oil, olive oil, spermaceti, ethyl oleate, or butyl stearate (pg. 121, white *General Formulations Section*). To find this entry one must first consult the index in the front of the General Formulations Section.

4. A 19-year-old female is brought to the emergency room with dilated and fixed pupils, shallow respirations and a slow respiratory rate. Examination of the arm shows needle tracks, and narcotic overdose is the preliminary diagnosis. The nurse and house officer frantically begin looking for the naloxone (Narcan). What basic principle of poisoning treatment are these two individuals ignoring?

A patient's breathing and other vital functions must be supported *before* an antidote is considered. Once this has been accomplished, a specific antidote such as naloxone can be given.

5. Young children have easy access to the area under the kitchen sink. What products commonly stored here are toxic? Describe their toxicity.

(a) *Drain cleaners* are commonly caustic and produce esophageal burns. The most common ingredient of the crystalline products is potassium hydroxide. The principle ingredient of some of the liquid preparations, 1,1,1-trichloroethane, is not caustic.

(b) *Automatic dishwasher detergents.* Several different formulations exist. Those which are highly alkaline may burn the mucous membranes of the mouth, esophagus, and stomach.

(c) *Furniture polishes* frequently contain petroleum distillates. Products containing mineral seal oil are the most toxic, as the chemical pneumonia produced when they are aspirated is more severe than that caused by other petroleum distillates (32).

(d) *Insecticide* toxicity depends on the individual agent. Many contain petroleum distillates which add the hazard of aspiration.

(e) *Household cleaning agents* are generally nontoxic, with the exception of those which contain petroleum distillates, eg, pine oil.

6. Many household products are relatively nontoxic in small amounts. List some of these (30).

After shave lotions *(a)*	Fish bowl additives
Airplane glue *(b)*	Fluoride tablets (60 tablets)
Ballpoint pen inks	Matches (20 wooden or
Battery (dry cell)	2 books)
Bleach (sodium	Model cement *(b)*
hypochlorite 5%) *(c)*	Pencils
Body conditioners *(a)*	Porous tip ink markers
Bubble bath soaps *(d)*	Play Doh
Candles	Putty
Caps for toy pistols	Roach tablets (1-2)
(up to one roll)	Sachets
Cigarettes *(e)*	Shaving creams
Colognes *(a)*	Silly Putty
Crayons marked AP or CP	Soaps
Contraceptive pills *(f)*	Teething ring fluid
Cosmetics and skin	Thermometers *(g)*
preparations	Toilet water *(a)*
Dehumidifying packets	Toothpaste
Deodorizer cakes	

a. Contains high concentrations of ethyl alcohol: may be toxic in large amounts.
b. Not harmful unless deliberately inhaled in high concentrations.
c. Stronger solutions (20%) found in some industrial bleaches are caustic. This concentration (5%) may produce gastrointestinal distress and vomiting.
d. May produce vomiting or diarrhea.
e. Nicotine is poorly absorbed and produces vomiting.
f. May produce nausea and occasionally vaginal bleeding in young girls.

g. Metallic mercury is not harmful.

7. A patient enters a pharmacy along with her two young children. While the pharmacist is taking a drug history from the mother, her two children are running up and down the aisles. While in hot pusuit of one of the children, the clerk notices the three-year-old drinking from a bottle of cologne. It is estimated that the child drank about 15 ml. What treatment is necessary?

The major toxic ingredient in this type of product is ethyl alcohol. Ingestion of 15 ml of cologne is not toxic, but large amounts of alcohol in young children may produce hypoglycemia (17,57). A glass of fruit juice will help combat the hypoglycemia and will replace the potassium and sodium that may be lost from alcohol's diuretic effect. If a large amount has been ingested, one may consider emetics or lavage, but they are not routinely advised. Small amounts of alcohol are often completely absorbed before an emetic or lavage would have its effect.

8. For many years salt was regarded as a reliable and safe emetic. It is universally available and is easily administered. Discuss why salt should not be used as an emetic.

Salt is not only unreliable as an emetic, but is in fact dangerous. Hysterical parents have been known to give their children large amounts of salt unnecessarily, resulting in death from salt intoxication (7). Five infants died when a kitchen employee accidentally substituted salt for sugar in their infant formulas (27). Fatality has also occurred in children lavaged with hypertonic saline solution (14). Ingestion of large amounts of salt may cause gastroenteritis, hypernatremia (serum sodium levels as high as 274 mEq/L have been reported) (27), severe thirst, anorexia, tachypnea, dyspnea, muscular twitching and rigidity, convulsions, and death.

9. How do fluid extract of ipecac and syrup of ipecac differ? Should fluid extract of ipecac be dispensed?

The fluid extract of ipecac contains approximately 14 times as much active ingredient as the syrup. The fluid extract should never be dispensed, because it is almost impossible to measure accurately and may be easily mistaken for the syrup. Severe toxicity and deaths have resulted when the fluid extract was mistakenly dispensed in place of the syrup (3,8,83).

10. Describe those patients who should not receive an emetic.

Unconscious or *deeply sedated* patients should not be given emetics, because vomiting can only be induced if medullary centers are responsive. Also, if vomiting is produced, these patients are likely to aspirate their gastric contents. Apomorphine may also further depress respiratory and central nervous system function.

Emetics may precipitate or worsen convulsions in patients who are *convulsing* or *have ingested a convulsant*.

Caustics such as strong acids and bases may cause severe esophageal burns. Induction of vomiting in these patients may further traumatize the esophagus through additional exposure to the caustic agent. Also, if the esophagus is badly burned, the trauma of vomiting may produce esophageal perforation.

Ingestion of *antiemetic* agents such as phenothiazines are a relative contraindication to the use of emetics. Emetics may be efficacious if administered within one hour of ingestion of an antiemetic (87). If an emetic is given and fails to produce vomiting, gastric lavage should be considered.

The use of emetics in *petroleum distillate* ingestions is controversial. If a small amount (less than one ounce or 1 ml/kg) has ben ingested, emptying the stomach is not necessary, and thus, emetics should not be considered. If a large amount has been taken, or if a potentially dangerous chemical such as a pesticide is dissolved in a petroleum distillate, emptying the stomach is necessary.

Traditionally, it was felt that administering an emetic would increase the likelihood of aspiration. Thus, vomiting was not recommended, and gastric lavage was the preferred method of emptying the stomach. In a retrospective study of petroleum distillate ingestion, aspiration pneumonitis occurred less frequently when vomiting was induced than when patients were lavaged or vomited spontaneously (55). Furthermore, radiographic evidence of aspiration is less likely to be observed when petroleum distillate ingestions are treated with ipecac as opposed to lavage. The pneumonitis that did develop was less severe in the ipecac treated group (59). Thus, administration of syrup of ipecac is the method of choice for emptying the stomach of a petroleum distillate. To reduce the possibility of aspiration, ipecac should only be administered to those patients under medical supervision.

11. A parent telephones and says his two-year-old daughter has taken 20 children's aspirin tablets. It is determined that the dose is sufficiently toxic to warrant the administration of syrup of ipecac. What directions should be given to the parent?

(a) Give the child one tablespoonful (½ of the 1 oz. container) of the syrup.

(b) Immediately thereafter give her at least 8 oz. of a clear liquid, such as water, Kool-Aid, or fruit juice, but not milk. Although milk has been recommended in the past, it has recently been shown that this practice delays the onset of vomiting (89). Warm water is thought to be more effective than cold. The administration of too much fluid may cause some of the poison to be pushed past the pylorus.

(c) Emesis should occur in 15 to 20 minutes.

12. The same parent telephones 35 minutes later. The child took the ipecac and drank part of the fluid, but still has not vomited. What further suggestions should be given to the parent?

Give the child more fluid. Wait 5 minutes. If vomiting does not occur, give the child another tablespoonful of ipecac syrup.

If after another ten minutes vomiting does not occur, the parent should attempt to gag the child with his finger. Patients who ambulate tend to vomit more quickly than those who do not. If emesis does not occur, the decision to lavage should be based on the toxicity of the ingested product.

One ounce, the maximum recommended dose of ipecac is not toxic to young children even if emesis does not occur. Some cases of toxicity from larger doses of syrup of ipecac have been reported. A 23-month-old child who was given 90 ml of syrup (5 ml every 5 minutes) developed symptoms of ipecac intoxication despite lavage, but did recover (46).

13. Forty-five minutes after the original aspirin ingestion, the same parent calls back to report success. Orange tablets were seen in the vomitus. The child now complains that she is hungry and sleepy. Is it all right to feed her and let her take a nap?

If the child is allowed to eat or drink anything shortly after vomiting, she will probably vomit again. Both the ipecac and the trauma of vomiting often cause sedation in children. It is acceptable for the child to sleep if the parent checks on her frequently. One should be certain that the sedation is not a direct effect of the ingested agent.

14. Syrup of ipecac and apomorphine are the most commonly used emetics. Compare the advantages and disadvantages of both.

See Table 1.

15. A father discovered his four-year-old eating berries from a Japanese yew tree. Knowing that yew berries can be poisonous, he gave his son two tablespoonfuls of prepared mustard in a glass of water as an emetic. After 45 minutes the child had not vomited. Why?

An aqueous solution of dry mustard powder is sometimes effective as an emetic; however, prepared table mustard has no emetic properties. Because much better emetics such as syrup of ipecac are available for home use, mustard is not recommended.

16. Copper and zinc sulfate have been used as emetics. Are they effective? Safe?

Both of these sulfate salts induce emesis by direct gastric irritation. Hopefully, vomiting occurs before

significant absorption of the salts occurs. However, only 54 - 67% of administered copper sulfate is recovered in the vomitus, and significant increases in serum copper levels have occurred following the administration of copper sulfate (37). Copper sulfate administered to a patient with a partial gastrectomy has been fatal (85). Since safer, more effective emetics are available, copper or zinc sulfate are not recommended.

17. Of the two procedures commonly employed to empty the stomach, gastric lavage and emesis, which is more efficacious?

Early reports comparing ipecac with lavage concluded that ipecac removes more gastric contents than does lavage (1, 6, 10, 33). In all of these reports a lavage tube considerably smaller than the 26-50 French (Fr) (8.7 - 16.7 mm) orogastric tubes currently recommended was used. Although objective evidence is not available, the larger tubes should empty the stomach much more thoroughly than the smaller tubes. The administration of syrup of ipecac is easier and less traumatic than lavage, and until objective evidence is available to demonstrate the superiority of lavage with a large bore tube over ipecac induced emesis, it is the preferred method of emptying gastric contents.

Table 1
COMPARISON OF IPECAC AND APOMORPHINE

	IPECAC	APOMORPHINE
AVAILABILITY:	OTC	Requires a prescription. Generally available only in a hospital.
COST:	Low	High. Requires administration under supervision of a physician.
ROUTE:	Oral	Parenteral. (Unsterile.)
TIME OF ONSET:	Slow (15-20 minutes)	Fast (3-5 minutes)
TOXICITY:	Cardiovascular toxicity in high doses.	May produce protracted vomiting and worsen respiratory and CNS depression. This may be reversed with narcotic antagonists.*
STABILITY:	Stable in oral solution	Unstable in solution. Must be prepared immediately prior to injection from a hypodermic tablet.
EFFICACY:	Excellent	Excellent

* Recent evidence suggests that narcotic antagonists do not always reverse the adverse effects of apomorphine (79a).

18. When is gastric lavage indicated?

Lavage is indicated in the comatose or deeply sedated patient. These patients must have their airway protected with a cuffed endotracheal tube to prevent gastric contents from entering the lungs. Patients who are seizing can be lavaged after their seizures are controlled.

19. Lavage or emesis may be useful several hours after ingestion. Explain why.

A large number of tablets ingested over a short period of time may mass to form a concretion in the stomach. Even soluble drugs may form such a mass. Examples of drugs whose ingestion has caused concretions include glutethimide, barbiturates, aspirin, and meprobamate (5, 39). Since such a mass of tablets dissolves and is absorbed slowly, gastric emptying may be useful even several hours after ingestion. If lavage is to be useful in this situation, a large bore lavage tube must be used.

Certain agents, such as methyl salicylate and anticholinergics decrease stomach emptying time. This effect delays absorption so that tablets remain in the stomach for a longer period of time. Thus, lavage may be effective long after the ingestion of these agents.

20. Various fluids have been used for gastric lavage. Discuss the advantages and disadvantages of distilled water, normal saline, and sodium bicarbonate.

Distilled water. In most cases, the composition of the lavage fluid is not as important as the amount of fluid instilled. For this reason, tap water is commonly used. Children have a limited tolerance to electrolyte-free solutions; a 5% increase in total body fluid with electrolyte-free solutions is sufficient to produce water intoxication and seizures (5). In most instances, water is a safe, useful lavage fluid; however it may be safer to use normal saline or half normal saline solution in young children.

Normal saline is the preferred solution for routine use. It is as effective as distilled water and safer. A patient who has taken a large amount of salt as an emetic and has not vomited should be lavaged with distilled water. If silver nitrate is the toxin, normal saline is especially useful, because it precipitates the silver as silver chloride, an insoluble non-corrosive salt.

Sodium bicarbonate should not be used to neutralize an acid ingestion. A 5% solution of sodium bicarbonate or sodium dihydrogen phosphate may be useful for ferrous salt ingestions, since the less corrosive, more insoluble salts, ferrous carbonate and ferrous phosphate, are produced.

21. *Adsorbents* are used clinically to bind unabsorbed poisons in the gastrointestinal tract. Although other substances have been used, activated charcoal

is the most effective. To be effective, it must have a large surface area (usually around 1,000 m²/gm), be of vegetable origin, and have a low ash content (5). Charcoal tablets are ineffective, as their particle size is too large; thus, their surface area is too small. Discuss the adsorptive spectrum of activated charcoal.

Although some experts feel activated charcoal is an effective local antidote for virtually all organic or inorganic compounds and cite cyanide as the only exception (5), recent evidence suggests that it is relatively ineffective in poisonings due to ethanol, methanol, caustic alkalies, and mineral acids (62).

22. What is the proper dose of activated charcoal? How should it be administered?

The proper dose is five to ten times, by weight, the amount of the ingested agent (62). Generally, two or more ounces of activated charcoal is mixed with water and administered as a slurry by mouth or via a lavage tube. One ounce of activated charcoal is approximately five or six tablespoonfuls. A recently developed suspension of activated charcoal is easier to use, more palatable and equally effective (48).

23. A mother gave her son, who took some iron tablets, a slurry of activated charcoal, followed by 15 cc of syrup of ipecac and 8 oz. of water. Twenty minutes later vomiting had not occurred, so another tablespoonful of ipecac and more fluid were administered. Thirty minutes later he still had not vomited. Why?

Activated charcoal effectively adsorbs ipecac. This renders the ipecac completely ineffective and decreases the adsorptive capacity of the activated charcoal. If activated charcoal and ipecac are to be used together, the charcoal must be given after vomiting has been induced by the ipecac.

24. Discuss the following *cathartics* as they are used in the treatment of poisoning: magnesium sulfate, cathartic oils, sodium sulfate, and vegetable cathartics.

Magnesium sulfate (Epsom Salts) is an effective saline cathartic which is renally excreted. It should not be used if renal function is impaired as magnesium intoxication may occur. An appropriate dose is 250 mg/kg for children and approximately 15 grams for adults. The dose must be diluted to prevent vomiting.

Cathartic oils (such as castor oil) may increase the absorption of fat soluble agents such as the chlorinated insecticides, and therefore should be avoided. One to four ounces of castor oil is useful in phenol poisoning because phenol is highly soluble in oil. A saline cathartic may be given after the administration of the castor oil.

Sodium sulfate (Glauber's Salts), a saline cathartic, is the safest available agent for routine use. Hypernatremia or fluid imbalances may develop secondary to its use, but overall, it is less toxic than magnesium sulfate. The dosage is the same as magnesium sulfate. Alternatively, one-half to one ounce of Fleets Phospho-Soda (sodium phosphate/sodium biphosphate) may be diluted in a 1:4 solution. The onset of catharsis is 30-60 minutes.

Vegetable cathartics, such as cascara and aloes should never be used in poisoning cases, because they are slower in onset and are generally less effective. Sorbitol may be used if saline cathartics are unavailable. Cathartics should not be used in patients who have ingested caustics or in those who have electrolyte imbalances.

25. Administration of large volumes of fluid or osmotic diuretics, such as mannitol and urea, are useful for increasing the urinary excretion of some toxins. Compare the efficacy of these methods.

Water diuresis is only minimally effective in most cases. A water load only increases flow through the distal renal tubules and the collecting ducts. However, since passive solute resorption occurs primarily in the proximal tubules, water resorption must be minimized at this site. Osmotic diuretics are far more efficacious, because they increase the excretion rate of many compounds that are passively reabsorbed, eg, salicylates, phenobarbital. Mannitol is the most commonly recommended osmotic diuretic. Fluids and osmotic diuretics must be used with caution. Care must be taken not to volume overload the patient and produce pulmonary or cerebral edema.

Following a test dose, adults are usually given mannitol 25 gm IV rapidly to start diuresis. Diuresis is maintained by administering 1.5 gm/kg/day of a 20% solution, up to a maximum dose of 100 gm. (Also see chapter on *Edema*.)

26. *Manipulation of urinary pH* is sometimes useful as a method of enhancing excretion. Acidification is appropriate for some weak bases and alkalinization for some weak acids. Discuss why a pH change would affect urinary excretion in the example cited below. Use the Henderson-Hasselbach equation in your explanation. For phenobarbital (pK$_a$ = 7.24) describe the effect of increasing urinary pH from 6.24 to 8.24.

For tubular reabsorption to occur, the substance must be in the unionized form. If the urinary pH were changed so that more of the compound was in the ionized form, reabsorption would be decreased and excretion would be increased. For phenobarbital, approximately 9% is in the unionized, reabsorbable form at pH 6.24.

pH = pK$_a$ + log (A-)/(HA)

(Henderson-Hasselbach eq.)

6.24 = 7.24 + log (A-)/(HA)

(A-)/(HA) = 0.1

However, approximately 90% of the phenobarbital is in the ionized non-reabsorbable form when the urine pH is 8.24, since the ratio of (A-)/(HA) is 10.

This manipulation of urinary pH should increase the excretion significantly.

27. Discuss the use of tromethamine (THAM) in poisoning situations.

Tromethamine, a weak base, combines with hydrogen ions and acid anions. The salts generated from this reaction are excreted in the urine. Dissolved carbon dioxide is decreased and the concentration of bicarbonate increased. The decreased carbon dioxide tension removes a stimulus to breathing which may result in hypoventilation and hypoxia. Tromethamine is also a weak osmotic diuretic and may be useful in long acting barbiturate intoxications as it causes an alkaline diuresis. If tromethamine is used, equipment for supporting respiration must be available in case apnea develops. It is for this reason that tromethamine is not recommended.

28. In *dialysis,* unwanted plasma solutes diffuse across a semipermeable membrane into a dialysis solution. The dialysis fluid is formulated to allow diffusion of the unwanted agents, nonessential electrolytes and chemicals. Two basic types of dialysis exist. In peritoneal dialysis, the patient's peritoneum is utilized as the dialysis membrane. In extracorporeal hemodialysis, cellulose servies as the membrane. When should dialysis be used in the treatment of poisoning?

Dialysis should not be used unless a potentially fatal dose of a dialyzable drug has been ingested by a patient who would not be expected to survive with less heroic measures. Dialysis is also indicated when metabolism of the ingested compound yields a more toxic substance (for example, methanol to formaldehyde; ethylene glycol to oxalic acid) and rapid removal will decrease the amount metabolized.

29. Compare extracorporeal and peritoneal dialysis.

The main differences between these two methods involve efficiency, availability and complexity. Peritoneal dialysis is available at most treatment centers and can be performed by health professionals with little special training. Clearance rates for peritoneal dialysis are at best 20% of those achieved by extracorporeal hemodialysis. Although hemodialysis is more efficient, it is generally only available at large referral centers.

30. What is *hemoperfusion?* Is it effective?

Hemoperfusion is a procedure in which blood is passed through adsorbent materials including charcoal and resins. Blood is pumped through a column where it comes in direct contact with the adsorbent material and is then returned to the patient.

Charcoal emboli, thrombocytopenia and leukopenia have been associated with charcoal adsorbents, however, coating the charcoal with various substances has successfully prevented many of these problems. Charcoal hemoperfusion may be three times more efficient than hemodialysis in clearing glutethimide and long acting barbiturates and six times more efficient in clearing short acting barbiturates (88).

IRON

A three-year-old male was brought to the emergency department about six hours after ingesting an unknown amount of his mother's ferrous sulfate. On arrival the child was mildly lethargic with spontaneous vomiting and profuse watery diarrhea. Vital signs were normal. Intravenous fluids were started, and the child was given 3 ounces of a 5% sodium dihydrogen phosphate solution orally. An abdominal x-ray showed iron tablets in the child's stomach, and he was then given syrup of ipecac to try to remove them. The child vomited several times with the emesis containing many partially disintegrated iron tablets. A repeat x-ray showed no remaining tablets. A serum iron level was 625 mcg%. The child was admitted and deferoxamine therapy was begun. His symptoms abated and the deferoxamine was stopped after 24 hours with a serum iron of 173 mcg%. The recovery was uneventful.

31. What are the toxic effects of iron and how are these efforts expressed as symptoms?

The clinical features of this poisoning are independent of the age of the patient and progress through five distinct phases (38).

Stage one occurs in the first six hours following the ingestion. Diarrhea, vomiting and melena dominate this stage due to the direct irritative effect of the iron on the gastrointestinal tract. This, along with the vasodilation produced by ferritin which is released from the gastrointestinal mucosa may lead to shock. A direct depressant effect of the iron on the brain or decreased brain perfusion may produce central nervous system depression, lethargy, or coma (12).

Stage two, a period of apparent improvement, occurs 6 to 24 hours after ingestion. The patient may fully recover or may progress to Stage three.

Stage three is characterized by numerous metabolic derangements. Profound metabolic acidosis, secondary to interference with metabolism of organic acids, occurs and may be accentuated by loss of large amounts of bicarbonate in diarrheal fluids (70). Fever and leukocytosis result from the extensive gastrointestinal mucosa damage. Alterations in hemodynamics secondary to fluid loss may produce renal failure.

Death occurs as a result of this multiplicity of factors. Stage three generally lasts from 12 to 48 hours.

If the patient survives Stage three, he may progress to **Stage four,** characterized by hepatic necrosis. This Stage is seen two to four days after ingestion. Two to four weeks after ingestion, the **fifth** phase is observed and is characterized by scarring of the pylorus and stomach.

32. How much elemental iron is present in common iron-containing products?

The elemental iron content of each product varies according to the iron salt it contains. These are shown in Table 2.

Table 2
IRON CONTENT OF VARIOUS
IRON-CONTAINING PRODUCTS

Iron Product	Elemental Iron Content per Tablet
Ferrous sulfate 325 mg	60 mg.
Ferrous gluconate 325 mg	40 mg.
Ferrous fumarate 325 mg	105 mg.
Prenatal vitamins with iron	40-60 mg.
Adult multi-vitamins with iron	10-100 mg.
Children's multi-vitamins with iron	3-25 mg.

33. A two-year-old child was found playing with his mother's prenatal iron tablets (each tablet containing 325 mg of ferrous fumarate). After counting the tablets, the mother concluded that approximately 10 tablets were missing. Is this a dangerous situation?

Each 325 mg ferrous fumarate tablet contains 105 mg of elemental iron. This child, therefore, ingested 1050 mg of elemental iron. The toxic dose of iron has not been well established, but it is generally accepted that 1-2 grams of elemental iron will produce severe poisoning in a two-to-five-year-old child (35). Children have been symptomatic after ingesting 300-400 mg of elemental iron, and a fatality has been reported at 65 mg/kg (49,74). This ingestion is potentially life-threatening and must be treated as such.

34. The two-year-old child described in the above question has now arrived in the emergency room. What can be done to retard the absorption of the iron?

If no contraindication exists, emesis should be induced with syrup of ipecac. As part of the fluids given with ipecac, 2-3 ounces of a 5% solution of either sodium dihydrogen phosphate or sodium bicarbonate should be given (28). The phosphate solution can be prepared by diluting one part of the contents of a Fleets Enema with four parts of water. The phosphate solution converts the iron salt in the stomach to ferrous phosphate; the bicarbonate solution converts it to ferrous carbonate, both of which are more insoluble and poorly absorbed. If contraindications to emesis exist, lavage can be performed by either using a lavage fluid made by further dilution of the phosphate solution to approximately 2% or a sodium bicarbonate solution. This fluid should be used for the first three or four fluid exchanges. Following emesis or lavage, 2-3 ounces of the solution should be allowed to remain in the stomach. The phosphate solution also acts as a cathartic which will hasten the movement of any unabsorbed iron through the gastrointestinal tract.

35. Is there any way that the extent of removal of the iron from the stomach can be determined?

Iron tablets are radiopaque and will, therefore visualize on x-ray. An abdominal x-ray should be taken following emesis or lavage to determine the extent of removal. If iron is seen in the small bowel, cathartics should be given. If the tablets appear clumped and stuck in the stomach, surgical removal should be considered. Other radiopaque agents include chloral hydrate, heavy metals, and phenothiazines. These radiopaque drugs can more easily be remembered by utilization of the mnemonic CHIP which represents Chloral hydrate, Heavy metals, Iron, and Phenothiazines.

36. How useful is the serum iron level in determining the potential seriousness of the ingestion?

If possible, a serum iron and a total iron binding capacity (TIBC) should be performed in all iron cases. Since it is the unbound or "free" iron that is toxic, both tests are useful. However, because only a serum iron is available on an emergency basis in most hospitals, guidelines for therapy based on this parameter alone have been established. Patients with levels greater than 300 mcg/100 ml should be admitted to the hospital for observation. It is highly probable, in these cases, that the TIBC has been exceeded. Patients who have levels greater than 500 mcg/100 ml or who are in Stage 3 of intoxication should be admitted and started on immediate chelation therapy with deferoxamine. Patients with levels between 300 and 500 mcg/100 ml may require only fluid replacement therapy (50).

37. What is the proper dose of deferoxamine and how should it be given?

Children and adults are usually given an initial dose of deferoxamine 1 gram followed by 500 mg every four hours for two doses. More may be given, but no more than 6 grams should be given in a 24 hour period. Deferoxamine is generally given intramuscularly unless the patient is in shock. In such cases, intravenous administration is the route of choice at a rate not to exceed 15 mg/kg/hour. A brick red urine indicates the presence of the iron-deferoxamine complex. Although orally administered deferoxamine will bind with iron in the stomach, this complex is absorbable. Even though it is probably not toxic, there is no evidence that it is

superior to the phosphate or bicarbonate solutions. In addition, large amounts of deferoxamine must be given, for example 5000 mg per liter, representing a cost of approximately $40 per liter.

38. Should deferoxamine be administered to a pregnant woman who has ingested iron?

Fetal abnormalities have been produced in animals from administration of deferoxamine. However, in a potentially life threatening iron ingestion by a pregnant woman, the use of deferoxamine should be considered.

39. Is hemodialysis or peritoneal dialysis useful in the treatment of iron poisoning?

Dialysis is useful only as an adjunct to supportive care, particularly if renal failure has resulted. It does not remove iron at a rate faster than chelation therapy. Exchange transfusion may be useful (41).

SALICYLATES

40. A mother telephones for help after finding her two-year-old child with an open bottle of children's aspirin in his hand. Upon questioning it is determined that at least six of the original 36 tablets were used previously and 10 tablets remain. The ingestion occurred approximately 10 minutes ago; the child weighs 10 kg, has been in good health, and is not demonstrating any symptoms. What should be done?

One must assume that the child ingested 20 children's aspirin or 1215 mg. A minimum toxic dose for this child is estimated to be approximately 1620 mg (based on 150 mg/kg or 1 grain/lb). Because this dose is expected to produce minimal toxicity and the ingestion is recent, treatment at home with syrup of ipecac is appropriate. At this dose the need for further treatment would not be anticipated. Had the child been dehydrated as a result of fever, vomiting, or diarrhea, or had he been receiving aspirin recently, the minimum toxic dose would be about half of that indicated above. The lethal dose of aspirin is estimated to be 400 to 500 mg/kg.

41. Describe the expected symptomatology of a salicylate ingestion in children and adults. Discuss the basis for these symptoms when known.

Young children and adults differ in their response to high doses of salicylates. Infants and young children are generally acidotic, whereas adults are generally alkalotic (56). The most common initial signs of salicylate intoxication are tinnitus and vomiting, neither of which appear until hours after ingestion. Tinnitus, of course, is not recognized in infants and young children. Other common symptoms include hyperventilation and acid-base disturbances, vomiting, hyperthermia, hypoglycemia, convulsions, coma and death.

Pulmonary edema, renal damage and bleeding disorders are rare.

The metabolic rate is markedly increased and hyperpnea is common. Salicylates stimulate ventilation through a direct effect on the medulla. The increased metabolic rate may be due to salicylate-induced uncoupling of oxidative phosphorylation and an enhanced rate of catabolism (82). Hyperventilation results in a respiratory alkalosis (decreased serum pCO_2 and increased pH). Generally, this is the only acid-base imbalance observed in older children and adults. Infants and children less than two years of age commonly proceed from alkalosis to acidosis 20 hours or so following the ingestion. Several factors are responsible for this change to an acidotic state, including accumulation of organic anions in the plasma, renal retention of hydrogen ions, and respiratory depression.

Depletion of the infant's liver glycogen stores, as well as an increased glucose requirement, produce hypoglycemia and ketosis. While hypoglycemia is most common, hyperglycemia is also occasionally associated with salicylate ingestion (see *Diabetes* chapter) (82).

Vomiting is common and is caused by a central and local action of the salicylate.

Hyperpyrexia is another consequence of the uncoupling of oxidative phosphorylation. Energy derived from oxidation cannot be used for ATP formation and is liberated as heat. Loss of hypotonic sweat produces further dehydration. Hyperpyrexia occurs much more frequently in infants than in older individuals.

Respiratory failure is commonly reported as the cause of death. Convulsions are frequently seen in terminal salicylate intoxication.

42. A four-year-old, 38 lb female arrived at the emergency room at 10:00 p.m. Her respirations were shallow and rapid (48/min); her pulse was 136/min; the blood pressure was 84/46 mm Hg and her temperature was 102.4°F. The mother stated that her child had been playing "hospital" around 1:00 p.m. and that an empty adult aspirin bottle was found in the vicinity. At 4:30 p.m. she appeared restless; she vomited twice around 6:00 p.m. A serum salicylate level drawn at 10:00 p.m. was 60 mg%. Evaluate this situation. What other information is needed? Describe appropriate treatment of this individual.

The patient's symptomatology and history are consistent with aspirin intoxication. Before the results of a serum salicylate level are known, the presence of salicylate may be qualitatively determined by testing the urine with either ferric chloride or Phenistix. Either of these tests can be performed quite rapidly in the emergency room, however, they are not always accurate and false positive reactions can occur.

A nomogram developed by Done may be used to estimate the severity of the intoxication (asymptomatic,

mild, moderate or severe) if the serum salicylate level and time since ingestion are known. This nomogram is only useful in patients whose ingestion occurred at least 6 hours before the serum salicylate level was drawn and who were not pretreated with aspirin (22). This patient fits both of these criteria. A 60 mg% salicylate level, 9 hours after ingestion is indicative of a moderately severe intoxication.

Gastric removal may be useful as long as 10 hours after the ingestion of aspirin (even longer for methyl salicylate) (53). Emesis is the treatment of choice unless the patient is deeply sedated or convulsing. If either of these symptoms is present or if syrup of ipecac has been given and emesis has not occurred, the patient should be lavaged with normal saline solution until returns are clear by the ferric chloride test. Activated charcoal effectively adsorbs aspirin and should be administered (20) and followed by a saline cathartic.

In addition to a serum salicylate level, other basic laboratory tests such as pCO_2, serum pH, and electrolytes should be ordered. In all cases of salicylate poisoning patients should not be released from the hospital until at least two salicylate levels have been performed and the second level is lower than the first.

Intravenous fluids should be given in all but the mildest salicylate intoxications. Specific treatment must of course be individualized to the patient's acid-base and electrolyte status. D-5-½ NS is recommended for initial hydration.

Diuretics such as furosemide or mannitol may be added to enhance excretion. Once urine flow has been established, approximately 50 mEq of sodium bicarbonate should be added to each liter of intravenous fluid to alkalinize the urine to a pH of 7-8.

THAM (Tromethamine) has occasionally been used to alkalinize the urine but is not currently recommended. (Also see Question 27.)

Acetazolamide (Diamox), a carbonic anhydrase inhibitor, effectively alkalinizes the urine. Acetazolamide should not be used for salicylate intoxication, especially in young children, because it produces a metabolic acidosis which may be additive with that produced by the salicylate (58).

Dialysis should be considered in severely intoxicated patients who are not responding to conservative measures. Both peritoneal and extracorporeal hemodialysis are effective. A dialysis solution containing 5% human albumin is particularly effective (5). Clearance values of salicylate with hemoperfusion are comparable to those seen with hemodialysis (11).

43. A two-year-old girl is found playing with a tube of Ben-Gay. The tube still appears full, but there is some ointment on her face and around her mouth. What is the principal toxic ingredient?

Ben-Gay contains 18% methyl salicylate. On a weight

basis, methyl salicylate is far more toxic than aspirin. One teaspoonful of pure methyl salicylate is equivalent to approximately 4,000 mg of aspirin, or twelve adult aspirin tablets (60 grains). Methyl salicylate has been fatal in children at a dose of 4 ml (32). Many external products contain methyl salicylate as approximately 20% of the total weight. If a child were to consume a one ounce tube of such a product, a potentially fatal dose, equivalent to 5 ml of oil of wintergreen, would have been ingested.

Symptomatology and treatment of methyl salicylate and aspirin ingestions are similar. Absorption of methyl salicylate from the gastrointestinal tract is, however, considerably slower than that of other salicylates. Therefore, lavage or emesis may be useful many hours after ingestion.

ACETAMINOPHEN

RJ, a 15-year-old 50 kg white female is brought to a local emergency room at 1:00 a.m. complaining of nausea, vomiting and anorexia. These symptoms began approximately two hours earlier. She admits to taking 35 five grain acetaminophen tablets at approximately 7:00 p.m. the evening prior to admission. The patient appeared slightly lethargic and all vital signs were within normal limits. Pertinent laboratory findings (normals in parenthesis) on admission were:

SGOT	309 units/ml (5-40)
SGPT	606 units/ml (5-35)
LDH	143 units/100 ml (200-450)
Total Bilirubin	0.5 mg/dl (0.3-1.1)

At 2:00 a.m. blood for a serum acetaminophen level was drawn and sent to the lab and was later reported to be 320 mcg/ml.

Throughout the day she became progressively more lethargic until approximately 18 hours after admission when her state of consciousness began to improve.

At 11:00 p.m. on day 1, the acetaminophen level was reported as 6.2 mcg/ml.

Day 2: **The patient was alert, coherent and well oriented.**

SGOT	378 units/ml
LDH	119 units/100 ml

The blood level of acetaminophen at 5:00 p.m. on day 2 was 0.0.

Day 3: **Scleral jaundice and epigastric tenderness were noted.**

Total bilirubin	2.0 mgm/dl
SGOT	2712 units/ml
SGPT	2664 units/ml
LDH	502 units/100 ml

Day 4: **Coagulation studies within normal limits. Anorexia, epigastric discomfort and jaundice gradually disappeared following peak levels reported**

below and liver function tests began to return towards normal.

Total bilirubin	5.3 mgm/dl
SGOT	7050 units/ml
SGPT	10,230 units/ml
LDH	650 units/100 ml
Serum ammonia	38 mcg/dl
Day 8:	
Total bilirubin	0.9 mg/dl
SGOT	213 units
SGPT	1240 units
LDH	192 units

Day 14: **Liver biopsy was done and was consistent with toxic hepatitis. Necrosis was not massive.**

Day 19: **Patient was discharged from the hospital. All tests of hepatic function were within normal limits.**

44. What is the mechanism of acetaminophen hepatic toxicity?

Acetaminophen (N-acetyl-p-aminophenol) is metabolized in the liver by non-cytochrome P450 enzyme systems and excreted. The major pathway, which is responsible for about 80% of metabolism, involves conjugation as the glucuronide or sulfate (92). A small percentage is metabolized by the hepatic cytochrome P450 mixed function oxidase system to an active intermediate metabolite, perhaps the N-hydroxyl or N-oxime that is normally conjugated with glutathione and excreted (54). When large doses of acetaminophen are taken, more of the active intermediate is formed, and stores of glutathione are not sufficient to allow for conjugation and excretion. Levels of the intermediate metabolite increase, and this metabolite binds covalently to hepatocytes and produces hepatic necrosis (63).

45. Is the dose of acetaminophen that was taken by this patient consistent with the hepatic toxicity observed?

Acute ingestions of greater than 200 mg/kg of acetaminophen in adults are thought to be consistent with the production of hepatic necrosis (72). It must be stressed that considerable variability exists. This patient weighs 50 kg and by history took 35 five grain tablets. This is a total dose of 11.3 gm or approximately 227 mg/kg, an amount consistent with the production of hepatic necrosis.

46. Could one have predicted whether this patient would develop hepatic necrosis from her acetaminophen blood levels?

Blood levels can be used to predict outcome. Patients who four hours after ingestion had blood levels of 300 mcg/ml or greater consistently developed hepatic necrosis; those with levels less than 120 mcg/ml did not develop hepatic damage (64). Prediction of outcome was difficult at levels between 120 and 300 mcg/ml.

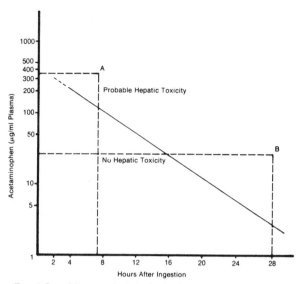

Figure 1: Rumack Nomogram for Acetaminophen Poisoning (modified from Ref 72).

The nomogram in Figure 1 provides useful information from a single blood determination. This patient's first two acetaminophen blood levels (320 mcg/ml at approximately 7 hours after the ingestion and 26.2 mcg/ml at approximately 28 hours after ingestion) are plotted as points A and B. As one can clearly see, both of these points fall in the probable hepatic toxicity range, a finding one would expect from the case presentation.

In general, the determination of acetaminophen excretion half-life is a more accurate prognostic indication. Those patients whose half-life of excretion is greater than four hours are likely to develop hepatotoxicity (64). The excretion half life in this patient is approximately 6¾ hours, a finding consistent with the development of hepatic toxicity.

47. What immediate emergency room treatment would have been appropriate for this patient early on the morning of her admission?

The methods for decreasing absorption discussed earlier in this chapter are appropriate. Since significant CNS depression and loss of gag reflex are absent in this patient, administration of syrup of ipecac as an emetic would be appropriate. Activated charcoal effectively binds acetaminophen if given soon after ingestion and should be considered (45a). After vomiting is successfully produced, a saline cathartic should follow the administration of the activated charcoal.

48. Discuss the role of cysteamine, methionine and N-acetylcysteine in preventing acetaminophen induced hepatic necrosis. Should one of these agents have been given to this patient?

Since it is the lack of glutathione that prevents metabolism and excretion of the toxic metabolite, administration of glutathione would be expected to decrease the toxicity of large doses of acetaminophen. However, administered glutathione does not enter cells readily, and thus, will not prevent the hepatic necrosis (65). Glutathione precursors, such as cysteine, and other necleophilic sulfhydryl containing compounds, such as cysteamine, have been investigated as potential glutathione substitutes. Intravenously administered cysteamine has been shown to be quite effective in preventing hepatic necrosis from large doses of acetaminophen if given within 10 hours of ingestion (65). Cysteamine has been approved by the FDA for investigational use.

Methionine, another glutathione precursor, has been shown to be effective in preventing acetaminophen induced hepatic necrosis (16a,65a). It too should be given within 10 hours after the ingestion. Methionine has two major advantages over cysteamine; first, it can be given orally, and second, it is more readily available for use in the United States. L-methionine is available in power form and dl-methionine is available commercially in capsules and as a liquid (Pedameth). Since only the l-isomer is effective, a higher dose must be given if the racemic mixture is used. The use of methionine for the treatment of acetaminophen overdose is not yet FDA approved.

Another investigational agent, N-acetylcysteine, also appears promising for the treatment of acetaminophen overdose. Seven-day survival rates in mice were better at all times than either a cysteamine group or control (62a). Seven-day survival rate was near zero for cysteamine and 90% for N-acetyleysteine when they were administered four and a half hours after the ingestion. This is particularly noteworthy since the onset of hepatic damage occurs far more quickly with mice than with humans. In the first reported human case, a 32-year-old 75 kg man who had taken 60 gm of acetaminophen 15 hours earlier was given N-acetylcysteine and survived (45b). His extrapolated four hour blood level was 350 mcg/ml and his excretion half-life was seven hours. N-acetylcysteine is given orally or by lavage tube in an initial dose of 140 mg/kg and then 70 mg/kg every four hours for 68 hours (72a). An IND for this agent has been issued. Contact the Rocky Mountain Poison Center (303) 893-7771, for further information.

Although BAL and d-penicillamine, two other sulfhydryl containing compounds, are also available for use in the United States and have been suggested for use in acetaminophen poisoning, their effectiveness in preventing acetaminophen-induced hepatic necrosis has not been demonstrated.

Since by history and initial blood level determination one could predict that this patient would be likely to develop hepatic necrosis, and she was first seen less than ten hours after the ingestion, the administration of either cysteamine, methionine, or N-acetyleysteine should have been considered.

49. What is the role of hemodialysis in acetaminophen intoxications?

Although hemodialysis decreases the acetaminophen excretion half life (24), there is no evidence that this decreases mortality. This is not unexpected since both the toxic metabolite and damage to the liver are produced quickly and thus the possibility of removing enough acetaminophen quickly enough to decrease production of the metabolite is unlikely. In addition, since the toxic metabolite is produced intracellularly, it is not removed by dialysis.

SEDATIVE HYPNOTICS

A 23-year-old white female was brought to the emergency room by a paramedic crew after being found on the floor in a motel room. On arrival in the emergency room, she was unconscious with an esophageal airway in place with assisted ventilation. Vital signs were BP 60/0 palpable and pulse 110. Her pupils were dilated and sluggishly responsive to light. Neurologic examination showed absence of spinal and corneal reflexes. Pressure sores were present on the patient's forehead, left arm and left leg. The paramedic crew brought in an empty bottle labeled as pentobarbital 100 mg, 30 capsules which was dispensed two days previously.

Intravenous fluids and dopamine drip were started with a resultant increase in BP to 100/80. The esophageal airway was removed after placement of an endotracheal tube. Tracheal suction removed vomitus from the trachea. The patient was then transferred to the medical intensive care unit where she was treated with supportive care including meticulous pulmonary toilet. Chest X-ray showed a left upper lobe infiltrate and intravenous penicillin G was started. Her serum pentobarbital level was 3.6 mg%. The patient made an uneventful recovery and awoke approximately 18 hours after admission.

50. What is the fatal dose of a barbiturate?

The fatal dose of a barbiturate depends upon its duration of action. The fatal dose is estimated to be 5 grams for the long-acting barbiturates and 3 grams for the short- and intermediate-acting compounds. There is tremendous variability of response, however, and individuals tolerant to the effects of barbiturates can survive following much higher doses. This factor must also be considered when interpreting blood level information. For non-tolerant patients a potentially fatal blood level is 3.5 mg% for short-acting barbiturates and 8-12 mg% for long-acting barbiturates (5,80).

51. Describe the differences in elimination patterns for short- and long-acting barbiturates. How does this affect therapy?

The following is the general structure for barbiturates:

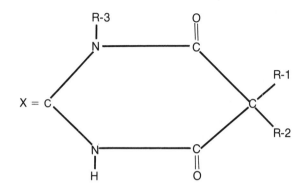

Substitution at R-1 and R-2 determines the duration of action of the compound. In general, those with shorter side chains (for example, barbital with two ethyl groups), are less fat soluble and have a longer duration of action. Those with longer side chains (for example, pentobarbital with an ethyl and a 1-methylbutyl), are more lipid soluble and have a shorter duration of action.

Metabolic degradation is the primary means of elimination for the short-acting barbiturates. A significant fraction of the longer-acting compounds are excreted unchanged by the kidneys. Enhancing elimination through diuresis or dialysis is thus more likely to be useful for the long-acting compounds.

The pKa values of different barbituates are useful in determining whether urinary alkalinization will be effective. All the barbiturates are weak acids with pKa's in the range of 7.0-8.0. Phenobarbital has one of the lowest pKa's (7.24), and secobarbital, one of the highest (7.90). At a physiologic pH of 7.4, approximately 41% of the phenobarbital is unionized, as opposed to approximately 76% of the secobarbital. Raising the urinary pH to a high enough level to produce a clinically significant increase in excretion of a compound with a pKa in the 7.90 range is impractical. Therefore, alkalinization is only useful for phenobarbital. Also, many of the agents with higher pKa's are not extensively excreted by the kidney; thus, osmotic diuretics with or without alkalinization, are not particularly useful.

52. Methaqualone abuse and overdoses are quite common. How do intoxications with this agent differ from other sedative hypnotics? Is forced diuresis indicated to enhance excretion?

In mild intoxications, symptoms are very similar to those seen with other sedative hypnotics. In severe overdoses, several differences are apparent. Hyperexcitability, hyper-reflexia and convulsions are common.

Hypotension and respiratory depression are rare. Pulmonary edema has been reported and may be related to forced diuresis. Since forced diuresis only minimally enhances the clearance of methaqualone and since it may produce pulmonary edema in these patients, it is clearly contraindicated.

53. What symptoms are unique to *glutethimide* intoxications? What is the role of hemodialysis and hemoperfusion in the treatment of glutethimide overdose?

Glutethimide is highly lipid soluble and partitions into body fat. Cyclical coma for periods up to 100 hours after ingestion has been reported and may be related to the anticholinergic effects of the drug. As tissue levels increase, anticholinergic effects increase, and gastric motility and absorption are decreased. As metabolism and excretion occur, tissue levels decrease, the depth of coma decreases, and gastric absorption increases. This cycle continues as long as absorbable glutethimide remains in the gastrointestinal tract. For this reason emptying the stomach and administration of charcoal and cathartics are very important.

Aqueous hemodialysis removes little glutethimide and does not shorten the duration of coma, lessen complications or improve survival (15); however, the effectiveness of hemodialysis in removal of the active metabolite (see below) requires more study. Although lipid dialysis successfully removes more glutethimide than does aqueous dialysis, its ability to decrease mortality or morbity is questionable. In addition, lipid dialysis is generally unavailable. Glutethimide is removed very well by both charcoal and resin hemoperfusion devices (88). This procedure is simpler than either lipid or aqueous dialysis and may be useful in the treatment of severe glutethimide intoxications.

Correlation of glutethimide blood levels with clinical status has been disappointing. However, the existence of a previously unknown active metabolite, 4-hydroxy-2-ethyl-2-phenylglutarimide (4-HG), has recently been demonstrated (36a). This metabolite is approximately twice as potent as glutethimide, and clinical course correlates well with combined glutethimide and 4-HG blood levels when the greater potency of the latter is taken into account. The effectiveness of hemodialysis and hemoperfusion must be re-evaluated in light of these findings.

54. Discuss the use of analeptics in the management of CNS depressant intoxication.

Clinical experience with analeptics in the management of CNS depressant poisonings has been disappointing. Analeptics do not decrease either the morbidity or mortality of sedative hypnotic poisonings and in fact may do just the opposite (16). Analeptics are not indicated in the treatment of any overdose.

OPIATES

55. A 28-year-old 55 kg female was brought into the emergency room after a narcotic overdose. She was apneic, hypotensive and unconscious. After being given one ampule of naloxone (0.4 mg) IV she began to breathe on her own and responded to painful stimuli. Five minutes later an additional 0.4 mg of naloxone was given. At this point she woke up and her respiratory rate increased to 20/minute. Upon awaking the patient admitted to taking her normal daily methadone dose (80 mg) plus two take-home doses, a total of 240 mg, orally. After initial stabilization she was moved from the emergency room to an adult medicine ward. Approximately two hours after the last dose of naloxone, a nurse found her apneic and unresponsive. What happened? Comment on the appropriateness of her naloxone doses.

Naloxone injected intravenously acts within minutes and usually within a few seconds. At best, its duration of action is from one to four hours (38a). Clinically, it is frequently necessary to repeat administration as frequently as every 20-60 minutes to prevent symptoms from recurring (73).

The methadone that this patient had ingested was still present after the naloxone had been eliminated. It is critical that all patients receiving naloxone be carefully monitored and that doses be repeated as needed.

Naloxone should be given in an initial dose of 0.005 - 0.01 mg/kg IV. An initial dose of 0.275 - 0.55 mg would be appropriate for this patient. One ampule of naloxone contains 0.4 mg; thus the initial dose of one ampule was appropriate for this patient. The initial dose should be repeated at least once within five minutes if no response is seen; response is diagnostic of narcotic overdose.

56. What are the characteristic clinical effects of an acute opiate intoxication?

Acute opiate exposure may produce coma and apnea. The degree of central nervous system and respiratory depression depends upon dose and tolerance. Although pinpoint pupils are common, anoxic patients may have dilated pupils. Hypotension, bradycardia, urinary retention, muscle spasm hyperpyrexia and leukocytosis may be seen (73). Pulmonary edema has been reported following parenteral or oral ingestions of narcotics including morphine, methadone, propoxyphene and heroin (45,47,86).

57. How does naloxone (Narcan) differ from nalorphine and levallorphan?

Naloxone is a narcotic antagonist that effectively reverses the effects of morphine, heroin, codeine, meperidine, propoxyphene, pentazocine, methadone, dextromethorphan and similar agents. Unlike nalorphine and levallorphan, naloxone is a pure narcotic antagonist. Levallorphan and nalorphine have both narcotic antagonist and agonist properties; and administered to a patient who had not taken a narcotic, or had taken a narcotic and other non-narcotic CNS depressants, the depression could be worsened. For this reason naloxone is the narcotic antagonist of choice. (Also see chapter on **Drug Abuse.**)

ANTICHOLINERIC AND RELATED INGESTIONS

58. A 17-year-old male was brought to the hospital 45 minutes after ingesting 72 Sominex tablets. What symptoms might be expected from this patient?

Sominex is a commercial, non-prescription sleep-aid that contains scopolamine, methapyrilene and salicylamide. Scopolamine and methapyrilene produce the "anticholinergic syndrome" (75) which is characterized by the following symptoms: dry mucous membranes, decreased gastrointestinal motility, dilated pupils which are unreactive to light, blurred vision, photophobia, urinary retention, vasodilitation, tachycardia, hyperpyrexia, elevations in blood pressure, restlessness, excitement, confusion, hallucinations and delirium. Severe poisoning may lead to coma, respiratory depression, circulatory collapse, and death (51).

59. What other drugs are capable of producing the "anticholinergic syndrome?"

Any drug with anticholinergic effects or side effects can produce this clinical picture. These drugs include: antihistamines, antiparkinsonians (benztropine, trihexyphenidyl, etc.), tricyclic antidepressants, non-prescription sleep aids (Sominex, Nytol, etc.), non-prescription cold remedies, non-prescription tranquilizers, antispasmodics and plants that contain atropine-like alkaloids.

60. What additional problem is commonly associated with the ingestion on large amounts of the tricylic antidepressants that make them particularly hazardous?

The tricyclic antidepressants produce a high incidence of cardiac arrhythmias which are the usual cause of death. These arrhythmias are usually present early in the course of the ingestion but may be delayed as long as six days after ingestion (52). The types of arrhythmias observed usually include, but are not limited to, atrial tachycardia, nodal tachycardia, atrioventricular block, intraventricular conduction delays, and asystole (81). Spiker and associates (84), showed a strong correlation between the duration of the QRS complex on electrocardiogram and plasma tricyclic antidepressant levels. Patients with high plasma levels had QRS durations of greater than 100 msec.

61. A 23-year-old female was brought to the

emergency room after ingesting an unknown amount of amitriptyline. She was comatose with an irregular heart rate of 190 beats per minute and a blood pressure of 170/120. EKG showed a sinus tachycardia with incomplete right bundle branch block. While the EKG was being done the patient had a grand mal seizure. How should this situation be treated?

This patient has developed several indications for the use of the anticholinesterase drug, physostigmine (76). An initial dose of physostigmine should be given to patients who have central of peripheral signs of anticholinergic toxicity plus one or more of the following: coma, convulsions, hallucinations, arrhythmias and severe hypertension. This initial dose provides diagnostic assistance in that a positive response reinforces the diagnosis. Moreover, patients responding to this initial dose will continue to respond if repeat doses are deemed necessary. Repeated doses should be given to those patients who are experiencing seizures, arrhythmias of hypertension. Coma and hallucinations are not indications for repeated administration of physostigmine. Coma, in these patients, usually lasts no longer than 24 hours and is not life-threatening. Hallucinations and delirium should be treated with physostigmine only if the patient becomes uncontrollable to the point of threatening injury to himself or others.

Because the antidotal action of physostigmine requires the accumulation of acetylcholine, the maximal effect is not seen for five to ten minutes following the administration of the drug. The effect of physostigmine typically lasts from one to three hours, and therefore, repeated doses of the drug may be necessary.

Physostigmine is not innocuous and carries the risk of inducing seizures and cholinergic crisis. It should not be used routinely.

62. A decision is made to use physostigmine. What is the dose of physostigmine and how should it be administered to this patient?

The dose of physostigmine is (75):

Adult: Initial dose: 2 mg IV injected slowly (over at least 2 minutes). 1-2 mg is repeated until a desired positive response is achieved or cholinergic signs develop. Repeat dose: 1-2 mg IV as needed.

Pediatric: Initial dose: 0.5 mg IV injected slowly (over at least 2 minutes). 0.5 mg is repeated every 5 minutes until the desired positive response is achieved, cholinergic signs develop, or 2 mg has been given. Repeat dose: The effective dose can be given as needed.

Atropine in a dose one-half the amount of injected physostigmine should be kept on hand and administered if excessive cholinergic symptoms develop.

63. What other measures are occasionally successful in the treatment of these arrhythmias?

Increasing the systemic blood pH to 7.50 to 7.55 appears to enhance the effect of physostigmine on these arrhythmias. The mechanism of this enhancement is unclear. Vasopressors should be avoided whenever possible, because they enhance the risk of development of arrhythmias (75). Arrhythmias unresponsive to physostigmine and alkalinization should be treated with traditional antiarrhythmic drugs such as lidocaine, phenytoin or propranolol.

64. Why is physostigmine preferred over neostigmine?

Physostigmine is a tertiary amine which will cross the blood brain barrier and reverse both central and peripheral anticholinergic effects. Neostigmine, a quaternary amine, will not cross the blood brain barrier and, thus, will only reverse the peripheral effects.

PETROLEUM DISTILLATES

65. A one-year-old boy is found with a bottle of Old English Furniture Polish that has approximately one ounce missing. The child gagged and choked when he first swallowed it but is now asymptomatic except for an occasional cough. What is the hazard with this product? How should this child be managed?

This product contains mineral seal oil which is a petroleum distillate of low viscosity. This product, as well as many other petroleum distillates, are easily aspirated and can produce a severe chemical pneumonitis. This occurs in 25-40% of children who ingest kerosene and other petroleum distillates (25). Ingestions of large amounts (more than one ounce or 1 ml/kg) may result in CNS depression by an unknown mechanism. The management of this type of patient is controversial (see Question 68). However, aspiration has occurred as evidenced by the gagging, choking and coughing. Therefore, a chest x-ray should be performed and he should be monitored closely in the hospital.

66. What properties of a petroleum distillate influence its toxicity?

The three properties which influence petroleum distillate toxicity are viscosity, surface tension, and volatility. Agents with low viscosity are more likely to be aspirated into the lungs and penetrate further and more quickly than petroleum distillates with higher viscosity. Those agents with a viscosity of less than 45 SSU are more likely to pose an aspiration hazard (typical examples are naptha, gasoline, and kerosene). More viscous compounds, such as mineral oil and vegetable oil, do not normally pose a significant aspiration hazard. Those agents with low surface tension have a greater tendency to spread in the lung and are thus more toxic. An example of a petroleum distillate with low surface tension is mineral seal oil. Those petroleum distillates

with high volatility tend to be more toxic than those with low volatility.

67. Describe the usual clinical course in petroleum distillate ingestion.

There is usually an initial burning sensation in the mouth and throat followed by gagging and choking. Dyspnea and cyanosis may result if large amounts are aspirated. Continued coughing is common. The child may be lethargic and in respiratory distress with minimal auscultatory findings. Fever may develop within 30 minutes to several hours after ingestion. In severe cases pulmonary edema, hemoptysis, cyanosis and death occur, usually within 24 hours. In milder cases symptoms generally plateau at about 24 hours and subside over several days (29). Chest x-ray findings may be apparent after 30 minutes but often take several hours to materialize (18). Approximately 75% of patients ingesting petroleum distillates develop x-ray changes; however, only 25-50% of these develop symptoms (18, 29, 61, 66).

68. Under what circumstances should the stomach be emptied in petroleum distillate ingestions?

This is a very controversial issue. What cannot be agreed upon is if emptying of the stomach provides any therapeutic benefit. There are no well controlled, large population clinical trials that demonstrate whether stomach emptying is a necessary technique. If emptying of the stomach is deemed necessary, emesis is preferred to lavage unless other contraindications exist. (See Question 10). Therefore, if very large amounts of a petroleum distillate have been ingested, emesis with syrup of ipecac should be performed unless other contraindications exist.

CAUSTICS

69. When corrosive substances are ingested what is their toxic hazard? How do acids and alkalies differ in their effects?

Alkaline corrosives produce a reaction on the gastrointestinal tract referred to as "liquefaction necrosis." This is a penetrating necrosis that may involve all layers of the gastrointestinal tract, leading to perforation. Upon initial ingestion intense pain occurs which often makes swallowing and further ingestion difficult. The granular drain cleaner products usually produce severe oral and pharyngeal burns, and in 40-60% of these cases esophageal burns are present (2, 13), however, the presence or absence of burns in the mouth is not a reliable indicator of esophageal involvement, and therefore, each patient must be thoroughly evaluated (2, 13). About 50% of patients with documented esophageal burns will develop esophageal strictures (2).

The liquid drain cleaners produce a more severe reaction in that the damage often is not limited to the oral, pharyngeal and esophageal areas but may include the stomach and upper portions of the small bowel (68). These products are also more likely to damage adjacent thoracic and abdominal organs (69). Death may occur as a result of hemorrhage, shock, asphyxia due to laryngeal or glottic edema, infection or damage to thoracic organs (i.e., heart and major vessels). Aspiration of the corrosive has been reported resulting in severe pulmonary necrosis (19).

Acids, such as sulfuric, hydrochloric, nitric and phosphoric (found in rust removers, toilet bowel cleaners and similar products) produce an immediate, severe sensation of pain when ingested. They appear to have only a superficial effect on the esophageal mucosa, resulting in burns in only 6-20% of cases (9,34). In such cases the acid produces pylorospasm, trapping the acid in the antrum where it produces its destructive effect. Acids produce a "coagulation necrosis" which differs from "liquefaction necrosis" in that the supporting tissue structures are usually left intact. Strictures in the pyloric region are late complications which may occur in as many as 80% of cases (40). Death usually occurs from the same complications as with the alkaline corrosives.

70. On the labels of many products containing strong alkalies the suggested first-aid therapy commonly includes the oral administration of dilute vinegar or citric acid solutions. Discuss why such action is undesireable.

The combination of an acid (citric or acetic) with an alkali produces an exothermic reaction. The heat produced from this reaction can be severe enough to produce thermal damage to the already damaged esophageal and oral mucosa. The first-aid treatment for this type of ingestion is immediate dilution of the chemical with milk. If milk is unavailable, then water can be used (77). Additionally, it has been shown experimentally that the damage to the mucosa occurs in the first 30-60 seconds after exposure. Therefore, dilution with a weak acid is at best a questionably effective treatment which can produce more severe damage as a result of the exothermic reaction (31, 44).

71. How effective are steroids in reducing the complications of corrosive ingestion?

In the 1950's it was shown both experimentally and in clinical trials that steroids, 1-2 mg/kg of prednisone or equivalent, if started within 48 hours of the ingestion of an alkaline agent, decreased the incidence of stricture formation in cases where esophageal burns were demonstrated by esophagoscopy (42, 67). Steroids will not stop stricture formation in severe cases but will make the esophagus more pliable and therefore, make dilitation by bougienage easier (36). The use of steroids, however, increases the risk of infection, and therefore, patients must be closely monitored for signs of infection and receive appropriate antibiotic therapy when necessary (67).

The effectiveness of steroids in acid corrosive ingestion has not been studied.

SNAKE AND INSECT BITES

72. What types of snakes are considered poisonous in the United States?

In the United States, only four types of poisonous snakes are found. These include the pit vipers (rattlesnakes, water moccasins and copperheads), coral snakes, California lyre snakes and mangrove snakes. The majority of bites are caused by pit vipers and coral snakes (60).

73. By examining the bite, how can it be determined if the bite was caused by a poisonous snake?

Harmless snakes produce a bite characterized by two rows of tiny, shallow teeth wounds, while poisonous snakes produce bites with deep fang punctures connected by a row of very small teeth wounds. Fang marks from the pit vipers may vary from one to four in number. The pit vipers have long, retractable fangs that allow the snake to attach to varying shaped surfaces and therefore are very effective at producing envenomation. The coral snakes have short nonretractable fangs and cannot bite flat surfaces. Most coral snake bites result in no envenomation. The California lyre snake and the mangrove snake have rear fixed fangs that rarely produce severe or venomous bites (60).

74. How should venomous snake bites be treated?

Pit viper bites that show signs of envenomation (rapid swelling, discoloration and pain) should be treated with immediate steps to retard venom absorption, remove as much venom as possible and to neutralize the effects. A light constriction band should be applied 2 to 10 cm above the bite. The band should be tight enough to inhibit the lymphatic flow which carries the venom, but not tight enough to constrict blood flow. Cold packs can be applied to the wound, but care should be taken not to freeze the wound. If the bite has occurred within the previous hour, then incision of the fang marks and suction of the venom may reduce the potential severity. This procedure should be performed by trained personnel and not laymen in the field. Surgical excision of the wound area to remove the venom has been used, but this approach is considered controversial and is not widely accepted.

Administration of antivenin is the single most effective therapy available. The most severe complication of its use is the precipitation of an anaphylactic reaction, because the antivenin is prepared from horse serum. Therefore, the patient must be given a test dose of horse serum prior to administration of the antivenin to determine any sensitivity. This is a conjunctival or skin test. The amount of antivenin required depends upon the seriousness of the envenomation. Severe cases may require more than 15 vials of antivenin. Antivenin should be given intravenously. Administration of antivenin into or around the bite is no longer suggested. Additional therapy aimed at maintenance of a patent airway, control of pain and infection, and local wound care are also necessary (60,78,79). Serum sickness following antivenin therapy is also seen.

Coral snake bites produce symptoms in a very short period of time; usually 20 minutes. The bite produces minimal pain and usually no local reaction. The venom is a neurotoxin that produces paralysis. Death occurs as a result of respiratory paralysis. Because of the rapid onset of symptoms, local therapy of the bite is not useful. Administration of the specific coral snake antivenin is the only effective treatment (60,78,79).

75. The bite of which insects commonly found in the United States pose a significant hazard to life?

Although many insects are venomous, only a small number have significantly potent venom, produce large enough quantities of venom, or have venom injecting apparatus strong enough to pose a serious threat to humans.

Of the spiders, only two species, the black widow and the brown recluse, are capable of producing severe toxicity. The **black widow** venom is neurotoxic, producing ascending paralysis and destruction of peripheral nerve endings. Severe poisonings are characterized by coma, respiratory paralysis and cardiovascular collapse. Treatment includes supportive care and administration of the specific antivenin in the following patients: victims under 16 years of age or over 60 years of age, victims with hypertension, or those with symptoms of severe envenomization. These patients should be given one ampule of antivenin intramuscularly or, in severe cases, intravenously (79).

The **brown recluse** spider venom has hemolytic and necrotizing properties. The wound that develops following a bite is an ulcerating wound that does not heal for weeks or months. Treatment is symptomatic and is aimed at treating local infections that may prolong healing (79).

Bees, wasps and ants are also venomous insects, but their threat to humans is primarily due to allergic reactions to the venom leading to anaphylaxis. Direct venom toxicity is extremely rare but has occurred following attacks by swarms of bees.

Scorpions are the other group of venomous insects that produce significant problems. In the United States only two species are dangerous. All others are relatively harmless. These two species are *Centuroides sculpturatus* and *Vejovis spinigerus,* and they are found only in southwestern Arizona. The venom of *Centuroides sculpturatus* is extremely toxic with an LD_{50} in mice of 0.096 mg per kilogram of body weight. The adult venom gland contains 0.5 mg of venom. The *Vejovis spinigerus* venom is less toxic but similar in effects. The sting of these insects provokes a reaction characterized by erythma and swelling at the site of the sting, flushing, fasiculations, increased parasympathetic activity, hyperirritability, hypertonicity, hypertension, weakness, and paraesthesias of the affected extremity. In severe cases paralysis and respiratory distress can be seen. Treatment involves supportive care and the use of the specific antivenin in the young and very old or those patients with hypertension. Healthy adult patients may only require muscle relaxants along with supportive care.

REFERENCES

1. Abdallah AH et al: A comparison of the efficacy of emetics and stomach lavage. Am J Dis Child 113:571, 1967.
2. Alford BR et al: Chemical burns of the mouth, pharynx, and esophagus. Ann Otol Rhinol Laryngol 68:122, 1959.
3. Allport RB: Ipecac not innocuous. Am J Dis Child 98:786, 1959.
4. Anon: Natl Clgh Poison Control Cent Bull (May-June) 1974.
5. Arena J: *Poisoning*, Chas C Thomas, Springfield, Ill, 1970.
6. Arnold FJ et al: Evaluation of the efficacy of lavage and induced emesis in treatment of salicylate poisoning. Pediatrics 23:286, 1959.
7. Barer J et al: Fatal salt poisoning from salt used as an emetic. Am J Dis Child 125:889, 1973.
8. Bates T et al: Ipecac poisoning. Am J Dis Child 103:169, 1962.
9. Boikan WS: Gastric sequelae of corrosive poisoning. Arch Int Med 46:342, 1930.
10. Boxer L et al: Comparison of ipecac-induced emesis with gastric lavage in the treatment of acute salicylate ingestion. Pediat Pharmacol Ther 84:800, 1969.
11. Brookings C et al: Salicylate removal by charcoal hemoperfusion in experimental intoxication in dogs; assessment of efficacy and safety. Arch Toxicol 34:243, 1975.
12. Brown RK et al: Mechanism of acute ferrous sulfate poisoning. Can Med Assoc J 73:192, 1955.
13. Cardona JC et al: Current management of corrosive esophagitis: An evaluation of results in 239 cases. Ann Otol Rhinol Laryngol 80:521, 1971.
14. Carter RF et al: Fatal salt poisoning due to gastric lavage with hypertonic saline. Med J Aust 1:539, 1971.
15. Chazan J et al: Clinical spectrum of glutethimide intoxication. JAMA 208:837, 1969.
16. Clemesen C et al: Therapeutic tends in the treatment of barbiturate poisoning — the Scandinavian method, Clin Pharmacol Ther 2:220, 1961.
16a. Crome P et al: Oral methionine in the treatment of severe paracetamol (acetaminophen) overdose. Lancet 2:829, 1976.
17. Cummins L: Hypoglycemia and convulsions in children following alcohol ingestion. J Pediatr 58:23, 1961.
18. Daeschner CW et al: Hydrocarbon pneumonitis, Pediatric Clin North Amer 4:423, 1957.
19. Danrigal A et al: Necrose totale du poumon par caustique. Med Leg Domm Corpor 42:68, 1962.
20. Decker W et al: Inhibition of aspirin absorption by activated charcoal and apomorphine Clin Pharmacol Therap 10:710, 1969.
21. DeGenaro F et al: Salt — a dangerous antidote. J Pediatr 78:1048, 1971.
22. Done AK: Salicylate intoxication. Significance of measuring salicylate in blood. Pediatrics 26:800, 1960.
23. Done AK: Salicylate poisoning. JAMA 192:770, 1965.

24. Done AK: Treatment of salicylate poisoning. Clin Toxicol 1:451, 1968.
25. Eade NR et al: Hydrocarbon pneumonitis. Pediatrics for the Clinician 54:351, 1974.
26. Farid NR: Haemodialysis in paracetamol self-poisoning. Lancet 2:396, 1972.
27. Finberg LF et al: Mass accidental salt poisoning in infancy. JAMA 184:187, 1963.
28. Fischer DS et al: Acute iron poisoning in children; the problem of appropriate therapy. JAMA 218:1179, 1971.
29. Foley JC et al: Kerosene poisoning in children. Radiology 62:817, 1954.
30. Furth MS: Toxicity of common household items. Maryland Poison Information Center Treatment Protocols, unpublished, July 1969, Baltimore MD.
31. Gago O et al: Aggressive surgical treatment for caustic injury of the esophagus and stomach. Ann Thorac Surg 13:243, 1972.
32. Gosselin R et al: Clinical Toxicology of Commercial Products, 4th ed, Williams and Wilkins, Baltimore, MD, 1976.
33. Goldstein LI: Emesis vs lavage for drug ingestion. JAMA 208:2162, 1969.
34. Gray HK et al: Pyloric stenosis caused by ingestion of corrosive substances. Surg Clin North Am 28:1041, 1948.
35. Greengard J: Iron poisoning in children. Clin Toxicol 8:575, 1975.
36. Haller JA et al: The comparative effect of current therapy on experimental caustic burns of the esophagus. Pediatrics 34:236, 1964.
36a. Hansen AR et al: Glutethimide poisoning. NEJM 292:250, 1975.

37. Holtzman NA et al: Evaluation of serum copper following copper sulfate as an emetic. Pediatrics 42:189, 1968.
38. Jacobs J et al: Acute iron intoxication. NEJM 273:1124, 1965.
38a. Jaffe JH et al: Narcotic analgesics and antagonists, in The Pharmacological Basis of Therapeutics, 5th ed, edited by Goodman L and Gilman A, MacMillan Co, New York 1975.
39. Jenis EH et al: Acute meprobamate poisoning. JAMA 207:361, 1969.
40. Karon AB: The delayed gastric syndrome with pyloric stenosis and achlorhydria following the ingestion of acid — a definite clinical entity. Am J Dig Dis 7:1041, 1962.
41. Knepshield JH et al: Dialysis of poisons and drugs; annual review. Trans Am Soc Artif Int Org 19:590, 1973.
42. Krey H: On treatment of corrosive lesions in esophagus: experimental study. Acta Otolaryngol suppl 102:1, 1952.
43. Laurence BH et al: Hypernatremia following a saline emetic. Med J Aust 1:1301, 1969.
44. Leape LL: New liquid drain cleaners. Clin Toxicol 7:109, 1974.
45. Levine SB: Pulmonary edema and heroin overdose in Vietnam. Arch Pathol 95:330, 1973.
45a. Levy G et al: Effect of activated charcoal on acetaminophen absorption. Pediactrics 58:432, 1976.
45b. Lyons L et al: Treatment of acetaminophen overdose with N-acetyl-cysteine. NEJM 296:174, 1977.
46. MacLeod J: Ipecac intoxication — use of cardiac pacemaker in management. NEJM 268:1467, 1963.
47. Malek SK et al: Pulmonary edema and oral ingestion of methadone. JAMA 221:915, 1972.
48. Manes M: Easily swallowed formulations of antidote charcoals. Clin Toxicol 7:355, 1974.
49. Manoguerra AS: Iron poisoning cases treated in a metropolitan general hospital. Presented at the American Association of Poison Control Centers — American Academy of Clinical Toxicology Annual Meeting, Kansas City, Aug. 9, 1975.
50. Manoguerra AS: Treatment protocol for Iron Poisoning, Hennepin County Poison Center, Minneapolis, 1976.
51. Manoguerra AS et al: Physostigmine treatment of anticholinergic poisoning. J Amer Coll Emer Phys 5:125, 1976.
52. Masters AB: Delayed death in imipramine poisoning. Brit Med J 3:30, 1967.
53. Matthew H: Gastric aspiration and lavage. Clin Toxicol 3:179, 1970.
54. Mitchell J et al: Acetaminophen induced hepatic necrosis. I. Role of drug metabolism. J Pharmacol Exper Ther 187:185, 1973.
55. Molinas: Natl Clgh Poison Control Cent Bull (March-April) 1966.
56. Morrelli HF: Rational therapy of drug overdosage, in Clinical Pharmacology, edited by Melmon K and Morrelli H, MacMillan Co, New York 1972.
57. Moss M: Alcohol induced hypoglycemia caused by alcohol sponging. Pediatrics 46:445, 1970.
58. Mudge GH: Diuretics and other agents employed in the mobilization of edema fluid, in The Pharmacological Basis of Therapeutics, 5th ed, edited by Goodman L and Gilman A, MacMillan Co, New York 1975.
59. Ng RC et al: Emergency treatment of petroleum distillate and turpentine ingestion. Can Med Assoc J 111:537, 1974.
60. Oehme FW et al: Toxins of animal origin, in Toxicology, the Basic Science of Poisons, edited by Casarett L and Doull J, MacMillan Co, New York 1975.
61. Olstad RB et al: Kerosene intoxication. Amer J Dis Child 79:623, 1950.
62. Picchioni AL: Activated charcoal — a neglected antidote. Pediatric Clin North Am 17:535, 1970.
62a. Piperno E et al: Reversal of experimental paracetamol toxicosis with N-acetylcysteine. Lancet 2:738, 1976.
63. Potter W et al: Acetaminophen induced hepatic necrosis. III. Cytochrome p-450 mediated covalent binding in vitro. J Pharmacol Exper Ther 187:203, 1973.
64. Prescott LF et al: Plasma paracetamol half-life and hepatic necrosis in patients with paracetamol overdosage. Lancet 1:519, 1971.
65. Prescott LF et al: Successful treatment of severe paracetamol overdosage with cysteamine. Lancet 1:588, 1974.
65a. Prescott LF et al: Cysteamine, methionine, and penicillamine in the treatment of paracetamol poisoning. Lancet 2:109, 1976.
66. Press E et al: Co-operative kerosene study: evaluation of gastric lavage and other factors in the treatment of accidental ingestion of petroleum distillate products. Pediatrics 29:648, 1962.
67. Ray ES: Cortisone therapy of lye burns of the esophagus. J Pediatr 49:394, 1956.
68. Ray JF et al: Lye ingestion. JAMA 229:765, 1974.
69. Ray JF et al: The natural history of liquid lye ingestions. Arch Surg 109:436, 1974.
70. Reissman KR et al: Acute intestinal iron intoxication. II. Metabolic, circulatory and respiratory effects of absorbed iron salts. Blood 10:46, 1955.
71. Robertson W: A further warning on the use of salt as an emetic agent. J Pediatr 79:877, 1971.
72. Rumack BH et al: Acetaminophen poisoning and toxicity. Pediatrics 55:871, 1975.
72a. Rumack BH: Poisindex management on acetaminophen. Micromedex, Denver 1977.
73. Rumack BH: Poisindex management on opiates. Micromedex, Denver 1977.
74. Rumack BH: Poisindex management on iron. Micromedex, Denver 1977.
75. Rumack BH: Anticholinergic poisoning, treatment with physostigmine. Pediatrics 52:449, 1973.
76. Rumack BH: Physostigmine: rational use. J Amer Coll Emer Phys 5:541, 1976.
77. Rumack BH: Poisindex management on alkaline corrosives. Micromedex, Denver 1976.
78. Rumack BH: Poisindex management on snake bite. Micromedex, Denver 1976.
79. Russell FE: Venom poisoning. Ration Drug Ther 5:1, 1971.
79a. Schofferman JA: A clinical comparison of syrup of ipecac and apomorphine; use in adults. J Amer Coll Emer Phys 5:22, 1976.
80. Schreiner GH: Barbiturate intoxication evaluation of therapy including dialysis in a large series selectively referred because of severity. Arch Int Med 117:224, 1966.
81. Slovis DG et al: Physostigmine therapy in acute tricyclic antidepressant poisoning. Clin Toxicol 4:451, 1971.
82. Smith MJ: The metabolic basis of the major symptoms in acute salicylate intoxication. Clin Toxicol 1:387, 1968.
83. Speer J et al: Ipecacuanha poisoning — another fatal case. Lancet 1:475, 1963.
84. Spiker DG et al: Tricyclic antidepressant overdose: clinical presentation and plasma levels. Clin Pharmacol Ther 18:539, 1975.
85. Stein RS et al: Death after use of cupric sulfate as an emetic. JAMA 235:801, 1976.
86. Tenant F: Complications of propoxyphene abuse. Arch Int Med 132:191, 1973.

87. Thoman ME et al: Ipecac syrup in antiemetic ingestion. JAMA 196:433, 1966.

88. Vale J et al: Use of charcoal hemoperfusion in the management of severely poisoned patients. Brit Med J 1:5, 1975.

89. Varipapa R et al: Effect of milk on pecac-induced emesis. NEJM 296:112, 1977.

90. Viscomi CJ et al: An evaluation of early esophagoscopy and corticosteroid therapy in the management of corrosive injury of the esophagus. J Pediatr 59:356, 1961.

91. Ward DJ: Fatal hypernatremia after a saline emetic. Brit Med J 2:432, 1963.

92. Woodbury DM et al: Analgesic-antipyretics, anti-inflammatory agents, and drugs employed in the therapy of gout, in *The Pharmacological Basis of Therapeutics*, 5th ed, edited by Goodman L and Gilman A, MacMillan Co, New York 1975.